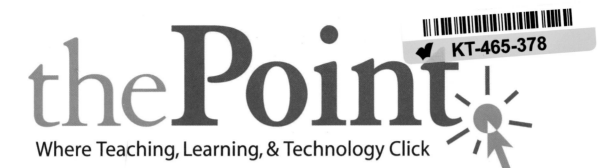
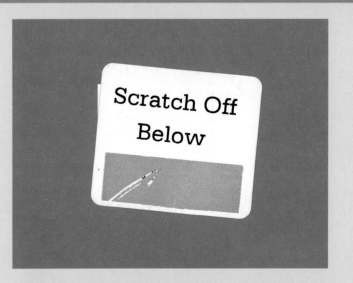

Exercise Physiology

Energy, Nutrition, and Human Performance

Sixth Edition

William D. McArdle

Professor Emeritus, Department of Family, Nutrition,
and Exercise Science
Queens College of the City University of New York
Flushing, New York

Frank I. Katch

International Research Scholar
Faculty of Health and Sport, Agder University College
Kristiansand, Norway
Instructor and Board Member
Certificate Program in Fitness Instruction
UCLA Extension, Los Angeles, California
Former Professor and Chair of Exercise Science
University of Massachusetts, Amherst, Massachusetts

Victor L. Katch

Professor, Department of Movement Science
Division of Kinesiology
Associate Professor, Pediatrics
School of Medicine
University of Michigan
Ann Arbor, Michigan

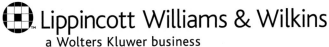

a Wolters Kluwer business

Philadelphia · Baltimore · New York · London
Buenos Aires · Hong Kong · Sydney · Tokyo

Acquisitions Editor: Emily Lupash
Managing Editor: Rebecca Keifer, Rebecca Kerins
Marketing Manager: Christen Murphy
Production Editor: Julie Montalbano
Design Coordinator: Risa Clow
Illustrator: Rob Duckwall
Compositor: Maryland Composition
Printer: R.R. Donnelley & Sons—Willard

Printed in the United States of America.

First Edition, 1981; Second Edition, 1986; Third Edition, 1991; Fourth Edition, 1996; Fifth Edition, 2001.

Library of Congress Cataloging-in-Publication Data
McArdle, William D.
    Exercise physiology : energy, nutrition, and human performance /
William D. McArdle, Frank I. Katch, Victor L. Katch.— 6th ed.
      p. ; cm.
    Includes bibliographical references and index.
    ISBN 0-7817-4990-5
    1. Exercise—Physiological aspects. I. Katch, Frank I. II. Katch, Victor L. III. Title.
    [DNLM: 1. Exercise—physiology. 2. Nutrition. 3. Sports Medicine. QT 260 M478e 2006]
QP301.M375 2006
612'.044—dc22

2005029306

The publishers have made every effort to trace the copyright holders for borrowed material. If they have inadvertently overlooked any, they will be pleased to make the necessary arrangements at the first opportunity.

To purchase additional copies of this book, call our customer service department at **(800) 638-3030** or fax orders to **(301) 223-2320**. International customers should call **(301) 223-2300**.

Visit Lippincott Williams & Wilkins on the Internet: http://www.LWW.com. Lippincott Williams & Wilkins customer service representatives are available from 8:30 am to 6:00 pm, EST.

06 07 08 09 10
1 2 3 4 5 6 7 8 9 10

In the mid-1970s while attending an ACSM conference and contemplating what direction our careers might take, we tried to convince each other what exercise physiology textbook to adopt for our classes. Admittedly, the choices were limited because the "big name" authors of that time pretty much dominated the field. Each of us had used different early texts in our own undergraduate and graduate education in the 1960s. Being naive but full of enthusiasm, we soon began to wonder about writing our own text. We did have limited experience in writing one textbook (*Nutrition, Weight Control, and Exercise*), so we thought, "how tough could it be?" A year passed, and the more we thought about it, the more we became convinced we should try.

The mid-1970s were not exactly a "hot time" for promotion of the physiology of exercise and physical fitness, particularly because there were only several dozen academically oriented "exercise science-type" undergraduate and graduate programs that might adopt a new textbook. But we pressed on with one goal in mind—to create the best possible book in the field without mimicking the outline and content of the prior, established texts. We decided it would make sense to begin with the concept of nutrition as energy for exercise (a unique approach to the current exercise physiology textbooks) and then proceed to mechanisms of energy transfer at rest and during exercise, followed by the physiologic–anatomic systems and their response to short- and long-term physical activity. Our focus was to produce a text to best prepare the next generation of physical education and exercise science students for diverse careers including the expanding health-related exercise sciences. We also wanted to include an "upscale" art and graphics program to make the text the best it could be. That in a nutshell is why we wrote the first edition of this textbook.

Now in its sixth edition, *Exercise Physiology* continues a tradition of excellence by providing a comprehensive, up-to-date, and visually appealing introduction to the subject. The new edition retains our nutrition-based approach to the study of exercise physiology and continues exploration of the concept that nutrition is the source of energy for exercise. Another distinguishing characteristic of our text is our belief that the serious student of exercise physiology should be aware of the "roots" of the field. Thus we devote an introductory chapter to the early history of our discipline in considerably more detail (with reference citations) than other texts. The inclusion of more than 600 high-quality figures, charts, tables, and photographs should enhance student learning and help to make exercise physiology come alive.

We conclude the text with a look to the future—molecular biology—that now plays such a vital role in unraveling the secrets about the dynamics and interactions of physical activity, health, and disease. Current and future developments about molecular biology basics will be the key to unlocking so many current mysteries related to our field—obesity, muscular force dynamics, athletic potential, gender differences in human performance, debilitating diseases (diabetes, cancer, cardiovascular complications), and adaptation to heat, cold, prolonged microgravity, and altitude. The science of exercise physiology will depend on the future contributions from the new breed of exercise physiology students, well-versed in the basic and applied sciences (including molecular biology)

ORGANIZATION

This sixth edition maintains the same seven-section structure as previous editions, including an introductory section on the origins of exercise physiology, and a concluding "On the Horizons" section that deals with a maturing effort in exercise physiology to incorporate molecular biology to human performance and the many interrelated aspects of health and disease.

FEATURES

Many features throughout the text are included to engage the student and facilitate learning. These include the following:

Introduction: A View of the Past. The text's introduction, "Exercise Physiology: Roots and Historical Perspectives," reflects our interest and respect for the earliest underpinnings of the field, and the direct and indirect contributions of the men and women physicians/scientists who contributed to the field.

In a Practical Sense. This element in every chapter highlights practical applications that include:

- Lowering high blood pressure with dietary intervention: the DASH diet
- Leveraging nutrition to prevent chronic athletic fatigue
- Predicting $\dot{V}O_{2max}$ during pregnancy from submaximum exercise heart rate and oxygen consumption
- Predicting energy expenditure during treadmill walking and running
- Determining anaerobic power and capacity: the Wingate cycle ergometer test
- Predicting pulmonary function variables in males and females
- Measuring lactate threshold
- Blood pressure measurement, classifications, and recommended follow-up

- Placing electrodes of bipolar and 12-lead ECG recordings
- Diabetes, hypoglycemia, and exercise
- Protecting the lower back
- Assessing heat quality of the environment: how hot is too hot?

Focus on Research. Each chapter's Focus on Research features a key research article from a renowned scientist. These well-designed studies illustrate how "theory comes to life" via the dynamics of research.

Integrative Questions. Another element in each chapter, "Integrative Questions," poses open-ended questions to encourage students to consider complex concepts without a single "correct" answer.

Expanded Art Program. The full-color art program continues to be an important feature of the textbook. New figures have been added to enhance the new and updated content.

Up-Close and Personal Interviews. The text features nine contemporary scientists whose important research contributions and visionary leadership continue the tradition of the scientists of prior generations—Steven Blair, Frank Booth, Claude Bouchard, David Costill, Barbara Drinkwater, John Holloszy, Loring Rowell, Bengt Saltin, and Charles Tipton. These individuals clearly merit recognition, not only for expanding knowledge through their many scientific contributions, but also for elucidating mechanisms that underlie responses and adaptations to exercise and health enhancement. Each person has been placed within a section linked to his or her main scholarship interests, yet all of them span one or more sections in terms of scientific contributions. Appendix E, which is available on the Student CD and online at http://connection.lww.com/mkk6e, lists individual honors and awards for each of these distinguished and meritorious scientist–researchers. The intimate insights from the "superstars" should inspire current exercise physiology students to actualize their potential, whether through accomplishments in graduate school, teaching, research, or numerous other exciting opportunities to achieve excellence.

References and Appendices Available on Student CD and Online. All references and appendices are now available on the Student CD that accompanies this text and online at http://connection.lww.com/mkk6e or http://thepoint.lww.com/mkk6e. Appendices feature valuable information on nutritive values, energy expenditures, metabolic computations in open-circuit spirometry, and more.

NEW TO THE SIXTH EDITION

In addition to an expanded art program, components of the entire text have been upgraded to reflect current research findings, applications, and updated recommendations related to the broad areas of exercise physiology. Chapters remain similar to those of the fifth edition, although some additions, deletions, and rearrangement of sections have occurred to enhance the flow of chapter material.

Significant Additions and Modifications to the Text

- Expanded discussion on the effects of different carbohydrate forms on insulin release and the risk of type 2 diabetes, weight gain, and metabolic syndrome.
- Inclusion of the latest Dietary Reference Intakes, a radically new and more comprehensive approach to nutritional recommendations in planning and assessing diets for healthy people that considers gender and life stages of growth and development based on age and, when appropriate, pregnancy and lactation.
- Inclusion of the latest information and recommendations from the *Dietary Guidelines for Americans,* the Institute of Medicine, and the American Heart Association concerning diet and lifestyle choices to promote health, support physically active lives, reduce chronic disease risks, and combat the obesity epidemic.
- Current epidemiologic and clinical findings from the flourishing field of exercise immunology concerning the effects of moderate and strenuous physical activity on immune function.
- Analysis of the nutrient composition of commercially prepared liquid and prepackaged nutrition bars, powders, and liquid meals as an alternative approach in precompetition feeding or as supplemental feedings during periods of competition.
- Presentation of the latest (2005) visual illustration of recommended food intake, the MyPyramid—a personalized approach to choosing a healthier lifestyle that balances nutrition and exercise. Recognizing the diverse demographic backgrounds of individuals in terms of culture and dietary preferences, we also present Mediterranean and Near-Vegetarian Diet Pyramids.
- Expanded discussion of potential ergogenic effects of androstenedione and modified variations of this hormone, including risk of testing positive for the standard marker for the banned anabolic steroid nandrolone.
- Discussion of gender differences in the response to carbohydrate loading and possible gender-related differences in glucose catabolism in exercise before and following endurance training.
- Expanded discussion of Atkins-type low-carbohydrate ketogenic diets on health-related variables and body-weight loss.
- Contemporary information about the optimal number of sets and repetitions, including frequency and relative intensity, of progressive resistance training for optimal strength improvement.
- Added sections on ginseng and ephedrine, two herbal and botanical remedies promoted to improve health,

boost energy, control body weight, and enhance exercise performance.

- The most recent data on the status of overweight and obesity in the United States and worldwide, the health risks and economic burden of obesity-related medical problems, and the government's actions (or lack thereof) to thwart this potential and expanding epidemic.
- Latest information about coronary heart disease rehabilitation programs and the role of exercise as treatment.
- Expanded sections on aging and exercise throughout the text, particularly highlighting research that shows the positive effects of regular exercise on the aging process.

ANCILLARIES: THE TOTAL TEACHING PACKAGE

The carefully developed supplementary material for this text will help instructors and students maximize the benefits of core contents.

Instructor's Resource CD-ROM: Includes Brownstone test generator software offering more than 1200 questions, a complete set of PowerPoint presentations composed of more than 1000 slides presenting key lecture points and images from each chapter of the text, a searchable Image Bank containing every figure from the text downloadable in either .jpg or .pdf format, Chapter Objectives in Microsoft Word format, and a complete package of all these materials pre-prepared for use in your school's Learning Management System (e.g., Desire2Learn, Blackboard, etc.).

Student CD-ROM: Includes an interactive Quiz Bank that provides self-test questions with immediate feedback on material from each of the chapters, in addition to a complete student workbook with 500 pages of questions and exercises covering every aspect of the text, formatted for use in either electronic or hardcopy form. References and Appendices can also be found on this CD

Companion Website: Offers all of the materials from the student and instructor CDs, as well as a Syllabus Conversion Guide. Go to http://connection.lww.com/mkk6e or http://thepoint.lww.com/mkk6e

LiveAdvise Exercise Physiology: LiveAdvise, online teaching advice and student tutoring, is also available with this textbook. Tutors are handpicked educators who are trained to help you. They are very familiar with this book and its ancillary package. You can connect live with a tutor during certain hours of the week, or send e-mail style messages to which the tutor will respond quickly—often within 24 hours. This service is free with the purchase of your textbook!

Instructors: To use this service, please visit http://connection.LWW.com/liveadvise.

Students: See the codebook in the front of this book for more details. You will find instructions for using the service, along with a personal code to log on and get started.

Exercise Physiology, Sixth Edition, offers comprehensive coverage of exercise physiology uniting the topics of physical conditioning, sports nutrition, body composition, weight control, and more. To help your comprehension of the material, the authors have included numerous features that reinforce concepts and enhance your learning experience. This guide will introduce you to these features.

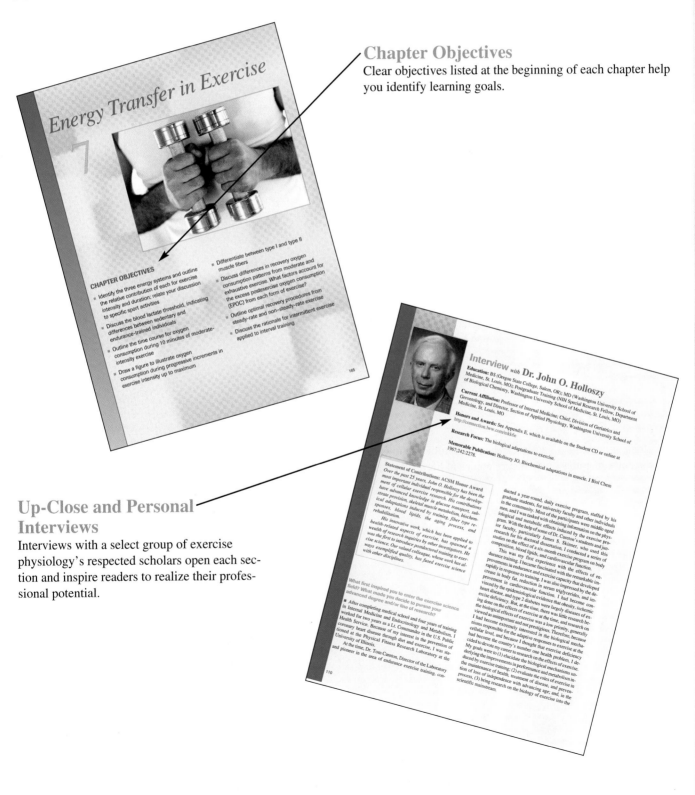

Chapter Objectives

Clear objectives listed at the beginning of each chapter help you identify learning goals.

Up-Close and Personal Interviews

Interviews with a select group of exercise physiology's respected scholars open each section and inspire readers to realize their professional potential.

Vivid Illustrations

More than 600 high-quality figures, charts, tables, and photographs enhance the learning process and make exercise physiology come

Focus on Research

This element presents a key research article from a renowned scientist and illustrates how "theory comes to life."

In a Practical Sense

These boxes connect theoretical concepts to practical skills.

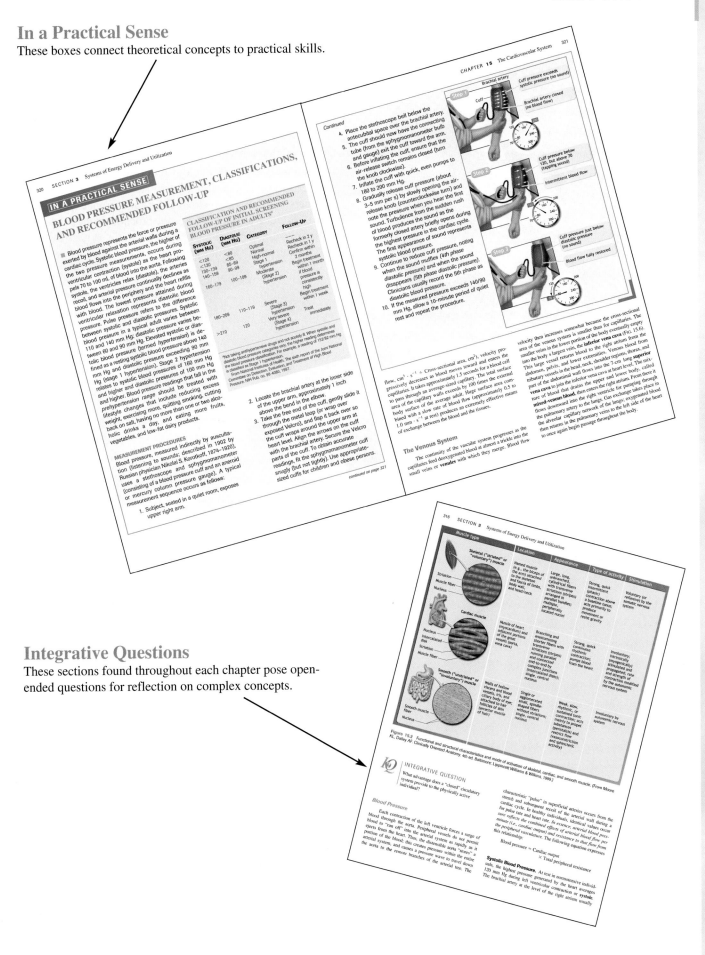

Integrative Questions

These sections found throughout each chapter pose open-ended questions for reflection on complex concepts.

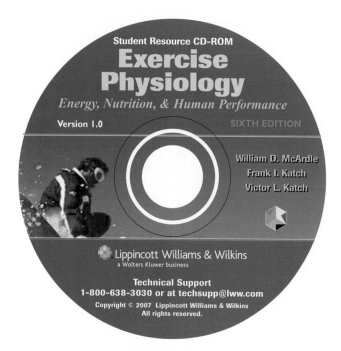

Bonus Student CD-ROM

The CD-ROM packaged with the book includes a robust student workbook with over 500 pages of additional questions and activities. Plus the CD-ROM offers a quiz tool with numerous multiple choice and true/false questions to allow you to test your knowledge of text material and better prepare for exams. The materials from the CD-ROM are also available at http://connection.lww.com/mkk6e or http://thepoint.lww.com/mkk6e.

LiveAdvise

Online Tutoring and Assistance Service

LiveAdvise Exercise Physiology online tutoring and course assistance service is free with this textbook. Students and faculty members will have access to live assistance from experts in the field of exercise physiology. See the brochure in the front of the book or visit http://connection.LWW.com/liveadvise for more information and to try this free service.

acknowledgments

We wish to thank many individuals. First, to Dr. Loring Rowell for his constructive comments on the chapters related to pulmonary and cardiovascular dynamics during rest and exercise, particularly the sections related to the possible role of the venous system as an active vasculature. We thank Drs. Victor Convertino and Charles Tipton for insightful comments and suggestions on the microgravity chapter.

Stephen Lee (Exercise Physiology Laboratory, Johnson Space Center, Houston) kindly supplied original NASA photos and documents, and Mission Specialist Astronaut Dr. Martin Fettman (Colorado State University, Ft. Collins, CO) provided original slides he took during his Skylab 2 Mission, and Dr. Helen Lane (Chief Nutritionist, Johnson Space Center, Houston), provided prepublication documents and resource materials. Dr. Ron White, National Space Biomedical Research Institute allowed us to use charts he helped to create from *Human Physiology In Space Teacher's Manual*. We sincerely appreciate the expertise of Drs. Frank Booth, University of Missouri, Kristin Steumple, Department of Health and Exercise Science at Gettysburg College, and Marvin Balouyt, Division of Kinesiology, University of Michigan, for their expert opinions and suggestions for improving the chapter on molecular biology. Shaun Wallace, Hypoxico Inc., provided photos of the Wallace altitude tent (altitudetent.com). Mr. John Selby (www.hyperlite.co.uk) kindly provided timely information and photos of the portable, collapsible decompression chamber. Gerald J. Nolan, Glenn Research Center and Jim Eckles, White Sands Missile Range, provided original NASA photographs. Many competent staff associates, web curators, and research scientists at various NASA facilities helped to direct us to original documents and photographs. Dr. Alex Knight, York University, UK, graciously provided information about molecular biology techniques he has pioneered (in vitro motility assay) and other information and a photograph about myosin, muscle, and single molecules. Yakl Freedman (www.dna2z.com) was supportive in supplying recent information about DNA and molecular biology. Sue Hilt of the American College of Sports Medicine staff headquarters did a superb job of securing the text of the Citation and Honor Awards reproduced in Appendix E. Dr. Martine Thomis, Leuven University, kindly sent original information from his research group's studies about muscular strength in twins. Dr. Sam Case, Western Maryland College, generously supplied original photos of the Iditarod competition. Dr. James A. Freeman, professor of English, University of Massachusetts, unselfishly lent his expertise to make words sing. Dr. Barry Franklin, Beaumont Hospital, Detroit, MI, supplied original information about cardiac rehabilitation. Paul Petrich, Goleta, CA, provided photos of scuba expeditions. The Trustees of Amherst College and Archival Library gave permission to reproduce the photographs and materials of Dr. Hitchcock. Magnus Mueller, the University of Geisen, kindly provided the photo of Liebig's Geisen lab on p. xx.

We are collectively indebted to the nine researchers/scholars who took time from their busy schedules to answer our interview questions and provide personal photos. Each of those individuals, in his or her own unique way, inspired the three of us in our careers by their work ethic, scientific excellence, and generosity of time and advice with colleagues and students. Over the years, we have had the good fortune to come to know these individuals both socially and in the academic arena. We must admit, however, that the interviews provided insights previously unknown to us. We hope you too are as impressed as we are by all they have accomplished and given back to the profession. Frank Katch also wishes to thank Dr. Drinkwater, who served on his MS thesis at UC Santa Barbara. He now 'fesses up after 40 years that she provided much needed statistical and grammatical assistance beyond the call of duty with that project!

We also acknowledge the following Master's and senior honors students who contributed so much to our research and personal experiences: Pedro Alexander, Christos Balabinis, Margaret Ballantyne, Brandee Black, Michael Carpenter, Steven Christos, Roman Czula, Gwyn Danielson, Toni Denahan, Marty Dicker, Sadie Drumm, Peter Frykman, Scott Glickman, Marion Gurry, Carrie Hauser, Margie King, Peter LaChance, Jean Lett, Maria Likomitrou, Robert Martin, Cathi Moorehead, Susan Novitsky, Joan Perry, Sharon Purdy, Michelle Segar, Debra Spiak, Lorraine Turcotte, Lori Waiter, Stephen Westing, and Howard Zelaznik.

Finally, we would like to thank all of the individuals at LWW who helped bring this sixth edition to fruition.

William D. McArdle
Sound Beach, NY

Frank I. Katch
Santa Barbara, CA

Victor L. Katch
Ann Arbor, MI

contents

Section 3 Systems of Energy Delivery and Utilization

Interview with Dr. Loring B. Rowell

PART TWO: APPLIED EXERCISE PHYSIOLOGY

Section 4 Enhancement of Energy Capacity

Interview with Dr. Bengt Saltin

Section 7 Exercise, Successful Aging, and Disease Prevention

Interview with Dr. Steven N. Blair

On the Horizon

Interview with Dr. Frank Booth

Introduction: A View of the Past

Exercise Physiology: Roots and Historical Perspectives

Since the first edition of our textbook 25 years ago in 1981, knowledge concerning the physiologic effects of exercise in general, and the body's unique and specific responses to training in particular has exploded. Tipton's search of the 1946 English literature for the terms *exercise* and *exertion* yielded 12 citations in 5 journals.[59] Tipton also cited a 1984 analysis by Booth, who reported that in 1962, the number of yearly citations of the term *exertion* increased to 128 in 51 journals, and by 1981, there were 655 citations to the word *exertion* in 224 journals. The accompanying figure reveals the number of entries for the words *exercise* or *exertion* referred to above from an Internet search of *Index Medicus* (Medline) and for the years 2000 to October 11, 2005, using PubMed (www.ncbi.nlm.nih.

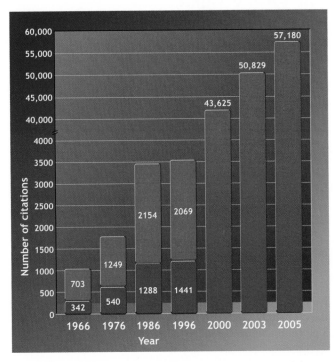

Exercise or *exertion* as a topic *(top bars)* and frequency of the word *exercise* appearing in a scientific journal *(bottom bars)* for the years 1966 to 1996 (from Index Medicus). The last three columns used PubMed via an Internet search for citations with the terms *exercise* or *exertion*.

gov/entrez/query.fcgi). In just a two-year period, the number of citations has increased another 12.5%, and since 2000, 31.1%. At the time of the fourth edition, we stated that the greatest increases occurred between 1976 and 1986, and that citation frequency appeared to level off from 1986 and 1996. From that time, the rate of increase has been even greater. Obviously, we misjudged how greatly exercise-related topics would affect research productivity in biologic sciences research. With expanding interest in molecular biology related to some facet of exercise and physical activity, the rate of citations devoted to these topics should continue to accelerate.

As graduate students in the late 1960s, we never dreamed that interest in exercise physiology would increase so dramatically. A new generation of scholars committed to studying the scientific basis of exercise set to work. Some studied the physiologic mechanisms involved in adaptations to regular exercise; others evaluated individual differences in exercise and sports performance. Collectively, both approaches contributed knowledge to the growing field of exercise physiology. At our first scientific conference (American College of Sports Medicine [ACSM] in Las Vegas, 1967), we rubbed elbows with the "giants" of the field, many of whom were themselves students of the leaders of their era. Sitting under an open tent in the Nevada desert with one of the world's leading physiologists, Dr. David Bruce Dill (then age 74), we listened to his researcher—a high school student—lecture about temperature regulation in the desert burro. Later, one of us (FK) sat next to a white-haired gentleman and chatted about a Master's thesis project. Only later did an embarrassed FK learn that this gentleman was Captain Albert R. Behnke, MD (1898–1993; ACSM Honor Award, 1976), the modern-day "father" of human body composition assessment and whose crucial experiment in diving physiology established standards for decompression and use of mixed gases. His pioneering studies of hydrostatic weighing in 1942, the development of a reference man and reference woman model, and creation of the somatogram based on anthropometric measurements underlie much current work in body composition assessment (see Chapter 28 and its "Focus on Research"). That timely meeting began a lasting personal and fulfilling professional friendship until Dr. Behnke's death in 1993. Several hundred ACSM members listened attentively as the superstars of exercise

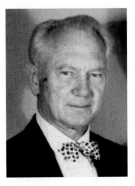

Albert R. Behnke

physiology and physical fitness (Per-Olof Åstrand, Erling Asmussen, Bruno Balke, Elsworth Buskirk, Thomas Cureton, Lars Hermansen, Steven Horvath, Henry Montoye, Bengt Saltin, Charles Tipton) presented their research and fielded penetrating questions from an audience of young graduate students eager to savor the latest scientific information.

Over the years, the three of us were fortunate to work with the very best in our field. William McArdle studied for his PhD at the University of Michigan with Dr. Henry Montoye (charter member of ACSM, President of ACSM 1962–1963, Citation Award, 1973) and Dr. John Faulkner (President of ACSM, 1971–1972, Citation Award, 1973, and ACSM Honor Award, 1992). At the University of California, Berkeley, Victor Katch completed his MS thesis in physical education under the supervision of Dr. Jack Wilmore (ACSM President, 1978–1979, Citation Award 1984, and first editor of *Exercise and Sport Science Reviews*, 1973–1974) and was a doctoral student of Dr. Franklin Henry (ACSM Honor Award, 1975, originator of the "Memory-Drum Concept" about the specificity of exercise, and author of the seminal paper "Physical Education—an Academic Discipline," *JOHPER* 1964;35:32). Frank Katch completed his MS degree at the University of California, Santa Barbara, under the supervision of Dr. Ernest Michael, Jr., (former PhD student of pioneer exercise physiologist–physical fitness scientist Dr. Thomas Kirk Cureton, ACSM Honor Award, 1969) and Dr. Barbara Drinkwater (President of ACSM, 1988–1989; ACSM Honor Award, 1996), and then also completed doctoral studies at the University of California, Berkeley with Professor Henry.

As the three of us examine those earlier times, we realize, like many of our colleagues, that our academic good fortunes prospered because our professors and mentors shared an unwavering commitment to study sport and exercise from a strong scientific and physiologic perspective. These scholars demonstrated why it was crucial that physical educators be well grounded in both the scientific basics and underlying concepts and principles of exercise physiology.

We are so pleased to acknowledge the pioneers who created exercise physiology, realizing full well the difficult task in an introduction to adequately chronicle the history of exercise physiology from its origins in ancient Asia to the present. Instead, our brief review presents a historical tour regarding topics not normally covered in prior exercise physiology textbooks or history texts. Our discussion begins with an acknowledgment of the ancient but tremendously influential Greek physicians; along the way, we highlight some milestones (and ingenious experiments), including the many contributions from Sweden, Denmark, Norway, and Finland that fostered the study of sport and exercise as a respectable field of scientific inquiry.

A treasure of information about the early beginnings of exercise physiology in America was uncovered in the archives of Amherst College, Massachusetts, in an anatomy and physiology textbook (incorporating a student study guide) written by the first American father-and-son writing team. The father, Edward Hitchcock, was President of Amherst College; the son, Edward Hitchcock, Jr., an Amherst graduate and Harvard-trained physician, made detailed anthropometric and strength measurements of almost every student enrolled at Amherst College from 1861 to 1889. A few years later in 1891, much of what forms current college curricula in exercise physiology, including evaluation of body composition by anthropometry and muscular strength by dynamic measurements, began in the first physical education scientific laboratory at Harvard University's Lawrence Scientific School. Even before the creation of this laboratory, another less formal but still tremendously influential factor affected the development of exercise physiology: the publication during the 19th century of American textbooks on anatomy and physiology, physiology, physiology and hygiene, and anthropometry. TABLE 1 lists a sampling of 45 textbooks published between 1801 and 1899 containing information about the muscular, circulatory, respiratory, nervous, and digestive systems—including the influence of exercise and its effects—that eventually shaped the content area of exercise physiology during the next century. Additional textbooks from 1900 to 1947 deal with exercise, training, and exercise physiology.[a]

IN THE BEGINNING: ORIGINS OF EXERCISE PHYSIOLOGY FROM ANCIENT GREECE TO AMERICA IN THE EARLY 1800s

Exercise physiology arose mainly in early Greece and Asia Minor, although the topics of exercise, sports, games, and health concerned even earlier civilizations. These included the Minoan and Mycenaean cultures, the great biblical empires of David and Solomon, Assyria, Babylonia, Media, and Persia, including the Empires of Alexander. Other early references to sports, games, and health practices (personal hygiene, exercise, and training) were recorded in the ancient civilizations of Syria, Egypt, Macedonia, Arabia, Mesopotamia and Persia, India, and China. The greatest influence on Western Civilization, however, came from the Greek physicians of antiquity—Herodicus (5th century BC); Hippocrates (460–377 BC), and Claudius Galenus or Galen (AD 131–201[b]).

Herodicus, a physician and athlete, strongly advocated proper diet in physical training. His early writings and devoted followers influenced the famous physician Hippocrates ("father of preventive medicine"), credited with producing 87 treatises on medicine—several on health and hygiene—during the influential Golden Age of Greece.[7] Hippocrates espoused a profound understanding of human suffering, emphasizing a

---

[a] Buskirk[11] provides a bibliography of books and review articles on exercise, fitness, and exercise physiology from 1920 to 1979. Berryman[7] lists many textbooks and essays from the time of Hippocrates through the Civil War period in the United States.
[b] According to Green, the dates for Galen's birth are estimates based on a notation Galen made when at age 38 he served as personal physician to the Roman emperors Marcus Aurelius and Lucius Verus.[24] Siegel's bibliography contains an excellent source for references to Galen.[57]

TABLE 1 ■ SAMPLING OF TEXTBOOKS ON ANATOMY AND PHYSIOLOGY, ANTHROPOMETRY, EXERCISE AND TRAINING, AND EXERCISE PHYSIOLOGY (1801–1947)

YEAR	AUTHOR AND TEXT	YEAR	AUTHOR AND TEXT
1801	Willich AFM. *Lectures on Diet and Regimen: Being a Systematic Inquiry into the Most Rational Means of Preserving Health and Prolonging Life: Together with Physiological and Chemical Explanations, Calculated Chiefly for the Use of Families, in Order to Banish the Prevailing Abuses and Prejudices in Medicine.* New York: T and J Sworos, 1801.	1866	Flint A. *The Physiology of Man; Designed to Represent the Existing State of Physiological Science as Applied to the functions of the Human Body. Vol. 1. Introduction; The Blood; Circulation; Respiration.* 1866. *Vol II. Digestion; Absorption;* Lymph and Chyle (1867). *Vol. III. Secretion; Excretion; Ductless Glands; Nutrition; Animal Heat; Movement; Voice and Speech* (1870). *Vol. IV. Nervous System* (1873). *Vol. V. Special Senses; Generation* (1874). New York: D. Appleton and Company.
1831	Hitchcock E. *Dyspepsy Forestalled and Resisted, or, Lectures on Diet, Regimen, and Employment.* 2nd ed. Northampton: J.S. & C. Adams, 1831.	1866	Huxley TH. *Lessons in Elementary Physiology.* London: Macmillan and Co., 1866.
1833	Beaumont W. *Experiments and Observations on the Gastric Juice and the Physiology of Digestion.* Pittsburgh: F.P. Allen, 1883.	1866	Lewis D. *Weak Lungs and How to Make them Strong.* Boston: Ticknor and Fields, 1866.
1839	Carpenter WB. *Principles of Physiology, General and Comparative.* London: John Churchill, 1839. 4th ed. 1854.	1869	Dalton JC. *A Treatise on Physiology and Hygiene; for Schools, Families, and Colleges.* New York: Harper & Brothers, 1869.
1842	Carpenter WB. *Principles of Human Physiology.* London: Churchill, 1842.	1869	Gould BA. *Investigations in the Military and Anthropological Statistics of American Soldiers. Published for the U.S. Sanitary Commission.* New York: Hurd and Houghton, 1869.
1843	Carpenter WB. *Principles of Human Physiology, with Their Chief Applications to Pathology, Hygiene, and Forensic Medicine. Especially Designed for the Use of Students.* Philadelphia: Lea & Blanchard, 1843, Numerous reprints and editions; 9th ed, 1881 (London): 4th American ed., 1890.	1871	Flint A. *On the Physiological Effects of Severe and Protracted Muscular Exercise; with Special Reference to Its Influence Upon the Excretion of Nitrogen.* New York: D. Appleton & Co., 1871.
1843	Combe A. *The Principles of Physiology Applied to the Preservation of Health, and to the Improvement of Physical and Mental Education.* New York: Harper & Brothers, 1843.	1873	Huxley TH, Youmans WJ. *The Elements of Physiology and Hygiene for Educational Institutions.* New York: D. Appleton & Co., 1873.
1844	Dunglison R. *Human Health: The Influence of Atmosphere and Locality; Change of Air and Climate; Seasons; Food; Clothing: Bathing and Mineral Springs; Exercise; Sleep; Corporeal and Intellectual Pursuits, on Healthy Man; Constituting Elements of Hygiene.* Philadelphia: Lea & Blanchard, 1844.	1873	Morgan JE. *University Oars.* London: MacMillan, 1873.
1846	Warren JC. *Physical Education and the Preservation of Health.* Boston: William D. Ticknor, 1846.	1875	Baxter JH. *Statistics, Medical and Anthropological, of the Provost-Marshal-General's Bureau, Derived from Records of the Examination for Military Service in the Armies of the United States During the Late War of the Rebellion, of Over a Million Recruits, Drafted Men, Substitutes, and Enrolled Men. Vol. 1.* Washington, DC: U.S. Government Printing Office, 1875.
1848	Cuder C. *Anatomy and Physiology Designed for Academies and Families.* Boston: Benjamin B. Mussey and Co., 1848.		
1852	Ehickwell E. *The Laws of Life, with Special Reference to the Physical Education of Girls.* New York: George P. Putnam, 1852.	1876	Hitchcock E. A part of the course of instruction given in the Department of Physical Education and Hygiene in Amherst College. First issued by the class of 1877 while juniors. Amherst, MA, 1876.
1854	Stokes W. *Diseases of the Heart and Aorta.* Philadelphia: Lindsay, 1854.	1877	Flint A. *A Text-Book of Human Physiology; Designed for the Use of Practitioners and Students of Medicine.* New York: D. Appleton, 1877. (2nd ed., rev. and cor. 1879; 3rd ed., rev. and cor. 1881, 1882, 1884, 1888; 4th ed., entirely rewritten 1888 and published 1889, 1891, 1892, 1893, 1895, 1896, 1897, 1901.)
1855	Combe A. *The Physiology of Digestion, Considered with the Relation to the Principles of Dietetics.* Philadelphia: Harper and Brothers, 1855.		
1856	Beecher C, *Physiology and Calisthenics for Schools and Families.* New York: Harper and Brothers, 1856.	1877	Flint A. *The Source of Muscular Power, as Deduced from Observations Upon the Human Subject Under Conditions of Rest, and of Muscular Exercise.* London: 1877.
1859	Flint A. *The Clinical Study of the Heart Sounds in Health and Disease.* Philadelphia: Collins, 1859.	1878	Flint A. *On the Sources of Muscular Power, Arguments and Conclusions Drawn from Observations Upon the Human Subject, Under Conditions of Rest and of Muscular Exercise.* New York: D. Appleton and Company, 1878.
1860	Hitchcock E, Hitchcock E Jr. *Elementary Anatomy and Physiology for Colleges, Academies, and Other Schools.* New York: Ivison, Phinney & Co., 1860.		
1863	Ordronaux J. *Manual of Instruction for Military Surgeons, on the Examination of Recruits and Discharge of Soldiers.* New York: D. Van Nostrand, 1863.	1878	Foster M. *A Text-Book of Physiology.* London: Macmillan and Co. 1878.
1866	Flint A. *A Treatise on the Principles and Practice of Medicine; Designed for the Use of Practitioners and Students of Medicine.* Philadelphia: H.C. Les, 1866; 5th edition, 1884.	1881	Huxley TH, Youmans WJ. *The Elements of Physiology and Hygiene: A Text-Book for Educational Institutions.* New York: Appleton and Co., 1881.

continued on page xxvi

TABLE 1 ■ *continued*

YEAR	AUTHOR AND TEXT
1884	Martin HN, Martin HC. *The Human Body. A Beginner's Text-book of Anatomy, Physiology and Hygiene.* New York: H. Holt and Company, 1884 (261 p); revised, 1885.
1885	Martin HN, Martin HC. *The Human Body. A Beginner's Text-book of Anatomy, Physiology and Hygiene, with Directions for Illustrating Important Facts of Man's Anatomy from That of the Lower Animals, and with Special References to the Effects of Alcoholic and Other Stimulants, and of Narcotics.* New York: Henry Holt and Son, 1885.
1888	Huxley TH, Martin HN. *A Course of Elementary Instruction in Practical Biology.* Rev. ed. London: Macmillan and Co., 1888.
1888	Lagrange F. *Physiology of Bodily Exercise.* New York: D. Appleton and Company, 1890.
1889	Hitchcock E, Seelye HH. *An Anthropometric Manual, Giving the Average and Mean Physical Measurements and Tests of Male College Students and Method of Securing Them.* 2nd ed. Amherst, MA: Williams, 1889.
1893	Kolb G. *Physiology of Sport.* London: Krohne and Sesemann, 1893.
1895	Galbraith AM. *Hygiene and Physical Culture for Women.* New York: Dodd, Mead and Company, 1895.
1896	Atkinson E. *The Science of Nutrition.* 7th edition. Boston: Damrell & Upham, 1896.
1896	Martin H.N. *The Human Body. An Account of Its Structure and Activities and the Conditions of Its Healthy Working.* New York: Holt & Co., 1881; 3rd ed. rev., 1864; 4th ed. rev. 1885; 5th ed. rev., 1888, 1889 (621 p); 6th ed. rev., 1890, 1894 (621 p); 7th ed., 1896 (685 p); 8th ed. rev., 1896 (685 p).
1896	Seaver, JW. *Anthropometry and Physical Examination. A Book for Practical Use in Connection with Gymnastic Work and Physical Education.* New Haven, CN: Press of the O.A. Dorman Co., 1896.
1898	Martin H.N. *The Human Body. A Text-book of Anatomy, Physiology and Hygiene; with Practical Exercises.* 5th ed., rev. by George Wells Fitz. New York: H. Holt and Company. 1898 (408 p), 1899 (408 p); 5 editions 1900, 1902, 1911, 1912, 1930.
1900	Atwater WO, Bryant AP. Dietary Studies of University Boat Crews. U.S. Department of Agriculture, Office of Experiment Stations, Bulletin no. 25. Washington, DC: U.S. Government Printing Office, 1900.
1900	Howell WH, ed. *An American Text-Book of Physiology. Vol. 1. Blood Lymph, and Circulation; Secretion, Digestion, and Nutrition; Respiration and Animal Heat; Chemistry of the Body.* 2nd. rev. Philadelphia: W.B. Saunders & Company, 1900.
1901	Howell WH, ed. *An American Text-Book of Physiology. Vol. 2. Muscle and Nerve; Central Nervous System; The Special Senses; Special Muscular Mechanisms; Reproduction.* 2nd. rev. Philadelphia: W.B. Saunders & Company, 1901.
1902	Hastings WW. *A Manual for Physical Measurements for Use in Normal Schools, Public and Preparatory Schools, Boys Clubs, Girls Clubs, and Young Men's Christian Associations.* Springfield: Young Men's Christian Association Training School, 1902.

YEAR	AUTHOR AND TEXT
1903	Demeny G. *Les Bases Scientifiques de Education Physique.* Paris. Felix Alcan, Editeur, 1903.
1903	Flint A. *Collected Essays and Articles on Physiology and Medicine,* 2 volumes. New York: D. Appleton and Company, 1903
1904	Butts EL. *Manual of Physical Drill. United States Army.* New York: D. Appleton and Company, 1904.
1904	Mosso A. *Fatigue.* New York: G.P. Putnam's Sons, 1904.
1905	Atwater WO, Benedict FG. *A Respiration Calorimeter with Appliances for the Direct Determination of Oxygen.* Washington, DC: Carnegie Institution of Washington, 1905.
1905	Flint A. *Handbook of Physiology; for Students and Practitioners of Medicine.* New York: The Macmillan Company, 1905.
1906	Hough T, Sedgewick WT. *The Human Mechanism, Its Physiology and Hygiene and the Sanitation of Its Surroundings.* New York: Ginn and Company, 1906.
1906	Sargent DA. *Physical Education.* Boston: Ginn and Company, 1906.
1906	Sherrington SC. *The Integrative Action of the Nervous System.* New Haven, CT: Yale University Press, 1906.
1906	Stevens AW, Darling ED. *Practical Rowing and the Effects of Training,* Boston: Little, Brown and Company, 1906.
1908	Fisher I. *The Effect of Diet on Endurance: Based on an Experiment with Nine Healthy Students at Yale University, January-June, 1906.* New Haven, CT: Tuttle, Morehouse and Taylor Press, 1908.
1908	Fitz GW. *Principles of Physiology and Hygiene* 2nd ed. rev. New York: H. Holt and Company, 1908; 2nd ed. rev., 1908.
1909	McKenzie RT. *Exercise in Education and Medicine.* Philadelphia: W.B. Saunders Company, 1909.
1911	Cannon WB. *The Mechanical Factors of Digestion:* New York: Longmans, Green and Company, 1911.
1914	Barcroft J. *The Respiratory Function of the Blood.* Cambridge: Cambridge University Press, 1914.
1914	Goodman EH. *Blood Pressure in Medicine and Surgery.* Philadelphia: Lea & Febiger, 1914.
1915	Benedict F, Murchhauser J. *Energy Transformation During Horizontal Walking. Carnegie Institute Publication. No. 231.* Washington, DC: Carnegie Institute of Washington, 1915.
1915	Cannon WB. *Bodily Changes in Pain, Hunger, Fear and Rage.* New York: D. Appleton and Company, 1915.
1917	Haldane JS. *Organism and Environment as Illustrated by the Physiology of Breathing.* New Haven: Yale University Press, 1917.
1918	Fisher I. *The Effect of Diet on Endurance.* New Haven: Yale University Press, 1918.
1918	Lewis T. *The Soldier's Heart and the Effort Syndrome.* New York: P.B. Hoeber, 1918.
1918	Starling EH. *Linacare Lecture; The Law of the Heart.* London. Longmans, Green and Company, 1918.
1918	Wilbur WC. *The Koehler Method of Physical Drill.* Philadelphia: J.B. Lippincott Company, 1918.
1919	Bainbridge FA. *Physiology of Muscular Exercises.* New York: Longmans, Green and Company, 1919.

continued on page xxvii

TABLE 1 ■ *continued*

YEAR	AUTHOR AND TEXT	YEAR	AUTHOR AND TEXT
1919	Love AG, Davenport CB. *Physical Examination of the First Million Draft Recruits: Methods and Results.* Washington, DC: U.S. Government Printing Office, 1919.	1931	Schmidt FA, Kohlrasch W. *Physiology of Exercise.* (Translated by C.B. Sputh). Philadelphia: F.A. Davis and Company, 1931.
1920	Amar J. *The Human Motor.* New York: E.P. Dutton and Company, 1920.	1932	Boas EP, Goldschmidt EF. *The Heart Rate.* Springfield, IL: Charles C. Thomas, 1932.
1920	Burton-Ovitz R. *A Textbook of Physiology.* Philadelphia: W.B. Saunders Company, 1920.	1932	Creed R.S., et al. *Reflex Activity of the Spinal Cord.* Oxford, Oxford University Press, 1932.
1920	Dreyer G. *The Assessment of Physical Fitness.* New York: P.B. Hoeber, 1920.	1932	Gould AG, Dye JA. *Exercise and Its Physiology.* New York: A.S. Barnes and Company, 1932.
1920	Gaskell WH. *The Involuntary Nervous System.* New York: Longmans, Green and Company, 1920.	1932	Grollman A. *The Cardiac Output of Man in Health and Disease.* Springfield, IL: Charles C Thomas, 1932.
1920	Jansen M. *On Bone Formation: Its Relation to Tension and Pressure.* New York: Longmans, Green and Company, 1920.	1932	McCloy CH. *The Measurement of Athletic Power.* New York: A.S. Barnes and Company, 1932.
1921	Martin EG. *Tests of Muscular Efficiency.* Physiological Reviews 1921;1:454.	1933	Haggard HW, Greenberg LA. *Diet and Physical Efficiency.* New Haven, CT: Yale University Press, 1933.
1922	Haldane JS. *Respiration.* New Haven, CT: Yale University Press, 1922.	1933	Schneider EC. *Physiology of Muscular Activity.* Philadelphia: WB Saunders Company, 1933.
1922	Krogh A. *The Anatomy and Physiology of Capillaries.* New Haven, CT: Yale University Press, 1922.	1934	Konradi, Slonim D, Farfel VS. *Work Physiology.* Moscow: Medgiz Publishing, 1934.
1923	MacKenzie RT. *Exercise in Education and Medicine.* Philadelphia: W.B. Saunders Company, 1923.	1935	Boorstein SW. *Orthopedics for the Teacher of Crippled Children.* New York: Aiden, 1935.
1924	Douglas CG, Priestley JG. *Human Physiology.* Oxford: The Clarendon Press, 1924.	1935	Dawson PM. *The Physiology of Physical Education.* Baltimore: Williams & Wilkins, 1935.
1926	Fulton JF. *Muscular Contraction and Reflex Control of Movement.* Baltimore: Williams & Wilkins Company, 1926.	1935	Haggard HW, Greenberg LA. *Diet and Physical Efficiency.* New Haven, CT: Yale University Press, 1935.
1926	Hill AV. *Muscular activity.* Lectures on the Herter Foundation, 16th course. "Muscles," 1924. Baltimore: Williams & Wilkins (for the Johns Hopkins University), 1926.	1935	Haldane JS, Priestly JG. *Respiration.* New York: Oxford Univesity Press, 1935.
1927	Deutsch F, Kauf E. *Heart and Athletics.* Translation by L.M. Warfield. St. Louis C. V. Mosby Company, 1927.	1937	Griffin FWW. *The Scientific Basis of Physical Education.* London: Oxford University Press, 1937.
1927	DuBois EF. *Basal Metabolism in Health and Disease.* Philadelphia: Lea and Febiger, 1927.	1938	Benedict FG. *Vital Energetics. A Study in Comparative Basal Metabolism.* Washington, DC: Carnegie Institute of Washington, 1938.
1927	Hill AV. *Living Machinery.* New York: Harcourt, Brace and Company, 1927.	1938	Dill DB. *Life, Heat, and Altitude. Physiological Effects of Hot Climates and Great Heights.* Cambridge: Harvard University Press, 1938.
1927	Hill AV. *Muscular Movement in Man.* New York: McGraw-Hill Book Company, 1927.	1939	Hrdlicka A. *Practical Anthropometry.* Philadelphia: Wistar Institute of Anatomy and Biology, 1939.
1928	Henderson LJ. *Blood: A Study in General Physiology.* New Haven, CT: Yale University Press, 1928.	1939	Krestovnikoff A. *Fiziotologia Sporta.* Moscow: Fizkultura and Sport, 1939.
1928	McCurdy HG, McKenzie RT. *The Physiology of Exercise.* Philadelphia: Lea & Febiger, 1928.	1939	McCurdy JH, Larson LA. *The Physiology of Exercise.* Philadelphia: Lea and Febiger, 1939.
1928	Schwartz L, et al. *The Effect of Exercise on the Physical Condition and Development of Adolescent Boys.* U.S. Public Health Service Bulletin 179, Washington, DC: U.S. Government Printing Office, 1928.	1939	Schneider EC. *Physiology of Muscular Activity.* 2nd ed. Philadelphia: W.B. Saunders Company, 1939.
1929	Krogh A. *The Anatomy and Physiology of Capillaries.* 2nd ed. New Haven, CT: Yale University Press, 1929.	1942	Cureton TK. *Physical Fitness Workbook.* Champaign, IL: Stipes Publishing Company, 1942.
1929	Macklin CC. The Musculature of the bronchi and lungs. *Physiological Reviews* 1929;9:1 (492 references).	1945	Cureton TK, et al. *Endurance of Young Men.* Washington, DC: National Research Council, National Society for Research in Child Development, 1945.
1930	Starling EH. *Human Physiology.* Philadelphia: Lea and Febiger, 1930.	1947	Adolph EF, et al. *Physiology of Man in the Desert.* New York: Wiley, 1947.
1931	Bainbridge FA. *The Physiology of Muscular Exercise.* 3rd edition. Rewritten by AV Bock, DB Dill. London: Longmans, Green and Company, 1931.	1947	Cureton TK, et al. *Physical Fitness Appraisal and Guidance.* St. Louis: The C.V. Mosby Company, 1947.
1931	Hill, A. V. *Adventures in Biophysics.* London: Oxford University Press, 1931.		

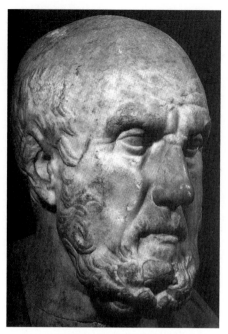

Hippocrates (460–377 BC)

doctor's place at the patient's bedside. Today, physicians take the Hippocratic Oath based on Hippocrates' "Corpus Hippocratum."

Five centuries after Hippocrates, during the early decline of the Roman Empire, Galen emerged as perhaps the most well-known and influential physician that ever lived. The son of a wealthy architect, Galen was born in the city of Pergamos[c] and educated by scholars of the time. He began studying medicine at approximately age 16. During the next 50 years, he implemented and enhanced current thinking about health and scientific hygiene, an area that some might consider "applied" exercise physiology. Throughout his life, Galen taught and practiced the "laws of health": breathe fresh air, eat proper foods, drink the right beverages, exercise, get adequate sleep, have a daily bowel movement, and control one's emotions.[7] A prolific writer, Galen produced at least 80 sophisticated treatises (and perhaps 500 essays) on numerous topics, many of which addressed human anatomy and physiology, nutrition, growth and development, the beneficial effects of exercise, the deleterious consequences of sedentary living, and a variety of diseases and their treatment. One of the first "bench physiologists," Galen conducted original experiments in physiology, comparative anatomy, and medicine, including dissections of humans and a variety of animals (e.g., goats, pigs, cows, horses, elephants). Also, as physician to the gladiators

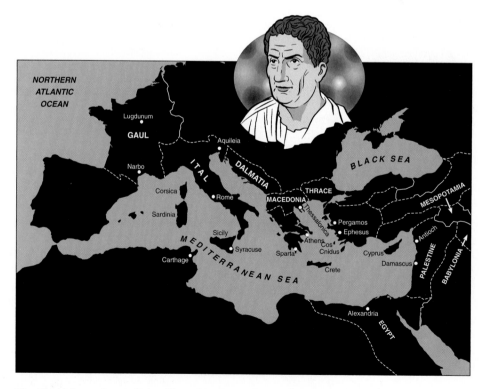

The World According to Galen. The *white dots* refer to the 14 major cities of that time period.

---

[c] An important city on the Mediterranean coast of Asia Minor, Pergamos influenced trade and commerce. From AD 152 to 156, Galen studied in Pergamos, renowned at the time for its library of 50,000 books (approximately one-fourth as many as in Alexandria, the greatest city for learning and education) and its famous medical center in the Temple of Asclepios.

of Pergamos, Galen treated torn tendons and muscles ripped apart in combat by using various surgical procedures he invented, including the procedure depicted in the 1544 woodcut of shoulder surgery shown at the bottom with commentaries from his Greek text *De Fascius*. Galen formulated rehabilitation therapies and exercise regimens, including treatment for a dislocated shoulder. He followed the Hippocratic school of medicine that believed in logical science grounded in experimentation and observation.

Galen wrote detailed descriptions about the forms, kinds, and varieties of "swift" and vigorous exercises, including their proper quantity and duration. The following definition of exercise is from the first complete English translation by Green[24] of Hygiene (*De Sanitate Tuenda*, pages 53–54) (see TABLE 2), Galen's insightful and detailed treatise on healthful living:

> To me it does not seem that all movement is exercise, but only when it is vigorous. But since vigor is relative, the same movement might be exercise for one and not for another. The criterion of vigorousness is change of respiration; those movements that do not alter the respiration are not called exercise. But if anyone is compelled by any movement to breathe more or less or faster, that movement becomes exercise from him. This therefore is what is commonly called exercise or gymnastics, from the gymnasium or public-place to which the inhabitants of a city come to anoint and rub themselves, to wrestle, throw the discus, or engage in some other sport. . . . The uses of exercise, I think are twofold, one for the evacuation of the excrements, the other for the production of good condition of the

TABLE 2 ■ TABLE OF CONTENTS FOR BOOKS 1 AND 2ᵃ OF GALEN'S *DE SANITATE TUENDA (HYGIENE)*	
BOOK 1 **THE ART OF PRESERVING HEALTH**	
Chapter	
I	Introduction
II	The Nature and Sources of Growth and of Disease
III	Production and Elimination of Excrements
IV	Objectives and Hypothesis of Hygiene
V	Conditions and Constitutions
VI	Good Constitution: A Mean Between Extremes
VII	Hygiene of the Newborn
VIII	The Use and Value of Exercise
IX	Hygiene of Breast-Feeding
X	Hygiene of Bathing and Massage
XI	Hygiene of Beverages and of Fresh Air
XII	Hygiene of the Second Seven Years
XIII	Causes and Prevention of Excrementary Retardation
XIV	Evacuation of Retained Excrements
XV	Summary of Book I
BOOK 2 **EXERCISE AND MASSAGE**	
I	Standards of Hygiene Under Individual Conditions
II	Purposes, Time, and Methods of Exercise and Massage
III	Techniques and Varieties of Massage
IV	Theories of Theon and Hippocrates
V	Definitions of Various Terms
VI	Further Definitions About Massage
VII	Amount of Massage and Exercise
VIII	Forms, Kinds, and Varieties of Exercise
IX	Varieties of Vigorous Exercises
X	Varieties of Swift Exercises
XI	Effects, Exercises, Functions, and Movements
XII	Determination of Diet, Exercise, and Regime

ᵃ Book III. Apotherapy, Bathing, and Fatigue. Book IV. Forms and Treatment of Fatigue. Book V. Diagnosis, Treatment, and Prevention of Various Diseases. Book VI. Prophylaxis of Pathological Conditions.

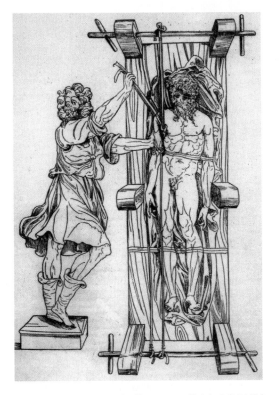

Woodcut by Renaissance artist Francesco Salviati (1544) based on Galen's *De Fascius* from the first century BC. The woodcut showing shoulder surgery provides a direct link with Hippocratic surgical practice that continued through the Byzantine period.

firm parts of the body. For since vigorous motion is exercise, it must needs be that only these three things result from it in the exercising body—hardness of the organs from mutual attrition, increase of the intrinsic warmth, and accelerated movement of respiration. These are followed by all the other individual benefits which accrue to the body from exercise; from hardness of the organs, both insensitivity and strength for function; from warmth, both strong attraction for things to be eliminated, readier metabolism, and better nutrition and diffusion of all substances, whereby it results that solids are softened, liquids diluted, and ducts dilated. And from the vigorous movement of respiration the ducts must be purged and the excrements evacuated.

During the early Greek period, the Hippocratic school of physicians devised ingenious methods to treat common maladies; these methods included procedures to reduce pain from dislocated lower lumbar vertebrae. The illustration from

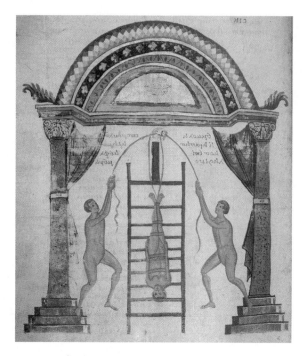

Ancient treatment for low-back pain.

the 11th-century *Commentairies of Apollonius of Chitiron* on the Periarthron of Hippocrates (*top left*) provided details about early Greek surgical "sports medicine" interventions to treat athletes and the common citizen.

The era of more "modern-day" exercise physiology includes the periods of Renaissance, Enlightenment, and Scientific Discovery in Europe. It was then that Galen's ideas affected the writings of the early physiologists, anatomists, doctors, and teachers of hygiene and health.[45,49] For example, in Venice in 1539, the Italian physician Hieronymus Mercurialis (1530–1606) published *De Arte Gymnastica Apud Ancientes* (The Art of Gymnastics Among the Ancients). This text, heavily influenced by Galen and other early Greek and Latin authors, profoundly affected subsequent writings about physical training and exercise (then called gymnastics) and health (hygiene), not only in Europe (influencing the Swedish and Danish gymnastic systems), but also in early America (the 19th-century gymnastic–hygiene movement). The panel in Figure 1, redrawn from *De Arte Gymnastica*, acknowledges the early Greek influence of one of Galen's famous essays, *Exercise with the Small Ball,* and his technical regimen of specific strengthening exercises (discus throwing and rope climbing).

RENAISSANCE PERIOD TO NINETEENTH CENTURY

New ideas formulated during the Renaissance exploded almost every idea inherited from antiquity. Johannes Gutenberg's (ca. 1400–1468 AD) printing press disseminated both classic and newly acquired knowledge. The commoner could learn about local and world events. Education became more available because universities sprang up in Oxford, Cambridge, Cologne, Heidelberg, Prague, Paris, Angiers, Orleans, Vienna,

Padua, Bologna, Siena, Naples, Pisa, Montpellier, Toulouse, Valencia, Lisbon, and Salamanca. Art broke with past forms, emphasizing spatial perspective and realistic depictions of the human body (FIG. 1).

Although the supernatural still influenced discussions of physical phenomena, many persons turned from dogma to experimentation as a source of knowledge. For example, medicine had to confront the new diseases spread by commerce with distant lands. Plagues and epidemics decimated at least 25 million people throughout Europe in just two years (1348–1350). New towns and expanding populations in confined cities led to environmental pollution and pestilence, forcing authorities to cope with new problems of community sanitation and care for the sick and dying. Science had not yet solved the medical problems from disease carriers such as insects and rats.

As populations expanded throughout Europe and elsewhere, medical care became more important for all levels of society. Unfortunately, medical knowledge failed to keep pace with need. For roughly 12 centuries, few advances had been made since the advances in Greek and Roman medicine. The writings of the early physicians had either been lost or preserved only in the Arab world. Thanks to the prestige of classical authors, Hippocrates and Galen still dominated medical education until the end of the 15th century. Renaissance discoveries greatly modified these men's theories, however. New

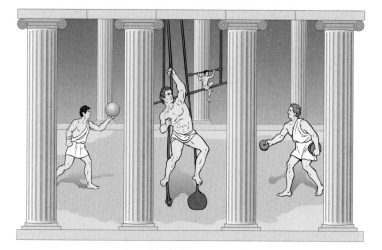

Figure 1   The early Greek influence of Galen's famous essay *Exercise with the Small Ball* and specific strengthening exercises (throwing the discus and rope climbing) appeared in Mercurialis's *De Arte Gumnastica,* a treatise about the many uses of exercise for preventive and therapeutic medical and health benefits. Mercurialis favored discus throwing to aid patients suffering from arthritis and to improve the strength of the trunk and arm muscles. He advocated rope climbing because it did not pose health problems, and he was a firm believer in walking (a mild pace was good for stimulating conversation, and a faster pace would stimulate appetite and help with digestion). He also believed that climbing mountains was good for those with leg problems, long jumping was desirable (but not for pregnant women), but tumbling and handsprings were not recommended because they would produce adverse effects from the intestines pushing against the diaphragm! The *three panels* above represent the exercises as they might have been performed during the time of Galen.

anatomists went beyond simplistic notions of four humors (fire, earth, water, air) and their qualities of hot, dry, cold, and wet when they discovered the complexities of circulatory, respiratory, and excretory mechanisms.[1]

Once rediscovered, these new ideas caused turmoil. The Vatican seemed to ban human dissections, but a number of "progressive" medical schools continued to conduct them, usually sanctioning one or two cadavers a year or with official permission to perform an "anatomy" (the old name for a dissection) every 3 years. Performing autopsies helped physicians solve legal questions about a person's death, or determine the cause of a disease. In the mid-1200s at the University of Bologna (founded in 1088 as a law school), every medical student had to attend one dissection each year, with 20 students assigned to a male cadaver and 30 students to a female cadaver. The first sanctioned dissection in Paris took place in 1407. In Rembrandt's first major portrait commission, the 1632 *The Anatomy Lesson of Dr. Nicholas Tulp*, shown *below*, medical students listen intensely to the renowned Dr. Tulp as he dissects the arm of a recently executed criminal. The pioneering efforts of Vesalius (p. xxxiii) and Harvey (p. xxxiv) made anatomic study a central focus of medical education, yet conflicted with the Church's strictures against violation of the individual rights of the dead because of the doctrine concerning the eventual resurrection of each person's body. In fact, the Church considered anatomic dissections a disfiguring violation of bodily integrity, despite the dismemberment of criminals as an extension of punishment. Nevertheless, the art of the period reflected close collaboration between artists and medical school physicians to portray anatomic dissections, essential for medical education, and to satisfy a public thirst for new information in the emerging fields of physiology and medicine.

In 1316, Mondino de Luzzio (ca. 1275–1326), professor of anatomy at Bologna, published *Anathomia,* the first book of human anatomy. He based his teaching on human cadavers, not Greek and Latin authorities or studies of animals. The 1513 edition of *Anathomia* presented the same drawing as the original edition of the heart with three ventricles, a tribute to his accuracy in translation of the original inaccuracies! Certainly by the turn of the 15th century, anatomic dissections for postmortems were common in the medical schools of France and Italy; they paved the way for the Golden Age of the Renaissance anatomists whose careful observations accelerated understanding of human form and function. Two women from the University of Bologna achieved distinction in the field of anatomy. Laura Bassi (1711–1778), the first woman to earn a doctor of philosophy degree, and the university's first female professor, specialized in experimental physics and basic sciences but had to conduct her experiments at home. Soon after, female scholars were allowed to teach in university classrooms.

At the time, Bassi gave her yearly public lectures on topics related to physics (including electricity and hydraulics, correction distortion in telescopes, hydrometry, and relation between a flame and "stable air"). Anna Morandi Manzolini (1717–1774), also a professor at the University of Bologna, was an expert at creating wax models of internal organs and became the anatomy department's chief model maker. She produced an ear model that students took apart and reassembled to gain a better understanding of the ear's internal structures. Her wax and wood models

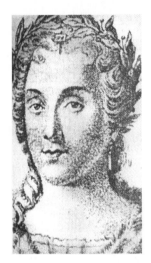

Professor Laura Bassi

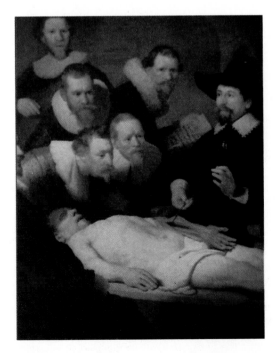

Rembrandt's 1632 *The Anatomy Lesson of Dr. Nicholas Tulp.*

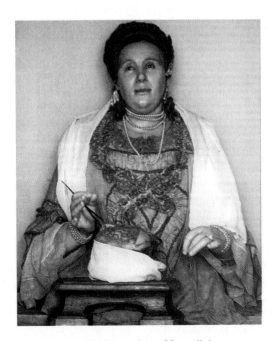

Professor Anna Manzolini

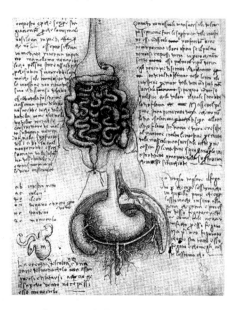

Anatomical sketch by Da Vinci.

of the abdomen and uterus were used didactically in the medical school for several hundred years. The wax self-portrait (*bottom right*, page xxxi) in the Anatomical Museum of the University of Bologna shows Manzolini performing an anatomical dissection, clad in the traditional white lab coat, but also dressed in silks with diamonds and pearl jewelry—the manner expected of a woman of her high social and economic status.

Progress in understanding human anatomic form paved the way for specialists in physical culture and hygiene to design specific exercises to improve overall body strength, and training regimens to prepare for rowing, boxing, wrestling, competitive walking, and track and field activities and competitions.

Notable Achievements by European Scientists

An explosion of new knowledge in the physical and biologic sciences helped prepare the way for future discoveries about human physiology during rest and exercise.

Leonardo da Vinci (1452–1519)

Da Vinci dissected cadavers at the hospital of Santa Maria Nuova in Florence and made detailed anatomic drawings. Accurate as the sketches were, they still preserved Galenic ideas. Although he never saw the pores in the septum of the heart, he included them, believing they existed because Galen had "seen" them. Da Vinci first accurately drew the heart's inner structures and

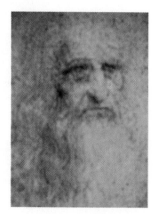

constructed models of valvular function that showed how the blood flowed in only one direction. This observation contradicted Galen's notion about the ebb and flow of blood between the heart's chambers. Because many of Da Vinci's drawings were lost for nearly two centuries, they did not influence later anatomic research.

Da Vinci's work built on and led to discoveries by two fellow artists. Leon Battista Alberti (1404–1472), an architect who perfected three-dimensional perspectives, which influenced Da Vinci's concepts of internal relationships. Da Vinci's drawings no doubt inspired the incomparable Flemish anatomist Andreas Vesalius (1514–1564). These three exemplary Renaissance anatomists empowered physiologists to understand the systems of the body with technical accuracy, not theoretical bias.

Albrecht Dürer (1471–1528)

Dürer, a German contemporary of Da Vinci, extended the Italian's concern for ideal dimensions as depicted in Da Vinci's famous "1513 Vitruvian Man" by illustrating age-related differences in body segment ratios formulated by 1st century BC Roman architect Marcus Vitruvivus Pollio (*De architectura libri decem* [Ten books on architecture]). Dürer created a canon of proportion, considering total height as unity. For example, in his schema, the length of the foot was one-sixth of this total, the head one-seventh, and the hand one-tenth. Relying on his artistic skills rather than objective comparison, Dürer made the ratio of height between men and women as 17 to 18 (soon thereafter proved incorrect). Nonetheless, Dürer's work inspired Behnke[23] in the 1950s to quantify body proportions into reference standards to evaluate body composition in men and women (see Chapter 28).

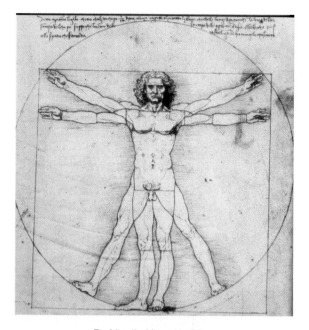

Da Vinci's *Vitruvian Man*.

Michelangelo Buonarroti (1475–1564)

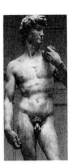

Michelangelo, like Da Vinci, was a superb anatomist. Body segments appear in proper proportion in his accurate drawings. The famous "David" (right) clearly shows the veins, tendons, and muscles enclosing a realistic skeleton. Although his frescos on the Sistine ceiling often exaggerate musculature, they still convey a scientist's vision of the human body.

Andreas Vesalius (1514–1564)

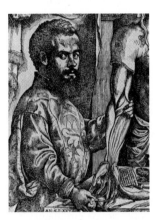

Belgian anatomist and physician Vesalius learned Galenic medicine in Paris, but after making careful human dissections, he rejected the Greek's ideas about bodily functions. At the start of his career, Vesalius authored books on anatomy, originally relying on Arabic texts, but then incorporating observations from his own dissections including a self-portrait (*right*) from *Fabrica* published at age 29 showing the anatomic details of an upper and lower right arm. His research culminated in the exquisitely illustrated text first published in Basel, Switzerland in 1543, *De Humani Corporis Fabrica* (On the Fabric of the Human Body). Many consider Vesalius' drawings the best anatomical renderings ever made, ushering in the age of modern medicine. The same year, he published *Epitome,* a popular version of *De Fabrica* without Latin text.

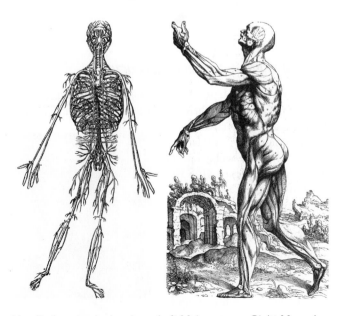

Vesalius' anatomic drawings. *Left,* Major nerves. *Right,* Muscular system in action. Note the graveyard crypts.

Some physicians and clergymen became outraged, fearful that the new science was overturning Galen's time-honored speculations. Vesalius' treatise accurately rendered bones, muscles, nerves, internal organs, blood vessels (including veins for blood-letting), and the brain, but he differed from Galenic tradition by ignoring what he could not see. His remarkably detailed record of the muscular and skeletal architecture of the human body pared away one muscle layer at a time to reveal the hidden structures underneath.

Despite his attempt at accuracy, some of Vesalius' drawings contain curious inaccuracies. For example, he drew the inferior vena cava as a continuous vessel; he inserted an extra muscle to move the eyeball; and added an extra neck muscle present only in apes. Despite these minor discrepancies, Vesalius attempted to connect form with function. He showed that a muscle contracted when a longitudinal slice was made along the muscle's belly, but a transverse cut prevented contraction. Vesalius substantiated that nerves controlled muscles and stimulated movement. His two texts profoundly influenced medical education. They demolished traditional theories about human anatomy and emboldened later researchers to explore circulation and metabolism unburdened by past misconceptions. The illuminating work of Vesalius hastened the subsequent important discoveries in physiology and the beginning of modern science.

Santorio Santorio (1561–1636)

A friend of Galileo and professor of medicine at Padua, Italy, Santorio used innovative tools for his research. He recorded changes in daily body temperature with the first air thermometer as a temperature measuring device he crafted in 1612. Accuracy was poor because scientists had not yet discovered the effects of differential air pressures on temperature. Santorio also measured pulse rates with Galileo's pulsilogium (pulsiometer). Ever inventive, Santorio, a pioneer in the science of physical measurement, studied digestion and changes in metabolism by constructing a wooden frame that supported a chair, bed, and worktable (see illustration below). Suspended from the ceiling with scales, the frame recorded changes in body weight.

For 30 years, Santorio slept, ate, worked, and made love in the weighing contraption to record how much his weight changed as he ate, fasted, or excreted. He invented the term "insensible perspiration" to account for differences in body weight because he believed that weight was gained or lost through the pores during respiration. Often depriving himself of food and drink, Santorio determined that the daily change in body mass approached 1.25 kg. Santorio's book of medical aphorisms, *De Medicina Statica Aphorismi* (1614), drew worldwide attention. Although this scientifically trained Italian instrument inventor did not explain the role of nutrition in weight gain or loss, Santorio nevertheless inspired

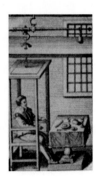

later 18th century researchers in metabolism by quantifying metabolic effects.

William Harvey (1578–1657)

Harvey discovered that blood circulates continuously in one direction and, just as Vesalius had done, overthrew 2000 years of medical dogma. Animal vivisection disproved the ancient supposition that blood moved from the right to left side of the heart through pores in the septum—pores that even Da Vinci and Vesalius acknowledged. Harvey announced his discovery during a 3-day dissection–lecture on April 16, 1616, at the oldest medical institution in England—the Royal College of Physicians in London, originally founded in 1518 by a small 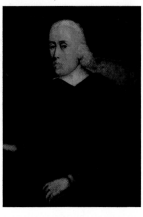 group of distinguished physicians. Twelve years later, Harvey published the details in a 72-page monograph, *Exercitatio Anatomica de Motu Cordis et Sanguinis in Animalibus* (An Anatomical Treatise on the Movement of the Heart and Blood in Animals).

By combining the new technique of experimentation on living creatures with mathematical logic, Harvey deduced that contrary to conventional wisdom, blood flowed in only one direction—from the heart to the arteries and from the veins

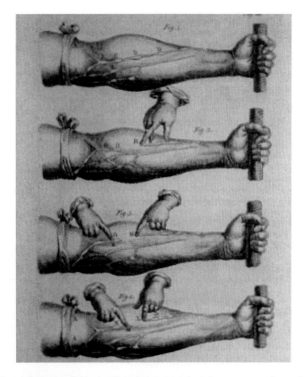

Harvey's famous illustration demonstrating the one-way flow of the circulation.

back to the heart. It then traversed to the lungs before completing a circuit and reentering the heart. Harvey publicly demonstrated the one-way flow of blood by placing a tourniquet around a man's upper arm that constricted arterial blood flow to the forearm and stopped the pulse (see illustration *below left*). By loosening the tourniquet, Harvey allowed some blood into the veins. Applying pressure to specific veins forced blood from a peripheral segment where there was little pressure into the previously empty veins. Thus, Harvey proved that the heart pumped blood through a closed, unidirectional (circular) system, from arteries to veins and back to the heart. As he put it:

> It is proved by the structure of the heart that the blood is continuously transferred through the lungs into the aorta as by two clacks of a water bellows to raise water. It is proved by a ligature that there is a passage of blood from the arteries to the veins. It is therefore demonstrated that the continuous movement of the blood in a circle is brought about by the beat of the heart.[21]

Harvey's experiments with sheep proved mathematically that the mass of blood passing through the sheep's heart in a fixed time was greater than the body could produce—a conclusion identical to that concerning the human heart. Harvey reasoned that if a constant mass of blood exists, then the large circulation volumes would require a one-way, closed circulatory system. Harvey did not explain why the blood circulated, only that it did. However, he correctly postulated that circulation might distribute heat and nourishment throughout the body. Despite the validity of Harvey's observations, distinguished scientists criticized them. Jean Riolan, an ardent Galenist who chaired the anatomy and botany departments at the University of Paris in the 1640s, maintained that if anatomic findings differed from Galen's, then the body in question must be abnormal and the results faulty. Nevertheless, Harvey's epic discovery governed subsequent research on circulation and demolished 1500 years of dogma.

Giovanni Alfonso Borelli (1608–1679)

Borelli, a protégé of Galileo and Benedetto Castelli (1578–1643) and a mathematician at the University of Pisa, Italy, used mathematical models to explain how muscles enabled animals to walk, fish to swim, and birds to fly. His ideas explaining how air entered and exited the lungs, though equally important, were less well known. Borelli's accomplished student, Marcello Malpighi (1628–1694), described blood flowing through microscopic structures (capillaries) around the lung's terminal air sacs (alveoli). Borelli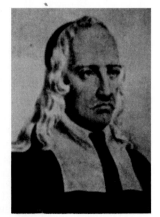

observed that lungs filled with air because chest volume increased as the diaphragm moved downward. He concluded that air passed through the alveoli and into the blood, a sharp contrast to Galen's notion that air in the lungs cooled the heart, and an advance on Harvey's general observation concerning blood flow.

Robert Boyle (1627–1691)

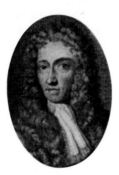

Working at Gresham College, London, with his student Robert Hooke (1635–1703), Boyle devised experiments with a vacuum pump and bell jar to show that combustion and respiration required air. Boyle partially evacuated air from the jar containing a lit candle. The flame soon died. When he removed air from a jar containing a rodent or bird, it became unconscious; recirculating air back into the jar often revived the animal. Compressing the air produced the same results: animals and flames survived longer.

Boyle removed the diaphragm and ribs from a living dog and forced air into its lungs with a bellows. Although the experiment did not prove that air was essential for life, it demonstrated that air pressure (and volumes) alternately contracted and expanded the lungs. He repeated the experiment, this time pricking the lungs so air could escape. Boyle kept the animal alive by forcing air into its lungs, proving that chest movement maintained airflow and disproving the earlier assertion that the lungs effected circulation.

Scientific societies and journals broadcasted these discoveries. Boyle belonged to the Royal Society of London, chartered in 1662 by Charles II. Four years later in France, Louis XIV sponsored the Académie Royale des Sciences so its salaried members could conduct a variety of studies. Both societies established journals (*Philosophical Transactions of the Royal Society* and *Journal des Scavans*, respectively) to disseminate information in chemistry, physics, medicine, nutrition, and metabolism to scientists and an increasingly educated lay public.

Stephen Hales (1677–1761)

A renowned English plant physiologist and Fellow of the Royal Society, Hales amassed facts from his experiments with animals about blood pressure, the heart's capacity, and velocity of blood flow in *Vegetable Statics: Or, an Account of Some Statical Experiments on the Sap in Vegetables* (1727). In this venerable text, Hales tells how water absorbed air when phosphorus and melted brimstone (sulfur) burned in a closed glass vessel (see illustra-

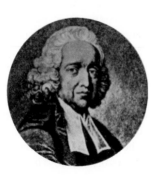

tion [right] that shows the transfer of "air" released from substances burned in a closed vessel). Hales measured the volume of air either released or absorbed, and he demonstrated that air was a constituent of many common substances. His experiments proved that chemical changes occurred in solids and liquids during calcination (oxidation during combustion). Hales developed an idea suggested by Newton in 1713 that provided the first experimental evidence that the nervous system played a role in muscular contraction.

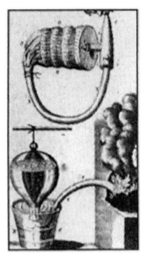

James Lind (1716–1794)

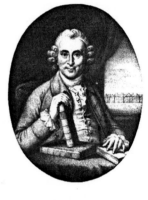

Trained in Edinburgh, Lind entered the British Navy as a Surgeon's Mate in 1739 (www.sportsci.org/news/history/lind/lind_sp.html). During an extended trip in the English Channel in 1747 on the 50-gun, 960-ton H.M.S. *Salisbury,* Lind carried out a decisive experiment (the first planned, controlled clinical trial) that changed the course of naval medicine. He knew that scurvy ("the great sea plague") often killed two thirds of a ship's crew. Their diet included 1 lb 4 oz of cheese biscuits daily, 2 lb of salt beef twice weekly, 2 oz of dried fish and butter thrice weekly, 8 oz of peas 4 days per week, and 1 gallon of beer daily. Deprived of vitamin C, sailors fell prey to scurvy. By adding fresh fruit to their diet, Lind fortified their immune systems so that British sailors no longer perished on extended voyages. From Lind's *Treatise on the Scurvy* (1753) comes the following poignant excerpt:[35]

> On the 20th of May, 1747, I selected 12 patients in the scurvy, on board the Salisbury at sea. Their cases were as similar as I could have them. They all in general had putrid gums, the spots and lassitude, with weakness of their knees. . . . The consequence was, that the most sudden and visible good effects were perceived from the use of oranges and lemons; one of those who had taken them, being at the end of 6 days fit for duty. The spots were not indeed at that time quite off his body, nor his gums sound; but without any other medicine than a gargle for his mouth he became quite healthy before we came into Plymouth which was on the 16th of June. The other was the best recovered in his condition; and being now pretty well, was appointed nurse to the rest of the sick. . . Next to oranges, I thought the cyder had the best effects. It was indeed not very sound. However, those who had taken it, were in a

fairer way of recovery than the others at the end of the fort-night, which was the length of time all these different courses were continued, except the oranges. The putrification of their gums, but especially their lassitude and weakness, were somewhat abated, and their appetite increased by it.

Lind published two books[58]: *An Essay on Preserving the Health of Seamen in the Royal Navy* (1757) and *Essay on Diseases Incidental to Europeans in Hot Climates* (1768). Easily available, his books were translated into German, French, and Dutch. Lind's landmark emphasis on the crucial importance of dietary supplements antedates modern prac-tices. His treatment regimen defeated scurvy, but 50 years had to pass with many more lives lost before the British Admiralty required fresh citrus fruit on all ships.

Joseph Black (1728–1799)

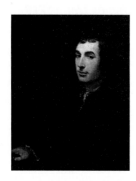

After graduating from the medical school in Edinburgh, Black became professor of chemistry at Glasgow. *Experiments Upon Magnesia Alba, Quicklime, and Some Other Alcaline Substances* (1756) determined that air con-tained carbon dioxide gas. He ob-served that carbonate (lime) lost half its weight after burning. Black reasoned that removing air from lime treated with acids produced a new substance he named "fixed air," or carbon dioxide ($CaCO_3 = CaO + CO_2$). Black's dis-covery that gas existed either freely or combined with other substances encouraged later experiments on the chemical composition of gases.

Joseph Priestley (1733–1804)

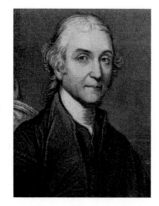

Although Priestley discov-ered oxygen by heating red ox-ide of mercury in a closed ves-sel, he stubbornly clung to the phlogiston theory that had mis-led other scientists. Dismissing Lavoisier's (1743–1794) proof that respiration produced car-bon dioxide and water, Priestley continued to believe in an im-material constituent (phlogis-ton) that supposedly escaped from burning substances. He told the Royal Society about oxygen in 1772 and published *Observations on Different Kinds of Air* in 1773. Elated by his discovery, Priestley failed to grasp two facts that later research confirmed: (1) the body needs oxygen and (2) cellular respiration produces carbon dioxide.

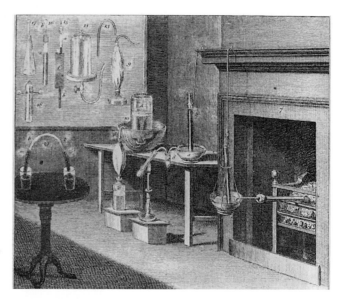

Priestley's London laboratory.

Carl Wilhelm Scheele (1742–1786)

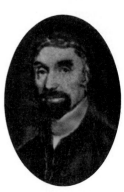

In one of history's great coin-cidences, Scheele, a Swedish phar-macist, discovered oxygen inde-pendently of Priestley. Scheele noted that heating mercuric oxide released "fire-air" (oxygen); burn-ing other substances in fire-air pro-duced violent reactions. When dif-ferent mixtures contacted air inside a sealed container, the air volume decreased by 25% and could not support combustion. Scheele named the gas that extinguished fire "foul air." In a memorable experiment, he added two bees to a glass jar im-mersed in lime water containing fire-air (illustration at *right*). After a few days, the bees remained alive, but the level of lime water had risen in the bottle and be-come cloudy. Scheele concluded that fixed air replaced the fire-air to sustain

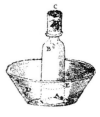

the bees. At the end of 8 days, the bees died despite ample honey inside the container. Scheele blamed their demise on phlogiston, which he felt was hostile to life. What Scheele called foul-air (phlogisticated air in Priestley's day) was later identified as nitrogen.

Just like Priestley, Scheele refused to accept Lavoisier's explanations concerning respiration. Although Scheele ad-hered to the phlogiston theory, he discovered, in addition to oxygen, chlorine, manganese, silicon, glycerol, silicon tetra-fluoride, hydrofluoric acid, and copper arsenite (named Scheele's green in his honor). Scheele also experimented with silver salts and how light influenced them (which became the basis of modern photography). He was the first and only student of pharmacy elected in 1775 into the prestigious Swedish Royal Academy of Sciences.

Henry Cavendish (1731–1810)

Cavendish and his contemporaries Black and Priestley began to identify the constituents of carbohydrates, lipids, and proteins. *On Factitious Air* (1766) describes a highly flammable substance, later identified as hydrogen, which was liberated when acids combined with metals. *Experiments in Air* (1784) showed that "inflammable air" (hydrogen) combined with "deflogisticated air" (oxygen) produced water. Cavendish performed meticulous calculations using a sensitive torsion balance to measure the value of the gravitational constant G that allowed him to compute the mass of the earth (5.976×10^{24} kg). His work eventually played an important role in the development of the space sciences, especially modern rocketry that led to space exploration (see Chapter 27).

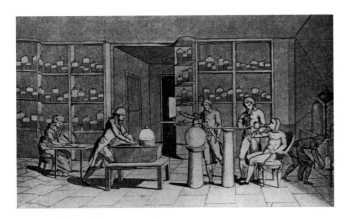

Lavoisier supervises the first "true" exercise physiology experiment (heart rate and oxygen consumption measured as the seated subject at the right breathes through a copper pipe while pressing a foot pedal to increase external work). Sketched by Madame Lavoisier (sitting at the left taking notes).

Antoine Laurent Lavoisier (1743–1794)

Lavoisier ushered in modern concepts of metabolism, nutrition, and exercise physiology (http://www.sportsci.org /news/history/lavoisier/ lavoisier.html). His discoveries in respiration chemistry and human nutrition were as essential to these fields as Harvey's discoveries were to circulatory physiology and medicine. Lavoisier paved the way for studies of energy balance by recognizing for the first time

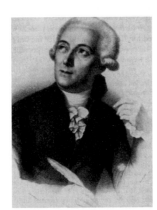

that the elements carbon, hydrogen, nitrogen, and oxygen involved in metabolism neither appeared suddenly nor disappeared mysteriously. He supplied basic truths: only oxygen participates in animal respiration, and the "caloric" liberated during respiration is itself the source of the combustion. In the early 1770s, Lavoisier was the first person to conduct experiments on human respiration. According to Lusk,[43] Lavoisier told of his experiments in a letter written to a friend dated November 19, 1790, as follows:

> The quantity of oxygen absorbed by a resting man at a temperature of 26°C is 1200 pouces de France (1 cubic pouce = 0.0198 L) hourly. (2) The quantity of oxygen required at a temperature of 12°C rises to 1400 pouces. (3) During the digestion of food the quantity of oxygen amounts to from 1800 to 1900 pouces. (4) During exercise 4000 pouces and over may be the quantity of oxygen absorbed.

These discoveries, fundamental to modern concepts of energy balance, could not protect Lavoisier from the intolerance of his revolutionary countrymen. The Jacobean tribunal beheaded him in 1794. Yet once more, thoughtless resistance to innovative science temporarily delayed the triumph of truth.

Lazzaro Spallanzani (1729–1799)

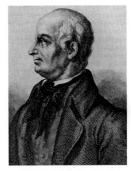

An accomplished Italian physiologist, Spallanzani debunked spontaneous generation as he studied fertilization and contraception in animals. In a famous study of digestion, he refined regurgitation experiments similar to those of the French scientist, René-Antoine Fercault de Réaumur (1683–1757). Réaumur's *Digestion in Birds* (1752) told how he recovered partially digested food from the gizzard of a kite. Spallanzani swallowed a sponge tied to the end of a string and then regurgitated it. He found that the sponge had absorbed a substance that dissolved bread and various animal tissues, thus indirectly observing how gastric juices function. His experiments with animals showed that the tissues of the heart, stomach, and liver consume oxygen and liberate carbon dioxide, even in creatures without lungs.

Spallanzani's idea that respiration and combustion took place within the tissues was novel and appeared posthumously in 1804. A century later, this phenomenon would be called *internal respiration*.

Nineteenth Century Metabolism and Physiology

The untimely death of Lavoisier did not terminate fruitful research in nutrition and medicine. During the next half century, scientists discovered the chemical composition of carbohydrates, lipids, and proteins and further clarified the energy balance equation.

Claude Louis Berthollet (1748–1822)

A French chemist and contemporary of Lavoisier, Berthollet (in white lab coat in illustration at *right*) identified the "volatile substances" associated with animal tissues. One of these "substances," nitrogen, was produced when ammonia gas burned in oxygen. Berthollet showed that normal tissues did not contain ammonia. He believed that hydrogen united with nitrogen during fermentation to produce ammonia. In 1865, Berthollet took exception to Lavoisier's ideas concerning the amount of

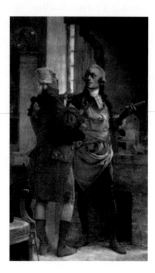

heat liberated when the body oxidized an equal weight of carbohydrate or fat. According to Berthollet, "the quantity of heat liberated in the incomplete oxidation of a substance equaled the difference between the total caloric value of the substance and that of the products formed."

Joseph Louis Proust (1755–1826)

Proust proved that a pure substance isolated in the laboratory or found in nature would always contain the same elements in the same proportions. Known as the "Law of Definite Proportions," Proust's ideas about the chemical constancy of substances provided an important milestone for future nutritional explorers, helping them analyze the major nutrients and calculate energy metabolism as measured by oxygen consumption.

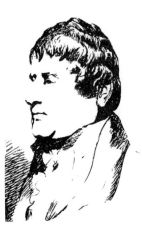

Louis-Joseph Gay-Lussac (1778–1850)

In 1810, Gay-Lussac, a pupil of Berthollet, analyzed the chemical composition of 20 animal and vegetable substances. He placed the vegetable substances into one of three categories depending on their proportion of hydrogen to oxygen atoms. One class of compounds he called saccharine (later identified as carbohydrate) was accepted by William Prout (1785–1850) in

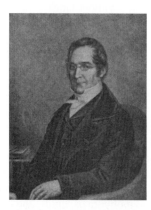

his classification of the three basic macronutrients.

William Prout (1785–1850)

Following up the studies of Lavoisier and Séguin on muscular activity and respiration, Prout, an Englishman, measured the carbon dioxide exhaled by men exercising to fatigue (*Annals of Philosophy* 1813;2:328). Moderate exercise such as walking raised carbon dioxide production to an eventual

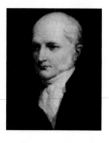

plateau. This observation heralded the modern concept of steady-state gas exchange kinetics in exercise. Although Prout could not determine the exact amount of carbon dioxide respired because there were no instruments to measure respiration rate, he nevertheless observed that carbon dioxide concentration in expired air decreased dramatically in fatiguing exercise.

François Magendie (1783–1855)

In 1821, Magendie founded the first journal for the study of experimental physiology (*Journal de Physiologie Expérimentale*), a field he literally created. The next year, he showed that anterior spinal nerve roots control motor activities and posterior roots control sensory functions.

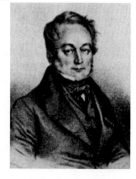

Magendie's accomplishments were not limited to neural physiology. Unlike others who claimed that the tissues derived their nitrogen from the air, Magendie argued that the food they consumed provided the nitrogen. To prove his point, he studied animals subsisting on nitrogen-free diets. He described his 1836 experiment as follows:

> . . . I took a dog of three years old, fat, and in good health, and put it to feed upon sugar alone, and gave it distilled water to drink: it had as much as it chose of both. . . It appeared to thrive very well in this way of living the first 7 or 8 days; it was brisk, active, ate eagerly, and drank in its usual manner. It began to get meagre upon the second week, though it had always a good appetite, and took about 6 or 8 ounces of sugar in 24 hours. . . In the third week its leanness increased, its strength diminished, the animal lost its liveliness, and its appetite was much lessened. At this period there was developed, first upon one eye, and then upon the other, a small ulceration in the center of the transparent cornea; it increased very quickly, and in a few days it was more than a line in diameter; its depth increased in the same proportion; the cornea was very soon entirely perforated, and the humours of the eye ran out. This singular phenomenon was accompanied with an abundant secretion of the glands of the eyelids.

It, however, became weaker and weaker, and lost its strength; and though the animal took from 3 to 4 ounces of sugar every day, it became at length so weak that it could neither chew nor swallow; for the same reason every other motion was impossible. It expired the 32nd day of the experiment. I opened it with every suitable precaution; I found a total want of fat; the muscles were reduced by more than five-sixths of their ordinary size; the stomach and the intestines were also much diminished in volume, and strongly contracted.

The excrements, that were also examined by M. Chevreul, contained very little azote (nitrogen), whilst they generally present a great deal. . . A third experiment produced similar results, and thence I considered sugar incapable of supporting dogs of itself.

William Beaumont (1785–1853)

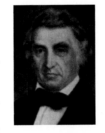

One of the most fortuitous experiments in medicine began on June 6, 1822 at Fort Mackinac on the upper Michigan peninsula (www.sportsci.org/news/history/beaumont/beaumont.html). As fort surgeon, Beaumont tended the accidental shotgun wound that perforated the abdominal wall and stomach of a young French Canadian, Samata St. Martin, a voyageur for the American Fur Company.

The wound healed after 10 months but continued to provide new insights concerning digestion. Part of the wound formed a small natural "valve" that led directly into the stomach. Beaumont turned St. Martin on his left side, depressing the valve, and then inserted a tube the size of a large quill five or six inches into the stomach. He began two kinds of experiments on the digestive processes from 1825 to 1833. First, he observed the fluids discharged by the stomach when different foods were eaten (in vivo); second, he extracted samples of the stomach's content and put them into glass tubes to determine the time required for "external" digestion (in vitro).

Beaumont revolutionized concepts about digestion. For centuries, the stomach was thought to produce heat that somehow "cooked" foods. Alternatively, the stomach was portrayed as a mill, a fermenting vat, or a stew pan.[d]

Beaumont published the first results of his experiments on St. Martin in the *Philadelphia Medical Recorder* in January 1825 and full details in his "Experiments and Observations on the Gastric Juice and the Physiology of Digestion" (1833).[21] Beaumont ends his treatise with a list of 51 inferences based on his 238 separate experiments. Although working away from the centers of medicine, Beaumont used findings from Spallanzini, Carminiti, Viridet, Vauquelin, Tiedemann and Gmelin, Leuret and Lassaigne, Montegre, and Prout. Even with their information, he still obeyed the scientific method, basing all his inferences on direct experimentation. Beaumont concluded:

> Pure gastric juice, when taken directly out of the stomach of a healthy adult, unmixed with any other fluid, save a portion of the mucus of the stomach with which it is most commonly, and perhaps always combined, is a clear, transparent fluid; inodorous; a little saltish; and very perceptibly acid. Its taste, when applied to the tongue, is similar to thin mucilaginous water, slightly acidulated with muriatic acid. It is readily diffusible in water, wine or spirits; slightly effervesces with alkalis; and is an effectual solvent of the materia alimentaria. It possess the property of coagulating albumen, in an eminent degree; is powerfully antiseptic, checking the putrefaction of meat; and effectually restorative of healthy action, when applied to old, fetid sores, and foul, ulcerating surfaces.

Beaumont's accomplishment is even more remarkable because the United States, unlike England, France, and Germany, provided no research facilities for experimental medicine. Little was known about the physiology of digestion. Yet Beaumont, a "backwoods physiologist,"[12] inspired future studies of gastric emptying, intestinal absorption, electrolyte balance, rehydration, and nutritional supplementation with "sports drinks."

Michel Eugene Chevreul (1786–1889)

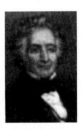

During his long life, Chevreul carried on a 200-year family tradition of studying chemistry and biology. His *Chemical Investigations of Fat* (1823) described different fatty acids. In addition, he separated cholesterol from biliary fats, coined the term *margarine,* and was first to show that lard consisted of two main fats (a solid he called *stearine* and the other a liquid called *elaine*). Chevreul also demonstrated that sugar from a diabetic's urine resembled cane sugar.

Jean Baptiste Boussingault (1802–1884)

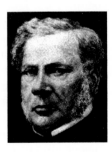

Boussingault's studies of animal nutrition paralleled later studies of human nutrition. He calculated the effect of calcium, iron, and other nutrient intake (particularly nitrogen) on energy balance. His pioneering work among Columbians formed the basis for his recommendations that they receive

---

[d] Jean Baptise van Helmont (1577–1644), a Flemish doctor, is credited with being first to prescribe an alkaline cure for indigestion.[24] Observing the innards of birds, he reasoned that acid in the digestive tract could not alone decompose meats and that other substances ("ferments," now known as digestive enzymes) must break down food.

iodine to counteract goiter. Boussingault also turned his attention to plants. He showed that the carbon within a plant came from atmospheric carbon dioxide. He also determined that a plant derived most of its nitrogen from the nitrates in the soil, not from the atmosphere, as previously believed.

Gerardus Johannis Mulder (1802–1880)

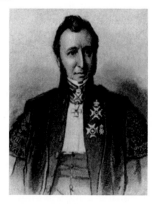

Professor of chemistry at Utrecht, Netherlands, Mulder analyzed albuminous substances he named "proteine." He postulated a general protein radical identical in chemical composition to plant albumen, casein, animal fibrin, and albumen. This protein would contain substances other than nitrogen available only from plants. Because animals consume plants, substances from the plant kingdom, later called amino acids, served to build their tissues. Unfortunately, an influential German chemist, Justus von Liebig (1803–1873) attacked Mulder's theories about protein so vigorously that they fell out of favor.

Despite the academic controversy, Mulder strongly advocated society's role in promoting quality nutrition. He asked, "Is there a more important question for discussion than the nutrition of the human race?" Mulder urged people to observe the "golden mean" by eating neither too little nor too much food. He established minimum standards for his nation's food supply that he believed should be compatible with optimum health. In 1847, he gave these specific recommendations: laborers should consume 100 g of protein daily; those doing routine work about 60 g. He prescribed 500 g of carbohydrate as starch and included "some" fat without specifying an amount.

Justus von Liebig (1803–1873)

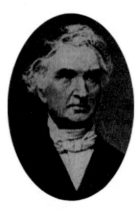

Embroiled in professional controversies, Liebig nevertheless established a large, modern chemistry laboratory that attracted numerous students (www. sportsci.org/news/history/ liebig/liebig.html). He developed unique equipment to analyze inorganic and organic substances. Liebig restudied protein compounds (alkaloids discovered by Mulder) and concluded that muscular exertion (by horses or humans) required mainly proteins, not just carbohydrates and fats. Liebig's influential *Animal Chemistry* (1842) communicated his ideas about energy metabolism.

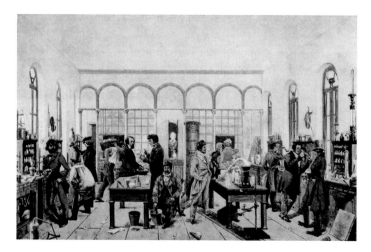

Hundreds of chemists trained at Liebig's Geisen laboratory, many achieving international reputations for pioneering discoveries in chemistry. (Photo courtesy of Magnus Mueller, Liebig Museum, Giessen, Germany.)

Liebig dominated chemistry; his theoretical pronouncements about the relation of dietary protein to muscular activity were usually accepted without critique by other scientists until the 1850s. Despite his pronouncements, Liebig never carried out a physiologic experiment or performed nitrogen balance studies on animals or humans. Liebig demeaned physiologists, believing them incapable of commenting on his theoretic calculations unless they themselves achieved his level of expertise.

By midcentury, physiologist Adolf Fick (1829–1901) and chemist Johannes Wislicenus (1835–1903) challenged Liebig's dogma concerning protein's role in exercise. Their simple experiment measured changes in urinary nitrogen during a mountain climb. The protein that broke down could not have supplied all the energy for the hike. The result discredited Liebig's principle assertion regarding the importance of protein metabolism in supplying energy for vigorous exercise.

Although erroneous, Liebig's notions about protein as a primary exercise fuel worked their way into popular writings. By the turn of the 20th century, an idea that survives today seemed unassailable: athletic prowess requires a large protein intake. He lent his name to two commercial products; *Liebig's Infant Food*, advertised as a replacement for breast milk, and *Liebig's Fleisch Extract* (meat extract) that supposedly conferred special benefits to the body. Liebig argued that consuming his extract and meat would help the body perform extra "work" to convert plant material into useful substances. Even today, fitness magazines tout protein supplements for peak performance with little except anecdotal confirmation. Whatever the merit of Liebig's claims, debate continues, building on the metabolic studies of W. O. Atwater (1844–1907), F. G. Benedict (1870–1957), and R. H. Chittenden (1856–1943) in the United States and M. Rubner (1854–1932) in Germany.

Henri Victor Regnault (1810–1878)

With his colleague Jules Reiset, Henri Regnault, professor of chemistry and physics at the University of Paris, used closed-circuit spirometry to determine the respiratory quotient (RQ; carbon dioxide ÷ oxygen) in dogs, insects, silkworms, earthworms, and frogs (1849). Animals were placed in a sealed, 45-L bell jar surrounded by a water jacket (see illustration below). A potash solution filtered the carbon dioxide gas produced during respiration. Water rising in a glass receptacle forced oxygen into the bell jar to replace the quantity consumed during energy metabolism. A thermometer recorded temperature, and a manometer measured variations in chamber pressure. For dogs, fowl, and rabbits deprived of food, the RQ was lower than when the same animals consumed meat. Regnault and Reiset reasoned that starving animals subsist on their own tissues. Foods never were completely destroyed during metabolism because urea and uric acid were recovered in the urine.

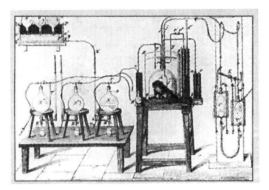

Regnault established relationships between different body sizes and metabolic rates. These ratios preceded the law of surface area and allometric scaling procedures now used in exercise science. Regnault and Reiset related oxygen consumption to heat production and body size in animals:

> The consumption of oxygen absorbed varies greatly in different animals per unit of body weight. It is ten times greater in sparrows than in chickens. Since the different species have the same body temperature, and the smaller animals present a relatively larger area to the environmental air, they experience a substantial cooling effect, and it becomes necessary that the sources of heat production operate more energetically and that respiration increase.

Claude Bernard (1813–1878)

Claude Bernard, typically acclaimed as the greatest physiologist of all time, succeeded Magendie as professor of medicine at the Collège de France (www.sportsci.org/news/history/bernard/bernard.html). Bernard interned in medicine and surgery before serving as laboratory assistant (préparateur) to Magendie in 1839. Three years later, he followed Magendie to the Hôtel-Dieu (hospital) in Paris. For the next 35 years, Bernard discovered fundamental properties concerning

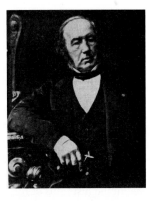

physiology. He participated in the explosion of scientific knowledge in the midcentury. Bernard indicated his single-minded devotion to research by producing a doctorate thesis on gastric juice and its role in nutrition (*Du sac gastrique et de son rôle dans la nutrition*; 1843). Ten years later, he received the Doctorate in Natural Sciences for his study entitled *Recherches*

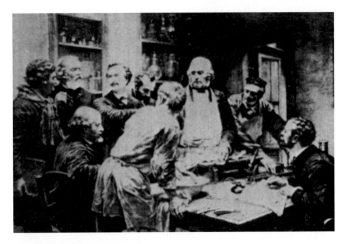

Students observing Bernard perform a dissection as part of their medical training.

sur une nouvelle fonction du foie, consideré comme organe producteur de matière sucrée chez l'homme et les animaux (Research on a new function of the liver as a producer of sugar in man and animals). Before this seminal research, scientists assumed that only plants could synthesize sugar, and that sugar within animals must derive from ingested plant matter. Bernard disproved this notion by documenting the presence of sugar in the hepatic vein of a dog whose diet lacked carbohydrate.

Bernard's experiments that profoundly affected medicine include:

1. Discovery of the role of the pancreatic secretion in the digestion of lipids (1848)
2. Discovery of a new function of the liver—the "internal secretion" of glucose into the blood (1848)
3. Induction of diabetes by puncture of the floor of the fourth ventricle (1849)
4. Discovery of the elevation of local skin temperature upon section of the cervical sympathetic nerve (1851)
5. Production of sugar by washed excised liver (1855) and the isolation of glycogen (1857)
6. Demonstration that curare specifically blocks motor nerve endings (1856)
7. Demonstration that carbon monoxide blocks the respiration of erythrocytes (1857)

Bernard's work also influenced other sciences. His discoveries in chemical physiology spawned physiological chemistry and biochemistry, which in turn a century later spawned molecular biology. His contributions to regulatory physiology helped the next generation of scientists understand how metabolism and nutrition affected exercise. Bernard's influential *Introduction à l'étude de la médecine expérimentale* (*The Introduction to the Study of Experimental Medicine*, 1865) illustrates the self-control that enabled him to succeed despite external disturbances. Bernard urged researchers to vigorously observe, hypothesize, and then test their hypothesis. In the last third of the book, Bernard shares his strategies for verifying results. His disciplined approach remains valid, and exercise physiologists would profit from reading this book.

Edward Smith (1819–1874)

Edward Smith, physician, public health advocate, and social reformer, promoted better living conditions for Britain's lower class, including prisoners (www.sportsci.org/news/history/smith/smith.html). He believed those in prison were maltreated because they received no additional food while toiling on the exhausting "punitive treadmill." Smith had observed prisoners climbing up a treadwheel, whose steps resem-

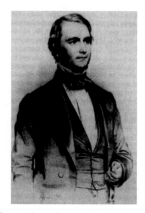

bled the side paddle wheels of a Victorian steamship. Prisoners climbed for 15 minutes, after which they were allowed a 15-minute rest, for a total of 4 hours of work three times a week. To overcome resistance from a sail on the prison roof attached to the treadwheel, each man traveled the equivalent of 1.43 miles up a steep hill.

Curious about this strenuous exercise, Smith conducted studies on himself. He constructed a closed-circuit apparatus (facemask with inspiratory and expiratory valves; see *below*) to measure carbon dioxide production while climbing at Brixton prison.[21] He expired 19.6 more grams of carbon while climbing for 15 minutes and resting for 15 minutes than he expired while resting. Smith estimated that if he climbed and rested for 7.5 hours, his daily total carbon output would

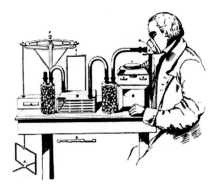

increase 66%. Smith analyzed the urine of four prisoners over a 3-week period to show that urea output was related to the nitrogen content of the ingested foods, while carbon dioxide related more closely to exercise intensity.

Smith inspired two German researchers to validate the prevailing idea that protein alone powered muscular contraction. Adolf Eugen Fick (1829–1901), a physiologist at the University of Zurich, and Johannes Wislicenus (1835–1903), professor of chemistry at Zurich, questioned whether protein oxidation or oxidation of carbohydrates and fats supplied energy for muscular work. In 1864, they climbed Mt. Faulhorn in the Swiss Alps. Prior to the climb, they eliminated protein from their diet, reasoning that nonprotein nutrients would have to supply them energy. They collected their urine before and immediately after the ascent and the following morning. They calculated the external energy equivalent of the 1956-m climb by multiplying body mass by the vertical distance. This external energy requirement exceeded protein catabolism reflected by nitrogen in the urine. Therefore, they concluded that the energy from protein breakdown hardly contributed to the exercise energy requirement. Again, these findings posed a serious challenge to Liebig's claim that protein served as the primary source of muscular power.

Health and Hygiene Influence in the United States

By the early 1800s in the United States, ideas about health and hygiene were strongly promoted by European science-oriented physicians and experimental anatomists and physiologists. Prior to 1800, only 39 first edition American-authored medical books had been published, a few medical schools had been started (Harvard Medical School was founded in 1782), seven medical societies existed (the New Jersey State Medical Society being the first in 1766[8]), and only one medical journal was available (*Medical Repository* published in 1797). Outside of the United States, 176 medical journals were being published, but by 1850 the number in the United States had increased to 117.

Medical journal publications in the United States had increased tremendously during the first half of the 19th century, concurrent with a steady growth in the number of scientific contributions, yet European influences still affected the thinking and practice of U.S. medicine.[56] This influence was particularly apparent in the "information explosion" that reached the public through books, magazines, newspapers, and traveling "health salesmen" who peddled an endless array of tonics, elixirs, and other products for purposes of optimizing health and curing disease. The "hot topics" of the early 19th century (also true today) included nutrition and dieting (slimming), general information concerning exercise, how to best develop overall fitness, training (or gymnastic) exercises for recreation and sport preparation, and all matters relating to personal health and hygiene.

By the middle of the 19th century, fledgling medical schools in the United States began to graduate their own students, many of whom assumed positions of leadership in the academic world and allied medical sciences. Interestingly, physicians had the opportunity either to teach in medical school and conduct research (and write textbooks) or become associated with departments of physical education and hygiene. There, they would oversee programs of physical training for students and athletes.

Within this framework, we begin our discussion of the early physiology and exercise physiology pioneers with Austin Flint, Jr., MD, a respected physician, physiologist, and successful textbook author (Table 1, page xxv, lists his texts). His writings provided reliable information for those wishing to place their beliefs about exercise on a scientific footing.

Austin Flint, Jr., MD: American Physician–Physiologist

Austin Flint, Jr., MD (1836–1915) was one of the first influential American pioneer physician–scientists whose writings contributed significantly to the burgeoning literature in physiology. Flint served as professor of physiology and physiological anatomy in the Bellevue Hospital Medical College of New York, and chaired the Department of Physiology and Microbiology from 1861 to 1897. In 1866, he published a series of five classic textbooks, the first titled *The Physiology of Man; Designed to Represent the Existing State of Physiological Science as Applied to the Functions of the Human Body. Vol. 1; Introduction; The Blood; Circulation; Respiration.* Eleven years later, Flint published *The Principles and Practice of Medicine*, a synthesis of his first five textbooks, which consisted of 987 pages of meticulously organized sections with supporting documentation. The text included 4 lithograph plates and 313 woodcuts of detailed anatomic illustrations of the body's major systems, along with important principles of physiology. In addition, there were illustrations of equipment used to record physiologic phenomena, such as Etienne-Jules Marey's (1830–1904) early cardiograph for registering the wave form and frequency of the pulse and a refinement of one of Marey's instruments, the sphygmograph, for making pulse measurements—the forerunner of modern cardiovascular instrumentation (FIG. 2).

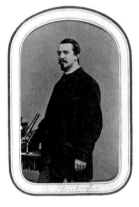

Dr. Flint, one of six generations of physicians spanning the years 1733 to 1955, was well trained in the scientific method. In 1858, he received the American Medical Association's prize for basic research on the heart, and his medical school thesis titled, "The Phenomena of Capillary Circulation," was published in 1878 in the *American Journal of the Medical Sciences.* A characteristic of Flint's textbooks was his admiration for the work of other scholars. These included the noted French physician Claude Bernard (1813–1878); the celebrated observations of Dr.

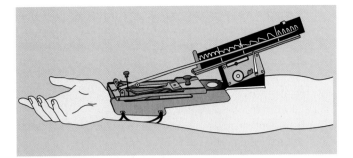

Figure 2   Marey's advanced sphygmograph, including portions of four original tracings of the pulse under different conditions. It was not until the next century in 1928 that Boas and Goldschmidt (cited in the 1932 Boas and Goldschmidt text; see Table 1) reported on their human experiments with the first electronic cardiotachometer. (Goldschmidt had invented the pulse resonator for recording pulse rate in 1927.)

William Beaumont; and William Harvey's momentous discoveries.

Dr. Flint was a careful writer. This was a refreshing approach, particularly because so many "authorities" in physical training, exercise, and hygiene in the United States and abroad were uninformed and unscientific about exercise and its possible role in health care. In his 1877 textbook, Flint wrote about many topics related to exercise. The following sample passages are quoted from Flint's 1877 book to present the flavor of the emerging science of exercise physiology in the late 19th century:

1. Influence of posture and exercise on pulse rate (pp. 52–53)

It has been observed that the position of the body has a very marked influence upon the rapidity of the pulse. Experiments of a very interesting character have been made by Dr. Guy and others, with a view to determine the difference in the pulse in different postures. In the male, there is a difference of about ten beats between standing and sitting, and fifteen beats between standing and the recumbent posture. In the female, the variations with position are not so great. The average given by Dr. Guy is, for the male standing, 81; sitting, 71; lying, 66;-for the female: standing, 91; sitting, 84; lying, 80. This is given as the average of a large number of observations.

Influence of age and sex. In both the male and female, observers have constantly found a great difference in the rapidity of the heat's action at different periods of life.

During early life, there is no marked and constant difference in the rapidity of the pulse in the sexes; but, toward the age of puberty, the development of the sexual peculiarities is accompanied with an acceleration of the heart's action in the female, which continues even into old age. The differences at different ages are shown in the following table, compiled from the observations of Dr. Guy:

Influence of Exercise, etc.—It is a fact generally admitted that muscular exertion increases the frequency of the pulsations of the heart; and the experiments just cited show that the difference in rapidity, which is by some attributed to change in posture (some positions, it is fancied, offering fewer obstacles

| AGES | AVERAGE PULSATIONS | |
YEARS	MALES	FEMALES
2 to 7	97	98
8 to 14	84	94
14 to 21	76	82
21 to 28	73	80
28 to 35	70	78
35 to 42	68	78
42 to 49	70	77
49 to 56	67	76
56 to 63	68	77
63 to 70	70	78
70 to 77	67	81
77 to 84	71	82

to the current of blood than others), is mainly due to muscular exertion. Everyone knows, indeed, that the action of the heart is much more rapid after violent exertion, such as running, lifting, etc. Experiments on this point date from quite a remote period. Bryan Robinson, who published a treatise on the *"Animal Economy"* in 1734, states, as the result of observation, that a man in the recumbent position has 64 pulsations per minute; sitting, 68; after a slow walk, 78; after walking four miles in one hour, 100; and 140 to 150 after running as fast as he could. This general statement, which has been repeatedly verified, shows the powerful influence of the muscular system on the heart. The fact is so familiar that it need not be farther dwelt upon.

2. Influence of muscular activity on respiration (pp. 150–151)

Nearly all observers are agreed that there is a considerable increase in the exhalation of carbonic acid during and immediately following muscular exercise. In insects, Mr. Newport has found that a greater quantity is sometimes exhaled in an hour of violent agitation than in twenty-four hours of repose. In a drone, the exhalation in twenty-four hours was 0.30 of a cubic inch, and during violent muscular exertion the exhalation in one hour was 0.34. Lavoisier recognized the great influence of muscular activity upon the respiratory changes. In treating of the consumption of oxygen, we have quoted his observations on the relative quantities of air vitiated in repose and activity.

The following results of the experiments of Dr. Edward Smith on the influence of exercise are very definite and satisfactory:

In walking at the rate of two miles an hour, the exhalation of carbonic acid during one hour was equal to the quantity produced during 1⅚ hour of repose with food, and 2½ hours with, and 3½ hours without food.

One hour's labor at the tread-wheel, while actually working the wheel, was equal to 4½ of rest with food, and 6 hours without food.

The various observers we have cited have remarked that, when muscular exertion is carried so far as to produce great fatigue and exhaustion, the exhalation of carbonic acid is notably diminished.

3. Influence of muscular exercise on nitrogen elimination (pp. 429–430)

We have had an opportunity of settling definitely the vexed question of the influence of muscular exercise upon elimination of nitrogen.[e] In 1871, we made an exceedingly elaborate series of observations upon Mr. Weston, the pedestrian. Of these we can only give here a brief summary. Mr. Weston walked for five consecutive days as follows: First day, 92 miles; second day, 80 miles; third day, 57 miles; fourth day, 48 miles; fifth day, 40.5 miles. The nitrogen of the food was compared with the nitrogen excreted for three periods; viz, five days before the walk, five days walking, and five days after the walk. A trusty assistant was with Mr. Weston day and night for the fifteen days; the food was weighted and analyzed; the excreta were collected; and other observations were made during the entire period. The analyses were made independently, under the direction of Prof. R.O. Doremus, who had no idea of the results until we had classified and tabulated them. The conclusions were most decided, and, as far as possible, all the physiological conditions were fulfilled. As regards the proportion of nitrogen eliminated to the nitrogen of the food, the general results were as follows:

For the 5 days before the walk, with an average exercise of about 8 miles daily, the nitrogen eliminated was 92:82 parts for 100 parts of nitrogen ingested. For the five days of the walk, for every hundred parts of nitrogen ingested, there were discharged 153:99 parts. For the five days after the walk, when there was hardly any exercise, for every hundred parts of nitrogen ingested, there were discharged 84:63 parts. During the walk, the nitrogen excreted was in direct ratio to the amount of exercise; and, what was still more striking, the excess of nitrogen eliminated over the nitrogen of food almost exactly corresponded with a calculation of the nitrogen of the muscular tissue wasted, as estimated from the loss of weight of the body. Full details of the method of investigation, the processes employed, etc., are given in our original paper.

Through his textbooks, Austin Flint, Jr., influenced the first medically trained and scientifically oriented professor of physical education, Edward Hitchcock, Jr., MD. Hitchcock quoted Flint about the muscular system in his syllabus of Health Lectures, required reading for all students enrolled at Amherst College between 1861 and 1905.

---

[e] Flint A Jr. On the physiological effects of severe and protracted muscular exercise, with special reference to its influence upon the excretion of nitrogen. New York Medical Journal, 1871;xiii:609, et seq.

The Amherst College Connection

Two physicians, father and son, pioneered the American sports science movement. Edward Hitchcock, DD, LLD (1793–1864), was a professor of chemistry and natural history at Amherst College and also served as president of the college from 1845–1854. He convinced the college president in 1861 to allow his son Edward [(1828–1911); Amherst undergraduate (1849); Harvard medical degree (1853)] to assume the duties of his anatomy course. Subsequently, Edward Hitchcock, Jr., was officially appointed on August 15, 1861, as Professor of Hygiene and Physical Education with full academic rank in the Department of Physical Culture at an annual salary of $1000, a position he held almost continuously until 1911. This was the second such appointment in physical education to an American college in the United States.[f]

The Hitchcocks geared their textbook to college physical education (Hitchcock E., Hitchcock E., Jr. *Elementary Anatomy and Physiology for Colleges, Academies, and Other Schools.* New York: Ivison, Phinney & Co., 1860; Edward Hitchcock, Sr., had previously published a textbook on hygiene in 1831). The Hitchcock and Hitchcock anatomy and physiology book predated Flint's anatomy and physiology text by six years. Topics covered were listed in numerical order by subject, and considerable attention was devoted to the physiology of species other than humans. The text included questions at the bottom of each page concerning the topics under consideration, making the textbook a "study guide" or "workbook," not an uncommon pedagogic feature (Cutter, 1848; see Table 1). FIGURE 3 shows sample pages on muscle structure and function from the Hitchcock and Hitchcock text.

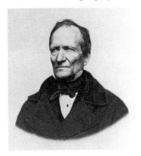

Dr. Edward Hitchcock
(1793–1864)

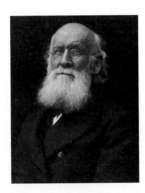

Dr. Edward Hitchcock, Jr., MD (1828–1911)

From 1865 to approximately 1905, Hitchcocks' syllabus of Health Lectures (a 38-page pamphlet titled *"The Subjects and Statement of Facts Upon Personal Health Used for the Lectures Given to the Freshman Classes of Amherst College"*) was part of the required curriculum. The topics included hygiene and physical education, with brief quotations about the topic, including a citation for the quote. In addition to quoting Austin Flint, Jr., regarding care of the muscles, "The condition of the muscular system is an almost unfailing evidence of the general state of the body," other quotations peppered each section of the pamphlet, some from well-known physiologists such as Englishman Thomas Huxley (1825–1895: www.lexicorps.com/Huxley.htm) and Harvard's Henry Pickering Bowditch (1840–1911; cofounder of the American Physiological Society in 1887 and American editor of the *Journal of Physiology*). For example, with regard to physical education and hygiene, Huxley posited "The successful men in life are those who have stored up such physical health in youth that they can in an emergency work sixteen hours in a day without suffering from it." Concerning food and digestion, Bowditch stated: "A scientific or physiological diet for an adult, per day, is two pounds of bread, and three-quarters of a pound of lean meat," and in regard to tobacco use, "Tobacco is nearly as dangerous and deadly as alcohol, and a man with tobacco heart is as badly off as a drunkard." Other quotations were used for such tissues as skin. Dr. Dudley A. Sargent (1849–1924: pioneer Harvard physical educator) told readers "Wear dark clothes in winter and light in summer. Have three changes of underclothing—heavy flannels for winter, light flannels for spring and fall, lisle thread, silk or open cotton for summer."

Anthropometric Assessment of Body Build

During the years 1861 to 1888, Dr. Hitchcock, Jr., obtained 6 measures of segmental height, 23 girths, 6 breadths, 8 lengths, 8 measures of muscular strength, lung capacity, and pilosity (amount of hair on the body) from almost every student who attended Amherst College. From 1882 to 1888, according to Hitchcock, his standardization for measurement was improved based on suggestions of Dr. W. T. Brigham of Boston and Dr. Dudley A. Sargent (Yale medical degree, 1878; assistant professor of physical training and director of Harvard's Hemenway Gymnasium).

In 1889, Dr. Hitchcock and his colleague in the Department of Physical Education and Hygiene, Hiram H. Seelye, MD (who also served as college physician from 1884–1896), published a 37-page anthropometric manual that included five tables of anthropometric statistics of students from 1861 to 1891. This resource compendium provided detailed descriptions for taking measurements that also included

---

[f] Edward Hitchcock, Jr., often is accorded the distinction of being the first professor of physical education in the United States, whereas, in fact, John D. Hooker was first appointed to this position at Amherst College in 1860. Because of poor health, Hooker resigned in 1861, and Hitchcock was appointed in his place. The original idea of a Department of Physical Education with a professorship had been proposed in 1854 by William Agustus Stearns, DD, the fourth president of Amherst College, who considered physical education instruction essential for the health of the students and useful to prepare them physically, spiritually, and intellectually. Other institutions were slow to adopt this innovative concept; the next department of physical education in America was not created until 1879. In 1860, the Barrett Gymnasium at Amherst College was completed and served as the training facility where all students were required to perform systematic exercises for 30 minutes, 4 days a week. The gymnasium included a laboratory with scientific instruments (e.g., spirometer, strength and anthropometric equipment) and also a piano to provide rhythm during the exercises. Hitchcock reported to the Trustees that in his first year, he recorded the students' "vital statistics—including age, weight, height, size of chest and forearm, capacity of lungs, and some measure of muscular strength."

108   HITCHCOCK'S ANATOMY

FIG. 121.

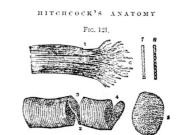

A View of the Fragments of Striped elementary Fibers, showing a cleavage in opposite directions—magnified 300 Diameters. 1, The Longitudinal Cleavage. 2, The Transverse Cleavage, the Longitudinal Lines being scarcely visible. 3, Incomplete Fracture, following the opposite surfaces of a Disc which stretches across the Interval and retains the two Fragments in connexion. The Edge and Surface of this Disc are seen to be minutely granular, the Granules corresponding in size to the thickness of the Disc and to the distance between the faint Longitudinal Lines. 4, Another Disc nearly detached. 5, A detached Disc more highly magnified, showing the Sarcous Elements. 6, Fibrillæ separated by violence from each other at the broken end of the Fiber. 7, 8, The two appearances commonly presented by the separated single Fibrillæ; more highly magnified, at 7 the spaces are rectangular, at 8 the borders are scalloped and the spaces bead-like.

CHAPTER SECOND.

THE MOVING POWERS OF THE SYSTEM.—MYOLOGY, OR THE HISTORY OF THE MUSCLES.

DEFINITIONS AND DESCRIPTIONS.

228. **Microscopic Structure of Muscle.**—The Muscles, known as flesh or lean meat, compose a large part of the extremities, and the covering of the trunk. To the naked eye they appear to be fibrous, and, with the assistance of the microscope, these fibers are found to be bundles—called Fasciculi—of still smaller fibers, called Ultimate Fibers. These seem to be polygonal in form, and with an average diameter of $\frac{1}{125}$th of an inch in man, though in some of the lower animals their size is much less.

View of the stages of development of Muscular Fiber. 1, A Muscular Fiber of Animal life enclosed in its Sheath or Myolemma. 2, An Ultimate Fibril of the same. 3, A more highly magnified View of Fig. 1, showing the true nature of the Longitudinal Striæ, as well as the mode of formation of the Transverse Striæ. The Myolemma is here so thin as to permit the Ultimate Fibrils to be seen through it. 4, A Muscular Fibre of Organic life with two of its Nuclei; taken from the Urinary Bladder, and magnified 600 Diameters. 5, A Muscular Fibre of Organic life from the Stomach, magnified the same.

FIG. 120.

229. **Fibrils.**—The ultimate fibers are still further divisible into what are termed Fibrils. These have an average diameter of about $\frac{1}{10000}$th

of an inch, and number about 650 in each ultimate fiber. They are unprotected by any covering, while both the fasciculus and ultimate fiber are everywhere protected by a delicate sheath called the Sarcolemma.

230. **Organic, or Unstriped, and Animal, or Striped Fibers.**—All the muscles of the body are divided into two classes, according to their function. Those necessary for carrying on the vital functions, such as breathing and digestion, are called Organic, and those under the control of the will Animal Fibers. In addition to their use as a means of distinction, they may be known by their appearance under the micro-

FIG. 122.

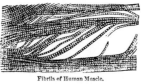

Fibrils of Human Muscle.

228. What is lean meat? How does muscle appear to the naked eye? What are the three microscopic elements? Describe each. 229. What is the diameter of the Fibrils?

What is the Sarcolemma? On what element of muscle is this wanting? 230. Give the two functional classes of the muscles.

Figure 3   Examples from the Hitchcocks' text on structure and function of muscles. (Reproduced from Hitchcock E, Hitchcock E Jr. Elementary anatomy and physiology for colleges, academies, and other schools. New York: Ivison, Phinney & Co., 1860:132, 137. Materials courtesy of Amherst College Archives and permission of the Trustees of Amherst College, 1995.)

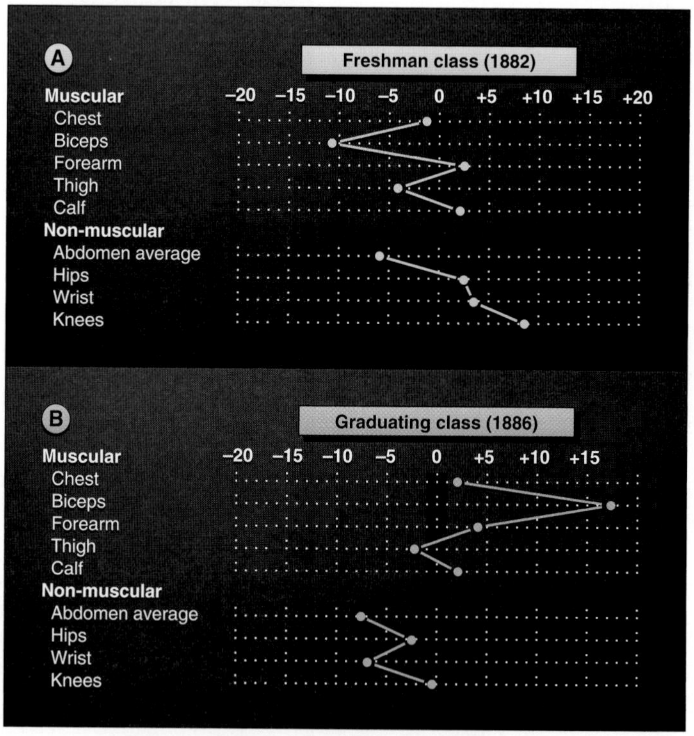

Figure 4   Changes in selected girth measurements of Amherst College men over 4 years of college using Behnke's reference man standards (presented in Chapter 28). **A.** The average body mass of the freshman class in 1882 was 59.1 kg (stature, 171.0 cm). **B.** Four years later, average body mass increased 5.5 kg (11.3 lb) and stature increased by 7.4 cm (2.9 in).

eye testing and an examination of the lungs and heart before testing subjects for muscular strength. In the last section of the manual, Dr. Seelye wrote detailed instructions for using the various pieces of gymnasium apparatus for "enlarging and strengthening the neck, to remedy round or stooping shoulders, to increase the size of the chest and the capacity of the lungs, to strengthen and enlarge the arm, abdominal muscles, and weak back, and to enlarge and strengthen the thighs, calves, legs and ankles." The Hitchcock and Seelye manual, the first of its kind devoted to an analysis of anthropometric and strength data based on detailed measurements, influenced other departments of physical education in the United States (e.g., Yale, Harvard, Wellesley, Mt. Holyoke) to include anthropometric measurements as part of the physical education and hygiene curriculum.[g]

One reason for the early interest in anthropometric measurement was to demonstrate that engaging in daily, vigorous exercise produced desirable results, particularly for muscular development. Although none of the early physical education scientists used statistics to evaluate the outcomes of exercise programs, it is instructive to apply modern methods of anthropometric analysis to the original data of Hitchcock on entering students at Amherst College in 1882 and on their graduation in 1886. FIGURE 4 shows how the average student changed in anthropometric dimensions throughout 4 years of college in relation to Behnke's reference standards presented in Chapter 28. Note the dramatic increase in biceps girth and decreases in the nonmuscular abdomen and hip regions. Although data for a nonexercising "control" group of students were not available, these changes coincided with daily resistance training prescribed in the Hitchcock and Seelye *Anthropometric Manual.* This training used Indian club or barbell swinging exercises (FIG. 5) and other strengthening modalities (horizontal bar, rope and ring exercises, parallel bar exercises, dipping machine, inclined presses with weights, pulley weights, and rowing machine workouts). The Hitchcock data presentation, a first of its kind initially reported in the *Anthropometric Manual* in March, 1892, used "bodily stature" as the basis of comparison "from measurements of 1322 students between 17 and 26 years of age. The strength tests are derived from 20,761 items." The Hitchcock anthropometric and strength studies were acknowledged in the first formal American textbook on

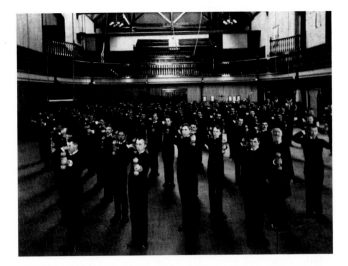

Figure 5   Dr. Edward Hitchcock, Jr., (second from right, with beard) observing the students perform barbell exercises in the Pratt Gymnasium of Amherst College. (Photo courtesy of Amherst College Archives and by permission of the Trustees of Amherst College, 1995.)

anthropometry published in 1896 by Jay W. Seaver, MD (1855–1915), physician and lecturer on personal hygiene at Yale University. TABLE 3 presents a sample of the average and "best" anthropometric values at Amherst College from 1861 to 1900.

While Hitchcock was performing pioneering anthropometric studies at the college level, the military was making the first detailed anthropometric, spirometric, and muscular strength measurements on Civil War soldiers in the early 1860s published in 1869 by Gould (cited in Table 1). The specially trained military anthropometrists used a unique device, the andrometer (FIG. 6), to secure the physical dimensions to the nearest 1/10th of an inch of soldiers for purposes of fitting uniforms. The andrometer was originally devised in 1855 by a tailor in Edinburgh, Scotland, commissioned by the British government to determine the proper size for British soldiers' clothing. This device was set by special gauges to adjust "sliders" for measurement of total height; breadth of the neck, shoulders, and pelvis; and the length of the legs and height to the knees and crotch. Each examiner

---

[g] Probably unknown to Hitchcock was the 1628 manuscript of the Flemish fencing instructor at the French Royal Court, Gerard Thibault, who studied optimal body proportions and success in fencing.[53] This early text, *L'Académie de l'Espée,* appeared at a time when important discoveries were being made by European scientists, particularly anatomists and physiologists, whose contributions played such an important role in laboratory experimentation and scientific inquiry. Had Hitchcock known about this early attempt to link anthropometric assessment with success in sport, the acceptance of anthropometry in the college curriculum might have been easier. Nevertheless, just 67 years after Hitchcock began taking anthropometric measurements at Amherst, and 37 years following the creation of Harvard's physical education scientific laboratory in 1891, anthropometric measurements were made of athletes at the 1928 Amsterdam Olympic Games. One of the athletes measured in Amsterdam, Ernst Jokl from South Africa, became a physician and then professor of physical education at the University of Kentucky. Jokl was a charter member and founder of the American College of Sports Medicine. Thus, Hitchcock's visionary ideas about the importance of anthropometry finally caught on, and such assessment techniques are now used routinely in exercise physiology to assess physique status and the dynamics between physiology and performance. The more modern application of anthropometry is now known as *kinanthropometry.* This term, first defined at the International Congress of Physical Activity Sciences in conjunction with the 1976 Montreal Olympic Games,[52] was refined in 1980[53] as follows: "Kinanthropometry is the application of measurement to the study of human size, shape, proportion, composition, maturation, and gross function. Its purpose is to help us to understand human movement in the context of growth, exercise, performance, and nutrition. We see its essentially human-enobling purpose being achieved through applications in medicine, education, and government."

TABLE 3 ■ AVERAGE AND BEST ANTHROPOMETRIC RECORDS OF AMHERST COLLEGE FROM 1861 TO 1900 INCLUSIVE

ITEMS	AVERAGE		MAXIMA		HELD BY	DATE OF RECORD
	METRIC	ENGLISH	METRIC	ENGLISH		
Weight	61.2	134.9	113.7	250.6	K. R. Otis, '03	Oct. 2, '99
Height	1725	67.9	1947	76.6	B. Matthews '99	Oct. 28, '95
Girth, head	572	22.5	630	24.8	W. H. Lewis '92	Feb. '92
Girth, neck	349	13.7	420	16.5	D. R. Knight '91	Feb. '91
Girth, chest, repose	880	34.6	1140	44.9	K. R. Otis '03	Oct. 2 '99
Girth, belly	724	28.5	1017	40.1	G. H. Colman '99	May '97
Girth, hips	893	35.1	1165	45.9	K. R. Otis '03	Oct. 2, '99
Girth, right thigh	517	20.3	745	29.3	K. R. Otis '03	Oct. 2, '99
Girth, right knee	361	14.2	460	18.1	K. R. Otis '03	Oct. 2, '99
Girth, right calf	359	14.1	452	17.8	K. R. Otis '03	Oct. 2, '99
Girth, upper-right arm	257	10.1	396	15.6	K. R. Otis '03	Oct. 2, '99
Girth, right forearm	267	10.5	327	12.8	K. R. Otis '03	Oct. 2, '99
Girth, right wrist	166	6.5	191	7.5	H. B. Haskell '94	April '92
Strength, chest, dip	6	—	45	—	H. W. Lane '95	March '95
Strength, chest, pull up	9	—	65	—	H. W. Seelye '79	Oct. '75
Strength, right forearm	41	90	86	189.6	A. J. Wyman '98	April '96
Strength, left forearm	38	84	73	160.9	A. J. Wyman '98	April '96
Capacity of lungs	377	230	6.66	406	E. D. Blodgett '87	June '87

From Hitchcock E, et al. An anthropometric manual, 4th ed. Amherst, MA: Carpenter and Morehouse, 1900.

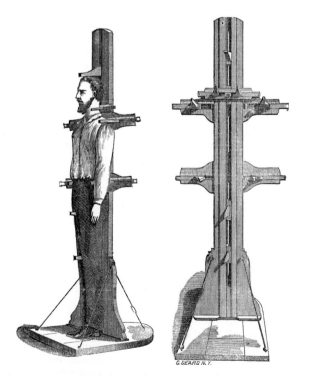

Figure 6 The andrometer, first used by the United States Sanitary Commission at numerous military installations along the Atlantic seaboard during the early 1860s, sized soldiers for clothing.

received 2 days of practice to perfect measurement technique before assignment to different military installations (e.g., Fort McHenry in Baltimore, Naval Rendezvous in New York City, Marine Barracks at the Brooklyn Navy Yard, and bases in South Carolina; Washington, DC; Detroit; and New Orleans). Data were compiled on the actual and relative proportions of 15,781 men ("Whites, Blacks, Indians") between the ages of 16 and 45 years. One purpose of these military studies was to determine relationships among the anthropometric and other physical measurements, and to gather demographic and anthropologic statistics on enlisted and commissioned soldiers in the infantry, cavalry, and artillery. These early investigations about muscular strength and body dimensions served as prototypical studies whose measurement techniques led the way to many later studies conducted in the military about muscular strength and human performance per se. Most laboratories in exercise physiology today include assessment procedures to evaluate aspects of muscular strength and body composition.[48]

The *top* of FIGURE 7 shows two views of the instrument used to evaluate muscular strength in the military studies; the *bottom* of the figure shows the early spirometers used to evaluate pulmonary dimensions. The strength device predates the various strength-measuring instruments shown in FIGURE 8 used by Hitchcock (Amherst), Sargent (Harvard), and Seaver (Yale), as well as anthropometric measuring instruments used in their batteries of physical measurements. The *inset* shows the price list of some of the equipment from the 1889 and 1890 Hitchcock manuals on anthropometry. Note the progression in complexity of the early spirometers and strength devices used in the 1860 military studies (Fig. 7), and the more "modern" equipment of the 1889–1905 period displayed in Figure 8. FIGURE 9 includes three uncovered photographs (circa 1897–1901) of the strength testing equipment (Kellogg's Universal Dynamometer) acquired by Dr. Hitchcock in 1897 to assess the strength of arms *(panel A)*, anterior trunk and forearm supinators *(panel B)*, and leg extensors, flexors, and adductors *(panel C)*.[h]

The First Exercise Physiology Laboratory and Associated Degree Program in the United States

The first formal exercise physiology laboratory in the United States was established in 1891 at Harvard University and housed in a newly created Department of Anatomy, Physiology, and Physical Training at the Lawrence Scientific School.[22,41] Several instructors in the initial undergraduate BS degree program in Anatomy, Physiology, and Physical Training started at the same time were Harvard-trained physicians; others—including Henry Pickering Bowditch, professor of physiology who discovered the all-or-none principle of cardiac contraction and treppe, the staircase phenomenon of muscular contraction, and William T. Porter, also a physiologist in the Harvard Medical School—were respected for their rigorous scientific and laboratory training.

George Wells Fitz, MD: A Major Influence

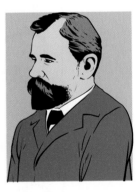

An important influence in creating the new departmental major and recruiting top scientists as faculty in the Harvard program was George Wells Fitz, MD (1860–1934). Fitz vociferously supported a strong, science-based curriculum in preparing the new breed of physical educators. The archival records show that the newly formed major was grounded in the basic sciences, including formal coursework in exercise physiology, zoology, morphology (animal and human), anthropometry, applied anatomy and animal mechanics, medical chemistry, comparative anatomy, remedial exercises, physics, gymnastics and athletics, history of physical education, and English. Physical education students took general anatomy and physiology courses in the medical school; after 4 years of study, graduates could enroll as second-year medical students and graduate in 3 years with an MD degree. Dr. Fitz taught the physiology of

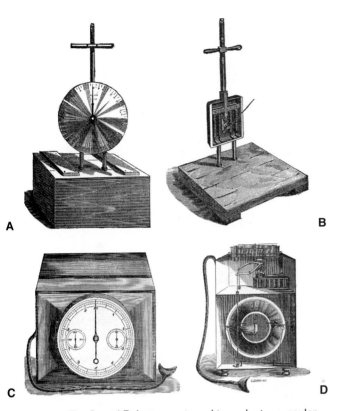

A **B**

C **D**

Figure 7 *Top* **A.** and **B.** Instrument used to evaluate muscular strength in the military studies of Gould in 1869. The illustration on the *left* shows the general look of the device, while the *right side* shows the internal arrangement without face-plate. Gould described the procedure for measuring muscular strength as follows: "The man stands upon the movable lid of the wooden packing box, to which the apparatus is firmly attached, and grasps with both hands the rounded extremities of a wooden bar, of convenient shape and adjustable in height. The handle is conveniently shaped for firm and easy grasp, its height well suited for application and the full muscular power, and the mechanism such as to afford results which are to all appearance very trustworthy." This was not the first dynamometer; Gould cites Regnier (no date given), who published a description of a dynamometer to measure the strength of Parisians; and Péron, who carried a dynamometer on an expedition to Australia. Other researchers in Europe had also used dynamometers to compare the muscular strength of men of different races. Figure 22.1C (Chapter 22) shows the modern back-leg lift dynamometer still used for assessing muscular strength as part of physical fitness test procedures. *Bottom* **C** and **D.** Spirometers (or dry gas meters), manufactured by the American Meter Company of Philadelphia, were used to measure vital capacity. According to Gould, the spirometers needed to be rugged ". . . to undergo the rough usage inseparable from transportation by army trains or on military railroads, which are in danger of being handled roughly at some unguarded moment by rude men. . . ." The spirometers were graduated in cubic centimeters and were "furnished with a mouth-piece of convenient form, connected with the instrument by flexible tubing."

---

[h] According to Hitchcock and Selye's *Anthropometric Manual*, the device consisted "of a lever acting by means of a piston and cylinder on a column of mercury in a closed glass tube. Water keeps the oil in the cylinder from contact with the mercury and various attachments enable the different groups of muscles to be brought to bear on the lever. By means of this apparatus, the strength of most of the large muscles may be tested fairly objectively"(p. 25). In the photographs, note the attachment of the tube to each device. Interestingly, Hitchcock determined an individual's total strength as a composite of body weight multiplied by dip and pull tests, strength of the back, legs, and average of the forearms, and the lung strength. Hitchcock stated, "The *total strength* is purely an arbitrary, and relative, rather than an actual test of strength as its name would indicate. And while confessedly imperfect, it seems decidedly desirable that there should be some method of comparison which does not depend entirely on lifting a dead weight against gravity, or steel springs."

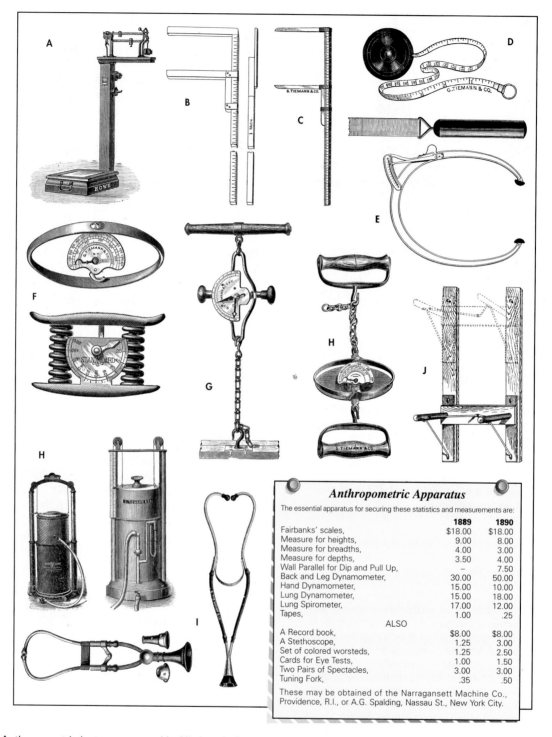

Anthropometric Apparatus

The essential apparatus for securing these statistics and measurements are:

	1889	1890
Fairbanks' scales,	$18.00	$18.00
Measure for heights,	9.00	8.00
Measure for breadths,	4.00	3.00
Measure for depths,	3.50	4.00
Wall Parallel for Dip and Pull Up,	–	7.50
Back and Leg Dynamometer,	30.00	50.00
Hand Dynamometer,	15.00	10.00
Lung Dynamometer,	15.00	18.00
Lung Spirometer,	17.00	12.00
Tapes,	1.00	.25
ALSO		
A Record book,	$8.00	$8.00
A Stethoscope,	1.25	3.00
Set of colored worsteds,	1.25	2.50
Cards for Eye Tests,	1.00	1.50
Two Pairs of Spectacles,	3.00	3.00
Tuning Fork,	.35	.50

These may be obtained of the Narragansett Machine Co., Providence, R.I., or A.G. Spalding, Nassau St., New York City.

Figure 8 Anthropometric instruments used by Hitchcock, Seaver, and Sargent. Sargent, also an entrepreneur, constructed and sold specialized strength equipment used in his studies. **A.** Metric graduated scale. **B.** Height meter. **C.** Sliding anthropometer. **D.** Cloth tape measure, with an instrument made by the Narragansett Machine Co. at the suggestion of Dr. Gulick (head of the Department of Physical Training of the YMCA Training School, Springfield, MA) in 1887. The modern version of this tape, now sold as the "Gulick tape," was "for attachment to the end of a tape to indicate the proper tension, so that the pressure may be always alike." **E.** Calipers for taking body depths. **F.** Several types of hand dynamometers, including push holder and pull holder instruments. **G.** Back and leg dynamometer, also used to measure the strength of the pectoral and "retractor" muscles of the shoulders. **H.** Vital capacity spirometer and Hutchinson's wet spirometer. **I.** Two stethoscopes. The soft rubber bell was used to "secure perfect coaptation to the surface of the chest." The Albion Stethoscope was preferred because it could be conveniently carried in the pocket. **J.** Parallel bars for testing arm extensors during push-ups and testing of flexors in pull-ups. In special situations, physiology laboratories used Marey's cardiograph to record pulse, but the preferred instrument was a pneumatic kymograph (or sphygmograph; see Fig. 2). The *inset table* shows a price comparison for the testing equipment from the 1889 and 1890 Hitchcock manuals. Note the yearly variation in prices. (Inset courtesy of Amherst College Archives, reproduced by permission of the Trustees of Amherst College, 1995.)

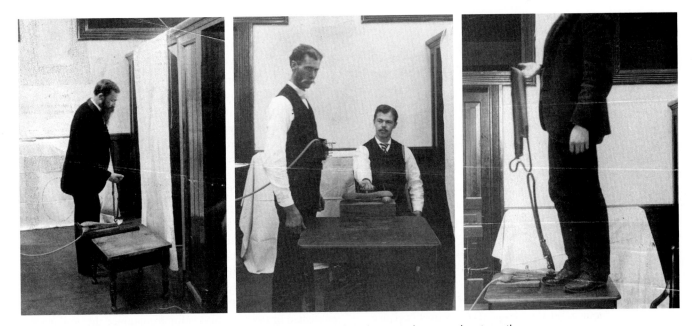

Figure 9   Kellogg's Universal Dynamometer acquired by Dr. Hitchcock to test the muscular strength of Amherst College students. From 1897 to 1900, strength measurements were taken on 328 freshmen, 111 sophomores, and 88 seniors, including retests of 58 individuals. Arm strength was measured bilaterally for the forearms and for the latissimus dorsi, deltoid, pectoral, and shoulder "retractor" muscles. Trunk measurements included the anterior trunk, and anterior and posterior neck. The leg measurements included the leg extensors and flexors and thigh adductors. **A.** "Arm pull." **B.** Anterior trunk (standing) and forearm supinators (sitting). **C.** Legs. (Photos courtesy of Amherst College Archives and by permission of the trustees of Amherst College, 1995.)

exercise course; thus, we believe he was the first person to formally teach such a course. It included experimental investigation and original work and thesis, including 6 hours a week of laboratory study. The course prerequisites included general physiology at the medical school or its equivalent. The purpose of the course was to introduce the student to the fundamentals of physical education and provide training in experimental methods related to exercise physiology. Fitz also taught a more general course titled The Elementary Physiology of The Hygiene of Common Life, Personal Hygiene, Emergencies. The course included one lecture and one laboratory section a week for a year (or three times a week for one-half year). The official course description stated: "This is a general introductory course intended to give the knowledge of human anatomy, physiology and hygiene which should be possessed by every student; it is suitable also for those not intending to study medicine or physical training." Fitz also taught a course Remedial Exercises. The Correction of Abnormal Conditions and Positions. Course content included observations of deformities such as spinal curvature (and the corrective effects of specialized exercises), and the "selection and application of proper exercises, and in the diagnosis of cases when exercise is unsuitable." Several of Fitz's scientific publications dealt with spinal deformities. In addition to the remedial exercise course, students took a required course, Applied Anatomy and Animal Mechanics. Action of Muscles in Different Exercises. This thrice-weekly course taught by Dr. Dudley Sargeant was the forerunner of

modern biomechanics courses. Its prerequisite was general anatomy at the medical school or its equivalent. Sargeant designed numerous exercise machines with pulleys and weights (www.ihpra.org/imagesa/sargentex.jpg), many of which he sold to individuals and schools.

Nine men graduated with BS degrees from the Department of Anatomy, Physiology, and Physical Training up to 1900. The aim of the major was to prepare students to become directors of gymnasia or instructors in physical training, to provide students with the necessary knowledge about the science of exercise, and to offer suitable training for entrance to the medical school. The stated purpose of the new exercise physiology research laboratory was as follows:

> A large and well-equipped laboratory has been organized for the experimental study of the physiology of exercise. The object of this work is to exemplify the hygiene of the muscles, the conditions under which they act, the relation of their action to the body as a whole affecting blood supply and general hygienic conditions, and the effects of various exercises upon muscular growth and general health.

With the activities of the department in full operation, its outspoken and critical director Dr. Fitz was not afraid to speak his mind about academic topics. For example, Fitz reviewed a new physiology text (*American Text-Book of Physiology*, edited by William H. Howell, PhD, MD) in the March 1897 issue of the *American Physical Education Review* (Vol II, No. 1, p. 56). The review praised Dr. Howell's collection of contributions from outstanding physiologists (such as Bowditch, Lee, Lusk, and Sewall), and attacked an 1888 French book by Lagrange that some historians consider the first important text in exercise physiology.[i] The following is Fitz's review:

> No one who is interested in the deeper problems of the physiology of exercise can afford to be without this book [referring to Howell's Physiology test], and it is to be hoped it may be used as a text-book in the normal schools of physical training. These schools have been forced to depend largely on Lagrange's "physiology of exercise" for the discussion of specific problems, or at least for the basis of such discussions. The only value Lagrange has, to my mind, is that he seldom gives any hint of the truth, and the student is forced to work out his own problems. This does very well in well-taught classes, but, Alas! for those schools and readers who take his statements as final in matters physiological. We have a conspicuous example of the disastrous consequences in Treve's contribution of the "Cyclopaedia of Hygiene on Physical Education," in which he quotes freely from Lagrange and rivals him in the absurdity of his conclusions.
>
> The time has surely come for a thoroughly scientific investigation of the physiological problems involved in physical exercise and the promulgation of the exact and absolute. It is not too much to hope that the use of the American Text-Book of Physiology by training schools and teachers, may aid to bring about this much needed consummation.

For unknown reasons, but coinciding with Fitz's untimely departure from Harvard in 1899,[j] the department changed its curricular emphasis (the term *physical training* was dropped from the department title), thus terminating at least temporarily this unique experiment in higher education.

One of the legacies of the Fitz-directed "Harvard experience" between 1891 and 1899 was the training it provided to the cadre of young scholars who began their careers with a strong scientific basis in exercise and training and its relationship to health. Unfortunately, it would take about another quarter century before the next generation of science-oriented physical educators (led by such world-class physiologists as Nobel laureate A. V. Hill and 1963 ACSM Honor Award recipient David Bruce Dill, not physical educators) would once again exert a strong influence on the physical education curriculum.

Exercise Studies in Research Journals

Another notable event in the growth of exercise physiology occurred in 1898: the appearance of three articles dealing with physical activity in the first volume of the *American Journal of Physiology*.[k] This was followed in 1921 with the publication of the prestigious journal *Physiological Reviews* (physrev.physiology.org/). TABLE 4 lists the articles in this journal (and two from the *Annual Review of Physiology*) from the first review of the mechanisms of muscular contraction by A. V. Hill (www.sportsci.org/news/history/hill/hill.html) in 1922, to Professor Francis Hellebrandt's classic review of exercise in 1940. The German applied physiology publication *Internationale Zeitschrift fur angewandte Physiologie einschliesslich Arbeitsphysiologie* (1929–1973) was a significant journal for research in exercise physiology. The current title of this journal is *European Journal of Applied Physiology and Occupational Physiology*. The *Journal of Applied Physiology* (jap.physiology.org/)was first published in 1948. Its first volume contained the now-classic paper on ratio expressions of physiologic data with reference to body size and function by J. M. Tanner, a must-read for exercise physiologists. The journal *Medicine and Science in Sports* was first published in 1969. Its aim was to integrate both medical and physiologic aspects of the emerging fields of sports medicine and exercise science. The official name of this journal was changed in 1980 (Volume 12) to *Medicine and Science in Sports and Exercise*.

The First Textbook in Exercise Physiology: The Debate Continues

What was the first textbook in exercise physiology? Several recent exercise physiology texts give the distinction of being "first" to the English translation of Fernand Lagrange's book, *The Physiology of Bodily Exercise*, originally published in French in 1888.[6,51,60] To deserve such historical recognition, we believe the work should meet the following three criteria:

1. Provide sound scientific rationale for major concepts
2. Provide summary information (based on experimentation) about important prior research in a

---

[i] We disagree with Berryman's[6] assessment of the relative historical importance of the translation of the original Lagrange text. We give our reasons for this disagreement in a subsequent section titled "First Textbook in Exercise Physiology: The Debate Continues."

[j] The reasons for Fitz's early departure from Harvard have been discussed in detail in Park's scholarly presentation of this topic.[46] His leaving was certainly unfortunate for the next generation of students of exercise physiology. In his 1909 textbook *Principles of Physiology and Hygiene* (New York, Henry Holt and Co.), the title page listed the following about Fitz's affiliation: Sometime Assistant Professor Physiology and Hygiene and Medical Visitor, Harvard University.

[k] The originator of the *American Journal of Physiology* was physiologist William T. Porter of the St. Louis College of Medicine and Harvard Medical School, who remained editor until 1914.[10] Porter's research focused on cardiac physiology. The three articles in volume 1 concerned (1) spontaneous physical activity in rodents and the influence of diet (C. C. Stewart, Department of Physiology, Clark University), (2) neural control of muscular movement in dogs (R. H. Cunningham, College of Physicians and Surgeons, Columbia University), and (3) perception of muscular fatigue and physical activity (J. C. Welch, Hull Physiological Laboratory, University of Chicago). As pointed out by Buskirk,[10] the next four volumes of the *American Journal of Physiology* (1898–1901) contained six additional articles about exercise physiology from experimental research laboratories at Harvard Medical School, Massachusetts Institute of Technology, the University of Michigan, and the Johns Hopkins University.

TABLE 4 ■ REVIEW ARTICLES ABOUT EXERCISE, 1922–1940

YEAR	AUTHOR AND ARTICLE
1922	Hill AV. The mechanism of muscular contraction. Physiol Rev 1922;2:310.
1925	Cathcart EP. The influence of muscle work on protein metabolism. Physiol Rev 1925;5:225.
1925	Cobb S. Review on the tonus of skeletal muscle. Physiol Rev 1925;5:518.
1928	Vernon HM. Industrial fatigue in relation to atomospheric conditions. Physiol Rev 1928;8:1.
1929	Eggleton P. The position of phosphorus in the chemical mechansim of muscle contraction. Physiol Rev 1929;9:432.
1929	Richardson HB. The respiratory quotient (including: The source of energy used for muscular exertion). Physiol Rev 1929;9:61.
1930	Gasset HS. Contracture of skeletal muscle. Physiol Rev 1930;10:35.
1931	Milroy TH. The present status of the chemistry of skeletal muscular contraction. Physiol Rev 1931;11:515.
1932	Baetzer AM. The effect of muscular fatigue upon resistance. Physiol Rev 1932;12:453.
1932	Hill AV. The revolution in muscle physiology. Physiol Rev 1932;12:56.
1933	Jordan HE. The structural changes in striped muscle during contraction. Physiol Rev 1933;13:301.
1933	Steinhaus AH. Chronic effects of exercise. Physiol Rev 1933;13:103.
1934	Hinsey JC. The innervation of skeletal muscle. Physiol Rev 1934;14:514.
1936	Dill DB. The economy of muscular exercise. Physiol Rev 1936;16:263,.
1936	Fenn WO. Electrolytes in muscle. Physiol Rev 1936;16:450.
1937	Anderson WW, Williams HH. Role of fat in diet. Physiol Rev 1937;17:335.
1939	Bozler E. Muscle. Annu Rev Physiol 1939;1: 217.
1939	Dill DB. Applied Physiology. Annu Rev Physiol 1939;1:551.
1939	Millikan GA. Muscle hemoglobin. Physiol Rev 1939;19:503.
1939	Tower SS. The reaction of muscle to denervation. Physiol Rev 1939;19:1.
1940	Hellebrandt FA. Exercise. Annu Rev Physiol 1940;2:411.

particular topic area (e.g., contain scientific references to research in the area)

3. Provide sufficient "factual" information about a topic area to give it academic legitimacy

After reading the Lagrange book in its entirety, we came to the same conclusion as George Wells Fitz. Specifically, it was a popular book about health and exercise with a "scientific" title. It is our opinion that the book is *not* a legitimate scientific textbook of exercise physiology based on any reasonable criteria of the time. Despite Lagrange's assertion that the focus of his book assessed physiology applied to exercise and not hygiene and exercise, it is informed by a 19th century hygienic perspective, not science. We believe Fitz would accept our evaluation.

There was much information available to Lagrange from existing European and American physiology textbooks about the digestive, muscular, circulatory, and respiratory systems, including some limited information on physical training, hormones, basic nutrition, chemistry, and the biology of muscular contraction. Admittedly, this information was relatively scarce, but well-trained physiologists Flint, Howell, Martin,

Huxley, Dalton, Carpenter, and Combe had already produced high-quality textbooks that contained relatively detailed information about physiology in general, with some reference to muscular exercise. We now understand why Fitz was so troubled by the Lagrange book. By comparison, the two-volume text by Howell titled *An American Text-Book of Physiology* was impressive; this edited volume contained articles from acknowledged American physiologists at the forefront of physiologic research. This textbook was a high-level physiology text even by today's standards. In his quest to provide the best possible science for his physical education students, Fitz could not tolerate a book that did not live up to his expectations for excellence. In fact, the Lagrange book contained fewer than 20 reference citations, and most of these were ascribed to French research reports or were based on observations of friends performing exercise. This plethora of anecdotal reports must have given Fitz "fits."

Lagrange, an accomplished writer, wrote extensively on exercise. Despite the titles of several of his books,[1] Lagrange was not a scientist but probably a practicing "physical culturist." Bibliographic information about Lagrange is limited in

---

[1] The following books (including translations, editions, and pages) were published by Lagrange beginning in 1888: *Physiologie des Exercices du Corps.* Paris: Alcan, 1888, 372 pp. (6th ed., 1892); *L'Hygiene de l'Exercice Chez les Enfants et les Jeunes Gens.* Paris: Alcan, 1890, 312 pp. (4th ed., 1893; 6th ed, 1896; 7th ed, 1901, 8th ed, 1905); *Physiology of Bodily Exercise.* New York: D. Appleton, 1890, 395 pp.; *De l'Exercice Chez les Adultes.* Paris: Alcan, 1891, 367 pp. (2nd ed., 1892, 367 pp.; 4th ed., 1900, 367 pp.; Italian translation, *Fisiologia degli Esercizj del Corpo.* Milano: Dumolard, 1889; Hungarian translation, 1913); *La Medication par l'Exercice.* Paris: Alcan, 1894, 500 pp.

the French and American archival records of the period—a further indication of his relative obscurity as a thinker of distinction. As far as we know, there have been no citations to his work in any physiology text or scientific article. For these reasons, we contend the Lagrange book does not qualify as the first exercise physiology textbook.[m]

Other Early Exercise Physiology Research Laboratories

The Nutrition Laboratory at the Carnegie Institute in Washington, DC, had been created in 1904 to study nutrition and energy metabolism, and the first research laboratories established in physical education in the United States to study exercise physiology were at George Williams College (1923), the University of Illinois (1925), and Springfield College (1927). However, the real impact of laboratory research in exercise physiology (along with many other research specialties) occurred in 1927 with the creation of the 800-square foot Harvard Fatigue Laboratory in the basement of Morgan Hall of Harvard University's Business School.[33] The outstanding work of this laboratory during the next two decades established the legitimacy of exercise physiology on its own merits as an important area of research and study. Another exercise physiology laboratory started before World War II was the Laboratory of Physiological Hygiene at the University of California, Berkeley, in 1934. The syllabus for the Physiological Hygiene course (taught by professor Frank Kleeberger), the precursor of contemporary exercise physiology courses, contained 12 laboratory experiments.[47] Several years later, Dr. Franklin M. Henry (isb.ri.ccf.org/biomch-l/archives/biomch-l-1993-09/00050.html) assumed responsibility for the laboratory. Dr. Henry began publishing the results of different experiments in various physiology-oriented journals including the *Journal of Applied Physiology, Annals of Internal Medicine, Aviation Medicine, War Medicine,* and *Science.* Henry's first research project as a faculty member in the Department of Physical Education (published in 1938) concerned the validity and reliability of the pulse–ratio test of cardiac efficiency;[26,27] a later paper dealt with predicting aviators' bends. Henry applied his training in experimental psychology to exercise physiology topics, including individual differences in the kinetics of the fast and slow components of the oxygen uptake and recovery curves during light- and moderate-cycle ergometer exercise; muscular strength; cardiorespiratory responses during steady-rate exercise; assessment of heavy-work fatigue; determinants of endurance performance; and neural control factors related to human motor performance (FIG. 10).

Contributions of the Harvard Fatigue Laboratory (1927–1946)

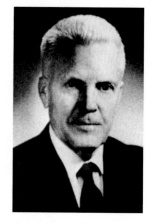

Many of the great scientists of the 20th century with an interest in exercise were associated with the Harvard Fatigue Laboratory. This research facility was established by Lawrence J. Henderson, MD (1878–1942), renowned chemist and professor of biochemistry at the Harvard Medical School. The first and only scientific director of the Fatigue Laboratory was David Bruce Dill (1891–1986: www.the-aps.org/about/pres/introdbd.htm), a Stanford PhD in physical chemistry. Dill was transformed from a biochemist to an experimental physiologist while at the Fatigue Laboratory, and an influential driving force behind the laboratory's numerous scientific accomplishments. His early academic association with Boston physician Arlen Vernon Bock (a student of famous high-altitude physiologist Dr. Barcroft at Cambridge, England,[5] and Dill's closest friend for 59 years) and contact with 1922 Nobel laureate Archibald Vivian (A. V.) Hill (for his discovery related to heat production in muscles) provided Dill with the confidence to successfully coordinate the research efforts of dozens of scholars from 15 different countries. A. V. Hill convinced Bock to write a third edition of Bainbridge's text *Physiology of Muscular Activity.* Bock, in turn, invited Dill to coauthor the book republished in 1931.[17]

Over a 20-year period, at least 352 research papers, numerous monographs, and a book[18] were published in areas of basic and applied exercise physiology, including methodologic refinements concerned with blood chemistry analysis and simplified methods for analyzing the fractional concentrations of expired air. Research at the Fatigue Laboratory included many aspects of short-term responses and chronic physiologic adaptations to exercise under environmental stresses produced by exposure to altitude, heat, and cold. Most of the key human exercise experiments were conducted using treadmill and bicycle ergometer exercise, but several important studies used animals. The human and animal studies framed the cornerstone for research in modern laboratories of exercise physiology, particularly those related to the assessment of physical working capacity and fitness, cardiovascular and hemodynamic responses during maximal exercise, kinetics of oxygen consumption and substrate use, metabolism during exercise and recovery, and maximal oxygen consumption.

---

[m] Possible pre-1900 candidates for "first" exercise physiology textbook listed in Table 1 also include Combe's 1843 text "*The Principles of Physiology Applied to the Preservation of Health, and to the Improvement of Physical and Mental Education*"; Hitchcock and Hitchcock's *Elementary Anatomy and Physiology for Colleges, Academies, and Other Schools* (1860); Kolb's 1887 German monograph, translated into English in 1893 as *Physiology of Sport*; and the 1898 Martin text, *The Human Body. An Account of Its Structure and Activities and the Conditions of Its Healthy Working.*

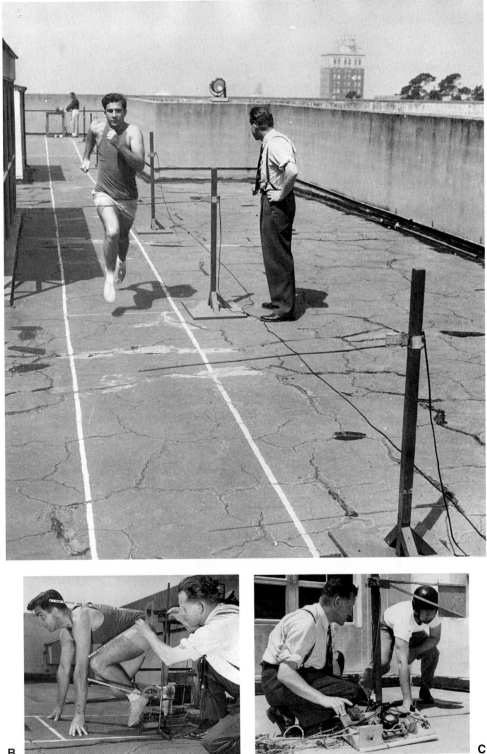

A

B   C

Figure 10   **A.** Professor Franklin Henry supervising 50-yard sprints (at 5-yd intervals) on the roof of Harmon Gymnasium. Henry's study[28] was prompted by A. V. Hill's 1927 observations concerning the "viscosity" factor of muscular contraction that at first helped to explain the large decline in metabolic efficiency at fast rates of movement and that the oxygen requirement of running increased with the cube of speed. Henry verified that metabolic efficiency was not correlated with a muscle viscosity factor. **B.** Henry making limb and trunk anthropometric measurements on a sprinter during continuous studies of the force-time characteristics of the sprint start[29] to further evaluate A. V. Hill's theoretical equation for the velocity of sprint running. **C.** Henry recording the timing of the initial movements of blocking performance in football players.[44]

Detailed discussions of each of these topics appear in various chapters of this 6th edition.

Like the first exercise physiology laboratory established at Harvard's Lawrence Scientific School in 1892, the Harvard Fatigue Laboratory demanded excellence in research and scholarship. Particularly noteworthy was the cooperation among scientists from around the world that fostered lasting collaborations. Furthermore, many of the scientists who had contact with the Fatigue Laboratory profoundly affected a new generation of exercise physiologists in the United States and abroad. Noteworthy were Ancel Keys (1904–: mbbnet.umn. edu/firsts/blackburn_h.html and www.epi.umn.edu/about/history/ancelkeys.shtm), who established the Laboratory of Physiology and Physical Education (later renamed the Laboratory of Physiological Hygiene) at the University of Minnesota; Henry L. Taylor (Keys and Taylor were mentors to exercise physiologist Elsworth R. Buskirk [www.noll.psu.edu/users/buskirk/ eb_bio.html], formerly at the NIH and later the Noll Laboratory at Pennsylvania State University); Robert E. Johnson at the Human Environmental Unit at the University of Illinois; Sid Robinson at Indiana University; Robert C. Darling at the Department of Rehabilitation Medicine at Columbia University; Harwood S. Belding, who started the Environmental Physiology Laboratory at the University of Pittsburgh; C. Frank Consolazio of the U.S. Army Medical Research and Nutrition Laboratory at Denver; Lucien Brouha, who headed the Fitness Research Unit at the University of Montreal, and then went to the Dupont Chemical Company in Delaware; and Steven M. Horvath, who established the Institute of Environmental Stress at the University of California, Santa Barbara, where he worked with visiting scientists and mentored graduate students in the Biology Department and Department of Ergonomics and Physical Education. After the Fatigue Laboratory was unfortunately forced to close in 1946, Dill continued as the deputy director of the U.S. Army Chemical Corps Medical Laboratory in Maryland for 13 years (1948–1961). Thereafter, he worked with Sid Robinson at Indiana University's physiology department. He then started the Desert Research Institute (connected with the University of Nevada at Las Vegas), where he studied the physiologic responses of men and animals to hot environments, a topic that culminated in a book on the subject.[20]

The group of scholars associated with the Harvard Fatigue Laboratory mentored the next generation of students who continue to make significant contributions to the field of exercise physiology. The monograph by Horvath and Horvath[33] and the chronology by Dill[19] are the best direct sources of historical information about the Harvard Fatigue Laboratory. Exercise physiology continued to expand after the closing of the Fatigue Laboratory. Subsequent efforts probed the full range of physiologic functions. The depth and breadth of these early investigations summarized in TABLE 5 provided much of the current knowledge base for establishing exercise physiology as a respectable academic field of study.

TABLE 5 ■ AREAS OF INVESTIGATION AT THE HARVARD FATIGUE LABORATORY THAT HELPED TO ESTABLISH EXERCISE PHYSIOLOGY AS AN ACADEMIC DISCIPLINE

1. Specificity of the exercise prescription
2. Genetic components of an exercise response
3. Selectivity of the adaptive responses by diseased populations
4. Differentiation between central and peripheral adaptations
5. The existence of cellular thresholds
6. Actions of transmitters and the regulation of receptors
7. Feed-forward and feedback mechanisms that influence cardiorespiratory and metabolic control
8. Matching mechanisms between oxygen delivery and oxygen demand
9. The substrate utilization profile with and without dietary manipulations
10. Adaptive responses of cellular and molecular units
11. Mechanisms responsible for signal transduction
12. The behavior of lactate in cells
13. The plasticity of muscle fiber types
14. Motor functions of the spinal cord
15. The ability of hormonally deficient animals to respond to conditions of acute exercise and chronic exercise
16. The hypoxemia of severe exercise

From Tipton CM. Personal communication to F. Katch, June 12, 1995. From a presentation made to the American Physiological Society Meetings, 1995.

Research Methodology Textbook Focusing on Physiologic Research

In 1949, the Research Section of the Research Council of the Research Section of the American Association for Health, Physical Education, and Recreation, or AAHPER (an outgrowth of the American Association for the Advancement of Physical Education created in 1885), sponsored publication of the first textbook devoted to research methodology in physical education.[1] Thomas Cureton (1901–1992; 1969 ACSM Honor Award), PhD, a pioneer researcher in physical fitness evaluation and director of the exercise physiology research laboratory he established at the University of Illinois in 1944, appointed Dr. Henry to chair the committee to write the chapter on physiologic research methods. The other committee members were respected scientists in their own right and included the following: Anna Espenshade (PhD in psychology from Berkeley, specialist in motor development and motor performance during growth); Pauline Hodgson (Berkeley PhD in physiology who did postdoctoral work at the Harvard Fatigue Laboratory); Peter V. Karpovich, MD (originator of the Physiological Research Laboratory at Springfield College); Arthur H. Steinhaus, PhD (director of the research laboratory at George Williams College, one of the eleven founders of the American College of Sports Medicine and research physiologist who authored an important review article [*Physiological Reviews*, 1933] about chronic effects of exercise); and distinguished Berkeley physiologist Hardin Jones, PhD (Donner Research Laboratory of Medical Physics at Berkley).

The book chapter by this distinguished committee stands as a hallmark of research methodology in exercise physiology. The 99 references, many of them key articles in this then-embryonic field, covered such exercise-related topics as the "heart and circulation, blood, urine and kidney function, work, lung ventilation, respiratory metabolism and energy exchange, and alveolar air."

Another masterful compendium of research methodologies published 14 years later, *Physiological Measurements of Metabolic Functions in Man*, by C. F. Consolazio and colleagues provided complete details about specific measurements in exercise physiology.[16] Several sections in this book contained material previously published from the Harvard Fatigue Laboratory one year before its closing in 1946[34] and from another book dealing with metabolic methods[15] published in 1951.

THE NORDIC CONNECTION (DENMARK, SWEDEN, NORWAY, AND FINLAND)

Denmark and Sweden have made a significant historical impact on physical education as an academic field. In 1800, Denmark was the first European country to include physical training (military-style gymnastics) as a requirement in the public school curriculum. Since that time, Danish and Swedish scientists have made outstanding contributions to research in both traditional physiology and exercise physiology.

Danish Influence

In 1909, the University of Copenhagen endowed the equivalent of a Chair in Anatomy, Physiology, and Theory of Gymnastics.[42] The first docent was Johannes Lindhard, MD (1870–1947). He later teamed with August Krogh (1874–1949; www.sportsci.org/news/history/krogh/krogh.html), PhD, an eminent scientist specializing in

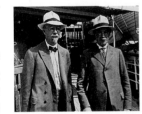

Professors August Krogh and Johannes Lindhard in the early 1930s.

physiological chemistry and research instrument design and construction, to conduct many of the now classic experiments in exercise physiology. For example, Krogh and Lindhard investigated gas exchange in the lungs, pioneered studies of the relative contribution of fat and carbohydrate oxidation during exercise (see "Focus on Research," Chapter 8), measured the redistribution of blood flow during different exercise intensities, and measured cardiorespiratory dynamics in exercise (including cardiac output using nitrous oxide gas, a method described by a German researcher in 1770).

By 1910, Krogh and his wife Marie (a physician) had proven through a series of ingenious, decisive experiments[54] that diffusion was how pulmonary gas exchange occurred—not by secretion of oxygen from lung tissue into the blood during exercise and exposure to altitude, as postulated by

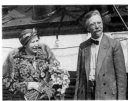

Marie and August Krogh

Scottish physiologist Sir John Scott Haldane 1860–1936) and Englishman James Priestley.[25] By 1919, Krogh had published reports of a series of experiments (with three appearing in the *Journal of Physiology*, 1919) concerning the mechanism of oxygen diffusion and transport in skeletal muscles. The details of these early experiments are included in Krogh's 1936 textbook,[37] but he also was prolific in many other areas of science.[36,38–40] In 1920, Krogh received the Nobel Prize in physiology or medicine for discovering the mechanism of capillary control of blood flow in resting and exercising muscle (in frogs). To honor the achievements of this renowned scientist (which included 300 scientific articles), an institute for physiologic research in Copenhagen was named for him.

Three other Danish researcher–physiologists, Erling Asmussen (1907–1991; ACSM Citation Award, 1976 and ACSM Honor Award, 1979), Erik Hohwü-Christensen (1904–1996; ACSM Honor Award, 1981), and Marius Nielsen (1903–2000) conducted pioneering studies in exercise physiology. These "three musketeers," as Krogh referred to them, published numerous research papers from the 1930s to the 1970s. Asmussen, initially an assistant in Lindhard's laboratory, became a productive researcher specializing in muscle fiber architecture and mechanics. He also published papers with Nielsen and Christensen as coauthors on many applied topics including muscular strength and performance, ventilatory and cardiovascular response to changes in posture and exercise intensity, maximum working capacity during arm and leg exercise, changes in oxidative response of muscle during exercise, comparisons of positive and negative work, hormonal and core temperature response during different intensities of exercise, and respiratory function in response to decreases in oxygen partial pressure. As evident in his classic review article[2] of muscular exercise that cites many of his own studies (plus 75 references from other Scandinavian researchers), Asmussen's grasp of the importance of the study of biologic functions during exercise is as relevant today as it

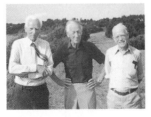

The "three musketeers," Drs. Erling Asmussen *(left)*, Erik Hohwü-Christensen *(center)*, and Marius Nielsen *(right)* (1988 photo).

was more than 41 years ago when the article was published.

He clearly defines exercise physiology within the context of biologic science:

> The physiology of muscular exercise can be considered a purely descriptive science: it measures the extent to which the human organism can adapt itself to the stresses and strains of the environment and thus provides useful knowledge for athletes, trainers, industrial human engineers, clinicians, and workers in rehabilitation on the working capacity of humans and its limitations. But the physiology of muscular exercise is also part of the general biological science, physiology, which attempts to explain how the living organism functions, by means of the chemical and physical laws that govern the inanimate world. Its important role in physiology lies in the fact that muscular exercise more than most other conditions, taxes the functions to their uttermost. Respiration, circulation, and heat regulation are only idling in the resting state. By following them through stages of increasing work intensities, a far better understanding of the resting condition is also achieved. Although the physiology of muscular exercise must be studied primarily in healthy subjects, the accumulated knowledge of how the organism responds to the stresses of exercise adds immensely to the understanding of how the organism adapts itself to disease or attempts to eliminate its effects by mobilizing its regulatory mechanisms.

Christensen became Lindhard's student in Copenhagen in 1925. Together with Krogh and Lindhard, Christensen published an important review article in 1936 that described physiologic dynamics during maximal exercise.[14] In his 1931 thesis, Christensen reported on studies of cardiac output with a modified Grollman acetylene method; body temperature and blood sugar concentration during heavy cycling exercise; comparisons of arm and leg exercise; and the effects of training. Together with Ové Hansen, he used oxygen consumption and the respiratory quotient to describe how diet, state of training, and exercise intensity and duration affected carbohydrate and fat use. Interestingly, the concept of "carbohydrate loading" was first discovered in 1939! Other notable studies included core temperature and blood glucose regulation during light-to-heavy fatiguing exercise at various ambient temperatures. A study by Christensen and Nielsen in 1942 used finger plethysmography to study regional blood flow (including skin temperature) during brief periods of constant-load cycle ergometer exercise.[13] Experiments published in 1936 by physician Olé Bang, inspired by his mentor Ejar Lundsgaard, described the fate of blood lactate during exercise of different intensities and durations.[4] The experiments of Christensen, Asmussen, Nielsen, and Hansen were conducted at the Laboratory for the Theory of Gymnastics at the University of Copenhagen. Today, the August Krogh Institute (www.aki.ku.dk/index.asp?sprog5EN&level5&page5&indhold5) carries on the tradition of basic and applied research in exercise physiology. Since 1973, Swedish-trained scientist Bengt Saltin (the only Nordic researcher besides Erling Asmussen to receive the ACSM Citation Award [1980] and ACSM Honor Award [1990]; former student of Per-Olof Åstrand, discussed in the next section) has been a professor and continues his significant scientific

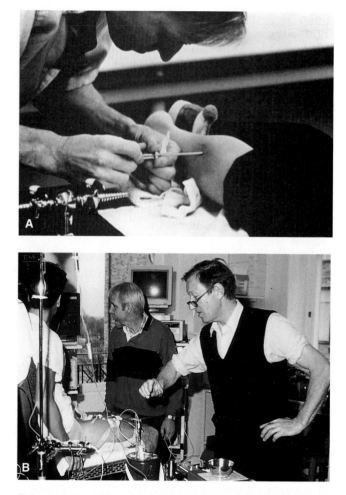

A. Bengt Saltin taking muscle biopsy of gastrocnemius muscle. (Photo courtesy of Dr. David Costill.) **B.** Saltin (hand on hip) during an experiment at the August Krogh Institute, Copenhagen. (Photo courtesy Per-Olof Åstrand.)

studies as professor and director of the Copenhagen Muscle Research Centre, University of Copenhagen, Denmark.

Swedish Influence

Modern exercise physiology in Sweden can be traced to Per Henrik Ling (1776–1839) who in 1813 became the first director of Stockholm's Royal Central Institute of Gymnastics.[42] Ling, a specialist in fencing, developed a system of "medical gymnastics." This system, which became part of the school curriculum of Sweden in 1820, was based on his studies of anatomy and physiology.

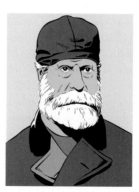

Hjalmar Ling

Ling's son Hjalmar also had a strong interest in medical gymnastics and physiology and anatomy, in part owing to his attendance at lectures by French physiologist Claude Bernard in

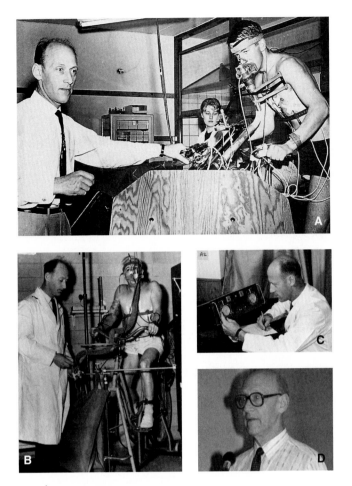

P-O. Åstrand, Department of Physiology. Karolinska Institute, Stockholm. **A.** Measuring maximal performance of Johnny Nilsson, Olympic Gold Medal speed skater, 1964. **B.** Maximal oxygen consumption measured during cycle ergometer exercise, 1958. **C.** Laboratory experiment, 1955. **D.** Invited lecture, 1992 International Conference on Physical Activity, Fitness and Health, Toronto.

Paris in 1854. Hjalmar Ling published a book on the kinesiology of body movements in 1866. As a result of the Lings' philosophy and influence, the physical educators who graduated from the Stockholm Central Institute were well schooled in the basic biologic sciences, in addition to being highly proficient in sports and games. Currently, the College of Physical Education (Gymnastik-Och Idrottshögskolan) and Department

of Physiology in the Karolinska Institute Medical School in Stockholm continue to sponsor studies in exercise physiology.

Per-Olof Åstrand, MD, PhD (1922–) is the most famous graduate of the College of Physical Education (1946); in 1952, he presented his thesis to the Karolinska Institute Medical School. Åstrand taught in the Department of Physiology in the College of Physical Education from 1946 to 1977. When the College of Physical Education became a department of the Karolinska Institute, Åstrand served as professor and department head from 1977 to 1987. Christensen was Åstrand's mentor and supervised his doctoral dissertation, which included data on the physical working capacity of both sexes aged 4 to 33 years. This important study—along with collaborative studies with his wife Irma Ryhming—established a line of research that propelled Åstrand to the forefront of experimental exercise physiology for which he achieved worldwide fame.[n] Four papers published by Åstrand in 1960, with Christensen as one of the authors, stimulated further studies on the physiologic responses to intermittent exercise. Åstrand has mentored an impressive group of exercise physiologists, including such "superstars" as Bengt Saltin and Björn Ekblom. TABLE 6 is a sampling of contributions to the exercise physiology literature by Åstrand and Saltin in books, book chapters, monographs, and research articles. As further evidence of their phenomenal international influence, the bottom part of the table includes the number of times each was cited in the scientific literature from 1996 through April 2001.

Two Swedish scientists at the Karolinska Institute, Drs. Jonas Bergström and Erik Hultman, performed important experiments with the needle biopsy procedure that have provided a new vista from which to study exercise physiology. With this procedure, it became relatively easy to conduct invasive studies of muscle under various exercise conditions, training, and nutritional status. Collaborative work with other Scandinavian researchers

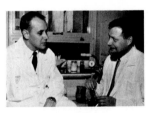

Drs. Jonas Bergström *(left)* and Eric Hultman, Karolinska Institute, mid-1960s.

(Saltin and Hultman from Sweden and Lars Hermanson from Norway) and researchers in the United States (e.g., Phillip Gollnick at Washington State University and David Costill at Ball State University) contributed a unique new dimension to the study of muscular exercise.

[n] Personal communication to F. Katch, June 13, 1995, from Dr. Åstrand regarding his professional background. Recipient of five honorary doctorate degrees (Université de Grenoble [1968], University of Jyväskylä [1971], Institut Superieur d'Education Physique, Université Libre de Bruxelles [1987], Loughborough University of Technology [1991], Aristoteles University of Thessaloniki [1992]). Åstrand is an honorary Fellow of nine international societies, a Fellow of the American Association for the Advancement of Science (for "outstanding career contributions to understanding of the physiology of muscular work and applications of this understanding"), and has received many awards and prizes for his outstanding scientific achievements, including the ACSM Honor Award in 1973. Åstrand served on a committee for awarding the Nobel Prize in physiology or medicine from 1977 to 1988 and is coauthor with Kaare Rodahl of *Textbook of Work Physiology*, 3rd edition, 1986 (translated in Chinese, French, Italian, Japanese, Korean, Portuguese, and Spanish). His English publications number about 200 (including book chapters, proceedings, a history of Scandinavian scientists in exercise physiology[3] and monographs), and he has given invited lectures in approximately 50 countries and 150 different cities outside of Sweden. His classic 1974 pamphlet *Health and Fitness* has an estimated distribution of 15 to 20 million copies (about 3 million copies in Sweden)—unfortunately, all without personal royalty!

TABLE 6 ■ SELECTED CONTRIBUTIONS TO THE EXERCISE PHYSIOLOGY LITERATURE BY SWEDISH EXERCISE PHYSIOLOGISTS PER-OLOF ÅSTRAND AND BENGT SALTIN

Åstrand P-O Experimental studies of physical working capacity in relation to sex and age. Copenhagen: Munksgaard, 1952.

Åstrand P-O, Ryhming I. A nomogram for calculation of aerobic capacity (physical fitness) from pulse rate during submaximal work. J Appl Physiol 1954;7:218.

Åstrand P-O, Saltin B. Maximal oxygen uptake and heart rate in various types of muscular activity. J Appl Physiol 1961;16:977.

Åstrand P-O, et al. Girl swimmers. Acta Paediatr 1963;(Suppl 147).

Åstrand P-O, Grimby G, eds. Physical activity in health and disease: Proceedings of the Second Acta Medica Scandinavica International Symposium. Goteborg, Sweden, June 10–12, 1985.

Åstrand P-O, Rodahl K. Textbook of work physiology. 3rd ed. New York: McGraw-Hill, 1986.

Åstrand P-O, et al. A 33-year followup of peak oxygen uptake and related variables of former physical education students. J Appl Physiol 1997;82:844.

Ekblom B, Åstrand P-O. Role of physical activity on health in child and adolescents. Acta Paediatr 2000;89:762.

Saltin B. Aerobic work capacity and circulation of man. Acta Physiol Scand 1964;(Suppl 230).

Saltin B, Åstrand P-O. Maximal oxygen uptake in athletes. J Appl Physiol 1967;23:353.

Saltin B, et al. Physical training in sedentary middle-aged and older men. Scand J Clin Lab Invest 1967;24:323.

Saltin B, Hermansen L. Glycogen stores and prolonged severe exercise. In Blix G, ed. Nutrition and physical activity. Symposia of the Swedish Nutrition Foundation. Stockholm: Almqvist & Wiksell, 1967.

Saltin B, et al. Response to submaximal and maximal exercise after bedrest and training. Circulation 1968;38(Suppl 7).

Saltin B, ed. International Symposium on Biochemistry of Exercise. Champaign, IL: Human Kinetics, 1986.

Saltin B, et al. Skeletal muscle blood flow in humans and its regulation during exercise. Acta Physiol Scand 1998;162:421.

Bouvier F, Saltin B, et al. Left ventricular function and perfusion in elderly endurance athletes. Med Sci Sports Exerc 2001;33:735.

NUMBER OF CITATIONS IN THE SCIENTIFIC LITERATURE (1996–2001)

YEAR	1996	1997	1998	1999	2000	2001[a]
Åstrand	7526	6502	6485	7834	8523	3822
Saltin	20,332	16,780	17,272	21,441	18,060	14,524

Source: Science Citation Index. Numbers refer to the total number of citations ("hits") in the published literature (including books).
[a] Through April 30, 2001.

Norwegian and Finnish Influence

The new generation of exercise physiologists trained in the late 1940s analyzed respiratory gases by means of a highly accurate sampling apparatus that measured relatively small quantities of carbon dioxide and oxygen in expired air. The method of analysis (and also the analyzer) was developed in 1947 by Norwegian scientist Per Scholander (1905–1980). A diagram of Scholander's micrometer gas analyzer[55] is presented in Chapter 8, Figure 8.7, along with its larger counterpart, the Haldane analyzer.

Another prominent Norwegian researcher was Lars A. Hermansen (1933–1984; ACSM Citation Award, 1985) from the Institute of Work Physiology, died prematurely. Nevertheless, his many contributions include a classic 1969 article entitled "Anaerobic Energy Release" that appeared in the first volume of *Medicine and Science in Sports*.[30] Other papers included work with exercise physiologist K. Lange Andersen.[31]

In Finland, Martti Karvonen, MD, PhD (ACSM Honor Award, 1991) from the Physiology Department of the Institute of Occupational Health, Helsinki, is best known for a method to predict optimal exercise training heart rate, the so-called "Karvonen formula" (see "Focus on Research," Chapter 15). He also conducted studies dealing with exercise performance and the role of exercise in longevity. In 1952, Lauri Pikhala, a physiologist, suggested that obesity was the consequence and not the cause of physical "unfitness." Ilkka Vuori, starting in the early 1970s, reported on hormone responses to exercise. Paavo Komi, from the Department of Biology of Physical Activity, University of Jyväskylä, has been Finland's most prolific researcher, with numerous experiments published in the combined areas of exercise physiology and sport biomechanics. TABLE 7 lists the Nordic researchers who

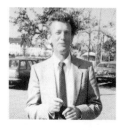

Lars A. Hermansen (1933–1984). Institute of Work Physiology, Oslo.

TABLE 7 ■ NORDIC RESEARCHERS[a] AWARDED THE ACSM HONOR AWARD AND ACSM CITATION AWARD

ACSM HONOR AWARD	ACSM CITATION AWARD
Per-Olof Åstrand, 1973	Erling Asmussen, 1976
Erling Asmussen, 1979	Bengt Saltin, 1980
Erik Hohwü-Christensen, 1981	Lars A. Hermansen, 1985
Bengt Saltin, 1990	C. Gunnar Blomqvist, 1987
Martti J. Karvonen, 1991	

[a] Born and educated in a Nordic country.

have received the prestigious ACSM Honor Award or ACSM Citation Award.

OTHER CONTRIBUTORS TO THE KNOWLEDGE BASE IN EXERCISE PHYSIOLOGY

In addition to the distinguished American and Nordic applied scientists profiled earlier, there have been many other "giants" in the field of physiology and experimental science[o] who have made monumental contributions that indirectly added to the knowledge base in exercise physiology. The list includes:

Sir Joseph Barcroft (1872–1947). High-altitude research physiologist who pioneered fundamental work concerning the functions of hemoglobin, later confirmed by Nobel laureate August Krogh. Barcroft also performed experiments to determine how cold affected the central nervous system. For up

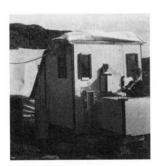

Marie Krogh collects data at Barcroft's high-altitude experimental station to assess oxygen tension of gases.

to one hour, he would lie without clothing on a couch in subfreezing temperature and record his subjective reactions.

Christian Bohr (1855–1911). Professor of physiology in the medical school at the University of Copenhagen who mentored August Krogh, and father of nuclear physicist Niels Bohr. Bohr studied with Carl Ludwig in Leipzig in

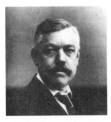

1881 and 1883, publishing papers on the solubility of gases in various fluids, including oxygen absorption in distilled water and in solutions containing hemoglobin. Krogh's careful experiments using advanced instruments (microtonometer) disproved Bohr's secretion theory that both oxygen and carbon dioxide were secreted across the lung epithelium in opposite directions based on the time required for equalization of gas tension in blood and air.

John Scott Haldane (1860–1936). Conducted research in mine safety, investigating principally the action of dangerous gases (carbon monoxide), the use of rescue equipment, and the incidence of pulmonary disease. He devised a decompression apparatus for the safe ascent of deep-sea divers. The British Royal Navy and the United States Navy adopted tables based on this work. In 1905, he discovered

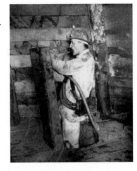

Haldane investigating carbon monoxide gas in an English coal mine at the turn of the 20th century.

that carbon dioxide acted on the brain's respiratory center to regulate breathing. In 1911, he and several other physiologists organized an expedition to Pikes Peak, Colorado to study the effects of low oxygen pressures at high altitudes. Haldane also showed that the reaction of oxyhemoglobin with ferricyanide rapidly and quantitatively released oxygen and formed methemoglobin. The amount of liberated oxygen could be accurately calculated from the increased gas pressure in the closed reaction system at constant temperature and volume. Haldane devised a microtechnique to fractionate a sample of a mixed gas into its component gases (see Chapter 8, Haldane apparatus). Haldane founded the *Journal of Hygiene.*

Otto Meyerhof (1884–1951). Meyerhof's experiments on the energy changes during cellular respiration led to discoveries on lactic acid related to muscular activity, research that led to the Nobel Prize (with A.V. Hill in 1923). In 1925, Meyerhof extracted from muscle the enzymes that convert glycogen to lactic acid. Subsequent research confirmed work done by

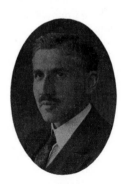

---

[o] There are many excellent sources of information about the history of science and medicine, including the following: Bettman O. *A Pictorial History of Medicine.* Springfield, IL: Charles C Thomas, 1956; Clendening L. *Source Book of Medical History.* New York: Dover Publications/Henry Schuman, 1960; Coleman W. *Biology in the Nineteenth Century.* New York: Cambridge University Press, 1977; Franklin K. *A Short History of Physiology,* 2nd ed. London: Staples Press, 1949; Fye WB, *The Development of American Physiology. Scientific Medicine in the Nineteenth Century.* Baltimore: Johns Hopkins University Press, 1987; Guthrie D. *A History of Medicine.* London: T. Nelson & Sons, 1945; Haskins T. *Science and Enlightenment.* New York: Cambridge University Press, 1985; Holmes FL. *Lavoisier and the Chemistry of Life.* Madison: University of Wisconsin Press, 1985; Knight B. *Discovering the Human Body.* London: Bloomsbury Books; Lesch JE. *Science and Medicine in France. The Emergence of Experimental Physiology,* 1790–1855. Cambridge, MA: Harvard University Press, 1984; Vertinsky PA. *The Eternally Wounded Woman: Women, Exercise, and Doctors in the Late Nineteenth Century.* Urbana: University of Illinois Press; Walker K. *The Story of Medicine.* London: Arrow Books, 1954.

Gustav Embden in 1933; together they discovered the pathway that converts glucose to lactic acid (the Embden-Meyerhof pathway).

Nathan Zuntz (1847–1920). Devised the first portable metabolic apparatus to assess respiratory exchange in animals and humans at different altitudes; proved that carbohydrates were precursors for lipid synthesis. He maintained that dietary lipids and carbohydrates should not be consumed equally for proper nutrition. He 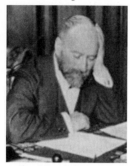 produced 430 articles concerning blood and blood gases, circulation, mechanics and chemistry of respiration, general metabolism and metabolism of specific foods, energy metabolism and heat production, and digestion.

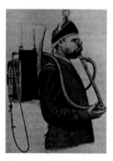

Zuntz tests his portable, closed-circuit spirometer carried on his back. This device made it possible for the first time to measure O_2 consumed and CO_2 produced during ambulation.

Carl von Voit (1831–1908) and his student Max Rubner (1854–1932). Discovered the isodynamic law and the calorific heat values of proteins, lipids, and carbohydrates; Rubner's surface area law states 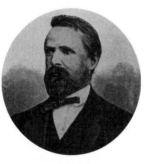 that resting heat production is proportional to body surface area and that consuming food increases heat production. Voit disproved Liebig's assertion that protein was a primary energy fuel by showing that protein breakdown does not increase in proportion to exercise duration or intensity.

Max Joseph von Pettenkofer (1818–1901). Perfected the respiration calorimeter to study human and animal metabolism; discovered creatinine, an amino acid in urine. The top chamber of the figure below shows the entire calorimeter. The cut-away image shows a human experiment where fresh air was pumped into the sealed chamber and vented air sampled for carbon dioxide.

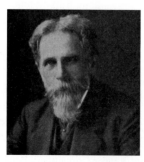

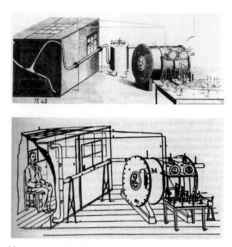

Human respiration calorimeter.

Eduard F. W. Pflüger (1829–1910). First demonstrated that minute changes in the partial pressure of blood gases affect the rate of oxygen release across capillary membranes, thus proving that blood flow alone does not govern how tissues receive oxygen.

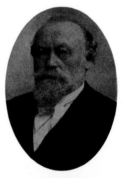

Wilbur Atwater (1844–1907). Published data about the chemical composition of 2600 American foods currently used in databases of food composition (www.sportsci.org/news/history/atwater/atwater.html). 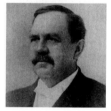 Also performed human calorimetric experiments and confirmed that the law of conservation of energy governs transformation of matter in the human body.

Russel Henry Chittenden (1856–1943). Refocused attention on the minimal protein requirement of humans while resting or exercising; concluded that no debilitation occurred if protein intake equaled $1.0 \, g \cdot kg$ body mass^{-1} in either normal or athletic young men (www.sportsci. 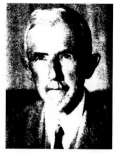 org/news/history/chittenden/chittenden.html). Chittenden received the first PhD in physiological chemistry given by an American University. Some scholars[10] regard Chittenden as the father of biochemistry in the United States—he believed that physiological chemistry would provide basic tools for researchers to study important aspects of physiology and provided the impetus for incorporating biochemical analyses in exercise physiology.

Frederick Gowland Hopkins (1861–1947: www.sportsci.org/news/history/hopkins/hopkins.html). Nobel Prize in 1929 for isolating and identifying the structure of the amino acid tryptophan. Hopkins collaborated with W. M. Fletcher (mentor to A. V. Hill) to study muscle chemistry. Their classic

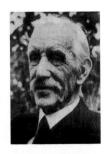

1907 paper in experimental physiology used new methods to isolate lactic acid in muscle. Fletcher and Hopkins' chemical methods reduced the muscle's enzyme activity prior to analysis to isolate the reactions. They found that a muscle contracting under low oxygen conditions produced lactate at the expense of glycogen. Conversely, oxygen in muscle suppressed lactate formation. The researchers deduced that lactate forms from a nonoxidative (anaerobic) process during contraction; during recovery in a noncontracted state, an oxidative (aerobic) process removes lactate with oxygen present.

Francis Gano Benedict (1870–1957). Conducted exhaustive studies of energy metabolism in newborn infants, growing children and adolescents, starving persons, athletes, and vegetarians (www.sportsci.org/news/history/benedict/benedict.html).

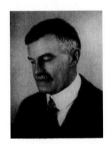

Devised "metabolic standard tables" based on sex, age, height, and weight to compare energy metabolism in normals and patients. His last monograph, "Vital Energetics, A Study in Comparative Basal Metabolism" (*Carnegie Institution Monograph* no. 503, 1938), refers to many of his approximately 400 publications.

CONTRIBUTIONS OF WOMEN TO SCIENCE AT THE DAWN OF THE 20TH CENTURY

The triumphs and accomplishments during the evolution of exercise physiology reveal a glaring absence of credit to the contributions of women from the 1850s and continuing for the next 100 years. Many reasons can explain this occurrence—but it was not from women's lack of interest in pursuing a career in the sciences. Rather, females who wished to stand with male colleagues found the going difficult. Opposition included hostility, ridicule, and professional discrimination, typically in chemistry, physics, and medicine, but also in related fields such as botany, biology, and mathematics. A few women did break through the almost exclusively male-dominated fields to make significant contributions despite such considerable hurdles.

The leadership at the "top" of the scientific culture (college presidents, academic deans, curriculum and personnel committees, governing bodies, heads of departments, and review boards for grants and journals) subtly and directly repressed women's attempts to even enter some fields, let alone achieve parity with male scientists. Subtle discrimination included assignment to underequipped, understaffed, and substandard laboratory facilities; having to teach courses without proper university recognition; disallowing membership on graduate thesis or dissertation committees; and having a male colleague's name appear first (or only) on research publications, regardless of his involvement. Male "supervisors" typically presented the results of joint work at conferences and seminars when the woman clearly worked as the lead scientist. Direct suppression included outright refusal to hire women to teach at the university or college level. For those who were hired, many could not directly supervise graduate student research projects. Women also routinely experienced shameful inequity in salary received or were paid no salary as "assistants."

The Nobel Prize in the sciences, the most prestigious award for discoveries in physics, chemistry, and physiology or medicine, has honored 300 men but only 10 women since the award originated in 1901. The Karolinska Institute in Stockholm selects the Nobel laureates in physiology or medicine, and the Swedish Academy of Sciences awards the prizes in chemistry and physics. Considerable controversy has emerged over the years about the role of "in-fighting and politics" in the selection process. The difference in the gender-specific pool of outstanding scientists cannot adequately explain the disparity between male and female Nobel winners. However, reading about the lives and times of the 10 female winners, including others who by all accounts probably deserved the honor, gives a better appreciation for the inequity. Each of the 10 female laureates and the other 3 world-class scientists we chronicle in TABLE 8 overcame huge "nonscientific" issues before achieving their eventual scientific triumphs.

In a way, some of the same problems faced by women in academia and the private sector over the years help to explain the relatively slow ascendance of women to positions of prominence during the first 100 years of modern exercise physiology. A salient example comes from reviewing the historical record of the ACSM from its inception on January 8, 1955, to the present. Of the 11 founders, one was a woman (Josephine L. Rathbone, PhD, specialist in physical education and rehabilitation). Eighteen months later, three other women joined Dr. Rathbone (Dorothy Ainsworth, PhD, from Smith College, MA; Anna Espenshare, PhD, from UC Berkeley; and Clair Langdon, EdD, from Oregon State College) as part of the 54 original Charter ACSM members.

From ACSM's founding, it would take 33 years before a woman was elected the organization's president. Barbara L. Drinkwater, PhD, from the Institute of Environmental Stress at UC Santa Barbara, became ACSM's first woman president (see "Interview with Barbara L. Drinkwater" in Section 5). Dr. Drinkwater was followed in 1997 to 1998 by Charlotte A. "Toby" Tate, PhD, Dean of the College of Health and Human

TABLE 8 ■ SCIENTIFIC CONTRIBUTIONS OF THIRTEEN OUTSTANDING FEMALE SCIENTISTS

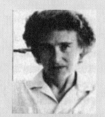

Gerty Radnitz Cori
(1896–1954)

Gerty Cori, with her husband, received international recognition for discovering how glucose converts to glycogen (Cori cycle). This husband and wife team won the 1947 Nobel Prize in physiology or medicine for "discovering the course of the catalytic conversion of glycogen" (mechanism for blood glucose regulation). Cori's later studies on enzymes and hormones advanced research in diabetes treatment, contributing new understandings that missing enzymes resulted from defective genes. This laid the foundation for future studies of genetic defects in humans. Her research profoundly affected diabetes treatment, allowing physicians to understand how the body stores glucose by converting it predominantly into glycogen, which the body then uses for energy. Despite her significant research, she fought discrimination and nepotism within the scientific community. In 1947, the same year she became the first American woman and the third worldwide to receive a Nobel Prize in the sciences, she achieved full professor status in biochemistry at Washington University, St. Louis. In 1950, President Harry Truman appointed her to the Board of Directors of the National Science Foundation.

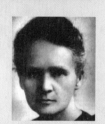

Marie Sklodowska Curie
(1867–1934)

Considered the most famous of all women scientists, this Polish researcher "extraordinaire" was the first person (male or female) to win two Nobel Prizes. At age 16, she had already won a gold medal at the Russian lycée in Poland upon completion of her secondary education. In 1891, almost penniless, she began her education at the Sorbonne in Paris and later became the first woman professor to teach there. Marie Curie (with her husband Pierre) discovered that the source of natural radioactivity did not result from a chemical reaction but rather from a property of the element's specific atoms. This led to the discovery in 1898 of two highly radioactive elements, radium and polonium, for which they were awarded the 1903 Nobel Prize in physics. Madame Curie continued her work on radioactive elements and again won the Nobel Prize in chemistry in 1911 for isolating radium and studying its chemical properties. In 1914, she helped found the Radium Institute in Paris and was the Institute's first director. When World War I broke out, Madame Curie believed that x-rays would help to locate metal fragments and bullets and facilitate surgery. It was also important not to move the wounded, so she invented mobile x-ray vans and trained female attendants. Curie died of leukemia, presumably from extensive exposure to high radiation levels in her research. After her death, the Radium Institute was renamed the Curie Institute in her honor.

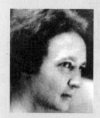

Irene Joliot-Curie
(1897–1956)

Daughter of Marie Curie, Irene continued her mother's work in radioactivity with her husband Frédéric (1900–1958). In 1933, they made the important discovery that radioactive elements can be artificially prepared from stable elements. Their experiments bombarded boron with alpha particles, creating an "artificially" radioactive element, an isotope of nitrogen. The Joliot-Curies were awarded the 1935 Nobel Prize in chemistry "for their synthesis of new radioactive elements." In later years, they extended their work to identifying products of nuclear fission. Although Joliot-Curie won many awards for contributions to science, the French Academy of Science never admitted her to membership. In 1911, the Institute de France voted to maintain its all-male status, a policy maintained for the next 40 years, even denying Curie membership after she died in 1956. A social activist who lobbied hard for gender equality, Joliet-Curie planned a fund-raising tour of the United States. Even with a valid visa, she was denied entry and kept in a detention center until the French Embassy in Washington intervened.

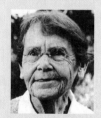

Barbara McClintock
(1902–1992)

America's most distinguished cytogeneticist, McClintock studied genetic mutations by examining changes in the color and texture of kernels and leaf pigments of growing plants. In 1951, McClintock first reported that genetic information could transpose from one chromosome to another. Other scientists didn't believe this unorthodox view of genes, assuming instead that genes remained in place in the chromosome like a necklace of beads. By the early 1970s, scientists finally acknowledged McClintock's view of gene transpositions. Her prodigious research accomplishments clarified our understanding of human disease. The concept of "jumping genes" helped to explain how bacteria develop antibiotic resistance and provided insight as to how these genes play a role in transforming normal cells to cancerous ones. By the late 1970s, her work with transposable elements (i.e., that mobile genetic elements play important roles in inherited birth defects, resistance to antibiotics, and incidence of cancer) became recognized by the scientific–medical community. During 1980 and 1981, McClintock received eight major awards including the Albert Lasker Basic Medical Research Award, Israel's Wolf Prize in Medicine, and McArthur Foundation Fellowship. In 1983, she was the sole recipient of the Nobel Prize in medicine or physiology. The Nobel Committee called her work "one of the two great discoveries of our times in genetics," the other being the structure of DNA.

continued on page lxv

TABLE 8 ■ *continued*

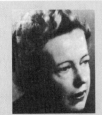

Maria Goeppert Mayer
(1906–1972)

The first American woman and the second woman ever to win the Nobel Prize in physics, Maria Mayer made extensive contributions to several different technical fields in physics. Mayer calculated the probability that an electron orbiting an atom's nucleus would emit not one but two photons (quantum units of light) as it jumps to an orbit closer to the nucleus. Because the Johns Hopkins University had strict nepotism rules that forbade her employment (her husband had been hired), she worked without pay or formal academic status. She produced 10 papers in 9 years applying quantum mechanics to chemistry. She and her husband coauthored *Statistical Mechanics,* a textbook in print for over four decades. At the University of Chicago, Mayer worked part time, supported by a federal grant as senior physicist at the Argonne National Laboratory. There she began her eventual Nobel Prize-winning project elucidating the basic shell model of an atom's nucleus. In 1956, Mayer was elected to the National Academy of Sciences. In 1959, at age 53, after a 30-year career, she was finally appointed full time professor (with pay), at the University of California, San Diego. In 1963, she received the Nobel Prize in physics for her pioneering research.

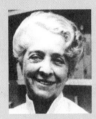

Rita Levi-Montalcini
(1909–)

Rita Levi-Montalcini's first studies between 1938 and 1944 investigated the mechanisms controlling vertebrate nervous system development. In 1952, she showed that when tumors from mice were transplanted to chick embryos, they induced potent growth of the embryo's nervous system, specifically the sensory and sympathetic neurons. Since this outgrowth did not require direct contact between tumor and embryo, Levi-Montalcini concluded that the tumor released a nerve growth-promoting factor (NGF) that selectively acted on specific neurons. Following this discovery, Levi-Montalcini focused on a more sensitive cell culture model to measure NGF activity in various extracts. NGF proved to be an extremely potent biologic substance in that a sensory or sympathetic nerve cell reacted within 30 seconds to minute quantities of NGF. More specifically, one-billionth of a gram of NGF per milliliter of culture medium exerted a powerful effect on growth. The biologic assay to detect NGF paved the way for the next step of discovery—identification of the active nerve growth-promoting substance. The discovery of NGF opened new fields related to pathology such as developmental malformations, degenerative changes in senile dementia, delayed wound healing, and tumor diseases. Levi-Montalcini received the 1986 Nobel Prize in medicine or physiology (with Stanley Cohen) for their discovery of NGF. From 1993 to 1998, she served as President of the Institute of the Italian Encyclopedia. She is a member of prestigious scientific academies: Accademia Nazionale dei Lincei, Pontifical Academy, Accademia delle Scienze detta dei XL, U.S. National Academy of Sciences, and the Royal Society.

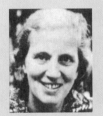

Dorothy Crowfoot Hodgkin
(1910–1994)

Applying her expertise as an x-ray crystallographer, Dorothy Hodgkin developed the analytical methods to identify the structures of penicillin (previously discovered in 1929): cholesteryl iodide (cholesterol), vitamin B_{12} (used to treat pernicious anemia), vitamin B_{12} coenzyme, and the protein hormone insulin. Hodgkin studied more than 100 steroid crystals, reporting on their unit-cell dimensions and refractive indices relative to their crystallographic axes. Her monumental studies of crystalline steroids showed their probable crystal packing and hydrogen-bonding arrangements. Her later studies involved three-dimensional calculations and established the relative stereochemistry at each carbon atom of the steroids. Hodgkin took the first x-ray diffraction photographs of insulin in 1935 and ultimately resolved this crystal's full structure 34 years later. Hodgkin and colleagues reported the structure of insulin in August 1969. She singly won the 1964 Nobel Prize in chemistry "for her determination by x-ray techniques of the structures of biologically important molecules." In addition to pioneering work in chemistry, she applied computer algorithms to help unravel insulin's complex structure.

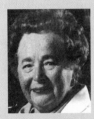

Gertrude B. Elion
(1918–1999)

In 1944, with a master's degree in chemistry, Burroughs-Wellcome (now Glaxo-Wellcome) pharmaceutical company hired Gertrude Elion as a $50-a-week research assistant. Prior to that, female scientists had difficulty finding jobs in either academia or the private sector. At Wellcome, however, her strong scientific training paid off. The strategy was to create new medicines by studying the chemical composition of diseased cells. Her research developed acyclovir (Zovirax) for herpes; azathioprine (Imuran) to help prevent rejection of transplanted organs among nonrelated donors and to treat severe rheumatoid arthritis; allopurinol (Zyloprim) for gout; pyriemthamine (Daraprim) for malaria; and trimethoprim (a component of Septra) for bacterial infections. Elion never completed her PhD (she took courses at night, commuting 3 hours round-trip). Eventually she had to quit because she was told the PhD program at Brooklyn's Polytechnic Institute required full-time attendance, and she could not afford to give up her job. Nonetheless, Gertrude Elion received 25 honorary degrees from prestigious universities, including Duke, Columbia, Brown, Michigan, and Rochester Institute of Technology. In 1988, she shared the Nobel Prize in physiology or medicine with George Hitchings (coworker at Glaxo-Wellcome) for "important principles of drug development." After retirement in 1983, she helped to oversee development of AZT as the first drug against HIV, the AIDS virus. Elion is the only woman inducted into the Inventors Hall of Fame. Her 45 drug patents have provided wide-ranging benefits in many areas; for example, a drug that helps the body suppress its immune response to foreign tissue—most important, that of transplanted organs. This drug has thus made relatively routine kidney transplants between nonrelated donors and patients. In addition to the Nobel Prize, Elion received many top awards: 1991 National Medal of Science presented by President George Bush, who said that her work had "transformed the world;" Garvan Medal from the

continued on page lxvi

TABLE 8 ■ *continued*

American Chemical Society; President's Medal from Hunter College; Judd Award from Memorial-Sloan Kettering Institute; Cain Award from the American Association for Cancer Research; Ernst W. Bertner Memorial Award from the M. D. Anderson Cancer Center; City of Medicine Award in Durham, NC; Discoverers Award from the Pharmaceutical Manufacturers Association; Medal of Honor from the American Cancer Society; Ronald H. Brown Innovator Award; and the Lemelson/MIT Lifetime Achievement Award. Elion served as past president of the American Association for Cancer Research, and presidential appointee on the National Cancer Advisory Board. She belonged to the National Academy of Sciences, the Royal Society, the Institute of Medicine, the American Academy of Arts and Sciences, the National Women's Hall of Fame, and the Engineering and Science Hall of Fame.

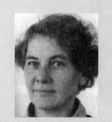

Rosalyn Sussman Yalow
(1921–)

Rosalyn Sussman Yalow was the first American woman to win the Albert Lasker Prize for Medicine (1976) and Nobel Prize for physiology or medicine (1977) for developing radioimmunoassay (RIA). This procedure uses radioactive isotopes to "tag" previously undetected concentrations of hormones, viruses, vitamins, enzymes, and drugs to study disease and biochemical reactions. In essence, RIA provided the technique that unlocked the field of endocrinology. On accepting her Nobel Prize, Yalow spoke about women in science careers: "We must believe in ourselves or no one else will believe in us. We must feel a personal responsibility to ease the path for those who come after us. The world cannot afford the loss of the talents of half its people if we are to solve the many problems that beset us." Yalow holds the title of Distinguished Service Professor from the Mount Sinai School of Medicine. She is a member of the National Academy of Sciences. Honors include Albert Lasker Basic Medical Research Award, A. Cressy Morrison Award in Natural Sciences of the New York Academy of Sciences, Scientific Achievement Award of the American Medical Association, Koch Award of the Endocrine Society, Gairdner Foundation International Award, American College of Physicians Award for distinguished contributions in science related to medicine, Eli Lilly Award of the American Diabetes Association, First William S. Middleton Medical Research Award, and 39 honorary degrees.

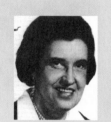

Christiane Nüsslein-Volhard
(1942–)

During the 1970s, developmental biologist Christiane Nüsslein-Volhard's research focused on the genetics of mutated fruit-fly embryos. In 1984, she expanded her research by cataloguing 120 well-defined genes that affected the entire embryonic pattern of the fruit fly's development. She received the 1995 Nobel Prize in medicine or physiology (with colleague Eric Wieschaus) for pioneering molecular biology and genetics studies of specific areas of a gene that contributes to mammalian immune system development. Her discoveries had universal application because the same genetic parts that govern gene activity in different cells also similarly operate in plants and many animal organisms, including humans. Defective parts in genes that modulate early growth and development trigger congenital disorders such as spina bifida and cleft palate in humans. Because genes encoding the same protein affect a variety of conditions (e.g., arteriosclerosis, organ rejection, AIDS, and other maladies), the scope of her discoveries had wide-ranging applications. Her awards include membership in the National Academy of Sciences and Royal Society and honorary degrees from Harvard, Yale, and Princeton.

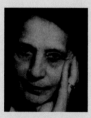

Lise Meitner
(1878–1968)

Lise Meitner was the first woman to earn a doctoral degree in physics at the University of Vienna in 1906, which had previously awarded only 14 doctorates to women in the prior 541 years. Meitner worked at the Kaiser-Wilhelm Institute with radiochemist Otto Hahn (eventual Nobel Prize winner). They discovered the 91st element, *protactinium,* and studied neutron bombardment of uranium. Meitner became joint director of the Institute and head of the Physics Department in 1917. After fleeing Nazi Germany in 1938, she worked at the Nobel Physical Institute in Stockholm, continuing her research with nephew Otto Frisch. Meitner predicted that the atom's nucleus captures neutrons, causing enough instability to pinch it in two, much like a water droplet splitting into two parts. According to Einstein's equation $E = mc^2$, an observed loss of mass must unleash energy. Meitner, combining Bohr's liquid-drop model of the nucleus and Einstein's equation, predicted that a proposed experiment by Hahn should yield barium, krypton, and energy. Within days, she and Frisch worked out a theoretical model for nuclear fission. Frisch, hastily working in Bohr's institute in Copenhagen to test Meitner's expectations, quickly verified the theory. The Meitner-Frisch paper introducing nuclear fission appeared in early 1939. Their momentous discovery (they had split the uranium nucleus) was termed "fission" and predicted the existence of the chain reaction that contributed to the development of the atomic bomb.

During World War II, Meitner refused to work on the atomic bomb. In 1947, the Swedish Atomic Energy Commission established a laboratory where she continued to work on an experimental nuclear reactor. She received the Max Planck Medal, the Leibnitz Medal, and in 1966 she shared the Fermi Award. In 1946, Otto Hahn received the Nobel Prize for his work on fission. Interestingly, he failed to acknowledge that Mietner's ideas had stimulated his research—contributions that many in science believed were considerable. Though denied the Nobel Prize, an international commission in 1994 named element 109, artificially created by slamming bismuth with iron ions, meitnerium.

continued on page lxvii

TABLE 8 ■ *continued*

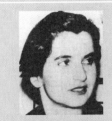

Rosalind Franklin
(1920–1958)

A graduate of Cambridge University who specialized in chemistry, Franklin's expertise focused on understanding the chemical (atomic) structure of complex organic compounds. She perfected the technique of x-ray crystallography that locates atoms in any crystal by precisely mapping the image of the crystal under an x-ray beam. Using an extremely fine beam of x-rays, Franklin produced high-resolution photographs of single DNA fibers. These fibers, finer than ever seen before, were then arranged in parallel bundles. Her results showed that DNA's sugar-phosphate backbone lies on its outside; in essence, she elucidated the basic helical structure of the molecule. Unfortunately, Franklin's notes and photographs about the discovery were made available (without her permission) to Watson and Crick at Cambridge University, who were rushing to determine DNA's final structure. Within days, Watson and Crick applied Franklin's data to complete their own detailed and ultimately correct description of DNA's structure. The strained relationship with her immediate supervisor (Maurice Wilkins) and other aspects about King's College where she worked (women scientists were forbidden to eat lunch in the common room with men) led Franklin to seek employment elsewhere. She turned her attention to tobacco mosaic viruses, publishing 17 papers in 5 years—a body of knowledge that formed the basis for structural virology. Franklin began work on the polio virus before succumbing to ovarian cancer in 1958. Ten years after deciphering the double-helix structure (and following Franklin's death), Watson, Crick, and Wilkins received the Nobel Prize in physiology or medicine, thus forever denying Franklin formal credit she richly deserved for her crucial discovery of DNA's helical structure.

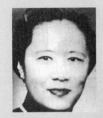

Wu-Chien-Shiung Wu
(1912–1997)

A pioneering physicist, Wu radically altered modern physical theory by changing the accepted view of the structure of the universe. Her experiments helped to demolish a proposed "law" of nature concerning the conservation of parity. Wu was the first woman to receive the prestigious Research Corporation Award and the Comstock Prize—given once every 5 years from the National Academy of Sciences—for her contributions to atomic research (understanding of beta decay and the weak interactions) on the Manhattan Project. Wu became the first woman to receive an honorary Doctorate of Science from Princeton University (and 10 other doctorates, including ones from Harvard and Yale), was elected first woman president of the American Physical Society, received the first Wolf Prize from the State of Israel, was awarded a full-professorship and endowed chair (Pupin Professor of Physics) at Columbia University, became the seventh woman elected to the National Academy of Sciences, and was awarded the National Medal of Science prize, the nation's highest science award. And complementing her accomplishments, she was the first living scientist to have an asteroid named after her.

Development Sciences at the University of Illinois at Chicago; in 1999 to 2000 by Priscilla M. Clarkson, PhD, Associate Dean of the School of Public Health and Heath Sciences at the University of Massachusetts at Amherst; and in 2000 to 2001 by Angela D. Smith, MD, Philadelphia's Children's Hospital Sports Medicine & Performance Center. From 1955 to 1980, only Drs. Rathbone and Drinkwater served as officers of the College (as vice presidents); from 1981 to 1992, three additional women achieved elective office (Christine Wells, PhD, Arizona State University; Betty Atwater, PhD, University of Arizona; Mona Shangold, MD, Georgetown Medical Center). Since 2000, five women have served as vice presidents: Janet Walberg Rankin (2000–2002) Connie Lebrun (2001–2003), Susan Hall (2002–2004) Linda Pescatello (2003–2005) and Milinda Millard Stafford (2005–2007). Until 1996, no woman received the prestigious ACSM Honor Award, delivered the Wolffe Memorial Lecture, or won a New Investigator or Scholar Award. The 1996 Honor Award winner was Barbara Drinkwater; nine years later, Priscilla M. Clarkson was the 2005 Honor Award recipient. Between 1955 and 2004, women received ACSM's Citation Award (Francis Hellebrandt, 1966; Josephine L. Rathbone, 1974; Barbara L. Drinkwater, 1984; Christine Wells, 1995; Emily M. Haymes, 1996; Priscilla M. Clarkson, 1997; and Charlotte A. Tate, 2000).

The ACSM has bestowed other honors on outstanding female scholars; Barbara Drinkwater (1994) and Nanette Wenger (2001) delivered the Joseph B. Wolffe Memorial Lecture at the national ACSM meeting, Gretchen Von Loewe Kreuter (1992), Roberta J. Park (1995), Jan Todd (1998), and Maria T.E. Hopman (2005), have given the ACSM D. B. Dill Historical Lecture at the national ACSM meeting. In addition to the four female ACSM presidents, many women currently hold key positions as deans, associate deans, chairs of departments of exercise science and kinesiology, principal investigators on major research grants, and directors of exercise physiology laboratories.

We hope the legacy of the 13 women we profile in Table 8 inspires students to strive for excellence in their particular specialty related to exercise physiology. Each scientist surmounted many obstacles in her path to achieve success and recognition. They all shared common traits—an unyielding passion for science and uncompromising quest to explore new ground where others had not ventured. As you progress in your own careers, we hope that you too will experience the pure joy of discovering new truths in exercise physiology. Perhaps the achievements of the 13 women scientists from outside our field will serve as a gentle reminder to support the next generation of scientists from their accomplishments and passion for the field.

SUMMARY

This introductory section on the historical development of exercise physiology illustrates that interest in exercise and health had its roots with the ancients. During the next 2000 years, the field we now call exercise physiology evolved from a symbiotic (albeit, sometimes rocky) relationship between the classically trained physicians, the academically based anatomists and physiologists, and a small cadre of physical educators who struggled to achieve their identity and academic credibility through research and experimentation in the basic and applied sciences. The physiologists used exercise to study the dynamics of human physiology, and the early physical educators often adapted the methodology and knowledge of physiology to study human responses to exercise.

Beginning in the mid-1850s in the United States, there was a small but slowly growing effort to raise standards for the scientific training of physical education and hygiene specialists who were primarily involved in teaching at the college and university level. The creation of the first exercise physiology laboratory at Harvard University in 1891 contributed to an already burgeoning knowledge explosion in basic physiology. Originally, medically trained physiologists made the significant scientific advances in most of the subspecialties now included in the exercise physiology course curriculum. They studied oxygen metabolism, muscle structure and function, gas transport and exchange, mechanisms of circulatory dynamics, and neural control of voluntary and involuntary muscular activity.

The field of exercise physiology also owes a debt of gratitude to the pioneers of the physical fitness movement in the United States, notably Thomas K. Cureton (1901–1993; ACSM charter member, 1969 ACSM Honor Award) at the University of Illinois, Champaign—a prolific, insightful researcher who trained four generations of physical educators beginning in 1941. Many of these pioneers assumed leadership positions as professors with teaching and research responsibilities in exercise physiology at numerous colleges and universities in the United States and throughout the world.

Although we have focused on the contributions of selected early American scientists and physical educators and their counterparts from the Nordic countries to the development of modern-day exercise physiology, we would be neglectful not to acknowledge the numerous contributions from many scholars in other countries. The group of foreign contributors, many still active, includes but certainly is not limited to the following individuals: Roy Shephard, School of Physical and Health Education, University of Toronto (ACSM Citation Award, 1991; ACSM Honor Award, 2001); Claude Bouchard, Pennington Biomedical Research Center, Baton Rouge, LA (ACSM Citation Award, 1992; ACSM Honor Award, 2002); Oded Bar-Or, McMaster University, Hamilton, Ontario, Canada (ACSM 1997 Citation Award; ACSM President's Lecture); Rodolfo Margaria and P. Cerretelli, Institute of Human Physiology, Medical School of the University of Milan; M. Ikai, School of Education, University of Japan; Wildor Holloman, Director of the Institute for Circulation, Research and Sports Medicine, and L. Brauer and H. W. Knipping, Institute of Medicine, University of Cologne, Germany (in 1929, they described the "vita maxima" now called the maximal oxygen consumption); L. G. C. E. Pugh, Medical Research Council Laboratories, London; Z. I. Barbashova, Sechenov Institute of Evolutionary Physiology, Leningrad, U.S.S.R.; Sir Cedric Stanton Hicks, Human Physiology Department, University of Adelaide, Australia; Otto Gustaf Edholm, National Institute for Medical Research, London, England; John Valentine George Andrew Durnin, Department of Physiology, Glasgow University, Scotland; Reginald Passmore, Department of Physiology, University of Edinburgh, Scotland; Ernst F. Jokl (ACSM founder and charter member), Witwatersrand Technical College, Johannesburg, South Africa, and later the University of Kentucky; C. H. Wyndham and N. B. Strydom, University of the Witwatersrand, South Africa. There were also many early German scientific contributions to exercise physiology and sports medicine.[32]

CONCLUDING COMMENT

One theme unites the history of exercise physiology: the value of mentoring by those visionaries who spent an extraordinary amount of their careers "infecting" students with love for hard science. These demanding but inspiring relationships developed researchers who, in turn, nurtured the next generation of productive scholars. This applies not only to the current group of exercise physiologists, but also to scholars of previous generations. Siegel[57] cites Payne,[50] who in 1896 wrote the following about Harvey's 1616 discovery of the mechanism of the circulation, acknowledging the discoveries of the past:

> No kind of knowledge has ever sprung into being without an antecedent, but is inseparably connected with what was known before. . . . We are led back to Aristotle and Galen as the real predecessors of Harvey in his work concerning the heart. It was the labors of the great school of Greek anatomists. . . . that the problem though unsolved, was put in such a shape that the genius of Harvey was enabled to solve it. . . . The moral is, I think, that the influence of the past on the present is even more potent than we commonly suppose. In common and trivial things, we may ignore this connection; in what is of enduring worth we cannot.

We end our overview of the history of exercise physiology with a passage from an American physiology and hygiene textbook written more than 137 years ago by J. C. Dalton, MD, a professor of physiology in the College of Physicians and Surgeons in New York City. It shows how current themes in exercise physiology share a common bond with what was known and advocated at that time (the benefits of moderate physical activity, walking as an excellent exercise, the appropriate exercise intensity, the specificity of training, the importance of mental well-being). Even the "new" thoughts and ideas of Dalton penned in 1869 had their roots in antiquity—reinforcing to us the importance of maintaining a healthy respect for the past.

Exercise. The natural force of the muscular system requires to be maintained by constant and regular Exercise. If all of the muscles, or those of any particular part, be allowed to remain for a long time unused they diminish in size, grow softer, and finally become sluggish and debilitated. By use and exercise, on the contrary, they maintain their vigor, continue plump and firm to the touch, and retain all the characters of their healthy organization. It is very important, therefore, that the muscles should be trained and exercised by sufficient daily use. Too much confinement by sedentary occupation, in study, or by simple indulgence in indolent habits, will certainly impair the strength of the body and injuriously affect the health. Every one who is in a healthy condition should provide for the free use of the muscles by at least two hours' exercise each day; and this exercise can not be neglected with impunity, any more than the due provision of clothing and food.

The muscular exercise of the body, in order to produce its proper effect, should be regular and moderate in degree. It will not do for any person to remain inactive during the greater part of the week, and then take an excessive amount of exercise on a single day. An unnatural deficiency of this kind cannot be compensated by an occasional excess. It is only a uniform and healthy action of the parts that stimulates the muscles and provides for their nourishment and growth. Exercise that is so violent and long-continued as to produce exhaustion or unnatural fatigue is an injury instead of an advantage, and creates a waste and expenditure of the muscular force instead of its healthy increase.

Walking is therefore one of the most useful kinds of exercise, since it calls into easy and moderate action nearly all the muscles of the body, and may be continued for a long time without fatigue. Riding on horseback is also exceedingly efficacious, particularly as it is accompanied by a certain amount of excitement and interest that acts as an agreeable and healthy stimulus to the nervous system. Running and leaping, being more violent should be used more sparingly. For children, the rapid and continuous exercise that they spontaneously take in their various games and amusements in the open air is the best. The exact quantity of exercise to be taken is not precisely the same for different persons, but should be measured by its effect. It is always beneficial when it has fully employed the muscular powers without producing any sense of excessive fatigue or exhaustion.

In all cases, also, the exercise that is taken should be regular and uniform in degree, and should be repeated as nearly as possible for the same time every day.

As a student of Exercise Physiology, you are about to embark on an exciting journey into the world of human physiologic response and adaptation to physical activity. We hope our tour of the beginnings of exercise physiology inspires you in your studies to begin your own journey to new discoveries.

References are available on the Student CD and online at http://connection.lww.com/mkk6e.

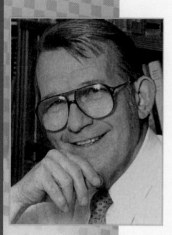

Interview *with* **Dr. Tipton**

Education: BA (Springfield College in Springfield, MA); MA, PhD in Physiology, with minors in Biochemistry and Anatomy (University of Illinois, Champaign, IL).

Current Affiliation: Professor Emeritus of Physiology and Surgery at the College of Medicine at the University of Arizona.

Honors and Awards: See Appendix E, which is available on the Student CD and online at http://connection.lww.com/mkk6e.

Research Focus: The physiologic effects of short- and long-term exercise and their responsible mechanisms.

Memorable Publication: Tipton CM, et al. The influence of exercise, intensity, age, and medication on resting systolic blood pressure of SHR populations. J Appl Physiol 1983;55:1305.

Statement of Contributions: ACSM Honor Award
Dr. Tipton is well known for his contributions as an investigator in exercise physiology, his educational vision in establishing the "gold standard" for graduate training in the exercise sciences, and his leadership and driving energy. For almost 25 years, Professor Tipton has excelled as an investigator by using animal models to study the acute and chronic effects of exercise on connective tissue, hormones, metabolism, and the cardiovascular system. This broad scope of knowledge has enabled him to build a graduate training program with an international reputation that has produced researchers and educators who have subsequently achieved prominence in the exercise sciences.

What first inspired you to enter the exercise science field? What made you decide to pursue your degree and/or line of research?

■ My experiences in athletics and as a Physical Fitness Instructor in an infantry division convinced me that I should secure an education on the G.I. Bill of Rights to be able to teach health and physical education while coaching in a rural high school. Once I realized that I did not enjoy my chosen career, I returned to the University of Illinois for more education in health education. To support a growing family, I secured a summer and part-time position as a 4-H Club Fitness Specialist who conducted fitness tests and clinics through the state of Illinois. When it became apparent that I had to have more physiology and biochemistry to explain what I was testing and advocating, I knew I had to be a physiologist with an expertise in exercise physiology. So I

transferred to the Physiology Department, and the rest is history.

What influences did your undergraduate education have on your final career choice?

■ Very little. Although I had the late Peter V. Karpovich as my exercise physiology instructor at Springfield College, he did not stimulate, motivate, or encourage me to become one. My mind set was to teach and coach in a rural high school, and everything in the undergraduate curriculum or experience was to help me achieve that goal.

Who were the most influential people in your career, and why?

■ The drive to learn and acquire more education was imprinted by my father, who had to leave school in the eighth grade to help support the family. Early in graduate school at the University of Illinois, I became interested in the physiological and biochemical foundations of physical fitness by the interesting and evangelical lectures of Thomas K. Cureton of the Physical Education Department However, my interest in physiological research and its scientific foundations was stimulated, developed, and perfected by Darl M. Hall, who was a critical and caring research scientist in the Illinois Extension Service who had the responsibility of testing the fitness levels of 4-H Club members. He made me recognize that functional explanations require in-depth scientific knowledge and encouraged me to transfer into the physiology department to secure such information. Once in physiology, I became exposed to the unique scholarship of Robert E. Johnson and to his example of the scientific attributes necessary to become a productive exercise physiologist. Inherent in this profile of recognition is the fact that without the love and support of my wife, Betty, and our four children, my transition to the various departments — and survival of a poverty state — would have never occurred.

What has been the most interesting/enjoyable aspect of your involvement in science? What was the least interesting/enjoyable aspect

■ To me, the most interesting and stimulating aspect of exercise physiology was the planning, testing and evaluation of one's hypotheses. The least enjoyable were the administrative aspects of supervising a laboratory and in the conduct of research.

What is your most meaningful contribution to the field of exercise science, and why is it so important?

■ Exercise science evolved from the discipline of physical education and includes exercise physiology. My most meaningful contribution to the field was the planning and implementation of a rigorous, science-based Ph.D. graduate program in exercise physiology at the University of Iowa, which served as a model for other departments of physical education to follow. It was important to me because it attracted many outstanding individuals to the University of Iowa who became dear friends and help paved the way for exercise science to become an academic entity.

What advice would you give to students who express an interest in pursuing a career in exercise science research?

■ Research requires more than intellectual curiosity and infectious enthusiasm. It is an exciting occupation that demands hard work, while requiring an individual to be disciplined, dedicated, and honest. A future researcher must acquire an education that enables him/her to be well prepared in mathematics, the biological and physical sciences, and the ability to communicate by written and verbal means. Lastly, seek a mentor whose research interests you and one who is concerned about you as a future researcher and not as a contributor to their vitae.

What interests have you pursued outside of your professional career?

■ Becoming a civil war "buff," enjoying the pleasures of dancing and listening to Dixieland jazz, exercising regularly, participating in road races, reading nonfiction, learning about

poetry, being a member of a book club, watching televised sports, cheering for the Washington Redskins football team, and observing our grandchildren as they grow up.

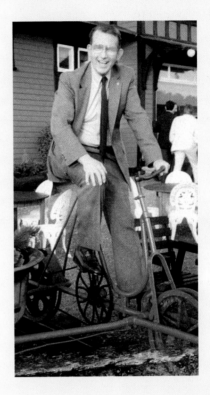

Where do you see the exercise science field (particularly your area of greatest interest) heading in the next 20 years?

■ It is my speculation that during the next 20 years exercise physiologists will be emphasizing and investigating molecular mechanisms in all of the known systems. Since the genome will have been characterized during this interval, exercise physiology genomics will have become a well-defined subdiscipline, and countless studies will be under way to determine the interactions between the genome and the exercise response in normal and diseased populations.

You have the opportunity to give a "last lecture." Describe its primary focus.

■ It would be entitled "Exercise Physiology in the Last Frontier," and would pertain to what is known and unknown about exercising in a microgravity environment.

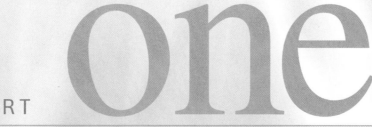

PART **ONE**

Exercise Physiology

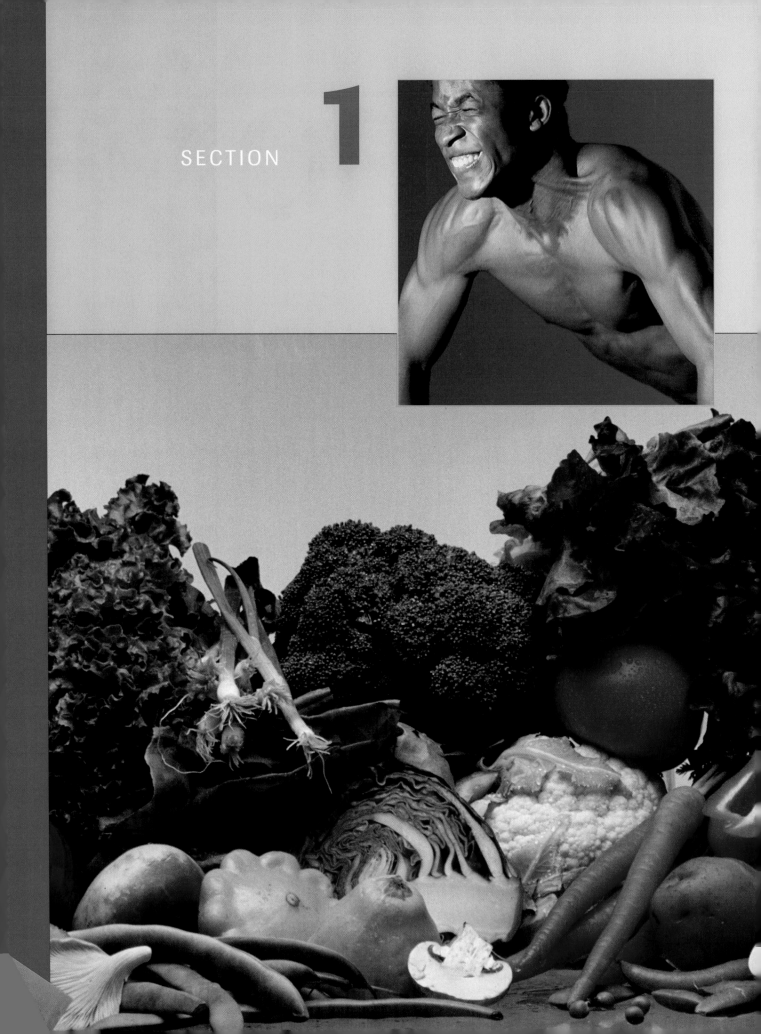

SECTION 1

Nutrition: The Base for Human Performance

OVERVIEW

Nutrition and exercise physiology share a natural linkage. Proper nutrition forms the foundation for physical performance; it provides fuel for biologic work and chemicals for extracting and using the potential energy within this fuel. Nutrients from food also furnish essential elements for repairing existing cells and synthesizing new tissues.

Some may argue that a well-balanced diet readily provides adequate nutrients for exercise, so in-depth nutrition knowledge offers little value to exercise physiologists. We maintain, however, that the study of exercise, viewed within the framework of energy capacities and performance, must include an understanding of energy sources and the role diverse nutrients play in energy release and transfer. With this perspective, the exercise specialist critically evaluates claims about special nutritional supplements, including dietary modifications to enhance physical performance. Because nutrients provide energy and regulate physiologic processes in exercise, improved athletic performance often links with dietary modification. Too often, individuals devote considerable time and effort striving to optimize exercise performance, only to fall short because of inadequate, counterproductive, and sometimes harmful nutritional practices. Finally, food nutrients affect diseases for which regular exercise makes important, protective contributions. The three chapters that follow present the six broad categories of nutrients—carbohydrates, lipids, proteins, vitamins, minerals, and water—and explore the following questions: What are they? Where are they found? What are their functions? What is their specific role in physical activity? We also discuss optimal nutrition for exercise and training.

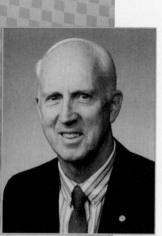

Interview *with* Dr. David L. Costill

Education: BS (Ohio University, Athens, OH); MEd (Miami University, Oxford, OH); PhD (Physiology, Ohio State University, Columbus, OH)

Current Affiliation: Professor Emeritus, John and Janice Fisher Chair in Exercise Science. Ball State University

Honors and Awards: See Appendix E, which is available on the Student CD and online at http://connection.lww.com/mkk6e.

Research Focus: My research interest was aimed at several areas: body fluid balance, carbohydrate metabolism in human muscle, thermal regulation during exercise, physiologic characteristics of runners and swimmers, aging distance runners, and changes in muscle fiber function during bed rest and space flight.

Memorable Publication: Costill DL, et al. Skeletal muscle enzymes and fiber composition in male and female track athletes. J Appl Physiol 1976;40:149.

Statement of Contributions: ACSM Honor Award
In recognition of his lifetime of distinguished scientific achievement in the applied, basic and clinical aspects of exercise physiology, and sports medicine through his research, teaching, lecturing, mentoring of students and colleagues, and professional leadership.

Professor Costill has been one of the pioneers in researching the areas of human performance and sports nutrition. He provided the scientific community with the first complete assessment of the physiological factors, which determine distance-running perform-ance. His early studies on carbohydrate metabolism and fluid replacement were foundational to under-standing the fuel and fluid needs of the endurance athlete, and have provided the stimulus to what has become one of the most active areas in exercise re-search today. His studies of environmental limitation to endurance performance have contributed greatly to our understanding of how to best prepare individuals to exercise and compete in the heat. His personal in-terest in and dedication to distance running or swim-ming led him to conduct an unprecedented series of studies in both sports. The results of these studies have provided the physiologist, coach, and athlete with better understanding of the physiological basis for these sports.

His most recent research in the area of over-train-ing has made major contributions to the training of elite athletes.

Professor Costill has dedicated considerable time and energy to the education of scientists, clinicians, coaches and athletes, through his professional articles, books, and lecturing. No single scientist has impacted the sports community nationally or internationally more than Professor Costill, due largely to his ability to effectively communicate the results of his research and those of others.

Professor Costill has also had a tremendous im-pact on those who have trained with him as under-graduate students, graduate students, post-doctoral fellows, or visiting colleagues.

Professor Costill's national and international professional leadership is widely acknowledged. He has served the American College of Sports Medicine in many ways, but most importantly as President during a critical time in the growth of the College. He has served as Editor-in-Chief of the International Journal of Sports Medicine.

Professor Costill's unceasing search for new in-sights into the mechanism underlying exercise and sports medicine has received the respect and admira-tion of the international scientific community. His pro-lific career has brought honor to his university, his stu-dents, his colleagues, and the American College of Sports Medicine.

What first inspired you to enter the exercise science field?

■ Growing up in Ohio, I was always interested in biology and physiology, although I never thought of it in those terms. Even as an 8-year-old I needed to know why animals differed and what made them work.

In college, I was more interested in anatomy and physi-ology than in physical education. But I was a poor student who was satisfied with taking all the activities classes and easy grades that I was able to attain. My primary interest was staying eligible for swimming. During my senior year at OSU, I signed up for an independent study and was assigned a research project with 30 rats. The project never amounted to much, but I was left on my own and learned that the research process was challenging.

My first introduction to exercise physiology was as a graduate student at Miami University in Ohio. A faculty member (Fred Zeckman) in the Department of Zoology offered an exercise physiology class to about six students. Again, the class project involved data collection, a process I'd already found interesting. After teaching high school general science and biology for three years, as well as coaching three teams, I decided it was time to see if I could get the credentials to become a coach at a small college. I began working toward a doctorate in higher education. At the same time, I became close friends with Dick Bowers and Ed Fox, fellow graduate students who were majoring in exercise physiology under the direction of Dr. D. K. Mathews. It wasn't long before they persuaded me to switch over to work in the laboratory with them.

What influence did your undergraduate education have on your final career choice?

■ It enabled me to get a degree and a teaching job. It was not until I had been teaching for several years that I identified what I really wanted to do. After one year at OSU, I moved to Cortland (SUNY), where I coached cross-country track and swimming for 2 years. Although I enjoyed coaching, I just couldn't take the recruiting and continual exposure to 18-year-olds. So I decided to focus my energy on research. Exercise physiology gave me a chance to do research in an area that held numerous practical questions. My early studies with runners were a natural, considering the experience I'd had in coaching runners at Cortland. Interestingly, a few of those runners (e.g., Bob Fitts and Bob Gregor) have become well known in the exercise science field.

Who were the most influential people in your career, and why?

■ Dr. Bob Bartels: Bob was my college swimming coach. First, he kept me on the freshman team, even though I was one of the least talented. There were moments during my senior year (as co-captain) when I'm sure he had second thoughts! Bob was also instrumental in getting me admitted to Miami University and OSU. Without his efforts, I'd probably still be teaching junior high science in Ohio.

Dr. David Bruce (D. B.) Dill: I worked with Bruce in the summer of 1968. His words of wisdom and advice headed me in the right direction. Drs. Bengt Saltin and Phil Gollnick: Since I received my PhD after only one year at OSU, I had little research background and no postdoctoral experience. In 1972, I spent 6 months with Bengt and Phil in Bengt's laboratory in Stockholm. I learned a great deal working with them and the "gang" (Jan Karlsson, Björn Ekblom, E. H. Christensen, P. O. Åstrand, and others), which I consider to be my postdoctoral experience.

What has been the most interesting/enjoyable aspect of your involvement in science?

■ Most interesting: Meeting people! The professional contact and friendships I had with other scientists (Charles Tipton, Skip Knuttgen, Jack Wilmore, Lars Hermansen, Harm Kuipers, Mark Hargreaves, Reggie Edgerton, Bill Fink, Clyde Williams, Per Blom, George Sheehan, astronauts from STS-78 flight, and others).

Most enjoyable: Following the success of my former students. Since I was a student with little talent but a good work ethic, I tended to recruit those types as graduate students. They were not always the ones with the high GPAs, but they were motivated and knew how to work. A number of them have become well known in our field, including Bill Evans, Ed Coyle, Mike Sherman, Mark Hargreaves, Bob Fitts, Bob Gregor, Paul Thompson, Carl Foster, Joe Houmard, Rick Sharp, Larry Armstrong, Rob Robergs, John Ivy, Hiro Tanaka, Mike Flynn, Scott and Todd Trappe, Abe Katz, Pete Van Handel, Darrell Neufer, Matt Hickey, and others.

One of the most enjoyable aspects of my research has been the opportunity to work with some very interesting subjects such as Bill Rogers, Steve Prefontaine, Alberto Salazar, Matt Biondi, Derek Clayton, Shella Young, Frank Shorter, Kenny Moore, and Ken Sparks.

What was the least interesting/enjoyable aspect?

■ I have never liked writing books or chasing after grant money, but I knew that was essential to expand the laboratory and upgrade facilities to continue to do research. Also, seeing students with great talent fail to live up to full potential. Not every student achieved the level of success I expected, but their lives were often altered by events outside the laboratory. I always view my students as a part of my family, so when they had troubles and/or were unsuccessful, it was like watching my own kids' struggle.

What advice would you give to students who express an interest in pursuing a career in exercise science research?

■ There are six keys to success as a researcher: (1) Identify a worthy question; (2) Design a protocol that will give you the best possible answer; (3) Make sure the question is fundable, i.e., it must be a problem that an outside source is willing to support financially; (4) Be good at and enjoy collecting data. Precision in the laboratory is essential if you want to generate a clear answer to your question; (5) Be capable of reducing the data to an intelligible form and writing a clear/concise paper that is publishable in a creditable journal; and (6) Be capable of presenting your research at scientific forums, as this helps to establish your scientific creditability.

What interests have you pursued outside of your professional career?

■ Photography (1949–1955): I went to college to study photography (won three national photo contests in HS), but switched to physical education during my sophomore year.

Distance running (1965–1982): I started running for fitness and eventually ran 16 marathons in the late 1970s and early 1980s. Knee injuries forced me back to swimming in 1982. Masters Swimming (1982–present): After training for six months, Doc Counsilman, the famed Indiana University swim coach, talked me into entering a Masters meet, where he promptly beat me in a 500-yard freestyle event. My graduate students Rick Sharp and John Troup convinced me to "shave down" and compete in one more meet. Subsequently, I performed almost as well as I had in college, so I was hooked. At the age of 60 I could still beat my best college times and set six age-group national records.

I have two passions: aviation and auto restoration. I also enjoy fishing, camping, and canoeing. We have a cottage in northern Wisconsin where we spend as much time in the summer as possible. But I always like to come back to the small town of Muncie where there is no traffic, a nice house, good airport, and all the activities of the University.

Where do you see the exercise physiology field heading in the next 20 years?

■ This field has moved from whole body measurements (handgrip and vital capacity) to molecular biology (single muscle fiber physiology). To fully understand the physiology of exercise, the answers lie at the subcellular level. Students need solid training in chemistry and molecular biology in order to contribute to knowledge over the next 20 years.

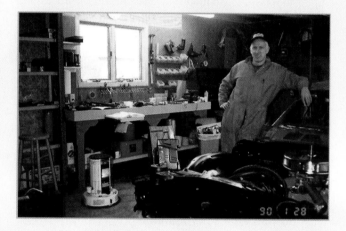

Carbohydrates, Lipids, and Proteins

1

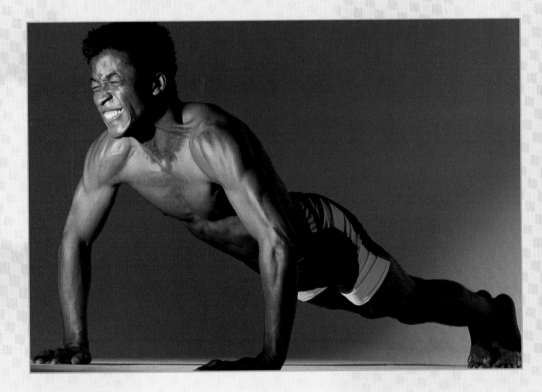

CHAPTER OBJECTIVES

- Distinguish among monosaccharides, disaccharides, and polysaccharides

- Identify the two major classifications of dietary fiber and their roles in overall health

- Discuss physiologic responses to different dietary carbohydrates in the development of type 2 diabetes and obesity

- Quantify the amount, energy content, and distribution of carbohydrate within an average-sized person

- Summarize carbohydrate's role as an energy source, protein sparer, metabolic primer, and central nervous system fuel

- Outline the dynamics of carbohydrate metabolism during physical activity of various intensities and durations

- Contrast the speed of energy transfer from carbohydrate and fat combustion

- Discuss how diet affects muscle glycogen levels and endurance exercise performance

- Give an example of a food source of each of the diverse fatty acids (including trans- and omega-3 fatty acids), its physiologic functions, and its possible role in coronary heart disease

- List major characteristics of high- and low-density lipoprotein cholesterol and discuss

- the role of each cholesterol form in coronary heart disease development

- Make prudent recommendations for dietary lipid intake, including cholesterol and fatty acids

- Quantify the amount, energy content, and distribution of fat within an average-sized man

- Outline the dynamics of fat metabolism during physical activity of different intensities and durations

- List four functions of fat in the body

- Discuss how aerobic training affects fat and carbohydrate catabolism during exercise

- Explain how aerobic training affects fat-burning adaptations within skeletal muscle

- Define the terms *essential amino acid* and *nonessential amino acid* and give food sources for each

- Discuss the advantages and potential limitations of a mainly vegetarian diet in maintaining good health and a physically active lifestyle

- Outline the dynamics of protein metabolism during physical activity of various intensities and durations

- Provide a rationale for increasing protein intake above the Recommended Dietary Allowance (RDA) for individuals who perform strenuous endurance or resistance exercise training

- Describe the alanine–glucose cycle and how the body uses amino acids for energy during exercise

The carbohydrate, lipid, and protein nutrients provide energy to maintain bodily functions during rest and physical activity. Aside from their role as biologic fuel, these nutrients, called **macronutrients**, preserve the structural and functional integrity of the organism. This chapter discusses each macronutrient's general structure, function, and dietary source. We emphasize their importance in sustaining physio-logic function during physical activities of differing intensity and duration.

PART 1 • *Carbohydrates*

KINDS AND SOURCES OF CARBOHYDRATES

Atoms of carbon, hydrogen, and oxygen combine to form a basic carbohydrate (sugar) molecule in the general formula $(CH_2O)_n$, where n ranges from 3 to 7 carbon atoms with hydrogen and oxygen atoms attached by single bonds. Except for lactose and a small amount of glycogen from animal origin, plants provide the carbohydrate source in the human diet. Carbohydrates generally classify as monosaccharides, oligosaccharides, and polysaccharides. The number of simple sugars linked within each of these molecules distinguishes each carbohydrate form.

Monosaccharides

*The **monosaccharide** represents the basic unit of carbohydrates.* **Glucose**, also called dextrose or blood sugar, consists of a 6-carbon (hexose) compound that forms naturally in food or in the body through digestion of more complex carbohydrates. **Gluconeogenesis** also synthesizes glucose, primarily in the liver, from the carbon residues of other compounds (generally amino acids, but also glycerol, pyruvate, and lactate). After absorption by the small intestine, glucose either (1) becomes available as an energy source for cellular metabolism, (2) forms glycogen for storage in the liver and muscles, or (3) converts to fat (triacylglycerol) for later use as energy. FIGURE 1.1 illustrates the most typical sugar, glucose, along with other carbohydrates formed in plants from photosynthesis. Glucose consists of 6 carbon, 12 hydrogen, and 6 oxygen atoms, with the chemical formula $C_6H_{12}O_6$. Each carbon atom has four bonding sites that can link to other atoms, including carbons. Carbon bonds not linked to other carbons are "free" to hold hydrogen (with only one bond site), oxygen (with two bond sites), or an oxygen–hydrogen combination termed a hydroxyl (OH). Fructose and galactose, two other simple sugars with the same chemical formula as glucose, have a slightly different C-H-O linkage. The alteration in atomic arrangement makes fructose, galactose, and glucose different substances with distinct biochemical characteristics.

Fructose (fruit sugar or levulose), the sweetest sugar, occurs in large amounts in fruits and honey. Some fructose moves directly from the digestive tract into the blood, but all eventually converts to glucose in the liver. **Galactose** does not exist freely in nature; rather, it combines with glucose to form milk sugar in the mammary glands of lactating animals. The body converts galactose to glucose for use in energy metabolism.

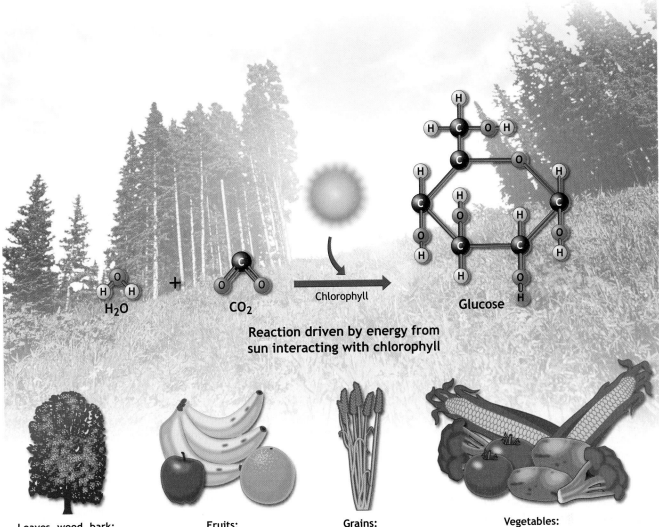

H_2O + CO_2 → Chlorophyll → Glucose

Reaction driven by energy from sun interacting with chlorophyll

Leaves, wood, bark:
cellulose, hemicellulose

Fruits:
sugars, starch, cellulose

Grains:
starch, cellulose

Vegetables:
starch, cellulose

Figure 1.1 Three-dimensional ring structure of the simple sugar glucose molecule formed during photosynthesis when energy from sunlight interacts with water, carbon dioxide, and the green pigment chlorophyll.

Oligosaccharides

Oligosaccharides (from the Greek *oligo,* meaning a few) form when 2 to 10 monosaccharides bond chemically. The major oligosaccharides, the **disaccharides** or double sugars, form when two monosaccharide molecules combine. Monosaccharides and disaccharides collectively make up the **simple sugars**. These sugars are packaged commercially under a variety of guises—brown sugar, corn syrup, fruit syrup, molasses, barley malt, invert sugar, honey, and "natural sweeteners."

Disaccharides all contain glucose. The three principal disaccharides are the following:

- **Sucrose** (glucose + fructose), the most common dietary disaccharide, contributes up to 25% of the total calories consumed in the United States. It occurs naturally in most foods that contain carbohydrates, especially beet and cane sugar, brown sugar, sorghum, maple syrup, and honey. Honey, while sweeter than table sugar because of its greater fructose content, is not superior to table sugar either nutritionally or as an energy source.

- **Lactose** (glucose + galactose), a sugar *not* found in plants, exists in natural form only in milk as milk sugar. The least sweet of the disaccharides, lactose when artificially processed often becomes an ingredient in carbohydrate-rich, high-calorie liquid meals.

- **Maltose** (glucose + glucose) occurs in beer, breakfast cereals, and germinating seeds. Also called malt sugar, this sugar readily cleaves into two glucose molecules but makes only a small contribution to the carbohydrate content of the diet.

Polysaccharides

The term **polysaccharide** describes the linkage of three to thousands of sugar molecules. Polysaccharides form during the chemical process of **dehydration synthesis**, a water-losing reaction that forms a more complex molecule. Both plant and animal sources provide these large chains of linked monosaccharides.

Plant Polysaccharides

Starch and fiber are the common forms of plant poly-saccharides.

Starch, the storage form of carbohydrate in plants, occurs in seeds, corn, and various grains of bread, cereal, pasta, and pastries. Large amounts also exist in peas, beans, potatoes, and roots, in which starch serves as an energy store for future use. Starch exists in two forms: (1) **amylose**, a long straight chain of glucose units twisted into a helical coil, and (2) **amylopectin**, a highly branched monosaccharide linkage. The relative proportion of each form of starch in a particular plant species determines the characteristics of the starch, including its "digestibility." *Starches with a relatively large amount of amylopectin digest and absorb rapidly, whereas starches with high amylose content break down (hydrolyze) at a slower rate.*

Starch still represents the most important dietary source of carbohydrate in the American diet, accounting for approximately 50% of the total carbohydrate intake. The term **complex carbohydrate** describes dietary starch.

Fiber, classified as a nonstarch, structural polysaccharide, includes cellulose, the most abundant organic molecule on earth, first recognized by French chemists Anselm Payen and Jean-François Persoz in 1834 (www.fibersource.com/f-tutor/cellulose.htm). Fibrous materials resist chemical breakdown by human digestive enzymes, although a small portion ferments by action of intestinal bacteria and ultimately participates in metabolic reactions following intestinal absorption. *Fibers occur exclusively in plants; they make up the structure of leaves, stems, roots, seeds, and fruit coverings.* Fibers differ widely in physical and chemical characteristics and physiologic action. Cell walls contain different kinds of fibers (cellulose, hemicellulose, pectin, and the noncarbohydrate lignin); mucilage and gums occur within the plant cell itself.

Health Implications of Fiber Deficiency. Dietary fiber has received considerable attention from researchers and the lay press. Much of this interest originates from studies that link high fiber intake, particularly whole-grain cereal fibers, with a lower occurrence of obesity, diabetes, digestive disorders (including cancers of the mouth, pharynx, larynx, esophagus, and stomach), and heart disease.[37,41,60,64,69,70] The Western diet contains significant fiber-free animal foods and loses much of its natural plant fiber through processing. Americans typically consume about 12 to 15 g of fiber daily, far short of the recommendations of the Food and Nutrition Board of the National Academy of Sciences of 38 g for men and 25 g for women up to age 50, and 30 g for men and 21 g for women over age 50.[25] (*Note:* Appendix A is available on the Student CD or online at

http://connection.lww.com/mkk6e and shows the relationship between metric units and U.S. units, including common expressions of work, energy, and power.)

Fibers hold considerable water and thus give "bulk" to the food residues in the intestinal tract. They may aid gastrointestinal function by (1) exerting a scraping action on the cells of the gut wall, (2) binding or diluting harmful chemicals or inhibiting their activity, and (3) shortening the transit time for food residues (and possibly carcinogenic materials) to pass relatively unhindered through the digestive tract. The potential protective effect of fiber on colon cancer risk remains a hotly debated topic.[9,27,76]

Fiber intake *modestly* reduces serum cholesterol in humans by lowering the low-density lipoprotein component of the cholesterol profile. Particularly effective are the **water-soluble**, mucilaginous fibers such as psyllium seed husk, β-glucan, pectin, and guar gum present in oats, beans, brown rice, peas, carrots, corn husk, and many fruits.[11,17,42] Dietary fiber exerts no effect on high-density lipoproteins. The **water-insoluble fibers** cellulose, hemicellulose, and lignin and cellulose-rich products (wheat bran) do not lower cholesterol.

Precisely how water-soluble dietary fibers favorably affect serum cholesterol remains unknown. Possibly, added fiber simply replaces cholesterol-laden items in the diet. Additionally, some fibers may hinder cholesterol absorption, while others reduce cholesterol synthesis in the gut. These actions would depress cholesterol synthesis and facilitate excretion of existing cholesterol bound to fiber in the feces. Heart disease and obesity protection may relate to dietary fiber's regulatory role in reducing insulin secretion by slowing nutrient absorption by the small intestine following a meal. Fiber consumption may also confer heart disease protection through beneficial effects on blood pressure, insulin sensitivity, and blood clotting characteristics.[62,107] On the negative side, excessive fiber intake inhibits intestinal absorption of the minerals, calcium, phosphorus, and iron.

Present nutritional wisdom advocates a diet that contains 20 to 40 g of fiber (depending on age) per day (ratio of 3:1 for water-insoluble to soluble fiber) by following the recommendations of the MyPyramid from the U.S. Department of Agriculture (see Chapter 3, p. 88). TABLE 1.1 lists the fiber content of common foods and TABLE 1.2 presents a sample daily 2200-kCal menu that includes 31 g of fiber (21 g of insoluble fiber). Total lipid calories equal 30% (saturated fat 10%), protein equals 16%, and carbohydrate equals 54% of total calories ingested.

Some Confusion Concerning Dietary Carbohydrates

Controversy exists concerning the potential effects of high-carbohydrate diets on increased risk for obesity, diabetes, and coronary heart disease, particularly among sedentary and obese adults and children.[6,58,59,68,86,96] For example, the dietary patterns of women chronicled over 6 years showed that those who ate a low-fiber, starchy diet (potatoes and processed white rice, pasta, and white bread, along with

TABLE 1.1 ■ FIBER CONTENT OF COMMON FOODS (LISTED IN ORDER OF TOTAL FIBER CONTENT)

	SERVING SIZE	TOTAL FIBER (g)	SOLUBLE FIBER (g)	INSOLUBLE FIBER (g)
100% bran cereal	1/2 cup	10.0	0.3	9.7
Peas	1/2 cup	5.2	2.0	3.2
Kidney beans	1/2 cup	4.5	0.5	4.0
Apple	1 small	3.9	2.3	1.6
Potato	1 small	3.8	2.2	1.6
Broccoli	1/2 cup	2.5	1.1	1.4
Strawberries	3/4 cup	2.4	0.9	1.5
Oats, whole	1/2 cup	1.6	0.5	1.1
Banana	1 small	1.3	0.6	0.7
Pasta	1/2 cup	1.0	0.2	0.8
Lettuce	1/2 cup	0.5	0.2	0.3
White rice	1/2 cup	0.5	0	0.5

nondiet soft drinks) had a rate of diabetes 2.5 times that of women who ate less of those foods and more fiber-containing, unrefined whole-grain cereals, fruits, and vegetables.[83] Participants who became diabetic developed type 2 diabetes, the most common form of the disease that afflicts nearly 17 million individuals in the United States (approximately 90 to 95% of Americans diagnosed with diabetes have type 2 diabetes, with 20.1 million having prediabetes; www.diabetes. org). Chapter 20 discusses in detail diabetes and the associated risk of the metabolic syndrome.

Not All Carbohydrates Are Physiologically Equal. Digestion rates of different carbohydrate sources possibly explain the link between carbohydrate intake and diabetes and excess body fat. Foods containing dietary fiber slow carbohydrate digestion, minimizing surges in blood glucose. In contrast, low-fiber processed starches (and simple sugars in soft drinks) digest quickly and enter the blood at a relatively rapid rate (high glycemic index foods; see Chapter 3). The blood glucose surge after consuming refined, processed starch and simple sugar stimulates overproduction of insulin by the pancreas to accentuate hyperinsulinemia, elevate plasma triacylglycerol concentrations, and accelerate fat synthesis. Consistently eating such foods may eventually reduce the body's sensitivity to insulin (i.e., peripheral tissues become more resistant to insulin's effects), thus requiring progressively more insulin to control blood sugar levels. *Type 2 diabetes results when the pancreas cannot produce sufficient insulin to regulate blood glucose, causing it to rise.* In contrast, fiber-rich, low-glycemic carbohydrate diets lower blood glucose and insulin response following eating, improve blood lipid profiles, and increase insulin sensitivity.[29,57,78,98] Intake of high-fiber whole-grain foods also thwarts the tendency for weight gain among middle-aged individuals compared with intake of refined-grain foods.[61]

TABLE 1.2 ■ SAMPLE DAILY MENU FOR BREAKFAST, LUNCH, AND DINNER (2200 kCal) CONTAINING 31 g OF DIETARY FIBER[a]

BREAKFAST	LUNCH	DINNER
Whole-grain cereal (3/4 cup)	Bran muffin (1)	Green salad (3.5 oz)
Whole-wheat toast (2 slices)	Milk, 2% (1 cup)	Broccoli, steamed (1/2 cup)
Butter (2 tsp)	Hamburger on bun, lean	Roll, whole wheat (1)
Jelly, strawberry (1 Tbsp)	beef patty (3 oz) with	Butter (2 tsp)
Milk, 2% (1 cup)	2 slices tomato and	Brown rice (1/2 cup)
Raisins (2 Tbsp)	lettuce, catsup (1 Tbsp)	Chicken breast, skinless,
Orange juice (1/2 cup)	and mustard (1 Tbsp)	broiled (3 oz)
Coffee (or tea)	Whole-wheat crackers	Salad dressing, vinegar and
	(4 small)	oil (1 Tbsp)
	Split-pea soup (1 cup)	Pear, medium (1)
	Coffee (or tea)	Yogurt, vanilla, lowfat
		(1/2 cup)

[a] The diet's total cholesterol content is less than 200 mg, and total calcium equals 1242 mg.

A Role in Obesity? Some have speculated that insulin-resistant individuals experience greater risk for weight gain if they consistently eat carbohydrates with a rapid absorption rate. This occurs because excessive insulin facilitates glucose oxidation at the expense of fatty acid oxidation; it also stimulates synthesis of very-low-density lipoprotein (VLDL) cholesterol by the liver and fat storage in adipose tissue. Consequently, obese persons become most affected by diets high in simple sugars and processed starches because they exhibit the greatest insulin resistance and exaggerated insulin response to a glucose challenge. However, long-term comparisons of low-glycemic index and high-glycemic index diets and weight gain have not been conducted. *Regular exercise exerts a potent influence to improve insulin sensitivity, independent of body fat levels, thereby reducing the insulin requirement for a given glucose uptake.*[51]

To reduce type 2 diabetes and obesity risks, one strategy advocates consuming more slowly absorbed, unrefined, complex carbohydrate foods with a lower glycemic index. These foods provide "slow-release" carbohydrates without triggering rapid fluctuations in blood sugar. If rice, pasta, and bread remain the carbohydrate sources of choice, consume them in unrefined form as brown rice, whole-grain pastas, and multigrain breads. *The same dietary modification benefits individuals involved in intense physical training and endurance competition.* In such cases, daily dietary carbohydrate intake should approach 800 g or 8 to 10 g per kg of body mass.

Animal Polysaccharides

Glycogen is the storage carbohydrate peculiar to mammalian muscle and liver. It forms as a large polysaccharide polymer synthesized from glucose in the process of **glucogenesis** (catalyzed by the enzyme **glycogen synthase**). Irregularly shaped, glycogen ranges from a few hundred to 30,000 glucose molecules linked together, much like links in a chain of sausages, with branch linkages for joining additional glucose units (see inset Stage 4, FIG. 1.2). Its compact structure produces the dense glycogen granules within cells, which vary in composition, subcellular location, and metabolic regulation and responsiveness. These glycosomes contain glycogen and the proteins that regulate its metabolism.[85]

Figure 1.2 shows that glycogen biosynthesis involves adding individual glucose units to an existing glycogen polymer. Stage 4 of the figure shows an enlarged view of the chemical configuration of the glycogen molecule. Overall, glycogen synthesis progresses in an irreversible manner. Also, glycogen synthesis requires energy, as one adenosine triphosphate (ATP; stage 1) and one uridine triphosphate (UTP; stage 3) degrade during glucogenesis.

FIGURE 1.3 shows that a well-nourished 80-kg person stores approximately 500 g of carbohydrate. Of this, muscle glycogen accounts for the largest reserve (approximately 400 g), followed by 90 to 110 g as liver glycogen (highest concentration, representing 3 to 7% of the liver's weight), with only about 2 to 3 g as blood glucose. Because each gram of either glycogen or glucose contains approximately 4 calories (kCal) of energy, the average person stores 1500 to 2000 kCal as carbohydrate—enough total energy to power a 20-mile run at high intensity.

Several factors determine the rate and quantity of glycogen breakdown and resynthesis. During exercise, intramuscular glycogen provides the *major* carbohydrate energy source for active muscles. In addition, liver glycogen rapidly reconverts to glucose (regulated by a specific **phosphatase** enzyme) for release into the blood as an extramuscular glucose supply for exercise. The term **glycogenolysis** describes this reconversion of glycogen to glucose. In essence, glycogen breakdown involves the cleavage of glucose units, one at a time, from the glycogen molecule through the introduction of high-energy phosphates (see Chapter 6). Depletion of liver and muscle glycogen by dietary restriction of carbohydrates or intense exercise stimulates glucose synthesis. This occurs through gluconeogenic metabolic pathways from the structural components of other nutrients, particularly proteins.

Hormones play a key role in regulating liver and muscle glycogen stores by controlling circulating blood sugar levels. Elevated blood sugar causes the beta (β) cells of the pancreas to secrete additional insulin; this facilitates cellular glucose uptake and inhibits further insulin secretion. This type of feedback regulation maintains blood glucose at an appropriate physiologic concentration. In contrast, when blood sugar falls below normal, the pancreas's alpha (α) cells secrete **glucagon** to normalize blood sugar concentration. Known as the "insulin antagonist" hormone, this 29-amino acid peptide elevates blood glucose by stimulating the liver's glycogenolytic and gluconeogenic pathways (www.glucagon.com). Chapter 20 contains further discussion of hormonal regulation in exercise.

Figure 1.2 Glycogen synthesis consists of a four-stage process. *Stage 1.* ATP donates a phosphate to glucose to form glucose 6-phosphate. This reaction involves the enzyme hexokinase. *Stage 2.* The enzyme phosphoglucomutase catalyzes the isomerization of glucose 6-phosphate to glucose 1-phosphate. *Stage 3.* The enzyme uridyl transferase reacts with glucose 1-phosphate to form UDP-glucose (a pyrophosphate forms in the degradation of uridine triphosphate [UTP]). *Stage 4.* UDP-glucose attaches to one end of an already existing glycogen polymer chain. This forms a new bond (known as a glycoside bond) between the adjacent glucose units, with concomitant release of UDP. For each glucose unit added, two molecules of high-energy phosphate (ATP and UDP) convert to two molecules of ADP and inorganic phosphate. The inset at the *upper right* of Stage 4 shows a low-resolution view of glycogen; the atomic arrangement of the *circled area of the inset* appears beneath the inset.

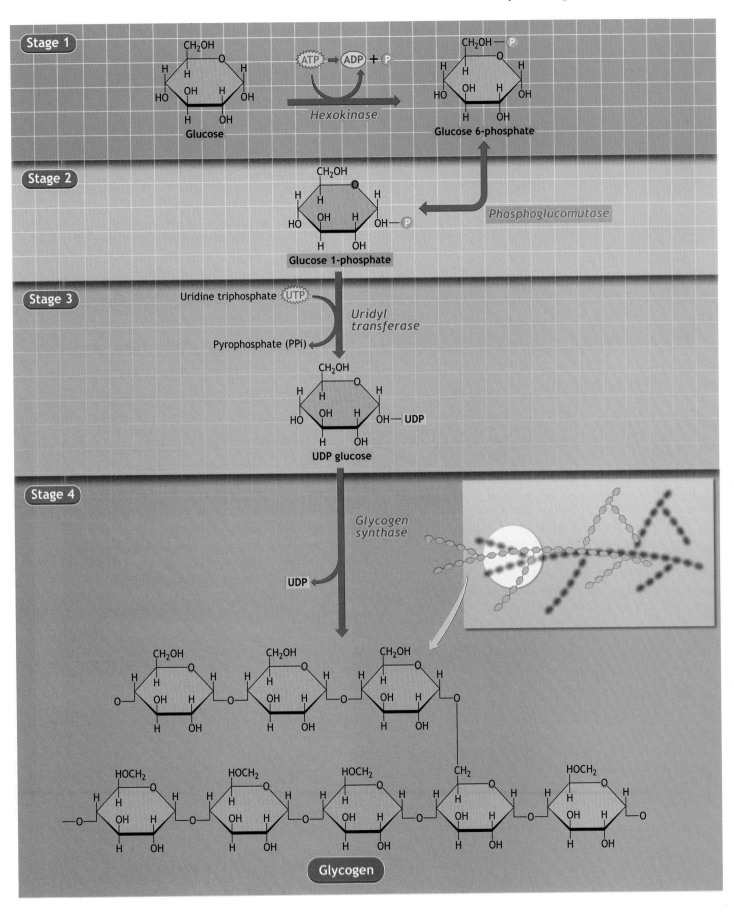

Stage 1

Glucose

Hexokinase

ATP → ADP + P

Glucose 6-phosphate

Stage 2

Glucose 1-phosphate

Phosphoglucomutase

Stage 3

Uridine triphosphate UTP

Uridyl transferase

Pyrophosphate (PPi)

UDP glucose

Stage 4

Glycogen synthase

UDP

Glycogen

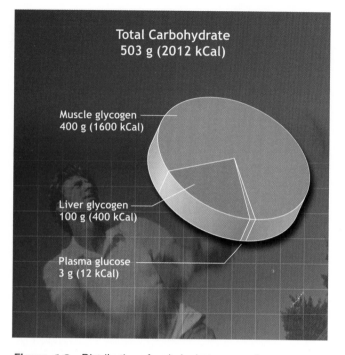

Figure 1.3   Distribution of carbohydrate energy in an average 80-kg person.

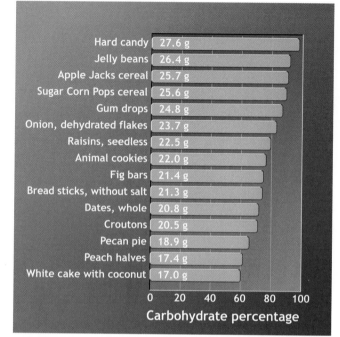

Figure 1.4   Percentage of carbohydrate (relative to food's total weight) common foods arranged by food type. The insert in each bar displays the number of grams of carbohydrate per ounce (28.4 g) of the food.

The body stores comparatively little glycogen, so its quantity fluctuates considerably through dietary modifications. For example, a 24-hour fast or low-carbohydrate, normal-calorie diet nearly depletes glycogen reserves. On the other hand, maintaining a carbohydrate-rich diet for several days almost doubles the body's carbohydrate stores compared with levels attained with a normal, well-balanced diet. *The body's upper limit for glycogen storage averages about 15 g per kilogram (kg) of body mass, equivalent to 1050 g for a 70-kg man and 840 g for a 56-kg woman.* On p. 18, we discuss how enhanced carbohydrate storage affects exercise performance.

RECOMMENDED INTAKE OF CARBOHYDRATES

FIGURE 1.4 lists the carbohydrate content of selected foods. Cereals, cookies, candies, breads, and cakes provide rich carbohydrate sources. Thus, fruits appear as less valuable carbohydrate sources because of their large water content. However, the dried portion of these foods, sold as a dehydrated product, contains almost pure or concentrated carbohydrate.

The typical American diet contains between 40 and 50% of total calories as carbohydrates. For a sedentary 70-kg person, this amounts to a daily carbohydrate intake of about 300 g. *For more physically active people and those involved in exercise training, carbohydrates should represent about 60% of daily calories (400 to 600 g), predominantly as unrefined, fiber-rich fruits, grains, and vegetables. During peri-* *ods of intense training, we recommend that carbohydrate intake increase to 70% of total calories consumed (8 to 10 g per kg of body mass).*

Nutritious dietary carbohydrate sources consist of fruits, grains, and vegetables, yet this does not represent the typical source of carbohydrate intake for all people. The typical American consumes about 50% of carbohydrate as simple sugars whose intake comes primarily from sugars added in food processing as sucrose and high-fructose corn syrup (formed commercially by enzyme action on cornstarch that emphasizes fructose formation). These sugars do not come in a nutrient-dense package typical of the simple sugars found naturally in fruits and vegetables. Sodas represent the largest single source of added sugars (33%) in the American diet (a 12-oz soft drink contains about 40 g or 10 tsp of sugar). Over the course of a year, the average American drinks 54 gallons of soft drinks, 2.5 times the amount of coffee consumed. Substituting fructose (a monosaccharide about twice as sweet as table sugar) for sucrose provides equal sweetness with fewer calories. Furthermore, fructose does not stimulate pancreatic insulin secretion; thus, adding fructose to the diet helps to stabilize blood glucose and insulin levels.

ROLE OF CARBOHYDRATES IN THE BODY

Carbohydrates serve four important functions related to energy metabolism and exercise performance.

1. Energy Source

Carbohydrates primarily serve as an energy fuel, particularly during high-intensity exercise. Energy derived from the catabolism of blood-borne glucose and muscle glycogen ultimately powers the contractile elements of muscle and other forms of biologic work.

Daily carbohydrate intake for physically active individuals must achieve levels that maintain the body's relatively limited glycogen stores. Once cells reach their maximum capacity for glycogen storage, excess sugars convert to and store as fat. This biologic "fact of life" should be made crystal clear to individuals who believe that consuming unlimited carbohydrate (in lieu of lipids) confers an advantage for weight control. The interconversion of macronutrients for energy storage explains how body fat can increase when dietary carbohydrate exceeds energy requirements, even if the diet is hypolipidic (contains little lipid).

2. Protein Sparer

Adequate carbohydrate intake helps to preserve tissue protein. Normally, protein serves a vital role in tissue maintenance, repair, and growth and to a considerably lesser degree as a nutrient energy source. Depletion of glycogen reserves—readily occurring with starvation, reduced energy and/or carbohydrate intake, and strenuous exercise—dramatically affects the metabolic mixture for energy. In addition to stimulating fat catabolism, glycogen depletion triggers glucose synthesis from the labile pool of amino acids (protein). This gluconeogenic conversion offers a metabolic option for augmenting carbohydrate availability (and maintaining plasma glucose levels) even with insufficient glycogen stores. The price paid, however, strains the body's protein levels, particularly muscle protein. In the extreme, this reduces lean tissue mass and adds a solute load on the kidneys, forcing them to excrete the nitrogen-containing byproducts of protein catabolism.

INTEGRATIVE QUESTION

Discuss the rationale for recommending adequate carbohydrate intake rather than an excess of protein to increase muscle mass through heavy resistance training.

3. Metabolic Primer

Components of carbohydrate catabolism serve as "primer" substrate for fat oxidation. Insufficient carbohydrate breakdown—either through limitations in glucose transport into the cell (e.g., diabetes where insulin production wanes or insulin resistance increases) or glycogen depletion through inadequate diet or prolonged exercise—causes fat mobilization to exceed fat oxidation. The lack of adequate byproducts of glycogen breakdown produces incomplete fat breakdown with accumulation of **ketone bodies** (acetoacetate and β-hydroxybutyrate, acetone-like byproducts of incomplete fat breakdown). Ketone formation takes place in hepatic mitochondria from an excess of acetyl-CoA formed during β-oxidation. That is, acetyl-CoA accumulates beyond its capacity for oxidation or to participate in fatty acid synthesis. In excess, ketone bodies increase body fluid acidity to produce a potentially harmful condition called acidosis or, specifically with regard to fat breakdown, **ketosis**. Chapter 6 continues the discussion of carbohydrate as a primer for fat catabolism.

4. Fuel for the Central Nervous System

The central nervous system requires an uninterrupted stream of carbohydrate to function properly. Under normal conditions, the brain uses blood glucose almost exclusively as its fuel. In poorly regulated diabetes, during starvation, or with a prolonged low carbohydrate intake, the brain adapts after about 8 days and metabolizes relatively large amounts of fat (as ketones) for alternative fuel. Chronic low-carbohydrate, high-fat diets also induce adaptations in skeletal muscle that increase fat use during low-to-moderate exercise levels, thus sparing muscle glycogen.

Blood sugar usually remains regulated within narrow limits for two main reasons: (1) glucose serves as a primary fuel for nerve tissue metabolism and (2) glucose represents the sole energy source for red blood cells. At rest and during exercise, liver glycogenolysis maintains normal blood glucose levels, usually at $100 \text{ mg} \cdot \text{dL}^{-1}$ (5.5 mM). In prolonged, intense exercise such as marathon running, blood glucose concentration eventually falls below normal levels because liver glycogen depletes, and active muscle continues to catabolize the available blood glucose. Symptoms of significantly reduced blood glucose (**hypoglycemia:** <45 mg glucose per deciliter [dL] of blood) include weakness, hunger, and dizziness. This ultimately impairs exercise performance and can contribute to central nervous system fatigue associated with prolonged exercise. Sustained and profound hypoglycemia triggers unconsciousness and produces irreversible brain damage.

CARBOHYDRATE DYNAMICS IN EXERCISE

Biochemical and biopsy techniques and labeled nutrient tracers assess the energy contribution of nutrients during physical activity. For example, needle biopsies permit serial sampling of specific muscles to assess the kinetics of intramuscular nutrient metabolism with little interruption during exercise. Data from such research indicate that the intensity and duration of effort and the fitness and nutritional status of the exerciser largely determine the fuel mixture in exercise.[14,28]

The liver increases glucose release to active muscle as exercise progresses from low to high intensity. Simultaneously, muscle glycogen supplies the predominant carbohydrate energy source during the early stages of exercise and as intensity increases.[33,81] Compared with fat and protein, carbohydrate remains the preferential fuel in high-intensity aerobic exercise because it rapidly supplies energy (ATP) via oxidative processes. In anaerobic effort (requiring glycolysis reactions; see Chapter 6), carbohydrate becomes the *sole* macronutrient contributor of ATP. Just 3 days of maintaining a diet containing only 5% of its energy as carbohydrate depresses all-out exercise capacity.[54]

Carbohydrate availability in the metabolic mixture controls its use for energy. In turn, carbohydrate intake dramatically affects its availability. The concentration of blood glucose provides feedback regulation of the liver's glucose output; an increase in blood glucose inhibits hepatic glucose release during exercise.[38] Carbohydrate availability during exercise also helps regulate fat mobilization and its use for energy.[16,18] For example, increasing carbohydrate oxidation by ingesting high-glycemic carbohydrates prior to exercise (with accompanying hyperglycemia and hyperinsulinemia) inhibits two processes: (1) long-chain fatty acid oxidation by skeletal muscle and (2) free fatty acid (FFA) liberation from adipose tissue. Some speculate that adequate carbohydrate availability (and resulting increased catabolism) inhibits transport of long-chain fatty acids into the mitochondria, thus controlling the exercise metabolic mixture. This proposition directly opposes the classic notion that fatty acid availability and breakdown inhibit carbohydrate metabolism, as described by the glucose–fatty acid cycle.[30,105]

Intense Exercise

During strenuous exercise, neural–humoral factors increase the output of epinephrine, norepinephrine, and glucagon and decrease insulin release. These hormonal responses activate **glycogen phosphorylase** (indirectly via activation of cyclic AMP; see Chapter 20), the enzyme that facilitates glycogenolysis in the liver and active muscles. Think of glycogen phosphorylase as the controller of the glycogen-glucose interconversion. Thus, this important enzyme regulates the concentration of circulating glucose in the bloodstream. Because muscle glycogen provides energy without oxygen, it contributes the most energy in the early minutes of exercise when oxygen use does not meet oxygen demands. As exercise continues, blood-borne glucose increases its contribution as a metabolic fuel. For example, blood glucose may supply up to 30% of the total energy required by vigorously active muscles, with the remaining carbohydrate energy supplied by muscle glycogen.[81]

An hour of high-intensity exercise decreases liver glycogen by about 55%; a 2-hour strenuous workout almost depletes glycogen in the liver and specifically exercised muscles. FIGURE 1.5 illustrates that the muscles' uptake of circulating blood glucose increases sharply during the initial stage of exercise and continues to increase with further exercise. By the 40th minute, glucose uptake rises 7 to 20 times the uptake at rest, depending on exercise intensity. *During intense aerobic exercise, the advantage of a selective dependence on carbohydrate metabolism lies in its rate of energy*

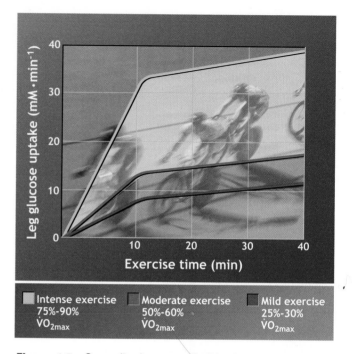

Figure 1.5 Generalized response for blood glucose uptake by the leg muscles during cycling in relation to exercise duration and intensity. Exercise intensity is expressed as a percentage of $\dot{V}O_{2max}$.

transfer, which is twice that of fat and protein. [94] In addition, per unit oxygen consumed, carbohydrate generates almost 6% more energy than fat. Chapter 6 presents the specifics of energy release from carbohydrate under anaerobic and aerobic conditions.

Moderate and Prolonged Exercise

Glycogen stored in active muscles supplies almost all of the energy in the transition from rest to moderate exercise. During the next 20 minutes or so, liver and muscle glycogen supply between 40 and 50% of the energy requirement, with the remainder provided by fat catabolism and a limited amount of protein. The nutrient mixture for energy depends on the relative intensity of exercise. During light-intensity exercise, fat remains the main energy substrate throughout exercise (see Fig. 1.19). As exercise continues and muscle glycogen stores decrease, blood glucose becomes the major supplier of carbohydrate energy, while fat catabolism furnishes an increasingly greater percentage of total energy. Eventually, the liver's glucose output fails to keep pace with glucose use by muscle, and plasma glucose concentration decreases. In such cases, the level of circulating blood glucose may fall toward hypoglycemic levels.

FIGURE 1.6 depicts the metabolic profile during prolonged exercise in the glycogen-depleted and glycogen-loaded states. As submaximal exercise progresses in the glycogen-depleted state, blood glucose levels fall and circulating fat (predominantly as free fatty acids, or FFA) increases dramatically compared with exercise under glyco-

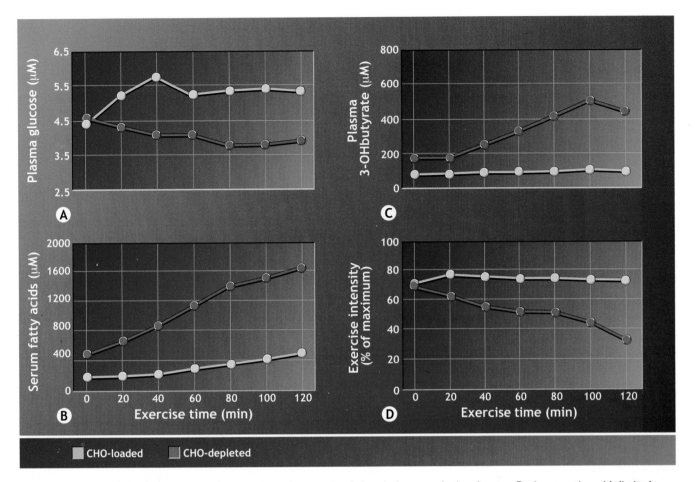

Figure 1.6 Dynamics of nutrient metabolism in the glycogen-loaded and glycogen-depleted states. During exercise with limited carbohydrate availability, plasma glucose levels (**A**) progressively decrease, while fat metabolism (**B**) progressively increases compared with similar exercise when glycogen loaded. In addition, protein use for energy (**C**), as indicated by plasma levels of 3-OH butyrate, remains considerably higher with glycogen depletion. After 2 hours, exercise capacity (**D**) decreases to about 50% of maximum in exercise begun in the glycogen-depleted state. (From Wagenmakers AJM, et al. Carbohydrate supplementation, glycogen depletion, and amino acid metabolism. Am J Physiol 1991;260:E883.)

gen-loaded conditions. Concurrently, the contribution of protein to energy expenditure increases. Exercise intensity (expressed as percentage of maximum) also progressively decreases under the glycogen-depleted condition. At the end of 2 hours, an exerciser can only maintain about 50% of the initial exercise intensity. Reduced power output results directly from the relatively slow rate of aerobic energy release from fat oxidation, which now becomes the primary energy source. Any of the following potential rate-limiting metabolic processes that precede the citric acid cycle could explain the relatively slower rate of fat oxidation compared with that of carbohydrate:

- FFA mobilization from adipose tissue
- FFA transport to skeletal muscle via circulation
- FFA uptake by the muscle cell
- FFA uptake by the muscle from triacylglycerols in chylomicrons and lipoproteins
- Fatty acid mobilization from intramuscular triacylglycerols and cytoplasmic transport

- Fatty acid transport into the mitochondria
- Fatty acid oxidation within the mitochondria

Fatigue occurs when exercise continues to the point that compromises liver and muscle glycogen supply. This occurs despite sufficient oxygen availability to muscle and almost unlimited energy supply from stored fat. Endurance athletes commonly refer to this sensation of fatigue as "bonking" or "**hitting the wall**." Because skeletal muscle lacks the phosphatase enzyme, which allows glucose exchange between cells, the relatively inactive muscles maintain their full glycogen content. What remains unclear is why muscle glycogen depletion coincides with the point of fatigue. The answer may relate in some way to the following:

- Use of blood glucose for optimal central nervous system function
- Muscle glycogen's role as a "primer" in fat breakdown
- Significantly slower rate of energy release from fat than from carbohydrate breakdown

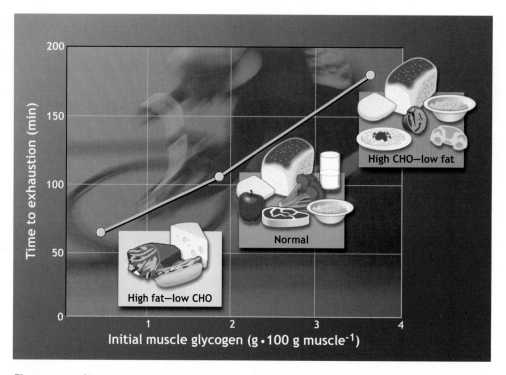

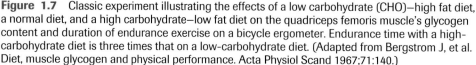

Figure 1.7   Classic experiment illustrating the effects of a low carbohydrate (CHO)–high fat diet, a normal diet, and a high carbohydrate–low fat diet on the quadriceps femoris muscle's glycogen content and duration of endurance exercise on a bicycle ergometer. Endurance time with a high-carbohydrate diet is three times that on a low-carbohydrate diet. (Adapted from Bergstrom J, et al. Diet, muscle glycogen and physical performance. Acta Physiol Scand 1967;71:140.)

Effect of Diet on Muscle Glycogen Stores and Endurance

Diet composition profoundly affects glycogen reserves. FIGURE 1.7 shows the effects of dietary manipulation on muscle glycogen and endurance performance. In this classic experiment, six subjects maintained normal caloric intake for 3 days but consumed most of their calories as lipid and 5% or less as carbohydrate (high-fat diet). In the second condition (normal diet), the 3-day diet contained the recommended daily percentages of carbohydrate, lipid, and protein. The third diet provided 82% of the calories as carbohydrates (high-carbohydrate diet). The glycogen content of the quadriceps femoris muscle, determined from needle biopsy specimens, averaged 0.63 g of glycogen per 100 g wet muscle with the high-fat diet, 1.75 g for the normal diet, and 3.75 g for the high-carbohydrate diet.

Endurance capacity during cycling exercise varied considerably, depending on what was consumed for 3 days before the exercise test. With the normal diet, exercise lasted an average of 114 minutes, whereas endurance averaged only 57 minutes with the high-fat diet. The high-carbohydrate diet improved endurance performance by more than three times the endurance on the high-fat diet. Interestingly, the point of fatigue coincided with the same low level of muscle glycogen under the three diet conditions. This classic experiment conclusively demonstrated the importance of muscle glycogen to sustain high-intensity exercise lasting more than 1 hour. The research emphasized the important role played by nutrition in establishing appropriate energy reserves for long-term exercise and strenuous training.

A carbohydrate-deficient diet rapidly depletes muscle and liver glycogen and negatively affects performance in short-term anaerobic exercise and prolonged high-intensity aerobic activities. These observations relate particularly to individuals who modify their diets by reducing carbohydrate intake below recommended levels. Reliance on starvation diets or other extreme diet forms (e.g., high-fat, low-carbohydrate diets or "liquid-protein" diets) proves counterproductive for optimizing exercise performance. Reliance on low-carbohydrate diets makes it particularly difficult from an energy supply standpoint to engage regularly in longer-duration, vigorous physical activities. Chapter 3 discusses optimal provision for carbohydrate needs prior to, during, and in recovery from strenuous exercise.

Summary

1. Carbon, hydrogen, oxygen, and nitrogen represent the primary structural units for most bioactive substances within the body. Specific combinations of carbon with oxygen and hydrogen form carbohydrates and lipids. Proteins form when combinations of carbon, oxygen, and hydrogen bind with nitrogen and minerals.
2. Simple sugars consist of chains of 3 to 7 carbon atoms, with hydrogen and oxygen in the ratio of 2:1. Glucose, the most common simple sugar, contains a 6-carbon chain as $C_6H_{12}O_6$.
3. Three major classifications of carbohydrates include monosaccharides (sugars such as glucose and

fructose), oligosaccharides (disaccharides such as sucrose, lactose, and maltose), and polysaccharides that contain three or more simple sugars to form plant starch and fiber and glycogen, the large glucose polymer from the animal kingdom.

4. Glycogenolysis describes the reconversion of glycogen to glucose; gluconeogenesis refers to glucose synthesis, particularly from protein sources.

5. Americans typically consume 40 to 50% of total caloric intake as carbohydrates, often as simple sugars and refined starches. Excess consumption of simple sugars and other rapidly absorbed carbohydrates may have negative health implications.

6. Carbohydrate, stored in limited quantity in liver and muscle, has four important functions: (1) provides a major source of energy, (2) spares protein breakdown, (3) functions as a metabolic primer for fat catabolism, and (4) provides the required, uninterrupted fuel supply for the central nervous system.

7. Muscle glycogen provides the primary energy substrate (fuel) during intense anaerobic exercise. The body's glycogen stores (muscle glycogen and glucose from the liver) also contribute substantially to energy metabolism in longer-duration endurance-type activities.

8. Fat contributes about 50% of the energy requirement during light and moderate exercise. Stored intramuscular fat and fat derived from adipocytes becomes important during prolonged exercise. In this situation, the fatty acid molecules (mainly as circulating FFAs) supply more than 80% of the exercise energy requirements.

9. A carbohydrate-deficient diet quickly depletes muscle and liver glycogen. This profoundly affects both all-out exercise capacity and the capacity to sustain high-intensity endurance exercise.

10. Individuals who train intensely should consume between 60 and 70% of daily calories as carbohydrates, predominantly in unrefined, complex form (400 to 800 g; 8 to 10 g per kg of body mass).

11. With muscles depleted of carbohydrate, exercise intensity decreases to a level determined by the body's ability to mobilize and oxidize fat.

PART 2 • *Lipids*

THE NATURE OF LIPIDS

A lipid (from the Greek *lipos,* meaning fat) molecule has the same structural elements as carbohydrate, but it differs significantly in its linkage of atoms. Specifically, the lipid's ratio of hydrogen to oxygen considerably exceeds that of carbohydrate. For example, the formula $C_{57}H_{110}O_6$ describes the common lipid stearin with an H:O ratio of 18.3:1; for carbohydrate, the ratio remains constant at 2:1.

Lipid, the general term for a heterogeneous group of compounds, includes oils, fats, waxes, and related compounds. Oils become liquid at room temperature, whereas fats remain solid. Approximately 98% of dietary lipid exists as triacylglycerol (see next section), while about 90% of the body's total fat resides in the adipose tissue depots of the subcutaneous tissues.

KINDS AND SOURCES OF LIPIDS

Plants and animals contain lipids in long hydrocarbon chains. Lipids, generally greasy to the touch, remain insoluble in water but soluble in the nonpolar organic solvents acetone, ether, chloroform, and benzene. According to common classification, lipids belong to one of three main groups: **simple lipids**, **compound lipids**, and **derived lipids**.

Simple Lipids

The simple lipids or "neutral fats" consist primarily of **triacylglycerols**—a more preferred term than triglycerides among biochemists because it describes glycerol acylated by three fatty acids. The fats are "neutral" because at the pH of the cell. They carry no electrically charged groups. These completely nonpolar molecules have no affinity for water Triacylglycerols constitute the major storage form of fat in fat cells (**adipocytes**). This molecule contains two different clusters of atoms. One cluster, **glycerol**, consists of a 3-carbon molecule that itself does not qualify as a lipid because of its high solubility in water. Three clusters of unbranched carbon-chained atoms, termed **fatty acids**, attach to the glycerol molecule. A carboxyl (-COOH) cluster at one end of the fatty acid chain gives the molecule its acidic characteristics. Fatty acids have straight hydrocarbon chains with as few as 4 carbon atoms or more than 20, although chain lengths of 16 and 18 carbons prevail. As the chain length of the fatty acid increases, it becomes less water-soluble and thus more oily with fatty characteristics.

Three molecules of water form when glycerol and fatty acids join in the synthesis (**condensation**) of the triacylglycerol molecule. Conversely, during hydrolysis, when **lipase** enzymes cleave the molecule into its constituents, three molecules of water attach at the points where the fat molecule splits. FIGURE 1.8 illustrates the basic structure of a **saturated fatty acid** and an **unsaturated fatty acid** molecule. All lipid-containing foods consist of a mixture of different proportions of saturated and unsaturated fatty acids. Fatty acids are so named because the organic acid molecule (COOH) forms part of their chemical structure. Body fat contains both forms of fatty acids.

Saturated Fatty Acids

A saturated fatty acid contains only single covalent bonds between carbon atoms; all of the remaining bonds attach to hydrogen. If the carbon within a fatty acid chain binds the maximum possible number of hydrogens, the fatty acid

Saturated Fatty Acid

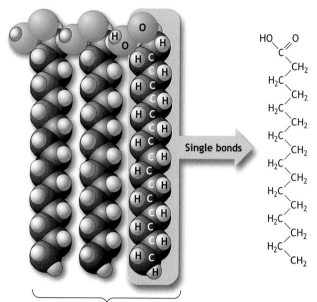

Carbon atoms linked by single bonds enable close packing of these fatty acids

A No double bonds; fatty acid chains fit close together

Unsaturated Fatty Acid

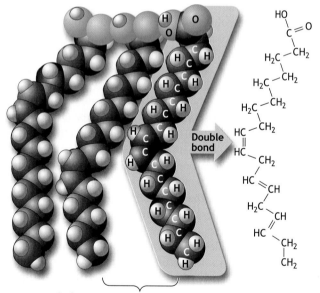

Carbon atoms linked by double bonds increases distance between fatty acids

B Double bonds present; fatty acid chains do not fit close together

Figure 1.8 The presence or absence of double bonds between the carbon atoms is the major structural difference between saturated and unsaturated fatty acids. **A.** The saturated fatty acid palmitic acid has no double bonds in its carbon chain and thus contains the maximum number of hydrogen atoms. Without double bonds, the three saturated fatty acid chains fit together closely to form a "hard" fat. **B.** The three double bonds in linoleic acid, an unsaturated fatty acid, reduce the number of hydrogen atoms along the carbon chain. Insertion of double bonds into the carbon chain prevents close association of the fatty acids; this produces a "softer" fat, or an oil.

molecule becomes saturated with respect to hydrogen, and hence the name saturated fatty acid.

Saturated fatty acids occur primarily in animal products such as beef (52% saturated fatty acids), lamb, pork, chicken, egg yolk, and dairy fats of cream, milk, butter (62% saturated fatty acids), and cheese. Saturated fatty acids from the plant kingdom include coconut and palm oil, vegetable shortening, and hydrogenated margarine; commercially prepared cakes, pies, and cookies contain plentiful amounts of these fatty acids.

Unsaturated Fatty Acids

Unsaturated fatty acids contain one or more double bonds along their main carbon chain. Each double bond along the chain reduces the number of potential hydrogen-

	Saturated	Polyunsaturated	Monounsaturated
Canola oil	6	36	58
Safflower oil	9	78	13
Sunflower oil	11	69	20
Avocado oil	12	14	74
Corn oil	13	62	25
Olive oil	15	11	73
Soybean oil	15	61	24
Peanut oil	18	34	48
Cottonseed oil	27	54	19
Lard	41	12	47
Palm oil	51	10	39
Beef tallow	52	2	44
Butter fat	66	4	30
Coconut oil	92	2	6

Percent of fatty acid

☐ Saturated fatty acids   ☐ Polyunsaturated fatty acids   ☐ Monounsaturated fatty acids

Hidden fat percentage of total calories			
Food	**Fat %**	**Food**	**Fat %**
Brazil nuts	67	Lamb roast	19
Walnuts	61	Avocado	16
Almonds	54	Ice cream	13
Peanuts	50	Herring	12
Sunflower seeds	47	Poached eggs	11
Pork sausage	44	Tuna, canned	8
Pork roast	30	Poultry, dark meat	7
Cheese	30	Oatmeal, dry	7
Bologna	28	Salmon	6
Beef roast	25	Whole milk	4
Ham, cured	22	Poultry, light meat	4
Hamburger	20	Shredded wheat cereal	2

Figure 1.9 The *upper graph* shows the composition of diverse fatty acids (g per 100 g) in common lipid sources in the diet. The *lower table* shows the hidden total fat percentage of total calories in popular foods. (Data from Food Composition Tables, United States Department of Agriculture.)

binding sites; the molecule, therefore, remains unsaturated with respect to hydrogen. A **monounsaturated fatty acid** contains *one* double bond along the main carbon chain; examples include canola oil, olive oil (77% monounsaturated fatty acids), peanut oil, and the oil in almonds, pecans, and avocados. A **polyunsaturated fatty acid** contains *two or more* double bonds along the main carbon chain; safflower, sunflower, soybean, and corn oil serve as examples. FIGURE 1.9 lists the contents of saturated, monounsaturated, and polyunsaturated fatty acids in common fats and oils (expressed in g per 100 g of the lipid). The insert table shows the hidden fat percentage in some popular foods. Several polyunsaturated fatty acids, most notably **linoleic acid** (an 18-carbon fatty acid with two double bonds; present in cooking and salad oils), must originate from dietary sources because they serve as precursors of other fatty acids the body cannot synthesize (called **essential fatty acids**). Linoleic acid maintains the integrity of plasma membranes and sustains growth, reproduction, skin maintenance, and general body functioning.

Fatty acids from plant sources generally remain unsaturated and liquefy at room temperature. In contrast, lipids containing longer (more carbons in the chain) and more saturated fatty acids exist as solids at room temperature; those with shorter and more unsaturated fatty acids remain soft. Oils exist as liquids and contain unsaturated fatty acids. The chemical process of **hydrogenation** changes oils to semisolid fats by bubbling liquid hydrogen under pressure into vegetable oil (with the addition of the mineral catalyst nickel at a temperature of 120 to 210°C). This reduces the unsaturated fatty acids' double bonds to single bonds so more hydrogens can attach to carbons along the chain. Firmer fat forms because adding hydrogen increases the lipid's melting temperature. Hydrogenated oil thus behaves like a saturated fat; the most common hydrogenated fats include lard substitutes and margarine.

Triacylglycerol Formation

FIGURE 1.10 outlines the sequence of reactions in triacylglycerol synthesis, a process termed **esterification**. Initially, a fatty acid substrate attached to coenzyme A forms fatty acyl-CoA, which then transfers to glycerol (as glycerol 3-phosphate). In subsequent reactions, two additional fatty acyl-CoAs link to the single glycerol backbone as the composite triacylglycerol molecule forms. Triacylglycerol synthesis increases following a meal for the following two reasons: (1) increased blood levels of fatty acids and glucose from food absorption and (2) relatively high level of circulating insulin, which facilitates triacylglycerol synthesis.

Triacylglycerol Breakdown

The term hydrolysis (more specifically **lipolysis**) describes triacylglycerol catabolism to yield glycerol and the energy-rich fatty acid molecules. FIGURE 1.11 shows that lipolysis adds water in three distinct hydrolysis reactions, each catalyzed by hormone-sensitive lipase.[20] The mobiliza-

tion of fatty acids via lipolysis predominates under conditions of (1) low-to-moderate exercise, (2) low-calorie dieting or fasting, (3) cold stress, and (4) prolonged exercise that depletes glycogen reserves.

Both triacylglycerol esterification and lipolysis occur in the cytosol of the adipocytes. The fatty acids released during lipolysis can (1) reesterify to triacylglycerol following their conversion to a fatty acyl-CoA or (2) exit from the adipocyte, enter the blood, and combine with the blood protein albumin for transport to tissues throughout the body. The term **free fatty acid** (**FFA**) describes this albumin–fatty acid combination. The glycerol released in lipolysis cannot be reused by adipocytes; instead it exits the cell and circulates in the blood. For this reason, the plasma glycerol concentration provides a convenient index of the degree of lipolysis.

Lipolysis also proceeds in tissues other than adipocytes. Hydrolysis of dietary triacylglycerol occurs in the small intestine, catalyzed by pancreatic lipase; lipoprotein lipase, an enzyme located on the walls of capillaries, catalyzes the hydrolysis of the triacylglycerols carried by the blood's lipoproteins. Adjacent adipose tissue and muscle cells can "take up" the fatty acids released by the action lipoprotein lipase; these fatty acids can then be resynthesized to triacylglycerol for energy storage.

Butter Versus Margarine: A Health Risk in Trans-Fatty Acids?

Butter and margarine cannot be distinguished by caloric content, only by their fatty acid composition. The manufacture of margarine and some other vegetable shortenings involves the partial hydrogenation of unsaturated corn, soybean, or sunflower oil with the final product containing a **trans-fatty acid**. A *trans*-fatty acid forms when one of the hydrogen atoms along the restructured carbon chain moves from its naturally occurring position (*cis* position) to the opposite side of the double bond that separates 2 carbon atoms (*trans* position). From 17 to 25% of margarine's fatty acids exist as *trans*-fatty acids, compared with only 7% in butter. Margarine, consisting of vegetable oil, contains no cholesterol; butter, in contrast, originates from a dairy source and contains between 11 and 15 mg of cholesterol per teaspoon. Small amounts of naturally occurring *trans* fat can be found in some animal products such as butter, milk products, cheese, beef, and lamb. The richest sources comprise vegetable shortenings, some margarines, crackers, candies, cookies, snack foods, fried foods, baked goods, salad dressings, and other processed foods made with partially hydrogenated vegetable oils. *Trans*-fatty acids represent about 5 to 10% of the fat in the typical American diet.

Concern about margarine centers on the possible detrimental health effects of *trans*-fatty acids through their adverse effects on serum lipoproteins.[4,5,65,67] A diet high in margarine and commercial baked goods (cookies, cakes, doughnuts, pies) and deep-fried foods prepared with hydrogenated vegetable oils increases low-density lipoprotein cholesterol concentration by a similar amount as a diet high in

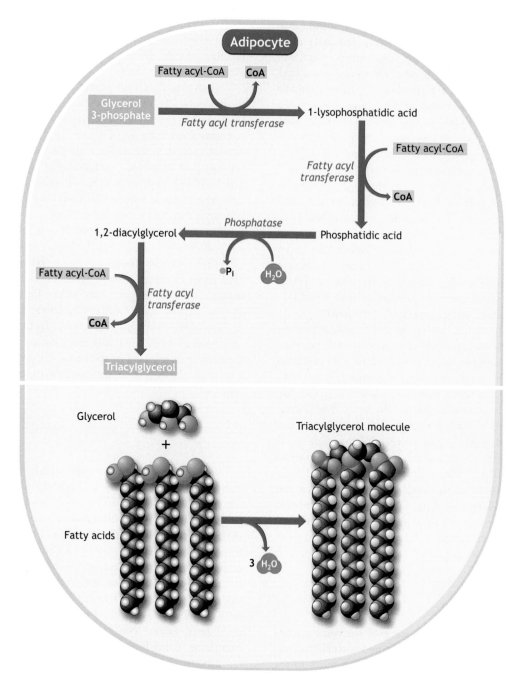

Figure 1.10   *Top.* Triacylglycerol formation in adipocytes (and muscle) tissue involves a series of reactions (dehydration synthesis) that link three fatty acid molecules to a single glycerol backbone. The *bottom portion* of the figure summarizes this linkage.

saturated fatty acids (e.g., butter). Unlike saturated fats, hydrogenated oils also decrease the concentration of beneficial high-density lipoprotein cholesterol. Dietary *trans*-fatty acids account for up to 30,000 deaths annually from heart disease.[101] FIGURE 1.12 shows heart disease risk associated with the type of fatty acid intake in a 14-year prospective study of 80,082 nurses. Women who consumed the largest amounts of *trans* fats had a 53% higher heart disease risk than those with lower *trans* fat intake. The lowest heart disease risk emerged among women with the lowest intake of *trans* fat and the

highest intake of polyunsaturated fat. In light of the strong evidence that *trans*-fatty acids do indeed place individuals at increased risk for heart disease, the Food and Drug Administration (FDA) announced on July 9, 2003 that it would require food processors to include the amount of *trans*-fatty acids on nutrition labels. This requirement does not go into effect until 2006. The FDA estimates that this change in regulations "will save between $900 million and $1.8 billion a year in medical costs, lost productivity, and pain and suffering."

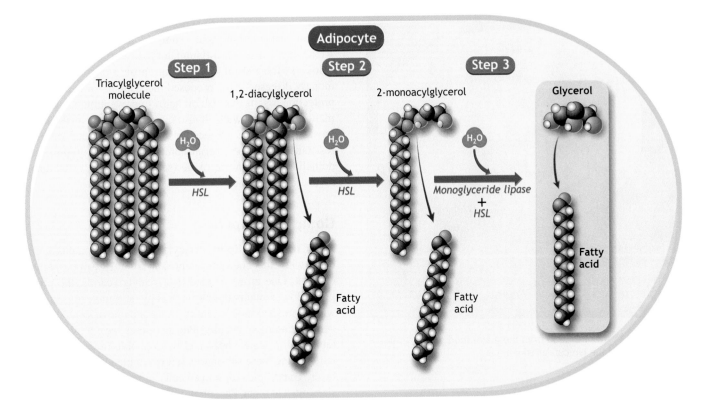

Figure 1.11   Triacylglycerol catabolism (hydrolysis or, more specifically, lipolysis) to its glycerol and fatty acid components involves a three-step process regulated by hormone-sensitive lipase *(HSL)*.

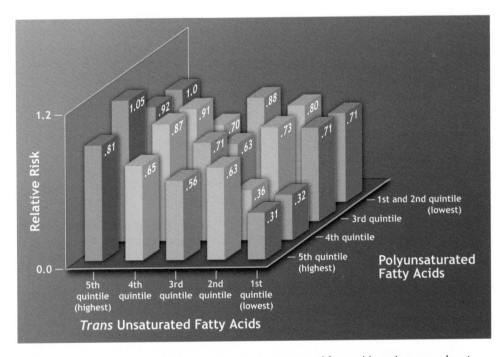

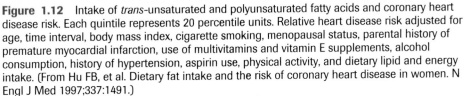

Figure 1.12   Intake of *trans*-unsaturated and polyunsaturated fatty acids and coronary heart disease risk. Each quintile represents 20 percentile units. Relative heart disease risk adjusted for age, time interval, body mass index, cigarette smoking, menopausal status, parental history of premature myocardial infarction, use of multivitamins and vitamin E supplements, alcohol consumption, history of hypertension, aspirin use, physical activity, and dietary lipid and energy intake. (From Hu FB, et al. Dietary fat intake and the risk of coronary heart disease in women. N Engl J Med 1997;337:1491.)

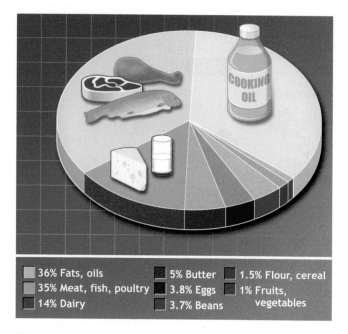

■ 36% Fats, oils	■ 5% Butter	■ 1.5% Flour, cereal
■ 35% Meat, fish, poultry	■ 3.8% Eggs	■ 1% Fruits,
■ 14% Dairy	■ 3.7% Beans	vegetables

Figure 1.13 Contribution from the major food groups to the lipid content of the typical American diet.

Lipids in the Diet

FIGURE 1.13 displays the approximate percentage contribution of some common food groups to the total lipid content of the typical American diet. Plant sources generally contribute about 34% to the daily lipid intake; the remaining 66% comes from animal sources.

The average person in the United States consumes about 15% of total calories as saturated fatty acids, the equivalent of over 23 kg of saturated fats per year. The relationship between saturated fatty acid intake and coronary heart disease risk has prompted health professionals to recommend (1) replacing at least a portion of the saturated fatty acids and all *trans*-fatty acids with nonhydrogenated monounsaturated and polyunsaturated oils and (2) balancing energy intake with regular physical activity to minimize weight gain and obtain the health benefits of regular exercise.[49,50] From a health perspective, individuals should consume no more than 10% of total daily energy intake as saturated fatty acids; this amounts to about 300 kCal or 30 to 35 g for the average young adult male who consumes 3000 kCal.

Fish Oils Are Healthful. The health profiles and dietary patterns of Greenland Eskimos, who consume large quantities of lipids from fish, seal, and whale, yet have a low incidence of heart disease, indicate that two essential long-chain polyunsaturated fatty acids, eicosapentaenoic acid and docosahexaenoic acid, confer positive health benefits. These oils belong to the **omega-3 fatty acid** family (also termed *n-3*; the last double bond begins 3 carbons from the end carbon), found primarily in the oils of shellfish and cold-water herring, sardines, and mackerel and sea mammals. Regular intake of fish (minimum 2 servings weekly) and fish oil benefits the blood lipid profile, particularly plasma triacylglycerols,[52]

overall heart disease risk and mortality rate (chance of ventricular fibrillation and sudden death),[1,2,19,22,39,40,55] Alzheimer's disease, inflammatory disease risk,[15] and (for smokers) the risk of contracting chronic obstructive pulmonary disease.[84] One proposed mechanism for heart attack protection asserts that fish oil helps to prevent blood clot formation on arterial walls. It also may inhibit the growth of atherosclerotic plaques, reduce pulse pressure and total vascular resistance (increase arterial compliance), and stimulate endothelial-derived nitric oxide (see Chapter 16) to facilitate myocardial perfusion.[73]

Compound Lipids

Compound lipids, triacylglycerol components combined with other chemicals, represent about 10% of the body's total fat. One group of modified triacylglycerols, the **phospholipids**, contains one or more fatty acid molecules joined with a phosphorus-containing group and one of several nitrogen-containing molecules. Phospholipids have a hydrophilic (attracted to water) head and hydrophobic (avoiding water) tail, making these substances self assemble in water into a bilayer. These lipids form in all cells, although the liver synthesizes most of them. Phospholipids interact with both water and lipid to modulate fluid movement across cell membranes. Phospholipids also maintain the structural integrity of the cell, play an important role in blood clotting, and provide structural integrity to the insulating sheath that surrounds nerve fibers

Other compound lipids include **glycolipids** (fatty acids bound with carbohydrate and nitrogen) and water-soluble **lipoproteins** (protein spheres formed primarily in the liver when a protein molecule joins with either triacylglycerols or phospholipids). *Lipoproteins provide the major avenue for transporting lipids in the blood.* If blood lipids did not bind to protein, they literally would float to the top like cream in nonhomogenized fresh milk, instead of circulating throughout the vascular system.

High-Density and Low-Density Lipoproteins

Lipoproteins can be categorized into types according to their size and density and whether they carry cholesterol or triacylglycerol. FIGURE 1.14 illustrates the general dynamics of cholesterol and lipoproteins in the body, including their transport among the small intestine, liver, and peripheral tissues. Four types of lipoproteins exist on the basis of their gravitational density. **Chylomicrons** form when emulsified lipid droplets (including long-chain triacylglycerols, phospholipids, and FFAs) leave the intestine and enter the lymphatic vessels. Normally, the liver metabolizes chylomicrons and sends them for storage in adipose tissue. Chylomicrons also transport the fat-soluble vitamins A, D, E, and K.

The liver and small intestine produce **high-density lipoprotein (HDL)**, which contains the highest percentage of protein (about 50%) and the least total lipid (about 20%) and cholesterol (about 20%) of the lipoproteins. Degradation in the

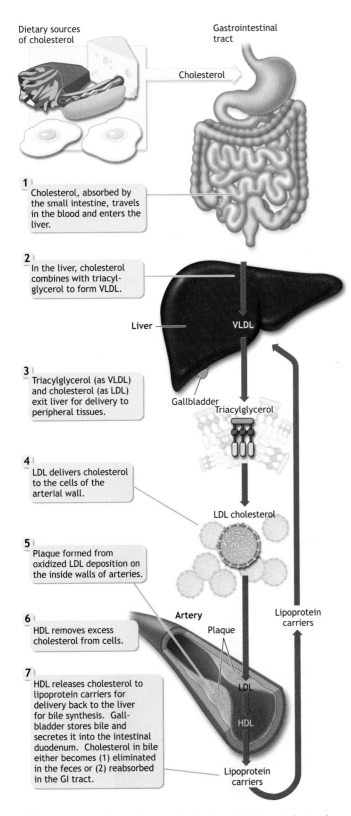

Dietary sources of cholesterol

Gastrointestinal tract

Cholesterol

1 Cholesterol, absorbed by the small intestine, travels in the blood and enters the liver.

2 In the liver, cholesterol combines with triacylglycerol to form VLDL.

Liver

VLDL

3 Triacylglycerol (as VLDL) and cholesterol (as LDL) exit liver for delivery to peripheral tissues.

Gallbladder

Triacylglycerol

4 LDL delivers cholesterol to the cells of the arterial wall.

LDL cholesterol

5 Plaque formed from oxidized LDL deposition on the inside walls of arteries.

6 HDL removes excess cholesterol from cells.

Artery

Plaque

Lipoprotein carriers

LDL

7 HDL releases cholesterol to lipoprotein carriers for delivery back to the liver for bile synthesis. Gallbladder stores bile and secretes it into the intestinal duodenum. Cholesterol in bile either becomes (1) eliminated in the feces or (2) reabsorbed in the GI tract.

HDL

Lipoprotein carriers

Figure 1.14 General interaction between dietary cholesterol and lipoproteins and their transport among the small intestine, liver, and peripheral tissues.

liver of a **very low-density lipoprotein** (**VLDL**) produces a **low-density lipoprotein** (**LDL**). VLDLs formed in the liver from fats, carbohydrates, alcohol, and cholesterol contain the highest percentage of lipid (95%), of which about 60% consists of triacylglycerol. VLDLs transport triacylglycerols to muscle and adipose tissue. Under the action of **lipoprotein lipase**, the VLDL molecule becomes a denser LDL molecule because it then contains fewer lipids. LDLs and VLDLs have the most lipid and fewest protein components.

"Bad" Cholesterol. Among the lipoproteins, LDL, which normally carries from 60 to 80% of the total serum cholesterol, has the greatest affinity for cells of the arterial wall. LDL delivers cholesterol to arterial tissue where the LDL particles are (1) oxidized to alter their physiochemical properties and (2) taken up by macrophages inside the arterial wall to initiate atherosclerotic plaque development. LDL oxidation ultimately contributes to smooth muscle cell proliferation and other unfavorable cellular changes that damage and narrow arteries.[88] A sedentary lifestyle, cigarette smoking, visceral fat accumulation, and a diet high in cholesterol and saturated fatty acids raise serum LDL concentration.

"Good" Cholesterol. Unlike LDL, HDL protects against heart disease. HDL acts as a scavenger in the **reverse transport of cholesterol** by removing it from the arterial wall and delivering it to the liver for incorporation into bile and subsequent excretion via the intestinal tract.

The amount of LDL and HDL and their specific ratios (e.g., HDL ÷ total cholesterol; LDL ÷ HDL) and subfractions provide more meaningful indicators of coronary artery disease risk than total cholesterol. Regular aerobic exercise and abstinence from cigarette smoking significantly increase HDL, lower LDL, and favorably alter the LDL:HDL ratio.[48,56,87,103] We discuss these effects more fully in Chapter 31. An online computer program calculates the risk and the appropriate cholesterol levels for adults (www.nhlbi.nih.gov/guidelines/cholesterol/index.htm).

Derived Lipids

Simple and compound lipids form **derived lipids**. **Cholesterol**, the most widely known derived lipid, exists *only* in animal tissue. Cholesterol does not contain fatty acids; instead it shares some of lipid's physical and chemical characteristics. From a dietary viewpoint, cholesterol classifies as a lipid. Cholesterol, widespread in the plasma membrane of all cells, originates either through the diet (*exogenous cholesterol*) or through cellular synthesis (*endogenous cholesterol*). Even with a "cholesterol-free" diet, endogenous daily cholesterol synthesis varies between 0.5 and 2.0 g. More endogenous cholesterol forms with a diet high in saturated fatty acids and *trans*-fatty acids, which facilitate LDL cholesterol synthesis in the liver.[21] The liver synthesizes about 70% of the body's cholesterol, but other tissues—including the walls of the arteries and intestines—also construct this compound. Endogenous cholesterol synthesis usually meets the body's needs; hence, severely reducing cholesterol intake, except in pregnant women and infants, probably has negligible health effects.

Functions of Cholesterol

Cholesterol participates in many bodily functions, including building plasma membranes and serving as a precursor in synthesizing vitamin D, adrenal gland hormones, and the sex hormones estrogen, androgen, and progesterone. Cholesterol furnishes a key component for the synthesis of bile (emulsifies lipids during digestion) and plays a crucial role in forming tissues, organs, and body structures during fetal development.

Egg yolk provides a rich source of cholesterol (average of about 213 mg per egg), as are red meats and organ meats (liver, kidney, and brains). Shellfish (particularly shrimp) and dairy products (ice cream, cream cheese, butter, and whole milk) contain relatively large amounts of cholesterol. *Foods of plant origin contain no cholesterol.* FIGURE 1.15 lists the cholesterol contents of different foods.

Cholesterol and Coronary Heart Disease Risk

Powerful predictors of increased risk for coronary artery disease include high levels of total serum cholesterol and the cholesterol-rich LDL molecule. These become particularly potent risks when combined with other risk factors of cigarette smoking, physical inactivity, excess body fat, and untreated hypertension. Patients with existing heart disease improve coronary blood flow (thus reducing myocardial ischemia during daily life) within 6 months by aggressively using drug and diet therapy that lower total blood cholesterol and LDL cholesterol. For example, statin can reduce cholesterol by up to $60 \text{ mg} \cdot \text{dL}^{-1}$ with the drug Lipitor significantly slowing disease progression.[3]

In "susceptible" individuals, a dietary cholesterol excess eventually produces **atherosclerosis**, a degenerative process that forms cholesterol-rich deposits (**plaque**) on the inner lining of the medium and larger arteries, causing them to narrow and eventually close. Reducing saturated fatty acid and cholesterol intake generally lowers serum cholesterol, although for most people the effect remains modest.[26,100] Similarly, in-

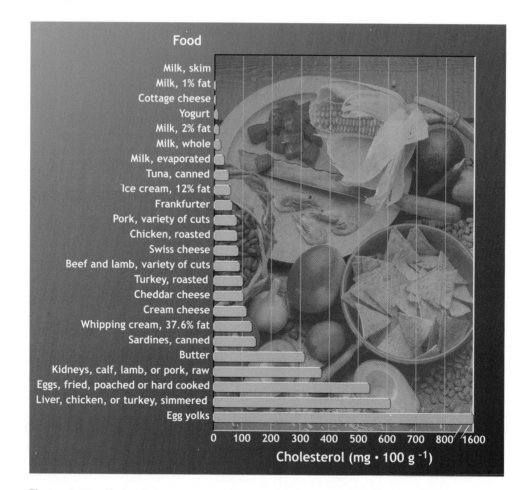

Figure 1.15   Cholesterol content of representative foods in the diet. (Data from Food Composition Tables, United States Department of Agriculture.)

creasing dietary intake of monounsaturated and polyunsaturated fatty acids lowers blood cholesterol, particularly LDL cholesterol.[31,80] Chapter 31 presents specific recommended values for "desirable," "borderline," and "undesirable" plasma lipid and lipoprotein levels.

RECOMMENDED DIETARY LIPID INTAKE

Recommendations for dietary lipid intake for physically active individuals generally follow prudent health-related recommendations for the general population. Dietary lipid represents between 34 and 38% of total caloric intake in the United States, or about 50 kg of lipid consumed per person each year. No firm standards for optimal lipid intake exist. Rather than providing a precise number for daily cholesterol intake, the American Heart Association (AHA; www.americanheart.org) encourages Americans to focus more on replacing high-fat foods with fruits, vegetables, unrefined whole grains, fat-free and low-fat dairy products, fish, poultry, and lean meat.[47] Other new components of the AHA guidelines include a focus on weight control and addition of two weekly servings of fish high in omega-3 fatty acids. The American Cancer Society (www.cancer.org) advocates a diet that contains only 20% of total calories from lipid to reduce risk of cancers of the colon and rectum, prostate, endometrium, and perhaps breast. More drastic lowering of total dietary fat intake toward the 10% level may produce even more pronounced cholesterol-lowering effects, accompanied by clinical improvement for patients with established coronary heart disease.[75]

The AHA has recommended a cholesterol intake of no more than 300 mg (0.01 oz) daily, limiting intake to 100 mg per 1000 calories of food consumed. The current main sources of dietary cholesterol include the same animal food sources rich in saturated fatty acids. Curtailing intake of these foods reduces preformed cholesterol intake and, more importantly, reduces intake of fatty acids known to stimulate endogenous cholesterol synthesis.

ROLE OF LIPID IN THE BODY

Important functions of lipids in the body include:

- Energy source and reserve
- Protection of vital organs
- Thermal insulation
- Vitamin carrier and hunger suppressor

Energy Source and Reserve

Fat constitutes the ideal cellular fuel because each molecule (1) carries a large quantity of energy per unit weight, (2) transports and stores easily, and (3) provides a ready source of energy. Fat provides as much as 80 to 90% of the energy requirement of a well-nourished individual at rest. One gram of pure lipid contains about 9 kCal (38 kJ) of energy, more than *twice* the energy available to the body from equal quantities of carbohydrate or protein. Recall that the synthesis of a tria-

cylglycerol molecule from glycerol and three fatty acid molecules produces three water molecules. In contrast, when glycogen forms from glucose, each gram of glycogen stores 2.7 g of water. *Fat exists as a relatively water-free, concentrated fuel, whereas glycogen remains hydrated and heavy relative to its energy content.*

INTEGRATIVE QUESTION

What benefit derives from storing carbohydrate and lipid within muscle cells and specific tissue depots for selective use under diverse exercise conditions?

For young adults, approximately 15% of the body mass of males and 25% of that of females consists of fat. FIGURE 1.16 illustrates the total mass (and energy content) of fat from various sources in an 80-kg man. The potential energy stored in the fat molecules of the adipose tissue translates to about 108,000 kCal (12,000 g body fat × 9.0 kCal · g^{-1}). A run from New York City to Madison, Wisconsin (assuming an energy expenditure of about 100 kCal per mile) would deplete the energy provided from adipose tissue and intramuscular triacylglycerols and a small amount of plasma FFAs. Contrast this with the limited 2000-kCal reserve of stored carbohydrate that would provide energy for only a 20-mile run. Viewed from a different perspective, the body's energy reserves from carbohydrate could power high-intensity running for about 1.6 hours, while exercise would continue for about 120 hours using the body's fat reserves! Fat used as a fuel also "spares" protein to carry out its important functions of tissue synthesis and repair.

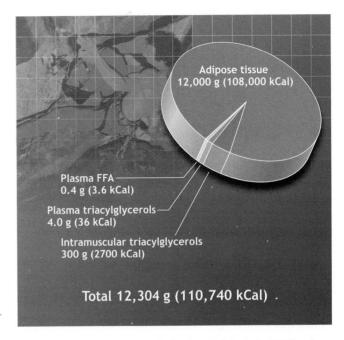

Figure 1.16 Distribution of quantity and energy stored as fat within an average 80-kg man (*FFA*, free fatty acids).

Protection of Vital Organs and Thermal Insulation

Up to 4% of the body's fat protects against trauma to vital organs (e.g., heart, liver, kidneys, spleen, brain, spinal cord). Fat stored just below the skin (subcutaneous fat) provides insulation, permitting individuals to tolerate extremes of cold.[91] This insulatory layer of fat benefits those who regularly engage in cold-related activities such as deep-sea divers, ocean or channel swimmers, or Arctic inhabitants. Excess body fat hinders temperature regulation during heat stress, most notably during sustained exercise in air, when the body's heat production can increase 20 times above resting levels. In this situation, the shield of insulation from subcutaneous fat retards heat flow from the body.

For large football linemen, for example, excess fat storage provides additional cushioning to protect the participant from the sport's normal traumas. Any possible protective benefit, however, must be weighed against the liability imposed by the "dead weight" of excess fat and its impact on exercise energy expenditure, thermal regulation, and subsequent exercise performance.

Vitamin Carrier and Hunger Depressor

Consuming approximately 20 g of dietary fat daily provides a sufficient source and transport medium for the fat-soluble vitamins A, D, E, and K. Thus, severely reducing lipid intake depresses the body's level of these vitamins and ultimately leads to vitamin deficiency. Dietary lipid also facilitates absorption of vitamin A precursors from nonlipid plant sources such as carrots and apricots. It takes about 3.5 hours after ingesting lipids for the stomach to empty them.

FAT DYNAMICS IN EXERCISE

Intracellular and extracellular fat (FFAs, intramuscular triacylglycerols, and circulating plasma triacylglycerols bound to lipoproteins as VLDL and chylomicrons) supply between 30 and 80% of the energy for physical activity, depending on nutritional and fitness status and exercise intensity and duration.[7,63,104,105] Increased blood flow through adipose tissue with exercise increases the release of FFAs for delivery to and use by muscle. The quantity of fat used for energy in light and moderate exercise is three times that used in resting conditions. With more intense exercise (greater percentage of aerobic capacity), adipose tissue release of FFAs fails to increase much above resting levels, which leads to a decrease in plasma FFAs. This in turn stimulates increased muscle glycogen use[82] and concurrently increases intramuscular triacylglycerol oxidation (see Fig. 1.20). The energy contribution from intramuscular triacylglycerols probably ranges between 15 and 35%, with endurance-trained athletes catabolizing the largest quantity and a substantial impairment in use among the obese and/or type 2 diabetics.[44,46,95] Long-term consumption of a high-fat diet induces enzymatic adaptations that enhance fat oxidation during submaximal exercise.[53,71] However, this adaptation does not translate to improved exercise performance.

Fatty acids released from triacylglycerol storage sites and delivered to muscle as FFAs and intramuscular triacylglycerols provide the major energy for light to moderate exercise. The start of exercise produces a transient initial drop in plasma FFA concentration because of increased FFA uptake by active muscles. An increased FFA release from adipose tissue follows (with concomitant suppression of triacylglycerol formation) owing to (1) hormonal stimulation by the sympathetic nervous system and (2) a decrease in plasma insulin levels. During moderate exercise, approximately equal amounts of carbohydrate and fat supply energy. When exercise continues for an hour or more, fat catabolism gradually supplies a greater percentage of energy; this coincides with the progression of glycogen depletion.

Carbohydrate availability also influences fat use for energy. With adequate glycogen reserves, carbohydrate becomes the preferred fuel during high-intensity aerobic exercise, owing to its more rapid rate of catabolism. Toward the end of prolonged exercise, when glycogen reserves become nearly depleted, fat (mainly as circulating FFAs) supplies up to 80% of the total energy requirement. FIGURE 1.17 shows this phenomenon, observed in the mid-1930s, for a subject who exercised continuously for 6 hours. Carbohydrate combustion (reflected by the RQ [respiratory quotient]; see Chapter 8) steadily de-

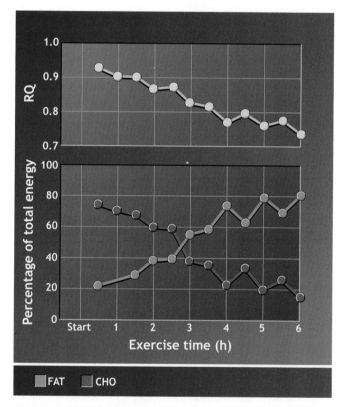

Figure 1.17 Classic study in 1934 showing the relationship between respiratory quotient (RQ) and substrate use during long-duration, submaximal exercise. *Top.* Progressive reduction in RQ at an oxygen consumption of 2.36 L · min⁻¹ during 6 hours of continuous exercise. *Bottom.* Percentage of energy derived from carbohydrate and fat (1 kCal = 4.2 kJ). (Modified from Edwards HT, et al. Metabolic rate, blood sugar and utilization of carbohydrate. Am J Physiol 1934;108:203.)

clined during exercise, with an associated increase in fat use. Toward the end of exercise, 84% of the total energy for exercise came from fat breakdown! This experiment, conducted more than 70 years ago, illustrates fat oxidation's important role as an energy substrate during extended exercise with glycogen depletion.

The increase in fat catabolism during prolonged exercise probably results from a small drop in blood sugar and a decrease in insulin (a potent inhibitor of lipolysis), with a corresponding increase in glucagon output by the pancreas. Such responses ultimately reduce glucose catabolism and its potential inhibitory effect on long-chain fatty acid breakdown, further stimulating FFA liberation for energy. FIGURE 1.18 shows that FFA uptake by active muscle rises during hours 1 and 4 of moderate exercise. In the first hour, fat (including intramuscular fat) supplied about 50% of the energy; by the third hour, fat contributed up to 70% of the total energy requirement. *With greater dependence on fat catabolism (e.g., with carbohydrate depletion), high-intensity exercise decreases to a level governed by the body's capacity to mobilize and oxidize fat.*

Exercise intensity governs fat's contribution to the metabolic mixture.[81,93,97] FIGURE 1.19 illustrates the dynamics of fat use by trained men who exercised between 25 and 85% of their maximum aerobic metabolism. During light-to-mild exercise ($\leq$40% of maximum), fat provided the main energy source, predominantly as plasma FFAs from adipose tissue depots. Increased exercise intensity produced an eventual *crossover* in the balance of fuel use—total energy from fat breakdown (all sources) remained essentially unchanged, but

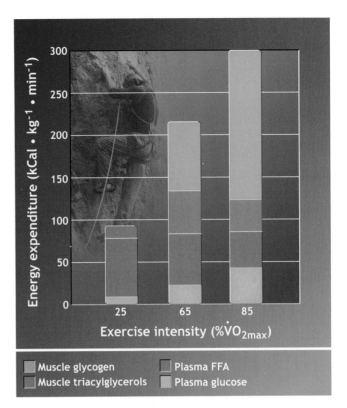

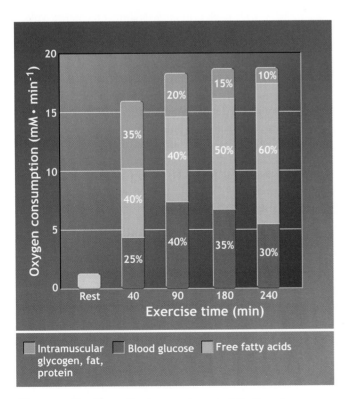

Figure 1.18 Generalized percentage contribution of macronutrient catabolism in relation to oxygen consumption of the leg muscles during prolonged exercise.

Figure 1.19 Steady-state substrate use calculated using three isotopes and indirect calorimetry in trained men performing cycle ergometer exercise at 25, 65, and 85% of $\dot{V}O_{2max}$. As exercise intensity increases, absolute use of glucose and muscle glycogen increases, while muscle triacylglycerol and plasma FFA use decreases. (From Romijn JA, et al. Regulation of endogenous fat and carbohydrate metabolism in relation to exercise intensity and duration. Am J Physiol 1993;265:E380.)

more intense exercise required added energy from blood glucose and muscle glycogen. Total energy from fats during exercise at 85% of maximum did not differ from exercise at 25%. *Such data highlight the major role that carbohydrate, primarily muscle glycogen, plays as a preferential fuel for high-intensity aerobic exercise.*

Exercise Training and Fat Use

Regular aerobic exercise profoundly improves long-chain fatty acid oxidation, particularly from triacylglycerols within active muscle during mild- to moderate-intensity exercise.[33,43,66,72] FIGURE 1.20 illustrates the contribution of various energy substrates during 2 hours of submaximal exercise in the trained and untrained state. For a total exercise energy expenditure of about 1000 kCal, intramuscular triacylglycerol combustion supplied 25% of total energy expenditure before training; this increased to more than 40% following training. Energy from plasma FFA oxidation decreased from 18% pretraining to about 15% posttraining. Biopsy samples revealed a 41% reduction in muscle glycogen combustion in the trained state, which accounted for the overall decrease in total energy from all carbohydrate fuel sources (58% pretraining to 38% posttraining). The important point concerns the greater uptake

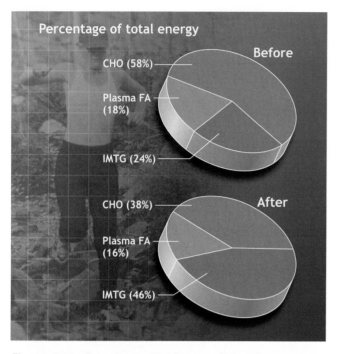

Percentage of total energy

CHO (58%) — Before

Plasma FA (18%)

IMTG (24%)

CHO (38%) — After

Plasma FA (16%)

IMTG (46%)

Figure 1.20 Percentage of total energy derived from carbohydrate *(CHO)*, intramuscular triacylglycerol *(IMTG)*, and plasma fatty acid *(FA)* fuel sources during prolonged exercise (8.3 kCal · min⁻¹) before and after endurance training. (From Martin WH III, et al. Effect of endurance training on plasma free fatty acid turnover and oxidation during exercise. Am J Physiol 1993;265:E708.)

of FFAs and concurrent conservation of glycogen reserves by the trained than by untrained limbs at the same moderate absolute exercise level. These training-induced changes in substrate metabolism in exercise may result from:

- Facilitated fatty acid mobilization from adipose tissue through increased rate of lipolysis within adipocytes
- Proliferation of capillaries in trained muscle to increase the total number and density of these microvessels for energy substrate delivery
- Improved transport of FFAs through the muscle fiber's plasma membrane
- Increased fatty acid transport within the muscle cell, mediated by carnitine and carnitine acyltransferase
- Increased size and number of mitochondria
- Increased quantity of enzymes involved in β-oxidation, citric acid cycle metabolism, and electron-transport chain within specifically trained muscle fibers
- Maintenance of cellular integrity and function, which enhances endurance performance regardless of conservation of glycogen reserves

Enhanced responsiveness of adipocytes to lipolysis allows endurance athletes to exercise at a higher absolute submaximal exercise level before experiencing the fatiguing effects of glycogen depletion. Improved capacity for fat oxidation does *not* sustain the level of aerobic metabolism generated when oxidizing glycogen for energy. Consequently,

near-maximal sustained aerobic effort in well-nourished endurance athletes still requires almost total reliance on oxidation of stored glycogen.[7]

INTEGRATIVE QUESTION

Explain why a high level of daily physical activity requires regular carbohydrate intake. Additionally, give two "nonexercise" benefits from a diet rich in foods that contain unrefined, complex carbohydrates.

Summary

1. Lipids contain carbon, hydrogen, and oxygen atoms, but with a higher ratio of hydrogen to oxygen. The lipid stearin has the formula $C_{57}H_{110}O_6$. Lipid molecules consist of 1 glycerol molecule and 3 fatty acid molecules.
2. Lipids, synthesized by plants and animals, classify into one of three groups: simple lipids (glycerol plus three fatty acids), compound lipids (phospholipids, glycolipids, and lipoproteins) composed of simple lipids combined with other chemicals, and derived lipids such as cholesterol, synthesized from simple and compound lipids.
3. Saturated fatty acids contain as many hydrogen atoms as chemically possible; saturated describes this molecule with respect to hydrogen. Saturated fatty acids exist primarily in animal meat, egg yolk, dairy fats, and cheese. A large saturated fatty acid intake elevates blood cholesterol concentration and promotes coronary heart disease.
4. Unsaturated fatty acids contain fewer hydrogen atoms attached to the carbon chain. Unlike saturated fatty acids, double bonds connect carbon atoms; these fatty acids are either monounsaturated or polyunsaturated with respect to hydrogen. Increasing the diet's proportion of unsaturated fatty acids protects against coronary heart disease.
5. Lowering blood cholesterol, especially that carried by LDL cholesterol, provides significant heart disease protection.
6. Dietary lipid provides between 34 and 38% of total caloric intake. Prudent recommendations suggest a level of 30% or less for dietary lipid, of which 70 to 80% should consist of unsaturated fatty acids.
7. Lipids provide the largest nutrient store of potential energy for biologic work. They also protect vital organs, provide insulation from the cold, and transport the fat-soluble vitamins A, D, E, and K.
8. Fat contributes 50 to 70% of the energy requirement during light and moderate exercise. Stored fat (intramuscular and derived from adipocytes) plays an increasingly important role during prolonged exercise. Fatty acid molecules (mainly circulating

FFAs) provide more than 80% of the exercise energy requirements.

9. Carbohydrate depletion reduces exercise intensity to a level determined by the body's ability to mobilize and oxidize fatty acids.

10. Aerobic training increases long-chain fatty acid oxidation, primarily fatty acids from triacylglycerols within active muscle, during mild- to moderate-intensity exercise.

11. Enhanced fat oxidation with training spares glycogen; this allows trained individuals to exercise at a higher absolute level of submaximal exercise before experiencing the fatiguing effects of glycogen depletion.

PART 3 • *Proteins*

THE NATURE OF PROTEINS

Combinations of linked amino acids form proteins. An average-sized adult contains between 10 and 12 kg of protein, with the largest quantity (6 to 8 kg or 60 to 75% of all proteins) located within skeletal muscle. Additionally, approximately 210 g of amino acids exist in free form, largely as glutamine, a key amino acid with functions that include serving as fuel for immune system cells. Humans typically ingest about 10 to 15% of their total calories as protein. During digestion, protein hydrolyzes to its amino acid constituents for absorption by the small intestine. The protein content of most adults remains remarkably stable, and no amino acid "reserves" exist in the body. Amino acids not used to synthesize protein or other compounds (e.g., hormones) or for energy metabolism provide substrate for gluconeogenesis or convert to triacylglycerol for storage in adipocytes.

Structurally, proteins (from the Greek word meaning "of prime importance") resemble carbohydrates and lipids because they contain atoms of carbon, oxygen, and hydrogen. Protein molecules also contain about 16% nitrogen, along with sulfur and occasionally phosphorus, cobalt, and iron. Just as glycogen forms from many simple glucose subunits linked together, the protein molecule polymerizes from its **amino acid** "building-block" constituents in numerous complex arrays. **Peptide bonds** link amino acids in chains that take on diverse forms and chemical combinations; two joined amino acids produce a **dipeptide**, and linking three amino acids produces a **tripeptide**, and so on. A **polypeptide** chain contains 50 to more than 1000 amino acids. Combination of more than 50 amino acids forms a **protein** of which humans can synthesize about 80,000 different kinds. Single cells contain thousands of different protein molecules; some have a linear configuration, some are folded into complex shapes having three-dimensional properties. In total, approximately 50,000 different protein-containing compounds exist in the body. The biochemical

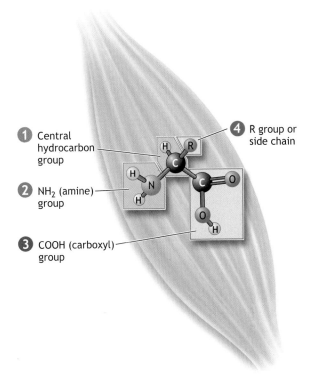

Figure 1.21 lists the following:
1. Central hydrocarbon group
2. NH₂ (amine) group
3. COOH (carboxyl) group
4. R group or side chain

Figure 1.21 Four common features of all amino acids.

functions and properties of each protein depend on the sequence of specific amino acids as discussed more fully in the final chapter, "On the Horizon."

The 20 different amino acids required by the body each have a positively charged **amine group** at one end and a negatively charged **organic acid group** at the other end. The amine group has two hydrogen atoms attached to nitrogen (NH_2), whereas the organic acid group (technically termed a carboxylic acid group) contains 1 carbon atom, 2 oxygen atoms, and 1 hydrogen atom (COOH). The remainder of the amino acid, referred to as the **R group** or **side chain**, takes on a variety of forms. *The R group's specific structure dictates the amino acid's particular characteristics.* FIGURE 1.21 shows the four common features that constitute the general structure of all amino acids. The potential for combining the 20 amino acids produces an almost infinite number of possible proteins, depending on their amino acid combinations. For example, linking just three different amino acids could generate 20^3, or 8000, different proteins.

KINDS OF PROTEIN

The body cannot synthesize eight amino acids (nine in children and some older adults), so one must consume foods containing them. These make up the **essential amino acids**—isoleucine, leucine, lysine, methionine, phenylalanine, threonine, tryptophan, and valine. In addition, the body synthesizes cystine from methionine and tyrosine from phenylalanine. Infants cannot synthesize histidine, and children have reduced capability for synthesizing arginine. The body manufactures the remaining nine **nonessential** amino acids. The term nonessential does not indicate a lack of importance; rather, they are synthesized from other compounds already in the body at a rate that meets demands for normal growth and tissue repair.

Animals and plants manufacture proteins that contain essential amino acids. An amino acid derived from an animal has no health or physiologic advantage over the same amino acid from vegetable origin. Plants synthesize amino acids by incorporating nitrogen from the soil (along with carbon, oxygen, and hydrogen from air and water). In contrast, animals have no broad capability for amino acid synthesis; instead, they consume most of their protein.

Synthesizing a specific protein requires the availability of appropriate amino acids. **Complete proteins**, or higher-quality proteins, come from foods containing all of the essential amino acids in the quantity and correct ratio to maintain nitrogen balance and to allow tissue growth and repair. An **incomplete protein**, or lower-quality protein, lacks one or more essential amino acids. A diet of incomplete protein eventually leads to protein malnutrition, whether or not the food sources contain an adequate amount of energy or protein.

Protein Sources

Sources of complete protein include eggs, milk, meat, fish, and poultry. High-quality protein sources in nutritional supplements include whey, colostrum, casein, and milk and egg proteins. Eggs provide the optimal mixture of essential amino acids among food sources; hence, eggs receive the highest quality rating (100) for comparison with other foods. TABLE 1.3 rates some common sources of protein in the diet. Animal sources provide almost two thirds of dietary protein in the United States; 80 years ago plant and animal sources contributed equally to protein consumption. Reliance on animal sources for dietary protein accounts for the relatively high cholesterol and saturated fatty acid intake in the major industrialized nations.

TABLE 1.3 ■ COMMON SOURCES OF DIETARY PROTEIN RATED FOR PROTEIN QUALITY	
FOOD	**PROTEIN RATING**
Eggs	100
Fish	70
Lean beef	69
Cow's milk	60
Brown rice	57
White rice	56
Soybeans	47
Brewer's hash	45
Whole-grain wheat	44
Peanuts	43
Dry beans	34
White potato	34

The **biologic value** of a food refers to how well it supplies essential amino acids. High-quality protein foods come from animal sources; vegetables (lentils, dried beans and peas, nuts, and cereals) remain incomplete in one or more essential amino acids; thus, their proteins have a lower biologic value. *Eating a variety of grains, fruits, and vegetables supplies all of the essential amino acids.* See "In a Practical Sense," p. 33, for information about reading food labels.

The Vegetarian Approach

True vegetarians, or **vegans**, consume nutrients from only two sources—the plant kingdom and dietary supplements. Vegans constitute less than 1% of the U.S. population, although between 5 and 7% of Americans consider themselves "almost" vegetarians. Nutritional diversity remains the key for these individuals. For example, a vegan diet contains all the essential amino acids if the RDA for protein contains 60% of protein from grain products, 35% from legumes, and 5% from green leafy vegetables. A 70-kg person would satisfy the essential amino acid requirement by consuming about 56 g of protein from approximately 1 1/4 cups of beans, 1/4 cup of seeds or nuts, 4 slices of whole-grain bread, 2 cups of vegetables (1 cup leafy green), and 2 1/2 cups from grain sources (brown rice, oatmeal, and cracked wheat).

An increasing number of competitive and champion athletes consume diets consisting predominately of nutrients from varied plant sources, including some dairy and meat products.[74] Vegetarian athletes often encounter difficulty in planning, selecting, and preparing nutritious meals from only plant sources without relying on supplementation. In contrast to diets that rely heavily on animal sources for protein, well-balanced vegetarian and vegetarian-type diets provide abundant carbohydrate, crucial in intense training. Such diets contain little or no cholesterol, abundant fiber, and rich fruit and vegetable sources of diverse phytochemicals and antioxidant vitamins. A **lactovegetarian diet** provides milk and related products as ice cream, cheese, and yogurt. The lactovegetarian approach minimizes the problem of consuming sufficient high-quality protein and increases the intake of calcium, phosphorus, and vitamin B_{12} (produced by bacteria in the digestive tract of animals). Good meatless sources of iron include fortified ready-to-eat cereals, soybeans, and cooked farina, while cereals and wheat germ contain relatively high zinc levels. Adding an egg to the diet (**ovolactovegetarian diet**) ensures intake of high-quality protein.

FIGURE 1.22 displays the contribution of various food groups to the protein content of the American diet. By far, the greatest protein intake comes from animal sources, with only about 30% from plant sources.

RECOMMENDED DIETARY PROTEIN INTAKE

Despite the beliefs of many coaches, trainers, and athletes, little benefit accrues from consuming excessive protein. *Muscle mass does not increase simply by eating high-protein foods.*

IN A PRACTICAL SENSE

HOW TO READ FOOD LABELS

■ In 1990, the United States Congress passed the Nutrition Labeling and Education Act, which brought sweeping changes to regulations for food labeling. The act (including 1993–1998 updates) aimed to (1) help consumers choose more healthful diets and (2) offer an incentive to food companies to improve the nutritional qualities of their products. All foods except those containing only a few nutrients, such as plain coffee, tea, and spices, now provide consistent nutrition information. Leading health and nutrition authorities have petitioned the FDA (*www.FDA.gov*) to list the grams of added sugars in a serving of the food and to indicate how this amount compares with intakes recommended by other organizations (food labels now only list total sugars—sugars naturally in food plus those added by processing). Currently, the food label must display the following information prominently and in words an average person can understand (the numbers in the figure on p. 34 relate to the numbered information below):

1. Product's common or usual name
2. Name and address of manufacturer, packer, or distributor
3. Net contents for weight, measure, or count
4. All ingredients, listed in descending order of predominance by weight
5. Serving size, number of servings per container, and calorie information
6. Quantities of specified nutrients and food constituents, including total food energy in calories, total fat (g), saturated fat (g), *trans* fat (g), cholesterol (mg), sodium (mg), and total carbohydrate including starch, sugar, fiber (g), and protein (g)
7. Descriptive terms of content
8. Approved health claims stated in terms of the total diet

The figure displays the current food label generated as an outgrowth of regulations from the FDA, the United States Department of Agriculture, and the Nutrition Labeling and Education Act of 1990.

TERMS ON FOOD LABELS

Common Terms and What They Mean
Free: Nutritionally trivial and unlikely to have physiologic consequences; synonyms include "without," "no," and "zero"

High: 20% or more of the Daily Value (DV) for a given nutrient per serving; synonyms include "rich in" or "excellent in"

Less: At least 25% less of a given nutrient or calories than the comparison food

Low: An amount that allows frequent consumption of the food without exceeding the nutrient's DV

Good source: Product provides between 10 and 19% of a given nutrient's DV per serving

Cholesterol Terms
Cholesterol-free: Less than 2 mg per serving and 2 g or less saturated fat per serving

Low cholesterol: 20 mg or less of cholesterol per serving and 2 g or less of saturated fat per serving

Less cholesterol: 25% or less cholesterol per serving and 2 g or less saturated fat per serving

Fat Terms
Extra lean: Less than 5 g of fat, 2 g of saturated fat, and 95 mg of cholesterol per serving and per 100 g of meat, poultry, and seafood

Fat-free: Less than 0.5 g of fat per serving (no added fat or oil)

Lean: Less than 10 g of fat, 4.5 g of saturated fat, and 95 mg of cholesterol per serving and per 100 g of meat, poultry, and seafood

Less fat: 25% or less fat than the comparison food

Low-fat: 3 g or less of fat per serving

Light: 50% or less fat than comparison food (e.g., "50% less fat than our regular cookies")

Less saturated fat: 25% or less saturated fat than the comparison food

Energy Terms
Calorie-free: Fewer than 5 calories per serving

Light: One third fewer calories than the comparison food

Low-calorie: 40 calories or fewer per serving

continued on page 34

Continued

Reduced calorie: At least 25% fewer calories per serving than the comparison food

Fiber Terms
High-fiber: 5 g or more of fiber per serving

Sodium Terms
Sodium-free and salt-free: Less than 5 mg of sodium per serving
Low sodium: 140 mg or less of sodium per serving
Light: Low-calorie food with 50% sodium reduction

Light in sodium: No more than 50% of the sodium of the comparison food
Very low sodium: 35 mg or less of sodium per serving.

From the Nutrition Labeling Act of 1990. Federal Register 58(3), 1993. U.S. Government Printing Office, Superintendent of Documents, Washington, DC, and updated November, 2004 (*www.cfsan.fda.gov/~dms/foodlab.html*). (This site provides a complete description of the new Nutrition Facts label and relevant terms and materials related to the label, including Daily Values [DV].)

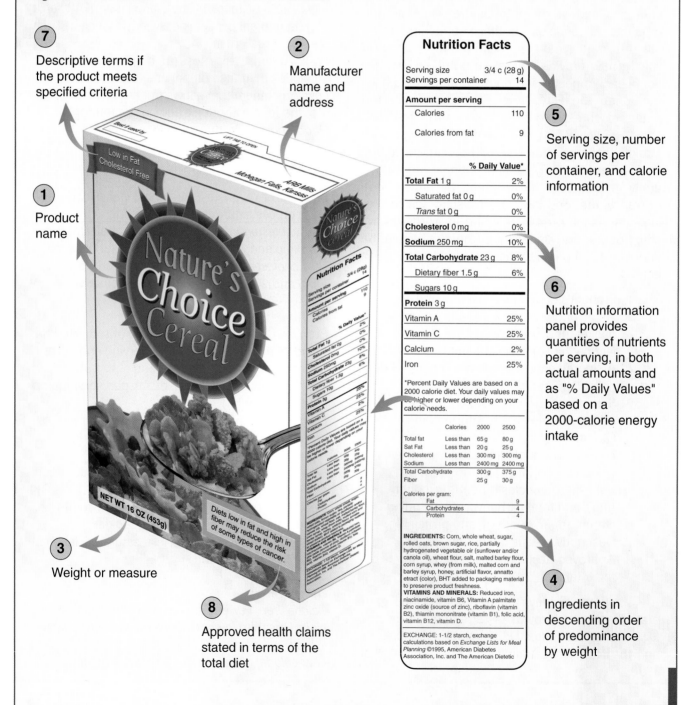

7 Descriptive terms if the product meets specified criteria

2 Manufacturer name and address

1 Product name

3 Weight or measure

8 Approved health claims stated in terms of the total diet

Nutrition Facts

| Serving size | 3/4 c (28 g) |
| Servings per container | 14 |

Amount per serving

| Calories | 110 |
| Calories from fat | 9 |

	% Daily Value*
Total Fat 1 g	2%
Saturated fat 0 g	0%
Trans fat 0 g	0%
Cholesterol 0 mg	0%
Sodium 250 mg	10%
Total Carbohydrate 23 g	8%
Dietary fiber 1.5 g	6%
Sugars 10 g	
Protein 3 g	
Vitamin A	25%
Vitamin C	25%
Calcium	2%
Iron	25%

*Percent Daily Values are based on a 2000 calorie diet. Your daily values may be higher or lower depending on your calorie needs.

		Calories	2000	2500
Total fat	Less than	65 g	80 g
Sat Fat	Less than	20 g	25 g
Cholesterol	Less than	300 mg	300 mg
Sodium	Less than	2400 mg	2400 mg
Total Carbohydrate		300 g	375 g
Fiber		25 g	30 g

Calories per gram:
Fat	9
Carbohydrates	4
Protein	4

INGREDIENTS: Corn, whole wheat, sugar, rolled oats, brown sugar, rice, partially hydrogenated vegetable oir (sunflower and/or canola oil), wheat flour, salt, malted barley flour, corn syrup, whey (from milk), malted corn and barley syrup, honey, artificial flavor, annatto etract (color), BHT added to packaging material to preserve product freshness.
VITAMINS AND MINERALS: Reduced iron, niacinamide, vitamin B6, Vitamin A palmitate zinc oxide (source of zinc), riboflavin (vitamin B2), thiamin mononitrate (vitamin B1), folic acid, vitamin B12, vitamin D.

EXCHANGE: 1-1/2 starch, exchange calculations based on *Exchange Lists for Meal Planning* ©1995, American Diabetes Association, Inc. and The American Dietetic

5 Serving size, number of servings per container, and calorie information

6 Nutrition information panel provides quantities of nutrients per serving, in both actual amounts and as "% Daily Values" based on a 2000-calorie energy intake

4 Ingredients in descending order of predominance by weight

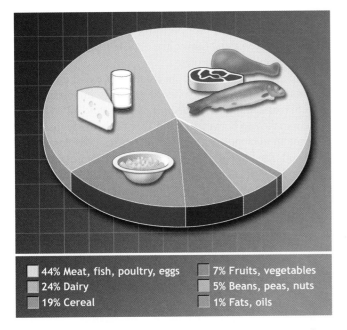

Figure 1.22 Contribution from the major food sources to the protein content of the typical American diet.

- 44% Meat, fish, poultry, eggs
- 24% Dairy
- 19% Cereal
- 7% Fruits, vegetables
- 5% Beans, peas, nuts
- 1% Fats, oils

The diets of endurance- and resistance-trained athletes often exceed two to three times the recommended intake, usually as meat. This occurs because athletes' diets normally emphasize high-protein foods. Furthermore, an athlete's caloric intake and energy output usually surpass those of a sedentary counterpart. If lean tissue synthesis resulted from all of the extra protein consumed by the typical athlete, then muscle mass would increase tremendously. For example, consuming an extra 100 g of protein (400 kCal) daily would translate to a daily 500-g (1.1-lb) increase in muscle mass. This obviously does not happen. Excessive dietary protein is catabolized directly for energy (following deamination) or recycled as components of other molecules, including fat stored in subcutaneous depots. Excessive dietary protein intake above recommended values can trigger harmful side effects, particularly strained liver and kidney function from elimination of urea and other compounds.

The RDA: A Liberal Standard

The **Recommended Dietary Allowance (RDA)** for protein, vitamins, and minerals represents a standard for nutrient intake expressed as a daily average. These guidelines, initially developed in 1943 by the Food and Nutrition Board of the National Research Council/National Academy of Science (www2.nas.edu/iom), have been revised 11 times. RDA levels represent a liberal yet safe excess to prevent nutritional deficiencies in practically all healthy persons. In the 11th edition (1999), RDA recommendations included 19 nutrients, energy intake, and the Estimated Safe and Adequate Daily Dietary Intakes (ESADDIs) for seven additional vitamins and minerals and three electrolytes.[24] The ESADDI recommendation for certain essential micronutrients (e.g., vitamins biotin and pantothenic acid and trace elements copper, manganese, fluoride, selenium, chromium, and molybdenum) required sufficient scientific data to formulate a range of intakes considered adequate and safe, yet insufficient for a precise RDA value. No RDA or ESADDI exists for sodium, potassium, and chlorine; instead, recommendations refer to a minimum requirement for health.

We emphasize that the RDA reflects nutritional needs of a *population* over a long time; one only can assess a specific individual's requirement by laboratory measurements. Malnutrition occurs from cumulative weeks, months, and even years of inadequate nutrient intake. Also, someone who regularly consumes a diet containing nutrients below the RDA standards may not become malnourished. *The RDA represents a probability statement for adequate nutrition; as nutrient intake falls below the RDA, the statistical probability for malnourishment increases for that person and the probability progressively increases with lower nutrient intake.* In Chapter 2, we discuss the **Dietary Reference Intakes** that represent the current set of standards for recommended intakes of nutrients and other food components.[23,92]

TABLE 1.4 lists the protein RDAs for adolescent and adult males and females. On average, 0.83 g of protein per kg body mass represents the recommended daily intake. To determine the protein requirement for men and women ages 18 to 65, multiply body mass in kg by 0.83. Thus, for a 90-kg man, total protein requirement equals 75 g (90 × 0.83). The

---

TABLE 1.4 ▪ PROTEIN RECOMMENDED DIETARY ALLOWANCE (RDA) FOR ADOLESCENT AND ADULT MEN AND WOMEN				
RECOMMENDED AMOUNT	**MEN**		**WOMEN**	
	Adolescent	Adult	Adolescent	Adult
Grams of protein per kg body mass	0.9	0.8	0.9	0.8
Grams of protein per day based on average body mass[a]	59.0	56.0	50.0	44.0

[a] Average body mass based on a "reference" man and woman. For adolescents (ages 14–18), body mass averages 65.8 kg (145 lb) for males and 55.7 kg (123 lb) for females. For adult men, average mass equals 70 kg (154 lb); for adult women, mass averages 56.8 kg (125 lb).

protein RDA holds even for overweight persons; it includes a reserve of about 25% to account for individual differences in the protein requirement for about 98% of the population. Generally, the protein RDA (and the quantity of the required essential amino acids) decreases with age. In contrast, the protein RDA for infants and growing children equals 2.0 to 4.0 g per kg body mass. Pregnant women should increase total daily protein intake by 20 g, and nursing mothers should increase their intake by 10 g. *A 10% increase in the calculated protein requirement, particularly for a vegetarian-type diet, accounts for dietary fiber's effect in reducing the digestibility of many plant-based protein sources* Stress, disease, and injury usually increase the protein requirement.

Debate has focused on the need for a larger protein requirement for athletes. These include still-growing adolescent athletes, athletes involved in resistance training programs that stimulate muscle growth and endurance training programs that increase protein breakdown, and athletes subjected to recurring tissue microtrauma like wrestlers and football players.[12,36,90] Inadequate protein and energy intake can induce muscle protein loss, with concomitant performance deterioration. If athletes require additional protein, this need can be met by increased food intake, which compensates for increased energy expenditure in training. This may not pertain to athletes with poor nutritional habits or those who reduce energy intake to achieve a desired aesthetic "look" or compete at a lower weight-class category to gain a competitive advantage. We present additional information about protein balance in exercise and training in subsequent sections of this chapter and in the "Focus on Research" section, p. 37.

Preparations of Simple Amino Acids

Male and female weight lifters, body builders, and other power athletes regularly consume up to four times the RDA for protein. Much of the excess takes the form of liquids, powders, or pills of "purified" protein. The usual reasons for using protein and amino supplements include stimulation of muscle growth and strength, enhanced energy capacity, and increased growth hormone output.[106] Supplementation often includes proteins "predigested" to simple amino acids through chemical action in the laboratory. Advocates believe the intestinal tract absorbs the simple amino acid molecule more readily to (1) optimize the expected muscle growth brought on by training or (2) improve strength, power, or "vigor" in the short term for a heavy workout. Unfortunately for the athlete, this does not occur. The small intestine readily absorbs amino acids when they exist in more complex di- and tripeptide forms rather than only in simple amino acid form. A concentrated amino acid solution draws water into the intestine. This can precipitate intestinal irritation, cramping, and diarrhea. Provided caloric intake balances energy output by consuming a wide variety of foods, no need exists to consume supplements of protein or amino acids.

ROLE OF PROTEIN IN THE BODY

Blood plasma, visceral tissue, and muscle represent the three major sources of body protein.

No "reservoirs" of this macronutrient exist; all protein contributes to tissue structures or exists as important constituents of metabolic, transport, and hormonal systems. Protein makes up between 12 and 15% of the body mass, but the protein content of different cells varies considerably. A brain cell, for example, consists of about 10% protein, while red blood cells and muscle cells include up to 20% of their total weight as protein. The protein content of skeletal muscle can increase to varying degrees with the systematic application of resistance training.

Amino acids provide the major building blocks for synthesizing tissue. They also incorporate nitrogen into (1) coenzyme electron carriers nicotinamide adenine dinucleotide (NAD) and flavin adenine dinucleotide (FAD) (see Chapter 5), (2) heme components of hemoglobin and myoglobin compounds, (3) catecholamine hormones epinephrine and norepinephrine, and (4) the serotonin neurotransmitter. Amino acids activate vitamins that play a key role in metabolic and physiologic regulation. **Anabolism** refers to tissue-building processes; the amino acid requirement for anabolism can vary considerably. Tissue anabolism accounts for about one third of the protein intake during rapid growth in infancy and childhood. As growth rate declines, so does the percentage of protein retained for anabolic processes. A continual turnover of tissue protein occurs (with no net protein gain or loss) when a person attains a stable body size and growth ceases; normal protein dynamics for adults require adequate protein intake simply to replace the amino acids continually degraded in the turnover process.

Proteins serve as primary constituents for plasma membranes and internal cellular material. As the final chapter, "On the Horizon," discusses in considerable detail, the cell nucleus contains the genetically coded nucleic acid material deoxyribonucleic acid (DNA). DNA replicates itself before the cell divides to ensure that each new cell contains identical genetic material. It also provides the instructions, or "master plan," for the cellular manufacture of all the body's proteins via its control over cytoplasmic ribonucleic acid (RNA). Collagenous structural proteins compose the hair, skin, nails, bones, tendons, and ligaments. Globular proteins make up the nearly 2000 different enzymes that speed up chemical reactions and regulate the catabolism of fats, carbohydrates, and proteins for energy release. Blood plasma also contains the specialized proteins thrombin, fibrin, and fibrinogen required for blood clotting. Within red blood cells, the oxygen-carrying compound hemoglobin contains the large globin protein molecule. Proteins help to regulate the acid–base characteristics of bodily fluids. Buffering neutralizes excess acid metabolites formed during vigorous exercise. The structural proteins actin and myosin play the predominant role in muscle action as they slide past each other as muscle fibers shorten and lengthen during movement.

PROTEIN AND EXERCISE: HOW MUCH IS ENOUGH?

Tarnopolsky MA, et al. Influence of protein intake and training status on nitrogen balance and lean body mass. J Appl Physiol 1988;64:187.

▲ The question of how much dietary protein a physically active person requires to support training and optimize improvements continues to intrigue nutritionists and exercise physiologists. In the mid-1800s, initial studies of human protein needs postulated that muscular contraction destroyed a portion of the muscle's protein content to provide energy for biologic work. Based on this belief, overzealous entrepreneurs and "physical culturists" (the early predecessors of health club fitness trainers) recommended high-protein diets to those doing intense physical labor and exercise training.

In some ways, many modern-day athletes who devote considerable time and effort to training with resistance equipment mimic the older beliefs and practices. They too believe that a significant excess of dietary protein is the most important macronutrient to build bigger muscles and increase strength. They believe resistance training in some way damages or "tears down" a muscle's inherent structure. This drain on body protein would require additional dietary protein (above the 0.83 g of protein per kg body mass supplied by the RDA) for tissue resynthesis to a new, larger, and more powerful state. Many endurance athletes believe arduous training increases protein catabolism (and consequently its dietary requirement) to sustain the energy requirements of exercise. To some extent, both lines of reasoning have merit. The relevant question, however, concerns whether the protein RDA provides sufficient reserve should 4 to 6 hours of daily heavy training add demands for protein synthesis and/or catabolism. While the debate continues and sales of protein supplements soar, researchers have attempted to quantify any added protein requirements of intense exercise training.

In one of the earlier attempts to study this problem systematically, Tarnopolsky and colleagues determined the effects of aerobic and resistance training on nitrogen balance in subjects fed a high-protein (HP) or relatively lower-protein (LP) diet. Subjects were placed into three groups of six men each: sedentary controls (S), elite endurance athletes (EA), and competitive body builders (BB). Ten-day measurements during training included nitrogen balance evaluation (N-Bal; daily dietary nitrogen-intake vs. nitrogen excretion) under HP and LP diets. Quantification of total nitrogen excretion required three sequential 24-hour urine collections, 72-hour fecal collec-

tions, and representative samplings of resting and exercise sweat secretion.

The figure shows N-Bal (g of N per day) related to protein intake for each group receiving HP and LP diets. The *white horizontal line* at the zero point on the *y* axis represents the condition when nitrogen intake equals the body's nitrogen requirement. The three lines that intersect the zero point of nitrogen balance theoretically represent a sufficient protein intake: $0.73 \text{ g} \cdot \text{kg}^{-1} \cdot \text{d}^{-1}$ for the S group, $0.82 \text{ g} \cdot \text{kg}^{-1} \cdot \text{d}^{-1}$ for the BB group, and $1.37 \text{ g} \cdot \text{kg}^{-1} \cdot \text{d}^{-1}$ for the EA group. These findings showed that endurance exercise training increased net protein catabolism and protein requirement not evident for the BB group. The researchers recommended that body builders could reduce their abnormally high protein intakes, while endurance athletes could possibly benefit from increased protein intake above the RDA level.

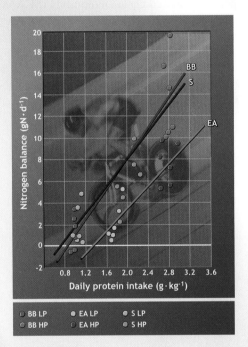

Positive and negative nitrogen balance plotted in relation to daily protein intake of sedentary men *(S)* and groups of elite athletes undergoing either endurance training *(EA)* or resistance training *(BB)*. Subjects consumed either a high-protein *(HP)* diet or a relatively lower-protein *(LP)* diet during the 10-day training period. The *white horizontal line* at zero nitrogen balance represents the point at which nitrogen intake equals excretion (i.e., nitrogen balance). The point at which each of the three lines crosses the "zero line" indicates the necessary daily protein intake for the group.

DYNAMICS OF PROTEIN METABOLISM

Dietary protein's main contribution is supplying amino acids to numerous anabolic processes. In addition, some protein is catabolized for energy. In well-nourished individuals at rest, protein catabolism contributes between 2 and 5% of the body's total energy requirement. During catabolism, protein first degrades into its component amino acids. The amino acid molecule then loses its nitrogen (amine group) in the liver (**deamination**) to form **urea** (H_2NCONH_2). The remaining deaminated amino acid then either converts to a new amino acid, converts to carbohydrate or fat, or catabolizes directly for energy. Urea formed in deamination (including some ammonia) leaves the body in solution as urine. Excessive protein catabolism promotes fluid loss because urea must be dissolved in water for excretion.

Enzymes in muscle facilitate nitrogen removal from certain amino acids (usually α-keto acid or glutamate; FIG. 1.23), with nitrogen passed to other compounds in the reversible reactions of **transamination**. Transamination occurs when an amine group from a donor amino acid transfers to an acceptor acid to form a new amino acid. A specific transferase enzyme accelerates the transamination reaction. In muscle, transamination incorporates branched-chain amino acids (BCAAs) that generate branched-chain ketoacids (mediated by BCAA transferase). This allows amino acid formation from nonnitrogen-carrying organic compounds such as pyruvate formed in metabolism. In both deamination and transamination, the resulting carbon skeleton of the nonnitrogenous amino acid residue undergoes further degradation during energy metabolism.

Fate of Amino Acids After Nitrogen Removal

After deamination, the remaining carbon skeletons of α-keto acids such as pyruvate, oxaloacetate, or α-ketoglutarate follow diverse biochemical routes that include the following:

- *Gluconeogenesis*—18 of the 20 amino acids serve as a source for glucose synthesis

- *Energy source*—the carbon skeletons oxidize for energy because they form intermediates in citric acid cycle metabolism or related molecules
- *Fat synthesis*—all amino acids provide a potential source of acetyl-CoA and thus furnish substrate to synthesize fatty acids

FIGURE 1.24 shows the commonality of the carbon sources from amino acids and the major metabolic paths taken by their deaminated carbon skeletons.

NITROGEN BALANCE

Nitrogen balance occurs when nitrogen intake (protein) equals nitrogen excretion as follows:

$$\text{Nitrogen balance} = N_t - N_u - N_f - N_s = 0$$

where N_t = total nitrogen intake from food; N_u = nitrogen in urine; N_f = nitrogen in feces; and N_s = nitrogen in sweat.

In **positive nitrogen balance**, nitrogen intake exceeds nitrogen excretion with new tissues synthesized by the additional protein. Positive nitrogen balance often occurs in growing children, during pregnancy, in recovery from illness, and during resistance exercise training when muscle cells promote protein synthesis. The body does not develop a protein reserve as it does with fat storage in adipose tissue and to some extent storage of carbohydrate as muscle and liver glycogen. Nevertheless, individuals who consume the recommended protein intake have a higher content of muscle and liver protein than individuals fed a subpar protein diet. Also, research using labeled protein (injecting protein with one or several of its carbon atoms "tagged") indicates that a significant amount of muscle protein is recruited for energy metabolism. In contrast, proteins in neural and connective tissues remain relatively "fixed" as cellular constituents and cannot be mobilized for energy without harming tissue functions.

Greater nitrogen output than intake, or **negative nitrogen balance**, indicates protein use for energy and possible encroachment on amino acids, primarily from skeletal muscle.

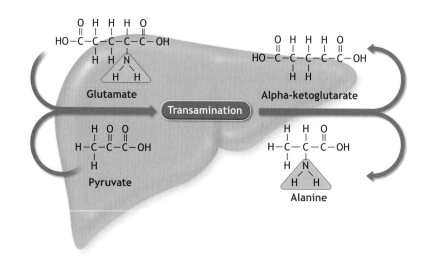

Figure 1.23   Transamination provides for the intramuscular synthesis of amino acids from nonprotein sources. Enzyme action facilitates removal of an amine group from a donor amino acid for transfer to an acceptor, nonnitrogen-containing acid to form a new amino acid.

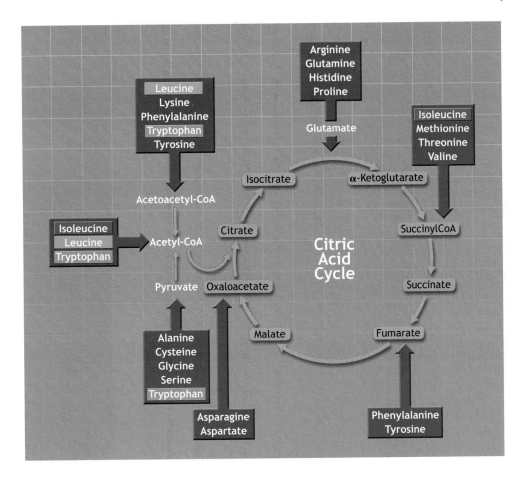

Figure 1.24 Major metabolic pathways for amino acids following removal of the nitrogen group by deamination or transamination. Upon removal of their amine group, all amino acids form reactive citric acid cycle intermediates or related compounds. Some of the larger amino acid molecules (e.g., leucine, tryptophan, and isoleucine—colored *gold*, *green*, and *red*, respectively) generate carbon-containing compounds that enter metabolic pathways at different sites.

Interestingly, a negative nitrogen balance can occur even when protein intake exceeds the recommended standard if the body catabolizes protein because of a lack of other energy nutrients. For example, an individual who participates regularly in heavy training may consume adequate or excess protein but inadequate energy from carbohydrate or lipid. In this scenario, protein becomes a primary energy fuel, which creates a negative protein (nitrogen) balance that produces a loss of lean tissue mass. The protein-sparing role of dietary carbohydrate and lipid previously discussed becomes important during tissue growth periods and the high-energy output and/or tissue synthesis requirements of intensive exercise training. A negative nitrogen balance can occur during diabetes, fever, burns, dieting, growth, steroid administration, and recovery from severe illness. The greatest negative nitrogen balance takes place during starvation. *Starvation diets, or diets with reduced carbohydrate and/or energy, deplete glycogen reserves and trigger a protein deficiency with accompanying loss of lean tissue.*

While protein breakdown increases only modestly with exercise, muscle protein synthesis rises substantially following endurance and resistance-type exercise.[12,77] FIGURE 1.25 shows that muscle protein synthesis (determined from labeled leucine incorporation into muscle) increased between 10 and 80% within 4 hours following termination of aerobic exercise. It then remained elevated for at least 24 hours. Thus, two factors justify reexamining protein intake recommendations for those involved in intense training: (1) increased protein breakdown during long-term exercise and protracted training and (2) increased protein synthesis in recovery from exercise.

 INTEGRATIVE QUESTION

Discuss whether consuming extra protein above the RDA can facilitate muscle enlargement if muscle growth with resistance training occurs primarily from deposition of additional protein within the cell.

PROTEIN DYNAMICS IN EXERCISE AND TRAINING

Current understanding of protein dynamics in exercise comes from studies that expanded the classic method of determining protein breakdown through urea excretion. For example, release of labeled CO_2 from amino acids injected or ingested increases during exercise in proportion to the metabolic rate.[100] As exercise progresses, the concentration of plasma urea also increases, coupled with a dramatic rise in nitrogen excretion in sweat, often without any change in urinary nitrogen excretion.[34,79] These observations account for prior conclusions concerning minimal protein breakdown during endurance exercise because the early studies only measured nitrogen in urine. FIGURE 1.26 shows that the sweat mechanism serves an

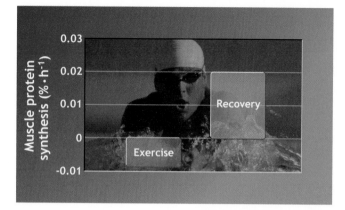

Figure 1.25 Stimulation of human protein synthesis during recovery from aerobic exercise. Values refer to differences between the exercise group and the control group that received the same diet for each time interval. (From Carraro F, et al. Whole body and plasma protein synthesis in exercise and recovery in human subjects. Am J Physiol 1990;258:E821.)

important role in excreting nitrogen from protein breakdown during exercise. Furthermore, urea production may not reflect all aspects of protein breakdown because the oxidation of plasma and intracellular leucine (an essential BCAA) increases significantly during moderate exercise independent of changes in urea production.[10,99]

Figure 1.26 illustrates that protein use for energy reached its highest level during exercise in the glycogen-depleted state. This emphasizes the important role of carbohydrate as a protein sparer and indicates that carbohydrate availability affects the demand on protein "reserves" in exercise. Protein breakdown and gluconeogenesis undoubtedly play a role in endurance exercise (or in frequent high-intensity training) when glycogen reserves diminish.

Increases in protein catabolism during endurance exercise and intense training often mirror the metabolic mixture in acute starvation. With depleted glycogen reserves, gluconeogenesis from carbon skeletons of amino acids largely sustains the liver's glucose output. Augmented protein breakdown reflects the body's attempt to maintain blood glucose for central nervous system functioning. *Athletes in protracted and intense training should consume a high-carbohydrate diet with adequate energy to conserve muscle protein.* The potential for increased protein use for energy and depressed protein synthesis during intense exercise may explain why individuals who resistance train to build muscle size generally refrain from glycogen-depleting, endurance workouts.

Some Modification Required for Recommended Protein Intake

A continuing area of controversy concerns whether the initial increased protein demand when training commences creates a true long-term increase in protein requirement above the RDA. *A definitive answer remains elusive, but protein breakdown above the resting level does occur during intense endurance training and resistance training to a greater degree*

than previously believed. Increased protein catabolism occurs to a greater extent when exercising with low carbohydrate reserves and/or low energy intakes. Unfortunately, research has not pinpointed protein requirements for individuals who train 4 to 6 hours daily by resistance exercise. Their protein needs may average only slightly more than those for sedentary individuals (see "Focus on Research," p. 37). In addition, despite increased protein use for energy during intense training, adaptations may augment the body's efficiency in using dietary protein to enhance amino acid balance. *Until research clarifies this issue, we recommend that athletes who train intensely consume between 1.2 and 1.8 g of protein per kg of body mass daily.* This protein intake falls within the range typically consumed by physically active men and women, thus obviating the need to consume supplementary protein. With adequate protein intake, consuming animal sources of protein does not facilitate muscle strength or size gains with resistance training compared with protein intake from plant sources.[35]

 INTEGRATIVE QUESTION

Outline reasons why exercise physiologists debate the adequacy of the current protein RDA for individuals involved in intense exercise training.

The Alanine–Glucose Cycle

Some proteins do not readily metabolize for energy, yet muscle proteins can provide energy for exercise.[13,32] For example, alanine *indirectly* participates in energy metabolism

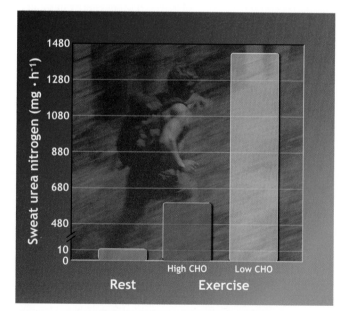

Figure 1.26 Excretion of urea in sweat at rest and during exercise after carbohydrate loading *(High CHO)* and carbohydrate depletion *(Low CHO).* The largest use of protein (as reflected by sweat urea) occurs when glycogen reserves are low. (From Lemon PWR, Nagel F. Effects of exercise on protein and amino acid metabolism. Med Sci Sports Exerc 1981;13:141.)

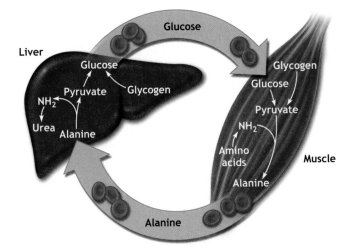

Figure 1.27 The alanine–glucose cycle. Alanine, synthesized in muscle from glucose-derived pyruvate via transamination, enters the blood where the liver converts it to glucose and urea. Glucose release into the blood coincides with its subsequent delivery to the muscle for energy. During exercise, increased production and output of alanine from muscle helps to maintain blood glucose for nervous system and active muscle needs. Exercise training augments hepatic gluconeogenesis.

when the exercise energy demand increases; its release from active leg muscle increases proportionately to the severity of exercise.[102]

Active skeletal muscle synthesizes alanine (during transamination) from the glucose intermediate pyruvate (with nitrogen derived in part from the amino acid leucine). The residual carbon fragment from the amino acid that formed alanine oxidizes for energy within skeletal muscle. The newly formed alanine leaves the muscle and enters the liver for deamination. Alanine's remaining carbon skeleton converts to glucose via gluconeogenesis and enters the blood for delivery to active muscle. FIGURE 1.27 summarizes the sequence of the **alanine–glucose cycle**. After 4 hours of continuous light exercise, the liver's output of alanine-derived glucose accounts for about 45% of the liver's total glucose release. *The alanine–glucose cycle generates from 10 to 15% of the total exercise energy requirement.* Regular exercise training enhances the liver's synthesis of glucose from the carbon skeletons of noncarbohydrate compounds.[89] This facilitates blood glucose homeostasis during prolonged exercise.

Summary

1. Proteins differ chemically from lipids and carbohydrates because they contain nitrogen in addition to sulfur, phosphorus, and iron.
2. Protein forms from subunit amino acids. The body requires 20 different amino acids, each containing an amine group (NH_2) and an organic acid group (carboxylic acid group; COOH). Amino acids contain a side chain (R group) that determines the amino acid's particular chemical characteristics.
3. The number of possible protein structures is enormous because of the tremendous number of combinations of 20 different amino acids.
4. Regular exercise training enhances the liver's synthesis of glucose from the carbon skeletons of noncarbohydrate compounds, particularly amino acids.
5. The body cannot synthesize 8 of the required 20 amino acids; these essential amino acids must be consumed in the diet.
6. All animal and plant cells contain protein. Complete (higher-quality) proteins contain all the essential amino acids; incomplete (lower-quality) proteins represent the others. Examples of higher-quality, complete proteins include animal proteins found in eggs, milk, cheese, meat, fish, and poultry.
7. Physically active people and competitive athletes usually obtain the required nutrients predominantly from a broad array of plant sources.
8. Proteins provide the building blocks for synthesizing cellular material during anabolic processes. Their amino acids also contribute "carbon skeletons" for energy metabolism.
9. The Recommended Dietary Allowance (RDA) represents a liberal yet safe level of excess to meet the nutritional needs of practically all healthy persons. For adults, the protein RDA equals 0.83 g per kg of body mass.
10. Depleting carbohydrate reserves significantly increases protein catabolism during exercise. Athletes who regularly train vigorously must maintain optimal levels of muscle and liver glycogen to minimize deterioration in athletic performance.
11. Protein serves as an energy fuel to a much greater extent than previously believed. This applies particularly to BCAAs, oxidized in skeletal muscle rather than in the liver.
12. Reexamining the current protein RDA seems justified for athletes who engage in intense exercise training. This examination must account for increased protein breakdown during exercise and augmented protein synthesis in recovery. Increasing protein intake to 1.2 to 1.8 g per kg body mass daily seems reasonable.
13. Proteins in neural and connective tissues generally do not participate in energy metabolism. The muscle-derived amino acid alanine plays a key role via gluconeogenesis in supporting carbohydrate availability during prolonged exercise. The alanine—glucose cycle accounts for up to 45% of the liver's release of glucose during long-duration exercise.

References are available on the Student CD and online at http://connection.lww.com/mkk6e.

Vitamins, Minerals, and Water

2

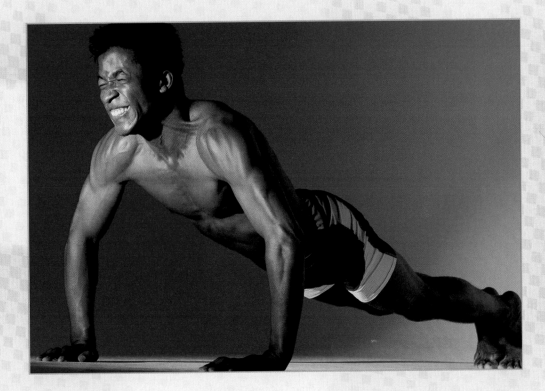

CHAPTER OBJECTIVES

- List one function for each fat- and water-soluble vitamin and potential risks of consuming it in excess

- Discuss how free radicals form in the body, particularly during physical activity, and the mechanisms to defend against oxidative stress

- Respond to those who advocate vitamin supplementation above the Recommended Dietary Allowance (RDA) for individuals involved in heavy exercise training

- Outline three broad roles of minerals in the body

- Define the terms *osteoporosis, exercise-induced anemia,* and *sodium-induced hypertension*

- Describe how regular physical activity affects bone mass and the body's iron stores

- Present a possible explanation for "sports anemia"

- Outline factors related to the "female athlete triad"

- Argue for or against mineral supplementation above the RDA with heavy exercise training

- List water's diverse functions in the body

- Quantify the volumes of the body's three water compartments

- List five predisposing factors to hyponatremia with prolonged exercise

The effective regulation of all metabolic processes requires a delicate blending of food nutrients in the watery medium of the cell. The **micronutrients**—the small quantities of vitamins and minerals—play highly specific roles in facilitating energy transfer and tissue synthesis. For example, over the course of a year, the body requires only about 350 g (12 oz) of vitamins from the 862 kg of food consumed in well-balanced meals by the average adult. With proper nutrition from a variety of food sources, the physically active person or competitive athlete need not consume vitamin and mineral supplements; such practices usually prove physiologically and economically wasteful. Furthermore, consuming some micronutrients in excess poses a significant risk to health and safety.

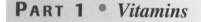

PART 1 • *Vitamins*

THE NATURE OF VITAMINS

The formal discovery of vitamins revealed that they were organic substances needed by the body in minute amounts. Vitamins have no particular chemical structure in common and as such are considered accessory nutrients because they neither supply energy nor contribute substantially to the body's mass. With the exception of vitamin D, the body cannot manufacture vitamins; they must be supplied in the diet or through supplementation.

Some foods contain an abundance of vitamins. For example, the green leaves and roots of plants manufacture vitamins during photosynthesis. Animals obtain vitamins from the plants, seeds, grains, and fruits they eat or from the meat of animals that previously consumed these nutrients. Several vitamins, notably vitamins A and D, niacin, and folic acid, are activated from their inactive precursor or **provitamin** form. Carotenes, the best-known provitamins, are the yellow and yellow-orange pigmented precursors of vitamin A that give color to vegetables (e.g., carrots, squash, corn, and pumpkins) and fruits (e.g., apricots and peaches).

KINDS OF VITAMINS

Thirteen different vitamins have been isolated, analyzed, classified, synthesized, and assigned RDAs. Vitamins are classified as **fat soluble**—vitamins A, D, E, and K—or **water soluble**—vitamin C and the B-complex vitamins: thiamine (B_1), riboflavin (B_2), vitamin B_6 (pyridoxine), niacin (nicotinic acid), pantothenic acid, biotin, folic acid (folacin or folate, its active form in the body), and cobalamin (B_{12}).

Fat-Soluble Vitamins

Fat-soluble vitamins dissolve and remain in the body's fatty tissues, obviating the need to ingest them daily. In fact, years may pass before symptoms emerge denoting a fat-soluble

vitamin deficiency. The liver stores vitamins A and D, whereas vitamin E is distributed throughout the body's fatty tissues. Vitamin K is stored only in small amounts, mainly in the liver. Dietary lipid is the source of fat-soluble vitamins; these vitamins, transported as part of lipoproteins in the lymph, travel to the liver for dispersion to various tissues. Consuming a true "fat-free" diet would certainly accelerate a fat-soluble vitamin insufficiency.

Fat-soluble vitamins should not be consumed in excess without medical supervision. Toxic reactions to excessive fat-soluble vitamin intake occur at a lower multiple of the RDA than with water-soluble vitamins. For example, consuming vitamin A (as retinol but not in carotene form) in amounts not much greater than recommended values (RDA of 700 $\mu g \cdot d^{-1}$ for females and 900 $\mu g \cdot d^{-1}$ for males) precipitates bone fractures later in life.[132] Also, high doses of vitamin A early in pregnancy significantly increase the risk of birth defects in utero. In young children, excessive vitamin A accumulation (called hypervitaminosis A) causes irritability, swelling of bones, weight loss, and dry, itchy skin. In adults, symptoms can include nausea, headache, drowsiness, hair loss, diarrhea, and calcium loss from bones. Discontinuing the high vitamin A intake reverses these symptoms. Regular but excessive vitamin D consumption can cause kidney damage. An "overdose" from vitamins E and K is rare, and intakes above the recommended level yield no known health benefits.

Water-Soluble Vitamins

Water-soluble vitamins act largely as **coenzymes**—small molecules combined with a larger protein compound (apoenzyme) to form an active enzyme that accelerates the interconversion of chemical compounds (see Chapter 5). Coenzymes participate directly in chemical reactions; after the reaction runs its course, coenzymes remain intact and participate in additional reactions. Water-soluble vitamins, like their fat-soluble counterparts, consist of carbon, hydrogen, and oxygen atoms. They also contain nitrogen and metal ions including iron, molybdenum, copper, sulfur, and cobalt.

Water-soluble vitamins disperse in the bodily fluids without being stored to any appreciable extent. If the diet regularly contains less than 50% of the recommended amounts of water-soluble vitamins, marginal deficiencies may develop within 4 weeks. Generally, an excess intake of water-soluble vitamins is voided in the urine. Water-soluble vitamins exert their influence for 8 to 14 hours after ingestion; thereafter, their potency decreases. For maximum benefit, vitamin C supplements should be consumed at least every 12 hours. Some researchers recommend increasing vitamin C intake for healthy persons from the recommended daily value of 75 mg for women and 90 mg for men to 200 mg (not in supplement form but in 2 to 4 daily servings of fruits and 3 to 5 servings of vegetables) to ensure optimal cellular saturation.[117] FIGURE 2.1 illustrates various food sources for vitamin C and its diverse biologic and biochemical functions. These include

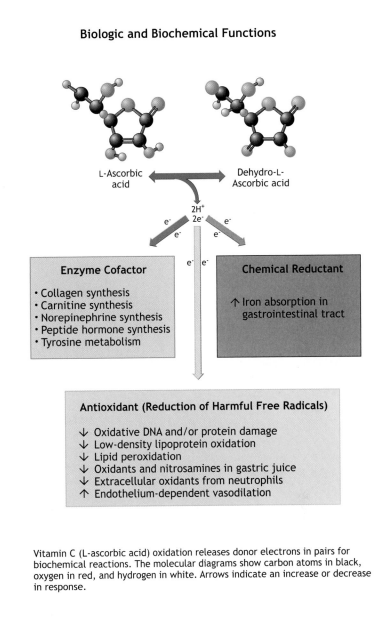

Food Sources

Source (Portion Size)	Vitamin C (mg)
Fruit	
Cantaloupe (1/4 Medium)	60
Fresh grapefruit (1/2 Fruit)	40
Honeydew melon (1/8 Medium)	40
Kiwi (1 Medium)	75
Mango (1 Cup, sliced)	45
Orange (1 Medium)	70
Papaya (1 Cup, cubes)	85
Strawberries (1 Cup, sliced)	95
Tangerines or tangelos (1 Medium)	25
Watermelon (1 Cup)	15
Juice	
Grapefruit (1/2 Cup)	35
Orange (1/2 Cup)	50
Fortified Juice	
Apple (1/2 Cup)	50
Cranberry juice cocktail (1/2 Cup)	45
Grape (1/2 Cup)	120
Vegetables	
Asparagus, cooked (1/2 Cup)	10
Broccoli, cooked (1/2 Cup)	60
Brussels sprouts, cooked (1/2 Cup)	50
Cabbage	
Red, raw, chopped (1/2 Cup)	20
Red, cooked (1/2 Cup)	25
Raw, chopped (1/2 Cup)	10
Cooked (1/2 Cup)	15
Cauliflower, raw or cooked (1/2 Cup)	25
Kale, cooked (1/2 Cup)	55
Mustard greens, cooked (1 Cup)	35
Pepper, red or green	
Raw (1/2 Cup)	65
Cooked (1/2 Cup)	50
Plantains, sliced, cooked (1 Cup)	15
Potato, baked (1 Medium)	25
Snow peas	
Fresh, cooked (1/2 Cup)	40
Frozen, cooked (1/2 Cup)	20
Sweet potato	
Baked (1 Medium)	30
Vacuum can (1 Cup)	50
Canned, syrup-pack (1 Cup)	20
Tomato	
Raw (1/2 Cup)	15
Canned (1/2 Cup)	35
Juice (6 Fluid oz)	35

Biologic and Biochemical Functions

L-Ascorbic acid ⟷ Dehydro-L-Ascorbic acid

$2H^+$ $2e^-$

Enzyme Cofactor

- Collagen synthesis
- Carnitine synthesis
- Norepinephrine synthesis
- Peptide hormone synthesis
- Tyrosine metabolism

Chemical Reductant

↑ Iron absorption in gastrointestinal tract

Antioxidant (Reduction of Harmful Free Radicals)

↓ Oxidative DNA and/or protein damage
↓ Low-density lipoprotein oxidation
↓ Lipid peroxidation
↓ Oxidants and nitrosamines in gastric juice
↓ Extracellular oxidants from neutrophils
↑ Endothelium-dependent vasodilation

Vitamin C (L-ascorbic acid) oxidation releases donor electrons in pairs for biochemical reactions. The molecular diagrams show carbon atoms in black, oxygen in red, and hydrogen in white. Arrows indicate an increase or decrease in response.

Figure 2.1 Various food sources for vitamin C and diverse biologic and biochemical functions. (Modified from Levine M, et al. Criteria and recommendations for vitamin C intake. JAMA 1999;281:1415.)

serving as an electron donor for eight enzymes and as a chemical reducing agent (antioxidant) in intracellular and extracellular reactions.

ROLE OF VITAMINS

FIGURE 2.2 summarizes the major biologic functions of vitamins. Vitamins contain no useful energy for the body; instead they serve as essential links and regulators in metabolic reactions that release energy from food. Vitamins also control tissue synthesis and protect the integrity of the cells' plasma membrane. The water-soluble vitamins play important roles in energy metabolism (TABLES 2.1 and 2.2). For example:

- Vitamin B_1 facilitates the conversion of pyruvate to acetyl-coenzyme A (CoA) in carbohydrate breakdown
- Niacin and vitamin B_2 regulate mitochondrial energy metabolism
- Vitamins B_6 and B_{12} catalyze protein synthesis
- Pantothenic acid, part of CoA, participates in the aerobic breakdown of the carbohydrate, fat, and protein macronutrients

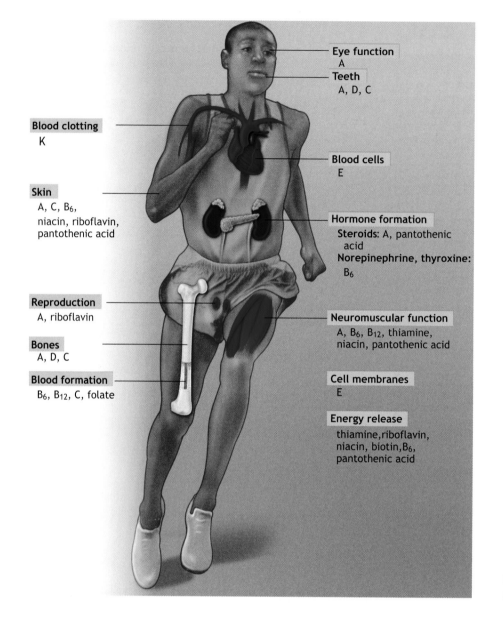

Figure 2.2 Biologic functions of vitamins.

TABLE 2.1 ■ THE MAJOR COENZYMES, THEIR VITAMIN SOURCE AND FUNCTION

NAME	ABBREVIATION	VITAMIN SOURCE	FUNCTION
Biotin		Biotin	CO_2 fixation
Coenzyme A	CoA	Pantothenic acid	Acyl transfer reactions
Flavin adenine dinucleotide	FAD	B_2 (riboflavin)	Oxidation–reduction reactions
Nicotinamide adenine dinucleotide	NAD	Niacin	Oxidation–reduction reactions
Pyridoxal phosphate	PLP	B_6 (pyridoxine)	Amino acid metabolism (transamination)
Tetrahydrofolic acid		Folate	Transfer of single-carbon units
Thiamine pyrophosphate	TPP	B_1 (thiamine)	Aldehyde transfer

Many vitamins function as coenzymes in metabolic reactions. For example, vitamin B_1 (thiamine) is involved in carbohydrate metabolism and citric acid cycle (Krebs cycle). The active coenzyme of thiamine is thiamine diphosphate. Vitamin C is a cofactor in some hydroxylation reactions (e.g., dopamine to noradrenalin), and pantothenic acid is involved in fatty acid synthesis.

TABLE 2.2 ■ FOOD SOURCES, MAJOR BODILY FUNCTIONS, AND SYMPTOMS OF DEFICIENCY OR EXCESS OF THE FAT-SOLUBLE AND WATER-SOLUBLE VITAMINS FOR HEALTHY ADULTS (19–50 YEARS)

VITAMIN	DIETARY SOURCES	MAJOR BODILY FUNCTIONS	DEFICIENCY	EXCESS
Fat-soluble				
Vitamin A (retinol)	Provitamin A (β-carotene) widely distributed in green vegetables; retinol present in milk, butter, cheese, fortified margarine	Constituent of rhodopsin (visual pigment) Maintenance of epithelial tissues; role in mucopolysaccharide synthesis	Xerophthalmia (keratinization of ocular tissue), night blindness, permanent blindness	Headache, vomiting, peeling of skin, anorexia, swelling of long bones
Vitamin D	Cod-liver oil, eggs, dairy products, fortified milk and margarine	Promotes growth and mineralization of bones Increases absorption of calcium	Rickets (bone deformities) in children Osteomalacia in adults	Vomiting, diarrhea, loss of weight, kidney damage
Vitamin E (tocopherol)	Seeds, green leafy vegetables, margarines, shortenings	Functions as an antioxidant to prevent cell damage	Possible anemia	Relatively nontoxic
Vitamin K (phylloquinone)	Green leafy vegetables; small amounts in cereals, fruits, and meats	Important in blood clotting (involved in formation of active prothrombin)	Conditioned deficiencies associated with severe bleeding; internal hemorrhages	Relatively nontoxic Synthetic forms at high doses may cause jaundice
Water-soluble				
Vitamin B$_1$ (thiamine)	Pork, organ meats, whole grains, nuts, legumes, milk, fruits, and vegetables	Coenzyme (thiamine prophosphate) in reactions involving the removal of carbon dioxide	Beriberi (peripheral nerve changes, edema, heart failure)	None reported
Vitamin B$_2$ (riboflavin)	Widely distributed in foods; meats, eggs, milk products, whole-grain and enriched cereal products, wheat germ, green leafy vegetables	Constituent of two flavin nucleotide coenzymes involved in energy metabolism (FAD and FMN)	Reddened lips, cracks at mouth corner (cheilosis), eye lesions	None reported
Niacin (nicotinic acid)	Liver, lean meats, poultry, grains, legumes, peanuts (can be formed from tryptophan)	Constituent of two coenzymes in oxidation reduction reactions (NAD and NADP)	Pellagra (skin and gastrointestinal lesions, nervous mental disorders)	Flushing, burning and tingling around neck, face, and hands
Vitamin B$_6$ (pyridoxine)	Meats, fish, poultry, vegetables, whole grains, cereals, seeds	Coenzyme (pyridoxal phosphate) involved in amino acid and glycogen metabolism	Irritability, convulsions, muscular twitching, dermatitis, kidney stones	None reported
Pantothenic acid	Widely distributed in foods, meat, fish, poultry, milk products, legumes, whole grains	Constituent of coenzyme A, which plays a central role in energy metabolism	Fatigue, sleep disturbances, impaired coordination, nausea	None reported
Folate	Legumes, green vegetables, whole-wheat products, meats, eggs, milk products, liver	Coenzyme (reduced form) involved in transfer of single-carbon units in nucleic acid and amino acid metabolism	Anemia, gastrointestinal disturbances, diarrhea, red tongue	None reported
Vitamin B$_{12}$ (cobalamin)	Muscle meats, fish, eggs, dairy products (absent in plant foods)	Coenzyme involved in transfer of single-carbon units in nucleic acid metabolism	Permicious anemia, neurologic disorders	None reported

continued on page 48

TABLE 2.2 ■ *continued*

VITAMIN	DIETARY SOURCES	MAJOR BODILY FUNCTIONS	DEFICIENCY	EXCESS
Biotin	Legumes, vegetables, meats, liver, egg-yolk, nuts	Coenzymes required for fat synthesis, amino acid metabolism, and glycogen (animal starch) formation	Fatigue, depression, nausea, dermatitis, muscle pain	None reported
Vitamin C (ascorbic acid)	Citrus fruits, tomatoes, green peppers, salad greens	Maintains intercellular matrix of cartilage, bone, and dentine; important in collagen synthesis	Scurvy (degeneration of skin, teeth, blood vessels, epithelial hemorrhages)	Relatively nontoxic Possibility of kidney stones

• Vitamin C acts as a cofactor in enzymatic reactions, as a scavenger of free radicals in antioxidative processes, and as a component in hydroxylation reactions that provide connective tissue stability and wound healing

Vitamins participate repeatedly in metabolic reactions; thus, the vitamin needs of physically active persons do not exceed those of sedentary counterparts.

INTEGRATIVE QUESTION

If vitamins play such an important role in energy release, should athletes "supercharge" with vitamin supplements to enhance exercise performance and training responsiveness?

Table 2.2 lists the major bodily functions, dietary sources, and symptoms of a deficiency or excess for the water-soluble and fat-soluble vitamins. Well-balanced meals provide an adequate quantity of all vitamins, regardless of age and physical activity level. Indeed, individuals who expend considerable energy exercising generally need not consume special foods or supplements that increase vitamin intake above recommended levels. At high levels of daily physical activity, food intake generally increases to sustain the added exercise energy requirements. Additional food through a variety of nutritious meals proportionately increases vitamin and mineral intakes.

Several exceptions exist concerning the possible need for vitamin supplementation because of difficulty obtaining the recommended amounts. First, vitamin C and folic acid in foods usually make up only a small part of most Americans' total caloric intake; the availability of such foods also varies by season. Second, different athletic groups have relatively low intakes of vitamins B_1 and B_6, two vitamins prevalent in fresh fruit, grains, and uncooked or steamed vegetables.[51,176] Individuals on meatless diets should consume a small amount of milk, milk products, or eggs because vitamin B_{12} exists *only* in foods of animal origin. A relatively high daily intake of the B vitamins folate (400 μg) and B_6 (3 mg) reduces a woman's heart attack risk by nearly 50%, in a manner equivalent to quit-

ting smoking, lowering blood cholesterol, or reducing blood pressure.[165] Rich sources of these vitamins include fortified cold cereals, orange juice, spinach and other leafy greens, whole grains, nuts and seeds, bananas, legumes, potatoes, chicken, and fish. The possible protective mechanism of vitamins B_6 and folate may lie in their lowering effects on plasma homocysteine, an amino acid related to increased heart attack risk (see Chapter 31).

DEFINING NUTRIENT NEEDS

Controversy surrounding the RDAs caused the Food and Nutrition Board and scientific nutrition community to reexamine the usefulness of a single standard. This process, begun in 1997, led the National Academies' Institute of Medicine (in cooperation with Canadian scientists) to develop the **Dietary Reference Intakes** (www.nal.usda.gov/fnic/etext/000105. html).

Dietary Reference Intakes

Dietary Reference Intakes (DRIs) represent a radically new and more comprehensive approach to nutritional recommendations for individuals.[210] Think of the DRIs as the umbrella term that encompasses the array of new standards— RDAs, Estimated Average Requirements, Adequate Intakes, and the Tolerable Upper Intake Levels—for nutrient recommendations in planning and assessing diets for healthy persons.

Recommendations encompass not only daily intakes intended for health maintenance but also upper intake levels that reduce the likelihood of harm from nutrient intake excess. The DRIs differ from their predecessor RDAs by focusing more on promoting health maintenance and risk reduction for nutrient-dependent diseases (e.g., heart disease, diabetes, hypertension, osteoporosis, various cancers, and age-related macular degeneration), rather than the traditional criterion of preventing the deficiency diseases scurvy or beriberi. In addition to including values for energy, protein, and the micronutrients, DRIs also provide values for macronutrients and food components of nutritional importance, such as phytochemicals. Whenever possible, nutrient intakes are recommended in four categories instead of one.

Unlike its RDA predecessor, the DRI value also includes recommendations that apply to gender and life stages of growth and development based on age and, when appropriate, pregnancy and lactation. The goal of a complete revision every 5 years as with the RDAs was abandoned, with the new modification of making immediate changes in the DRI as new scientific data become available. The National Academy Press presents up-to-date reports on the DRIs (www.nap.edu/; search for Dietary Reference Intakes).

The following definitions apply to the four different sets of values for the intake of nutrients and food components in the DRIs:

- **Estimated Average Requirement (EAR):** Average level of daily nutrient intake to meet the requirement of one half of the healthy individuals in a particular life stage and gender group. The EAR provides a useful value for determining the prevalence of inadequate nutrient intake by the proportion of the population with intakes below this value.
- **Recommended Dietary Allowance (RDA):** The average daily nutrient intake level sufficient to meet the requirement of nearly 98% of healthy individuals in a particular life-stage and gender group. For most nutrients, this value represents the EAR plus two standard deviations of the requirement.
- **Adequate Intake (AI):** The AI provides an assumed adequate nutritional goal when no RDA exists. It represents a recommended average daily nutrient intake level based on observed or experimentally determined approximations or estimates of nutrient intake by a group (or groups) of apparently healthy persons—used when an RDA cannot be determined. Low risk exists with intakes at or above the AI level.
- **Tolerable Upper Intake Level (UL):** The highest average daily nutrient intake level likely to pose no risk of adverse health effects to almost all individuals in the specified gender and life-stage group of the general population. As intake increases above the UL, the potential risk of adverse effects increases.

The DRI report indicates that fruits and vegetables yield about one half as much vitamin A as previously believed. Thus, individuals who do not eat vitamin A–rich, animal-derived foods should upgrade their intake of carotene-rich fruits and vegetables. The report also sets a daily maximum intake level for vitamin A, in addition to boron, copper, iodine, iron, manganese, molybdenum, nickel, vanadium, and zinc. Specific recommended intakes are provided for vitamins A and K, chromium, copper, iodine, manganese, molybdenum, and zinc. The report concludes that an individual can meet the daily requirement for the nutrients examined without need for additional supplementation. The exception is the mineral iron; most pregnant women need supplements to obtain their increased daily requirement. TABLE 2.3 presents the RDA, AI, and UL values for vitamins.

Antioxidant Role of Vitamins

Most of the oxygen consumed within the mitochondria during energy metabolism combines with hydrogen to produce water. Normally, 2 to 5% of oxygen forms the reactive oxygen- and nitrogen-containing **free radicals** superoxide (O_2^-), hydrogen peroxide (H_2O_2), hydroxyl (OH^-), and nitric oxide ($ONOO^-$) radicals owing to electron "leakage" along the electron transport chain. *A free radical, a highly unstable, chemically reactive molecule or molecular fragment, contains at least one unpaired electron in its outer orbital or valence shell.* These are the same free radicals produced by external heat and ionizing radiation and carried in cigarette smoke, environmental pollutants, and even some medications. Once formed, free radicals interact with other compounds to create new free radical molecules. The new molecules frequently damage the electron-dense cellular components DNA and lipid-rich cell membranes. By contrast, paired electrons represent a far more stable state.

Fortunately, cells possess enzymatic and nonenzymatic mechanisms that work in concert to immediately counter potential oxidative damage from the challenge of chemical and enzymatic mutagens. Antioxidants scavenge the oxygen radicals or chemically eradicate them by reducing oxidized compounds. For example, when O_2^- forms, the enzyme **superoxide dismutase** catalyzes its dismutation to form hydrogen peroxide. This enzyme catalyzes the reaction of two identical molecules to produce two molecules in different states of oxidation as follows:

$$O_2^- + O_2^- \xrightarrow[\text{superoxide dismutase}]{2\,H^+} H_2O_2 + O_2$$

The hydrogen peroxide produced in this reaction breaks down further to water and oxygen in a reaction catalyzed by the widely distributed enzyme catalase as follows:

$$2\,H_2O_2 \xrightarrow[\text{catalase}]{} 2\,H_2O + O_2$$

Protection from Disease

An accumulation of free radicals increases the potential for cellular damage (**oxidative stress**) to many biologically important substances through processes that add oxygen to cellular components. These substances include DNA, proteins, and lipid-containing structures, particularly the polyunsaturated fatty acid–rich bilayer membrane that isolates the cell from noxious toxins and carcinogens. During unchecked oxidative stress, the plasma membrane's fatty acids deteriorate through a chain-reaction series of events termed **lipid peroxidation**. These reactions incorporate abnormal amounts of oxygen into lipids and increase the vulnerability of the cell and its constituents. Free radicals also facilitate peroxidation of low-density lipoprotein (LDL) cholesterol, thus leading to cytotoxicity and enhanced plaque formation in the coronary arteries.[124,200] Oxidative stress ultimately increases the likelihood of cellular deterioration associated with advanced aging, many diseases, and a general decline in central nervous system and immune functions.

TABLE 2.3 ■ DIETARY REFERENCE INTAKES (DRIs): RECOMMENDED VITAMIN INTAKES AND TOLERABLE UPPER INTAKE LEVELS (UL)

RECOMMENDED INTAKES FOR INDIVIDUALS

Life Stage Group	Vitamin A (µg/D)[a]	Vitamin C (mg/D)	Vitamin D (µg/D)[b,c]	Vitamin E (mg/D)[d]	Vitamin K (µg/D)	Thiamin (mg/D)	Riboflavin (mg/D)	Niacin (mg/D)[e]	Vitamin B₆ (mg/D)	Folate (µg/D)[f]	Vitamin B₁₂ (µg/D)	Pantothenic Acid (mg/D)	Biotin (µg/D)	Choline (mg/D)[g]
INFANTS														
0–6 mo	400*	40*	5*	4*	2.0*	0.2*	0.3*	2*	0.1*	65*	0.4*	1.7*	5*	125*
7–12 mo	500*	50*	5*	5*	2.5*	0.3*	0.4*	4*	0.3*	80*	0.5*	1.8*	6*	150*
CHILDREN														
1–3 y	**300**	**15**	5*	**6**	30*	**0.5**	**0.5**	**6**	**0.5**	**150**	**0.9**	2*	8*	200*
4–8 y	**400**	**25**	5*	**7**	55*	**0.6**	**0.6**	**8**	**0.6**	**200**	**1.2**	3*	12*	250*
MALES														
9–13 y	**600**	**45**	5*	**11**	60*	**0.9**	**0.9**	**12**	**1.0**	**300**	**1.8**	4*	20*	375*
14–18 y	**900**	**75**	5*	**15**	75*	**1.2**	**1.3**	**16**	**1.3**	**400**	**2.4**	5*	25*	550*
19–30 y	**900**	**90**	5*	**15**	120*	**1.2**	**1.3**	**16**	**1.3**	**400**	**2.4**	5*	30*	550*
31–50 y	**900**	**90**	5*	**15**	120*	**1.2**	**1.3**	**16**	**1.3**	**400**	**2.4**	5*	30*	550*
51–70 y	**900**	**90**	10*	**15**	120*	**1.2**	**1.3**	**16**	**1.7**	**400**	**2.4**[h]	5*	30*	550*
>70 y	**900**	**90**	15*	**15**	120*	**1.2**	**1.3**	**16**	**1.7**	**400**	**2.4**[h]	5*	30*	550*
FEMALES														
9–13 y	**600**	**45**	5*	**11**	60*	**0.9**	**0.9**	**12**	**1.0**	**300**	**1.8**	4*	20*	375*
14–18 y	**700**	**65**	5*	**15**	75*	**1.0**	**1.0**	**14**	**1.2**	**400**[f]	**2.4**	5*	25*	400*
19–30 y	**700**	**75**	5*	**15**	90*	**1.1**	**1.1**	**14**	**1.3**	**400**[f]	**2.4**	5*	30*	425*
31–50 y	**700**	**75**	5*	**15**	90*	**1.1**	**1.1**	**14**	**1.3**	**400**[f]	**2.4**	5*	30*	425*
51–70 y	**700**	**75**	10*	**15**	90*	**1.1**	**1.1**	**14**	**1.5**	**400**	**2.4**[h]	5*	30*	425*
>70 y	**700**	**75**	15*	**15**	90*	**1.1**	**1.1**	**14**	**1.5**	**400**	**2.4**[h]	5*	30*	425*
PREGNANCY[i,j]														
≤18 y	**750**	**80**	5*	**15**	75*	**1.4**	**1.4**	**18**	**1.9**	**600**[f]	**2.6**	6*	30*	450*
19–30 y	**770**	**85**	5*	**15**	90*	**1.4**	**1.4**	**18**	**1.9**	**600**[f]	**2.6**	6*	30*	450*
31–50 y	**770**	**85**	5*	**15**	90*	**1.4**	**1.4**	**18**	**1.9**	**600**[f]	**2.6**	6*	30*	450*
LACTATION														
≤18 y	**1200**	**115**	5*	**19**	75*	**1.4**	**1.6**	**17**	**2.0**	**500**	**2.8**	7*	35*	550*
19–30 y	**1300**	**120**	5*	**19**	90*	**1.4**	**1.6**	**17**	**2.0**	**500**	**2.8**	7*	35*	550*
31–50 y	**1300**	**120**	5*	**19**	90*	**1.4**	**1.6**	**17**	**2.0**	**500**	**2.8**	7*	35*	550*

NOTE: This table (taken from the DRI reports, see www.nap.edu) presents Recommended Dietary Allowances (RDAs) in **bold type** and Adequate Intakes (AIs) in ordinary type followed by an asterisk (*). RDAs and AIs may both be used as goals for individual intake. RDAs are set to meet the needs of almost all (97 to 98%) individuals in a group. For healthy breastfed infants, the AI is the mean intake. The AI for other life stage and gender groups is believed to cover needs of all individuals in the group, but lack of data or uncertainty in the data prevent being able to specify with confidence the percentage of individuals covered by this intake.

[a]As retinol activity equivalents (RAEs). 1 RAE = 1 µg retinol, 12 µg β-carotene, 24 µg α-carotene, or 24 µg β-cryptoxanthin. To calculate RAEs from REs of provitamin A carotenoids in foods, divide the REs by 2. For preformed vitamin A in foods or supplements and for provitamin A carotenoids in supplements, 1 RE = 1 RAE.

[b]Calciferol. 1 µg calciferol = 40 IU vitamin D.

[c]In the absence of adequate exposure to sunlight.

[d]As α-tocopherol. α-Tocopherol Includes *RRR*-α-tocopherol, the only form of α-tocopherol that occurs naturally in foods, and the 2*R*-stereoisometric forms of α-tocopherol (*RRR-, RSR-, RRS-,* and *RSS*-α-tocopherol) that occur in fortified foods and supplements. It does not include the 2*S*-stereoisomeric forms of α-tocopherol (*SRR-, SSR-, SR-,* and *SSS*-α-tocopherol), also found in fortified foods and supplements.

[e]As niacin equivalents (NE). 1 mg of niacin = 60 mg of tryptophan; 0–6 months = preformed niacin (not NE).

[f]As dietary folate equivalents (DFE). 1 DFE = 1 µg food folate = 0.6 µg of folic acid from fortified food or as a supplement consumed with food = 0.5 µg of a supplement taken on an empty stomach.

[g]Although AIs have been set for choline, there are few data to assess whether a dietary supply of choline is needed at all stages of the life cycle, and it may be that the choline requirement can be met by endogenous synthesis at some of these stages.

[h]Because 10 to 30% of older people may malabsorb food-bound B₁₂, it is advisable for those older than 50 years to meet their RDA mainly by consuming foods fortified with B₁₂ or a supplement containing B₁₂.

[i]In view of evidence linking folate intake with neural tube defects in the fetus, it is recommended that all women capable of becoming pregnant consume 400 µg from supplements or fortified foods in addition to intake of food folate from a varied diet.

[j]It is assumed that women will continue consuming 400 µg from supplements or fortified food until their pregnancy is confirmed and they enter prenatal care, which ordinarily occurs after the end of the periconceptional period—the critical time for formation of the neural tube.

continued on page 51

TABLE 2.3 ■ *continued*

TOLERABLE UPPER INTAKE LEVELS (UL[a])

LIFE STAGE GROUP	VITAMIN A (µG/D)[b]	VITAMIN C (MG/D)	VITAMIN D (MG/D)	VITAMIN E (MG/D)[a,d]	VITAMIN K	THIAMIN	RIBOFLAVIN	NIACIN (MG/D)[d]	VITAMIN B$_6$ (MG/D)[d]	FOLATE (µG/D)[d]	VITAMIN B$_{12}$	PANTOTHENIC ACID	BIOTIN	CHOLINE (G/D)	CAROTENOIDS[e]
INFANTS															
0–6 mo	600	ND[f]	25	ND	ND	ND	ND	ND	ND	ND	ND	ND	ND	ND	ND
7–12 mo	600	ND	25	ND	ND	ND	ND	ND	ND	ND	ND	ND	ND	ND	ND
CHILDREN															
1–3 y	600	400	50	200	ND	ND	ND	10	30	300	ND	ND	ND	1.0	ND
4–8 y	900	650	50	300	ND	ND	ND	15	40	400	ND	ND	ND	1.0	ND
MALES, FEMALES															
9–13 y	1700	1200	50	600	ND	ND	ND	20	60	600	ND	ND	ND	2.0	ND
14–18 y	2800	1800	50	800	ND	ND	ND	30	80	800	ND	ND	ND	3.0	ND
19–70 y	3000	2000	50	1000	ND	ND	ND	35	100	1000	ND	ND	ND	3.5	ND
>70 y	3000	2000	50	1000	ND	ND	ND	35	100	1000	ND	ND	ND	3.5	ND
PREGNANCY[i,j]															
≤18 y	2800	1800	50	800	ND	ND	ND	30	80	800	ND	ND	ND	3.0	ND
19–50 y	3000	2000	50	1000	ND	ND	ND	35	100	1000	ND	ND	ND	3.5	ND
LACTATION															
≤18 y	2800	1800	50	800	ND	ND	ND	30	80	800	ND	ND	ND	3.0	ND
19–50 y	3000	2000	50	1000	ND	ND	ND	35	100	1000	ND	ND	ND	3.5	ND

[a]UL = The maximum level of daily nutrient intake that is likely to pose no risk of adverse effects. Unless otherwise specified, the UL represents total intake from food, water, and supplements. Due to lack of suitable data, ULs could not be established for vitamin K, thiamin, riboflavin, vitamin B$_{12}$, pantothenic acid, biotin, or carotenoids. In the absence of ULs, extra caution may be warranted in consuming levels above recommended intakes.
[b]As preformed vitamin A only.
[c]As α-tocopheral; applies to any form of supplemental α-tocopheral.
[d]The ULs for vitamin E, niacin, and folate apply to synthetic forms obtained from supplements, fortified foods, or a combination of the two.
[e]β-carotene supplements are advised only to serve as a provitamin A source for individuals at risk of vitamin A deficiency.
[f]ND, not determinable due to lack of data of adverse effects in this age group and concern with regard to lack of ability to handle excess amounts. Source of intake should be from food only to prevent high levels of intake.
SOURCES: Dietary Reference Intakes for Calcium, Phosphorus, Magnesium, Vitamin D, and Fluoride (1997); Dietary Reference Intakes for Thiamin, Riboflavin, Niacin, Vitamin B$_6$, Folate, Vitamin B$_{12}$, Pantothenic Acid, Biotin, and Choline (1998); Dietary Reference Intakes for Vitamin C, Vitamin E, Selenium, and Carotenoids (2000); and Dietary Reference Intakes for Vitamin A, Vitamin K, Arsenic, Boron, Chromium, Copper, Iodine, Iron, Manganese, Molybdenum, Nickel, Silicon, Vanadium, and Zinc (2001). These reports may be accessed via www.nap.edu. Copyright 2001 by the National Academy of Sciences. All rights reserved.

No way exists to stop oxygen reduction and free radical production, but the body does provide an elaborate natural defense against their damaging effects. This defense includes the antioxidant scavenger enzymes catalase, glutathione peroxidase, superoxide dismutase (produced in the cell and cannot be obtained through dietary supplementation), and metal-binding (metalloenzyme) proteins.[90] In addition, the nutritive, nonenzymatic reducing agents vitamins A, C, and E and the vitamin A precursor β-carotene (a "carotenoid" in dark green and orange vegetables) serve important protective functions.[83,111,158,201] Antioxidant vitamins protect the plasma membrane by reacting with and removing free radicals, thus quenching the chain reaction; these vitamins also blunt the damaging effects to cellular constituents of high serum homocysteine levels.[141]

Maintaining a diet with appropriate quantities of antioxidant vitamins and other chemoprotective agents reduces the occurrence of cardiovascular disease, diabetes, osteoporosis, cataracts, premature aging, and diverse cancers including those of the breast, distal colon, prostate, pancreas, ovary, and endometrium.[50,84,133,166,226] A normal to above normal intake of dietary vitamin E (in α- and γ-tocopherol forms) and β-carotene and/or high serum levels of carotenoids may blunt the progression of coronary artery narrowing and reduce risk for heart attack and possibly diabetes in men and women.[60,72,80] Unfortunately, the heart disease protection from vitamin E is not always observed in diverse populations, high-risk patients, and those with congestive heart failure.[99,131,205,222,232] In fact, the latest research indicates that for patients with vascular disease or diabetes mellitus, long-term vitamin E supplementation does not prevent cancer or major cardiovascular events and may increase the risk for heart failure.[121]

One model for heart disease protection proposes that the antioxidant vitamins inhibit oxidation of LDL cholesterol and its subsequent uptake into foam cells embedded in the arterial wall. In this "**oxidative-modification hypothesis**," the mild oxidation of LDL cholesterol—similar to butter turning rancid—contributes to the plaque-forming, artery-clogging process of atherosclerosis.[41,91,119,199] Almost 30% of adults in the United States have low blood levels of vitamin E.[58]

Nutritional guidelines focus more on the consumption of a broad array of foods than on isolated chemicals within these foods. The current recommendation is to increase the consumption of fruits, vegetables, and whole grains, and include lean meat or meat substitutes and low-fat dairy foods to gain substantial health benefits and reduce risk of early mortality. Disease protection from diet can be linked to the myriad of accessory nutrients and substances (e.g., the numerous "chemoprotectant" phytochemicals and zoochemicals) within the vitamin-containing foods in a healthful diet.[82] Three potential mechanisms for antioxidant health benefits include:

1. Influencing molecular mechanisms and gene expression
2. Providing enzyme-inducing substances that detoxify carcinogens
3. Blocking uncontrolled growth of cells

According to the director of the Division of Cancer Prevention and Control at the National Cancer Institute (NCI; www.cancer.gov/), "more than 150 studies have clearly shown that groups of people who eat plenty of fruits and vegetables get less cancer at a number of cancer sites." The NCI encourages consumption of five or more servings (nine recommended for men) of fruits and vegetables daily, while the USDA's *Dietary Guidelines* recommend two to four servings of fruits and three to five servings of vegetables daily. Rich dietary sources of antioxidants include:

- **β-carotene** (pigmented compounds, or carotenoids, that give color to yellow and green, leafy vegetables): carrots; dark-green leafy vegetables such as spinach, broccoli, turnips, beet and collard greens; sweet potatoes; winter squash; apricots; cantaloupe; mangos; papaya
- **Vitamin C:** citrus fruits and juices, cabbage, broccoli, turnip greens, cantaloupe, tomatoes, strawberries, apples with skin
- **Vitamin E:** vegetable oils, wheat germ, whole-grain bread and cereals, dried beans, green leafy vegetables

EXERCISE, FREE RADICALS, AND ANTIOXIDANTS

The benefits of physical activity are well known, but the possibility for negative effects remains controversial. Potentially negative effects occur because elevated aerobic exercise metabolism increases free radical production.[97,115,152,216] Increased free radicals could possibly overwhelm the body's natural defenses and pose a health risk from increased oxidative stress. Free radicals also play a role in muscle injury and soreness from eccentric muscle actions and unaccustomed exercise (see Chapter 22). Muscle damage of this nature releases muscle enzymes and initiates inflammatory cell infiltration into the damaged tissue.

The opposing position maintains that while free radical production increases during exercise, the body's normal antioxidant defenses are either adequate or concomitantly improve. Improvement occurs as natural enzymatic defenses (e.g., superoxide dismutase and glutathione peroxidase) "upregulate" through training adaptations.[64,76,157,185,218] Upregulation of antioxidant defenses accompanies reduced exercise-induced lipid peroxidation in red blood cell membranes, which increases their resistance to subsequent oxidative stress.[136] *Research supports this latter position because the beneficial effects of regular exercise decrease the incidence of various cancers and heart disease, whose occurrences relate to oxidative stress.* Regular exercise training also protects against myocardial injury from lipid peroxidation induced by short-term tissue ischemia followed by reperfusion.[39] In humans, free radical production and tissue damage are not directly measured but, rather, inferred from markers of free radical byproducts.

Increased Metabolism in Exercise and Free-Radical Production

Exercise produces reactive oxygen in at least two ways. The first occurs via an electron leak in the mitochondria, probably at the cytochrome level to produce superoxide radicals. The second occurs during alterations in blood flow and oxygen supply—underperfusion during intense exercise followed by substantial reperfusion in recovery—which trigger excessive free radical generation. The reintroduction of molecular oxygen in recovery produces reactive oxygen species that magnify oxidative stress. Some argue that the potential for free-radical damage also increases during trauma, stress, and muscle damage and from environmental pollutants, including smog.

The risk of oxidative stress with exercise increases with high-intensity physical effort.[160] The aerobic and anaerobic nature of the physical activity (e.g., prolonged running versus isometric exercise) also influences the type of oxidative stress.[2] Exhaustive endurance exercise by untrained persons produces oxidative damage in the active muscles. In addition, high-intensity resistance exercise of the body's major muscle groups increases free radical production, indirectly measured by malondialdehyde, the lipid peroxidation byproduct.[130] Variations in estrogen levels during the menstrual cycle do not affect the mild oxidative stress that accompanies moderate-intensity exercise.[28] FIGURE 2.3 illustrates how regular aerobic exercise affects oxidative response and potential for tissue damage, including protective adaptive responses.

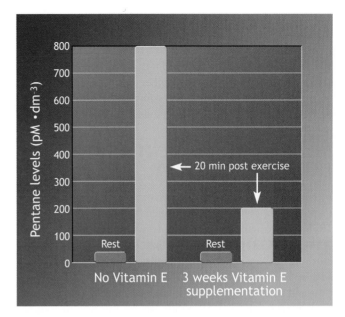

Figure 2.4 Pentane levels before and after 20 minutes of exercise at 100% $\dot{V}O_{2max}$ with and without vitamin E supplementation. (Adapted from Pincemail J, et al. Pentane measurement in man as an index of lipoperoxidation. Bioelectronchem Bioenerg 1987;18:117.)

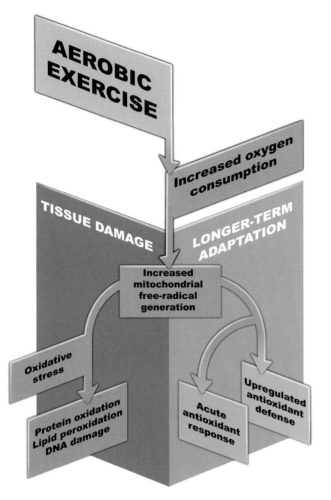

Figure 2.3 Cascade of events and adaptations produced by regular aerobic exercise that lessen the likelihood of tissue damage.

Important Questions

Two questions arise about the potential for oxidative stress with exercise: (1) are physically active individuals more prone to free-radical damage, and (2) are protective agents with antioxidant properties required in increased quantities in the diets of physically active people?

In answer to the first question, research indicates that the natural antioxidant defenses in well-nourished humans respond adequately to increased physical activity.[220] A single bout of submaximal exercise increased oxidant production, yet antioxidant defenses coped effectively in healthy individuals and trained heart transplant recipients.[92] Even with multiple bouts of exercise on consecutive days, the various indices of oxidative stress showed no depletion of the body's antioxidant system. The answer to the second question remains equivocal.[217] Some evidence indicates that consuming exogenous antioxidant compounds either slows exercise-induced free radical formation or augments the body's natural defense system.[89,90]

If supplementation proves beneficial, vitamin E may be the most important antioxidant related to exercise.[32,66,86] Vitamin E–deficient animals begin an exercise program with

plasma membrane function compromised from oxidative damage and thus reach exhaustion earlier than animals with recommended vitamin E levels. In animals fed a normal diet, vitamin E supplements diminished oxidative damage to skeletal muscle fibers and myocardial tissue caused by exercise.[66,67] FIGURE 2.4 shows that 3 weeks of a daily 200 International Unit (IU) vitamin E supplement dramatically reduced free radical production as measured by pentane elimination in men after maximal exercise. Humans fed a daily antioxidant vitamin mixture of β-carotene, vitamin C, and vitamin E had lower serum and breath markers of lipid peroxidation at rest and following exercise than subjects not receiving supplements.[97] Five months of vitamin E supplementation in racing cyclists reduced markers of oxidative stress induced by extreme endurance exercise. For intense whole-body resistance training, 2 weeks of daily supplementation with 120 IU of vitamin E decreased free radical interaction with cellular membranes and blunted muscle tissue disruption caused by a bout of intense exercise.[130] In contrast, 30 days of vitamin E supplementation ($1200 \text{ IU} \cdot \text{d}^{-1}$) produced a 2.8-fold increase in serum vitamin E concentration without affecting contraction-induced indices of muscle damage (including postexercise force decrement) or inflammation caused by eccentric muscle actions.[16] Similarly, a 4-week daily vitamin E supplement of 1000 IU produced no effect on biochemical or ultrastructural indices of muscle damage in experienced runners after a half marathon.[38] Differences in exercise severity and oxidative stress could account for discrepancies in research findings.

Recommended vitamin E supplementation ranges between 100 and 400 IU per day. IU is the common unit of measurements on supplement labels. If vitamin E comes from isolated food sources, 1 mg equals 1.5 IU; if taken in supplement form, 1 mg equals 1 IU. This lower conversion reflects a higher concentration of a less active form of vitamin E. Daily supplements of vitamin E containing up to 800 IU probably pose no risk for most persons. Higher amounts have produced harmful effects (e.g., internal bleeding) by inhibiting vitamin K metabolism, particularly in persons taking anticoagulants.

VITAMIN SUPPLEMENTS: THE COMPETITIVE EDGE?

FIGURE 2.5 illustrates the progressive increase in money spent on dietary supplements in the United States between 1990 and 1996 with growth rate exceeding 10% per year (also true from 1996–2000). Reports estimate that 158 million Americans currently take dietary supplements, spending an estimated $18 billion annually.[68,159,214] Of this total, vitamin–mineral pills and powders represent the most common form of supplement used by the general public, accounting for 70% of the total annual supplement sales. Worldwide sales of dietary supplements exceeded $50 billion in 2004, with an expected increase to $55 billion by 2010. Estimates indicate that more than 40% of men and 50% of women age 60 and older use at least one vitamin or mineral supplement. Particularly susceptible marketing targets include the exercise enthusiast, the competitive athlete, and coaches and personal trainers who try to get individuals to achieve peak performance. More than 50% of competitive athletes in some sports consume supplements on a regular basis, either to ensure adequate micronutrient intake or to achieve an excess with the hope of enhancing performance and training responsiveness.[30,31,103] When vitamin–mineral deficiencies appear in active people, they often occur among (1) vegetarians or groups with low energy intake (e.g., dancers, gymnasts, and weight-class sport athletes who strive to maintain or reduce body weight), (2) those that eliminate one or more food groups from their diet, or (3) individuals who consume large amounts of processed foods and simple sugars with low micronutrient density (e.g., endurance athletes). For these individuals, a multivitamin–mineral supplement at recommended dosages can upgrade the micronutrient density of their daily diet.

Vitamins synthesized in the laboratory are no less effective for bodily functions than vitamins from food sources. When deficiencies exist, vitamin supplements can reverse the deficiency symptoms. However, when vitamin intake achieves recommended levels, supplements have not been shown to improve exercise performance. Testimonials from coaches and elite athletes who attribute their success to level, a particular dietary modification (usually includes specific vitamin supplements) only cloud the issue. *More than 50 years of research does not support the wisdom of using vitamin (and mineral) supplements to improve exercise performance, the hormonal and metabolic responses to exercise, or ability to train arduously in healthy persons with nutritionally adequate diets.*[128,207,215,224]

Megavitamins

Most nutritionists believe little harm occurs from taking a multivitamin capsule containing the recommended quantity of each vitamin. However, some athletes take **megavitamins**, or doses at least 10 times and up to 1000 times the RDA, hoping to improve exercise performance by "supercharging" with vitamins. However, Such practice warrants concern and may cause harm, except in serious medical illness requiring a pharmacologic dose of vitamins.

INTEGRATIVE QUESTION

Respond to an athlete who asks: "What's wrong with taking megadoses of vitamin and mineral supplements to ensure I'm getting an adequate intake on a daily basis?"

Excess Vitamins Behave as Chemicals

Once the enzyme systems with specific vitamin cofactors become saturated, any excess vitamins taken in megadose function as chemicals (drugs) in the body. A megadose of water-soluble vitamin C, for example, can raise serum uric acid levels and precipitate gout in persons predisposed to this disease. At intakes above 1000 mg daily, urinary excretion of oxalate (a breakdown product of vitamin C) increases, accelerating kidney stone formation in susceptible individuals.[117] Also, some American blacks, Asians, and Sephardic Jews have a genetic metabolic deficiency that transforms to hemolytic anemia with excessive vitamin C intake. In iron-deficient individuals, megadoses of vitamin C may destroy significant amounts of vitamin B_{12}. In healthy persons, vitamin C supplements frequently irritate the bowel and cause diarrhea.

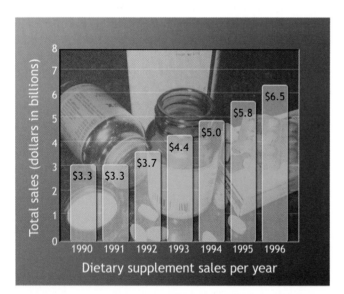

Figure 2.5 Expansion of the dietary supplement industry. (From Packaged Facts Inc., NYC. U.S. Food and Drug Administration. FDA consumer: an FDA guide to dietary supplements. Sep–Oct, 1998.)

Excess vitamin B_6 can induce liver disease and nerve damage, while riboflavin (B_2) excess can impair vision. A megadose of nicotinic acid (niacin) functions as a potent vasodilator and inhibits fatty acid mobilization during exercise. This could more rapidly deplete glycogen reserves. Folic acid excess in supplement form can trigger an allergic response, producing hives, light-headedness, and breathing difficulties. Possible side effects of vitamin E megadose include headache, fatigue, blurred vision, gastrointestinal disturbances, internal bleeding, muscular weakness, and low blood sugar.

Vitamin C May Protect Against URTI. Consuming vitamin C above recommended levels does not protect the general population against upper respiratory tract infection (URTI). However, daily supplements of 500 to 1500 mg may confer some benefit to individuals engaged in strenuous exercise who experience frequent viral infections.[77,154,155]

Moderate exercise heightens immune function, whereas a prolonged period of intense physical activity (marathon running or an intense training session) transiently suppresses the body's first line of defense against infectious agents. This increases the risk of URTI within 1 or 2 weeks of the exercise stress. For these individuals, additional vitamin C and E and perhaps carbohydrate ingestion before, during, and following a workout may boost the normal immune mechanisms for combating infection.[89,143,149]

Vitamins and Exercise Performance

FIGURE 2.6 illustrates that B-complex vitamins play key roles as coenzymes to regulate energy-yielding reactions during carbohydrate, fat, and protein catabolism. They also contribute to hemoglobin synthesis and red blood cell production. The belief that "if a little is good, more must be better" has led many coaches, athletes, fitness enthusiasts, and even some scientists to advocate using vitamin supplements above recommended levels. Research findings and the overwhelming majority of professional nutritionists simply do not support this approach for individuals who consume an adequate diet.

Supplementing with vitamin B_6, an essential cofactor in glycogen and amino acid metabolism, did not benefit the metabolic mixture metabolized by women during high-intensity aerobic exercise. In general, athletes' status for this vitamin equals reference standards for the population[128] and does not decrease with strenuous exercise to a level warranting supplementation.[174] For endurance-trained men, 9 days of vitamin B_6 supplementation (20 mg per day) provided no ergogenic effect on cycling to exhaustion performed at 71% of aerobic capacity.[221]

Chronic high-potency, multivitamin–mineral supplementation for well-nourished, healthy individuals does not augment aerobic fitness, muscular strength, and athletic performance.[187] In addition to the B-complex group, no exercise benefit exists for excess vitamins C and E on stamina, circulatory function, or energy metabolism. For example, short-term daily supplementation with vitamin E (400 IU) produced no effect on normal neuroendocrine and metabolic responses to strenuous exercise or performance time to exhaustion.[188] Vitamin C status, assessed by serum concentrations and urinary ascorbate levels, in trained athletes does not differ from that in untrained subjects despite large differences in daily physical activity level.[177] Other investigators report similar findings for this and other vitamins.[57,71,175] Active persons generally increase their energy intake to match the increased energy requirement of physical activity; thus, a proportionate increase also occurs in micronutrient intake, often in amounts greatly exceeding recommended levels.

Summary

1. Vitamins, organic compounds that neither supply energy nor contribute to body mass, serve crucial functions in almost all bodily processes. They must be obtained from food or dietary supplementation.
2. Plants synthesize vitamins; animals also produce them from precursor substances known as provitamins.
3. Thirteen known vitamins are classified as either water soluble or fat soluble. The fat-soluble vitamins include A, D, E, and K; vitamin C and the B-complex vitamins constitute the water-soluble vitamins.
4. Excess fat-soluble vitamins accumulate in body tissues and can increase to toxic concentrations. Except in relatively rare instances, excess water-soluble vitamins remain nontoxic and are eventually excreted in the urine.
5. Vitamins regulate metabolism, facilitate energy release, and play key functions in bone and tissue synthesis.
6. Vitamins A, C, E, and the provitamin β-carotene serve important protective functions as antioxidants. A diet with appropriate levels of these micronutrients can reduce the potential for free radical damage (oxidative stress) and may offer protection against heart disease and some types of cancer.
7. The Dietary Reference Intakes (DRIs) differ from their predecessor RDAs by focusing more on promoting health maintenance and risk reduction for nutrient-dependent diseases rather than the traditional criterion of preventing deficiency diseases.
8. The new DRIs serve as the umbrella term that encompasses the new standards—the RDAs, Estimated Average Requirements, Adequate Intakes, and the Tolerable Upper Intake Levels—for nutrient recommendations for use in planning and assessing diets for healthy persons. DRI values include recommendations that apply to gender and life stages of growth and development based on age and, when appropriate, pregnancy and lactation.

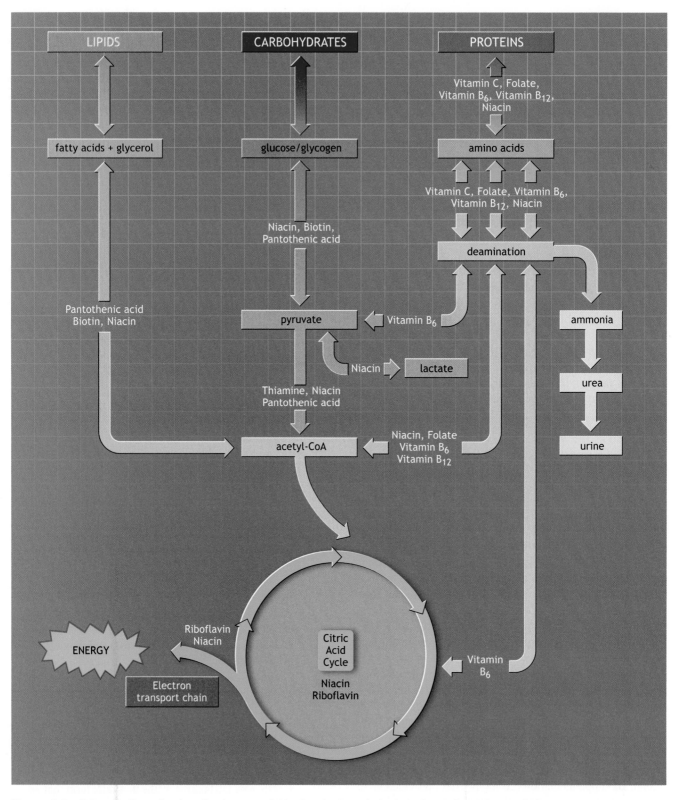

Figure 2.6   General schema for the role of water-soluble vitamins in carbohydrate, fat, and protein metabolism.

9. Physical activity elevates metabolism and increases the production of potentially harmful free radicals. The daily diet should contain foods rich in antioxidant vitamins and minerals to lessen oxidative stress.
10. For well-nourished individuals, the body's natural antioxidant defenses upregulate in response to increased physical activity.
11. Vitamin supplementation above the RDA does not improve exercise performance or the potential for intense physical training.

PART 2 • *Minerals*

THE NATURE OF MINERALS

Approximately 4% of the body's mass (about 2 kg for a 50-kg woman), consists of 22 mostly metallic elements collectively called **minerals**. Minerals serve as constituents of enzymes, hormones, and vitamins; they combine with other chemicals (e.g., calcium phosphate in bone, iron in the heme of hemoglobin) or exist singularly (e.g., free calcium and sodium in body fluids).

The minerals essential to life include seven **major minerals** (required in amounts >100 mg daily) and 14 minor or **trace minerals** (required in amounts <100 mg daily). Trace minerals account for less than 15 g (approximately 0.5 oz), or 0.02% of the total body mass. Like consuming excess vitamins, excess mineral intake serves no useful physiologic purpose and can produce toxic effects. DRIs have been established for many minerals; if the diet supplies these requirements, this ensures an adequate intake of the remaining minerals.

Most minerals, major or trace, occur freely in nature—mainly in the waters of rivers, lakes, and oceans; in topsoil; and beneath the earth's surface. Minerals exist in the root systems of plants and the body structure of animals that consume plants and water containing minerals.

KINDS AND SOURCES OF MINERALS

TABLE 2.4 lists the major bodily functions, dietary sources, and symptoms of deficiency or excess for the minerals, while TABLE 2.5 presents the RDA, UL, and AI values for these minerals. Mineral supplements, like vitamin supplements, generally confer little benefit because a well-balanced diet readily supplies the recommended quantities. The National Institutes of Health (NIH) coordinates the Office of Dietary Supplements, a rich repository of research dealing with dietary supplements. We highly recommend their Internet site and the excellent database. (http://ods.od.nih.gov/).

ROLE OF MINERALS

Whereas vitamins catalyze chemical processes without becoming part of the reaction's byproducts, some minerals become part of the body's structures and existing chemicals. Minerals serve three broad roles in the body:

1. Minerals provide *structure* in forming bones and teeth.
2. In terms of *function*, minerals help maintain normal heart rhythm, muscle contractility, neural conductivity, and acid-base balance.
3. Minerals *regulate* cellular metabolism by becoming constituents of enzymes and hormones that modulate cellular activity.

FIGURE 2.7 lists the minerals that participate in catabolic and anabolic cellular processes. Minerals activate reactions that release energy during carbohydrate, fat, and protein catabolism. In addition, minerals participate in the biosynthesis of nutrients—glycogen from glucose, triacylglycerols from fatty acids and glycerol, and proteins from amino acids. A lack of one or more essential minerals often disrupts the fine balance between catabolism and anabolism. Minerals also form important constituents of hormones. Inadequate thyroxine production from iodine insufficiency, for example, slows the body's resting metabolism. In extreme cases, this could predispose a person to develop obesity. Synthesis of insulin, the hormone that facilitates glucose uptake by the cells, requires zinc (as do approximately 100 enzymes), whereas the mineral chlorine forms the digestive acid hydrochloric acid:

Mineral Bioavailability

The body varies considerably in its capacity to absorb and use the minerals in food. For example, spinach contains considerable calcium, but only about 5% of it becomes absorbed. The same holds true for dietary iron, which the intestine absorbs with an average efficiency of 5 to 10%. Factors that affect the bioavailability of minerals in food include:

- *Type of food:* The small intestine readily absorbs minerals contained in animal products because they do not contain plant binders and dietary fibers that hinder digestion and absorption. With the exception of magnesium, foods from the animal kingdom generally have a high mineral concentration.
- *Mineral–mineral interaction:* Many minerals have the same molecular weight and thus compete for intestinal absorption. This makes it unwise to consume an excess of any one mineral because it can retard another mineral's absorption.
- *Vitamin–mineral interaction:* Various vitamins interact with minerals in a manner that affects mineral bioavailability. From a positive perspective, vitamin D facilitates calcium absorption, while vitamin C improves intestinal absorption of iron.
- *Fiber–mineral interaction:* High fiber intake blunts the absorption of calcium, iron, magnesium, and

TABLE 2.4 ■ THE IMPORTANT MAJOR AND TRACE MINERALS FOR HEALTHY ADULTS (AGE 19–50 YEARS) AND THEIR FOOD SOURCES, FUNCTIONS, AND THE EFFECTS OF DEFICIENCIES AND EXCESSES

MINERAL	DIETARY SOURCES	MAJOR BODILY FUNCTIONS	DEFICIENCY	EXCESS
Major				
Calcium	Milk, cheese, dark green vegetables, dried legumes	Bone and tooth formation, blood clotting, nerve transmission	Stunted growth, rickets, osteoporosis, convulsions	Not reported in humans
Phosphorus	Milk, cheese, yogurt, meat, poultry, grains, fish	Bone and tooth formation, acid-base balance, helps prevent loss of calcium from bone	Weakness, demineralization	Erosion of jaw (phossy jaw)
Potassium	Leafy vegetables, canteloupe, lima beans, potatoes, bananas, milk, meats, coffee, tea	Fluid balance, nerve transmission, acid-base balance	Muscle cramps, irregular cardiac rhythm, mental confusion, loss of appetite; can be life threatening	None if kidneys functon normally; poor kidney function causes potassium buildup and cardiac arrythmias
Sulfur	Obtained as part of dietary protein; present in food preservatives	Acid-base balance, liver function	Unlikely to occur with adequate dietary intake	Unknown
Sodium	Common salt	Acid-base balance, body water balance, nerve function	Muscle cramps, mental apathy, reduced appetite	Contributes to high blood pressure
Chlorine (chloride)	Chloride part of salt-containing food; some vegetables and fruits	Important part of extra-cellular fluids	Unlikely to occur with adequate dietary intake	Contributes to high blood pressure
Magnesium	Whole grains, green leafy vegetables	Activates enzymes involved in protein synthesis	Growth failure, behavioral disturbances	Diarrhea
Trace				
Iron	Eggs, lean meats, legumes, whole grains, green leafy vegetables	Constituent of hemoglobin and enzymes involved in energy metabolism	Iron deficiency anemia (weakness, reduced resistance to infection)	Siderosis; cirrhosis of liver
Fluoride	Drinking water, tea, seafood	May be important in maintenance of bone structure	Higher frequency of tooth decay	Mottling of teeth, increased bone density
Zinc	Widely distributed in foods	Constituent of enzymes involved in digestion	Growth failure, small sex glands	Fever, nausea, vomiting, diarrhea
Copper	Meats, drinking water	Constituent of enzymes associated with iron metabolism	Anemia, bone changes (rare)	Rare metabolic condition (Wilson's disease)
Selenium	Seafood, meats, grains	Functions in close association with vitamin E	Anemia (rare)	Gastrointestinal disorders, lung irritations
Iodine (iodide)	Marine fish and shell-fish, dairy products, vegetables, iodized salt	Constituent of thyroid hormones	Goiter (enlarged thyroid)	High intake depresses thyroid activity
Chromium	Legumes, cereals, organ meats, fats, vegetable oils, meats, whole grains	Constituent of some enzymes; involved in glucose and energy metabolism	Not reported in humans; impaired ability to metabolize glucose	Inhibition of enzymes Occupational exposures: skin and kidney damage

phosphorus by binding to them and causing them to pass unabsorbed through the digestive tract.

In the sections that follow, we describe specific functions for several of the more important minerals related to physical activity.

CALCIUM

Calcium, the body's most abundant mineral, combines with phosphorus to form bones and teeth. These two minerals represent about 75% of the body's total mineral content, or about

TABLE 2.5 ■ DIETARY REFERENCE INTAKES (DRIS): RECOMMENDED MINERAL INTAKES AND TOLERABLE UPPER INTAKE LEVELS (UL^a)

RECOMMENDED MINERAL INTAKES

LIFE STAGE GROUP	CALCIUM (mg/d)	CHROMIUM (µg/d)	COPPER (µg/d)	FLUORIDE (mg/d)	IODINE (µg/d)	IRON (mg/d)	MAGNESIUM (mg/d)	MANGANESE (mg/d)	MOLYBDENUM (µg/d)	PHOSPHORUS (mg/d)	SELENIUM (µg/d)	ZINC (mg/d)
Infants												
0–6 mo	210*	0.2*	200*	0.01*	110*	0.27*	30*	0.003*	2*	100*	15*	2*
7–12 mo	270*	5.5*	220*	0.5*	130*	11*	75*	0.6*	3*	275*	20*	3
Children												
1–3 y	500*	11*	340	0.7*	90	7	80	1.2*	17	460	20	3
4–8 y	800*	15*	440	1*	90	10	130	1.5*	22	500	30	5
Males												
9–13 y	1,300	25*	700	2*	120	8	240	1.9*	34	1,250	40	8
14–18 y	1,300*	35*	890	3*	150	11	410	2.2*	43	1,250	55	11
19–30 y	1,000*	35*	900	4*	150	8	400	2.3*	45	700	55	11
31–50 y	1,000*	35*	900	4*	150	8	420	2.3*	45	700	55	11
51–70 y	1,200*	30*	900	4*	150	8	420	2.3*	45	700	55	11
>70 y	1,200*	30*	900	4*	150	8	420	2.3*	45	700	55	11
Females												
9–13 y	1,300*	21*	700	2*	150	8	240	1.6*	34	1,250	40	8
14–18 y	1,300*	24*	890	3*	150	15	360	1.6*	43	1,250	55	9
19–30 y	1,000*	25*	900	3*	150	18	310	1.8*	45	700	55	8
31–50 y	1,000*	25*	900	3*	150	18	320	1.8*	45	700	55	8
51–70 y	1,200*	20*	900	3*	150	8	320	1.8*	45	700	55	8
>70 y	1,200*	20*	900	3*	150	8	320	1.8*	45	700	55	8
Pregnancy												
≤18 y	1,300*	29*	1,000	3*	220	27	400	2.0*	50	1,250	60	13
19–30 y	1,000*	30*	1,000	3*	220	27	350	2.0*	50	700	60	11
31–50 y	1,000*	30*	1,000	3*	220	27	360	2.0*	50	700	60	11
Lactation												
≤18 y	1,300*	44*	1,300	3*	290	10	360	2.6*	50	1,250	70	14
19–30 y	1,000*	45*	1,300	3*	290	9	310	2.6*	50	700	70	12
31–50 y	1,000*	45*	1,300	3*	290	9	320	2.6*	50	700	70	12

Table presents Recommended Dietary Allowances (RDAs) in **bold type** and Adequate Intakes (AIs) in ordinary type followed by an asterisk (*). RDAs and AIs may both be used as goals for individual intake. RDAs are set to meet the needs of almost all (97 to 98 percent) individuals in a group. For healthy breastfed infants, the AI is the mean intake. The AI for other life stage and gender groups is believed to cover needs of all individuals in the group, but lack of data or uncertainty in the data prevent being able to specify with confidence the percentage of individuals covered by this intake.

Source: Dietary Reference Intakes for Calcium, Phosphorous, Magnesium. Vitamin D and Fluoride (1997); Dietary Reference Intakes for Thiamin, Riboflavin, Niacin, Vitamin B₅ Folate, Vitamin B₁₂, Pantothenic Acid, Biotin, and Choline (1998): Dietary reference Intakes for Vitamin C, Vitamin E, Selenium, and Carotenoids (2000); and Dietary Reference Intakes for Vitamin A, Vitamin K, Arsenic, Boron, Chromium, Copper, Iodine, Iron, Manganese, Molybdenum, Nickel, Silicon, Vanadium, and Zinc (2001). These reports may be accessed via www.nap.edu.

Copyright 2001 by the National Academy of Sciences. Reprinted with permission.

continued on page 60

TABLE 2.5 ■ *continued*

TOLERABLE UPPER INTAKE LEVELS[a]

LIFE STAGE GROUP	ARSENIC[b] (mg/d)	BORON (mg/d)	CALCIUM (g/d)	CHROMIUM	COPPER (µg/d)	FLUORIDE (mg/d)	IODINE (µg/d)	IRON (mg/d)	MAGNESIUM (mg/d)[c]	MANGANESE (mg/d)	MOLYBDENUM (µg/d)	NICKEL (mg/d)	PHOSPHORUS (g/d)	SELENIUM (µg/d)	SILICON[d]	VANADIUM (mg/d)[e]	ZINC (mg/d)
Infants																	
0–6 mo	ND[f]	ND	ND	ND	ND	0.7	ND	40	ND	ND	ND	ND	ND	45	ND	ND	4
7–12 mo	ND	ND	ND	ND	ND	0.9	ND	40	ND	ND	ND	ND	ND	60	ND	ND	5
Children																	
1–3 y	ND	3	2.5	ND	1,000	1.	200	40	65	2	300	0.2	3	90	ND	ND	7
4–8 y	ND	6	2.5	ND	3,000	2.2	300	40	110	3	600	0.3	3	150	ND	ND	12
Males, females																	
9–13 y	ND	11	2.5	ND	5,000	10	600	40	350	6	1,100	0.6	4	280	ND	ND	23
14–18 y	ND	17	2.5	ND	800	10	900	45	350	9	1,700	1.0	4	400	ND	ND	34
19–70 y	ND	20	2.5	ND	10,000	10	1,100	45	350	11	2,000	1.0	4	400	ND	1.8	40
>70 y	ND	20	2.5	ND	10,000	10	1,100	45	350	11	2,000	1.0	3	400	ND	1.8	40
Pregnancy																	
≤18 y	ND	17	2.5	ND	8,000	10	900	45	350	9	1,700	1.0	3.5	400	ND	ND	34
19–50 y	ND	20	2.5	ND	10,000	10	1,100	45	350	11	2,000	1.0	3.5	400	ND	ND	40
Lactation																	
≤18 y	ND	17	2.5	ND	8,000	10	900	45	350	9	1,700	1.0	4	400	ND	ND	34
19–50 y	ND	20	2.5	ND	10,000	10	1,100	45	350	11	2,000	1.0	4	400	ND	ND	40

Sources: Dietary Reference Intakes for Calcium, Phosphorous, Magnesium, Vitamin D and Fluoride (1997); Dietary Reference Intakes for Thiamin, Riboflavin, Niacin, Vitamin B6, Folate, Vitamin B12, Pantothenic Acid, Biotin, and Choline (1998); Dietary Reference Intakes for Vitamin C, Vitamin E, Selenium, and Carotenoids (2000); and Dietary Reference Intakes for Vitamin A, Vitamin K, Arsenic, Boron, Chromium, Copper, Iodine, Iron, Manganese, Molybdenum, Nickel, Silicon, Vanadium, and Zinc (2001). These reports may be accessed via www.nap.edu.

Copyright 2001 by the National Academy of Sciences. Reprinted with permission.

[a]UL = The maximum level of daily nutrient intake that is likely to pose no risk of adverse effects. Unless otherwise specified, the UL represents total intake from food, water, and supplements. Due to lack of suitable data, ULs could not be established for arsenic, chromium, and silicon. In the absence of ULs, extra caution may be warranted in consuming levels above recommended intakes.

[b]Although the UL was not determined for arsenic, there is no justification for adding arsenic to food or supplements.

[c]The ULs for magnesium represent intake from a pharmacologic agent only and do not include intake from food and water.

[d]Although silicon has not been shown to cause adverse effects in humans, there is no justification for adding silicon to supplements.

[e]Athough vanadium in food has not been shown to cause adverse effects in humans, there is no justification for adding vanadium to food and vanadium supplements should be used with caution. The UL is based on adverse effects in laboratory animals and this data could be used to set a UL for adults but not children and adolescents.

[f]ND = not determinable due to lack of data of adverse effects in this age group and concern with regard to lack of ability to handle excess amounts. Source of intake should be from food only to prevent high levels of intake.

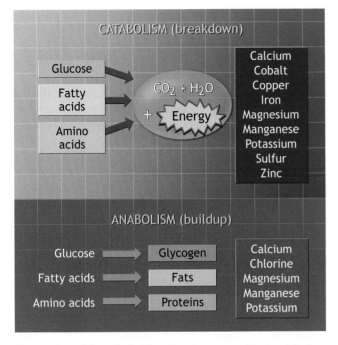

Figure 2.7 Minerals that function in macronutrient catabolism and anabolism.

2.5% of body mass. In its ionized form (about 1% of 1200 mg of endogenous calcium), calcium functions in muscle stimulation, blood clotting, transmission of nerve impulses, activation of several enzymes, synthesis of calcitriol (active form of vitamin D), and transport of fluids across cell membranes. It also may contribute to easing premenstrual syndrome, preventing colon cancer, and optimizing blood pressure regulation,[47,129] although its role in reducing heart disease risk remains unclear.[1,87]

> **BONE HEALTH DIAGNOSTIC CRITERIA BASED ON VARIATION (STANDARD DEVIATION [SD]) OF OBSERVED BONE DENSITY VALUES COMPARED TO VALUES FOR SEX-MATCHED YOUNG ADULT POPULATION**
>
> | | |
> |---|---|
> | Normal | < 1.0 SD below mean |
> | Osteopenia | 1.0 to 2.5 SD below mean |
> | Osteoporosis | > 2.5 SD below mean |
> | Severe osteoporosis | > 2.5 SD below mean plus one or more fragility fractures |

Osteoporosis: Calcium, Estrogen, and Exercise

Bone, a dynamic tissue matrix of collagen and minerals, exists in a continual state of flux, or **remodeling**. In fact, most of the adult skeleton is replaced about every 10 years. Bone-destroying cells (osteoclasts), under the influence of parathyroid

hormone, cause the breakdown (resorption) of bone by enzyme action, while bone-forming osteoblast cells induce bone synthesis. Calcium availability significantly affects the dynamics of bone remodeling. The two broad categories of bone are:

1. **Cortical bone**: dense, hard outer layer of bone such as the shafts of the long bones of the arms and legs
2. **Trabecular bone**: spongy, less dense, and relatively weaker bone, most prevalent in the vertebrae and ball of the femur

Calcium from food or calcium derived from bone resorption maintains plasma calcium levels. As a general guideline, adolescents and young adults require 1300 mg of calcium daily (1000 mg for adults ages 19 to 50 and 1200 mg for those older than 50) or about as much calcium as in five 8-oz glasses of milk. Unfortunately, calcium remains one of the most frequent nutrients lacking in the diet of sedentary and physically active individuals, particularly adolescent girls. For a typical adult, daily calcium intake ranges between 500 and 700 mg. *Among athletes, female dancers, gymnasts, and endurance competitors are most prone to calcium dietary insufficiency.*[18,138]

Inadequate calcium intake or low levels of calcium-regulating hormones cause withdrawal of calcium "reserves" in bone to restore any deficit. Prolonging this restorative imbalance promotes one of two conditions: (1) **osteoporosis**, literally meaning "porous bones," with bone density more than 2.5 standard deviations below normal for gender, or (2) **osteopenia**—from the Greek words *osteo,* meaning bone, and *penia,* meaning poverty—a midway condition in which bones weaken with increased risk of fractures. Osteoporosis develops progressively as bone loses its calcium mass (bone mineral content) and calcium concentration (bone mineral density). This causes bone to become progressively more porous and brittle (FIG. 2.8). Eventually, the stresses of normal living often cause bone to break, with compression fracture of the spine occurring most frequently.

> **RISK FACTORS FOR OSTEOPOROSIS**
>
> - History of fracture as an adult, regardless of cause
> - History of fracture in a parent or sibling
> - Cigarette smoking
> - Slight build or tendency toward underweight
> - White or Asian female
> - Sedentary lifestyle
> - Early menopause
> - Eating disorder
> - High protein intake (particularly animal protein)
> - Excess sodium intake
> - Alcohol abuse
> - Calcium-deficient diet before and after menopause
> - High caffeine intake (equivocal)
> - Vitamin D deficiency, either through inadequate exposure to sunlight or dietary insufficiency (prevalent in about 40% of adults)

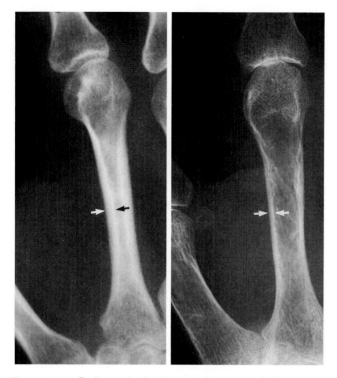

Figure 2.8 Radiograph of mid-second metacarpal of person with normal mineralization *(left)* and of patient with severe osteoporosis *(right)*. Under normal conditions, cortical width *(arrows)* is more than one third of the total width of the metacarpal, whereas osteoporosis produces extreme cortical narrowing. Note the intracortical tunneling that occurs in more aggressive forms of osteoporosis. (From Brant W, Helms C. Fundamentals of diagnostic radiology. 2nd ed. Baltimore: Williams & Wilkins, 1998.)

INTEGRATIVE QUESTION

Discuss the interactions between physical activity and calcium intake and bone health.

A Disease of Significant Prevalence

Osteoporosis currently afflicts 28 million Americans, of whom 80 to 90% are women, with another 18 million individuals with low bone mass and at risk for developing the disease. Fifty percent of all women eventually develop osteoporosis. Men are not immune from osteoporosis, as about 2 million men suffer from this disease. The devastation of this disease shows up most dramatically in fracture rates. Osteoporosis accounts for more than 1.5 million fractures (the clinical manifestation of the disease) yearly, including about 700,000 vertebral fractures, 300,000 hip fractures, 250,000 wrist fractures, and 300,000 fractures at other sites. On average, 24% of hip fracture patients aged 50 and over die in the year following their fracture.

Estimates from the largest study to date indicate that nearly one half of postmenopausal women with no previous osteoporosis diagnosis have low bone mineral density, including 7% with osteoporosis.[190] This indicates that one of two women and one of eight men over age 50 will experience an osteoporosis-

related fracture in their lifetime. National direct expenditures (hospitals and nursing homes) for osteoporotic and associated fractures equaled $21 billion in 2005 ($51 million each day); this cost may exceed $250 billion by the mid-21st century. Increased susceptibility to osteoporosis among older women coincides with menopause and the marked decrease in estradiol secretion, the most potent naturally occurring human estrogen. Exactly how estrogen exerts its protective effects on bone remains unknown (see p. 67 for estrogen's possible actions). Most men normally produce some estrogen into old age—a major reason why they exhibit a relatively lower prevalence of osteoporosis. A portion of circulating testosterone converts to estradiol, which also promotes positive calcium balance. Osteoporosis risk factors for men include low testosterone levels, cigarette smoking, and steroid use.

A Progressive Disease

Between 60 and 80% of an individual's susceptibility to osteoporosis links to genetic factors, while 20 to 40% remains lifestyle related. Adequate intake of calcium and vitamin D (maintains normal blood levels of calcium and bone mineralization)[116,206] and regular physical activity (with a synergistic effect of both variables on bone mass in children[178]) enable women to gain bone mass throughout the third decade of life. *The early teens serve as the prime years to maximize bone mass.*[17,137,204] Osteoporosis for many women begins early in life because the average teenager consumes suboptimal calcium to support growing bones. This creates an irreversible deficit that cannot be fully eliminated after achieving skeletal maturity. Calcium imbalance worsens into adulthood, particularly among women with genetic predisposition toward the disease.[55,63,120,212] Estrogen therapy, although increasing bone mineral density and reducing risk of fracture,[27] dramatically increases risk for blood clots, strokes, heart attacks, and cancers of the uterus, breast, and other organs.[230] Consequently, hormone treatment for osteoporosis should be viewed as a more dramatic approach requiring medical consultation and supervision. The NIH Osteoporosis and Related Bone Diseases–National Resource Center maintains an active web presence (www.osteo.org/) concerning bone diseases.

Prevention Through Diet

FIGURE 2.9A illustrates that the variation in bone mass results from a complex interaction among the factors rather than the separate influence of each factor.[127,150,193] That portion of bone mass variation attributable to diet may actually reflect how diet interacts with genetic factors, physical activity patterns, body weight, and drug or medication use (e.g., estrogen therapy). *Despite these interactive effects, adequate calcium intake throughout life remains the prime defense against bone loss with age.*[17,93] For example, calcium supplementation in postmenarchal girls with suboptimal calcium intake significantly enhances bone mineral acquisition.[179] The NIH consensus panel recommends that adolescent girls consume 1500 mg

green leafy vegetables. Calcium supplements, best absorbed on an empty stomach, can also correct dietary deficiencies regardless of whether the extra calcium comes from fortified foods or commercial supplements. Calcium citrate causes less stomach upset than other supplement forms; it also enhances iron absorption better than calcium gluconate, calcium carbonate, or other commercial products. Adequate availability of vitamin D (currently estimated at 400 IU daily for persons 51 to 70 and 600 IU for those over 70) facilitates calcium uptake, while excessive consumption of meat, salt, coffee, and alcohol inhibits absorption. For individuals who live and train (primarily indoors) in northern latitudes, a vitamin D supplement of 200 IU is recommended.[7] Bone matrix production also depends on vitamin K, prevalent in leafy green vegetables. The RDA for vitamin K is 90 μg for women and 120 μg for men, although some researchers suggest increasing this to 250 μg for adequate bone health.

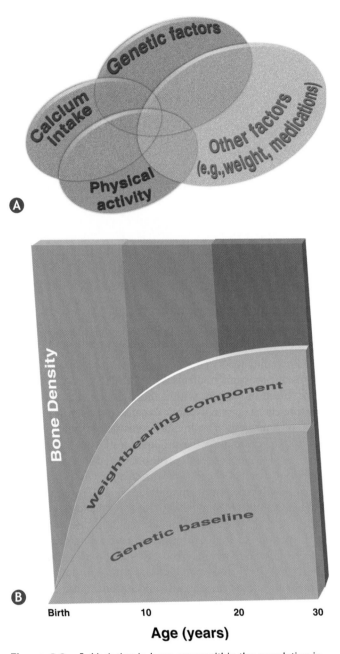

Figure 2.9 **A.** Variation in bone mass within the population is likely a function of how the different factors that affect bone mass interact with each other. (Modified from Specker BL. Should there be dietary guidelines for calcium intake. Am J Clin Nutr 2000;71:663.) **B.** Weight-bearing exercise augments skeleton mass during growth above the genetic baseline. The degree of augmentation depends largely on the amount of mechanical loading on a particular bone. (Modified from Turner CH. Site-specific effects of exercise: importance of interstitial fluid pressure. Bone 1999;24:161.)

SIX PRINCIPLES FOR PROMOTING BONE HEALTH THROUGH EXERCISE

1. *Specificity:* Exercise provides a local osteogenic effect.
2. *Overload:* Progressively increasing exercise intensity promotes continued bone deposition.
3. *Initial values:* Individuals with the smallest total bone mass show the greatest potential for bone deposition.
4. *Diminishing returns:* As one approaches the biologic ceiling for bone density, further density gains require greater effort.
5. *More Not Necessarily Better:* Bone cells become desensitized in response to prolonged mechanical-loading sessions.
6. *Reversibility:* Discontinuing exercise overload reverses the positive osteogenic effects gained through appropriate exercise stress.

Exercise Provides Benefits. Mechanical loading through regular dynamic exercise slows the rate of skeletal aging. Regardless of age or gender, children and adults who maintain an active lifestyle have significantly greater bone mass than sedentary counterparts.[4,5,19,52,74,100,106,147,153,198,213] Benefits of regular exercise on bone mass accretion (and perhaps bone shape and size) are greatest during childhood and adolescence when peak bone mass can increase to the greatest extent (Fig. 2.9B).[6,95,108,144] These benefits often accrue into the seventh and even eighth decades of life.[202,219] The decline in vigorous exercise with a sedentary lifestyle with aging closely parallels the age-related bone mass loss. In this regard, regular moderate physical activity associates with substantially lower risk of hip fracture in postmenopausal women.[53,180]

The osteogenic effect of exercise and everyday amounts of physical activity becomes particularly effective during the growth periods of childhood and adolescence and may reduce fracture risk later in life.[17,88,98] Short bouts of intense mechanical loading of bone with dynamic exercise three to five

of calcium daily. Increasing daily calcium intake for middle-aged women, particularly estrogen-deprived women following menopause, to 1200 to 1500 mg improves the body's calcium balance.[75,162]

Good dietary calcium sources include milk and milk products, sardines and canned salmon, kidney beans, and dark

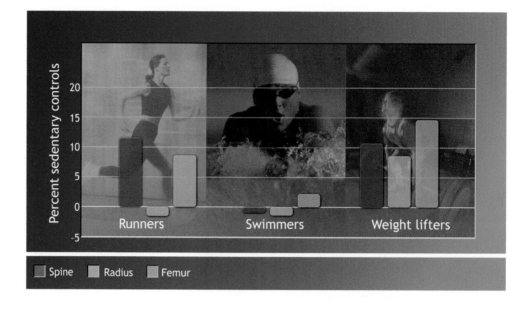

Figure 2.10 Bone mineral density expressed as a percentage of sedentary control values at three skeletal sites for runners, swimmers, and weight lifters. (From Drinkwater BL. Physical activity, fitness, and osteoporosis. In: Bouchard C, et al., eds. Physical activity, fitness, and health. Champaign, IL: Human Kinetics, 1994.)

times a week provides a potent stimulus to maintain or increase bone mass. FIGURE 2.10 illustrates the beneficial effects of heavy resistance exercises and circuit-resistance training or weight-bearing walking, running, dancing, rope skipping, or gymnastics. These exercises generate a significant impact load and/or intermittent force against the long bones of the body.[46,48,118,203,227] Activities with relatively high impact and high strain on the skeletal mass (e.g., volleyball, basketball, and gymnastics) induce the greatest increases in bone mass, particularly at weight-bearing sites.[9,36,42,189] Men and women in strength and power activities have as much or more bone mass than endurance athletes.[170] The exercise effects are site specific to the working muscles and bones to which they attach.[114] Bone mineral density relates directly to measures of muscular strength and regional lean tissue mass.[146] For example, lumbar spine and proximal femur bone masses of elite teenage weight lifters exceed representative values for fully mature bone of reference adults.[34] Eccentric exercise training provides a more potent site-specific osteogenic stimulus than concentric muscle training because greater forces usually occur with eccentric muscle loading.[73] Prior exercise and sports experience offers residual effects on an adult's bone mineral density. Exercise-induced increases in bone mass achieved during teenage and young-adult years remain despite cessation of active competition.[104,107]

Site-Specific Effects. In a normal hormonal milieu, muscle forces acting on specific bones during physical activity (particularly intermittent compression and tension mechanical loading) modify bone metabolism at the point of stress.[14,85,101] For example, the lower limb bones of older cross-country runners have greater bone mineral content than the bones of less active counterparts. The throwing arm of baseball players also shows greater bone thickness than the less-used, nondominant arm. Likewise, the bone mineral content of the humeral shaft and proximal humerus of the playing arm of tennis players averages 20 to 25% more than the nondominant arm; side-to-side difference in the arms of nonplayers generally averages

only 5%.[107] For females, this response is most noticeable in players who begin training before menarche.[96]

Prevailing theory considers that dynamic loading creates hydrostatic pressure gradients within a bone's fluid-filled network. Fluid movement within this network in response to pressure changes from dynamic exercise generates fluid shear stress on bone cells. This initiates a cascade of cellular events to ultimately stimulate the production of bone matrix protein.[211] Mechanosensitivity of bone and its subsequent buildup of calcium depends on two factors: (1) magnitude of the applied force (strain magnitude) and (2) frequency or number of cycles of application. Owing to the transient sensitivity of bone cells to mechanical stimuli, shorter, more frequent periods of high-frequency force (mechanical strain) with rest periods interspersed facilitate bone mass accretion.[70,112,113,171,172] As applied force and strain increase, the number of cycles required to initiate bone formation decrease.[37] Chemicals produced in bone itself also contribute to bone formation. Alterations in bone's geometric configuration to long-term exercise training enhance its mechanical properties.[12] FIGURE 2.11 illustrates the anatomic structure and cross-sectional view of a typical long bone and depicts the dynamics of bone growth and remodeling.

THE FEMALE ATHLETE TRIAD: UNEXPECTED PROBLEM FOR WOMEN WHO TRAIN INTENSELY

A paradox exists between exercise and bone dynamics for athletic premenopausal women, particularly young athletes who have yet to attain peak bone mass (see "Focus on Research"). Women who train intensely and emphasize weight loss often engage in disordered eating behaviors. This decreases energy availability, reducing body mass and body fat to a point that (1) creates menstrual irregularities (**oligomenorrhea**; 35 to 90 days between periods) or (2) causes cessation of menstruation (**secondary amenorrhea**). Clinicians define secondary amen-

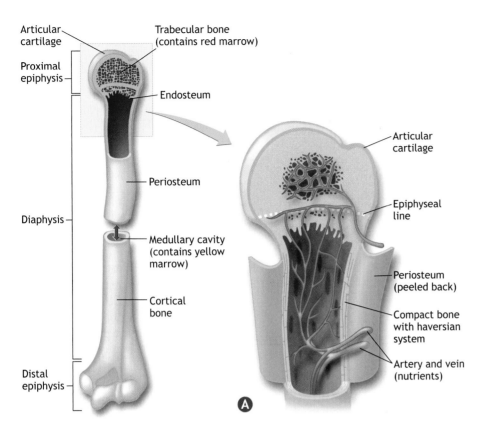

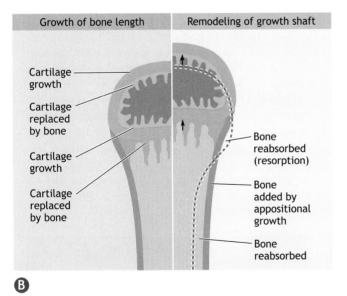

Figure 2.11 Anatomic structure (**A**) and longitudinal view of a typical long bone, and (**B**) bone dynamics during growth and continual remodeling.

orrhea as cessation of menstrual cycles for at least three consecutive months after regular cycles have begun. A tightly bound continuum generally begins with disordered eating—a serious ailment that in the extreme causes life-threatening complications.[33] Disordered eating behaviors eventually lead to the **female athlete triad** (FIG. 2.12)—energy drain, amenorrhea, and osteoporosis.[123,142,191,231] Some prefer the term *female triad* because the syndrome of disorders also afflicts physically active women in the general population who do not fit the typical profile of the competitive athlete.

INTEGRATIVE QUESTION

Why do resistance exercises for the body's major muscle groups offer unique benefits to bone mass compared with a typical weight-bearing program of brisk walking?

Many young women who play sports likely suffer from at least one of the triad's disorders, particularly disordered eating behaviors and accompanying energy deficit. This mal-

FEMALE ATHLETES WITH OSTEOPOROSIS

Drinkwater BL, et al. Menstrual history as a determinant of current bone density in young athletes. JAMA 1990;263:545.

▲ Research on female athletes has focused on their reduced bone mineral density associated with menstrual dysfunctions (oligomenorrhea, irregular menstrual cycle; amenorrhea, menstrual cessation). Persistent amenorrhea often minimizes the benefits of exercise on bone mass, increasing risk of repeated stress fractures during exercise because osteoporosis develops at an early age.

A pioneering 1984 study by Drinkwater and colleagues linked amenorrhea in 14 female athletes with a statistically significant 13.8% decrease in spinal bone mineral density compared with age-matched eumenorrheic athletes. The researchers hypothesized that early onset and repeated menstrual dysfunction produced permanent suboptimal bone mass throughout life. The condition increased these women's risk for developing early osteoporosis and stress fractures, even after competitive athletics ceased and normal menstruation resumed.

A subsequent study by Drinkwater (6 years later and presented here), demonstrated that women with regular menstrual cycles maintained higher lumbar bone densities (1.27 g $\cdot$ cm^{-2}) than athletic women with oligomenorrhea/amenorrhea interspersed with regular cycles (1.18 g $\cdot$ cm^{-2}). Moreover, the density of the lumbar bone region of both groups exceeded that of athletic women who never had regular cycles (1.05 g $\cdot$ cm^{-2}).

The researchers studied 97 active women aged 18 to 38 years. No woman smoked, and all exercised regularly at least 4 days per week for 45 minutes or longer per session. None of the women used oral contraceptives, and none experienced medical problems with bone metabolism. The following definitions defined current menstrual status: *regular* (10 to 13 periods per year), *oligomenorrheic* (3 to 6 periods per year at intervals longer than 36 days), or *amenorrheic* (no more than 2 periods per year or no period during the last 6 months). Assays for estradiol and progesterone levels confirmed menstrual status. Menstrual history included one of three categories: always had regular menses (R), had episodes of oligomenorrhea (O), or amenorrhea (A). Two reproductive endocrinologists ranked subjects on a scale from 1 to 9 on their expectations for bone mass for all combinations of reported present and past menstrual patterns. A pattern of always maintaining regular menses (R/R) ranked first as the most positive effect on bone. Current amenorrheics who also exhibited previous amenorrhea (A/A) received the lowest rank (ninth) for the physician's expectation of identifying women with the most negative bone pattern.

The main figure displays vertebral bone density versus menstrual history for the 97 women. The plot includes the averages and variability for the menstrual groupings (only means with 5 or more subjects plotted) containing the following numbers of subjects per grouping: 1, R/R ($n = 21$); 2, R/O ($n = 7$); 3, O/R ($n = 2$); 4, O/O ($n = 5$); 5, R/A ($n = 22$); 6, A/R ($n = 9$); 7, O/A ($n = 10$); 8, A/O ($n = 10$); 9, A/A ($n = 11$). Statistical analyses revealed significant bone mineral density differences between group 1 and groups 8 and 9, but no statistically significant differences among groups 2 through 7. Thus, the researchers merged the nine groups into three subgroups: group 1, women who always maintained regular menses (R/R); group 2, women with bouts of oligomenorrhea or amenorrhea interspersed with regular menses and women with current oligomenorrhea (R/O/A); and group 3, women with current amenorrhea who experienced previous amenorrhea or oligomenorrhea (O/A). The inset figure relates the three subgroups to bone mineral density. Women who always menstruated regularly had the highest bone density values, women with occasional irregularity averaged 6% less bone density, and women who never menstruated regularly averaged 17% less. The third group was younger, weighed less, and experienced menarche at an older age. They also began to train seriously earlier in life, they trained more frequently and for longer durations each day and traversed more miles than women who always maintained regular menses (group 1).

These studies suggest that prolonged oligomenorrhea/amenorrhea may irreversibly decrease vertebral bone density; the condition becomes exacerbated in women with persistently low body weight.

The work of Drinkwater and colleagues also increased awareness in the research and medical communities about the importance of understanding interactions among bone mineral density and intense physical training, estrogen levels, menstrual dysfunction, low body weight, and suboptimal energy and nutrient intake. The research paved the way for more clinically relevant treatment of female athletes at increased risk of irreversible loss of bone mass.

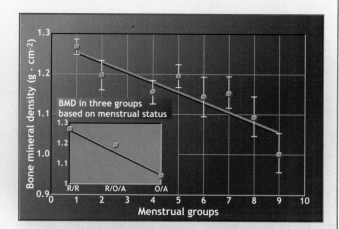

Relationship between vertebral bone mineral density (BMD) and menstrual history for 97 young women. (Inset) Bone mineral densities in three groups based on menstrual status.

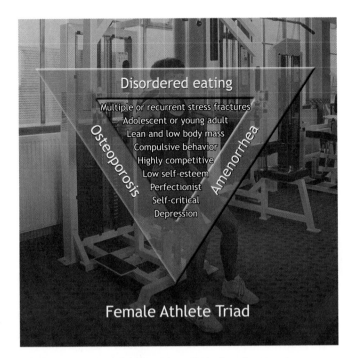

Figure 2.12 The female athlete triad: disordered eating, amenorrhea, and osteoporosis.

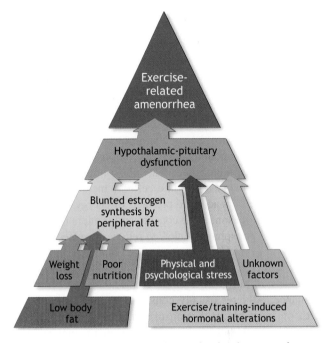

Figure 2.13 Factors contributing to the development of exercise-related amenorrhea.

ady afflicts 15 to 60% of female athletes, particularly those involved in leanness-related sports.[29] FIGURE 2.13 illustrates the contributing factors associated with exercise-related amenorrhea, considered the "red flag," or most recognizable symptom for the triad's presence. Female athletes of the 1970s and 1980s believed the loss of normal menstruation reflected hard training and was the inevitable consequence of athletic success. The prevalence of amenorrhea among female athletes in body weight–related sports (distance running, gymnastics, ballet, cheerleading, figure skating, body building) probably ranges between 25 and 65%; no more than 5% of the general population of women of menstruating age experience this condition.

INTEGRATIVE QUESTION

Advise a group of high school females about strategies to achieve weight loss to compete successfully and healthfully in competitive gymnastics.

Bone density relates closely to (1) menstrual regularity and (2) the total number of menstrual cycles. Premature cessation of menstruation removes estrogen's protective effect on bone, making these young women more vulnerable to calcium loss with concomitant decrease in bone mass.[69,229] The most severe menstrual disorders produce the greatest negative effect on bone mass.[208] Lowered bone density from extended amenorrhea often occurs at multiple sites, including bone areas regularly subjected to increased force and impact loading during exercise.[163] Concurrently, the problem worsens in individuals undergoing an energy deficit accompanied by low protein, lipid, and energy intakes,[233] in such cases, a poor diet also provides inadequate

calcium intake. Persistent amenorrhea that begins at an early age diminishes the benefits of exercise on bone mass; it also increases the risk of musculoskeletal injuries, particularly repeated stress fractures during exercise.[140] For example, a 5% loss in bone mass increases the risk of stress fractures by nearly 40%. Reestablishing normal menses causes some regain in bone mass but not to levels achieved with normal menstruation. Bone mass often remains *permanently* at suboptimal levels throughout adult life—leaving the woman at increased risk for osteoporosis and stress fractures, even years after competitive athletic participation.[44,134] Professional organizations recommend that intervention begin within 3 months of the onset of amenorrhea. Some colleges and universities maintain a web page that deals directly with the triad (www.bc.edu/bc_org/svp/uhs/eating/eating-femaleathletes.htm; www.ianr.unl.edu/pubs/foods/nf361.htm). Successful treatment of athletic amenorrhea uses a nonpharmacologic, behavioral approach plus diet and training interventions as follows[43]:

• Reduce training level by 10 to 20%
• Gradually increase total energy intake
• Increase body weight by 2 to 3%
• Maintain daily calcium intake at 1500 mg

ESTROGEN'S ROLE IN BONE HEALTH

■ Increases intestinal calcium absorption
■ Reduces urinary calcium excretion
■ Inhibits bone resorption
■ Decreases bone turnover

PHOSPHORUS

Phosphorus combines with calcium to form hydroxyapatite and calcium phosphate—compounds that give rigidity to bones and teeth. Phosphorus also serves as an essential component of the intracellular mediator cyclic adenosine monophosphate (cAMP) and the intramuscular high-energy compounds adenosine triphosphate (ATP) and phosphocreatine (PCr). Phosphorus combines with lipids to form phospholipid compounds, integral components of the cells' bilayer plasma membrane. The phosphorous-containing phosphatase enzymes regulate cellular metabolism; phosphorus also buffers acid end products of energy metabolism. For this latter reason, some coaches and trainers recommend consuming "phosphate drinks" to reduce the effects of acid production in intense exercise and perhaps enhance oxygen release from red blood cells.[31] In Chapter 23, we discuss the usefulness of buffering agents for augmenting exercise performance. Athletes usually consume adequate phosphorus, with the possible exception of female dancers and gymnasts.[18,138] Rich dietary sources of phosphorus include meat, fish, poultry, milk products, and cereals.

MAGNESIUM

Only about 1% of the body's 20 to 30 g of magnesium is found in blood, with about one half of the stores present inside cells of body tissues and organs and the remainder combined with calcium and phosphorus in bone. About 400 enzymes that regulate metabolic processes contain magnesium. Magnesium plays an important role in glucose metabolism by facilitating muscle and liver glycogen formation from blood-borne glucose. It also participates as a cofactor in glucose, fatty acid, and amino acid breakdown during energy metabolism. Magnesium affects lipid and protein synthesis and contributes to optimal neuromuscular functioning. It acts as an electrolyte, which along with potassium and sodium helps to maintain blood pressure

By regulating deoxyribonucleic acid (DNA) and ribonucleic acid (RNA) synthesis and structure, magnesium affects cell growth, reproduction, and plasma membrane structure. Because of its role as a Ca^{+2} channel blocker, inadequate magnesium could lead to hypertension and cardiac arrhythmias. Only small losses of magnesium occur with sweating.

Conflicting data exist concerning the possible effects of magnesium supplements on exercise performance and the training response. In one study, magnesium supplementation did not affect quadriceps muscle strength or measures of fatigue in the 6-week period following a marathon.[209] Subsequent research showed that 4 weeks of a 212 mg per day magnesium oxide supplement increased resting magnesium levels but not anaerobic or aerobic exercise performance compared with a placebo.[54] In contrast, other research shows that untrained men and women who supplemented with magnesium increased quadriceps power compared with a placebo treatment during 7 weeks of resistance training.[21]

The magnesium intake of athletes generally attains recommended levels, although female dancers and gymnasts have relatively low intakes.[18,138] Green leafy vegetables, legumes, nuts, bananas, mushrooms, and whole grains provide a rich source of magnesium. The magnesium content of refined foods is usually low. Whole-wheat bread, for example, contains twice the magnesium of white bread because industrial processing removes the magnesium-rich germ and bran. In addition, the nation's water supply provides a ready source of magnesium, but the amount varies according to the water source. "Hard" water contains more magnesium than "soft" water. We do not recommend taking magnesium supplements because these often are mixed with dolomite $(CaMg(CO_3)_2$, an extract from dolomitic limestone and marble), which often contains the toxic elements mercury and lead.

IRON

The body normally contains between 2.5 and 4.0 g (about 1/6 oz) of the trace mineral iron. Seventy to 80% exists in functionally active compounds, predominantly combined with **hemoglobin** in red blood cells (85% of functional iron). This iron–protein compound increases the blood's oxygen-carrying capacity 65 times. Iron serves other important exercise-related functions besides its role in oxygen transport. It is a structural component of **myoglobin** (12% of functional iron), a compound similar to hemoglobin, which aids in oxygen storage and transport within the muscle cell. Small amounts of iron also exist in **cytochromes**, the specialized substances that facilitate energy transfer within the cell. About 20% of the body's iron does not combine in functionally active compounds and exists as **hemosiderin** and **ferritin** stored in the liver, spleen, and bone marrow. These stores replenish iron lost from the functional compounds; they also provide the iron reserve during periods of insufficient dietary iron intake. An iron-binding plasma glycoprotein, **transferrin**, transports iron from ingested food and damaged red blood cells to tissues in need, particularly the liver, spleen, bone marrow, and skeletal muscles. *Plasma levels of transferrin often reflect the adequacy of the current iron intake.*

Physically active individuals should include normal amounts of iron-rich foods in their daily diet. Persons with inadequate iron intake or with limited rates of iron absorption or high rates of iron loss often develop a reduced concentration of hemoglobin in red blood cells. The result of the extreme condition of iron insufficiency, commonly called **iron deficiency anemia**, produces general sluggishness, loss of appetite, skin pale or gray (pallor), sore tongue, brittle nails, frontal headaches, dizziness, and reduced capacity to sustain even mild exercise. "Iron therapy" normalizes the blood's hemoglobin content and exercise capacity. TABLE 2.6 gives recommendations for iron intake for children and adults.

Females: A Population at Risk

Inadequate iron intake frequently occurs among young children, teenagers, and females of childbearing age, including many physically active women.[15,31,161] In the United States, estimates place between 10 and 13% of premenopausal

TABLE 2.6 ■ RECOMMENDED DIETARY ALLOWANCES FOR IRON

	AGE (YEARS)	IRON (mg)
Children	1–10	10
Males	11–18	12
	19	10
Females	11–50	15
	51	10
	Pregnant	30[a]
	Lactating	15[a]

Food and Nutrition Board, National Academy of Sciences–National Research Council, Washington, DC.
[a]Generally, this increased requirement cannot be met by ordinary diets; therefore, the use of 30 to 60 mg of supplemental iron is recommended.

women as deficient in iron intake; between 3 and 5% are anemic by conventional diagnostic criteria.[49,122] In addition, pregnancy can trigger a moderate iron deficiency anemia from the increased iron demand for both mother and fetus.

Iron loss from the 30 to 60 mL of blood generally lost during a menstrual cycle ranges between 15 and 30 mg. This requires an additional 5 mg of dietary iron daily for premenopausal females and increases the average monthly dietary iron requirement by 150 mg for synthesizing red blood cells lost during menstruation. Not surprisingly, 30 to 50% of American women experience dietary iron insufficiency from menstrual blood loss and limited dietary iron intake. The typical iron intake averages 6 mg of iron per 1000 calories of food consumed, with heme iron providing about 15% of the total iron.

Importance of Iron Source

The healthy small intestine absorbs about 10 to 15% of the total ingested iron, depending on one's iron status, the form of iron ingested, and the meal's composition. For example, the intestine usually absorbs 2 to 5% of iron from plants (trivalent ferric or **nonheme** elemental iron), whereas iron absorption from animal (divalent ferrous or **heme**) sources increases to 10 to 35%. The presence of heme iron, which represents between 35 and 55% of iron in animal sources, also increases iron absorption from nonheme sources. Increased iron loss or requirement also induces increased intestinal iron absorption.

The relatively low bioavailability of nonheme iron places women on vegetarian-type diets at risk for developing iron insufficiency. Female vegetarian runners have a poorer iron status than counterparts who consume the same quantity of iron from predominantly animal sources.[192] Including foods rich in vitamin C in the diet upgrades dietary iron bioavailability (see Fig. 2.1). This occurs because ascorbic acid prevents oxidation of ferrous iron to the ferric form, thus increasing nonheme iron's solubility for absorption at the alkaline pH of the small intestine. The ascorbic acid in one glass of orange juice

stimulates a 3-fold increase in nonheme iron absorption from a breakfast.[182] Heme sources of iron include beef, beef liver, pork, tuna, and clams; oatmeal, dried figs, spinach, beans, and lentils are good nonheme sources. Fiber-rich foods, coffee, and tea contain compounds that interfere with the intestinal absorption of iron (and zinc).

Exercise-Induced Anemia: Fact or Fiction?

Interest in endurance sports, combined with increased participation of women in these activities, has focused research on the influence of intense training on the body's iron status. The term **sports anemia** frequently describes reduced hemoglobin levels approaching clinical anemia (12 g per dL of blood for women and 14 g per dL for men) attributable to training. Some maintain that *strenuous* training creates an added demand for iron that often exceeds its intake. This taxes iron reserves and eventually leads to depressed hemoglobin synthesis and/or reduction in iron-containing compounds within the cell's energy transfer system. Individuals susceptible to an "iron drain" could experience reduced exercise capacity because of iron's crucial role in oxygen transport and use.

Intense physical training theoretically creates an augmented iron demand from three sources:

1. Small loss of iron in sweat[223]
2. Loss of hemoglobin in urine from red blood cell destruction with increased temperature, spleen activity, and circulation rates and from jarring of the kidneys and mechanical trauma from feet pounding on the running surface (called foot-strike hemolysis)[94]
3. Gastrointestinal bleeding with distance running that is unrelated to age, gender, or performance time[25,168]

Real Anemia or Pseudoanemia?

Apparent suboptimal hemoglobin concentrations and hematocrits occur more frequently among endurance athletes, thus supporting the possibility of an exercise-induced anemia. Reductions in hemoglobin concentration are transient, occurring in the early phase of training and then returning toward pretraining values. FIGURE 2.14 illustrates the general response for hematologic variables for high-school female cross-country runners during a competitive season. The decrease in hemoglobin concentration generally parallels the disproportionately large expansion in plasma volume (compared with total hemoglobin) with both endurance and resistance training (see Fig. 13.5).[40,65,184,186] Just several days of exercise training increase plasma volume by 20%, while total red blood cell volume remains unchanged. Consequently, *total* hemoglobin (an important factor in endurance performance) remains the same or increases slightly with training, while hemoglobin *concentration* decreases in the expanding plasma volume. Despite this

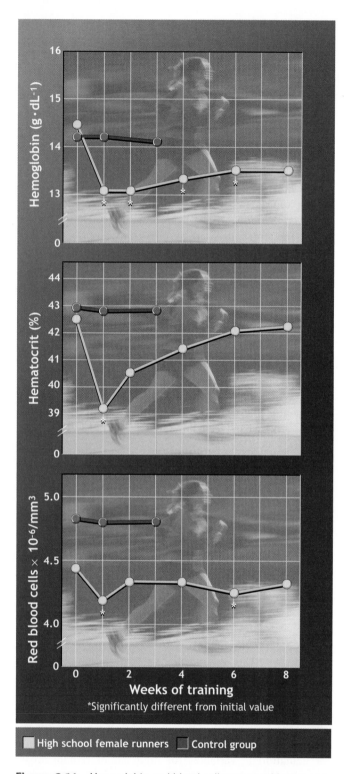

Figure 2.14 Hemoglobin, red blood cell count, and hematocrit in female high school cross-country runners and a comparison group during the competitive season. (Adapted from Puhl JL, et al. Erythrocyte changes during training in high school women cross-country runners. Res Q Exerc Sport 1981;52:484.)

hemoglobin dilution, aerobic capacity and exercise performance improve with training.

Mechanical destruction of red blood cells occurs with vigorous exercise, along with some loss of iron in sweat.[223] However, no evidence indicates that these factors strain an athlete's iron reserves and precipitate clinical anemia if iron intake remains at recommended levels. Applying stringent criteria for both anemia and insufficiency of iron reserves makes sports anemia much less prevalent than generally believed.[225] For male collegiate runners and swimmers, no indications of the early stages of anemia were noted despite large changes in training volume and intensity during the competitive season.[156] For female athletes, the prevalence of iron deficiency anemia did *not* differ in comparisons among specific athletic groups or with nonathletic controls.[167]

FACTORS AFFECTING IRON ABSORPTION

Increase iron absorption
- Acid in the stomach
- Iron in heme form
- High body demand for red blood cells (blood loss, high altitude exposure, physical training, pregnancy)
- Low body iron stores
- Presence of mean protein factor (MPF)
- Presence of vitamin C in small intestine

Decrease iron absorption
- Phytic acid (in dietary fiber)
- Oxalic acid
- Polyphenols (in tea and coffee)
- High body iron stores
- Excess of other minerals (Zn, Mg, Ca), particularly when taken as supplements
- Reduction in stomach acid
- Antacids

Should Athletes Take an Iron Supplement?

Any increase in iron loss with exercise training (coupled with poor dietary habits) in adolescent and premenopausal women could strain an already limited iron reserve. This does not mean that all individuals in training should supplement with iron or that dietary iron insufficiency or iron loss caused by exercise produces sports anemia. It does suggest the importance of monitoring an athlete's iron status by periodic evaluation of hematologic characteristics and iron reserves, particularly athletes who supplement with iron.[125,126] Measuring serum ferritin concentration provides useful information about iron reserves; values below $20 \ \mu g \cdot L^{-1}$ for females and $30 \ \mu g \cdot L^{-1}$ for males indicate depleted reserves.

Potential harm exists from overconsumption or overabsorption of iron (particularly with the widespread use of vitamin C supplements, which facilitate iron absorption).[56] Iron supplements should not be used indiscriminately because excessive iron can accumulate to toxic levels and contribute significantly to diabetes, liver disease, and heart and joint damage; it may even promote the growth of latent cancers and infectious organisms.[145]

Functional Anemia

For an individual whose diet contains the recommended iron intake or who shows no clinical signs of iron deficiency, iron supplementation does not increase hemoglobin or hematocrit concentrations or other measures of iron status.[11] Low values for hemoglobin within the "normal" range could reflect **functional anemia** or **marginal iron deficiency**, a condition characterized by depleted iron stores, reduced iron-dependent protein production (e.g., oxidative enzymes) but a relatively *normal* hemoglobin concentration. The ergogenic effects of iron supplementation on aerobic exercise performance and training responsiveness have been noted for iron-deficient athletes.[22,23,59] For example, physically active but untrained women classified as iron depleted (serum ferritin < 16 µg · L^{-1}) but not anemic (Hb > 12 g · dL^{-1}) received either iron therapy (50 mg ferrous sulfate) or a placebo twice daily for 2 weeks.[79] All subjects then completed 4 weeks of aerobic training. The iron-supplemented group significantly increased serum ferritin levels with only a small (nonsignificant) increase in hemoglobin concentration. The improvement in 15-km endurance cycling time in the supplemented group was twice that of the women who consumed the placebo (3.4 vs. 1.6 min faster). These findings suggest that women with low serum ferritin levels but hemoglobin concentrations above 12 g · dL^{-1},

although not clinically anemic, might still be functionally anemic and thus benefit from iron supplementation to augment exercise performance. Similarly, iron-depleted but nonanemic women received either a placebo or 20 mg of elemental iron as ferrous sulfate twice daily for 6 weeks. FIGURE 2.15 shows that the iron supplement attenuated the rate of decrease in maximal force measured sequentially during 8 minutes of dynamic knee extension exercise.[24]

These findings support current recommendations to use an iron supplement for nonanemic physically active women with low serum ferritin levels.[148] Supplementation in this case exerts little effect on hemoglobin concentration and red blood cell volume. Any improved exercise capacity most likely comes from increased muscle oxidative capacity, not increases in the blood's oxygen transport capacity.

SODIUM, POTASSIUM, AND CHLORINE

Sodium, potassium, and chlorine, collectively termed **electrolytes**, remain dissolved in the body fluids as electrically charged particles, or **ions**. Sodium and chlorine represent the chief minerals contained in blood plasma and extracellular fluid. Electrolytes modulate fluid exchange within the body's fluid compartments, promoting a constant, well-regulated exchange of nutrients and waste products between the cell and its external fluid environment. Potassium is the chief intracellular mineral.

Sodium and potassium ions establish the proper electrical gradient across cell membranes. The difference in

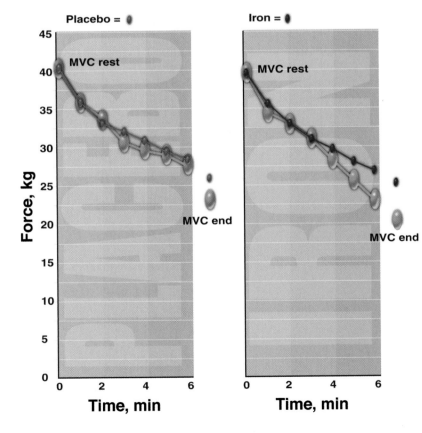

Figure 2.15 Maximal voluntary static contractions (MVCs) over the first 6 minutes of a progressive fatigue test of dynamic knee extensions before ( ) and after ( ) supplementation with either a placebo or iron. MVC_{end} represents the last MVC of the protocol and occurred at different times (average $\approx$ 8 min) for each subject. (From Brutsaert TD, et al. Iron supplementation improves progressive fatigue resistance during dynamic knee extensor exercise in iron-depleted, nonanemic women. Am J Clin Nutr 2003;77:441.)

electrical balance between the cell's interior and exterior surfaces facilitates nerve impulse transmission, stimulation and action of muscle, and proper gland functioning. Electrolytes also maintain plasma membrane permeability and regulate the acid and base qualities of bodily fluids, particularly blood. TABLE 2.7 lists normal values for serum and sweat electrolyte concentrations and the electrolyte and carbohydrate concentrations of common beverages.

Optimal Sodium Intake

Aldosterone conserves sodium in the kidneys under conditions of low-to-moderate dietary sodium intake. In contrast, high dietary sodium blunts this hormone's release, with excess sodium voided in the urine. This maintains sodium balance throughout a wide range of intakes. Some individuals cannot adequately regulate excessive sodium intake. Abnormal sodium accumulation in bodily fluids increases fluid volume and elevates blood pressure to levels that may pose a health risk.

Sodium distributes naturally in foods that one can readily maintain the daily requirement without adding salt to the diet. Sodium intake in the United States regularly exceeds the daily level recommended for adults of 2400 mg, or the amount of one heaping teaspoon of table salt (sodium makes up about 40% of salt). The typical Western diet contains about 4500 mg of sodium (8 to 12 g of salt) each day with three quarters coming from processed food and restaurant meals. This represents 10 times the 500 mg of sodium the body actually needs. Reliance on table salt in processing, curing, cooking, seasoning, and preserving common foods accounts for the large sodium intake. Common sodium-rich dietary sources include monosodium glutamate (MSG), soy sauce, condiments, canned foods, baking soda, and baking powder.

Sodium-Induced Hypertension. For decades, the first line of defense in treating high blood pressure eliminated excess sodium from the diet. Reducing sodium intake can lower blood pressure via reduced plasma volume. However, considerable variation exists in blood pressure responsiveness to NaCl intake.[109] For "salt-sensitive" individuals (30% of hypertensive adults, 30% with prehypertension, and the nearly 90% who will eventually get hypertension if they live to age 75) and middle-age and older normotensive individuals, reducing dietary sodium to the low end of the recommended range and upgrading the quality of the diet reduces blood pressure (see "In a Practical Sense," p. 73).[20,197,228] If dietary constraints prove ineffective in lowering blood pressure, drugs that induce water loss (diuretics) become the next line of defense. Unfortunately, diuretics also produce losses in other minerals, particularly potassium. Patients who use diuretics should consume a potassium-rich diet (e.g., potatoes, bananas, oranges, tomatoes, and meat).

MINERALS AND EXERCISE PERFORMANCE

Consuming mineral supplements above recommended levels on a long- or short-term basis does not benefit exercise performance or enhance training responsiveness.

Mineral Loss in Sweat

Excessive water and electrolyte loss impairs heat tolerance and exercise performance. It also can lead to severe dysfunction culminating in heat cramps, heat exhaustion, or heat stroke. The yearly toll of heat-related deaths during spring and summer football practice provides a tragic illustration of the importance of fluid and electrolyte replacement. During practice or an athletic event an athlete may lose up to 5 kg of water from sweating. This corresponds to about 8.0 g of salt depletion, because each kg (1 L) of sweat contains about 1.5 g of salt. Despite this potential for mineral loss, replacement of water lost through sweating becomes the crucial and immediate need.

TABLE 2.7 ■ ELECTROLYTE CONCENTRATIONS IN BLOOD SERUM AND SWEAT, AND CARBOHYDRATE AND ELECTROLYTE CONCENTRATIONS OF SOME POPULAR BEVERAGES

SUBSTANCE	NA+ (mEq · L⁻¹)ᵃ	K+ (mEq · L⁻¹)	CA++ (mEq · L⁻¹)	MG++ (mEq · L⁻¹)	CL⁻ (mEq · L⁻¹)	OSMOLALITY (mOsm · L⁻¹)ᵇ	CHO (g · L⁻¹)ᶜ
Blood serum	140	4.5	2.5	1.5–2.1	110	300	—
Sweat	60–80	4.5	1.5	3.3	40–90	170–220	—
Coca Cola	3.0	—	—	—	1.0	650	—
Gatorade	23.0	3.0	—	—	14.0	280	107
Fruit juice	0.5	58.0	—	—	—	690	62
Pepsi Cola	1.7	Trace	—	—	—	568	118
Water	Trace	Trace	—	—	Trace	10–20	81

ᵃMilliequivalents per liter.
ᵇMilliosmoles per liter.
ᶜGrams per liter.

IN A PRACTICAL SENSE

LOWERING HIGH BLOOD PRESSURE WITH DIETARY INTERVENTION: THE DASH DIET

■ Nearly 50 million Americans have hypertension, a condition that if left untreated increases the risk of stroke, heart attack, and kidney failure. Fifty percent of hypertensives actually seek treatment. Only about one half of these individuals achieve long-term success. One reason for the lack of compliance concerns possible side effects of readily available antihypertensive medication. For example, fatigue and impotence often discourage patients from maintaining a chronic medication schedule required by pharmacologic treatment of hypertension.

THE DASH APPROACH

Research using **DASH** (Dietary Approaches to Stop Hypertension) to treat hypertension shows that this diet lowers blood pressure in some individuals to the same extent as pharmacologic therapy and often more than other lifestyle changes. Two months of the diet reduced systolic pressure by an average of 11.4 mm Hg; diastolic pressure decreased by 5.5 mm Hg. Every 2-mm Hg reduction in systolic pressure lowers heart disease risk by 5% and stroke risk by 8%. Further good news emerges from recent research that indicates that the standard DASH diet combined with a daily dietary salt intake of 1500 mg produced even greater blood pressure reductions than achieved with the DASH diet only.

Table 1 shows the general nature of the DASH diet with its high content of fruits, vegetables, and dairy products and low fat composition.

SAMPLE DASH DIET

Table 2 shows a sample DASH diet consisting of approximately 2100 calories (kCal). This level of energy intake provides a stable body weight for a typical 70-kg person. More physically active and heavier individuals should boost portion size or the number of individual items to maintain weight. Individuals desiring to lose weight or who are lighter and/or sedentary should eat less, but not less than the minimum number of servings for each food group shown below.

Sacks FM, et al. Rationale and design of the Dietary Approaches to Stop Hypertension trial (DASH): a multicenter controlled feeding study of dietary patterns to lower blood pressure. Ann Epidemiol 1995;108:118.

Bray GA, et al, A further subgroup analysis of the effect of the DASH diet and three sodium levels on blood pressure: results of the Dash-Sodium Trial. Am J Cardiol 2004; 94:222.

TABLE 1 ■ DIETARY APPROACHES TO STOP HYPERTENSION (DASH)

FOOD GROUP	EXAMPLE OF ONE SERVING	SERVINGS
Vegetables	1/2 cup of cooked or raw chopped vegetables; 1 cup of raw leafy vegetables; or 6 oz of juice	8 to 12 daily
Fruit	1 medium apple, pear, orange, or banana; 1/2 grapefruit; 1/3 cantaloupe; 1/2 cup of fresh frozen or canned fruit; 1/4 cup of dried fruit; or 6 oz of juice	8 to 12 daily
Grains	1 slice of bread; 1/2 cup of cold, dry cereal; 1/2 cup cooked rice or pasta	6 to 12 daily
Dairy	1 cup of no-fat or low-fat milk or 1 1/2 oz of low-fat or part-skim cheese	2 to 4 daily
Nuts, seeds, and beans	1/3 cup (1 1/2 oz) of nuts; 2 Tbsp of seeds; or 1/2 cup of cooked beans	4 to 7 weekly
Meat, poultry, or fish	3 oz serving (roughly the size of a deck of cards)	1 to 2 daily
Oil or other fats	1 tsp vegetable oil, butter, salad dressings, soft margarine	2 to 4 daily

continued on page 74

Continued

TABLE 2 ■ SAMPLE DASH DIET (2100 kCal)

FOOD	AMOUNT	FOOD	AMOUNT
Breakfast		*Dinner*	
Orange juice	6 oz	Herbed baked cod	3 oz
1% low-fat milk	8 oz (used with corn flakes)	Scallion rice	1 cup [equals 2 servings of grain]
Corn flakes	1 cup (dry) [equals 2 servings of	Steamed broccoli	1/2 cup
(1 tsp sugar)	grains]	Stewed tomatoes	1/2 cup
Banana	1 medium	Spinach salad	1/2 cup
Whole-wheat bread	1 slice	(raw spinach)	
Solf margarine	1 tsp	Cherry tomatoes	2
Lunch		Cucumber	2 slices
Low-fat chicken salad	3/4 cup	Light Italian salad	1 Tbsp [equals 1/2 fat serving]
Pita bread	1/2 large	dressing	
Raw vegetable medley		Whole-wheat dinner	1
Carrot and celery sticks	3–4 sticks each	roll	
Radishes	2	Soft margarine	1 tsp
Lettuce	2 leaves	Melon balls	1/2 cup
Part-skim mozzarella	1 1/2 slices (1.5 oz)	*Snack*	
1% low-fat milk	8 oz	Dried apricots	1 oz (1/4 cup)
Fruit cocktail	1/2 cup	Mixed nuts, unsalted	1.5 oz (1/3 cup)
		Mini-pretzels, unsalted	1 oz (3/4 cup)
		Diet ginger ale	12 oz [does not count as a serving of any food]

Svetkey LP, et al. Effects of dietary patterns on blood pressure: subgroup analysis of the Dietary Approaches to Stop Hypertension (DASH) randomized clinical trial. Arch Intern Med 1999;159:285.

INTEGRATIVE QUESTION

Many young girls and women engaged in sports likely suffer from at least one of the disorders of the female athlete triad. Discuss factors related to this syndrome and how a coach might guard against their occurrence.

Defense Against Mineral Loss

Sweat loss during vigorous exercise triggers a rapid, coordinated release of the hormones vasopressin and aldosterone and the enzyme renin, which reduce sodium and water loss through the kidneys. An increase in sodium conservation occurs even under such extreme conditions as running a marathon in warm, humid weather when sweat output often reaches 2 L per hour. Adding a "pinch" of salt to the fluid or food ingested usually replenishes electrolytes lost in sweat. During a 20-day road race in Hawaii, runners maintained plasma minerals at normal levels when they consumed an unrestricted diet without mineral supplements.[43] Salt supplements may be beneficial in prolonged exercise in the heat when fluid loss exceeds 4 or 5 kg. This can be achieved by drinking a 0.1 to 0.2% salt solution (adding 0.3 tsp of table salt per liter of water).[3] A mild potassium deficiency can occur with intense exercise during heat stress, but a diet containing normal amounts of this mineral usually ensures adequate potassium levels.[35] An 8-oz glass of orange or tomato juice replaces almost all of the calcium, potassium, and magnesium lost in 3 L (3 kg) of sweat.

Trace Minerals and Exercise

Many individuals believe that supplementing with certain trace minerals enhances exercise performance and counteracts the demands of intense training. Strenuous exercise may increase excretion of the following trace elements:

- *Chromium:* required for carbohydrate and lipid catabolism and proper insulin function and protein synthesis
- *Copper:* required for red blood cell formation; influences gene expression and serves as a cofactor or prosthetic group for several enzymes
- *Manganese:* component of superoxide dismutase in the body's antioxidant defense system
- *Zinc:* component of lactate dehydrogenase, carbonic anhydrase, superoxide dismutase, and enzymes related to energy metabolism, cell growth and differentiation, and tissue repair

Urinary losses of zinc and chromium were 1.5- to 2.0-fold higher after a 6-mile run than on a rest day.[8] Sweat loss of copper and zinc also can attain relatively high levels.

Documentation of trace mineral losses with exercise does not necessarily mean athletes should supplement with these micronutrients. For example, short-term zinc supplementation ($25 \text{ mg} \cdot \text{d}^{-1}$) did not benefit metabolic and endocrine responses or endurance performance during intense exercise by eumenorrheic women.[188] Men and women who train intensely (with large sweat production) and have marginal nutrition (e.g., wrestlers, endurance runners, ballet dancers, and female gymnasts) should monitor trace mineral intake to prevent an overt deficiency. Collegiate football players who supplemented with 200 µg of chromium (as chromium picolinate) daily for 9 weeks experienced no beneficial changes in body composition and muscular strength during intense weight lifting compared with a control group that received a placebo.[29] Power and endurance athletes had significantly higher plasma levels of copper and zinc than nontraining controls.[173] An excessive intake of one mineral may cause a deficiency in the other because iron, zinc, and copper interact with each other and compete for the same carrier during intestinal absorption. *For most athletes, trace mineral deficiency does not compromise exercise performance or overall health.*

Summary

1. Approximately 4% of body mass consists of 22 elements called minerals distributed in all body tissues and fluids.

2. Minerals occur freely in nature in the waters of rivers, lakes, and oceans, and in soil. The root system of plants absorbs minerals; they eventually incorporate into the tissues of animals that consume plants.

3. Minerals function primarily in metabolism as important parts of enzymes. Minerals provide structure to bones and teeth and serve in synthesizing the biologic macronutrients—glycogen, fat, and protein.

4. A balanced diet generally provides adequate mineral intake, except in some geographic locations lacking a mineral in the soil such as iodine.

5. Osteoporosis has reached near-epidemic proportions among older individuals, particularly women. Adequate calcium intake and regular weight-bearing exercise and/or resistance training provide an effective defense against bone loss at any age.

6. Women who train intensely often do not match energy intake to energy output. This reduces body weight and body fat to a point that adversely affects menstruation, which contributes to significant bone loss at an early age. Restoration of normal menstruation does not fully restore bone mass.

7. About 40% of American women of childbearing age suffer from dietary iron insufficiency. This could lead to iron deficiency anemia, which negatively affects aerobic exercise performance and ability to train intensely.

8. For women on vegetarian-type diets, the relatively low bioavailability of nonheme iron increases the risk for developing iron insufficiency. Vitamin C in food or supplement form increases intestinal absorption of nonheme iron.

9. Regular physical activity probably does not significantly drain the body's iron reserves. If it does, females, with the greatest iron requirement and lowest iron intake increase their risk for anemia. Periodic assessment of the body's iron status should evaluate hematologic characteristics and iron reserves.

10. Significant losses of body water and related minerals occur with excessive sweating during exercise; these should be replaced during and following exercise. Sweat loss during exercise usually does not increase the mineral requirement above recommended values.

PART 3 • *Water*

THE BODY'S WATER CONTENT

Water makes up from 40 to 70% of body mass, depending on age, gender, and body composition; it constitutes 65 to 75% of the weight of muscle and about 10% of the fat mass. Consequently, differences in total body water between individuals largely result from variations in body composition (i.e., differences in lean versus fat tissue). Body fat has a low water content, so individuals with more total fat have a smaller overall percentage of their body weight as water.

FIGURE 2.16 depicts the fluid compartments of the body, the normal daily body water variation, and specific terminology to describe the various states of human hydration. The body contains two fluid "compartments." The first compartment, **intracellular**, refers to fluid inside the cells. The second compartment, **extracellular**, includes the fluid that flows within the microscopic spaces between cells (**interstitial fluid**) in addition to lymph, saliva, fluid in the eyes, fluid secreted by glands and the digestive tract, fluid that bathes the spinal cord nerves, and fluid excreted from the skin and kidneys. Blood plasma accounts for nearly 20% of the extracellular fluid (3 to 4 L). *Extracellular fluid provides most of the fluid lost through sweating, predominantly from blood plasma.* Of the total body water, an average of 62% (26 L of the body's 42 L of water for an average 80-kg man) represents intracellular water, and 38% comes from extracellular sources. These volumes represent averages from a dynamic exchange of fluid between compartments, particularly in physically active men and women.[181] Exercise training often increases the percentage of water distributed within the intracellular compartment because muscle mass increases, with its accompanying large water content. In contrast, an acute bout of exercise temporarily shifts fluid from plasma to interstitial and intracellular spaces from the increased hydrostatic (fluid) pressure within the circulatory system.

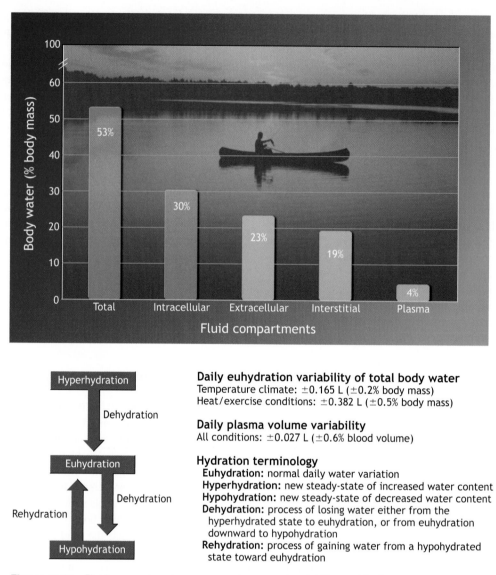

Figure 2.16 Fluid compartments, average volumes and variability, and hydration terminology. Volumes represent an 80-kg man. Approximately 55% of the body mass consists of water in striated muscle, skeleton, and adipose tissue. For a man and woman of similar body mass, the woman contains less total water because of her larger ratio of adipose tissue (low water content) to lean body mass (striated muscle and skeleton). (Adapted from Greenleaf JE. Problem: thirst, drinking behavior, and involuntary dehydration. Med Sci Sports Exerc 1992;24:645.)

Functions of Body Water

Water is a ubiquitous, remarkable nutrient. Without water, death occurs within days. It serves as the body's transport and reactive medium; diffusion of gases always takes place across surfaces moistened by water. Nutrients and gases travel in aqueous solution; waste products leave the body through the water in urine and feces. Water, in conjunction with various proteins, lubricates joints and cushions a variety of "moving" organs such as the heart, lungs, intestines, and eyes. Because water is noncompressible, it gives structure and form to the body through the turgor it provides for body tissues. Water has tremendous heat-stabilizing qualities because it absorbs considerable heat with only small changes in temperature. This quality, combined with water's high heat of vapor-

ization, maintains a relatively stable body temperature during (1) environmental heat stress and (2) the increased internal heat load generated by exercise. More is presented in Chapter 25 on the dynamics of thermoregulation during heat stress and exercise, particularly water's vital role.

WATER BALANCE: INTAKE VERSUS OUTPUT

The body's water content remains relatively stable over days, weeks, months, and even years. Considerable water output occurs in physically active individuals, but appropriate fluid intake rapidly restores any imbalance in the body's fluid level. FIGURE 2.17 displays the sources of water intake and output.

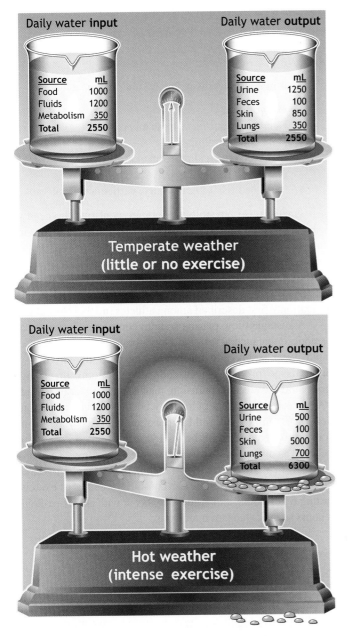

Figure 2.17 Water balance in the body. *Top.* Little or no exercise with thermoneutral ambient temperature and humidity. *Bottom.* Moderate-to-intense exercise in a hot, humid environment.

Water Intake

A sedentary adult in a thermoneutral environment requires about 2.5 L of water daily. For an active person in a warm, humid environment, the water requirement often increases to between 5 and 10 L daily. Three sources provide this water: (1) foods, (2) liquids, and (3) metabolism.

Water in Foods

Fruits and vegetables contain considerable water; in contrast, butter, oils, dried meats, and chocolate, cookies, and cakes have a relatively low water content. As examples of low water

content, peanut butter and shelled peanuts contain a trace of water, walnuts contain 4% water, and dried coconuts and pecans 7%. The percentage then increases for molasses (25%), whole wheat bread (35%), hamburger beef (54%), and whole milk (87%), while following foods exceed 90%—lettuce, raw strawberries, cucumbers, and watercress, Swiss chard, boiled squash, green peppers, bean sprouts, boiled collards, watermelon and cantaloupe, canned pumpkin, celery, and raw peaches.

Water from Liquids

The average individual normally consumes 1200 mL or 41 oz of water each day. Exercise and thermal stress increase the need for fluid by five or six times this amount. At the extreme, an individual lost 13.6 kg of water weight during a 2-day, 17-hour, 55-mile run across Death Valley, California.[169] With proper fluid ingestion, including salt supplements, the actual body weight loss amounted to only 1.4 kg. In this example, fluid loss and replenishment represented nearly 4 gallons of liquid!

Metabolic Water

The breakdown of macronutrient molecules in energy metabolism forms carbon dioxide and water. Termed **metabolic water**, this fluid provides about 14% of the daily water requirement of a sedentary person. When glucose breaks down, it liberates 55 g of metabolic water. A larger amount of water forms from protein (100 g) and fat (107 g) catabolism. Additionally, each gram of glycogen joins with 2.7 g of water as its glucose units link together; glycogen liberates this bound water during its catabolism for energy.

Water Output

Water loss from the body occurs in four ways: (1) in urine, (2) through the skin, (3) as water vapor in expired air, and (4) in feces.

Water Loss in Urine

Under normal conditions, the kidneys reabsorb about 99% of the 140 to 160 L of renal filtrate formed each day; consequently, the volume of urine excreted daily by the kidneys ranges from 1000 to 1500 mL, or about 1.5 quarts. Elimination of 1 g of solute by the kidneys requires about 15 mL of water. Thus, a portion of water in urine becomes "obligated" to rid the body of metabolic byproducts such as urea, an end product of protein breakdown. Large quantities of protein used for energy (as occurs with a high-protein diet) accelerate dehydration during exercise.

Water Loss Through the Skin

On a daily basis, perhaps 350 mL of water continually seeps from the deeper tissues through the skin to the body's surface as **insensible perspiration**. Water loss also occurs through the skin in the form of sweat produced by specialized sweat glands beneath the skin. Evaporation of sweat provides the refrigeration mechanism to cool the body. Each day under normal thermal and physical activity conditions the body produces 500 to 700 mL of sweat. This by no means reflects sweating capacity because a well-acclimatized person produces up to 12 L of sweat (at a rate of 1 L per hour) during prolonged, intense exercise in a hot environment.

Water Loss as Water Vapor

Insensible water loss through small water droplets in exhaled air amounts to between 250 and 350 mL per day from the complete moistening of inspired air as it passes down the pulmonary airways. Exercise affects this source of water loss. For physically active persons, the respiratory passages release 2 to 5 mL of water each minute during strenuous exercise, depending on climatic conditions. Ventilatory water loss is least in hot, humid weather and greatest in cold temperatures (inspired air contains little moisture) and at altitude. The latter occurs because inspired air volumes (which require humidification) are significantly larger than at sea level.

Water Loss in Feces

Intestinal elimination produces between 100 and 200 mL of water loss because water constitutes approximately 70% of fecal matter. The remainder comprises nondigestible materials including bacteria from the digestive process and the residues of digestive juices from the intestine, stomach, and pancreas. With diarrhea or vomiting, water loss increases up to 5000 mL, a potentially dangerous situation that can create fluid and electrolyte imbalance.

WATER REQUIREMENT IN EXERCISE

The loss of body water represents the most serious consequence of profuse sweating. The severity of physical activity, environmental temperature, and humidity determine the amount of water lost through sweating. **Relative humidity** (water content of the ambient air) affects the efficiency of the sweating mechanism in temperature regulation. Ambient air completely saturates with water vapor at 100% relative humidity. This blocks any evaporation of fluid from the skin surface to the air, minimizing this important avenue for body cooling. Under such conditions, sweat beads on the skin and eventually rolls off without providing a cooling effect. On a dry day, air can hold considerable moisture, and fluid evaporates rapidly from the skin. Thus, the sweat mechanism functions at optimal efficiency and body temperature remains regulated within a narrow range. Chapters 3 and 25 present a more detailed discussion of fluid replacement with exercise. Importantly, plasma volume decreases when sweating causes a fluid loss equal to 2 or 3% of body mass. Fluid loss from the vascular compartment strains circulatory function, which ultimately impairs exercise capacity and thermoregulation. *Monitoring changes in body weight (after urination) conveniently assesses fluid loss during exercise*

and/or heat stress. Each 0.45 kg (1 lb) of body weight loss corresponds to 450 mL (15 oz) of dehydration.

Hyponatremia

Four major concerns in hot-weather exercise include:

1. Dehydration
2. Decreased plasma volume and resulting hemoconcentration
3. Impaired physical performance and thermoregulatory capacity
4. Increased risk of heat injury, particularly heat stroke

The exercise physiology literature confirms the need to consume fluid before, during, and after exercise. In many instances, the recommended beverage remains plain, hypotonic water. However, excessive fluid intake under certain exercise conditions can be counterproductive, producing the potentially serious medical complication of **hyponatremia**, or "water intoxication," first described among athletes in 1985 (FIG. 2.18).

A sustained low plasma sodium concentration creates an osmotic imbalance across the blood–brain barrier that causes rapid water influx into the brain. The resulting swelling of brain tissue produces a cascade of symptoms that range from mild (headache, confusion, malaise, nausea, cramping) to severe (seizures, coma, pulmonary edema, cardiac arrest, and death).[10,62] In general, mild hyponatremia exists when serum sodium concentration falls below 135 mEq / L^{-1}; serum sodium below 125 mEq / L^{-1} triggers severe symptoms. The most conducive conditions for hyponatremia include water overload during high-intensity, ultramarathon-type, continuous exercise lasting 6 to 8 hours, although it may occur with exercise of only 4 hours such as standard marathons.[13,78,81,139]

PREDISPOSING FACTORS TO HYPONATREMIA

- Prolonged, high-intensity exercise in hot weather
- Augmented sodium loss associated with sweat production containing high sodium concentration, which often occurs in poorly conditioned individuals
- Beginning physical activity in a sodium-depleted state because of "salt-free" or "low-sodium" diet
- Use of diuretic medication for hypertension
- Frequent intake of large quantities of sodium-free fluid during prolonged exercise

---

Mild-to-severe hyponatremia has been reported with increasing frequency in ultraendurance athletes competing in hot weather.[196] For example, nearly 30% of the athletes competing in the 1984 Ironman Triathlon had symptoms of hyponatremia, most frequently observed late in the race or in the recovery period. In a large study of more than 18,000 ultraendurance athletes (including triathletes), approximately 9% of collapsed athletes during or following competition had symptoms of

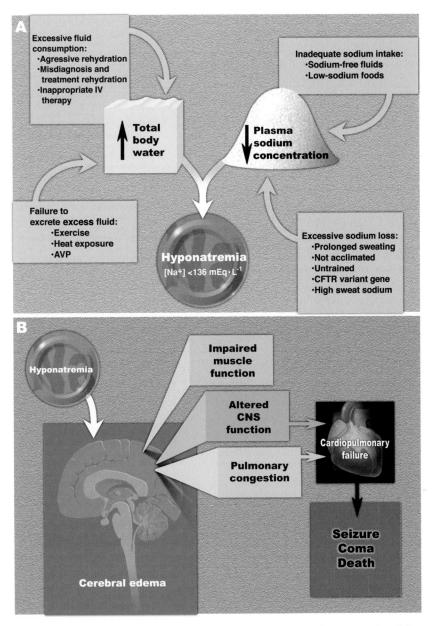

Figure 2.18 **A.** Factors that contribute to the development of hyponatremia. *AVP,* arginine vasopressin; *CFTR,* cystic fibrosis transmembrane regulatory gene. **B.** Physiologic consequences of hyponatremia. *CNS,* central nervous system. (Modified from Montain SJ, et al. Hyponatremia associated with exercise: risk factors and pathogenesis. Exerc Sport Sci Rev 2001;29:113.)

hyponatremia.[151] The athletes, on average, drank fluids with low sodium chloride content (<6.8 mmol $\cdot$ L^{-1}). The runner with the most severe hyponatremia (serum Na level = 112 mEq $\cdot$ L^{-1}) excreted more than 7.5 L of dilute urine during the first 17 hours of hospitalization.

INTEGRATIVE QUESTION

In what way would knowledge about hyponatremia modify your recommendations concerning fluid intake prior to, during, and in recovery from long-duration exercise?

Medical personnel monitored 95 athletes receiving medical care and 169 athletes not requiring care in the 1996 New Zealand Ironman Triathlon for changes in body mass and blood sodium concentration.[194] For athletes with clinical evidence of fluid or electrolyte disturbance, body mass declined 2.5 kg versus a decline of 2.9 kg in athletes not requiring medical care. Hyponatremia accounted for 9% of medical abnormalities. One athlete with hyponatremia (serum Na = 130 mEq $\cdot$ L^{-1}) drank 16 L of fluid during the race and gained 2.5 kg of body mass—consistent with the hypothesis that fluid overload causes hyponatremia. In an ultradistance multisport triathlon (kayak 67 km, cycle 148 km, run 23.8 km), average body mass of the competitors declined 2.5 kg (3% of initial body mass).[195] None of the athletes gained weight, and six weighed the same; the one athlete who became hyponatremic (serum Na = 134 mEq · L^{-1}) maintained weight and did not seek medical attention. Serum sodium concentration at the end of the race for the 47 athletes averaged 139.3 mEq · L^{-1}.

The level of acclimatization affects sodium loss. For example, sodium concentration in sweat ranges from 5 to 30 mmol · L^{-1} (115–690 mg · L^{-1}) in individuals fully acclimatized to the heat to 40 to 100 mmol · L^{-1} (920–2300 mg · L^{-1}) in the unacclimatized. In addition, some individuals produce relatively highly concentrated sweat regardless of their degree of acclimatization. *Development of hyponatremia involves extreme sodium loss through prolonged sweating, coupled with dilution of existing extracellular sodium (reduced osmolality) from consuming fluids with low or no sodium* (Fig. 2.18A). A reduced extracellular solute concentration moves water into the cells (Fig. 2.18B). Water movement of sufficient magnitude congests the lungs, swells brain tissue, and adversely affects central nervous system function.

Several hours of exercise in the heat can produce significant sodium loss. Exercise in hot, humid weather often produces a sweating rate of more than 1 L per hour, with sweat sodium concentrations ranging from 20 to 100 mEq · L^{-1}. Also, frequently ingesting large volumes of plain water draws sodium from the extracellular fluid compartment into the unabsorbed intestinal water, further diluting serum sodium concentration. Exercise compounds the problem because urine production declines during exercise from significantly reduced renal blood flow. This reduces ability to excrete excess water. Competitive athletes, recreational participants, and occupational workers should be aware of the dangers of excessive hydration and that fluid intake should not exceed fluid loss. To reduce overhydration and hyponatremia risk in prolonged exercise, we recommend the following four steps:

1. Drink 400 to 600 mL (14 to 22 oz) of fluid 2 to 3 hours before exercise.
2. Drink 150 to 300 mL (5 to 10 oz) of fluid about 30 minutes before exercise.
3. Drink no more than 1000 mL · h^{-1} (33 oz) of plain water spread over 15-minute intervals during or after exercise.
4. Add a small amount of sodium (approximately 1/4 to 1/2 teaspoon per 32 oz) to the ingested fluid.
5. Do not restrict salt in the diet.

Including some glucose in the rehydration drink facilitates intestinal water uptake via the glucose–sodium transport mechanism (see Chapters 3 and 25).

Summary

1. Water makes up 40 to 70% of the total body mass. Muscle contains 70% water by weight, whereas water represents only about 10% of the weight of body fat.
2. Of the total body water, roughly 62% occurs intracellularly (inside the cells) and 38% extracellularly in the plasma, lymph, and other fluids.
3. The typical average daily water intake of 2.5 L comes from (1) liquid (1.2 L), (2) food (1.0 L), and (3) metabolic water produced during energy-yielding reactions (0.35 L).
4. Water loss from the body each day occurs from (1) urine (1 to 1.5 L), (2) skin, as insensible perspiration and sweat (0.85 L), (3) water vapor in expired air (0.35 L), and (4) feces (0.10 L).
5. Food and oxygen always are supplied in aqueous solution, and waste products leave via a watery medium. Water also helps to provide structure and form to the body and plays a vital role in temperature regulation.
6. Exercise in hot weather greatly increases the body's water requirement. Extreme conditions increase fluid needs five or six times above normal requirements.
7. Excessive sweating combined with consuming large volumes of plain water during prolonged exercise set the stage for hyponatremia or water intoxication. This potentially dangerous condition relates to a significant decrease in serum sodium concentration.

References are available on the Student CD and online at http://connection.lww.com/mkk6e.

Optimal Nutrition for Exercise

3

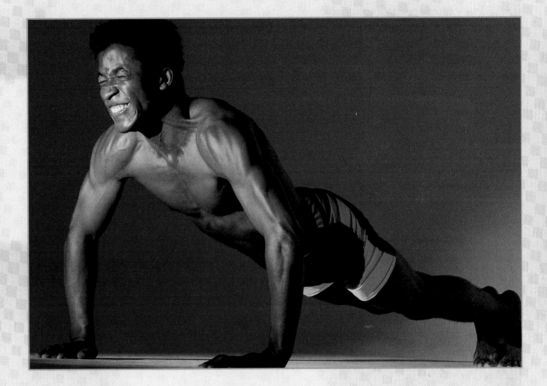

CHAPTER OBJECTIVES

- Compare nutrient and energy intakes of the physically active with sedentary counterparts

- Provide recommendations for carbohydrate, lipid, and protein intake for individuals who (1) maintain a physically active lifestyle and (2) regularly engage in intense physical training

- Outline the MyPyramid recommendations

- Give examples of the energy intakes of athletes who train for competitive sports

- Advise an athlete concerning timing and composition of the precompetition meal

- Advise endurance athletes about (1) the potential negative effects of consuming a concentrated sugar drink within 30 minutes of competition and (2) the rationale and

recommended carbohydrate intake during intense endurance exercise

- Provide examples of high-, moderate-, and low-glycemic index foods.

- Describe the role of the glycemic index in pre- and postexercise glycogen replenishment

- Outline an optimal glycogen replenishment schedule following high-intensity endurance exercise

- Describe the ideal sports drink and give the rationale for its composition

- Give recommendations for fluid and carbohydrate replacement during exercise

- Discuss the controversy concerning high-fat diets for training and endurance performance

An optimal diet supplies required nutrients in adequate amounts for tissue maintenance, repair, and growth without excess energy intake. Less than optimal fluid, nutrient, and energy intakes profoundly affect thermoregulatory function, substrate availability, exercise capacity, recovery from exercise, and training responsiveness. As the understanding of human nutrition evolves, a reasonable estimate of nutritional needs of men and women considers normal variation in nutrient digestion, absorption, and assimilation and daily energy expenditure. Dietary recommendations for physically active individuals must account for the energy requirements of a particular activity or sport and its training demands, including individual dietary preferences. No "one" food or diet exists for optimal health and exercise performance, but careful planning and evaluation of food intake should follow sound nutritional guidelines. The physically active person must obtain sufficient energy and macronutrients to replenish liver and muscle glycogen, provide amino acid building blocks for tissue growth and repair, and maintain a desirable body weight. Lipid intake must also provide essential fatty acids and fat-soluble vitamins. *The large number of teenagers and adults, including competitive athletes, who exercise regularly to keep fit do not require*

additional nutrients beyond those obtained through the regular intake of a nutritionally well-balanced diet.

NUTRIENT INTAKE AMONG THE PHYSICALLY ACTIVE

Inconsistencies exist among studies that relate diet quality to physical activity level or physical fitness. Part of the discrepancy relates to relatively crude and imprecise self-reported measures of physical activity, unreliable dietary assessments, and/or small sample size.[8,34,40,47,57,74] TABLE 3.1 contrasts the nutrient and energy intakes with national dietary recommendations of a large population-based cohort of about 7000 men and 2500 women classified as low, moderate, and high for cardiorespiratory fitness. The most significant findings indicate:

- A progressively lower body mass index with increasing levels of physical fitness for men and women
- Remarkably small differences in energy intake related to physical fitness classification for women (≤94 kCal per day) and men (≤82 kCal per day); the

TABLE 3.1 ■ AVERAGE VALUES FOR NUTRIENT INTAKE BASED ON 3-DAY DIET RECORDS BY LEVELS OF CARDIORESPIRATORY FITNESS IN 7059 MEN AND 2453 WOMEN

VARIABLE			LOW FITNESS (*N* = 786)	MODERATE FITNESS (*N* = 2457)	HIGH FITNESS (*N* = 4716)
Demographic and health data					
Age (y)			47.3 ± 11.1[a,b]	47.3 ± 10.3[c]	48.1 ± 10.5
Apparently healthy (%)	51.5[a,b]	69.1[c]	77.0		
Current smokers (%)	23.4[a,b]	15.8[c]	7.8		
BMI (kg · m^{-2})			30.7 ± 5.5[a,b]	27.4 ± 3.7[c]	25.1 ± 2.7
Nutrient data					
Energy (kCal)			2378.6 ± 718.6[a]	2296.9 ± 661.9[c]	2348.1 ± 664.3
kCal · kg^{-1} · d^{-1}			25.0 ± 8.1[a]	26.7 ± 8.4[c]	29.7 ± 9.2
Carbohydrate (% kCal)			43.2 ± 9.4[b]	44.6 ± 9.1[c]	48.1 ± 9.7
Protein (% kCal)			18.6 ± 3.8	18.5 ± 3.8	18.1 ± 3.8
Total fat (% kCal)			36.7 ± 7.2[b]	35.4 ± 7.1[c]	32.6 ± 7.5
SFA (% kCal)			11.8 ± 3.2[b]	11.3 ± 3.2[c]	10.0 ± 3.2
MUFA (% kCal)			14.5 ± 3.2[a,b]	13.8 ± 3.1[c]	12.6 ± 3.3
PUFA (% kCal)			7.4 ± 2.2[a,b]	7.5 ± 2.2	7.4 ± 2.3
Cholesterol (mg)			349.5 ± 173.2[b]	314.5 ± 147.5[c]	277.8 ± 138.5
Fiber (g)			21.0 ± 9.5[b]	22.0 ± 9.7[c]	26.2 ± 11.9
Calcium (mg)			849.1 ± 371.8[a,b]	860.2 ± 360.2[c]	924.4 ± 386.8
Sodium (mg)			4317.4 ± 1365.7	4143.0 ± 1202.3	4133.2 ± 1189.4
Folate (mcg)			336.4 ± 165.2[b]	359.5 ± 197.0[c]	428.0 ± 272.0
Vitamin B$_6$ (mg)			2.4 ± 0.9[b]	2.4 ± 0.9[c]	2.8 ± 1.1
Vitamin B$_{12}$ (mcg)			6.6 ± 5.5[a]	6.8 ± 6.0	6.6 ± 5.8
Vitamin A (RE)			1372.7 ± 1007.3[a,b]	1530.5 ± 1170.4[c]	1766.3 ± 1476.0
Vitamin C (mg)			117.3 ± 80.4[b]	129.2 ± 108.9[c]	166.0 ± 173.2
Vitamin E (AE)			11.5 ± 9.1[b]	12.1. ± 8.6[c]	13.7 ± 11.4

From Brodney S, et al. Nutrient intake of physically fit and unfit men and women. Med Sci Sports Exerc 2001;33:459.
BMI, body mass index; SFA, saturated fatty acid; PUFA, polyunsaturated fatty acid; MUFA, monounsaturated fatty acid; RE, retinol equivalents; AE, α-tocopherol units.
[a] Significant difference between low and moderate fit, *P* < .05.
[b] Significant difference between low and high fit, *P* < .05.
[c] Significant difference between moderate and high fit, *P* < .05.

moderate fitness group consumed the fewest calories for both sexes

- A progressively higher dietary fiber intake and lower cholesterol intake across fitness categories
- Men and women with higher fitness levels generally consumed diets that more closely approached dietary recommendations (with respect to dietary fiber, percentage energy from total fat, percentage energy from saturated fat, and dietary cholesterol) than peers of lower levels of fitness

 INTEGRATIVE QUESTION

In what ways might nutritional and energy intake goals for training differ from the requirements for actual competition?

Recommended Nutrient Intake

FIGURE 3.1 illustrates the recommended intakes for protein, lipid, and carbohydrate and the food sources for these macronutrients for a resting daily energy requirement of about 1200 kCal. A total daily energy requirement of 2000 kCal for women and 3000 kCal for men represents the average values for typical young adults. *After meeting basic nutrient requirements (as recommended in Fig. 3.1), a variety of food sources based on individual preference can supply the extra energy demands for physical activity.*

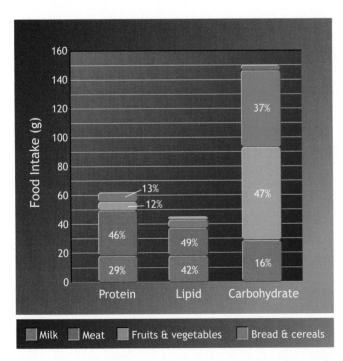

Figure 3.1 Basic recommendations for carbohydrate, lipid, and protein components and the general categories of food sources in a balanced diet to meet resting daily energy requirement of about 1200 kCal. Values within bars represent percentage of that group's contribution to the specific macronutrient intake.

Protein

As discussed in Chapter 1, 0.83 g per kg of body mass represents the Recommended Dietary Allowance (RDA) for protein intake. A person weighing 77 kg (170 lb) would therefore require about 64 g, or 2.2 oz, of protein daily. Even if relatively little protein catabolism occurs through energy metabolism during physical activity (an assumption not entirely correct), this protein recommendation remains adequate for most physically active individuals. Also, the protein intake of the typical American significantly exceeds protein's RDA. For athletes who train intensely, a protein intake between 1.2 and 1.8 g per kg body mass should meet any added protein-related nutrient demands. This does not necessarily require protein supplementation as an athlete's diet typically exceeds the protein RDA by two to four times.

 INTEGRATIVE QUESTION

In what situations might a protein intake representing twice the RDA still prove inadequate for an individual involved in intense exercise training?

Lipid

Standards for optimal lipid intake have not been firmly established. The amount of dietary lipid varies widely depending on personal taste, money spent on food, geographic influences, and availability of lipid-rich foods. For example, lipid furnishes only about 10% of the energy in the average diet of people living in Asia, whereas in many Western countries it accounts for 40 to 45% of the total energy intake. To promote good health, lipid intake should not exceed 30% of the diet's energy content. Of this, at least 70% should be in the form of unsaturated fatty acids. For those who consume a Mediterranean-type diet, rich in monounsaturated fatty acids, a somewhat higher total fat percentage of 35 to 40% remains reasonable.

High-Fat Versus Low-Fat Diets for Exercise Training and Performance

High-Fat Diets. Debate centers on the wisdom of maintaining a high-fat diet (or even fasting) during training or prior to endurance competition.[24,68,81,123] Adaptations to high-fat diets have consistently shown a shift in substrate use toward higher fat oxidation during exercise.[18,51,126] Proponents of high-fat diets argue that a long-term increased dietary fat intake stimulates fat burning and augments the capacity to mobilize and catabolize this energy nutrient during high-intensity aerobic exercise. Any fat-burning metabolic enhancement should conserve glycogen reserves and/or contribute to improved endurance capacity under conditions of low glycogen reserves.[52] To investigate possible benefits, endurance capacity was compared in two groups of 10 young men

IN A PRACTICAL SENSE

NUTRITION TO PREVENT CHRONIC ATHLETIC FATIGUE

■ Endurance runners, swimmers, cross-country skiers, and cyclists frequently experience chronic fatigue as successive days of hard training become progressively more difficult. Normal exercise performance deteriorates because the individual experiences increasing difficulty recovering from each training session. The overtraining syndrome (see Chapter 21) also relates to frequent infections, general malaise, and loss of interest in sustaining high-level training. Injuries occur more frequently in the overtrained, stale state.

DEPLETED CARBOHYDRATE PLAYS A ROLE

Gradually depleting carbohydrate reserves with repeated strenuous training most likely contributes to the overtraining syndrome. It requires at least 1 to 2 days of rest or lighter exercise combined with a high carbohydrate intake to reestablish preexercise muscle glycogen levels after exhaustive training or competition. Unduly heavy exercise performed regularly requires an upward adjustment of daily carbohydrate intake to optimize glycogen resynthesis and high-quality training.

The following table provides nutritional recommendations to reduce the likelihood of athletic fatigue or staleness.

PRACTICAL NUTRITIONAL GUIDELINES TO PREVENT CHRONIC FATIGUE

1. Consume easily digested, high-carbohydrate drinks or solid foods 1 to 4 h before training or competition. Consume about 1 g carbohydrate/kg body mass 1 h before exercise and up to 5 g carbohydrate/kg body mass if the feeding occurs 4 h prior to exercise. For example, a 70-kg swimmer could drink 350 mL (12 oz) of a 20% carbohydrate beverage 1 h before exercise or eat 14 "energy bars," each containing 25 g carbohydrate, spread over the 4-h period before exercise.
2. Consume a readily digested, high-carbohydrate liquid or solid food containing 0.35–1.5 g carbohydrate/kg body mass/h immediately after exercise and for the first 4 h after exercise. Thus, a 70-kg swimmer could drink 100–450 mL (3.6–16 oz) of a 25% carbohydrate beverage or 1 to 4 energy bars, each containing 25 g of carbohydrate immediately after exercise and every hour thereafter for 4 h.
3. Consume a 15–25% carbohydrate drink or a solid, high-carbohydrate supplement with each meal. For example, reduce consumption of normal foods by 250 kCal and consume a high-carbohydrate beverage or solid food containing 250 kCal of carbohydrate with each meal.
4. Stabilize body weight during all phases of training by matching energy consumption to training's energy demands. This also helps to maintain body glycogen reserves.

From Sherman WJ, Maglischo EW. Minimizing chronic athletic fatigue among swimmers: special emphasis on nutrition. Sports Science Exchange. Gatorade Sports Science Institute. 1991;35(4).

matched for aerobic capacity and fed either a high-carbohydrate diet (65% kCal from carbohydrate) or high-fat diet (62% kCal from lipid) for 7 weeks. Each group trained for 60 to 70 minutes at 50 to 85% of aerobic capacity, 3 days a week during weeks 1 to 3 and 4 days a week during weeks 4 to 7. Following 7 weeks of training, the group consuming the high-fat diet switched to the high-carbohydrate diet. FIGURE 3.2 displays the performance of both groups. The results for endurance were clear—the group consuming the high-carbohydrate diet performed significantly longer after training for 7 weeks than the group consuming the high-fat diet (102.4 min vs. 65.2 min). When the high-fat diet group switched to

the high-carbohydrate diet during week 8 of the experiment, only a small improvement in endurance of 11.5 minutes occurred. Consequently, total overall improvement in endurance over the 8-week period reached 115% for the high-fat diet group, and endurance for the group receiving the high-carbohydrate diet while training improved by 194%. The inset table shows daily intakes of energy and nutrients prior to the experimental treatment (habitual diet) and during the 7-week experimental diet. The authors concluded that the high-fat diet produced *suboptimal* adaptations in endurance performance, which did not become fully remedied by switching to a high-carbohydrate diet. Subsequent research

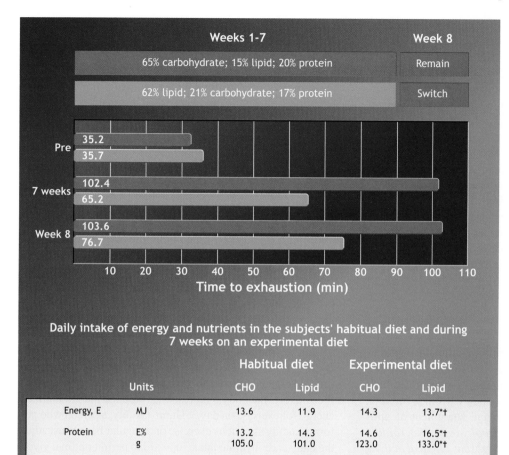

Weeks 1-7	Week 8
65% carbohydrate; 15% lipid; 20% protein	Remain
62% lipid; 21% carbohydrate; 17% protein	Switch

Time to exhaustion (min) — Pre: 35.2 / 35.7; 7 weeks: 102.4 / 65.2; Week 8: 103.6 / 76.7

Daily intake of energy and nutrients in the subjects' habitual diet and during 7 weeks on an experimental diet

		Habitual diet		Experimental diet	
	Units	CHO	Lipid	CHO	Lipid
Energy, E	MJ	13.6	11.9	14.3	13.7*†
Protein	E%	13.2	14.3	14.6	16.5*†
	g	105.0	101.0	123.0	133.0*†
Carbohydrate	E%	48.2	53.4	65.0	22.0*†
	g	386.0	373.0	546.0	177.0*†
	g · kg body wt^{-1}	4.7	5.0	6.8	2.4*†
Simple sugars	E%	11.0	10.0	7.0	2.2*†
Dietary fiber	g · MJ^{-1}	2.3	2.6	4.3	2.2†
Lipid	E%	34.3	39.0	20.4	62.0*†
	g	118.0	94.0	75.0	217.0*†
Cholesterol	mg · MJ^{-1}	31.0	29.0	26.0	44.0*†
Essential FA	E%	4.4	4.3	4.0	11.2*†
P/S ratio		0.39	0.43	0.53	0.62*†

Values are means; *significantly different between the habitual and the experimental diet; †significantly different between the two experimental diets; MJ, megajoule; E%, percent of total energy

Figure 3.2 Effects of a high-carbohydrate (CHO) versus a high-fat diet on endurance performance. The group consuming the high-fat diet for 7 weeks switched to the high CHO diet during week 8. The endurance test consisted of pedaling a bicycle ergometer at the desired rate. The inset table compares the average daily energy and nutrient intake during the habitual and experimental diets. *P/S ratio*, polyunsaturated-to-saturated fatty acid ratio. (From Helge JW, et al. Interaction of training and diet on metabolism and endurance during exercise in man. J Physiol 1996;492:293.)

from the same laboratory failed to demonstrate any endurance-enhancing effect of a high-fat diet containing only moderate carbohydrate (15% total calories) in rats, regardless of their current training status. For sedentary humans, maintaining a low or high dietary fat intake for 4 weeks produced no differences in maximal or submaximal aerobic exercise performance.[89]

A high-fat diet may stimulate adaptive responses that augment fat use, but reliable research has yet to demonstrate consistent exercise or training benefits from this dietary modification. Compromised training capacity and symptoms of lethargy, increased fatigue, and higher ratings of perceived exertion usually accompany exercise when subsisting on a high-fat diet.[18,108,126] Furthermore, one must carefully consider recommending a diet consisting of 60% of total calories from lipid from the standpoint of potential detrimental health risks. This concern may prove unwarranted for athletes with high daily levels of energy expenditure. Increasing the percentage of total lipid calories in the diet to 50% for physically active individuals who maintain a stable body weight and body composition does not adversely affect selected heart disease risk factors, including plasma lipoprotein profiles.[13,71] Considered in total, available research does *not* support the popular notion that reducing carbohydrate while increasing fat intake above a 30% level produces a more optimal metabolic "zone" for endurance performance.[100,122]

Low-Fat Diets. Significantly restricting dietary fat below recommended levels can impair exercise performance.[51,81,122] For example, a diet of 20% lipid produced poorer endurance performance scores than a diet of identical caloric value containing about 40% lipid.[86] A low-fat diet also blunts the normal rise in plasma testosterone following an acute bout of resistance exercise.[127] If additional research verifies these findings, and if changes in the hormonal milieu actually diminish training responsiveness and tissue synthesis, a low-fat intake may be contraindicated for optimal resistance training responses. Consuming low-fat diets during strenuous training creates difficulty in increasing carbohydrate and protein intake enough to furnish energy to maintain body weight and muscle mass. Essential fatty acids and fat-soluble vitamins enter the body in dietary lipids, so sustaining a low-fat or "fat-free" diet could create a relative state of malnutrition for these nutrients.

Carbohydrate

The negative end of the nutrition continuum includes low-calorie "semi-starvation" diets and other potentially harmful high-fat, low-carbohydrate diets, "liquid-protein" diets, or single-food-centered diets. Such extremes threaten good health, exercise performance, and attainment of optimum body composition. *A low-carbohydrate diet rapidly compromises glycogen reserves for vigorous physical activity or regular training.* Excluding sufficient carbohydrate energy from the diet causes an individual to train in a state of relative glycogen depletion; this may eventually produce "staleness" that hinders exercise performance.

The prominence of dietary carbohydrates varies widely throughout the world, depending on availability and relative cost of lipid-rich and protein-rich foods. Carbohydrate-rich unrefined grains, starchy roots, and dried peas and beans usually cost less relative to their energy value. In the Far East, carbohydrates (rice) contribute 80% of the total energy intake, whereas in the United States only about 40 to 50% of total energy comes from carbohydrates. *No hazard to health exists when subsisting chiefly on a variety of fiber-rich complex unrefined carbohydrates, with adequate intake of essential amino acids, fatty acids, minerals, and vitamins.* The diet of the Tarahumara Indians of Mexico (see "Focus on Research," p. 87) consists of high-fiber and complex-carbohydrate foods and correspondingly low cholesterol, lipid, and saturated fat.[22] The Tarahumaras exhibit little or no hypertension, obesity, or death from cardiac and circulatory complications.

Dietary carbohydrate intake takes on additional importance for individuals involved in physical activity on the job or in exercise training and sports competition. Muscle glycogen becomes the prime energy contributor during exercise with inadequate oxygen supply to active muscles. In addition to its anaerobic energy role, muscle glycogen and blood glucose provide substantial energy during intense aerobic exercise. *Considering the body's limited glycogen reserves, the diet of physically active individuals should contain at least 55 to 60% of calories in the form of carbohydrates, predominantly starches from fiber-rich, unprocessed grains, fruits, and vegetables.* For many competitive athletes (e.g., swimmers, rowers, and speed skaters), the importance of maintaining a relatively high daily carbohydrate intake relates more to the considerable energy demands of training than to the short-term demands of competition.

Carbohydrate Needs in Intense Training

Athletes training for endurance activities such as distance running, ocean swimming, cross-country skiing, or cycling frequently experience a state of chronic fatigue in which successive days of hard training become progressively more difficult. This **staleness** often relates to the gradual depletion of the body's glycogen reserves, even though the diet contains the typical percentage of carbohydrate. FIGURE 3.3 shows that three successive days of running 16.1 km (10 miles) nearly depleted the glycogen in the thigh muscle. This occurred even though the runners' diet contained 40 to 60% carbohydrates. By the third day, the quantity of glycogen used during the run averaged considerably lower than on the first day. Presumably, the body's fat reserves supplied the predominant energy for exercise on day 3. Unmistakably, a person who performs unduly strenuous exercise on a regular basis must adjust the daily carbohydrate intake upward to permit optimal glycogen resynthesis to maintain high-quality training. The need for optimal replenishment of depleted glycogen reserves provides nutritional justification to gradually reduce, or taper, the intensity of exercise routines several days prior to competition.[114]

Carbohydrate intake recommendations for physically active individuals assume that daily energy intake balances daily energy expenditure. Unless this condition exists, even consuming a relatively large *percentage* of carbohydrate calories will not adequately replenish this important energy macronutrient. General recommendations for carbohydrate intake range between 6 and 10 g per kg of body mass per day. This amount varies with an individual's daily energy expenditure and type of exercise performed. *Glycogen synthesis relates to carbohydrate intake, so individuals who undergo intense training should consume 10 g of carbohydrate per kg of body mass each day to induce protein sparing and ensure adequate glycogen reserves.*[11,12] The daily carbohydrate intake for a small 46-kg (100-lb) athlete who expends about 2800 kCal each day should average 450 g, or 1800 kCal. A 68-kg (150-lb) athlete should consume 675 g of carbohydrate (2700 kCal) daily to sustain an energy requirement averaging 4200 kCal. In both examples, carbohydrates exceed the minimum recommendation of 55 to 60% to represent 65% of total energy intake. This relatively high level of carbohydrate intake better maintains physical performance and mood state over the course of training.[1] Even with a high-carbohydrate diet, complete glycogen replenishment does not occur rapidly following prolonged effort, particularly in the type I (slow-twitch) muscle fibers.

FOCUS On Research

POTENTIAL EFFECT OF DIET ON HEALTH STATUS

Connor WE, et al. The plasma lipids, lipoproteins, and diet of the Tarahumara Indians of Mexico. Am J Clin Nutr 1978;31:1131.

▲ The Tarahumara Indians compose a group of about 50,000 farmers who inhabit the rugged Sierra Madre Occidental Mountains in the north-central state of Chihuahua, Mexico. These individuals, renowned for their endurance capacity, reportedly run distances of up to 200 miles in the competitive sport of "kickball" that lasts 2 days.

Conner and colleagues assessed the diet, blood lipid status, and blood pressure of these 20th-century Spartans. Measurements of 523 Tarahumaras over a 3-year period included plasma cholesterol and triacylglycerol, lipoprotein fractions, body stature and mass, triceps skinfold, resting blood pressure, and nutrient intake by dietary history and observation of food intake. The most striking findings included extremely low values for total cholesterol, LDL- and VLDL-cholesterol, blood pressure, skinfold thickness, and dietary lipid intake. The average blood cholesterol levels (136 mg · dL^{-1} for men; 117 mg · dL^{-1} for women; and 116 mg · dL^{-1} for children) contrast sharply with typical U.S. values of more than 200 mg · dL^{-1}.

The low plasma cholesterol of the Tarahumaras largely relates to their unique dietary patterns. Their diet averaged a low cholesterol intake of 71 mg · d^{-1} (typical U.S. cholesterol intake ranges from 500 to 700 mg · d^{-1}). Additionally, lipid intake averaged only 11% of total energy intake, compared with nearly 40% for the U.S. diet. Corn and beans accounted for 95% of total lipid consumption, mainly from polyunsaturated and monounsaturated fatty acids. Saturated fat constituted only 2% of total calories, compared with 15% in the U.S. Thus, the healthful polyunsaturated-to-saturated fat ratio exceeded 2.0, compared with only 0.35 for the U.S. diet.

Simple sugars provided only 5% of total energy intake, compared with 25% for the typical North American diet. No obesity or hypertension occurred in the Tarahumara. Vegetable sources provided more than 96% of all dietary protein, while protein intake ranged from 79 to 96 g · d^{-1} and accounted for 236 to 1221% of the total essential amino acid requirements based on the U.S. RDA. The Tarahumaras' high level of physical activity coincided with favorable blood lipid and blood pressure profiles and other low coronary risk factors. Overall, the results illustrated that diet and increased physical activity linked to the group's relatively good health status.

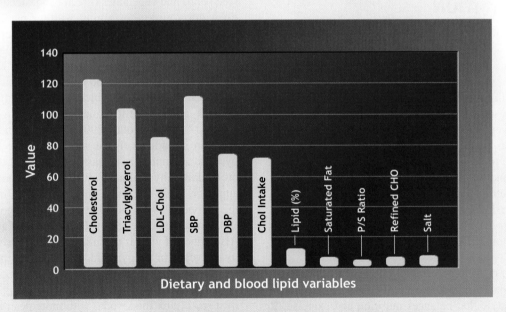

Dietary and blood lipid variables for the Tarahumara Indians of Mexico. Plasma *cholesterol, triacylglycerol,* and *LDL-Chol* in mg per dL. *Chol Intake* is cholesterol intake in mg per day. Lipid intake (*Lipid %*) and saturated fat intake (*Saturated Fat*) expressed as percentage of total caloric intake; *P/S Ratio* represents ratio of polyunsaturated to saturated fatty acid intake; *Refined CHO* is the percentage of total calories from refined sugar; *Salt* is salt intake in g per day; *SBP* and *DBP* represent systolic and diastolic blood pressure in mm Hg.

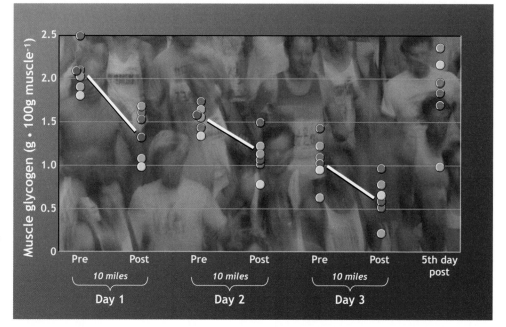

Figure 3.3 Changes in muscle glycogen concentration for six male subjects before and after each 10-mile (16.1-km run performed on 3 successive days. Muscle glycogen measured 5 days after the last run is referred to as "5th day post." (From Costill DL, et al. Muscle glycogen utilization during prolonged exercise on successive days. J Appl Physiol 1971;31:834.)

INTEGRATIVE QUESTION

From a nutritional perspective, how can a reduced total volume of daily training improve training responsiveness and competitive performance?

MYPYRAMID: **THE ESSENTIALS OF GOOD NUTRITION**

Key principles of good eating include *variety, balance,* and *moderation.* Lobbyists for the beef and dairy industries greatly influenced earlier approaches to formulating recommendations for sound nutrition, as the Four-Food-Group Plan developed by the U.S. Department of Agriculture (USDA; www.usda.com). Research in nutrition, cancer, and heart disease over the past 45 years uncovered the shortcomings of this plan, with its emphasis on meat and milk products, as a guide to healthful eating. In the typical American diet, energy-dense but nutrient-poor foods frequently substitute for more nutrient-rich foods. This pattern of food intake increases the risk for obesity, marginal micronutrient intakes, low high-density lipoprotein (HDL) and high low-density lipoprotein (LDL) cholesterol, and elevated levels of homocysteine.[66]

In April 2005, the federal government unveiled its latest attempt to personalize the approach of Americans to choose a healthier lifestyle that balances nutrition and exercise. It replaces the 1992 pyramid criticized as being broad and vague; it recommended, for example, that people eat 6 to 12 servings of grains but gave no explanation as to who should eat 6 versus 12 and did not define a serving size. The new color-coded food pyramid (FIG. 3.4A), termed **MyPyramid**, offers a fresh look and a complementary Web site

(www.mypyramid.gov) to provide personalized and supplementary materials on food intake guidance (e.g., the recommended number of cups of vegetables) based on age, sex, and level of daily exercise. The pyramid is based on the 2005 *Dietary Guidelines for Americans* published by the Department of Health and Human Services and the Department of Agriculture (www.healthierus.gov/dietaryguidelines/). It provides a series of vertical color bands of varying widths with the combined bands for fruits (red band) and vegetables (green band) occupying the greatest width, followed by grains, with the narrowest bands occupied by fats, oils, meats, and sugars. A personalized pyramid is obtained by logging on to the Web site. For example, a 40-year-old man who exercises less than 30 minutes a day should consume about 2200 kCal daily, which includes 7 oz of grains, 3 cups of vegetables, 2 cups of fruit, 3 cups of low-fat milk, and 6 oz of lean meat. He can also consume 6 teaspoons of oil and another 290 kCal of fats and sweets. A new addition includes a figure walking up the left side of the pyramid to emphasize at least 30 minutes of moderate to vigorous daily physical activity. Critics maintain that the new approach shifts too much of the burden of responsibility to the individual, who must have access to a computer and the skills to navigate the relatively complicated government site. Also, much of what is contained in the guidelines is not readily conveyed in the pyramid. For example, the pyramid only hints about the necessity for eating fewer foods such as fats, sugars, and salt, and the concept of replacing unhealthy food (fast food, junk food, soda) with more desirable food is difficult to discern. The *Guidelines*, revised every 5 years, with sixth edition evidence-based revisions due out in 2006, are formulated for the general population but also provide a sound framework for meal planning for physically active individuals. The principle message advises consuming a varied but balanced diet. To maintain a healthful body

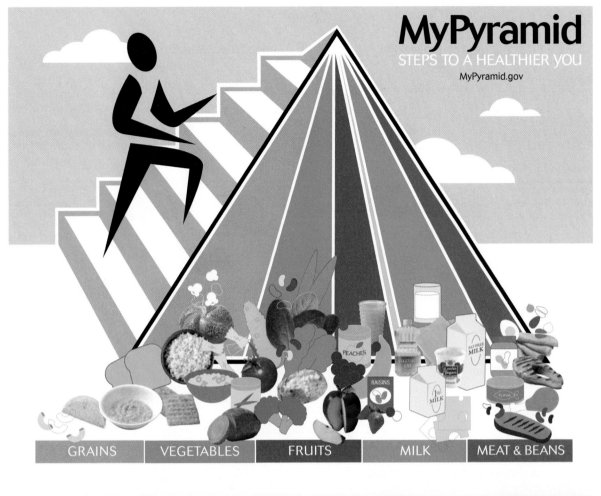

GRAINS Make half your grains whole	VEGETABLES Vary your veggies	FRUITS Focus on fruits	MILK Get your calcium-rich foods	MEAT & BEANS Go lean with protein
Eat at least 3 oz. of whole-grain cereals, breads, crackers, rice, or pasta every day 1 oz. is about 1 slice of bread, about 1 cup of breakfast cereal, or ¹⁄₂ cup of cooked rice, cereal, or pasta	Eat more dark-green veggies like broccoli, spinach, and other dark leafy greens Eat more orange vegetables like carrots and sweetpotatoes Eat more dry beans and peas like pinto beans, kidney beans, and lentils	Eat a variety of fruit Choose fresh, frozen, canned, or dried fruit Go easy on fruit juices	Go low-fat or fat-free when you choose milk, yogurt, and other milk products If you don't or can't consume milk, choose lactose-free products or other calcium sources such as fortified foods and beverages	Choose low-fat or lean meats and poultry Bake it, broil it, or grill it Vary your protein routine — choose more fish, beans, peas, nuts, and seeds

For a 2,000-calorie diet, you need the amounts below from each food group. To find the amounts that are right for you, go to MyPyramid.gov.

Eat 6 oz. every day	Eat 2¹⁄₂ cups every day	Eat 2 cups every day	Get 3 cups every day; for kids aged 2 to 8, it's 2	Eat 5¹⁄₂ oz. every day

Find your balance between food and physical activity

- Be sure to stay within your daily calorie needs.
- Be physically active for at least 30 minutes most days of the week.
- About 60 minutes a day of physical activity may be needed to prevent weight gain.
- For sustaining weight loss, at least 60 to 90 minutes a day of physical activity may be required.
- Children and teenagers should be physically active for 60 minutes every day, or most days.

Know the limits on fats, sugars, and salt (sodium)

- Make most of your fat sources from fish, nuts, and vegetable oils.
- Limit solid fats like butter, stick margarine, shortening, and lard, as well as foods that contain these.
- Check the Nutrition Facts label to keep saturated fats, *trans* fats, and sodium low.
- Choose food and beverages low in added sugars. Added sugars contribute calories with few, if any, nutrients.

MyPyramid.gov

U.S. Department of Agriculture
Center for Nutrition Policy and Promotion
April 2005
CNPP-15

USDA

Figure 3.4 A. MyPyramid: A more comprehensive and personalized guide to sound nutrition. *(Continued on p. 90.)*

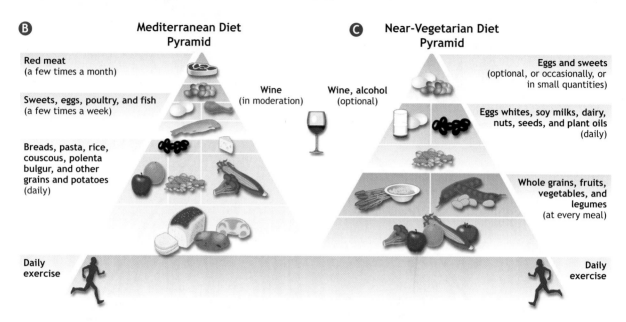

	MyPyramid	**Food Guide Pyramid**
Calories	Individualized amounts from each food group based on age, gender, and physical activity	Broad range designed to fit the needs of the majority of people
Physical activity	Balance activity with food intake. Physical activity for at least 30 min/d, and more for those trying to lose weight or prevent weight gain	No recommendations made
Grains	7-oz equivalents for a 2200 kCal diet; half the choices from whole grains	9 servings for a 2200 kCal diet (1 serving = 1 slice of bread or a 1/2 cup rice or pasta), choose whole grain bread, cereals and grains; limit high-fat and high-sugar baked foods
Vegetables	3 cups/d for a 2200 kCal diet; choose a variety of veggies each day. 3 cups/wk from dark green veggies; 2 cups/wk from orange veggies; 3 cups/wk from legumes; 6 cups/wk from starchy veggies, 7 cup/wk from other veggies	4 servings per day for 2200 kCal diet (1 serving = about 2 cups/d); eat a variety of vegetables, including dark green leafy vegetables, deep yellow vegetables, starchy vegetables, and other vegetables
Fruits	2 cups/d for a 2200 kCal diet; choose a variety of fruits; choose fresh, frozen, dried or canned; fruit juice should be less than 1/2 of total fruit intake	3 servings/d for a 2200 kCal diet (1 serving = about 1.5 cups); choose fresh frut, frozen without sugar, dried, or fruit canned in water or juice; eat whole fruits more often than juices; regularly eat citrus fruits, melons, and berries
Milk, yogurt, cheese	3 cups/d for a 2200 kCal diet; choose fat-free or low-fat products	2–3 servings for a 2000 kCal diet (1 serving = 2–3 cups/d); use low-fat or nonfat milk and yogurt and part skim and low-fat cheeses
Meat, poultry, fish, dry beans, eggs, nuts	6-oz equivalents/d for a 2200 kCal diet; choose low-fat or lean; baked, broil, or grill; choose more fish, beans, peas, nuts, and seeds	6 oz for a 2200 kCal diet; eat lean meat, poultry without skin, and dry beans; trim fat and cook by broiling, roasting, grilling, or boiling; limit egg yolks (high cholesterol), and nuts and seeds (high kCal)
Oils	6 teaspoons/d on a 2200 kCal diet; choose from fish, nuts, and vegetable oils; limit solid fats (stick margarine, butter, shortening, and lard	Limit amount consumed; use unsaturated vegetable oils, and margarines that list liquid vegetable oils as first ingredients on label
Sugars and sweets	Choose foods and beverages with little added sugars	Limit amount consumed; limit high-sugar baked goods, sugar added as toppings and spreads, rinse fruits canned in heavy syrup

Figure 3.4 *Continued* **B.** Mediterranean Diet Pyramid. **C.** Near-Vegetarian Diet Pyramid. **D.** Comparing MyPyramid and the 1992 Food Guide Pyramid. (From U.S. Department of Agriculture, 2005.)

weight, attention must focus on portion size and number. Importance is placed on consuming a diet rich in fruits and vegetables, cereals and whole grains, nonfat and low-fat dairy products, legumes, nuts, fish, poultry, and lean meats.[6,23,40,59,73,120]

Figures 3.4B and C present modifications of the basic pyramid. These apply to individuals whose diet consists largely of (1) foods from the plant kingdom (**Near-Vegetarian Diet Pyramid**) or (2) fruits, nuts, vegetables, fish, beans, and all manner of grains, with dietary fat composed mostly of monounsaturated fatty acids with mild ethanol consumption (**Mediterranean Diet Pyramid**). A Mediterranean-style diet protects individuals at high risk of death from heart disease.[30] Its high content of monounsaturated fatty acids (generally olive oil with its associated phytochemicals[107]) helps delay age-related memory loss, cancer, and overall mortality rate in healthy, elderly people.[70,104,116] Dietary focus of all three pyramids on fruits and vegetables, particularly cruciferous and green leafy vegetables and citrus fruit and juice, also reduces risk for ischemic stroke[63,64] and enhances the benefits of cholesterol-lowering drugs.[65]

INTEGRATIVE QUESTION

How would you advise a high school soccer team with individuals from diverse ethnic backgrounds with unique food intake patterns about sound nutrition?

AN EXPANDING EMPHASIS ON HEALTHFUL EATING AND REGULAR PHYSICAL ACTIVITY

Scientists have responded to the rapidly rising number of overweight and obese adults and children and the increasing incidence of comorbidities associated with these conditions. In September, 2002, the Institute of Medicine (www.iom.edu), the medical division of the National Academies, issued Guidelines as part of their *Dietary Reference Intakes* (see Chapter 2).[36] They recommend that Americans spend at least *1 hour* over the course of each day in moderately intense physical activity (about 400 to 500 kCal of brisk walking, swimming, or cycling) to maintain health and normal body weight. This amount of regular physical activity—based on an assessment of the amount of exercise healthy persons engage in each day—represents twice as much as previously recommended in 1996 in a report from the United States Surgeon General! The advice agrees with the 2003 recommendations by the World Health Organization (WHO; www.who.int) and the Food and Agriculture Organization of the United Nations (and most recently, the International Association for the Study of Obesity[96]) and the findings of recent research that points to the health and weight-loss benefits of longer duration weekly physical activity.[56,59] The advice represents a bold increase in exercise duration considering that (1) 30 minutes of similar type exercise on most days significantly decreases disease risk and (2) more than 60% of the U.S. population fails to incorporate even a moderate level of exercise into their lives, and 25% perform no exercise at all. Underlying the Institute's 60-minute exercise recommendation is the belief that 30 minutes of daily exercise burns insufficient calories to prevent weight gain; thus, a greater amount of regular exercise becomes necessary.

The team of 21 experts also recommended for the first time a range for macronutrient intake plus how much dietary fiber to consume daily. These recommendations are intended for professional nutritionists and the general public. To meet daily energy and nutrient needs and minimize risk for chronic diseases such as heart disease and type 2 diabetes, adults should consume between 45 and 65% of their total calories from carbohydrates. This wide range offers flexibility that recognizes that the high-carbohydrate, low-fat diet of Asians and the higher-fat diet of peoples from the Mediterranean region, with its high monounsaturated fatty acid olive oil content, contribute to good health. The maximum intake of added sugars—the caloric sweeteners in manufactured foods and beverages, such as soda, candy, fruit drinks, cakes, cookies, and ice cream—is placed at 25% of total calories. The panel suggested that this relatively high 25% level represented the threshold above which a significant decline would occur for several im-

LATEST REVISIONS

On January 12, 2005, a government panel of prominent experts in nutrition and health issued the latest evidence-based version of the *Dietary Guidelines for Americans*, which has been translated into a pyramid, for the public to use for advice on diet (see Fig. 3.4). The recommendations center around the following nine major "messages":

- Control caloric intake to manage body weight.
- Consume a variety of foods within and among the basic food groups while staying within energy needs.
- Increase daily intake of fruits, vegetables, whole grains, and nonfat or low-fat milk and milk products.
- Choose fats wisely for good health; limit saturated fats (dairy, fatty meats, and other animal products) and *trans*-fats (packaged baked goods and fried foods).
- Choose carbohydrates wisely for good health; select fiber-rich foods: whole fruits rather than juices; whole grains (wheat bread, oatmeal, brown rice) rather than refined grains.
- Choose and prepare foods with little salt; reduce daily salt intake to 2300 mg.
- If you drink alcoholic beverages, do so in moderation; up to one drink a day for women, two for men.
- Be physically active every day; at least 30 minutes of moderate activity a day, although children and adolescents need at least 60 minutes a day for healthy growth.
- Keep food safe to eat; wash and cook foods properly to avoid foodborne illnesses; refrigerate perishable items promptly.

TABLE 3.2 ■ MACRONUTRIENT COMPOSITION OF A 2500-kCal DIET BASED ON RECOMMENDATIONS OF THE INSTITUTE OF MEDICINE

	COMPOSITION OF 2500 KCAL INTAKE		
	Carbohydrate	Lipid	Protein
Percentage	60	15	25
kCal	1500	375	625
Grams	375	94	69
Ounces	13.2	3.3	2.4

portant micronutrients such as vitamin A and calcium. Acceptable lipid intake ranges between 20 and 35% of caloric intake, a range lower at the lower end of most recommendations and higher at the upper end of the 30% limit set by the American Heart Association (AHA; www.americanheart.org), American Cancer Society (ACS; www.cancer.org), and National Institutes of Health (NIH; www.nih.gov/). The panel noted that very low fat intake combined with high carbohydrate intake tends to lower HDL cholesterol and raise triacylglycerol levels. Conversely, high intake of dietary fat (and accompanying increased caloric intake) contributes to obesity and related medical complications. Moreover, high-fat diets usually associate with an increased saturated fatty acid intake This raises plasma LDL cholesterol concentration, which potentiates further coronary heart disease risk. "As low as possible" saturated fat intake was recommended; the panel also recognized that no safe level exist for *trans*-fatty acid intake.

Recommended protein intake ranges between 10 and 35% of calories, which remains consistent with prior recommendations. For the first time, age-based recommendations are provided for all of the essential amino acids contained in dietary protein. TABLE 3.2 presents an example of the macronutrient composition for a 2500-kCal diet based on these new guidelines.

The panel's recommendations for intake of dietary fiber were discussed in Chapter 1. Particularly important is the consumption of water-soluble fibers (pectin from fruits and oat and rice bran); these lower plasma cholesterol and reduce the risk of overeating.

EXERCISE AND FOOD INTAKE

Balancing energy intake with energy expenditure represents a primary goal for the physically active individual of normal body weight. Energy balance not only optimizes physical performance but it helps to maintain lean body mass, training responsiveness, and immune and reproductive function. The level of physical activity is the most important factor that affects daily energy expenditure.

FIGURE 3.5 illustrates that average energy intakes for males and females in the United States peak between ages 16 and 29 years and then decline for succeeding age groups. A similar pattern occurs for males and females, although males report higher daily energy intakes than females at all ages. Between ages 20 and 29 years, women consume on average 35% fewer kCal than men on a daily basis (3025 kCal vs. 1957 kCal). Thereafter, gender difference in energy intake becomes smaller; at age 70 years, women consume about 25% fewer kCal than men.

Physical Activity Makes a Difference

Individuals who engage regularly in moderate-to-intense physical activity eventually increase daily energy intake to match their higher energy expenditure level. Lumber workers, who expend approximately 4500 kCal daily, unconsciously adjust energy intake to closely balance energy output. Consequently, body mass remains stable despite a seemingly large food intake. The daily food intake of ath-

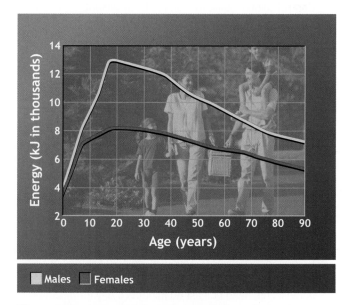

Figure 3.5 Average daily energy intake for males and females by age in the U.S. population during the years 1988 to 1990. Multiply by 0.239 to convert kJ to kCal. (From Briefel RR, et al. Total energy intake of the US population: the third National Health and Nutrition Examination Survey, 1988–1991. Am J Clin Nutr 1995;62(suppl):1072S.)

letes in the 1936 Olympics reportedly averaged more than 7000 kCal, or roughly three times the average daily intake. These oft-quoted energy values justify what many believe to be an enormous food requirement of athletes in training. However, these figures probably depict inflated estimates because objective dietary data do not appear in the original report. Distance runners who train upward of 100 miles per week (6-min mile pace at 15 kCal per min) probably do not expend more than 800 to 1300 "extra" kCal each day above their normal energy requirements to balance the increased energy expenditure. FIGURE 3.6 presents energy intake data from a large sample of elite male and female endurance, strength, and team sport athletes in the Netherlands. Daily

energy intake for males ranged between 2900 and 5900 kCal, whereas female competitors consumed between 1600 and 3200 kCal. With the exception of the large energy intakes of athletes at extremes of performance and training, daily energy intake generally did not exceed 4000 kCal for men and 3000 kCal for women.

To complement these observations, daily energy expenditure of elite female swimmers increased to 5593 kCal during high-volume training.[115] This value represents the highest level of sustained daily energy expenditure reported for female athletes but energy intake did not increase to match training demands. It averaged only 3136 kCal, implying a negative energy balance of 43%. A negative energy balance in the transition from moderate to intense training may ultimately compromise an athlete's full potential to train and compete.

Tour de France and Other Endurance Activities

FIGURE 3.7 outlines the variation in daily energy expenditure for a male competitor during the Tour de France professional cycling race. In this most grueling of sporting events, energy expenditure averaged 6500 kCal daily for nearly 3 weeks. Large variation occurred depending on activity level for a particular day; the daily energy expenditure decreased to about 3000 kCal on a "rest" day and increased to 9000 kCal cycling over a mountain pass. By combining liquid nutrition with normal meals, this cyclist nearly matched daily energy expenditure with energy intake.

Other sport and training activities also require extreme energy output and correspondingly high energy intake, sometimes in excess of 1000 kCal per hour in elite marathoners. Daily energy requirements of world class cross-country skiers during 1 week of intense training averaged 3740 to 4860 kCal for women and 6120 to 8570 kCal for men.[102] The values for women agree with the average 3957 kCal daily energy expenditure over a 14-day training period reported for seven elite lightweight female rowers.[55] In another study, the doubly labeled water technique evaluated the energy balance for two men who pulled sledges with starting weights of 222 kg (10 h · d^{-1} for 95 days) for 2300 km across Antarctica.[109] During a 10-day period, one man averaged a daily energy expenditure of 10,654 kCal, while his counterpart averaged an extraordinary output of 11,634 kCal. These values approach the 13,975-kCal theoretical daily energy expenditure ceiling attained by ultra long-distance runners.[19]

Ultraendurance Running Competition

Energy balance was studied during a 1000-km (approximately 600-mile) race from Sidney to Melbourne, Australia. The Greek ultramarathon champion Kouros completed the race in 5 days, 5 hours, and 7 minutes, finishing 24 hours and 40 minutes ahead of the next competitor. TABLE 3.3 provides relevant features of race conditions, distance covered, average daily speed, and rest and sleep patterns. Kouros did not sleep

Daily Energy Expenditure (kCal)

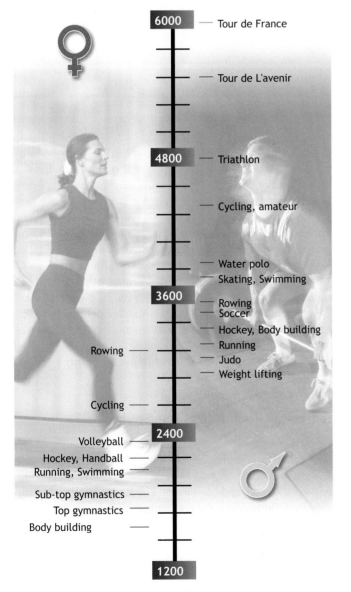

Figure 3.6 Daily energy intake (kCal) of elite male and female endurance, strength, and team sport athletes. (Modified from van Erp-Baart AMJ, et al. Nationwide survey on nutritional habits in elite athletes. Int J Sports Med 1989;10:53.)

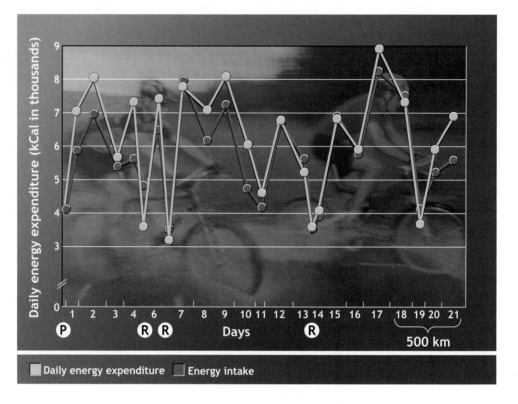

Figure 3.7 Daily energy expenditure *(yellow circles)* and energy intake *(red circles)* for a cyclist during the Tour de France competition. For 3 weeks in July, nearly 200 cyclists ride over and around the perimeter of France, covering 2405 miles, more than 100 miles daily (only 1 day of rest), at an average speed of 24.4 mph. Note the extremely high energy expenditure values and ability to achieve energy balance with liquid nutrition plus normal meals. *P,* stage; *R,* rest day. (Modified from Saris WHM, et al. Adequacy of vitamin supply under maximal sustained workloads; the Tour de France. In: Walter P, et al., eds. Elevated dosages of vitamins. Toronto: Huber Publishers, 1989.)

during the first 2 days of competition. He covered 463 km (287.8 miles) at an average speed of 11.4 km · h^{-1} during day 1 and 8.3 km · h^{-1} on day 2. During the remaining days, he took frequent rest periods, including periodic breaks for short "naps." Weather ranged from spring to winter conditions (30 to 8°C), and terrain varied. The bottom of TABLE 3.3 lists the pertinent details of food and water intake.

The near equivalence between Kouros' estimated total energy intake (55,970 kCal) and energy expenditure (59,079 kCal) represents a remarkable aspect of energy balance homeostasis in response to extremes of physical activity. Of the total energy intake, carbohydrates represented 95.3% and lipids 3%, with the remaining 1.7% from proteins. Protein intake from food averaged considerably below recommended levels, but Kouros did take protein supplements in tablet form. The unusually large daily energy intake, which ranged from 8,600 to 13,770 kCal, came from Greek sweets (baklava, cookies, and doughnuts), some chocolate, dried fruit and nuts, various fruit juices, and fresh fruits. Every 30 minutes after the first 6 hours of running, Kouros replaced sweets and fruit with a small biscuit soaked in honey or jam. He consumed a small amount of roasted chicken on day 4 and drank coffee every morning. He took a 500-mg vitamin C supplement every 12 hours and a protein tablet twice daily.

The exceptional achievement by Kouros exemplifies a highly conditioned athlete's exquisite regulatory control for energy balance during this most demanding exercise. He performed at a pace that required an energy metabolism averaging 49% of aerobic capacity during the first 2 days of competition and 38% for days 3 through 5. He also finished the competition without compromising overall health (no

muscular injuries or thermoregulatory problems, and body mass remained unchanged); reported difficulties included a severe bout of constipation during the run and frequent urination that persisted for several days postrace.

Another case study of a 37-year-old male ultramarathoner further demonstrates the tremendous capacity for prolonged, high daily energy expenditure. The doubly labeled water technique evaluated energy expenditure during a 2-week period of a 14,500-km run around Australia in 6.5 months (average 70–90 km · d^{-1}) with no days for rest.[54] Daily energy expenditure over the measurement period averaged 6321 kCal; daily water turnover equaled 6.1 L. The athlete ran about the same distance each day over the study period as in the entire race period. As such, these data likely represent energy dynamics for the entire run.

Extreme Ultraendurance Sports

The Iditasport ultramarathon consists of a choice of one race event from among the following options: run 120 km, snowshoe 120 km, bicycle 259 km, cross-country ski 250 km, or snowshoe, ski, and bicycle 250 km. Begun in 1983 as a single-event (Iditaski), a parallel competition emerged in 1987 consisting of long-distance cycling (Iditabike). In 1991, the two races merged along with foot, snowshoe, and triathlon events. The triathlon was discontinued in 1997, and the lengths of all other races changed to 160 km. The competition begins in late February, and the athletes traverse varied terrain, mostly in the wilderness over frozen rivers and lakes; wooded, rolling hills; and packed snow trails. On any given day, racers can experience extremes in weather conditions,

TABLE 3.3 ■ *TOP.* RACE CONDITIONS, DISTANCE COVERED, AVERAGE DAILY SPEED, REST AND SLEEP PATTERNS, AND NUTRIENT BALANCE DURING AN ELITE ULTRAENDURANCE PERFORMANCE. *BOTTOM.* DAILY AND TOTAL ENERGY BALANCE, NUTRIENT DISTRIBUTIONS IN FOOD, AND WATER INTAKE DURING THE RACE[a]

Course topography	SYDNEY			CANBERRA							MELBOURNE
Distance (km)	0	100	200	300	400	500	600	700	800	900	960

| Road conditions | Continuous uphill | Level ground | Continuous hills | Plateau uphill course | Flat terrain |

| Weather | Temperature 26°C + Humidity 60% Spring weather | 30°C + Summer weather | Gradual temp. drop (8–10°C) Drizzle + opposing winds Autumn weather | Rain | Winter conditions |

Accumulated distance covered: 270 km 463 km 615 km 780 km 915 km

days (d): d1 d2 d3 d4 d5

| Average daily speed km · h⁻¹ (m · s⁻¹) | 11.74 (3.26) | 8.3 (2.31) | 8.07 (2.24) | 8.9 (2.47) | 6.21 (1.72) |

Rest (min): 60 30 15 75 10 10 60 10 10 10 10 15 10 / 30 15 10 10 15 90 10 90

Sleep (min): 30 20 60 30 20 120

RACE DAY	DISTANCE COVERED (km)	ESTIMATED ENERGY EXPENDITURE (kCal)	ESTIMATED ENERGY INTAKE (kCal)	CARBOHYDRATES (g)	(%)	(kCal)	LIPIDS (g)	(%)	(kCal)	PROTEINS (g)	(%)	(kCal)	H₂O (L)
1	270	15,367	13,770	3375	98.0	13,502	20	1.3	180	22	0.7	88	22.0
2	193	10,741	8600	1981	92.2	7923	53	5.6	477	50	2.3	200	19.2
3	152	8919	12,700	3074	96.8	12,297	27	1.9	243	40	1.3	160	22.7
4	165	9780	7800	1758	90.1	7032	56	6.5	504	66	3.4	264	14.3
5	135	7736	12,500	3014	96.4	12,058	30	2.2	270	43	1.4	172	18.3
5 h	45	2536	550	138	100.0	550	—	—	—	—	—	—	3.2
Total	960	55,079	55,970	13,340		53,362	186		1674	221		734	99.7

Modified from Rontoyannis GP, et al. Energy balance in ultramarathon running. Am J Clin Nutr 1989;49:976.
[a]The runner Kouros weighed 65 kg, stature 171 cm, percentage body fat 8%, and $\dot{V}O_{2max}$ 62.5 mL · kg⁻¹ · min⁻¹

ranging from calm, "balmy" 30°F to "harsh" −40°F with blizzard conditions. During the 48-hour time limit for the event, racers carry a minimum of 15 pounds of survival gear; this includes a sleeping bag rated to −20°F, insulated sleeping pad, bivy sack or tent, stove and 8 ounces of fuel with fire starter (matches or lighter), pot to melt snow, insulated water containers to carry 2 quarts of water, headlamp or flashlight, and a minimum of 1 day's supply of emergency food. The supplies are carried in a backpack or pulled by sled (weighing from 15 to 30 lb).

Researchers estimated the total energy and macronutrient requirements for 14 participants (13 males, 1 female) in the 1995 race with 49 entrants. FIGURE 3.8 displays the total energy intake and percentage intake of carbohydrate, protein, and fat by runners and snowshoers, bikers, skiers, and triathletes. The bikers consumed the most total calories (8458 kCal), 74.1% as carbohydrate, 9.4% as protein, and 16.5% as fat. A comparison study between 1997–1998 Iditasport athletes and their 1995 counterparts showed only small differences in energy and nutrient contents except for higher intakes of carbohydrate (78.5%) and less fat (14.5%) and protein (7.3%) for skiers. The authors concluded that even though the length of the events differed in 1994–1996 and 1997–1998, few differences existed in the energy content and macronutrient percentages of the diets among the four categories of competitors from the two time periods.

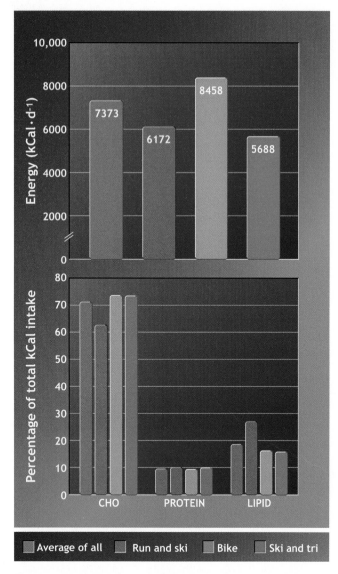

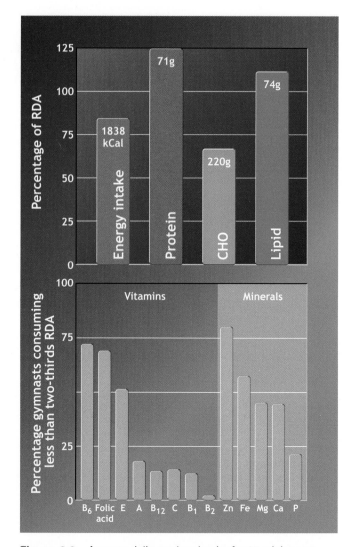

Figure 3.8 Energy and macronutrient content of the diets of Iditasport competitors. Multiply kCal value by 4.182 to convert to kJ. (Data for 1995 from Case D, et al. Dietary intakes of participants in the Iditasport human powered ultra-marathon. Alaska Med 1995;37:20. Data reported in the text for 1997–1998 from Stuempfle K, et al. Dietary factors of participants in the 1994–1998 Iditasport human powered ultra-marathon. Med Sci Sports Exerc 1999;31:S80.)

Figure 3.9 Average daily nutrient intake for 97 adolescent female gymnasts (11 to 14 y) related to recommended values. The RDA on the y axis *(top)* reflects only protein, while energy, CHO, and lipid reflect "recommended" values. Percentage of gymnasts consuming less than two thirds of the RDA for micronutrients *(bottom)*. Mean age, 13.1 years; mean stature, 152.4 cm (60 in.); mean body mass, 43.1 kg (94.8 lb). (Modified from Loosli AR, Benson J. Nutritional intake in adolescent athletes. Sports Med 1990;37:1143.)

High-Risk Sports for Marginal Nutrition

Gymnasts, ballet dancers, ice dancers, and weight-class athletes in boxing, wrestling, and judo engage in arduous training. Owing to the nature of their sport, these men and women continually strive to maintain a lean, relatively light body mass dictated by either esthetic or weight-class considerations. Energy intake often intentionally falls short of energy expenditure, and a relative state of malnutrition develops.[111] Nutritional supplementation for these athletes may prove beneficial as suggested by the data in FIGURE 3.9 for daily nutrient intake (% of RDA) of 97 competitive female gymnasts aged 11 to 14 years. Twenty-three percent of the girls consumed less than 1500 kCal daily, and more than 40%

consumed less than two thirds of the RDA for vitamins E and folic acid and the minerals iron, magnesium, calcium, and zinc. Clearly, many of these adolescent gymnasts needed to upgrade the nutritional quality of their diets or consider supplementation. For athletes like these, carbohydrate intake often fails to match the energy requirements of heavy training. Unfortunately, training and competition occur in a carbohydrate-depleted state.

Eat More, Weigh Less

Physically active individuals generally consume more calories per kg of body mass than sedentary counterparts. The extra energy required for exercise accounts for the larger caloric intake. Paradoxically, the most active men and women, who eat more on a daily basis, weigh less than those who exercise at a lower total caloric expenditure. Thus, regular exercise allows a person to "eat more yet weigh less" while maintaining a lower percentage of body fat, despite the age-related tendency toward weight gain in middle age.[14] *Physically active persons maintain a lighter and leaner body and a healthier heart disease risk profile, despite increased intake of the typical American diet.* TABLE 3.4 presents a sample model for food intake for active athletes and an example of a 2500-kCal menu with 350 g of carbohydrates. Chapter 30 discusses the important role of exercise for weight control in more detail.

PRECOMPETITION MEAL

Athletes often compete in the morning following an overnight fast. As pointed out in Chapter 1, significant depletion occurs in the body's carbohydrate reserves over an 8- to 12-hour period without eating. This occurs even if the person previously follows appropriate dietary recommendations. Consequently, precompetition nutrition takes on considerable importance. *The precompetition meal provides adequate carbohydrate energy and ensures optimal hydration.* Fasting before competition or training makes no sense physiologically because it rapidly depletes liver and muscle glycogen and impairs exercise performance.[32,75,98] If a person trains or competes in the afternoon, breakfast becomes the important meal to optimize glycogen reserves. For late afternoon training or competition, lunch becomes the important source for topping off glycogen stores. Consider the following three factors when individualizing the precompetition meal plan: (1) food preference of the athlete, (2) "psychological set" of competition, and (3) digestibility of foods.

As a general rule, competition day should exclude foods high in lipid and protein. Such foods digest slowly and remain in the digestive tract longer than foods containing similar energy content as carbohydrate. Precompetition meal timing also deserves consideration. The increased stress and tension that usually accompany competition significantly reduce blood flow to the digestive tract, causing depressed intestinal

TABLE 3.4 ■ SAMPLE TRAINING DIET[a]

Body Weight(50 kg)	110 LB 60 (kg)	132 LB 70 (kg)	154 LB 80 (kg)	176 LB
Total kCal 2500[b]	**3000**	**3500**	**4000**	
Milk group (90 kCal) Skim milk, 1 cup Plain, low-fat yogurt, 1 cup	4	4	4	4
Meat group (55–75 kCal) Cooked, lean meat (fish, poultry), 1 oz Egg, 1 Peanut butter, 1 Tbsp Low-fat cheese, 1 oz Cottage cheese, 1/4 cup	5	5	6	6
Fruits	7	9	10	12
Vegetables	3	5	6	7
Grains	16	18	20	24
Lipids	5	6	8	10

SAMPLE HIGH-CARBOHYDRATE 2500-KCAL MENU (350 G)

Breakfast	Lunch	Dinner	Snack 1	Snack 2
1 cup bran cereal	3 oz lean roast beef	Chicken stir-fry:	3 cups popcorn	8 oz apple cider
8 oz low-fat milk	1 hard roll	3 oz chicken		
1 English muffin	2 tsp mayonnaise or mustard,	1 cup diced vegetables		
	lettuce and tomato	2 tsp oil		
1 tsp margarine	1/2 cup cole slaw	2 cup rice		
4 oz orange juice	2 fresh plums	1 cup orange and grapefruit		
	2 oatmeal cookies	sections		
	8 oz seltzer water with lemon	1 cup vanilla yogurt		

[a] An active athlete requires approximately 50 kCal of food per kg (23 kcal per lb) of body mass each day to provide enough calories for optimal athletic performance. A training diet ideally consists of approximately 60% carbohydrates, 15 to 20% proteins, and less than 25% lipids.
[b] Numbers below total kCal values are recommended number of daily servings.
Modified from Carbohydrates and Athletic Performance. Sports Science Exchange, vol. 7. Chicago: Gatorade Sports Science Institute, 1988.

absorption. *It takes 3 to 4 hours to digest, absorb, and store a carbohydrate-rich, precompetition meal as muscle and liver glycogen.* However, extending the time for eating beyond this period may negatively affect glycogen replenishment and subsequent endurance exercise.[77]

Protein or Carbohydrate?

Many athletes look forward to the classic "steak and eggs" precompetition meal. Such foods may satisfy the athlete, coach, and restaurateur, yet their benefits to exercise performance remain undemonstrated. A meal of this type, with its low carbohydrate content, actually thwarts optimal performance.

The following five reasons justify modifying or even abolishing the high-protein precompetition meal in favor of one high in carbohydrates:

1. Dietary carbohydrates replenish the significant depletion of liver and muscle glycogen from the overnight fast.
2. Carbohydrate digestion and absorption are more rapid than either protein or lipid. Thus, carbohydrate provides energy faster and reduces the feeling of fullness following a meal.
3. A high-protein meal elevates resting metabolism more than a high-carbohydrate meal because of protein's greater energy requirements for digestion, absorption, and assimilation. This additional thermic effect could strain the body's heat-dissipating mechanisms and impair exercise performance in hot weather.
4. Protein catabolism for energy facilitates dehydration during exercise because the byproducts of amino acid breakdown require water for urinary excretion. About 50 mL of water "accompanies" the excretion of each gram of urea.
5. Carbohydrate, not protein, serves as the main energy nutrient for short-term anaerobic activity and high-intensity aerobic exercise.

The ideal precompetition meal maximizes muscle and liver glycogen storage and provides glucose for intestinal absorption during exercise. The meal should:

- Contain 150 to 300 g of carbohydrate (3 to 5 g per kg body mass in either solid or liquid form)
- Be consumed 3 to 4 hours before exercising
- Contain relatively little fat and fiber to facilitate gastric emptying and minimize gastrointestinal distress

The benefits of proper precompetition feeding occur only if the athlete maintains a nutritionally sound diet throughout training. Preexercise feedings cannot correct existing nutritional deficiencies or inadequate nutrient intake during the weeks before competition. Chapter 23 discusses how endurance athletes can augment precompetition glycogen storage in conjunction with specific exercise/diet modifications using "carbohydrate-loading" techniques.

INTEGRATIVE QUESTION

Outline your presentation to a high school class about how to eat well to establish a physically active and healthy lifestyle.

Liquid and Prepackaged Bars, Powders, and Meals

Commercially prepared nutrition bars, powders, and liquid meals offer an alternative approach in precompetition feeding or as supplemental feedings during periods of competition. These supplements also effectively enhance energy and nutrient intake in training, particularly if energy output exceeds energy intake from lack of interest or mismanagement of feedings.

Liquid Meals

Liquid meals provide high carbohydrate content but contain enough lipid and protein to contribute to satiety. They also supply the person with fluid because they exist in liquid form. The liquid meal digests rapidly, leaving essentially no residue in the intestinal tract. Liquid meals prove particularly effective during daylong swimming and track meets, or during tennis, soccer, and basketball tournaments. In these situations, the person usually has little time for (or interest in) food. Liquid meals offer a practical approach to supplementing caloric intake during the high-energy–output phase of training. Athletes can also use liquid nutrition if they have difficulty maintaining body weight, and as a ready source of calories to gain weight.

Nutrition Bars

Nutrition bars (also called "energy bars," "protein bars," and "diet bars") contain a relatively high protein content that ranges between 10 and 90 g per bar. The typical 60-g bar contains 25 g (100 kCal) of carbohydrate (equal amounts of starch and sugar), 15 g (60 kCal) of protein, and 5 g (45 kCal) of lipid (3 g or 27 kCal of saturated fat), with the remaining weight as water. Thus, 49% of the bar's total 205 calories are from carbohydrates, 29% from protein, and 22% from lipid. Nutrition bars often include vitamins and minerals (30 to 50% of recommended values) and some contain dietary supplements such as β-hydroxy-β-methylbutyrate (HMB). These bars must be labeled as dietary supplements rather than as foods.

The composition of nutrition bars generally varies with their purpose. For example, so-called "energy bars" contain a greater proportion of carbohydrates while "diet" or "weight loss" bars are lower in carbohydrate content and higher in protein. "Meal-replacement bars" have the largest energy content (240 to 900 kCal) with proportionately more of the three macronutrients. "Protein bars" simply contain a larger amount of protein. While nutrition bars provide a relatively easy way to obtain important nutrients, they should not totally substitute for normal food intake. They lack the broad array of plant fibers and phytochemicals found in food and contain a relatively high level of saturated fatty acids. As an added warning, because these bars are generally sold as dietary supplements, no independent assessment by the FDA or other federal or state agency exists to validate the labeling claims for macronutrient content and composition.

Nutrition Powders and Drinks

A high protein content between 10 and 50 g per serving represents a unique aspect of nutrition powders and drinks. They also contain added vitamins, minerals, and other dietary supplement ingredients. The powders come in canisters or packets that readily mix with water (or other liquid), while the drinks come premixed in cans. These products often serve as an alternative to nutrition bars; they are marketed as meal replacements, dieting aids, energy boosters, or concentrated protein sources.

The composition of nutrition powders and drinks varies considerably from nutrition bars. For one thing, nutrition bars contain at least 15 g of carbohydrates to provide texture and taste, whereas powders and drinks do not. This accounts for the relatively high protein content of powders and drinks. Nutrition powders and drinks generally contain fewer calories per serving than bars, but this can vary for a powder depending on the liquid used for mixing.

The recommended serving of a powder averages about 45 g, the same amount as a nutrition bar (minus its water content), but wide variation exists in this recommendation. A typical serving of a high-protein powder mix contains about 10 g of carbohydrate (two thirds as sugar), 30 g of protein, and 2 g of lipid. This amounts to a total of 178 kCal or 23% of calories from carbohydrate, 67% from protein, and 10% from lipid. When mixed in water, the powdered nutrient supplements far exceed the recommended protein intake percentage and fall below recommended lipid and carbohydrate percentages. The nutrient composition of a drink typically contains slightly more carbohydrate and less protein than does a powder.

Do not use powders and drinks to substitute for regular food because of their relatively high protein content and lack of the broad array of plant fibers and phytochemicals in a well-balanced diet. As with nutrition bars, the FDA or other federal or state agency makes no independent assessment about the validity of labeling claims for nutrient content and composition. Prudent use of some of these supplements can replenish glycogen reserves before and after high-intensity exercise and competition, especially because an athlete's appetite for "normal" food wanes.

CARBOHYDRATE FEEDINGS PRIOR TO, DURING, AND IN RECOVERY FROM EXERCISE

High-intensity aerobic exercise for 1 hour decreases liver glycogen by about 55%, whereas a 2-hour strenuous workout almost depletes the glycogen content of the liver and active muscle fibers. Even supermaximal, repetitive 1- to 5-minute bouts of exercise interspersed with brief rest intervals (e.g., soccer, ice hockey, field hockey, European handball, and tennis) dramatically lower liver and muscle glycogen. The vulnerability of the body's glycogen stores during strenuous exercise has focused research on the potential benefits of carbohydrate feedings immediately before and during exercise. Scientists also study ways to optimize carbohydrate replenishment in the postexercise recovery period.

Prior to Exercise

Confusion exists regarding the potential endurance benefits of preexercise ingestion of simple sugars. Some researchers argue that consuming rapidly absorbed high-glycemic carbohydrates within 1 hour before exercising accelerates glycogen depletion. This negatively affects endurance performance by the following mechanisms:

- A rapid rise in blood sugar triggers an overshoot in insulin release. An excess of insulin causes a relative hypoglycemia (also called **rebound hypoglycemia**, or reactive hypoglycemia). Significant blood sugar reduction impairs central nervous system function during exercise.
- A large insulin release facilitates the influx of glucose into muscle, which disproportionately increases glycogen catabolism in exercise. At the same time, high insulin levels *inhibit* lipolysis, which reduces fatty acid mobilization from adipose tissue. Augmented carbohydrate breakdown and depressed fat mobilization contribute to premature glycogen depletion and early fatigue.

Research in the late 1970s indicated that drinking a highly concentrated sugar solution before exercise precipitated early fatigue in endurance activities. For example, when young men and women consumed a 300-mL solution containing 75 g of glucose 30 minutes before cycling exercise, endurance was 19% lower than in similar trials preceded by 300 mL of plain water or a liquid meal of protein, lipid, and carbohydrate.[38] Paradoxically, the concentrated sugar drink depleted muscle glycogen reserves prematurely compared with drinking plain water. The researchers hypothesized that the dramatic rise in blood sugar within 5 to 10 minutes after consuming the concentrated preevent sugar drink caused the pancreas to oversecrete insulin (accentuated hyperinsulinemia). This, in turn, triggered rebound hypoglycemia as glucose moved rapidly into muscle.[49,133] At the same time, insulin inhibited mobilization and use of fat for energy (lipolysis suppression).[105] Consequently, intramuscular glycogen catabolized to a much greater extent, causing early glycogen depletion and fatigue compared with control conditions. Subsequent research has *not* corroborated these negative effects of concentrated preexercise sugar feedings on endurance.[3,35,105] The discrepancy in research findings has no clear explanation. One way to eliminate any potential for negative effects of preexercise simple sugars is to ingest them at least 60 minutes before exercising.[45,98] This provides sufficient time to reestablish hormonal balance before exercise begins.

Debate Concerning Fructose

The small intestine absorbs fructose more slowly than either glucose or sucrose. This causes a minimal insulin response with essentially no decline in blood glucose.[29] The theoretical rationale for fructose use appears plausible, but its exercise benefits remain inconclusive. From a practical standpoint, gastrointestinal distress (vomiting and diarrhea) often accompanies high-fructose beverage consumption, which itself negatively affects exercise performance. After absorption, the liver must first convert the fructose to glucose; this further limits the rapidity of fructose availability as an energy source.

During Exercise

Physical and mental performance improves with carbohydrate supplementation *during* exercise.[2,27,82,121,124,128,131] The addition of protein to the carbohydrate-containing beverage (4:1 ratio of carbohydrate to protein) may delay fatigue and reduce muscle damage compared with supplementation during exercise with carbohydrate only.[58,97] When a person consumes carbohydrates during endurance exercise, the carbohydrate form exerts little negative effect on hormonal response, exercise metabolism, or endurance performance.[17] The reason is straightforward: increased levels of sympathetic nervous system hormones (catecholamines) in exercise inhibit insulin release. Concurrently, exercise increases a muscle's absorption of glucose, so any exogenous glucose moves into the cells with a lower insulin requirement.

Ingested carbohydrate provides a readily available energy nutrient for active muscles during intense exercise. *Consuming about 60 g of liquid or solid carbohydrates each hour during exercise benefits high-intensity, long-duration (≥ 1 h) aerobic exercise and repetitive short bouts of near-maximal effort.*[28,62,79,80] Supplemental carbohydrate during protracted intermittent exercise to fatigue also facilitates skill performance, such as improved stroke quality during the final stages of prolonged tennis play.[124] Little benefit comes from carbohydrate feedings during low-intensity exercise because fat oxidation fuels exercise with little demand on carbohydrate breakdown.[2] Mixtures of combinations of glucose, fructose, and sucrose ingested at a high rate (about 1.8 g·min^{-1}) results in 20 to 55% higher exogenous carbohydrate oxidation rates (with reduced oxidation of endogenous carbohydrate), compared with ingestion of an isocaloric amount of glucose.[61,94]

Exogenous carbohydrate intake during intense exercise provides the following benefits:

- Spares muscle glycogen, particularly in the type I, slow-twitch muscle fibers because the ingested glucose powers exercise.[117–119]
- Maintains a more optimal blood glucose level. This lowers the rating of perceived exertion; elevates plasma insulin; lowers cortisol and growth hormone levels; prevents headache, lightheadedness, and nausea; and attenuates other symptoms of central nervous system distress and diminished muscular performance.[15,84,134]

- Blood glucose maintenance also supplies muscles with glucose when glycogen reserves deplete in the later stages of prolonged exercise.[21,48]

Carbohydrate feedings during exercise at 60 to 80% of aerobic capacity postpone fatigue by 15 to 30 minutes.[26] This effect contributes to performance in endurance competition because well-nourished athletes without supplementation usually fatigue within 2 hours. A single concentrated carbohydrate feeding about 30 minutes before anticipated fatigue (about 2 hours into exercise) proves as effective as periodic carbohydrate ingestion throughout exercise. This later feeding restores the blood glucose level (FIG. 3.10), which delays fatigue by increasing carbohydrate availability to active muscles.

The greatest benefits from carbohydrate feedings emerge during prolonged exercise at about 75% of aerobic capacity. When exercise begins above this level, subjects must reduce exercise intensity to about the 75% level to attain the benefits from carbohydrate feedings.[21] Fat provides the primary energy fuel in light-to-moderate exercise below 50% of maximum; at this intensity, glycogen reserves do not decrease to a level that limits endurance. Repeated feedings of carbohydrate in solid form (43 g sucrose with 400 mL water) at the beginning and at 1, 2, and 3 hours of exercise maintain blood glucose and slow glycogen depletion during 4 hours of cycling. Glycogen conservation not only extends endurance but also enhances sprint performance to exhaustion at the end of exercise.[5,7,92,106,110] *These findings demonstrate that carbohydrate feeding during prolonged, high-intensity exercise either conserves muscle glycogen for later use or maintains blood glucose for use as exercise progresses and muscle glycogen*

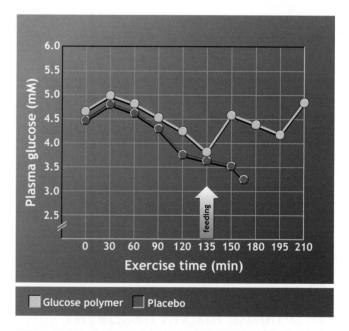

Figure 3.10 Average plasma glucose concentration during prolonged high-intensity aerobic exercise when subjects consumed a placebo or glucose polymer (3 g per kg body mass in a 50% solution). (Modified from Coggan AR, Coyle EF. Metabolism and performance following carbohydrate ingestion late in exercise. Med Sci Sports Exerc 1989;21:59.)

depletes, or both. Oxidation of exogenous carbohydrates supplied during exercise can reach values as high as 1.3 $g \cdot min^{-1}$.[93] The end result is as follows: (1) improved endurance at a high steady pace or during intense intermittent exercise and (2) augmented sprint capacity toward the end of prolonged physical efforts. In a marathon run, a sustained high-energy output and final sprint to the finish contribute greatly to a winning performance.

Replenishing Glycogen Reserves: Refueling for the Next Bout of Intense Training or Competition

All carbohydrates and carbohydrate-containing foods do not digest and absorb at the same rate. Plant starch composed primarily of amylose is a resistant carbohydrate because of its relatively slow hydrolysis rate. Conversely, starch, with a relatively high amylopectin content digests more rapidly. The **glycemic index** provides a relative measure of the increase in blood glucose concentration in the 2 hours after ingestion of a food containing 50 g of carbohydrate compared with a "standard" for carbohydrate (usually white bread or glucose) with an assigned value of 100 (FIG. 3.11).[39] Ingesting 50 g of a food with a glycemic index of 45 raises blood glucose concentrations to levels that reach 45% of the value for 50 g of glucose. The glycemic index is a function of glucose appearance in the systemic circulation and its uptake by peripheral tissues, which is influenced by the properties of the carbohydrate-containing food. For example, the food's amylose-to-amylopectin ratio and its fiber and fat content influence intestinal glucose absorption, whereas the protein content of the food may augment insulin release to facilitate tissue glucose uptake.[99] FIGURE 3.12 presents a sample from the more than 600 foods classified by their glycemic index. This includes high- and low-glycemic index meals of similar calorie and macronutrient composition (see inset table).

Differences in glycemic index values exist depending on the laboratory and exact food type evaluated (e.g., slight variations in type of white bread, rice, and potatoes used as the standard of comparison). The glycemic index should not be viewed as an unwavering standard because variability exists among individuals in their response to consuming a specific carbohydrate-containing food. A high-glycemic index rating does not necessarily indicate poor nutritional quality.[87,132] For example, carrots, brown rice, and corn (high-glycemic index values) contain rich quantities of health-protective micronutrients, phytochemicals, and dietary fibers.

Interestingly, a food's index rating does not depend simply on its grouping as simple (monosaccharides and disaccharides) or complex (starch and fiber) carbohydrate. The plant starch in white rice and potatoes has a higher glycemic index than the simple sugars (particularly fructose) in apples and peaches. Because a food's fiber content slows digestion, peas, beans, and other legumes have a low glycemic index. Dietary lipids and proteins slow food passage into the intestine. This reduces the glycemic index of the meal's accompanying carbohydrate content. *A food with a moderate- to high-glycemic index rating offers more benefit for rapid replenishment of carbohydrate following prolonged exercise than one rated low,*[25,129] *even if the replenishment meal contains a small amount of lipid and protein.*[16]

The revised glycemic index listing also includes the **glycemic load** associated with the consumption of specified serving sizes of different foods. Whereas the glycemic index compares equal quantities of a carbohydrate-containing food, the glycemic load quantifies the overall glycemic effect of a typical *portion* of food. This represents the product of the amount of available carbohydrate in that serving and the glycemic index of the food. A high glycemic load indicates a greater elevation in blood glucose and a greater insulin release. An increased risk for type 2 diabetes and coronary heart disease coincides with the chronic consumption of a diet with a high glycemic load.[60,73]

Optimal glycogen replenishment benefits individuals involved in (1) regular intense training, (2) tournament competition with qualifying rounds, or (3) events scheduled with only 1 or 2 days for recuperation. An intense bout of resistance training also significantly reduces muscle glycogen reserves. For athletes, acute weight loss by energy restriction without dehydration impairs anaerobic exercise capacity.[90] When these athletes then consumed a diet containing 75% carbohydrate (21 kCal per kg body mass) over the next 5 hours, anaerobic performance recovered to near-baseline values. No improvement occurred if the refeeding diet contained only 45% carbohydrate. Even without full glycogen replenishment, some restoration in recovery provides beneficial effects in the next exercise bout. For example, consuming carbohydrate for

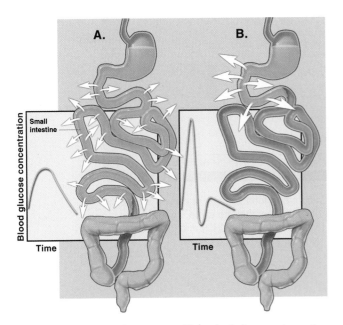

Figure 3.11 General response of intestinal glucose absorption following feeding of foods with either (**A**) low or (**B**) high-glycemic index.

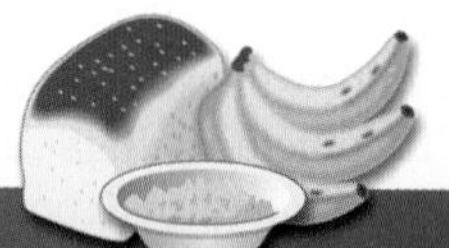

High glycemic		Moderate glycemic		Low glycemic	
Glucose	100	Corn	59	Apples	39
Carrots	92	Sucrose	59	Fish sticks	38
Honey	87	All-Bran	51	Butter beans	36
Corn flakes	80	Potato chips	51	Navy beans	31
Whole-meal bread	72	Peas	51	Kidney beans	29
White rice	72	White pasta	50	Lentils	29
New potatoes	70	Oatmeal	49	Sausage	28
White bread	69	Sweet potatoes	48	Fructose	20
Shredded wheat	67	Whole-wheat pasta	42	Peanuts	13
Brown rice	66	Oranges	40		
Beets	64				
Raisins	64				
Bananas	62				

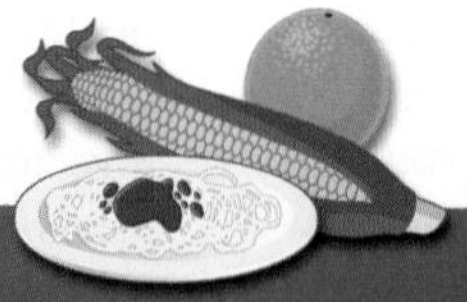

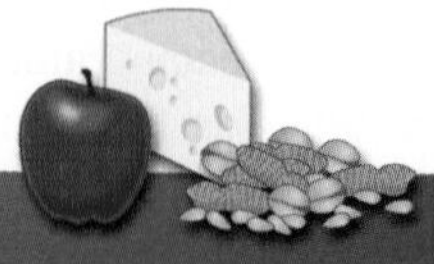

High GI Diet	CHO (g)	Contribution to Total GI	Low GI Diet	CHO (g)	Contribution to Total GI
Breakfast			**Breakfast**		
30 g Corn Flakes	25	9.9	30 g All-Bran	24	4.7
1 banana	30	7.8	1 diced peach	8	1.1
1 slice whole meal bread	12	3.8	1 slice grain bread	14	2.2
1 tsp margarine			1 tsp margarine		
			1 tsp jelly		
Snack			**Snack**		
1 crumpet	20	6.4	1 slice grain fruit loaf	20	4.1
1 tsp margarine			1 tsp margarine		
Lunch			**Lunch**		
2 slices whole-meal bread	23.5	7.6	2 slices grain bread	28	4.5
2 tsp margarine			2 tsp margarine		
25 g cheese			25 g cheese		
1 cup diced cantaloupe	8	10.4	1 apple	20	3.6
Snack			**Snack**		
4 plain sweet biscuits	28	10.4	200 g low-fat fruit yogurt	26	4.1
Dinner			**Dinner**		
120 g lean steak			120 g lean minced beef		
1 cup of mashed potatoes	32	12.1	1 cup boiled pasta	34	6.4
1/2 cup of carrots	4	1.7	1 cup of tomato and onion sauce	8	2.5
1/2 cup of green beans	2	0.6	Green salad with vinaigrette	1	0.6
50 g broccoli					
Snack			**Snack**		
290 g watermelon	15	5.1	1 orange	10	2.1
1 cup of reduced-fat milk throughout day	14	1.9	1 cup of reduced-fat milk throughout day	14	1.9
Total	212	69.8	**Total**	212	39.0

For each diet, the carbohydrate choices are maximized for differences between the two diets.

Figure 3.12 Categorization for glycemic index (GI) of common food sources of carbohydrates. The *inset table* presents high- and low-glycemic index diets that contain the same amounts of energy and macronutrients and derive 50% of energy from carbohydrate (CHO) and 30% of energy from lipid. (Diets from Brand-Miller J, Foster-Powell K. Nutr Today 1999;34:64.)

only 4 hours in recovery from a glycogen-depleting exercise bout significantly improves endurance capacity in subsequent exercise compared with performance when no carbohydrate is eaten in the 4-hour recovery.

 INTEGRATIVE QUESTION

Explain why foods with different glycemic index values dictate the nutritional recommendations for immediate preexercise versus immediate postexercise feedings.

Glycogen depletion of previously exercised muscle augments the resynthesis of glycogen during recovery.[135] In addition, endurance-trained individuals restore more muscle glycogen than untrained counterparts.[53] Consuming food after exercising facilitates glucose transport into muscle cells by:

1. Enhanced hormonal milieu, particularly higher insulin and lower catecholamine levels
2. Increased tissue sensitivity to insulin and intracellular glucose transporter proteins (e.g., GLUT 1 and GLUT 4, members of a family of facilitative monosaccharide transporters that mediate much of glucose transport activity; see Chapter 20)
3. Increased activity of a specific form of the glycogen-storing enzyme glycogen synthase

Practical Recommendations

Consuming carbohydrate-rich, high-glycemic foods immediately following intense training or competition speeds glycogen replenishment. One strategy is to consume about 50 to 75 g (2 to 3 oz) of high- to moderate-glycemic carbohydrates every 2 hours until reaching 500 to 700 g (7 to 10 g per kg of body mass) or until eating a large, high-carbohydrate meal. If immediately ingesting carbohydrate after exercise proves impractical, an alternative strategy entails eating meals containing 2.5 g of high-glycemic carbohydrate per kg body mass at 2, 4, 6, 8, and 22 hours postexercise. This replenishes glycogen to levels similar to those with the same protocol begun immediately postexercise.[85] Legumes, fructose, and milk products have a slow rate of digestion and/or intestinal absorption and should be avoided. Adding protein to an isocaloric postexercise supplement does not facilitate carbohydrate replenishment.[93] Glycogen resynthesis occurs more rapidly if the person remains inactive during the recovery period.[20]

Glycogen Replenishment Takes Time

Optimal carbohydrate intake replenishes glycogen stores at about 5 to 7% per hour. Even under the best of circumstances, it takes at least 20 hours to reestablish glycogen stores following glycogen-depleting exercise. Postexercise consumption of high-glycemic carbohydrates also may speed recovery by facilitating removal of free ammonia that forms at an increased rate during strenuous exercise. This occurs because consuming glucose enhances glutamine and alanine synthesis in skeletal muscle; these compounds provide the primary vehicle to transport ammonia out of muscle tissue.[44]

Cellular Uptake of Glucose

Normal blood glucose concentration (**euglycemia**) approximates 5 mM, equivalent to 90 mg of glucose per dL (100 mL) of blood. Blood glucose can rise above the hyperglycemic level to about 9 mM (162 mg $\cdot$ dL^{-1}) following a meal. A decrease in blood glucose concentration well below normal to 2.5 mM ($<$45 mg $\cdot$ dL^{-1}) classifies as hypoglycemia; it can occur during starvation or extremes of prolonged exercise.

Glucose entry into red blood cells, brain cells, and kidney and liver cells depends on the maintenance of a positive concentration gradient of glucose across the cell membrane (termed *unregulated glucose transport*). In contrast, large tissue masses such as skeletal and heart muscle and adipose tissue require glucose transport via regulated uptake, with insulin and GLUT 4, the predominant intracellular glucose transporter protein, as the regulating compounds.[76] Active skeletal muscle also increases its ability to take up glucose from the blood, independent of the effect of insulin. This effect persists into the early postexercise period and helps to replenish glycogen stores. Maintaining an adequate level of blood glucose during exercise and in recovery decreases possible negative effects from a low blood glucose concentration.

The Glycemic Index and Preexercise Feedings

The ideal meal immediately before exercising should provide a source of carbohydrate to sustain blood glucose and muscle metabolism while minimizing any increase in insulin release. Maintaining a relatively normal plasma insulin level should theoretically preserve blood glucose availability, optimize fat mobilization and catabolism, and at the same time spare liver and muscle glycogen reserves.

Use the glycemic index to formulate the immediate preexercise feeding.[4,31,35] Consuming simple sugars (concentrated high-glycemic carbohydrates) immediately before exercising causes blood sugar to rise rapidly (**glycemic response**), triggering an excessive insulin release (**insulinemic response**).[9,37] Endurance performance could be compromised by rebound hypoglycemia, depressed fat catabolism, and possible earlier-than-expected depletion of glycogen reserves. In contrast, consuming low-glycemic, carbohydrate-rich foods (starch with high amylose content or moderate-glycemic carbohydrate with high dietary fiber content) in the immediate 45- to 60-minute preexercise period allows a slower rate of glucose absorption; this reduces the potential rebound glycemic response. This strategy would eliminate the insulin surge, while a steady supply of "slow-release" glucose becomes available from the digestive tract throughout exercise. This effect should prove beneficial during prolonged, high-intensity exercise (such as ocean swimming), where it often becomes impractical to consume carbohydrate during the activity.

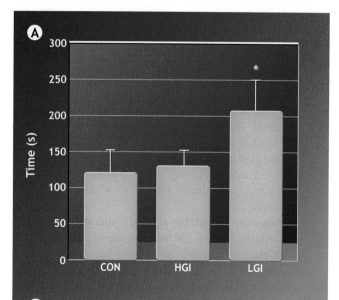

B Calculation of mixed-meal GI*a*

	Percent of Total Meal Available Carbohydrate	Food GI	Meal GI
High GI meal (HGI)			
Cornflakes	55	84	46.2
Banana	30	60	18.0
Low-fat Milk	15	34	05.1
Total	100	–	69.3
Low GI meal (LGI)			
All-Bran	55	42	23.1
Apple	30	36	10.8
Low-fat yogurt (unsweetened)	15	14	02.1
Total	100	–	36.0

a The glycemic index (GI) of mixed meals is expressed as the weighted mean of the GI values of each of the component foods, with the weighting based on the percentage of the total meal carbohydrate provided by each food.

C Mean dietary composition of meals*a*

	High GI Meal (HGI)	Low GI Meal (LGI)
Available CHO (g)	113	113
Protein (g)	18	33
Fat (g)	6	9
Dietary fiber (g)	5	57
Total energy		
kJ/meal	2418	2782
kCal/meal	578	665

a Data from United States Department of Agriculture, *Home and Garden Bulletin*, No. 72. *Nutritive Value of Foods*. Washington, D.C., U.S. Government Printing Office. 1988.

Figure 3.13 **A**. All-out cycling time to exhaustion (after 2 h high-intensity exercise) for control *(CON)*, moderately high-glycemic index meal *(HGI)*, and low-glycemic index meal *(LGI)* trials. Values represent the average cycling times for 10 trained cyclists. *Indicates LGI significantly longer than HGI and CON. Inset boxes indicate (**B**) calculation of mixed-meal glycemic index and (**C**) average dietary composition of the meals. (From DeMarco HM, et al. Pre-exercise carbohydrate meals: application of glycemic index. Med Sci Sports Exerc 1999;31:164.)

Several studies compared the effects of preexercise, low-glycemic versus high-glycemic carbohydrate ingestion on endurance performance and blood glucose levels during sustained exercise. For trained cyclists who performed high-intensity aerobic exercise, a preexercise low-glycemic meal of lentils significantly extended endurance compared with feedings of glucose or a high-glycemic meal of potatoes of equivalent carbohydrate content.[113] A moderate-glycemic index breakfast cereal with added dietary fiber eaten 45 minutes before moderately intense exercise increased time to fatigue by 16% over control conditions or a high-glycemic meal without fiber.[67]

Maintaining relatively high plasma glucose levels during prolonged exercise following a preexercise meal of low-glycemic carbohydrate also enhances subsequent performance at maximal effort (FIG. 3.13). Ten trained cyclists consumed either a low-glycemic or high-glycemic meal 30 minutes before bicycling for 2 hours at 70% $\dot{V}O_{2max}$ followed by bicycling to exhaustion at 100% $\dot{V}O_{2max}$.[29] The low-glycemic meal produced significantly lower plasma insulin levels after 20 minutes of exercise. At the end of 2 hours, carbohydrate oxidation and plasma glucose levels remained higher and ratings of perceived exertion lower than under the high-glycemic conditions. Thereafter, time to exhaustion exercising at $\dot{V}O_{2max}$ averaged 59% longer than the high-glycemic maximal effort. All research, however, does not support the wisdom of preexercise low-glycemic feedings for enhancing endurance performance.[35,46,129] Further study of the topic certainly seems warranted.

INTEGRATIVE QUESTION

Advise an endurance athlete whose preevent nutrition consists of a fast-food hamburger and high-protein shake consumed one hour before competition.

GLUCOSE FEEDINGS, ELECTROLYTES, AND WATER UPTAKE

As we discuss in Chapter 25, ingesting fluid before and during exercise minimizes the detrimental effects of dehydration on cardiovascular dynamics, temperature regulation, and exercise performance. Adding carbohydrate to an **oral rehydration solution** provides additional glucose energy for exercise. Adding electrolytes to the rehydration beverage maintains the thirst mechanism and reduces the risk of hyponatremia. Determining the optimal fluid/carbohydrate mixture and volume becomes important to minimize fatigue and prevent dehydration. Concern centers on the dual observations that (1) a large fluid volume intake impairs carbohydrate uptake, while (2) a concentrated sugar solution impairs fluid replenishment.

Important Considerations

The rate the stomach empties greatly affects absorption of fluid and nutrients by the small intestine. FIGURE 3.14 shows the important factors that influence gastric emptying. Little

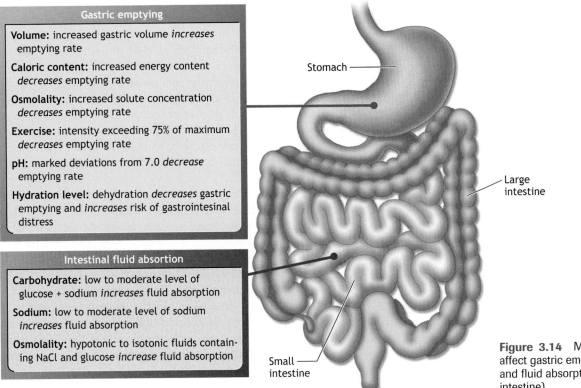

Gastric emptying

Volume: increased gastric volume *increases* emptying rate

Caloric content: increased energy content *decreases* emptying rate

Osmolality: increased solute concentration *decreases* emptying rate

Exercise: intensity exceeding 75% of maximum *decreases* emptying rate

pH: marked deviations from 7.0 *decrease* emptying rate

Hydration level: dehydration *decreases* gastric emptying and *increases* risk of gastrointesinal distress

Intestinal fluid absorption

Carbohydrate: low to moderate level of glucose + sodium *increases* fluid absorption

Sodium: low to moderate level of sodium *increases* fluid absorption

Osmolality: hypotonic to isotonic fluids containing NaCl and glucose *increase* fluid absorption

Stomach

Large intestine

Small intestine

Figure 3.14 Major factors that affect gastric emptying (stomach) and fluid absorption (small intestine).

negative effect of exercise on gastric emptying occurs up to an intensity of about 75% of maximum, after which the emptying rate slows. Gastric volume, however, greatly influences gastric emptying; the emptying rate increases exponentially as fluid volume increases. *A major factor to speed gastric emptying (and compensate for any inhibitory effects of the beverage's carbohydrate content) involves maintaining a relatively high fluid volume in the stomach.* Consuming 400 to 600 mL of fluid immediately before exercise optimizes the beneficial effect of increased stomach volume on fluid and nutrient passage into the intestine. Then, regularly drinking 150 to 250 mL of fluid at 15-minute intervals throughout exercise continually replenishes fluid passed into the intestine.[33,69,72] This protocol produces a fluid delivery rate of about 1 L per hour, a volume sufficient to meet the fluid needs of most endurance athletes. Moderate hypohydration of up to 4% body mass does not impair the gastric emptying rate.[95] Fluid temperature does not exert a major effect during exercise, but highly carbonated beverages retard gastric emptying.[88] Beverages containing alcohol or caffeine induce a diuretic effect (alcohol most pronounced) that facilitates water loss from the kidneys, making them inappropriate for fluid replacement.

Particles in Solution

Gastric emptying slows when ingested fluids contain a high concentration of particles in solution (**osmolality**) or possess high caloric content.[10,95,125] Whether rehydration beverages hypertonic to plasma (≥ 280 mOsm $\cdot$ L^{-1}) retard net fluid uptake by the intestine remains unclear. If this does occur, it

could negatively affect prolonged exercise in hot weather, when adequate fluid intake, absorption, *and* retention play prime roles in the participant's health and safety.

The negative effect of concentrated sugar solutions on gastric emptying diminishes (and plasma volume maintained) when the drink contains a short-chain glucose polymer (**maltodextrin**) rather than simple sugars.[103] Short-chain polymers (3 to 20 glucose units) derived from cornstarch breakdown reduce the number of particles in solution. Fewer particles facilitate water movement from the stomach for intestinal absorption. Adding small amounts of glucose and sodium (glucose the more important factor) to the oral rehydration solution creates little negative effect on gastric emptying.[41,42,50] Glucose plus sodium actually facilitates fluid uptake by the intestinal lumen because of the rapid, active cotransport of glucose–sodium across the intestinal mucosa. Absorption of these particles stimulates water's passive uptake by osmotic action.[42,72] Extra glucose uptake also helps to preserve blood glucose. The additional glucose then spares muscle and liver glycogen and/or maintains blood glucose should glycogen reserves decrease as prolonged exercise continues.

Adding sodium (the most abundant ion in the extracellular space) to a fluid aids in maintaining plasma sodium concentrations. Extra sodium benefits the ultraendurance athlete at risk for hyponatremia from a large sweat–sodium loss coupled with drinking copious amounts of plain water (see Chapter 2). Maintaining plasma osmolality by adding sodium to the rehydration beverage also reduces urine output and sustains the sodium-dependent osmotic drive to drink (see Chapter 25).[91] A normal plasma and extracellular fluid osmolality promotes continued fluid intake *and* fluid retention during recovery.

RECOMMENDATIONS FOR FLUID AND CARBOHYDRATE REPLENISHMENT DURING EXERCISE

- Monitor dehydration rate from changes in body weight; require urination before postexercise body weight measurement for precise determination of the body's total fluid loss. Each pound of weight loss corresponds to 450 mL (15 oz) of dehydration.
- Drink fluids at the same rate as their estimated depletion (or at least drink at a rate close to 80% of sweating rate) during prolonged exercise that increases cardiovascular stress, metabolic heat load, and dehydration.
- Achieve carbohydrate (30 to 60 g $\cdot$ h^{-1}) and fluid requirements by drinking a 4 to 8% carbohydrate beverage each hour (625 to 1250 mL; average 250 mL every 15 min).

Recommended Oral Rehydration Solution

A 5 to 8% carbohydrate–electrolyte beverage consumed during exercise in the heat contributes to temperature regulation and fluid balance as effectively as plain water. As an added bonus, the drink provides intestinal energy delivery of approximately 5.0 kCal $\cdot$ min^{-1}; this helps maintain glucose metabolism and glycogen reserves in prolonged exercise.[33,101] Consuming this solution in recovery from prolonged exercise in a warm environment also improves endurance capacity for subsequent exercise. To determine a drink's percentage carbohydrate, divide the carbohydrate content (g) by the fluid volume (mL) and multiply by 100. For example, 80 g of carbohydrate in 1 L (1000 mL) of water represents an 8% solution. Effective fluid absorption during prolonged exercise

occurs over a wide range of osmolalities. For example, total fluid absorption of carbohydrate–electrolyte beverages with osmolalities of 197 (hypotonic), 295 (isotonic), and 414 (hypertonic) mOsm per liter of H_2O did not differ from the absorption rate of a plain water placebo.[43]

Do not confuse the conventional fluid replacement beverage with more-concentrated carbohydrate beverages designed to provide significant carbohydrate without concern for rapid fluid replenishment. These products, composed of 20 to 25% carbohydrates (largely as maltodextrins to prevent excessive sweetness), are well suited as carbohydrate sources for use during recovery from heavy training or competition.

Environmental and exercise conditions interact to influence the rehydration solution's optimal composition. Fluid replenishment becomes crucial to health and safety when intense aerobic effort performed under high thermal stress lasts 30 to 60 minutes. Under these conditions, the individual should consume a more dilute carbohydrate–electrolyte solution ($\leq$5% carbohydrate). In cooler weather, when dehydration does not pose a problem, a more-concentrated 15% carbohydrate beverage would suffice. Little difference exists among liquid glucose, sucrose, or starch as the ingested carbohydrate fuel source during exercise. Fructose is undesirable because of its potential to cause gastrointestinal distress. Furthermore, fructose absorption by the gut does not involve the active cotransport process required for glucose–sodium. This makes fructose absorption relatively slow and promotes less fluid uptake than an equivalent amount of glucose. *The optimal carbohydrate replacement rate during intense aerobic exercise ranges from 30 to 60 g (about 1 to 2 oz) per hour.*

FIGURE 3.15 presents a general guideline for fluid intake each hour during exercise for a given amount of carbohydrate replenishment. A tradeoff exists between how much carbohydrate to consume and gastric emptying. The stomach still empties up to 1700 mL of water per hour, even when drinking an 8% carbohydrate solution. Approximately 1000 mL (about 1 qt) of fluid consumed each hour probably represents the optimal volume to offset dehydration, because larger fluid volumes often produce gastrointestinal discomfort.

		Carbohydrate replenishment				
		30 g·h^{-1}	40 g·h^{-1}	50 g·h^{-1}	60 g·h^{-1}	
CHO concentration in drink (g · dL^{-1})	2%	1500 mL	2000 mL	2500 mL	3000 mL	Volume too large: greater than 1200 mL · h^{-1}
	4%	750	1000	1250	1500	
	6%	500	667	833	1000	Adequate fluid replacement: 600-1250 mL · h^{-1}
	8%	375	500	625	750	
	10%	300	400	300	600	
	15%	200	267	333	400	Low fluid replacement: less than 600 mL · h^{-1}
	20%	150	200	250	300	
	25%	120	160	200	240	
	50%	60	80	100	120	

Figure 3.15 Volume of fluid to ingest each hour to obtain the noted amount of carbohydrate (g · h^{-1}). (Modified from Coyle EF, Montain SJ. Benefits of fluid replacement with carbohydrate during exercise. Med Sci Sports Exerc 1992;24:S324.)

Summary

1. Within rather broad limits, a balanced diet provides the nutrient requirements of athletes and other individuals who train regularly. Well-planned daily menus with as few as 1200 kCal provide the vitamin, mineral, and protein requirements.

2. The recommended protein intake of 0.83 g per kg body mass represents a liberal requirement believed adequate for nearly all persons, regardless of physical activity level.

3. A protein intake between 1.2 and 1.8 g per kg of body mass should adequately meet the possibility of added protein need during intense exercise training. Athletes generally consume two to four times the protein RDA because their greater caloric intake usually provides proportionately more protein.

4. No precise recommendations exist for daily lipid and carbohydrate intake. Prudent advice recommends no more than 30% of daily calories from lipids; of this amount, most should be unsaturated fatty acids. For physically active persons, unrefined polysaccharides should provide 60% or more of the daily calories (400 to 600 g on a daily basis).

5. A high-fat diet stimulates adaptative responses that augment fat catabolism. However, reliable research has not demonstrated consistent exercise or training benefits from this dietary modification.

6. Successive days of hard training gradually deplete the body's liver and muscle glycogen reserves and could lead to training staleness, making continued training more difficult.

7. MyPyramid provides a comprehensive and personalized approach for Americans to choose a healthier lifestyle that balances sound nutrition and regular exercise.

8. Intensity of daily physical activity largely determines energy intake requirements. The daily caloric needs of athletes in strenuous sports do not consistently exceed 4000 kCal; exceptions include individuals with a large body mass or those involved in extreme levels of training or competition.

9. The precompetition meal should include foods high in carbohydrates and relatively low in lipids and proteins. Three hours provides sufficient time to digest and absorb the precompetition meal.

10. Commercially prepared liquid meals offer well-balanced nutritive value, contribute to fluid need, and absorb rapidly, leaving little residue in the digestive tract.

11. Consuming carbohydrate-containing rehydration solutions during exercise enhances high-intensity endurance performance by maintaining blood glucose concentration.

12. Glucose supplied via the blood can (1) spare existing glycogen in active muscles during exercise or (2) serve as reserve blood glucose for later use should muscle glycogen become depleted.

13. The glycemic index provides a relative measure of blood glucose increase after consuming a specific carbohydrate food. For rapid carbohydrate replenishment after exercise, individuals should consume 50 to 75 g of moderate- to high-glycemic index, carbohydrate-containing foods each hour.

14. With optimal carbohydrate intake, glycogen stores replenish at a rate of about 5 to 7% per hour. It takes about 20 hours for full replenishment of liver and muscle glycogen following a glycogen-depleting exercise bout.

15. Foods with a low glycemic index digest and absorb at a relatively slow rate to provide a steady supply of slow-release glucose during prolonged exercise.

16. Consuming 400 to 600 mL of fluid immediately before exercise, followed by regular fluid ingestion during exercise (250 mL every 15 minutes) optimizes gastric emptying by maintaining a relatively large fluid volume in the stomach.

17. The ideal oral rehydration solution to maintain fluid balance during exercise and heat stress contains between 5 and 8% carbohydrates.

18. Adding a moderate amount of sodium to fluid stabilizes plasma sodium concentrations, which benefits the ultraendurance athlete at risk for hyponatremia. Added sodium in the rehydration beverage also reduces urine production and sustains the sodium-dependent osmotic drive to drink.

References are available on the Student CD and online at http://connection.lww.com/mkk6e.

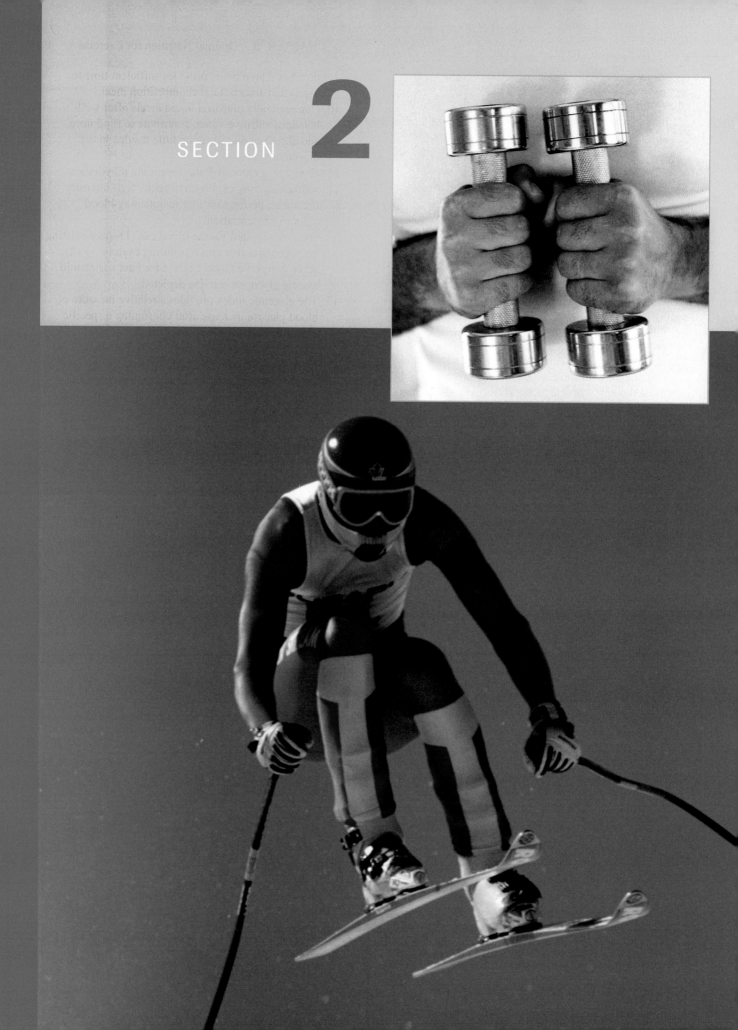

SECTION **2**

Energy for Physical Activity

Biochemical reactions that do not consume oxygen generate considerable energy for short durations. The rapid generation of energy remains crucial in maintaining a high standard of performance in sprint activities and other bursts of all-out exercise. In comparison, longer-duration aerobic exercise extracts energy more slowly from food through reactions that require oxygen. For greatest effectiveness, training the various physiologic systems requires an understanding of how the body generates energy to sustain exercise, the sources that provide energy, and the energy requirements of diverse physical activities.

This section presents a broad overview of how cells extract chemical energy bound within the food molecules and use it to power all forms of biologic work. We emphasize the importance of the food nutrients and processes of energy transfer to sustain physiologic function during light, moderate, and strenuous exercise.

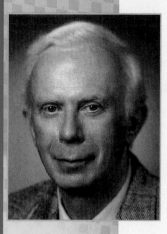

Interview *with* **Dr. John O. Holloszy**

Education: BS (Oregon State College, Salem, OR); MD (Washington University School of Medicine, St. Louis, MO); Postgraduate Training (NIH Special Research Fellow, Department of Biological Chemistry, Washington University School of Medicine, St. Louis, MO)

Current Affiliation: Professor of Internal Medicine; Chief, Division of Geriatrics and Gerontology, and Director, Section of Applied Physiology, Washington University School of Medicine, St. Louis, MO

Honors and Awards: See Appendix E, which is available on the Student CD and online at http://connection.lww.com/mkk6e.

Research Focus: The biological adaptations to exercise.

Memorable Publication: Holloszy JO. Biochemical adaptations in muscle. J Biol Chem 1967;242:2278.

Statement of Contributions: ACSM Honor Award
Over the past 25 years, John O. Holloszy has been the most important individual responsible for the development of cellular exercise research. His contributions have advanced knowledge in glucose transport, substrate provision, skeletal muscle metabolism, biochemical adaptations induced by training, fiber type responses, blood lipids, the aging process, and rehabilitation.

His innovative work, which has been applied to health-related aspects of exercise, has spawned a wealth of research inquiries by other investigators. He was the first to introduce postdoctoral training to exercise science. Our valued colleague, whose work has always exemplified quality, has fused exercise science with other disciplines.

What first inspired you to enter the exercise science field? What made you decide to pursue your advanced degree and/or line of research?

■ After completing medical school and four years of training in Internal Medicine and Endocrinology and Metabolism, I worked for two years as a Lt. Commander in the U.S. Public Health Service. Because of my interest in the prevention of coronary heart disease through diet and exercise, I was stationed at the Physical Fitness Research Laboratory at the University of Illinois.

At the time, Dr. Tom Cureton, Director of the Laboratory and pioneer in the area of endurance exercise training, conducted a year-round, daily exercise program, staffed by his graduate students, for university faculty and other individuals in the community. Most of the participants were middle-aged men, and I was tasked with obtaining information on the physiological and metabolic effects induced by the exercise program. With the help of some of Dr. Cureton's students and junior faculty, particularly James S. Skinner, who used this research for his doctoral dissertation, I conducted a series of studies on the effect of a six-month exercise program on body composition, blood lipids, and cardiovascular function.

This was my first experience with the effects of endurance training. I became fascinated with the remarkable improvements in endurance and exercise capacity that developed rapidly in response to training. I was also impressed by the decrease in body fat, reduction in serum triglycerides, and improvement in cardiovascular function. I had become convinced by the epidemiological evidence that obesity, ischemic heart disease, and type 2 diabetes were largely diseases of exercise deficiency. But, at the time, there was little research being done on the effects of exercise at the time, and research on the biological effects of exercise was a low priority, generally viewed as unimportant and not prestigious. Therefore, because I had become extremely interested in the biological mechanisms responsible for the adaptive responses to exercise at the cellular level, and because I thought that exercise deficiency had become the country's number one health problem, I decided to devote my career to research on the effects of exercise. My goals were to (1) elucidate the biological mechanisms underlying the improvements in performance and metabolism induced by exercise training; (2) evaluate the roles of exercise in the maintenance of health, treatment of disease, and prevention of loss of independence with advancing age; and, in the process, (3) bring research on the biology of exercise into the scientific mainstream.

Who were the most influential people in your career, and why?

■ The only person who had a major influence on my career was Dr. Hiro Narahara, my mentor during my two years of postdoctoral research training in biochemistry. Like many physicians who come to basic research relatively late in their careers, I tended to be sloppy in laboratory work. Hiro forced me to become careful and accurate in my technical work, although, because of a lack of natural aptitude, I never did become a skilled bench researcher. My other mentors generally tried to dissuade me from devoting my research career to the biology of exercise because they thought that I would ruin my academic career by working in what was at the time a low-prestige area of science.

What has been the most interesting/enjoyable aspect of your involvement in science? What was the least interesting/enjoyable aspect?

■ The most interesting and enjoyable aspects of my involvement in science have been the excitement and intellectual stimulation that comes from making new discoveries.

What is your most meaningful contribution to the field of exercise science, and why is it so important?

■ Although it is difficult to single out, the most meaningful contribution that I have made to exercise science—the one that has probably had the greatest impact—is the discovery that endurance training induces an increase in muscle mitochondria. The importance of this finding is that it plays a major role in explaining how endurance training improves endurance and alters the metabolic response to exercise.

What advice would you give to students who express an interest in pursuing a career in exercise science research?

■ A career in research in any area of biology can be extremely exciting and rewarding. This is particularly true of exercise science, a field in which there are still so many interesting, unanswered questions. However, biological research is extremely competitive in terms of coming up with novel, important ideas; obtaining research funding; keeping current with new methodology; and getting papers published. I would, therefore, strongly discourage students from pursuing a research career if they are not (1) highly intelligent, able to think independently and originally, with the ability to identify important problems and devise approaches for solving them; (2) highly motivated; (3) persevering and not easily discouraged; and (4) able to write well. There is probably nothing more discouraging than having to struggle for support and advancement, yet to be unsuccessful in one's chosen profession, but the chance for both is extremely high in biological research. A sensible approach for individuals who have an interest in exercise science but are not sure that they can succeed in a research career is to get a professional degree (MD, DO, PT, RN, RD, etc.), preferably along with a PhD. This way, one can remain associated with the research area and yet still be assured of making a good *living*.

What interests have you pursued outside of your professional career?

■ My interests unrelated to my professional career include literature, particularly historical novels, opera, and gourmet food.

Where do you see the exercise science field (particularly your area of greatest interest) heading in the next 20 years?

■ The most discouraging aspect of working in the field of exercise science is that, despite the now rather general perception that exercise is necessary for maintenance of health and functional capacity, the majority of people in North America are sedentary. Therefore, it seems likely to me that the major emphasis during the next 20 years will be (1) from a practical aspect, trying to get people to exercise, and (2) from a basic research perspective, trying to find pharmacological and other approaches that induce some of the same health benefits as exercise.

You have the opportunity to give a "last lecture." Describe its primary focus.

■ The adaptive response of muscle mitochondria to endurance exercise.

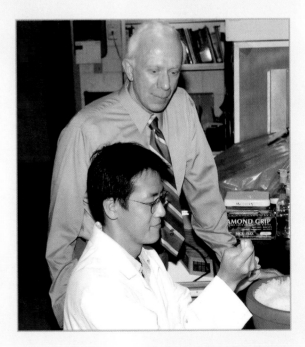

Energy Value of Food

4

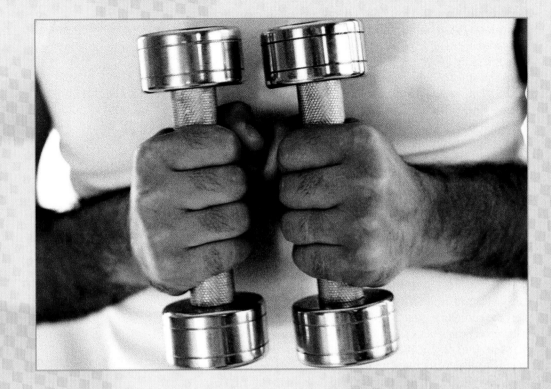

CHAPTER OBJECTIVES

- Describe the method to directly determine the energy content of the macronutrients

- Discuss three factors that influence the difference between a food's gross energy value and its net physiologic energy value

- Define the following: (1) heat of combustion, (2) digestive efficiency, and (3) Atwater general factors

- Compute the energy content of a meal from its macronutrient composition

MEASUREMENT OF FOOD ENERGY

The Calorie as a Measurement Unit

For food energy, 1 calorie expresses the quantity of heat needed to raise the temperature of 1 kg (1 L) of water 1°C (specifically from 14.5 to 15.5°C). Thus, a kilogram calorie or **kilocalorie (kCal)** more accurately defines the calorific value of food. For example, if a particular food contains 400 kCal, then releasing the potential energy trapped within this food's chemical structure increases the temperature of 400 L of water 1°C. Different foods contain different amounts of potential energy. One-half cup of peanut butter with a caloric value of 759 kCal contains the equivalent heat energy to increase the temperature of 759 L of water 1°C.

A corresponding unit of heat using Fahrenheit degrees is the British thermal unit, or BTU. One BTU represents the quantity of heat required to raise the temperature of 1 pound (weight) of water 1°F from 63 to 64°F. A clear distinction exists between temperature and heat. **Temperature** reflects a quantitative measure of an object's hotness or coldness. **Heat** describes energy transfer or exchange from one body or system to another.

The joule (J), or **kilojoule (kJ)**, reflects the standard international unit to express food energy. To convert kCal to kJ, multiply the kilocalorie value by 4.184. The kilojoule value for one-half cup of peanut butter, for example, would equal 759 kCal × 4.184 or 3176 kJ. The **megajoule (MJ)** equals 1000 kJ; its use avoids unmanageably large numbers. The following conversions apply: 1000 cal = 1 kCal = 4184 J or 0.004184 kJ; 1 BTU = 778 ft-lb = 252 cal = 1055 J. Appendix A (available on Student CD or online at http://connection.lww.com/mkk6e) lists metric system transpositions and conversion constants commonly used in exercise physiology.

Gross Energy Value of Foods

Laboratories use bomb calorimeters similar to the one illustrated in FIGURE 4.1 to measure the total or **gross energy value** of various food macronutrients. Bomb calorimeters operate on the principle of **direct calorimetry**, measuring the heat liberated as the food completely burns.

Figure 4.1 shows food within a sealed chamber charged with oxygen at high pressure. An electrical current moving through the fuse at the tip ignites the food–oxygen mixture. As the food burns, a water jacket surrounding the bomb absorbs the heat (energy) liberated. Because the calorimeter remains fully insulated from the ambient environment, the increase in water temperature directly reflects the heat released during a food's oxidation (burning).

Heat of combustion refers to the heat liberated by oxidizing a specific food; it represents the food's total energy value. For example, a teaspoon of margarine releases 100 kCal of heat energy when burned completely in a bomb calorimeter. This equals the energy required to raise 1.0 kg (2.2 lb) of ice water to the boiling point. The oxidation pathways of the intact organism and the bomb calorimeter differ, yet the quantity of energy liberated in the complete breakdown of a food remains the same.

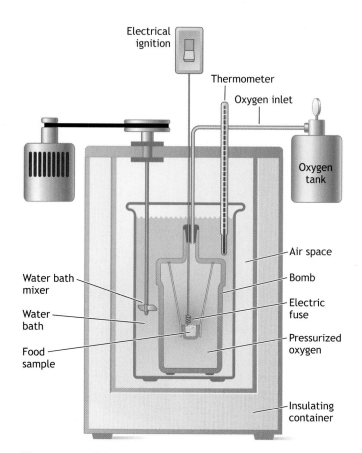

Figure 4.1. A bomb calorimeter directly measures the energy value of food.

Heat of Combustion: Lipid

The heat of combustion for lipid varies with the structural composition of the triacylglycerol molecule's fatty acids. For example, 1 g of either beef or pork fat yields 9.50 kCal, whereas oxidizing 1 g of butterfat liberates 9.27 kCal. The average caloric value for 1 g of lipid in meat, fish, and eggs equals 9.50 kCal. In dairy products, the calorific equivalent amounts to 9.25 kCal per gram and in vegetables and fruits, 9.30 kCal. *The average heat of combustion for lipid equals 9.4 kCal per gram.*

Heat of Combustion: Carbohydrate

The heat of combustion for carbohydrate also varies, depending upon the arrangement of atoms in the particular carbohydrate molecule. The heat of combustion for glucose equals 3.74 kCal per gram, whereas larger values result for glycogen (4.19 kCal) and starch (4.20 kCal). *A value of 4.2 kCal generally represents the heat of combustion for one gram of carbohydrate.*

Heat of Combustion: Protein

Two factors affect energy release during combustion of a food's protein component: (1) the type of protein in the food and (2) the relative nitrogen content of the protein. Common proteins in eggs, meat, corn (maize), and beans (jack, lima, navy, soy) contain approximately 16% nitrogen and have corresponding heats of combustion that average 5.75 kCal per gram. Proteins in other foods have a somewhat higher nitrogen content (e.g., most nuts and seeds [18.9%] and whole-kernel wheat, rye, millets, and barley [17.2%]). Other foods contain a slightly lower nitrogen percentage, for example, whole milk (15.7%) and bran (15.8%). *The heat of combustion for protein averages 5.65 kCal per gram.*

Comparing the Energy Value of Macronutrients

The average heats of combustion for the three macronutrients (carbohydrate, 4.2 kCal $\cdot$ g^{-1}; lipid, 9.4 kCal $\cdot$ g^{-1}; protein, 5.65 kCal $\cdot$ g^{-1}) demonstrate that the complete oxidation of lipid in the bomb calorimeter liberates about 65% more energy per gram than protein oxidation and 120% more energy than the oxidation of carbohydrate. Recall from Chapter 1 that lipid molecules contain more hydrogen atoms than either carbohydrate or protein molecules. The common fatty acid palmitic acid, for example, has the structural formula $C_{16}H_{32}O_2$. The ratio of hydrogen atoms to oxygen atoms in fatty acids always exceeds the 2:1 ratio in carbohydrates. Simply stated, lipid molecules have more hydrogen atoms available for cleavage and subsequent oxidation for energy than carbohydrates and proteins.

INTEGRATIVE QUESTION

Respond to a friend who asks: "How can the oxygen required to burn food indicate the number of calories in a meal?"

One can conclude from the above discussion that lipid-rich foods have a higher energy content than relatively fat-free foods. One cup of whole milk, for example, contains 160 kCal, whereas the same quantity of skim milk contains only 90 kCal. If a person who normally consumes 1 quart of whole milk each day switches to skim milk, the total calories ingested each year would decrease by the equivalent of the calories in 25 pounds of body fat. In 3 years, all other things remaining constant, the loss of body fat would approximate 75 pounds! Such a theoretical comparison merits serious consideration because of the almost identical nutrient composition between whole milk and skim milk except for lipid content. Drinking skim rather than whole milk also significantly reduces saturated fatty acid intake (0.4 vs. 5.1 g; 863%) and cholesterol (0.3 vs. 33 mg; 910%).

Net Energy Value of Foods

Differences exist in the energy value of foods when the heat of combustion (gross energy value) determined by direct calorimetry contrasts with the **net energy** available to the body. This pertains particularly to protein because the body cannot oxidize the nitrogen component of this nutrient. In the body, nitrogen atoms combine with hydrogen to form urea (NH_2CONH_2), which the kidneys excrete in the urine. Elimination of hydrogen in this manner represents a loss of

approximately 19% of the protein molecule's potential energy. This hydrogen loss reduces protein's heat of combustion to approximately 4.6 kCal per gram instead of 5.65 kCal per gram released during oxidation in the bomb calorimeter. In contrast, the physiologic fuel values of carbohydrates and lipids (which contain no nitrogen) are *identical* to their heats of combustion in the bomb calorimeter.

Coefficient of Digestibility. The efficiency of the digestive process influences the ultimate energy yield from the food macronutrients. Numerically defined as the **coefficient of digestibility**, digestive efficiency indicates the percentage of ingested food actually digested and absorbed to meet the body's metabolic needs. The food remaining unabsorbed in the intestinal tract is voided in the feces. Dietary fiber reduces the coefficient of digestibility; a high-fiber meal has less total energy absorbed than does a fiber-free meal of equivalent caloric content. This variance occurs because fiber moves food through the intestine more rapidly, reducing time for absorption. Fiber also may cause mechanical erosion of the intestinal mucosa, which is then resynthesized through energy-requiring processes.

TABLE 4.1 shows different digestibility coefficients, heats of combustion, and net energy values for nutrients in the various food groups. *The relative percentage of the macronutrients digested and absorbed averages 97% for carbohydrate, 95% for lipid, and 92% for protein.* Little difference exists in digestive efficiency between obese and lean individuals. However, considerable variability exists in efficiency percentages for any food within a particular category. Proteins in particular have digestive efficiencies ranging from a low of about 78% for protein in legumes to a high of 97% for protein from animal sources. Some advocates promote the use of vegetables in weight-loss diets because of plant protein's relatively low coefficient of digestibility. From the data in Table 4.1, one can round the average net energy values to whole numbers referred to as **Atwater general factors**. Named for Wilbur Olin Atwater (1844–1907), the 19th-century chemist who pioneered human nutrition and energy balance studies at Wesleyan College, these values indicate the net metabolizable energy available to the body from ingested foods. If precise energy values for experimental or therapeutic diets are not required, the Atwater general factors provide a good estimate of the energy content of the daily diet (see "In a Practical Sense"). For alcohol, 7 kCal (29.4 kJ) represents each g (mL) of pure (200-proof) alcohol ingested. In terms of potential energy available to the body, alcohol's efficiency of use equals that of other carbohydrates.

ATWATER GENERAL FACTORS

- 4 kCal per gram for dietary carbohydrate
- 9 kCal per gram for dietary lipid
- 4 kCal per gram for dietary protein

TABLE 4.1 ■ FACTORS FOR DIGESTIBILITY, HEATS OF COMBUSTION, AND NET PHYSIOLOGIC ENERGY VALUES[a] OF PROTEIN, LIPID, AND CARBOHYDRATE

FOOD GROUP	DIGESTIBILITY (%)	HEAT OF COMBUSTION (kCal·g^{-1})	NET ENERGY (kCal·g^{-1})
Protein			
Animal food	97	5.65	4.27
Meats, fish	97	5.65	4.27
Eggs	97	5.75	4.37
Dairy products	97	5.65	4.27
Vegetable food	85	5.65	3.74
Cereals	85	5.80	3.87
Legumes	78	5.70	3.47
Vegetables	83	5.00	3.11
Fruits	85	5.20	3.36
Average protein	92	5.65	4.05
Lipid			
Meat and eggs	95	9.50	9.03
Dairy products	95	9.25	8.79
Animal food	95	9.40	8.93
Vegetable food	90	9.30	8.37
Average lipid	95	9.40	8.93
Carbohydrate			
Animal food	98	3.90	3.82
Cereals	98	4.20	4.11
Legumes	97	4.20	4.07
Vegetables	95	4.20	3.99
Fruits	90	4.00	3.60
Sugars	98	3.95	3.87
Vegetable food	97	4.15	4.03
Average carbohydrate	97	4.15	4.03

From Merrill AL, Watt BK. Energy values of foods: basis and derivation. Agricultural Handbook no. 74, Washington, DC: USDA, 1973.
[a] Net physiologic energy values are computed as the coefficient of digestibility times the heat of combustion adjusted for energy loss in urine.

Use of Tabled Values

Computing the kCal content of foods requires considerable time and labor. Various governmental agencies in the United States and elsewhere have evaluated and compiled nutritive values for thousands of foods. The most comprehensive data bank resources include the United States Nutrient Data Bank (USNDB; www.nal.usda.gov/fnic/foodcomp/), maintained by the U.S. Department of Agriculture's Consumer Nutrition Center, and a computerized data bank maintained by the Bureau of Nutritional Sciences of Health and Welfare Canada. Appendix B (available on Student CD or online at http://connection.lww.com/mkk6e) presents the energy and nutritive values for common foods and lists resources for finding values of specialty and fast-food items.

A brief review of Appendix B indicates that large differences exist between the energy values of various foods. Consuming an equal number of calories from different foods often requires a tremendous intake of a particular food or relatively little of another. For example, to consume 100 kCal from each of six common foods—carrots, celery, green peppers, grapefruit, medium-sized eggs, and mayonnaise—one must eat 5 carrots, 20 stalks of celery, 6.5 green peppers, 1 large grapefruit, 1 1/4 eggs, but only 1 tablespoon of mayonnaise. Consequently, a typical sedentary adult female who expends 2100 kCal each day must consume about 420 celery stalks, 105 carrots, 136 green peppers, 26 eggs, yet only 1 1/2 cup of mayonnaise or 8 oz of salad oil to meet daily energy needs. These examples illustrate dramatically that foods high in lipid content contain considerably more calories than foods low in lipid and correspondingly higher in water content.

IN A PRACTICAL SENSE

DETERMINING A FOOD'S MACRONUTRIENT COMPOSITION AND ENERGY CONTRIBUTION

■ Food labels must indicate a food's macronutrient content (g) and total calories (kCal). Knowing the energy value per gram for carbohydrate, lipid, and protein in a food allows one to readily compute the percentage kCal derived from each macronutrient. The net energy value, referred to as Atwater general factors, equals 4 kCal for carbohydrate, 9 kCal for lipid, and 4 kcal for protein.

CALCULATIONS

The table shows the macronutrient composition for one large serving of McDonald's French fries (weight, 122.3 g [4.3 oz]). [*Note:* McDonald's publishes the weight of each of the macronutrients for one serving along with the total kCal value.]

1. Calculate kCal value of each macronutrient (column 4).
   Multiply the weight of each nutrient (column 2) by the appropriate Atwater general factor (column 3).
2. Calculate percentage weight of each nutrient (column 5).
   Divide weight of each macronutrient (column 2) by the food's total weight.

3. Calculate percentage kCal for each macronutrient (column 6).
   Divide kCal value of each macronutrient (column 4) by food's total kCal value.

LEARN TO READ FOOD LABELS

Computing the percentage weight and kCal of each macronutrient in a food promotes wise decisions in choosing foods. Manufacturers must state the absolute and percentage weights for each macronutrient, but computing their absolute and percentage energy contributions completes the more important picture. In the example for French fries, lipid represents only 17% of the food's total weight. However, the percentage of total calories from lipid jumps to 48.3%, or about 195 kCal of this food's 402 kCal energy content. This information becomes crucial for those interested in maintaining a low-fat diet.

Similar computations can estimate the caloric value of any food serving. Of course, increasing or decreasing portion sizes, adding lipid-rich sauces or creams, or using fruits or calorie-free substitutes affects the caloric content accordingly.

MACRONUTRIENT ENERGY CONTENT AND PERCENTAGE COMPOSITION OF McDONALD'S FRENCH FRIES, LARGE (TOTAL WEIGHT, 122.3 G [4.3 OZ])

(1) NUTRIENT	(2) WEIGHT	(3) ATWATER GENERAL FACTOR	(4) KCAL	(5) % OF WEIGHT	(6) % OF KCAL
Protein	6	4 kCal·g^{-1}	24	4.9	6.0
Carbohydrate	45.9	4 kCal·g^{-1}	183.6	37.5	45.7
Lipid	21.6	9 kCal·g^{-1}	194.4	17.7	48.3
Ash	3.2		0	2.6	0
Water	45.6		0	37.3	0
Total	122.3		402	100	100

OBESITY-RELATED THERMOGENIC RESPONSE

Segal KR, Gutin B. Thermic effects of food and exercise in lean and obese women. Metabolism 1983;32:581.

▲ Considerable research links obesity and impaired thermogenesis—a diminished capacity to increase metabolism in response to different stimuli. These studies note a lower rise in metabolism for obese individuals than for lean individuals after ingestion of a meal, exposure to cold, infusion of noradrenaline, or the combination of eating and exercising. A diminished thermogenic response probably plays an accessory role in total energy conservation, contributing to the onset and persistence of obesity.

The research of Segal and Gutin evaluated the thermogenic difference between overfat (obese) and lean women in response to food intake, two levels of exercise, and the possible potentiation of the thermic effect of food with physical activity. Subjects included 10 obese (%fat, 37; body mass, 77.9 kg) and 10 lean (%fat, 18.8; body mass, 53.2 kg) women, measured under six different conditions: *(a)* resting metabolism ($\dot{V}O_2$) for 4 hours; *(b)* $\dot{V}O_2$ for 4 hours following consumption of a 910-kCal meal (14% protein, 46% carbohydrate, 40% lipid); *(c)* $\dot{V}O_2$ during exercise at a constant submaximal intensity of 300 kg-m · min^{-1} (cycling for 5 min every 0.5 h for 4 h); *(d)* $\dot{V}O_2$ during exercise at an intensity equal to the subject's lactate threshold (cycling for 5 min every 0.5 h for

4 h); and *(e)* and *(f)* same as protocols c and d, except the subjects consumed the test meal before exercising.

The figure indicates that consumption of the 910-kCal meal increased exercise $\dot{V}O_2$ more for the lean than for the obese women. Stated somewhat differently, a greater difference emerged between the fed and fasting conditions for the lean group at both exercise intensities. The postprandial exercise $\dot{V}O_2$ for the lean group also remained elevated above the corresponding fasting value at the end of the 4 hours, while for the obese group, the postprandial value at 4 hours equaled their fasting exercise metabolism. Thus, using a 4-hour measurement underestimated the total amount that eating augmented energy expenditure during exercise for the lean women. These subjects exhibited a larger thermic effect of food during exercise than during rest. Obese subjects, on the other hand, showed similar thermic effects of food for exercise and rest conditions, with no thermogenic bonus from exercise after eating.

The researchers concluded that exercise significantly potentiated the thermic effect of food for lean but not for obese women. The large differences in response to the combination of food and subsequent exercise emerged despite similar thermogenic responses of the lean and obese women to food alone and exercise alone. Therefore, the cumulative effect of a lower metabolic rate of the obese (compared with lean subjects) during exercise that follows eating favors energy conservation rather than energy dissipation.

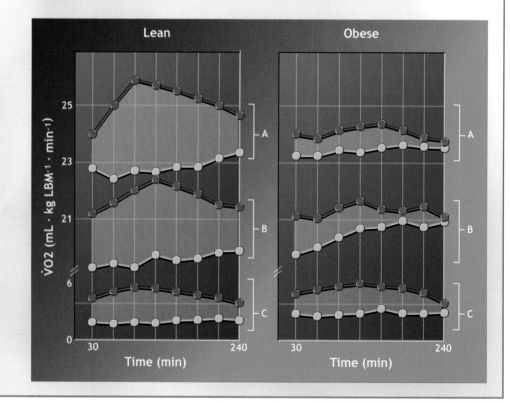

Effects of exercise and a 910-kCal meal on metabolic rates of lean and obese men and women. *A.* Exercise at lactate threshold; *(B)* exercise at 300 kg-m·min^{-1}; and *(C)* rest. *Red circles* represent postprandial (after the meal) data; *yellow circles* represent postabsorptive (after fasting) data. The *shaded areas* indicate the thermic effect of food under each condition.

INTEGRATIVE QUESTION

What factors account for a discrepancy between computations of the energy value of daily food intake using the Atwater general factors and direct measurement by bomb calorimetry?

Also note that a calorie reflects the food energy *regardless* of the food source. Thus, from an energy standpoint, 100 calories from mayonnaise equals the same 100 calories in 20 celery stalks. The more a person eats of any food, the more calories the person consumes. However, a small amount of fatty food represents a considerable number of calories; thus, the term *fattening* often describes these foods. An individual's caloric intake equals the sum of *all* energy consumed from either small or large quantities of foods. Celery would become a fattening food if consumed in excess!

Summary

1. A calorie or kilocalorie (kCal) is a measure of heat to express a food's energy value.
2. Burning food in the bomb calorimeter permits direct quantification of the food's energy content.
3. The heat of combustion quantifies the amount of heat liberated in the complete oxidation of a food. Average gross energy values equal 4.2 kCal per gram for carbohydrate, 9.4 kCal per gram for lipid, and 5.65 kCal per gram for protein.
4. The coefficient of digestibility represents the proportion of food consumed actually digested and absorbed.
5. Coefficients of digestibility average 97% for carbohydrates, 95% for lipids, and 92% for proteins. Thus, the net energy values equal 4 kCal per gram of carbohydrate, 9 kCal per gram of lipid, and 4 kCal per gram of protein. These values, known as Atwater general factors, provide an accurate estimate of the net energy value of typical foods a person consumes.
6. The Atwater calorific values allow one to compute the energy (caloric) content of any meal from the carbohydrate, lipid, and protein compositions of the food.
7. Calories represent heat energy regardless of the food source. From an energy standpoint, 500 kCal of peppermint ice cream topped with whipped cream and Brazil nuts is no more fattening than 500 kCal of watermelon, 500 kCal of cheese and pepperoni pizza, or 500 kCal of an egg bagel topped with salmon, onions, and sour cream.

Suggested Readings are available on the Student CD and online at http://connection.lww.com/mkk6e.

Introduction to Energy Transfer

5

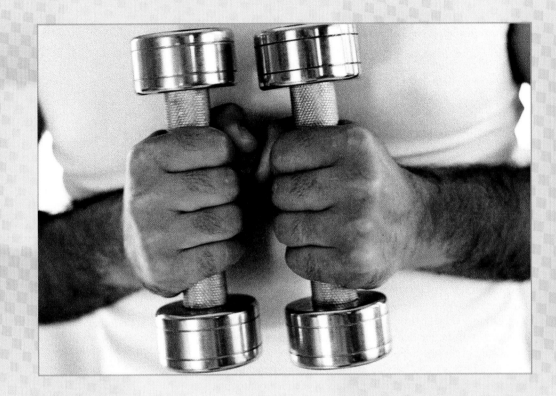

CHAPTER OBJECTIVES

- Describe the first law of thermodynamics related to energy balance and work within biologic systems

- Define potential energy and kinetic energy and give examples of each

- Discuss the role of free energy in biologic work

- Give examples of exergonic and endergonic chemical reactions within the body and indicate their importance

- State the second law of thermodynamics and give a practical application of this law

- Discuss the role of coupled reactions in biologic processes within the body

- Differentiate between photosynthesis and respiration and give the biologic significance of each

- Identify and give examples of the three forms of biologic work

- Describe how enzymes and coenzymes affect energy metabolism

- Differentiate between hydrolysis and condensation and explain their importance in physiologic function

- Discuss the role of redox chemical reactions in energy metabolism

Bioenergetics refers to the flow of energy within a living system. The capacity to extract energy from food macronutrients and continually transfer it at a high rate to the contractile elements of skeletal muscle determines one's capacity for swimming, running, or skiing long distances. Likewise, specific energy-transferring capacities that demand all-out, "explosive" power output for brief durations determine success in weight lifting, sprinting, jumping, and football line play. Although muscular activity represents the main frame of reference in this text, *all* forms of biologic work require power generated from the direct transfer of chemical energy.

The sections that follow introduce general concepts about bioenergetics. They provide the basis for understanding energy metabolism during physical activity.

ENERGY—THE CAPACITY FOR WORK

Extracting energy from the stored macronutrients and transferring it to the contractile proteins of skeletal muscle greatly influence exercise performance. But unlike the physical properties of matter, one cannot define energy in concrete terms of size, shape, or mass. Rather the term *energy* reflects a dynamic state related to change; thus, energy emerges only when a change occurs. Within this context, energy relates to the performance of work—as work increases so also does energy transfer, thus producing a change.

The **first law of thermodynamics** describes an immutable principle related to biologic work. The basic tenet states that energy cannot be created or destroyed but, instead, transforms from one form to another without being depleted. In essence, this law describes the important **conservation of energy principle** that applies to both living and nonliving systems. In the body, chemical energy within the bonds of the macronutrients does not immediately dissipate as heat during energy metabolism; instead, a large portion remains as chemical energy, which the musculoskeletal system then changes into mechanical energy (and ultimately to heat energy). *The first law of thermodynamics dictates that the body does not produce, consume, or use up energy; instead it transforms it from one state into another as physiologic systems undergo continual change.*

 INTEGRATIVE QUESTION

Based on the first law of thermodynamics, why is it imprecise to refer to energy "production" in the body?

Potential and Kinetic Energy

Potential energy and **kinetic energy** *constitute the total energy of a system.* FIGURE 5.1 shows potential energy as energy of position, similar to a boulder tottering atop a cliff or water before it flows downstream. In the example of flowing water, the energy change is proportional to the water's vertical drop—the greater the vertical drop, the greater the potential energy at the top. The waterwheel harnesses a portion of the energy from the falling water to produce useful work. In the

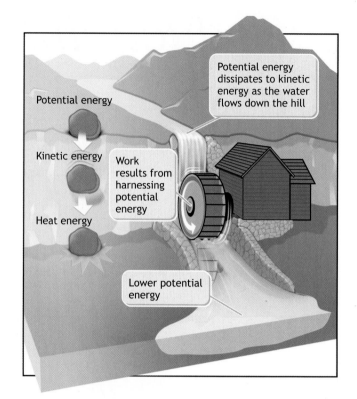

Figure 5.1   High-grade potential energy capable of performing work degrades to a useless form of kinetic energy. In the example of falling water, the water wheel harnesses potential energy to perform useful work. For the falling boulder, all of the potential energy dissipates to kinetic energy (heat) as the boulder crashes to the surface below.

case of the falling boulder, *all* potential energy transforms to kinetic energy and dissipates as unusable heat.

Other examples of potential energy include bound energy within the internal structure of a battery, a stick of dynamite, or a macronutrient before releasing its stored energy in metabolism. *Releasing potential energy transforms it into kinetic energy of motion.* In some cases, bound energy in one substance directly transfers to other substances to increase their potential energy. Energy transfers of this type provide the necessary energy for the body's chemical work of **biosynthesis**. In this process, specific building-block atoms of carbon, hydrogen, oxygen, and nitrogen become activated and join other atoms and molecules to synthesize important biologic compounds and tissues. Some newly created compounds provide structure as in bone or the lipid-containing plasma membrane that encloses each cell. Other synthesized compounds such as adenosine triphosphate (ATP) and phosphocreatine (PCr) serve the cell's energy requirements.

Energy-Releasing and Energy-Conserving Processes

The term **exergonic** describes any physical or chemical process that releases (frees) energy to its surroundings. Such reactions represent "downhill" processes because of a decline in free energy—"useful" energy for biologic work that encompasses all of the cell's energy-requiring, life-sustaining processes. Within a cell, where pressure and volume remain relatively stable, free energy (denoted by the symbol G to honor Willard Gibbs [1839–1903], whose research provided the foundation of biochemical thermodynamics) equals the potential energy within a molecule's chemical bonds (called *enthalpy* or H) minus the energy unavailable because of randomness (S), times the absolute temperature (°C + 273). The equation $G = H - TS$ describes free energy quantitatively.

Chemical reactions that store or absorb energy are **endergonic**; these reactions represent "uphill" processes and proceed with an increase in free energy for biologic work. Exergonic processes sometimes link or *couple* with endergonic reactions to transfer some energy to the endergonic process. In the body, such coupled reactions conserve in usable form a large portion of the chemical energy stored within the macronutrients.

FIGURE 5.2 illustrates the flow of energy in exergonic and endergonic chemical reactions. Changes in free energy occur when the bonds in the reactant molecules form new product molecules with different bonding. The equation that expresses these changes, under conditions of constant temperature, pressure, and volume, takes the following form:

$$\Delta G = \Delta H - T\Delta S$$

The symbol Δ designates change. The change in free energy represents a keystone of chemical reactions. In exergonic reactions, ΔG is negative; the products contain *less* free energy than the reactants, with the energy differential released as heat. For example, the union of hydrogen and oxygen to form water releases 68 kCal per mole (molecular weight of a substance in grams) of free energy in the following reaction:

$$H_2 + O \rightarrow H_2O - \Delta G\ 68\ kCal \cdot mole^{-1}$$

In the reverse endergonic reaction, ΔG is positive because the product contains *more* free energy than the reactants. The infusion of 68 kCal of energy per mole of water causes the chemical bonds of the water molecule to split apart, freeing the original hydrogen and oxygen atoms. This "uphill" process of energy transfer provides the hydrogen and oxygen atoms with their original energy content to satisfy the principle of the first law of thermodynamics—the conservation of energy.

$$H_2 + O \leftarrow H_2O^+ + \Delta G\ 68\ kCal \cdot mole^{-1}$$

Energy transfer in cells follows the same principles as those in the waterfall–waterwheel example. Carbohydrate, lipid, and protein macronutrients possess considerable potential energy. The formation of product substances progressively reduces the nutrient molecule's original potential energy with a corresponding increase in kinetic energy. Enzyme-regulated transfer systems harness or conserve a portion of this chemical energy in new compounds for use in biologic work. In essence, living cells serve as transducers with the capacity to extract and use chemical energy stored within a compound's atomic structure. Conversely, and equally important, cells also bond atoms and molecules together, raising them to a higher level of potential energy.

The transfer of potential energy in any spontaneous process always proceeds in a direction that *decreases* the capacity to perform work. The tendency of potential energy to degrade to kinetic energy of motion with a lower capacity for work (i.e., increased **entropy**) reflects the **second law of thermodynamics**. A flashlight battery provides a good illustration. The electrochemical energy stored within its cells slowly dissipates, even if the battery remains unused. The energy from sunlight also continually degrades to heat energy when light strikes and becomes absorbed by a surface. Food and other chemicals represent excellent stores of potential energy, yet this energy continually decreases as the compounds decompose through normal oxidative processes. Energy, like water, always runs downhill so potential energy decreases. *Ultimately, all of the potential energy in a system degrades to the unusable form of kinetic or heat energy.*

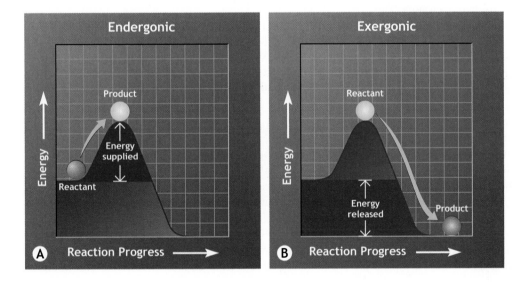

Figure 5.2 Energy flow in chemical reactions. **A.** Energy supply prepares an endergonic reaction to proceed because the reaction's product contains *more* energy than the reactant. **B.** Exergonic reaction releases energy, resulting in *less* energy in the product than in the reactant.

INTERCONVERSIONS OF ENERGY

The total energy in an isolated system remains constant, so a decrease in one form of energy matches an equivalent increase in another form. During energy conversions, a loss of potential energy from one source often produces a temporary increase in the potential energy of another source. In this way, nature harnesses vast quantities of potential energy for useful purposes. But even under such favorable conditions, the net flow of energy in the biologic world moves toward entropy, ultimately producing a loss of potential energy.

In 1877, Austrian physicist Ludwig Boltzmann (1844–1906) established the relationship between entropy and the statistical analysis of molecular motion. Entropy reflects the continual process of energy change. All chemical and physical processes proceed in a direction in which total randomness or disorder *increases* and the energy available for work *decreases*. In coupled reactions during biosynthesis, part of a system may show a decrease in entropy while another part shows an increase. However, no way exists to circumvent the second law—the entire system always shows a net increase in entropy. In a more global sense, the biochemical reactions within the body's trillions of cells (as within the universe as a whole) "tilt" in the direction of spontaneity that favors disorder and randomness of an irreversible process (i.e., entropy) as originally theorized by Boltzmann.

Forms of Energy

FIGURE 5.3 shows energy categorized into one of six forms: chemical, mechanical, heat, light, electric, and nuclear.

Examples of Energy Conversions

The conversion of energy from one form to another occurs readily in the inanimate and animate worlds. **Photosynthesis** and **respiration** represent the most fundamental examples of energy conversion in living cells.

Photosynthesis. In the sun, where effective temperature averages 5800° Kelvin, nuclear fusion releases part of the potential energy stored in the nucleus of the hydrogen atom. This energy, in the form of gamma radiation, then converts to radiant energy.

FIGURE 5.4 depicts the dynamics of photosynthesis, an endergonic process powered by energy from sunlight. The pigment chlorophyll, contained in large chloroplast organelles within the leaf's cells, absorbs radiant (solar) energy to synthesize glucose from carbon dioxide and water, while oxygen flows to the environment. The plant also converts carbohydrates to lipids and proteins for storage as a future reserve for energy and growth. Animals then ingest plant nutrients to serve their own energy and growth needs. *In essence, solar energy coupled with photosynthesis powers the animal world with food and oxygen.*

Respiration. FIGURE 5.5 shows that the exergonic reactions of respiration are the reverse of photosynthesis, as the plant's

stored energy is recovered for biologic work. In the presence of oxygen, the cells extract the chemical energy stored in the carbohydrate, lipid, and protein molecules. For glucose, respiration releases 689 kCal per mole (180 g) oxidized. *A portion of the energy released during cellular respiration becomes conserved in other chemical compounds for use in energy-requiring processes; the remaining energy flows to the environment as heat.*

INTEGRATIVE QUESTION

From the perspective of human bioenergetics, discuss the significance of a bumper sticker that reads: "Have you thanked a green plant today?"

BIOLOGIC WORK IN HUMANS

Figure 5.5 also illustrates that biologic work takes one of three forms:

- **Mechanical work** of muscle contraction
- **Chemical work** that synthesizes cellular molecules
- **Transport work** that concentrates substances in the intracellular and extracellular fluids

Mechanical Work

Mechanical work generated by muscle contraction and subsequent movement provides the most obvious example of energy transformation. The molecular motors in a muscle fiber's protein filaments directly convert chemical energy into mechanical energy. This does not represent the body's only form of mechanical work. In the cell nucleus, for example, contractile elements literally tug at the chromosomes to facilitate cell division. Specialized structures (such as cilia) also perform mechanical work in many cells. The "In a Practical Sense" article located on p. 128 shows the method for quantifying work (and power) on three common exercise modes.

Chemical Work

All cells perform chemical work for maintenance and growth. Continuous synthesis of cellular components takes place as other components break down. The extreme muscle tissue synthesis that occurs in response to chronic overload in resistance training vividly illustrates chemical work.

Transport Work

The biologic work of concentrating substances in the body (transport work) progresses much less conspicuously than mechanical or chemical work. Cellular materials normally flow from an area of high concentration to one of lower concentration. This passive process of **diffusion** does not require energy. For proper physiologic functioning, certain chemicals require transport "uphill" against their normal concentration gradients from an area of lower to one of higher

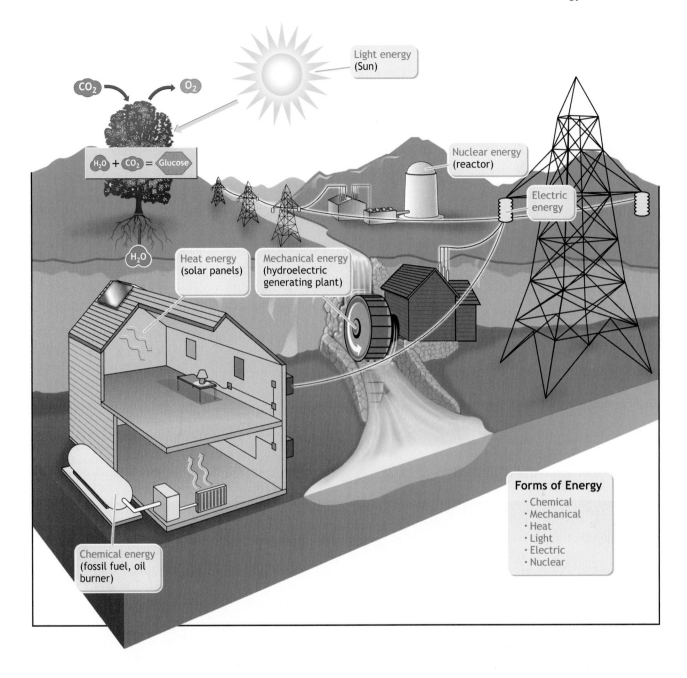

Figure 5.3 Interconversions of six forms of energy.

concentration. **Active transport** describes this energy-requiring process. Secretion and reabsorption in the kidney tubules rely on active transport mechanisms, as does neural tissue to establish the proper electrochemical gradients about its plasma membranes. These "quiet" forms of biologic work require a continual expenditure of stored chemical energy.

FACTORS THAT AFFECT THE RATE OF BIOENERGETICS

The upper limits of exercise intensity ultimately depend on the rate that cells extract, conserve, and transfer chemical energy in the food nutrients to the contractile filaments of skeletal

muscle. *The sustained pace of the marathon runner at close to 90% of maximum aerobic capacity, or the rapid speed achieved by the sprinter in all-out exercise, directly reflects the body's capacity to transfer chemical energy into mechanical work.* Enzymes and coenzymes significantly alter the rate of energy release during chemical reactions.

Enzymes as Biologic Catalysts

*An **enzyme**, a highly specific and large protein catalyst, accelerates the forward and reverse rates of chemical reactions without being consumed or changed in the reaction.* Enzymes only govern reactions that would normally take

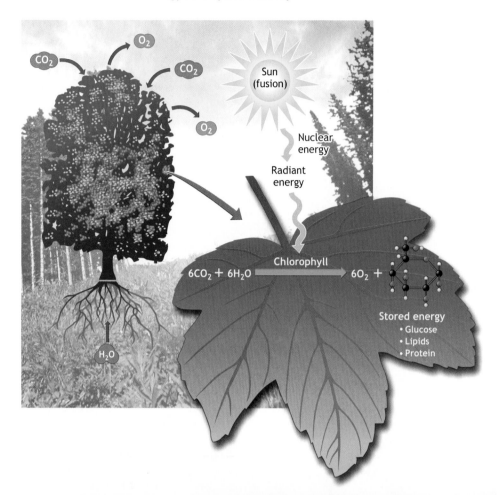

Figure 5.4   The endergonic process of photosynthesis in plants, algae, and some bacteria serves as the mechanism to synthesize carbohydrates, lipids, and proteins. In this example, a glucose molecule forms when carbon dioxide binds with water with a positive free energy (useful energy) change ($+\Delta G$).

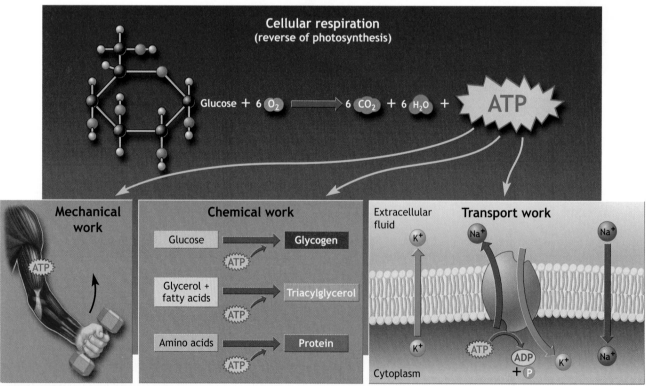

Figure 5.5   The exergonic process of cellular respiration. Exergonic reactions, such as the burning of gasoline or the oxidation of glucose, release potential energy. This produces a negative standard free energy change (i.e., reduction in total energy available for work or $-\Delta G$). In this illustration, cellular respiration harvests the potential energy in food to form ATP. Subsequently, the energy in ATP powers all forms of biologic work.

place but at a much slower rate. In a way, enzymes reduce the required **activation energy**—the energy input to initiate a reaction—so its rate changes. Enzyme action takes place without altering the equilibrium constants and total energy released (free energy change or ΔG) in the reaction. FIGURE 5.6 contrasts the effectiveness of a catalyst in initiating a chemical reaction with initiation in the uncatalyzed state. The vertical axis represents the energy required to activate each reaction; the horizontal axis plots the reaction's progress. Clearly, initiation (activation) of an uncatalyzed reaction requires considerably more energy than a catalyzed one. The rate of a catalyzed reaction can be 10^6 to 10^{20} times faster than the uncatalyzed reaction under similar conditions. Biochemists estimate that without enzyme action, the complete digestion of a breakfast meal might take 50 years!

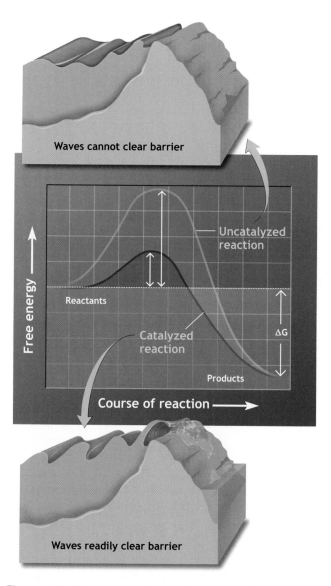

Figure 5.6 The presence of a catalyst greatly reduces the activation energy to initiate a chemical reaction compared with the energy for an uncatalyzed reaction. For the uncatalyzed reaction to proceed, the reactant must have a higher free uncatalyzed energy level than the product.

In its simplest form, an enzyme-catalyzed reaction occurs when a single reactant converts to a single product. The reaction proceeds in one direction so that all substrate (substance acted upon by an enzyme) molecules convert into product molecules. Most enzyme-catalyzed reactions proceed in discrete steps. The enzyme first combines with its substrate to form an enzyme–substrate complex. This complex then converts to an enzyme–intermediate complex, which then changes to an enzyme–product complex that quickly dissociates into free product with the enzyme released unchanged.

Enzymes possess the unique property of not being readily altered by the reactions they affect. Consequently, enzyme turnover in the body remains relatively slow, and the specific enzymes are continually reused. A typical mitochondrion may contain up to 10 billion enzyme molecules, each carrying out millions of operations within a brief time. During all-out exercise, the rate of enzyme activity increases tremendously, as energy demands increase some 100 times above the resting level. A single cell contains thousands of different enzymes, each with a specific function that catalyzes a distinct cellular reaction. For example, glucose breakdown to carbon dioxide and water requires 19 different chemical reactions, each catalyzed by its own specific enzyme. Enzymes contact precise locations on the surfaces of cell structures; they also operate within the structure itself. Many enzymes operate outside the cell—in the bloodstream, digestive mixture, or intestinal fluids.

Except for older enzyme names such as renin, trypsin, and pepsin, the suffix -*ase* appends to the enzyme based on its mode of operation or substance with which it interacts. For example, hydro*lase* adds water during hydrolysis reactions, prote*ase* interacts with protein, oxid*ase* adds oxygen to a substance, isomer*ase* rearranges atoms within a substrate to form structural isomers such as glucose and fructose, and ribonucle*ase* splits apart ribonucleic acid (RNA).

Reaction Rates

Enzymes do not all operate at the same rate; some operate slowly, others much more rapidly. Consider the enzyme carbonic anhydrase, which catalyzes the hydration of carbon dioxide to form carbonic acid. Its maximum **turnover number**—number of moles of substrate that react to form product per mole of enzyme per unit time—is 800,000. On the other hand, the turnover number is only 2 for tryptophan synthetase, which catalyzes the final step in tryptophan synthesis. Enzymes often work cooperatively among their binding sites. While one substance "turns on" at a particular site, its neighbor "turns off" until the process completes. The operation then can reverse, with one enzyme becoming inactive and the other active. Enzymes also act along small regions of the substrate, each time working at a different rate than previously. Some enzymes delay initiating their work. The precursor digestive enzyme trypsinogen, manufactured by the pancreas in inactive form, serves as a good example. Trypsinogen enters the small intestine where, upon activation by intestinal enzyme action, it becomes the active enzyme trypsin to digest complex proteins

IN A PRACTICAL SENSE

MEASUREMENT OF WORK ON A TREADMILL, CYCLE ERGOMETER, AND STEP BENCH

■ An ergometer is an exercise apparatus that quantifies and standardizes physical exercise in terms of work and/or power output. The most common ergometers include treadmills, cycle and arm-crank ergometers, stair steppers, and rowers.

Work (W) represents application of force (F) through a distance (D):

$$W = F \times D$$

For example, for a body mass of 70 kg and vertical jump score of 0.5 m, work accomplished equals 35 kilogram-meters (70 kg × 0.5 m). The most common units of measurement to express work include kilogram-meters (kg-m), foot-pounds (ft-lb), joules (J), Newton-meters (Nm), and kilocalories (kCal).

Power (P) represents W performed per unit time (T):

$$P = F \times D \div T$$

CALCULATION OF TREADMILL WORK

Consider the treadmill as a moving conveyor belt with variable angle of incline and speed. Work performed on a treadmill equals the product of the weight (mass) of the person *(F)* and the vertical distance *(vert dist)* the person achieves walking or running up the incline. Vert dist equals the sine of the treadmill angle (theta or θ) multiplied by the distance traveled *(D)* along the incline (treadmill speed × time).

$$W = \text{body mass (force)} \times \text{vertical distance}$$

EXAMPLE

For an angle θ of 8° (measured with an inclinometer or determined by knowing the percent grade of the treadmill), the sine of angle θ equals 0.1392 (see table). The *vert dist* represents treadmill speed multiplied by exercise duration multiplied by sine θ. For example, *vert dist* on the incline while walking at 5000 m·h^{-1} for 1 hour equals 696 m (5000 ×

0.1392). If a person with a body mass of 50 kg walked on a treadmill at an incline of 8° (grade approximately 14%) for 60 minutes at 5000 m · h^{-1}, work accomplished computes as:

$$W = F \times \text{vert dist (sine } \theta \times D)$$
$$= 50 \text{ kg} \times (0.1392 \times 5000 \text{ m})$$
$$= \textbf{34,800 kg-m}$$

The value for power equals 34,800 kg-m ÷ 60 minutes or 580 kg-m·min^{-1}.

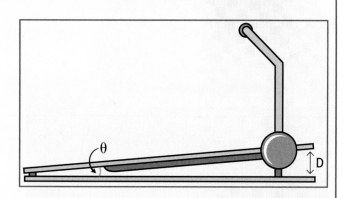

Angle (°)	Sine θ	Grade (%)
1	0.0175	1.75
2	0.0349	3.49
3	0.0523	5.23
4	0.0698	6.98
5	0.0872	8.72
6	0.1045	10.51
7	0.1219	12.28
8	0.1392	14.05
9	0.1564	15.84
10	0.1736	17.63
15	0.2588	26.80
20	0.3420	36.40

CALCULATION OF CYCLE ERGOMETER WORK

The mechanically braked cycle ergometer contains a flywheel with a belt around it connected by a small spring at one end and an adjustable tension lever at the other end. A pendulum balance indicates the resistance against the flywheel as it turns. Increasing the tension on the belt increases

continued on page 129

Continued

flywheel friction, which increases resistance to pedaling. The force (flywheel friction) represents braking load in kg or kilopounds (kp = force acting on 1-kg mass at the normal acceleration of gravity). The distance traveled equals number of pedal revolutions times flywheel circumference.

EXAMPLE

A person pedaling a bicycle ergometer with a 6-m flywheel circumference at 60 rpm for 1 minute covers a distance (D) of 360 m each minute (6 m × 60). If the frictional resistance on the flywheel equals 2.5 kg, total work computes as

$$W = F \times D$$
$$= \text{frictional resistance} \times \text{distance traveled}$$
$$= 2.5 \text{ kg} \times 360 \text{ m}$$
$$= 900 \text{ kg-m}$$

Power generated by the effort equals 900 kg-m in 1 minute or 900 kg-m·min^{-1} (900 kg-m ÷ 1 min).

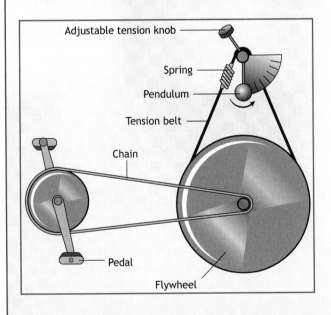

CALCULATION OF WORK DURING BENCH STEPPING

Only the vertical (positive) work can be calculated in bench stepping. Distance (D) computes as bench height times the number of times the person steps; force (F) equals the person's body mass (kg).

EXAMPLE

If a 70-kg person steps on a bench 0.375-m high at a rate of 30 steps per minute for 10 minutes, total work computes as:

$$W = F \times D$$
$$= \text{body mass, kg} \times (\text{vertical distance [m]} \times \text{steps per min} \times 10 \text{ min})$$
$$= 70 \text{ kg} \times (0.375 \text{ m} \times 30 \times 10)$$
$$= 7875 \text{ kg-m}$$

Power generated during stepping equals 787 kg-m·min^{-1} (7875 kg-m ÷ 10 min).

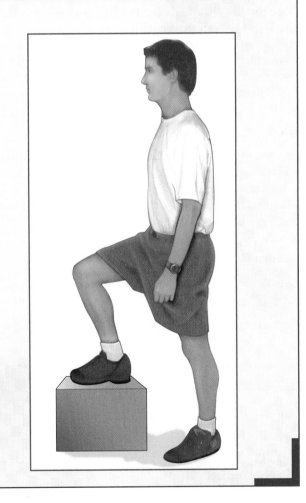

into simple amino acids. **Proteolytic action** describes this catabolic process. Without the delay in activity, trypsinogen would literally digest the pancreatic tissue that produced it.

FIGURE 5.7 shows that pH and temperature dramatically alter enzyme activity. For some enzymes, peak activity requires relatively high acidity, while others function optimally on the alkaline side of neutrality. Note that the two enzymes pepsin and trypsin exhibit different pH profiles that modify their activity rates and determine optimal function. Pepsin operates optimally at a pH between 2.4 and 2.6,

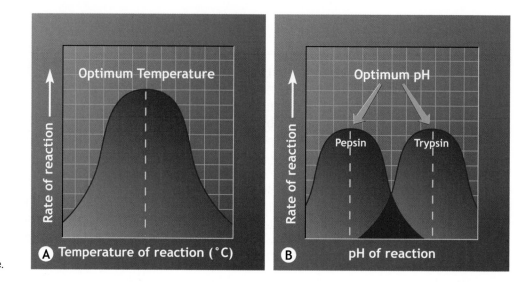

Figure 5.7 Effects of (**A**) temperature and (**B**) pH on the enzyme action turnover rate.

whereas trypsin's optimum range is close to that of saliva and milk (6.2 to 6.6). This pH effect on enzyme dynamics takes place because changing a fluid's hydrogen ion concentration alters the balance between positively and negatively charged complexes in the enzyme's amino acids. Increases in temperature generally accelerate enzyme reactivity. As temperature rises above 40 to 50°C, however, the protein enzymes permanently denature, and their activity ceases.

Mode of Action

Interaction with its specific substrate represents a unique characteristic of an enzyme's three-dimensional globular protein structure. Interaction works like a key fitting a lock as illustrated in FIGURE 5.8. The enzyme turns on when its **active**

site (usually a groove, cleft, or cavity on the protein's surface) joins in a "perfect fit" with the substrate's active site. Upon forming an **enzyme–substrate complex**, the splitting of chemical bonds forms a new product with new bonds. This frees the enzyme to act on additional substrate. The example depicts the interaction sequence of the enzyme maltase as it disassembles (hydrolyzes) maltose into its component two glucose building blocks:

Step 1: The active site of the enzyme and substrate line up to achieve a perfect fit, forming an enzyme–substrate complex.

Step 2: The enzyme catalyzes (greatly speeds up) the chemical reaction with the substrate. Note that the hydrolysis reaction adds a water molecule.

Step 3: An end-product forms (two glucose molecules) releasing the enzyme to act on another substrate.

First proposed in the early 1890s by the German chemist and Nobel laureate Emil Fischer (1852–1919), a "**lock and key mechanism**" describes the enzyme–substrate interaction. This process ensures that the correct enzyme "mates" with its specific substrate to perform a particular function. Once the enzyme and substrate join, a conformational change in enzyme shape takes place as it molds to the substrate. Even if an enzyme links with a substrate, unless the specific conformational change occurs in the enzyme's shape, it will not interact chemically with the substrate. A more contemporary hypothesis considers the lock and key more of an "induced fit" because of the required conformational characteristics of enzymes.

The lock-and-key mechanism serves a protective function so only the correct enzyme activates a given substrate. Consider the enzyme hexokinase, which accelerates a chemical reaction by linking with a glucose molecule. When this occurs, a phosphate molecule transfers from ATP to a specific binding site on one of glucose's carbon atoms. Once the two binding sites join to form a glucose–hexokinase complex, the substrate begins its stepwise degradation (controlled by other specific enzymes) to form less complex molecules during energy metabolism.

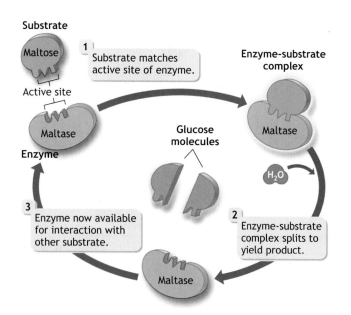

Figure 5.8 Sequence of steps in the "lock and key" mechanism of an enzyme with its substrate. The example shows how two monosaccharide glucose molecules form when maltase interacts with its disaccharide substrate maltose.

Coenzymes

Some enzymes remain totally dormant unless activated by additional substances termed **coenzymes**. These nonprotein, organic substances facilitate enzyme action by binding the substrate with its specific enzyme. Coenzymes then regenerate to assist in further similar reactions. The metallic ions iron and zinc play coenzyme roles, as do the B vitamins or their derivatives. Oxidation–reduction reactions use the B vitamins riboflavin and niacin, while other vitamins serve as transfer agents for groups of compounds in different metabolic processes (see Table 2.1). Some advertisements for vitamins imply that taking vitamin supplements provides immediate usable energy for exercise. This simply does not occur. Vitamins serve as coenzymes to "make the reactions go," but they contain *no* chemical energy for biologic work.

A coenzyme requires less specificity in its action than an enzyme because the coenzyme affects a number of different reactions. It either acts as a "cobinder" or serves as a temporary carrier of intermediary products in the reaction. For example, the coenzyme **nicotinamide adenine dinucleotide** (**NAD$^+$**) forms NADH in transporting hydrogen atoms and electrons released from food fragments during energy metabolism. The electrons then pass to other special transporter molecules in another series of chemical reactions that ultimately deliver the electrons to oxygen.

Enzyme Inhibition. A variety of substances inhibit enzyme activity to slow the rate of a reaction. **Competitive inhibitors** closely resemble the structure of the normal substrate for an enzyme. They bind to the enzyme's active site but cannot be changed by the enzyme. The inhibitor repetitively occupies the active site and blunts the enzyme's interaction with its substrate. **Noncompetitive inhibitors** do not resemble the enzyme's substrate and do not bind to its active site. Instead, they bind to the enzyme at a site other than the active site. This changes the enzyme's structure and ability to catalyze the reaction because of the presence of the bound inhibitor. Many drugs act as noncompetitive enzyme inhibitors.

HYDROLYSIS AND CONDENSATION: THE BASIS FOR DIGESTION AND SYNTHESIS

In general, hydrolysis reactions digest or break down complex molecules into simpler subunits; condensation reactions build larger molecules by bonding their subunits together.

Hydrolysis Reactions

Hydrolysis catabolizes complex organic molecules— carbohydrates, lipids, and proteins—into simpler forms the body easily absorbs and assimilates. This basic decomposition process splits chemical bonds by adding H$^+$ and OH$^-$ (constituents of water) to the reaction byproducts. Examples of hydrolytic reactions include digestion of starches and disaccharides to monosaccharides, proteins to amino acids,

and lipids to glycerol and fatty acids. Specific enzymes catalyze each step of the breakdown process. For disaccharides, the enzymes are lactase (lactose), sucrase (sucrose), and maltase (maltose). The lipid enzymes (lipases) degrade the triacylglycerol molecule by adding water. This cleaves the fatty acids from their glycerol backbone. During protein digestion, protease enzymes accelerate amino acid release when the addition of water splits the peptide linkages. The following represents the general form for all hydrolysis reactions:

$$AB + HOH \rightarrow A\text{-}H + B\text{-}OH$$

Water added to the substance AB causes the chemical bond that joins AB to decompose to produce the breakdown products A-H (H refers to a hydrogen atom from water) and B-OH (OH refers to the remaining hydroxyl group from water). FIGURE 5.9A illustrates the hydrolysis reaction for the disaccharide sucrose to its end-product molecules, glucose and fructose. The figure also shows the hydrolysis of a dipeptide (protein) into its two constituent amino acid units. Intestinal absorption occurs quickly following hydrolysis of the carbohydrate, lipid, and protein macronutrients.

Condensation Reactions

The general reaction illustrated for hydrolysis can occur in the opposite direction as the compound AB synthesizes from A-H and B-OH. A water molecule also forms in this building process of **condensation** (also termed *dehydration synthesis*). The structural components of the nutrients bind together in condensation reactions to form more complex molecules and compounds. Figure 5.9B shows the condensation reactions for maltose synthesis from two glucose units and the synthesis of a more complex protein from two amino acid units. During protein synthesis, a hydroxyl removed from one amino acid and a hydrogen from the other amino acid join to create a water molecule. **Peptide bond** describes the new bond that forms for the protein. Water also forms in the synthesis of more complex carbohydrates from simple sugars; for lipids, water forms when glycerol and fatty acid components combine to form a triacylglycerol molecule.

Oxidation and Reduction Reactions

Literally thousands of simultaneous chemical reactions that involve the transfer of electrons from one substance to another occur in the body. *Oxidation reactions transfer oxygen atoms, hydrogen atoms, or electrons.* A loss of electrons always occurs in oxidation reactions, with a corresponding net gain in valence. For example, removing hydrogen from a substance yields a net gain of valence electrons. *Reduction involves any process in which the atoms in an element gain electrons, with a corresponding net decrease in valence.*

The term **reducing agent** describes the substance that donates or loses electrons as it oxidizes. The substance being reduced or gaining electrons is called the electron acceptor or **oxidizing agent**. Electron transfer requires both oxidizing and

A Hydrolysis

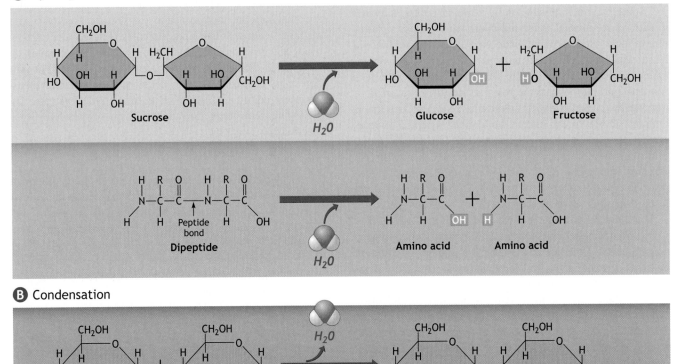

B Condensation

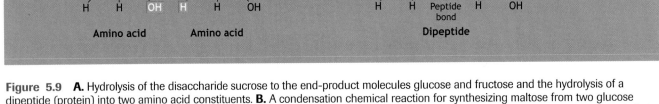

Figure 5.9   A. Hydrolysis of the disaccharide sucrose to the end-product molecules glucose and fructose and the hydrolysis of a dipeptide (protein) into two amino acid constituents. **B.** A condensation chemical reaction for synthesizing maltose from two glucose units and creation of a protein dipeptide from two amino acid subunits. Note that the reactions in **B** illustrate the reverse of the hydrolysis reaction for the dipeptide. The symbol *R* represents the remainder of the molecule.

reducing agents. Oxidation and reduction reactions become characteristically **coupled**. Whenever oxidation occurs, the reverse reduction also takes place; when one substance loses electrons, the other substance gains them. The term **redox reaction** commonly describes a coupled oxidation–reduction reaction.

An excellent example of a redox reaction involves the transfer of electrons within the mitochondria. Here, special carrier molecules transfer oxidized hydrogen atoms and their removed electrons for delivery to oxygen, which becomes reduced. The carbohydrate, fat, and protein substrates provide a ready source of hydrogen atoms. Dehydrogenase (oxidase) enzymes speed up the redox reactions. Two hydrogen-accepting

dehydrogenase coenzymes are the vitamin B–containing NAD^+ and flavin adenine dinucleotide (FAD). Transferring electrons from NADH and $FADH_2$ harnesses energy in the form of ATP.

Energy release in glucose oxidation occurs when electrons reposition (shift) as they move closer to their final destination—oxygen atoms. The close-up illustration of a mitochondrion in FIGURE 5.10 shows the various chemical events that take place on the outer and inner mitochondrial membranes and matrix. The inset table summarizes the mitochondrion's molecular reactions related to its structures. Most of the energy-generating "action," including the redox reactions, takes place within the mitochondrial matrix. The inner membrane is rich in protein

Cell

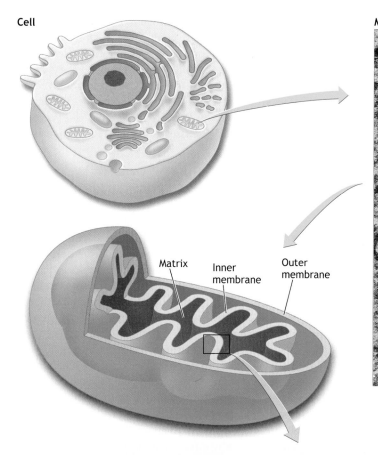

Mitochondrion

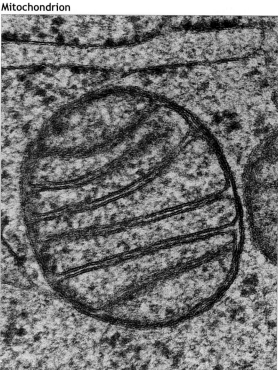

Matrix

Inner membrane

Outer membrane

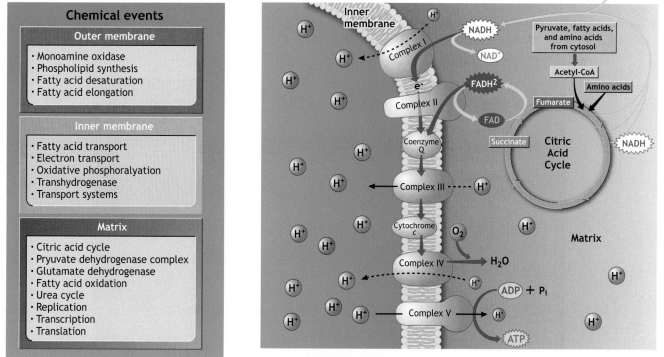

Chemical events

Outer membrane

· Monoamine oxidase
· Phospholipid synthesis
· Fatty acid desaturation
· Fatty acid elongation

Inner membrane

· Fatty acid transport
· Electron transport
· Oxidative phosphoralyation
· Transhydrogenase
· Transport systems

Matrix

· Citric acid cycle
· Pryuvate dehydrogenase complex
· Glutamate dehydrogenase
· Fatty acid oxidation
· Urea cycle
· Replication
· Transcription
· Translation

Inner membrane

H^+ NADH from cytosol

NADH   Pyruvate, fatty acids, and amino acids from cytosol

Complex I   NAD$^+$ Acetyl-CoA   Amino acids

e$^-$ FADH^2 Fumarate

Complex II   FAD   Succinate   Citric Acid Cycle   NADH

Coenzyme Q

Complex III   H$^+$

Cytochrome c   O$_2$ Matrix

Complex IV   H$_2$O

ADP + P$_i$

Complex V   ATP

Figure 5.10 The mitochondrion, its intramitochondrial structures, and primary chemical reactions. The inset table summarizes the different chemical events in relation to mitochondrial structures.

(70%) and lipid (30%), two key macromolecules whose configurations encourage transfer of chemicals through membranes.

INTEGRATIVE QUESTION

What biologic benefit comes from the characteristic coupling of oxidation and reduction reactions?

*The transport of electrons by specific carrier molecules constitutes the **respiratory chain**.* **Electron transport** represents the final common pathway in aerobic (oxidative) metabolism. For each pair of hydrogen atoms, two electrons flow down the chain and reduce one oxygen atom. The process ends when oxygen accepts two hydrogens and forms water. This coupled redox process constitutes hydrogen oxidation and subsequent oxygen reduction. Chemical energy trapped (conserved) during cellular oxidation–reduction forms ATP, the energy-rich molecule that powers all biologic work.

Figure 5.10 illustrates a redox reaction during vigorous physical activity. As exercise intensifies, hydrogen atoms are stripped from the carbohydrate substrate faster than their oxidation in the respiratory chain. To continue energy metabolism, a substance other than oxygen must "accept" the nonoxidized excess hydrogens. This occurs when a pyruvate molecule, an intermediate compound formed in the initial phase of carbohydrate catabolism, temporarily accepts a pair of hydrogens (electrons). A new compound, lactate (ionized form of lactic acid as exists in body), forms when reduced pyruvate accepts additional hydrogens. FIGURE 5.11 illustrates that as more intense exercise produces a greater flow of excess hydrogens to pyruvate, lactate concentration rises rapidly within the active muscle and blood. During recovery, the excess hydrogens in lactate oxidize (electrons removed and passed to NAD^+) to re-form a pyruvate molecule. The enzyme lactate dehydrogenase (LDH) accelerates this reversal. Chapter 6 more fully discusses oxidation–reduction reactions in energy metabolism.

The Mass Action Effect

The effect of the concentration of chemicals in solution on the occurrence of a particular chemical reaction embodies the law of mass action, often referred to as the **mass action effect**. In essence, a chemical reaction progresses to the right with the addition of reactants and to the left with the addition of byproducts. In a simple chemical reaction, product formation increases linearly with the concentration of chemicals available to enter the reaction. In an enzyme-mediated reaction, the rate of product formation increases dramatically with a small change in substrate concentration. This generally produces a relatively large effect on product formation. Certain substances in the body frequently link to several reactions; thus, the products of one reaction become reactant substances for other reactions. Simply changing the concentration of one substance profoundly affects a number of different reactions. Also, some molecules play key roles in a whole chain of chemical events. Oxygen, for example, exerts a significant mass action effect on reactions required for energy transfer. If oxygen

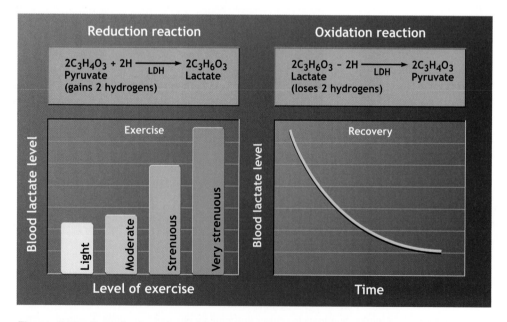

Figure 5.11   Example of a redox (oxidation–reduction) reaction. During progressively more strenuous exercise when oxygen supply (or use) becomes inadequate, some pyruvate formed in energy metabolism gains two hydrogens (two electrons) and becomes *reduced* to a new compound, lactate. In recovery, when oxygen supply (or use) becomes adequate, lactate loses two hydrogens (two electrons) and *oxidizes* back to pyruvate. This example shows how a redox reaction continues energy metabolism, despite limited oxygen availability (or use) in relation to exercise energy demands.

VALID DETERMINATION OF OXYGEN CONSUMPTION

Wilmore JH, Costill DL. Adequacy of the Haldane transformation in the computation of exercise $\dot{V}O_2$ in man. J Appl Physiol 1973;35:85.

▲ Oxygen consumption using open-circuit spirometry represents a fundamental measurement in exercise physiology. This methodology assumes no nitrogen production or retention by the body, so the nitrogen volume remains equal in the inspired and expired air. Because of this intrinsic relationship, no need exists to collect and analyze both inspired and expired air volumes during measurement of oxygen consumption and carbon dioxide production. The following mathematical relationship, known as the *Haldane transformation*, exists between inspired and expired air volumes:

$$V_I = V_E \times F_{E}N_2 \div F_{I}N_2$$

where V_I equals air volume inspired, V_E equals air volume expired, and $F_{E}N_2$ and $F_{I}N_2$ equal the fractional concentrations of nitrogen in the expired and inspired air. Because the fractional concentrations for inspired oxygen, carbon dioxide, and nitrogen are known, only V_E (or V_I) and the concentrations in expired air of CO_2 ($F_{E}CO_2$) and O_2 ($F_{E}O_2$) are required to calculate the oxygen consumed each minute ($\dot{V}O_2$):

$$\dot{V}O_2 = \dot{V}_E \times F_{E}N_2/F_{I}N_2 \times F_{I}O_2 - \dot{V}_E \times F_{E}O_2$$

In this formula, $F_{E}N_2$ usually equals $1.00 - (F_{E}O_2 + F_{E}CO_2)$.

The study by Wilmore and Costill determined any nitrogen retention or production and how it influenced the accuracy of oxygen consumption computations using the traditional *Haldane transformation* during light-to-intense exercise. Six subjects completed treadmill exercise by walking on the level at 4 mph; a 5-minute jog followed at 6.0 mph, followed again by a 5-minute run at 7.5 mph. Oxygen consumption, continuously monitored using open-circuit spirometry, included measurement of inspired and expired ventilation volumes. Measurements also included barometric pressure, inspired and expired gas temperatures, relative humidity, and $F_{E}O_2$, $F_{E}CO_2$, $F_{I}O_2$, and $F_{I}CO_2$.

The figure shows $\dot{V}O_2$ calculated from the inspired and expired air volumes (actual) for all subjects compared with the values estimated from the *Haldane transformation*. The slope of the regression line deviates only 0.003 units from unity (the intercept equals nearly zero), demonstrating the closeness between the actual oxygen consumption and that predicted by the *Haldane transformation*. The largest difference between the 68 actual and estimated $\dot{V}O_2$ values was 230 mL, an error of 7.3%. The average difference of 0.8% for all subjects fell within the measurement error of the instruments. For the nitrogen data, a difference of 1.6% occurred between the minute volume of nitrogen

inspired and expired for any subject at any exercise intensity; 11 of 17 subjects' work rates exhibited less than 1% difference. The largest difference, 1099 mL of $N_2 \cdot min^{-1}$, occurred during intense exercise (2.1% difference).

The researchers noted that the major sources of variation in assessing $\dot{V}O_2$ included the measurement of ventilation volume, gas meter calibration, and determination of the inspired air's water vapor pressure (P_{H_2O}). Ventilation volume posed a problem because accuracy depended on the subject being "switched in" and "switched out" at the same phase of the tidal volume at the beginning and end of the collection period. This remains difficult (if not impossible) to achieve, so an inspired-to-expired volume differential nearly always occurs. Also, a 10 percentage point difference in inspired P_{H_2O} (e.g., from 50 to 60% relative humidity) produces more than a 100-mL difference between the inspired and expired N_2 volumes.

This study supported the continued use of the *Haldane transformation* to calculate exercise $\dot{V}O_2$. While production and/or retention of N_2 can occur during exercise, it exerts little or no effect on the $\dot{V}O_2$ computation.

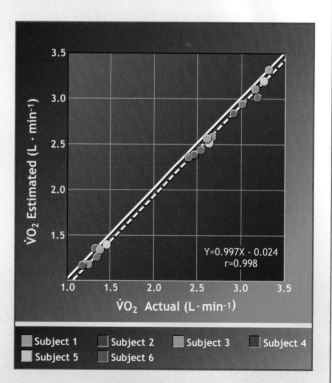

Y=0.997X - 0.024
r=0.998

| Subject 1 | Subject 2 | Subject 3 | Subject 4 |
| Subject 5 | Subject 6 | | |

Actual versus estimated exercise oxygen consumption for six subjects. The *solid line* represents the line of identity, and the *dashed line* represents the regression line that predicts oxygen consumption estimated from the *Haldane transformation* (*y* axis) from the actual oxygen consumption (*x* axis). Note the slope of nearly 1.00 and intercept of 0. *Colored data points* indicate the same subjects measured under each condition.

supply to tissues diminishes, several chemical processes cease, and the net energy available for biologic work decreases dramatically.

Measuring Energy Release in Humans

The gain or loss of heat in a biologic system provides a simple way to determine the energy dynamics of any chemical process. In food catabolism within the body, a human calorimeter (see Fig. 8.1), similar to the bomb calorimeter described in Chapter 4, measures the energy change directly as heat (kCal) liberated from the reactions.

The complete combustion of food takes place at the expense of molecular oxygen, so the heat generated in these exergonic reactions can be inferred readily from measurements of oxygen consumption. Oxygen consumption measurement forms the basis of indirect calorimetry to determine the energy expended by humans during rest and diverse physical activities (see "Focus on Research," p. 135). Chapter 8 discusses how direct calorimetry and indirect calorimetry determine heat production (energy metabolism) in humans.

IQ   INTEGRATIVE QUESTION

Discuss the implications of the second law of thermodynamics for measuring energy expenditure.

Summary

1. Energy, defined as the ability to perform work, emerges only when a change takes place.
2. Energy exists in either potential or kinetic form. *Potential energy* refers to energy associated with a substance's structure or position; *kinetic energy* refers to energy of motion. Potential energy can be measured when it transforms into kinetic energy.
3. The six forms of energy are chemical, mechanical, heat, light, electric, and nuclear. Each energy form can convert or transform to another form.
4. Exergonic energy reactions release energy to the surroundings. Endergonic energy reactions store, conserve, or increase free energy. All potential energy ultimately degrades into kinetic (heat) energy.
5. Living organisms, temporarily conserve a portion of potential energy within the structure of new compounds, some of which power biologic work.
6. Entropy describes the tendency of potential energy to degrade to kinetic energy with a lower capacity for work.
7. Plants transfer the energy of sunlight to the potential energy bound within carbohydrates, lipids, and proteins through the endergonic process of photosynthesis.
8. Respiration, an exergonic process, releases stored energy in plants for coupling to other chemical compounds for biologic work.
9. Energy transfer in humans supports three forms of biologic work: chemical (biosynthesis of cellular molecules), mechanical (muscle contraction), or transport (transfer of substances among cells).
10. Enzymes represent highly specific protein catalysts that tremendously accelerate chemical reaction rates without being consumed or changed in the reaction.
11. Coenzymes consist of nonprotein organic substances that facilitate enzyme action by binding a substrate to its specific enzyme.
12. Hydrolysis (catabolism) of complex organic molecules performs critical functions in macronutrient digestion and energy metabolism. Condensation (anabolism) reactions synthesize complex biomolecules for tissue maintenance and growth.
13. The linking (coupling) of oxidation–reduction (redox) reactions enables oxidation (in which a substance loses electrons) to coincide with the reverse reaction of reduction (in which a substance gains electrons). Redox reactions provide the basis for the body's energy-transfer processes.
14. The transport of electrons by specific carrier molecules constitutes the respiratory chain. Electron transport represents the final common pathway in aerobic metabolism.

Suggested Readings are available on the Student CD and online at http://connection.lww.com/mkk6e.

Energy Transfer in the Body

6

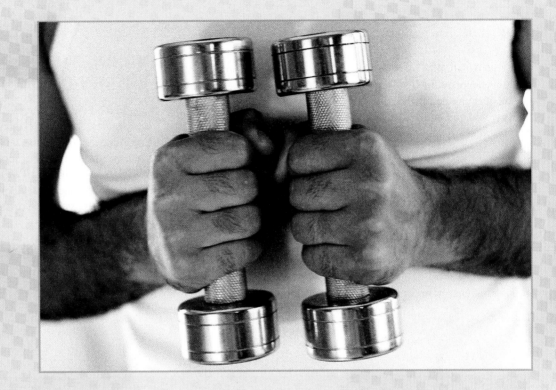

CHAPTER OBJECTIVES

- Identify the high-energy phosphates and discuss their contributions to powering biologic work

- Quantify the body's reserves of adenosine triphosphate (ATP) and phosphocreatine (PCr) and give examples of physical activities in which each of these energy sources predominates

- Outline electron transport–oxidative phosphorylation

- Discuss the role of oxygen in energy metabolism

- List the important functions of carbohydrate in energy metabolism

- Describe cellular energy release during anaerobic metabolism

- Contrast the energy-conserving efficiencies of aerobic and anaerobic metabolism

- Discuss the dynamics of lactate formation and its accumulation in the blood during increasing exercise intensity

- Indicate the role of the citric acid cycle in energy metabolism

- Outline the general pathways for energy release during macronutrient catabolism

- Contrast ATP yield from the catabolism of a molecule of carbohydrate, fat, and protein

- Discuss the role of the Cori cycle in exercise energy metabolism

- Outline the interconversions among carbohydrate, fat, and protein

- Discuss the statement: "Fats burn in a carbohydrate flame"

The human body demands a continual supply of chemical energy to perform its many complex functions. Energy derived from the oxidation of food does not release suddenly at some kindling temperature (FIG. 6.1A) because the body, unlike a mechanical engine, cannot use heat energy. If it could, body fluids would boil and tissues would burst into flames. *Instead, human energy dynamics involve transferring energy by chemical bonds.* Potential energy within carbohydrate, fat, and protein bonds releases stepwise in small quantities when bonds split. A portion of this energy is conserved when new bonds form during enzymatically controlled reactions in the relatively cool, watery medium of the cell (Fig. 6.1B). In essence, some energy lost by one molecule transfers to the chemical structure of other molecules without appearing as heat. This provides a relatively high efficiency in energy transformations. Biologic work occurs when compounds relatively low in potential energy become "juiced up" from energy transfer

via high-energy phosphate bonds. In a sense, the cells receive energy as needed.

The story of how the body maintains its continuous energy supply begins with ATP, the special carrier molecule of free energy.

Part 1 • Phosphate Bond Energy

ADENOSINE TRIPHOSPHATE: THE ENERGY CURRENCY

The energy in food does not transfer directly to the cells for biologic work. Rather, energy from macronutrient oxidation is harvested and funneled through the energy-rich compound **adenosine triphosphate** (**ATP**). The potential energy within this nucleotide molecule powers *all* of the cell's energy-requiring processes. In essence, the energy donor–energy receiver role of ATP represents the cells' two major energy-transforming activities:

1. Extract potential energy from food and conserve it within the bonds of ATP
2. Extract and transfer the chemical energy in ATP to power biologic work

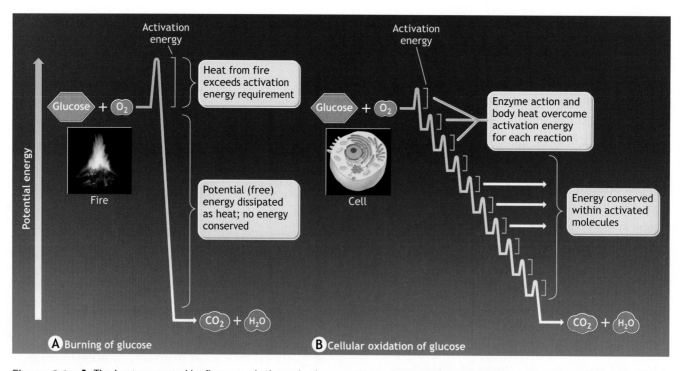

Figure 6.1   **A.** The heat generated by fire exceeds the activation energy requirement of a macronutrient (e.g., glucose), causing all of the molecule's potential energy to release suddenly at kindling temperature and dissipate as heat. **B.** Human energy dynamics involve release of the same amount of potential energy from carbohydrate in small quantities when bonds split during enzymatically controlled reactions. The formation of new molecules conserves energy.

ATP serves as the ideal energy-transfer agent. In one respect, ATP's phosphate bonds "trap" a large portion of the original food molecule's potential energy. ATP also readily transfers this energy to other compounds to raise them to a higher activation level. The cell contains other high-energy compounds, but ATP is by far the most important. FIGURE 6.2 shows how ATP forms from a molecule of adenine and ribose (called adenosine) linked to three phosphates, each consisting of phosphorus and oxygen atoms. The bonds that link the two outermost phosphates (symbolized ◎) represent high-energy bonds because they release considerable useful energy during hydrolysis. A new compound, **adenosine diphosphate (ADP)** forms when ATP joins with water, catalyzed by the enzyme **adenosine triphosphatase (ATPase)**. The reaction cleaves ATP's outermost phosphate bond to release a phosphate ion (inorganic phosphate) and approximately 7.3 kCal of free energy (i.e., energy available for work) per mole of ATP hydrolyzed to ADP. The value $7.3 \text{ kCal} \cdot \text{mol}^{-1}$ represents the standard free energy change under standard conditions. In the intracellular environment, the value may actually approach 10 $\text{kCal} \cdot \text{mol}^{-1}$.

$$\text{ATP} + \text{H}_2\text{O} \xrightarrow{\text{ATPase}} \text{ADP} + \text{P}_i - \Delta G \ 7.3 \text{ kCal} \cdot \text{mol}^{-1}$$

The free energy liberated in ATP hydrolysis reflects the energy difference between the reactant and end products. This reaction generates considerable free energy, making ATP known as a **high-energy phosphate** compound. Infrequently, additional energy releases when another phosphate splits from ADP. In some reactions of biosynthesis, ATP donates its two terminal phosphates simultaneously to construct new cellular material. Adenosine monophosphate (AMP) is the new molecule with a single phosphate group.

The energy liberated during ATP breakdown directly transfers to other energy-requiring molecules. In muscle, the energy stimulates specific sites on the contractile elements to activate the molecular motors that power muscle fibers to shorten. *Energy from ATP hydrolysis powers all forms of biologic work; thus, ATP constitutes the cell's "energy currency."* FIGURE 6.3 illustrates the role of ATP as energy currency for biologic work and its subsequent reconstruction from ADP and a phosphate ion (P_i) via oxidation of the stored macronutrients.

An ATP molecule splits almost instantly without oxygen. This capability to hydrolyze ATP anaerobically generates energy for rapid this would not occur if energy metabolism required oxygen at all times. For this reason, any body movement can happen immediately without consuming oxygen; examples include sprinting for a bus, lifting an object, swinging a golf club, spiking a volleyball, or performing a pull-up or push-up. In sports, the well-known practice of holding one's breath

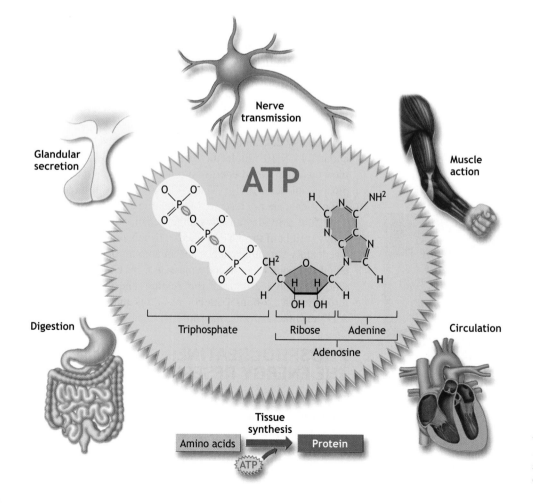

Figure 6.2 Structure of ATP, the energy currency that powers *all* forms of biologic work. The symbol ◎ represents high-energy bonds.

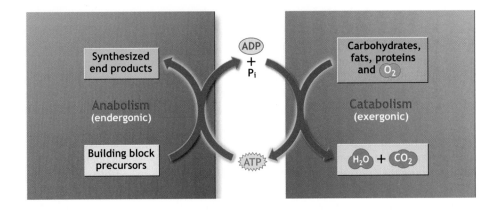

Figure 6.3 Catabolism–anabolism interactions. Continual recycling of ATP for biologic work from intracellular ADP, P$_i$, and energy released from stored macronutrients.

during a sprint swim provides a clear example of ATP splitting (and subsequent resynthesis) without consuming atmospheric oxygen. Withholding air (oxygen) would not preclude a 50-yard sprint on the track, lifting a barbell, or a dash up several flights of stairs. In each case, energy metabolism proceeds uninterrupted because the energy required for the activity derives almost exclusively from intramuscular anaerobic sources.

The body maintains a continuous ATP supply through different metabolic pathways; some are located in the cell's cytosol, while others operate within the mitochondria (FIG. 6.4). For example, the cytosol contains the pathways for ATP production from the anaerobic breakdown of PCr, glucose, glycerol, and the carbon skeletons of deaminated amino acids. Reactions that harness cellular energy to generate ATP aerobically—the citric acid cycle, β-oxidation, and respiratory chain—reside within the mitochondria.

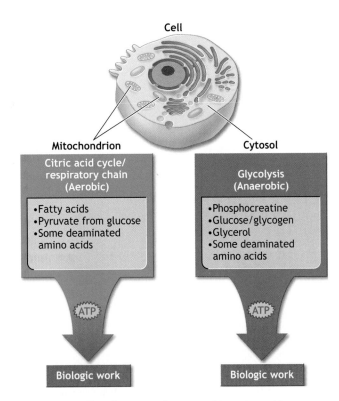

Figure 6.4 Contributors to the anaerobic and aerobic resynthesis of ATP.

A Limited Currency

Cells store a small quantity of ATP and must therefore continually resynthesize it at its rate of use. Only under extreme exercise conditions do ATP levels in skeletal muscle decrease. A limited ATP supply provides a biologically useful mechanism to regulate energy metabolism. By maintaining only a small amount of ATP, its relative concentration (and the corresponding concentration of ADP) changes rapidly in response to only a small increase in cellular metabolism. Any increase in energy requirement immediately disrupts the balance between ATP and ADP. An imbalance stimulates the breakdown of other stored energy-containing compounds to resynthesize ATP. In this way, several systems for energy transfer increase rapidly when movement begins. As one might expect, increases in energy transfer depend on exercise intensity. Energy transfer increases about fourfold in the transition from sitting in a chair to slow walking. Changing from a walk to an all-out sprint almost immediately accelerates the rate of energy transfer within active muscles about 120-fold.

The body stores only 80 to 100 g (about 3.0 oz) of ATP at any time. This quantity makes available each second approximately 2.4 mmol of ATP per kg wet muscle weight, or about 1.44×10^{10} molecules of ATP. This represents enough intramuscular stored energy to power several seconds of explosive, all-out exercise. Thus, ATP alone does not represent a significant energy reserve. Maintaining a limited quantity of ATP fuel provides an advantage because of the relatively heavy weight of the ATP molecule. Biochemists estimate that a sedentary person resynthesizes an amount of ATP each day equal to about 75% of body mass. For an endurance athlete who generates 20 times the resting energy expenditure throughout a 2.5-hour marathon race, this amounts to 80 kg of ATP resynthesis during the run!

PHOSPHOCREATINE: THE ENERGY RESERVOIR

To overcome its storage limitation, ATP resynthesis proceeds uninterrupted to continuously supply energy for biologic work. Fat and glycogen represent the major energy sources for maintaining an as-needed ATP resynthesis. Some energy for ATP resynthesis also comes directly from the anaerobic splitting of a phosphate from **phosphocreatine (PCr)**, another intracellu-

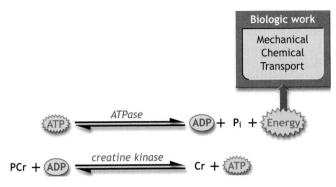

Figure 6.5 ATP and PCr provide anaerobic sources of phosphate-bond energy. The energy liberated from the hydrolysis (splitting) of PCr rebonds ADP and P_i to form ATP.

lar high-energy phosphate compound. FIGURE 6.5 schematically illustrates the release and use of phosphate-bond energy in ATP and PCr. The term **high-energy phosphates** describes these compounds.

The PCr and ATP molecules share a similar characteristic; a large amount of free energy releases when the bond cleaves between the creatine and phosphate molecules in PCr. The arrow in the reaction that points in both directions indicates a reversible reaction. In other words, phosphate (P) and creatine (Cr) rejoin to form PCr. This also applies to ATP; ADP plus P re-forms ATP. Because PCr has a larger free energy of hydrolysis than ATP, its hydrolysis (catalyzed by the enzyme **creatine kinase**—4 to 6% on the outer mitochondrial membrane, 3 to 5% in the sarcomere, and 90% in the cytosol) drives ADP phosphorylation to ATP. Cells store approximately four to six times more PCr than ATP.

Transient increases in ADP within the muscle's contractile unit during exercise shift the creatine kinase reaction toward PCr hydrolysis and ATP production; the reaction does not require oxygen and reaches a maximum energy yield in about 10 seconds.[38] Thus, PCr serves as a "reservoir" of high-energy phosphate bonds. Its rapidity of ADP phosphorylation considerably exceeds anaerobic energy transfer from stored muscle glycogen because of the high activity rate of creatine kinase.[19] If maximal effort continues beyond 10 seconds, energy for continual ATP resynthesis must originate from less-rapid catabolism of the stored macronutrients.[15] Chapter 23 discusses the potential for exogenous creatine supplementation to enhance short-term, explosive exercise performance.

The **adenylate kinase reaction** represents another single-enzyme–mediated reaction for ATP regeneration. The reaction uses two ADP molecules to produce one molecule of ATP and AMP as follows:

$$2\ ADP \xrightarrow{\text{adenylate kinase}} ATP + AMP$$

The creatine kinase and adenylate kinase reactions not only augment the muscle's ability to rapidly increase energy output (ATP availability), they also produce the molecular byproducts AMP, P_i, and ADP that activate the initial stages of glycogen and glucose catabolism and the respiration pathways of the mitochondrion.

CELLULAR OXIDATION

Most energy for phosphorylation derives from the oxidation ("biologic burning") of the dietary carbohydrate, lipid, and protein macronutrients. Recall from Chapter 5 that a molecule becomes reduced when it accepts electrons from an electron donor. In turn, the molecule that gives up the electron becomes oxidized. Oxidation reactions (those that donate electrons) and reduction reactions (those that accept electrons) remain coupled, because every oxidation coincides with a reduction. *In essence, cellular oxidation–reduction constitutes the biochemical mechanism that underlies energy metabolism.* This process continually provides hydrogen atoms from the catabolism of stored macronutrients. The mitochondria, the cell's "energy factories," contain carrier molecules that remove electrons from hydrogen (oxidation) and eventually pass them to oxygen (reduction). ATP synthesis occurs during oxidation–reduction (redox) reactions.

Electron Transport

FIGURE 6.6 illustrates the general schema for hydrogen oxidation and accompanying electron transport to oxygen. During cellular oxidation, hydrogen atoms are not merely turned loose in intracellular fluids. Rather, substrate-specific **dehydrogenase enzymes** catalyze hydrogen's release from the nutrient substrate. The coenzyme component of the dehydrogenase (usually the niacin-containing **nicotinamide**

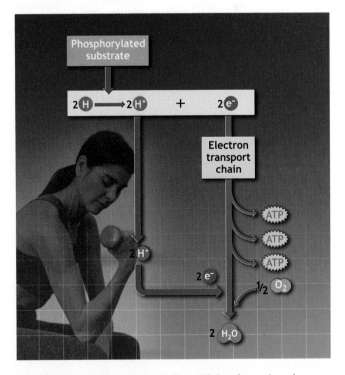

Figure 6.6 A general scheme for oxidizing (removing electrons) hydrogen and the accompanying electron transport. In this process, oxygen is reduced (gain of electrons) and water forms. The liberated energy powers the synthesis of ATP from ADP.

adenine dinucleotide [**NAD**$^+$]) accepts pairs of electrons (energy) from hydrogen. While the substrate oxidizes and gives up hydrogens (electrons), NAD$^+$ gains hydrogen and two electrons and reduces to NADH; the other hydrogen appears as H$^+$ in the cell fluid. The riboflavin-containing coenzyme, **flavin adenine dinucleotide** (**FAD**) serves as the other important electron acceptor in oxidizing food fragments. Like NAD$^+$, FAD catalyzes dehydrogenation and accepts electron pairs. Unlike NAD$^+$, FAD becomes FADH$_2$ by accepting both hydrogens. *NADH and FADH$_2$ provide energy-rich*

molecules because they carry electrons with a high energy-transfer potential.

The **cytochromes**, a series of iron-protein electron carriers dispersed on the inner membranes of the mitochondrion, then pass (in "bucket brigade" fashion) pairs of electrons carried by NADH and FADH$_2$. The iron portion of each cytochrome exists in either its oxidized (ferric, or Fe^{3+}) or reduced (ferrous, or Fe^{2+}) ionic state. By accepting an electron, the ferric portion of a specific cytochrome reduces to its ferrous form. In turn, ferrous iron donates its electron to the next

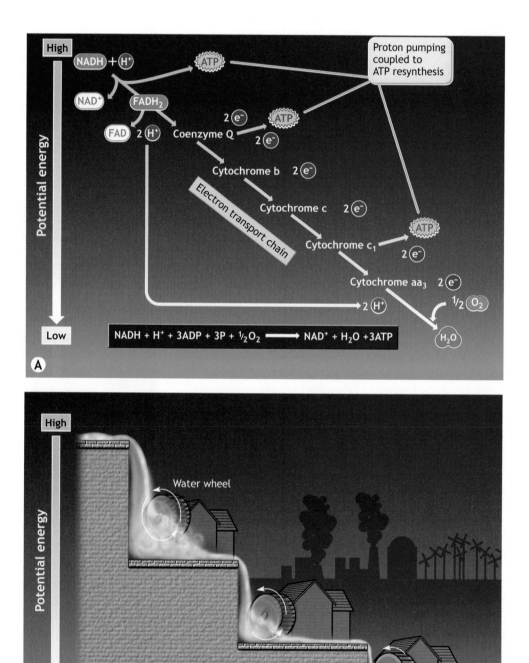

Figure 6.7 Examples of harnessing potential energy. **A.** *In the body,* the electron transport chain removes electrons from hydrogens for ultimate delivery to oxygen. In oxidation–reduction, much of the chemical energy stored within the hydrogen atom does not dissipate to kinetic energy, but instead becomes conserved within ATP. **B.** *In industry,* energy from falling water becomes harnessed to turn the waterwheel, which in turn performs mechanical work.

cytochrome, and so on down the line. By shuttling between these two iron forms, the cytochromes transfer electrons to their ultimate destination, where they reduce oxygen to form water. NAD$^+$ and FAD then recycle for subsequent use in energy metabolism.

Electron transport by specific carrier molecules constitutes the **respiratory chain**, the final common pathway where electrons extracted from hydrogen pass to oxygen. For each pair of hydrogen atoms, two electrons flow down the chain and reduce one atom of oxygen to form one water molecule. Of the five specific cytochromes, only the last, cytochrome oxidase (cytochrome aa$_3$, with strong affinity for oxygen), discharges its electron directly to oxygen. FIGURE 6.7A shows the route for hydrogen oxidation, electron transport, and energy transfer in the respiratory chain that releases free energy in relatively small amounts. In several of the electron transfers, the formation of high-energy phosphate bonds conserves energy. Each electron acceptor in the respiratory chain has a progressively greater affinity for electrons. In biochemical terms, this affinity represents a substance's **reduction potential**. Oxygen, the last electron receiver in the transport chain, pos-

sesses the largest reduction potential. Thus, mitochondrial oxygen ultimately drives the respiratory chain and other catabolic reactions that require continual availability of NAD$^+$ and FAD.

Oxidative Phosphorylation

Oxidative phosphorylation synthesizes ATP by transferring electrons from NADH and FADH$_2$ to oxygen. FIGURE 6.8 illustrates that the energy generated in the reactions of electron transport pumps protons across the inner mitochondrial membrane into the intermembrane space. The electrochemical gradient generated by this reverse flow of protons represents stored potential energy. It provides the coupling mechanism that binds ADP and a phosphate ion to synthesize ATP. The mitochondrion's inner membrane remains impermeable to ATP, so the protein complex ATP/ADP translocase exports the newly synthesized ATP molecule. In turn, ADP and P$_i$ move into the mitochondrion for subsequent synthesis to ATP. Biochemists refer to this union as **chemiosmotic coupling**, the cell's primary endergonic means to extract and trap chemical

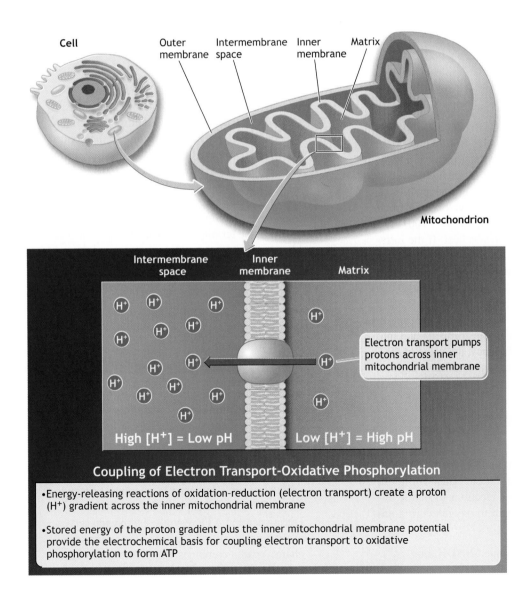

Coupling of Electron Transport-Oxidative Phosphorylation

- Energy-releasing reactions of oxidation-reduction (electron transport) create a proton (H$^+$) gradient across the inner mitochondrial membrane

- Stored energy of the proton gradient plus the inner mitochondrial membrane potential provide the electrochemical basis for coupling electron transport to oxidative phosphorylation to form ATP

Figure 6.8 The mitochondrion: the site for aerobic energy metabolism. Electron transport creates a proton (H$^+$) gradient across the inner mitochondrial membrane. This produces a net flow of protons to provide the coupling mechanism to drive ATP resynthesis.

energy in the high-energy phosphates. *More than 90% of ATP synthesis takes place in the respiratory chain by oxidative reactions coupled with phosphorylation.*

In a way, oxidative phosphorylation can be likened to a waterfall divided into several separate cascades by the intervention of waterwheels at different heights. Figure 6.7B depicts the waterwheels harnessing the energy of the falling water; similarly, electrochemical energy generated in the electron transport chain becomes harnessed and transferred (coupled) to ADP. Energy transfer from NADH to ADP to re-form ATP happens at three distinct coupling sites during electron transport (Fig. 6.7A). Oxidation of hydrogen and subsequent phosphorylation occurs as follows:

$$NADH + H^+ + 3 ADP + 3 P_i + 1/2 O_2 \rightarrow NAD^+ + H_2O + 3 ATP$$

The ratio of phosphate bonds formed to oxygen atoms consumed (**P/O ratio**) reflects quantitatively the coupling of ATP production to electron transport. Note in the above reaction that the P/O ratio equals 3 for each NADH plus H^+ oxidized. However, if $FADH_2$ originally donates hydrogen, only two ATP molecules form (P/O ratio = 2) for each hydrogen pair oxidized. This occurs because $FADH_2$ enters the respiratory chain at a lower energy level at a point beyond the site of the first ATP synthesis (Fig. 6.7A).

Efficiency of Electron Transport–Oxidative Phosphorylation

Each mole of ATP formed from ADP conserves approximately 7 kCal of energy. Because 3 moles of ATP regenerate from the total of 52 kCal of energy released to oxidize 1 mole of NADH, about 21 kCal (7 kCal · mol^{-1} × 3) is conserved as chemical energy. This represents a relative efficiency of 40% for harnessing chemical energy via electron transport-oxidative phosphorylation (21 kCal ÷ 52 kCal × 100). The remaining 60% of the energy dissipates as heat. If the intracellular energy change for ATP synthesis approaches 10 kCal · mol^{-1}, then efficiency of energy conservation approximates 60%. The number of ATPs synthesized per NADH oxidized is not necessarily an integral number (probably closer to 2.5), so some biochemists estimate energy transfer efficiency at nearly 50%. Considering that a steam engine transforms its fuel into useful energy at only about 30% efficiency, the value of 40% or above for the human body represents a remarkably high efficiency rate.

OXYGEN'S ROLE IN ENERGY METABOLISM

Three prerequisites exist for the continual resynthesis of ATP during coupled oxidative phosphorylation. Satisfying these three conditions causes hydrogen and electrons to shuttle uninterrupted down the respiratory chain to oxygen during energy metabolism.

1. Availability of the reducing agent NADH (or $FADH_2$) in the tissues

2. Presence of the oxidizing agent oxygen in the tissues
3. Sufficient concentration of enzymes and mitochondria to ensure that energy transfer reactions proceed at their appropriate rate

In strenuous exercise, inadequacy in oxygen delivery (condition 2) or its rate of use (condition 3) creates a relative imbalance between hydrogen release and its final acceptance by oxygen. If either of these deficiencies exists, electron flow down the respiratory chain "backs up" and hydrogens accumulate bound to NAD^+ and FAD. On p. 150, we describe how the compound pyruvate, a product of carbohydrate breakdown, temporarily binds excess hydrogens (electrons) to form lactate. Lactate formation allows electron transport–oxidative phosphorylation to continue to provide energy.

Aerobic metabolism refers to energy-generating catabolic reactions in which oxygen serves as the final electron acceptor in the respiratory chain and combines with hydrogen to form water. In one sense, the term *aerobic* seems misleading because oxygen does not participate directly in ATP synthesis. On the other hand, oxygen's presence at the "end of the line" largely determines the capacity for aerobic ATP production and sustainability of high-intensity endurance exercise.

Summary

1. Energy within the molecular structure of carbohydrate, fat, and protein does not suddenly release in the body at some kindling temperature. Rather, energy releases slowly in small amounts during complex, enzymatically controlled reactions. This enables more efficient energy transfer and conservation.
2. About 40% of the potential energy in food nutrients transfers to the high-energy compound ATP.
3. Splitting the terminal phosphate bond from ATP liberates free energy to power all forms of biologic work. This makes ATP the body's energy currency despite its limited quantity of only about 3.0 ounces.
4. PCr interacts with ADP to form ATP; this nonaerobic, high-energy reservoir replenishes ATP almost instantaneously.
5. Phosphorylation refers to energy transfer via phosphate bonds as ADP and creatine continually recycle into ATP and PCr.
6. Cellular oxidation occurs on the inner lining of the mitochondrial membranes; it involves transferring electrons from NADH and $FADH_2$ to oxygen.
7. Electron transport–oxidative phosphorylation produces coupled transfer of chemical energy to form ATP from ADP plus phosphate ion.
8. During aerobic ATP resynthesis, oxygen serves as the final electron acceptor in the respiratory chain; oxygen combines with hydrogen to form water.

PART 2 • *Energy Release from Macronutrients*

Energy release in macronutrient catabolism serves one crucial purpose—to phosphorylate ADP to re-form the energy-rich compound ATP. FIGURE 6.9 outlines three broad stages that ultimately lead to the release and conservation of energy by the cell for biologic work. *Stage 1* involves the digestion, absorption, and assimilation of relatively large food macromolecules into smaller subunits for use in cellular metabolism. Within the cytosol, *stage 2* degrades amino acid, glucose, and fatty acid and glycerol units into acetyl-coenzyme A (CoA) (formed within the mitochondrion), with limited ATP and NADH production. In *stage 3* within the -mitochondrion, acetyl-CoA degrades to CO_2 and H_2O with considerable ATP production. The specific pathways of degradation differ, depending on the nutrient substrate catabolized. In the sections that follow, we show how ATP resynthesis occurs from extraction of the potential energy in carbohydrate, fat, and protein.

FIGURE 6.10 outlines the macronutrient fuel sources that supply substrate for oxidation and subsequent formation of ATP. These sources consist of (1) triacylglycerol and glycogen molecules stored within muscle cells, (2) blood glucose (derived from liver glycogen), (3) free fatty acids (derived from triacylglycerols in liver and adipocytes), and (4) intramuscular- and liver-derived carbon skeletons of amino acids. A small amount of ATP also forms from (5) anaerobic reactions in the cytosol in the initial phase of glucose or glycogen breakdown, and (6) phosphorylation of ADP by PCr under enzymatic control by creatine kinase and adenylate kinase.

Energy Release from Carbohydrate

Carbohydrate's primary function is to supply energy for cellular work. Our discussion of macronutrient energy metabolism begins with carbohydrate for four reasons:

1. Carbohydrate provides the only macronutrient substrate whose stored energy generates ATP anaerobically. This takes on importance in maximal exercise that requires rapid energy release above levels supplied by aerobic metabolism. In such a case, intramuscular glycogen supplies most of the energy for ATP resynthesis.
2. During light and moderate aerobic exercise, carbohydrate supplies about one third of the body's energy requirements.
3. Processing a large quantity of fat for energy requires some carbohydrate catabolism.
4. Aerobic breakdown of carbohydrate for energy occurs more rapidly than energy generation from fatty acid breakdown. Thus, depleting glycogen reserves significantly reduces exercise power output. In prolonged aerobic exercise such as marathon

running, athletes often experience nutrient-related fatigue—a state associated with muscle and liver glycogen depletion.

The complete breakdown of one mole of glucose to carbon dioxide and water yields a maximum of 686 kCal of chemical free energy available for work.

$$C_6H_{12}O_6 + 6 O_2 \rightarrow 6 CO_2 + 6 H_2O - \Delta G\ 686\ \text{kCal} \cdot \text{mol}^{-1}$$

Complete glucose breakdown conserves only some of the released energy as ATP. Recall that the synthesis of 1 mole of ATP from ADP and a phosphate ion requires 7.3 kCal of energy. Coupling all of the energy from glucose oxidation to phosphorylation could theoretically form 94 moles of ATP per mole of glucose (686 kCal ÷ 7.3 kCal · mol^{-1} = 94 mol). In the muscle, phosphate bond formation conserves only 38%, or 263 kCal of energy with the remainder dissipated as heat. Consequently, glucose breakdown regenerates 36 moles of ATP (263 kCal ÷ 7.3 kCal · mol^{-1} = 36 mol) with an accompanying free energy gain of 263 kCal.

Glucose degradation occurs in two stages. In stage one, glucose breaks down relatively rapidly into two molecules of pyruvate. Energy transfer for phosphorylation occurs without oxygen (anaerobic). In stage two, pyruvate degrades further to carbon dioxide and water. Energy transfers from these reactions require electron transport and accompanying oxidative phosphorylation (aerobic).

Glycolysis Generates Anaerobic Energy from Glucose

FIGURE 6.11 illustrates the first stage of glucose degradation in a series of fermentation reactions collectively termed **glycolysis**, or the Embden-Meyerhof pathway for its discoverers. Glycolysis occurs in the watery medium of the cell outside the mitochondrion. In a sense, the reactions represent a more primitive form of rapid energy transfer highly developed in amphibians, reptiles, fish, and marine mammals. In humans, the cells' capacity for glycolysis remains crucial during physical activities that require maximal effort for up to about 90 seconds.

In reaction 1, ATP acts as a phosphate donor to phosphorylate glucose to glucose 6-phosphate. In most tissues, this "traps" the glucose molecule in the cell. The liver and, to a small extent, kidney cells contain the enzyme **phosphatase**, which splits the phosphate from glucose 6-phosphate. This frees glucose from the cell for transport throughout the body. In the presence of the enzyme **glycogen synthase**, glucose can now link or become polymerized with other glucose molecules to form the large glycogen molecule (see Fig. 1.2). During energy metabolism, glucose 6-phosphate changes to fructose 6-phosphate. At this stage, energy is not yet extracted, yet some energy incorporates into the original glucose molecule at the expense of one ATP molecule. In a sense, phosphorylation "primes the pump" for continuation of energy metabolism. The fructose 6-phosphate molecule gains an additional phosphate and changes to fructose 1,6-diphosphate under control of **phosphofructokinase (PFK)**. The activity level of this enzyme probably limits the rate of glycolysis during maximum-effort exercise. Fructose

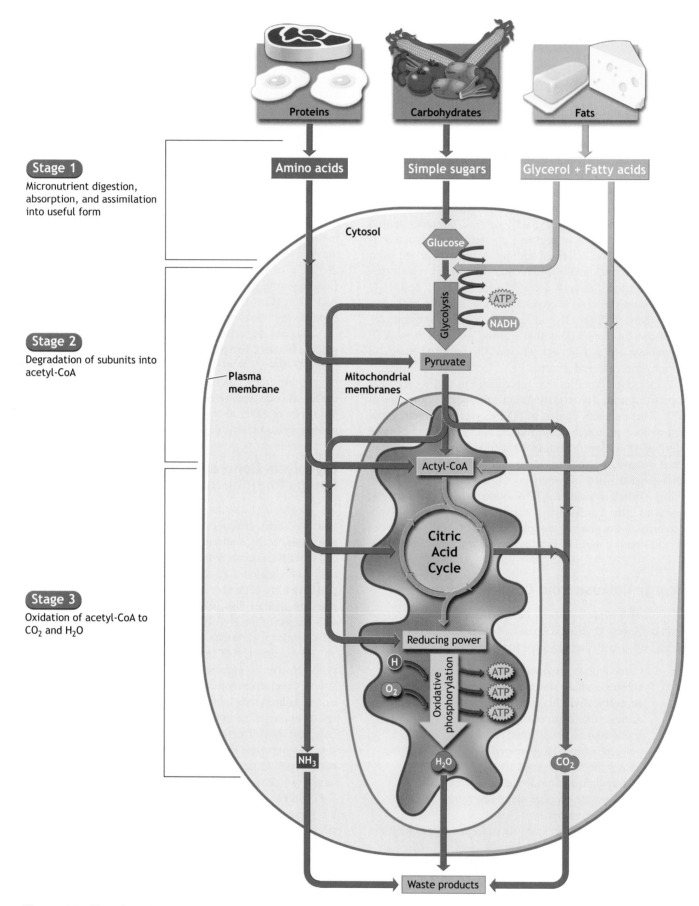

Figure 6.9 Three broad stages for macronutrient use in energy metabolism.

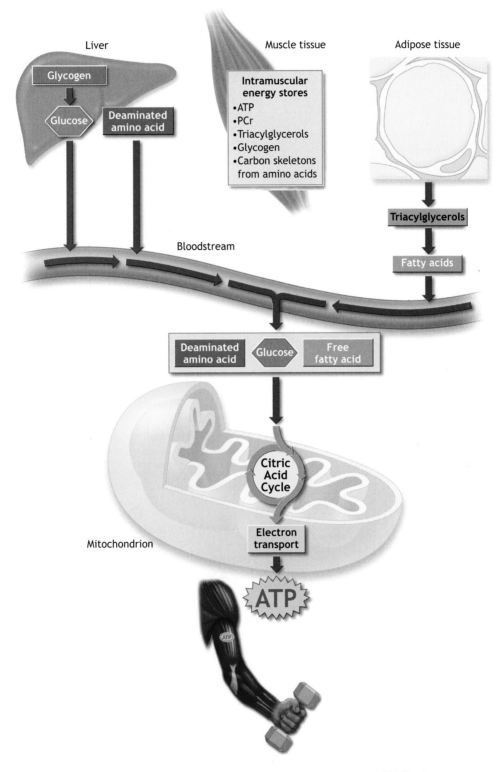

Figure 6.10 Macronutrient fuel sources that supply substrates to regenerate ATP. The liver provides a rich source of amino acids and glucose, while adipocytes generate large quantities of energy-rich fatty acid molecules. After their release, the bloodstream delivers these compounds to the muscle cell. Most of the cells' energy production takes place within the mitochondria. Mitochondrial proteins carry out their roles in oxidative phosphorylation in the inner membranous walls of this architecturally elegant complex. The intramuscular energy sources consist of the high-energy phosphates ATP and PCr and triacylglycerols, glycogen, and amino acids.

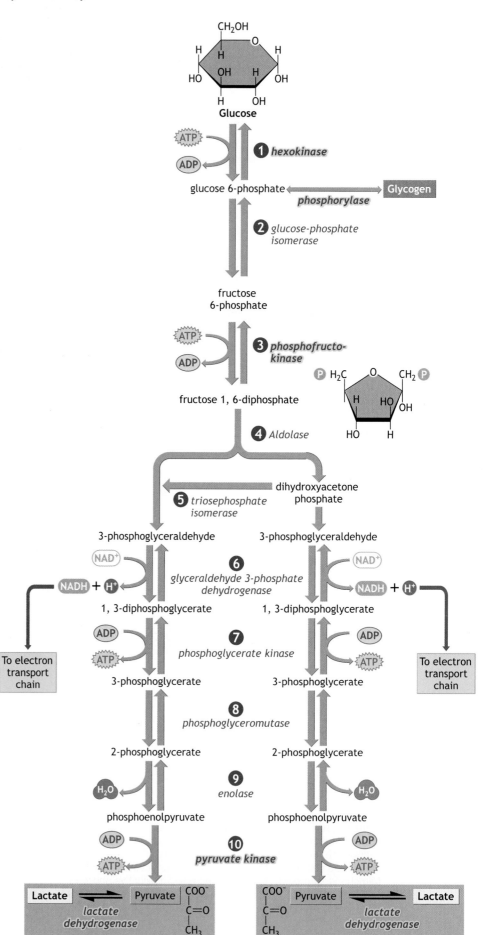

Figure 6.11 Glycolysis: a series of 10 enzymatically controlled chemical reactions create two molecules of pyruvate from the anaerobic breakdown of glucose. Lactate forms when NADH oxidation does not keep pace with its formation in glycolysis. Enzymes colored *yellow/purple* play a key regulatory role in these metabolic reactions.

1,6-diphosphate then splits into two phosphorylated molecules with three carbon chains; these further decompose to pyruvate in five successive reactions. Fast-twitch (type II) muscle fibers (see Chapter 7, p. 174) contain relatively large quantities of PFK; this makes them ideally suited for generating anaerobic energy via glycolysis.

Metabolism of Glucose to Glycogen and Glycogen to Glucose

The cytoplasm of liver and muscle cells contains glycogen granules and the enzymes for glycogen synthesis (glycogenesis) and glycogen breakdown (glycogenolysis). Under normal conditions following a meal, glucose does not accumulate in the blood. Rather, surplus glucose either enters the pathways of energy metabolism or stores as glycogen or converts to fat. In high cellular activity, available glucose oxidizes via the glycolytic pathway, citric acid cycle, and respiratory chain to form ATP. In contrast, low cellular activity and/or depleted glycogen reserves inactivate key enzymes in glycolysis. This causes surplus glucose to form glycogen.

Glycogenolysis describes the cleavage of glucose from the glycogen molecule. The glucose residue then reacts with a phosphate ion to produce glucose 6-phosphate, bypassing step 1 of the glycolytic pathway. Thus, when glycogen provides a glucose molecule for glycolysis, a net gain of three ATPs occurs rather than two ATPs during glucose breakdown.

Regulation of Glycogen Metabolism. In the liver, **glycogen phosphorylase** enzymes become inactive following a meal, while glycogen synthase activity increases to facilitate storage of the glucose obtained from food. Conversely, between meals when glycogen reserves decrease, liver phosphorylase becomes active (concurrent depression of glycogen synthase activity) to maintain stability in blood glucose for use by body tissues. Skeletal muscle at rest shows higher synthase activity, while physical activity induces increased phosphorylase activity with a concomitant blunting of the synthase enzyme. **Epinephrine**, a sympathetic nervous system hormone, accelerates the rate that phosphorylase cleaves one glucose component at a time from the glycogen molecule.[7,11]

Epinephrine's action has been termed the **glycogenolysis cascade** because the hormone affects progressively greater phosphorylase activation to ensure rapid glycogen mobilization. Thus, phosphorylase activity remains most active during intense exercise when sympathetic activity increases and carbohydrate represents the optimum fuel. Sympathetic outflow and subsequent glycogen catabolism decrease considerably during low- to moderate-intensity exercise when the slower rate of fatty acid oxidation adequately maintains ATP concentrations in active muscle.

Substrate-Level Phosphorylation in Glycolysis

Most of the energy generated in glycolysis (44 kCal · mol^{-1}) does not result in ATP resynthesis but instead dissipates as heat. Note that in reactions 7 and 10 in Figure 6.11, the energy released from the glucose intermediates stimulates the direct transfer of phosphate groups to four ADP molecules, generating four ATP molecules. *Because two molecules of ATP contribute to the initial phosphorylation of the glucose molecule, glycolysis generates a net gain of two ATP molecules. This represents an endergonic conservation of 14.6 kCal · mol^{-1}, all without the need for oxygen.* Instead, the energy transferred from substrate to ADP by phosphorylation in glycolysis occurs via phosphate bonds in the anaerobic reactions called **substrate-level phosphorylation**. Energy conservation during glycolysis operates at an efficiency of about 30%.

Glycolysis generates only about 5% of the total ATP during the glucose molecule's complete degradation. Significant energy for muscle action occurs rapidly during glycolysis because of the high concentration of glycolytic enzymes and speed of the reactions. Examples of activities that rely heavily on ATP generated by glycolysis include sprinting at the end of a mile run, swimming all-out from start to finish in a 50- and 100-m swim, routines on gymnastics apparatus, and sprint running up to 200 m. Note that anaerobic energy transfer from macronutrients occurs *only* from carbohydrate breakdown during glycolytic reactions.

Regulation of Glycolysis

Three factors regulate glycolysis:

1. Concentrations of the key glycolytic enzymes hexokinase, phosphofructokinase, and pyruvate kinase.
2. Levels of the substrate fructose 1,6-disphosphate.
3. Oxygen, which in abundance inhibits glycolysis.

In addition, glucose delivery to cells influences its subsequent use in energy metabolism.

Glucose locates in the surrounding extracellular fluid for transport across the cell's plasma membrane. A family of five proteins, collectively termed *facilitative glucose transporters,* mediates this process of **facilitative diffusion**. Muscle fibers and adipocytes contain an insulin-dependent transporter known as Glu T4, or simply **GLUT 4**. This transporter, in response to insulin and physical activity (independent of insulin), migrates from vesicles within the cell to the plasma membrane.[31] Its action facilitates glucose transport into the sarcoplasm where it subsequently catabolizes to form ATP. Another glucose transporter, GLUT 1, accounts for basal levels of glucose transport into muscle.

Hydrogen Release in Glycolysis

Glycolytic reactions strip two pairs of hydrogen atoms from the glucose substrate and pass their electrons to NAD^+ to form NADH (Fig. 6.11, reaction 6). Normally, if the respiratory chain processed these electrons directly, three ATP molecules would form for each NADH molecule oxidized (P/O ratio = 3). Within heart, kidney, and liver cells, extramitochondrial hydrogen (NADH) appears as NADH in the mitochondrion (via a mechanism termed the **malate–aspartate shuttle**). This produces three ATP molecules from the oxidation of each NADH molecule. The mitochondria in skeletal muscle and brain cells remain impermeable to cytoplasmic NADH formed during glycolysis. Consequently, electrons from extramitochondrial NADH shuttle indirectly into the mitochondria. This route ends when electrons pass to FAD to form $FADH_2$ (via a mechanism termed the **glycerol-phosphate shuttle**) at a point below the first formation of ATP (see Fig. 6.7A). *Thus two, rather than three, ATP molecules form when the respiratory chain oxidizes cytoplasmic NADH (P/O ratio = 2). Because two molecules of NADH form in glycolysis, four molecules of ATP generate aerobically by subsequent electron transport–oxidative phosphorylation in skeletal muscle.*

Lactate Formation

Sufficient oxygen bathes the cells during light-to-moderate levels of energy metabolism. The hydrogens (electrons) stripped from the substrate and carried by NADH oxidize within the mitochondria, forming water when they join with oxygen. In a biochemical sense, a "steady state," or more precisely a "steady rate," exists because hydrogen oxidizes at about the same *rate* that it becomes available. Biochemists frequently refer to this relatively steady dynamic condition as **aerobic glycolysis**, with pyruvate as the end product.

In strenuous exercise, when energy demands exceed either oxygen supply or its rate of use, the respiratory chain cannot process all of the hydrogen joined to NADH. Continued release of anaerobic energy in glycolysis depends on NAD^+ availability to oxidize 3-phosphoglyceraldehyde (see reaction 6, Fig. 6.11); otherwise, the rapid rate of glycolysis "grinds to a halt." During **anaerobic glycolysis**, NAD^+ "frees up" when pairs of "excess" nonoxidized hydrogens combine temporarily with pyruvate to form lactate. Lactate formation requires one additional step, catalyzed by **lactate dehydrogenase**, in a reversible reaction (FIG. 6.12).

Lactate accumulation, not simply its production, signifies the onset of anaerobic energy metabolism. During rest and moderate exercise, some lactate continually forms in two ways: (1) energy metabolism of red blood cells that contain no mitochondria and (2) limitations posed by enzyme activity in muscle fibers with high glycolytic capacity. Any lactate that forms in this manner readily oxidizes in neighboring muscle fibers with high oxidative capacity or in more distant tissues such as the heart. Consequently, lactate does not *accumulate* because its removal rate equals its rate of production. Endurance athletes show an enhanced ability for lactate clearance (or turnover) during exercise.[22]

The temporary storage of hydrogen with pyruvate represents a unique aspect of energy metabolism because it provides a ready "collector" for temporary storage of the end product of anaerobic glycolysis. Once lactate forms in muscle, it diffuses into the interstitial space and blood for buffering and removal from the site of energy metabolism. In this way, glycolysis continues to supply anaerobic energy for ATP resynthesis. This avenue for extra energy remains temporary

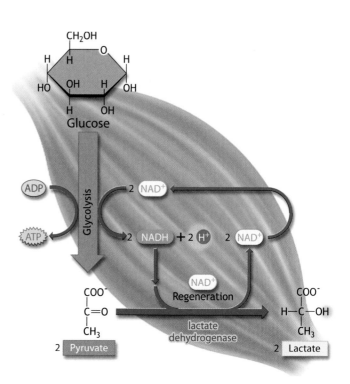

Figure 6.12 Under physiologic conditions within muscle, lactate forms when hydrogens from NADH combine temporarily with pyruvate. This frees up NAD to accept additional hydrogens generated in glycolysis.

because blood lactate and muscle lactate levels increase and ATP regeneration fails to keep pace with its rate of use. Fatigue soon sets in and exercise performance diminishes. Increased intracellular acidity and other disruptions under anaerobic conditions mediate fatigue by inactivating various enzymes in energy transfer and impairing the muscle's contractile properties.[2,6,18,23] However, increased acidity (decreased pH) does not singularly explain the decrement in exercise capacity during heavy physical effort.[20]

A Valuable "Waste Product." Lactate should not be viewed as a metabolic waste product. To the contrary, it provides a valuable source of chemical energy that accumulates from intense exercise.[14] When sufficient oxygen once again becomes available during recovery, or when exercise pace slows, NAD^+ scavenges hydrogens attached to lactate for subsequent oxidation to form ATP. The carbon skeletons of the pyruvate molecules re-formed from lactate during exercise become either oxidized for energy or synthesized to glucose (gluconeogenesis) in the **Cori cycle** (FIG. 6.13). The Cori cycle not only removes lactate but also uses it to replenish glycogen reserves depleted in intense exercise.[36]

In strenuous exercise with elevated carbohydrate catabolism, the glycogen within inactive tissues can supply the needs of active muscle. Such active glycogen turnover through the **exchangeable lactate pool** progresses because inactive tissues release lactate into the circulation. The lactate provides a gluconeogenic precursor to synthesize carbohydrate (via the Cori cycle in liver and kidneys) to support

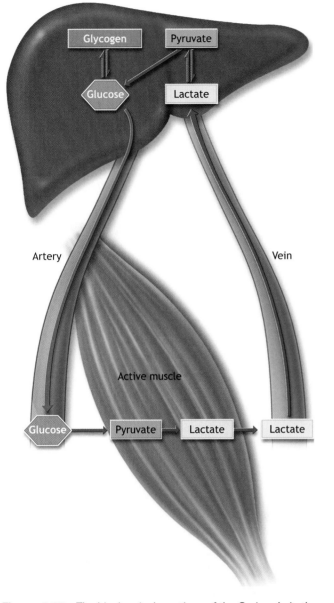

Figure 6.13 The biochemical reactions of the Cori cycle in the liver synthesize glucose from the lactate released from active muscles. This gluconeogenic process helps to maintain carbohydrate reserves.

blood glucose homeostasis and the energy requirements of exercise.[3,22]

Lactate Shuttle: Blood Lactate as an Energy Source.

Isotope tracer studies show that lactate produced in fast-twitch muscle fibers circulates to other fast-twitch or slow-twitch fibers for conversion to pyruvate. Pyruvate, in turn, converts to acetyl-CoA for entry into the citric acid cycle for aerobic energy metabolism. Such **lactate shuttling** among cells enables glycogenolysis in one cell to supply other cells with fuel for oxidation. *This makes muscle not only a major site of lactate production, but also a primary tissue for lactate removal via oxidation.*[4]

Citric Acid Cycle

The anaerobic reactions of glycolysis release only about 5% of the energy within the original glucose molecule. Extraction of the remaining energy continues when pyruvate *irreversibly* converts to **acetyl-CoA**, a form of acetic acid. Acetyl-CoA enters the **citric acid cycle** (also termed Krebs cycle or tricarboxylic acid cycle), the second stage of carbohydrate breakdown. This sequence of metabolic events often bears the name of its discoverer, 1953 Nobel chemist Sir Hans Krebs. As shown schematically in FIGURE 6.14, the citric acid cycle degrades the acetyl-CoA substrate to carbon dioxide and hydrogen atoms within the mitochondria. ATP forms when hydrogen atoms oxidize during electron transport–oxidative phosphorylation.

FIGURE 6.15 shows pyruvate preparing to enter the citric acid cycle by joining with coenzyme A (*A* for acetic acid) to form the 2-carbon compound acetyl-CoA. The two released hydrogens transfer their electrons to NAD^+ to form one molecule of carbon dioxide as follows:

$$Pyruvate + NAD^+ + CoA \rightarrow Acetyl\text{-}CoA$$
$$+ CO_2 + NADH^+ + H^+$$

The acetyl portion of acetyl-CoA joins with **oxaloacetate** to form **citrate** (the same 6-carbon citric acid compound found in citrus fruits), which then proceeds through the citric acid cycle. This cycle continues to operate because it retains the original oxaloacetate molecule to join with a new acetyl fragment that enters the cycle.

Each acetyl-CoA molecule entering the citric acid cycle releases two carbon dioxide molecules and four pairs of hydrogen atoms. One molecule of ATP also regenerates directly by substrate-level phosphorylation from citric acid cycle reactions (reaction 7, Fig. 6.15). As summarized at the bottom of Figure 6.15, the formation of two acetyl-CoA molecules from two pyruvate molecules created in glycolysis releases four hydrogens, while the citric acid cycle releases 16 hydrogens. *Generating electrons (H^+) for passage in the respiratory chain to NAD^+ and FAD represents the primary function of the citric acid cycle.*

Oxygen does not participate directly in citric acid cycle reactions. The major portion of the chemical energy within pyruvate transfers to ADP through the subsequent aerobic process of electron transport–oxidative phosphorylation. With adequate oxygen, including enzymes and substrate, NAD^+ and FAD regenerate, and citric acid cycle metabolism proceeds unimpeded. *The citric acid cycle, electron transport, and oxidative phosphorylation represent the three components of aerobic metabolism.*

Total Energy Transfer from Glucose Catabolism

FIGURE 6.16 summarizes the pathways for energy transfer during glucose catabolism in skeletal muscle. Two ATPs (net gain) form from substrate-level phosphorylation in glycolysis; similarly, two ATPs emerge from acetyl-CoA

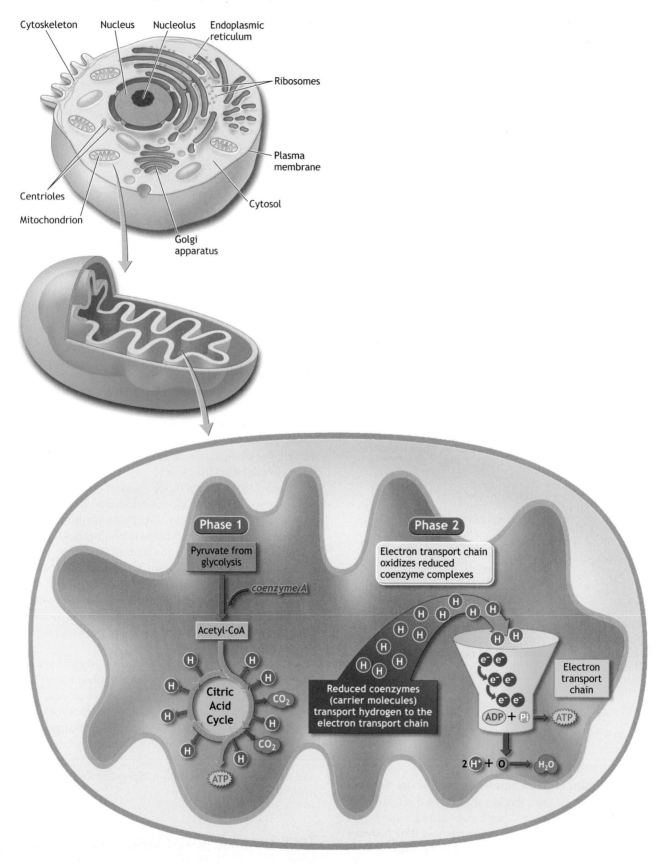

Figure 6.14 Aerobic energy metabolism. *Phase 1*. In the mitochondria, the citric acid cycle generates hydrogen atoms during acetyl-CoA breakdown. *Phase 2*. Significant quantities of ATP regenerate when these hydrogens oxidize via the aerobic process of electron transport–oxidative phosphorylation (electron transport chain).

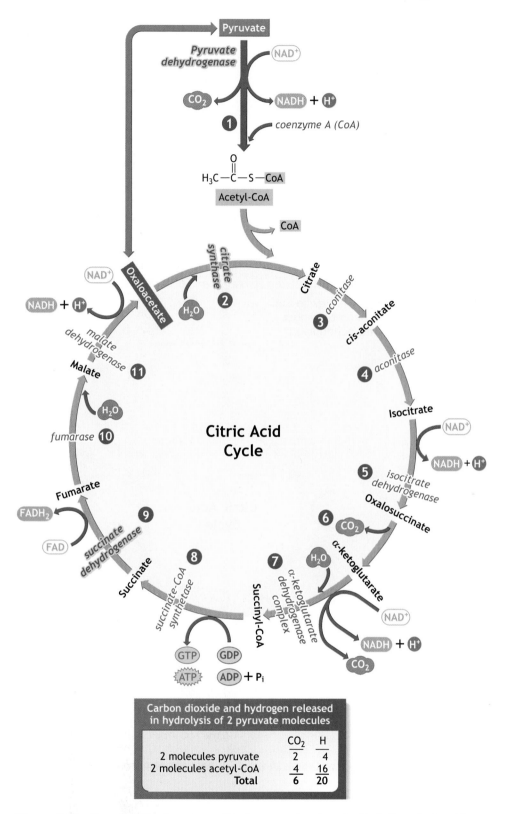

Figure 6.15 Flow sheet for the release of hydrogen and carbon dioxide in the mitochondrion during the breakdown of one pyruvate molecule. All values are doubled when computing the net gain of hydrogen and carbon dioxide because two molecules of pyruvate form from one glucose molecule in glycolysis. Enzymes colored *yellow/purple* are key regulatory enzymes.

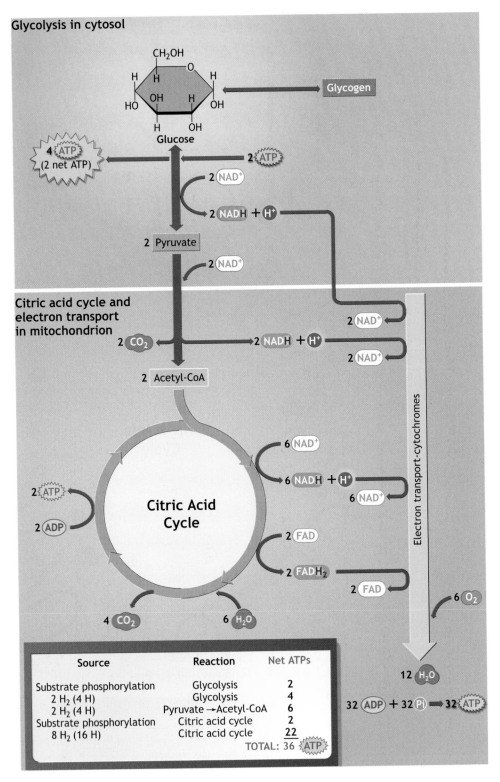

Figure 6.16 A net yield of 36 ATPs from energy transfer during the complete oxidation of one glucose molecule in glycolysis, citric acid cycle, and electron transport.

degradation in the citric acid cycle. The 24 released hydrogen atoms can be accounted for as follows:

1. Four extramitochondrial hydrogens (2 NADH) generated in glycolysis yield 4 ATPs during oxidative phosphorylation (6 ATPs in heart, kidney, and liver).
2. Four hydrogens (2 NADH) released in the mitochondrion when pyruvate degrades to acetyl-CoA yield 6 ATPs.

3. Twelve of the 16 hydrogens (6 NADH) released in the citric acid cycle yield 18 ATPs.
4. Four hydrogens joined to FAD (2 FADH$_2$) in the citric acid cycle yield 4 ATPs.

The complete breakdown of glucose yields a total of 38 ATPs. Because 2 ATPs initially phosphorylate glucose, 36 ATP molecules equal the net ATP yield from glucose catabolism in skeletal muscle. Four ATP molecules form directly from substrate-level phosphorylation (glycolysis and citric acid cycle), whereas 32 ATP molecules regenerate during oxidative phosphorylation.

Some textbooks quote 38 while others give 36 as the net ATP yield from glucose catabolism. The disparity depends on which shuttle system (the glycerol–phosphate or malate–aspartate) transports NADH + H$^+$ into the mitochondrion. One must temper the *theoretical* values for ATP yield in energy metabolism in light of biochemical information that suggests they overestimate because only 30 to 32 ATP *actually* enter the cell's cytoplasm. The differentiation between theoretical versus actual ATP yield may result from the added energy cost required to transport ATP out of the mitochondria.[12] As discussed previously, 4 ATPs represent the final yield from the glycerol–phosphate shuttle (skeletal muscle and brain) as opposed to 6 ATPs from the malate–aspartate shuttle (myocardium, liver, and kidneys) during the complete breakdown of a single glucose molecule.

What Regulates Energy Metabolism?

Under normal conditions, electron transfer and subsequent energy release tightly couple to ADP phosphorylation. Without ADP availability for phosphorylation to ATP, electrons generally do not shuttle down the respiratory chain to oxygen. *Metabolites that either inhibit or activate enzymes at key control points in the oxidative pathways modulate regulatory control of glycolysis and the citric acid cycle.*[15–17,20,26,29] Each pathway contains at least one enzyme considered rate limiting because the enzyme controls the overall speed of that pathway's reactions. *Cellular ADP concentration exerts the greatest effect on the rate-limiting enzymes controlling the energy metabolism of macronutrients.* This mechanism for respiratory control makes sense because any increase in ADP signals a need to supply energy to restore ATP levels. Conversely, high cellular ATP levels indicate a relatively low energy requirement. From a broader perspective, ADP concentrations function as a cellular feedback mechanism to maintain a relative constancy (homeostasis) in the level of energy currency required for biologic work. Other rate-limiting modulators include cellular levels of phosphate, cyclic AMP, AMP-activated protein kinase (AMPK), calcium, NAD$^+$, citrate, and pH. More specifically, ATP and NADH act as enzyme inhibitors, while intracellular calcium, ADP, and NAD$^+$ function as activators. Such chemical feedback allows rapid metabolic adjustment to the cells' energy needs. Within the resting cell, the ATP concentration considerably exceeds the concentration of ADP by about 500:1. However, a decrease in the ATP/ADP ratio and intramitochondrial NADH/NAD$^+$ ratio, as occurs in the beginning of exercise, signals a need for increased metabolism of stored nutrients. In contrast, relatively low levels of energy demand maintain high ratios of ATP/ADP and NADH/NAD$^+$, which depress the rate of energy metabolism.[1]

Independent Effects. No single chemical regulator dominates in affecting mitochondrial ATP production. In vitro and in vivo experiments show that changes in each of these compounds independently alter the rate of oxidative phosphorylation. All exert regulatory effects, each contributing differently depending on energy demands, cellular conditions, and the specific tissue involved.

ENERGY RELEASE FROM FAT

Stored fat represents the body's most plentiful source of potential energy. Relative to carbohydrate and protein, stored fat provides almost unlimited energy. The fuel reserves from fat in a typical young adult male come from two main sources: (1) between 60,000 and 100,000 kCal from triacylglycerol in fat cells (**adipocytes**) and (2) about 3000 kCal from intramuscular triacylglycerol (12 mmol · kg muscle^{-1}). In contrast, carbohydrate energy reserves generally amount to less than 2000 kCal. Specific energy sources for fat catabolism include:

- Triacylglycerols stored directly within the muscle fiber in close proximity to the mitochondria (more in slow-twitch than in fast-twitch muscle fibers)
- Circulating triacylglycerols in lipoprotein complexes that become hydrolyzed on the surface of a tissue's capillary endothelium
- Circulating free fatty acids mobilized from triacylglycerols in adipose tissue

Prior to energy release from fat, hydrolysis (**lipolysis**) in the cell's cytosol splits the triacylglycerol molecule into a glycerol molecule and three water-insoluble fatty acid molecules. **Hormone-sensitive lipase** (activated by cyclic AMP; see p. 156) catalyzes triacylglycerol breakdown as follows:

$$\text{Triacylglycerol} + 3\ H_2O \xrightarrow{\text{lipase}} \text{Glycerol} + 3\ \text{Fatty acids}$$

INTEGRATIVE QUESTION

Discuss the claim that regular low-intensity exercise stimulates greater body fat loss than high-intensity exercise of equal total caloric expenditure.

Adipocytes: The Site of Fat Storage and Mobilization

FIGURE 6.17 outlines the dynamics of fatty acid mobilization (lipolysis) in adipose tissue and delivery for use by skeletal muscle. Although all cells store some fat, adipose tissue serves as an active, major supplier of fatty acid molecules. Adipocytes specialize in synthesizing and storing triacylglycerols. Triacylglycerol fat droplets occupy up to 95% of the adipocyte cell's volume. Once hormone-sensitive lipase stimulates fatty acids to diffuse from the adipocyte into the circulation, nearly all of them bind to plasma albumin for transport to active tissues as **free fatty acids (FFAs)**.[10,32] Hence, FFAs are not truly "free" entities. At the muscle site, the albumin–FFA complex releases FFAs for transport by diffusion and/or a protein-mediated carrier system across the plasma membrane.

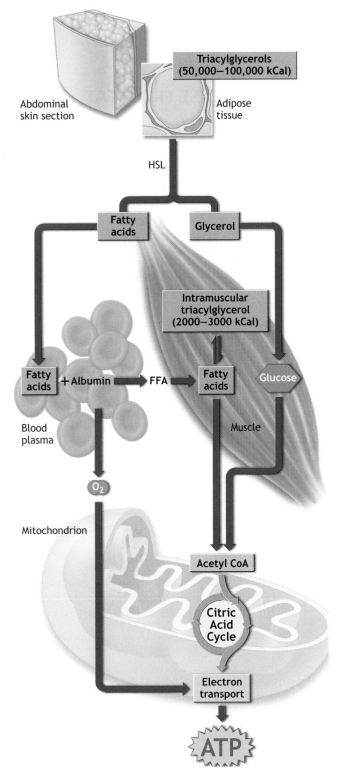

Figure 6.17 Dynamics of fat mobilization and fat use. Hormone-sensitive lipase *(HSL)* stimulates triacylglycerol breakdown into its glycerol and fatty acid components. The blood transports free fatty acids *(FFAs)* released from adipocytes and bound to plasma albumin. Triacylglycerols stored within the muscle fiber also degrade to glycerol and fatty acids to provide energy.

Once inside the muscle fiber, FFAs can (1) reesterify to form triacylglycerols or (2) bind with intramuscular proteins and enter the mitochondria for energy metabolism by action of **carnitine acyltransferase** located on the inner mitochondrial membrane. This enzyme catalyzes the transfer of an acyl group to carnitine to form acyl carnitine, a compound that readily crosses the mitochondrial membrane. Medium- and short-chain fatty acids do not depend on this enzyme-mediated transport. Instead, most diffuse freely into the mitochondria.

The water-soluble glycerol molecule formed during lipolysis readily diffuses from the adipocyte into the circulation. This allows plasma glycerol levels to reflect the level of triacylglycerol catabolism.[30] When delivered to the liver, glycerol serves as a gluconeogenic precursor for glucose synthesis. The relatively slow rate of this process explains why supplementing with exogenous glycerol contributes little as an energy substrate (or glucose replenisher) during exercise.[25]

Adipose tissue release of FFAs and their subsequent use for energy in light and moderate exercise increase directly with blood flow through adipose tissue (threefold increase not uncommon) and active muscle. FFA catabolism increases principally in slow-twitch muscle fibers whose ample blood supply and large numerous mitochondria make them ideal for fat breakdown.

Circulating triacylglycerols carried in lipoprotein complexes also provide an energy source. **Lipoprotein lipase (LPL)**, an enzyme synthesized within the cell and then localized on the surface of its surrounding capillaries, catalyzes the hydrolysis of these triacylglycerols. LPL also facilitates a cell's uptake of fatty acids for energy metabolism or for resynthesis (reesterification) of triacylglycerols stored within muscle and adipose tissues.[32,34]

INTEGRATIVE QUESTION

If an average person stores enough energy as body fat to power a 750-mile run, why do athletes often experience impaired performance toward the end of a 26.2-mile marathon performed under high-intensity, steady-rate aerobic metabolism?

Hormonal Effects

Epinephrine, norepinephrine, glucagon, and growth hormone augment lipase activation and subsequent lipolysis and FFA mobilization from adipose tissue. Plasma concentrations of these lipogenic hormones increase during exercise to continually supply active muscles with energy-rich substrate. An intracellular mediator, **adenosine 3′,5′-cyclic monophosphate**, or **cyclic AMP**, activates hormone-sensitive lipase and thus regulates fat breakdown. The various lipid-mobilizing hormones, which themselves do not enter the cell, activate cyclic AMP.[33] Circulating lactate, ketones, and particularly insulin inhibit cyclic AMP activation.[10] Exercise training-induced increases in the activity level of skeletal muscle and adipose tissue lipases, including biochemical and vascular

AEROBIC METABOLISM AND EXERCISE

Hill AV, Lupton H. Muscular exercise, lactic acid and the supply and utilization of oxygen. Q J Med 1923;16:135.

▲ Perhaps no scientist has contributed more to the field of exercise physiology than Archibald Vivian Hill. He won the Nobel Prize in physiology or medicine for studies of energy metabolism using mostly frog muscle, but also pioneered studies of the physiology of running in humans. His careful experiments on oxygen consumption ($\dot{V}O_2$) during exercise and recovery enhanced understanding of the dynamics of exercise energy metabolism and mechanical efficiency. Hill and Lupton's 1923 research investigated interrelationships among exercise intensity, lactate production, and recovery $\dot{V}O_2$. This lengthy article reported the results of many experiments on several individuals (including the researchers) performing different athletic events like running, continuous jumping, and "violent" gymnastics for 10 to 40 minutes. Measurements included $\dot{V}O_2$ and blood lactate during exercise and recovery, using what currently seem crude techniques.

The subject finished the exercise in front of a stand carrying a wide pipe with nine projecting tubes. To one of these tubes the valves and mouth piece were fixed: to the others were attached rubber bags through single-way stopcocks. The subject on cessation of exercise adopted the standard resting position adjusted the valves, and nose clip, and commenced to expire into the first bag. At the end of about one-half minute (end of nearest expiration) the first bag was turned off, and the second one turned on for a like interval. This process was continued, the intervals of collection being gradually increased.

Topics covered in this article included the following: role of lactate in muscle; heat release in exercise; metabolic efficiency and speed of recovery from different levels of exercise; lactate production in humans; interrelation between lactate formation and oxygen debt; maximal lactate accumulation in exercise; exercise steady state; maximal $\dot{V}O_2$; relation between exercise intensity and $\dot{V}O_2$; and acid–base balance during exercise.

The inclusion of a detailed description of the $\dot{V}O_2$ in recovery from different exercise intensities represents a notable feature of this pioneering article in exercise physiology. The figure shows that the time course of recovery of $\dot{V}O_2$ related to the intensity of previous exercise and accompanying lactate accumulation (not shown). Nearly 80 years of subsequent research has confirmed most of Hill and Lupton's astute observations.

The researchers also presented data for near-maximal (peak) oxygen consumption ($\dot{V}O_{2peak}$). Prior to 1923, little information existed on oxygen consumption in individuals "of athletic disposition" during high-intensity exercise. Hill and Lupton reported $\dot{V}O_{2peak}$ for five men during running (last row of values in table inset). We also include other $\dot{V}O_{2peak}$ data for high-intensity exercise, collected between 1913 and 1934. Compare the average value of $3.95 \text{ L} \cdot \text{min}^{-1}$ for the Hill and Lupton data with the $\dot{V}O_{2max}$ data presented in Figure 11.9 (assume 70-kg body mass to convert data to mL $O_2 \cdot \text{kg}^{-1} \cdot \text{min}^{-1}$). How might you account for the discrepancy in the values?

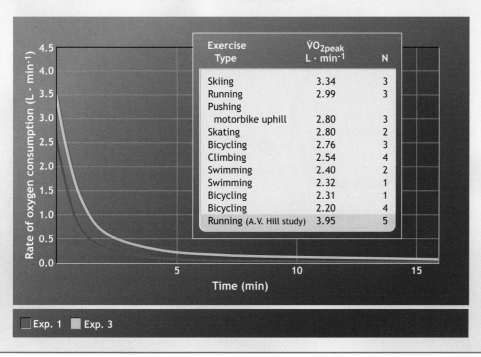

Exercise Type	$\dot{V}O_{2peak}$ L · min⁻¹	N
Skiing	3.34	3
Running	2.99	3
Pushing motorbike uphill	2.80	3
Skating	2.80	2
Bicycling	2.76	3
Climbing	2.54	4
Swimming	2.40	2
Swimming	2.32	1
Bicycling	2.31	1
Bicycling	2.20	4
Running (A.V. Hill study)	3.95	5

Exp. 1 ▢ Exp. 3 ▪

Postexercise oxygen consumption ($\dot{V}O_2$) during recovery from moderate *(Exp. 1)* and intense *(Exp. 3)* exercise. Note the elevated and more prolonged duration of recovery from the intense exercise bout. The inset table presents average values for $\dot{V}O_2$ in diverse forms of intense exercise obtained by A. V. Hill's group *(last row)* and other researchers between 1913 and 1934.

adaptations in the muscles themselves, enhance fat use for energy during moderate exercise.[8,9,21,34] Chapter 20 presents a more detailed evaluation of hormone regulation in exercise and training.

Fat breakdown or synthesis depends on the availability of fatty acid molecules. After a meal, when energy metabolism remains relatively low, digestive processes increase FFA and triacylglycerol delivery to cells; this in turn stimulates triacylglycerol synthesis. In contrast, moderate exercise increases fatty acid use for energy, which reduces their cellular concentration. The decrease in intracellular FFAs stimulates triacylglycerol breakdown into glycerol and fatty acid components. Concurrently, hormonal release triggered by exercise stimulates adipose tissue lipolysis to further augment FFA delivery to active muscle.

Catabolism of Glycerol and Fatty Acids

FIGURE 6.18 summarizes the pathways for degrading the glycerol and fatty acid fragments of the triacylglycerol molecule.

Glycerol

The anaerobic reactions of glycolysis accept glycerol as 3-phosphoglyceraldehyde. This molecule then degrades to pyruvate to form ATP by substrate-level phosphorylation. Hydrogen atoms pass to NAD^+, and the citric acid cycle oxidizes pyruvate. *The complete breakdown of the single glycerol molecule synthesizes 19 ATP molecules.* Glycerol also provides carbon skeletons for glucose synthesis (see "In a Practical Sense"). The gluconeogenic role of glycerol becomes important when glycogen reserves deplete from either dietary restriction of carbohydrates, long-term exercise, or intense training.

INTEGRATIVE QUESTION

Respond to a person who asks: "If elite marathoners run at an exercise intensity that does not cause appreciable accumulation of blood lactate, why do some athletes appear disoriented and fatigued and forced to slow down toward the end of the race?"

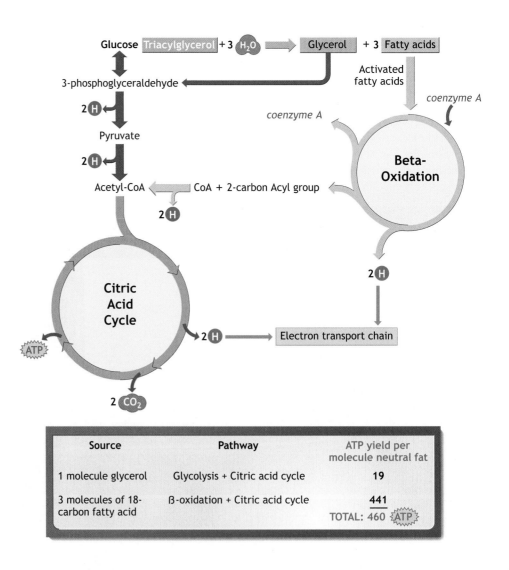

Figure 6.18 General schema for the breakdown of the glycerol and fatty acid components of a triacylglycerol molecule. Glycerol enters the energy pathways during glycolysis. Fatty acids prepare to enter the citric acid cycle through β-oxidation. The electron transport chain accepts hydrogens released during glycolysis, β-oxidation, and citric acid cycle metabolism.

Source	Pathway	ATP yield per molecule neutral fat
1 molecule glycerol	Glycolysis + Citric acid cycle	19
3 molecules of 18-carbon fatty acid	ß-oxidation + Citric acid cycle	441
		TOTAL: 460 ATP

Fatty Acids

The fatty acid molecule transforms to acetyl-CoA in the mitochondrion during **beta (β)-oxidation**. This involves successive splitting of 2-carbon acyl fragments from the long chain of the fatty acid. ATP phosphorylates the reactions, water is added, hydrogens pass to NAD^+ and FAD, and the acyl fragment joins with coenzyme A to form acetyl-CoA. *β-oxidation provides the same acetyl unit as that generated from glucose catabolism.* β-oxidation continues until the entire fatty acid molecule degrades to acetyl-CoA for direct entry into the citric acid cycle. The hydrogens released during fatty acid catabolism oxidize through the respiratory chain. *Note that fatty acid breakdown relates directly to oxygen consumption.* For β-oxidation to proceed, oxygen must join with hydrogen. Under anaerobic conditions, hydrogen remains with NAD^+ and FAD, thus halting fat catabolism.

Total Energy Transfer from Fat Catabolism

The breakdown of a fatty acid molecule progresses as follows:

1. β-oxidation produces NADH and $FADH_2$ by cleaving the fatty acid molecule into 2-carbon acyl fragments.
2. Citric acid cycle degrades acetyl-CoA into carbon dioxide and hydrogen atoms.
3. Hydrogen atoms oxidize via electron transport–oxidative phosphorylation.

For each 18-carbon fatty acid molecule, 147 molecules of ADP phosphorylate to ATP during β-oxidation and citric acid cycle metabolism. Each triacylglycerol molecule contains 3 fatty acid molecules, forming 441 ATP molecules from the fatty acid components (3 × 147 ATP). Also, 19 ATP molecules form during glycerol breakdown, generating a total of 460 molecules of ATP for each triacylglycerol molecule catabolized. This represents a considerable energy yield compared to the 36 ATPs formed when a skeletal muscle catabolizes a glucose molecule. The efficiency of energy conservation for fatty acid oxidation amounts to about 40%, a value similar to that with glucose oxidation.

Intracellular and extracellular lipid molecules usually supply between 30 and 80% of the energy for biologic work depending on a person's nutritional status and level of training and the intensity and duration of physical activity.[37] Fat becomes the *primary* energy fuel for exercise and recovery when high-intensity, long-duration exercise depletes glycogen.[21] Furthermore, enzymatic adaptations occur with prolonged exposure to a high-fat, low-carbohydrate diet because this dietary regimen enhances one's capacity for fat oxidation during exercise.[24]

ENERGY RELEASE FROM PROTEIN

Chapter 1 emphasized that protein plays a contributory role as an energy substrate during endurance activities and intense training. When used for energy, the amino acids, primarily the branched-chain amino acids leucine, isoleucine, valine, glutamine, and aspartate, first convert to a form that readily enters pathways for energy release. This conversion requires nitrogen removal (**deamination**) from the amino acid molecule. Whereas the liver serves as the main site for deamination, skeletal muscle also contains enzymes that remove nitrogen from an amino acid and pass it to other compounds during **transamination** (see Fig. 1.23). For example, the citric acid cycle intermediate α-ketoglutarate accepts a nitrogen-containing amine group (NH_2) to form a new amino acid, glutamate. The muscle cell then uses the carbon-skeleton byproducts of donor amino acids to form ATP. The levels of enzymes for transamination increase with exercise training, which further facilitates protein's use as an energy substrate.

Some amino acids are **glucogenic**; when deaminated, they yield pyruvate, oxaloacetate, or malate—all intermediates for glucose synthesis via gluconeogenesis. For example, pyruvate forms when alanine loses its amino group and gains a double-bonded oxygen. The gluconeogenic role of certain amino acids provides an important component of the Cori cycle for furnishing glucose during prolonged exercise. Regular exercise training enhances the liver's capacity for glucose synthesis from alanine.[36] Other amino acids such as glycine are **ketogenic**; when deaminated, they yield the intermediates acetyl-CoA or acetoacetate. These compounds cannot be used to synthesize glucose; instead, they synthesize to triacylglycerol or catabolize for energy in the citric acid cycle.

INTEGRATIVE QUESTION

Give examples of how the amount of ATP produced varies depending on where a deaminated amino acid enters the catabolic pathways.

Protein Breakdown Facilitates Water Loss. When protein provides energy, the body must eliminate the nitrogen-containing amine group and other solutes produced from protein breakdown. These waste products leave the body dissolved in "obligatory" fluid (urine). For this reason, excessive protein catabolism increases the body's water needs.

THE METABOLIC MILL: INTERRELATIONSHIPS AMONG CARBOHYDRATE, FAT, AND PROTEIN METABOLISM

The "metabolic mill" depicts the citric acid cycle as the vital link between food (macronutrient) energy and chemical energy in ATP (FIG. 6.19). The citric acid cycle also serves as a metabolic hub to provide intermediates that cross the mitochondrial membrane into the cytosol for synthesis to bionutrients for maintenance and growth. For example, excess carbohydrates provide the glycerol and acetyl fragments to synthesize triacylglycerol. Acetyl-CoA functions as the starting point for synthesizing cholesterol and many hormones. Fatty acids *cannot* con-

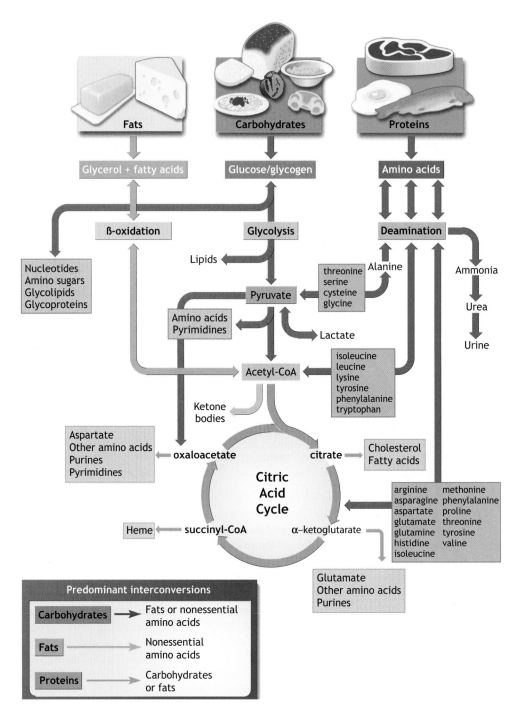

Figure 6.19 The "metabolic mill" allows important interconversions for catabolism and anabolism among carbohydrates, fats, and proteins.

tribute to glucose synthesis because the conversion of pyruvate to acetyl-CoA does not reverse (notice the one-way arrow in Fig. 6.18). Many of the carbon compounds generated in citric acid cycle reactions also provide the organic starting points to synthesize nonessential amino acids.

Glucose Conversion to Fat

Lipogenesis describes the formation of fat, mostly in the cytoplasm of liver cells. It occurs when ingested glucose or protein not used to sustain energy metabolism converts into stored triacylglycerol. For example, when muscle and liver glycogen stores fill, as after a large carbohydrate-containing

meal, insulin release from the pancreas causes a 30-fold increase in glucose transport into adipocytes. Insulin initiates the translocation of a latent pool of GLUT 4 transporters from the adipocyte cytosol to the plasma membrane. GLUT 4 action facilitates glucose transport into the cytosol for synthesis to triacylglycerols and subsequent storage within the adipocyte. This lipogenic process requires ATP energy and the B vitamins biotin, niacin, and pantothenic acid.

Lipogenesis begins with carbons from glucose and the carbon skeletons from amino acid molecules that metabolize to acetyl-CoA (see section on protein metabolism). Liver cells bond the acetate parts of the acetyl-CoA molecules in a series of steps to form the 16-carbon saturated fatty acid palmitic

POTENTIAL FOR GLUCOSE SYNTHESIS FROM TRIACYLGLYCEROL COMPONENTS

■ Circulating glucose provides vital fuel for brain and red blood cell functions. Maintaining blood glucose homeostasis becomes a challenge during prolonged starvation or high-intensity endurance exercise when muscle and liver glycogen reserves rapidly deplete. When this occurs, the central nervous system eventually metabolizes ketone bodies as an energy fuel. Concurrently, muscle protein (amino acids) degrades to gluconeogenic constituents to sustain plasma glucose levels. Excessive muscle protein catabolism eventually produces a muscle-wasting effect. Reliance on protein catabolism, coincident with depleted glycogen, continues because fatty acids from triacylglycerol hydrolysis in muscle and adipose tissue fail to provide gluconeogenic substrates.

NO GLUCOSE SYNTHESIS FROM FATTY ACIDS

The figure illustrates why humans cannot convert fatty acids (palmitate in example) from triacylglycerol breakdown to glucose. Fatty acid oxidation within the mitochondria produces acetyl-CoA. Because the *pyruvate dehydrogenase* and *pyruvate kinase* reactions proceed irreversibly, acetyl-CoA cannot simply form pyruvate by carboxylation and synthesize glucose by reversing glycolysis. Instead, the 2-carbon acetyl group formed from acetyl-CoA degrades further when it enters the citric acid cycle. Hence, in humans, fatty acid hydrolysis produces *no* net synthesis of glucose.

LIMITED GLUCOSE FROM TRIACYLGLYCEROL-DERIVED GLYCEROL

The figure also shows that triacylglycerol hydrolysis via hormone-sensitive lipase (HSL) produces a single 3-carbon glycerol molecule. Unlike fatty acids, the liver can use glycerol for glucose synthesis. After delivery of glycerol in the blood to the liver, *glycerol kinase* phosphorylates it to glycerol 3-phosphate. Further reduction produces dihydroxyacetone phosphate, a substance that provides the carbon skeleton for glucose synthesis.

There is a clear "practical application" to sports and exercise nutrition from an understanding of the limited metabolic pathways available for glucose synthesis from the body's triacylglycerol

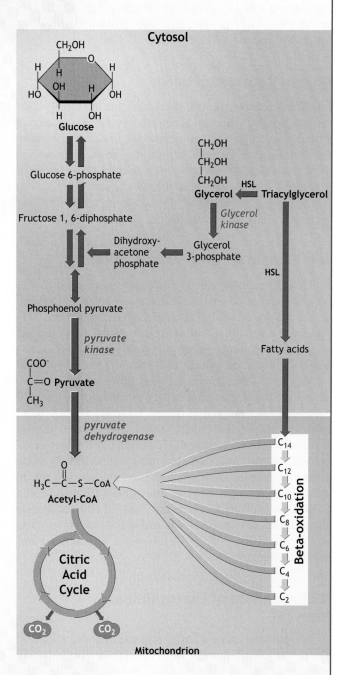

energy depots. Replenishment and maintenance of liver and muscle glycogen reserves intimately depend on exogenous carbohydrate intake. The physically active person must make a concerted effort to regularly consume nutritious, low to moderate glycemic sources of this macronutrient.

acid. This molecule then lengthens to an 18- or 20-carbon chain fatty acid in either the cytosol or the mitochondria. Three fatty acid molecules ultimately join (esterify) with one glycerol molecule (produced during glycolysis) to yield one triacylglycerol molecule. Triacylglycerol releases into the circulation as a very-low-density lipoprotein (VLDL); cells may use VLDL for ATP production or store it in adipocytes along with other fats from dietary sources.

Protein Conversion to Fat

Surplus dietary protein (like carbohydrate) readily converts to fat. The amino acids absorbed by the small intestine after protein's digestion are transported in the circulation to the liver. Figure 6.19 illustrates that the carbon skeletons derived from these amino acids after deamination convert to pyruvate. Pyruvate then enters the mitochondrion for conversion to acetyl-CoA for either (1) catabolism in the citric acid cycle or (2) fatty acid synthesis.

Fats Burn in a Carbohydrate Flame

In metabolically active tissues, fatty acid breakdown depends somewhat on continual background levels of carbohydrate catabolism. Recall that acetyl-CoA enters the citric acid cycle by combining with oxaloacetate to form citrate. Oxaloacetate, in turn, regenerates from pyruvate during carbohydrate breakdown under enzymatic control of pyruvate carboxylase, which adds a carboxyl group to the pyruvate molecule. The degradation of fatty acids in the citric acid cycle continues only if sufficient oxaloacetate and other intermediates combine with acetyl-CoA formed during β-oxidation. These intermediates are continually lost or removed from the cycle and need to be replenished. Pyruvate formed during glucose metabolism plays an important role in maintaining a proper level of oxaloacetate (Figs. 6.15 and 6.19). Low pyruvate levels reduce levels of citric acid cycle intermediates (oxaloacetate and malate), which slows citric acid cycle activity.[5,13,28,35,39] In this sense, "fats burn in a carbohydrate flame."

A Slower Rate of Energy Release from Fat

A rate limit exists for fatty acid use by active muscle.[40] The power generated solely by fat breakdown represents only about one half that achieved with carbohydrate as the chief aerobic energy source. Thus, depleting muscle glycogen must decrease a muscle's maximum aerobic power output. Just as the hypoglycemic condition coincides with a "central" or neural fatigue, muscle glycogen depletion probably causes "peripheral" or local muscle fatigue during exercise.[27]

Gluconeogenesis provides a metabolic option for synthesizing glucose from noncarbohydrate sources. This process, however, does not replenish or even maintain glycogen stores without adequate carbohydrate consumption. Appreciably reducing carbohydrate availability seriously limits energy

transfer capacity. Glycogen depletion can occur in one of five ways: (1) prolonged exercise (marathon running), (2) consecutive days of intense training, (3) inadequate energy intake, (4) dietary elimination of carbohydrates (as advocated with high-fat, low-carbohydrate "ketogenic diets"), or (5) diabetes. Depletion of glycogen depresses aerobic exercise intensity, even if large amounts of fatty acid substrate still circulate to muscle. With extreme carbohydrate depletion, the acetate fragments produced in β-oxidation (acetoacetate and β-hydroxybutyrate) accumulate in extracellular fluids because they cannot enter the citric acid cycle. The liver readily converts these compounds to ketone bodies, some of which pass in the urine. If ketosis persists, the acid quality of the body fluids can increase to potentially toxic levels.

Summary

1. Food macronutrients provide the major sources of potential energy to form ATP when ADP and a phosphate ion rejoin.
2. The complete breakdown of 1 mole of glucose liberates 689 kCal of energy. Of this, ATP bonds conserve about 263 kCal (38%), with the remaining energy dissipated as heat.
3. During glycolytic reactions in the cell's cytosol, a net of two ATP molecules forms during anaerobic substrate-level phosphorylation.
4. Pyruvate converts to acetyl-CoA during the second stage of carbohydrate breakdown within the mitochondrion. Acetyl-CoA then progresses through the citric acid cycle.
5. Hydrogen atoms released during glucose breakdown oxidize via the respiratory chain; a portion of the released energy couples with ADP phosphorylation.
6. The complete oxidation of a glucose molecule in skeletal muscle yields a total (net gain) of 36 ATP molecules.
7. Oxidation of hydrogen atoms at their rate of formation establishes a biochemical steady state or "steady rate" of aerobic metabolism.
8. During intense exercise, when hydrogen oxidation does not keep pace with its production, pyruvate temporarily binds hydrogen, and lactate forms. This allows progression of anaerobic glycolysis for an additional time.
9. Compounds that either inhibit or activate enzymes at key control points in the oxidative pathways modulate regulatory control of glycolysis and citric acid cycle.
10. Cellular ADP concentration exerts the greatest effect on the rate-limiting enzymes that control energy metabolism.
11. The complete oxidation of a triacylglycerol molecule yields about 460 ATP molecules. Fatty acid catabolism requires oxygen; the term *aerobic* describes such reactions.

12. Protein serves as a potentially important energy substrate. After nitrogen removal from the amino acid molecule during deamination, the remaining carbon skeleton enters metabolic pathways to produce ATP aerobically.

13. Numerous interconversions take place among the food nutrients. Fatty acids represent a noteworthy exception; they cannot yield glucose.

14. Fats require intermediates generated in carbohydrate breakdown for their continual catabolism for energy in the metabolic mill.

To this extent, "fats burn in a carbohydrate flame."

15. The power generated solely by fat breakdown represents only about one half of that achieved with carbohydrate as the chief aerobic energy source. Thus, depleting muscle glycogen significantly decreases a muscle's maximum aerobic power output.

References and Suggested Readings are available on the Student CD and online at http://connection.lww.com/mkk6e.

Energy Transfer in Exercise

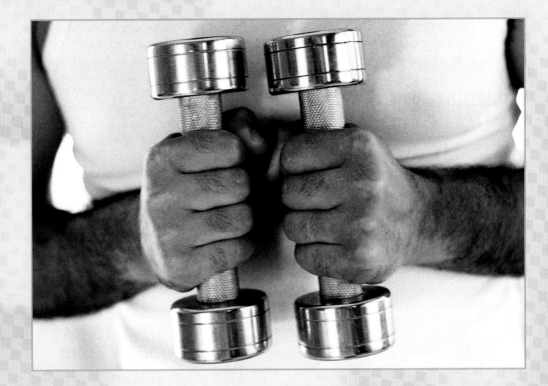

CHAPTER OBJECTIVES

- Identify the three energy systems and outline the relative contribution of each for exercise intensity and duration; relate your discussion to specific sport activities

- Discuss the blood lactate threshold, indicating differences between sedentary and endurance-trained individuals

- Outline the time course for oxygen consumption during 10 minutes of moderate-intensity exercise

- Draw a figure to illustrate oxygen consumption during progressive increments in exercise intensity up to maximum

- Differentiate between type I and type II muscle fibers

- Discuss differences in recovery oxygen consumption patterns from moderate and exhaustive exercise. What factors account for the excess postexercise oxygen consumption (EPOC) from each form of exercise?

- Outline optimal recovery procedures from steady-rate and non–steady-rate exercise

- Discuss the rationale for intermittent exercise applied to interval training

Physical activity provides the greatest demand for energy. In sprint running and swimming, for example, energy output from active muscles exceeds their resting value by 120 times or more. During less-intense but sustained exercise such as marathon running, the whole-body energy requirement increases 20 to 30 times above resting levels. The relative contribution of the different energy transfer systems differs markedly depending on intensity and duration of exercise and the participant's specific fitness status.

IMMEDIATE ENERGY: THE ATP–PCr SYSTEM

High intensity exercise of short duration (100-m dash, 25-m swim, or lifting a heavy weight) requires an immediate energy supply. This comes almost exclusively from the intramuscular high-energy phosphates, or phosphagens, adenosine triphosphate (ATP) and phosphocreatine (PCr). Each kilogram of skeletal muscle contains 3 to 8 mmol of ATP and 4 to 5 times more PCr. For a 70-kg person with a muscle mass of 30 kg, this represents between 570 and 690 mmol of high-energy phosphates. Assuming that 20 kg of muscle becomes active during "big-muscle" exercise, sufficient stored phosphagen energy can power brisk walking for 1 minute, running at marathon pace for 20 to 30 seconds, or sprint running for 5 to 8 seconds. The maximum rate of energy transfer from the intramuscular high-energy phosphates exceeds by 4 to 8 times the maximal energy transfer from aerobic metabolism. In a world record 100-m sprint (9.84 s or 27.1 mph), the runner cannot maintain maximum speed throughout the run. During the last few seconds, the runner begins to slow, often with the winner slowing down least. In this situation, the quantity of intramuscular high-energy phosphates significantly affects performance.

All sports use the high-energy phosphates, but many rely almost exclusively on this means of energy transfer. For example, success in football, weight lifting, field events, baseball, and volleyball requires brief but maximal efforts during the performance. Visualize a breakaway for the goal in ice hockey or soccer, driving for a lay-up in basketball, thrusting upward in a pole vault, or an end run in football without the capability for generating energy rapidly from the stored phosphagens. Sustaining exercise beyond a brief period and recovering from all-out effort requires an additional energy source to replenish ATP. If this does not occur, the "fuel" supply diminishes and high-intensity movement ceases. As we discuss, the carbohydrate, fat, and protein macronutrients within the cellular fluids and tissue depots remain ready to continually recharge the available pool of high-energy phosphates to sustain muscular activity.

Nuclear Magnetic Resonance Spectroscopy to Study Exercise Muscle Metabolism

Nuclear magnetic resonance (**NMR**) spectroscopy provides a noninvasive means to study intracellular metabolism. NMR applies radio-frequency energy to identify the content of chemical elements and compounds within living tissue. The technique continuously monitors the relative concentrations and turnover rates of phosphorylated high-energy compounds and other metabolic events within muscle during exercise.[7,38,39] Measurements take place at regular intervals without the disruptive consequences of the muscle biopsy technique. FIGURE 7.1A illustrates the NMR method during wrist flexion exercise. The active muscles are placed over a superconducting magnet while the subject exercises under conditions that control for power output, contraction speed, and exercise duration. Application of specific radio-frequency pulses within a strong magnetic field determines concentrations of diverse bioactive compounds. Figure 7.1B shows the results for ATP, PCr, and inorganic phosphate during rest and low- and moderate-intensity exercise. The areas under the peaks correspond to relative concentrations of free phosphorus compounds, including the three phosphorus atoms of ATP. Such elegant studies of the ratio of inorganic phosphate (phosphate ion) to PCr provide insight into the rate of mitochondrial respiration. With this methodology, investigators have studied muscle injury, glycolytic metabolism, and the effects of training on the intricacies of muscle metabolism, including the relationships among local muscle substrate catabolism, cardiovascular functional capacity, and exercise performance.[8,34]

SHORT-TERM ENERGY: THE LACTIC ACID SYSTEM

Resynthesis of the high-energy phosphates must proceed at a rapid rate to continue strenuous exercise. The energy to phosphorylate ADP during intense exercise comes mainly from stored muscle glycogen through anaerobic glycolysis (maximal energy transfer rate is 45% that of the high-energy phosphates), with resulting lactate formation. In a way, anaerobic glycolysis with lactate formation buys time. It allows ATP to form rapidly by substrate-level phosphorylation, even though the oxygen supply remains inadequate and/or energy demands outstrip the muscle's capacity to resynthesize ATP aerobically. Anaerobic energy for ATP resynthesis in glycolysis can be viewed as reserve fuel activated when a person accelerates at the start of exercise or during the last few hundred yards of a mile run or performs all-out from start to finish during a 440-m run or 100-m swim. *Rapid and large accumulations of blood lactate occur during maximal exercise that lasts between 60 and 180 seconds.* Decreasing the intensity of such arduous exercise to extend the exercise period correspondingly decreases (1) the rate of lactate accumulation and (2) the final level of blood lactate.

Lactate Accumulation

Blood lactate does not accumulate at all levels of exercise. FIGURE 7.2 illustrates for endurance athletes and untrained subjects the general relationship between oxygen consumption, expressed as a percentage of maximum, and blood lactate during light, moderate, and strenuous exercise. Oxygen-consuming reactions adequately meet the energy demands of the trained and untrained during relatively light exercise (<50% aerobic

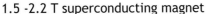

1.5 -2.2 T superconducting magnet

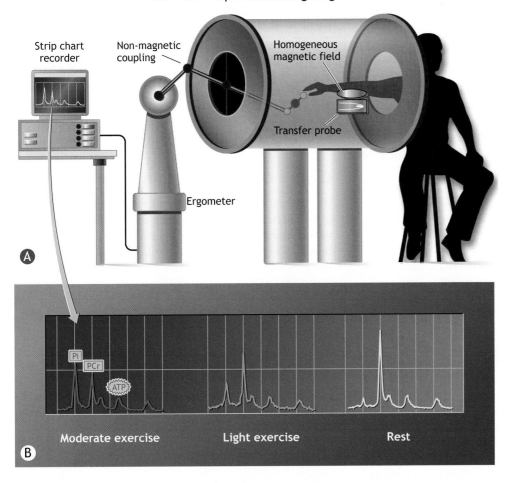

Figure 7.1 NMR spectroscopy. **A.** The wrist flexor muscles are placed on a surface coil in a superconducting magnet. The subject grasps a handle attached to an isokinetic dynamometer (constant velocity, variable force output) while observing a recorder that provides feedback on force production. **B.** Example of NMR spectroscopy spectra for *ATP, PCr,* and inorganic phosphate *(Pi)* during rest and two levels of exercise. (From McCully KK, et al. Application of ^{31}P magnetic resonance spectroscopy to the study of athletic performance. Sports Med 1988;5:312.)

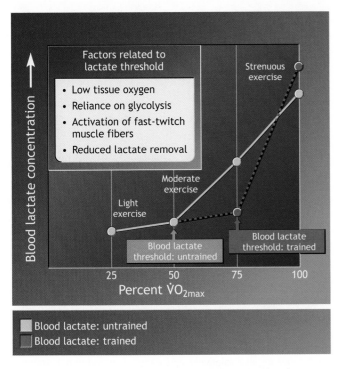

Figure 7.2 Blood lactate concentration for trained and untrained subjects at different levels of exercise expressed as a percentage of maximal oxygen consumption ($\dot{V}O_{2max}$).

capacity). In biochemical terms, energy generated from the oxidation of hydrogen provides the predominant ATP for muscular activity. Any lactate formed in one part of a working muscle becomes rapidly oxidized by muscle fibers with high oxidative capacity (heart and other fibers in the same muscle or less active nearby muscles).[11,32] When lactate oxidation equals its production, blood lactate level remains stable even though increases occur in exercise intensity and oxygen consumption.

For healthy, untrained persons, blood lactate begins to accumulate and rise in an exponential fashion at about 55% of the individual's maximal capacity for aerobic metabolism. The usual explanation for blood lactate accumulation in exercise assumes a relative tissue hypoxia. When glycolytic metabolism predominates, nicotinamide adenine dinucleotide (NADH) production exceeds the cell's capacity for shuttling its hydrogens (electrons) down the respiratory chain because insufficient oxygen exists at the tissue level. The imbalance in hydrogen release and subsequent oxidation (more precisely, the cytoplasmic NAD^+/NADH ratio) causes pyruvate to accept the excess hydrogens (i.e., 2 hydrogen ions attach to the pyruvate molecule). The original pyruvate with 2 additional hydrogens forms a new molecule, lactic acid, which begins to accumulate.[33]

Research with radioactive tracers to label the carbon in the glucose molecule provides an alternate explanation for lactate buildup in muscle and its subsequent appearance in blood.[10] These studies reveal that lactate continuously forms during rest and moderate exercise. Under aerobic conditions, lactate removal by other tissues matches its rate of formation, resulting in no *net* lactate accumulation (i.e., blood lactate concentration remains stable). Only when removal does not match production does blood lactate accumulate. Adaptations within muscle from aerobic training allow high rates of lactate turnover; thus, lactate accumulates at higher exercise levels than in the untrained state.[45] Another explanation for lactate buildup during exercise might include the tendency for the enzyme lactate dehydrogenase (LDH) in fast-twitch muscle fibers to favor the conversion of pyruvate to lactate. In contrast, the LDH level in slow-twitch fibers favors conversion of lactate to pyruvate. Recruitment of fast-twitch fibers with increasing exercise intensity therefore favors lactate formation, independent of tissue oxygenation.

Lactate production and accumulation accelerate as exercise intensity increases and the muscle cells can neither meet the additional energy demands aerobically nor oxidize lactate at its rate of production. A similar pattern exists for untrained subjects and endurance athletes, except the threshold for lactate buildup, termed the **blood lactate threshold**, occurs at a higher percentage of the athlete's aerobic capacity.[21,51,52] Trained endurance athletes, for example, perform steady-rate aerobic exercise at intensities between 80 and 90% of their maximum capacity for aerobic metabolism.[49] This favorable aerobic response relates to one of three factors: (1) the athletes' specific genetic endowment (e.g., muscle fiber type, muscle blood flow responsiveness), (2) specific local training adaptations that favor less lactate production,[14,20] and/or (3) a more rapid rate of lactate removal (greater lactate clearance or turnover) at any exercise intensity.[11,37] For example, capillary density and the size and number of mitochondria increase with endurance training, as does the concentration of enzymes and transfer agents in aerobic metabolism.[30,46,47] The training response remains unimpaired with aging.[15] Such training adaptations enhance cellular capacity to generate ATP aerobically through glucose and fatty acid catabolism. Maintaining a low lactate level also conserves glycogen reserves, which extends the duration of high-intensity aerobic effort. Chapter 14 further develops the concept of the blood lactate threshold, its measurement, and its relation to endurance performance. In Chapter 21 we discuss adaptations in the blood lactate threshold with exercise training.

Lactate-Producing Capacity

Generating high blood lactate levels during maximal exercise increases with specific sprint-power anaerobic training and decreases when training ceases. Sprint-power athletes often achieve 20 to 30% higher blood lactate levels than untrained counterparts during maximal short-duration exercise. One or more of the following three mechanism helps to explain this response: (1) improved motivation accompanying the trained state, (2) increased intramuscular glycogen stores that accompany training (which probably allow a greater contribution of energy via anaerobic glycolysis), and (3) training-induced increase in enzymes that regulate glycolysis,

particularly phosphofructokinase. However, the 20% increase in glycolytic enzymes falls well below the two- to threefold increase in aerobic enzymes with endurance training.

LONG-TERM ENERGY: THE AEROBIC SYSTEM

The reactions of glycolysis produce relatively little ATP. Consequently, aerobic metabolism provides most of the energy transfer when intense exercise exceeds several minutes.

Oxygen Consumption During Exercise

FIGURE 7.3 illustrates oxygen consumption—also referred to as **pulmonary oxygen uptake** because oxygen measurements occur at the lung and not the active muscles—during each minute of a steady, relatively slow 10-minute run. Oxygen consumption rises exponentially during the first minutes of exercise (fast component of exercise oxygen consumption) to achieve a plateau between the third and fourth minutes. It then remains relatively stable for the duration of the effort. The term **steady state** or **steady rate** generally describes the flat portion (plateau) of the oxygen consumption curve. Steady rate reflects a balance between energy required by the working muscles and ATP production in aerobic metabolism. Within this region, oxygen-consuming reactions supply the energy for exercise; any lactate produced either oxidizes or reconverts to glucose via the Cori cycle in the liver and possibly the kidneys. *No appreciable blood lactate accumulates under steady-rate metabolic conditions.*

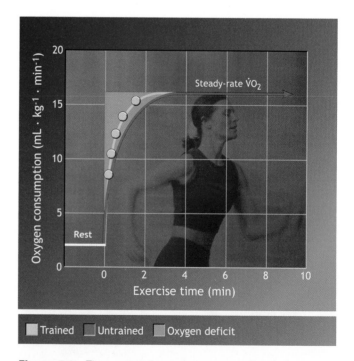

Figure 7.3 Time course for oxygen consumption during a continuous jog at a relatively slow pace by an endurance-trained and untrained individual. The *orange region* indicates the oxygen deficit—the quantity of oxygen that would have been consumed had oxygen consumption reached steady rate immediately.

Once a steady rate of aerobic metabolism occurs, exercise could theoretically progress indefinitely if the individual possessed the will to continue. This assumes that steady-rate aerobic metabolism singularly determines one's capacity to sustain submaximal exercise. Fluid loss and electrolyte depletion often pose significant limiting factors, especially during exercise in hot weather. In addition, maintaining adequate reserves of both liver glycogen for central nervous system function and muscle glycogen to power exercise takes on added significance at high intensities of prolonged aerobic effort. Glycogen depletion dramatically reduces exercise capacity.

Individuals possess many steady-rate levels of exercise. For some, the spectrum might range from sitting and watching TV to pushing a power lawn mower for 40 minutes. An elite endurance runner maintains a steady rate of aerobic metabolism throughout a 26.2-mile marathon, averaging slightly less than 5 minutes per mile, or during a 658-mile ultramarathon, averaging 118 miles a day over 5.6 days! These magnificent endurance accomplishments result from (1) high capacity of the central circulation to *deliver* oxygen to the working muscles and (2) high capacity of those muscles to *use* the oxygen available to them.

Oxygen Deficit

At the onset of exercise, the oxygen consumption curve shown in Figure 7.3 does not increase instantaneously to steady rate. In the beginning transitional stage of constant-load exercise, oxygen consumption remains considerably below the steady-rate level, even though the energy requirement remains unchanged throughout the exercise period. A lag in oxygen consumption early in exercise should not be surprising because the energy for muscle contraction comes directly from the immediate anaerobic breakdown of ATP. Even with experimentally increased oxygen availability and increased oxygen diffusion gradients at the tissue level, the initial increase in exercise oxygen consumption always lags behind energy expenditure.[24,25] Owing to the interaction of (1) intrinsic inertia in cellular metabolic signals and enzyme activation and (2) sluggishness of oxygen delivery to the mitochondria, the hydrogens produced in energy metabolism do not immediately oxidize and combine with oxygen.[41,48] Oxygen consumption becomes evident in subsequent energy transfer reactions when oxygen combines with the hydrogens liberated in glycolysis, β-oxidation of fatty acids, or the reactions of the citric acid cycle. In other words, oxygen is not consumed without substrate (hydrogens). After several minutes of submaximal exercise, hydrogen production and subsequent oxidation becomes proportional to exercise intensity and oxygen consumption attains a steady rate.

*The **oxygen deficit** quantitatively expresses the difference between the total oxygen consumed during exercise and the total that would have been consumed had steady-rate aerobic metabolism been reached from the start.* The energy derived in the early stage of exercise represents immediate energy transfer from hydrolysis of intramuscular high-energy phosphates and glycolysis until steady-rate oxygen consumption matches energy demands. Oxygen consumption kinetics at the onset of exercise do not differ in children and adults.[27]

FIGURE 7.4 depicts the relationship between the size of the oxygen deficit and the contribution of energy from the ATP–PCr and lactate energy systems. The high-energy phosphates are substantially depleted in exercise that generates about a 3- to 4-L oxygen deficit. Consequently, further exercise progresses only on a "pay-as-you-go" basis. Continual ATP resynthesis occurs through either anaerobic glycolysis or the aerobic breakdown of macronutrients. Interestingly, lactate begins to increase in active muscle well before the high-energy phosphates reach their lowest levels. This indicates that glycolysis also contributes anaerobic energy in the early stages of vigorous exercise, before full use of the high-energy phosphates. *Energy for exercise does not simply occur from activating a series of energy systems that "switch on" and "switch off," but rather from smooth blending with considerable overlap of one mode of energy transfer to another.*[26,45]

Oxygen Deficit in the Trained and Untrained

Trained and untrained individuals attain similar steady-rate oxygen consumption values. The endurance-trained person, however, reaches steady rate more rapidly, with a smaller

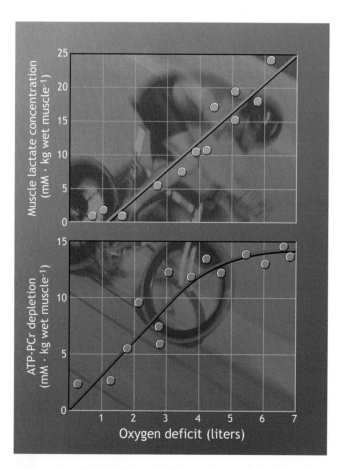

Figure 7.4 Muscle ATP and PCr depletion and muscle lactate concentration in relation to the oxygen deficit. (Adapted from Pernow B, Karlsson J. Muscle ATP, PCr and lactate in submaximal and maximal exercise. In: Pernow B, Saltin B, eds. Muscle metabolism during exercise. New York: Plenum, 1971.)

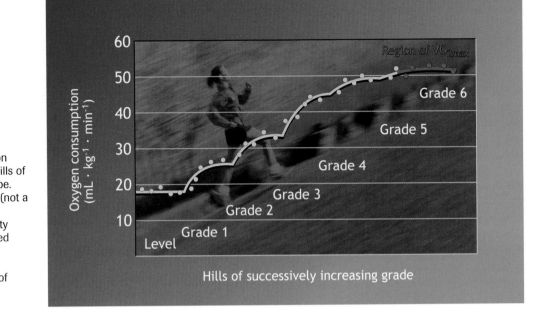

Figure 7.5 Attainment of maximal oxygen consumption ($\dot{V}O_{2max}$) while running up hills of progressively increasing slope. $\dot{V}O_{2max}$ occurs in the region (not a single point) where further increases in exercise intensity produce a less-than-expected increase (or no increase) in oxygen consumption. *Dots* represent measured values of oxygen consumption while traversing the hills.

oxygen deficit than sprint-power athletes, cardiac patients, older adults, or untrained individuals (Fig. 7.3).[13,16,18,31,35,36] Consequently, the aerobically trained person consumes a greater total amount of oxygen during steady-rate exercise. This makes the anaerobic component of exercise energy transfer becomes proportionately smaller. *A facilitated rate of aerobic metabolism in the early stages of exercise occurs from a more rapid increase in overall blood flow (cardiac output) and/or a disproportionately large regional blood flow to active muscle complemented by training-induced cellular adaptations. Many of these adaptations increase cellular capacity to generate ATP aerobically (see Chapter 21).*

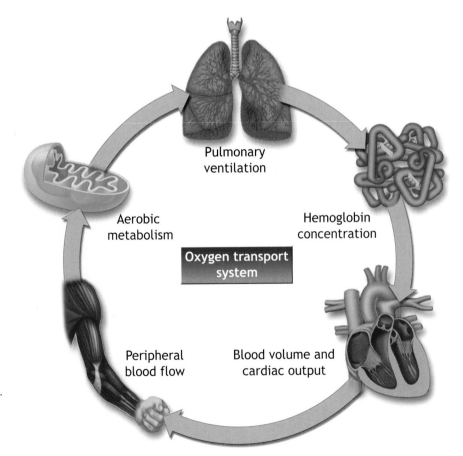

Figure 7.6 The oxygen transport system. The physiologic significance of $\dot{V}O_{2max}$ depends on the functional capacity and integration of systems required for oxygen supply, transport, delivery, and use.

INTEGRATIVE QUESTION

Respond to a student who asks: "At what exercise level does the body switch to anaerobic energy metabolism?"

Maximal Oxygen Consumption

FIGURE 7.5 depicts oxygen consumption during a series of constant-speed runs up six progressively steeper hills. The laboratory simulates these hills by increasing treadmill or step bench elevation or increasing the resistance to pedaling a bicycle ergometer. Each successive hill requires a greater energy output that places an additional demand on the capacity for aerobic ATP resynthesis. During the first several hills, oxygen consumption increases rapidly, with each new steady-rate value in direct proportion to exercise severity. The runner maintains speed up the two last hills, but oxygen consumption fails to increase as rapidly or to the same extent as with the previous hills. No increase in oxygen consumption occurs during the run up the last hill. *The region where oxygen consumption plateaus or increases only slightly with additional increases in exercise intensity represents the **maximal oxygen consumption**—also called maximal oxygen uptake, maximal aerobic power, aerobic capacity, or, simply $\dot{V}O_{2max}$.* Performing more-intense exercise results only from energy transfer in glycolysis, with resulting lactate accumulation. Under these conditions, the runner soon becomes exhausted and unable to continue.

The $\dot{V}O_{2max}$ provides a quantitative measure of a person's *capacity* for aerobic ATP resynthesis. This makes the $\dot{V}O_{2max}$ an important determinant of how well a person can sustain high-intensity exercise for longer than 4 or 5 minutes. Attainment of a high $\dot{V}O_{2max}$ has important physiologic meaning in addition to its role in sustaining energy metabolism. High aerobic power requires the integrated and high-level response of physiologic support systems illustrated in FIGURE 7.6. In subsequent chapters, we discuss various aspects of $\dot{V}O_{2max}$, including its physiologic significance, measurement, and role in exercise performance and cardiovascular health.

IN A PRACTICAL SENSE

INTERPRETING $\dot{V}O_{2max}$—ESTABLISHING CARDIOVASCULAR FITNESS CATEGORIES

■ Cardiovascular fitness reflects the maximal amount of oxygen consumed during each minute of near-maximal exercise. Values for maximal oxygen consumption, or $\dot{V}O_{2max}$, generally are expressed in milliliters of oxygen per kilogram of body mass per minute ($mL \cdot kg^{-1} \cdot min^{-1}$). Individual values can range from about $10 \; mL \cdot kg^{-1} \cdot min^{-1}$ in cardiac patients to 80 or $90 \; mL \cdot kg^{-1} \cdot min^{-1}$ in world-class runners and cross-country skiers. Men and women distance runners, swimmers, cyclists, and cross-country skiers generally attain $\dot{V}O_{2max}$ values nearly double those of sedentary persons (see Fig. 11.8).

Researchers have measured the $\dot{V}O_{2max}$ of thousands of individuals of different ages. The average values and respective ranges for men and women of different ages establish category values to classify individuals for cardiovascular fitness. The table presents a five-part classification based on data from the literature for non-athletes.

CARDIOVASCULAR FITNESS CLASSIFICATIONS

GENDER	AGE	POOR	FAIR	AVERAGE	GOOD	EXCELLENT
Men	≤29	≤24.9	25–33.9	34–43.9	44–52.9	≥53
	30–39	≤22.9	23–30.9	31–41.9	42–49.9	≥50
	40–49	≤19.9	20–26.9	27–38.9	39–44.9	≥45
	50–59	≤17.9	18–24.9	25–37.9	38–42.9	≥43
	60–69	≤15.9	16–22.9	23–35.9	36–40.9	≥41
Women	≤29	≤23.9	24–30.9	31–38.9	39–48.9	≥49
	30–39	≤19.9	20–27.9	28–36.9	37–44.9	≥45
	40–49	≤16.9	17–24.9	25–34.9	35–41.9	≥42
	50–59	≤14.9	15–21.9	22–33.9	34–39.9	≥40
	60–69	≤12.9	13–20.9	21–32.9	33–36.9	≥37

Fast- and Slow-Twitch Muscle Fibers

Extracting about 20 to 40 mg of tissue (the size of a grain of rice) during surgical biopsy gives exercise physiologists the means to study functional and structural characteristics of human skeletal muscle. Two distinct types of muscle fiber exist in humans. A **fast-twitch (FT)** or **type II** fiber has two primary subdivisions, type IIa and type IIb; each possesses rapid contraction speed and high capacity for anaerobic ATP production in glycolysis. The type IIa fiber also possesses somewhat high aerobic capacity. Type II fibers become active during change-of-pace and stop-and-go activities such as basketball, field hockey, lacrosse, soccer, and ice hockey. They also contribute increased force output when running or cycling up a hill while maintaining a constant speed or during all-out effort that requires rapid, powerful movements that depend almost exclusively on energy from anaerobic metabolism.

The second fiber type, the **slow-twitch (ST)** or **type I** muscle fiber, generates energy primarily through aerobic pathways. This fiber possesses a relatively slow contraction speed compared with its fast-twitch counterpart. Its capacity to generate ATP aerobically intimately relates to numerous large mitochondria and high levels of enzymes required for aerobic metabolism, particularly fatty acid catabolism. Slow-twitch muscle fibers primarily sustain continuous activities requiring a steady rate of aerobic energy transfer. Fatigue in prolonged running is associated with glycogen depletion in the leg muscles' type I and type IIa muscle fibers.[2,22] This selective glycogen depletion pattern also occurs in the arms of wheelchair-dependent athletes during extended exercise durations.[44] More than likely, the predominance of slow-twitch muscle fibers greatly contributes to high blood lactate thresholds observed among elite endurance athletes. FIGURE 7.7 illustrates the muscle fiber type composition of two athletes in sports that rely on distinctly different energy transfer systems favored by a specific fiber type predominance. For the 50-m sprint swim champion, type II fibers represent nearly 80% of the total muscle fibers, whereas the endurance cyclist possesses 80% type I fibers. From a practical perspective, most sports require relatively slow, sustained muscle actions interspersed with short

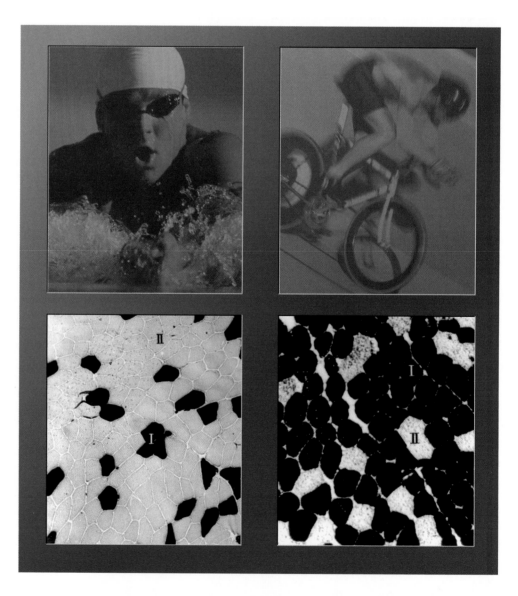

Figure 7.7 Differences in muscle-fiber type composition between a sprint swimmer and endurance cyclist. The type I and type II muscle fibers were sampled from the vastus lateralis muscle and stained for myofibrillar ATPase after incubation at pH 4.3. Type I fibers stain dark, while type II fibers remain unstained. (Photos and photomicrographs courtesy of Dr. R. Billeter, Department of Anatomy, University of Bern, Switzerland.)

bursts of powerful effort (e.g., basketball, soccer, field hockey). These activities require activation of both muscle fiber types.

The preceding discussion suggests that a muscle's predominant fiber type significantly contributes to success in certain sports or physical activities. Chapter 18 explores this idea more fully, including other considerations concerning metabolic, contractile, and fatigue characteristics of each fiber type, the various subdivisions, proposed classification system, and effects of exercise training.

ENERGY SPECTRUM OF EXERCISE

FIGURE 7.8 illustrates the relative contribution of anaerobic and aerobic energy sources related to maximal exercise duration. TABLE 7.1 also shows the relative contributions of the major energy fuels during various running competitions. These data based on laboratory experiments involving all-out running readily transpose to other activities by drawing the appropriate time relationships. For example, a 100-m sprint run corresponds to any all-out exercise for 10 seconds, while an 800-m run and 200-m swim last about 2 minutes. All-out 1-minute exercise includes the 400-m run, the 100-m swim, and repeated full-court presses at the end of a basketball game.

The allocation of energy for exercise from each form of energy transfer progresses along a continuum. At one extreme, the intramuscular high-energy phosphates supply almost all of the energy for exercise. The ATP–PCr and lactic acid systems supply about one half the energy for intense exercise lasting 2 minutes; aerobic reactions supply the remainder. To excel under these conditions requires a well-developed capacity for both anaerobic and aerobic metabolism. Intense exercise of intermediate duration performed for 5 to 10 minutes (e.g., middle-distance running and swimming, or

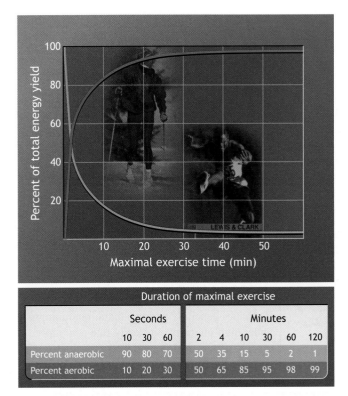

Duration of maximal exercise								
	Seconds			Minutes					
	10	30	60	2	4	10	30	60	120
Percent anaerobic	90	80	70	50	35	15	5	2	1
Percent aerobic	10	20	30	50	65	85	95	98	99

Figure 7.8 Relative contribution of aerobic and anaerobic energy metabolism during maximal physical effort of various durations. Note that 2 minutes of maximal effort requires about 50% of the energy from combined aerobic and anaerobic processes. A world-class 4-minute-mile pace derives approximately 65% of its energy from aerobic metabolism, with the remainder generated from anaerobic processes. A 2-hour and 30-minute marathon, in contrast, generates almost all of its energy from aerobic processes. (Adapted from Åstrand PO, Rodahl K. Textbook of work physiology. New York: McGraw-Hill, 1977.)

TABLE 7.1 ■ ESTIMATE OF THE PERCENT CONTRIBUTION OF DIFFERENT FUELS TO ATP GENERATION IN VARIOUS RUNNING EVENTS

	PERCENT CONTRIBUTION TO ATP GENERATION				
		GLYCOGEN		BLOOD GLUCOSE	TRIACYLGLYCEROL
EVENT	PHOSPHOCREATINE	ANAEROBIC	AEROBIC	(LIVER GLYCOGEN)	(FATTY ACIDS)
100 m	50	50	—	—	—
200 m	25	65	10	—	—
400 m	12.5	62.5	25	—	—
800 m	6	50	44	—	—
1500 m	a	25	75	—	—
5000 m	a	12.5	87.5	—	—
10,000 m	a	3	87	—	—
Marathon	—	—	75	5	20
Ultramarathon (80 km)	—	—	35	5	60
24-h race	—	—	10	2	88
Soccer game	10	70	20	—	—

a In such events phosphocreatine is used for the first few seconds and, if it has been resynthesized during the race, in the sprint to the finish. From Newsholme EA, et al. Physical and mental fatigue: metabolic mechanisms and importance of plasma amino acids. Br Med Bull 1992;48:477.

basketball) places greater demand on aerobic energy transfer. Long-duration marathon running, distance swimming, cycling, recreational jogging, and hiking and trekking require a constant aerobic energy supply with little reliance on energy from anaerobic sources.

An understanding of the energy demands of diverse physical activities helps to explain why a world-record holder in the 1-mile run does not necessarily excel in distance running. Conversely, premier marathon runners rarely run 1 mile in less than 4 minutes yet complete 26.2 miles at a 5-minute-per-mile pace. The appropriate approach to exercise training analyzes an activity for its specific energy components and then formulates training strategies to ensure optimal adaptations in physiologic and metabolic function. *Improved capacity for energy transfer usually translates into improved exercise performance.*

INTEGRATIVE QUESTION

If athletes generally perform marathon running under high-intensity but steady-rate conditions, explain why some have reduced capacity to sprint to the finish at race end.

OXYGEN CONSUMPTION DURING RECOVERY

Following exercise, bodily processes do not immediately return to resting levels. Following relatively light, short-duration physical effort, recovery proceeds rapidly and unnoticed. In contrast, stressful exercise such as running a one-half mile race or swimming 200 yards as fast as possible, requires considerable time for resting metabolism to recover. How well an individual responds in recovery from light, moderate, and strenuous exercise depends upon specific metabolic and physiologic processes during and in recovery from each form of effort.

FIGURE 7.9 illustrates oxygen consumption during exercise and recovery from different exercise intensities. Light exercise (A), with rapid attainment of steady-rate oxygen consumption, produces a small oxygen deficit. The magnitude of recovery oxygen consumption approximates the size of the oxygen deficit at the beginning of exercise. Recovery proceeds rapidly. Oxygen consumption follows a logarithmic curve, decreasing by about 50% over each subsequent 30-second period until reaching the preexercise level.

Oxygen consumption during steady-rate and non-steady-rate (intense) exercise and recovery plot as a logarithmic function in relation to time.[6,50] The function increases in exercise or decreases in recovery by some constant fraction for each unit of time as oxygen consumption approaches an asymptote, or level value. Consider the example of recovery from 10 minutes of light, steady-rate exercise at an oxygen consumption of 2000 mL · min^{-1}. If recovery oxygen consumption decreased by one half over 30 seconds, then oxygen consumption would equal 1000 mL · min^{-1} at 30-seconds recovery and 500 mL · min^{-1} at 60 seconds, with the resting value of 250 mL · min^{-1} achieved in about 90 seconds.

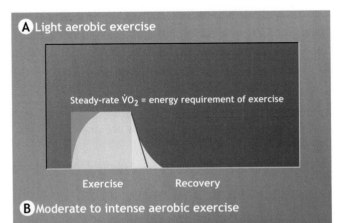

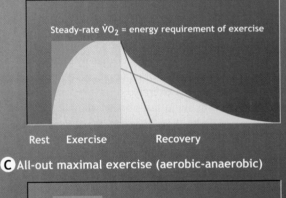

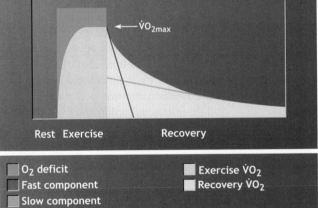

Figure 7.9 Oxygen consumption during exercise and in recovery from (**A**) light steady-rate exercise, (**B**) moderate-to-intense steady-rate exercise, and (**C**) exhaustive exercise that does not produce a steady rate of aerobic metabolism. Note that in exhaustive exercise, the exercise oxygen requirement significantly exceeds the actual exercise oxygen consumption.

Moderate-to-intense aerobic exercise (Fig. 7.9B) requires a longer time to achieve steady rate, which creates a larger oxygen deficit than less-intense exercise. Consequently, it takes longer for oxygen consumption to return to the resting recovery level. The oxygen consumption recovery curve demonstrates an initial rapid decline (similar to recovery from light exercise) followed by a more gradual decline to baseline resting levels. In Figure 7-9A and B, the oxygen deficit and recovery oxygen consumption are computed by using the steady-rate oxygen consumption to represent the oxygen (energy) requirement of exercise. Figure 7.9C shows that exhaustive exercise does not produce a steady rate of aerobic metabolism. Such exercise demands a larger energy requirement than supplied by aerobic processes. Under these conditions, anaerobic energy transfer increases and blood lactate accumulates, with considerable time required to achieve complete recovery. Failure to achieve steady-rate oxygen consumption makes it unfeasible to quantify the true oxygen deficit accurately.

Each of the curves in Figure 7.9 shows that oxygen consumption in recovery always exists in excess of the resting value, regardless of exercise intensity. The excess has classically been termed the **oxygen debt** or more appropriately, **recovery oxygen consumption** (indicated by the yellow shaded area under each recovery curve). It computes as the total oxygen consumed in recovery minus the total oxygen theoretically consumed at rest during the recovery period. For example, if a total of 5.5 L of oxygen was consumed in recovery until attaining the resting value of $0.310 \text{ L} \cdot \text{min}^{-1}$, and recovery required 10 minutes, the recovery oxygen consumption would equal 5.5 L minus 3.1 L ($0.310 \text{ L} \times 10$ min) or 2.4 L. This indicates that the preceding exercise caused physiologic alterations during exercise *and* recovery that required an additional 2.4 L of oxygen before oxygen consumption returned to the preexercise resting level. The inference assumes that resting oxygen consumption remains unchanged during exercise and recovery. As we discuss below, this assumption is not entirely correct, particularly following strenuous exercise.

The curves in Figure 7.9 illustrate two important characteristics of recovery oxygen consumption:

1. With mild aerobic exercise of relatively short duration (little disruption in body temperature and hormonal milieu), about one half of the total recovery oxygen consumption occurs within 30 seconds, with complete recovery within several minutes. The decline in oxygen consumption follows a single-component exponential curve termed the **fast component** of recovery oxygen consumption.

2. Recovery from strenuous exercise presents a different picture because blood lactate, body temperature, and thermogenic hormone levels increase substantially. In addition to the fast component of the recovery phase, a second phase of recovery, termed the **slow component,** exists. Depending on the intensity and duration of the previous exercise, the slow component can take up to 24 hours to return to preexercise oxygen consumption.[5,23,42] Even with shorter, intermittent bouts of "supermaximal" exercise (e.g., three 2-min bouts at 108% $\dot{V}O_{2max}$ interspersed with a 3-min rest), recovery oxygen consumption remains elevated for 1 hour or longer.[4]

Aerobic training accelerates the recovery rate. Trained subjects show a faster rate of recovery oxygen consumption to baseline when exercising at either the same absolute or relative exercise intensities as untrained counterparts.[43] More than likely, training adaptations that facilitate the rapid achievement of steady rate also facilitate recovery.

Metabolic Dynamics of Recovery Oxygen Consumption

A precise biochemical explanation for the recovery oxygen consumption, particularly the role of lactate, remains elusive because no comprehensive explanation exists about specific contributory factors.

Traditional Concepts

In 1922, Nobel laureate Archibald Vivian Hill and colleagues first coined the term *oxygen debt*. These scientists discussed energy metabolism during exercise and recovery in financial–accounting terms.[28] Within this framework, the body's carbohydrate stores were likened to energy "credits." Expending stored credits during exercise incurred an energy "debt." The greater the energy "deficit" (use of available stored energy credits), the larger the energy debt. Hill believed that the recovery oxygen consumption represented the cost of repaying this debt—hence the term *oxygen debt*.

Lactate accumulation from the anaerobic component of exercise represented use of glycogen, the stored energy credit. The ensuing oxygen debt served two purposes: (1) reestablishing the original glycogen stores (credits) by synthesizing approximately 80% of the lactate back to glycogen in the liver (Cori cycle) and (2) catabolizing the remaining lactate through the pyruvate–citric acid cycle pathway. The ATP generated in this process presumably powered glycogen resynthesis from lactate. This early explanation of the dynamics of recovery oxygen consumption was subsequently termed the "lactic acid theory of oxygen debt."

In 1933, following the work of Hill, researchers at the Harvard Fatigue Laboratory explained their observation that the initial phase of recovery oxygen consumption ended before blood lactate began to decline.[38] They showed that one could incur an oxygen debt of almost 3 L without any appreciable blood lactate accumulation. To resolve these findings, they proposed two phases of oxygen debt: (1) **alactic (or alactacid) oxygen debt** (without lactate buildup) and (2) **lactic acid** or (**lactacid**) **oxygen debt** associated with elevated blood lactate levels. They based these two explanations on speculation because they could not measure ATP and PCr replenishment or the relationship between blood lactate and glucose and glycogen levels. For nearly 65 years, the following model served to explain the energetics of oxygen debt:

- **Alactacid debt:** The alactacid portion of the oxygen debt depicted in the recovery from light, steady-rate exercise in Figure 7.9A or rapid phase of recovery from more strenuous exercise (Fig. 7.9B and C), resulted from restoration of the intramuscular high-energy phosphates ATP and PCr depleted during exercise. This restoration came from the aerobic breakdown of the stored macronutrients during recovery. A small portion of the recovery oxygen consumption also reloaded muscle myoglobin and hemoglobin in blood returning from previously active tissues.

- **Lactacid debt:** In keeping with A. V. Hill's explanation, most of the lactacid oxygen debt represented the reconversion of lactate to glycogen in the liver.

Controversy with Traditional Explanation of Oxygen Debt. Several relationships must exist to support the contention that (1) anaerobic energy sources temporarily compensate for an aerobic energy deficit during exercise and (2) the recovery oxygen consumption reflects the magnitude of the anaerobic energy contribution in exercise. For example, only a moderate relationship exists between the oxygen deficit and the excess oxygen consumption in recovery (oxygen debt). To accept the traditional explanation for the lactacid phase of the oxygen debt, one must show that most lactate accumulated in exercise actually contributes to glycogen resynthesis in recovery as Hill and others had speculated. This has never been shown. In experiments with humans, no substantial replenishment of glycogen occurred 10 minutes following strenuous exercise, even though blood lactate levels decreased significantly. *This suggests that most lactate oxidizes for energy* (see "Focus on Research"). This occurs because heart, liver, kidney, and skeletal muscle tissues use lactate as an energy substrate during exercise *and* recovery.

Contemporary Concepts

The elevated aerobic metabolism in recovery restores the body to its preexercise condition. In short-duration, light-to-moderate exercise, recovery oxygen consumption generally replenishes the high-energy phosphates depleted by exercise. Recovery typically proceeds rapidly within several minutes. In longer-duration (>60 min), high-intensity aerobic exercise, recovery oxygen consumption remains elevated considerably longer.[9] FIGURE 7.10 clearly illustrates the effect of exercise duration on the magnitude of recovery oxygen consumption. Eight trained women walked at 70% of $\dot{V}O_{2max}$ for 20, 40, or 60 minutes. Recovery oxygen consumption, also termed **excess postexercise oxygen consumption** (EPOC), totaled 8.6 L for the 20-minute exercise period and 9.8 L for the 40-minute session, while the cost of recovery from the 60-minute workout nearly doubled to 15.2 L. The increase in EPOC in each bout of steady-rate exercise did not relate to lactate accumulation. Rather, other disequilibriums in physiologic function elevate the recovery metabolism.

In exhaustive exercise with its significant anaerobic component and lactate accumulation, a small portion of EPOC resynthesizes lactate to glycogen. This gluconeogenic mechanism also progresses during exercise, particularly among trained individuals.[17,37] As expected, the main source for replenishing glycogen remains dietary carbohydrate, not

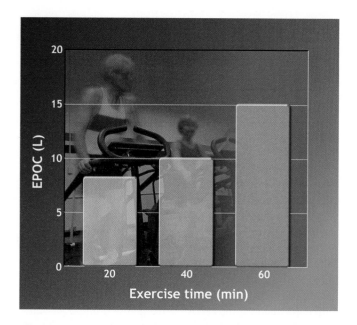

Figure 7.10 Total excess postexercise oxygen consumption (EPOC) during a 3-hour recovery from 20, 40, and 60 minutes of treadmill walking at 70% $\dot{V}O_{2max}$. EPOC for the 60-minute exercise significantly exceeded the 20- or 40-minute workouts. (From Quinn TJ, et al. Postexercise oxygen consumption in trained females: effect of exercise duration. Med Sci Sports Exerc 1994;26:908.)

resynthesized lactate. A significant component of EPOC relates to physiologic processes that take place *during* recovery, in addition to metabolic events during exercise. Such factors likely account for the considerably larger oxygen debt than oxygen deficit in prolonged aerobic exercise and exhaustive anaerobic exercise. Body temperature, for example, rises about 3°C (5.4°F) during a long bout of intense aerobic exercise and can remain elevated for several hours in recovery. Elevated body temperature directly stimulates metabolism to increase recovery oxygen consumption.

Other factors also affect EPOC. Up to 10% of the recovery oxygen consumption reloads the blood returning to the lungs from the previously active muscles. An additional 2 to 5% restores oxygen dissolved in bodily fluids and bound to myoglobin within the muscle. Ventilation volumes in recovery from intense exercise remain 8 to 10 times above the resting requirement, a cost that can equal 10% of the EPOC. The heart also works harder and requires a greater oxygen supply during recovery. Tissue repair and redistribution of calcium, potassium, and sodium ions within muscle and other body compartments also require additional energy. The residual effects of the thermogenic hormones epinephrine, norepinephrine, and thyroxine and the glucocorticoids released in exercise keep metabolism elevated for a considerable time in recovery. In essence, all of the physiologic systems activated in exercise increase their own particular need for oxygen during recovery (FIG. 7.11). EPOC is not affected by different phases of the menstrual cycle.[19] *The recovery oxygen consumption, or EPOC, reflects two factors: (1) the level of anaerobic metabolism in previous*

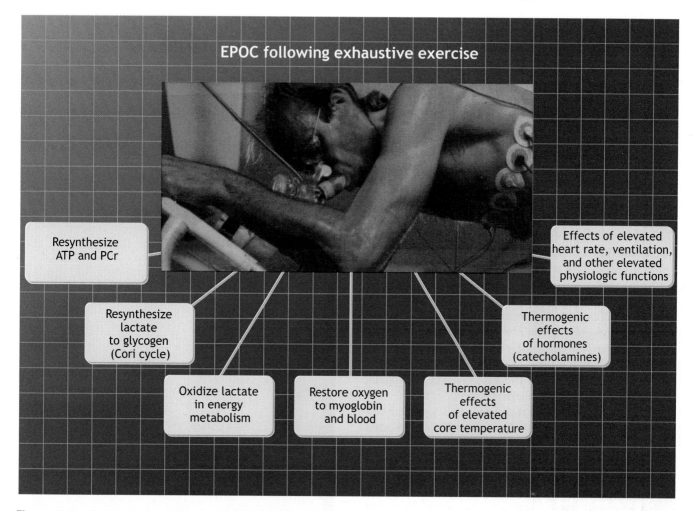

Figure 7.11   Factors that contribute to the EPOC following exhaustive exercise.

exercise and (2) the respiratory, circulatory, hormonal, ionic, and thermal adjustments that exert a metabolic influence during recovery.

Implications of EPOC for Exercise and Recovery

Understanding the dynamics of EPOC provides a basis for structuring exercise intervals and optimizing recovery. No appreciable lactate accumulates either with steady-rate aerobic exercise or with brief 5- to 10-second bouts of all-out effort powered by the intramuscular high-energy phosphates. Consequently, recovery progresses rapidly (fast component predominantly), and exercise can begin again with only a short rest period. In contrast, longer periods of anaerobic exercise produce considerable lactate buildup (in active muscles and blood), with significant disruption in physiologic functions. In such cases, EPOC consists of both a fast component and a slower component that often requires considerable time to return to baseline. Prolonged recovery between exercise intervals would impair performance in basketball, hockey, soccer, tennis, and badminton. An athlete

pushed to a high level of anaerobic metabolism may not fully recover during brief time-out periods or intermittent intervals of less-intense exercise.

Procedures for speeding recovery from exercise generally are either active or passive. In **active recovery** (often termed "cooling-down" or "tapering-off"), the individual performs submaximal exercise, believing that continued physical activity in some way prevents muscle cramps and stiffness and facilitates overall recovery. With **passive recovery**, the person usually lies down, presuming that total inactivity reduces the resting energy requirements and thus "frees" oxygen for the recovery process. Modifications of passive recovery have included massage, cold showers, specific body positions, and consuming cold liquids.

Optimal Recovery from Steady-Rate Exercise

Most persons generally perform exercise in steady rate with little lactate accumulation at oxygen consumptions below 55 to 60% of $\dot{V}O_{2max}$. Recovery entails resynthesis of high-energy phosphates; replenishment of oxygen in the blood,

FOCUS On Research

A CHALLENGE TO CONVENTIONAL WISDOM

Brooks GA, et al. Glycogen synthesis and metabolism of lactic acid after exercise. Am J Physiol 1973; 224:1162.

▲ The early research of A. V. Hill and colleagues postulated that the elevated oxygen consumption ($\dot{V}O_2$) in recovery from exercise (so-called oxygen debt) resulted from oxidation of about one fifth of the lactate produced in exercise. Lactate oxidation provided the necessary energy to resynthesize the remaining lactate to glycogen. Subsequent research by Margaria (see "Focus on Research," Chapter 9) retained this traditional "lactic acid interpretation" of the elevated $\dot{V}O_2$ in recovery from exercise. Until the 1973 publication by Brooks and coworkers, few investigators had directly challenged the conventional wisdom that lactate produced in strenuous exercise caused significant glycogen resynthesis during the postexercise repayment of the oxygen debt.

Female rats served in two experiments to test the lactic acid–oxygen debt theory. *Experiment 1* placed animals into either a sedentary group or an exercise group that ran at intensities that produced significant lactate buildup and a large postexercise $\dot{V}O_2$. Following exercise, the researchers periodically sacrificed some animals and measured glycogen, glucose, and lactate in muscle, liver, and blood during a 24-hour recovery. The *top figure* displays liver and muscle glycogen concentrations during recovery from exercise. Compared with sedentary controls *(purple and blue squares)* little glycogen remained in the muscles and liver at the end of exhaustive exercise (0 min). Furthermore, no significant glycogen resynthesis occurred in the postexercise period; liver and muscle glycogen concentrations after 24 hours' recovery did not exceed the immediate postexercise values. These findings did not support the hypothesis proposed by Hill and colleagues that the elevated postexercise $\dot{V}O_2$ largely related to glycogen resynthesis from lactate produced during exhaustive exercise.

In a parallel experiment *(experiment 2, bottom figure)*, the researchers infused ^{14}C-labeled lactate into exercise-exhausted and pair-fasted sedentary control rats. Measurements included release of labeled CO_2 in recovery to assess the fate of the infused ^{14}C-labeled lactate. If lactate resynthesized to glycogen in recovery—as proposed by the "lactic acid theory of oxygen debt"—then little of the injected isotope should have appeared in expired CO_2. Conversely, if oxidation explains the primary fate of lactate then most of the labeled carbon in the infused lactate should indeed appear as $^{14}CO_2$ in expired air. The experiment produced unequivocal results: 70 to 90% of the isotope appeared as CO_2.

Under the conditions of Brooks' experiment, glycogen resynthesis from elevated lactate did not represent a predominant process to explain the oxygen debt proposed by Hill and colleagues in the 1920s. Subsequent research by Brooks and other investigators continues to redefine and expand the biochemical and physiologic factors that affect recovery $\dot{V}O_2$.

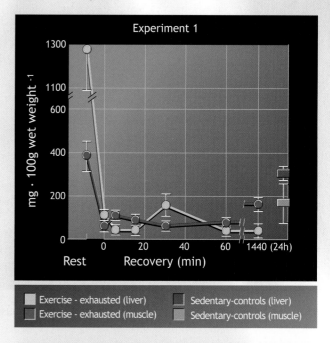

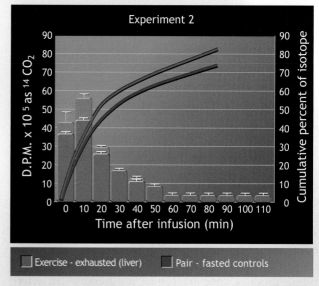

Experiment 1. Liver and muscle glycogen concentrations over time after exhaustive exercise in rats previously fasted for 10 to 12 hours. *Experiment 2.* Production of labeled CO_2 after infusion of ^{14}C-labeled lactate in exercise-exhausted and pair-fasted rats *(bar graph, left ordinate)*. Expiration of labeled CO_2 is also expressed as a cumulative percentage of ^{14}C-labeled lactate *(line graph, right ordinate)*.

bodily fluids, and muscle myoglobin; and a small energy cost to sustain elevated circulation and ventilation. Under these circumstances, passive procedures facilitate recovery because any additional exercise only serves to elevate total metabolism and delay recovery.

Optimal Recovery from Non–Steady-Rate Exercise

When exercise intensity exceeds the maximum steady-rate level, lactate formation in muscle exceeds its removal rate, and blood lactate accumulates. As exercise intensity increases, blood lactate levels rise sharply and the exerciser soon becomes exhausted. Although the precise mechanisms for exhaustion during anaerobic exercise remain unclear, blood lactate levels provide an objective indication of the relative strenuousness of exercise; they also reflect the adequacy of recovery. Because the lactate anion induces a fatiguing effect

on skeletal muscle, independent of associated reductions in pH,[29] any procedure that accelerates lactate removal probably augments subsequent exercise performance.[1]

Performing aerobic exercise in recovery accelerates blood lactate removal.[12,21] The optimal level of recovery exercise ranges between 30 and 45% $\dot{V}O_{2max}$ for bicycle exercise and 55 to 60% $\dot{V}O_{2max}$ when the recovery involves running.[40] This difference between exercise modes reflects the more localized muscle involvement in bicycling that lowers the threshold for blood lactate accumulation.

FIGURE 7.12 illustrates blood lactate recovery patterns for trained men who performed 6 minutes of supermaximal exercise on a bicycle ergometer. Active recovery involved 40 minutes of continuous exercise at either 35 or 65% $\dot{V}O_{2max}$. A combination of 65% $\dot{V}O_{2max}$ (7 min) followed by 35% $\dot{V}O_{2max}$ (33 min) evaluated whether a higher-intensity exercise interval early in recovery would expedite lactate removal. These data clearly reveal that moderate aerobic exercise performed in recovery

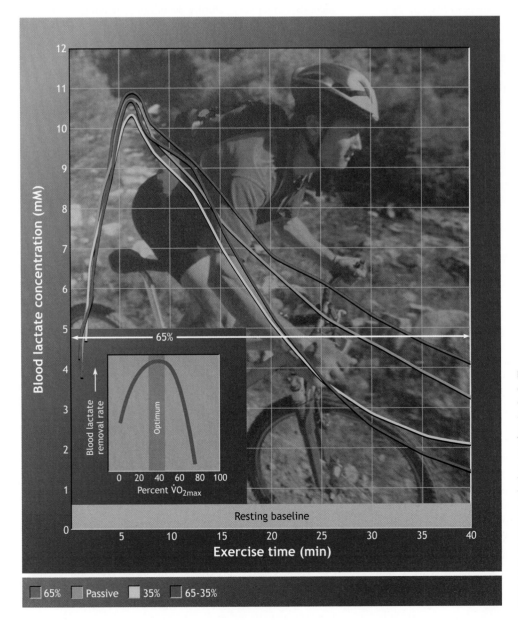

Figure 7.12 Blood lactate concentration following maximal exercise using passive recovery and active recoveries at 35%, 65%, and a combination 35 and 65% $\dot{V}O_{2max}$. The *horizontal white line* indicates the blood lactate level produced by exercise at 65% $\dot{V}O_{2max}$ without previous exercise. The *inset curve* depicts the generalized relationship between exercise intensity and rate of lactate removal. (Adapted from Dodd S, et al. Blood lactate disappearance at various intensities of recovery exercise. J Appl Physiol: Respir Environ Exerc Physiol 1984;57:1462.)

TABLE 7.2 ■ **RESULTS OF CLASSIC STUDY WITH INTERMITTENT EXERCISE**

EXERCISE–REST PERIODS	TOTAL DISTANCE RUN (YARDS)	AVERAGE OXYGEN CONSUMPTION ($L \cdot min^{-1}$)	BLOOD LACTATE LEVEL (MG $\cdot$ DL BLOOD^{-1})
4 min continuous	1422	5.6	150
10 s exercise 5 s rest	7294	5.1	44
10 s exercise 10 s rest	5468	4.4	20
15 s exercise 30 s rest	3642	3.6	16

From data of Christenson EH, et al. Intermittent and continuous running. Acta Physiol Scand 1960;60:269.

facilitates lactate removal, compared with passive recovery procedures. Combining higher-intensity followed by lower-intensity exercise provided no greater benefit than a single exercise level at moderate intensity. Performing recovery exercise above the lactate threshold offers no advantage and may even prolong recovery by initiating lactate formation and accumulation. In a practical sense, if left to their own choice, most individuals select the optimal recovery exercise intensity.

The facilitated lactate removal with active recovery likely results from increased perfusion of blood through the "lactate-using" liver and heart.[3] In addition, increased blood flow through the muscles in active recovery enhances lactate removal because this tissue readily oxidizes lactate via citric acid cycle metabolism.

Intermittent (Interval) Exercise

An approach to performing exercise that normally causes exhaustion within several minutes if performed continuously requires exercising *intermittently* using a preestablished spacing of exercise and rest intervals. The physical conditioning program of **interval training** characterizes this approach. This training applies various work-to-rest intervals, using supermaximal exercise to overload the energy transfer systems. For example, with all-out exercise of up to 8 second's duration, the intramuscular high-energy phosphates provide most of the energy with minimal reliance on the glycolytic pathway. This produces rapid recovery (alactic, fast component), enabling a subsequent bout of heavy exercise to begin, following a brief recovery.

TABLE 7.2 summarizes the results of a classic series of experiments that combined exercise and rest intervals. On one day, the subject ran at a speed that would normally exhaust him within 5 minutes. The continuous run covered about 0.8 mile, and the runner attained a $\dot{V}O_{2max}$ of 5.6 L $\cdot$ min^{-1}. A high blood lactate level (last column of the table), owing to substantial anaerobic metabolism, verified a relative state of exhaustion. On another day, he ran at the same fast speed but intermittently with periods of 10 seconds of exercise and 5

seconds of recovery. During 30 minutes of intermittent exercise, the time running amounted to 20 minutes and the distance covered equaled 4 miles, compared with less than 5 minutes and 0.8 miles with a continuous run! The effectiveness of the intermittent exercise protocol becomes even more impressive considering that the blood lactate remained low, even though oxygen consumption averaged 5.1 L $\cdot$ min^{-1} (91% $\dot{V}O_{2max}$) during the 30-minute period. Thus, a relative balance existed between the energy requirements of exercise and aerobic energy transfer within the muscles throughout the exercise and rest intervals.

Manipulating the duration of exercise and rest intervals can effectively overload a specific energy-transfer system. When the rest interval increased from 5 to 10 seconds, oxygen consumption averaged 4.4 L $\cdot$ min^{-1}; 15-second work and 30-second recovery intervals produced only a 3.6-L oxygen consumption. For each 30-minute bout of intermittent exercise, however, the runner achieved a longer distance and a substantially lower blood lactate level than when exercising continuously at the same intensity. Chapter 21 focuses on the specific application of the principles of intermittent exercise for aerobic and anaerobic training and sports performance.

Summary

1. The relative contribution of the pathways for ATP production differs, depending on exercise intensity and duration.
2. In short-duration, intense exercise (100-m dash, repetitive lifting of heavy weights), the intramuscular stores of ATP and PCr (immediate energy system) provide the energy for exercise.
3. For less intense exercise of longer duration (1 to 2 min), anaerobic reactions of glycolysis (short-term energy system) generate most of the energy.
4. As exercise progresses beyond several minutes, the aerobic system (long-term energy system) predominates.

5. Humans possess two distinct types of muscle fibers, each with unique metabolic and contractile properties: (1) low glycolytic–high oxidative, slow-twitch fibers (type I) and (2) low oxidative–high glycolytic, fast-twitch fibers (type II). Intermediate fibers of the fast-twitch type also exist, with overlapping metabolic characteristics.

6. Understanding the energy spectrum of exercise makes it possible to train for specific improvement in each of the body's energy transfer systems.

7. A steady rate of oxygen consumption represents a balance between the energy requirements of the active muscles and aerobic ATP resynthesis.

8. Oxygen deficit defines the difference between the oxygen requirement of exercise and the oxygen consumed during exercise.

9. Maximum oxygen consumption ($\dot{V}O_{2max}$) quantitatively defines a person's maximum capacity to resynthesize ATP aerobically and serves as an important indicator of physiologic functional capacity to sustain high-intensity exercise.

10. Oxygen consumption remains elevated above the resting level following exercise. Recovery oxygen consumption reflects the metabolic demands of exercise and the exercise-induced physiologic imbalances that last into recovery.

11. Moderate physical activity performed following intense exercise (active recovery) facilitates recovery, compared with passive procedures.

12. Proper spacing of the work-to-rest intervals provides a way to significantly augment exercise at an intensity that would normally prove fatiguing if performed continuously.

References are available on the Student CD and online at http://connection.lww.com/mkk6e.

Measurement of Human Energy Expenditure

8

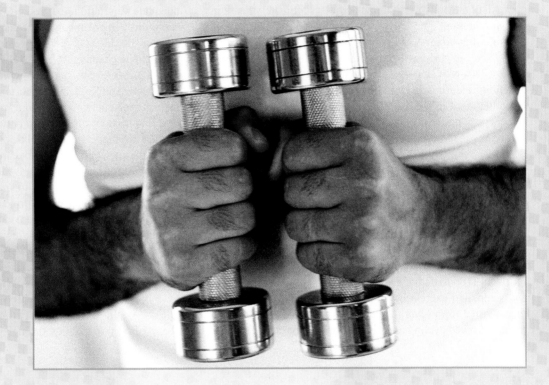

CHAPTER OBJECTIVES

- Define direct calorimetry, indirect calorimetry, closed-circuit spirometry, and open-circuit spirometry

- Diagram the closed-circuit spirometry system for oxygen consumption determinations

- Describe portable spirometry, bag technique, and computerized instrumentation systems of open-circuit spirometry

- Outline the basics of the micro-Scholander and Haldane techniques to chemically analyze expired air samples

- Discuss how the doubly labeled water technique estimates human energy expenditure and give advantages and limitations of the method

- Define respiratory quotient (RQ), and discuss its use to quantify (1) energy release in metabolism and (2) composition of the food mixture metabolized during rest and steady-rate exercise

- Discuss the difference between RQ and respiratory exchange ratio (R) and factors that affect each

METHODS OF MEASURING THE BODY'S HEAT PRODUCTION

Two different approaches, **direct calorimetry** and **indirect calorimetry**, accurately quantify human energy expenditure during rest and physical activity.

Direct Calorimetry

All of the body's metabolic processes ultimately result in heat production. The early experiments of French chemist Antoine Lavoisier (1743–1794) and his contemporaries (http://scienceworld.wolfram.com/biography/Lavoisier.html) in the 1770s provided the impetus to directly measure energy expenditure during rest and physical activity. The idea, similar to that used in the bomb calorimeter described in Chapter 4 to determine food energy, provides a convenient (though elaborate) methodology to measure heat production in humans.

In the 1890s at Wesleyan University, professors W. O. Atwater (a chemist) and E. B. Rosa (a physicist) used the first human calorimeter of major scientific importance.[1,30] Their elegant calorimetric experiments relating energy input (food consumption) to energy expenditure verified the law of the conservation of energy and established the validity of indirect calorimetry. The calorimeter, diagramed schematically in FIGURE 8.1, consisted of a chamber where a subject could live, eat, sleep, and exercise on a bicycle ergometer. The experiments lasted from several hours to 13 days, and some experiments involved cycling exercise performed for up to 16 hours

with total energy expenditure exceeding 10,000 kCal! A staff of 16, working in teams for 8- to 12-hour shifts, operated the airtight, thermally insulated calorimeter. A known volume of water at a specified temperature circulated through a series of coils at the top of the chamber; this water absorbed the heat produced and radiated by the subject. Insulation protected the entire chamber so that any change in water temperature (measured in 0.01°C with a microscope mounted alongside a thermometer) reflected the subject's energy metabolism. For adequate ventilation, exhaled air continually passed from the room through chemicals that removed moisture and absorbed carbon dioxide. Oxygen was added to the air recirculated through the chamber.

In the 100 years since the publication of the seminal papers by Atwater and Rosa, other calorimetric methods have emerged for inferring energy expenditure from metabolic gas exchange (see next section) for extended periods in respiration chambers, and via metabolic and thermal balance with water flow and airflow calorimeters.[4,7,13,19–21] For example, the modern space suit worn by astronauts during extravehicular activities represents a "suit calorimeter" designed to maintain respiratory gas exchange, thermal balance, and protection from a potentially hostile ambient environment. These suits have application for performing extended work outside an orbiting space vehicle, on the lunar surface, and, eventually, while constructing space stations or revisiting the moon in the next decade and eventually Mars.[23]

Over the years, various other heat-measuring devices have been developed, each based on a different principle of operation. In an **airflow calorimeter**, the temperature change in air that flows through an insulated space, multi-

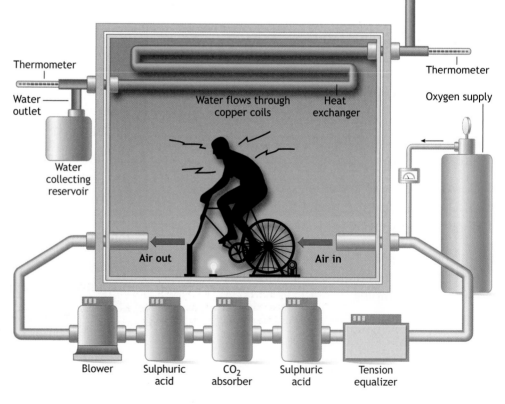

Figure 8.1 A human calorimeter directly measures the body's rate of energy metabolism (heat production). In the Atwater-Rosa calorimeter depicted, a thin sheet of copper lines the interior wall to which heat exchangers attach overhead and through which cold water passes. Water cooled to 2°C moves at a high flow rate, rapidly absorbing the heat radiated from the subject during exercise. As the subject rests, warmer water flows at a slower rate. In the original bicycle ergometer shown in the schematic, the rear wheel contacts the shaft of a generator that powers a light bulb. In later versions of ergometers, copper composed part of the rear wheel. The wheel rotated through the field of an electromagnet to produce an electric current for accurately determining power output.

Water inlet

Thermometer

Water outlet

Thermometer

Oxygen supply

Water collecting reservoir

Water flows through copper coils

Heat exchanger

Air out

Air in

Blower

Sulphuric acid

CO$_2$ absorber

Sulphuric acid

Tension equalizer

plied by the air's mass and specific heat (including calculations for evaporative heat loss), determines heat production. A **water flow calorimeter** operates similarly, except that a change in temperature occurs in water flowing through coils that make up part of an environmentally self-contained body suit worn by astronauts. **Gradient layer calorimetry** measures body heat that flows from the subject through a sheet of insulating materials (with appropriate piping and cooler water flowing on the outside of the gradient). In **storage calorimetry**, the subject sits in an insulated tank surrounded by a known mass of water at a constant temperature. The heat given off by the subject changes the temperature of the surrounding water.

Direct measurement of heat production in humans has considerable theoretical implications but limited practical applications. Accurate measurements of heat production in the calorimeter require considerable time and expense and formidable engineering expertise. Thus, calorimeters remain inapplicable for energy determinations for most sport, occupational, and recreational activities.

Indirect Calorimetry

All energy-releasing reactions in the body ultimately depend on oxygen use. Measuring a person's oxygen consumption during physical activities provides researchers with an indirect yet highly accurate estimate of energy expenditure. Compared with direct calorimetry, indirect calorimetry remains simpler and less expensive.

Studies with the bomb calorimeter show the release of approximately 4.82 kCal of energy when a mixed-diet blend of carbohydrate, lipid, and protein burns with 1 L of oxygen. Even with large variations in the metabolic mixture, this **calorific value for oxygen** varies only slightly, generally within 2 to 4%. A rounded value of 5.0 kCal per liter of oxygen consumed is an appropriate conversion factor to estimate energy expenditure under steady-rate conditions of aerobic metabolism. This energy–oxygen equivalent of 5.0 kCal per liter provides a suitable yardstick to express any aerobic physical activity in energy units (see Appendix C).

Indirect calorimetry yields results comparable to direct measurement in the human calorimeter. **Closed-circuit spirometry** and **open-circuit spirometry** represent the two applications of indirect calorimetry.

 INTEGRATIVE QUESTION

What rationale underlies early experiments that quantified energy metabolism of small animals by measuring the rate that ice melted in a container surrounding the animal?

Closed-Circuit Spirometry

FIGURE 8.2 illustrates the technique of closed-circuit spirometry developed in the late 1800s and currently used in hospitals and research laboratories to estimate resting energy expenditure. The subject breathes 100% oxygen from a prefilled container (spirometer). The equipment is a closed system because the subject rebreathes only the gas in the spirometer. A canister of potassium hydroxide (soda lime) placed in the breathing circuit absorbs the carbon dioxide in the exhaled air. A drum attached to the spirometer revolves at a known speed to record the oxygen removed (oxygen consumption) from changes in the system's total volume.

During exercise, closed-circuit spirometry measurement becomes problematic. The subject must remain close to the bulky equipment, the circuit offers considerable resistance to accommodate the large breathing volumes during exercise, and carbon dioxide removal lags behind its production rate during intense exercise. For these reasons, open-circuit spirometry remains the most widely used laboratory procedure to measure exercise oxygen consumption.

Open-Circuit Spirometry

The open-circuit method provides a relatively simple way to measure oxygen consumption. A subject inhales ambient air with a constant composition of 20.93% oxygen, 0.03% carbon dioxide, and 79.04% nitrogen (includes a small quantity of inert gases). The changes in oxygen and carbon dioxide percentages in expired air compared with the percentages in inspired ambient air indirectly reflect the ongoing process of energy metabolism. Thus, analysis of two factors—the volume of air breathed during a specified time and the composition of exhaled air—provides a practical way to measure oxygen consumption and infer energy expenditure.

Three common indirect calorimetry procedures measure oxygen consumption during physical activity:

- Portable spirometry
- Bag technique
- Computerized instrumentation

Portable Spirometry

Two German scientists in the early 1940s perfected a lightweight, portable system (first devised by German respiratory physiologist Nathan Zuntz [1847–1920] at the turn of the century) to determine energy expenditure indirectly during physical activity.[15] The activities included war-related operations such as traveling over different terrain with full battle gear, operating transportation vehicles including tanks and aircraft, and performing physical tasks that soldiers encounter during combat operations. With this system, the subject carries the 3-kg box-shaped apparatus shown in FIGURE 8.3 on the back like a backpack. The subject inspires ambient air through a two-way breathing valve, while expired air exits through a gas meter. The meter measures the total expired air volume and simultaneously collects a small gas sample for later analysis of oxygen and carbon dioxide content. These values determine oxygen consumption and energy expenditure for the measurement period.

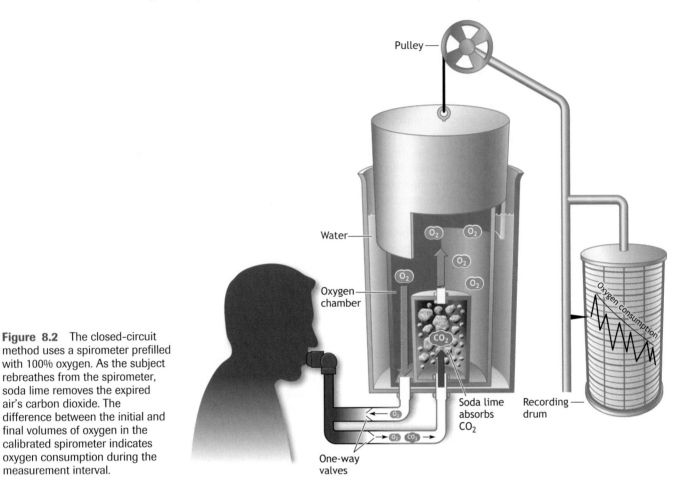

Figure 8.2 The closed-circuit method uses a spirometer prefilled with 100% oxygen. As the subject rebreathes from the spirometer, soda lime removes the expired air's carbon dioxide. The difference between the initial and final volumes of oxygen in the calibrated spirometer indicates oxygen consumption during the measurement interval.

Carrying the portable spirometer allows considerable freedom of movement in physical activities as diverse as mountain climbing, downhill skiing, sailing, golf, and common household activities (Appendix C). The equipment becomes cumbersome during vigorous activity, and the meter begins to underrecord airflow volume during intense exercise with rapid breathing.[17]

Bag Technique

FIGURE 8.4A and B depicts the classic bag technique. The subject in Figure 8.4A rides a stationary bicycle ergometer, wearing headgear attached to a two-way, high-velocity, low-resistance breathing valve. He breathes ambient air through one side of the valve and expels it through the other side. The expired air then passes into either large plastic or canvas Douglas bags (named for the distinguished British respiratory physiologist Claude G. Douglas [1882–1963]) or rubber meteorological balloons or directly through a gas meter that continually measures expired air volume. The meter draws off a small sample of expired air for subsequent analysis of O_2 and CO_2 composition. Figure 8.4B illustrates oxygen consumption measured by the bag technique while the subject lifts boxes of different weights and sizes to evaluate the energy requirement of a specific occupational task. The technique also has determined energy expenditure during common household and garden tasks.[10]

Computerized Instrumentation

With advances in computer and microprocessor technology, the exercise scientist can rapidly measure metabolic and physiologic responses to exercise, although questions have recently been raised concerning the accuracy of a widely used computerized breath-by-breath system.[9] A computer interfaces with at least three instruments: a system to continuously sample the subject's expired air, a flow-measuring device to record air volume breathed, and oxygen and carbon dioxide analyzers to measure the expired gas mixture's composition. The computer performs metabolic calculations based on electronic signals it receives from the instruments. A printed or graphic display of the data appears throughout the measurement period. More-advanced systems include automated blood pressure, heart rate, and temperature monitors, including preset instructions to regulate speed, duration, and exercise intensity with a treadmill, bicycle ergometer, stepper, rower, swim flume, or other exercise apparatus. FIGURE 8.5 depicts a computerized system to assess and monitor metabolic and physiologic responses during exercise.

Computerized systems offer tremendous advantages in ease of operation and speed of data analysis, but distinct disadvantages also exist.[3,32] These include the high cost of equipment and delays from system breakdowns. Of course, good results require good data. *Regardless of the apparent sophistication of a particular automated system, the output data still reflect the accuracy of the measuring device.*

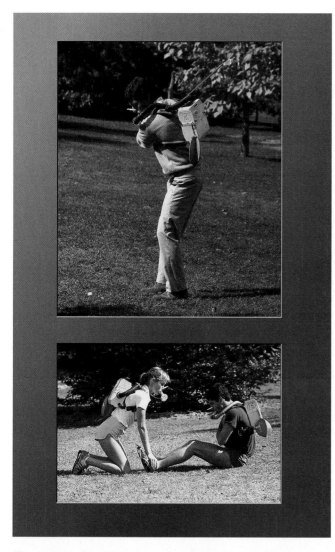

Figure 8.3 Portable spirometer to measure oxygen consumption via the open-circuit method during golf and calisthenics exercise.

Therefore, accuracy and validity of measurement devices require careful and frequent calibration using established reference standards.

INTEGRATIVE QUESTION

Discuss the common energy basis to equate food intake and physical activity.

Chemical Gas Analyzers for Calibration Purposes.

FIGURE 8.6 illustrates two common chemical procedures to analyze gas mixtures for oxygen, carbon dioxide, and nitrogen and for calibrating and/or validating electronic analyzers. The **micro-Scholander** technique measures oxygen and carbon dioxide concentration in expired air to an accuracy of ± 0.015 mL per 100 mL of gas.[22] A skilled technician can perform one analysis of a 0.5-mL microsample of the gas in about 10 minutes. The **Haldane** method provides another technique for gas analysis.[11] It uses a larger air sample and requires between 10 and 15 minutes to complete one analysis.

Before the conversion to electronic and computerized instrumentation, oxygen consumption determinations used either the Scholander or Haldane gas analysis methods. These methods involved hundreds of time-consuming separate analyses for a single experiment, with frequent duplicate measurements to verify results. This partly explains why energy metabolism studies from the early exercise physiology literature often only relied on one or two subjects and took so long to complete. When performed properly with attention to detail, these chemical analyzers produced highly accurate and reliable data. Chemical gas analyzers should verify the accuracy of the more modern electronic gas analyzers.

INTEGRATIVE QUESTION

Justify measuring only CO_2 production to estimate energy expenditure during steady-rate exercise.

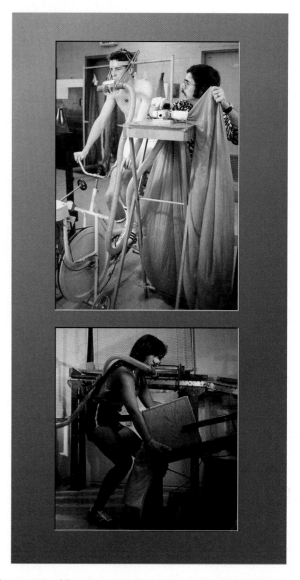

Figure 8.4 Measurement of oxygen consumption with open-circuit spirometry (classic bag technique) during (**A**) stationary cycle-ergometer exercise and (**B**) box loading and unloading.

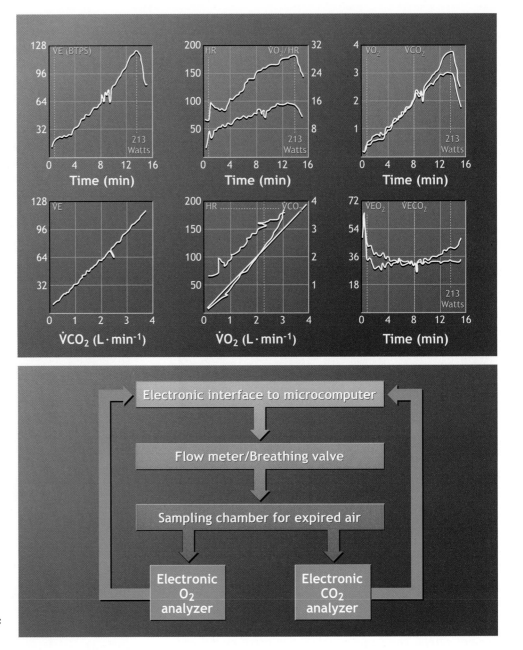

Figure 8.5 Computer systems approach to collect, analyze, and monitor physiologic and metabolic data.

Direct Versus Indirect Calorimetry

Comparisons of energy metabolism with direct and indirect calorimetry provide convincing evidence for the validity of the indirect method. Research in the early part of the 19th century compared the two methods of calorimetry over 40 days on three men who lived in a calorimeter similar to the one shown in Figure 8.1. Daily energy expenditure averaged 2723 kCal when measured directly by heat production and 2717 kCal when computed indirectly by closed-circuit oxygen consumption measures. Other experiments with animals and humans, using moderate (steady-rate) exercise, also showed close agreement between direct and indirect methods; in most instances, the difference averaged less than ± 1%. In Atwater and Rosa's calorimetry experiments, the error of the method averaged only ± 0.2%. This remarkable achievement, using

mostly handmade instruments, resulted from these scientists' dedication to precise calibration methods long before the availability of electronic instrumentation.

DOUBLY LABELED WATER TECHNIQUE

The doubly labeled water technique provides an isotope-based method to estimate total daily energy expenditure of groups of children and adults in free-living conditions without the normal constraints imposed by laboratory procedures.[6,24,25,27,33] Because of the expense in using doubly labeled water and the need for sophisticated measurement equipment, few studies routinely use this method and subject number remains small. Nevertheless, its measurement does serve as a criterion or standard to validate other methods that estimate total daily energy expenditure over prolonged periods.[2,5,8,17,23,28]

The subject consumes a quantity of water with a known concentration of the stable isotopes of hydrogen (^2H or deuterium) and oxygen (^{18}O or oxygen-18)—hence the term **doubly labeled water**. The isotopes distribute throughout all bodily fluids. Labeled hydrogen leaves the body as water (^2H_2O) in sweat, urine, and pulmonary water vapor, while labeled oxygen leaves as both water ($H_2^{18}O$) and carbon dioxide ($C^{18}O_2$) produced during macronutrient oxidation in energy metabolism. Differences between elimination rates of the two isotopes (determined by an isotope ratio mass spectrometer) relative to the body's normal background levels estimate total CO_2 production during the measurement period. Oxygen consumption is easily estimated on the basis of CO_2 production and an assumed (or measured) RQ value of 0.85 (see next section).

Under normal circumstances, analysis of the subject's urine or saliva before consuming the doubly labeled water serves as the control baseline values for ^{18}O and ^2H. Ingested isotopes require about 5 hours to distribute throughout the body water. The researchers then measure the enriched urine or saliva sample initially and then every day (or week) thereafter for the study's duration, which is usually up to 3 weeks. The progressive decrease in the sample concentrations of the two isotopes permits computation of the CO_2 production rate.[26] Accuracy of the doubly labeled water technique versus directly measured energy expenditure in controlled settings averages between 3 and 5%. This magnitude of error probably increases in field studies, particularly among physically active individuals.[31]

The doubly labeled water technique provides an ideal way to assess total energy expenditure of individuals over prolonged periods including bed rest and extreme activities like climbing Mt. Everest, cycling the Tour de France, trekking across Antarctica, military activities, extravehicular activities in space, and endurance running and swimming.[12,18,29] Drawbacks to the method include the cost of enriched ^{18}O and expense incurred in spectrometric analysis of both isotopes.

RESPIRATORY QUOTIENT

Research in the early part of the 20th century uncovered a way to evaluate the metabolic mixture metabolized during rest and exercise from measures of pulmonary gas exchange (see "Focus on Research").[16] Because of inherent chemical differences in carbohydrate, fat, and protein composition, they require different amounts of oxygen for complete oxidation of each molecule's carbon and hydrogen atoms to the carbon dioxide and water end products. Thus, carbon dioxide produced per unit of oxygen consumed varies with the type of substrate (carbohydrate, fat, protein) catabolized. The **respiratory quotient (RQ)** describes this ratio of metabolic gas exchange as follows:

$$RQ = CO_2 \text{ produced} \div O_2 \text{ consumed}$$

The RQ provides a convenient guide to approximate the nutrient mixture catabolized for energy during rest and aerobic

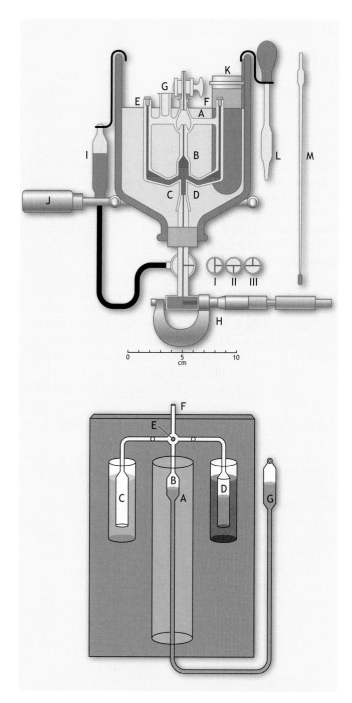

Figure 8.6 General schematic for two common analytical procedures for gas analysis. *Top.* Micro-Scholander gas analyzer. *A*, Compensating chamber; *B*, reaction chamber; *C*, side arm for CO_2 absorber; *D*, side arm for O_2 absorber; *E* and *F*, solid vaccine bottle stoppers; *G*, receptacle for stopcock; *H*, micrometer burette; *I*, leveling bulb containing mercury; *J*, handle for tilting apparatus; *K*, tube for storing the acid rinsing solution; *L*, pipette for the rinsing acid; *M*, transfer pipette. *Bottom.* Haldane gas analyzer. *A*, Water jacket surrounding the measuring burette; *B*, calibrated measuring burette containing a gas sample for measurement; *C*, vessel containing CO_2 absorber (potassium hydroxide); *D*, vessel containing O_2 absorber (pyrogallate); *E*, glass valve; *F*, entry for gas sample; *G*, mercury-leveling bulb. The gas introduced into the burette is exposed to the O_2 and CO_2 absorbers by alternately lowering and raising the mercury-leveling bulb. The O_2 and CO_2 gas volumes are determined by subtraction from the initial volume.

RESPIRATORY GAS EXCHANGE IMPLIES METABOLIC MIXTURE

Krogh A, Lindhard J. The relative value of fat and carbohydrate as sources of muscular energy. Biochem J 1920;14:290.

▲ In this 73-page research report, Nobel laureate August Krogh and colleague Johannes Lindhard made 220 determinations of respiratory gas exchange on 6 subjects (including themselves) who consumed varied diets to determine macronutrient combustion during rest and exercise. For 2 days prior to testing, subjects maintained a high-carbohydrate, low-protein diet or a high-fat, low-protein diet. Krogh and Lindhard believed that different respiratory quotients (RQs) for the same exercise under different diets would indicate the preferential use of a particular fuel substrate.

The researchers made careful energy expenditure measurements during rest and 2 hours of cycling, with a closed-circuit, air current flow-through apparatus common to that time. Subjects rode the stationary bicycle within the chamber, with appropriate tubing placed between the subject and a gas collection system outside the chamber (see figure). Typical of Krogh's research, extreme care in data collection ensured high accuracy and reliability of data. Respiratory gas exchange measurements achieved accuracy to within ± 1.0%, a remarkable figure considering his equipment was handmade.

The major research finding was that the energy expended to perform a standard physical effort varied inversely with RQ. This meant that different energy values existed for fat and carbohydrate oxidation; specifically, fat

released less energy than carbohydrate per liter of oxygen consumed during exercise. Although subjects consumed exclusively either lipid or carbohydrate (with protein held constant), RQ values did not indicate combustion of fat only or carbohydrate only. This permitted quantifying the relationship between RQ and the relative amounts of fat and carbohydrate oxidized. The researchers discovered that the percentage of total energy derived from fat oxidation approximated a straight-line function of RQ.

In a second series of experiments performed on two trained athletes during rest and exercise, the proportion of carbohydrate to fat catabolized varied with the relative availability of the two substrates. Krogh and Lindhard hypothesized that neither fat nor carbohydrate exclusively supplied energy during exercise, but that a blend of the macronutrients probably served simultaneously as fuel.

Overall, this important 1920 experiment revealed the following:

1. Efficiency of constant-load exercise is higher with carbohydrate as the energy fuel than with fat.
2. Performance deteriorates in high-intensity exercise when fat (not carbohydrate) serves as the preferential energy nutrient.
3. Preexercise nutrition influences the metabolic mixture during rest and exercise.
4. The RQ changes in the transition from rest to moderate exercise and increases with higher-intensity exercise, indicating greater reliance on carbohydrate oxidation.
5. Fat oxidation predominates during the latter portion of 1 hour of constant-intensity exercise.

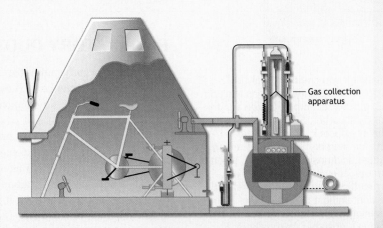

Gas collection apparatus

Unique enclosed chamber containing a cycle ergometer and two fans. The gas collection apparatus, situated outside the chamber, connects to the chamber via small-bore tubing. The chamber sits in water to ensure an airtight seal.

exercise. Also, because the caloric equivalents for oxygen differ somewhat depending on the nutrient oxidized, *precise determination of the body's heat production by indirect calorimetry requires measuring both RQ and oxygen consumption.*

RQ for Carbohydrate

The complete oxidation of one glucose molecule requires six oxygen molecules and produces six molecules of carbon dioxide and water as follows:

$$C_6H_{12}O_6 + 6\,O_2 \rightarrow 6\,CO_2 + 6\,H_2O$$
$$RQ = 6\,CO_2 \div 6\,O_2$$
$$= 1.00$$

Gas exchange during glucose oxidation produces a number of CO_2 molecules equal to the number of O_2 molecules consumed; therefore, the RQ for carbohydrate equals 1.00.

RQ for Fat

The chemical composition of fats differs from carbohydrates because fats contain considerably more hydrogen and carbon atoms than oxygen atoms. Consequently, fat catabolism requires more oxygen in relation to carbon dioxide production. For example, palmitic acid, a typical fatty acid, oxidizes to carbon dioxide and water, producing 16 carbon dioxide molecules for every 23 oxygen molecules consumed. The following equation summarizes this exchange to compute the RQ:

$$C_{16}H_{32}O_2 + 23\,O_2 \rightarrow 16\,CO_2 + 16\,H_2O$$
$$RQ = 16\,CO_2 \div 23\,O_2$$
$$= 0.696$$

Generally, a value of 0.70 represents the RQ for fat, with values ranging between 0.69 and 0.73 depending on the oxidized fatty acid's carbon-chain length.

RQ for Protein

Proteins do not simply oxidize to carbon dioxide and water during energy metabolism in the body. Rather, the liver first deaminates the amino acid molecule. The body then excretes the nitrogen and sulfur fragments in the urine, sweat, and feces. The remaining keto acid fragment oxidizes to carbon dioxide and water to provide energy for biologic work. To achieve complete combustion, these short-chain keto acids, as in fat catabolism, require more oxygen in relation to carbon dioxide produced. The protein albumin oxidizes as follows:

$$C_{72}H_{112}N_2O_{22}S + 77\,O_2 \rightarrow 63\,CO_2$$
$$+ 38\,H_2O + SO_3 + 9\,CO(NH_2)_2$$
$$RQ = 63\,CO_2 \div 77\,O_2$$
$$= 0.818$$

The general value 0.82 characterizes the RQ for protein.

Nonprotein RQ

The RQ computed from the compositional analysis of expired air usually reflects the catabolism of a blend of carbohydrates, fats, and proteins. One can determine the precise contribution of each of these nutrients to the metabolic mixture. For example, the kidneys excrete approximately 1 g of urinary nitrogen for every 5.57 (modern value) to 6.25 g (classic value) of protein metabolized for energy.[14] Each gram of excreted nitrogen represents a carbon dioxide production of approximately 4.8 L and an oxygen consumption of about 6.0 L. Within this framework, the following example illustrates the stepwise procedure to calculate the elements in the **nonprotein RQ**; that is, that portion of the respiratory exchange attributed not to the combustion of protein, but *only* to carbohydrate and fat.

This example considers data from a subject who consumes 4.0 L of oxygen and produces 3.4 L of carbon dioxide during a 15-minute rest period. During this time, the kidneys excrete 0.13 g of nitrogen in the urine.

Step 1. 4.8 L CO_2 per g protein metabolized $\times$ 0.13 g = 0.62 L CO_2 produced in protein catabolism

Step 2. 6.0 L O_2 per g protein metabolized $\times$ 0.13 g = 0.78 L O_2 consumed in protein catabolism

Step 3. Nonprotein CO_2 produced = 3.4 L CO_2 − 0.62 L CO_2 = 2.78 L CO_2

Step 4. Nonprotein O_2 consumed = 4.0 L O_2 − 0.78 L O_2 = 3.22 L O_2

Step 5. Nonprotein RQ = 2.78 ÷ 3.22 = 0.86

TABLE 8.1 presents the thermal of energy equivalents for oxygen consumption for different nonprotein RQ values and the actual percentage of fat and carbohydrate used for energy. For the nonprotein RQ of 0.86 computed in the previous example, each liter of oxygen consumed liberates 4.875 kCal. Also, for this RQ, 54.1% of the nonprotein calories derive from carbohydrate, and 45.9% come from fat. The total 15-minute heat production at rest attributable to fat and carbohydrate catabolism equals 15.70 kCal (4.875 kCal $\cdot$ L$^{-1} \times$ 3.22 L O_2); the energy from the breakdown of protein equals 3.51 kCal (4.5 kCal $\cdot$ L$^{-1} \times$ 0.78 L O_2). Consequently, the total energy from the combustion of protein and nonprotein macronutrients during the 15-minute period equals 19.21 kCal (15.70 kCal nonprotein + 3.51 kCal protein).

Interestingly, if the thermal equivalent for a mixed diet (RQ = 0.82) had been used in the caloric transformation, or if RQ had been computed from total respiratory gas exchange and applied to Table 8.1 without considering the protein component, the estimated energy expenditure would be 19.3 kCal (4.825 kCal $\cdot$ L$^{-1} \times$ 4.0 L O_2; assuming a mixed diet). This corresponds to a difference of only 0.5% from the value obtained with the more elaborate and time-consuming method requiring urinary nitrogen analysis. *In most cases, the gross metabolic nonprotein RQ calculated from pulmonary gas exchange and applied to Table 8.1 without measures of urinary and other nitrogen sources introduces only minimal error because the contribution of protein to energy metabolism usually remains small.*

TABLE 8.1 ■ THERMAL EQUIVALENTS OF OXYGEN FOR THE NONPROTEIN RQ, INCLUDING PERCENTAGE KILOCALORIES AND GRAMS DERIVED FROM CARBOHYDRATE AND FAT

NONPROTEIN RQ	kCAL PER LO$_2$	PERCENTAGE kCAL DERIVED FROM		GRAMS PER LO$_2$	
		CARBOHYDRATE	FAT	CARBOHYDRATE	FAT
0.707	4.686	0.0	100.0	0.000	0.496
0.71	4.690	1.1	98.9	0.012	0.491
0.72	4.702	4.8	95.2	0.051	0.476
0.73	4.714	8.4	91.6	0.090	0.460
0.74	4.727	12.0	88.0	0.130	0.444
0.75	4.739	15.6	84.4	0.170	0.428
0.76	4.750	19.2	80.8	0.211	0.412
0.77	4.764	22.8	77.2	0.250	0.396
0.78	4.776	26.3	73.7	0.290	0.380
0.79	4.788	29.9	70.1	0.330	0.363
0.80	4.801	33.4	66.6	0.371	0.347
0.81	4.813	36.9	63.1	0.413	0.330
0.82	4.825	40.3	59.7	0.454	0.313
0.83	4.838	43.8	56.2	0.496	0.297
0.84	4.850	47.2	52.8	0.537	0.280
0.85	4.862	50.7	49.3	0.579	0.263
0.86	4.875	54.1	45.9	0.621	0.247
0.87	4.887	57.5	42.5	0.663	0.230
0.88	4.899	60.8	39.2	0.705	0.213
0.89	4.911	64.2	35.8	0.749	0.195
0.90	4.924	67.5	32.5	0.791	0.178
0.91	4.936	70.8	29.2	0.834	0.160
0.92	4.948	74.1	25.9	0.877	0.143
0.93	4.961	77.4	22.6	0.921	0.125
0.94	4.973	80.7	19.3	0.964	0.108
0.95	4.985	84.0	16.0	1.008	0.090
0.96	4.998	87.2	12.8	1.052	0.072
0.97	5.010	90.4	9.6	1.097	0.054
0.98	5.022	93.6	6.4	1.142	0.036
0.99	5.035	96.8	3.2	1.186	0.018
1.00	5.047	100.0	0	1.231	0.000

From Zuntz N. Ueber die Bedeutung der verschiedenen Nährstoffe als Erzeuger der Muskelkraft. Arch Gesamte Physiol, Bonn, Germany: 1901; LXXXIII:557–571; Pflügers Arch Physiol,1901;83:557.

How Much Food Metabolizes for Energy?

The last two columns of Table 8.1 present conversions for the nonprotein RQ to grams of carbohydrate and fat metabolized per liter of oxygen consumed. For the subject with an RQ of 0.86, this represents approximately 0.62 g of carbohydrate and 0.25 g of fat. For the 3.22 L of oxygen consumed during the 15-minute rest period, this represents 2.0 g of carbohydrate (3.22 L O$_2$ × 0.62) and 0.80 g of fat (3.22 L O$_2$ × 0.25) metabolized for energy.

RQ for a Mixed Diet

The RQ seldom reflects the oxidation of pure carbohydrate or pure fat during activities ranging from complete bed rest to mild aerobic exercise (walking or slow jogging). Instead, catabolism of a mixture of these nutrients occurs with an RQ intermediate between 0.70 and 1.00. *For most purposes, we assume an RQ of 0.82 (metabolism of a mixture of 40% carbohydrate and 60% fat) and apply the caloric equivalent of 4.825 kCal per liter of oxygen for energy transformations.* In using 4.825, the maximum error possible in estimating energy expenditure from steady-rate oxygen consumption averages about 4%. When requiring greater precision, one must compute the actual RQ and consult Table 8.1 to obtain the exact caloric transformation and percentage contribution of carbohydrate and fat to the metabolic mixture.

INTEGRATIVE QUESTION

How have exercise physiologists determined that between 70% and 80% of the energy during the last phases of a marathon run comes from the combustion of fat?

RESPIRATORY EXCHANGE RATIO

The RQ assumes that the exchange of O_2 and CO_2 measured at the lungs reflects gas exchange from macronutrient catabolism in the cell. This assumption remains reasonably valid during rest and steady-rate exercise conditions with little reliance on anaerobic metabolism. However, several factors spuriously alter the exchange of oxygen and carbon dioxide in the lungs. When this occurs, the ratio of gas exchange no longer reflects only the substrate mixture in energy metabolism. Respiratory physiologists refer to the ratio of carbon dioxide produced to oxygen consumed under such conditions as the **respiratory exchange ratio** (**R** or **RER**). In this case, the pulmonary exchange of oxygen and carbon dioxide no longer reflects cellular oxidation of specific foods. One computes this exchange ratio in exactly the same manner as RQ.

For example, carbon dioxide elimination increases during hyperventilation because breathing increases to disproportion-

---

IN A PRACTICAL SENSE

THE WEIR METHOD TO CALCULATE ENERGY EXPENDITURE

■ In 1949, J. B. Weir, a Scottish physician and physiologist from Glasgow University, presented a simple method to estimate caloric expenditure (kCal · min^{-1}) from measures of pulmonary ventilation and expired oxygen percentage, accurate to within ±1% of the traditional respiratory quotient (RQ) method.

BASIC EQUATION

Weir showed that the following formula could calculate energy expenditure if total energy production from protein breakdown equaled 12.5% (a reasonable percentage for most people):

$$kCal \cdot min^{-1} = \dot{V}_{E(STPD)} \times (1.044 - 0.0499 \times \%O_{2E})$$

where $\dot{V}_{E(STPD)}$ represents expired minute ventilation (L · min^{-1}) corrected to STPD conditions, and $\%O_{2E}$ represents expired oxygen percentage. The value in parentheses $(1.044 - 0.0499 \times \%O_{2E})$ represents the "Weir factor." The table displays Weir factors for different $\%O_{2E}$ values.

To use the table, locate the $\%O_{2E}$ and corresponding Weir factor. Compute energy expenditure in kCal · min^{-1} by multiplying the Weir factor by $\dot{V}_{E(STPD)}$.

EXAMPLE

A person runs on a treadmill and $\dot{V}_{E(STPD)}$ = 50 L·min^{-1} and $\%O_{2E}$ = 16.0%. Compute energy expenditure by the Weir method as follows:

$$kCal \cdot min^{-1} = \dot{V}_{E(STPD)} \times (1.044 - [0.0499 \times \%O_{2E}])$$
$$= 50 \times (1.044 - [0.0499 \times 16.0])$$
$$= 50 \times 0.2456$$
$$= 12.3$$

Weir also derived the following equation to calculate kCal · min^{-1} from RQ and $\dot{V}O_2$ in L · min^{-1}:

$$kCal \cdot min^{-1} = ([1.1 \times RQ] + 3.9) \times \dot{V}O_2.$$

WEIR FACTORS

$\%O_{2E}$	Weir Factor	$\%O_{2E}$	Weir Factor
14.50	0.3205	17.00	0.1957
14.60	0.3155	17.10	0.1907
14.70	0.3105	17.20	0.1857
14.80	0.3055	17.30	0.1807
14.90	0.3005	17.40	0.1757
15.00	0.2955	17.50	0.1707
15.10	0.2905	17.60	0.1658
15.20	0.2855	17.70	0.1608
15.30	0.2805	17.80	0.1558
15.40	0.2755	17.90	0.1508
15.50	0.2705	18.00	0.1468
15.60	0.2656	18.10	0.1408
15.70	0.2606	18.20	0.1368
15.80	0.2556	18.30	0.1308
15.90	0.2506	18.40	0.1268
16.00	0.2456	18.50	0.1208
16.10	0.2406	18.60	0.1168
16.20	0.2366	18.70	0.1109
16.30	0.2306	18.80	0.1068
16.40	0.2256	18.90	0.1009
16.50	0.2206	19.00	0.0969
16.60	0.2157	19.10	0.0909
16.70	0.2107	19.20	0.0868
16.80	0.2057	19.30	0.0809
16.90	0.2007	19.40	0.0769

If $\%O_{2E}$ does not appear in the table, compute individual Weir factors as $1.044 - 0.0499 \times \%O_{2E}$. From Weir JB. New methods for calculating metabolic rates with special reference to protein metabolism. J Physiol 1949;109:1.

ately higher levels compared with metabolic demands (see Chapter 14). Overbreathing decreases the blood's normal level of carbon dioxide because this gas "blows off" from the lungs in the expired air without a corresponding increase in oxygen consumption. This creates a rise in the respiratory exchange ratio (usually above 1.00) that does not reflect macronutrient oxidation.

Exhaustive exercise presents another situation in which R rises above 1.00. Sodium bicarbonate in the blood buffers or neutralizes the lactate generated during anaerobic metabolism to maintain proper acid–base balance. Lactate buffering produces carbonic acid, a weaker acid. In the pulmonary capillaries, carbonic acid degrades to its component carbon dioxide and water molecules. Carbon dioxide readily exits the lungs in the reaction:

$$HLa + NaHCO_3 \rightarrow NaLa + H_2CO_3 \rightarrow$$
$$H_2O + CO_2 \rightarrow Lungs$$

The R increases above 1.00 because buffering adds "extra" carbon dioxide to the expired air above the quantity normally released during energy metabolism. In rare instances, the exchange ratio exceeds 1.00 when a person gains body fat through excessive dietary carbohydrate intake. In this lipogenic situation, the conversion of carbohydrate to fat liberates oxygen as the excess calories accumulate in adipose tissue. The released oxygen then supplies energy metabolism; this reduces the lungs' uptake of atmospheric oxygen despite the normal carbon dioxide production.

Relatively low R values also can occur. For example, following exhaustive exercise the cells and bodily fluids retain carbon dioxide to replenish the sodium bicarbonate that buffered the accumulating lactate. This action to replenish alkaline reserve decreases the expired carbon dioxide level without affecting oxygen consumption and may cause the respiratory exchange ratio to dip below 0.70.

METABOLIC CALCULATIONS

Much of the study of exercise physiology involves assessment of energy metabolism. Measurement of the oxygen and carbon dioxide content of expired air, together with either the inspired or expired breathing volume, provides the basic data to determine respiratory gas exchange and oxygen consumption to infer energy expenditure. Appendix D presents the step-by-step method and rationale for metabolic calculations based on experimental data obtained from open-circuit spirometry.

Summary

1. Direct calorimetry and indirect calorimetry represent two methods to determine human energy expenditure.
2. Direct calorimetry measures heat production in an appropriately insulated calorimeter. Indirect calorimetry infers energy expenditure from oxygen consumption and carbon dioxide production, using either closed-circuit spirometry or open-circuit spirometry.
3. The doubly labeled water technique estimates energy expenditure in free-living conditions without the normal constraints imposed by laboratory procedures. It serves as a "gold standard" to validate other long-term energy expenditure estimates.
4. The complete oxidation of each macronutrient requires a different quantity of oxygen consumption for comparable carbon dioxide production. The ratio of carbon dioxide produced to oxygen consumed, the respiratory quotient (RQ), quantifies the macronutrient mixture catabolized for energy.
5. The RQ equals 1.00 for carbohydrate, 0.70 for fat, and 0.82 for protein.
6. For each RQ, a corresponding caloric value exists per liter of oxygen consumed. The RQ–kCal relationship can accurately determine energy expenditure during exercise.
7. The respiratory exchange ratio (R) reflects the pulmonary exchange of carbon dioxide and oxygen under differing physiologic and metabolic conditions; R does not fully mirror the gas exchange of the macronutrient mixture catabolized.

References are available on the Student CD and online at http://connection.lww.com/mkk6e.

Human Energy Expenditure During Rest and Physical Activity

9

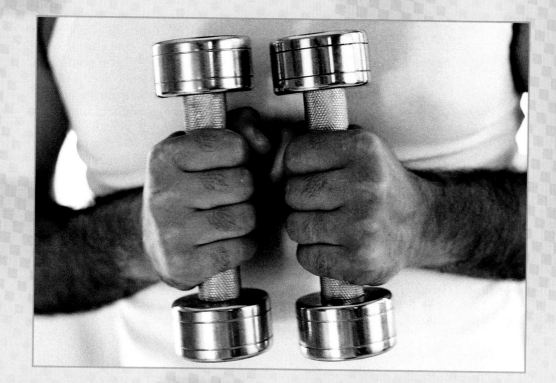

CHAPTER OBJECTIVES

- Define basal metabolic rate and list factors that affect it

- Discuss important factors that affect total daily energy expenditure

- Outline different classification systems to rate the strenuousness of physical activity

- Explain the role of body weight in the energy cost of different physical activities

- Present the rationale (including advantages and limitations) for using heart rate to estimate exercise energy expenditure

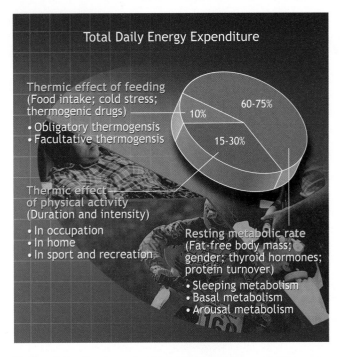

Figure 9.1 Components of total daily energy expenditure (TDEE).

Metabolism involves all of the chemical reactions of biomolecules within the body that encompass both synthesis (anabolism) and breakdown (catabolism). FIGURE 9.1 illustrates the three general factors that determine **total daily energy expenditure** (**TDEE**):

1. Resting metabolic rate, consisting of basal and sleeping conditions plus the added metabolic cost of arousal
2. Thermogenic effect of food consumed
3. Energy expended during physical activity and recovery

PART 1 • *Energy Expenditure at Rest*

BASAL METABOLIC RATE

Each person requires a minimum level of energy to sustain vital functions in the waking state. This energy requirement—termed **basal metabolic rate**, or simply **BMR** (also referred to as basal energy expenditure [BEE])—reflects the body's heat production. Measuring oxygen consumption under stringent conditions indirectly determines the BMR. For example, measurement takes place while the subject rests in the postabsorptive state, having eaten no food for at least the 12 previous hours to avoid increases in metabolism from digestion, absorption, and assimilation of ingested nutrients. To reduce

other calorigenic influences, the subject cannot perform any physical activity for a minimum of 2 hours prior to the test. The subject rests supine for about 30 minutes in a comfortable, thermoneutral environment; then oxygen consumption is measured for 10 minutes. Oxygen consumption values for BMR usually range between 160 and 290 mL · min^{-1} (0.8 to 1.43 kCal · min^{-1}), depending on gender, age, overall body size, and fat-free body mass (FFM).

Knowledge of BMR establishes the important energy baseline for constructing a sound program of weight control through food restriction, regular exercise, or a combination of both. In most instances, basal values measured under controlled laboratory conditions fall only slightly below values for **resting metabolic rate** (**RMR**) measured 3 to 4 hours after a light meal without prior physical activity. For this reason, the term RMR substitutes for BMR in many situations. When measured under standardized conditions, RMR shows high reproducibility and stability.[8] Essentially, RMR refers to the sum of the metabolic processes of the active cell mass required to maintain normal regulatory balance and body functions at rest. For the typical person, RMR accounts for about 60 to 75% of TDEE, while thermic effects from eating account for approximately 10%, and physical activity accounts for the remaining 15 to 30%.

An equation to predict TDEE in older women (67 ± 6 y) and men (70 ± 7 y) uses estimated resting daily energy expenditure (RDEE; see p. 199) and $\dot{V}O_{2peak}$ as follows:

$$\text{TDEE (kCal} \cdot \text{d}^{-1}) = [1.95 \times \text{RDEE (kCal} \cdot \text{d}^{-1})]$$
$$+ [217.3 \times \dot{V}O_{2peak} \text{ (L} \cdot \text{min}^{-1})] - 825.5$$

The equation, formulated from doubly labeled water determinations of the actual daily energy expenditure of 51 women and 48 men, explained 62% of the total variance in TDEE with a standard error of estimate of ± 348 kCal · d^{-1}.[27]

METABOLISM AT REST

Experiments in the late 1800s indicated that resting energy metabolism varied in proportion to the body's surface area. This led to a "surface area law" to account for individual differences in energy metabolism. A series of careful experiments determined energy metabolism of a dog and a man over a 24-hour period. The total heat generated by the larger man exceeded the energy metabolism of the dog by about 200%. Expressing heat production in relation to surface area reduced the metabolic difference between man and dog to only about 10%. This provided the basis for the common practice of expressing basal metabolic rate (energy expenditure) by body surface area per hour (kCal · m^{-2} · h^{-1}).

Later research in the 1920s provided solid evidence that the surface area formulation did not apply universally to different species of temperature-regulating animals (homeotherms). One classic monograph proposed the concept of *metabolic size* that related basal metabolism to body mass raised to the 0.75 power (body mass$^{0.75}$). BMR expressed relative to body mass$^{0.75}$ holds true for humans and a wide

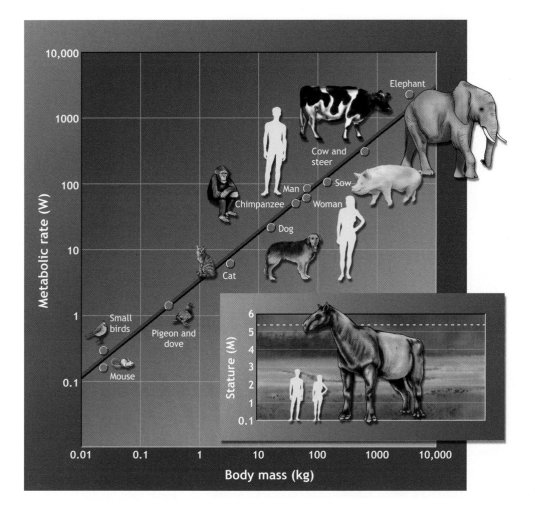

Figure 9.2   Metabolic rate (in watts) from mouse to elephant. Logarithmic plot of body mass and metabolic rate for a variety of birds and mammals differing considerably in body size and shape. Numerous experiments have confirmed the "mouse-to-elephant curve" for metabolism using body mass to the 0.75 power, whereas metabolic rate relates to body surface area to the 0.67 power. The schematic inset figure compares the body size of the world's tallest male (2.89 m [9 ft 5 3/4 in]) and female (2.48 m [8 ft 1 3/4 in]) with the world's largest land mammal (*Baluchitherium,* predecessor of the rhinoceros), whose body mass approximated 30 tons at a stature of 5.26 m (17 ft 3 in). Comparisons between a microorganism (amoeba; mass, 0.1 mg) and a 100-ton blue whale (or the smallest shrew at one tenth the size of a mouse or one millionth the size of an elephant) illustrate the importance of appropriate scaling procedures when relating oxygen consumption, heart size, and blood volume to body mass.

variety of mammals and birds that differ considerably in size and shape. FIGURE 9.2 illustrates the logarithmic plot of body mass (range, 0.01–10,000 kg) and metabolic rate expressed in watts (W), where $1W = 0.01433$ kCal $\cdot$ m^{-2} (range, 0.1–1000 W). The best-fitting straight line describing this relationship truly represents one of the more striking biologic observations related to animal size and metabolic and physiologic functions. Chapter 22 discusses the use of allometric scaling as a mathematical procedure to establish a proper relationship between a body size variable (e.g., stature, body mass, FFM) and some other variable of interest, such as muscular strength or aerobic capacity. This "correction" permits comparisons among individuals or groups that exhibit large individual differences in body size.

Many subsequent studies have shown that indexing RMR to lean body mass (representing the nonadipose tissue component of the body) or the FFM (representing nonlipid mass) provides the overall best method to account for gender differences in energy expenditure (see inset FIG. 9.3). For an individual or group of individuals of the same gender, body surface area provides as good an index of RMR as FFM because of the strong within-gender association between body surface area and FFM.

Numerous experiments have provided data on average BMR values for men and women over a wide range of age and body weight. Figure 9.3 presents BMR data expressed as kCal $\cdot$ m^{-2} $\cdot$ h^{-1}. Whereas the values represent averages from measurements of large numbers of men and women, an individual's BMR (RMR) estimated from the curves generally falls within ±10% of the actual value obtained from laboratory measurements. The inset figure illustrates the relatively strong association between FFM and daily RMR for men and women.

Figure 9.3 also reveals that BMR averages 5 to 10% lower in women than in men. This does not necessarily reflect true "sex differences" in the metabolic rate of specific tissues. Rather, it results largely because women possess more body fat (and less fat-free tissue) than men of similar size; fat tissue has lower metabolic activity than muscle. Changes in body composition, either a decrease in FFM and/or increase in body fat during adulthood, usually explain the 2 to 3% per decade BMR reduction observed for adult men and women.[2,7,22] Some depression of the metabolic activity of the lean tissue components also may progress as one ages;[19] this could contribute to an age-related increase in body fat.

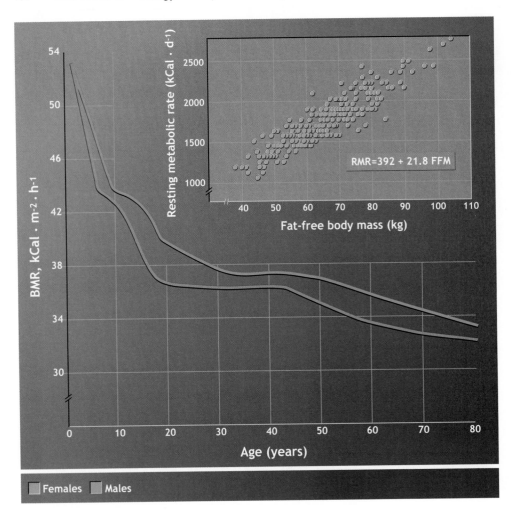

Figure 9.3 Basal metabolic rate (BMR) as a function of age and gender. (Data from Altman PL, Dittmer D. Metabolism. Bethesda, MD: Federation of American Societies for Experimental Biology, 1968.) Inset graph shows the relatively strong relationship between fat-free body mass (FFM) and daily resting metabolic rate (RMR) for men and women. (From Ravussin E, et al. Determination of 24-hour energy expenditure in man. Methods and results using a respiratory chamber. J Clin Invest 1986;78:1568.)

Effects of Regular Exercise

Remarkably similar BMR measures emerged in comparisons of young and middle-aged endurance-trained men who showed no group difference for FFM.[16] Moreover, resting metabolism increased by 8% when 50- to 65-year-old men increased their FFM with heavy resistance training.[23] In addition, an 8-week aerobic training program for older individuals produced a 10% increase in resting metabolism without a change in FFM.[20] This suggests that regular exercise affects factors in addition to body composition to stimulate resting metabolism. *Regular endurance and resistance exercise offsets the decrease in resting metabolism that usually accompanies aging. Each 1-pound gain in FFM increases RMR by 7 to 10 kCal per day.*

The curves in Figure 9.3 adequately estimate a person's resting metabolic rate. For example, between ages 20 and 40 years, the BMR of men averages about 38 kCal per m² per hour, whereas for women the corresponding value equals 35 kCal. For greater precision, read the specific age-related value directly from the appropriate curve. To estimate total metabolic rate per hour, multiply the BMR value by the person's surface area. This hourly total provides important information for estimating the daily energy baseline requirement for caloric intake.

FIGURE 9.4 illustrates a simple method to determine body surface area from stature and body mass. To determine surface area from the nomogram, locate stature on scale I and body mass on scale II. Connect these two points with a straightedge; the intersection on scale III gives the surface area in square meters (m²). For example, if stature equals 185 cm and body mass equals 75 kg, surface area from scale III on the nomogram equals 1.98 m².

Accurate measurement of the body's surface area poses a considerable challenge. Experiments in the early 1900s provided the data to formulate Figure 9.4. The studies clothed 8 men and 2 women in very tight whole-body underwear and applied melted paraffin and paper strips to prevent modification of the surface. The treated cloth was then removed and cut into flat pieces to allow precise measurements of body surface area (length × width). The close relationship between height (stature) and body weight (mass) and body surface area enabled derivation of the following empirical formula to predict body surface area (BSA):

$$BSA = H^{0.725} \times W^{0.425} \times 71.84$$

where H = stature in cm and W = mass in kg. This formula yields results similar to the nomogram values in Figure 9.4.

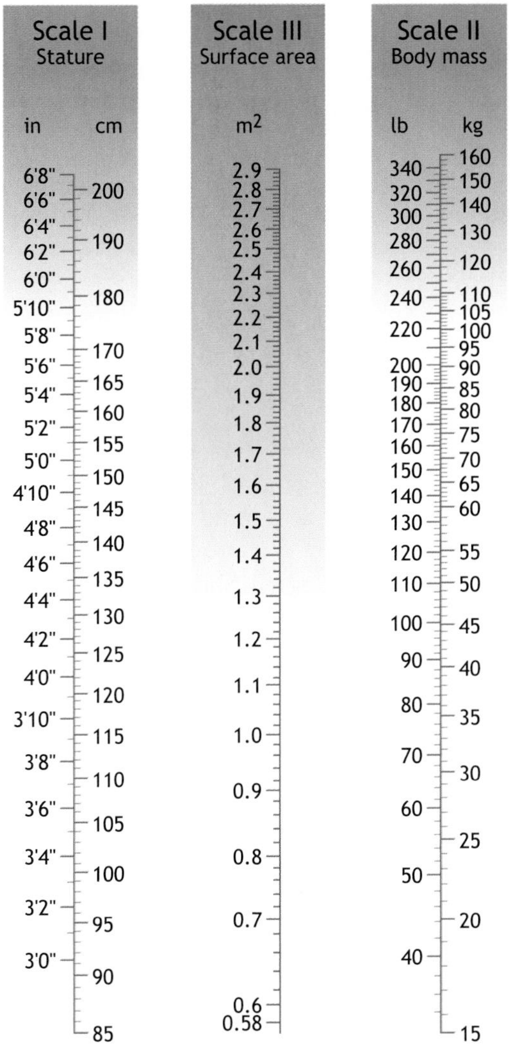

Scale I Stature		Scale III Surface area	Scale II Body mass	
in	cm	m²	lb	kg

Figure 9.4 Nomogram to estimate body surface area from stature and body mass. (Reproduced from Clinical spirometry, prepared by Boothby and Sandiford of the Mayo Clinic, through the courtesy of Warren E. Collins, Inc., Braintree, MA; based on work of Dubois, EF. Basal metabolism in health and disease. Philadelphia: Lea & Febiger, 1936.)

"Normalcy" of BMR Values

Classical assessment of the normalcy of thyroid function compares a person's measured BMR with "standard metabolic rates" based on age and gender (TABLE 9.1 and Fig. 9.3). Any value within ±10% of the standard represents a normal BMR. The following formula computes the deviation expressed as a percentage:

$$\Delta BMR = (\text{measured BMR} - \text{standard BMR}) \times 100 \div \text{standard BMR}$$

For example, a BMR of 35 kCal · m² · h⁻¹ for a 19-year-old male, determined by indirect calorimetry falls 10.7% below the standard BMR.

$$\Delta BMR = (35 - 39.2) \times 100 \div 39.2$$
$$= -10.7\%$$

Estimating Resting Daily Energy Expenditure

To estimate a person's resting daily energy expenditure, multiply the appropriate BMR value in Table 9.1 by the surface area computed from stature and mass. For a 50-year-old woman, for example, the estimated BMR equals 34 kCal per m^2 per hour. For a surface area of 1.40 m^2, the hourly energy expenditure equals 47.6 kCal per hour (34 kCal $\times$ 1.40 m^2). On a daily basis, this amounts to an energy expenditure of 1142 kCal (47.6 kCal $\times$ 24).

TABLE 9.2 provides an estimate of RDEE from FFM estimated from several indirect procedures described in Chapter 28. The data in the table were computed from the following generalized equation, applicable to males and females over a wide range of body weights:

$$\text{RDEE (kCal)} = 370 + 21.6 \text{ (FFM, kg)}$$

TABLE 9.1 ■ STANDARD BASAL METABOLIC RATES

	kCal · m⁻² · h⁻¹		kJ · m⁻² · h⁻¹	
AGE (YEARS)	MEN	WOMEN	MEN	WOMEN
1	53.0	53.0	222	222
2	52.4	52.4	219	219
3	51.3	51.2	215	214
4	50.3	49.8	211	208
5	49.3	48.4	206	203
6	48.3	47.0	202	197
7	47.3	45.4	198	190
8	46.3	43.8	194	183
9	45.2	42.8	189	179
10	44.0	42.5	184	178
11	43.0	42.0	180	176
12	42.5	41.3	178	173
13	42.3	40.3	177	169
14	42.1	39.2	176	164
15	41.8	37.9	175	159
16	41.4	36.9	173	154
17	40.8	36.3	171	152
18	40.0	35.9	167	150
19	39.2	35.5	164	149
20	38.6	35.3	162	148
25	37.5	35.2	157	147
30	36.8	35.1	154	147
35	36.5	35.0	153	146
40	36.3	34.9	152	146
45	36.2	34.5	152	144
50	35.8	33.9	150	142
55	35.4	33.3	148	139
60	34.9	32.7	146	137
65	34.4	32.2	144	135
70	33.8	31.7	141	133
75+	33.2	31.3	139	131

From Fleish A. Le metabolisme basal standard et sa determination au moyen du "Metabocalculator." Helv Med Acta 1951;18:23.

TABLE 9.2 ■ ESTIMATION OF RESTING DAILY ENERGY EXPENDITURE (RDEE) BASED ON FAT-FREE BODY MASS (FFM)

FFM (KG)	RDEE[a] (KCAL)[b]	FFM (KG)	RDEE (KCAL)	FFM (KG)	RDEE (KCAL)
30	1018	58	1623	86	2228
31	1040	59	1644	87	2249
32	1061	60	1666	88	2271
33	1083	61	1688	89	2292
34	1104	62	1709	90	2314
35	1126	63	1731	91	2336
36	1148	64	1752	92	2357
37	1169	65	1774	93	2379
38	1191	66	1796	94	2400
39	1212	67	1817	95	2422
40	1234	68	1839	96	2444
41	1256	69	1860	97	2465
42	1277	70	1882	98	2487
43	1299	71	1904	99	2508
44	1320	72	1925	100	2530
45	1342	73	1947	101	2552
46	1364	74	1968	102	2573
47	1385	75	1990	103	2595
48	1407	76	2012	104	2616
49	1428	77	2033	105	2638
50	1450	78	2055	106	2660
51	1472	79	2076	107	2681
52	1493	80	2098	108	2703
53	1515	81	2120	109	2724
54	1536	82	2141	110	2746
55	1558	83	2163	111	2768
56	1580	84	2184	112	2789
57	1601	85	2206	113	2811

[a] Prediction equation for RDEE derived as the weighted mean of regression constants from studies of large samples of males and females.
[b] To convert kCal to kJ, multiply by 4.18; to convert kCal to MJ, multiply by 0.0042.

For example, a male who weighs 90.9 kg at 21% body fat has an estimated FFM of 71.7 kg. Rounding to 72 kg translates to an RDEE of 1925 kCal, or 8047 kJ (8.08 MJ).

Contribution of Diverse Tissues

TABLE 9.3 shows estimates of the absolute and relative energy needs, expressed as oxygen consumption, of various organs and tissues of adults at rest. Note that the brain and skeletal muscles consume about the same total quantity of oxygen, even though the brain weighs only 1.6 kg (2.3% of body mass), while muscle constitutes almost 50% of the body mass. For children, brain metabolism represents nearly 50% of total resting energy expenditure. This similarity in metabolism, however, does not transfer to maximal exercise because

TABLE 9.3 ■ OXYGEN CONSUMPTION OF VARIOUS BODY TISSUES AT REST FOR A 65-KG MAN

ORGAN	OXYGEN CONSUMPTION (ML · MIN^{-1})	PERCENTAGE OF RESTING METABOLISM
Liver	67	27
Brain	47	19
Heart	17	7
Kidneys	26	10
Skeletal muscle	45	18
Remainder	48	19
	250	100

the energy generated by active muscle increases nearly 100 times; the total energy expended by the brain increases only marginally.

 INTEGRATIVE QUESTION

Discuss why middle-aged men and women should try to maintain or increase muscle mass for purposes of weight control.

FACTORS THAT AFFECT ENERGY EXPENDITURE

Important factors that affect TDEE include physical activity, diet-induced thermogenesis, climate, and pregnancy and lactation.

Physical Activity

As we discuss and illustrate throughout this text, *physical activity has by far the most profound effect on human energy expenditure.* World-class athletes nearly double their TDEE with 3 or 4 hours of intense training. Most persons can sustain metabolic rates 10 times the resting value during continuous "big muscle" exercise such as fast walking, running, bicycling, and swimming. Under typical circumstances, physical activity accounts for between 15 and 30% of a person's TDEE.

Diet-Induced Thermogenesis

Food consumption generally increases energy metabolism. **Diet-induced thermogenesis** (**DIT**) consists of two components. One component, called **obligatory thermogenesis** (formerly called specific dynamic action or SDA), results from the energy required to digest, absorb, and assimilate food nutrients. The second component, called **facultative thermogenesis**, relates to the activation of the sympathetic nervous system and its stimulating influence on metabolic rate.

The first experiment on DIT to our knowledge was performed by Max Rubner in 1891 using indirect calorimetry. This classic work established the 24-hour energy expenditure of a fasting dog at 742 kCal.[13] Rubner then fed the dog 2 kg of meat that contained 1926 kCal. Food consumption increased the dog's daily energy expenditure to 1046 kCal. Rubner attributed the 41% increase of 304 kCal to the "chemical work of glands in metabolizing absorbed nutrients" or the "work of digestion." The increased metabolism represented 16% of the total energy ingested. Numerous subsequent experiments indicate that the meal's size and macronutrient composition time elapsed since the previous meal, nutritional status, and health status differentially affect the magnitude of DIT.

The thermic effect of food generally reaches maximum within 1 hour following a meal. Considerable variability exists among individuals; the magnitude of DIT usually varies between 10 and 30% of the ingested food energy, depending on the quantity and type of food consumed. A meal of pure protein, for example, elicits a thermic effect nearly 25% of the meal's total caloric value. This large thermic effect results largely from activation of digestive processes. It also includes extra energy required by the liver to assimilate and synthesize protein and/or to deaminate amino acids and convert them to glucose or triacylglycerols.

Advocates of consuming a high-protein diet for weight reduction base their argument on the relatively large calorigenic effect of ingested protein. In this scenario, protein's relatively high thermic effect would cause fewer calories to ultimately become available to the body than a meal of similar caloric value consisting mainly of lipid or carbohydrate. This point has some merit, but one must consider other factors in formulating a prudent and effective program for weight loss—not to mention the potentially harmful strain on kidney and liver function from high protein intake. Well-balanced nutrition requires a blend of carbohydrate, lipid, and protein combined with an appropriate intake of vitamins and minerals. When physical activity combines with dietary modification for weight loss, adequate carbohydrate intake maintains glycogen reserves to power diverse forms of exercise.

Overweight individuals often have a blunted thermic response to eating that contributes to excess body fat accumulation.[24–26] Interestingly, the magnitude of DIT also may be lower in endurance-trained individuals than in untrained counterparts.[11,21,29] Any "training effect" probably reflects a calorie-sparing adaptation to conserve energy and glycogen during periods of increased physical activity. Energy conservation in any form seems counterproductive to the potential of increased physical activity for weight control. For a physically active person, however, DIT represents only a small portion of TDEE compared with the energy expended through regular physical activity.

Calorigenic Effect of Food on Exercise Metabolism

DIT has been compared in resting and exercising subjects after consuming meals of identical macronutrient composition and caloric content. In one study, six men performed moderate exercise on a bicycle ergometer before breakfast on 1 day; then on separate days, they performed exercise for 30 minutes after a breakfast containing either 350, 1000, or 3000 kCal.[3] The results indicated that (1) breakfast increased resting metabolism by 10%, (2) variations in the caloric value of the meal exerted no influence on the thermic effect, and (3) performing exercise following a meal of 1000 or 3000 kCal produced a larger energy expenditure than exercise without prior food. The calorigenic effect of food on exercise metabolism nearly doubled the food's thermic effect at rest. Apparently, exercise augments DIT. This agrees with previous findings in which the thermic response to a 1000-kCal meal averaged 28% of the basal requirement at rest, yet increased to 56% of the basal requirement when subjects exercised following eating.[17] Like their response during rest, some obese men and women exhibit a depressed DIT when they exercise after eating (see Chapter 4, "Focus on Research").[25,31] For most individuals, it seems reasonable to encourage moderate exercise after eating to possibly augment a diet-induced increase in caloric expenditure for weight control.

Climate

Environmental factors influence resting metabolic rate. For example, the resting metabolism of people in a tropical climate generally is 5 to 20% higher than for counterparts living in more temperate areas. Exercise performed in hot weather also imposes a small additional metabolic load; it causes about 5% higher oxygen consumption than in a thermoneutral environment. This probably results from the thermogenic effect of an elevated core temperature per se, including additional energy required for sweat gland activity and altered circulatory dynamics during work in the heat.

Cold environments significantly increase energy metabolism during rest and exercise. The magnitude of the effect depends largely on a person's body fat content and effectiveness of the clothing ensemble. Metabolic rate can increase up to fivefold at rest during extreme cold stress because shivering generates body heat to maintain a stable core temperature. The effects of cold stress during exercise become most evident in cold water because of the great difficulty maintaining a stable core temperature in such a stressful environment.[28]

Pregnancy

One area of interest concerns the degree that pregnancy affects the metabolic cost and physiologic strain imposed by exercise.[4] One investigation studied 13 women from the sixth month of pregnancy to 6 weeks after gestation.[9] Physiologic measures taken every 4 weeks included heart rate and oxygen consumption during bicycle and treadmill exercise. Heart rate and oxygen consumption during walking (weight-bearing exercise) increased progressively during the measurement period. Exercise heart rate and oxygen consumption remained unchanged during

IN A PRACTICAL SENSE

PREDICTING $\dot{V}O_{2MAX}$ DURING PREGNANCY FROM SUBMAXIMUM EXERCISE HEART RATE AND OXYGEN CONSUMPTION

■ Authorities recommend that a woman participate in regular physical activity during an uncomplicated pregnancy. Most agree that an individualized exercise prescription should guide exercise because of concern for fetal well-being. The exercise prescription typically specifies intensity, duration, and frequency of activity. Exercise intensity usually represents some percentage of the maximal oxygen consumption ($\%\dot{V}O_{2max}$) obtained from equations relating heart rate (HR) to $\%\dot{V}O_{2max}$. The direct determination of $\dot{V}O_{2max}$ requires that subjects perform near-exhaustive exercise, an unacceptable requirement for most pregnant women.

PREDICTING $\dot{V}O_{2MAX}$ FROM SUBMAXIMAL EXERCISE
Predicting $\dot{V}O_{2max}$ during pregnancy involves a three-stage, submaximum cycle-ergometer exercise test. Oxygen consumption ($\dot{V}O_2$) and HR, measured toward the end of the final exercise stage, predict $\dot{V}O_{2max}$ via regression analyses.

SUBMAXIMUM CYCLE ERGOMETER TEST
Subject rests for 10 minutes and then performs a continuous three-stage, 6-minute per stage, cycle ergometer test as follows:
Stage 1: 0 watts (W) (unloaded cycling)
Stage 2: 30 W (184 kg-m · min^{-1})
Stage 3: 60 W (367 kg-m · min^{-1})

PREDICTION EQUATIONS
Measure $\dot{V}O_2$ (L · min^{-1}) and HR (b · min^{-1}) for each of the last 3 minutes of the final exercise stage. Average the three HR values to predict $\%\dot{V}O_{2max}$ in the following equation:

Predicted $\%\dot{V}O_{2max}$
$$= (0.634 \times HR \ [b \cdot min^{-1}]) - 30.79$$

Use the predicted $\dot{V}O_{2max}$ and the measured $\dot{V}O_2$ (L · min^{-1}) during the last exercise stage to predict $\dot{V}O_{2max}$ (L · min^{-1}) in the following equation:

Predicted $\dot{V}O_{2max}$
$$= \dot{V}O_2 \div \text{predicted} \ \%\dot{V}O_{2max} \times 100$$

EXAMPLE
A woman 20 weeks pregnant, weighing 70.4 kg, performs the three-stage cycle-ergometer test. The average value for final-stage exercise HR equals 155 b · min^{-1}; the average value for $\dot{V}O_2$ equals 1.80 L · min^{-1}.

Predicted $\%\dot{V}O_{2max}$
$$= (0.634 \times HR \ [b \cdot min^{-1}]) - 30.79$$
$$= (0.634 \times 155) - 30.79$$
$$= 67.5\%$$

Predicted $\dot{V}O_{2max}$
$$= \dot{V}O_2 \div \text{predicted} \ \%\dot{V}O_{2max} \times 100$$
$$= 1.80 \div 67.5 \times 100$$
$$= 2.67 \ L \cdot min^{-1} \ (2670 \ mL \cdot min^{-1})$$
$$= 2670 \ mL \cdot min^{-1} \div 70.4 \ kg$$
$$= 37.9 \ mL \cdot kg^{-1} \cdot min^{-1}$$

Sady SP, et al. Prediction of $\dot{V}O_{2max}$ during cycle exercise in pregnant women. J Appl Physiol 1988;65:657.

weight-supported bicycle exercise at a constant intensity. These findings indicate that the added energy cost to weight-bearing locomotion such as walking, jogging, and stair climbing during pregnancy results *primarily* from the additional weight transported (and reduced economy of effort from encumbrance of fetal tissue) with a relatively small effect from the developing fetus per se. Chapter 21 more fully discusses the physiologic and metabolic impact of exercise on both mother and fetus during pregnancy.

Summary

1. Total daily energy expenditure equals the sum of resting metabolism, thermogenic influences (e.g., thermic effect of food), and the energy generated in physical activity.

2. The BMR represents the minimum energy required

to maintain vital functions in the waking state measured under controlled laboratory conditions. The BMR averages only slightly lower than the resting metabolic rate (RMR) and relates closely to body surface area.

3. RMR (like BMR) decreases with age, owing to variations in fat-free body mass (FFM). The RMR for men generally exceeds values for women of similar body size. One can accurately predict RMR from FFM in men and women who vary considerably in body size.

4. Different organs expend different amounts of energy during rest and exercise. At rest, muscles generate about 20% of the body's total energy expenditure. In contrast, the energy expended by skeletal muscles during all-out exercise can increase more than 100 times above its resting value.

5. Five major factors affect a person's metabolic rate: body size, physical activity, DIT, climate, and pregnancy. The greatest influence comes from physical activity.

PART 2 • *Energy Expenditure in Physical Activity*

CLASSIFICATION OF PHYSICAL ACTIVITIES BY ENERGY EXPENDITURE

Most individuals have performed some type of physical work they would classify as "exceedingly difficult." This might include walking up a long flight of stairs, shoveling snow for 60 minutes, running to catch a bus, digging a deep trench, skiing through a blizzard, or hiking up a steep mountain. *Intensity and duration represent two important factors affecting the strenuousness of a particular physical task.* It requires about the same net number of calories to complete a 26.2-mile marathon at various running speeds. One person might expend a considerable rate of energy expenditure running at maximum steady-rate pace (e.g., 80% $\dot{V}O_{2max}$) and complete the distance in a little more than 2 hours. Another runner of equal fitness might select a slower, more comfortable pace (e.g., 55% $\dot{V}O_{2max}$) and complete the run in 3 hours. In this example, the *intensity* of effort distinguishes the physical demands of the task. In another example, two persons of equal fitness may run at the same speed, but one person runs for twice as long as the other. In this situation, exercise *duration* becomes the important consideration in classifying the strenuousness of physical effort.

Several classification systems rate sustained physical activity for its strenuousness. One system recommends classification of work by the ratio of energy required for the task to the resting energy requirement.[1] This system uses the **physical activity ratio** (**PAR**). **Light work** for men elicits an oxygen consumption (or energy expenditure) up to 3 times the resting requirement. **Heavy work** encompasses physical activity requiring 6 to 8 times resting metabolism, whereas **maximal work** includes any task that requires metabolism to increase 9 times or more above rest. As a frame of reference, most industrial jobs and household tasks require less than 3 times resting energy expenditure. These work classifications (in multiples of resting metabolism) average slightly lower for women because of their generally lower aerobic capacity. Work classification based on the PAR model rates the strenuousness of occupational tasks at a somewhat lower level than typical classifications for general exercise. Occupational and industrial work usually extends for much longer periods than exercise training, often requiring the use of a small muscle mass and performed under varying and often stressful environmental conditions and physical constraints.

THE MET

TABLE 9.4 presents a five-level classification system based on the energy (kCal) required by untrained men and women who perform different physical activities including a broad range of occupational tasks.[6] Because 5 kCal equals approximately 1 L of oxygen consumed, one can transpose these values into liters of oxygen consumed per minute (L · min^{-1}) or milliliters of oxygen per kilogram of body mass per minute (mL · kg^{-1} · min^{-1}), or **METs**, *defined as multiples of the resting metabolic rate.* One MET equals resting oxygen consumption, or about 250 mL · min^{-1} for an average man and 200 mL · min^{-1} for an average woman. Exercise performed at 2 METs requires twice the resting metabolism (about 500 mL · min^{-1} for a man), 3 METs equals three times rest, and so on. For a different but usually more accurate classification that considers variations in body size, one should express the MET in terms of oxygen consumption per unit body mass: *1 MET equals 3.5 mL · kg^{-1} · min^{-1}.*

TABLE 9.5 presents a classification system for characterizing the intensity of leisure-time physical activity in absolute (METs) and relative (%$\dot{V}O_{2max}$) intensity for various age categories. Categories for exercise intensity in METs adjust lower with age to account for the general aging effect on aerobic capacity.

DAILY RATES OF AVERAGE ENERGY EXPENDITURE

TABLE 9.6 shows averages for stature and body mass and daily energy expenditure for males and females living in the United States. The average man aged 19 to 50 years expends 2900 kCal per day, whereas his female counterpart expends 2200 kCal. As shown at the bottom of the table, these individuals spend nearly 75% of the day in activities requiring only light energy expenditure. Energy expenditure for most individuals rarely rises substantially above the resting level, with walking the most prevalent physical activity. The term *homo sedentarius* all too appropriately describes most of our citizens. This descriptor is compelling, as physical inactivity in industrial-

TABLE 9.4 ■ FIVE-LEVEL CLASSIFICATION OF PHYSICAL ACTIVITY BASED ON EXERCISE INTENSITY

LEVEL	ENERGY EXPENDITURE[a]			
	$KCAL \cdot MIN^{-1}$	$L \cdot MIN^{-1}$	$ML \cdot KG^{-1} \cdot MIN^{-1}$	METs
Men				
Light	2.0–4.9	0.40–0.99	6.1–15.2	1.6–3.9
Moderate	5.0–7.4	1.00–1.49	15.3–22.9	4.0–5.9
Heavy	7.5–9.9	1.50–1.99	23.0–30.6	6.0–7.9
Very heavy	10.0–12.4	2.00–2.49	30.7–38.3	8.0–9.9
Unduly heavy	≥12.5	≥2.50	≥38.4	≥10.0
Women				
Light	1.5–3.4	0.30–0.69	5.4–12.5	1.2–2.7
Moderate	3.5–5.4	0.70–1.09	12.6–19.8	2.8–4.3
Heavy	5.5–7.4	1.10–1.49	19.9–27.1	4.4–5.9
Very heavy	7.5–9.4	1.50–1.89	27.2–34.4	6.0–7.5
Unduly heavy	≥9.5	≥1.90	≥34.5	≥7.6

[a]$L \cdot min^{-1}$ based on 5 kCal per liter of oxygen; $mL \cdot kg^{-1} \cdot min^{-1}$ based on 65-kg man and 55-kg woman; one MET equals the average resting oxygen consumption (250 mL · min^{-1} for men, 200 mL · min^{-1} for women).

ized nations has become a pandemic despite the admonitions of scientists, educators, and governmental agencies. The Centers for Disease Control and Prevention (www.cdc.gov) estimates that some 300,000 deaths each year in the United States likely result from physical inactivity and poor eating habits. Deaths range across a number of diseases—from heart disease and stroke to colon cancer and diabetes.

ENERGY COST OF HOUSEHOLD, INDUSTRIAL, AND RECREATIONAL ACTIVITIES

Appendix C (available on the Student CD or online at http://connection.lww.com/mkk6e) lists examples of energy expenditures expressed by body mass for common household activities, selected industrial tasks, and popular recreational and sports activities. These data illustrate the large variation in energy expenditure with participation in diverse physical activ-

ities. The caloric values also represent averages, with values for an individual varying considerably depending on skill, pace, and fitness level.

The values listed in the column for body mass represent the activity's caloric cost for 1 minute. This equals the gross energy value (see Chapter 10) because it includes the cost of rest for the 1-minute period. Estimate the total cost of performing an activity by multiplying the caloric value in the table by the number of minutes of participation. For example, if a 70-kg man spends 30 minutes vacuuming (carpet sweeping), his total energy expenditure for this household task equals 102 kCal (3.4 kCal × 30 min). The same individual expends approximately 690 kCal during a 50-minute judo workout, but only 90 kCal while sitting quietly watching television for 2 hours. Golf requires about 6.0 kCal each minute, or 360 kCal · h^{-1} The same person expends almost twice this energy, or 708 kCal · h^{-1}, while swimming backstroke. Viewed somewhat differently, 25 minutes of swimming backstroke

TABLE 9.5 ■ CHARACTERIZATION OF THE INTENSITY OF LEISURE-TIME PHYSICAL ACTIVITY RELATED TO AGE

CATEGORIZATION	RELATIVE INTENSITY ($\%VO_{2MAX}$)	ABSOLUTE INTENSITY (METs)			
		YOUNG	MIDDLE-AGED	OLD	VERY OLD
Rest	<10	1.0	1.0	1.0	1.0
Light	<35	<4.5	<3.5	<2.5	<1.5
Fairly light	<50	<6.5	<5.0	<3.5	<2.0
Moderate	<70	<9.0	<7.0	<5.0	<2.8
Heavy	>70	>9.0	>7.0	>5.0	>2.8
Maximal	100	13.0	10.0	7.0	4.0

From Bouchard C, et al. Exercise, fitness, and health: a consensus of current knowledge. Champaign, IL: Human Kinetics, 1990.

TABLE 9.6 ■ REFERENCE HEIGHTS, WEIGHTS, AND ENERGY EXPENDITURES OF CHILDREN AND ADULTS LIVING IN THE UNITED STATES

HEIGHT, WEIGHT, AND BODY MASS INDEX

GENDER	AGE	MEDIAN BODY MASS INDEX[a]	REFERENCE HEIGHT (CM [IN])	REFERENCE WEIGHT,[b] (KG [LB])
Male, female	2–6 mo	—	64 (25)	7 (16)
	7–11 mo	—	72 (28)	9 (20)
	1–3 y	—	91 (36)	13 (29)
	4–8 y	15.8	118 (46)	22 (48)
Male	9–13 y	18.5	147 (58)	40 (88)
	14–18 y	21.3	174 (68)	64 (142)
	19–30 y	24.4	176 (69)	76 (166)
Female	9–13 y	18.3	148 (58)	40 (88)
	14–18 y	21.3	163 (64)	57 (125)
	19–30 y	22.8	163 (64)	61 (133)

[a] In kg per m^2.
[b] Calculated from median body mass index and median heights for ages 4 to 8 years and older.
Adapted from Dietary reference intakes: a risk assessment model for establishing upper intake levels for nutrients. Food and Nutrition Board. Institute of Medicine. Washington, DC: National Academy Press, 1998.

GENDER, AGE, AND ENERGY EXPENDITURE

	AGE (Y)	ENERGY EXPENDITURE (KCAL)
Males	15–18	3000
	19–24	2900
	25–50	2900
	51+	2300
Females	15–18	2200
	19–24	2200
	25–50	2200
	50+	1900

AVERAGE TIME SPENT DURING THE DAY

ACTIVITY	TIME (H)
Sleeping and lying down	8
Sitting	6
Standing	6
Walking	2
Recreational activity	2

Data from Food and Nutrition Board, National Research Council. Recommended dietary allowances, revised. Washington, DC: National Academy of Sciences, 1989.

requires about the same number of calories as playing golf for 1 hour. Increasing the pace of either the swim or the golf game proportionally increases the intensity of energy expenditure.

Effect of Body Mass

Body mass increases the energy expended in many physical activities (see Appendix C), particularly in **weight-bearing exercise** such as walking and running, in which a person transports body mass during the activity. FIGURE 9.5 clearly illustrates that the energy cost of walking increases directly with body mass. For persons with the same body mass, such a small variation in oxygen consumption exists that body mass will accurately predict the energy expended walking.

The influence of body mass on energy metabolism in weight-bearing exercise occurs whether the person gains weight naturally as body fat or FFM or as a short-term added load from sports equipment or weighted vest on the torso.[5,30] With **weight-supported exercise** (e.g., stationary cycling), the influence of body mass on energy cost decreases consider-

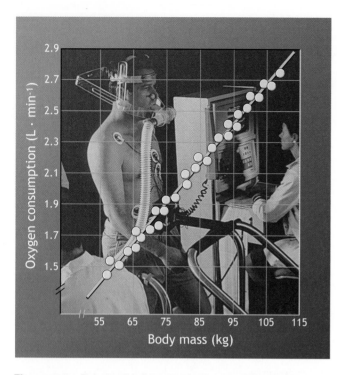

Figure 9.5 Relationship between body mass and oxygen consumption measured during submaximal, brisk treadmill walking. (From Laboratory of Applied Physiology, Queens College, NY.)

during aerobic exercise. This approach has proved useful when the oxygen consumption could not be measured during the actual activity.

FIGURE 9.6 presents data for two members of a women's basketball team during a laboratory treadmill running test. For each woman, heart rate increased linearly with oxygen consumption—a proportionate increase in exercise heart rate (HR) accompanied each increase in oxygen consumption ($\dot{V}O_2$). Both HR–$\dot{V}O_2$ lines display linearity, but the same heart rate does not correspond to the same oxygen consumption for both women because the slopes (rate of change) of the lines differ. Heart rate for subject B increases less than that for subject A for a given increase in oxygen consumption. Chapters 11, 17, and 21 discuss the significance of the difference in heart rate increase with exercise and its relation to cardiovascular fitness. For the current discussion, exercise heart rate can estimate exercise oxygen consumption with reasonable accuracy. For player A, an exercise heart rate of 140 b · min^{-1} corresponds to an oxygen consumption of 1.08 L · min^{-1}, whereas the same heart rate for player B corresponds to a 1.60 L · min^{-1} oxygen consumption. Heart rates obtained by radiotelemetry during basketball competition were then applied to each player's HR–$\dot{V}O_2$ line to estimate energy expenditure under game conditions.[15]

Heart rate to estimate energy expenditure appears practical but is limited for research purposes because it has been validated for only a few general activities. One major problem

ably. It averages only about 5% higher in stationary cycling among heavy people, because of extra energy required to lift heavier lower limbs.[10,12] The body weight effect in stationary cycling exercise slightly lowers energy cost values for women compared with men. For overweight persons desiring to use exercise for weight loss, weight-bearing exercise generates a considerable caloric expenditure simply from the added cost of transporting a heavier body weight.

Appendix C also shows that the energy cost for cross-country running ranges between 8.2 kCal per minute for a 50-kg person and almost twice as much (16.0 kCal) for a person weighing 98 kg. Expressing the energy requirement by body mass as kCal · kg^{-1} · min^{-1} essentially eliminates this variation. In this case, energy cost averages about 0.164 kCal · kg^{-1} · min^{-1}. Expressing energy cost per unit body mass reduces differences between individuals, regardless of age, race, gender, and body mass. The heavier person still expends more *total* calories than a lighter person for an equivalent exercise period. This occurs mainly because the activity requires the transport of body mass—and this requires proportionately more energy.

HEART RATE TO ESTIMATE ENERGY EXPENDITURE

For each person, heart rate and oxygen consumption relate linearly throughout a large range of aerobic exercise intensities. From this relationship, the exercise heart rate provides an estimate of oxygen consumption (and thus energy expenditure)

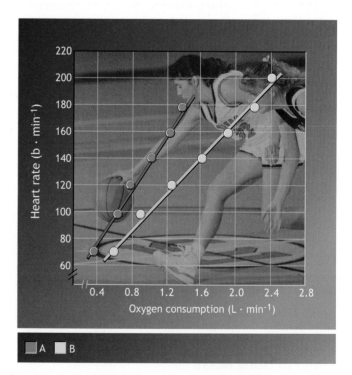

Figure 9.6 Linear relationship between heart rate and oxygen consumption for two women collegiate basketball players of different aerobic fitness levels. Measurements made during a graded exercise test on a motor-driven treadmill. (From Laboratory of Applied Physiology, Queens College, NY.)

FOCUS On Research

FACTORS THAT AFFECT RECOVERY OXYGEN CONSUMPTION

Margaria R, et al. The possible mechanisms of contracting and paying the oxygen debt and the role of lactic acid in muscular contraction. Am J Physiol 1933;106:689.

▲ A. V. Hill and colleagues had theorized that the increased oxygen consumption in recovery from exhaustive exercise (the so-called "oxygen debt") resulted largely from the delayed oxidation of a portion of the lactic acid (LA) that accumulated during exercise. Unfortunately, these researchers did not provide direct evidence to confirm their hypothesis by quantifying the relationship between the oxygen debt and LA accumulation.

Margaria and his group at the prestigious Harvard Fatigue Laboratory provided the first quantitative assessment of Hill's theory. The researchers determined the time-course characteristics of LA removal, described as an exponential function of time. They also related LA removal rate to recovery oxygen consumption ($\dot{V}O_2$). The $\dot{V}O_2$ recovery curve subdivided into two parts that the researchers attributed to distinctly different metabolic events during exercise. The terms *alactacid* and *lactacid* described these components of recovery $\dot{V}O_2$.

One subject, observed during 10-minute runs on different occasions at varied exercise intensities, provided the experimental data. LA, measured from the femoral vein and brachial artery at different times throughout exercise, indicated rapid and uniform diffusion of LA throughout the body. Blood LA concentration varied directly with the body's total LA content. The figure illustrates the relationship between exercise blood LA concentration and the magnitude of recovery $\dot{V}O_2$. Note that the curve does not deviate from baseline LA until the oxygen debt reaches 3 to 4 L. This coincided with the subject's exercise $\dot{V}O_2$ of about 3.0 L · min^{-1}. Blood LA concentration (and corresponding oxygen debt) then increased linearly with exercise intensity ($\dot{V}O_2$). The researchers reasoned that when the total oxygen debt remained below 3.0 L, the LA mechanism in exercise remained inactive. They termed this level of exercise *alactic* to signify work production without significant LA accumulation. Under these conditions, re-

covery $\dot{V}O_2$ proceeds rapidly to the resting level. LA began to accumulate with exercise at about 65% of the maximum aerobic metabolism ($\dot{V}O_{2max}$), accumulating rapidly thereafter. LA removal, a slow process, progressed at a velocity constant of 0.02—one half removed each 15 minutes.

Margaria and colleagues concluded that LA production became important only during strenuous exercise. They postulated that the total recovery $\dot{V}O_2$ consisted of the combined effects of two distinct components: (1) lactacid oxygen debt attributable to oxidation of LA produced in exercise and (2) alactacid oxygen debt, unrelated to LA accumulation and repaid early and rapidly in recovery. This important experiment in the early history of exercise physiology provided insight into why different $\dot{V}O_2$ recovery patterns emerged for different exercise intensities.

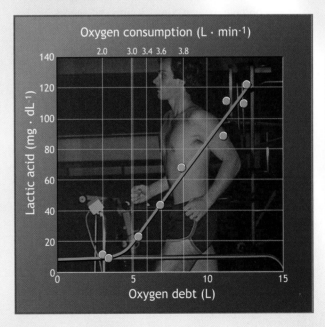

Relation between blood lactic acid concentration and oxygen debt (calculated after A. V. Hill) and oxygen consumption at various levels of exercise. Exercise duration equaled 10 minutes in each case.

concerns the degree of similarity between the laboratory exercise test to establish the HR–$\dot{V}O_2$ line and the specific activities to which it applies. For example, factors other than oxygen consumption influence the exercise heart rate response. These include environmental temperature, emotions, previous food intake, body position, muscle groups exercised, continuous or discontinuous (stop-and-go) exercise, or whether the muscles act statically or more dynamically. In aerobic dance, for example, heart rates while dancing at a specific oxygen consumption significantly exceed heart rates at the same oxygen consumption during treadmill exercise.[18] Consistently higher heart rates occur in upper-body exercise; they are also higher when muscles act statically in straining-type exercises than in dynamic exercise at any submaximal oxygen consumption. Consequently, applying heart rate during upper-body or static exercise to a HR–$\dot{V}O_2$ line developed during running or cycling *overpredicts* the measured oxygen consumption.[14]

INTEGRATIVE QUESTION

A high-tech computer company asks you to validate a wrist-mounted device to measure exercise energy expenditure. The person exhales one breath onto the top of the instrument while exercising. The device's electronic components and microprocessor analyze expired air to compute oxygen consumption and energy expenditure. Outline the steps to establish the instrument's validity.

Summary

1. Different classification systems rate the strenuousness of physical activities. These include ratings based on (1) ratio of the energy cost of the task to the resting energy requirement, (2) oxygen requirement in $mL \cdot kg^{-1} \cdot min^{-1}$, or (3) multiples of resting metabolism as METs.

2. Total daily energy expenditure averages 2900 kCal for men and 2200 kCal for women ages 19 to 50 years. Considerable variability among persons exists for daily energy expenditure, with the largest variation determined by one's physical activity level.

3. Daily energy expenditure provides a framework for classifying different occupations. Within any classification, energy expended during leisure time recreational pursuits often contributes considerable additional variability.

4. Heavier individuals generally expend more total energy in physical activity than lighter counterparts, particularly in weight-bearing walking and running activities.

5. Heart rate serves as a valid indicator of the relative strenuousness of physical activity. An array of factors affect heart rate independent of oxygen consumption. Consequently, heart rate has only limited use in predicting oxygen consumption and caloric expenditure in diverse forms of physical activities.

References are available on the Student CD and online at *http://connection.lww.com/mkk6e.*

Energy Expenditure During Walking, Jogging, Running, and Swimming

10

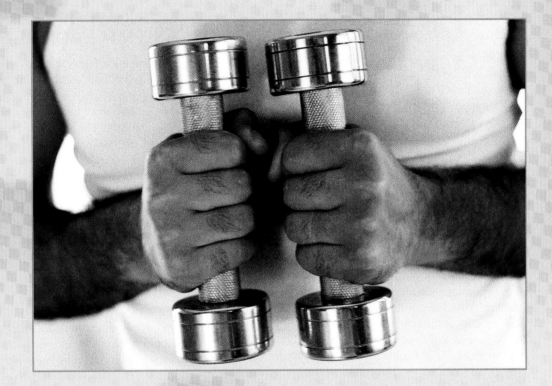

CHAPTER OBJECTIVES

- Differentiate between gross energy expenditure and net energy expenditure

- Explain exercise economy and mechanical efficiency

- Describe differences in running economy between trained and untrained children and adults

- Graph the relationship between walking velocity and energy expenditure up to velocities achieved during competitive race-walking

- Discuss the influence of body mass, exercise surface, and footwear on energy expenditure during walking and running

- Describe advantages and disadvantages of ankle and handheld weights to increase energy expenditure during walking and running

- Graph the relationship between running velocity and energy expenditure

- Explain the association between running velocity and energy cost per unit distance traveled

- Outline the interactions between stride length and stride frequency and linear velocity during running versus competitive race-walking

- Quantify how drafting influences energy expenditure during running, swimming, and bicycling

- Identify factors that contribute to a lower exercise economy swimming compared with running

The following sections detail energy expenditure for walking, running, and swimming. These popular activities take on special significance to the general population for their roles in weight control, physical conditioning, and health maintenance and rehabilitation.

GROSS VERSUS NET ENERGY EXPENDITURE

The following example illustrates the use of oxygen consumption to estimate the energy expenditure in swimming. A 25-year-old man swimming for 40 minutes at a moderate, steady pace requiring 2.0 L per minute oxygen consumption consumes a total of 80 L of oxygen. One can transpose this oxygen consumption to an energy value by using the approximate calorific transformation of 5.0 kCal per liter of oxygen consumed (assuming carbohydrate as sole energy fuel). Thus, the swimmer expends about 400 kCal (80 L O_2 × 5 kCal) during the swim. This computation does not assess the energy cost of the swim per se. The measured total or **gross energy expenditure** also includes energy that would have been expended if the person only rested and did not swim for the same time period. To obtain the true requirement of just exercise—the **net energy expenditure**—one must subtract resting metabolism from the gross energy expenditure of the exercise as follows:

Net energy expenditure = Gross energy expenditure
− Resting energy expenditure (for equivalent time)

Knowing the swimmer's size (mass, 65 kg; stature, 174 cm) permits computation of the surface area of 1.78 m² from the nomogram in Figure 9.4. Multiplying this value by the average basal metabolic rate (BMR) for young men, 38 kCal · m^{-2} · h^{-1} (Fig. 9.3), gives an estimated resting energy expenditure of 67.6 kCal per hour (1.78 m² × 38 kCal), or about 45 kCal for the 40-minute swim. The energy expended solely for the swim computes as gross energy expenditure (400 kCal) minus the 40-minute resting value (45 kCal), resulting in a net energy expenditure of 355 kCal just for swimming.

In Figure 7.3 of Chapter 7, we show that oxygen consumption during constant-load light to moderate exercise rises rapidly during the first several minutes, then levels off and remains stable thereafter. This permits estimating total energy expenditure from only one or two oxygen consumption measures during steady-rate exercise. Activities with considerable variation in pace such as tennis, soccer, lacrosse, field hockey, or basketball require more frequent measures for accurate estimates of total energy expenditure. Strenuous exercise, when energy requirements considerably exceed aerobic energy transfer, derives considerable energy anaerobically with accompanying blood lactate accumulation. Estimating energy expenditure in such situations becomes virtually impossible.

ECONOMY OF HUMAN MOVEMENT AND MECHANICAL EFFICIENCY

The concept of **mechanical efficiency** considers the relationship between energy input and output. In a figurative comparison to economics, efficiency of operation parallels the cost required to produce goods relative to the money generated from the sale of such goods. We might also liken human efficiency of operation to the auto industry that strives to optimize vehicle aerodynamic design to improve efficiency of operation and the important miles-per-gallon rating. Efficiency of human movement relates the amount of energy required to perform a particular task to the actual work accomplished. **Movement economy**, in contrast, refers to the energy required (usually measured as oxygen consumption) to maintain a constant velocity of movement.

Economy of Movement

Assessing economy of movement requires evaluating oxygen consumed while a subject exercises at a set power output or velocity. This approach only applies to steady-rate exercise where oxygen consumption closely mirrors energy expenditure. For example, at an established submaximal speed of running, cycling, or swimming, an individual with greater movement economy consumes *less* oxygen (lower steady-rate $\dot{V}O_2$). African women who balance heavy loads on their heads have mastered a subtle adjustment in walking technique that allows them to carry up to 20% of their body weight with no increase in energy expenditure. A group of Europeans, in contrast, exerted proportionately more effort (increased oxygen consumption) as the added weight on their head increased. Economy takes on added importance during longer-duration exercise where success largely depends on the individual's aerobic capacity and ability to maintain the lowest oxygen consumption relative to the work rate. Data obtained on a six-time Grand Champion of the Tour de France over the age of 21 to 28 years indicates an 8% improvement in muscular efficiency (and thus power production when cycling at a given oxygen uptake), perhaps due to changes in muscle myosin type stimulated from years of training intensely for 3 to 6 hours on most days.[19] For children and adults, any training adjustment that improves the economy of effort usually improves exercise performance.[22,36] FIGURE 10.1 displays the strong association between running economy and endurance performance in elite athletes

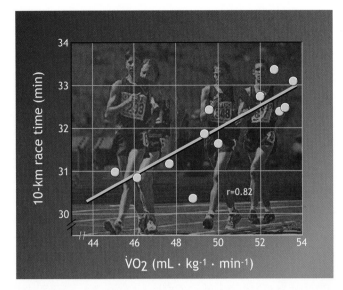

Figure 10.1 Relationship between submaximal oxygen consumption while running at 268 m · min⁻¹ and 10-km race time in elite male runners of comparable aerobic capacity. (From Morgan DW, Craib M. Physiological aspects of running economy. Med Sci Sports Exerc 1992;24:456.)

of comparable aerobic fitness. Clearly, athletes with greater running economies achieve better race times. Variation in running economy among this homogeneous group explains approximately 64% of the total variation in 10-km running performance.

No single biomechanical factor accounts for individual differences in running economy, although muscle structural and compositional factors play a role.[41] Even among trained runners, notable variation in economy emerges at a submaximal running speed.[52,56,69] In general, long-term programs of run training improve running economy, due partly to training-induced reductions in pulmonary ventilation during submaximal exercise.[13,30,73] It remains unclear whether the first 6 weeks of run training affect running mechanics or economy despite improvements in performance and physiologic function.[30,42] Short-term training emphasizing "proper" running technique (i.e., arm movements and body alignment) does not enhance running economy.[38] In contrast, distance runners with an uneconomical stride-length pattern benefit from a short-term audiovisual feedback program that focuses on optimizing stride length,[55] including biofeedback and relaxation psychophysiologic interventions.[13]

Indirect evidence from studies of cyclists indicates that muscle fiber-type distribution affects the economy of physical effort. During submaximal cycling, exercise economies of well-trained cyclists vary by 15%.[20] Differences in muscle fiber type in the active muscles represent an important component of the variation in economy. Cyclists with greater economy possessed a larger percentage of slow-twitch (type I) muscle fibers in their vastus lateralis muscle. Aerobic, type I muscle fibers act with greater mechanical efficiency than faster-contracting, highly anaerobic type II muscle fibers.[21]

Mechanical Efficiency

Mechanical efficiency represents another component for evaluating the relationship between energy input and exercise power output. *Mechanical efficiency reflects the percentage of total chemical energy expended that contributes to external work, with the remainder lost as heat.*

Mechanical efficiency (%) = External work
  accomplished (energy output) ÷ Energy input × 100

The external work accomplished (energy output) equals force acting through a vertical distance (F × D), usually recorded as foot-pounds (ft-lb) or kilogram-meters (kg-m) and then expressed in kCal units (1 kCal = 3087 ft-lb, or 426.4 kg-m in a perfect machine without loss in efficiency). External work is easily determined during cycle ergometry or an exercise task such as stair climbing or bench stepping—both requiring lifting the body mass a given distance (see "In A Practical Sense," Chapter 5). One cannot compute mechanical efficiency during horizontal walking or running because technically no external work is accomplished; reciprocal arm and leg movements negate each other without a net gain in vertical distance. If a person walks or runs up a grade, the work component can be estimated from body mass and the vertical distance (lift) achieved during the movement. Total oxygen consumed provides the means to infer the denominator (energy input) of the efficiency equation. Oxygen consumption converts to energy units—roughly 1.0 L O_2 = 5.0 kCal (see Table 8.1 for precise calorific transformations).

Suppose a 15-minute ride on a stationary bicycle generates 13,300 kg-m of work, with the net oxygen consumed to produce the work totaling 25 L (RQ = 0.88). To create common units of measurement, convert the oxygen consumed to a corresponding kCal value. For an RQ of 0.88, each liter of oxygen consumed generates an energy equivalent of 4.9 kCal (Table 8.1). Therefore, 25 L of oxygen consumption during the 15-minute ride generates 122.5 kCal of energy (25 × 4.9 kCal). The energy equivalent of 13,300 kg-m of external work equals 31.19 kCal (13,300 kg-m ÷ 426.4 kg-m per kCal). Mechanical efficiency computes as follows:

Mechanical efficiency = 31.19 kCal
  ÷ 122.5 kCal × 100
  = 25.5%

As with all machines, the efficiency of the human body for mechanical work falls considerably below 100%. The energy required to overcome internal and external friction represents the largest factor to affect efficiency. This constitutes wasted energy because it does not accomplish work; consequently, work input *always* exceeds work output.

Extensive research permits estimates of mechanical efficiencies for different large-muscle physical activities. On average, efficiency ranges between 20 and 25% for walking, running, and stationary cycling. Body size, gender, fitness level, and skill affect individual differences in efficiency. For activities with substantial drag force that resists movement (e.g., road cycling, cross-country skiing, ice skating, rowing, and swimming), mechanical efficiency falls below 20%.

Competitors in these sports focus attention on reducing drag by improving aerodynamics and/or hydrodynamics through alterations in clothing, equipment, and technique. A small improvement in efficiency for an elite athlete increases the likelihood of success.

Delta Efficiency

An alternative approach to determining mechanical efficiency (not affected by body mass or changes in body weight) involves calculating **delta efficiency** as follows[5,61]:

$$\text{Delta efficiency} = \frac{\Delta \text{ Work production}}{\Delta \text{ Energy expenditure}} \times 100$$

Where Δ work production equals the calculated difference in work output at two different exercise levels, and Δ energy expenditure equals the difference in the energy expenditure between the two exercise levels.

Suppose an individual cycles at 100 W at a $\dot{V}O_2$ of 1.50 L · min^{-1} and RQ of 0.89. Work intensity then increases to 200 W, with a corresponding $\dot{V}O_2$ of 2.88 L · min^{-1} and RQ of 0.95. Delta efficiency computes as follows, where 1 W = 0.014 kCal · min^{-1}; RQ of 0.89 = 4.911 kCal · LO$_2$$^{-1}$; RQ of 0.95 = 4.985 kCal · LO$_2$$^{-1}$:

$$
\begin{aligned}
\text{Delta} \\
\text{efficiency}
\end{aligned}
\quad
\begin{aligned}
&= 200\,\text{W} - 100\,\text{W} \div 2.88\,\text{L} \cdot \text{min}^{-1} \\
&\quad - 1.50\,\text{L} \cdot \text{min}^{-1} \times 100 \\
&= (200 \times 0.014) - (100 \times 0.014) \\
&\quad \div (2.88 \times 4.985) - (1.50 \times 4.911) \times 100 \\
&= 1.4\,\text{kCal} \cdot \text{min}^{-1} \div 6.99\,\text{kCal} \cdot \text{min}^{-1} \times 100 \\
&= 0.2003 \times 100 \\
&= 20.0\%
\end{aligned}
$$

ENERGY EXPENDITURE DURING WALKING

Walking represents the major daily physical activity for most persons. FIGURE 10.2 displays research from five countries on the energy expenditure of men who walked at speeds from 1.5 to 9.5 km · h^{-1} (0.9 to 5.9 mph). The relationship between walking speed and oxygen consumption remains approximately linear between speeds of 3.0 and 5.0 km · h^{-1} (1.9 and 3.1 mph); at faster speeds, walking economy decreases, and the relationship curves upward, indicating a disproportionate increase in energy expenditure with increasing speed. This explains the reason why, per unit distance traveled, faster, less-efficient walking speeds expend more total calories.

Influence of Body Mass

One can accurately predict energy expenditure of horizontal walking at speeds between 3.2 and 6.4 km · h^{-1} (2.0 and 4.0 mph) for men and women who differ in body mass, using an equation based on the combined data in Figure 10.2 and additional studies.[1,28] These values, listed in TABLE 10.1, achieve accuracy to within 15% of the measured energy

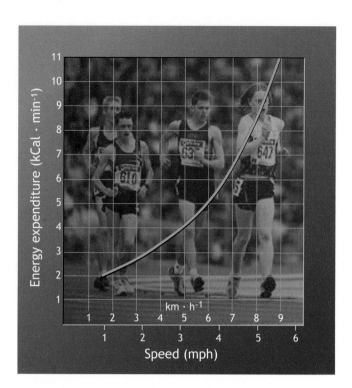

Figure 10.2 Energy expenditure while walking on a level surface at different speeds. The *yellow line* represents a compilation of average values from various studies reported in the literature.

expenditure. On a daily basis, error estimates of energy expended in walking generally range from 50 to 100 kCal (assuming the person walks 2 hours daily). Extrapolation for light (<36 kg) and heavy individuals (>91 kg) is possible but with some loss in accuracy.

Terrain and Walking Surface

TABLE 10.2 summarizes the influence of terrain and different surfaces on the energy cost of walking. Similar economies exist for level walking on a grass track or paved surface. In contrast, walking in the sand requires almost twice the energy of walking on a hard surface. This is explained by sand's hindering effects on the forward movement of the foot and the added force required by the calf muscle to compensate for foot slippage. Walking in soft snow triples metabolic cost compared with similar walking on a treadmill.[72] A brisk walk (or run) along a beach or in freshly fallen snow provides excellent exercise stress to "burn" additional calories or improve physiologic fitness.[70]

Another series of experiments revealed no differences between the energy cost of treadmill walking at 2.93 km · h^{-1} and 5.86 km · h^{-1} and normal walking on a hard surface at the same speeds.[65] Persons generate essentially the same physiologic stress by walking on a level surface or walking on a treadmill at an equivalent speed and distance. Such results lend support to the use of laboratory data to quantify human energy expenditure in real-life situations.

TABLE 10.1 ■ **PREDICTION OF ENERGY EXPENDITURE (KCAL · MIN^{-1}) FROM SPEED OF LEVEL WALKING AND BODY MASS**[a]

| WALKING SPEED | | BODY MASS | | | | | | |
MPH	KM · H^{-1}	KG 36 LB 80	45 100	54 120	64 140	73 160	82 180	91 200
2.0	3.22	1.9	2.2	2.6	2.9	3.2	3.5	3.8
2.5	4.02	2.3	2.7	3.1	3.5	3.8	4.2	4.5
3.0	4.83	2.7	3.1	3.6	4.0	4.4	4.8	5.3
3.5	5.63	3.1	3.6	4.2	4.6	5.0	5.4	6.1
4.0	6.44	3.5	4.1	4.7	5.2	5.8	6.4	7.0

Data from Passmore R, Durnin JVGA. Human energy expenditure. Physiol Rev 1955;35:801.
[a] How to use the table: A 120-lb (54-kg) person who walks at 3.0 mph (4.83 km · h^{-1}) expends 3.6 kCal · min^{-1}. This person expends 216 kCal in a 60-minute walk (3.6 × 60).

Downhill Walking

Walking the downhill portion of a mountain hike or golf course provides welcome relief compared with the uphill segment of the exercise. Downhill walking (or running) represents a form of **negative work** because the body's center of mass moves in a downward vertical direction with each step cycle. This decreases the total potential energy of the system. Consequently, at the same speed and elevation, it requires less energy to perform eccentric muscle actions (negative work) than the concentric actions of positive work.

FIGURE 10.3 illustrates the net oxygen requirement of both level and negative grade walking at constant speeds of either 6.3 or 5.4 km · h^{-1}. Compared with walking on level ground, progressive negative grade walking decreases oxygen cost down to a −9% grade for speeds of 5.4 km · h^{-1}

and −12% for speeds of 6.3 km · h^{-1}. Energy cost begins to increase at the more severe negative grades. The increase in oxygen cost for walking down the steeper grades probably results from additional energy to resist or "brake" the body from gravity's pull while trying to achieve a proper and safe walking rhythm.

Footwear

It requires considerably more energy to carry weight on the feet or ankles than to carry the same weight on the torso. A weight equal to 1.4% of body mass placed on the ankles

TABLE 10.2 ■ **EFFECT OF DIFFERENT TERRAIN ON THE ENERGY EXPENDITURE OF WALKING BETWEEN 5.2 AND 5.6 KM · H^{-1}**

TERRAIN	CORRECTION FACTOR[a]
Paved road (similar to grass track)	0.0
Plowed field	1.5
Hard snow	1.6
Sand dune	1.8

[a] The correction factor is a multiple of the energy expenditure for walking on a paved road or grass track. For example, the energy cost of walking in a plowed field equals 1.5 times that of walking on a paved road. Divide by 1.61 to convert to mph.
First entry from Passmore R, Durnin JVGA. Human energy expenditure. Physiol Rev 1955;35:801. Last three entries from Givoni B, Goldman RF. Predicting metabolic energy cost. J Appl Physiol 1971;30:429.

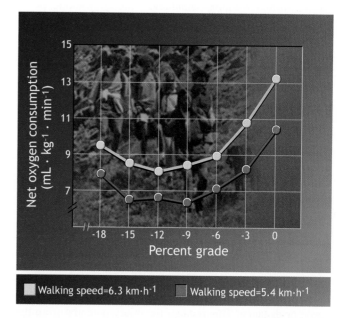

Figure 10.3 Net oxygen costs of level (0% grade) and downhill walking at grades between −3 and −18% and speeds between 5.4 and 6.3 km · h^{-1}. *Percent grade* reflects the vertical distance moved downward per unit horizontal distance traversed. (From Wanta DM, et al. Metabolic response to graded downhill walking. Med Sci Sports Exerc 1993;25:159.)

increases the energy cost of walking an average of 8%, or nearly 6 times more than with the same weight on the torso.[35] In a practical sense, wearing boots increases the energy cost of walking and running disproportionately compared with the energy cost when wearing lighter running shoes. Adding an additional 100 g to each shoe increases oxygen consumption during moderate running by 1%. Clear implications exists for these findings in the design of running shoes, hiking and climbing boots, and work boots traditionally required in mining, forestry, fire fighting, and the military—small changes in shoe weight produce meaningful changes in movement economy.[33] The cushioning properties of shoes also affect exercise economy.[59] A softer-soled running shoe reduces the oxygen cost (increased economy) of running at a moderate speed by 2.4% compared with a similar shoe with a firmer cushioning system, even though the pair of softer-soled shoes weighed an additional 31 g.[31]

Handheld and Ankle Weights

The impact force on the legs during running averages about three times body mass, whereas the level of leg shock walking equals only 30% of this value. Individuals desiring to increase energy expenditure using only walking as a "low-impact" exercise mode often add extra weight to the body. This modification also has been applied to running activities.

Walking

Ankle weights increase the energy expenditure of walking to values usually observed for running.[49] The effect benefits individuals who use only walking as a low-impact training modality, yet require greater energy expenditures than occur during normal walking. Handheld weights, walking poles (simulate arm action in cross-country skiing), power belts (worn around waist with resistance cords with handles for arm action), and upper-body exercise (swinging the arms) all increase the energy expenditure of walking.[12,27,62,66,80] However, handheld weights and walking poles may disproportionately increase exercise systolic blood pressure, perhaps from the blood pressure–elevating effects of (1) upper-body exercise (see Chapter 15, p. 328) and (2) increased intramuscular tension from gripping the object. An augmented blood pressure response contraindicates use of handheld weights for individuals with existing hypertension or coronary heart disease.

Running

Considering the relatively small increase in energy expenditure with hand or ankle weights in running, it seems more practical to simply increase the unweighted running speed or distance. This reduces the injury potential from the added impact force imparted by the weights and eliminates discomfort from carrying them. For individuals with orthopedic limitations that could worsen with leg impact shock from running, in-line skating offers a less-stressful alternative for an equivalent aerobic demand.[43,48]

INTEGRATIVE QUESTION

What recommendations would you make for exercise mode–specific physical activities for aerobic training of individuals with osteoarthritis of the knees?

Competition Walking

Researchers studied the treadmill energy expenditures of five Olympic-caliber walkers at various walking and running speeds. Walking speed during competition averaged 13.0 km · h^{-1} (11.5 to 14.8 km · h^{-1} [7.1 to 9.2 mph]) over distances from 1.6 to 50 km. This represents a relatively fast speed; the world record for the 20-km walk (12.6-mile) of 1:17:21 (Jefferson Perez, 2003) equals a speed of 15.51 km · h^{-1} (9.64 mph)! FIGURE 10.4 illustrates that the break point in the economy of locomotion between walking and running ranged between 8.0 and 9.0 km · h^{-1}. These data, plus biomechanical evidence, indicate about the same crossover speed—when running becomes more economical than walking—for conventional and competitive styles of walking (FIG. 10.5). In addition, treadmill walking at competition speeds produced only slightly lower oxygen consumptions for race-walkers than their highest oxygen consumptions during treadmill running. A linear relationship existed between oxygen consumption and walking at speeds above 8 km per hour (5.0 mph), but the slope of the line was *twice* as steep as that for running at the same speeds. The athletes could walk at velocities of nearly 16 km · h^{-1} (9.9 mph). *The economy of walking faster than 8 km · h^{-1} equaled only one half the economy for running at the*

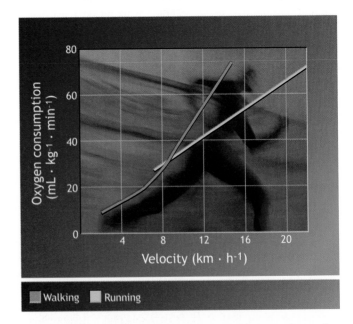

Figure 10.4   Relationship between oxygen consumption and horizontal velocity for walking and running in competition walkers. (Adapted from Menier DR, Pugh LGCE. The relation of oxygen intake and velocity of walking and running in competition walkers. J Physiol 1968;197:717.)

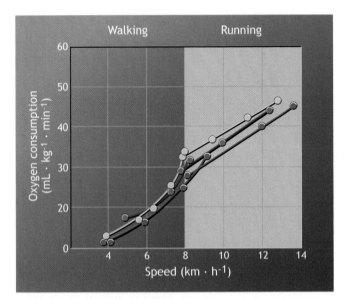

Figure 10.5   Relationship between oxygen consumption and speed of horizontal walking and running in men and women. Different *colored lines* represent values from various research studies. (From Falls HB, Humphrey LD. Energy cost of running and walking in young women. Med Sci Sports 1976;8:9.)

same speeds. The attainment of similar values for $\dot{V}O_{2max}$ during race-walking and running by elite competitors further supports the model for aerobic training specificity because $\dot{V}O_{2max}$ in untrained subjects during walking generally remains 5 to 15% below running values.[32,46]

Competition walkers achieve high yet uneconomical rates of movement, unattainable with conventional walking, with a distinctive modified walking technique that constrains the athlete to certain movement patterns regardless of walking speed. The athlete must maintain this gait despite progressive decreases in walking economy as exercise duration progresses and fatigue increases.[10,11] Among elite race-walkers, variations in walking economy contribute more to successful performance than in competitive running.[32]

ENERGY EXPENDITURE DURING RUNNING

Primary biomechanical factors that determine the energy cost of running related to velocity among mammals include the magnitude and rate of muscular force generation to counteract gravity and to operate the springlike properties of the muscle-tendon system.[39] Energy expenditure for running has been quantified in two ways: (1) during performance of the actual activity and (2) on a treadmill with precise control of speed and grade. The terms *jogging* and *running* reflect qualitative assessments related to speed and strenuousness. At identical submaximal speeds, an endurance athlete runs at a lower percentage of $\dot{V}O_{2max}$ than an untrained person, even though both maintain similar oxygen consumptions while running. The demarcation between a jog and a run relates more to the participant's fitness level; a jog for one person represents a run for another.

Independent of fitness, it becomes more economical from an energy standpoint to discontinue walking and begin running at speeds above about 8 km · h⁻¹. Figure 10.5 illustrates the relationship between oxygen consumption and horizontal walking and running for men and women at speeds between 4 and 14 km · h⁻¹. For the data depicted in purple and yellow, the lines relating oxygen consumption and speed intersect at a running speed of 8.0 km · h⁻¹; the breakpoint in locomotion economy for competition walkers (shown in red) occurs at about 8.7 km · h⁻¹.

Economy of Running Fast or Slow

The data for running in Figure 10.5 illustrate an important principle about running speed and energy expenditure. *Because of the linear relationship between oxygen consumption and running speed, the total energy requirement for running a given distance (in steady rate) is about the same regardless of speed.* Simply stated, running a mile at 10 mph requires about twice the energy per minute as running a mile at 5 mph; at the faster speed, completing the mile requires 6 minutes, but running at the slower speed takes twice as long or 12 minutes. As such, the net energy cost to traverse the mile remains about the same. Equivalent energy costs per mile (regardless of running speed) occur not only for horizontal running but also for running at a specific grade that ranges from −45 to +15%.[23,44] *During horizontal running, the net energy cost (i.e., excluding the resting requirement) per kilogram of body mass per kilometer traveled averages 1 kCal or 1 kCal · kg⁻¹ · km⁻¹.* Thus, the net energy cost of running 1 km for individuals weighing 78 kg averages 78 kCal, regardless of running speed. Expressed in terms of oxygen consumption (5 kCal = 1 L O₂), this amounts to 15.6 L of oxygen consumed per kilometer. Comparisons of net energy cost of locomotion per unit distance traveled for walking and running indicate greater energy expenditure when running a given distance.[6]

INTEGRATIVE QUESTION

An elite 140-lb runner claims she consistently consumes 12,000 kCal daily simply to maintain body weight owing to the strenuousness of her training. Using examples of exercise energy expenditures, discuss whether this level of intake could reflect a plausible energy intake.

Net Energy Cost Values

TABLE 10.3 presents values for *net energy expenditure* during running for 1 hour at various speeds—expressed in kilometers per hour, miles per hour, and the number of minutes required to complete 1 mile at a specific speed. Bolded values indicate net calories expended running 1 mile for a given body mass. As mentioned above, the energy requirement per mile remains fairly constant regardless of

PREDICTING ENERGY EXPENDITURE DURING TREADMILL WALKING AND RUNNING

■ An almost linear relationship exists between oxygen consumption (energy expenditure) and walking speeds between 3.0 and 5.0 km $\cdot$ h^{-1} (1.9 and 3.1 mph), and running at speeds faster than 8.0 km $\cdot$ h^{-1} (5 to 10 mph; see Fig. 10.5). Adding the resting oxygen consumption to the oxygen requirements of the horizontal and vertical components of the walk or run makes it possible to estimate total (gross) exercise oxygen consumption ($\dot{V}O_2$) and energy expenditure.

BASIC EQUATION

$\dot{V}O_2$ (mL $\cdot$ kg^{-1} $\cdot$ min^{-1}) = Resting component (1 MET [3.5 mL O$_2$ $\cdot$ kg^{-1}·min^{-1}]) + Horizontal component (speed, [m $\cdot$ min^{-1}] × oxygen cost of horizontal movement) + Vertical component (percentage grade × speed [m $\cdot$ min^{-1}] × oxygen cost of vertical movement).

[To convert mph to m $\cdot$ min^{-1}, multiply by 26.82; to convert m $\cdot$ min^{-1} to mph, multiply by 0.03728.]

Walking

Oxygen cost of the horizontal component of movement equals 0.1 mL $\cdot$ kg^{-1} $\cdot$ min^{-1}, and 1.8 mL $\cdot$ kg^{-1} $\cdot$ min^{-1} for the vertical component.

Running

Oxygen cost of the horizontal component of movement equals 0.2 mL $\cdot$ kg^{-1} $\cdot$ min^{-1}, and 0.9 mL $\cdot$ kg^{-1} $\cdot$ min^{-1} for the vertical component.

PREDICTING ENERGY COST OF TREADMILL WALKING

Problem

A 55-kg person walks on a treadmill at 2.8 mph (2.8 × 26.82 = 75 m $\cdot$ min^{-1}) up a 4% grade. Calculate (1) $\dot{V}O_2$ (mL $\cdot$ kg^{-1} $\cdot$ min^{-1}), (2) METs, and (3) energy expenditure (kCal $\cdot$ min^{-1}). *[Note: express % grade as a decimal value; i.e., 4% grade = 0.04]*

Solution

1. $\dot{V}O_2$ (mL $\cdot$ kg^{-1} $\cdot$ min^{-1}) = Resting component + Horizontal component + Vertical component
   $\dot{V}O_2$ = Resting $\dot{V}O_2$ (mL $\cdot$ kg^{-1} $\cdot$ min^{-1})
       + [speed (m $\cdot$ min^{-1})
       × 0.1 mL $\cdot$ kg^{-1} $\cdot$ min^{-1}]
       + [% grade × speed (m $\cdot$ min^{-1})
       × 1.8 mL $\cdot$ kg^{-1} $\cdot$ min^{-1}]
   = 3.5 + (75 × 0.1) + (0.04 × 75 × 1.8)

= 3.5 + 7.5 + 5.4
= 16.4 mL $\cdot$ kg^{-1} $\cdot$ min^{-1}

2. METs = $\dot{V}O_2$ (mL $\cdot$ kg^{-1} $\cdot$ min^{-1})
       ÷ 3.5 mL $\cdot$ kg^{-1} $\cdot$ min^{-1}
   = 16.4 ÷ 3.5
   = 4.7

3. kCal $\cdot$ min^{-1} = $\dot{V}O_2$ (mL $\cdot$ kg^{-1} $\cdot$ min^{-1})
       × Body mass (kg)
       × 5.05 kCal $\cdot$ LO$_2$$^{-1}$
   = 16.4 mL $\cdot$ kg^{-1} $\cdot$ min^{-1}
       × 55 kg × 5.05 kCal $\cdot$ L^{-1}
   = 0.902 L $\cdot$ min^{-1}
       × 5.05 kCal $\cdot$ L^{-1}
   = 4.6

PREDICTING ENERGY COST OF TREADMILL RUNNING

Problem

A 55-kg person runs on a treadmill at 5.4 mph (5.4 × 26.82 = 145 m $\cdot$ min^{-1}) up a 6% grade. Calculate (1) $\dot{V}O_2$ in mL $\cdot$ kg^{-1} $\cdot$ min^{-1}, (2) METs, and (3) energy expenditure (kCal $\cdot$ min^{-1}).

Solution

1. $\dot{V}O_2$ (mL $\cdot$ kg^{-1} $\cdot$ min^{-1}) = Resting component + Horizontal component + Vertical component
   $\dot{V}O_2$ = Resting $\dot{V}O_2$ (mL $\cdot$ kg^{-1} $\cdot$ min^{-1})
       + [speed (m $\cdot$ min^{-1})
       × 0.2 mL $\cdot$ kg^{-1} $\cdot$ min^{-1}]
       + [% grade × speed (m $\cdot$ min^{-1})
       × 0.9 mL $\cdot$ kg^{-1} $\cdot$ min^{-1}]
   = 3.5 + (145 × 0.2) + (0.06 × 145 × 0.9)
   = 3.5 + 29.0 + 7.83
   = 40.33 mL $\cdot$ kg^{-1} $\cdot$ min^{-1}

2. METs = $\dot{V}O_2$ (mL $\cdot$ kg^{-1} $\cdot$ min^{-1})
       ÷ 3.5 mL $\cdot$ kg^{-1} $\cdot$ min^{-1}
   = 40.33 ÷ 3.5
   = 11.5

3. kCal $\cdot$ min^{-1} = $\dot{V}O_2$ (mL $\cdot$ kg^{-1} $\cdot$ min^{-1})
       × Body mass (kg)
       × 5.05 kCal $\cdot$ LO$_2$$^{-1}$
   = 40.33 mL $\cdot$ kg^{-1} $\cdot$ min^{-1}
       × 55 kg × 5.05 kCal $\cdot$ L^{-1}
   = 2.22 L $\cdot$ min^{-1}
       × 5.05 kCal $\cdot$ L^{-1}
   = 11.2

TABLE 10.3 ■ NET ENERGY EXPENDITURE PER HOUR OF HORIZONTAL RUNNING RELATED TO VELOCITY AND BODY MASS[a]

BODY MASS		$KM \cdot H^{-1}$[b] MPH MIN PER MILE	8 4.97 12:00	9 5.60 10:43	10 6.20 9:41	11 6.84 8:46	12 7.46 8:02	13 8.08 7:26	14 8.70 6:54	15 9.32 6:26	16 9.94 6:02
(KG)	(LB)	KCAL PER MILE									
50	110	**80**	400	450	500	550	600	650	700	750	800
54	119	**86**	432	486	540	594	648	702	756	810	864
58	128	**93**	464	522	580	638	696	754	812	870	928
62	137	**99**	496	558	620	682	744	806	868	930	992
66	146	**106**	528	594	660	726	792	858	924	990	1056
70	154	**112**	560	630	700	770	840	910	980	1050	1120
74	163	**118**	592	666	740	814	888	962	1036	1110	1184
78	172	**125**	624	702	780	858	936	1014	1092	1170	1248
82	181	**131**	656	738	820	902	984	1066	1148	1230	1312
86	190	**138**	688	774	860	946	1032	1118	1204	1290	1376
90	199	**144**	720	810	900	990	1080	1170	1260	1350	1440
94	207	**150**	752	846	940	1034	1128	1222	1316	1410	1504
98	216	**157**	784	882	980	1078	1176	1274	1372	1470	1568
102	225	**163**	816	918	1020	1122	1224	1326	1428	1530	1632
106	234	**170**	848	954	1060	1166	1272	1378	1484	1590	1696

[a] Interpret the table as follows: For a 50-kg person, the *net* energy expenditure for running for 1 hour at 8 km · h⁻¹ or 4.97 mph equals 400 kCal; this speed represents a 12-minute per mile pace. Thus, 5 miles would be run in 1 hour and 400 kCal would be expended. Increasing the pace to 12 km · h⁻¹ expends 600 kCal during the hour of running.
[b] Running speeds are expressed as kilometers per hour (km · h⁻¹), miles per hour (mph), and minutes required to complete each mile (min per mile). The values in **boldface type** are *net* calories expended to run 1 mile for a given body mass, independent of running speed.

running speed. *A person who weighs 62 kg requires approximately 2600 kCal (net) to run a 26.2-mile marathon regardless of whether the run takes just over 2 hours, 3 hours, or 4 hours!*

Table 10.3 also indicates that the energy cost per mile increases proportionately with body mass. A lower energy cost (less heat production) in lighter runners at any given speed partly explains why small stature (and relatively larger surface area for heat dissipation) provides an advantage in distance running, particularly in warm, humid environments.[26] The influence of body mass on exercise energy expenditure certainly supports the role of weight-bearing exercise as an additional caloric stressor for the overly fat person who should increase daily energy expenditure for weight loss (see "Focus on Research," p. 223). For example, a 102-kg person who runs 5 miles each day at a comfortable pace expends 163 kCal for each mile completed or 815 kCal for the 5-mile run. *Increasing or decreasing the speed (within the broad range of steady-rate paces) simply alters the duration of the 5-mile run; it has little effect on the total energy (kCal) expended.*

TABLE 10.4 summarizes data from various studies of energy expenditure for horizontal and grade walking and running on a firm surface. The energy requirement represents multiples of the resting metabolic rate or METs (1 MET = 3.5 mL O_2 kg⁻¹ · min⁻¹).

Stride Length, Stride Frequency, and Speed

Running

One can increase running speed in three ways: (1) increase the number of steps each minute (*stride frequency*), (2) increase the distance between steps (*stride length*), or (3) increase *both* the length and frequency of strides. The third option may seem obvious for increasing running speed, but several experiments have provided objective data concerning this alternative.

Research in 1944 evaluated the stride pattern for the Danish champion in the 5- and 10-km running events.[8] At a running speed of 9.3 km · h⁻¹, this athlete's stride frequency equaled 160 per minute, with a corresponding stride length of 97 cm. When running speed increased 91% to 17.8 km · h⁻¹, stride frequency increased only 10%, to 176 per minute, whereas stride length increased 83%, to 168 cm. FIGURE 10.6A displays the interaction between stride frequency and stride length as running speed increases. Doubling the speed from 10 to 20 km · h⁻¹ increases stride length by 85%, whereas stride frequency increases only about 9%. Running at speeds above 23 km · h⁻¹ occurs mainly by increasing stride frequency. *As a general rule, running speed increases mainly by lengthening the stride. Only at faster speeds does stride frequency become important.* Relying on increasing the length of the "stroke"

TABLE 10.4 ■ **ENERGY REQUIREMENTS (METs) FOR HORIZONTAL AND GRADE WALKING AND RUNNING ON A SOLID SURFACE**

HORIZONTAL AND GRADE WALKING

% GRADE	MPH	1.7	2.0	2.5	3.0	3.4	3.75
	M · MIN⁻¹	45.6	53.7	67.0	80.5	91.2	100.5
0		2.3	2.5	2.9	3.3	3.6	3.9
2.5		2.9	3.2	3.8	4.3	4.8	5.2
5.0		3.5	3.9	4.6	5.4	5.9	6.5
7.5		4.1	4.6	5.5	6.4	7.1	7.8
10.0		4.6	5.3	6.3	7.4	8.3	9.1
12.5		5.2	6.0	7.2	8.5	9.5	10.4
15.0		5.8	6.6	8.1	9.5	10.6	11.7
17.5		6.4	7.3	8.9	10.5	11.8	12.9
20.0		7.0	8.0	9.8	11.6	13.0	14.2
22.5		7.6	8.7	10.6	12.6	14.2	15.5
25.0		8.2	9.4	11.5	13.6	15.3	16.8

HORIZONTAL AND GRADE JOGGING/RUNNING

% GRADE	MPH	5	6	7	7.5	8	9	10
	M · MIN⁻¹	134	161	188	201	215	241	268
0		8.6	10.2	11.7	12.5	13.3	14.8	16.3
2.5		10.3	12.3	14.1	15.1	16.1	17.9	19.7
5.0		12.0	14.3	16.5	17.7	18.8		
7.5		13.9	16.4	18.9				
10.0		15.5	18.5					

Modified from ACSM guidelines for exercise testing and prescription, 7th ed. Baltimore: Lippincott Williams & Wilkins, 2006.

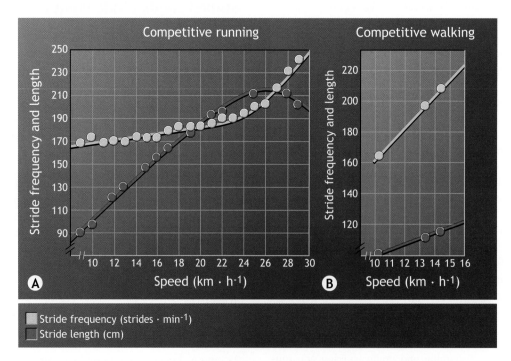

Figure 10.6 **A**. Stride frequency and stride length plotted as a function of running speed. **B.** Data for an Olympic walker during race-walking. (From Hogberg P. Length of stride, stride frequency, flight period and maximum distance between the feet during running with different speeds. Int Z Angew Physiol 1952;14:431.)

cycle, not the frequency. To achieve more rapid speeds in endurance performance also occurs among top-flight kayakers, rowers, cross-country skiers, and speed skaters.

Competition Walking

The competitive walker does not increase speed the same way a runner does. Figure 10.6B illustrates the stride length–stride frequency relationship for an Olympic 10-km medal winner who walked at speeds from 10 to 14.4 km · h^{-1}. When walking speed increased within this range, stride frequency increased by 27% and stride length increased by 13%. Faster speeds produced an even greater increase in stride frequency. Unlike running, in which the body glides through the air, competitive race-walking requires that the back foot remain on the ground until the front foot makes contact. Thus, lengthening the stride becomes a difficult and ineffective way to increase speed. Consequently, involving the trunk and arm musculature to move the leg forward rapidly requires additional energy expenditure; this explains the poorer economy for walking than for running at speeds above 8 or 9 km · h^{-1} (see Fig. 10.4).

Optimum Stride Length

Each person runs at a constant speed with an optimum combination of stride length and stride frequency. This optimum depends largely on the person's mechanics or "style" of running and cannot be determined from body measurements.[16] Nevertheless, energy expenditure increases more for overstriding than for understriding. FIGURE 10.7 relates oxy-gen consumption to different stride lengths altered by a subject running at the relatively fast speed of 14 km · h^{-1}.

For this runner, a stride length of 135 cm produced the lowest oxygen consumption (3.35 L · min^{-1}). When stride length decreased to 118 cm, oxygen consumption increased 8%; lengthening the distance between steps to 153 cm increased oxygen consumption by 12%. The inset graph shows a similar pattern for oxygen consumption when running speed increased to 16 km · h^{-1} and stride lengths varied between 135 and 169 cm. Decreasing this runner's stride length from the optimum of 149 cm to 135 cm increased oxygen consumption by 4.1%; lengthening the stride to 169 cm increased aerobic energy expenditure nearly 13%. As one might expect, the stride length selected by the subject (marked in the figure by the solid orange circle) produced the most economical stride length (lowest $\dot{V}O_2$). Lengthening the stride above the optimum caused a larger increase in oxygen consumption than a shorter-than-optimum length. Urging a runner who shows signs of fatigue to "lengthen your stride!" to maintain speed actually proves counterproductive in terms of economy of effort.

Well-trained runners should run at the stride length they have selected through years of running. In keeping with the concept that the body attempts to achieve a **level of minimum effort**, a self-selected length and frequency generally produce the most economical running performance. This reflects an individual's unique body size, inertia of limb segments, and anatomic development.[15,50,51] *No "best" style characterizes elite runners.* Biomechanical analysis may help the athlete correct minor irregularities in movement patterns while running. For the competitive runner, any minor improvement in movement economy generally improves performance.

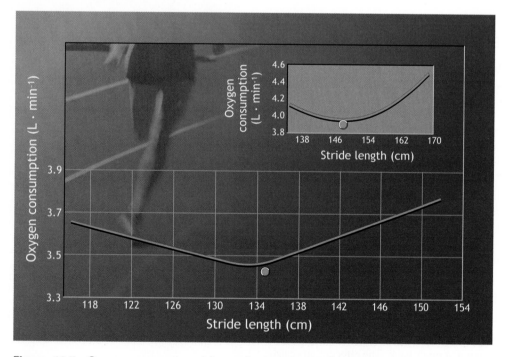

Figure 10.7 Oxygen consumption while running at 14 km · h^{-1} affected by different stride lengths. The *inset graph* plots oxygen consumption at a faster speed of 16 km · h^{-1}. (From Hogberg P. Length of stride, stride frequency, flight period and maximum distance between the feet during running with different speeds. Int Z Angew Physiol 1952;14:431.)

Running Economy: Children and Adults, Trained and Untrained

Boys and girls are less economical runners than adults because they require 20 to 30% more oxygen per unit body mass to run at a particular speed.[2,38,58] Consequently, adult models to predict energy cost in weight-bearing locomotion fails to account for the increased (and changing) energy costs in children and adolescents.[57]

FIGURE 10.8 illustrates the relationship between walking and running speeds (speeds between 2 and 8 mph) and oxygen consumption (A) and energy expenditure (B) in 47 male and 35 female adolescent volunteers. Despite the higher oxygen consumption and energy expenditure values during walking and running for adolescents than in adults (depicted in Figure 10.5), the shape of the curves for both groups remains remarkably similar.

Increased energy expenditure (reduced economy) among children and adolescents in weight-bearing exercise has been attributed to a larger ratio of surface area to mass, greater stride frequencies, and shorter stride lengths and to differences in anthropometric variables and body mechanics that reduce movement economy.[29,67] FIGURE 10.9B illustrates that running economy improves steadily during years 10 through 18. Poor running economy among young children partly explains their inferior performance in distance running compared with adults, and their progressive performance improvement through adolescence, while aerobic capacity (mL $O_2 \cdot kg^{-1} \cdot min^{-1}$; Fig. 10.9A) remains relatively constant throughout this period. Consequently, improvement during the growth years in scores in weight-bearing exercise tests like the 1-mile walk-run do not necessarily imply concomitant improvement in $\dot{V}O_{2max}$.[22]

INTEGRATIVE QUESTION

Discuss the practical implications of knowing that children demonstrate significantly lower economy for walking and running than adults.

When running at a particular speed, elite adolescent and adult endurance runners generally have lower oxygen consumptions than less trained or less successful age-matched counterparts.[36,56] Distance athletes as a group run 5 to 10% more economically than well-trained middle-distance runners. For trained runners, economy values and biomechanical characteristics during running remain fairly stable from day to day, even during high-intensity exercise, with probably no difference between genders.[24,53,54]

Air Resistance

Anyone who has run into a headwind knows that it requires greater energy to maintain a given pace than running in calm air or with the wind at one's back. The effect of air resistance on the energy cost of running varies with three factors: (1) air density, (2) runner's projected surface area, and (3) square of running velocity. Depending on speed, overcoming air resist-

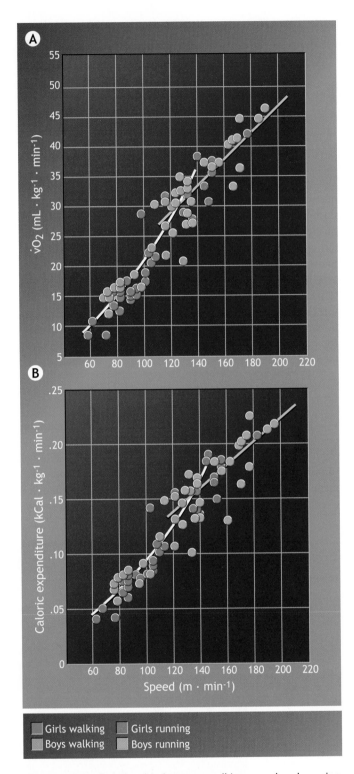

Figure 10.8   Relationship between walking speed and running speed and oxygen consumption (**A**) and energy expenditure (**B**) in adolescent boys and girls. The *white line* represents the curve-of-best-fit for walking; the *yellow line* represents the best-fit line for running. (From Walker JL, et al. The energy cost of horizontal walking and running in adolescents. Med Sci Sports Exerc 1999;31:311.)

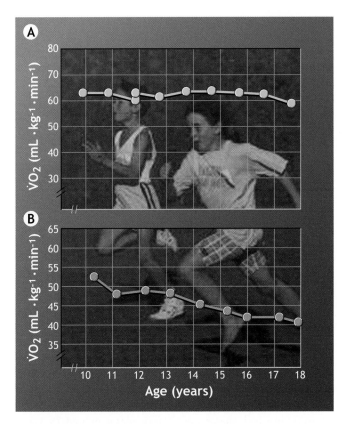

Figure 10.9 Effects of growth during childhood and adolescence on (**A**) aerobic capacity and (**B**) submaximal oxygen consumption during running at 202 m · min⁻¹. (Adapted from Daniels J, et al. Differences and changes in V̇O₂ among runners 10 to 18 years of age. Med Sci Sports 1978;10:200.)

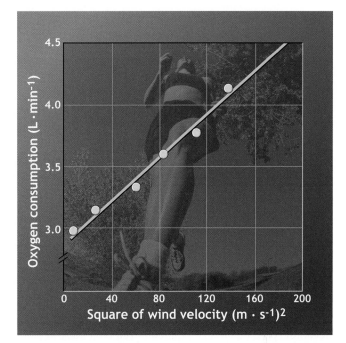

Figure 10.10 Oxygen consumption as a function of the square of the wind velocity while running at 15.9 km · h⁻¹ against various headwinds. (From Pugh LGCE. Oxygen intake and treadmill running with observations on the effect of air resistance. J Physiol 1970;207:823.)

ance requires 3 to 9% of the total energy cost of running in calm air.[63] Running into a headwind creates an additional energy "expense." FIGURE 10.10 shows that the oxygen consumption while running at 15.9 km · h⁻¹ in calm conditions averaged 2.92 L · min⁻¹. This increased 5.5% to 3.09 L · min⁻¹ against a 16-km · h⁻¹ headwind, and further to 4.1 L · min⁻¹ when running against the strongest wind (66 km · h⁻¹; 41 mph)—an additional 41% expenditure of energy to maintain running velocity!

Some may argue that the negative effects of running into a headwind become counterbalanced during one's return with the tailwind. This does not occur because the energy cost of cutting through a headwind exceeds the reduced oxygen consumption with an equivalent wind velocity at one's back. Wind tunnel tests show that clothing modification or even trimming one's hair improves aerodynamics and reduces the effects of air resistance up to 6%. A reduction of this magnitude translates into improved running performance. This fact has not escaped the elite athlete; wearing modern running suits takes advantage of any reduction in air resistance. At higher altitudes, wind velocity has less effect on energy expenditure than at sea level because of the lower air density at higher elevations. Moderate altitude always lowers the oxygen cost of competitive skating at a given speed compared with that at sea level.[3] An altitude effect probably also applies to the energy cost of running, cross-country skiing, and cycling.

Drafting: Often a Wise Position

The negative effect of air resistance and headwind on the energy cost of running confirms the wisdom of athletes who choose to run in a more aerodynamically desirable position directly behind a competitor. This technique, called **drafting**, maintains a sheltered position for the person taking advantage of it. Running 1 m behind another runner at a speed of 21.6 km · h⁻¹, for example, decreases total energy expenditure by about 7%.[61] The beneficial effect of drafting on economy of effort also occurs for cross-country skiing, short-track speed skating, and bicycling.[7,47,68] Bicycling at 40 km · h⁻¹ on a calm day requires generation of about 90% of the total exercise power simply to overcome air resistance. At this speed, energy expenditure decreases 26 to 38% when a competitor closely follows another cyclist.[40]

For elite cyclists, helmets now weigh 5.64 ounces, or less than a full can of soda. Helmet shape reduces drag by directing wind over the head and past the rider's back when leaning forward; adding dimples to the jersey reduces the drag, and the Dri-Fit microfiber polyester sucks moisture away from the body to facilitate a cooler and drier ride. When these economy-enhancing and thermal-optimizing modifications to equipment combine with a physiologic capacity of a seven-time Tour de France Champion with an oversized heart that pumps out nearly 34 L of blood per minute (versus 19 L for the average person) and V̇O₂max of 83 · mL · kg⁻¹ · min⁻¹ and an exceptionally high blood lactate threshold, the ingredients exist for world-class performance.[19]

For elite speed skaters, drafting (within 1 m of the leader) during controlled-pace 4-minute skating trials lowers exercise heart rate and blood lactate concentration.[68] A reduced level of exercise stress with drafting should theoretically give the competitor an additional energy reserve for the sprint to the finish. When triathletes maintain the drafting position during the cycling leg of a sprint-distance triathlon (0.75-km swim, 20-km bike, 5-km run), oxygen consumptions, heart rates, and blood lactate concentrations remain significantly lower than when the athletes cycle at the same speed without drafting.[34] These physiologic benefits translate into improved subsequent performance as maximal running speed after biking in the drafting situation is faster than running performance in no-draft trials.

Treadmill Versus Track Running

The treadmill provides the primary exercise mode to evaluate the physiology of running. One might question the validity of this procedure for determining energy metabolism during running and relating it to competitive track performance. For example, does the energy required to run at a given treadmill speed equal that required to run on a track in calm weather? To answer this question, eight distance runners ran on a treadmill and track under calm air conditions at three submaximal speeds of 180 m $\cdot$ min^{-1}, 210 m $\cdot$ min^{-1}, and 260 m $\cdot$ min^{-1}. Graded exercise tests determined possible differences between treadmill and track running on maximal oxygen consumption. TABLE 10.5 summarizes the results for one submaximal running speed and maximal exercise.

From a practical standpoint, no measurable differences emerged in the aerobic requirements of submaximal running (up to 286 m $\cdot$ min^{-1}) on the treadmill and track, either on level or up grade, or between the $\dot{V}O_{2max}$ in both forms of exercise. The possibility exists that at the faster speeds achieved by elite endurance runners, the impact of air resistance on a calm day increases the oxygen cost of track running compared with "stationary" treadmill running at the same fast speed.

This certainly occurs in activities requiring the athlete to move at high velocities as in cycling and speed skating, in which the retarding effects of air resistance become considerable. Factors that improve aerodynamics—clothing, equipment, and body position—can improve performance.

Marathon Running

The current (as of October 2005) world marathon record is 2h:04 min:55 s (P. Tergat of Kenya, September 28, 2003). This average speed of 4 min:46 s per mile over the 26.2-mile course represents a truly outstanding achievement in human exercise capacity. Not only does this blistering pace require a steady-rate oxygen consumption that exceeds the aerobic capacity of most male college students, it also demands that the marathoner sustain 80 to 90% of $\dot{V}O_{2max}$ for just over 2 hours!

Researchers measured two distance runners during a marathon to assess energy expenditure each minute and the total caloric cost of the run.[45] They determined oxygen consumption every 3 miles using open-circuit spirometry (Chapter 8). Marathon times were 2 h:36 min:34 s ($\dot{V}O_{2max} = 70.5$ mL $\cdot$ kg^{-1} $\cdot$ min^{-1}) and 2 h:39 min:28 s ($\dot{V}O_{2max} = 73.9$ mL $\cdot$ kg^{-1} $\cdot$ min^{-1}). The first runner maintained an average speed of 16.2 km $\cdot$ h^{-1} that required an oxygen consumption equal to 80% of $\dot{V}O_{2max}$. For the second runner, who averaged a slower speed of 16.0 km $\cdot$ h^{-1}, the aerobic component averaged 78.3% of maximum. For both men, the total energy required to run the marathon ranged between 2300 and 2400 kCal.

SWIMMING

Swimming differs in several important aspects from walking or running. One obvious difference entails the expenditure of energy to maintain buoyancy while simultaneously generating horizontal movement by using arms and legs, either in combination or separately. Other differences include the requirements for overcoming **drag forces** that impede a swimmer's forward movement. The amount of drag depends on the fluid medium and the swimmer's size, shape, and velocity. These factors contribute to a mechanical efficiency in front-crawl swimming that ranges between only 5 and 9.5%.[76] *A significantly lower mechanical efficiency makes the energy cost of swimming a given distance average about four times more than the energy cost of running the same distance.*

Methods of Measurement

For short swims of 25 yards at different velocities, subjects need not breathe. Estimates of energy expenditure can derive from oxygen consumption during a 20- to 40-minute recovery. For longer swims, including 12- to 14-hour endurance events, one can compute energy expenditure from oxygen consumption measured with open-circuit spirometry during portions of the swim. In studies conducted in the pool, pacer lights alongside the pool control swimming velocity, and the researcher walks alongside the swimmer and carries portable gas-collection equipment (FIG. 10.11E). For another form of swimming exercise, illustrated in Figure

TABLE 10.5 ■ COMPARISON OF AVERAGE METABOLIC RESPONSES DURING TREADMILL AND TRACK RUNNING			
MEASUREMENT	TREADMILL	TRACK	DIFFERENCE
Submaximal Exercise			
Oxygen consumption, mL $\cdot$ kg^{-1} $\cdot$ min^{-1}	42.2	42.7	0.5
Respiratory exchange ratio	0.89	0.87	−0.02
Running speed, m $\cdot$ min^{-1}	213.7	216.8	3.1
Maximal Exercise			
Oxygen consumption, L $\cdot$ min^{-1}	4.40	4.44	0.04
mL $\cdot$ kg^{-1} $\cdot$ min^{-1}	66.9	66.3	−0.6
Ventilation, L $\cdot$ min^{-1}, BTPS	142.5	146.5	4.0
Respiratory exchange ratio	1.15	1.11	−0.04

Adapted from McMiken DF, Daniels JT. Aerobic requirements and maximum aerobic power in treadmill and track running. Med Sci Sports 1976;8:14.

FOCUS On Research

IT COSTS MORE ENERGY TO MOVE MORE

Mahadeva K, et al. Individual variations in the metabolic cost of standardized exercises: the effects of food, age, sex and race. J Physiol 1953;121:225.

▲ Few early experiments in human energy metabolism dealt with energy requirements during exercise, particularly the influence of body size, age, gender, and skill. We now know that such contributing factors serve an important purpose for exercise prescription and estimating energy expenditure to adjust energy balance for weight loss and weight maintenance.

Mahadeva and colleagues conducted one of the first large-scale energy cost studies that focused attention on energy expenditure in two common exercise forms: (1) stepping that produces measurable external work in raising body mass and (2) walking on the level at a constant speed. The researchers made multiple observations on 50 men and women, aged 13 to 79 years, of diverse ethnic backgrounds, whose body mass ranged from 48 to 110 kg. Measurements included basal and resting metabolism with the Douglas bag method of open-circuit spirometry. Exercise studies used the portable Kofranyi-Michaelis spirometer (see Fig 8.3). Subjects stepped to a metronome cadence of 15 up-and-down cycles per minute for 10 minutes on a 25.4-cm stool and walked on an indoor track for 10 minutes at 4.8 km · h^{-1}.

The two graphs show the relationship and corresponding prediction (regression) line between energy expenditure and body mass for each activity (*C*, energy expenditure in kCal per 10 min; *W*, body mass in kg). Energy expenditure in walking and stepping varied directly with body mass. Separate analyses showed that age, gender, ethnicity, and previous diet contributed little to predicting energy cost of the activities. This pioneering work showed that body mass primarily determines the energy expended in nonskilled physical activities that require transporting one's body mass (i.e., weight-bearing

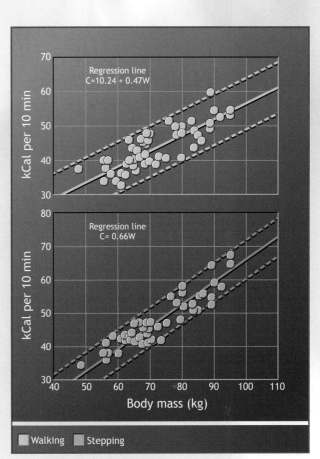

Top. Energy expenditure in kilocalories per 10 minutes as a function of body mass during walking at 3 mph. *Bottom.* Energy expenditure in kilocalories per 10 minutes as a function of body mass during stepping. The *dashed lines* show twice the standard error of estimate.

exercise). We now can accurately predict energy cost during steady-rate walking, running, and stepping exercise simply from knowledge of exercise intensity and body mass.

10.11A, the subject remains stationary, attached or tethered to a cable and pulley system by a belt worn around the waist. Periodic increases in the weight stack attached to the cable force the swimmer to exert greater effort to maintain a constant body position. Figure 10.11, B–D shows a swimmer in a flume or "swimming treadmill." Water circulates at velocities varying from a slow swimming speed to near-record pace for a freestyle sprint. Aerobic capacity measurements using tethered, free, or flume swimming produce essentially identical values.[9] Any of these modes of measurement objectively evaluate metabolic and physiologic dynamics during swimming.

Energy Cost and Drag

The total drag force encountered by a swimmer consists of three components:

- **Wave drag**—caused by waves that build up in front of, and form hollows behind, the swimmer moving through the water. This component of drag does not significantly affect swimming at slow velocities, but its influence increases at faster swimming speeds.
- **Skin friction drag**—produced as the water slides over the skin surface. Even at relatively fast

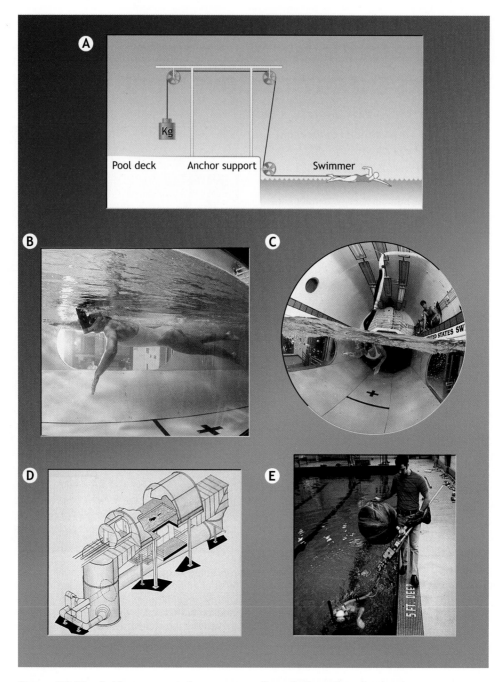

Figure 10.11   A. Measurement of energy expenditure during tethered swimming.
B–D. Swimming treadmill. An environmental chamber surrounding the swimming treadmill
controls atmospheric pressure (and other environmental conditions) during swimming. Using the
swimming treadmill, researchers conduct physiologic and biomechanical experiments during
swimming that simulate actual performance conditions. The underwater viewing area provides a
convenient means for directly observing swimming performance related to stroke mechanics.
E. Open-circuit spirometry (bag technique) to measure oxygen consumption during front-crawl
swimming. (Schematic and photos of the swimming treadmill courtesy of the United States
Swimming International Center for Aquatic Research, Colorado Springs, CO.)

swimming velocities, the quantitative contribution of
skin friction drag to the total drag remains small.
Research supports the common practice of swimmers
"shaving down" to reduce skin friction drag and
thereby decrease energy cost.[71]

- **Viscous pressure drag**—caused by the pressure differential created in front of and behind the swimmer,

which substantially counters propulsive efforts at slow
velocities. Viscous pressure drag, caused by the separation of the thin sheet of water or boundary layer, forms
adjacent to the swimmer. Its effect is reduced for highly
skilled swimmers who learn to streamline stroke mechanics. This reduces the separation region by moving
it closer to the trailing edge of the water, akin to an oar

slicing through water with the blade parallel rather than perpendicular to the water flow.

Ways to Reduce Effects of Drag Force

FIGURE 10.12 depicts a curvilinear relationship between body drag and velocity when towing a swimmer through the water. As velocity increases above 0.8 m · s⁻¹, drag decreases by supporting the legs with a flotation device that places the body in a more hydrodynamically desirable horizontal position. Generally, drag force averages 2 to 2.5 times more during swimming than passive towing.[75]

Variations in swim suit designs tend to reduce overall drag with a greater effect noted for suits that cover the shoulder to either the ankle or knee than for those that covered only the lower body or a conventional suit.[52] Wet suits worn by triathletes during swimming reduce body drag by about 14%, thus lowering oxygen consumption at a given speed.[76,78] Improved swimming economy largely explains the faster swim times of triathletes who use wet suits. As in running, cross-country skiing, and cycling, drafting in swimming (following up to 50 cm behind the toes of a lead swimmer) reduces drag force, metabolic cost (by 11 to 38%), and physiologic demand,[4,18] and also improves economy in a subsequent cycling session.[25] This effect enables an endurance swimmer (e.g., triathlete or ocean racer) to conserve energy and possibly improve performance toward the end of the competition. Triathletes swimming 400 m swam the total distance 3% faster in a drafting position with lower blood lactate levels and stroke rates than in the lead position.[17] Performance changes were related to large reductions in passive drag force in the drafting position; faster and leaner swimmers showed the greatest drag force reduction and performance improvement.

In the 2004 Athens Summer Olympic Games, swimmers wore neck-to-ankle body suits. Proponents maintain that the technology-driven approach to competitive swimming maximizes swimming economy and allows swimmers to achieve 3% faster times than those with standard swimsuits.

Kayaking. The energy demands of kayaking largely reflect the resistance provided by the water to the forward movement of the craft. Consequently, drafting (wash riding) behind the leader reduces the energy requirements of paddling between 18 and 32%.[60] Improved kayaking economy results from the assist to forward movement provided by the wash generated by the lead boat. This effect decreases resistance and water pressure through which the boat moves.

Energy Cost, Swimming Velocity, and Skill

Elite swimmers swim a particular stroke at a given velocity with lower oxygen consumption (greater economy) than relatively untrained or recreational swimmers. Highly skilled swimmers use more of the energy they generate per stroke to overcome drag forces. Consequently, they cover a greater distance per stroke than less skilled swimmers who waste considerable energy ineffectively moving water. FIGURE 10.13A compares the oxygen consumptions and velocities for the breaststroke, back crawl, and front crawl at three levels of swimming ability. One subject, a recreational swimmer, did not participate in swim training; the trained subject, a top Swedish swimmer, swam on a daily basis; the elite swimmer was a European champion. Except during the breaststroke, the elite swimmer had a lower oxygen consumption at a given speed than trained and untrained counterparts. Figure 10.13B illustrates that the breaststroke required greater oxygen consumption for the trained swimmers at any speed, followed by the backstroke, with the front crawl being the least "expensive" of the three strokes. The marked accelerations and decelerations within the stroke cycle cause the energy expended for the butterfly and breaststroke to nearly double that for the front and back crawl at the same speeds.[74] At comparable speeds that could be sustained aerobically, the energy cost of surface swimming with fins was about 40% lower than swimming without them.[79]

Effects of Water Temperature

Relatively cold water places the swimmer under thermal stress. This initiates metabolic and cardiovascular adjustments different from swimming in warmer water. These adaptive responses primarily maintain a stable core temperature by

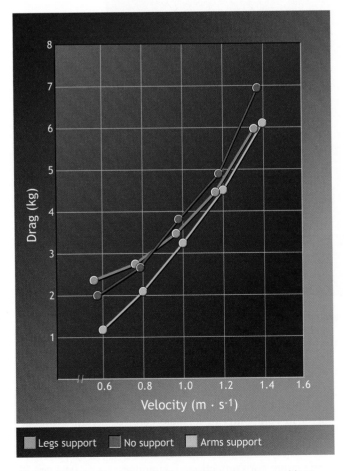

Figure 10.12 Drag force in three different prone positions related to towing velocity. (From Holmér I. Energy cost of arm stroke, leg kick, and the whole stroke in competitive swimming styles. Eur J Appl Physiol 1974;33:105.)

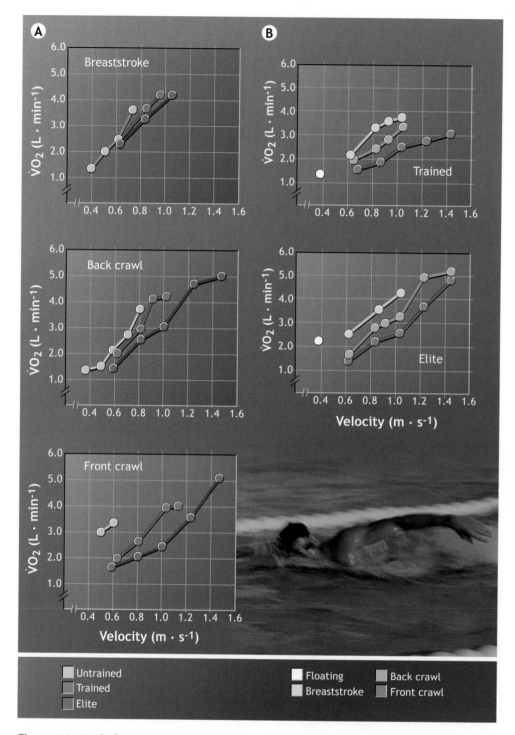

Figure 10.13   A. Oxygen consumption related to swimming velocity for the breaststroke, front crawl, and back crawl in subjects at three levels of skill ability. **B.** Oxygen consumption for two trained swimmers during three competitive strokes. (From Holmér I. Oxygen uptake during swimming in man. J Appl Physiol 1972;33:502.)

compensating for considerable heat loss from the body, particularly at water temperatures below 25°C (77°F). Body heat loss occurs most readily in lean swimmers, who lack the benefits from the insulatory effects of subcutaneous fat accumulation.

FIGURE 10.14 illustrates oxygen consumption during breaststroke swimming at water temperatures of 18, 26, and 33°C. Regardless of swimming speed, the highest oxygen

consumptions occurred in cold water. The body begins to shiver in cold water to regulate core temperature; this accounts for the extra oxygen cost of swimming in cold water. For individuals of average body composition, optimal water temperature for competitive swimming ranges between 28 and 30°C (82 to 86°F). Within this range, the metabolic heat generated during exercise transfers readily to the water.

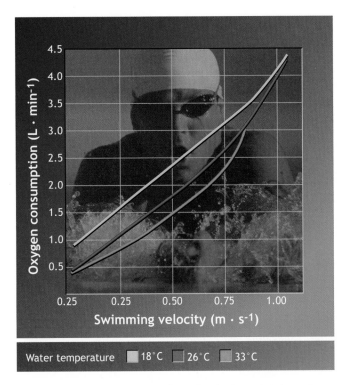

Water temperature ■ 18°C □ 26°C ■ 33°C

Figure 10.14 Energy expenditure for the breaststroke at three water temperatures related to swimming velocity. (From Nadel ER, et al. Energy exchanges of swimming man. J Appl Physiol 1974;36:465.)

However, the heat flow gradient from the body is not large enough to stimulate increased energy metabolism (shivering) or reduce core temperature from cold stress.

Effects of Buoyancy: Men Versus Women

Women of all ages possess, on average, a higher body fat percentage than men. Because fat floats and muscle and bone sink in water, the average woman gains a hydrodynamic lift and expends less energy to stay afloat than her male counterpart. More than likely, gender differences in percentage body fat and thus body buoyancy partially explain the greater swimming economy for women. For example, women swim a given distance at about a 30% lower total energy cost than do men. Expressed another way, women achieve higher swimming velocities than men for the same energy expenditure.

Women also show a greater peripheral body fat distribution. This causes their legs and arms to float relatively high in water, making them more streamlined. In contrast, the leaner legs of men tend to swing down and float lower in the water.[14] Lowering the legs to a deeper position increases body drag and reduces swimming economy (see Fig. 10.12). Enhanced flotation and the females' smaller body size, which also reduces drag, contribute to the gender difference in swimming economy.[74,75] The potential hydrodynamic benefits that women possess become noteworthy during longer distance ocean swims because swimming economy and body insulation contribute significantly to success. For example, the woman's

record for swimming the 21-mile English Channel from England to France equals 7 h 40 min (Penney Dean). The men's record (Chad Hundeby) equals 7 hr: 17 min, a difference of only 5.2%. In several instances, women swam faster than men. In fact, the first women to swim the Channel (1926) swam 35% faster than the first male to complete the swim (1875).

Endurance Swimmers

Distance swimming in ocean water poses a severe metabolic and physiologic challenge. A study of nine English Channel swimmers included measurements taken under race conditions in a salt-water pool at swimming speeds that ranged from 2.6 to 4.9 km $\cdot$ h^{-1}.[64] During the race, competitors maintained a constant stroke rate and pace until the last few hours when fatigue set in. From detailed observations of one male subject, the average speed of 2.85 km $\cdot$ h^{-1} during a 12-hour swim required an average oxygen consumption of 1.7 L $O_2 \cdot$ min^{-1}, or an equivalent energy expenditure of 8.5 kCal $\cdot$ min^{-1}. The gross caloric requirement for the 12-hour swim was about 6120 kCal (8.5 kCal $\times$ 60 min $\times$ 12 h). The net energy cost of swimming the English Channel, assuming a resting energy expenditure of 1.2 kCal $\cdot$ min^{-1} (0.260 L $O_2 \cdot$ min^{-1}), exceeded 5200 kCal, or approximately twice the number of calories expended running a marathon.

INTEGRATIVE QUESTION

Discuss whether swim training improves swimming economy more than run training improves running economy.

Summary

1. Total or gross energy expenditure includes the resting energy requirement; net energy expenditure represents the energy cost of the activity excluding the resting value.
2. Economy of movement refers to the oxygen consumed during steady-rate exercise; mechanical efficiency evaluates the relationship between work accomplished and energy expended doing the work.
3. Walking, running, and cycling produce mechanical efficiencies between 20 and 25%. Efficiencies decrease below 20% for activities with considerable resistance to movement (drag).
4. A linear relationship exists between walking speed and oxygen consumption at normal walking speeds. Walking surface also affects energy cost; walking on sand requires about twice the energy as walking on firm surfaces. A proportionately larger energy cost exists for heavier persons during such weight-bearing exercises.
5. Running becomes more economical than walking at speeds that exceed 8 km $\cdot$ h^{-1}.
6. Handheld and ankle weights can increase the energy cost of walking to values usually observed for running.

7. The total caloric cost of running a given distance at steady-rate oxygen consumption remains essentially the same regardless of running speed.

8. Net energy expenditure during horizontal running approximates $1 \; kCal \cdot kg^{-1} \cdot km^{-1}$.

9. It generally requires less energy to shorten running stride and increase stride frequency to maintain a constant running speed than to lengthen stride and reduce its frequency.

10. An individual subconsciously "selects" the combination of stride length and frequency that favors optimal economy of movement (i.e., a level of minimum effort).

11. Energy expended to overcome air resistance accounts for 3 to 9% of the energy cost of running in calm air. This percentage increases considerably if a runner attempts to maintain pace while running into a brisk headwind.

12. Children generally require more oxygen to transport their body mass while running than do adults. A relatively lower running economy accounts for the poor endurance performance of children, compared with adults of similar aerobic capacity.

13. Running a given distance or speed on a treadmill requires about the same energy as running on a track under identical environmental conditions.

14. A person expends about four times more energy to swim a given distance than to run the same distance. This occurs because the swimmer expends considerable energy to maintain buoyancy and overcome drag forces that impede forward movement.

15. Elite swimmers expend fewer calories to swim a given stroke at any velocity than less skilled counterparts.

16. Significant gender differences exist in body drag, mechanical efficiency, and net oxygen consumption during swimming. Women swim a given distance at about a 30% lower energy cost than men.

References are available on the Student CD and online at http://connection.lww.com/mkk6e.

Individual Differences and Measurement of Energy Capacities

11

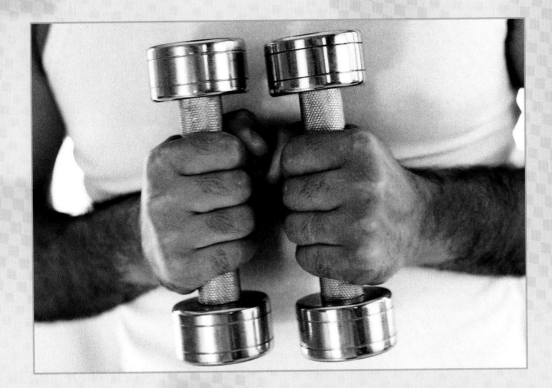

CHAPTER OBJECTIVES

- Explain specificity and generality applied to exercise performance and physiologic functions

- Outline the anaerobic-to-aerobic exercise energy transfer continuum

- Review procedures for administering two practical "field tests" to evaluate power output capacity of the immediate energy system

- Describe a common test to evaluate power output capacity of the short-term energy system

- Explain how motivation, buffering, and exercise training influence the glycolytic energy pathway

- Define maximal oxygen consumption and its physiologic significance

- Differentiate between maximal oxygen consumption and peak oxygen consumption

- Define graded exercise test and list criteria that indicate attainment of a "true" $\dot{V}O_{2max}$ during graded exercise testing

- Outline three common treadmill protocols to assess $\dot{V}O_{2max}$

- Indicate the influence of each of the following on $\dot{V}O_{2max}$: (1) mode of exercise, (2) heredity, (3) state of training, (4) gender, (5) body composition, and (6) age

- Describe procedures for administering a walking field test to predict $\dot{V}O_{2max}$

- List three assumptions when using submaximal exercise heart rate to predict $\dot{V}O_{2max}$

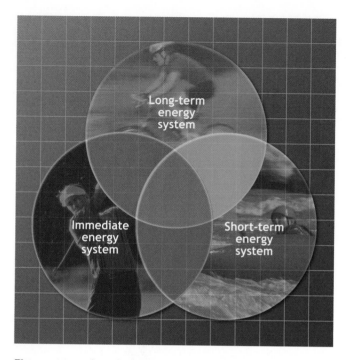

Figure 11.1 Specificity–generality of the three systems for energy transfer. When considering only two systems, their overlap represents generality and the remainder specificity.

The body derives useful energy from anaerobic and aerobic energy metabolic pathways, but the capacity for each form of energy transfer varies considerably. This between-person variability underlies the concept of **individual differences** in metabolic capacity for exercise. Highly specific physiologic and energy transfer capacities exist for such general fitness components as muscular strength versus joint flexibility versus endurance capacity but also the specific mode of exercise for training and evaluation. For example, **specificity** of metabolic capacity dictates that a high $\dot{V}O_{2max}$ in running does not necessarily ensure a similar $\dot{V}O_{2max}$ using different muscle groups required in swimming and rowing. Some individuals with high aerobic power in one activity do possess above average aerobic power in other activities. This illustrates the **generality** principle of metabolic function. Often, considerable specificity emerges when comparing the body's distinct energy transfer systems. The nonoverlapped areas in FIGURE 11.1 represent specificity of metabolic function, while the three overlapped portions represent generality. For each energy system, specificity exceeds generality. Most people do not possess high energy-generating capacity for activities as different as running (lower-body exercise) or swimming (upper-body exercise) or a particular sport's sprint, middle-distance, and long-distance competitions. It is unusual, for example, to identify an athlete who excels in sporting events like high jumping, 200-m swimming, and 3000-m steeplechase.

Based on the exercise specificity concept, training to achieve a high $\dot{V}O_{2max}$ contributes little to one's capacity to generate energy anaerobically, and vice versa. A high degree of specificity also exists for the effects of exercise training on neuromuscular patterning and demands. *Terms such as "speed," "power," and "endurance" must be applied precisely within the context of the specific movement patterns and specific metabolic and physiologic requirements of the activity.*

This chapter evaluates the capacity of the three energy-transfer systems discussed in Chapters 6 and 7, with emphasis on individual differences, specificity, and measurement.

INTEGRATIVE QUESTION

Respond to a potential triathlete who asks: "Why is it important to train in each of the sport's three events? Because they each require a high level of aerobic fitness, can't I just train aerobically for just one of the events?"

OVERVIEW OF ENERGY-TRANSFER CAPACITY DURING EXERCISE

The immediate and short-term energy systems largely power all-out exercise for up to 2 minutes. Both systems operate anaerobically because their transfer of chemical energy does not require molecular oxygen. A greater reliance on anaerobic energy exists for fast, short-duration movements, or when increasing resistance to movement at a given speed. FIGURE 11.2 illustrates the relative activation of the anaerobic and aerobic energy-transfer systems for different durations of all-out exercise. When movement begins at either fast or slow speed, the intramuscular high-energy phosphates adenosine triphosphate (ATP) and phosphocreatine (PCr) provide immediate, nonaerobic energy to power muscle actions. Following the first few seconds of movement, glycolytic pathways generate an increasingly greater percentage of energy for ATP resynthesis. Continued exercise places progressively greater demands on the long-term system of aerobic metabolism. All physical activities and sports lend themselves to classification on an anaerobic-to-aerobic

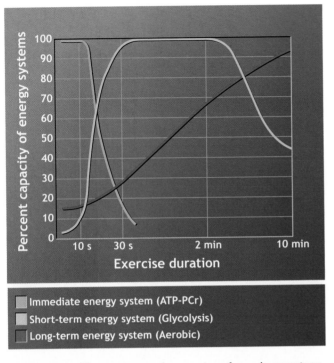

Figure 11.2 Three systems of energy transfer and percentage use of their total capacity during all-out exercise of different durations.

continuum. Some activities rely predominantly on a single system of energy transfer, whereas most require activation of more than one energy system, depending on exercise intensity and duration. Performing at a higher intensity but shorter duration of effort requires a markedly increased demand on anaerobic energy transfer.

ANAEROBIC ENERGY TRANSFER: THE IMMEDIATE AND SHORT-TERM ENERGY SYSTEMS

Evaluation of the Immediate Energy System: Performance Tests

Football, weight lifting, and other brief, maximal-effort physical activities that require an almost instantaneous energy release rely almost exclusively on energy from the intramuscular high-energy phosphates. Performance tests that maximally activate the ATP–PCr energy system serve as practical field tests to evaluate the capacity for "immediate" energy transfer. Two assumptions underlie the use of performance test scores to infer the power-generating capacity of the high-energy phosphates: (1) all ATP at maximal power output regenerates via ATP–PCr hydrolysis and (2) adequate ATP and PCr exist to support maximal performance for about 6 seconds duration. The term *power test* generally describes these measures of brief, maximal exercise capacity. *Power* in this context refers to the time-rate of accomplishing work computed as follows:

$$P = (FD) \div T$$

where F equals force generated, D equals distance the force moves, and T represents exercise duration. Power is often expressed in watts—1 watt equals 0.73756 ft-lb $\cdot$ s^{-1}, 0.01433 kCal $\cdot$ min^{-1}, 1.341 $\times$ 10^{-3} hp (or 0.0013 hp), or 6.12 kg-m $\cdot$ min^{-1}.

Stair-Sprinting Power Tests

Researchers have evaluated high-energy phosphate power output by the time required to run up a staircase as fast as possible taking three steps at a time (FIG. 11.3). External work accomplished consists of the total vertical distance traversed up the stairs; this distance for six stairs usually equals 1.05 m. For example, the power output of a 65-kg woman who traverses six steps in 0.52 second computes as follows:

$$F = 65 \text{ kg}$$
$$D = 1.05 \text{ m}$$
$$T = 0.52 \text{ s}$$
$$\text{Power} = (65 \text{ kg} \times 1.05 \text{ m}) \div 0.52 \text{ s}$$
$$= 131.3 \text{ kg-m} \cdot \text{s}^{-1} \text{ (1287 watts)}$$

Body mass significantly influences the power score in the stair-sprinting test; thus, a heavier person who achieves the same speed as a lighter counterpart necessarily achieves a higher power score. This implies that the heavier person pos-

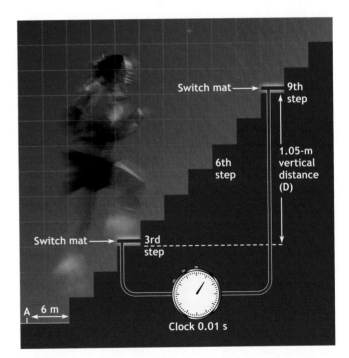

Figure 11.3 Stair-sprinting power test. The subject begins at point *A* and runs as fast as possible up a flight of stairs, taking three steps at a time. Electric switch mats placed on the steps record the time needed to cover the distance between stairs 3 and 9 to the nearest 0.01 second. Power output equals the product of the subject's mass *(F)* and vertical distance covered *(D)*, divided by the time *(T)*.

sesses a more highly developed immediate energy system. Unfortunately, no direct evidence justifies this conclusion, so one must use care interpreting differences in stair-sprinting power scores and inferring individual differences in ATP–PCr energy-transfer capacity. *The test should be used with individuals of similar body mass or the same individuals before and after specific training designed to develop leg power output from the immediate energy system (assuming no change in body mass).*

INTEGRATIVE QUESTION

Considering training specificity, describe how to test the power output capacity of the immediate energy system of (1) volleyball players, (2) swimmers, and (3) soccer players.

Jumping-Power Tests

Jump tests such as the popular Sargent jump-and-reach test or a standing broad jump often appear in physical fitness test batteries. The Sargent jump score reflects the difference between a person's standing reach and the maximum vertical jump-and-touch height. The broad jump score consists of the horizontal distance traversed in a leap from a semi-crouched position. Both tests purport to measure leg power, but they probably fail to achieve this goal. For example, jump tests generate power to propel the body from the crouched position *only* while the feet maintain contact with the surface. *This extremely brief period of muscle activation probably does not adequately evaluate a person's ATP and PCr energy transfer capacity.* Also, no data exist to show a relationship (correlation) between jump-test scores and actual ATP–PCr levels or depletion patterns in the primary muscles activated during the jump.

Attention should focus on the methodology to obtain such information when using jump tests to assess the immediate generation of nonaerobic power. FIGURE 11.4 displays data for subjects who performed consecutive multiple vertical jumps and standing broad jumps. Vertical jump trials consisted of 10 jumps with a 1-minute rest between jumps. Subjects stood with their hands on hips during the crouch before the jump to eliminate arm swing that augments vertical displacement. A significant underestimation of peak power occurs using the scores from only the first 2 or 3 jumps. Whether the progressive increase in power with repeated jumps results from a warming-up effect or improved neuromuscular activation has not been established. From a testing perspective, the important consideration requires administering enough trials to establish a person's true power score. This is best achieved by averaging 2 or 3 jumps after the performance curve plateaus.

Other Power Performance Tests

Figure 11.2 suggests that any all-out exercise of 6 to 8 seconds probably reflects a person's capacity for immediate power from the high-energy phosphates in the specific

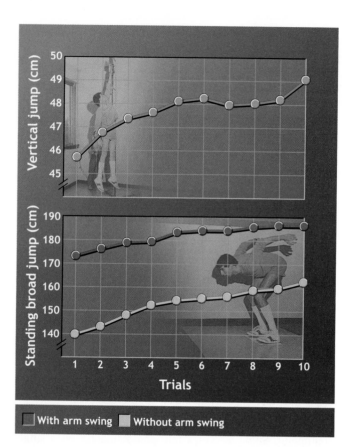

Figure 11.4 *Top.* Ten consecutive vertical jump trials (no arm swing) of male collegiate baseball players and (*bottom*) long-jump performances (with and without arm swing) of female collegiate soccer players. Prior to testing, subjects stretched for 3 minutes and performed light calisthenics. Subjects were exhorted to make a maximal effort in all jumps. A 7.5% improvement in vertical jump occurred between trials 1 and 10 (with no plateau in performance); improvement for the standing broad jump averaged 7.0% from trial 1 to trial 10 with arm swing and 15.5% without arm swing. (Vertical jump data courtesy of Jeff Smith; standing long-jump data courtesy of Jesse Sutella, Human Performance Laboratory, Exercise Science Department, University of Massachusetts, Amherst, 1996.)

muscles activated. Other tests include sprint running or cycling, brief shuttle runs, and localized movements produced by arm cranking.

Interrelationships Among Power Performance Tests

If the various power tests measure the same "general" metabolic capacity, then individuals who perform best on one test should rank correspondingly high on a second or third different test. Unfortunately, this does not usually occur to any great extent. While some individuals who score well on one power performance test tend to score well on another test, a poor relationship generally exists.[84] TABLE 11.1 shows the interrelationship (expressed statistically as a correlation coefficient) between several tests purported to measure immediate power output. The relationship ranges from poor to good, depending on the nature of the test. This indicates some

TABLE 11.1 ■ CORRELATIONS AMONG TESTS PURPORTED TO MEASURE IMMEDIATE ANAEROBIC POWER OUTPUT FROM THE INTRAMUSCULAR HIGH-ENERGY PHOSPHATES ATP AND PCR

VARIABLE	JUMP & REACH	STAIR-SPRINTING
40-yard dash	−0.48[a]	−0.88[a]
Jump and reach	—	−0.31[a]

From the Applied Physiology Laboratory, University of Michigan ($n = 31$ males).
[a] Negative correlations mean faster times (lower scores) associate with higher jumps or greater power outputs.

commonality among tests for measuring metabolic capacity. The fairly strong relationship between stair-sprinting power test scores and 40-yard dash scores (r = −0.88) indicates that one can obtain almost the same information on short-term power performance through sprint running on a track as in the more elaborate procedures required in the stair sprint.

Several factors explain the relatively low relationships among the other test scores. *First, human exercise performance remains highly task specific.* From a metabolic and performance perspective, this means that the best sprint runner does not necessarily rank as the best sprint swimmer, sprint cyclist, "stair sprinter," or "arm cranker." While identical metabolic reactions generate energy to power each performance, these reactions occur within the specific muscles activated by the exercise. Each specific test also requires different neuromuscular and skill components that introduce variability and specificity into test scores.

Power tests offer an excellent means for self-testing and motivation. The tests also can serve as exercise for training the immediate energy system. For example, football coaches often use the 40-yard dash both for power training and as a criterion to evaluate horizontal movement speed. Forty-yard dash test scores *may* provide relevant information concerning "speed" in football, even though no data exist to quantify how a 40-yard sprint in a straight line relates to all of the complex skills and movements involved in game performance, let alone some general factor of overall football ability. A run test of shorter distance (up to 20 yd) and/or with multiple changes in direction and pacing may provide a more appropriate, task-specific performance to assess football players.

Evaluation of the Immediate Energy System: Physiologic Tests

Several physiologic and biochemical measures evaluate the energy-generating capacity of the immediate energy system. These include estimating the (1) size of the intramuscu-

lar ATP–PCr pool, (2) depletion rates of ATP and PCr in all-out, short-duration exercise, (3) oxygen deficit calculated from the initial phase of the exercise oxygen consumption curve, and (4) alactic portion (fast component) of recovery oxygen consumption. Of these measures, ATP and PCr depletion rates provide the most direct estimate and correlate highly with physical performance assessments of the immediate energy system. For example, one experiment determined muscle PCr depletion at different intervals of a 100-m sprint using the muscle biopsy technique.[33] Compared with resting values (22 mmol · kg wet weight^{-1}), PCr decreased by 60% during the first 40 m (<6 s) and only another 20% for the remainder of the sprint. It remains nearly impossible with current technology to readily obtain precise biochemical data during all-out exercise of brief duration. Consequently, researchers must rely on the "face validity" of the various specific performance measures as satisfactory markers to evaluate capacity for ATP–PCr energy transfer.

Evaluation of the Short-Term Energy System

Figure 11.2 showed that when all-out exercise continues for longer than a few seconds, the short-term energy system (anaerobic glycolysis) generates increasingly more of the energy for ATP resynthesis. This does not mean that aerobic metabolism is unimportant at this stage of exercises or that oxygen-consuming reactions have not "switched on." To the contrary, the contribution of aerobic energy transfer increases early in the exercise (Fig. 11.2).[80] During short-duration maximal exercise, the energy requirement greatly exceeds the energy generated by hydrogen oxidation in the respiratory chain. Consequently, anaerobic glycolysis predominates, with large quantities of lactate accumulating in active muscle and ultimately in blood. *Blood lactate level provides the most common indicator of activation of the short-term energy system.*

Unlike tests for maximal oxygen consumption, no specific criteria exist to indicate that a person has attained maximal anaerobic effort. More than likely, self-motivation and the testing environment greatly influence performance on such tests.[102] Performance test scores show good reproducibility from day to day, particularly under standardized conditions, despite difficulty in validly assessing a person's true anaerobic power capacity.[4,50,62]

Anaerobic Power Performance and Capacity Tests

Performances that activate the short-term energy system require maximal exercise for up to 3 minutes. All-out runs and stationary cycling have usually assessed anaerobic capacity, as have shuttle runs and repetitive weight lifting of a certain percentage of maximum capacity. The influence of age, gender, skill, motivation, and body size creates difficulty selecting a suitable criterion test or developing appropriate norms to evaluate anaerobic power capacity. Above-normal intramuscular glycogen levels do not affect exercise test performance or final level of blood lactate accumulation.[88] Because of exercise specificity, one should not use a test that requires maximal activation of the leg musculature to assess short-term anaerobic capacity for an upper-body activity like rowing or swimming. *The performance test must closely resemble the activity that requires energy capacity assessment.* In most cases, the activity itself best serves as the performance test.

In 1973, the **Katch test** of all-out stationary cycling of short duration estimated the power and capacity of the anaerobic energy systems.[40] Subsequent extension of this work created a stationary bicycle test with frictional resistance against the flywheel preset at a high load (6 kg for men; 5 kg for women). Subjects turned as many revolutions as possible in 40 seconds with pedal rate continuously recorded with a microswitch assembly. Peak cycling power represented the subject's anaerobic power, while total work accomplished indicated anaerobic capacity. A later modification, the **Wingate test**, involves 30 seconds of supermaximal exercise on either an arm-crank or leg-cycle ergometer.[4,104] Body mass determines resistance to pedaling (originally set to 0.075 kg per kg body mass but now can exceed 0.12 kg in athletes) applied within 3 seconds after overcoming the initial inertia and unloaded frictional resistance of the ergometer. **Peak power** represents the highest mechanical power generated during any 3- to 5-second period of the test; **relative power** represents peak power divided by body mass. **Anaerobic fatigue** is the percentage decline in power output during the test and **anaerobic capacity** is the total work accomplished over the 30 seconds. **Rate of fatigue** represents the decline in power in relation to the peak value. The Katch and Wingate tests assume that peak power output reflects the energy-generating capacity of the high-energy phosphates, while average power reflects glycolytic capacity. "In a Practical Sense" on p. 235 provides the procedures to determine anaerobic power and capacity on the Wingate cycle ergometer test. Table 11.2 presents normative standards for average and peak power outputs in young, physically active men and women during the Wingate cycling test. Performance scores, blood lactate concentrations, and peak heart rates show high test–retest reproducibility and moderate validity compared with other anaerobic capacity criteria.[64,97] Elite volleyball and ice hockey players have achieved some of the highest Wingate power scores.

Figure 11.5A and B present the relative contributions of each energy system during three cycle ergometer anaerobic power tests of different durations. The lower figure (B) gives estimated kilojoules of total energy; the upper figure presents the percentage contribution of each system to total work accomplished. Note the progressive change in the percentage contribution of each energy system as a function of increasing duration of effort.

Lower in Children. The reason for the relatively poor performance of children on the Wingate test compared with adolescents and young adults remains unclear. Possible explanations include children's relatively lower intramuscular glycogen concentrations and their slower rate of glycogen use during exercise.

Gender Differences. Large gender differences exist in anaerobic power capacity when comparing test scores on an absolute basis.[21,75] These observations, as with most physiologic capacity and exercise performance tests, seem readily explained by the clear gender differences in factors that affect absolute anaerobic power-output capacity—body mass, active muscle mass, and fat-free body mass (FFM). Expressing power output capacity in relation to a component of body mass or composition should minimize or even eliminate the gender difference in anaerobic capacity. This adjustment should offer insight into whether true gender effects exist in a muscle's capacity to generate energy anaerobically.

Gender differences in body composition, physique, muscular strength, or neuromuscular factors do not fully explain the lower anaerobic performance of women.[51,65] For a given fat-free leg volume, the peak oxygen deficit (a measure of anaerobic capacity)[3,56] during supermaximal cycling remained higher in men than in women.[98] These differences averaged about 20%, even when adjusting for the estimated difference in active muscle mass between the genders. Similar gender differences in anaerobic exercise capacity exist for children and adolescents.[63,75] The gender effect among adolescents remains apparent for the lower body musculature, even when considering differences in body composition.[65] Males' superior anaerobic capacity may result from their greater relative area and metabolic capacity of the fast-twitch fiber type and larger catecholamine response to exercise.

Available evidence indicates a biologic gender difference in anaerobic exercise capacity. Physical testing that focuses on this fitness component would inflate the typically observed performance differences between men and women. Even adjusting the performance score to body size or body composition does not eliminate this difference. In the occupational setting, the justifiable concern when using all-out anaerobic exercise relates to the potential to exacerbate gender differences in performance scores and magnify any adverse impact on females. Variations in menstrual cycle phase do not affect maximal anaerobic performance.[28]

Maximally Accumulated Oxygen Deficit

Determination of the **maximally accumulated oxygen deficit** (**MAOD**) provides another indirect measure of anaerobic metabolic capacity.[56,57,78,95] MAOD determination relies on an extrapolation procedure using the linear exercise intensity–oxygen consumption relationship established from several levels of submaximal treadmill exercise. From these data, a regression line predicts the individual's supramaximal oxygen consumption, usually set at 125% of the subject's directly measured $\dot{V}O_{2max}$. MAOD calculates as the difference between the predicted supramaximal oxygen consumption from the exercise intensity–oxygen consumption relationship

IN A PRACTICAL SENSE

DETERMINING ANAEROBIC POWER AND CAPACITY: THE WINGATE CYCLE ERGOMETER TEST

■ Many sport and daily activities occur with rapid rest-to-exercise transitions or at high intensities using anaerobic metabolic processes. The Wingate cycle ergometer test represents the most popular test to assess anaerobic capacity. Developed at the Wingate Institute in Israel in the 1970s, test scores can reliably determine *peak anaerobic power, anaerobic fatigue,* and *total anaerobic capacity.*

THE TEST
A mechanically braked bicycle ergometer serves as the testing device. After warming up (3 to 5 min), the subject begins pedaling as fast as possible without resistance. Within 3 seconds, a fixed resistance is applied to the flywheel; the subject continues to pedal "all out" for 30 seconds. An electrical or mechanical counter continuously records flywheel revolutions in 5-second intervals.

RESISTANCE
Flywheel resistance equals 0.075 kg per kg body mass. For a 70-kg person, the flywheel resistance would equal 5.25 kg (70 kg × 0.075). Resistance often increases to 0.10 kg per kg body mass or higher (up to 0.12 kg) when testing power- and sprint-type athletes.

TEST SCORES
1. **Peak power output (PP)**—The highest power output, observed during the first 5-second exercise interval, indicates the energy-generating capacity of the immediate energy system (intramuscular high-energy phosphates ATP and PCr). PP, expressed in watts (1 W = 6.12 kg-m · min^{-1}), computes as Force × Distance (number of revolutions × distance per revolution) ÷ Time in minutes (5 s = 0.0833 min).
2. **Relative peak power output (RPP)**—Peak power output relative to body mass: PP ÷ Body mass (kg).
3. **Anaerobic fatigue (AF)**—Percentage decline in power output during the test;

AF represents the total capacity to produce ATP via the immediate and short-term energy systems. AF computes as (Highest 5-second PP − Lowest 5-s PP) ÷ Highest 5-second PP × 100.

4. **Anaerobic capacity (AC)**—Total work accomplished over 30 seconds; AC computes as the sum of each 5-second PP, or Force × Total distance in 30 seconds.

EXAMPLE
A male weighing 73.3 kg performs the Wingate test on a Monark cycle ergometer (6.0 m traveled per pedal revolution) with an applied resistance of 5.5 kg (73.3-kg body mass × 0.075 = 5.497, rounded to 5.5 kg); pedal revolutions for each 5-second interval equal 12, 10, 8, 7, 6, and 5 (48 total revolutions in 30 s).

CALCULATIONS
1. Peak power output
   PP = Force × Distance ÷ Time
   = 5.5 kg × (12 rev × 6 m) ÷ 0.0833 min
   = 396 kg-m ÷ 0.0833 min
   = 4753.9 kg-m · min^{-1} or 776.8 W
2. Relative peak power output
   RPP = PP ÷ Body mass, kg
   = 776.8 W ÷ 73.3 kg
   = 10.6 W · kg^{-1}

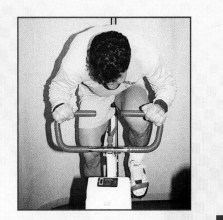

continued on page 236

Continued

3. Anaerobic fatigue

$\text{AF} = (\text{Highest PP} - \text{Lowest PP})$
$\div \text{Highest PP} \times 100$

[Highest PP = Force × Distance ÷ Time:

5.5 kg × (12 rev × 6 m)
÷ 0.0833 min
= 4753.9 kg-m · min⁻¹
or 776.8 W]

[Lowest PP = Force × Distance ÷ Time:

5.5 kg × (5 rev × 6 m)
÷ 0.0833 min
= 1980.8 kg-m · min⁻¹ or
323.7 W]

AF = 776.8 W − 323.7 W

÷ 776.8 W × 100
= 58.3%

4. Anaerobic capacity

AC = Force × Total Distance (in 30 s)
= 5.5 × [(12 rev + 10 rev + 8 rev
+ 7 rev + 6 rev + 5 rev) × 6 m]
= 1584 kg-m · min⁻¹ (258.8 W)

TABLE 11.2 ■ **PERCENTILE NORMS FOR AVERAGE POWER AND PEAK POWER FOR PHYSICALLY ACTIVE YOUNG ADULT MEN AND WOMEN**

%	AVERAGE POWER WATTS (W)		PEAK POWER WATTS (W)	
Rank	Male	Female	Male	Female
90	662	470	822	560
80	618	419	777	527
70	600	410	757	505
60	577	391	721	480
50	565	381	689	449
40	548	367	671	432
30	530	353	656	399
20	496	336	618	376
10	471	306	570	353

	W · KG BM⁻¹ᵃ		W · KG BM⁻¹	
	Male	Female	Male	Female
90	8.24	7.31	10.89	9.02
80	8.01	6.95	10.39	8.83
70	7.91	6.77	10.20	8.53
60	7.59	6.59	9.80	8.14
50	7.44	6.39	9.22	7.65
40	7.14	6.15	8.92	6.96
30	7.00	6.03	8.53	6.86
20	6.59	5.71	8.24	6.57
10	5.98	5.25	7.06	5.98

From Maud PJ, Schultz BB. Norms for the Wingate anaerobic test with comparisons in another similar test. Res Q Exerc Sport 1989;60:144.
ᵃ W · kg BM⁻¹, watts per kilogram of body mass.

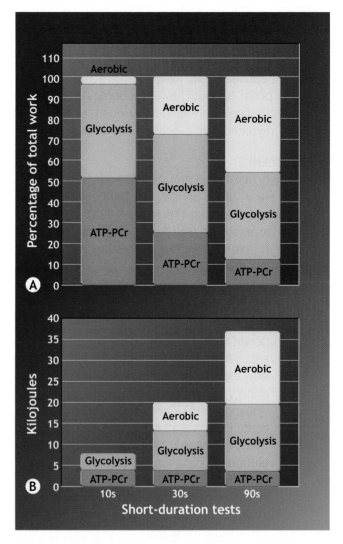

Figure 11.5 Relative contribution of each of the energy systems to total work accomplished in three short-duration exercise tests. **A.** Percentage of total work output. **B.** Total kilojoules of energy. Test results based on Katch test protocol (see p. 234). (Data from Applied Physiology Laboratory, University of Michigan, Ann Arbor.)

and oxygen consumption measured during a 2- to 3-minute all-out treadmill run to fatigue. The measure correlates positively with other popular anaerobic performance tests like the Wingate test, sprint running, and stair climbing; it demonstrates independence from aerobic energy estimates, differentiates between aerobically and anaerobically trained individuals, and remains unchanged with high-intensity exercise of varying durations.

Biologic Indicators for Anaerobic Power

Blood Lactate Levels

Physiologists have traditionally interpreted the appearance of "excess" lactate in muscle and blood following exercise to indicate the contribution of anaerobic metabolism to the exercise energy requirement. Measurements of muscle or venous blood lactate routinely served to verify steady-rate exercise or the magnitude of glycolytic activity consequent to non–steady-rate exercise. This view now appears overly simplified in light of research showing lactate's role as a metabolic intermediate rather than a metabolic "dead end," whose only fate involves reconversion to pyruvate. Up to 50% of glucose catabolized for energy converts to lactate. Lactate then serves as an important substrate in energy-storing *and* energy-generating pathways in different tissues. As such, lactate measured during or following exercise does not necessarily reflect absolute levels of anaerobic energy transfer via glycolysis.[11,18,29,30] Nevertheless, with increasing exercise intensity, including near-maximal and supramaximal levels, greater lactate production reflects increasing ATP resynthesis from anaerobic pathways.[81] About 70% of the total energy yield for 30 seconds of all-out exercise comes from anaerobic glycolysis and PCr degradation, with aerobic pathways generating the remaining energy (Fig. 11.5).

 INTEGRATIVE QUESTION

Explain why females score poorly when using absolute scores for "average power" and "peak power" on the Wingate leg-cycle ergometer test.

Glycogen Depletion

The pattern of glycogen depletion reveals the glycolytic contribution to exercise because glycogen stored in the specific muscles activated by exercise chiefly powers the short-term energy system. FIGURE 11.6 illustrates the close connection between glycogen depletion rate in the quadriceps femoris muscle during bicycle exercise and exercise intensity. During prolonged but relatively light exercise (30% $\dot{V}O_{2max}$), a considerable muscle glycogen reserve remains even after 180 minutes. Relatively large quantities of fatty acids provide fuel for exercise at this intensity with only minimal reliance on stored glycogen. The two heaviest supermaximal workloads produced the most rapid and pronounced

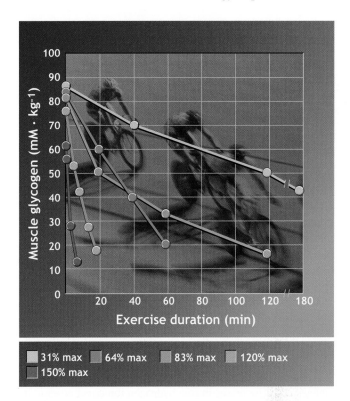

Figure 11.6 Glycogen depletion from the vastus lateralis of the quadriceps femoris muscles during bicycle exercise of different intensities and durations. Exercise at 31% of $\dot{V}O_{2max}$ (the lightest workload) caused some depletion of muscle glycogen, but the most rapid depletion occurred during exercise between 83 and 150% of $\dot{V}O_{2max}$. (Adapted from Gollnick PD. Selective glycogen depletion pattern in human muscle fibers after exercise of varying intensity and at varying pedaling rates. J Physiol 1974;241:45.)

glycogen depletion. This outcome makes sense from a metabolic standpoint because glycogen (1) provides the most rapid phosphorylation of ATP of the three macronutrients and (2) is the only stored macronutrient that anaerobically resynthesizes ATP. Clearly, glycogen serves as an important energy substrate in the "metabolic mill" during strenuous exercise.

Changes in *total* muscle glycogen, like those illustrated in Figure 11.6, do not necessarily indicate the precise degree of glycogen catabolism in specific fibers within an active muscle. Depending on exercise intensity, glycogen depletion progresses selectively in either fast- or slow-twitch muscle fibers. All-out exercise (e.g., repeated 1-min sprints on a bicycle ergometer at a heavy load) activates fast-twitch fibers to provide most of the power requirement. The glycogen content of these fibers becomes almost totally depleted because of the exercise's anaerobic nature. In contrast, during moderately intense but more prolonged aerobic exercise, the slow-twitch muscle fibers become glycogen depleted first. Specificity in glycogen use (and depletion) by specific fiber types makes it difficult to evaluate the anaerobic involvement of distinct fibers from changes in a muscle's total glycogen content before and after exercise.

Individual Differences in Anaerobic Energy-Transfer Capacity

Several factors contribute to differences among individuals in capacity to generate short-term anaerobic energy. These include (1) effects of previous training, (2) capacity to buffer acid metabolites, and (3) motivation.

Effects of Training

FIGURE 11.7 compares biochemical factors of anaerobic metabolism for trained and untrained subjects. Trained subjects always exhibited higher levels of muscle and blood lactate and greater depletion of muscle glycogen following short-term maximal bicycle ergometer exercise. Such cross-sectional comparisons suggest that training for short-term, all-out exercise enhances capacity to generate energy from anaerobic sources. In sprint- and middle-distance activities, individual differences in anaerobic capacity help to explain the considerable variations in exercise performance.

Buffering of Acid Metabolites

Buffering capacity refers to how well different substances resist increases in free hydrogen ion concentration by binding free protons to prevent a decrease in pH. When anaerobic energy transfer predominates, lactate accumulates and muscle and blood acidity increase to negatively affect the intracellular environment and the contractile capacity of active muscles. Anaerobic training might enhance short-term energy capacity by improving the body's alkaline reserve for buffering. Such a training adaptation would theoretically enable greater lactate production through more-effective buffering. Such reasoning seems appealing, yet athletes have only a slightly larger alkaline reserve than sedentary counterparts. Additionally, no appreciable change in alkaline reserve occurs following hard physical training. *Exercise training most likely confers a buffering capability within the range expected for healthy untrained individuals.*

Altering acid–base balance in the direction of alkalosis temporarily enhances high-intensity anaerobic exercise performance. Ingesting a buffering solution of sodium bicarbonate prior to an 800-m race significantly improved running performance.[100] Higher blood lactate levels and extracellular H^+ concentrations suggested an increased anaerobic energy transfer that contributed to the faster run times. Chapter 23 discusses the potential ergogenic effects of preexercise-induced alkalosis.

Motivation

Individuals with a higher "pain tolerance," "toughness," or ability to "push" beyond the discomforts of intense, fatiguing exercise can accomplish more work anaerobically. This coincides with higher blood lactate concentrations and greater glycogen depletion. Motivational factors that are sometimes difficult to categorize or quantify undoubtedly play an integral role in achieving superior performance at most levels of competition.

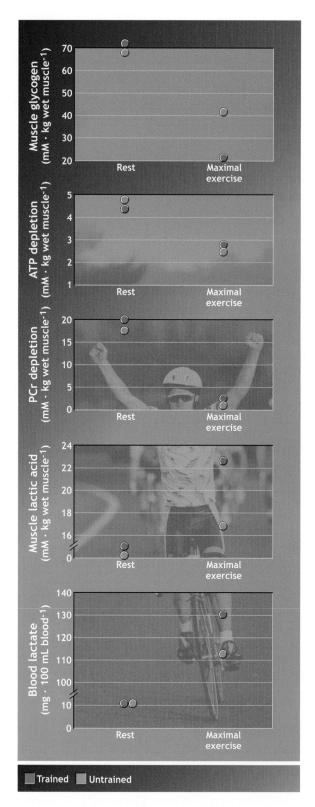

Figure 11.7 Depletion of the anaerobic substrates (ATP, PCr, and glycogen) and increases in muscle and blood lactate during short-term maximal exercise by trained and untrained subjects. Trained subjects exhibited a greater increase in anaerobic metabolism (higher lactate levels) and more pronounced muscle glycogen depletion; reductions in the intramuscular high-energy phosphates remained essentially the same as for the nontrained subjects. (From Karlsson J, et al. Muscle metabolites during submaximal and maximal exercise in man. Scand J Clin Invest 1971;26:382.)

AEROBIC ENERGY: THE LONG-TERM ENERGY SYSTEM

FIGURE 11.8 illustrates that athletes who excel in endurance sports generally have a superior capacity for aerobic energy transfer. The maximal oxygen consumption recorded for competitors in distance running, swimming, bicycling, and cross-country skiing exceeds that of sedentary men and women by almost twofold. This does not mean that $\dot{V}O_{2max}$ makes up the sole determinant of endurance performance. Other factors, principally those at the local tissue level, include improved capillary density, enzymes, mitochondrial size and number, and muscle fiber type. These intrinsic qualities strongly influence a muscle's capacity to sustain a high level of aerobic exercise.[34] However, $\dot{V}O_{2max}$ does provide important information about the capacity of the long-term energy system. This measure also conveys important physiologic meaning because attaining a high $\dot{V}O_{2max}$ requires integration of high levels of pulmonary, cardiovascular, and neuromuscular function (see Fig. 7.6). *This makes $\dot{V}O_{2max}$ a fundamental measure of physiologic functional capacity for exercise.*

Assessment of Maximal Oxygen Consumption

Over the past 65 years, considerable research effort has standardized methodology to assess maximal aerobic power. Normative standards exist related to age, gender, state of training, and body size.

Criteria for Maximal Oxygen Consumption

The plot in FIGURE 11.9 relates oxygen consumption and exercise intensity during progressive increases in treadmill effort. The test terminated when the subject would not complete the full duration of a particular exercise interval. The highest oxygen consumption (average of 18 subjects) occurred before subjects attained their maximum exercise level. *Demonstration of a leveling off or peaking over in oxygen consumption with increasing exercise intensity generally provides assurance that a person has reached maximum capacity for aerobic metabolism (i.e., achieved "true" $\dot{V}O_{2max}$; see "Focus on Research" on p. 242).* Agreement on a precise standard for the criterion remains controversial.[20,35] Less stringent criteria, besides failure for oxygen consumption to increase in graded exercise, also establish attainment of $\dot{V}O_{2max}$. Oxygen consumption that fails to increase by the value expected on the basis of previous observations with the specific test protocol often serves as an appropriate criterion.[1,35,83]

Oxygen consumption at the higher exercise levels does not readily plateau, particularly among children,[73] except in treadmill running. The term **peak oxygen consumption**, or **$\dot{V}O_{2peak}$**, applies when leveling off does not occur or test performance appears limited by local muscular factors rather than central circulatory dynamics. *$\dot{V}O_{2peak}$ refers to the high-*

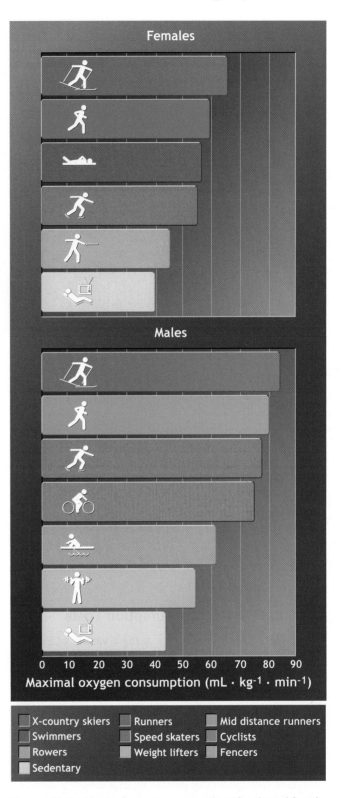

Figure 11.8 Maximal oxygen consumption of male and female Olympic-caliber athletes in different sports categories compared with healthy sedentary subjects. (Adapted from Saltin B, Åstrand PO. Maximal oxygen consumption in athletes. J Appl Physiol 1967;23:353.)

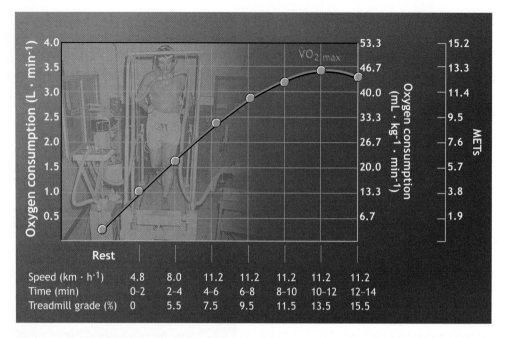

Figure 11.9 Peaking over in oxygen consumption with increasing treadmill exercise intensity. Each point represents the average oxygen consumption of 18 sedentary males. The region where oxygen consumption fails to increase the expected amount or even decreases slightly with increasing exercise intensity represents the $\dot{V}O_{2max}$. (Data from the Applied Physiology Laboratory, University of Michigan, Ann Arbor.)

est value of oxygen consumption measured during a graded exercise test. Often, the highest oxygen consumption occurs in the last minute of exercise. Secondary criteria that objectify $\dot{V}O_{2peak}$ include attainment of the age-predicted maximum heart rate (see Fig. 21.19) or respiratory exchange ratio (R) above 1.15. Some also argue that to accept an oxygen consumption value as near maximum, blood lactate should attain 70 or 80 mg per dL of blood (8 to 10 mmol) or above.[20]

Maximal Oxygen Consumption Tests

One can determine $\dot{V}O_{2max}$ using a variety of exercise tests that activate the body's large muscle groups provided exercise intensity and duration maximize aerobic energy transfer. The usual exercise modes include treadmill running or walking, bench stepping, and stationary cycling. Other forms of testing use free, tethered, and flume swimming[6,46]; swim-bench ergometry[27]; in-line skating[92]; roller skiing[74]; simulated arm-leg climbing[10]; rowing[14]; ice skating[23]; and arm-crank and wheelchair exercise.[77,87,89] Such performance tests generally remain unaffected by a subject's strength, speed, body size, and skill, with the exception of specialized tests that measure aerobic capacity in sport-specific activities.

The $\dot{V}O_{2max}$ test may require a single, continuous 3- to 5-minute supramaximal effort. In most cases, the test usually consists of progressive increments in effort (**graded exercise**) to a point at which the subject simply refuses to continue exercising. Some researchers have termed this end point "exhaustion." However, the person exercising terminates the test—a decision often influenced by motivational factors that do not necessarily reflect true physiologic strain. Bringing the subject to the point of acceptable criteria for either $\dot{V}O_{2max}$ or $\dot{V}O_{2peak}$ often requires considerable urging and prodding.[91] Practical experience indicates that attaining a plateau in oxygen consumption during a graded exercise test requires a high level of anaerobic energy output. This poses some difficulty, particularly for untrained and elderly persons who normally do not perform strenuous exercise with its associated discomforts.

INTEGRATIVE QUESTION

In what specific ways does $\dot{V}O_{2max}$ provide important insights about the functional capacities of different physiologic systems?

Test Comparisons

There are two popular maximal oxygen consumption test protocols:

1. Continuous—progressively increasing exercise increments without recovery or rest intervals
2. Discontinuous—progressively increasing exercise increments interspersed with recovery intervals

Both test protocols give similar $\dot{V}O_{2max}$ values.[20] The data in TABLE 11.3 show a systematic comparison of $\dot{V}O_{2max}$ scores measured using six common continuous and discontinuous treadmill and bicycle protocols. Only an 8-mL difference in $\dot{V}O_{2max}$ emerged between the continuous and discontinuous

AN IMPORTANT MEASURE OF CARDIORESPIRATORY FUNCTIONAL CAPACITY

Mitchell JH, et al. The physiological meaning of the maximal oxygen intake test. J Clin Invest 1958;37:538.

▲ In the 1920s, A. V. Hill and colleagues—and in latter years other scientists—considered maximal oxygen consumption ($\dot{V}O_{2max}$) the single best measure of cardiorespiratory capacity. Hill asserted that $\dot{V}O_{2max}$ "was physiologically restricted owing to the limitation of the circulatory and respiratory systems." This assertion, however, had not been tested experimentally because the interplay among physiologic parameters had not yet been established. Mitchell and coworkers directly examined the relationships among $\dot{V}O_{2max}$ and various cardiovascular–pulmonary measures to objectify the physiologic significance of $\dot{V}O_{2max}$.

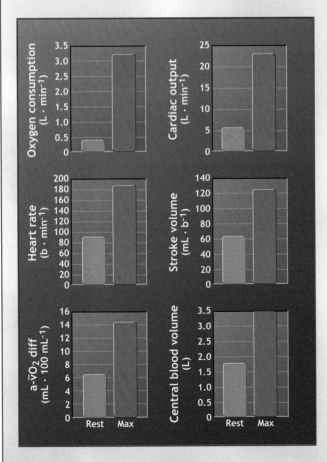

Magnitude of changes in cardiovascular dynamics (arteriovenous oxygen difference [a-$\bar{v}O_2$ diff], heart rate, oxygen consumption, stroke volume, and blood volume) in 15 normal subjects between rest and maximal exercise.

Sixty-five men performed graded, discontinuous treadmill exercise to $\dot{V}O_{2max}$. Subgroups ran in several different protocols to volitional exhaustion. Measurements included cardiac output and a-$\bar{v}O_2$ difference by the dye dilution technique, blood gas pressures, and central blood volume. Two significant findings emerged that related to test methodology. First, $\dot{V}O_{2max}$ provides a highly reproducible measure of aerobic capacity "if rigid criteria for determining the point at which the maximal value has been attained are applied." The reproducibility of test scores for 15 subjects was $r = 0.92$, with a standard error of measurement of $\pm7\%$ for the maximal values. Second, a "peaking over" or "plateauing" criterion (when relating $\dot{V}O_2$ to exercise intensity) provided an important conceptual standard to establish attainment of $\dot{V}O_{2max}$ in diverse forms of exercise as follows:

> Plots of oxygen intake against workload for the entire material showed that, until a maximal value was attained, oxygen intake rose 142 ± 44 mL with each increase in workload. If the rise was less than 142 minus 88 (twice the standard deviation), or 54 mL, the final value was accepted as the maximal oxygen intake, the assumption being that the subject had attained his true maximal value or had reached the beginning of a plateau and could not increase his intake very much more.

Findings from this study supported the view that the $\dot{V}O_{2max}$ depended almost exclusively on the functional capacity of the cardiovascular system (cardiac output and a-$\bar{v}O_2$ diff) and not accommodation of left ventricular output by the peripheral vascular bed. No significant change occurred in arterial oxygen pressure from rest to heavy work; the slight arterial desaturation often observed in intense exercise resulted from a blood pH decrease and the resulting Bohr effect on hemoglobin saturation. Maintenance of high arterial oxygen pressures during intense exercise argued against the possibility that pulmonary factors provided a "weak link" in limiting $\dot{V}O_{2max}$. The researchers maintained that in healthy individuals an adequate arterial oxygen diffusion gradient always exits from the alveoli to the blood and from the blood to active tissues.

This study confirmed the importance of $\dot{V}O_{2max}$ to indicate central circulatory function (cardiac capacity) and capacity of peripheral or local factors reflected by the a$\bar{v}O_2$ difference. This and subsequent research firmly established $\dot{V}O_{2max}$ as a "benchmark" to quantify cardiovascular functional capacity and aerobic fitness.

TABLE 11.3 ■ AVERAGE $\dot{V}O_{2MAX}$ FOR 15 MALE COLLEGE STUDENTS DURING CONTINUOUS AND DISCONTINUOUS TESTS ON THE TREADMILL AND BICYCLE ERGOMETER[a]

VARIABLE	BIKE, DISCONTINUOUS	BIKE, CONTINUOUS	TREADMILL, DISCONTINUOUS RUN-WALK	TREADMILL, CONTINUOUS WALK	TREADMILL, DISCONTINUOUS RUN	TREADMILL, CONTINUOUS RUN
$\dot{V}O_{2max}$, mL · min^{-1}	3691 ± 453	3683 ± 448	4145 ± 401	3944 ± 395	4157 ± 445	4109 ± 424
$\dot{V}O_{2max}$, mL · kg^{-1} · min^{-1}	50.0 ± 6.9	49.9 ± 7.0	56.6 ± 7.3	53.7 ± 7.6	56.6 ± 7.6	55.5 ± 6.8

Adapted from McArdle WD, et al. Comparison of continuous and discontinuous treadmill and bicycle tests for max $\dot{V}O_2$. Med Sci Sports 1973;5:156.
[a] Values are means ± standard deviations.

bicycle tests, but $\dot{V}O_{2max}$ during cycling averaged 6.4 to 11.2% below treadmill values. The largest difference among the three treadmill running tests equaled only 1.2%. In contrast, the walking test elicited $\dot{V}O_{2max}$ scores nearly 7% higher than values on the bicycle, but 5% lower than the three running tests.

Subjects commonly complained of intense local discomfort in the thigh muscles during intense exercise (limiting their ability to continue) in both continuous and discontinuous bicycle tests. They experienced discomfort in the lower back and calf muscles during treadmill walking, notably at the higher treadmill elevations. Running tests rarely produced local discomfort; subjects complained more of general fatigue, usually categorized as feeling "winded." For ease of administration, the continuous treadmill run provides a practical test of aerobic capacity for most healthy individuals. The total time to administer the test averaged about 12 minutes compared with 65 minutes for the discontinuous running test. Subjects tolerated the continuous test well and preferred the shorter time. Research also indicates achievement of $\dot{V}O_{2max}$ with a continuous protocol that increases exercise intensity progressively in 15-second intervals.[22] With this approach, total test time for either bicycle or treadmill exercise averages only about 5 minutes.

Common Treadmill Protocols. FIGURE 11.10 summarizes six common treadmill protocols to assess aerobic capacity in normal individuals and cardiac patients. Manipulation of exercise duration and treadmill speed and grade share common features. The Harbor treadmill test (example *F*), referred to as a ramp test, depicts a unique application. With this protocol, treadmill grade increases by a constant amount (between 1 and 4%) each minute for up to 10 minutes, depending on the person's fitness. This relatively quick procedure—well tolerated by both healthy subjects and cardiac patients—elicits a linear increase in oxygen consumption up to maximum.[12,17,68,94]

INTEGRATIVE QUESTION

Discuss why training studies should objectively demonstrate attainment of true $\dot{V}O_{2max}$ in both pre- and posttest measures. How can this goal be verified?

Factors That Affect Maximal Oxygen Consumption

The six most important factors that influence the maximal oxygen consumption score include (1) mode of exercise, (2) heredity, (3) state of training, (4) gender, (5) body size and composition, and (6) age.

Mode of Exercise

Variations in $\dot{V}O_{2max}$ with different forms of exercise generally reflect variations in the quantity of muscle mass activated. Studies that determined $\dot{V}O_{2max}$ for the same subjects during different exercise modes indicate that treadmill exercise usually produces the highest values. Bench stepping produces $\dot{V}O_{2max}$ scores similar to treadmill values and higher than values on a cycle ergometer.[37] During arm-crank exercise, aerobic capacity averages only about 70% of the treadmill score.[87] For skilled but untrained swimmers, the $\dot{V}O_{2max}$ during swimming usually equals about 80% of treadmill values.[46,54] A definite test specificity emerges for this form of exercise because trained collegiate swimmers achieve $\dot{V}O_{2max}$ values swimming only 11% below treadmill values.[52] Some elite swimmers equal or even exceed their treadmill scores during swimming tests.[46] Similarly, a distinct exercise specificity exists for competitive race-walkers who achieve similar $\dot{V}O_{2max}$ values during treadmill walking and treadmill running.[58] When competitive cyclists pedal at the rapid frequencies of competition, they too achieve $\dot{V}O_{2max}$ values equivalent to their treadmill $\dot{V}O_{2max}$ scores.[31,82]

Treadmill exercise proves highly desirable for determining $\dot{V}O_{2max}$ in healthy subjects in the laboratory. One can easily quantify and regulate exercise intensity. Compared with other forms of exercise, the treadmill allows subjects to more easily meet one or more of the criteria to attain $\dot{V}O_{2max}$ or $\dot{V}O_{2peak}$. In field experiments (outside the laboratory setting), bench stepping and cycle ergometry become suitable alternatives.

Heredity

The interaction between inherited factors (DNA sequence variation; see Section 8, "A Look to the Future") and exercise enhances our understanding of individual variations in training

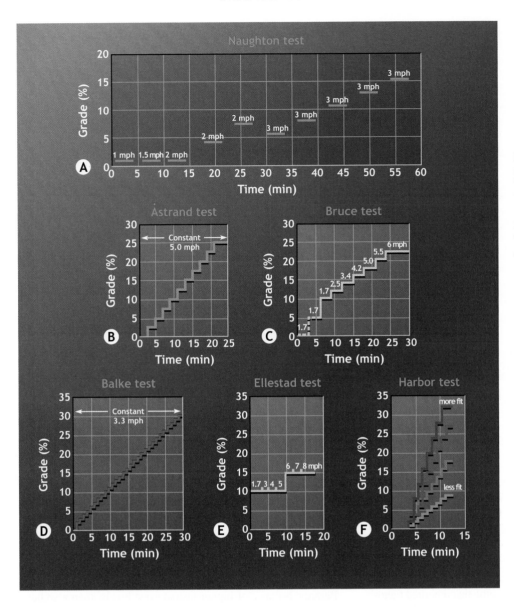

Figure 11.10 Six commonly used treadmill protocols to assess $\dot{V}O_{2max}$. **A.** Naughton protocol. Three-minute exercise periods of increasing intensity alternate with 3 minutes of rest. Exercise periods vary in % grade and speed. **B.** Åstrand protocol. Constant speed at 5 mph. After 3 minutes at 0% grade, the grade increases $2^{1}/_{2}$% every 2 minutes. **C.** Bruce protocol. Grade and/or speed change every 3 minutes. Omit the 0% and 5% grades for healthy subjects. **D.** Balke protocol. After 1 minute at 0% grade and 1 minute at 2% grade, the grade increases 1% per minute; speed is maintained at 3.3 mph. **E.** Ellestad protocol. Initial grade of 10% and later grade of 15%, while speed increases every 2 or 3 minutes. **F.** Harbor protocol. After 3 minutes of walking at a comfortable speed, the grade increases at a constant preselected amount each minute: 1%, 2%, 3%, or 4%, so that the subject achieves $\dot{V}O_{2max}$ in approximately 10 minutes. (From Wasserman K, et al. Principles of exercise testing and interpretation. 2nd ed. Philadelphia: Lea & Febiger, 1994.)

responsiveness, including anticipated health-related benefits derived from regular physical activity.[7,32,61,72] Frequent questions concern the relative contribution of natural endowment (**genotype**) to physiologic function, neuromuscular coordination, and exercise performance (**phenotype**).[25,45,60,71,101] For example, to what extent does heredity determine the extremely high aerobic capacities of the endurance athletes in Figure 11.8? Do these exceptionally high levels of functional capacity simply reflect intensive training? How does familial aggregation affect skeletal muscle capillary density and enzyme activity and their response to training? The answer remains incomplete, and researchers now focus on the genetic contribution to individual differences in physiologic and metabolic capacity.

In general, most physical fitness characteristics demonstrate high heritability. Earlier research studied 15 pairs of identical twins (monozygous; same heredity from a single fertilized ovum) and 15 pairs of fraternal twins (dizygous; like ordinary siblings, derived from two separate fertilized ovum) raised in the same city and with parents of similar socioeconomic backgrounds. Heredity alone accounted for up to 93%

of observed differences in $\dot{V}O_{2max}$. In addition, the capacity of the short-term glycolytic energy system indicated a genetic determination of approximately 81%, while maximum heart rate showed approximately 86% genetic determination.[43] Subsequent studies of larger groups of brothers, fraternal twins, and identical twins revealed a smaller effect of inherited factors on aerobic capacity and endurance performance.[8,9] FIGURE 11.11 presents data for $\dot{V}O_{2max}$ for identical twin and fraternal twin brothers. The least variation in aerobic capacity between brother pairs emerged for identical twins with identical genetic constitutions. Chapter 21 and "On the Horizon," the final chapter in this book, discuss the potential contribution of genetic makeup to one's responsiveness to aerobic exercise training.

Researchers estimate the genetic effect at about 20 to 30% for $\dot{V}O_{2max}$, 50% for maximum heart rate, and 70% for physical working capacity.[7,8,67] Combining the estimated effects of genetics and familial environment raises the upper limit of genetic determination to about 50% for $\dot{V}O_{2max}$ when adjusted for age, gender, and body mass and/or body composition.[9] Identical

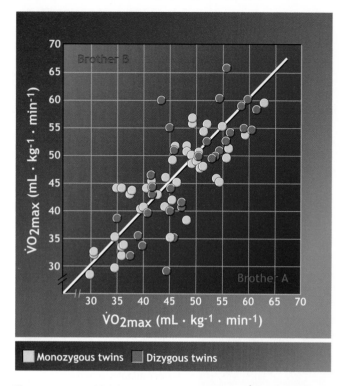

Monozygous twins **Dizygous twins**

Figure 11.11   Maximal oxygen consumptions ($\dot{V}O_{2max}$) for pairs of monozygotic (identical) and dizygotic (fraternal) twin brothers. (From Bouchard C, et al. Aerobic performance in brothers, dizygotic and monozygotic twins. Med Sci Sports Exerc 1986;18:639.)

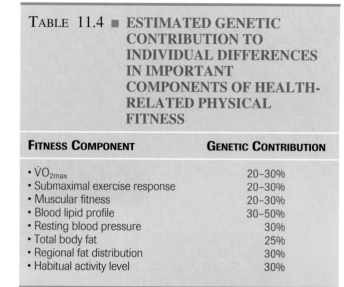

TABLE 11.4 ■ ESTIMATED GENETIC CONTRIBUTION TO INDIVIDUAL DIFFERENCES IN IMPORTANT COMPONENTS OF HEALTH-RELATED PHYSICAL FITNESS

FITNESS COMPONENT	GENETIC CONTRIBUTION
• $\dot{V}O_{2max}$	20–30%
• Submaximal exercise response	20–30%
• Muscular fitness	20–30%
• Blood lipid profile	30–50%
• Resting blood pressure	30%
• Total body fat	25%
• Regional fat distribution	30%
• Habitual activity level	30%

Modified from Bouchard C, Perusse L. Heredity, activity level, fitness, and health. In Physical activity, fitness, and health. Champaign, IL: Human Kinetics, 1994.

twins have similar muscle fiber type composition, whereas fiber type varies widely between fraternal twins and brothers.[44] Between 15 and 40% of the variation in muscular strength among individuals probably results from genetic factors.[66,86] TABLE 11.4 summarizes estimations of the genetic contribution to some important health-related physical fitness components. Future research may determine a precise upper limit of genetic determination; at this time, we can assume that inherited factors contribute significantly to physiologic function, exercise performance, training responsiveness, and specific components of health-related physical fitness.[25,45,70,72]

State of Training

A person's state of aerobic training contributes substantially to the $\dot{V}O_{2max}$, which normally varies between 5 and 20% depending on a person's fitness at the time of testing. Chapter 21 further discusses the influence of training on aerobic capacity.

Gender

Women typically achieve $\dot{V}O_{2max}$ scores 15 to 30% below values of male counterparts.[79,90] Even among trained endurance athletes, the gender difference ranges between 15 and 20%.[5] These differences remain considerably larger for $\dot{V}O_{2max}$ expressed in absolute units ($L \cdot min^{-1}$) rather than to body mass ($mL \cdot kg^{-1} \cdot min^{-1}$).[96] Among world-class cross-country skiers, for example, a 43% lower $\dot{V}O_{2max}$

absolute value for women (6.54 vs. 3.75 $L \cdot min^{-1}$) becomes 15% lower when expressed relative to body mass (83.8 vs. 71.2 $mL \cdot kg^{-1} \cdot min^{-1}$).

The gender difference in $\dot{V}O_{2max}$ has generally been ascribed to differences in body composition (discussed in the next section) and hemoglobin concentration. Untrained young adult women generally average about 25% body fat, whereas men average 15%. The average male generates more total aerobic energy simply because he possesses more muscle mass and has less fat than the average female. Trained athletes have lower percentages of fat than average individuals, yet trained women still possess more body fat than male counterparts. Perhaps because of higher testosterone levels, men also have a 10 to 14% greater hemoglobin concentration than women. This difference in the blood's oxygen-carrying capacity enables men to circulate more oxygen during exercise. This advantage increases their aerobic capacities above those of women.

Factors other than lower body fat and higher hemoglobin concentrations may also explain male–female aerobic capacity differences. For example, normal physical activity levels differ between the average male and average female. One could argue that social constraints reduce opportunities for females of all ages to participate in extracurricular athletic activities and recreational pursuits. Among prepubertal children, boys engage in more daily physical activity than do girls of the same age. Despite these fitness-inhibiting factors, the aerobic capacities of physically active females generally exceed those of sedentary males. The $\dot{V}O_{2max}$ of female cross-country skiers, for example, exceeds scores of untrained males by 40%.[5] Even among the so-called normal population, considerable variability exists within each gender, and the $\dot{V}O_{2max}$ scores for many women exceed average values for men.

Are Gender Differences Shrinking for Endurance Performance? FIGURE 11.12A illustrates the decline in running speed with increasing race distances for men and women in events that place a predominant demand on aerobic energy transfer. The average of the top 50 race times for the 1996 world rankings for the 1500-m, 10-km, and marathon events provided the data points to construct the curves.

Despite the decline in running speed with increasing race distance, a nearly identical gender difference emerged for each race. Men ran on average 14.5% faster than women, with no narrowing of the gender difference as race distance increased. This holds true despite a 37-fold greater duration for the marathon than for the 1500-m run. Clearly, this analysis does not support the contention that gender differences in endurance diminish as distance increases. In addition, analysis of annual world rankings (world best and 100th best times) from 1980 to 1996 (Fig. 11.12 B, C, and D, which includes world-best marathon times up to 2003) indicates that the gender difference in competitive distance running plateaued and remained stable for both the 1500-m and marathon for more than two decades. These findings run counter to current speculation that women's endurance should improve at a faster rate than men's to a point at which gender differences in performance vanish or reverse.[99]

Body Size and Composition

Variations in body mass explain nearly 70% of the differences in $\dot{V}O_{2max}$ scores among individuals. This limits interpretations of exercise performance or absolute values for oxygen consumption when comparing individuals who differ in body size or composition. The effect of body size on aerobic capacity has led to the common practice of expressing oxygen consumption related to surface area, body mass, FFM, or limb volume. TABLE 11.5 shows a 43% difference in $\dot{V}O_{2max}$ ($L \cdot min^{-1}$) for an untrained man and woman differing considerably in body size and composition. When expressed per unit of body mass ($mL \cdot kg^{-1} \cdot min^{-1}$), the $\dot{V}O_{2max}$ of the woman still remains about 20% lower than for the man. Expressing aerobic capacity by FFM reduces the between-subject difference even more (-9%). Adjusting for variation in muscle mass activated in exercise provides additional information to explain interindividual variation in $\dot{V}O_{2max}$. For example, adjusting oxygen consumption values obtained during maximal arm-cranking exercise for variations in estimated arm and shoulder size *eliminates* gender differences in $\dot{V}O_{2peak}$.[93] Expressing oxygen consumption per unit of appendicular skeletal muscle mass often negates the difference in $\dot{V}O_{2max}$ between men and women of similar training status.[13,67] *These findings suggest that the size of the contracting*

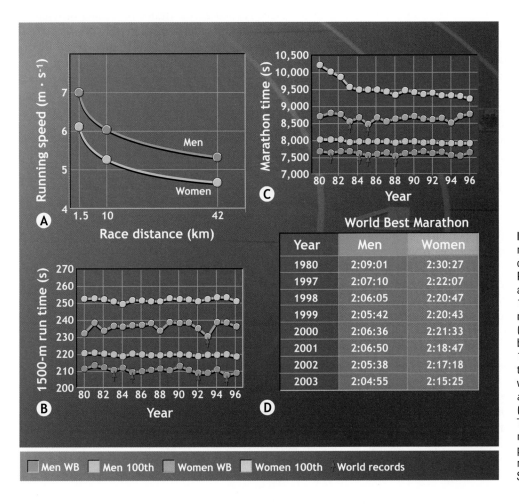

Figure 11.12 A. Decline in running pace over increasing race distance for men and women. Performance represents the average of the top 50 times for the 1996 world rankings for the 1500-m (1.5-km), 10-km, and marathon (42-km) events. Annual world best *(WB)* and 100th ranked 1500-m times (**B**) and marathon times (**C** and **D**) for men and women from 1980 to 2003. *Red arrows* indicate world records. (Modified from Sparling PB, et al. The gender difference in distance running performance has plateaued: an analysis of world rankings from 1980 to 1996. Med Sci Sports Exerc 1998;30:1725.)

TABLE 11.5 ■ DIFFERENT WAYS TO EXPRESS OXYGEN CONSUMPTION			
VARIABLE	**FEMALE**	**MALE**	**FEMALE VS. MALE % DIFFERENCE**
$\dot{V}O_{2max}$, $L \cdot min^{-1}$	2.00	3.50	−43
$\dot{V}O_{2max}$, $mL \cdot kg^{-1} \cdot min^{-1}$	40.0	50.0	−20
$\dot{V}O_{2max}$, $mL \cdot kg\,FFM^{-1} \cdot min^{-1}$	53.3	58.8	−9
Body mass, kg	50	70	−29
Percentage body fat	25	15	+67
Fat-free body mass, kg	37.5	59.5	−37

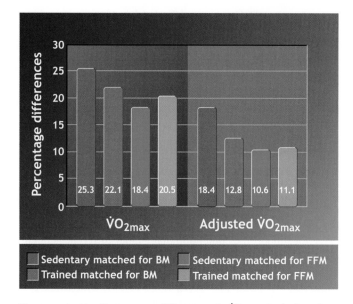

Figure 11.13   Percentage differences in $\dot{V}O_{2max}$, including the adjustment for hemoglobin *(adjusted $\dot{V}O_{2max}$)*, in sedentary and trained men and women matched for body mass *(BM)* and fat-free body mass *(FFM)*. (From Keller BA, Katch FI. It is not valid to adjust gender differences in aerobic capacity and strength for body mass or lean body mass. Med Sci Sports Exerc 1991;23:S167.)

muscle mass largely accounts for gender differences in aerobic capacity.

An Argument for Biologic Differences Between Genders. The traditional ways to express oxygen consumption presented in Table 11.5 do not necessarily answer whether gender differences in $\dot{V}O_{2max}$ remain biologically inherent or merely reflect differences in muscle mass and body composition.[103] Uncertainty exists because ratio adjustments may not "eliminate," "equate," or "normalize" gender differences: they simply express the criterion trait (e.g., aerobic capacity or muscular strength) relative to a specific divisor (e.g., body mass, FFM, or muscle cross-sectional area). Justification for which divisor best expresses an individual's $\dot{V}O_{2max}$ for comparison purposes makes certain assumptions. For example, creating the ratio score $\dot{V}O_2$ divided by FFM implies a direct and proportional relationship between the two variables, a condition not achieved for any of the variables mentioned above.[41] Any deviation in linearity in the relationship between the numerator and denominator in the ratio expression either underestimates or overestimates an individual's "true" $\dot{V}O_2$.

An experimental approach to this important topic would compare physiologic responses and capacities of men and women of near-similar body size, body composition, and training history. Such a comparison eliminates the need to express oxygen consumption as a ratio score relative to body size or body composition. If gender exerts no effect on aerobic capacity, then men and women should achieve similar $\dot{V}O_{2max}$ scores. One study tested this hypothesis in 10 pairs of sedentary and endurance-trained men and women matched for age, stature, body mass, FFM, and prior training history. The researchers also adjusted aerobic capacity for the gender difference in hemoglobin concentration. FIGURE 11.13 illustrates the effect of gender matching for body mass and FFM on the percentage difference in aerobic capacity during incremental treadmill running. The $\dot{V}O_{max}$ differences between men and women matched for body mass equaled

25.3% (sedentary) and 22.1% (trained). Gender differences persisted after adjustment for hemoglobin concentration *(adjusted $\dot{V}O_{2max}$)*; they decreased only slightly to 18.4% for the sedentary group and 12.8% for the trained group. Matching the groups for FFM did not minimize substantial gender differences that averaged 18.4% for the sedentary group and 20.5% for the trained group. Adjusting these differences in aerobic capacity further for hemoglobin concentration reduced the gender differences somewhat, but they still averaged about 11% for each group.

These findings suggest a biologically inherent and unalterable component to the gender difference in aerobic capacity. This does not mean that aerobic capacity cannot be significantly and equally affected for men and women by training or body composition alterations. Rather, an individual should not necessarily expect gender-free differences in aerobic capacity. Chapter 22 presents data on gender differences in muscular strength from experiments with equally trained men and women with the same body size and composition.

Age

Age does not spare its effect on maximal oxygen consumption.[38,55,69] Although one can draw only limited inferences from cross-sectional studies of persons of different ages, available data provide insight into the possible effects of aging on physiologic function. FIGURE 11.14 summarizes data from various studies on age trends in aerobic capacity of children and adults.

Children. Figure 11.14A and B illustrates age trends in the absolute and relative aerobic capacities of boys and girls aged 6 to 16 years.

- **Absolute values**—$\dot{V}O_{2max}$ values in $L \cdot min^{-1}$ (Fig. 11.14A) for boys and girls remain the same until about age 12; at age 14, $\dot{V}O_{2max}$ for boys averages 25% higher than that for girls, and by age 16 the difference exceeds 50%. The difference generally relates to the combined effect of a greater muscle mass in boys and their greater daily physical activity levels.
- **Relative values**—For boys, average aerobic capacity in $mL \cdot kg^{-1} \cdot min^{-1}$ (Fig. 11.14B) remains level at about 52 $mL \cdot kg^{-1} \cdot min^{-1}$ from ages 6 to 16; for girls, the line slopes downward with age, reaching about 40 $mL \cdot kg^{-1} \cdot min^{-1}$ at age 16, a value 32% below male counterparts. The greater accumulation of body fat in adolescent females partially accounts for the lower values; females must transport this extra fat that does not enhance the capacity for aerobic metabolism.

Adults. $\dot{V}O_{2max}$ declines steadily after age 25 at a rate of about 1% per year, so at age 55 it averages about 27% below values reported for 20-year-olds (Fig. 11.14C). The data in the inset graph indicate that active adults retain a relatively high $\dot{V}O_{2max}$ at all ages, yet it still progressively declines with advancing years. For eight women nearly 80 years of age, $\dot{V}O_{2max}$ averaged 13.4 $mL \cdot kg^{-1} \cdot min^{-1}$, or about 3.7 METs.[24] Despite this apparent significant aging effect, strong evidence indicates that a person's habitual physical activity level exerts far greater influence on aerobic capacity than chronological age per se.[59] Chapter 31 more fully discusses age-related influences on physiologic function.

Aerobic Capacity Prediction Tests

The direct measurement of $\dot{V}O_{2max}$ requires an extensive laboratory, specialized equipment, and considerable subject physical effort and motivation. Consequently, laboratory tests are impractical for assessing large groups of untrained subjects. In addition, strenuous exercise could prove risky to adults who do not receive proper medical clearance and appropriate supervision. These considerations increase the importance of submaximal exercise testing to *predict* $\dot{V}O_{2max}$ from performance during walking and running or from heart rate during or immediately postexercise.

A Word of Caution About Predictions

All predictions contain error, referred to as the **standard error of estimate** (**SEE**). Errors of estimate are expressed in measurement units of the predicted variable (e.g., kg, mL, s) or as a percentage. For example, suppose the $\dot{V}O_{2max}$ ($mL \cdot kg^{-1} \cdot min^{-1}$) predicted from time on a walking test equals 55 $mL \cdot kg^{-1} \cdot min^{-1}$, with SEE ± 10 $mL \cdot kg^{-1} \cdot min^{-1}$. This means that the actual $\dot{V}O_{2max}$ probably (68% confident) lies within ± 10 $mL \cdot kg^{-1} \cdot min^{-1}$ or between 45 and 65 $mL \cdot kg^{-1}$

$\cdot min^{-1}$ of the predicted value. This represents a large error ($\pm$ 18% of the absolute value).

Some predictions are associated with small errors (SEE $\pm 5\%$) and others with larger errors. Obviously, a larger error translates to a less useful predicted score because the likely true score encompasses such a large range of possible values. Without knowing the magnitude of the SEE, one cannot judge the usefulness of a predicted score. Using some prediction methods on repeated occasions for the same individual (e.g., pre-, mid-, and posttraining) can introduce large and sometimes unknown errors. Whenever predictions are made, one must interpret the predicted score in light of the magnitude of the prediction error. With a relatively small prediction error, prediction of $\dot{V}O_{2max}$ can be useful in appropriate situations in which direct measurement is not possible.

Walking Tests

Walking tests can predict $\dot{V}O_{2max}$. The following equation predicts $\dot{V}O_{2max}$ in $L \cdot min^{-1}$ from walking speed and other variables in men and women[42]:

$$\dot{V}O_{2max} = 6.9652 + (0.0091 \times Wt) - (0.0257 \times Age) + (0.5955 \times Gender) - (0.224 \times T1) - (0.0115 \times HR1\text{-}4)$$

where Wt is body weight in pounds; Age is in years; Gender is 0 for females, 1 for males; T1 is time for the 1-mile track walk, expressed as minutes and hundredths of a minute; and HR1-4 is heart rate in beats per minute measured immediately at the end of the last quarter-mile.

The following equation predicts $\dot{V}O_{2max}$ in $mL \cdot kg^{-1} \cdot min^{-1}$ using the same variables:

$$\dot{V}O_{2max} = 132.853 - (0.0769 \times Wt) - (0.3877 \times Age) + (0.5955(6.315 \times Gender) - (3.2649 \times T1) - (0.1565 \times HR1\text{-}4)$$

The multiple correlation is $r = 0.92$ for predicting $\dot{V}O_{2max}$ from 1-mile walking performance for both equations with a standard error of prediction of ± 0.335 $L \cdot min^{-1}$, or ± 4.4 $mL \cdot kg^{-1} \cdot min^{-1}$. This means that about 68% of the people tested have an actual $\dot{V}O_{2max}$ within ± 0.335 $L \cdot min^{-1}$ (± 4.4 $mL \cdot kg^{-1} \cdot min^{-1}$) of the predicted value. The group studied ranged in age from 30 to 69 years; thus, the prediction method applies to a large segment of the adult population.

The following data for a 30-year-old female illustrate the prediction method:

$$Body\ weight = 155.5\ lb$$
$$T1 = 13.56\ min$$
$$HR1\text{-}4 = 145\ b \cdot min^{-1}$$

Substituting in the equation to predict $\dot{V}O_{2max}$ in $mL \cdot kg^{-1} \cdot min^{-1}$:

$$\dot{V}O_{2max} = 132.853 - (0.0769 \times 155.5) - (0.3877 \times 30.0) + (6.315 \times 0) - (3.2649 \times 13.56) - (0.1565 \times 145)$$

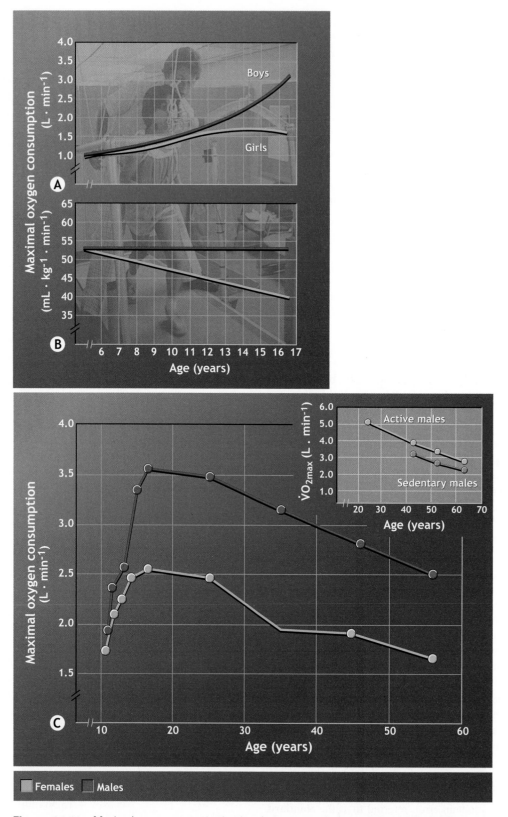

Figure 11.14   Maximal oxygen consumption in relation to age in boys and girls (**A** and **B**) and men and women (**C**). (**A** and **B** from Krahenbuhl GS, et al. Developmental aspects of maximal aerobic power in children. Exerc Sport Sci Rev. Terjung RL, ed. vol 13, New York: Macmillan, 1985, **C** modified from Hermansen L. Individual differences. In: Larson LA, ed. Fitness, health, and work capacity. International standards for assessment. New York: Macmillan, 1974. Inset graph in **C** redrawn from tabled data of Åstrand PO, Rodahl KR. Textbook of work physiology. New York: McGraw-Hill, 1970.)

$$\dot{V}O_{2max} = 132.853 - (11.96) - (11.63) + (0)$$
$$- (44.27) - (22.69)$$
$$\dot{V}O_{2max} = 42.3 \text{ mL} \cdot \text{kg}^{-1} \cdot \text{min}^{-1}$$

Endurance Runs

As with walking tests, runs of various durations or distances evaluate aerobic fitness. Test use reasonably assumes that a person's ability to maintain a high, steady-rate oxygen consumption largely determines the distance run over at least 5 minutes' duration. This ability depends on the maximum capacity to generate energy aerobically (i.e., $\dot{V}O_{2max}$). This rationale provided the framework for a field performance test devised in 1959 to evaluate aerobic fitness of military personnel.[2] The test required subjects to run as far as possible in 15 minutes. A 1968 study by Cooper shortened run time to 12 minutes.[15]

In his original validation of the 12-minute test, Cooper reported a strong association between $\dot{V}O_{2max}$ of Air Force personnel and distances run-walked in 12 minutes. The correlation coefficient was $r = 0.90$ between 12-minute run-walk distance and $\dot{V}O_{2max}$ (mL $\cdot$ kg^{-1} $\cdot$ min^{-1}) in 47 men who varied considerably in age (17 to 54 y), body mass (52 to 123 kg), and $\dot{V}O_{2max}$ (31 to 59 mL $\cdot$ kg^{-1} $\cdot$ min^{-1}). Other researchers reported the same correlation for 9 ninth-grade boys.[19] Subsequent studies have failed to demonstrate as strong a connection between "Cooper 12-minute run scores" and aerobic capacity. For example, one study measured 11- to 14-year-old boys and reported a correlation of $r = 0.65$.[47] For a group of 26 female athletes, the correlation between the run-walk scores and $\dot{V}O_{2max}$ was $r = 0.70$,[48] and for 36 untrained college women a similar correlation of $r = 0.67$ emerged.[39]

Importantly, a simple correlation between run-walk scores and $\dot{V}O_{2max}$ does not consider the interacting effects of age and body mass. These variables themselves relate to both run-walk times and $\dot{V}O_{2max}$ scores. When restricting Cooper's original data to the same age range as subjects in the preceding study of 36 untrained women, the computed correlation coefficient decreased dramatically from $r = 0.90$ to $r = 0.59$.

One must view with caution $\dot{V}O_{2max}$ predictions based on running performance. The need to establish a consistent level of motivation and effective pacing while running becomes critical with inexperienced subjects. Some individuals achieve an optimal pace throughout the run. Others may run too fast early in the run and be forced to slow down or even stop before completing the test. Other individuals may begin too slowly and continue this way, so that their final performance scores reflect inappropriate pacing or lack of motivation rather than poor physiologic capacity. In addition, $\dot{V}O_{2max}$ does not singularly determine endurance running performance. Body mass and fatness, running economy, and percentage of aerobic capacity sustained without blood lactate buildup contribute significantly to successful running. *Generally, the SEE of predicting $\dot{V}O_{2max}$ from walk-run performance averages about 8 to 10% of the predicted value.*

Limitations for Use with Children. Maximum 1-mile run or walk times serve only limited use for $\dot{V}O_{2max}$ prediction in growing children because the age-related exercise performance improvements in youth relate poorly to changes in aerobic capacity.[16] The largest contributions to test score improvement in children as they grow older result from two factors: (1) increased percentage of $\dot{V}O_{2peak}$ sustained during the exercise (i.e., increased blood lactate threshold) and (2) improved running economy. Both factors contribute significantly to faster times independent of any improvement in $\dot{V}O_{2max}$.

Predictions Based on Heart Rate

Tests to predict $\dot{V}O_{2max}$ use exercise or postexercise heart rate during a standardized regimen of submaximal exercise performed on either a bicycle ergometer, treadmill, or step test. These tests apply the essentially linear relationship between heart rate (HR) and oxygen consumption ($\dot{V}O_2$) during increasing intensities of light to relatively heavy aerobic exercise. The slope of the line describing the HR–$\dot{V}O_2$ relationship (i.e., rate of heart rate increase) reflects the adequacy of the cardiovascular response and aerobic fitness capacity. The $\dot{V}O_{2max}$ is estimated by drawing a best-fit straight line through several submaximal points that relate heart rate and oxygen consumption (or exercise intensity); the **HR–$\dot{V}O_2$ line** is then extended to an assumed maximum heart rate for the subject's age.

FIGURE 11.15 illustrates the **extrapolation procedure** for an untrained and an endurance-trained college student. Four submaximal measures during graded exercise provided the data points to construct the HR–$\dot{V}O_2$ line. Each person's HR–$\dot{V}O_2$ line tends toward linearity, although the slope of the line often differs considerably. A person of relatively high aerobic fitness performs more-intense exercise (achieves higher $\dot{V}O_2$) before reaching a heart rate of 140 or 160 b $\cdot$ min^{-1} than a less-fit person. Because heart rate increases linearly with exercise intensity ($\dot{V}O_2$), the person with the smallest heart rate increase tends to achieve the highest exercise capacity and, hence, the highest $\dot{V}O_{2max}$. Extrapolation of the HR–$\dot{V}O_2$ line to a heart rate of 195 b $\cdot$ min^{-1}—the assumed maximum heart rate for subjects of college age—predicted the $\dot{V}O_{2max}$ of the two subjects depicted in Figure 11.15.

The following four assumptions affect the accuracy of the $\dot{V}O_{2max}$ prediction from submaximal exercise heart rate:

1. *Linearity of heart rate–oxygen consumption (exercise intensity) relationship.* This assumption generally holds, particularly during light to moderate exercise. In some subjects, the HR–$\dot{V}O_2$ line curves (asymptotes) at more intense workloads in a direction that indicates a larger than expected increase in oxygen consumption per unit increase in heart rate. Oxygen consumption actually increases more than predicted by linear extrapolation of the HR–$\dot{V}O_2$ line. This *underestimates* the $\dot{V}O_{2max}$ of these subjects.

2. *Similar maximum heart rates for all subjects.* One standard deviation from the average maximum heart rate for individuals of the same age equals ± 10 b $\cdot$ min^{-1}. Extrapolating the HR–$\dot{V}O_2$ line of a young adult to 195 b $\cdot$ min^{-1}, for example, *overestimates* the $\dot{V}O_{2max}$ of a person whose actual maximum heart

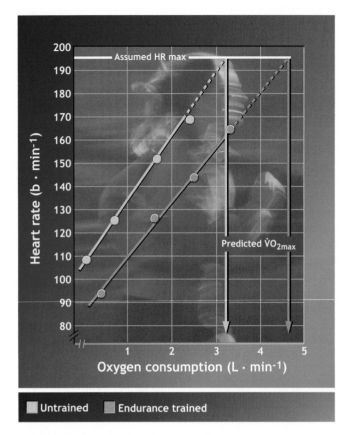

Figure 11.15 Extrapolating the linear relationship between submaximal heart rate and oxygen consumption up to an assumed maximum heart rate during graded exercise by an untrained subject and an endurance-trained subject.

rate is 185 b · min^{-1}. The opposite occurs for a subject with an actual maximum heart rate of 210 b · min^{-1}. Maximum heart rate also decreases with age. Failure to consider this age effect (i.e., extrapolating to a heart rate of 195 b · min^{-1}, the average heart rate for 25-year-olds) consistently *overestimates* $\dot{V}O_{2max}$ in older subjects. Chapter 31 discusses the effect of age on maximum heart rate.

3. *Assumed constant economy and mechanical efficiency during exercise.* Variations in exercise economy contribute to $\dot{V}O_{2max}$ prediction errors with tests that estimate submaximal oxygen consumption from the external workload (rather than measuring $\dot{V}O_2$ directly). More specifically, an underestimation of $\dot{V}O_{2max}$ occurs for a subject with poor exercise economy whose submaximal oxygen consumption increases more than assumed on the basis of estimates from exercise intensity. This occurs because of an elevated heart rate from the added oxygen cost of uneconomical exercise. Variation in walking or cycling economy among individuals usually does not exceed 6%; for bench stepping, the variation can equal about 10%, a value unrelated to age, leg length, aerobic fitness, or percentage body fat.[85] Seemingly small modifications in test procedures also profoundly affect exercise economy.

Simply allowing individuals to support themselves with the treadmill handrails reduces the oxygen cost of exercise by as much as 30%.[105]

4. *Day-to-day heart rate variation.* Even under highly standardized conditions, the day-to-day variation in heart rate averages about 5 b · min^{-1} during submaximal exercise.

Within the framework of these limitations, $\dot{V}O_{2max}$ predicted from submaximal heart rate generally falls within 10 to 20% of the person's actual value. This accuracy level remains unacceptable for research purposes, yet the prediction tests can effectively screen and classify individuals for aerobic fitness in a gymnasium or health-club setting. The technique also has proved useful to estimate aerobic capacity during pregnancy (see "In a Practical Sense," Chapter 9).[76]

The Step Test

A practical way to classify aerobic fitness uses heart rate during recovery from a standardized stepping exercise. "Prediction equations" applied to step-test results can estimate $\dot{V}O_{2max}$ with reasonable accuracy.

In our laboratories we used a 3-minute step test to evaluate exercise heart rate responses of thousands of college men and women.[53] The test used gymnasium bleachers (16$^{1}/_{4}$ in. high) to test large numbers of students at the same time. Subjects performed each stepping cycle to a four-step cadence, "up-up-down-down." The women performed 22 complete step-ups per minute, regulated by a metronome set at 88 beats per minute. Males tended to be "fitter" for step-up exercise than females, so their cadence was 24 step-ups per minute or 96 beats per minute on the metronome. The step test began after a brief demonstration and practice period. At the completion of stepping, students remained standing while pulse rate was measured for 15 seconds, 5 to 20 seconds into recovery. Recovery heart rate was converted to beats per minute (15-s HR × 4) and compared with the established percentile rankings presented in TABLE 11.6.

INTEGRATIVE QUESTION

Respond to a student who asks: "I've had my $\dot{V}O_{2max}$ measured directly in the laboratory and predicted with a 12-minute run. Why don't both values agree?"

Based on the essentially linear relationship between heart rate and oxygen consumption during submaximal exercise, one would expect a person with a low step-test heart rate (i.e., farther from maximum) to experience less exercise stress than someone of the same age performing the identical exercise with a relatively high heart rate. In other words, a lower heart rate during a standard exercise corresponds to a higher $\dot{V}O_{2max}$. To determine the validity of the step test to estimate aerobic capacity, we then measured the $\dot{V}O_{2max}$ for a group of untrained, young adult men and women who also performed

TABLE 11.6 ■ **PERCENTILE RANKINGS FOR STEP TEST RECOVERY HEART RATE (HR) AND PREDICTED $\dot{V}O_{2MAX}$ FOR UNTRAINED MALE AND FEMALE COLLEGE STUDENTS**

PERCENTILE RANKING	RECOVERY HR, FEMALE	PREDICTED $\dot{V}O_{2MAX}$ ($mL \cdot kg^{-1} \cdot min^{-1}$)	RECOVERY HR, MALE	PREDICTED $\dot{V}O_{2MAX}$ ($mL \cdot kg^{-1} \cdot min^{-1}$)
100	128	42.2	120	60.9
95	140	40.0	124	59.3
90	148	38.5	128	57.6
85	152	37.7	136	54.2
80	156	37.0	140	52.5
75	158	36.6	144	50.9
70	160	36.3	148	49.2
65	162	35.9	149	48.8
60	163	35.7	152	47.5
55	164	35.5	154	46.7
50	166	35.1	156	45.8
45	168	34.8	160	44.1
40	170	34.4	162	43.3
35	171	34.2	164	42.5
30	172	34.0	166	41.6
25	176	33.3	168	40.8
20	180	32.6	172	39.1
15	182	32.2	176	37.4
10	184	31.8	178	36.6
5	196	29.6	184	34.1

the step test. FIGURE 11.16 illustrates the relationship between $\dot{V}O_{2max}$ and the women's step-test scores. The results clearly indicated that step-test heart rate provided significant information about $\dot{V}O_{2max}$. Subjects with a high recovery heart rate tended to have a lower $\dot{V}O_{2max}$, whereas a faster recovery (lower heart rate) related to a relatively high $\dot{V}O_{2max}$. The following equations predict $\dot{V}O_{2max}$ ($mL \cdot kg^{-1} \cdot min^{-1}$) from step-test pulse rate (ST_{pulse}) results for similar groups of young adult men and women:

Men:

$$\dot{V}O_{2max} = 111.33 - (0.42 \times ST_{pulse} [b \cdot min^{-1}])$$

Women:

$$\dot{V}O_{2max} = 65.81 - (0.1847 \times ST_{pulse} [b \cdot min^{-1}])$$

To simplify these conversions, the "Predicted $\dot{V}O_{2max}$" columns of Table 11.6 present the maximal oxygen consumption values for men and women, based on recovery heart rate scores. For predictive accuracy, one can be 95% confidant that the predicted $\dot{V}O_{2max}$ falls within 16% of the person's true $\dot{V}O_{2max}$. For a high degree of accuracy, one must measure $\dot{V}O_{2max}$ directly in the laboratory with an appropriate graded exercise test. If this proves impractical or if accuracy can be compromised somewhat, prediction tests provide reasonable alternatives but *not* precise benchmarks.

Predictions from Nonexercise Data

A unique approach to $\dot{V}O_{2max}$ prediction for quick screening of large groups of individuals involves collecting specific nonexercise data from a questionnaire.[26,36] The SEE for a predicted score from the method described below equals ± 3.44 mL $O_2 \cdot kg^{-1} \cdot min^{-1}$.

Data input to predict $\dot{V}O_{2max}$ from nonexercise data:

1. **Sex** (female = 0; male = 1)

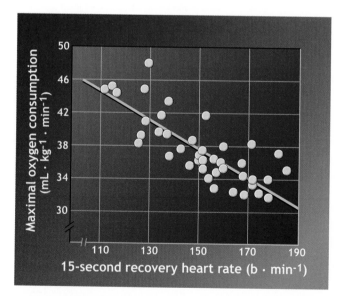

Figure 11.16 Scattergram and line of "best fit" that relates step-test heart rate score and maximal oxygen consumption in untrained college women.

TABLE 11.7 ■ INPUT INFORMATION ON LEVEL OF PHYSICAL ACTIVITY AND PERCEIVED FUNCTIONAL CAPACITY FOR PREDICTING $\dot{V}O_{2MAX}$ FROM NONEXERCISE DATA

A. PHYSICAL ACTIVITY RATING (PA-R)

SELECT THE NUMBER THAT BEST DESCRIBES YOUR OVERALL LEVEL OF PHYSICAL ACTIVITY FOR THE PREVIOUS 6 MONTHS:

Points	Description
0	**inactive:** avoid walking or exertion; e.g., always use elevator, drive when possible instead of walking
1	**light activity:** walk for pleasure, routinely use stairs, occasionally exercise sufficiently to cause heavy breathing or perspiration
2	**moderate activity:** 10 to 60 minutes per week of moderate activity such as golf, horseback riding, calisthenics, table tennis, bowling, weight lifting, yard work, cleaning house, walking for exercise
3	**moderate activity:** over 1 hour per week of moderate activity described above
4	**vigorous activity:** run less than 1 mile per week or spend less than 30 min per week in comparable activity such as running or jogging, lap swimming, cycling, rowing, aerobics, skipping rope, running in place, or engaging in vigorous aerobic-type activity such as soccer, basketball, tennis, racquetball, or handball
5	**vigorous activity:** run 1 mile to less than 5 miles per week or spend 30 min to less than 60 min per week in comparable physical activity as described above
6	**vigorous activity:** run 5 miles to less than 10 miles per week or spend 1 hour to less than 3 hours per week in comparable physical activity as described above
7	**vigorous activity:** run 10 miles to less than 15 miles per week or spend 3 hours to less than 6 hours per week in comparable physical activity as described above
8	**vigorous activity:** run 15 miles to less than 20 miles per week or spend 6 hours to less than 7 hours per week in comparable physical activity as described above
9	**vigorous activity:** run 20 to 25 miles per week or spend 7 to 8 hours per week in comparable physical activity as described above
10	**vigorous activity:** run over 25 miles per week or spend over 8 hours per week in comparable physical activity as described above

B. PERCEIVED FUNCTIONAL ABILITY (PFA) QUESTIONS

SUPPOSE YOU EXERCISE CONTINUOUSLY ON AN INDOOR TRACK FOR 1 MILE. WHICH EXERCISE PACE IS RIGHT FOR YOU—NOT TOO EASY OR NOT TOO HARD? CIRCLE THE APPROPRIATE NUMBER FROM 1 TO 13.

Points	Description
1	Walking at a slow pace (18-min mile or more)
2	
3	Walking at a medium pace (16-min mile)
4	
5	Walking at a fast pace (14-min mile)
6	
7	Jogging at a slow pace (12-min mile)
8	
9	Jogging at a medium pace (10-min mile)
10	
11	Jogging at a fast pace (8-min mile)
12	
13	Running at a fast pace (7-min mile or less)

HOW FAST COULD YOU COVER A DISTANCE OF 3 MILES AND NOT BECOME BREATHLESS OR OVERLY FATIGUED? BE REALISTIC. CIRCLE THE APPROPRIATE NUMBER FROM 1 TO 13.

Points	Description
1	I could walk the entire distance at a slow pace (18-min per mile or more)
2	
3	I could walk the entire distance at a medium pace (16-min per mile)
4	
5	I could walk the entire distance at a fast pace (14-min per mile)
6	
7	I could jog the entire distance at a slow pace (12-min per mile)
8	
9	I could jog the entire distance at a medium pace (10-min per mile)
10	
11	I could jog the entire distance at a fast pace (8-min per mile)
12	
13	I could run the entire distance at a fast pace (7-min per mile or less)

From George JD, et al. Non-exercise $\dot{V}O_{2max}$ estimation for physically active college students. Med Sci Sports Exerc 1997;29:415.

2. **Body mass index (BMI; kg · m^{-2})**. Self-reported body mass (kg) and stature (m) used to compute BMI as follows:

$$BMI = Body\ mass\ (kg) \div Stature\ (m^2)$$

3. **Physical activity rating (PA-R)**. A point value between 0 and 10 representing overall physical activity level for the previous 6 months (TABLE 11.7A)

4. **Perceived functional ability (PFA)**. Sum of the point values between 0 and 13 for questions about current level of perceived functional ability to maintain a continuous pace on an indoor track for 1 mile and perceived pace to cover a distance of 3 miles without becoming breathless or overly fatigued (Table 11.7B).

Equation

$$\dot{V}O_{2max}\ (mL \cdot kg^{-1} \cdot min^{-1}) = 44.895 + (7.042 \times Sex) - (0.823 \times BMI) + (0.738 \times PFA) + (0.688 \times PA\text{-}R)$$

Example

1. Sex, female
2. BMI = 22.66 (self-reported body mass = 136 lb [61.7 kg]; self-reported height = 5 feet 5 inches [1.65 m]); BMI = 61.7 ÷ (1.65 × 1.65) = 22.66
3. PA-R score = 5 (see Table 11.7A)
4. PFA score = 15 (sum of 7 scored on first set of questions and 8 on second set; see Table 11.7B.)

Computation

$$\dot{V}O_{2max} = 44.895 + (7.042 \times Sex) - (0.823 \times BMI) + (0.738 \times PFA) + (0.688 \times PA\text{-}R)$$

$$= 44.895 + (7.042 \times 0) - (0.823 \times 22.66) + (0.738 \times 15) + (0.688 \times 5)$$

$$= 44.895\ 0 - 18.65 + 11.07 + 3.77$$

$$= 41.1\ mL \cdot kg^{-1} \cdot min^{-1}$$

Summary

1. The concepts of individual differences and exercise specificity provide an important framework to understand anaerobic and aerobic power capacities.

2. Precise contributions of anaerobic and aerobic energy transfer depend largely on exercise intensity and duration. During strength and power–sprint activities, energy transfer primarily involves the immediate and short-term (anaerobic) energy systems. The long-term (aerobic) energy system becomes progressively more active during exercise lasting longer than 2 minutes

3. Appropriate physiologic measurements and performance tests evaluate the capacity of each energy-transfer system. These tests can (1) evaluate energy-transfer capacity at a particular point in time or (2) show changes consequent to a specific exercise-training program.

4. The stair-sprinting test commonly measures the power capacity of the intramuscular high-energy phosphates ATP and PCr. The 30-second, all-out Wingate test evaluates peak power and average power output capacity from the glycolytic pathway. Interpretations of test results must consider body size and the exercise specificity principle.

5. The maximal accumulated oxygen deficit (MAOD) correlates positively with other anaerobic performance tests; it demonstrates independence from aerobic energy sources and differentiates between aerobically and anaerobically trained individuals.

6. Training status, acid–base regulation, and motivation contribute to individual differences in the capacities of the immediate and short-term energy systems.

7. Maximal oxygen consumption ($\dot{V}O_{2max}$) provides important, reproducible information about the power capacity of the long-term energy system, including the functional capacity of the physiologic support systems.

8. Heredity, state and type of training, age, gender, and body composition contribute uniquely to an individual's $\dot{V}O_{2max}$

9. Expressing aerobic capacity by some ratio of body size or composition (e.g., mL · kg^{-1} · min^{-1} or mL · kg FFM^{-1} · min^{-1}) reduces the gender difference in $\dot{V}O_{2max}$.

10. Tests to predict $\dot{V}O_{2max}$ from submaximal physiologic and performance data often prove useful for fitness classification purposes.

11. Tests to predict $\dot{V}O_{2max}$ from submaximal physiologic and performance data rely on the validity of four assumptions: (1) linearity of the HR–$\dot{V}O_2$ relationship, (2) constancy in maximum heart rates, (3) relatively constant exercise economy, and (4) minimal day-to-day variation in exercise heart rate.

12. Field methods provide useful information about cardiovascular-aerobic function in the absence of more valid laboratory methods.

13. Nonexercise data predicts $\dot{V}O_{2max}$ accurately for screening and classification purposes.

References are available on the Student CD and online at http://connection.lww.com/mkk6e.

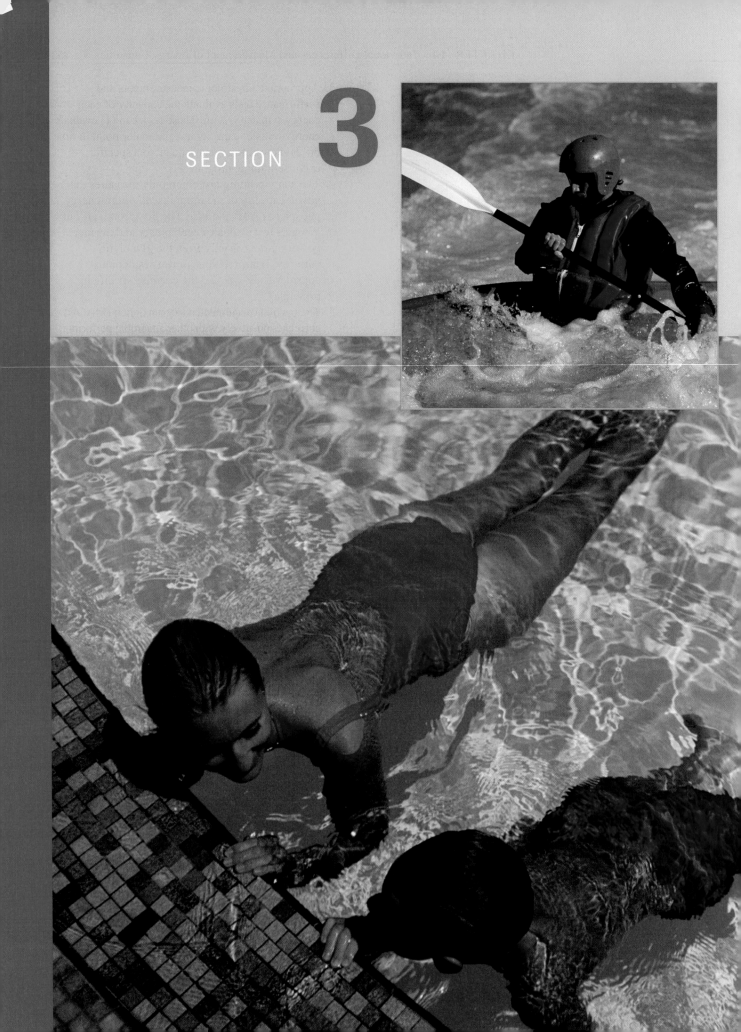

SECTION 3

Systems of Energy Delivery and Utilization

Many sports, recreational, and occupational activities require a moderately intense and sustained energy release. The aerobic breakdown of carbohydrates, fats, and proteins provides energy for such exercise by phosphorylating adenosine diphosphate (ADP) to adenosine triphosphate (ATP). An anaerobic–aerobic energy imbalance develops without a steady rate between the oxidative phosphorylation of ADP to ATP and the exercise energy requirements. When an imbalance occurs, tissue acidity increases and fatigue eventually ensues. Two factors influence how well individuals can sustain a high level of physical activity with minimal fatigue:

1. Capacity and integration of the physiologic systems for oxygen delivery
2. Capacity of specific muscle fibers activated in exercise to generate ATP aerobically

Individual differences in aerobic exercise capacity depend on the combined influence of the ventilatory, circulatory, muscular, and endocrine systems during exercise described in this section. Knowledge about the energy requirements and corresponding physiologic adjustments to exercise provides a solid basis to formulate an effective training program and evaluate its results.

Interview *with* Dr. Loring B. Rowell

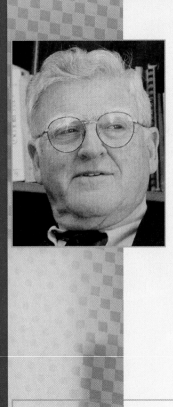

Education: BS (Springfield College, Springfield, MA); PhD (Physiology, University of Minnesota, MN); Postgraduate training (Senior Fellow, Department of Physiology and Biophysics, and of Medicine in Cardiology, University of Washington School of Medicine, St. Louis, MO)

Current Affiliation: Professor Emeritus, University of Washington

Honors and Awards: See Appendix E, which is available on the Student CD and online at http://connection.lww.com/mkk6e.

Research Focus: Human cardiovascular system control and adjustments to exercise

Memorable Publication: Rowell LB. Neural control of muscle blood flow. Importance during dynamic exercise. Clin Exp Pharm Physiol 1997;24:117.

Statement of Contributions: ACSM Honor Award

In recognition of his having achieved excellence in his contributions to cardiovascular physiology, as a scientist, as a teacher and mentor and as an author and editor.

Dr. Rowell's contributions have focused on the regulation of the human cardiovascular system in response to the stresses imposed by exercise, heat, gravity and hypoxia. Included among a long list of landmark findings:

Demonstration that decrements in visceral organ blood flow were proportionate to relative exercise intensity. Evidence that the sympathetically mediated redistribution of blood flow, blood volume and filling pressures was a critical regulatory response to exercise in the heat. Proof of the dominant reflex role of systemic baroreceptors in the regulation of blood pressure under stress. Evidence that muscle chemoreflexes and baroreceptors were reset during exercise and that this was crucial in the matching of cardiovascular responses to metabolic requirements.

Tracing Dr. Rowell's scientific achievements over the past three decades reveals a fascinating progression of discovery, with one study springing from the questions raised by its predecessor. The questions become more and more difficult and the methods and experimental designs more complex and ingenious. Thus, as the years progressed the risk of failure was often high, but this was overridden by the excitement of producing truly novel and significant advances. He demonstrated how important basic physiologic understandings could be uncovered in healthy human subjects, but did not hesitate to use animal or disease models when necessary to further knowledge. The same thoroughness in scientific inquiry has been perpetuated by the many leading scientists he has mentored.

Larry Rowell's writing has had a major impact on the field. He wrote the first Physiological Reviews on the topic of exercise physiology over twenty years ago. More recently he has provided two landmark reference texts concerned with human cardiovascular regulation and was editor in chief of the first APS sponsored Handbook of Exercise Physiology. As an author he was never merely an information broker; rather his writings constantly challenged the reader to criticize accepted dogma, to tackle the toughest questions and to advance the field.

Larry Rowell has been especially valuable to his students, his colleagues, his professional societies and his science, because he never trivialized any task or problem. His approach to life's challenges has always been intense and thorough, whether the problem was of a scientific or humanistic nature. Thus, he tackled the mysteries of baroreceptor resetting with the same zeal and dedication and work ethic that he applied to the editing of a handbook, or to traversing the steep terrain of a snow covered mountain, or in the preparation of a single lecture, or debating a controversial point of science, or in solving the predicaments of friends or colleagues whom he felt were dealt with unfairly. In short, Larry Rowell is indeed "good value"! He is well deserving of the College's highest distinction.

What first inspired you to enter the exercise science field? What made you decide to pursue your advanced degree and/or line of research?

■ Dr. Peter V. Karpovich at Springfield College (MA) provided my first exposure to the science of physiology. His precise and demanding teaching provided the motivation to seek an advanced degree in physiology and to do research in that field.

What influence did your undergraduate education have on your final career choice?

■ Again, the undergraduate teaching of Dr. Karpovich, my experience working in his laboratory, and his urging and support paved the way. His influence led me to the Department of Physiology at the University of Minnesota Medical School and the laboratories of Ancel Keys, Henry L. Taylor, and Francisco Grande and colleagues.

Who were the most influential people in your career, and why?

■ First, Drs. Henry L. Taylor and Francisco Grande guided my graduate education and taught me how to do research. They became lifelong models for an approach to research and scholarship that I admire greatly. Second, my scientific colleagues, students, and fellows have all provided me with constant stimulation and education, and have enriched my career.

What has been the most interesting/enjoyable aspect of your involvement in science? What was the least interesting/enjoyable aspect?

■ Regarding the most interesting and enjoyable aspects: First, are the wonderful colleagues from all over the world who became lifelong friends and enormous positive influences on my life. Second was the research, the excitement of developing methods to answer a scientific question, getting an answer, having it accepted by peers, and seeing it published. The least enjoyable aspects were not having our answers accepted by our peers and any breakdown or failure of our developed methods.

What is your most meaningful contribution to the field of exercise science, and why is it so important?

■ Time and history must judge. I think it is the collection of experiments (1964–1974) in which we quantified the reductions in regional organ blood flow, which were closely related to exercise intensity expressed as percent of $\dot{V}O_{2max}$ and heart rate. They revealed the quantitative significance of this regional vasoconstriction to blood pressure regulation and to the redistribution of oxygen from resting organs to active muscle. And they showed how this regional vasoconstriction determines the volume of blood available to fill the heart (and thus stroke volume) in exercising humans and how this crucial adjustment is upset by skin vasodilation during heat stress.

What advice would you give to students who express an interest in pursuing a career in exercise science research?

■ My advice is based on physiology, because that is what I do. I am a cardiovascular physiologist who has used exercise as a powerful precision tool to understand how the cardiovascular

system works. Acquisition of a strong background in general physics, mathematics, and chemistry (inorganic, analytical, organic, and especially basic physical chemistry) is essential. In as much as the physiology of exercise is actually the total physiology of a nonresting, nonsupine individual, all areas of physiology are essential because there is no physiological function, regulation, or control that is not vital (i.e., exercise physiology = physiology in toto). Thus, the broader and deeper the training in physiology, the more likely the research will yield basic new information. To quote Sir Joseph Barcroft (1934), "The condition of exercise is not a mere variant of the condition of rest, it is the essence of the machine."

What interests have you pursued outside your professional career?

■ Competitive and recreational Alpine skiing, plus coaching and instruction; Alpinism (glacier and rock climbing); road and mountain bicycling; tennis; landscape painting (oil); and historical literature.

Where do you see the exercise science field (particularly your area of greatest interest) heading in the next 20 years?

■ This field may play a more vital role in the biological sciences than we had once imagined. If the basic life scientist's rush to apply their expertise to provide functional meaning to the genetic code, as is expected, who will be left to teach basic human biology and physiology? Who will explore the functional consequences of aging, for example? Who will discover what controls breathing and the circulation during exercise? Who will do the systematic, integrative science that reveals how whole organ systems and organisms actually work? These questions are not likely to be answered by

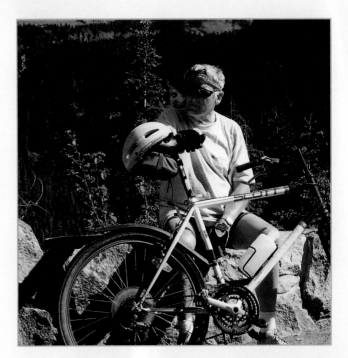

reductionists (e.g., molecular biologists) working upward from molecules to cells to systems–this is in the wrong direction!

You have the opportunity to give a "last lecture." Describe its primary focus.

■ Its primary focus would be on the question, "What reflexes govern cardiovascular function in exercise?" This century-old, unanswered question concerns what is being controlled (and how), and what signals or errors are being sensed (and how) and corrected (and how) by the autonomic nervous system. The lecture would present the currently dominant ideas and would argue which ones do not seem feasible (and why), and which ones seem feasible based on current knowledge. It would ask where we turn next. And, finally, it would warn us of the great danger of ignoring history–a danger now encouraged by exclusion of all literature published before 1970 from the computer indexing services.

Pulmonary Structure and Function

12

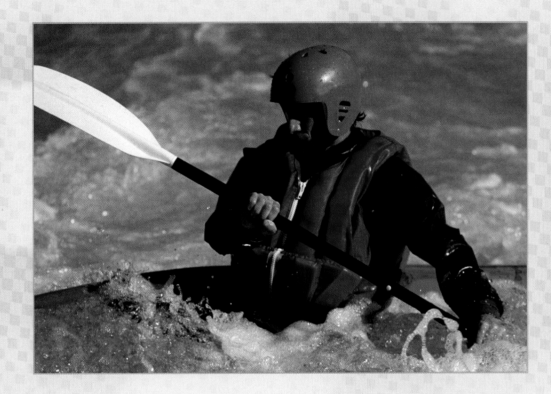

CHAPTER OBJECTIVES

- Diagram the ventilatory system—show the glottis, trachea, bronchi, bronchioles, and alveoli

- Discuss the mechanical and muscular aspects of inspiration and expiration during rest and exercise

- Define and quantify static and dynamic lung function measures and their relation to exercise performance

- Define *minute ventilation, alveolar ventilation, ventilation-perfusion ratio,* and *anatomic and physiologic dead space*

- Explain the four phases of the Valsalva and discuss the physiologic consequences of this maneuver

- Describe the effects of cold-weather exercise on the respiratory tract

SURFACE AREA AND GAS EXCHANGE

If oxygen supply to humans depended only on diffusion through the skin, one could not sustain the basal energy requirement, let alone the 4- to 5-L per minute oxygen consumption and carbon dioxide elimination required to run a world-class, 5-minute per mile marathon pace. The relatively compact and remarkably effective **ventilatory system** meets the requirements for gas exchange. This system, depicted in

FIGURE 12.1, regulates the gaseous state of the body's "external" pulmonary environment to effectively aerate body fluids.

ANATOMY OF VENTILATION

Pulmonary ventilation describes the process of moving and exchanging ambient air with air in the lungs. Air entering the nose and mouth flows into the conductive portions of the ventilatory system where it adjusts to body temperature, is

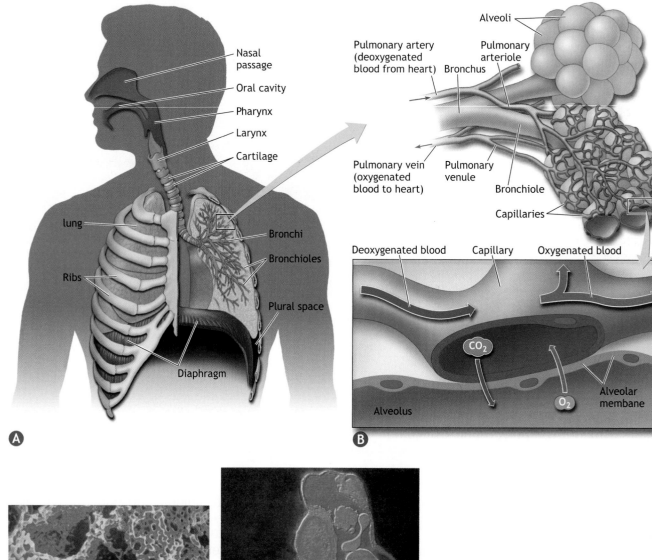

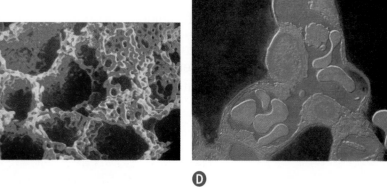

Figure 12.1 **A.** Major pulmonary structures within the thoracic cavity. **B.** General view of the ventilatory system showing the respiratory passages, alveoli, and gas exchange function in an alveolus. **C.** Section of lung tissue showing individual alveoli; the holes in the alveolar wall are the pores of Kohn. **D.** Pulmonary capillaries run within the walls of the alveoli. (Bottom images from West JB. Respiratory physiology—the essentials. 5th ed. Baltimore: Williams & Wilkins, 1995.)

filtered, and almost completely humidified as it travels through the **trachea**. Air conditioning continues as inspired air passes into two **bronchi**, the large first-generation of airways that serve as primary conduits into each of the lungs. The bronchi further subdivide into numerous **bronchioles** that conduct inspired air through a winding, narrow route until it eventually mixes with existing air in the alveolar ducts. Microscopic **alveoli**, the terminal branches of the respiratory tract, completely envelop these ducts.

The Lungs

The lungs provide the **gas exchange surface** that separates blood from the surrounding alveolar gaseous environment. Oxygen transfers from alveolar air into alveolar capillary blood; simultaneously, the blood's carbon dioxide moves into the alveolar chambers where it subsequently flows into ambient air. An average-sized adult's lungs weigh approximately 1 kg, and the volume varies between 4 and 6 L (the volume of air in a basketball). Lung tissue consists of about 10% solid tissue, with the remainder filled by air and blood. If spread out, lung tissue would cover an area of 50 to 100 m^2, an area 20 to 50 times larger than the body's external surface or about one half of a tennis court or an entire badminton court (FIG. 12.2).

The highly vascularized, moist surface of the lungs fits within the confines of the chest cavity, with numerous infoldings. The lung membranes fold over onto themselves to provide a considerable interface to aerate blood. At rest, a single red blood cell remains in a pulmonary capillary for only about 0.5 to 1.0 second as it traverses past two to three individual alveoli. During any 1 second of maximal exercise, no more than 1 pint of blood flows within the fine network of lung tissue blood vessels.

The Alveoli

The lungs contain more than 600 million **alveoli,** the final branching of the respiratory tree. These elastic, thin-walled membranous sacs (approximately 0.3 mm in diameter, composed of simple squamous epithelial cells) provide the vital surface for gas exchange between lung tissue and blood. Alveolar tissue receives the largest blood supply of any of the body's organs. Millions of short, thin-walled capillaries and alveoli lie side by side; air moves along one side and blood along the other. Gases diffuse across the extremely thin barrier of alveolar and capillary cells (~ 0.3 μm); the diffusion distance remains relatively constant throughout varying levels of exercise. For most individuals, the integrity of the thin pulmonary blood–gas barrier remains constant during sustained exercise. The surface remains as thin as possible (without compromising structural integrity) to facilitate rapid exchange of respiratory gases. In elite athletes, alveolar mechanical stress in near-maximal exercise (large ventilation and accompanying pulmonary blood flow) can impair the blood–gas barrier's permeability. Increased concentrations of red blood cells, total protein, and leukotriene B$_4$ (a potent chemotactic agent that initiates, coordinates, and amplifies the inflammatory response) in bronchoalveolar lavage fluid with maximal exercise reflect increased permeability in these athletes.[21,22,44]

Small **pores of Kohn** within each alveolus evenly disperse surfactant (see p. 264) over the respiratory membranes to reduce surface tension for easier alveolar inflation. The pores also provide for gas interchange between adjacent alveoli. Mixing in this manner sustains the indirect ventilation of alveoli damaged or blocked from emphysema, the chronic obstructive lung disease (see Chapter 32).

Each minute at rest, approximately 250 mL of oxygen leaves the alveoli and enters the blood, and 200 mL of carbon dioxide diffuses in the opposite direction. When endurance athletes exercise intensely, nearly 25 times this quantity of oxygen readily transfers across the alveolar–capillary membrane. Pulmonary ventilation primarily maintains a constant and favorable oxygen and carbon dioxide concentration in the alveolar chambers during rest and exercise. Adequate ventilation ensures complete gaseous exchange before the blood leaves the lungs for transport throughout the body.

MECHANICS OF VENTILATION

FIGURE 12.3 illustrates the physical principle that underlies breathing dynamics. Note the two lung-shaped balloons suspended in a jar with its glass bottom replaced by a thin rubber membrane. Pulling the membrane down increases jar volume. This reduces air pressure within the jar compared with ambient air outside the jar. This imbalance causes air to rush in and inflate the balloons. Conversely, as the elastic membrane recoils, pressure within the jar temporarily increases and air rushes out. Increasing the depth and rate of descent and ascent of the rubber membrane exchanges a considerable air volume within the balloons in a given time; this essentially illustrates how ambient air and alveolar air exchange within the lungs.

FIGURE 12.4 illustrates the ventilatory system subdivided into two parts: (1) **conducting zones** (zones 1–16) that includes the trachea and terminal bronchioles and

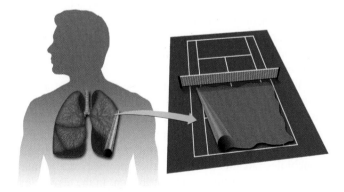

Figure 12.2 The lungs provide an exceptionally large surface for gas exchange.

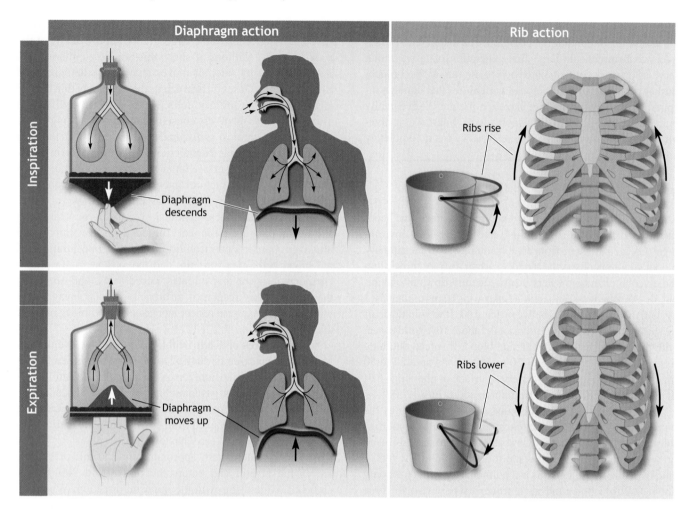

Figure 12.3 Mechanics of breathing. During *inspiration,* the chest cavity increases in size because the ribs raise and the diaphragm descends, causing air to flow into the lungs. Inhalation increases in the anterior–posterior (A-P) and vertical diameters of the rib cage. Approximately 70% of lung expansion results from A-P enlargement and 30% from diaphragmatic descent. In addition to diaphragmatic action, the external intercostal muscles become active and the internal intercostal muscles relax during inhalation. During *exhalation,* the ribs swing down and the diaphragm returns to a relaxed position. This reduces thoracic cavity volume and air rushes out. The movement of the jar's rubber bottom causes air to enter and exit the two balloons, simulating the action of the diaphragm. The movement of the bucket handle simulates rib action. The diaphragm, external intercostals, sternocleidomastoids, scapular elevators, anterior serrati scleni, and spinal erector muscles compose the inspiratory muscles that elevate and enlarge the thorax; muscles of expiration (rectus abdominis, internal intercostals, posterior inferior serrati muscles) depress the thorax and reduce its size.

(2) **transitional** and **respiratory zones** (zones 17–23) that comprise bronchioles, alveolar ducts, and alveoli. The structures of the conducting zone contain no alveoli, so the term *anatomic dead space* describes this area (see p. 269). The respiratory zone represents the site of gas exchange. It occupies about 2.5 to 3.0 L and constitutes the largest portion of the total lung volume. Air moving into the lungs literally flows down the trachea to the terminal bronchi, much like water flowing through a hose. As air reaches the smaller air passages in the transitional zone, the tremendous increase in surface area slows airflow into the alveoli.

The two ventilatory zones serve functions more diverse than the simple conduction and exchange of gases between blood and alveoli. Conducting-zone functions include air transport, humidification, warming, particle filtration,

vocalization, and immunoglobulin secretion. Respiratory zone functions encompass surfactant production (in the alveolar endothelium), molecule activation and inactivation (in the capillary endothelium), blood clotting regulation, and endocrine function.

FIGURE 12.5 depicts the relationship between airway generation (forward velocity) and total cross-sectional area of the conducting passages of various lung segments. Airway cross-section increases considerably (and velocity slows) as air moves through the conducting zone to the terminal bronchioles. At this stage, diffusion provides the primary means for gas movement and distribution. In the alveoli, gas pressures rapidly equilibrate on each side of the alveolar–capillary membrane. **Fick's law** governs gas diffusion through the alveolar membrane. This law states that a gas

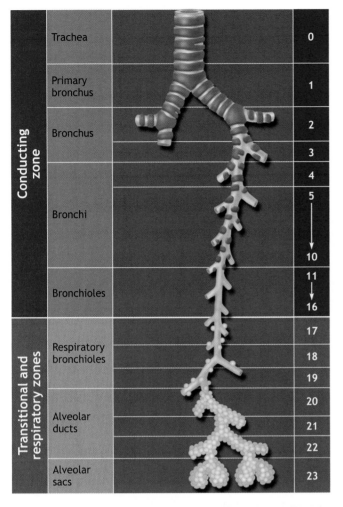

Figure 12.4 Separation of human lung tissue into a series of discrete *conduction zones* (zones 1 through 16) and *transitional* and *respiratory zones* (zones 17 through 23).

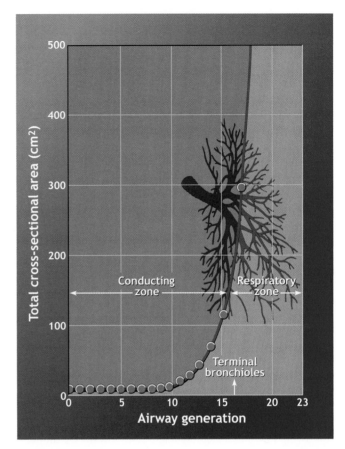

Figure 12.5 Airflow in the lungs in relation to the total cross-sectional tissue area. Forward airflow velocity during inspiration decreases considerably because of the large increase in tissue cross-sectional area beginning in the region of the terminal bronchioles. (Modified from West JB. Respiratory physiology—the essentials. 5th ed. Baltimore: Williams & Wilkins, 1995.)

diffuses through a sheet of tissue at a rate (1) directly proportional to the tissue area, a diffusion constant, and the pressure differential of the gas on each side of the membrane and (2) inversely proportional to the tissue's thickness. The diffusion constant (D) relates directly to gas solubility (S) and inversely to the square root of the molecular weight (MW) of the gas. On a per-molecule basis, carbon dioxide (MW = 44) diffuses about 20 times faster through thin membranous tissues than oxygen (MW = 32) because of carbon dioxide's higher solubility despite the relatively similar MWs of the two gases.

The lungs do not merely remain suspended in the chest cavity like the balloons in Figure 12.3. Instead, the pressure differential between the air in the lungs and the lung–chest wall interface causes them to adhere to the chest wall and literally follow its every movement. Thus, any change in thoracic cavity volume correspondingly alters lung volume. The lungs depend on accessory means to alter their volume because they contain no skeletal muscles. The action of a highly versatile, **multimuscle respiratory pump system** alters lung volume during inspiration and expiration.

Inspiration

The **diaphragm**, a large, dome-shaped sheet of striated, musculofibrous tissue, serves the same purpose as the jar's rubber membrane depicted in Figure 12.3. This primary ventilatory muscle creates an airtight separation between the abdominal and thoracic cavities. The diaphragm contains a series of openings through which the esophagus, blood vessels, and nerves pass. This separating membrane possesses high oxidative potential and the greatest capacity of all the respiratory muscles for shortening and volume displacement.[13,32] During **inspiration**, the diaphragm muscle contracts, flattens, and moves downward toward the abdominal cavity by as much as 10 cm. Elongation and enlargement of the chest cavity expands the air in the lungs, causing its **intrapulmonic pressure** to decrease to slightly below atmospheric pressure. The lungs inflate as air literally becomes sucked in through the nose and mouth. The degree of filling depends on the magnitude of inspiratory movements. Maximal activation of the inspiratory muscles of healthy individuals produces pressures that range between 80 and 140 mm Hg. Inspiration ends when thoracic cavity expansion ceases. This causes equality between intrapulmonic pressure and ambient atmospheric pressure.

During exercise, the highly efficient movements of the diaphragm, rib cage (ribs and sternum), and abdominal muscles synchronize to contribute to inspiration and expiration.[2,24] During inspiration, the **scaleni** and **external intercostal** muscles between the ribs contract, causing the ribs to rotate and lift up and away from the body. This action corresponds somewhat to the movement of the handle lifted up and away from the side of the bucket (see Fig. 12.3, *upper right*). Inspiratory action increases during exercise when the diaphragm descends, the ribs swing upward, and the sternum thrusts outward to increase the lateral and anterior–posterior diameter of the thorax. Athletes often bend forward from the waist to facilitate breathing following exhausting exercise. This serves two purposes: (1) promotes blood flow back to the heart and (2) minimizes antagonistic effects of gravity on the usual upward direction of inspiratory movements.

Expiration

Expiration during rest and light exercise represents a passive process of air movement out of the lungs. It results from two factors: (1) natural recoil of the stretched lung tissue and (2) relaxation of the inspiratory muscles. The sternum and ribs swing down and the diaphragm rises toward the thoracic cavity. These movements decrease chest cavity volume and compress alveolar gas so air moves from the respiratory tract to the atmosphere. Expiration ends when the compressive force of the expiratory musculature ceases and intrapulmonic pressure decreases to atmospheric pressure. During strenuous exercise, **internal intercostal** and **abdominal muscles** act powerfully on the ribs and abdominal cavity to reduce thoracic dimensions.[14] This makes exhalation rapid and more extensive.

No major differences exist in ventilatory mechanics between men and women of different ages. At rest in the supine position, most persons breathe diaphragmatically ("abdominal breathers"), whereas in the upright position rib and sternum actions become more apparent. Rib cage movement dictates the rapid alterations in thoracic volume in strenuous exercise. Distinct biochemical differences among muscles that compose the respiratory pump provide the evidence that the rib musculature acts more rapidly than the diaphragm and abdominal muscles.[33] The position of the head and back naturally adopted by distance runners—forward lean from the waist, neck flexed, and head extended forward with mandible parallel to the ground— favors pulmonary ventilation during intense exercise.

Surfactant

Pressures vary continually within the alveolar and pleural spaces throughout the ventilatory cycle. Resistance to normal expansion of the lung cavity and alveoli progressively increases during inspiration from the effect of **surface tension**, primarily in the alveoli. Surface tension relates to a resisting force created at the surface of a liquid in contact with a gas, structure, or another liquid. The tension or force created causes the liquid to assume a shape that presents the smallest surface area to the surrounding medium. The greater the surface tension surrounding a spherical object such as an alveolus, the greater the force required to overcome the pressure within the sphere and cause it to enlarge or inflate. **Surfactant** (a contraction of "surface active agent") consists of a lipoprotein mixture of phospholipids, proteins, and calcium ions produced by alveolar epithelial cells. It mixes with the fluid that encircles the alveolar chambers. Its action interrupts the surrounding water layer, reducing the alveolar membrane's surface tension to increase overall lung compliance. This effect reduces the energy required for alveolar inflation and deflation.

LUNG VOLUMES AND CAPACITIES

FIGURE 12.6 illustrates various lung volume measurements (including average values for men and women) that affect the ability to increase breathing depth. To obtain these measurements, the subject rebreathes through a water-sealed, volume-displacement recording spirometer similar to the one described in Chapter 8 (Fig. 8.2) for measuring oxygen consumption by the closed-circuit method. As with many anatomic and physiologic measures, lung volumes vary with age, gender, and body size and composition, but particularly with stature. Common practice evaluates lung volumes in relation to established standards that consider these factors.

Static Lung Volumes

The spirometer bell falls and rises during inhalation and exhalation to provide a record of ventilatory volume and breathing rate. **Tidal volume** (**TV**) describes air volume moved during either the inspiratory or expiratory phase of each breathing cycle (first portion of the record). Under resting conditions, TV usually ranges between 0.4 and 1.0 L of air per breath.

After recording several representative tracings for TV, the subject inspires as deeply as possible following a normal inspiration. The additional 2.5- to 3.5-L volume above inspired tidal air represents the reserve ability for inhalation, referred to as the **inspiratory reserve volume** (**IRV**). Following IRV measurement, the subject reestablishes the normal breathing pattern. After a normal exhalation, the subject continues to exhale and forces as much air as possible from the lungs. This additional volume represents **expiratory reserve volume** (**ERV**), which ranges between 1.0 and 1.5 L for an average-sized man. During exercise, encroachment on IRV and ERV, particularly IRV, considerably increases TV.

The total volume of air voluntarily moved in one breath, from full inspiration to maximum expiration, represents the vital capacity (VC), or, more precisely, **forced vital capacity** (**FVC**). FVC includes TV plus IRV and ERV. FVC usually ranges between 4 and 5 L in healthy young men and between 3 and 4 L in young women. Values of 6 to 7 L are not

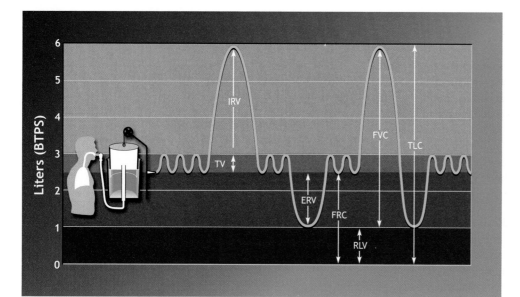

Lung volume/capacity	Definition	Average values (mL) Men	Women
Tidal Volume (TV)	Volume inspired or expired per breath	600	500
Inspiratory Reserve Volume (IRV)	Maximum inspiration at end of tidal inspiration	3000	1900
Expiratory Reserve Volume (ERV)	Maxium expiration at end of tidal expiration	1200	800
Total Lung Capacity (TLC)	Volume in lungs after maximum inspiration	6000	4200
Residual Lung Volume (RLV)	Volume in lungs after maximum expiration	1200	1000
Forced Vital Capacity (FVC)	Maximum volume expired after maximum inspiration	4800	3200
Inspiratory Capacity (IC)	Maximum volume inspired following tidal expiration	3600	2400
Functional Residual Capacity (FRC)	Volume in lungs after tidal expiration	2400	1800

Equation to predict RLV in normal-weight and overweight men and women*

	R	SEE
Normal-weight men and women		
RLV = 0.0275 AGE + 0.0189 HT - 2.6139	0.70	0.405
Overweight men and women		
RLV = 0.0277 AGE + 0.0048 WT + 0.0138 HT - 2.3967	0.65	0.404

R, multiple correlation coefficient; Age (y); HT, height (cm); WT, weight (kg); SEE, standard error or estimate.
*From Miller WC, et al. Derivation of prediction equations for RV in overweight men and women. Med Sci Sports Exerc 1998;30:322.

Figure 12.6 Static measurements of lung volumes.

uncommon for tall individuals, and unusually large FVC values have been reported for a professional football player (7.6 L) and an Olympic gold medalist in cross-country skiing (8.1 L).[3,45] These athletes' large lung volumes generally reflect genetic influences and body size characteristics because exercise training does not appreciably change static lung volumes.

Residual Lung Volume

The **residual lung volume** (**RLV**) represents the air volume remaining in the lungs after exhaling as deeply as possible This volume averages between 0.8 and 1.2 L for college-aged, healthy women and between 0.9 and 1.4 L for men. RLV for apparently healthy professional football players ranges between 0.96 and 2.46 L.[43] RLV increases with age, whereas IRV and ERV decrease proportionally. A decline in the elasticity of lung tissue components with aging probably decreases breathing reserve and concomitantly increases residual lung volume. Alterations in pulmonary function may not entirely reflect an aging phenomenon because regular aerobic training diminishes the typical age-related decline in static and dynamic lung functions.[16] *The RLV allows an uninterrupted exchange of gas between the blood and alveoli to prevent fluctuations in blood gases during phases of the breathing cycle including deep breathing.* RLV plus FVC constitutes **total lung capacity** (**TLC**).

Helium Dilution and Oxygen Dilution Methods. RLV cannot be measured directly from spirographic tracings. Instead, indirect determinations involve rebreathing a known gas volume containing either helium or pure oxygen. With the **helium dilution method**, the subject exhales normally. Air remaining in the lungs at this end-normal expiration position, termed the **functional residual capacity** (**FRC**), includes the known ERV and unknown RLV. The subject then rebreathes a known helium mixture for approximately 5 minutes. Absorbents remove expired carbon dioxide while an external oxygen supply continually replaces consumed oxygen to maintain a constant rebreathing volume within the spirometer. FRC is computed from the dilution of the original helium rebreathing mixture. FRC minus ERV equals RLV. FIGURE 12.7 illustrates the dilution principle to measure RLV by rebreathing a helium-containing gas mixture. The **oxygen dilution method** provides a more rapid RLV assessment than helium dilution. Oxygen dilution determines RLV from dilution of the lung's original nitrogen concentration, achieved by rapidly rebreathing a volume of approximately 5 L of 100% oxygen.

Effects of Previous Exercise. The RLV temporarily increases from an acute bout of either short-term or prolonged exercise. In one study, RLV increased during recovery from a maximal treadmill test by 21% after 5 minutes, 17% after 15 minutes, and 12% after 30 minutes.[5] RLV generally reverts to its original value within 24 hours. Possible factors that increase RLV with exercise include (1) closure of the small peripheral airways and (2) increase in thoracic blood volume. The added blood volume does not alter the lungs' mechanical properties, but it does displace air, thus preventing complete exhalation (reduced FVC).[8] Any temporary increase in RLV would affect subsequent computations of body volume by hydrostatic weighing for body composition studies (see Chapter 28). When RLV measurement is impractical, prediction equations based on the relation between RLV and age, stature, gender, and body mass provide reasonably accurate estimates (see inset table, Fig. 12.6).

Dynamic Lung Volumes

Adequacy of pulmonary ventilation depends how well an individual sustains high airflow levels rather than air movement in a single breath. Dynamic ventilation depends on two factors: (1) maximum "stroke volume" of the lungs (FVC) and (2) speed of moving a volume of air (breathing rate). In turn, airflow velocity depends on the resistance of the respiratory passages to the smooth flow of air and the "stiffness" imposed by the mechanical properties of the chest and lung tissue to a change in shape during breathing, termed **lung compliance**. Patients with lung disease rarely experience symptoms of distress until a large part of their ventilatory capacity decreases. Individuals with mild airway obstruction successfully engage in competitive distance running.[28]

FEV-to-FVC Ratio

Some individuals with severe lung disease achieve near-normal FVC values if measured with no time limit for this maneuver. For this reason, clinicians prefer a "dynamic" measurement of lung function such as the **forced expiratory volume** (**FEV**), usually measured over 1 second (**FEV$_{1.0}$**). FEV$_{1.0}$ divided by the FVC (**FEV$_{1.0}$ ÷ FVC**) indicates pulmonary airflow capacity. It reflects pulmonary expiratory power and overall resistance to air movement upstream in the lungs. Healthy individuals normally expel about 85% of the vital capacity in 1 second. Severe obstructive lung disease (emphysema or bronchial asthma)—with accompanying reduced airway caliber and loss of elastic recoil of lung tissue—considerably reduces FEV$_{1.0}$/FVC, often to values less than 40% of the vital capacity.[27,40] The demarcation point for airway obstruction during dynamic spirometry represents an FEV$_{1.0}$/FVC of 70% or less. FIGURE 12.8 presents pulmonary function test results for FEV$_{1.0}$ and FVC in individuals with normal lung function and those with obstructive and restrictive lung diseases. Clinicians also compute other values from portions of the curve generated in the forced spirometry maneuver (e.g., mid-50% of the expiratory curve or instantaneous flows at 25, 50, or 75% FVC) to assess airflow dynamics in the small airways of the pulmonary tract.[42]

Maximum Voluntary Ventilation

The **maximum voluntary ventilation** (**MVV**) evaluates ventilatory capacity with rapid and deep breathing for 15 seconds. The 15-second volume, extrapolated to the volume if the subject continued for 1 minute, represents MVV and typically ranges between 35 and 40 times the FEV$_{1.0}$.[43] MVV also averages 25% higher than ventilation during maximal exercise because exercise does not maximally stress how a healthy person breathes. For healthy, college-aged men, MVV ranges between 140 and 180 L · min^{-1}, with values for women ranging between 80 and 120 L · min^{-1}. MVV in male members of the United States Nordic Ski Team averaged 192 L · min^{-1}; the individual high was 239 L · min^{-1}.[17] Conversely, patients with obstructive lung disease achieve only about 40% of the MVV considered normal for their age and body size.

Specific exercise training of the ventilatory muscles improves their strength and endurance and increases both inspiratory muscle function and MVV.[1,35,40] Ventilatory training in patients with chronic pulmonary disease enhances exercise capacity and reduces physiologic strain.[9,37] Progressive

Before equilibration

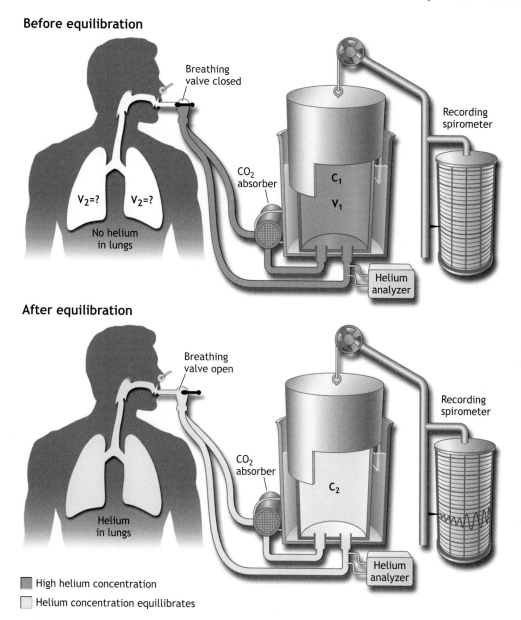

After equilibration

■ High helium concentration

□ Helium concentration equillibrates

Figure 12.7 Application of the dilution principle to assess residual lung volume. The subject exhales to the unknown functional residual capacity or residual lung volume and then breathes from a known volume and concentration of a gas such as oxygen or helium. In this example, a small concentration of helium represents the dilution gas. After a short period of deep, rapid breathing, the unknown, initially helium-free volume in the subject's lungs mixes with the known concentration of helium in the known volume the subject rebreathes. Equilibrium occurs between the gases in the spirometer and the gases in the subject's lung volume. During rebreathing, oxygen is continually added to the spirometer to replace that consumed by the subject. An absorbent continually removes carbon dioxide from the system. Residual lung volume computes from the concentration–volume relationship, in which initial helium volume (V_1) × initial helium concentration (C_1) = final gas volume (V_2) × final helium concentration (C_2). The residual lung volume (V_2) is determined from the relationship $V_1 (C_1 - C_2) \div C_2$. The final gas volume is corrected to body temperature and pressure saturated (BTPS; see Appendix D, available on the Student CD or online at http://connection.lww.com/mkk6e).

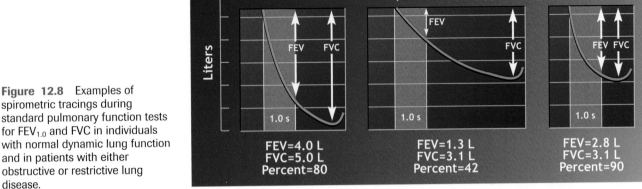

Figure 12.8 Examples of spirometric tracings during standard pulmonary function tests for $FEV_{1.0}$ and FVC in individuals with normal dynamic lung function and in patients with either obstructive or restrictive lung disease.

desensitization to the feeling of breathlessness and greater self-control of respiratory symptoms represent important benefits of ventilatory muscle training and regular exercise to patients with chronic obstructive lung disease.

INTEGRATIVE QUESTION

How does regular resistance and aerobic exercise training affect the typical aging decline in measures of lung function?

Exercise Implications of Gender Differences in Static and Dynamic Lung Function Measures

Adult women consistently have smaller static and dynamic lung function measures than men even after accounting for differences in stature. This disparity produces expiratory flow limitations and greater use of ventilatory reserve during maximal exercise. This is particularly true for highly trained women compared to trained men and less-fit women.[30] A relatively smaller lung volume plus a high expiratory flow rate requirement in trained women during intense exercise places considerable demand on the maximum flow–volume envelope of the airways (i.e., mechanical constraints of TV and pulmonary minute ventilation). This adversely affects how highly fit women maintain alveolar-to-arterial oxygen exchange, which could compromise arterial oxygen saturation.[19]

LUNG FUNCTION, AEROBIC FITNESS, AND EXERCISE PERFORMANCE

Dynamic lung function tests indicate the severity of obstructive and restrictive lung diseases, yet generally provide little information about aerobic fitness or exercise performance when values fall within the normal range. For example, no difference emerges when comparing the average FVC of prepubescent and Olympic wrestlers, middle-distance athletes, and untrained, healthy subjects.[34,36] Professional football players averaged only 94% of their predicted FVC; the defensive backs achieved only 83% of predicted "normal" values for body size (see "In a Practical Sense," p. 270). Somewhat surprisingly,

similar values emerged for static and dynamic lung function of accomplished marathon runners and other endurance-trained athletes compared with untrained controls of similar body size.[16,29]

Swimming and diving stimulate development of larger-than-normal static lung volumes. These sports strengthen the inspiratory muscles that work against additional resistance of the mass of water that compresses the thorax. Enhanced ventilatory muscle strength and power explain the relatively large FVC of skin divers and competitive swimmers.[4,6,10,11]

TABLE 12.1 ■ ANTHROPOMETRIC DATA, PULMONARY FUNCTION, AND RESTING MINUTE VENTILATION IN 20 MARATHON RUNNERS AND HEALTHY CONTROLS

MEASURE	RUNNERS	CONTROLS	DIFFERENCE[a]
ANTHROPOMETRIC			
Age, y	27.8	27.4	0.4
Stature, cm	175.8	176.7	0.9
Surface area, m^2	1.82	1.89	0.07
PULMONARY FUNCTION			
FVC, L	5.13	5.34	0.21
TLC, L	6.91	7.13	0.22
$FEV_{1.0}$, L	4.32	4.47	0.15
$FEV_{1.0}$ / FVC, %	84.3	83.8	0.5
MVV, $L \cdot min^{-1}$	179.8	176.0	3.8
RESTING VENTILATION			
$\dot{V}_E$, $L \cdot min^{-1}$	11.9	11.9	0.9
Breathing rate, breaths $\cdot min^{-1}$	10.9	11.1	0.2
Tidal volume, L	1.16	1.06	0.10

From Mahler DA, et al. Ventilatory responses at rest and during exercise in marathon runners. J Appl Physiol 1982;52:388.
[a] All differences not statistically significant.

Little relationship exists among diverse lung volumes and capacities and various track performances. This includes distance running for a large group of teenage boys and girls, even after adjusting for differences in body size.[12] For marathon runners versus sedentary subjects of similar body size, no difference existed for lung function values (TABLE 12.1).[23,28] For healthy, untrained individuals, no relationship exists between maximal oxygen consumption and FVC or MVV (adjusted for body size). Fatigue from strenuous exercise frequently relates to feeling "out of breath," or "winded," yet normal capacity for pulmonary ventilation for most individuals does not limit maximal aerobic exercise performance. The larger-than-normal lung volumes and breathing capacities of some athletes probably reflect genetic endowment. Specific exercise training can increase pulmonary function by strengthening the respiratory muscles.

PULMONARY VENTILATION

One can view pulmonary ventilation from two perspectives: (1) volume of air moved into or out of the total respiratory tract each minute and (2) air volume that ventilates only the alveolar chambers each minute.

Minute Ventilation

The normal breathing rate during quiet breathing at rest in a thermoneutral environment averages 12 breaths per minute and TV averages 0.5 L of air per breath. Consequently, the volume of air breathed each minute, referred to as **minute ventilation**, equals 6 L.

$$\text{Minute ventilation } (\dot{V}_E) = \text{Breathing rate} \times \text{Tidal Volume}$$
$$= 12 \times 0.5 \text{ L}$$
$$= 6 \text{ L} \cdot \text{min}^{-1}$$

An increase in either the rate or depth of breathing or both increases minute ventilation. During strenuous exercise, healthy young adults readily increase breathing rate to 35 to 45 breaths per minute. Some elite endurance athletes breathe as rapidly as 60 to 70 times each minute during maximal exercise. TVs of 2.0 L and higher commonly occur during exercise. Such increases in breathing rate and TV increase exercise minute ventilation to 100 L or more (about 17 to 20 times the resting value). In male endurance athletes, ventilation may increase to 160 L · min^{-1} during maximal exercise. Minute ventilation volumes of 200 L,

with a high volume of 208 L in a professional football player, have been observed during maximal bicycle exercise.[45] *Despite such large minute ventilations, TVs for trained and untrained individuals rarely exceed 60% of vital capacity.*

TYPICAL VALUES FOR PULMONARY VENTILATION DURING REST AND MODERATE AND INTENSE EXERCISE

CONDITION	BREATHING RATE (BREATHS · MIN^{-1})	TIDAL VOLUME (L · BREATH^{-1})	PULMONARY VENTILATION (L · MIN^{-1})
Rest	12	0.5	6
Moderate exercise	30	2.5	75
Intense exercise	50	3.0	150

Alveolar Ventilation

A portion of the air in each breath does not enter the alveoli and participate in gaseous exchange with the blood. The term **anatomic dead space** describes this air that fills the nose, mouth, trachea, and other nondiffusible conducting portions of the respiratory tract. The anatomic dead space generally ranges between 150 and 200 mL (about 30% of the resting TV) in healthy individuals. The composition of dead-space air remains almost identical to ambient air except for its full saturation with water vapor.

The dead-space volume permits about 350 mL of the 500 mL of inspired TV at rest to enter into and mix with existing alveolar air. This does not mean that only 350 mL of air enters and leaves the alveoli with each breath. Instead, if TV equals 500 mL, then 500 mL of air enters the alveoli but only 350 mL of this is fresh air. This represents about one seventh of total alveolar air. Such relatively small and seemingly inefficient **alveolar ventilation**—that portion of inspired air reaching the alveoli and participating in gas exchange—prevents drastic changes in alveolar air composition to ensure consistency in arterial blood gases throughout the breathing cycle.

TABLE 12.2 indicates that minute ventilation does not always reflect alveolar ventilation. The first example of shallow

TABLE 12.2 ■ RELATIONSHIPS AMONG TIDAL VOLUME, BREATHING RATE, AND BOTH TOTAL AND ALVEOLAR MINUTE VENTILATION

CONDITION	TIDAL VOLUME (mL)	×	BREATHING RATE (BREATHS · MIN^{-1})	=	TOTAL MINUTE VENTILATION (mL · MIN^{-1})	−	DEAD SPACE MINUTE VENTILATION (mL · MIN^{-1})	=	ALVEOLAR MINUTE VENTILATION (mL · MIN^{-1})
Shallow breathing	150		40		6000		(150 mL × 40)		0
Normal breathing	500		12		6000		(150 mL × 12)		4200
Deep breathing	1000		6		6000		(150 mL × 6)		5100

IN A PRACTICAL SENSE

PREDICTING PULMONARY FUNCTION VARIABLES IN MEN AND WOMEN

■ Pulmonary function variables do not directly relate to measures of physical fitness in healthy individuals. Instead, their measurement often forms part of a standard medical/health/fitness examination, particularly for individuals at risk for limited pulmonary function (e.g., chronic cigarette smokers, asthmatics). Measurement of pulmonary dimensions and lung functions with a water-filled spirometer (see figure) or electronic spirometer provides the framework for discussions of pulmonary dynamics during rest and exercise. Proper evaluation of measured values for pulmonary function requires comparison to "expected" values (norms) from the clinical literature.

EQUATIONS
Pulmonary function scores associate closely with stature (ST) and age (A), enabling these two variables to predict the expected average (normal) lung function value for an individual.

Data
Man: A, 22 y; ST, 182.9 cm (72 in)

Woman: A, 22 y; ST, 165.1 cm (65 in)

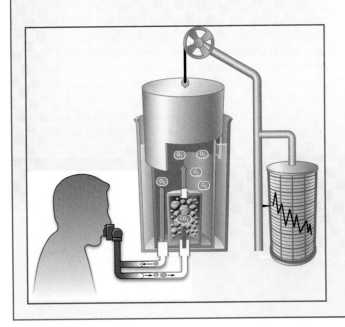

EXAMPLES
Woman
1. Forced vital capacity (FVC)
$$FVC\ (L) = (0.0414 \times ST\ [cm]) - (0.0232 \times A\ [y]) - 2.20$$
$$= 6.835 - 0.5104 - 2.20$$
$$= 4.12\ L$$

2. Forced expiratory volume in 1 s ($FEV_{1.0}$)
$$FEV_{1.0}\ (L) = (0.0268 \times ST\ [cm]) - 0.0251 \times A\ [y]) - 0.38$$
$$= 4.425 - 0.5522 - 0.38$$
$$= 3.49\ L$$

3. Percentage forced vital capacity in 1 s ($FEV_{1.0}/FVC$):
$$FEV_{1.0}/FVC\ (\%) = (-0.2145 \times ST\ [cm]) - 0.1523 \times A\ [y]) 124.5$$
$$= -35.41 - 3.35 \times 124.5$$
$$= 85.7\%$$

4. Maximum voluntary ventilation (MVV)
$$MVV\ (L \cdot min^{-1}) = 40 \times FEV_{1.0}$$
$$= 40 \times 3.49\ (from\ \#2)$$
$$= 139.6\ L \cdot min^{-1}$$

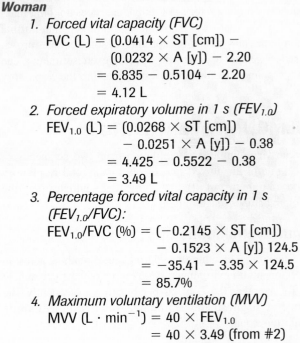

Man
1. Forced vital capacity (FVC)
$$FVC\ (L) = (0.0774 \times ST\ [cm] - (0.0212 \times A\ [y] - 7.75)$$
$$= 14.156 - 0.4664 - 7.75$$
$$= 5.49\ L$$

2. Forced expiratory volume in 1 s ($FEV_{1.0}$)
$$FEV_{1.0}\ (L) = (0.0566 \times ST\ [cm]) - 0.0233 \times A\ [y]) - 0.491$$
$$= 10.35 - 0.5126 - 4.91$$
$$= 4.93\ L$$

3. Percentage forced vital capacity in 1 s ($FEV_{1.0}/FVC$)
$$FEV_{1.0}/FVC\ (\%) = (-0.1314 \times ST\ [cm]) - 0.1490 \times A\ [y]) \times 110.2$$
$$= -24.03 - 3.35 \times 110.2$$
$$= 82.8\%$$

4. Maximum voluntary ventilation (MVV)
$$MVV\ (L \cdot min^{-1}) = 40 \times FEV_{1.0}$$
$$= 40 \times 4.93\ L\ (from\ \#2)$$
$$= 197.2\ L \cdot min^{-1}$$

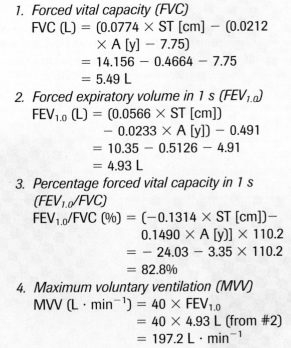

continued on page 271

Continued

EQUATIONS TO PREDICT PULMONARY FUNCTION VARIABLES

Variable	Men <25 Y	Men >25 Y	Female <25 Y	Female >25 Y
Forced vital capacity (FVC): Maximum volume expired following a maximum inspiration	FVC (L) = (0.0774 × ST) − (0.0212 × A) − 7.75	FVC (L) = (0.065 × ST) + (0.029 × A) − 5.459	FVC (L) = (0.0414 × ST) − (0.0232 × A) − 2.20	FVC (L) = (0.037 × ST) + (0.092 × A) − 3.469
Forced expiratory volume in 1 s (FEV$_{1.0}$): Volume forcibly expired in 1 s following a maximum inspiration	FEV$_{1.0}$(L) = (0.0566 × ST) − 0.0233 × A) − 0.491	FEV$_{1.0}$(L) = (0.052 × ST) + (0.027 × A) − 4.203	FEV$_{1.0}$(L) = (0.0268 × ST) − (0.0251 × A) − 0.38	FEV$_{1.0}$ (L) = (0.027 × ST) − (0.021 × A) − 0.794
FEV$_{1.0}$/FVC: Percentage of forced vital capacity expired in 1 s	FEV$_{1.0}$/FVC, (%) = (−0.1314 × ST) − (0.1490 × A) + 110.2	FEV$_{1.0}$/FVC (%) = 103.64 − (0.87 × ST) − (0.14 × A)	FEV$_{1.0}$/FVC (%) = (−0.2145 × ST) − (0.1523 × A) + 124.5	FEV$_{1.0}$/FVC (%) = 107.38 − (0.111 × ST) − (0.109 × A)
Maximum voluntary ventilation (MMV): Maximum amount of air forcibly breathed in 1 min	MMV (L · min^{-1}) = 40 × FEV$_{1.0}$	MMV (L · min^{-1}) = (1.15 × H) − (1.27 × A) + 14	MMV (L · min^{-1}) = 40 × FEV	MMV (L · min^{-1}) = (0.55 × ST) − (0.72 × A) + 50

ST, stature (height) in centimeters; A, age in years
Comroe JH, et al. The lung. Chicago: Year Book Medical Publishers, 1962.
Miller A. Pulmonary function tests in clinical and occupational disease. Philadelphia: Grune & Stratton, 1986.
Taylor AE, et al. Clinical respiratory physiology. Philadelphia: WB Saunders, 1989.
Wasserman K, et al. Principles of exercise testing. Baltimore: Lippincott Williams & Wilkins, 1999.

breathing shows that one can reduce TV to 150 mL, yet still maintain a 6-L minute ventilation by increasing breathing rate to 40 breaths per minute. The same 6-L minute volume results from decreasing breathing rate to 12 breaths per minute and increasing TV to 500 mL. In contrast, doubling TV and halving the breathing rate, as in the example of deep breathing, also produces a 6-L minute ventilation. Each of these ventilatory adjustments drastically affects alveolar ventilation. In the example of shallow breathing, dead-space air represents the *only* air volume moved without any alveolar ventilation. In the other examples, deeper breathing causes a larger portion of each breath to enter into and mix with alveolar air. Alveolar ventilation determines the gaseous concentrations at the alveolar–capillary membrane.

Dead Space Versus Tidal Volume

The preceding examples of alveolar ventilation represent oversimplifications because they assumed a constant dead space despite changes in TV. Actually, anatomic dead space increases as TV becomes larger; it often doubles during deep breathing from some stretching of the respiratory passages with a fuller inspiration. Importantly, any increase in dead space still represents proportionately less volume than the accompanying increase in TV. Consequently, deeper breathing provides more effective alveolar ventilation than a similar minute ventilation achieved through an increased breathing rate.

Ventilation–Perfusion Ratio

Adequate gas exchange between alveoli and blood requires effective matching of alveolar ventilation to the blood perfusing the pulmonary capillaries. Approximately 4.2 L of air normally ventilates the alveoli each minute at rest, and an average of 5.0 L of blood flows through the pulmonary capillaries. In this case, the ratio of alveolar ventilation to pulmonary blood flow, termed the **ventilation–perfusion ratio**, equals 0.84 (4.2 ÷ 5.0). This ratio means that alveolar ventilation of 0.84 L matches each liter of pulmonary blood flow. In light exercise, the ventilation–perfusion ratio remains approximately 0.8. In contrast, intense exercise produces a disproportionate increase in alveolar ventilation. In healthy individuals, the ventilation–perfusion ratio may exceed 5.0; in most instances, this response ensures adequate aeration of venous blood.

Physiologic Dead Space

Sometimes the alveoli may not function adequately in gas exchange because of two factors: (1) underperfusion of blood or (2) inadequate ventilation relative to the alveolar surface. The term **physiologic dead space** describes the portion of the alveolar volume with a ventilation–perfusion ratio that approaches zero. FIGURE 12.9 shows the negligible physiologic dead space in the healthy lung. In certain pathologic situations, physiologic dead space increases to

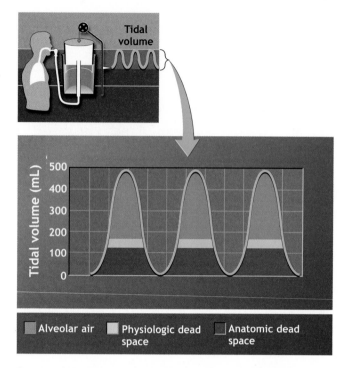

Figure 12.9 Distribution of tidal volume (TV) in a healthy subject at rest. TV includes about 350 mL of ambient air that mixes with alveolar air, 150 mL of ambient air that remains in the larger air passages (anatomic dead space), and a small portion of air distributed to either poorly ventilated or poorly perfused alveoli (physiologic dead space).

50% of the TV as with inadequate perfusion from hemorrhage or blockage of the pulmonary circulation by an embolism or inadequate ventilation in emphysema, asthma, and pulmonary fibrosis. An increased physiologic dead space from decreased functional alveolar surface in emphysema produces extreme ventilation even at low exercise intensities. Many patients cannot achieve maximal circulatory capacity from ventilatory muscle fatigue from excessive breathing. Adequate gas exchange becomes impossible when the dead space of the lung exceeds 60% of total lung volume.

Rate Versus Depth

Increasing the rate and depth of breathing increases alveolar ventilation in exercise. In moderate exercise, well-trained athletes maintain alveolar ventilation by increasing TV with only a small increase in breathing rate.[15] As breathing becomes deeper during exercise, alveolar ventilation increases from 70% of the total minute ventilation at rest to more than 85% of the exercise ventilation. FIGURE 12.10 shows that encroachment on the IRV, with a smaller decrease in the end-expiratory level, increases exercise TV. With more intense exercise, the increase in TV plateaus at approximately 60% of vital capacity; minute ventilation increases further through nonconscious increases in breathing rate. Each person develops a "style" of breathing in which breathing rate and TV blend to provide effective alveolar ventilation. Conscious manipulation of breathing usually disturbs the exquisitely

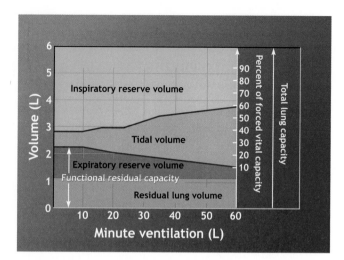

Figure 12.10 Tidal volume and subdivisions of pulmonary air during rest and exercise.

regulated physiologic adjustments to exercise. Attempts to modify breathing during running or other general physical activities offer no benefit to exercise performance. During rest and all levels of exercise, a healthy person should breathe in the manner that seems most natural.

INTEGRATIVE QUESTION

How can a person accelerate breathing rate at rest without disrupting normal alveolar ventilation?

VARIATIONS FROM NORMAL BREATHING PATTERNS

Breathing patterns during exercise generally progress in an effective and highly economical manner, yet some pulmonary responses can adversely affect exercise performance and/or physiologic balance.

Hyperventilation

Hyperventilation refers to an increase in pulmonary ventilation that exceeds the oxygen consumption and carbon dioxide elimination needs of metabolism. This "overbreathing" quickly lowers normal alveolar carbon dioxide concentration and causes excess carbon dioxide to leave bodily fluids via the expired air. An accompanying decrease in hydrogen ion concentration [H^+] increases plasma pH. Several seconds of hyperventilation generally produce lightheadedness; prolonged hyperventilation leads to unconsciousness from excessive carbon dioxide unloading.

Dyspnea

Dyspnea refers to an inordinate shortness of breath or subjective distress in breathing. The sense of breathing incapacity during exercise, particularly in novice exercisers, usually accompanies elevated arterial carbon dioxide and [H⁺]. Both conditions excite the inspiratory center to increase breathing rate and depth. Failure to adequately regulate arterial carbon dioxide and [H⁺] most likely relates to low aerobic fitness levels and poorly conditioned ventilatory musculature.

Valsalva Maneuver

The expiratory muscles, besides their normal role in pulmonary ventilation, provide for the ventilatory maneuvers of coughing and sneezing. They also contribute to stabilizing the abdominal and chest cavities during heavy lifting. In quiet breathing, intrapulmonic pressure decreases only about 3 mm Hg during inspiration and rises a similar amount above atmospheric pressure in exhalation (FIG. 12.11A). Closing the **glottis** (narrowest part of the larynx through which air passes into the trachea) following a full inspiration while maximally activating the expiratory muscles creates compressive forces that increase **intrathoracic pressure** more than 150 mm Hg above atmospheric pressure (Fig. 12.11B). Pressures increase to higher levels within the abdominal cavity during a maximal exhalation against a closed glottis.[18] Forced exhalation against a closed glottis, termed the **Valsalva maneuver**, occurs commonly in weight lifting and other activities that require a rapid, maximum application of force of short duration. The Valsalva stabilizes the abdominal and thoracic cavities to enhance muscle action.

Physiologic Consequences of the Valsalva Maneuver

A prolonged Valsalva maneuver produces an acute *drop* in blood pressure. Increased intrathoracic pressure during a Valsalva transmits through the thin walls of the veins that pass through the thoracic region. Because venous blood remains under relatively low pressure, thoracic veins collapse, which reduces blood flow to the heart. Reduced venous return sharply lowers the heart's stroke volume, triggering a fall in blood pressure below the resting level.[7,25] Performing a prolonged Valsalva maneuver during static, straining-type exercise dramatically reduces venous return and arterial blood pressure. These effects diminish the brain's blood supply, often producing dizziness, "spots before the eyes," or fainting. Once the glottis reopens and intrathoracic pressure normalizes, blood flow reestablishes with an "overshoot" in arterial blood pressure.[39,41]

Figure 12.11C illustrates four phases of the typical blood pressure response (heart beat by heart beat) during the Valsalva maneuver in a healthy subject. Aortic pulse pressure increases slightly as the Valsalva begins (phase I), probably from the mechanical effect of elevated intrathoracic pressure that expels blood from the left ventricle into the aorta. A biphasic response occurs within six heartbeats of Valsalva onset. This consists of a large reduction in aortic pulse pressure (phase IIa) followed by a relatively small gradual rise (phase IIb) and secondary decrease (phase III) during the continued Valsalva strain. When the maneuver ceases (release of strain), blood pressure rises rapidly and overshoots the resting value (phase IV).

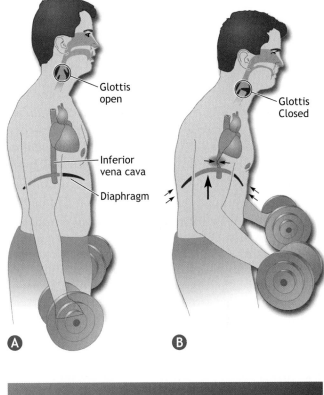

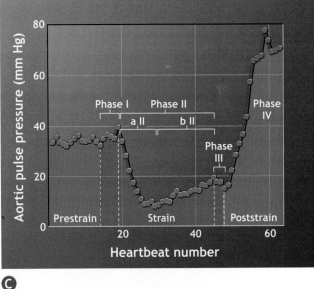

Figure 12.11 The Valsalva maneuver reduces the return of blood to the heart because increased intrathoracic pressure collapses the inferior vena cava that passes through the chest cavity. **A.** Normal breathing. **B.** Straining exercise with accompanying Valsalva maneuver. **C.** Typical normal response of aortic pulse pressure with a Valsalva maneuver during calibrated muscle strain. The figure illustrates 63 consecutive heartbeats (●). High-fidelity aortic pressure recordings were obtained at the aortic root level. Pulse pressure represents systolic pressure minus diastolic pressure. (Data from Hébert J-L, et al. Pulse pressure response to the strain of the Valsalva maneuver in humans with preserved systolic function. J Appl Physiol 1998;85:817.)

FOCUS On Research

PHYSIOLOGIC CONTROL OF PULMONARY VENTILATION

Dejours P. The regulation of breathing during muscular exercise in man. A neuro-humoral theory. In: Cunningham DJC, Lloyd BB, eds. The regulation of human respiration. Oxford, England: Blackwell, 1963.

▲ Early theories about pulmonary ventilation regulation during exercise centered singularly on arterial P_{CO_2}, arterial blood pH, or reflex stimulation originating from muscle receptors. Dejours believed that no factor by itself, but rather a multiplicity of interacting factors, regulated breathing during exercise. He hypothesized that exercise hyperpnea depended on humoral (chemical) and neurogenic stimuli that varied their contributions depending on the phase of exercise and recovery.

The figure presents Dejours' observations that the time course of pulmonary minute ventilation ($\dot{V}_E$) during the transitions from rest to exercise to recovery followed a consistent pattern. $\dot{V}_E$ increases within the same ventilatory cycle, coinciding with the start of exercise. Some 10 to 20 seconds later, ventilation volumes slowly increase to an eventual steady state. Minute ventilation declines abruptly when exercise stops, remains fairly constant for 20 to 30 seconds, and then decreases progressively to the resting value.

Dejours concluded that ventilatory dynamics in exercise combine rapid (fast component) and slow (slow component) responses that progress in defined stages during exercise and recovery. He proposed that different physiologic factors control the fast and slow components. Two factors contribute to the fast component:

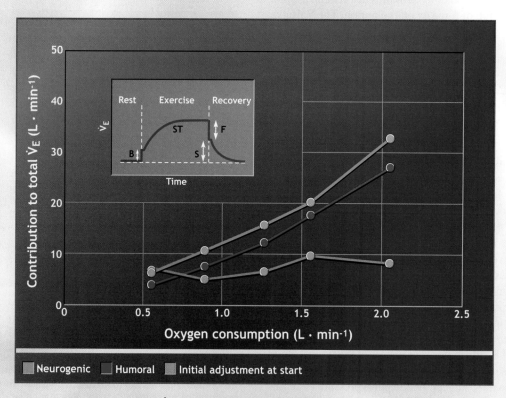

Pulmonary minute ventilation ($\dot{V}_E$) during mild exercise and recovery (inset graph). Portion *B* of inset represents the immediate, rapid increase when exercise begins; *ST* reflects the more gradual rise to a steady state; *F* indicates the quick fall when exercise stops; *S* represents the slower return of ventilation to the preexercise level. The main graph shows the contribution of these ventilatory response components to oxygen consumption. Neurogenic and humoral components both increase with the intensity of the preceding exercise; the fast component at the start of exercise increases with exercise intensity much less than the progressive increase in neurogenic and humoral controls.

continued on page 275

Continued

(1) cerebral input from afferent impulses from the brain's psychomotor area to the respiratory center in the medulla and (2) extrathoracic mechanoreceptor stimulation from "proprioceptors" in active body segments. Two mechanisms also modulate the slower component of the ventilatory response. The first, a reflex, originates from muscle chemoreceptors sensitive to progressive physiochemical changes within active muscle as exercise progresses. The second factor represents a humoral mechanism. Dejours' belief in humoral control developed from experiments that occluded leg blood flow. Restricting venous return during leg exercise caused $\dot{V}_E$ to decline below resting levels, thus demonstrating ventilatory dependence on blood-borne (humoral) chemicals produced in active tissues.

Dejours stressed the interrelationship between the fast and slow components in exercise ventilation. Reflex and cortical factors initiated the rapid rise in ventilation at exercise onset. Subsequently, humoral factors, and possibly progressive neurogenic output, modulated the slower rise in ventilation during the first minutes of exercise. The later steady-state response during exercise probably related to (1) increases in reflex drive through local physical and chemical changes at the peripheral mechanoreceptors and (2) positive interactions between neurogenic and humoral drives. Ventilation decreases precipitously when exercise stops and neurogenic input ceases. Ventilation then becomes regulated exclusively by humoral factors from the recovering musculature.

The studies of Dejours formed the basis for explaining pulmonary ventilation during exercise and recovery. Subsequent research (see Fig. 14.4) provides additional factors to explain exercise hyperpnea and provide a more comprehensive model for ventilatory control.

A Common Misconception. The Valsalva maneuver does not cause the relatively large increases in blood pressure during heavy resistance exercises. Recall from the preceding figure that a prolonged Valsalva dramatically reduces blood pressure. Confusion arises because a Valsalva maneuver of insufficient duration to lower blood pressure usually accompanies straining muscular efforts common during isometric and dynamic resistance exercise. These exercises (with or without Valsalva) greatly increase resistance to blood flow in active muscle with a resulting rise in systolic blood pressure.[20] For example, intramuscular fluid pressure increases linearly with all levels of isometric force to the maximum.[38] Increased peripheral vascular resistance increases the arterial blood pressure and workload of the heart throughout exercise. These responses pose potential danger to individuals with cardiovascular disease; they form the basis for advising cardiac patients to refrain from heavy resistance training. In contrast, performing rhythmic muscular activity, including moderate weight lifting, promotes a steadier blood flow and only modest increase in blood pressure and work of the heart. Chapter 15 more fully discusses the blood pressure response to different exercise modes.

INTEGRATIVE QUESTION

After completing a maximum-lift standing press, a person exclaims: "I feel slightly dizzy and see spots before my eyes." Provide a plausible physiologic explanation.

THE RESPIRATORY TRACT DURING COLD-WEATHER EXERCISE

Cold ambient air normally does not damage the respiratory passages. Even in extreme cold weather, the incoming air generally warms to 26.5 to 32.2°C by the time it reaches the bronchi. Nonetheless, values as low as 20°C can occur in the bronchi when breathing large volumes of cold, dry air.[31] Airway warming of inspired air greatly increases its capacity to hold moisture, which produces considerable water loss from the respiratory passages. In cold weather, the respiratory tract loses considerable water and heat, most notably during strenuous exercise with large ventilatory volumes. Fluid loss from the airways often contributes to overall dehydration, dry mouth, burning sensation in the throat, and generalized irritation of the respiratory passages. Wearing a scarf or cellulose mask-type "balaclava" that covers the nose and mouth traps the water in exhaled air and subsequently warms and moistens the next incoming breath of air. This effect reduces the symptoms of respiratory discomfort.

Postexercise Coughing

Exercise in cold weather can dry the throat and trigger coughing during the recovery period. The response becomes prevalent following exercise in cold weather when the respiratory tract loses considerable water. Postexercise coughing relates directly to the overall respiratory water loss (not respiratory heat loss) associated with the large ventilatory volumes breathed during exercise.

Summary

1. The lungs provide a large surface between the body's internal fluid environment and the gaseous external environment. During any 1 second of exercise, no more than 1 pint of blood flows in the pulmonary capillaries.
2. Normal regulation of pulmonary ventilation maintains a favorable concentration of alveolar oxygen and carbon dioxide to ensure adequate aeration of blood flowing through the lungs.

3. Pulmonary airflow depends on small pressure differentials between ambient air and air within the lungs. Muscle actions that alter thoracic cavity dimensions produce these pressure differences.

4. Lung volumes vary with age, gender, and body size (particularly stature) and should only be evaluated with established norms based on these factors.

5. The residual lung volume represents air remaining in the lungs following maximal exhalation. This air volume allows uninterrupted exchange of gas during all phases of the breathing cycle.

6. Forced expiratory volume and maximum voluntary ventilation dynamically measure the ability to sustain a high airflow level. These lung function measures serve as excellent screening tests to detect lung disease.

7. Measures of static and dynamic lung function within the normal range poorly predict aerobic fitness and exercise performance.

8. Breathing rate and tidal volume (TV) determine pulmonary minute ventilation. Minute ventilation averages $6 \, L \cdot min^{-1}$ at rest and can increase to $200 \, L \cdot min^{-1}$ during maximal exercise.

9. Alveolar ventilation reflects the portion of minute ventilation that enters the alveoli for gaseous exchange with the blood.

10. The ventilation–perfusion ratio reflects the association between alveolar minute ventilation and pulmonary blood flow. At rest, alveolar ventilation of 0.8 L matches each L of pulmonary blood flow. During intense exercise, alveolar ventilation increases disproportionately to increase the ventilation–perfusion ratio to 5.0.

11. TV increases during exercise by encroachment into inspiratory and expiratory reserve volumes. In intense exercise, TV plateaus at approximately 60% of the vital capacity; minute ventilation increases further through increases in breathing rate.

12. A healthy person should breathe in a manner that seems most natural during rest, exercise, and recovery.

13. Hyperventilation refers to increased pulmonary ventilation that exceeds gas exchange needs of metabolism. This "overbreathing" quickly lowers normal alveolar carbon dioxide concentration, causing excess carbon dioxide to leave body fluids via expired air.

14. A Valsalva maneuver describes a forced exhalation against a closed glottis. This action causes large pressure increases within the chest and abdominal cavities that compress the thoracic veins, thereby reducing venous return to the heart. This ultimately reduces arterial blood pressure.

15. The straining muscular effort that typically accompanies the Valsalva temporarily elevates blood pressure and adds to the heart's workload. Individuals with heart and vascular disease should refrain from heavy weight lifting and isometric muscle actions.

16. Breathing cold ambient air normally does not damage the respiratory passages.

References are available on the Student CD and online at http://connection.lww.com/mkk6e.

Gas Exchange and Transport

13

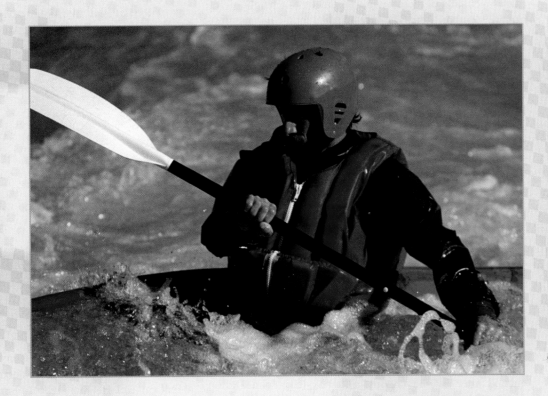

CHAPTER OBJECTIVES

- List the partial pressures of respired gases during rest and maximal exercise in the alveoli, arterial blood, active muscles, and mixed-venous blood

- Explain the impact of Henry's law on pulmonary gas exchange

- Quantify oxygen transport (1) in arterial plasma and (2) combined with hemoglobin under sea-level, ambient conditions

- Discuss the physiologic advantages of oxyhemoglobin's S-shaped dissociation curve

- Describe factors that produce the "Bohr effect" and outline its benefit in physical activity

- Explain the role of myoglobin during high-intensity, physical activity

- List and quantify three ways for carbon dioxide transport in blood

The body's supply of oxygen depends on its *concentration* and *pressure* in ambient air. Ambient air remains relatively constant in composition, containing 20.93% oxygen, 79.04% nitrogen (including small quantities of other inert gases that behave physiologically like nitrogen), 0.03% carbon dioxide, and usually small quantities of water vapor. The gas molecules move at relatively high speeds and exert a pressure against any surface they contact. At sea level, the pressure of air molecules raises a column of mercury in a barometer to a height of 760 mm (29.9 in) or 1 torr. The **torr**—named for the Italian physicist and mathematician Evangelista Torricelli (1608–1647) who invented the barometer—is not an SI unit but expresses gas pressure. One torr equals the pressure sufficient to raise a 1-mm column of mercury 1 mm high at 0°C against the standard acceleration of gravity at 45° north latitude (980.6 cm · s^{-2}). One standard atmosphere equals 760 torr. The barometric reading varies with changing weather conditions and is considerably lower at higher altitudes (see Chapter 24).

PART 1 • *Gaseous Exchange in the Lungs and Tissues*

CONCENTRATIONS AND PARTIAL PRESSURES OF RESPIRED GASES

The molecules of each specific gas in a mixture of gases exert their own **partial pressure**. The mixture's total pressure then equals the sum of the partial pressures of the individual gases in the mixture. This association, known as Dalton's law, is named after British chemist and physicist John Dalton (1766–1844) who also developed the atomic theory of matter. Partial pressure computes as follows:

Partial pressure = Percentage concentration of specific gas × Total pressure of gas mixture

Ambient Air

Table 13.1 lists the volumes, percentages, and partial pressures of the gases in dry ambient air at sea level. The partial pressure of oxygen equals 20.93% of the total 760 mm Hg pressure exerted by air or 159 mm Hg (20.93 ÷ 100 × 760 mm Hg). Carbon dioxide exerts a small pressure of only 0.23 mm Hg (0.03 ÷ 100 × 760 mm Hg), whereas the molecules of nitrogen exert a pressure that raises the mercury in a manometer about 600 mm (79.04 ÷ 100× 760 mm Hg). A *P* in front of the gas symbol denotes partial pressure. The partial pressures at sea level for the principal components of ambient air average as follows: oxygen (PO_2) = 159 mm Hg, carbon dioxide (PCO_2) = 0.2 mm Hg, and nitrogen (PN_2) = 600 mm Hg.

Tracheal Air

Air completely saturates with water vapor as it enters the nasal cavities and mouth and passes down the respiratory tract. The vapor dilutes the inspired air mixture somewhat. At a

COMMON SYMBOLS FOR GAS PRESSURE IN RESPIRATORY PHYSIOLOGY

- **$P_{A}O_2$**: Partial pressure of oxygen in alveolar chambers
- **Pao_2**: Partial pressure of oxygen in arterial blood
- **$Sao_2\%$**: Percent saturation of arterial blood with oxygen
- **Pvo_2**: Partial pressure of oxygen in venous blood
- **$P_{A}CO_2$**: Partial pressure of carbon dioxide in alveolar chambers
- **$Paco_2$**: Partial pressure of carbon dioxide in arterial blood
- **$Pvco_2$**: Partial pressure of carbon dioxide in venous blood
- **$Svo_2\%$**: Percent saturation of venous blood with oxygen
- **a-vO_2 diff**: Arteriovenous oxygen difference; difference between oxygen carried in arterial blood and carried in venous blood
- **a-$\bar{v}O_2$ diff**: Arterial–mixed-venous oxygen difference; difference between oxygen carried in arterial blood and carried in mixed-venous blood
- **$\bar{v}$**: mixed-venous blood

body temperature of 37°C, for example, the pressure of water molecules in humidified air equals 47 mm Hg; this leaves 713 mm Hg (760 − 47 mm Hg) as the total pressure exerted by the inspired dry air molecules. Consequently, the effective PO_2 in **tracheal air** decreases by about 10 mm Hg from its ambient value of 159 mm Hg to 149 mm Hg [0.2093 × (760 − 47 mm Hg)]. Humidification exerts little effect on inspired PCO_2 because of carbon dioxide's negligible contribution to inspired air.

Alveolar Air

Alveolar air composition differs considerably from the incoming breath of moist ambient air because carbon dioxide continually enters the alveoli from the blood; in contrast,

TABLE 13.1 ■ PARTIAL PRESSURE AND VOLUME OF GASES IN DRY AMBIENT AIR AT SEA LEVEL

GAS	PERCENTAGE	PARTIAL PRESSURE^a (MM HG)	GAS VOLUME (ML · L^{-1})
Oxygen	20.93	159	209.3
Carbon dioxide	0.03	0.2	0.4
Nitrogen	79.04^b	600	790.3

^{a} At 760 mm Hg ambient air pressure.
^{b} Includes 0.93% argon and other trace rare gases.

TABLE 13.2 ■ PARTIAL PRESSURE AND VOLUME OF DRY ALVEOLAR GASES AT SEA LEVEL (37°C)

GAS	PERCENTAGE	PARTIAL PRESSURE[a] (MM HG)	GAS VOLUME (ML · L⁻¹)
Oxygen	14.5	103	145
Carbon dioxide	5.5	39	55
Nitrogen[b]	80.0	571	800
Water vapor		47	

[a] At 760 − 47 mm Hg alveolar gas pressure.
[b] Nitrogen occupies a slightly greater percentage of alveolar air than ambient air because energy metabolism generally produces less carbon dioxide than oxygen consumed (i.e., the respiratory quotient [RQ = $\dot{V}CO_2$ ÷ $\dot{V}O_2$] equals less than 1.00). Because of this exchange imbalance, the nitrogen percentage increases.

oxygen flows from the lungs into the blood for transport throughout the body. TABLE 13.2 shows that alveolar air contains on average 14.5% oxygen, 5.5% carbon dioxide, and 80.0% nitrogen. After subtracting the vapor pressure from moist alveolar gas, the average alveolar P_{O_2} becomes 103 mm Hg [0.145 × (760 − 47 mm Hg)] and 39 mm Hg [0.055 × (760 − 47 mm Hg)] for P_{CO_2}. *These values represent average pressures exerted by oxygen and carbon dioxide molecules against the alveolar side of the alveolar–capillary membrane.* They do not remain physiologic constants; rather, they vary somewhat with the ventilatory cycle phase and the adequacy of ventilation in various lung regions. Recall that a relatively large volume of air remains in the lungs after each normal exhalation. This functional residual capacity serves as a damper, so each incoming breath exerts only a small effect on alveolar air composition. This explains why the partial pressures of alveolar gases remain relatively stable.

MOVEMENT OF GAS IN AIR AND FLUIDS

In accordance with **Henry's law** (named for English chemist and physician William Henry [1774–1836]), the mass of a gas that dissolves in a fluid at a given temperature varies in direct proportion to the pressure of the gas over the liquid, provided no chemical reaction takes place between the gas and liquid. The rate of gas diffusion into a fluid depends on two factors:

1. The **pressure differential** between the gas above the fluid and the gas dissolved in the fluid.
2. The **solubility** of the gas in the fluid.

Pressure Differential

Oxygen molecules continually strike the surface of the water in the three chambers illustrated in FIGURE 13.1. The pure water in chamber *A* contains no oxygen (P = 0 mm Hg), and a large number of oxygen molecules enter the water and dissolve in it. Dissolved gas molecules also move randomly, allowing some oxygen molecules to leave the water. In chamber *B*, oxygen still shows a *net* movement into the fluid from the gaseous state. Eventually, the number of molecules entering and leaving the fluid equalizes as occurs in chamber *C*. In this case, the gas pressures equilibrate without net oxygen diffusion into or out of the water. Conversely, if the pressure of dissolved oxygen molecules exceeds the pressure of the free gas in air, oxygen leaves the fluid until it attains a new pressure equilibrium. In humans, the pressure *difference* between alveolar and pulmonary blood gases creates the driving force for gas diffusion across the pulmonary membrane.

Solubility

For two different gases at identical pressure differentials, the solubility or dissolving power of each gas determines the number of molecules that move into or out of a fluid. Gas solubility is expressed as milliliters of a gas per 100 mL (dL) of a fluid. Oxygen, carbon dioxide, and nitrogen have different sol-

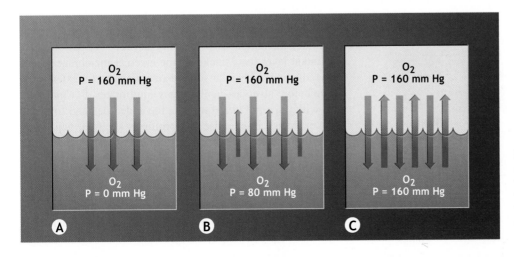

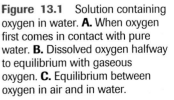

Figure 13.1 Solution containing oxygen in water. **A.** When oxygen first comes in contact with pure water. **B.** Dissolved oxygen halfway to equilibrium with gaseous oxygen. **C.** Equilibrium between oxygen in air and in water.

ubility coefficients in whole blood. Carbon dioxide dissolves most readily with a solubility coefficient of 57.03 mL of carbon dioxide per dL of fluid at 760 mm Hg and 37°C. Oxygen, with a solubility coefficient of 2.26 mL, remains relatively insoluble. Nitrogen is least soluble with a coefficient of 1.30 mL.

The amount of gas dissolved in a fluid computes as follows:

$$\text{Quantity of gas} = \text{Solubility coefficient} \times (\text{Gas partial pressure} \div \text{Total barometric pressure})$$

For example, the amount of oxygen dissolved in 1 dL of arterial whole blood ($P_{O_2} = 100$ mm Hg) at sea level (760 mm Hg) computes as:

$$\text{Quantity of gas} = 2.26 \times (100 \div 760)$$
$$= 0.3 \text{ mL} \cdot \text{dL}^{-1}$$

For each unit of pressure that favors diffusion, approximately 25 times more carbon dioxide than oxygen moves into (or out of) a fluid. Viewed another way, equal quantities of oxygen and carbon dioxide enter or leave a fluid under considerably different pressure gradients for each gas—precisely what occurs in the body.

Dissolved oxygen contributes about 4% of the total oxygen consumed by the body each minute during rest; in maximal exercise, it provides less than 2% of the total requirement. Even increasing arterial P_{O_2} by breathing 100% oxygen (ambient $P_{O_2} = 760$ mm Hg), dissolved oxygen (1.5 to 2.0 mL · dL of blood) still supplies only 40% of the total oxygen for rest and about 10% during maximal exercise. However, the physiologic significance of dissolved oxygen and carbon dioxide comes not from its role as a transport vehicle, but rather in determining the partial pressures of these gases. Partial pressure plays a central role in loading and unloading oxygen and carbon dioxide in the lungs and tissues.

GAS EXCHANGE IN THE LUNGS AND TISSUES

Exchange of gases between the lungs and blood and gas movement at the tissue level progress passively by diffusion, depending on their pressure gradients. FIGURE 13.2 illustrates the pressure gradients that favor gas transfer in different regions of the body at rest.

APPROXIMATE SOLUBILITY COEFFICIENTS OF GASES IN PHYSIOLOGIC FLUIDS			
GAS	WATER	PLASMA	BLOOD (QUANTITY DISSOLVED PER DL)
Oxygen	2.39	2.14	2.26 (0.3 mL)
Carbon dioxide	56.7	51.5	57.03 (3.0 mL)
Nitrogen	1.23	1.18	1.30 (0.8 mL)

Gas Exchange in the Lungs

At rest, the 100-mm Hg pressure of oxygen molecules in the alveoli exceeds by about 60 mm Hg the 40-mm Hg oxygen pressure in blood that enters the pulmonary capillaries. Consequently, oxygen dissolves and diffuses through the alveolar membranes into the blood. In contrast, carbon dioxide exists under a slightly greater pressure in returning venous blood than in the alveoli; this causes net diffusion of carbon dioxide from the blood into the lungs. Despite the relatively small pressure gradient of 6 mm Hg for carbon dioxide diffusion (compared with the 60-mm Hg diffusion gradient for oxygen), carbon dioxide transfer occurs rapidly because of its high solubility in plasma. Nitrogen, neither used nor produced in metabolic reactions, remains essentially unchanged in alveolar–capillary gas.

Gas exchange occurs so rapidly in the healthy lung that alveolar gas–blood gas equilibrium takes place in about 0.25 second, or within one third of the blood's transit time through the lungs. Even in high-intensity exercise, a red blood cell's velocity through a pulmonary capillary generally does not exceed by more than 50% its velocity at rest. With increasing exercise intensity, the pulmonary capillaries increase the blood volume within them by about 3 times the resting value.[2] The ability to accomodate larger blood volume helps to maintain a relatively slow pulmonary blood flow velocity during physical activity. With complete aeration, the blood leaving the lungs contains oxygen at an average pressure of 100 mm Hg and carbon dioxide at 40 mm Hg. For most healthy people, these values vary little during vigorous exercise.

The P_{O_2} of arterial blood usually remains slightly lower than alveolar P_{O_2} because some blood in the alveolar capillaries passes through poorly ventilated alveoli; also, the blood leaving the lungs joins venous blood from the bronchial and cardiac circulations. The term **venous admixture** defines this small amount of poorly oxygenated blood. Venous admixture exerts a small effect in healthy individuals and reduces the arterial P_{O_2} slightly below the value in pulmonary end-capillary blood.

Pulmonary Disease

Two factors impair gas transfer capacity at the alveolar–capillary membrane in pulmonary disease: (1) buildup of a pollutant layer that "thickens" the alveolar membrane and/or (2) reduction in alveolar surface area. Each factor extends the time before alveolar–capillary gas equilibrates. For individuals with impaired lung function, the added demand for rapid gas exchange in exercise compromises aeration, negatively affecting exercise performance.

 INTEGRATIVE QUESTION

Why do minute amounts of CO_2 and CO impurities in a breathing mixture exert such profound physiologic effects?

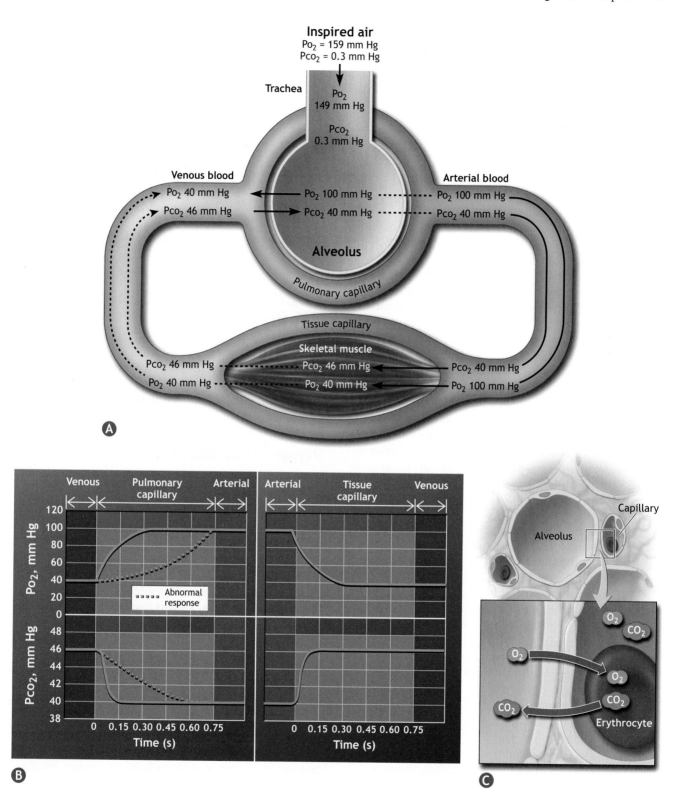

Figure 13.2 Pressure gradients for gas transfer within the body at rest. **A.** The Po₂ and Pco₂ of ambient, tracheal, and alveolar air and these gas pressures in venous and arterial blood and muscle tissue. Gas movement at the alveolar–capillary and tissue–capillary membranes always progresses from an area of higher partial pressure to lower partial pressure. **B.** Time required for gas exchange. At rest, blood remains in the pulmonary and tissue capillaries for about 0.75 seconds. Pulmonary disease *(dashed line)* impairs the rate of gas transfer across the alveolar–capillary membrane, thus prolonging the time for equilibration of gases. Blood's transit time through the pulmonary capillaries during maximal exercise decreases to about 0.4 seconds, but this still remains adequate for complete aeration in the healthy lung. **C.** Gas exchange (diffusion) between a pulmonary capillary and its adjacent alveolus.

Gas Transfer in Tissues

In tissues, where energy metabolism consumes oxygen and produces an almost equal amount of carbon dioxide, gas pressures differ considerably from those in arterial blood. At rest, the P_{O_2} in the fluid immediately outside a muscle cell averages 40 mm Hg, and intracellular P_{CO_2} averages 46 mm Hg. In vigorous exercise, oxygen pressure within muscle tissue falls toward 0 mm Hg, while the pressure of carbon dioxide approaches 90 mm Hg. *Pressure differences between gases in plasma and tissues establish diffusion gradients.* Oxygen leaves the blood and diffuses *toward* the cell, while carbon dioxide flows *from* the cell into the blood. Blood then passes into the venous circuit (venules and veins) for return to the heart and delivery to the lungs. Diffusion occurs rapidly as blood enters the dense pulmonary capillary network. The body does not attempt to rid itself completely of carbon dioxide. To the contrary, each liter of blood leaving the lungs with a P_{CO_2} of 40 mm Hg contains about 50 mL of carbon dioxide. As discussed in Chapter 14, this small "background level" of carbon dioxide provides the chemical basis for ventilatory control through its stimulating effect on the neurons of the pons and medullary centers of the brainstem. The term **respiratory center** describes this collection of neural tissue.

Alveolar ventilation couples tightly to metabolic demands to keep alveolar gas composition remarkably constant. Stability in alveolar gas concentrations persists even during strenuous exercise that increases oxygen consumption and carbon dioxide output 25 times the values at rest.

Summary

1. Gas molecules in the lungs and tissues diffuse down their concentration gradients from an area of higher concentration (higher pressure) to lower concentration (lower pressure).
2. The partial pressure of a specific gas in a mixture of gases varies directly with the concentration of the gas and the mixture's total pressure.
3. Henry's law states that pressure gradient and solubility determine how much gas dissolves in a fluid. Oxygen, carbon dioxide, and nitrogen exhibit different solubilities in whole blood. Carbon dioxide dissolves most readily while oxygen and nitrogen show relatively low solubility.
4. Carbon dioxide solubility in plasma exceeds oxygen solubility by 25 times, allowing carbon dioxide to move into and from body fluids down a relatively small diffusion (pressure) gradient.
5. Pulmonary ventilation adjusts during rest and exercise to maintain a remarkably constant alveolar gas composition. Alveolar ventilation maintains P_{O_2} at about 100 mm Hg and P_{CO_2} at 40 mm Hg.
6. Oxygen diffuses into the blood and carbon dioxide diffuses into the lungs because venous blood contains oxygen at lower pressure and carbon dioxide at higher pressure than alveolar gas.
7. Alveolar–blood gas exchange achieves equilibrium in the healthy lung at about the midpoint of the blood's transit through the pulmonary capillaries. Even in intense exercise, blood flow velocity through the lungs generally does not compromise full loading of oxygen and unloading of carbon dioxide.
8. Diffusion gradients favor oxygen movement from the capillaries to the tissues and carbon dioxide from the tissues to the blood. Oxygen and carbon dioxide diffuse rapidly as their pressure gradients widen during exercise.

PART 2 • *Oxygen Transport*

TRANSPORT OF OXYGEN IN THE BLOOD

The blood carries oxygen in two ways:

1. In physical solution dissolved in the fluid portion of blood
2. In loose combination with hemoglobin, the iron-protein molecule within the red blood cell

Oxygen in Physical Solution

Oxygen's relative insolubility in water keeps its concentration low in bodily fluids. At an alveolar P_{O_2} of 100 mm Hg, only about 0.3 mL of gaseous oxygen dissolves in each deciliter of blood (0.003 mL for each additional 1-mm Hg increase). This equals 3 mL of oxygen per liter of blood. The blood volume of a 70-kg person averages about 5 L; thus, 15 mL of oxygen dissolves in the fluid portion of the blood (3 mL per L $\times$ 5). This small amount of oxygen would sustain life for about 4 seconds. Viewed from a different perspective, if oxygen in physical solution provided the sole oxygen source to the body, about 80 L of blood would need to circulate each minute to supply the resting oxygen requirements—a blood flow about twice the maximum ever recorded for a world-class athlete!

As with carbon dioxide, the small quantity of oxygen transported in physical solution serves several important functions. The random movement of dissolved oxygen molecules establishes the P_{O_2} of the plasma and tissue fluids. The pressure of oxygen in solution helps to regulate breathing, particularly at higher altitudes when ambient P_{O_2} decreases considerably; it also determines oxygen loading of hemoglobin in the lungs and subsequent release in tissues.

Oxygen Combined with Hemoglobin

Metallic compounds exist in the blood of many animal species to augment the blood's oxygen-carrying capacity. FIGURE 13.3 illustrates the iron-containing globular protein pigment **hemoglobin** carried within the red blood cells of humans.

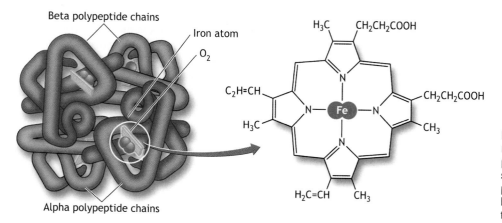

Figure 13.3 The hemoglobin molecule (*left*) consists of the protein globin, composed of four subunit polypeptide chains. Each polypeptide (*right*) contains a single heme group with its single iron atom that acts as a "magnet" for oxygen.

About 280 million hemoglobin molecules pack into each of the body's more than 25 trillion red blood cells. This concentration carries 65 to 70 times more oxygen than normally dissolves in plasma. Thus, hemoglobin temporarily "captures" and transports about 197 mL of oxygen in each liter of blood. Each of the four iron atoms in the hemoglobin molecule can loosely bind one oxygen molecule in the following reversible reaction:

$$Hb_4 + 4\,O_2 \leftrightarrow Hb_4O_8$$

The reaction requires no enzymes; it proceeds without a change in the valence of Fe^{2+}, as in the more permanent oxidation process. *The partial pressure of oxygen dissolved in physical solution dictates the oxygenation of hemoglobin to oxyhemoglobin.*

Oxygen-Carrying Capacity of Hemoglobin

In men, each dL of blood contains about 15 g of hemoglobin. The value decreases 5 to 10% for women and averages nearly 14 g per dL of blood. This gender difference partly explains the lower aerobic capacity of women relative to men, even when considering differences in body mass and body fat. The reason for higher hemoglobin concentrations in men relates to the stimulating effects on red blood cell production of the "male" hormone testosterone.

Each gram of hemoglobin combines loosely with 1.34 mL of oxygen. Thus, if one knows the hemoglobin content of the blood, its oxygen-carrying capacity computes as follows:

$$\begin{array}{ccc}
\text{Blood's oxygen} & & \\
\text{capacity} & \text{Hemoglobin} & \text{Oxygen capacity} \\
(\text{mL} \cdot \text{dL blood})^{-1} = (\text{g} \cdot \text{dL blood})^{-1} \times \text{of hemoglobin} \\
20\ \text{mL O}_2 = 15 \times 1.34\ \text{mL} \cdot \text{g}^{-1}
\end{array}$$

With full oxygen saturation (i.e., when all hemoglobin converts to HbO_2) and with normal hemoglobin levels, hemoglobin carries nearly 20 mL of oxygen in each dL of whole blood.

Anemia Affects Oxygen Transport. The blood's oxygen transport capacity changes only slightly with normal variations in hemoglobin content. On the other hand, a significant

decrease in the iron content of red blood cells reduces the blood's oxygen-carrying capacity. Such **iron deficiency anemia** diminishes a person's capacity to sustain even mild-intensity aerobic exercise.[1,5]

TABLE 13.3 presents data from 29 iron-deficient anemic men and women with low hemoglobin levels. They formed two groups; one received intramuscular iron injections over an 80-day period, while the placebo group received similar intramuscular injections of a colored saline solution. A third group with normal hemoglobin levels served as controls. The researchers tested all groups during exercise prior to the

TABLE 13.3 ■ HEMOGLOBIN (HB) LEVELS AND EXERCISE HEART RATES OF NORMAL AND ANEMIC SUBJECTS PRIOR TO AND FOLLOWING SUPPLEMENTAL IRON TREATMENT

SUBJECTS	HB (G PER DL BLOOD)	PEAK EXERCISE HEART RATE
Normal		
Men	14.3	119
Women	13.9	142
Iron-deficient men		
Pretreatment	7.1	155
Posttreatment	14.0	113
Iron-deficient women		
Pretreatment	7.7	152
Posttreatment	12.4	123
Iron-deficient men		
Preplacebo	7.7	146
Postplacebo	7.4	137
Iron-deficient women		
Preplacebo	8.1	154
Postplacebo	8.4	144

From Gardner GW, et al. Cardiorespiratory, hematological, and physical performance responses of anemic subjects to iron treatment. Am J Clin Nutr 1975;28:982.
Values represent group averages.

experiment and after 80 days of either iron therapy or placebo treatment. The results clearly show that the anemic group given iron supplements improved in exercise response compared with nonsupplemented counterparts. Peak heart rate during 5 minutes of stepping exercise decreased from 155 to 113 b · min^{-1} for men and from 152 to 123 b · min^{-1} for women. This translates into an average of 15% more oxygen delivered per heartbeat.

Po$_2$ and Hemoglobin Saturation

The term **cooperative binding** describes the union of oxygen with hemoglobin. The binding of an oxygen molecule to the iron atom in one of the four globin chains in Figure 13.3 progressively facilitates the binding of subsequent molecules. The cooperative binding phenomenon explains hemoglobin's sigmoid or S-shaped oxygen saturation curve.

The **oxyhemoglobin dissociation curve** (FIG. 13.4) illustrates the saturation of hemoglobin with oxygen at various Po$_2$ values, including alveolar–capillary gas at sea level (Po$_2$, 100 mm Hg). The right ordinate gives the quantity of oxygen carried in each deciliter of normal blood at a particular plasma Po$_2$ value. The term **volume percent** (**vol%**) describes blood's oxygen content. In this regard, volume percent refers to the milliliters of oxygen extracted (in a vacuum) from a deciliter sample of either whole blood (with plasma) or packed red blood cells (without plasma).

Physical chemists establish dissociation curves (oxygen content and percentage saturation) by exposing about 200 mL of blood in a sealed glass vessel (tonometer) to various pressures of oxygen at a given pH in a water bath of known temperature. Percentage saturation computes as follows:

$$\text{Percentage saturation} = \frac{\text{O}_2 \text{ combined with hemoglobin}}{\text{O}_2 \text{ capacity of hemoglobin}} \times 100$$

If an individual's hemoglobin oxygen-carrying capacity in whole blood equals 20 vol% and only 12 vol% oxygen actually combines with hemoglobin, then:

Percentage saturation = 12 vol% ÷ 20 vol% × 100 = 60%

One hundred percent saturation indicates that the oxygen combined with hemoglobin equals the oxygen-carrying capacity of hemoglobin.

Figure 13.4B depicts the **oxygen transport cascade** for oxygen partial pressure as oxygen moves from ambient air at sea level to the mitochondria of maximally active muscle tissue.

Po$_2$ in the Lungs

So far, we have assumed that hemoglobin fully saturates with oxygen when exposed to alveolar gas. *This does not occur because at the sea level alveolar Po$_2$ of 100 mm Hg, hemoglobin achieves 98% oxygen saturation.* The right ordinate of Figure 13.4A shows that at a Po$_2$ of 100 mm Hg, the hemoglobin in each deciliter of blood leaving the lungs carries about 19.7 mL of oxygen. Clearly, any additional increase in alveolar Po$_2$ contributes little to how much more

oxygen can combine with hemoglobin. In addition to the oxygen bound to hemoglobin, the plasma of each deciliter of arterial blood contains 0.3 mL of oxygen in solution. In healthy individuals who breathe ambient air at sea level, each deciliter of blood leaving the lungs carries approximately 20.0 mL of oxygen—19.7 mL bound to hemoglobin and 0.3 mL dissolved in plasma. FIGURE 13.5 shows the percentage composition of centrifuged whole blood for red blood cells (termed **hematocrit**) and plasma, including representative values for the quantity of oxygen carried in each component.

On television one frequently sees competitive athletes breathing a gas mixture of concentrated oxygen following strenuous exercise. This makes no sense from an oxygen-transport perspective. The oxyhemoglobin dissociation curve shows little or no potential for increased hemoglobin loading from additional pressure of supplemental oxygen inhaled at sea level or at relatively low altitude. We discuss the topic of breathing hyperoxic gas mixtures and exercise performance in more detail in Chapter 23.

Figure 13.4 also shows that hemoglobin saturation with oxygen changes little until the pressure of oxygen declines to about 60 mm Hg. This flat upper portion of the oxyhemoglobin dissociation curve provides a margin of safety to ensure adequate saturation of arterial blood with oxygen despite considerable fluctuations in ambient Po$_2$. Even if alveolar Po$_2$ decreases to 75 mm Hg, as occurs in lung disease or at higher altitudes, the saturation of hemoglobin decreases by only about 6%. At an alveolar Po$_2$ of 60 mm Hg, hemoglobin still remains 90% saturated with oxygen! Below this pressure, the quantity of oxygen combined with hemoglobin declines precipitously.

INTEGRATIVE QUESTION

Advise a coach who wants football players to breathe from an oxygen tank during time-outs or rest breaks to speed recovery.

Po$_2$ in the Tissues

At rest, the Po$_2$ in the cell fluids averages 40 mm Hg. This makes dissolved oxygen from the plasma diffuse across the capillary membrane through the tissue fluids into the cells. This reduces plasma Po$_2$ below the Po$_2$ in the red blood cell, causing hemoglobin to lower its oxygen saturation level. The released oxygen (HbO$_2$ → Hb + O$_2$) moves out of the blood cells through the capillary membrane into the tissues.

At the tissue–capillary Po$_2$ at rest of 40 mm Hg, hemoglobin holds about 70% of its original oxygen (Fig. 13.4). Thus, when blood leaves the tissues and returns to the heart, it carries about 15 mL of oxygen in each deciliter of blood, giving up 5 mL of oxygen to the tissues.

Arteriovenous Oxygen Difference

The **arteriovenous oxygen difference** (**a-v̄O$_2$ difference**) describes the difference in the oxygen content of arterial blood and mixed-venous blood. The a-v̄O$_2$ difference at rest normally averages 4 to 5 mL of oxygen per deciliter of blood. The large

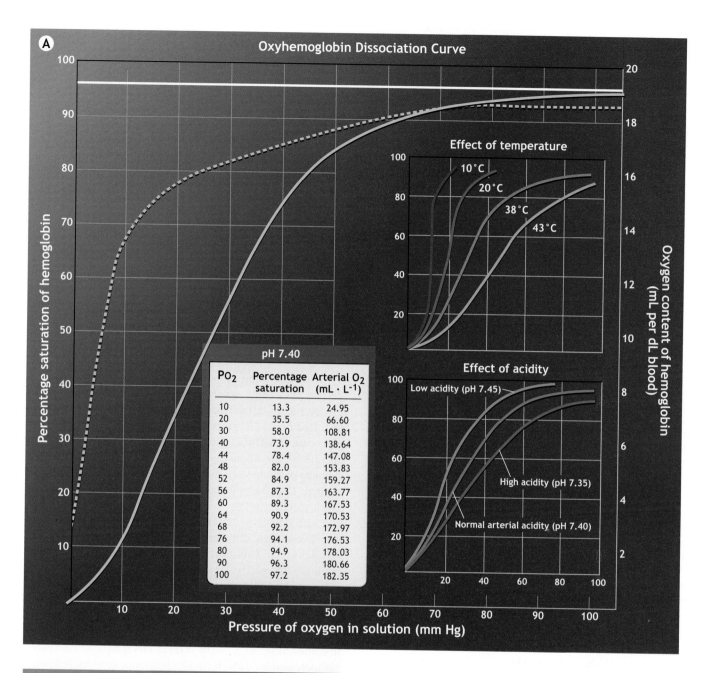

A. Oxyhemoglobin Dissociation Curve

pH 7.40		
PO_2	Percentage saturation	Arterial O_2 (mL · L^{-1})
10	13.3	24.95
20	35.5	66.60
30	58.0	108.81
40	73.9	138.64
44	78.4	147.08
48	82.0	153.83
52	84.9	159.27
56	87.3	163.77
60	89.3	167.53
64	90.9	170.53
68	92.2	172.97
76	94.1	176.53
80	94.9	178.03
90	96.3	180.66
100	97.2	182.35

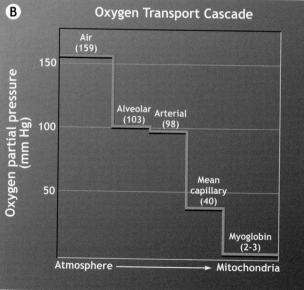

B. Oxygen Transport Cascade

Figure 13.4 A. Oxyhemoglobin dissociation curve. Lines indicate the percentage saturation of hemoglobin *(solid line)* and myoglobin *(dashed line)* in relation to oxygen pressure. The *right ordinate* shows the quantity of oxygen carried in each deciliter of blood under normal conditions. The *inset curves within the figure* illustrate the effects of temperature and acidity in altering hemoglobin's affinity for oxygen (Bohr effect). *Inset box* presents oxyhemoglobin saturation and arterial blood's oxygen-carrying capacity for different PO_2 values with hemoglobin concentration of 14 g · dL blood^{-1}. The *white horizontal line at the top of the graph* indicates percentage saturation of hemoglobin at the average sea-level alveolar PO_2 of 100 mm Hg. **B.** Partial pressures as oxygen moves from ambient air at sea level to the mitochondria of maximally active muscle tissue (oxygen transport cascade).

Centrifuged Whole Blood

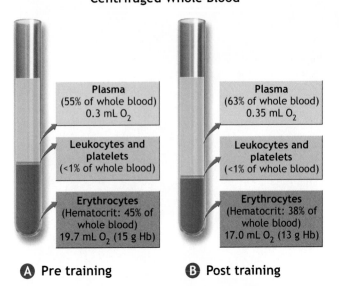

A Pre training   **B** Post training

Figure 13.5 A. Major components of centrifuged whole blood, including the quantity of oxygen carried in each deciliter of blood (*Hb*, hemoglobin) in an untrained individual. **B.** Changes in constituents of whole blood following 4 days of aerobic exercise training. Note that the increase in plasma volume (hemodilution) early in training decreases red blood cell concentration toward borderline anemia (see Chapters 2 and 21). Oxygen transport capacity does not decrease with training because total erythrocyte mass remains constant or increases slightly.

quantity of oxygen still attached to hemoglobin provides an "automatic" reserve so cells can immediately obtain oxygen should metabolic demands suddenly increase. Tissue P_{O_2} decreases as the cell's use of oxygen increases in exercise. This causes hemoglobin to immediately release a larger amount of oxygen. During intense exercise when extracellular P_{O_2} decreases to nearly 15 mm Hg, only about 5 mL of oxygen remains bound to hemoglobin. The a-$\bar{v}O_2$ difference increases to 15 mL of oxygen per 100 mL of blood. When active muscle P_{O_2} falls to 2 or 3 mm Hg during exhaustive exercise, the blood perfusing these tissues gives up virtually all its oxygen.[13] Oxygen release from hemoglobin can occur without any increase in local tissue blood flow. The amount of oxygen released to the muscles increases almost three times above that normally supplied at rest—just by a more complete unloading of hemoglobin, particularly as it flows through endurance-trained muscles (see "Focus on Research," p. 287). *An active muscle's uncompromising capacity to use available oxygen in its large blood flow supports the position that oxygen supply (blood flow), not muscle oxygen use, limits aerobic exercise capacity.*[11]

The Bohr Effect

The sigmoid, solid yellow line in Figure 13.4 represents the oxyhemoglobin dissociation curve under resting physiologic conditions at an arterial pH of 7.4 and tissue temperature of 37°C. The **inset curves** depict other important characteris-

tics of hemoglobin's affinity for oxygen. Any increase in plasma acidity (including carbon dioxide concentration) and temperature causes the dissociation curve to shift downward and to the right. This phenomenon, called the **Bohr effect** after its discoverer, Danish physiologist Christian Bohr (1855–1911; father of Nobel physicist Niels Bohr), indicates an altered hemoglobin molecular structure. It describes the reduced effectiveness of hemoglobin to hold oxygen, particularly in the P_{O_2} range between 20 and 50 mm Hg. The Bohr effect remains evident during intense exercise as even more oxygen releases to the tissues because of associated increases in metabolic heat, carbon dioxide, and increased acidity from blood lactate accumulation. At normal alveolar P_{O_2}, however, the Bohr effect exerts almost no effect on pulmonary capillary blood (even during maximal exercise), so hemoglobin loads (binds) fully with oxygen as blood flows through the lungs.

Red Blood Cell 2,3-DPG

Because a red blood cell contains no mitochondria, it derives its energy solely from the anaerobic reactions of glycolysis; this establishes the normal plasma lactate levels at rest. Red blood cells produce the compound **2,3-diphosphoglycerate** (**2,3-DPG**; also referred to as 2,3-biphosphoglycerate [2,3-BPG]) during glycolysis. 2,3-DPG binds loosely with subunits of the hemoglobin molecule, reducing its affinity for oxygen. This causes greater oxygen release to the tissues for a given decrease in P_{O_2}.[3]

Individuals with cardiopulmonary disorders and those who live at high altitudes have increased levels of red blood cell 2,3-DPG. This provides compensatory adjustments to facilitate oxygen release to the cells. During strenuous exercise, 2,3-DPG also aids in oxygen transfer to muscles.[6] Conflicting results emerge in comparison of 2,3-DPG levels of trained and untrained subjects.[4,7,10] One study reported higher resting levels of 2,3-DPG in two groups of athletes than in untrained subjects.[14] The level of this metabolic intermediate increased by 15% for middle-distance runners following short-duration maximal exercise. In contrast, prolonged steady-rate exercise in endurance athletes produced a small decrease in 2,3-DPG. These data support the proposition that increases in 2,3-DPG concentration with intense exercise (and perhaps training) reflect an adaptive response that augments oxygen delivery to more metabolically active tissues. More than likely, the effect of different types of exercise on erythrocyte 2,3-DPG levels reflects the specific metabolic demands of exercise. Females have higher levels of red blood cell 2,3-DPG than males of similar fitness status and physical activity level. This gender difference might compensate for the lower hemoglobin levels in females.[9]

Myoglobin, the Muscle's Oxygen Store

Myoglobin, an iron-containing globular protein in skeletal and cardiac muscle fibers, provides intramuscular oxygen storage. X-ray crystallography in 1960 revealed myoglobin's structural details. Austrian biochemist Max F. Perutz

(1914–2002; corecipient of the Nobel prize in Chemistry, 1962) took the first x-ray diffraction pictures of hemoglobin crystals at the same Cavendish laboratory in Cambridge, England, where researchers Watson and Crick decoded the final mystery of DNA's structure (see "On the Horizon", the final chapter in this book). The molecule contains a peptide backbone embedded with the heme group and its metallic Fe^{2+}. Reddish muscle fibers have a high concentration of this respiratory pigment, whereas myoglobin-deficient fibers appear pale or white.[8] Myoglobin resembles hemoglobin because it also combines reversibly with oxygen; however, each myoglobin molecule contains only one iron atom while hemoglobin contains four. Myoglobin adds additional oxygen to the muscle in the following chemical reaction:

$$Mb + O_2 \rightarrow MbO_2$$

FOCUS On Research

A REMARKABLY ADAPTABLE TISSUE

Holloszy JO. Biochemical adaptations in muscle: effects of exercise on mitochondrial oxygen uptake and respiratory enzyme activity in skeletal muscle. J Biol Chem 1967;242:2278.

▲ For years prior to the mid-1960s, conventional wisdom maintained that central cardiovascular adaptations exclusively increased capacity to deliver oxygen to active muscle and thus increased endurance performance with aerobic training. Proponents of this view argued that training-induced improvements in $\dot{V}O_{2max}$ resulted from increased maximal cardiac output from the heart's increased maximal stroke volume. Central to this concept was the belief that working muscle becomes hypoxic during high-intensity exercise, and improved oxygen delivery produced less hypoxia after training. Virtually no data were available to demonstrate adaptive changes in a muscle's metabolic machinery with regular exercise, although thyroxine feeding in rats had been shown to induce changes in mitochondrial composition and number.

The study by Holloszy was the first to show that endurance exercise training increased skeletal muscle mitochondrial content in rats. The author hypothesized that local (peripheral) changes in muscle (primarily in mitochondria) contribute to improved endurance performance with training. This study and subsequent research with colleagues ushered in a burgeoning new area in exercise biochemistry research.

In the exercise training program, rats ran on a treadmill 5 days per week for 12 weeks. Running speed and duration gradually increased so that after 12 weeks, the animals ran for 120 minutes daily on an 8% incline at $31 \text{ m} \cdot \text{min}^{-1}$, including 12, 30-second intervals at 42 $\text{m} \cdot \text{min}^{-1}$ interspersed at 10-minute intervals. The protocol was the most strenuous reported in the exercise literature of that time. The animals were placed into one of four groups of 12: (1) exercise trained; (2) exercise control–pair weighted, who performed only mild daily exercise (10 min, 5 days per week) with food intake adjusted to maintain the same body weight as group 1; (3) sedentary control–pair weighted, with food intake adjusted to maintain the same body weight as group 1; and (4) sedentary, freely eating.

The dependent variables were measured from the gastrocnemius and soleus muscles to show evidence for exercise training adaptations in muscle mitochondria and mitochondrial enzymes. These measures included succinate dehydrogenase, NADH dehydrogenase, NADH-cytochrome c reductase, level of respiratory control, mitochondrial protein, and succinate and cytochrome oxidase activity per gram of muscle.

The table shows that the capacity of the mitochondrial fraction from gastrocnemius muscle to oxidize pyruvate doubled in the trained rats. Succinate dehydrogenase, NADH dehydrogenase, NADH-cytochrome c reductase, and cytochrome oxidase activities per gram of muscle also increased approximately twofold. The near doubling of cytochrome c activity provided evidence that increases in respiratory chain enzyme activities resulted from increased mitochondrial enzyme activity. The total protein content of the mitochondrial fraction of trained muscle increased about 60%. The high level of mitochondrial respiratory control and tightly-coupled oxidative phosphorylation revealed that the increase in electron transport capacity with training accompanied rises in the capacity to generate ATP via oxidative phosphorylation.

Subsequent investigations with animals and humans soon confirmed the findings of increased respiratory capacity and mitochondrial enzyme levels in aerobically trained muscle. Holloszy's pioneering work served as a catalyst for further research concerning the profound effect of exercise training on muscle biochemistry. The research also helped to explain why regular aerobic overload increases ability to exercise at a higher percentage of $\dot{V}O_{2max}$ (i.e., increased blood lactate threshold) and provided an important cellular component to verify the specificity of training principle for aerobic exercise.

continued on page 288

Continued

EFFECTS OF ENDURANCE EXERCISE ON TRAINING RAT MUSCLE MITOCHONDRIA

VARIABLE	SEDENTARY TRAINED	CONTROL
Body mass, g	353 ± 17	491 ± 21.9
Gastrocnemius muscle weight, g	2.1 ± 0.06	2.62 ± 0.12
Treadmill run to exhaustion (min) at 31 m · min^{-1}	186 ± 18	29.0 ± 3
$\dot{V}O_2$, mL · h^{-1} · g^{-1}	1022 ± 118	506 ± 53
Respiratory control index	16.1 ± 2.2	14.7 ± 2.6
Cytochrome oxidase, mL O$_2$ · min^{-1} · g muscle^{-1}		
Gastrocnemius	551 ± 31	305 ± 15
Soleus	691 ± 52	427 ± 16
Succinate oxidase, mL O$_2$ · min^{-1} · g muscle^{-1}		
Gastrocnemius	117 ± 8	73 ± 5
Soleus	160 ± 8	95 ± 10
Succinate dehydrogenase activity, mmol · g muscle^{-1}	15.1 ± 1.4	8.3 ± 0.7
Cytochrome c concentration, mmol · g muscle^{-1}	6.46 ± 0.58	3.47 ± 0.18
DPNH dehydrogenase, mmol · g muscle^{-1}	11.8 ± 1.5	5.6 ± 0.6
Mitochondrial protein, mmol · min^{-1} · mg protein^{-1}	4.67 ± 0.30	2.97 ± 0.20
DPNH cytochrome c reductase, mmol · g muscle^{-1}	0.60 ± 0.09	0.25 ± 0.06

Oxygen Released at Low Pressures

Myoglobin facilitates the oxygen transfer of the mitochondria, particularly when exercise begins and during intense exercise when cellular PO_2 declines rapidly. The dissociation curve for myoglobin (Fig. 13.4; *dashed yellow line*) does not form an S-shaped line as does hemoglobin, but instead plots as a rectangular hyperbola. At the low end of PO_2 values, the curve form abruptly and significantly increases in percentage myoglobin saturation with a relatively small increase in PO_2 until the asymptote. Little further change in saturation occurs over a broad PO_2 range. Compared with the oxygen saturation curve for hemoglobin, the curve for myoglobin shows that it much more readily binds and retains oxygen at low oxygen pressures. During rest and moderate exercise, myoglobin maintains high oxygen saturation. For example, at a PO_2 of 40 mm Hg, myoglobin retains 95% of its oxygen. The greatest quantity of oxygen releases from MbO_2 when tissue PO_2 declines below 5 mm Hg.[12] Unlike hemoglobin, acidity, carbon dioxide, and temperature do not affect myoglobin's oxygen-binding affinity, so it does not exhibit a Bohr effect. Chapter 21 discusses the effects of aerobic exercise training on the muscles' myoglobin content.

Summary

1. Hemoglobin, the iron-protein pigment in the red blood cell, increases the amount of oxygen carried in whole blood about 65 times that carried in physical solution in the plasma.
2. The small amount of oxygen dissolved in plasma exerts molecular movement and establishes the partial pressure of oxygen (PO_2) in the blood. Plasma PO_2 determines the loading of hemoglobin at the lungs (oxygenation) and its unloading at the tissues (deoxygenation).
3. The blood's oxygen-transport capacity varies only slightly with normal variations in hemoglobin content. Iron deficiency anemia lowers hemoglobin concentration, thus decreasing the blood's oxygen-carrying capacity. Lowered hemoglobin concentration impairs aerobic exercise performance.

4. The shape of the oxyhemoglobin dissociation curve indicates that hemoglobin saturation changes little until P_{O_2} declines below 60 mm Hg. The quantity of oxygen bound to hemoglobin falls sharply as oxygen moves from capillary blood to the tissues when metabolic demands increase.

5. Arterial blood releases only about 25% of its total oxygen content to the tissues at rest; the remaining 75% returns "unused" to the heart in venous blood.

6. The difference in oxygen content of arterial and venous blood under resting conditions indicates an automatic reserve of oxygen for rapid use should metabolism suddenly increase.

7. The Bohr effect reflects alterations in the molecular structure of hemoglobin from increased acidity, temperature, carbon dioxide concentration, and red blood cell 2,3-DPG that reduce its effectiveness to hold oxygen. Exercise accentuates these factors, further facilitating oxygen's release to the tissues.

8. The iron-protein pigment myoglobin in skeletal and cardiac muscle provides an "extra" oxygen store to release oxygen at low P_{O_2}. During intense exercise, myoglobin facilitates oxygen transfer to the mitochondria when intracellular P_{O_2} in active skeletal muscle decreases dramatically.

PART 3 • *Carbon Dioxide Transport*

CARBON DIOXIDE TRANSPORT IN THE BLOOD

Once carbon dioxide forms in the cell, diffusion and subsequent transport in the venous blood provides the only means for its "escape" through the lungs. The blood carries carbon dioxide in three ways:

1. In physical solution in plasma (small amount).
2. Combined with hemoglobin within the red blood cell.
3. As plasma bicarbonate.

FIGURE 13.6 illustrates the three ways for transporting carbon dioxide from the tissues to the lungs.

Carbon Dioxide in Physical Solution

Approximately 5% of the carbon dioxide formed during energy metabolism moves into physical solution in the plasma as free carbon dioxide. *The random movement of this small quantity of dissolved carbon dioxide molecules establishes the P_{CO_2} of the blood.*

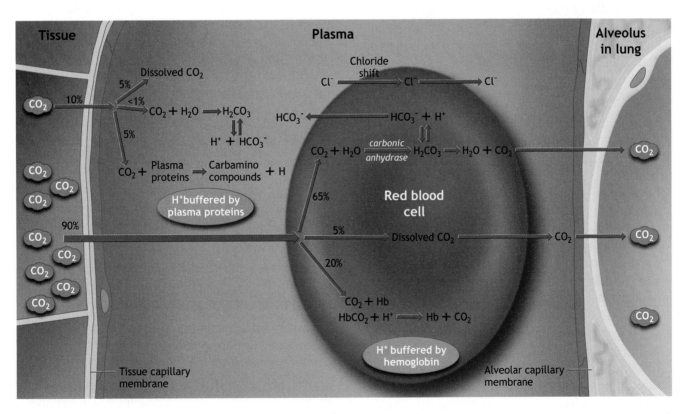

Figure 13.6 Transport of carbon dioxide in the plasma and red blood cells as dissolved CO_2, bicarbonate, and carbamino compounds. By far, the greatest amount of carbon dioxide combines with water to form carbonic acid.

IN A PRACTICAL SENSE

FACTORS THAT CONTRIBUTE TO THE SMOKING HABIT

■ Cigarette smoking represents the single greatest cause of death worldwide. Each year, more than 450,000 people in the United States die from smoking-related diseases—heart disease, cancer, stroke, aortic aneurysm, chronic bronchitis, emphysema, and peptic ulcers. Chronic cigarette smokers live an average of 18 years less than nonsmokers, and each cigarette smoked shortens life by 7 minutes! In addition to its adverse effects on health, cigarette smoking (both short and long term) has the potential to negatively affect exercise performance, which is discussed in greater detail in Chapter 14. Because of the potential for adverse effects on exercise and sports performance, we have included this "In a Practical Sense" in this chapter due to the fact it provides insight into factors related to the smoking habit.

WHY PEOPLE START SMOKING

People usually start smoking without realizing its detrimental effects. Cigarette smoking generally begins during the teen years or earlier. Health problems from smoking accrue quickly in young smokers. Three reasons generally explain why youths begin smoking: (1) peer pressure, (2) desire to appear "grown up," and (3) rebellion against authority.

CIGARETTES CAUSE ADDICTION

Tobacco smoke contains more than 1200 toxic chemicals; tar alone contains nearly 30 known carcinogens. Within seconds of inhalation, nicotine affects the central nervous system to act simultaneously as a tranquilizer *and* stimulant. Nicotine's stimulating effect produces a strong physiologic and psychologic dependency. Estimates place the physiologic addiction to nicotine at about 6 to 8 times the addictive power of alcohol. Psychologic dependency develops over a longer time and associates with calming and pleasurable activities such as drinking coffee or alcohol, participating in social gatherings, relaxing after a meal, talking on the telephone, driving, reading, and watching television.

THE "WHY-DO-YOU-SMOKE TEST"

The Why-Do-You-Smoke Test (see table) identifies reasons for smoking, which provides the important first step in behavioral approaches to smoking cessation.

The test lists 18 statements about why people smoke. A score between 1 and 5 indicates the strength of agreement with the statement, with 5 representing the strongest agreement. The responses to each of the statements provide input about one of six factors most frequently related to a person's smoking behavior. The information obtained provides (1) insight as to why a person smokes and (2) possible behavioral substitutes to aid in cessation.

■ Stimulation ("cigarettes are stimulating"): you feel that they help wake you up, organize your energies, and keep you going. Choose a safe substitute—a brisk walk or moderate exercise.
■ Handling ("keep my hands busy"): toy with a pen or pencil or doodle, play with a coin, piece of jewelry, or some other harmless object while quitting.
■ Accentuation of pleasure/pleasurable relaxation ("makes me feel good"): substitute social and physical activities or other relaxing activities to accentuate pleasure.
■ Reduction of negative feelings/crutch ("gets me through the tough times"): learning to handle stress helps with quitting.
■ Craving or dependence ("can't get through the day without them"): "cold turkey" is the most effective way to quit; biofeedback has shown some success.
■ Habit ("don't even know when I'm smoking"): need to break the habitual smoking pattern; being more aware of conditions and situations when smoking occurs aids in quitting.

Scores for each factor can vary between 3 and 15. A score of 11 or above indicates that for this factor smoking represents an important source of satisfaction. Scoring low (<7) on a factor indicates a greater likelihood of successful smoking cessation.

continued on page 291

Continued

WHY-DO-YOU-SMOKE TEST

QUESTION	ALWAYS	FREQUENTLY	OCCASIONALLY	SELDOM	NEVER
A. I smoke in order to keep myself from slowing down.	5	4	3	2	1
B. Handling a cigarette is part of the enjoyment of smoking it.	5	4	3	2	1
C. Smoking is pleasant and relaxing.	5	4	3	2	1
D. I light up when I feel angry about something.	5	4	3	2	1
E. When I have run out of cigarettes, I find it almost unbearable until I can get them.	5	4	3	2	1
F. I smoke automatically without even being aware of it.	5	4	3	2	1
G. I smoke to stimulate myself, to perk myself up.	5	4	3	2	1
H. Part of the enjoyment of cigarettes comes from the steps I take to light up.	5	4	3	2	1
I. I find cigarettes pleasurable.	5	4	3	2	1
J. When I feel uncomfortable or upset about something, I light up.	5	4	3	2	1
K. I am very much aware of the act when I am not smoking.	5	4	3	2	1
L. I light up without realizing I still have one burning in the ashtray.	5	4	3	2	1
M. I smoke to give myself a "lift."	5	4	3	2	1
N. When I smoke, part of the enjoyment is watching the smoke as I exhale it.	5	4	3	2	1
O. I want a cigarette most when I am comfortable and relaxed.	5	4	3	2	1
P. When I feel "blue" or want to take my mind off cares and worries, I smoke.	5	4	3	2	1
Q. I get a real gnawing hunger for a cigarette when I haven't smoked for a while.	5	4	3	2	1
R. I've found a cigarette in my mouth and didn't remember putting it there.	5	4	3	2	1

SCORING

Enter the number you circled on the test questions in the spaces provided below, putting the number you circled to question A on line A, to question B on line B, etc. Add the three scores on each line to get a total for each factor. For example, the sum of your scores over lines A, G, and M gives the score on "Stimulation"; lines B, H, and N give the score on "Handling," etc. Scores can vary between 3 and 15. Any score above 11 is high; any score 7 and below is low and indicates greater likelihood for successful smoking cessation.

```
A _____ + G _____ + M _____ = _____ Stimulation
B _____ + H _____ + N _____ = _____ Handling
C _____ + I _____ + O _____ = _____ Pleasure relaxation
D _____ + J _____ + P _____ = _____ Crutch: tension reduction
E _____ + K _____ + Q _____ = _____ Craving: psychologic addiction
F _____ + L _____ + R _____ = _____ Habit
```

From A self-test for smokers. U.S. Department of Health and Human Services, 1983.

Carbon Dioxide Transport As Bicarbonate

Carbon dioxide in solution slowly combines with water to form carbonic acid in the following reversible reaction:

$$CO_2 + H_2O \longleftrightarrow H_2CO_3$$

Little carbon dioxide transport as carbonic acid would occur without **carbonic anhydrase**, a zinc-containing enzyme within the red blood cell. One mole of this catalyst accelerates the union of a mole of carbon dioxide and water to a rate of about 800,000 times a second, or 5000 times faster than without enzymatic action. The reaction attains equilibrium as the blood cell moves through the tissue's capillary.

Once carbonic acid forms in the tissues, most of it ionizes into hydrogen ions (H^+) and bicarbonate ions (HCO_3^-) as follows:

In tissues

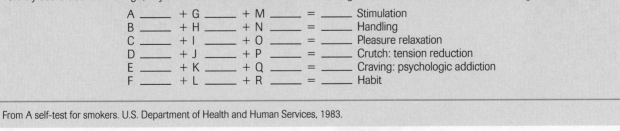

$$CO_2 + H_2O \xrightarrow{\text{carbonic anhydrase}}$$
$$H_2CO_3 \rightarrow H^+ + HCO_3^-$$

Buffering of the H^+ by the protein portion of hemoglobin maintains blood pH within relatively narrow limits (see "Acid-Base Regulation," Chapter 14). The HCO_3^- remains soluble, so it diffuses from the red blood cell into plasma. There it exchanges for a chloride ion (Cl^-) that moves into the blood cell to maintain ionic equilibrium. This phenomenon, termed the **chloride shift**, increases the Cl^- content of erythrocytes in venous blood more than in arterial red blood cells, particularly during exercise.

*Sixty to 80% of the total carbon dioxide exists as **plasma bicarbonate***. Bicarbonate forms in accordance with the law of mass action; carbonic acid formation accelerates as tissue P_{CO_2} increases. Plasma P_{CO_2} lowers as carbon dioxide leaves the blood via the lungs. This disturbs the equilibrium between carbonic acid and bicarbonate ion formation. The H^+ and HCO_3^- recombine to form carbonic acid. In turn, carbon dioxide and water re-form and carbon dioxide exits through the lungs as follows:

In lungs
$$H^+ + HCO_3^- \rightarrow H_2CO_3$$
$$\xrightarrow{\text{carbonic anhydrase}} CO_2 + H_2O$$

The Cl^- moves from the red blood cell back into the plasma because plasma HCO_3^- decreases in the pulmonary capillaries.

Carbon Dioxide Transport As Carbamino Compounds

At the tissue level, **carbamino compounds** form when carbon dioxide reacts directly with the amino acid molecules of blood proteins. The globin portion of hemoglobin, which carries about 20% of the body's carbon dioxide, forms a carbamino compound as follows:

$$CO_2 + \quad HbNH \quad \longrightarrow \quad HbNHCOOH$$
$$\text{(Hemoglobin)} \qquad \text{(Carbaminohemoglobin)}$$

Carbamino formation reverses as the plasma P_{CO_2} decreases in the lungs. This causes carbon dioxide to move into solution and enter the alveoli. Concurrently, oxygenation of hemoglobin reduces its ability to bind carbon dioxide. The interaction between oxygen loading and carbon dioxide release, termed the **Haldane effect** after English biologist J. S. Haldane (1860–1936), facilitates carbon dioxide removal in the lung.

Summary

1. About 5% of carbon dioxide travels in the plasma as free carbon dioxide in physical solution. Dissolved carbon dioxide establishes the P_{CO_2} of the blood, which modulates important physiologic functions.
2. The major quantity of carbon dioxide (80%) transports in chemical combination with water to form bicarbonate as follows:

$$CO_2 + H_2O \longrightarrow H_2CO_3 \longrightarrow H^+ + HCO_3^-$$

   In the lungs, the reaction reverses and carbon dioxide exits the blood into the alveoli.
3. About 20% of the body's carbon dioxide combines with blood proteins, including hemoglobin, to form carbamino compounds.

References are available on the Student CD and online at http://connection.lww.com/mkk6e.

Dynamics of Pulmonary Ventilation

14

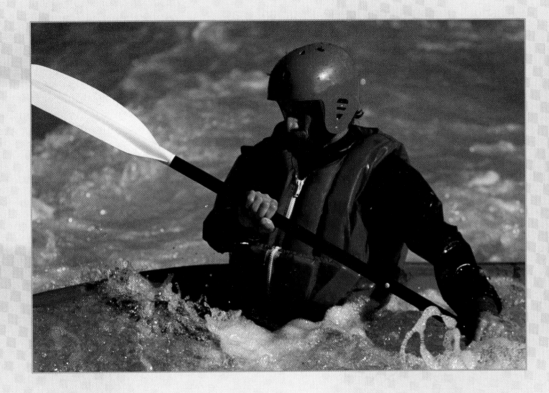

CHAPTER OBJECTIVES

- Describe how the hypothalamic neural command center controls pulmonary ventilation

- Identify major chemical and nonchemical factors that regulate pulmonary ventilation during rest and exercise

- Describe how hyperventilation extends breath-holding time but also poses a danger in sport diving

- Outline the dynamic phases of minute ventilation at the onset, early phase, and late stage of moderate exercise and recovery

- Graph the relationships among pulmonary ventilation, blood lactate, and oxygen consumption during incremental exercise, indicating the point of onset of blood lactate accumulation (OBLA)

- Explain the increase in ventilatory equivalent during the transition from steady-rate to non–steady-rate exercise

- Give the rationale for blood lactate threshold or OBLA rather than $\dot{V}O_{2max}$ to predict endurance performance

- Quantify the energy cost of breathing during rest and strenuous exercise in health and pulmonary disease

- Describe the acute effects of cigarette smoking on heart rate and energy cost of breathing during exercise

- Outline endurance training adaptations in pulmonary ventilation during submaximal and maximal exercise

- Discuss pros and cons to the argument that pulmonary ventilation represents the "weak link" in oxygen supply during maximal exercise

- Summarize how chemical and physiologic buffer systems regulate acid–base quality of body fluids during rest and exercise

PART 1 • *Regulation of Pulmonary Ventilation*

VENTILATORY CONTROL

Complex mechanisms exquisitely adjust breathing rate and depth in response to metabolic needs. Intricate neural circuits relay information from higher brain centers, the lungs, and other sensors throughout the body to coordinate ventilatory control.[7,64] The gaseous and chemical states of the blood that bathes the medulla and aortic and carotid artery chemoreceptors also mediate alveolar ventilation. In healthy individuals, these control mechanisms maintain relatively constant alveolar (and arterial) gas pressures throughout a broad range of exercise intensities. FIGURE 14.1 presents a schematic view of the input for ventilatory control.

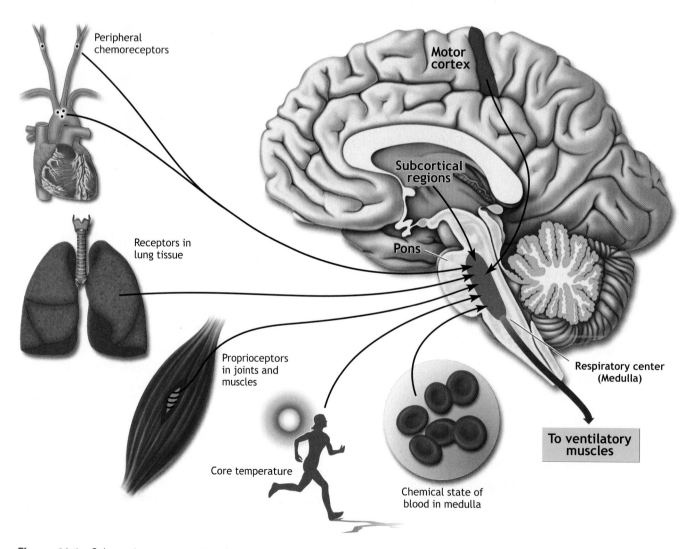

Figure 14.1   Schematic representation of factors that affect medullary control of pulmonary ventilation.

Neural Factors

The inherent activity of inspiratory neurons with cell bodies located in the medial portion of the **medulla** governs the normal respiratory cycle. These neurons activate the diaphragm and intercostal muscles causing the lungs to inflate. The inspiratory neurons cease firing because of self-limitations and the inhibitory influence of expiratory neurons also located in the medulla. Inhibitory and excitatory signals from throughout the body influence the normal rhythm of medullary neurons. For example, lung inflation stimulates stretch receptors, mainly in the bronchioles. These receptors act through afferent fibers to inhibit inspiration and stimulate expiration. As the inspiratory muscles relax, passive recoil of the stretched lung tissue and raised ribs produces exhalation. Activation of expiratory neurons and associated muscles that facilitate expiration synchronize with this passive phase. As expiration proceeds, the inspiratory center becomes progressively less inhibited and once again becomes active.

Inherent activity of the respiratory center alone cannot account for the smooth pattern of ventilatory adjustment to metabolic demands. A neural center in the hypothalamus integrates input from descending neurons in the higher locomotor areas of the cerebral hemispheres, the pons, and other brain regions to affect the duration and intensity of the inspiratory cycle. Simultaneously, ascending neural signals initiated by mechanical and/or chemical changes within active muscles and its vasculature provide peripheral feedback control from the cerebellum to the respiratory center to modulate ventilatory adjustments to exercise.

The lungs contain sensory receptors that communicate with the respiratory center through vagal nerve afferents. These receptors initiate a cough reflex when activated by various irritants. Irritation of the tracheal or bronchial mucosa by dust, air pollutants, cigarette smoke, noxious fumes, inhaled debris, or accumulated mucus promotes coughing, while the same irritants in the nasal cavity trigger sneezing. Both reflexes help keep the airways clear because bronchial irritation often constricts these conduits.

Humoral Factors

At rest, the chemical state of the blood exerts the greatest control of pulmonary ventilation. Variations in arterial P_{O_2}, P_{CO_2}, pH, and temperature activate sensitive neural units in the medulla and arterial system to adjust ventilation and maintain arterial blood chemistry within narrow limits.

Plasma Po_2 and Peripheral Chemoreceptors

Inhaling a gas mixture with 80% oxygen greatly increases alveolar P_{O_2} and reduces minute ventilation by 20%. Conversely, ventilation increases if the inspired oxygen concentration decreases below ambient levels, particularly if alveolar P_{O_2} falls below 60 mm Hg. Hemoglobin saturation at this P_{O_2} begins to decrease considerably (see Fig. 13.4).

Sensitivity to reduced oxygen pressure does not reside in the respiratory center. Instead, peripheral **chemoreceptors** provide the primary site to detect arterial hypoxia and reflexly initiate a ventilatory response.[53] FIGURE 14.2 shows these specialized neurons weighing only a few milligrams located in the arch of the aorta and branching of the carotid arteries in the neck. The strategic positioning of the **carotid bodies** monitors the state of arterial blood just before it perfuses the brain. Decreased arterial P_{O_2}, as occurs in pulmonary disease or ascent to high altitude, increases alveolar ventilation because of aortic and carotid chemoreceptor stimulation. These receptors *alone* protect the organism against reduced oxygen pressure in inspired air.

Peripheral chemoreceptor afferents also stimulate ventilation in exercise, even though reductions in arterial P_{O_2} do not normally occur.[49,51] The stimulating effects of exercise on carotid afferent chemoreceptor discharge mainly comes from increases in temperature, acidity, and carbon dioxide and potassium concentrations.[22,70]

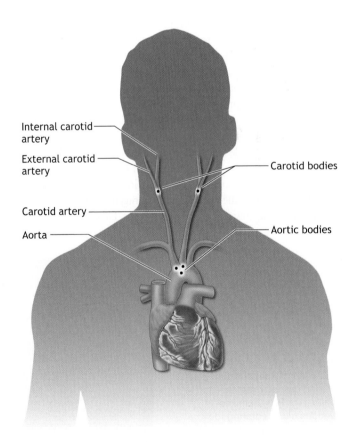

Internal carotid artery
External carotid artery
Carotid artery
Aorta
Carotid bodies
Aortic bodies

Figure 14.2 The aortic arch and bifurcation of the carotid arteries contain cell bodies sensitive to reduced P_{O_2} and increased P_{CO_2} and H^+ and potassium concentrations in arterial blood. The peripheral chemoreceptors defend the body against arterial hypoxia in pulmonary disease and ascent to high altitude. The chemoreceptors also help to regulate exercise hyperpnea through the stimulating effects of increased arterial carbon dioxide and H^+ concentrations.

Plasma Pco₂ and H⁺ Concentration

At rest, carbon dioxide pressure in arterial plasma provides the most important respiratory stimulus. Small increases in P_{CO_2} in inspired air trigger large increases in minute ventilation. For example, the resting ventilation nearly doubles by increasing inspired P_{CO_2} to just 1.7 mm Hg (0.22% CO_2 in inspired air).

Molecular carbon dioxide per se does not mediate the ventilatory response to arterial P_{CO_2}. Instead, plasma acidity, which varies directly with the blood's carbon dioxide content, exerts significant command over minute ventilation. A fall in blood pH signals acidosis and usually reflects carbon dioxide retention and subsequent carbonic acid formation. Lactate accumulation in strenuous exercise or fatty acid (ketone) accumulation in diabetes also can decrease blood pH. Regardless of cause, as arterial pH declines and hydrogen ions accumulate, inspiratory activity increases to eliminate carbon dioxide and reduce arterial levels of carbonic acid (see Chapter 13).

Hyperventilation and Breath Holding

If a person breath holds after a normal exhalation, it takes approximately 40 seconds before the urge to breathe strengthens enough to initiate inspiration. The stimulus to breathe comes primarily from increased arterial P_{CO_2} and H⁺ concentration, *not* decreased P_{O_2} in the breath-holding condition. The break point for breath holding corresponds to an increase in arterial P_{CO_2} to approximately 50 mm Hg.

If one consciously increases ventilation above the normal level (**hyperventilation**) before breath holding, alveolar air composition becomes more like ambient air. Alveolar P_{CO_2} decreases from its normal value of 40 mm Hg to a low of 15 mm Hg. This creates a considerable diffusion gradient for carbon dioxide runoff into the alveoli from venous blood that enters the pulmonary capillaries. Consequently, a larger-than-normal quantity of carbon dioxide leaves the blood and arterial P_{CO_2} decreases. Hyperventilation extends breath-holding duration until arterial P_{CO_2} and/or H⁺ concentration rises to levels that again stimulate the urge to breathe.

Swimmers and divers use hyperventilation and subsequent breath holding to improve performance. In sprint swimming, it is mechanically undesirable to roll the body and turn the head during the stroke's breathing phase. To avoid this pitfall, many sprinters hyperventilate on the starting blocks to prolong the breath-hold during the swim. In sport diving, hyperventilation offers a similar effect—to extend breath-holding time. In diving, however, extended breath holding from hyperventilation can be tragic. As the length and depth of a dive increase, the blood's oxygen content decreases to a critically low level before arterial P_{CO_2} rises enough to stimulate breathing and signal ascent. This can cause the diver to lose consciousness before surfacing. Chapter 26 discusses hyperventilation and other factors important to sport diving.

REGULATION OF VENTILATION DURING EXERCISE

Chemical Control

Neither chemical stimulation nor any other single mechanism entirely accounts for the increase in ventilation (hyperpnea) in physical activity. For example, the classic feedback control of resting ventilation via oxygen- and carbon dioxide–mediated mechanisms does not adequately explain exercise hyperpnea. Inducing maximum changes in plasma acidity and inspired P_{O_2} and P_{CO_2} does not increase minute ventilation to values during vigorous exercise.

FIGURE 14.3 illustrates the relationship between oxygen consumption during graded exercise and venous and alveolar P_{CO_2} and alveolar P_{O_2}. As exercise intensity increases, alveolar (arterial) P_{O_2} does not decrease to an extent that increases

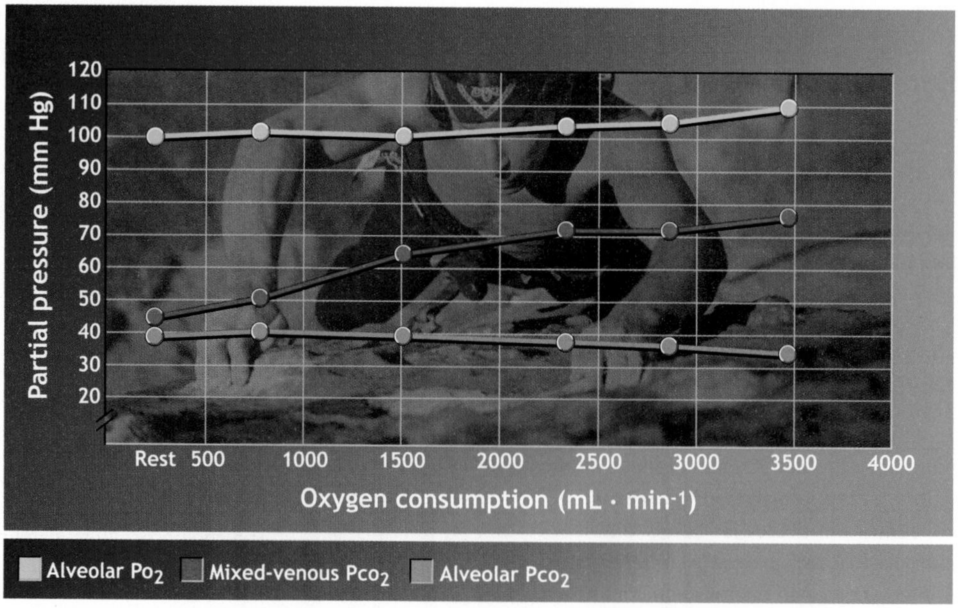

Figure 14.3 Relationship between oxygen consumption during graded exercise and (1) values for P_{CO_2} in mixed-venous blood entering the lungs and (2) alveolar P_{O_2} and P_{CO_2}. Alveolar P_{O_2} and P_{CO_2} remain near resting levels throughout a broad range of exercise intensities, despite relatively large increases in mixed-venous P_{CO_2}. (Data from the Laboratory of Applied Physiology, Queens College, Flushing, NY.)

■ Alveolar P$_{O_2}$ ■ Mixed-venous P$_{CO_2}$ ■ Alveolar P$_{CO_2}$

ventilation through chemoreceptor stimulation. In fact, the large ventilatory volumes during intense exercise cause alveolar PO_2 to rise *above* the average resting value of 100 mm Hg. Any increase in alveolar PO_2 in exercise hastens oxygenation of blood in the alveolar capillaries. Pulmonary ventilation during light and moderate exercise closely couples with metabolism in a manner proportional to oxygen consumption and carbon dioxide production. Under these conditions, alveolar (and arterial) PCO_2 generally averages 40 mm Hg. During strenuous exercise with its relatively large anaerobic component (lactate accumulation) increased carbon dioxide and subsequent H^+ concentrations provide an additional ventilatory stimulus. The resulting hyperventilation *reduces* alveolar and arterial PCO_2, sometimes as low as 25 mm Hg. Any reduction in arterial PCO_2 decreases the ventilatory drive from carbon dioxide during exercise.

On the basis of alterations in alveolar and arterial gas pressures during exercise, one might question how peripheral chemoreceptors exert their influence on exercise ventilation. A possible explanation considers the pattern of ventilation that causes alveolar–capillary PCO_2 to reach slightly lower values at the end of inhalation and higher values at the end of exhalation. Average levels of arterial oxygen, carbon dioxide, and pH remain well regulated during moderate exercise, yet the chemoreceptors may detect cyclic plasma oscillations in these variables during breathing to influence exercise ventilation. Any increase in chemoreceptor sensitivity also facilitates chemoreceptor control of exercise ventilation. Slow-conducting afferent fibers may sense local distension of the vascular network at the venular level of the active muscle. This regulatory system could "anticipate" chemical changes in arterial blood and minimize them by adjusting alveolar ventilation to the level of muscle perfusion.[26]

Nonchemical Control

The rapidity of the ventilatory response at the onset and cessation of exercise suggests that input other than from a change in arterial PCO_2 and H^+ concentration mediates these phases of exercise hyperpnea.

Neurogenic Factors

Neurogenic factors for ventilatory control include cortical and peripheral influences.

- *Cortical influence:* Neural outflow from regions of the motor cortex and cortical activation in anticipation of exercise stimulate respiratory neurons in the medulla to initiate the abrupt increase in exercise ventilation.
- *Peripheral influence:* Sensory input from joints, tendons, and muscles influences the ventilatory adjustments throughout exercise. Experiments involving passive limb movements, electrical muscle stimulation, and voluntary exercise with the muscle's blood flow occluded support the contribution of local mechanoreceptors and chemoreceptors to a reflex exercise hyperpnea.

Influence of Temperature

Except for extreme hyperthermia, an increase in body temperature exerts little effect on ventilatory regulation during exercise. In most exercise conditions, the rise in ventilation at exercise onset and its decline during recovery occurs too quickly to reflect control from core temperature changes.

Integrated Regulation

During Exercise

The combined and perhaps simultaneous effects of several chemical and neural stimuli initiate and modulate exercise alveolar ventilation. FIGURE 14.4 shows the dynamic phases of minute ventilation during moderate exercise and recovery. In **phase I** at the start of exercise, neurogenic stimuli from the cerebral cortex (**central command**), combined with feedback from the active limbs, stimulate the medulla to increase ventilation abruptly. Cortical and locomotor peripheral input continues throughout the exercise period. After a short plateau (approximately 20 s), minute ventilation then rises exponentially (in **phase II**) to reach a steady level related to the demands for metabolic gas exchange. Central command input, including factors intrinsic to neurons of the respiratory control system, regulates this phase of exercise ventilation. Continued activity

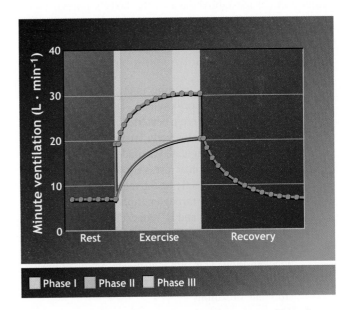

Figure 14.4 Three phases of exercise hyperpnea. *Phase I:* rapid increase from rest and brief plateau from central command drive and input from active muscles. *Phase II:* slower exponential rise begins approximately 20 seconds after exercise onset. Central command continues, along with feedback from active muscles plus the added effect of short-term potentiation of respiratory neurons. *Phase III:* major regulatory mechanisms reach stable values; added input from peripheral chemoreceptors fine-tunes the ventilatory response. The *lower graph* (red curve) depicts the contribution of central neuronal short-term potentiation and rising arterial H^+ concentration to the respiratory response. (Modified from Eldridge FL. Central integration of mechanisms in exercise hyperpnea. Med Sci Sports Exerc 1994;26:319.)

of respiratory neurons in the medulla causes short-term potentiation that augments their responsiveness to the same continuing stimulation. This brings minute ventilation to a new, higher level. In all likelihood, input from peripheral chemoreceptors in the carotid bodies also contributes to regulation during phase II.[70] The final phase of control (**phase III**) involves fine-tuning of the steady-state ventilation through peripheral sensory feedback mechanisms. Central and reflex stimuli from main byproducts of increased muscle metabolism—carbon dioxide and H^+ concentration—modulate alveolar gas pressures in this phase. These factors stimulate chemoreceptor group IV unmyelinated neurons that communicate with regions of the central nervous system to regulate cardiorespiratory function.[50] The lactate anion itself, apart from lactic acidosis, contributes an additional stimulus to increase ventilation in strenuous exercise.[27] Reflexes related to pulmonary blood flow and mechanical movement of the lung and respiratory muscles also provide regulatory input during exercise.

In Recovery

The abrupt decline in ventilation when exercise ceases reflects removal of both the central command drive and the sensory input from previously active muscles. More than likely, the slower recovery phase results from (1) gradual diminution of the short-term potentiation of the respiratory center and (2) reestablishment of the body's normal metabolic, thermal, and chemical milieu.

Summary

1. Inherent activity of neurons in the medulla regulates the normal respiratory cycle.
2. Input from higher brain centers, the lungs, and other sensors throughout the body interacts with medullary neural output to regulate ventilation.
3. Alveolar ventilation at rest is controlled by chemical factors that act directly on the respiratory center or modify its activity through peripheral chemoreceptors. Arterial PCO_2 and H^+ concentration are the most important regulatory factors.
4. Hyperventilation lowers arterial PCO_2 and H^+ concentration. This prolongs breath-holding time until levels of carbon dioxide and acidity increase to stimulate breathing.
5. Three nonchemical regulatory factors augment ventilatory adjustments to exercise: (1) cortical activation in anticipation of exercise and outflow from the motor cortex when exercise begins, (2) peripheral sensory input from chemoreceptors and mechanoreceptors in joints and muscles, and (3) increased body temperature.
6. The ventilatory response to exercise occurs in three phases. Phase I cortical stimulus plus feedback for active limbs causes the abrupt increase in ventilation as exercise begins. Phase II ventilation then rises exponentially to reach a steady level related to

exercise demands. Phase III involves fine-tuning of steady-state ventilation through peripheral sensory feedback mechanisms.

PART 2 • *Pulmonary Ventilation During Exercise*

VENTILATION AND ENERGY DEMANDS

Physical activity affects oxygen consumption and carbon dioxide production more than any other physiologic stress. With exercise, oxygen diffuses from the alveoli into the venous blood as it returns to the lungs, while about the same quantity of carbon dioxide moves from the blood into the alveoli. Concurrently, increased alveolar ventilation maintains the proper gas concentrations to facilitate rapid gas exchange.

Ventilation in Steady-Rate Exercise

FIGURE 14.5 relates oxygen consumption and minute ventilation during increasing levels of exercise up to maximal oxygen consumption ($\dot{V}O_{2max}$). During light-to-moderate exercise, ventilation increases *linearly* with oxygen consumption and carbon dioxide production, averaging between 20 and 25 L of air for each liter of oxygen consumed. Ventilation, in this case, increases mainly through increases in tidal volume; at higher exercise intensities, breathing frequency takes on a more important role. Such ventilatory adjustments provide complete aeration of blood because alveolar PO_2 and PCO_2 remain near resting levels. Transit time for blood in the pulmonary capillaries remains long enough for complete equilibration of the lung–blood gases (see Fig. 13.2).

The term **ventilatory equivalent** (symbolized $\dot{V}_E/\dot{V}O_2$) describes the ratio of minute ventilation to oxygen consumption. Healthy young adults usually maintain this ratio at 25 (i.e., 25 L of air breathed per liter of O_2 consumed) during submaximal exercise up to approximately 55% of the $\dot{V}O_{2max}$. Higher ventilatory equivalents occur in children, with values averaging 32 L of air breathed per liter of O_2 consumed. Exercise mode also affects the ventilatory equivalent. Prone swimming, for example, generates lower $\dot{V}_E/\dot{V}O_2$ ratios than running at all levels of energy expenditure. The restrictive nature of swimming on breathing lowers the ventilatory equivalent; this could constrain adequate gas exchange at maximal swimming velocities and partly explain the lower $\dot{V}O_{2max}$ during swimming than during running.

Ventilation in Non–Steady-Rate Exercise

At higher levels of progressively more intense submaximal exercise, minute ventilation moves sharply upward and increases disproportionately in relation to oxygen consumption.

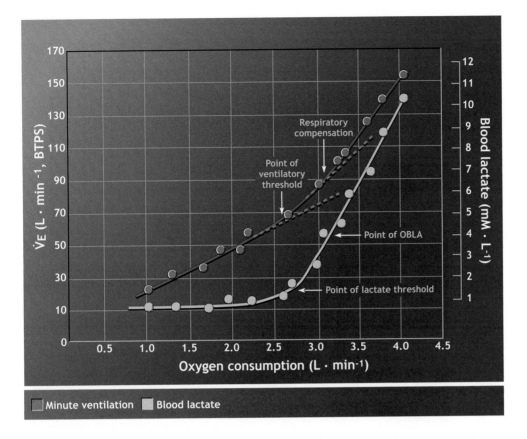

Figure 14.5 Pulmonary ventilation, blood lactate concentration, and oxygen consumption during graded exercise to maximum. The *dashed line* extrapolates the linear relationship between $\dot{V}_E$ and $\dot{V}O_2$ during submaximal exercise. The lactate threshold (not necessarily the threshold for anaerobic metabolism) represents the highest exercise intensity (oxygen consumption) not associated with elevated blood lactate concentration. It occurs at the point at which the relationship between $\dot{V}_E$ and $\dot{V}O_2$ deviates from linearity, indicated as the point of ventilatory threshold. OBLA represents the point of lactate increase just above a 4.0-mM baseline. Respiratory compensation represents a further increase in ventilation to counter the decrease in plasma pH in heavy exercise.

Ventilatory Threshold

The term **ventilatory threshold (V_T)** describes the point at which pulmonary ventilation increases disproportionately with oxygen consumption during graded exercise (see Fig. 14.5 and "In a Practical Sense," p. 303). At this exercise intensity, pulmonary ventilation no longer links tightly to oxygen demand at the cellular level. In fact, the "excess" ventilation (related to oxygen consumed) comes directly from carbon dioxide's increased output from buffering lactate that begins to accumulate from increased anaerobic glycolysis. Sodium bicarbonate in the blood buffers almost all of the lactate generated in anaerobic metabolism to sodium lactate in the following reaction:

$$Lactic\ acid + NaHCO_3 \longrightarrow Na\ Lactate + H_2CO_3$$
$$\Updownarrow$$
$$H_2O + CO_2$$

The excess nonmetabolic carbon dioxide released in the buffering reaction stimulates pulmonary ventilation that disproportionately increases $\dot{V}_E/\dot{V}O_2$. Additional carbon dioxide exhaled from acid buffering causes the respiratory exchange ratio (R; $\dot{V}CO_2/\dot{V}O_2$) to exceed 1.00. Traditionally, researchers believed that the disproportionate increase in $\dot{V}_E$ and

increase in R above 1.00 indicated that the oxygen demands of the active muscles exceeded mitochondrial oxygen supply with a resulting increase in anaerobic energy transfer. They maintained that $\dot{V}_T$ indicated the *threshold* for anaerobiosis and termed it the anaerobic threshold, or simply A_T, to indicate reliance on anaerobic glycolysis (see "Focus on Research," p. 301). FIGURE 14.6 outlines the underlying factors related to A_T detected from pulmonary gas exchange dynamics during graded exercise.

Attempts to validate a linkage between ventilatory changes and glycolytic events at the cellular level have proved elusive. Nevertheless, the ventilatory and anaerobic threshold concepts to target endurance exercise performance and physiologic responses to exercise and their changes over time remains popular and justifiable.[3]

Onset of Blood Lactate Accumulation

Researchers directly measure lactate's appearance in muscle and blood rather than ventilatory markers (such as $\dot{V}_T$) to indicate anaerobic metabolic events. During steady-rate exercise, aerobic metabolism matches the energy requirements of the active muscles. Little or no blood lactate accumulates because any lactate production equals lactate disappearance. *The term **lactate threshold** describes the highest oxygen consumption or exercise intensity achieved with less than a 1.0 mM increase in blood lactate concentra-*

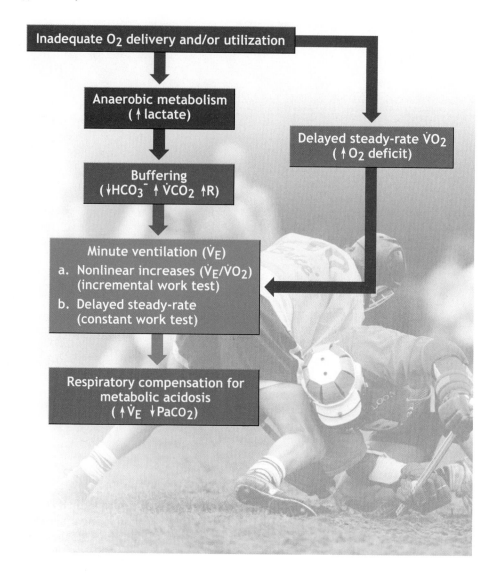

Figure 14.6 Factors that relate to pulmonary gas exchange dynamics for detecting the lactate threshold.

tion above the preexercise level.[67] By convention, blood lactate concentration is usually expressed in millimoles (mM) per liter of whole blood or as mg per dL^{-1} of whole blood, also termed volume percent (vol%); 1.0 mM equals 9.0 vol%.

Onset of blood lactate accumulation (**OBLA**) signifies when blood lactate concentration systematically increases to 4.0 mM.[58,67] The terms *lactate threshold* and *OBLA* are used interchangeably, although each represents an operationally different precise point for exercise intensity and blood lactate level. The 4.0-mM value for OBLA implies the maximum exercise intensity that a person can sustain for a prolonged duration. In reality, this maximum stable lactate level shows considerable variability among individuals.[15]

INTEGRATIVE QUESTION

In what ways are the terms *lactate threshold* and *onset of blood lactate accumulation* biochemically more precise than *anaerobic threshold*?

The exact cause of OBLA remains controversial. Some researchers assume that it represents a distinct point for the onset of muscle anaerobiosis. However, blood lactate values do not always reflect the lactate concentration in specific muscles. Lactate may accumulate not only from muscle anaerobiosis, but also from decreased total lactate clearance or increased lactate production in specific muscle fibers. A threshold of lactate appearance could result from (1) imbalance between the rate of glycolysis and mitochondrial respiration, (2) decreased redox potential (increased NADH relative to NAD^+), (3) lower blood oxygen content, or (4) lower blood flow to skeletal muscle. Caution should temper interpretations of the specific metabolic significance (and cause) of OBLA. It probably does signify initiation of an exponential accumulation of lactate in active muscle.[36]

Blood lactate accumulation reflects plasma changes in pH, bicarbonate and H^+ concentrations, and carbon dioxide production via buffering, so these variables provide an indirect assessment of OBLA.[37,38,65] Changes in these measures do indeed relate to OBLA, but they probably cannot serve independently to establish the onset of anaerobic metabolism in

FOCUS On Research

DETECTING THE ONSET OF ANAEROBIC METABOLISM

Wasserman K, McIlroy MB. Detecting the threshold of anaerobic metabolism in cardiac patients during exercise. Am J Cardiol 1964;14:844.

▲ The onset of anaerobiosis during exercise powerfully predicts a person's capability for sustained aerobic exercise. The pioneering work of Wasserman and colleagues presented their rationale and methodology with simple respiratory gas exchange data to detect the threshold of anaerobic metabolism; they named this point the "anaerobic threshold." These researchers argued that one could detect the threshold of anaerobic metabolism during exercise in one of three ways: (1) increased blood lactate concentration, (2) decreased arterial blood bicarbonate and pH, and (3) increased respiratory gas exchange ratio (R). A method that assesses R avoids blood-sampling procedures while using equipment common to exercise physiology, human performance, and medically related facilities.

Subjects performed a graded exercise test by either pedaling a cycle ergometer or walking on a treadmill for 4-minute exercise intervals. Measurements included heart rate, minute ventilation, oxygen consumption, and end-tidal CO_2 and N_2 concentrations. End-tidal oxygen and carbon dioxide concentrations provided data for computing R. The *upper figure* shows a sigmoid curve resulting from plotting R from the last 30 seconds of each exercise level against $\dot{V}O_2$. The inflection point at the onset of the steepest part of this curve, called by these researchers the *threshold* of anaerobic metabolism, indicated to them the $\dot{V}O_2$ level at which anaerobic metabolism became significant. The anaerobic threshold also corresponded to the exercise intensity at which arterial blood bicarbonate concentrations decreased and blood lactate increased.

The *lower figure* displays the anaerobic threshold data for 37 patients with heart disease. Subjects with the poorest fitness attained anaerobic threshold at a lower $\dot{V}O_2$ (i.e., lower exercise intensity). From a clinical perspective, the respiratory exchange ratio during exercise provides a useful measure of cardiovascular function to indicate how much exercise a patient performs before cardiovascular dynamics fail to meet the tissues' oxygen requirements. Current research indicates that factors other than the onset of exercise anaerobiosis affect

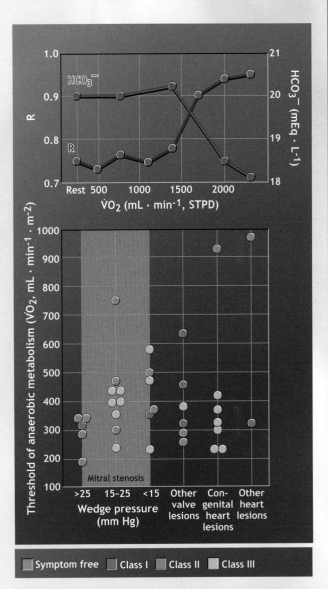

Top. Respiratory exchange ratio (R) and plasma bicarbonate (HCO_3^-) during rest and continuous graded exercise in one subject. *Bottom.* Threshold for anaerobic metabolism in 37 heart disease patients.

pulmonary and gas exchange dynamics. The initial research of Wasserman and coworkers, however, provided an important impetus to study interactions among pulmonary, cardiovascular, and metabolic dynamics during graded exercise.

muscle. Even if metabolic events and ventilatory dynamics in exercise do not relate causally, practical information about exercise performance results from these indirect evaluation procedures. "In a Practical Sense," p. 303 illustrates several common methods to indicate tissue hypoxia and an imbalance between lactate formation and its clearance during exercise.

Specificity of OBLA. Exercise task specificity characterizes OBLA, as it does many measures of physiologic function and exercise performance. Differences in OBLA relative to the level of oxygen consumption occur in comparing bicycle, treadmill, and arm-crank exercise.[71] These differences can be attributed to variations in muscle mass activated in each form of exercise. At a particular exercise intensity or submaximal oxygen consumption, a higher metabolic rate per unit of active muscle mass exists for arm-crank and bicycle exercise than treadmill walking or running. Therefore, OBLA occurs at a lower exercise level (oxygen consumption) during bicycling and arm-crank exercise. *Different exercise modes cannot interchangeably define the point of OBLA during graded exercise testing.*

Some Independence Between OBLA and $\dot{V}O_{2max}$. Chapter 7 indicated that blood lactate in trained individuals accumulates at higher submaximal oxygen consumptions and at higher percentages of $\dot{V}O_{2max}$ than in untrained individuals. For children and adults, endurance training often improves the exercise intensity at OBLA *without* concomitant increases in $\dot{V}O_{2max}$.[5,18,39,42] This indicates that different factors influence OBLA and $\dot{V}O_{2max}$. Muscle fiber type, capillary density, mitochondrial size and number, and enzyme concentrations play major roles in establishing the percentage of aerobic capacity sustainable without lactate accumulation.[13,34,66] In contrast, the functional capacity of the cardiovascular system for oxygen transport and the total muscle mass activated in exercise determine the $\dot{V}O_{2max}$.

A unique comparison among trained and untrained cardiac patients and trained healthy counterparts demonstrated the lack of close association between aerobic capacity and OBLA. The patients showed impaired cardiac function (i.e., a blunted capacity for maximal blood flow) that lowered $\dot{V}O_{2max}$ below levels attained by healthy individuals. However, trained patients could run at the same speed (and achieve essentially the same endurance performance) as healthy individuals, without accumulating blood lactate. FIGURE 14.7 shows these patients maintained a near-metabolic steady rate while running at a speed that elicited $\dot{V}O_{2max}$. In fact, the point of OBLA represented 100% of $\dot{V}O_{2max}$.

OBLA and Endurance Performance. FIGURE 14.8 illustrates the major variables that contribute to oxygen transport and use. They ultimately determine the maximum intensity a person can maintain in prolonged exercise. Two important factors influence endurance performance in a specific exercise mode:

1. Maximum capacity to consume oxygen ($\dot{V}O_{2max}$)
2. Maximum level for steady-rate exercise (OBLA)

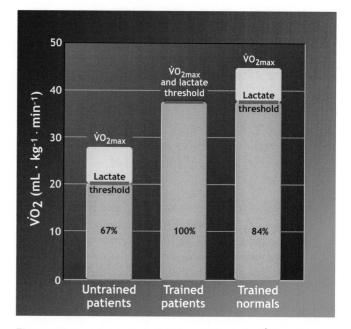

Figure 14.7 Lactate threshold in relation to the $\dot{V}O_{2max}$ in trained and untrained patients with coronary artery disease and in healthy, trained subjects. (Modified from Coyle EF, et al. Blood lactate threshold in some well-trained ischemic heart disease patients. J Appl Physiol 1983;54:18.)

Traditionally, exercise physiologists have used $\dot{V}O_{2max}$ as the yardstick to gauge capacity for endurance exercise. This measure generally relates to exercise performance, but it does not fully explain success because one does not perform endurance exercise at $\dot{V}O_{2max}$. *The exercise intensity at the point of OBLA consistently and powerfully predicts endurance exercise performance of men and women.*[8,16,48,61] For race-walkers, race-walking velocity at the point of OBLA predicted 20-km times to within 0.6% of the actual time.[25] Similar results occurred in elite cyclists. Cycling power output at lactate threshold showed a strong relationship ($r = 0.93$) to average absolute power output maintained during a 1-hour ride in the laboratory.[17] The laboratory measurement, in turn, accurately predicted performance in a 40-km road race. Improved endurance performance with training more closely relates to training-induced improvement in the exercise level for OBLA than to changes in $\dot{V}O_{2max}$.[72]

 INTEGRATIVE QUESTION

Give the rationale for measuring pulmonary ventilation and gas exchange dynamics during graded exercise to indicate the onset of lactate buildup at the cellular level.

Racial Differences. The overwhelming dominance of African athletes in competitive endurance running between 3000 and 10,000 m has stimulated research into the possibility of racial differences in resistance to fatigue, blood lactate accumulation, temperature regulation, and intramuscular

IN A PRACTICAL SENSE

MEASURING LACTATE THRESHOLD

■ Conceptually, the lactate threshold (LT) represents an exercise level (power output, $\dot{V}O_2$, or energy expenditure) where tissue hypoxia triggers an imbalance between lactate formation and its clearance, with a resulting increase in blood lactate concentration. All of the following terms refer essentially to the same LT phenomenon: *expiratory compensation threshold, anaerobic threshold, onset of blood lactate accumulation, optimal ventilatory efficiency, aerobic–anaerobic threshold, onset of plasma lactate accumulation, individual anaerobic threshold,* and *point of metabolic acidosis.*

The measurement of LT serves three important functions:

1. Provides a sensitive indicator of aerobic training status
2. Predicts endurance performance, often with greater accuracy than $\dot{V}O_{2max}$
3. Establishes an effective training intensity geared to the active muscles' aerobic metabolic dynamics

DIFFERENT INDICATORS OF LT

1. Fixed blood lactate concentration
2. Ventilatory threshold
3. Blood lactate–exercise $\dot{V}O_2$ response

1. FIXED BLOOD LACTATE CONCENTRATION

During low-intensity, steady-rate exercise, blood lactate concentration does not increase beyond normal biologic variation observed at rest. As exercise intensity increases, blood lactate levels exceed normal variation. Exercise intensity (or $\dot{V}O_2$) associated with a fixed blood lactate concentration that exceeds normal resting variation denotes the LT. This often coincides with a 2.5-millimole (mM) value. A 4.0-mM lactate value indicates the onset of blood lactate accumulation (OBLA). The *top figure* illustrates LT and OBLA computations from fixed blood lactate concentrations during incremental, 4-minute exercise stages on a bicycle ergometer. Interpolation from a visual plot of power output ($\dot{V}O_2$) versus blood lactate determines the exercise level associated with the fixed blood lactate con-

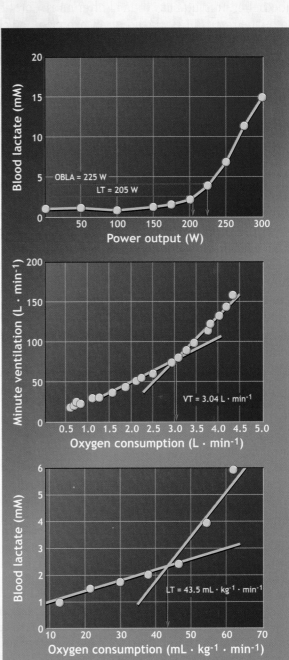

Top. Fixed blood lactate concentration method to determine lactate threshold (LT) and onset of blood lactate accumulation (OBLA). This example shows LT at a fixed blood lactate of 2.5 mM and OBLA at a fixed blood lactate of 4.0 mM. *Middle.* Determination of LT from the relationship between pulmonary minute ventilation and oxygen consumption during incremental exercise. *Bottom.* Determination of LT from relationship between blood lactate concentration and oxygen consumption during incremental exercise.

continued on page 304

Continued

centrations. The decision regarding stage duration, number of stages, and interval between stages becomes important. Stages 4 minutes or longer provide better predictability than shorter ones. For the data illustrated, LT occurred at an exercise power output of 205 W; 225 W predicted the fixed blood lactate concentration for OBLA.

2. VENTILATORY THRESHOLD

Pulmonary minute ventilation ($\dot{V}_E$) during exercise increases disproportionately in its relationship to oxygen consumption at about the same time blood lactate begins to accumulate. The ventilatory threshold (VT) predicts LT from the $\dot{V}_E$ response during graded exercise. The mechanistic link of lactate buffering by plasma bicarbonate to produce additional CO_2 (and respiratory stimulus unrelated to $\dot{V}O_2$) justifies the use of VT on a physiologic basis.

The test involves exercise with increments of short duration (a ramp test of 1- or 2-min increments) with continuous measurement of $\dot{V}_E$ (breath-by-breath or every 10, 20, or 30 s) to the point of fatigue (usually within 8 to 12 min). The point of nonlinear increase in $\dot{V}_E$ versus $\dot{V}O_2$ represents VT, expressed as a specific $\dot{V}O_2$ value rather than as running speed or power output common with the fixed blood lactate concentration method. The *middle figure* shows the relationship between $\dot{V}_E$ and $\dot{V}O_2$ during incremental exercise; VT occurs at an exercise $\dot{V}O_2$ of 3.04 L · min^{-1}. It is common to express the $\dot{V}O_2$ at LT as a percentage of $\dot{V}O_{2max}$ (71% in this example).

3. BLOOD LACTATE–EXERCISE $\dot{V}O_2$ RESPONSE

This protocol plots blood lactate concentration versus either $\dot{V}O_2$ or exercise intensity in a manner similar to determination of fixed blood lactate concentration. The person exercises for 3- or 4-minute increments on a bicycle ergometer or treadmill. With treadmill exercise, blood is sampled for lactate determination during a brief pause at the end of each stage, or without pause when using stationary cycling exercise. The *bottom figure* plots blood lactate versus oxygen consumption throughout the test. A best-fitting straight line depicts the linear portion of the curve; a second line describes the upward-trending curve after it "breaks" from linearity. The intersection of the two lines represents LT.

---

oxidative enzyme capacity. African and South African endurance runners consistently show greater resistance to fatigue at the same percentage of peak treadmill running velocity than Caucasian counterparts despite similar values for $\dot{V}O_{2max}$ and peak treadmill velocity.[12,67,68] The African athletes sustained a relatively higher percentage of maximal exercise capacity (i.e., superior fatigue resistance) from considerably higher oxidative enzyme profiles (citrate synthase and 3-hydroxyacyl-CoA dehydrogenase) and lower plasma lactate concentrations during sustained submaximal exercise.[57] In addition to a higher fractional use of $\dot{V}O_{2max}$, greater running economy probably contributes to superior endurance performance of elite African runners.[69] African runners also perform better in the heat than Caucasians, which partly contributes to their smaller size. This size "benefit" augments capacity to run faster in the heat while storing heat at the same rate as heavier Caucasian runners.[43]

 INTEGRATIVE QUESTION

What biochemical rationale exists for measuring oxygen consumption and carbon dioxide production to infer the onset of metabolic anaerobiosis (lactate accumulation) during exercise?

ENERGY COST OF BREATHING

FIGURE 14.9 specifies the oxygen cost of breathing during whole-body graded exercise up to maximum. The left panel indicates the effects of increasing minute ventilation on the oxygen cost of breathing expressed as a percentage of the total exercise oxygen consumption. The right panel illustrates the influence of increasing minute ventilation on the oxygen cost per liter of air breathed per minute. At rest and during light-to-moderate exercise, the oxygen requirement of breathing remains relatively small.[11] For exercise ventilations up to about 100 L · min^{-1}, oxygen cost averaged between 1.5 and 2.0 mL per liter of air breathed each minute (right panel). This represented from 3 to 5% of the total oxygen consumption in moderate exercise and 8 to 11% for minute ventilations at $\dot{V}O_{2max}$ values typical for most individuals (left panel). Among highly trained endurance athletes with maximum minute ventilations of 150 L · min^{-1} and higher, the cost of exercise hyperpnea can exceed 15% of the total oxygen consumption. At this level, the inspiratory muscles operate at 40 to 60% of maximum capacity to generate force.[1] The rate of blood flow to these muscles may equal that of the limb locomotor muscles.[21]

The metabolic demands of respiratory muscles during maximal exercise require a significant portion of total blood

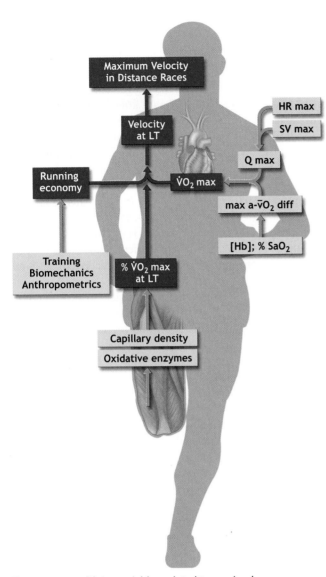

Figure 14.8 Major variables related to maximal oxygen consumption, onset of blood lactate accumulation, and maximal running velocity during endurance exercise. Q, cardiac output; [Hb], hemoglobin concentration; % SaO₂, percentage saturation with oxygen; max a-vO₂ diff, maximum arteriovenous oxygen difference; LT, lactate threshold. (Modified from Bassett DR Jr, Howley ET. Maximal oxygen uptake: "classical" versus "contemporary" viewpoints. Med Sci Sports Exerc 1997;29:591.)

flow. This musculature receives as much as 15% of the exercise cardiac output.[28,30] Evidence from healthy, fit individuals indicates a "competition" for blood flow and oxygen between respiratory and locomotor muscles during intense exercise. For example, altering respiratory muscle work during maximal exercise to increase the energy cost of breathing caused vasoconstriction in the locomotor muscles. Redirection of cardiac output to the respiratory musculature compromised perfusion of the active, nonrespiratory muscles. This reduced the total percentage of $\dot{V}O_{2max}$ used by the active locomotor muscles. Conversely, easing the work of breathing during maximal exercise with an assist ventilator elicited a corresponding increase in oxygen consumption (greater $\%\dot{V}O_{2max}$) of the active leg muscles.

Respiratory Disease

Even during moderate exercise, the healthy person rarely senses the effort to breathe. In respiratory disease, however, the work of breathing becomes an exhaustive exercise in itself. In chronic obstructive pulmonary disease (COPD), the added expiratory resistance can triple the normal cost of breathing at rest; during light exercise, ventilatory cost may reach 10 mL of oxygen for each liter of air breathed. In severe pulmonary disease, the cost of breathing easily attains 40% of the total exercise oxygen consumption. Competition between the oxygen–blood flow needs of locomotor and respiratory muscles encroaches on the oxygen available to the active, nonrespiratory muscle mass.[29] In COPD, the increased cost of breathing severely limits the exercise capacity of individuals with this debilitating medical condition. Unfortunately, only small improvements in measures of pulmonary function or disease status generally accrue from exercise training. Regular exercise, however, can improve exercise capacity, reduce dyspnea, decrease ventilatory equivalents for oxygen, improve respiratory and peripheral muscle function, and enhance psychologic state.[10,19,46,59] Chapter 32 more fully discusses the role of regular physical activity in rehabilitating COPD patients.

Figure 14.9 Oxygen cost of breathing during whole-body graded exercise up to maximum. *Left panel.* Effects of increasing minute ventilation ($\dot{V}_E$) on the total oxygen cost of breathing expressed as a percentage of total exercise oxygen consumption. *Right panel.* Effects of increasing minute ventilation on the oxygen cost per liter air breathed per minute. (From Dempsey JA, et al. Respiratory muscle perfusion and energetics during exercise. Med Sci Sports Exerc 1996;28:1123.)

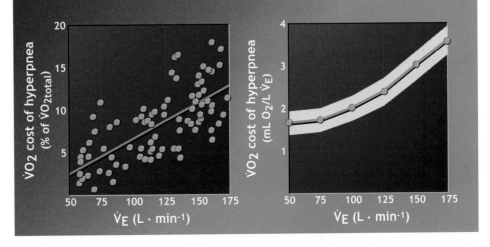

Cigarette Smoking

Research relating smoking habits to exercise performance remains meager, yet most endurance athletes avoid cigarettes for fear of hindering performance from a "loss of wind." Chronic cigarette smokers tend toward more-sedentary lifestyles and have lower fitness levels than nonsmoking counterparts.[6,56,60] For some unknown reason, cigarette smoking increases one's dependence on carbohydrate for energy during rest and sustained exercise.[14] Smokers also have lower dynamic lung function that, if severe, manifests in COPD. In adolescent smokers, chronic cigarette smoking obstructs the airways and slows normal lung function development, with greater deficits in girls than boys.[23] Children who smoked had higher rates of asthma and wheezing and reduced dynamic lung function capacity in a dose-response relationship to their smoking habits. Female smokers who trained vigorously for 12 weeks improved aerobic capacity and endurance performance compared with smokers who remained sedentary.[2] The females who exercised and quit smoking made greater fitness improvements than counterparts who trained similarly but continued to smoke. "In a Practical Sense," Chapter 13, provides an objective means to uncover factors that contribute to a person's smoking behavior.

Acute Effects

Airway resistance at rest increases as much as threefold in both chronic smokers and nonsmokers following 15 puffs on a cigarette during a 5-minute period.[47] The added resistance to breathing lasts an average of 35 minutes; it probably exerts only a minor effect during light exercise, when breathing cost remains small. The residual smoking effect could prove detrimental during vigorous exercise because of the additional oxygen cost to move larger air volumes. Increased peripheral airway resistance with smoking comes mainly from two sources: (1) vagal reflex—possibly triggered from sensory stimulation by minute particles in cigarette smoke and (2) stimulation of parasympathetic ganglia by nicotine.

Researchers determined the oxygen cost of breathing in six habitual smokers immediately after smoking two cigarettes and 1 day after tobacco abstinence. The subjects ran on a treadmill at a speed and grade requiring 80% of $\dot{V}O_{2max}$. Two methods increased ventilation during the "smoking" and "nonsmoking" runs: (1) subjects voluntarily hyperventilated during the run (voluntary HV) and (2) researchers induced hyperventilation by increasing alveolar PCO_2 by having subjects breathe through a large-diameter tube that increased anatomic dead space by 1400 mL (dead space HV). The oxygen cost of the "extra" breathing equaled the difference between the normal oxygen consumption and that in the hyperventilation experiments.

TABLE 14.1 indicates that the oxygen cost of breathing decreased between 13 and 79% with smoking abstinence. The energy requirement of breathing during exercise averaged 14% of the total exercise oxygen consumption after smoking, but only 9% in the nonsmoking trials for the heaviest smokers. Also, heart rate averaged 5 to 7% lower during exercise following 1 day of cigarette abstinence; all subjects reported feeling better when they exercised in the nonsmoking condition. These findings indicate a substantial reversibility of the increased cost of breathing with smoking in chronic smokers with only 1 day of abstinence. *From a practical standpoint, an athlete who cannot eliminate smoking completely should at least abstain the day before a competition.* Additional research complements these findings; a 7-day smoking abstinence period by young men reduced submaximal exercise heart rate and enhanced time to exhaustion during graded treadmill testing.[32]

TABLE 14.1 ■ OXYGEN COST OF HYPERVENTILATION (HV) IN "SMOKING" AND "NONSMOKING" EXERCISE AT APPROXIMATELY 80% OF $\dot{V}O_{2MAX}$

| | SMOKING | | | | NONSMOKING | | | |
| | VOLUNTARY HV | | DEAD SPACE HV | | VOLUNTARY HV | | DEAD SPACE HV | |
SUBJECT	$\dot{V}_E$ (L · MIN^{-1})	O_2 COST (mL · L^{-1})	$\dot{V}_E$ (L · MIN^{-1})	O_2 COST (mL · L^{-1})	$\dot{V}_E$ (L · MIN^{-1})	O_2 COST (mL · L^{-1})	$\dot{V}_E$ (L · MIN^{-1})	O_2 COST (mL · L^{-1})
1	26.4	15.1	18.9	12.7	22.7	11.4	23.0	6.5
2	39.0	10.3	28.1	5.9	42.6	11.3	41.3	4.8
3	22.8	7.9	27.2	7.0	23.8	7.2	22.8	5.7
4	36.3	5.0	28.7	5.6	44.7	3.8	18.6	−1.6[a]
5	52.7	13.5	26.7	12.4	75.2	6.1	22.8	5.7
6	22.4	8.5	27.3	1.1	23.2	3.4	30.1	3.0
Average	32.6	10.1	26.2	7.4	38.7	7.2	26.5	4.0

From Rode A, Shephard RJ. The influence of cigarette smoking upon the oxygen cost of breathing in near-maximal exercise. Med Sci Sports Exerc 1971;3:51.
[a] The implication of the "negative" cost of V_E in this subject is that the added dead space reduces the cost of the normal exercise ventilation.

Blunted Heart Rate Response

A paradox exists between the maximal exercise capacity of cigarette smokers and their submaximal heart rate response to exercise. Otherwise healthy chronic smokers exhibit significantly less endurance during graded exercise to maximum than nonsmokers.[6,40,60] Despite their poorer performance in maximal testing (i.e., shorter time to fatigue), the smokers spent more time to reach a heart rate of 130 b · min^{-1} during a graded exercise test. This indicates a *relatively higher* fitness level (i.e., more exercise accomplished before reaching the submaximal heart rate value). An altered sensitivity in autonomic neural control from cigarette smoking may inhibit the heart rate response of smokers to submaximal exercise.[41] These findings emphasize the need to consider smoking status when evaluating fitness data from submaximal heart rate response to a standard step test or a heart rate prediction test. Failure to account for cigarette smoking would inflate fitness estimates because the lower heart rate (blunted response) of smokers erroneously implies higher aerobic fitness.

DOES VENTILATION LIMIT AEROBIC POWER AND ENDURANCE?

Aerobic training produces considerably less adaptation in pulmonary structure and function than in cardiovascular and neuromuscular adaptations. Current interest concerns how the lack of pulmonary system "plasticity" affects aerobic exercise performance, particularly at the high exercise levels routinely performed by elite endurance athletes.

INTEGRATIVE QUESTION

Advise a person who performs specific breathing exercises rather than endurance training to increase "wind" and eliminate "breathlessness" when running continuously for 20 to 30 minutes.

If breathing during graded exercise becomes inadequate, the relationship between pulmonary ventilation and oxygen consumption would curve in a direction opposite to that indicated in Figure 14.5 (i.e., decreased ventilatory equivalent). Such a response, common in COPD patients, indicates a *failure* of ventilation to keep pace with oxygen consumption[4]; in this case, one truly would "run out of breath." During strenuous exercise, healthy individuals overbreathe at higher levels of oxygen consumption. The hyperventilation response generally *decreases* alveolar P_{CO_2} (see Fig. 14.3) and slightly *increases* alveolar P_{O_2}. Even during maximal exercise, a considerable **breathing reserve** exists because minute ventilation at $\dot{V}O_{2max}$ equals only 60 to 85% of a healthy person's maximum voluntary ventilation (MVV). Most individuals have a 20 to 40% MVV reserve during high-intensity exercise. *Pulmonary function does not form a "weak link" in the oxygen transport system of healthy individuals with average to moderately large aerobic capacities.*

An Important Exception

For endurance athletes, the pulmonary system lags behind their exceptional cardiovascular and aerobic muscular adaptations to training.[63] The potential for inequality in alveolar ventilation relative to pulmonary capillary blood flow (i.e., impaired ventilation–perfusion ratio) during high-intensity exercise may compromise arterial saturation and oxygen transport capacity—a condition termed **exercise-induced arterial hypoxemia (EIH)**.[20,31,35,44,45,52,54] EIH among trained individuals remains variable. It sometimes occurs at exercise levels as low as 40% $\dot{V}O_{2max}$ at sea level and mild to moderate altitudes.[9,24,55] When highly trained endurance athletes exercised near $\dot{V}O_{2max}$ (>65 mL·kg^{-1}·min^{-1}; FIG. 14.10), pressure differentials between alveolar and arterial oxygen widened to more than 30 mm Hg. This caused arterial oxygen saturation to fall below 90% with a corresponding arterial P_{O_2} below 75 mm Hg. Some elite endurance athletes cannot achieve complete aeration of the blood in the pulmonary capillaries in high-intensity exercise; in this situation, arterial desaturation becomes more apparent as exercise duration progresses. It does not appear that alterations in pulmonary structure at the alveolar–capillary interface produce EIH.[62]

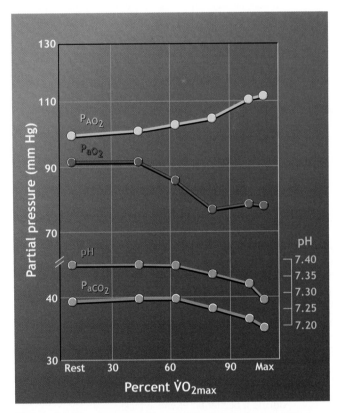

Figure 14.10 Average values for blood gas pressures (P_{aO_2} and P_{aCO_2}), acid–base status (pH), and difference between alveolar (P_{AO_2}) and arterial (P_{aO_2}) oxygen pressure in eight male athletes during graded exercise up to $\dot{V}O_{2max}$. Note the widening of the (A–a)O_2 gradient and the fall in P_{aO_2} during maximal exercise. (From Johnson BD, et al. Mechanical constraints on exercise hyperpnea in endurance athletes. J Appl Physiol 1992;73:874.)

Possible functionally based causes for arterial desaturation include:

1. Inequality in ventilation-perfusion ratio within the lungs or specific portions of the lungs
2. Shunting of blood between venous and arterial circulations, thus bypassing areas for diffusion
3. Failure to achieve end-capillary equilibrium between alveolar oxygen pressure and pressure of oxygen in blood perfusing the pulmonary capillaries

 INTEGRATIVE QUESTION

Discuss why pulmonary ventilation does not limit aerobic exercise performance for most healthy persons.

Summary

1. In light to moderate exercise, pulmonary ventilation increases linearly with oxygen consumption so the ventilatory equivalent ($\dot{V}_E/\dot{V}O_2$) averages 20 to 25 L of air breathed per liter of oxygen consumed.
2. In non–steady-rate exercise, ventilation increases disproportionately with increases in oxygen consumption, and the ventilatory equivalent can exceed 35 L.
3. A disproportionately sharp rise in minute ventilation during incremental exercise provides a "bloodless" way to estimate the onset of blood lactate accumulation (OBLA).
4. OBLA provides a submaximal exercise measure of aerobic fitness that relates to the beginning of anaerobiosis in the active muscles. OBLA occurs without significant metabolic acidosis or severe cardiovascular strain.
5. The oxygen cost of breathing for healthy individuals remains relatively small throughout a broad range of submaximal exercise. The work of breathing becomes excessive for individuals with respiratory disease, often producing inadequate alveolar ventilation.
6. Cigarette smoking causes airway resistance to rise considerably and increase the cost of breathing to adversely affect endurance performance.
7. Exercise training generally reduces the ventilatory equivalent in submaximal exercise. This "conserves" oxygen because the cost of breathing decreases during a particular exercise task.
8. For individuals of average aerobic fitness, maximal exercise does not tax pulmonary ventilation to a point that limits optimal alveolar gas exchange and arterial saturation.
9. Pulmonary function improvements for the endurance athlete can lag behind their exceptional adaptations in cardiovascular and muscle function, thereby

compromising aeration of blood during maximal effort.

PART 3 • *Acid–Base Regulation*

BUFFERING

Acids dissociate in solution and release H^+, whereas **bases** accept H^+ to form hydroxide ions (OH^-). The term **buffering** designates reactions that minimize changes in H^+ concentration; **buffers** refer to chemical and physiologic mechanisms that prevent this change.

The symbol **pH** designates a quantitative measure of acidity or alkalinity (basicity) of a liquid solution. Specifically, pH refers to the concentration of protons or H^+. Acid solutions have more H^+ than OH^- at a pH below 7.0, and vice versa for basic solutions whose pH exceeds 7.0. Chemically pure (distilled) water, considered neutral, has equal H^+ and OH^- and thus a pH of 7.0. The pH scale shown in FIGURE 14.11, devised in 1909 by Danish chemist Sören Sörensen (1868–1939; known for his work in amino acid synthesis and enzyme reactions at Carlsberg laboratory in Copenhagen, Denmark), ranges from 1.0 to 14.0. An inverse relation exists between pH and H^+ concentration. The logarithmic nature of the pH scale means a 1-unit change in pH produces a 10-fold change in H^+ concentration. For example, lemon juice and gastric juice (pH = 2.0) have 1000 times the H^+ concentration of black coffee (pH = 5.0), whereas hydrochloric acid (pH = 1.0) has approximately 1 million times the H^+ concentration of blood at a pH of 7.4.

The pH of bodily fluids ranges from a low of 1.0 for the digestive acid hydrochloric acid to a slightly basic pH between 7.35 and 7.45 for arterial and venous blood and most other bodily fluids. An increase in pH above the normal average of 7.4 results directly from decreased H^+ concentration (increased pH or **alkalosis**). Conversely, **acidosis** refers to increased H^+ concentration (decreased pH). The acid–base characteristics of bodily fluids fluctuate within narrow limits because metabolism remains highly sensitive to H^+ concentrations in the reacting medium. Three mechanisms regulate the pH of the internal environment:

1. Chemical buffers
2. Pulmonary ventilation
3. Renal function

Chemical Buffers

The chemical buffering system consists of a weak acid and the salt of that acid. Bicarbonate buffer, for example, consists of the weak acid **carbonic acid** and its salt, **sodium bicarbonate**. Carbonic acid forms when bicarbonate binds H^+. When the H^+ concentration remains elevated, the reaction produces the weak acid because the excess H^+ ions bind in accord with the general reaction:

$$H^+ + \text{Buffer} \rightarrow \text{H-Buffer}$$

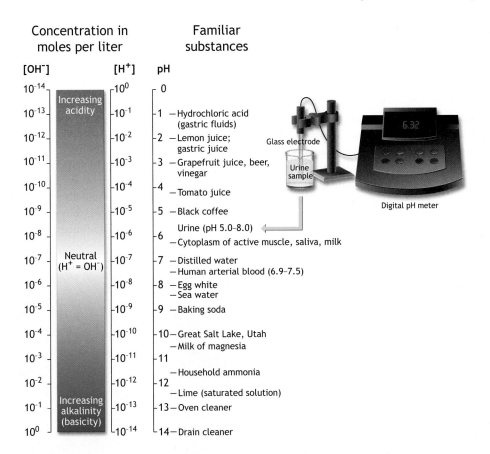

Figure 14.11 The pH scale provides a quantitative measure of the acidity or alkalinity (basicity) of a liquid solution. Blood pH normally stabilizes at the slightly alkaline pH of 7.4. Values for blood pH rarely fall below pH of 6.9, even during the most strenuous exercise, although values at the active muscle are lower. The digital pH meter accurately determines the pH of any substance. The example shows a pH of 6.32 for the urine sample.

In contrast, if the concentration of H^+ decreases—as occurs during hyperventilation, when plasma carbonic acid declines because carbon dioxide leaves the blood and exits through the lungs—the buffering reaction moves in the opposite direction and releases H^+:

$$H^+ + Buffer \longleftarrow H\text{-}Buffer$$

Most of the carbon dioxide generated in energy metabolism reacts with water to form the relatively weak carbonic acid that dissociates into H^+ and HCO_3^-. Likewise, the stronger lactic acid reacts with sodium bicarbonate to form sodium lactate and carbonic acid; in turn, carbonic acid dissociates and increases the H^+ concentration of the extracellular fluids. Other organic acids such as fatty acids dissociate and liberate H^+, as do sulfuric and phosphoric acids generated during protein catabolism. Bicarbonate, phosphate, and protein chemical buffers provide the rapid first line of defense to maintain consistency in the acid–base character of the internal environment.

Bicarbonate Buffer

The bicarbonate buffer system consists of carbonic acid and sodium bicarbonate in solution. During buffering, hy-

drochloric acid (a strong acid) converts to the much weaker carbonic acid by combining with sodium bicarbonate in the following reaction:

$$HCl + NaHCO_3 \rightarrow NaCl + H_2CO_3 \leftrightarrow H^+ + HCO_3^-$$

The buffering of hydrochloric acid produces only a slight reduction in pH. Sodium bicarbonate in plasma exerts a strong buffering action on lactic acid to form sodium lactate and carbonic acid. Any additional increase in H^+ concentration from carbonic acid dissociation causes the dissociation reaction to move in the opposite direction to release carbon dioxide into solution as follows:

Result of acidosis

$$H_2O + CO_2 \leftarrow H_2CO_3 \leftarrow H^+ + HCO_3^-$$

An increase in plasma carbon dioxide or H^+ concentration immediately stimulates ventilation to eliminate "excess" carbon dioxide.

Conversely, a decrease in plasma H^+ concentration inhibits the ventilatory drive and retains carbon dioxide that then combines with water to increase acidity (carbonic acid) and normalize pH.

Result of alkalosis

$$H_2O + CO_2 \rightarrow H_2CO_3 \rightarrow H^+ + HCO_3^-$$

Phosphate Buffer

The phosphate buffering system consists of phosphoric acid and sodium phosphate. These chemicals act similarly to the bicarbonate buffers. Phosphate buffer exerts an important effect on acid–base balance in the kidney tubules and intracellular fluids where phosphate concentration remains high.

Protein Buffer

Venous blood buffers the H^+ released from the dissociation of relatively weak carbonic acid (produced from H_2O + CO_2). *By far, hemoglobin provides the most important H^+ acceptor for this buffering function.* Hemoglobin is almost six times more potent in regulating acidity than the other plasma proteins. Hemoglobin's release of oxygen to the cells makes hemoglobin a weaker acid, thereby increasing its affinity to bind H^+. The H^+ generated when carbonic acid forms in the erythrocyte combines readily with deoxygenated hemoglobin (Hb^-) in the reaction:

$$H^+ + Hb^- \text{ (Protein)} \longrightarrow HHb$$

Intracellular tissue proteins also regulate plasma pH. Some amino acids possess free acidic radicals. When dissociated, they form OH^-, which readily reacts with H^+ to form water.

Relative Power of Chemical Buffers

TABLE 14.2 lists the relative power of the blood's chemical buffers and those in blood and interstitial fluids combined. As a frame of reference, the buffering power of the bicarbonate system receives the value 1.00.

PHYSIOLOGIC BUFFERS

The pulmonary and renal systems present the second line of defense in acid–base regulation. Their buffering function occurs only when a change in pH has already occurred.

TABLE 14.2 ■ RELATIVE BUFFERING POWER OF THE CHEMICAL BUFFERS

CHEMICAL BUFFER	BLOOD	BLOOD PLUS INTERSTITIAL FLUIDS
Bicarbonate	1.0	1.0
Phosphate	0.3	0.3
Proteins (excluding Hb)	1.4	0.8
Hemoglobin	5.3	1.5

Ventilatory Buffer

When the quantity of free H^+ in extracellular fluid and plasma increases, it directly stimulates the respiratory center to immediately increase alveolar ventilation. This rapid adjustment reduces alveolar P_{CO_2} and causes carbon dioxide to be "blown off" from the blood. Reduced plasma carbon dioxide levels accelerate the recombination of H^+ and HCO_3^-, lowering free H^+ concentration in plasma. For example, doubling alveolar ventilation by hyperventilation at rest increases blood alkalinity and pH by 0.23 units, from 7.40 to 7.63. Conversely, reducing normal alveolar ventilation (hypoventilation) by one half increases blood acidity by approximately 0.23 pH units. The potential magnitude of ventilatory buffer-

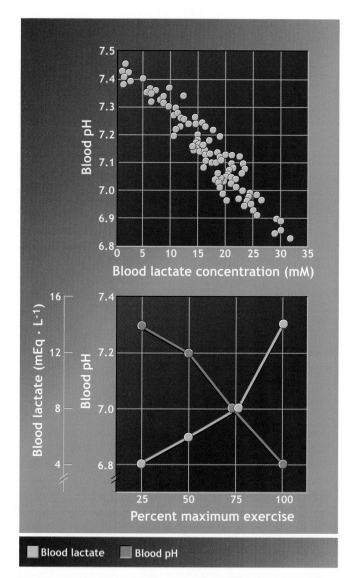

Figure 14.12 *Top.* Relationship between blood pH and blood lactate concentration during rest and increasing intensities of short-duration exercise up to maximum. *Bottom.* Blood pH and blood lactate concentration related to exercise intensity expressed as a percentage of the maximum. Decreases in blood pH accompany increases in blood lactate concentration. (From Osnes JB, Hermansen L. Acid–base balance after maximal exercise of short duration. J Appl Physiol 1972;32:59.)

ing equals twice the combined effect of all the body's chemical buffers.

Renal Buffer

Chemical buffers only temporarily affect excess acid buildup. Excretion of H^+ by the kidneys, although relatively slow, provides an important longer-term defense that maintains the body's buffer reserve (**alkaline reserve**). To this end, the kidneys stand as the final sentinel. The renal tubules regulate acidity through complex chemical reactions that secrete ammonia and H^+ into the urine and then reabsorb alkali, chloride, and bicarbonate.

EFFECTS OF INTENSE EXERCISE

Increased H^+ concentration from carbon dioxide production and lactate formation during strenuous exercise makes pH regulation progressively more difficult. Acid–base regulation becomes exceedingly difficult during repeated, brief bouts of all-out exercise that elevate blood lactate values to 30 mM (270 mg of lactate per dL of blood) or higher.[33] FIGURE 14.12 illustrates the inverse linear relationship between blood lactate concentration and blood pH. Blood lactate concentration in these experiments varied between 0.8 mM at rest (pH 7.43) and 32.1 mM during exhaustive exercise (pH 6.80). In active muscle, pH reaches even lower values than in blood, declining to 6.4 or lower at exhaustion.

The above data indicate that humans *temporarily* tolerate pronounced disturbances in acid–base balance during maximal exercise, at least to a blood pH as low as 6.80—one of the lowest blood lactate values ever reported. A plasma pH below 7.00 does not occur without consequences; this level of acidosis produces nausea, headache, and dizziness, in addition to discomfort and pain within active muscles.

Summary

1. The chemical and physiologic buffer systems normally regulate the acid–base quality of bodily fluids within narrow limits.
2. The bicarbonate, phosphate, and protein chemical buffers provide the rapid first line of defense in acid–base regulation. Buffers consist of a weak acid and the salt of that acid. Their action during acidosis converts a strong acid to a weaker acid and a neutral salt.
3. The lungs and kidneys also contribute to pH regulation. Changes in alveolar ventilation rapidly alter free H^+ concentration in extracellular fluids. The renal tubules act as the body's final defense by secreting H^+ into the urine and reabsorbing bicarbonate.
4. Anaerobic exercise increases the demand for buffering, making pH regulation progressively more difficult.

References are available on the Student CD and online at http://connection.lww.com/mkk6e.

The Cardiovascular System

15

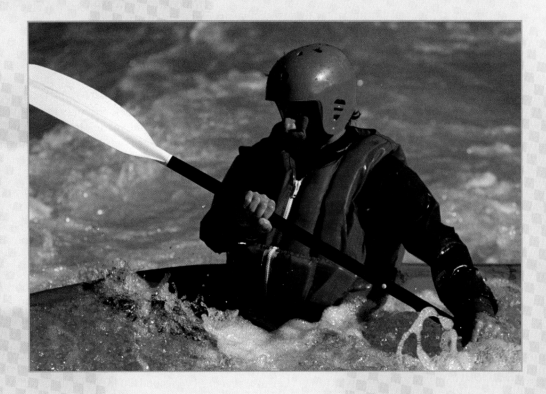

CHAPTER OBJECTIVES

- List four important functions of the cardiovascular system

- Describe the interactions among cardiac output, total peripheral resistance, and arterial blood pressure

- Discuss the role of the venous system as an active blood reservoir

- Describe the auscultatory method to measure blood pressure, and quantify the typical response for systolic and diastolic blood pressures during rest and moderate aerobic exercise

- Discuss the blood pressure response during (1) resistance exercise and (2) upper-body exercise

- Define the "hypotensive response" in recovery from exercise and provide possible explanations for its occurrence

- Diagram the major vessels of the coronary circulation

- Describe the pattern of myocardial blood flow, oxygen consumption, and substrate use during rest and various intensities of physical activity

- Explain the rate–pressure product and rationale for its use in clinical exercise physiology

The **cardiovascular system** integrates the body as a unit. It provides the active muscles with a continuous stream of nutrients and oxygen to sustain a high level of energy transfer. The circulation also removes byproducts of metabolism from the site of energy release.

Chapters 15, 16, and 17 explore the dynamics of circulation, particularly its role in oxygen delivery during exercise. Oxygen transport and delivery during exercise, coupled with the active muscles' capacity to generate adenosine triphosphate (ATP) aerobically, set the maximum level for aerobic energy transfer.

CARDIOVASCULAR SYSTEM COMPONENTS

The cardiovascular system consists of the continuous linkage of a pump, a high-pressure distribution circuit, exchange vessels, and a low-pressure collection and return circuit. If stretched out in a line, the 100,000 miles of blood vessels of an average-sized adult would encircle the earth four times. FIGURE 15.1 presents a schematic view of the cardiovascular system, including the major arteries. The table inset shows the distribution of blood in absolute and percentage terms. Note that small arteries, veins, and capillaries of the systemic circulation contain approximately 75% of the total blood volume, whereas the heart contains only 7%.

The Heart

The heart provides the impetus for blood flow. Situated in the midcenter of the chest cavity, about two thirds of its mass lies to the left of the body's midline. The four-chambered muscular organ weighs 11 oz for an average-size adult male and 9 oz for an average-size female and pumps about 2.4 oz, or 70 mL for each beat. At rest, the heart's output of blood averages 1900 gallons daily or 52 million gallons over a 75-year lifetime. For a person of average physical fitness, the maximum output of blood from this remarkable organ in 1 minute exceeds the fluid output from a household faucet turned wide open.

FIGURE 15.2 summarizes general functional and structural characteristics and mode of activation of the body's three types of muscle—skeletal, cardiac, and smooth. The heart muscle or **myocardium** represents a form of striated muscle similar to skeletal muscle. In contrast to skeletal muscle, however, the multinucleated, individual cells or fibers interconnect in latticework fashion. The stimulation or depolarization of one cell consequently spreads the action potential through the myocardium to all cells to make the heart function as a unit.

FIGURE 15.3 shows the structural details of the heart as a pump. Functionally, one can view the heart as two separate pumps. The hollow chambers on the right side of the heart (*right heart*) perform two crucial functions:

1. Receive blood returning from throughout the body
2. Pump blood to the lungs for aeration through the **pulmonary circulation**

The left side of the heart (*left heart*) also performs two crucial functions:

1. Receive oxygenated blood from the lungs
2. Pump blood into the thick-walled, muscular aorta for distribution throughout the body in the **systemic circulation**

A thick, solid muscular wall, or interventricular septum, separates the heart's left and right sides. The **atrioventricular valves** within the heart provide one-way blood flow from the right atrium to the right ventricle via the **tricuspid valve,** and from the left atrium to the left ventricle through the **mitral** or **bicuspid valve**. The **semilunar valves**, located in the arterial wall just outside the heart, prevent blood from flowing back into the heart between contractions. The relatively thin-walled, saclike atrial chambers serve as primer or "booster" pumps to receive and store blood during ventricular contraction. Approximately 70% of the blood returning to the atria flows directly into the ventricles before the atria contract. The simultaneous contraction of both atria then forces the remaining blood into their respective ventricles directly below. Almost immediately after atrial contraction, the ventricles contract and propel blood into the arterial system. Two excellent Internet sites (www.pbs.org/wgbh/nova/eheart/human.html; and www.new-media.co.uk/heart/) deal with many important aspects of heart function.

As ventricular pressure builds, the atrioventricular valves snap closed. All heart valves remain closed for 0.02 to 0.06 seconds. This brief interval of rising ventricular tension, during which heart volume and muscle fiber length remain unchanged, represents the heart's **isovolumetric contraction period**. Blood ejects from the heart when ventricular pressure exceeds arterial pressure. With each contraction, the spiral and circular arrangement of bands of cardiac muscle literally "wrings out" blood from the ventricles.

The Arterial System

The arteries compose the high-pressure tubing that propels oxygen-rich blood to the tissues. FIGURE 15.4 illustrates that arteries consist of layers of connective tissue and smooth muscle. No gaseous exchange takes place between arterial blood and surrounding tissues because of the thickness of these vessels. Blood pumped from the left ventricle into the highly muscular yet elastic **aorta** distributes in the body through an intricate network of arteries and smaller arterial branches called **arterioles**. The walls of arterioles contain circular layers of smooth muscle that either constrict or relax to regulate blood flow to the periphery. These "resistance vessels" dramatically alter their internal diameter to rapidly adjust blood flow through the vascular circuit. This redistribution function takes on added importance during exercise because blood rapidly diverts to active muscles from areas that temporarily compromise their blood supply. The inset table of Figure 15.4 lists average values for the diameter of blood vessels and corresponding velocities of blood flowing through them.

Body area	Blood volume	
	mL	Percentage
Heart	360	7.2
Lungs		
Arteries	130	2.6
Capillaries	110	2.2
Veins	200	4.0
Systemic		
Aorta, large arteries	300	6.0
Small arteries	400	8.0
Capillaries	300	6.0
Small veins	2300	46.0
Large veins	900	18.0
Total	**5000**	**100.0**

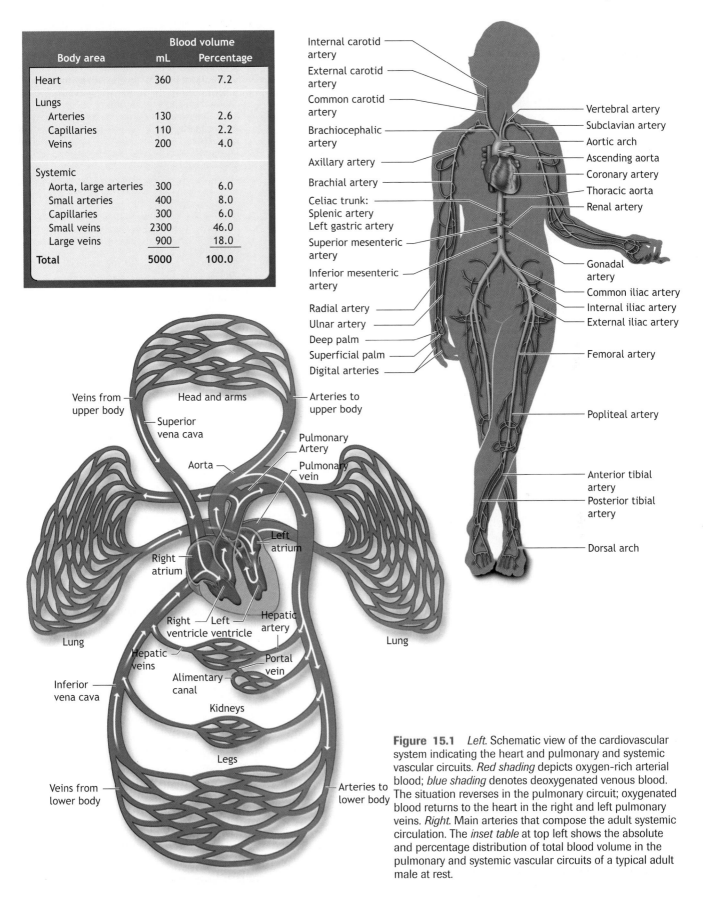

Figure 15.1 *Left.* Schematic view of the cardiovascular system indicating the heart and pulmonary and systemic vascular circuits. *Red shading* depicts oxygen-rich arterial blood; *blue shading* denotes deoxygenated venous blood. The situation reverses in the pulmonary circuit; oxygenated blood returns to the heart in the right and left pulmonary veins. *Right.* Main arteries that compose the adult systemic circulation. The *inset table* at top left shows the absolute and percentage distribution of total blood volume in the pulmonary and systemic vascular circuits of a typical adult male at rest.

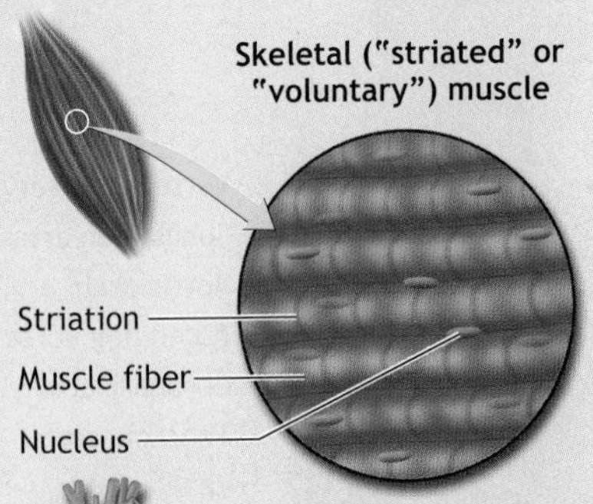

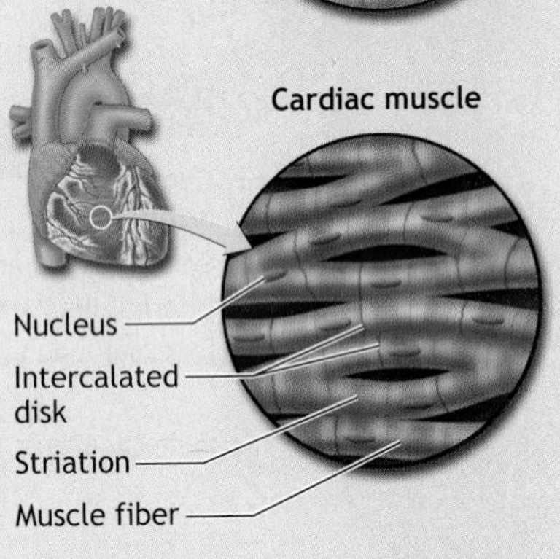

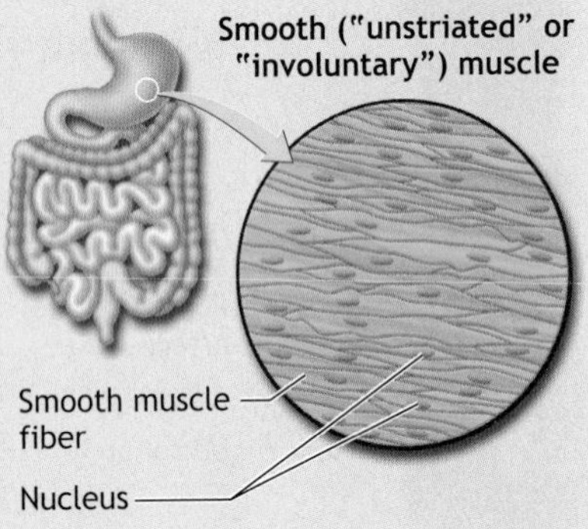

Muscle type	Location	Appearance	Type of activity	Stimulation
Skeletal ("striated" or "voluntary") muscle Striation Muscle fiber Nucleus	Named muscle (e.g., the biceps of the arm) attached to the skeleton and fascia of limbs, body wall, and head/neck	Large, long, unbranched, cylindrical fibers with transverse striations (stripes) arranged in parallel bundles; multiple, peripherally located nuclei	Strong, quick intermittent (phasic) contraction above a baseline tonus; acts primarily to produce movement or resist gravity	Voluntary (or reflexive) by the somatic nervous system
Cardiac muscle Nucleus Intercalated disk Striation Muscle fiber	Muscle of heart (myocardium) and adjacent portions of the great vessels (aorta, vena cava)	Branching and anastomosing shorter fibers with transverse striations (stripes) running parallel and connected end-to-end by complex junctions (intercalated disks); single, central nucleus	Strong, quick continuous rhythmic contraction; pumps blood from the heart	Involuntary; intrinsically (myogenically) stimulated and propagated; rate and strength of contraction modified by the autonomic nervous system
Smooth ("unstriated" or "involuntary") muscle Smooth muscle fiber Nucleus	Walls of hollow viscera and blood vessels, iris, and ciliary body of eye; attached to hair follicles of skin (arrector muscle of hair)	Single or agglomerated small, spindle-shaped fibers without striations; single, central nucleus	Weak, slow, rhythmic, or sustained tonic contraction; acts mainly to propel substances (peristalsis) and restrict flow (vasoconstriction and sphincteric activity)	Involuntary by autonomic nervous system

Figure 15.2 Functional and structural characteristics and mode of activation of skeletal, cardiac, and smooth muscle. (From Moore KL, Dalley AF. Clinically Oriented Anatomy. 4th ed. Baltimore: Lippincott Williams & Wilkins, 1999.)

INTEGRATIVE QUESTION

What advantage does a "closed" circulatory system provide to the physically active individual?

Blood Pressure

Each contraction of the left ventricle forces a surge of blood through the aorta. Peripheral vessels do not permit blood to "run off" into the arterial system as rapidly as it ejects from the heart. Thus, the distensible aorta "stores" a portion of the blood; this creates pressure within the entire arterial system, and causes a pressure wave to travel down the aorta to the remote branches of the arterial tree. The characteristic "pulse" in superficial arteries occurs from the stretch and subsequent recoil of the arterial wall during a cardiac cycle. In healthy individuals, identical values occur for pulse rate and heart rate. *In essence, arterial blood pressure reflects the combined effects of arterial blood flow per minute (i.e., cardiac output) and resistance to that flow from the peripheral vasculature.* The following equation expresses this relationship:

$$\text{Blood pressure} = \text{Cardiac output} \times \text{Total peripheral resistance}$$

Systolic Blood Pressure. At rest in normotensive individuals, the highest pressure generated by the heart averages 120 mm Hg during left ventricular contraction or **systole**. The brachial artery at the level of the right atrium usually

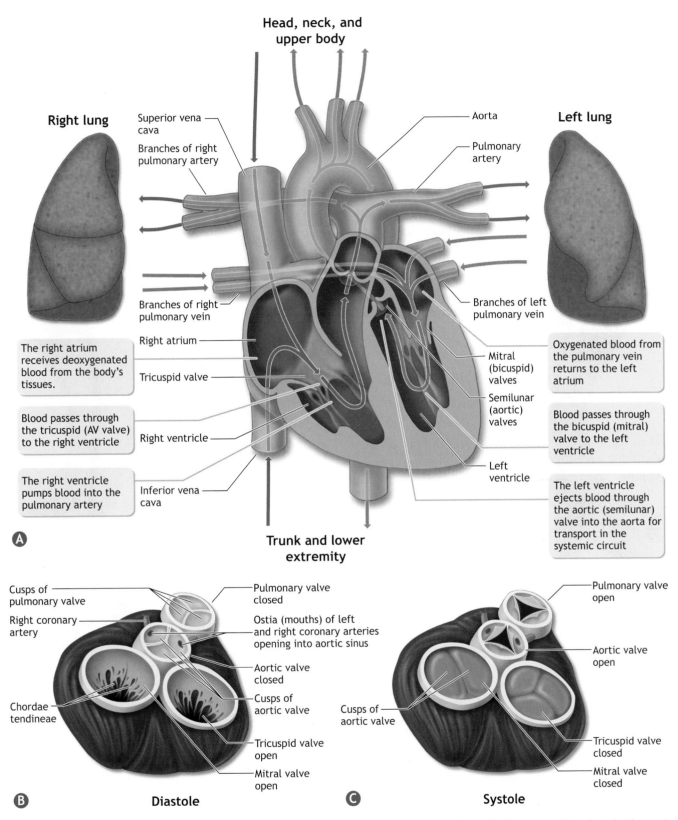

Head, neck, and upper body

Right lung

Superior vena cava

Branches of right pulmonary artery

Branches of right pulmonary vein

Right atrium

Tricuspid valve

Right ventricle

Inferior vena cava

The right atrium receives deoxygenated blood from the body's tissues.

Blood passes through the tricuspid (AV valve) to the right ventricle

The right ventricle pumps blood into the pulmonary artery

Aorta

Pulmonary artery

Left lung

Branches of left pulmonary vein

Mitral (bicuspid) valves

Semilunar (aortic) valves

Left ventricle

Oxygenated blood from the pulmonary vein returns to the left atrium

Blood passes through the bicuspid (mitral) valve to the left ventricle

The left ventricle ejects blood through the aortic (semilunar) valve into the aorta for transport in the systemic circuit

A

Trunk and lower extremity

Cusps of pulmonary valve

Right coronary artery

Chordae tendineae

Pulmonary valve closed

Ostia (mouths) of left and right coronary arteries opening into aortic sinus

Aortic valve closed

Cusps of aortic valve

Tricuspid valve open

Mitral valve open

B   **Diastole**

Pulmonary valve open

Aortic valve open

Cusps of aortic valve

Tricuspid valve closed

Mitral valve closed

C   **Systole**

Figure 15.3   A. The heart, its great vessels, and one-way blood flow through valves as indicated by the *arrows*. **B.** In diastole, the aortic and pulmonary valves snap closed; shortly thereafter, the mitral and tricuspid valves open and blood flows into the ventricular cavities. **C.** Initiation of systole and ventricular emptying closes the tricuspid and mitral valves, while the aortic and pulmonary valves open.

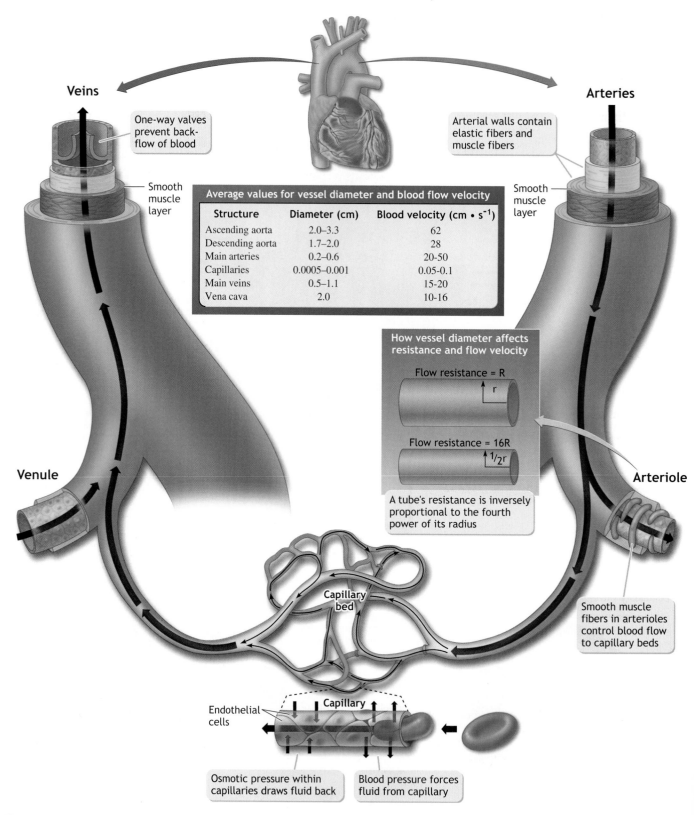

Figure 15.4   The structure of the walls of the blood vessels. A single layer of endothelial cells lines each vessel. Fibrous tissue wrapped in several layers of smooth muscle surrounds the arterial walls. A single layer of muscle cells sheathes the arterioles; capillaries consist of only one layer of rolled up endothelial cells often less than 1 micron (μm) thick with a flat surface area of 300 to 1200 μm^2. In the venule, fibrous tissue encases the endothelial cells; veins also possess a layer of smooth muscle. The *inset table* displays the average values for vessel diameter and corresponding values for blood flow velocity. A vessel's resistance (R) to flow depends on its radius. Decreasing vessel radius (r) by one half increases resistance 16-fold.

serves as the point of reference for this measurement. **Systolic blood pressure** provides an estimate of the work of the heart and force that blood exerts against the arterial walls during ventricular systole. During the heart's relaxation phase when aortic valves close, the natural elastic recoil of the arterial system maintains a continuous head of pressure. This provides a steady blood flow into the periphery until the next surge of blood.

Diastolic Blood Pressure. During the relaxation phase of the cardiac cycle or **diastole**, arterial blood pressure decreases to 70 or 80 mm Hg. **Diastolic blood pressure** indicates **peripheral resistance** or the ease that blood flows from the arterioles into the capillaries. With high peripheral resistance, pressure within the arteries after systole does not rapidly dissipate. Instead, it remains elevated for a larger portion of the cardiac cycle. The "In a Practical Sense" feature on p. 320 illustrates the measurement of systolic and diastolic blood pressure by the **auscultation method**.

Mean Arterial Pressure. Systolic blood pressure typically averages 120 mm Hg, and the diastolic pressure equals 80 mm Hg in young, healthy adults at rest. The average or **mean arterial pressure** (**MAP**) is slightly lower than the arithmetic average of systolic and diastolic pressures because the heart remains in diastole longer than in systole. MAP averages 93 mm Hg at rest; this represents the average force exerted by the blood against the arterial walls during the cardiac cycle. The following formula estimates MAP:

MAP = Diastolic BP + [0.333 (Systolic − Diastolic BP)]

For a person with a diastolic blood pressure of 89 mm Hg and a systolic pressure of 127 mm Hg, MAP equals 89 + [0.333 (127 − 89)] or 102 mm Hg.

Cardiac Output and Total Peripheral Resistance. The hemodynamic equation that relates blood pressure to cardiac output and total peripheral resistance rearranges as follows to illustrate factors that determine either cardiac output or total peripheral resistance:

Cardiac output = MAP ÷ Total peripheral resistance

Total peripheral resistance = MAP ÷ Cardiac output

MAP (computed from systolic and diastolic blood pressures) and cardiac output estimate the change in total resistance to blood flow in the transition from rest to exercise. Suppose systolic blood pressure at rest equals 120 mm Hg, diastolic pressure equals 80 mm Hg (MAP = 93.3 mm Hg), and cardiac output averages $5.0 \text{ L} \cdot \text{min}^{-1}$. Substituting these values in the formula for total peripheral resistance yields 18.7 mm Hg per liter of blood flow (93.3 mm Hg ÷ $5.0 \text{ L} \cdot \text{min}^{-1}$). Resistance to peripheral blood flow *decreases* dramatically during strenuous exercise, when systolic pressure increases considerably more than diastolic pressure and cardiac output increases six or seven times the resting value in an elite endurance athlete. For example, if exercise cardiac output equals $35.0 \text{ L} \cdot \text{min}^{-1}$ and MAP equals 130 mm Hg (systolic = 210 mm Hg; diastolic = 90 mm Hg), then resistance to blood flow in the systemic circulation averages 3.71 mm Hg per liter per minute, or five times *less* than the resting value.

Capillaries

The arterioles branch and form smaller and less muscular vessels 10 to 20 microns (μm) in diameter called **metarterioles**. These vessels end in a network of microscopically small blood vessels called **capillaries**, which generally contain 6% of the total blood volume. In skeletal muscle, with its widely varying oxygen requirements, each metarteriole interfaces with 8 to 10 capillaries. The average capillary diameter is 7 to 10 μm (approximately 1/100th of a millimeter). Figure 15.4 shows that the capillary wall usually consists of a single layer of rolled up endothelial cells. Some capillaries are so narrow (about 3–4 μm in diameter) that only one blood cell at a time can squeeze through. In many instances, the extensive proliferation of capillaries causes their walls to abut the membranes of the surrounding cells. Capillary density varies throughout the body, depending on the location and function of the particular tissue. Capillary density of human skeletal muscle averages between 2000 and 3000 capillaries per square millimeter of tissue. Capillary density is greater in heart muscle, where no cell lies farther than 0.008 mm from its nearest capillary.

Blood Flow in Capillaries

The **precapillary sphincter**, a ring of smooth muscle that encircles the vessel at its origin, controls capillary diameter. Sphincter constriction and relaxation provides an important local means of blood flow regulation within a specific tissue to meet metabolic requirements. Chapter 16 discusses specific factors for autoregulation of local blood supply.

FIGURE 15.5 depicts a generalized view of the dynamics of capillary blood flow within muscle during rest and exercise. Fewer capillaries function at rest than are available. In this example for the gastrocnemius muscle, blood flow each minute at rest averages 5 mL for every 100 g of muscle tissue. For a muscle that weighs 600 g, approximately 30 mL of blood flows through it each minute. During exercise, blood flow increases rapidly as previously "unused" capillaries open. Two factors trigger the relaxation of precapillary sphincters: (1) driving force of increased local blood pressure plus intrinsic neural control and (2) local metabolites produced in exercise. During strenuous exercise, a sustained local blood flow increases 15 to 20 times the resting value. For the gastrocnemius muscle, flow averages about 80 mL per 100 g of tissue each minute.

Branching of the capillary microcirculation increases its cross-sectional area to about 800 times the 1-inch diameter aorta. Because blood flow velocity relates inversely to the vasculature's cross section (Velocity, $\text{cm} \cdot \text{s}^{-1}$ = Volume of

IN A PRACTICAL SENSE

BLOOD PRESSURE MEASUREMENT, CLASSIFICATIONS, AND RECOMMENDED FOLLOW-UP

■ Blood pressure represents the force or pressure exerted by blood against the arterial walls during a cardiac cycle. Systolic blood pressure, the higher of the two pressure measurements, occurs during ventricular contraction (systole) as the heart propels 70 to 100 mL of blood into the aorta. Following systole, the ventricles relax (diastole), the arteries recoil, and arterial pressure continually declines as blood flows into the periphery and the heart refills with blood. The lowest pressure attained during ventricular relaxation represents diastolic blood pressure. Pulse pressure refers to the difference between systolic and diastolic pressures. Systolic blood pressure in a typical adult varies between 110 and 140 mm Hg; diastolic pressure varies between 60 and 90 mm Hg. Elevated systolic or diastolic blood pressure (termed *hypertension*) is defined as a resting systolic blood pressure above 140 mm Hg and diastolic pressure exceeding 90 mm Hg (stage 1 hypertension). Stage 2 hypertension relates to systolic blood pressures of 160 mm Hg and higher and diastolic pressures of 100 mm Hg and higher. Blood pressure readings that fall in the *prehypertension range* should be treated with lifestyle changes that include reducing excess weight, exercising more, quitting smoking, cutting back on salt, having no more than one or two alcoholic drinks a day, and eating more fruits, vegetables, and low-fat dairy products.

MEASUREMENT PROCEDURES

Blood pressure, measured indirectly by auscultation (listening to sounds; described in 1902 by Russian physician Nikolai S. Korotkoff, 1874–1920), uses a stethoscope and sphygmomanometer (consisting of a blood pressure cuff and an aneroid or mercury column pressure gauge). A typical measurement sequence occurs as follows:

1. Subject, seated in a quiet room, exposes upper right arm.

CLASSIFICATION AND RECOMMENDED FOLLOW-UP OF INITIAL SCREENING BLOOD PRESSURE IN ADULTS[a]

SYSTOLIC (MM HG)	DIASTOLIC (MM HG)	CATEGORY	FOLLOW-UP
<120	<80	Optimal	———
<130	<85	Normal	Recheck in 2 y
130–139	85–89	High-normal	Recheck in 1 y
140–159	90–99	Stage 1 hypertension	Confirm within 2 months
160–179	100–109	Moderate (Stage 2) hypertension	Begin treatment within 1 month if blood pressure is consistently high
180–209	110–119	Severe (Stage 3) hypertension	Begin treatment within 1 week
>210	120	Very severe (Stage 4) hypertension	Treat immediately

[a]Not taking antihypertensive drugs and not acutely ill. When systolic and diastolic blood pressure categories vary, the higher reading determines the blood pressure classification. For example, a reading of 152/82 mm Hg is classified as Stage 1 hypertension.

From National Institutes of Health. The sixth report of the Joint National Committee on Detection, Evaluation, and Treatment of High Blood Pressure. NIH Pub. no. 98-4080, 1997.

2. Locate the brachial artery at the inner side of the upper arm, approximately 1 inch above the bend in the elbow.
3. Take the free end of the cuff, gently slide it through the metal loop (or wrap over exposed Velcro), and flap it back over so the cuff wraps around the upper arm at heart level. Align the arrows on the cuff with the brachial artery. Secure the Velcro parts of the cuff. To obtain accurate readings, fit the sphygmomanometer cuff snugly (but not tightly). Use appropriate-sized cuffs for children and obese persons.

continued on page 321

Continued

4. Place the stethoscope bell below the antecubital space over the brachial artery.
5. The cuff should now have the connecting tube (from the sphygmomanometer bulb and gauge) exit the cuff toward the arm.
6. Before inflating the cuff, ensure that the air-release switch remains closed (turn the knob clockwise).
7. Inflate the cuff with quick, even pumps to 180 to 200 mm Hg.
8. Gradually release cuff pressure (about 3–5 mm per s) by slowly opening the air-release knob (counterclockwise turn) and note the pressure when you hear the first sound. Turbulence from the sudden rush of blood produces the sound as the formerly closed artery briefly opens during the highest pressure in the cardiac cycle. The first appearance of sound represents systolic blood pressure.
9. Continue to reduce cuff pressure, noting when the sound muffles *(4th phase diastolic pressure)* and when the sound disappears *(5th phase diastolic pressure).* Clinicians usually record the 5th phase as diastolic blood pressure.
10. If the measured pressure exceeds 140/90 mm Hg, allow a 10-minute period of quiet rest and repeat the procedure.

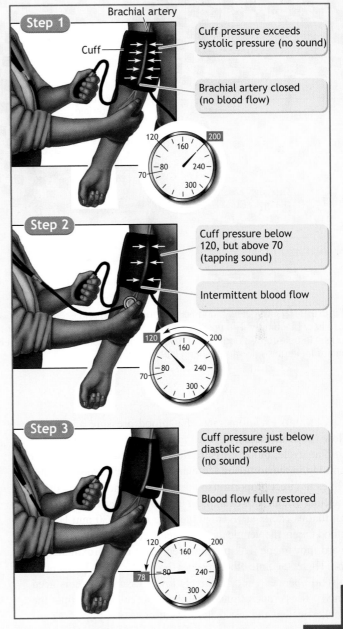

flow, cm³ · s⁻¹ ÷ Cross-sectional area, cm²), velocity progressively decreases as blood moves toward and enters the capillaries. It takes approximately 1.5 seconds for a blood cell to pass through an average-sized capillary. The total surface area of the capillary walls exceeds by 100 times the external body surface of the average adult. Huge surface area combined with a slow rate of blood flow (approximately 0.5 to 1.0 mm · s⁻¹ at rest) produces an extremely effective means of exchange between the blood and the tissues.

The Venous System

The continuity of the vascular system progresses as the capillaries feed deoxygenated blood at almost a trickle into the small veins or **venules** with which they merge. Blood flow velocity then increases somewhat because the cross-sectional area of the venous system is smaller than for capillaries. The smaller veins in the lower portion of the body eventually empty into the body's largest vein, the **inferior vena cava** (FIG. 15.6). This large vessel returns blood to the right atrium from the abdomen, pelvis, and lower extremities. Venous blood from tributary vessels in the head, neck, shoulder regions, thorax, and part of the abdominal wall flows into the 7-cm–long **superior vena cava** to join the inferior vena cava at heart level. The mixture of blood that drains the upper and lower body, called **mixed-venous blood**, then enters the right atrium. From there it flows downward into the right ventricle for pumping through the pulmonary artery to the lungs. Gas exchange takes place in the alveolar–capillary network of the lungs; oxygenated blood then returns in the pulmonary veins to the left side of the heart to once again begin passage throughout the body.

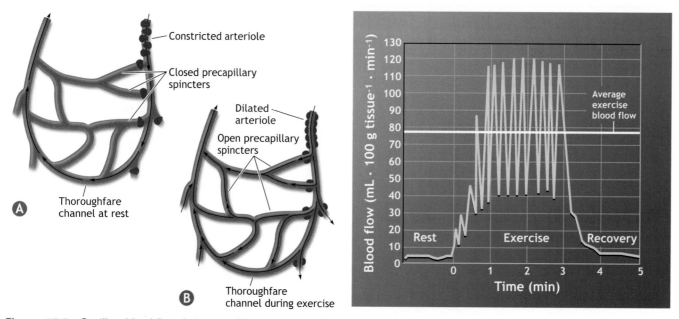

Figure 15.5 Capillary blood flow during rest (**A**) and exercise (**B**). Capillary diameter, red blood cell size, and blood viscosity all affect capillary blood flow. The position of the *dark red knobs* indicate closure or opening dormant capillaries. The *right figure* shows the pulsatile pattern of blood flow at rest, during exercise, and when exercise stops. Dilation of the active muscle's arterioles provides the major mechanism for augmenting local blood flow.

FIGURE 15.7 illustrates that blood pressure and blood flow vary considerably in the systemic circulation. During the cardiac cycle, blood pressure fluctuates between 120 and 80 mm Hg in the aorta and large arteries. The pressure then declines in direct proportion to the resistance encountered in the vascular circuit. For example, blood at the arteriole end of the capillaries exerts an average pressure of only 30 mm Hg. As blood enters the venules, it loses nearly all its impetus for forward movement. The pressure decreases to approximately 0 mm Hg by the time blood reaches the right atrium. The venous system operates under relatively low pressure, so veins need only possess much thinner and less muscular walls than the thicker-walled and less distensible arteries (see Fig. 15.4).

Venous Return

The low pressure of blood in the venous system poses a special problem that a unique characteristic of veins partly solves. FIGURE 15.8 shows that thin, membranous, flaplike **valves** spaced at short intervals within the vein allow blood to flow in only one direction toward the heart. This now seems so logical, but in 1759 when Harvey first proposed the idea, he was vilified for daring to contradict almost two thousand years of medical dogma since ancient physician Galen believed the blood "sloshed" back and fourth through the heart and blood vessels.

The low pressure in the venous circuit means that the smallest muscular contractions or even minor pressure changes within the thoracic cavity with breathing readily compress the veins.[14] The alternate compression and relaxation of veins and the one-way action of their valves provide a "milk-ing" or wringing action similar to heart action. Compressing the veins imparts considerable energy for blood flow, whereas "diastole" of these vessels lets them refill as blood flows to the heart. Without valves, blood would pool as it sometimes does in veins of the extremities. People would faint every time they stood up because of reduced venous return and cerebral blood flow. In ancient Rome when hanging people from a cross was the ultimate punishment, death mainly occurred from blood pooling and pulmonary edema, not necessarily the preceding physical torture.

A Question of an Active Vasculature

Physiologists have debated the role of the venous system as an active vasculature for mobilizing blood volume. The systemic venous vessels normally contain 65% of the total blood volume at rest; thus, the veins represent **capacitance vessels** that serve as blood reservoirs. This has led to speculation about the role of the veins as an active blood reservoir to either retard or facilitate blood delivery to the systemic circulation. Physiologists who take this position maintain that any increase in tension or tone of the vessels' smooth muscle layer alters the diameter of the venous tree. If true, this would initiate rapid redistribution of blood from peripheral veins toward the central blood volume that returns to the heart. Physiologists who oppose this position believe that only the veins in the splanchnic and cutaneous regions are innervated richly enough to contribute to blood mobilization. They posit that skeletal muscle veins do not receive neural input, and whatever brief venoconstriction occurs in other regions would do little to contribute to blood redistribution. Current opinion maintains that the major

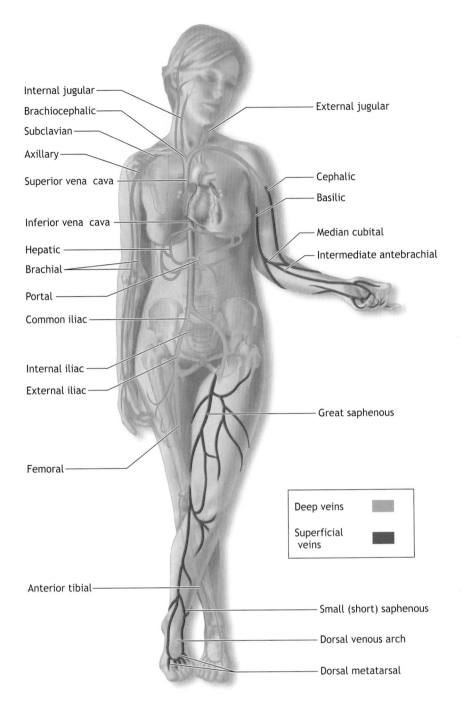

Internal jugular

Brachiocephalic

Subclavian

Axillary

Superior vena cava

Inferior vena cava

Hepatic

Brachial

Portal

Common iliac

Internal iliac

External iliac

Femoral

Anterior tibial

External jugular

Cephalic

Basilic

Median cubital

Intermediate antebrachial

Great saphenous

Small (short) saphenous

Dorsal venous arch

Dorsal metatarsal

Deep veins

Superficial veins

Figure 15.6 Distribution of the superficial (dark blue) and deep (light blue) veins.

contribution to blood mobilization in exercise occurs by action of the active **muscle pump** and passive effect of arterial vasoconstriction (not visceral venoconstriction), which reduces downstream venous pressure.[35]

Varicose Veins

Sometimes the valves within a vein fail to maintain their one-way blood flow, a defective condition termed **varicose veins**. This valvular deformity usually occurs in the surface veins of the lower extremities from the force of gravity that retards blood flow in the upright posture. The surface veins have little external support from surrounding tissues. Consequently, blood gathers in them and they become excessively distended and painful, impairing circulation from the affected area. In severe cases, the venous wall becomes inflamed and progressively deteriorates—a condition called **phlebitis**. This necessitates vessel removal either surgically or nonsurgically by injecting solutions that irritate the vessel's surface membranes (sclerotherapy). This procedure and laser ablation causes a portion of the vein to collapse, fuse, and eventually shrivel up. Blood then reroutes to the deeper veins.

Individuals with varicose veins should avoid straining-type exercises that often accompany resistance training.

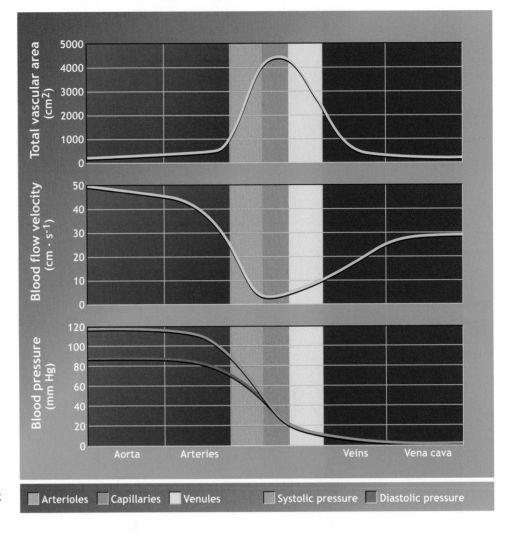

Figure 15.7 Blood flow and blood pressure in the systemic circulation. Note that blood pressure within each portion of the arterial system inversely relates to the total area (resistance) in that section of the vascular tree. For example, when total vascular area approaches 5000 cm², blood flow velocity is at its lowest level.

During sustained, nonrhythmic muscle actions, the muscle and ventilatory "pumps" contribute little to venous return. Increased intrathoracic and abdominal pressures (Valsalva maneuver) with straining also impede venous return. These factors act to pool blood in the veins of the lower body, which can aggravate an existing varicose vein condition. Exercise training does not prevent varicose veins; regular and rhythmic physical activity can minimize complications because repeated muscle actions continually propel blood toward the heart.

Venous Pooling

The rhythmic action of muscular activity and consequent compression of the vascular tree (i.e., the muscle pump) contribute so much to venous return that many people faint when forced to maintain an upright posture without movement. The classic "tilt table" experiment demonstrates this point. A subject lies supine, secured on a table that pivots to different positions from the horizontal. Heart rate and blood pressure stabilize if the person remains horizontal. When the table tilts vertically, an uninterrupted column of blood exists from the heart to toes. This creates a hydrostatic force of 80 to 100 mm Hg that causes blood to pool in the lower extremities. Fluid backs up in the capillary bed and seeps into the surrounding tis-

sues causing them to swell (**edema**). Reduced venous return simultaneously reduces cardiac output and arterial blood pressure; at the same time, heart rate accelerates and blood mobilizes from the splanchnic region by upstream vasoconstriction (causing passive mobilization from downstream veins). Some active venoconstriction to counter the effects of venous pooling also may occur. Forcing the person to maintain the upright position induces fainting from insufficient cerebral blood supply. Tilting the person either horizontally or head down immediately restores circulation and consciousness. In Chapter 27, we discuss a variation of the tilt table experiment applied in microgravity research to induce symptoms and responses to weightlessness when subjects remain in a slight tilt-down position for weeks at a time.

The pressurized suits worn by test pilots and special support stockings for individuals with varicose veins reduce hydrostatic shifts of blood to the veins of the lower extremities in the upright position. A swimming pool provides a similar supportive effect in upright exercise because the water's external support facilitates venous return.

The Active "Cool Down." The preceding discussion of venous pooling provides a sound rationale for continuing to walk or jog at a slow pace following strenuous exercise.

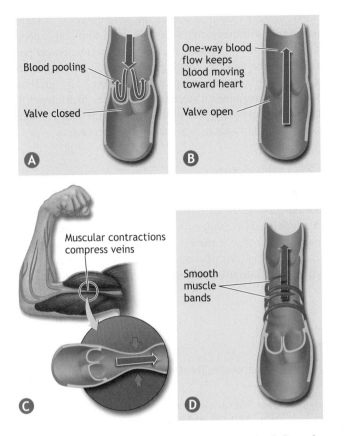

Figure 15.8 The valves in veins (**A**) prevent the back flow of blood, but (**B**) do not hinder the normal one-way flow of blood. (**C**) Blood moves through veins by the action of nearby active muscle or (**D**) contraction of smooth muscle bands within the veins.

Moderate exercise in recovery, popularly known as "**cooling down**," facilitates blood flow through the vascular circuit including myocardial vessels. In Chapter 7, we discuss how active recovery removes lactate from the blood. Continuation of mild exercise in recovery also may blunt potential deleterious effects on cardiac function from elevated catecholamines (epinephrine and norepinephrine) released during exercise.[6,7]

INTEGRATIVE QUESTION

The ancient Romans executed individuals by tying their arms and legs to a cross mounted in the vertical position. Discuss the physiologic responses that cause death under these circumstances.

HYPERTENSION

Systolic pressure at rest can exceed 300 mm Hg in individuals whose arteries (1) have become "hardened" with fatty materials deposited within their walls or because the vessel's connective tissue layer has thickened or (2) offer excessive resistance to peripheral blood flow because of neural hyperactivity or kidney malfunction. Diastolic pressure can also ex-

ceed 100 mm Hg under these conditions. Abnormally high blood pressure, termed **hypertension**, chronically strains the cardiovascular system. Untreated, chronic hypertension damages arterial vessels and leads to arteriosclerosis, heart disease, stroke, and kidney failure. FIGURE 15.9 shows the percentages of the United States population with hypertension (systolic pressure >140 mm Hg; diastolic pressure >90 mm Hg) and its increased prevalence with age. An elevated systolic blood pressure provides a more reliable and accurate predictor of the risk associated with hypertension (and need for treatment) than diastolic blood pressure, particularly in middle age.[21]

A Prevalent Disorder

As America ages and continues to become fatter, the rate of hypertension increases to alarmingly high levels. The number of hypertensive Americans has increased to 65 million from 50 million a decade ago (Fig. 15.9). One of every three to four Americans or a billion people worldwide experiences chronic, high blood pressure some time during their lifetime.

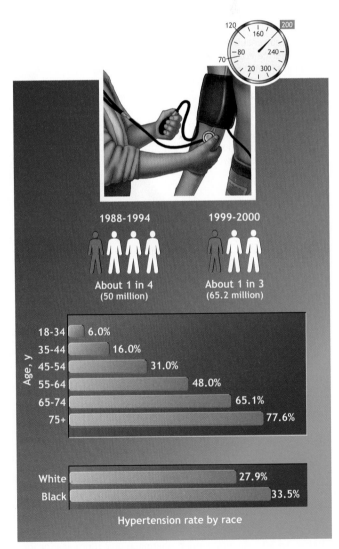

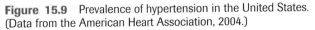

Figure 15.9 Prevalence of hypertension in the United States. (Data from the American Heart Association, 2004.)

A relatively high prevalence of hypertension exists among African Americans, who as a group exhibit a higher risk of hypertension and ischemic stroke than Caucasians.[33] Their predisposition for hypertension reflects reduced sensitivity to the vasodilating action of nitric oxide (see Chapter 16, p. 343).[5,36] Presently, about 65 million Americans have systolic pressures that exceed 140 mm Hg or diastolic pressures above 90 mm Hg. Only two thirds of hypertensive persons know of their disease, only one half are being treated, and only one quarter have their blood pressure under control. Each year, an additional 2 million people become hypertensive. An individual on medication for hypertension still classifies as hypertensive, even if blood pressure remains within the normal range. Uncorrected hypertension often leads to congestive heart failure, kidney disease, myocardial infarction, or stroke. Lowering systolic blood pressure just 2 mm Hg reduces deaths from stroke by 6% and heart disease by 4%. Lowering high blood pressure may also reduce the progression of dementia and cognitive impairment, which are more common in people with hypertension. FIGURE 15.10 shows recommended pharmacologic therapies for treating hypertension after initial nonpharmacologic approaches prove ineffective. Also presented is the renin–angiotensin mechanism. Chapter 20 discusses that a prolonged over-response of this mechanism with a resulting excess output of aldosterone causes hypertension.

Effectively Treated

Preventing a chronic rise in blood pressure serves a crucial function. Even when elevated blood pressure normalizes (through lifestyle changes or medication), the disease risk remains higher than if the person had never become hypertensive in the first place. Blood pressure should be checked periodically because hypertension progresses unnoticed for years.

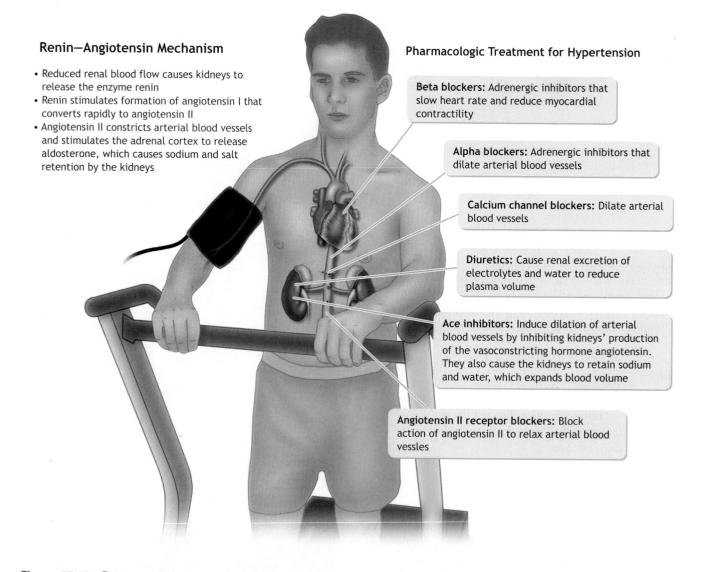

Renin–Angiotensin Mechanism

- Reduced renal blood flow causes kidneys to release the enzyme renin
- Renin stimulates formation of angiotensin I that converts rapidly to angiotensin II
- Angiotensin II constricts arterial blood vessels and stimulates the adrenal cortex to release aldosterone, which causes sodium and salt retention by the kidneys

Pharmacologic Treatment for Hypertension

Beta blockers: Adrenergic inhibitors that slow heart rate and reduce myocardial contractility

Alpha blockers: Adrenergic inhibitors that dilate arterial blood vessels

Calcium channel blockers: Dilate arterial blood vessels

Diuretics: Cause renal excretion of electrolytes and water to reduce plasma volume

Ace inhibitors: Induce dilation of arterial blood vessels by inhibiting kidneys' production of the vasoconstricting hormone angiotensin. They also cause the kidneys to retain sodium and water, which expands blood volume

Angiotensin II receptor blockers: Block action of angiotensin II to relax arterial blood vessles

Figure 15.10 Recommended pharmacologic therapies for the treatment of hypertension following an initial 6 to 12 months of treatment with diet, weight loss, reduced alcohol intake, and regular exercise. A chronically overactive renin–angiotensin mechanism also causes certain forms of high blood pressure.

Effective prevention strategies include lifestyle changes—regular physical activity (daily exercise for at least 30 minutes at a moderate level), modest weight loss (for the overweight and obese), stress management, smoking cessation, reduced sodium and alcohol consumption, and adequate potassium, calcium, and magnesium intake.[1,19,30,39,40] Hypertension treatment also applies medications that reduce either extracellular fluid volume or peripheral resistance to blood flow. A prudent diet, weight control, and regular, moderate exercise should precede pharmacologic treatment for **stage 1 hypertension** (140 to 159 mm Hg systolic; 90 to 99 mm Hg diastolic) and **stage 2 hypertension** (160 to 179 mm Hg systolic; 100 to 109 mm Hg diastolic). This is because of possible harmful side effects of drug therapy on other coronary artery disease risk factors.

The inset table in "In a Practical Sense" on p. 320 gives current classifications and recommended follow-up in initial blood pressure screening for adults. Chapter 32 discusses the role of regular aerobic exercise and resistance exercise to treat moderate hypertension.

BLOOD PRESSURE RESPONSE TO EXERCISE

The blood pressure response to exercise varies with the exercise mode.

Resistance Exercise

Straining exercise, particularly the concentric (shortening) and/or static phase of muscle actions, mechanically compresses the peripheral arterial vessels that supply active muscles. Arterial vascular compression dramatically increases total peripheral resistance and reduces muscle perfusion. Muscle blood flow decreases proportionally to the percentage of maximum force capacity exerted. In an attempt to restore muscle blood flow, substantial increases occur in sympathetic nervous system activity, cardiac output, and MAP. The magnitude of the hypertensive response relates directly to the intensity of effort and amount of muscle mass activated.[11,16,28] Young and older healthy adults have similar short-term hemodynamic responses to resistance exercise.[25,26]

A study from one of our laboratories measured blood pressure of normotensive subjects directly with a pressure transducer connected to a catheter inserted into the femoral artery. Measurements were made during three forms of exercise: (1) isometric bench press performed at 25, 50, 75, and 100% of the maximal voluntary contraction (MVC); (2) free-weight bench press performed at 25 and 50% of the isometric MVC; and (3) hydraulic resistance bench press exercise performed "all out" for 20 seconds at slow and fast speeds. The results, displayed in TABLE 15.1, show clearly that the three exercise modes substantially increased arterial blood pressure and the heart's corresponding workload (see "Rate–Pressure Product," p. 330). Other studies also show that exercise that activates a large muscle mass and requires relatively great muscle strain elicits dramatic blood pressure increases.[9,20,24,29] As we point out in Chapter 16, this exacerbated blood pressure response results from the combined effect of (1) greater stimulation of the cardiovascular center by the active areas of the motor cortex and (2) large peripheral feedback to this center from the contracting muscle mass.

The acute cardiovascular strain with heavy resistance exercise could prove harmful to individuals with heart and vascular disease, particularly individuals untrained in this form of exercise. For them, more rhythmic moderate exercise provides less strain and greater health-related benefits. FIGURE 15.11 presents generalized responses for blood pressure during rhythmic aerobic exercise and heavy resistance exercises that activate either a relatively small or relatively large muscle mass.

TABLE 15.1 ■ COMPARISON OF PEAK SYSTOLIC AND DIASTOLIC BLOOD PRESSURE AT VARIOUS PERCENTAGES OF A MAXIMUM VOLUNTARY CONTRACTION (MVC) DURING ISOMETRIC EXERCISE AND FREE-WEIGHT AND HYDRAULIC BENCH PRESS EXERCISE

Condition	Isometric[a] (% MVC)				Free-Weight Bench Press[b] (% MVC)		Hydraulic Bench Press[c]	
	25	50	75	100	25	50	Slow	Fast
Peak systolic, mm Hg	172	179	200	225	169	232	237	245
Peak diastolic, mm Hg	106	116	135	156	104	154	101	160

Values are averages for seven subjects. Data from Freedson PF, et al. Intra-arterial blood pressure during free weight and hydraulic resistive exercise. Med Sci Sports Exerc 1984;16:131 and unpublished data from the Human Performance Laboratory, Department of Exercise Science, University of Massachusetts, Amherst, MA.
[a] Open glottis (no Valsalva maneuver); average of two trials; contraction time, 2 to 3 seconds; arm position that of bench-press exercise with hands slightly above chest.
[b] The weight lifted was either 25 or 50% of previously determined isometric maximum action.
[c] Performed on Hydra-Fitness chest-press apparatus at dial setting 3 (slow) and 5 (fast) for 20 seconds of repeated maximal actions.

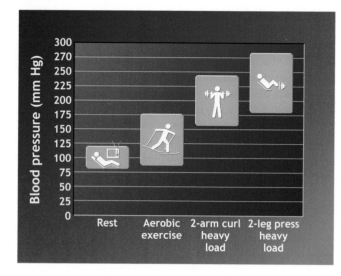

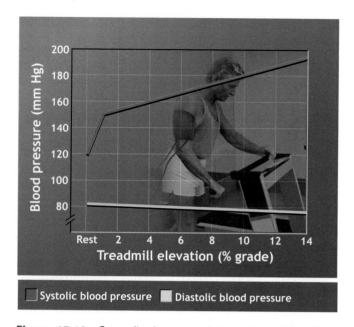

Figure 15.11 Heavy resistance exercise magnifies the exercise blood pressure response (higher with legs than arms) compared with rhythmic, continuous aerobic exercise. The height of the bar indicates pulse pressure.

■ Systolic blood pressure   ■ Diastolic blood pressure

Figure 15.12 Generalized response for systolic and diastolic blood pressures during continuous, graded treadmill exercise up to maximum.

Steady-Rate Exercise

During rhythmic muscular activity (e.g., jogging, swimming, bicycling), vasodilation in the active muscles reduces total peripheral resistance to enhance blood flow through large portions of the peripheral vasculature. Alternate muscle contraction and relaxation also provide an effective force to propel blood through the vascular circuit and return it to the heart. Increased blood flow during rhythmic, steady-rate exercise rapidly increases systolic pressure during the first few minutes of exercise. Blood pressure then levels off at 140 to 160 mm Hg for healthy men and women. As exercise continues, systolic pressure may gradually decline because the arterioles in the active muscles continue to dilate, further reducing peripheral resistance to blood flow. Diastolic blood pressure remains relatively unchanged throughout exercise.

 INTEGRATIVE QUESTION

How can regular resistance exercise training that disproportionately elevates blood pressure during exercise ultimately blunt the blood pressure response to performing a 2-arm curl with 80 pounds?

Graded Exercise

FIGURE 15.12 reveals the general pattern for systolic and diastolic blood pressures during continuous, graded treadmill exercise. After the initial rapid rise from the resting level, systolic blood pressure increases linearly with exercise intensity, while diastolic pressure remains stable or decreases slightly at the higher exercise levels. Healthy, sedentary and endurance-trained subjects demonstrate similar blood pressure responses. During maximum exercise by healthy, fit men and women, systolic blood pressure may increase to 200 mm Hg or higher, despite

significantly reduced total peripheral resistance.[28] This level of blood pressure most likely reflects the heart's large output of blood during maximal exercise by individuals with high aerobic capacity.

Blood Pressure in Upper-Body Exercise

Exercise with the arms produces considerably higher systolic and diastolic blood pressures than leg exercise performed at a given percentage of $\dot{V}O_{2max}$ in each form of exercise (TABLE 15.2).[31,37] This occurs because the smaller arm muscle mass and vasculature offer greater resistance to blood flow

TABLE 15.2 ■ COMPARISON OF SYSTOLIC AND DIASTOLIC BLOOD PRESSURE DURING DYNAMIC ARM AND LEG EXERCISE AT SIMILAR PERCENTAGES OF $\dot{V}O_{2max}$				
	SYSTOLIC PRESSURE (MM HG)		**DIASTOLIC PRESSURE (MM HG)**	
PERCENTAGE OF $\dot{V}O_{2MAX}$	**ARMS**	**LEGS**	**ARMS**	**LEGS**
25	150	132	90	70
40	165	138	93	71
50	175	144	96	73
75	205	160	103	75

From Åstrand PO, et al. Intra-arterial blood pressure during exercise with different muscle groups. J Appl Physiol 1965;20:253.

than the larger leg mass and blood supply. Upper-body exercise (and accompanying elevated blood pressure responses) produces a greater cardiovascular strain because the work requirement of the myocardium increases considerably from the exacerbated rise in blood pressure. Individuals with cardiovascular dysfunction should exercise relatively large muscle groups (walking, bicycling, and running) in contrast to exercise that engages a limited muscle mass (shoveling, overhead hammering, or arm-crank exercise).[10,27] Upper-body exercise to train coronary heart disease patients requires that the proper exercise levels be based upon the person's response to upper-body exercise and not an exercise stress test prescription based on bicycling or running. Chapter 17 further discusses the cardiovascular adjustments to upper-body exercise.

In Recovery

Upon completion of a single bout of submaximal exercise, blood pressure temporarily falls below preexercise levels for normotensive and hypertensive individuals from an unexplained peripheral vasodilation.[15,18,22] The **hypotensive response to previous exercise** can last up to 12 hours. It occurs in response to either low- and moderate-intensity aerobic exercise or resistance exercise.[23,31] One explanation for postexercise hypotension proposes that a significant quantity of blood remains pooled in the visceral organs and/or skeletal muscle vascular beds during recovery.[4] Venous pooling reduces central blood volume, which in turn decreases atrial filling pressure and lowers systemic arterial blood pressure. Recent evidence indicates that a prolonged increase in splanchnic, renal, or cutaneous blood flow in recovery probably plays only a limited contributory role in the postexercise hypotensive response.[32,41] Release of atrial natriuretic peptide hormone, a potent vasodilator, does not account for postexercise hypotension.[23] Postexercise reductions in blood pressure further support moderate exercise as a nonpharmacologic treatment for hypertension. Relatively prolonged reductions in postexercise blood pressure justify recommending multiple periods of physical activity interspersed throughout the day.

THE HEART'S BLOOD SUPPLY

Each day, nearly 2000 gallons of blood flow through the heart's chambers. However, none of the blood's nourishment passes directly into the myocardium because no direct circulatory channels lead from the chambers into the tissues. Instead, the heart muscle maintains its own elaborate circulatory network. FIGURE 15.13 shows that these vessels form a

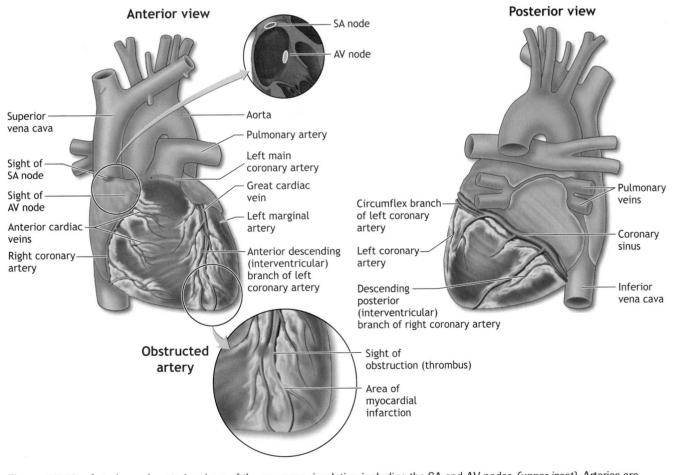

Figure 15.13 Anterior and posterior views of the coronary circulation including the SA and AV nodes *(upper inset).* Arteries are *shaded red* and veins *blue,* with the exception of the pulmonary circulation where colors reverse. The *lower inset* illustrates a myocardial infarction from the blockage of a coronary vessel.

visible, crownlike network, the **coronary circulation,** that arises from the top portion of the heart.

The right and left coronary arteries emerge from the upper part of the ascending aorta. Their openings form just above the semilunar valves at a point where oxygenated blood leaves the left ventricle. These arteries then curl around the heart's surface. The right coronary artery supplies predominantly the right atrium and ventricle. *The greatest volume of blood flows in the left coronary artery to the left atrium and left ventricle and small sections of the right ventricle.* These vessels divide and eventually form a dense capillary network within the myocardium. Blood leaves the tissues of the left ventricle through the **coronary sinus;** blood from the right ventricle exits via the **anterior cardiac veins,** which empty directly into the right atrium.

The driving force of each ventricular systole pushes some blood into the coronary arteries. Normal blood flow to the myocardium at rest equals 200 to 250 mL per minute; this represents approximately 5% of the heart's total output.

Myocardial Oxygen Use

At rest, the myocardium uses considerable oxygen relative to its blood flow; it extracts about 70 to 80% of the oxygen from the blood in the coronary vessels. The magnitude of myocardial oxygen extraction contrasts considerably to most other tissues, which use only about one fourth of their available oxygen at rest. Consequently, a proportionate increase in coronary blood flow in exercise essentially provides the *sole mechanism* to increase myocardial oxygen supply. During vigorous exercise, coronary blood flow increases four to six times above the resting level. Blood flow increases because elevated myocardial metabolism dilates coronary vessels. For example, tissue hypoxia provides a potent stimulus to myocardial blood flow. Sympathetic-mediated arteriolar vasodilation provides some contribution to increased coronary blood flow during exercise, but the local feedback control mechanism remains unknown.[38] Arterial blood pressure also facilitates coronary blood flow. Increased aortic pressure during exercise forces a proportionately greater volume of blood into the coronary circulation. The ebb and flow of blood in the coronary vessels fluctuates with each phase of the cardiac cycle. On average, about 2.5 times more blood flows during diastole than systole.

Effects of Impaired Blood Supply

The myocardium depends on an adequate oxygen supply because, unlike skeletal muscle, this tissue has limited anaerobic energy-generating capacity. Extensive vascular perfusion supplies at least one capillary to each of the heart's muscle fibers. Impaired coronary blood flow usually produces chest pains termed **angina pectoris.** More pronounced pain occurs during exercise because the heart's energy requirements increase considerably. Fortunately, the stress of exercise provides a unique way to evaluate adequacy of myocardial blood flow. A blood clot or **thrombus** lodged in a coronary vessel usually impairs normal heart function. This form of "heart attack," or more specifically **myocardial infarction,** may be mild; a more complete blockage severely damages the myocardium and causes death. Chapters 31 and 32 provide the details about coronary heart disease, stress testing, and the role of regular exercise as preventive and rehabilitative medicine.

Rate–Pressure Product: An Estimate of Myocardial Work

Interactions between several mechanical factors—most importantly, the development of tension within the myocardium and its contractility, and heart rate—determine myocardial oxygen consumption. With increases in each of these factors during exercise, myocardial blood flow adjusts to balance oxygen supply with demand. One common estimate of myocardial workload (and resulting oxygen consumption) uses the product of peak systolic blood pressure (SBP), measured at the brachial artery, and heart rate (HR). *This index of relative cardiac work, termed the double product or **rate–pressure product (RPP),** relates closely to directly measured myocardial oxygen consumption and coronary blood flow in healthy subjects over a wide range of exercise intensities.* RPP computes as follows:

$$RPP = SBP \times HR$$

Changes in heart rate and blood pressure contribute equally to changes in RPP. Typical values for RPP range from 6000 at rest (HR = 50 b · min^{-1}; SBP = 120 mm Hg) to 40,000 (HR = 200 b · min^{-1}; SBP = 200 mm Hg) or above, depending on intensity and exercise mode. Resistance training and upper-body exercise produce substantially higher heart rate and blood pressure responses (hence higher RPPs) than more rhythmic exercise with the lower body. This added myocardial work poses an unnecessary risk for coronary heart disease patients with compromised myocardial oxygen supply.

Research with heart disease patients shows a physiologic correlation between RPP and onset of angina pectoris and electrocardiographic abnormalities during exercise. The RPP thus provides an objective yardstick to evaluate the effects on cardiac performance of various clinical, surgical, or exercise interventions. The well-documented lowering of exercise heart rate and systolic blood pressure (hence lower RPP and myocardial oxygen requirement) with training helps to explain the improved exercise capacity of cardiac patients following exercise training. Prolonged, high-intensity aerobic training also allows cardiac patients to achieve a higher exercise RPP.[8,13] In nine patients followed over a 7-year training period, RPP increased by 11.5% before ischemic symptoms appeared during graded exercise testing.[34] These important findings provide *indirect* evidence for improved myocardial oxygenation, probably from greater coronary vascularization or reduced obstruction from the training adaptation.

INTEGRATIVE QUESTION

Why would a training-induced increase in the rate–pressure product before a patient experiences angina or electrocardiographic abnormalities during exercise imply enhanced myocardial oxygenation?

FOCUS On Research

REQUIRED EXERCISE INTENSITY TO IMPROVE FITNESS

Karvonen MJ, et al. The effects of training on heart rate: a longitudinal study. Ann Med Exp Biol Fenn 1957;35:307.

▲ For many years, research focused on the best ways to develop and maintain cardiorespiratory fitness. Exercise frequency, intensity, type, and time (FITT) all influence the exercise prescription, but the most important variable remains exercise intensity. Experts cannot agree about which method best determines optimal exercise intensity for inducing a training response. The study by Karvonen and colleagues provided a simple method based on heart rate to gauge the *minimum* training threshold.

The researchers used different exercise intensities to determine the influence of resting, exercise, and maximal heart rate on the training response of six young adult (20- to 23-year-old) male medical students. The study's unique aspect included constancy of exercise mode (treadmill running), duration (30 min), frequency (4 or 5 days per week), and length of training (4 weeks). Three different heart rates served as criterion measures: (1) training heart rate (THR), heart rate measured during each exercise session; (2) resting heart rate (RHR), measured every morning in bed before rising; and (3) maximal heart rate (MHR), determined before and after the 4-week training period.

The study aimed to keep relative training intensity constant by adjusting running speed so THR did not decrease as cardiovascular fitness improved (*top panel of figure*). The researchers' method for calculating THR, now known as the "**Karvonen method**" or "**HR reserve method**," applies the subject's exercise HR increase above RHR to the range between MHR and RHR. The following formula applies these data to establish THR at a percentage of training intensity (%T_{INT}):

$$THR = [(MHR - RHR) \times \%T_{INT}] + RHR$$

The following formula computes %T_{INT} at a known THR as follows:

$$\%T_{INT} = (THR - RHR) \div (MHR - RHR) \times 100$$

For example, if a woman wished to know her THR at %T_{INT} = 70% and knows that her MHR equals 170 b · min^{-1} and RHR equals 52 b · min^{-1}, then THR equals 135 b · min^{-1}: [(170 − 52) × 0.70] + 52 = 135. Conversely, knowing THR enables one to calculate the %T_{INT}: (135 − 52) ÷ (170 − 52) × 100 = 70%.

The researchers showed that when heart rate established training intensity, the "borderline" between effective and ineffective training slightly exceeded 60% of the percentage training intensity. The researchers recommended that THR must reach *at least* 60%T_{INT} and preferably 70%T_{INT}. The inset figure for a representative subject shows that THR averaged 136 b · min^{-1} or 71% of the available heart rate range. The *top panel* displays the change in running speed required to maintain a constant THR throughout the 4-week training period.

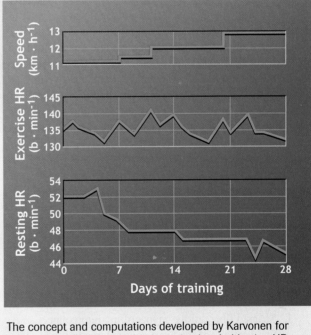

The concept and computations developed by Karvonen for establishing effective training intensity threshold using HR significantly affected the future study of exercise training.

MYOCARDIAL METABOLISM

Like all tissue, the myocardium uses the chemical energy stored in food to generate ATP to power its work. The myocardium relies almost exclusively on energy released in aerobic reactions; myocardial tissue therefore has a threefold higher oxidative capacity than skeletal muscle. Its muscle fibers contain the greatest mitochondrial concentration of all

tissues, with exceptional capacity for long-chain fatty acid catabolism as a primary means for ATP resynthesis.

FIGURE 15.14 shows the specific substrate use (on a percentage basis) by the myocardium during rest and moderate and intense exercise. Glucose, fatty acids, and lactate formed from glycolysis in skeletal muscle provide the energy for myocardial functioning.[3,17] At rest, these three substrates contribute to ATP resynthesis, with the most energy from free fatty

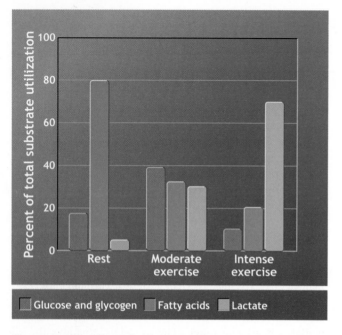

Figure 15.14 Generalized pattern of myocardial substrate use at rest and in relation to exercise intensity.

acid breakdown.[12] After a meal, however, glucose becomes the preferred energy substrate. In essence, the heart uses for energy whatever substrate it "sees" on a physiologic level. During intense exercise, for example, when lactate efflux from active skeletal muscle into the blood increases dramatically, the heart derives its major energy by oxidizing circulating lactate. In more moderate exercise, equal amounts of fat and carbohydrate provide the energy fuel. During prolonged submaximal exercise (not illustrated), myocardial metabolism of free fatty acids rises to almost 70% of the total energy requirement. Similar patterns of myocardial metabolism exist for trained and untrained individuals. An endurance-trained person, however, demonstrates considerably greater myocardial reliance on fat catabolism in submaximal exercise. This difference, similar to the effect for skeletal muscle, illustrates the "carbohydrate-sparing effect" of aerobic training.

Summary

1. Striated fibers of the myocardium interconnect so that portions of the heart contract in a unified manner.

2. The heart functions as two separate pumps: one pump receives blood from the body and pumps it to the lungs for aeration (pulmonary circulation), while the other receives oxygenated blood from the lungs and pumps it throughout the systemic circulation.

3. Pressure changes created during the cardiac cycle act on the heart's valves to provide one-way blood flow in the vascular circuit.

4. The surge of blood with ventricular contraction (and subsequent run-off of blood in relaxation) creates pressure changes within the arterial vessels.

Ventricular contraction generates systolic blood pressure, the highest pressure during the cardiac cycle. Diastolic pressure represents the lowest pressure before the next ventricular contraction.

5. The dense capillary network provides a large and effective surface for exchange between the blood and tissues. These minute-diameter blood vessels possess autoregulatory capacity to adjust blood flow in response to the tissue's metabolic activity.

6. The venous tree contains the largest portion of central blood volume at rest, but an increase in venous tone (venoconstriction) probably contributes little to the redistribution of blood during exercise.

7. Compression and relaxation of the veins by skeletal muscle action impart considerable energy to facilitate venous return. This "muscle pump" mechanism provides additional justification for active recovery immediately following vigorous exercise.

8. One of every three to four persons experiences chronic, abnormally high blood pressure sometime during his or her life. Hypertension imposes a chronic stress on the cardiovascular system that eventually damages arterial vessels and leads to arteriosclerosis, heart disease, stroke, and kidney failure.

9. Systolic blood pressure increases in proportion to oxygen consumption and blood flow during graded exercise, whereas diastolic pressure remains relatively unchanged or decreases slightly. At the same relative and absolute exercise levels, upper-body exercise produces a greater rise in systolic pressure than leg exercise.

10. After exercising, blood pressure decreases below the preexercise level and may remain lower for up to 12 hours.

11. During isometric, free-weight, and hydraulic resistance exercises, peak systolic and diastolic blood pressures mirror a hypertensive state. Performing high-intensity resistance exercises pose a risk to individuals with hypertension or heart disease.

12. At rest, the myocardium extracts approximately 80% of the oxygen flowing through the coronary arteries. An increase in coronary blood flow primarily provides for myocardial oxygen needs in exercise.

13. The myocardium requires a continual adequate supply of oxygen. Coronary blood flow impairment initiates chest (angina) pains; blockage of a coronary artery (myocardial infarction) causes irreversible damage to the heart muscle.

14. The product of heart rate and systolic blood pressure, termed rate–pressure product (RPP), estimates myocardial workload.

15. The myocardium metabolizes glucose, fatty acids, and circulating lactate for energy. Their percentage use varies with the severity and duration of exercise and the individual's training status.

References are available on the Student CD and online at http://connection.lww.com/mkk6e.

Cardiovascular Regulation and Integration

16

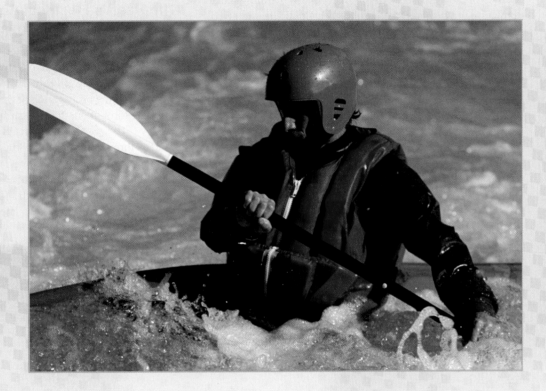

CHAPTER OBJECTIVES

- Discuss how intrinsic and extrinsic factors regulate heart rate during rest and exercise

- Draw a normal electrocardiogram (ECG) tracing, and identify and describe its major components

- Describe how local metabolic factors regulate blood flow during rest and exercise

- Explain the role of "central command" in cardiovascular regulation during exercise

- Describe the effects of aerobic exercise training on neural regulation of heart rate

- Outline the contributions of chemoreceptors, mechanoreceptors, and the metaboreflex in cardiovascular regulation during exercise

- Indicate how each component of Poiseuille's law affects blood flow

- Summarize the dynamics of blood flow to diverse tissues at exercise onset and as exercise progresses in duration and intensity

- Describe the proposed mechanisms for nitric oxide's regulation of local blood flow

- Outline the heart transplant patient's cardiovascular response to exercise

The vascular system demonstrates exceptional capacity for expansion. For example, the vessels of the skin, viscera, and skeletal muscles have the potential to conduct a blood volume three to four times the pumping capacity of the normal heart.[52] Complex mechanisms continually interact to maintain a dynamic balance between systemic blood pressure and blood flow to different tissues under various conditions. Neurochemical factors regulate heart rate and the internal opening of blood vessels. An exquisite level of cardiovascular regulation provides rapid control of heart function and effective distribution of blood flow throughout the body. When a person rests, for example, the skin receives approximately 5% of the 5 L of blood pumped by the heart each minute. This contrasts to exercise in a hot, humid environment when up to 20% of the total blood flow diverts to the body's surface to dissipate heat. "Shunting" of blood and maintenance of blood pressure occur only within a closed vascular system. This dynamic allows a near-immediate increase and redistribution of blood flow to meet changing metabolic and physiologic needs and environmental challenges.

INTRINSIC REGULATION OF HEART RATE

Cardiac muscle, unlike other tissues, maintains its own rhythm. If left to its inherent rhythmicity, the heart would beat steadily at about 100 times each minute. Situated within the posterior wall of the right atrium lies a small (3-mm wide and 1-cm long) mass of specialized muscle tissue called the **sinoatrial node** or **SA node**. This node spontaneously depolarizes and repolarizes to provide the innate stimulus for heart action. For this reason, the term **pacemaker** describes the SA node. FIGURE 16.1 (left) shows the normal route for impulse transmission within the myocardium.

The Heart's Electrical Activity

Electrochemical rhythms originating at the SA node spread across the atria to another small knot of tissue situated close to the tricuspid valve known as the **atrioventricular node** or **AV node**. Figure 16.1 (right) illustrates the time sequence of the propagation of the electrical impulse from the SA node throughout the myocardium.

A 0.10-second delay occurs after the electrical impulse spreads through the atria to allow them to contract and propel blood into the ventricles below. The AV node gives rise to the 1-cm long **AV bundle**, also called the **bundle of His** for Swiss cardiologist Wilhelm His, Jr. (1863–1934), who first described this tissue in 1893. The AV bundle transmits the impulse rapidly through the ventricles over specialized conducting fibers referred to as the **Purkinje system** (named for Bohemian anatomist–physiologist Johannes Evangelista von Purkinje [1787–1869]). These fibers form distinct bundle branches that penetrate the right and left ventricles. Purkinje

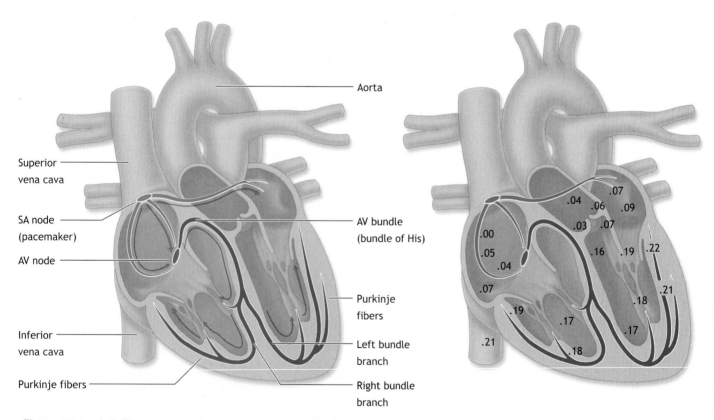

Figure 16.1 *Left.* The *red arrows* denote the normal route for excitation and conduction of the cardiac impulse. The impulse originates at the SA node, travels to the AV node, and then spreads throughout the ventricular mass. *Right.* Time sequence in seconds for electrical impulse transmission from the SA node throughout the myocardium.

system fibers transmit the impulse about 6 times faster than normal ventricular muscle fibers. The passage of the impulse into the ventricles stimulates each ventricular cell within 0.06 seconds. This allows a unified and simultaneous subsequent contraction of both ventricles. The transmission of the cardiac impulse flows as follows:

SA node → Atria → AV node → AV bundle
(Purkinje fibers) → Ventricles

Electrocardiogram

Like all nerve and muscle tissue, the outer surface of myocardial cells (fibers) maintains a more positive electrical charge than the inside. Upon stimulation prior to contraction, polarity reverses and the myocardial cells' inside becomes more positive than the outside. During the diastolic phase of the cardiac cycle, the membranes repolarize to reestablish the normal resting membrane potential.

The myocardium's electrical activity creates an electrical field throughout the body. Because the salty bodily fluids provide an excellent conducting medium, electrodes on the skin's surface readily detect voltage changes from the sequence of electrical events before and during each cardiac cycle. FIGURE 16.2 graphically displays the normal cycle of the heart's electrical activity by the **electrocardiogram**, or simply **ECG** (see also "In a Practical Sense," p. 336).

Recording the heart's electrical activity began in 1841 when Italian physicist Carlo Matteuci (1811–1868) documented the electrical properties of frog muscles proposed by biologist Luigi Galvani (1737–1798). Seven years later following considerable experiments also with frogs, world-renown German electrophysiologist Emil Dubois-Reymond (1818–1868) described the experimental set-ups, instruments, and frog preparations to explain the properties of electrical transmission through biologic tissues. In 1890, British physiologists Sir William Maddock Bayliss (1860–1924) and Edward Starling (1866–1927) of University College, London,

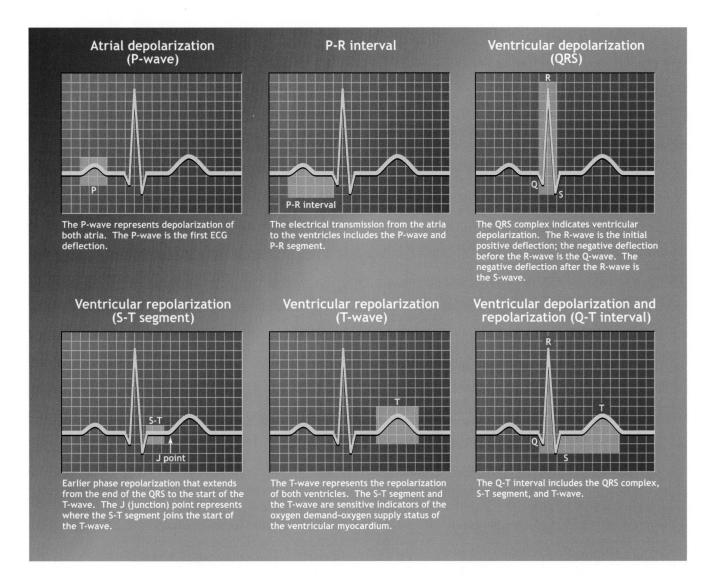

Figure 16.2 Different phases of the normal ECG from atrial depolarization *(upper left)* to ventricular repolarization *(lower middle)*.

IN A PRACTICAL SENSE

PLACING ELECTRODES FOR BIPOLAR AND 12-LEAD ECG RECORDINGS

■ The electrocardiogram (ECG) represents a composite record of the heart's electrical events during a cardiac cycle. These events provide a way to monitor heart rate during different physical activities and exercise stress testing. The ECG can detect contraindications to exercise, including previous myocardial infarction, ischemic S-T segment changes, conduction defects, and left ventricular enlargement (hypertrophy). A valid ECG tracing requires proper electrode placement. The term **ECG lead** indicates the specific placement of a *pair* of electrodes on the body that transmits the electrical signal to a recorder. The record of electrical differences across different ECG leads creates the composite electrical "picture" of myocardial activity.

SKIN PREPARATION
Proper skin preparation reduces extraneous electrical "noise" (interference and skeletal muscle artifact). Abrade the skin with fine sandpaper or commercially available pads and alcohol to remove surface epidermis and oil; the skin should appear red, slightly irritated, dry, and clean.

BIPOLAR (3-ELECTRODE) CONFIGURATION
The *top figure* shows the typical electrode placement for a 3-lead bipolar configuration. This positioning provides less sensitivity for diagnostic testing but proves useful for routine ECG monitoring in functional exercise testing and radiotelemetry of the ECG during physical activity. The ground (green or black) electrode attaches over the sternum, the positive (red) electrode attaches on the left side of the chest in the V_5 position (level of the 5th intercostal space adjacent to the midaxillary line), and the positive (white) electrode attaches on the right side of the chest just below the nipple at the level of the 5th intercostal space. Placement of the positive electrode can be altered to optimize the recording (e.g., 3rd and 4th intercostal spaces, anterior portion of the right shoulder, or near the clavicle). Correct electrode placement can be remembered as follows: *white to right, green to ground, red to left.*

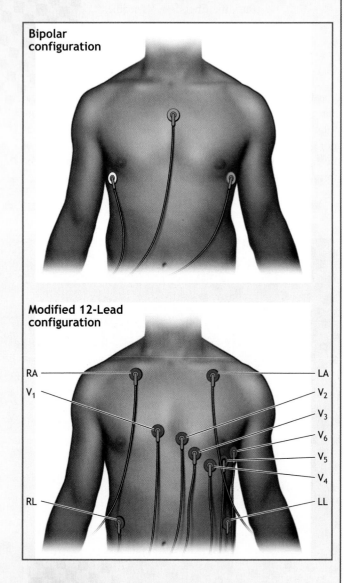

Bipolar configuration

Modified 12-Lead configuration

RA
V_1
RL
LA
V_2
V_3
V_6
V_5
V_4
LL

MODIFIED 12-LEAD (10-ELECTRODE TORSO-MOUNTED) CONFIGURATION FOR EXERCISE STRESS TESTING
The standard 12-lead ECG consists of three limb leads, three augmented unipolar leads, and six chest leads. For improved exercise ECG recordings, electrodes mounted on the torso (abdominal level) replace the conventional ankle (leg) and wrist electrodes. This "torso-mounted limb lead system" *(bottom figure)* reduces electrical artifact introduced by limb movement during exercise.

continued on page 337

Continued

ELECTRODE POSITIONING IN THE MODIFIED 10-ELECTRODE, TORSO-MOUNTED SYSTEM

1. RL (right leg): just above right iliac crest on midaxillary line
2. LL (left leg): just above left iliac crest on midaxillary line
3. RA (right arm): just below right clavicle medial to deltoid muscle
4. LA (left arm): just below left clavicle medial to deltoid muscle
5. V_1: on right sternal border in 4th intercostal space
6. V_2: on left sternal border in 4th intercostal space
7. V_3: at midpoint of a straight line between V_2 and V_4
8. V_4: on midclavicular line in 5th intercostal space
9. V_5: on anterior axillary line and horizontal to V_4
10. V_6: on midaxillary line and horizontal to V_4 and V_5

Phibbs B, Buckels L. Comparative yields of ECG leads in multistage stress testing. Am Heart J 1985;90:275.

---

connected the terminals from a capillary electrometer to the right hand and skin over the apex beat. This setup produced a pattern that showed a "triphasic variation accompanying (or rather preceding) each beat of the heart." These patterns of electrical deflections are now referred to as the P, QRS, and T waves.

The **P wave** represents depolarization of the atria. It lasts approximately 0.15 second and heralds atrial contraction. The relatively large **QRS complex** follows the P wave; it signals electrical changes from ventricular depolarization. At this point, the ventricles contract. Atrial repolarization follows the P wave; it produces a wave so small that the large QRS complex usually obscures it. The **T wave** represents ventricular repolarization that occurs during ventricular diastole. The heart's relatively long depolarization period of 0.20 to 0.30 seconds prevents initiation of the next myocardial impulse (and subsequent contraction). This rest or brief time-out **refractory period** allows sufficient time for ventricular filling between beats.

The ECG objectively monitors heart rate during exercise. Radiotelemetry (using wireless telephony) transmits the ECG while a person freely performs any physical activity from football, weight lifting, basketball, ice hockey, dancing, swimming and diving, to space extravehicular activity. As discussed in Chapter 31, electrocardiography furnishes a vital diagnostic tool to uncover abnormalities in heart function, particularly abnormalities related to cardiac rhythm, electrical conduction, myocardial oxygenation, and tissue damage.

EXTRINSIC REGULATION OF HEART RATE AND CIRCULATION

Changes in heart rate occur rapidly through nerves that directly supply the myocardium and chemical "messengers" that circulate in blood. These **extrinsic controls** of cardiac function accelerate the heart in anticipation before exercise

begins, and then rapidly adjust to the intensity of physical effort. To a large extent, extrinsic regulation can decrease heart rate to 25 to 30 b · min^{-1} under normal ambulatory conditions in highly trained endurance athletes[8] and exceed 200 b · min^{-1} in maximal exercise.

FIGURE 16.3 illustrates neural mechanisms for cardiovascular regulation before and during exercise. Input from the brain and peripheral nervous system continually bombards the cardiovascular control center in the **ventrolateral medulla**. This center regulates the heart's output of blood and blood's preferential distribution to all the body's tissues.

Sympathetic and Parasympathetic Neural Input

Neural influences can override the inherent rhythm of the myocardium. These influences originate in the cardiovascular center and flow through the **sympathetic** and **parasympathetic** components of the autonomic nervous system (see Chapter 19). These two divisions operate in parallel but act by distinctly different structural pathways and transmitter systems. FIGURE 16.4 illustrates the distribution of sympathetic and parasympathetic nerve fibers within the myocardium. Large numbers of sympathetic and parasympathetic neurons innervate the atria, whereas the ventricles receive sympathetic fibers almost exclusively.

Sympathetic Influence

Stimulation of the sympathetic cardioaccelerator nerves releases the **catecholamines** epinephrine and norepinephrine. These neuro hormones accelerate SA node depolarization, causing the heart to beat faster (**chronotropic effect**). The term **tachycardia** describes heart rate acceleration, usually to rates that exceed 100 b · min^{-1}. Catecholamines also increase

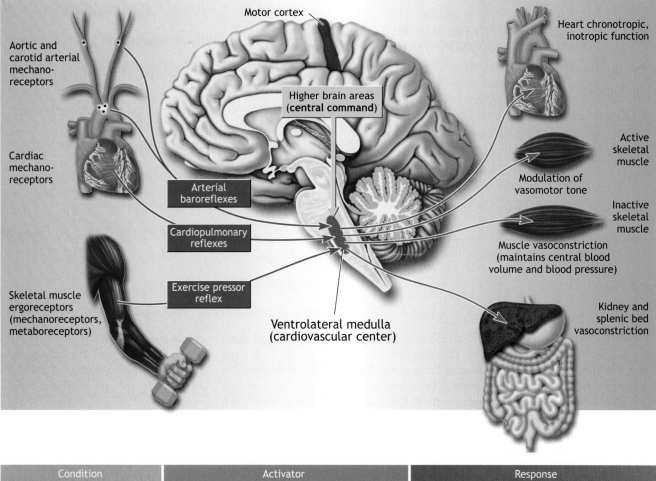

Condition	Activator	Response
Preexercise "anticipatory" response	Activation of central command from the motor cortex and higher areas of the brain cause an increase in sympathetic outflow and reciprocal inhibition of parasympathetic activity.	Acceleration of heart rate; increased myocardial contractility; vasodilation in skeletal and heart muscle (cholinergic fibers); vasoconstriction in other areas, especially skin, gut, spleen, liver, and kidneys (adrenergic fibers); increase in arterial blood pressure.
Exercise	Parasympathetic withdrawal at onset and during low-intensity exercise; progressive sympathetic stimulation in more intense exercise; reflex feedback from peripheral mechanical and chemical receptors that monitor muscle action; alterations in local metabolic conditions due to hypoxia, $\downarrow$pH, $\uparrow Pco_2$, $\uparrow$ADP, $\uparrow Mg^{2+}$, $\uparrow Ca^{2+}$, and $\uparrow$temperature cause autoregulatory vasodilation in active muscle.	Further dilation of muscle vasculature.
	Continued sympathetic adrenergic outflow in conjunction with epinephrine and norepinephrine from the adrenal medulla.	Concomitant constriction of vasculature in inactive tissues to maintain adequate perfusion pressure throughout arterial system. Action of the muscle pump and visceral vasoconstiction combine to facilitate venous return and maintain central blood volume.

Figure 16.3 Neural regulation of the cardiovascular system during exercise. (Modified from Mitchell JH, Raven PB. Cardiovascular adaptation to physical activity. (In: Bouchard C, et al., eds. Physical activity, fitness, and health. Champaign, IL: Human Kinetics, 1994.)

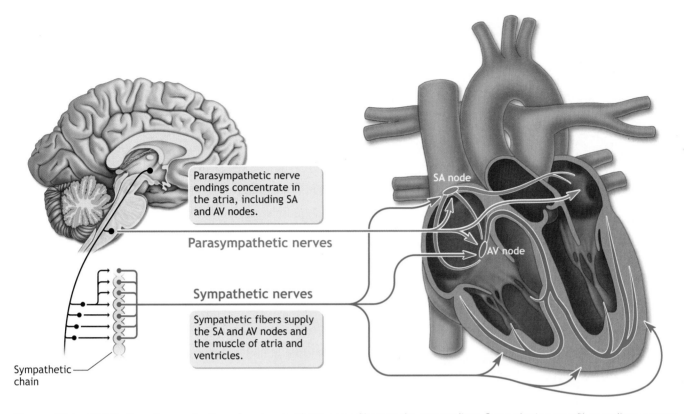

Figure 16.4 Distribution of sympathetic and parasympathetic nerve fibers to the myocardium. Sympathetic nerve fiber endings secrete epinephrine. Sympathetic fibers supply the SA and AV nodes and the muscle of the atria and ventricles. Parasympathetic nerve endings secrete acetylcholine. These fibers concentrate in the atria, including the SA and AV nodes.

myocardial contractility (**inotropic effect**) to augment how much blood the heart pumps with each beat. The force of ventricular contraction nearly doubles under maximum sympathetic stimulation. Epinephrine, released from the medullary portion of the adrenal glands during general sympathetic activation, produces a similar but slower acting tachycardia effect on cardiac function.

Sympathetic stimulation also profoundly affects blood flow throughout the body.[62] Sympathetic stimulation produces vasoconstriction except in the coronary vasculature. FIGURE 16.5 schematically depicts the distribution of sympathetic and parasympathetic outflow. The sympathetic system's preganglionic axons emerge *only* from the thoracic and lumbar segments of the spinal cord. The preganglionic neurons of the sympathetic nervous system lie within the cord's gray matter. Their axons emerge through the ventral roots and synapse in the ganglia of the sympathetic chain adjacent to the spinal column. Postganglionic sympathetic nerve fibers end in the smooth muscle layers of small arteries, arterioles, and precapillary sphincters. Norepinephrine acts as a general vasoconstrictor released by specific sympathetic neurons termed **adrenergic fibers**. Some adrenergic constrictor nerves remain continually active. This means that certain blood vessels always exhibit a state of constriction or **vasomotor tone** even within active muscle during intense exercise. Dilation of blood vessels under adren-

ergic influence results more from reduced vasomotor tone (decreased adrenergic activity) than from increased activity of either cholinergic sympathetic or parasympathetic dilator fibers (see next section). In addition, powerful vasodilation induced by byproducts of local metabolism rapidly overrides any sympathetically activated vasoconstriction in active tissue (see "Factors Within Active Muscle," p. 343). Humoral feedback from metabolites released to the circulation from active muscles accelerates heart rate during exercise.[32]

Parasympathetic Influence

Preganglionic axons of the parasympathetic division emerge *only* from the brainstem and the cord's sacral segments. Consequently, the parasympathetic and sympathetic systems complement each other anatomically. The preganglionic parasympathetic neurons lie within brainstem tissue and lower spinal cord. Their axons travel farther than sympathetic axons because their ganglia typically lie adjacent to or within target organs. Parasympathetic fibers distribute to the head, neck, and body cavities (except for erectile tissues of genitalia) and never emerge in the body wall and limbs. When stimulated, parasympathetic neurons release acetylcholine, which retards the rate of sinus discharge to slow heart rate. A reduced heart rate (**bradycardia**) results largely from stimulation of the pair of

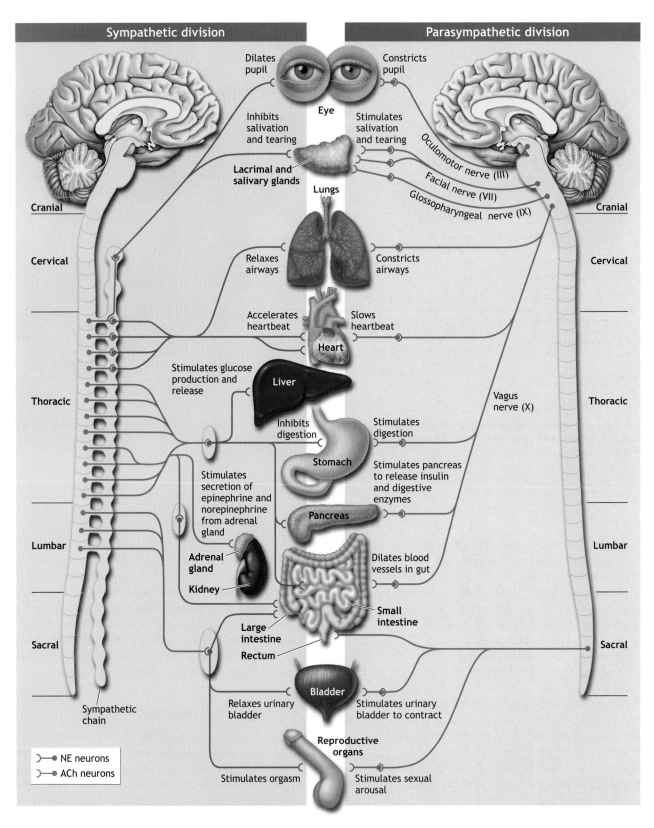

Figure 16.5 Schematic view of the chemical, anatomic, and functional organization of the sympathetic and parasympathetic divisions of the autonomic nervous system. The preganglionic inputs of both divisions use acetylcholine (ACh; *red*) as the neurotransmitter. The postganglionic parasympathetic innervation to the visceral organs also uses ACh, but postganglionic sympathetic innervation uses norepinephrine (NE; *blue*), with the exception that Ach innervates sweat glands. The adrenal medulla receives preganglionic sympathetic innervation and secretes epinephrine into the bloodstream when activated. In general, sympathetic stimulation produces catabolic effects that prepare the body to "fight" or "flee," while parasympathetic stimulation produces anabolic responses that promote normal function and conserve energy. (Modified from Bear MF, et al. Neuroscience: exploring the brain. Baltimore: Williams & Wilkins, 1996.)

vagus nerves whose cell bodies originate in the medulla's cardioinhibitory center. The vagus nerves are the only cranial nerves that exit the head and neck region and descend to the thorax and abdominal regions. These nerves carry approximately 80% of all parasympathetic fibers. Vagal stimulation exerts no effect on myocardial contractility. Parasympathetic nerve fibers leave the brainstem and spinal cord to affect diverse body areas. Like sympathetic function, parasympathetic stimulation excites some tissues (e.g., muscles of the iris, gallbladder and bile ducts, bronchi, and coronary arteries) and inhibits other tissues (muscles of gut sphincters, intestines, and skin vasculature). Except for sweat glands, parasympathetic stimulation induces glandular secretion.

At the start of and during low- to moderate-intensity exercise, heart rate increases by inhibiting of parasympathetic stimulation largely through central command activation (see next section). Heart rate in strenuous exercise increases by additional parasympathetic inhibition and direct activation of sympathetic cardioaccelerator nerves. The magnitude of heart rate acceleration relates directly to physical activity intensity and duration.[43,54]

Central Command: Input from Higher Centers

Impulses originating in the brain's higher somatomotor **central command** center continually modulate medullary activity. The motor center recruits muscles required for physical activity. Impulses from the "feed-forward" central command descend via small afferent nerves through the cardiovascular center in the medulla. This neural input coordinates the rapid adjustment of the heart and blood vessels to optimize tissue perfusion and maintain central blood pressure in relation to motor cortex involvement. This type of neural control operates during the preexercise anticipatory period and during the early stage of exercise. Motor cortex stimulation of the medulla increases with the size of the muscle mass activated in exercise. *Central command provides the greatest control over heart rate during exercise.*[25,44,68]

FIGURE 16.6 shows the influence of the central command on heart rate when exercise begins. Radiotelemetry continuously monitored the heart rate of trained sprint runners at rest, at the starting commands, and during 60-, 220-, and 440-yard races. Heart rate averaged 148 b·min^{-1} at the starting commands in anticipation of the 60-yard sprint; this represented 74% of the total heart rate adjustment to the run before exercise even began. The longer sprint events elicited successively lower anticipatory heart rates. This pattern also occurred for longer-duration events. For example, anticipatory heart rates of four athletes trained for the 880-yard run averaged 122 b · min^{-1}, whereas heart rates averaged 118 b · min^{-1} during the starting commands of the 1-mile run and 108 b · min^{-1} immediately before the 2-mile run. A high neural outflow from central command in anticipation of exercise and immediately at the start seems desirable for intense sprint activity to mobilize physiologic reserves rapidly. In contrast, "revving the body's engine" might prove wasteful before dis-

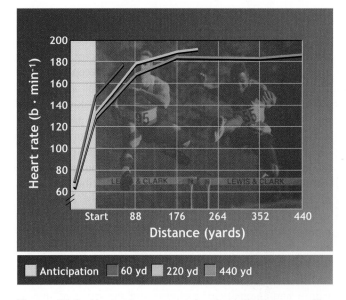

Figure 16.6 Heart rate response of sprint-trained runners. The largest increase in anticipatory heart rate (HR immediately before exercising) occured in the short-sprint events and was successively smaller before the longer sprints. (From McArdle WD, et al. Telemetered cardiac response to selected running events. J Appl Physiol 1967;23:566.)

tance events. Interestingly, muscle blood flow also increases in anticipation of exercise. The response demonstrates training specificity because the magnitude of the preexercise increases in mean arterial pressure and decreases in skeletal muscle vascular resistance varies with exercise intensity, duration, *and* specific mode of prior training.[3,16]

The heart rapidly "turns on" in exercise by decreasing parasympathetic inhibitory input and increasing stimulating input from the brain's central command. Accelerator input as exercise begins also comes from activation of receptors in active joints and muscles (see following section). The much slower contribution to heart rate increase from the sympathetic nervous system—triggered by reflex activity and *not* central command—does not occur until achieving a moderate exercise intensity. Even in so-called nonsprint events, heart rate reaches 180 b · min^{-1} within 30 seconds of 1- and 2-mile runs. Further heart rate increases progress gradually with several plateaus during the run. Almost identical results occur for heart rate measured by telemetry during competitive swimming events except for lower maximum heart rates during swimming.

Central command involvement in cardiovascular regulation also explains how variations in emotional state significantly affect cardiovascular response. Such neural input creates difficulty obtaining "true" resting values for heart rate and blood pressure.[6]

INTEGRATIVE QUESTIONS

Give a physiologic rationale for biofeedback and relaxation techniques to treat hypertension and stress-related disorders.

Peripheral Input

The cardiovascular center receives reflex sensory input (feedback) from peripheral receptors in blood vessels, joints, and muscles. **Chemoreceptors** and **mechanoreceptors** within muscle and its vasculature monitor its chemical and physical state. Afferent impulses from these receptors—slow-conducting, thin-fiber group III and IV afferents from pacinian corpuscles and unencapsulated nerve-ending receptors—provide rapid feedback. This input modifies either vagal (parasympathetic) or sympathetic outflow to bring about appropriate cardiovascular and respiratory responses to various intensities of physical activity.[1,21,22,24,52,59] Activation of chemically - sensitive afferents within the muscle's interstitium helps to regulate sympathetic neural activation of muscle during typical submaximal exercise. Metabolites produced primarily during the concentric phase of muscular activity stimulate this **metaboreflex**.[13] Three mechanisms continually assess the nature and intensity of exercise and the mass of muscle activated:

1. Reflex neural input from mechanical deformation of type III afferents within active muscles.
2. Chemical stimulation of type IV afferents within active muscles (exercise pressor reflex).
3. Feed-forward outflow from the motor areas of the central command.

Central nervous system's regulation of blood flow and blood pressure during dynamic exercise comes from specific mechanoreceptor feedback.[47,61] The aortic arch and carotid sinus contain pressure-sensitive **baroreceptors**, while cardiopulmonary mechanoreceptors assess mechanical activity in the left ventricle, right atrium, and large veins. These receptors function as negative feedback controllers to (1) inhibit sympathetic outflow from the cardiovascular center and (2) blunt an inordinate rise in arterial blood pressure.[49,53,69] As blood pressure increases, stretching of the arterial vessels activates the baroreceptors to slow the heart reflexly and dilate the peripheral vasculature. This *decreases* blood pressure toward more normal levels. During exercise, blood pressure becomes effectively regulated but at higher levels. This probably occurs from an override of the arterial baroreflex feedback mechanism or an upward resetting of its threshold and/or sensitivity (i.e., reduced baroreflex gain), partly from central command activation.[39,47,50] The baroreceptors more than likely act as a brake to curtail abnormally high blood pressure levels during exercise.

Carotid Artery Palpation

External pressure against the carotid artery sometimes slows the heart rate from direct baroreceptor stimulation at the bifurcation of the carotid artery. The potential for bradycardia from **carotid artery palpation** is important to exercise specialists because palpation routinely determines exercise heart rate. Consistently low heart rate estimation with carotid artery palpation in susceptible individuals would push the person to a higher exercise level—certainly an undesirable effect in exercise prescription for cardiac patients.

Research in the late 1970s showed that carotid artery palpation slowed postexercise heart rate and occasionally produced electrocardiographic abnormalities.[67] Several later reports indicated, rather convincingly for healthy adults and cardiac patients, that carotid artery palpation caused little or no heart rate alteration during rest or exercise and recovery.[46,55] However, vascular disease can affect carotid sinus sensitivity and produce falsely low heart rate values. An excellent substitute method uses pulse rate at the radial artery (thumb side of wrist) or temporal artery (side of head at temple) because even firm palpation of these vessels does not affect heart rate. Commercially available, wrist-worn monitors and watches provide accurate heart rate measurements under many exercise conditions, including space shuttle missions and earliest manned suborbital flights.[18,40]

Local Factors

The byproducts of energy metabolism provide an autoregulatory mechanism within the muscle to augment perfusion during physical activity. We discuss the local control of circulation in the following sections.

DISTRIBUTION OF BLOOD

If fully dilated, the body's blood vessels could hold approximately 20 L of blood, four times more than the total blood volume of 5 L. Thus, maintenance of blood flow and blood pressure, particularly during exercise, requires a finely regulated balance between vascular dilation and vascular constriction. *The capacity of large portions of the vasculature to constrict or dilate provides rapid blood redistribution to meet metabolic requirements. It also optimizes blood pressure throughout the vascular circuit.*

Physical Factors Affecting Blood Flow

Blood flows through the vascular circuit generally following physical laws of hydrodynamics applied to rigid, cylindrical vessels. However, blood is not a homogeneous fluid, and blood vessels are not rigid tubes; thus, such mathematical relationships exist mainly in a qualitative sense. The volume of flow in any vessel relates to two factors:

* *Directly* to the pressure gradient between the two ends of the vessels, *not* to the absolute pressure within the vessel
* *Inversely* to the resistance encountered to fluid flow

Friction between the blood and internal vascular wall creates resistance or force that impedes blood flow. Three factors determine resistance: (1) blood thickness or viscosity, (2) length of the conducting tube, and, most importantly, (3) blood vessel radius. An equation, referred to as **Poiseuille's law**, ties these factors together to express the general relationship among pressure differential, resistance, and flow as follows:

$$\text{Flow} = \text{Pressure gradient} \times \text{Vessel radius}^4$$
$$\div \text{Vessel length} \times \text{Fluid viscosity}$$

In the body, the transport vessel length remains constant, while blood viscosity varies only slightly under most circumstances. The radius of the conducting tube affects blood flow the most because resistance to flow changes with the vessel's radius raised to the fourth power. For example, halving a vessel's radius decreases flow 16-fold. Conversely, doubling the radius increases volume 16-fold. With pressure differential within the vascular circuit remaining constant, a small change in vessel radius dramatically alters blood flow. *Physiologically, constriction and dilation of the smaller arterial blood vessels provide the crucial mechanism for regulating regional blood flow.*

Effect of Exercise

Any increase in energy expenditure requires rapid adjustments in blood flow that affect the entire cardiovascular system. For example, nerves and local metabolites act on the smooth muscle bands of arteriole walls to alter their internal diameter almost instantaneously to meet blood flow demands. Visceral vasoconstriction and action of the muscle pump divert a large flow of blood into the central circulation.

At the onset of exercise, the vascular component of active muscles increases by dilation of local arterioles. These small feed arteries to skeletal muscle normally possess well-developed flow-mediated and myogenic regulatory mechanisms. They require little modification through exercise training to adequately supply the blood flow requirements of vigorous physical activity.[26] Concurrently, other vessels to tissues that can temporarily compromise their blood supply constrict or "shut down." Two examples include the splanchnic and renal areas. Here, blood flow decreases in proportion to relative exercise intensity (i.e., $\%\dot{V}O_{2max}$). Blood flow shifts from the abdominal viscera to active muscles even during relatively light exercise (HR $\leq$ 90 b·min^{-1}).[48] Two factors contribute to reduced blood flow to nonactive tissues: (1) increased sympathetic nervous system outflow (central and peripheral mechanisms) and (2) local chemicals that directly stimulate vasoconstriction or enhance the effects of other vasoconstrictors.[36,37,42]

The kidneys vividly illustrate regional blood flow adjustment and conservation of bodily fluids via sympathetic vasoconstriction of its vasculature.[70] Renal blood flow at rest normally averages 1100 mL per minute (20% of the total cardiac output), among the highest blood flow to any organ as either a percentage of cardiac output or relative to organ weight. During maximal exercise, renal blood flow decreases to 250 mL per minute or only 1% of the total exercise cardiac output. A large, temporary reduction in blood flow during strenuous exercise also occurs in the liver, pancreas, and gastrointestinal tract.[52]

Factors Within Active Muscle

Skeletal muscle blood flow closely couples to metabolic demands. Regulation occurs from the interaction of neural vasoconstriction activity and locally derived vasoactive substances within active tissues' vascular endothelium and red blood cells.[14] At rest, only one of every 30 to 40 capillaries in muscle tissue remains open. The opening of dormant capillaries in exercise serves three important functions:

1. Increases total muscle blood flow
2. Delivers a large blood volume with only a minimal increase in blood flow velocity
3. Increases the effective surface for gas and nutrient exchange between the blood and muscle fibers

Vasodilation occurs from local factors related to tissue metabolism that act directly on the smooth muscle bands of small arterioles and precapillary sphincters. This rapid response adjusts precisely to the muscle's force output and metabolic needs.[7] Decreased tissue oxygen supply serves as a potent local stimulus for vasodilation in skeletal and cardiac muscle. Additionally, local increases in blood flow, temperature, carbon dioxide, acidity, adenosine, magnesium and potassium ions, and nitric oxide production (see next section) by the endothelial cells lining the blood vessels trigger the discharge of relaxing factors that enhance regional blood flow.[17,34,35,58] The venous system may also increase local blood flow by "assessing" increases in the metabolic needs of active muscle and releasing vasodilatory factors (from venular endothelial cells) that diffuse to and dilate the adjacent arteriole.[23] The **autoregulatory mechanisms** for blood flow make sense physiologically because they reflect elevated tissue metabolism and increased oxygen need. Local regulation provides such strong control that it maintains adequate regional blood flow even for patients whose nerves to the blood vessels have been surgically removed. Local metabolite stimulation of chemoreceptors also provides the peripheral neural reflex input for medullary control of the heart and vasculature.

Nitric Oxide and Autoregulation of Tissue Blood Flow. **Nitric oxide** (**NO**) serves as an important signal molecule that dilates blood vessels and decreases vascular resistance.[28] This gas is a common, unstable industrial and automotive air pollutant formed when nitrogen burns. Most living organisms naturally produce it from its precursor *L-arginine*. Stimuli from diverse signal chemicals (including neurotransmitters) and sheering stress and vessel stretch from increased blood flow through the vessel lumen provoke NO synthesis and release by the vascular endothelium to serve its role as a vascular gatekeeper. Formerly termed *endothelium-derived relaxing factor* by 1998 physiology or medicine Nobel Prize recipient Robert F. Furchgott (1916–), NO rapidly spreads through underlying cell membranes to smooth muscle cells within the arterial wall. Here it binds with and activates *guanylyl cyclase,* an enzyme important in cellular communication and signal transduction. This initiates a cascade of reactions that attenuate sympathetic vasoconstriction and induce arterial smooth muscle relaxation to increase blood flow in neighboring blood vessels. NO exerts its potent vasodilator effect on skeletal muscle (including the diaphragm), spongelike vascular tissues, skin, and myocardial tissue (FIG. 16.7).[5,11,19,27,29,31,56,63]

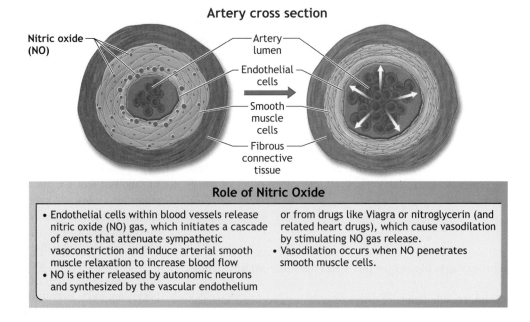

Figure 16.7 Mechanism for how nitric oxide regulates local blood flow.

NO mediates bodily functions as diverse as olfaction, inhibition of blood clot formation, and enhanced immune response regulation and acts as an interneuron or signaling messenger. It also contributes to cutaneous active vasodilation during heat stress[30] and rapidly dilates the coronary vasculature as an early adaptation to moderate exercise training.[57,60,66] The popular erectile dysfunction drug Viagra (sildenafil) potentiates NO's effect on blood vessel dilation, which augments blood flow into the penis. Vascular wall receptors for NO contribute to blood pressure regulation in response to central cardiovascular stimulation during emotionally stressful situations including exercise. Racial differences in resting blood pressure relate to a lower sensitivity to NO's dilating action in blacks than in whites.[12] In coronary artery disease, the endothelium produces less NO. Reduced NO bioavailability explains the potent beneficial effect of exogenous nitroglycerin treatment (which releases NO gas) to reverse chest discomfort or pain from coronary vessel disease (angina pectoris).

Research must determine how NO affects cardiovascular dynamics in exercise. FIGURE 16.8 illustrates a proposed mechanism for how hemoglobin molecules provide vascular control of blood flow to individual tissues via NO transport and release. The model proposes that hemoglobin oxygenation in the lungs changes the hemoglobin molecule's shape, enabling it to accept a different form of NO (S-nitrosohemoglobin, or SNO) that does not affix to hemoglobin's iron. Oxygen release in the local tissues again alters hemoglobin's shape, liberating NO and causing vasodilation. Greater oxygen release from hemoglobin (greater tissue oxygen need) induces greater NO release and more pronounced vasodilation and oxygen delivery. Hemoglobin thus plays an active role in autoregulation and homeostatic control of tissue blood flow in relation to oxygen needs. If the model proves correct, exogenous enriched SNO-hemoglobin could serve as a potent blood substitute to treat the oxygen-deficiency diseases atherosclerosis, stroke, septic shock, and sickle cell disease.

Hormonal Factors

Sympathetic nerves terminate in the medullary portion of the adrenal glands. With sympathetic activation, this glandular tissue secretes large quantities of epinephrine and a smaller amount of norepinephrine into the blood. These hormonal chemical messengers induce a generalized constrictor response, except in blood vessels of the heart and skeletal muscles. Hormonal control of regional blood flow plays a relatively minor role during exercise compared with the more local, rapid, and potent sympathetic neural drive.

INTEGRATED EXERCISE RESPONSE

The neural command center above the medullary region initiates cardiovascular changes immediately before and at the onset of exercise. Heart rate and myocardial contractility increase from feed-forward input from this center, which also suppresses parasympathetic activation. Concurrently, predictable alterations in regional blood flow occur in proportion to exercise severity. Modulation of vascular dilation and constriction optimizes blood flow to areas in need while maintaining blood pressure throughout the arterial system. As exercise continues, reflex feedback to the medulla from peripheral mechanical and chemical receptors in active tissue appraises tissue metabolism and circulatory needs. Local metabolic factors act directly to dilate resistance vessels in active muscles. Vasodilation reduces peripheral resistance to permit greater blood flow in these areas. Arterial blood flow through active muscles progresses in pulsatile oscillations that favor enhanced flow during eccentric (lengthening) muscle

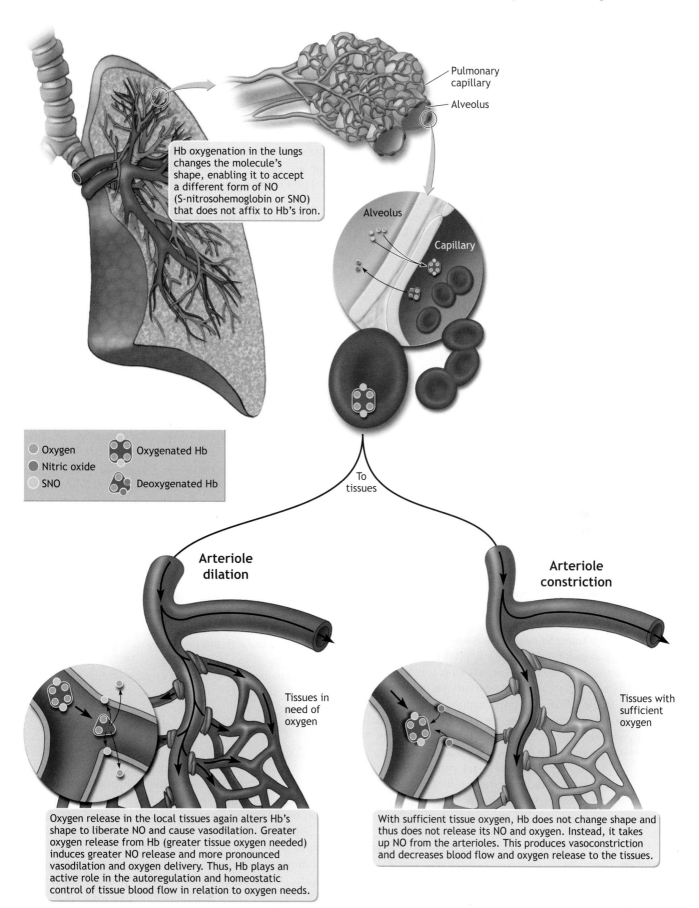

Hb oxygenation in the lungs changes the molecule's shape, enabling it to accept a different form of NO (S-nitrosohemoglobin or SNO) that does not affix to Hb's iron.

Pulmonary capillary

Alveolus

Alveolus

Capillary

● Oxygen
● Nitric oxide
○ SNO

Oxygenated Hb

Deoxygenated Hb

To tissues

Arteriole dilation

Arteriole constriction

Tissues in need of oxygen

Tissues with sufficient oxygen

Oxygen release in the local tissues again alters Hb's shape to liberate NO and cause vasodilation. Greater oxygen release from Hb (greater tissue oxygen needed) induces greater NO release and more pronounced vasodilation and oxygen delivery. Thus, Hb plays an active role in the autoregulation and homeostatic control of tissue blood flow in relation to oxygen needs.

With sufficient tissue oxygen, Hb does not change shape and thus does not release its NO and oxygen. Instead, it takes up NO from the arterioles. This produces vasoconstriction and decreases blood flow and oxygen release to the tissues.

Figure 16.8   Proposed mechanism for hemoglobin (Hb)–nitrous oxide (NO) interaction for vascular control of blood flow to individual tissues.

actions and/or the recovery phases of concentric (shortening) actions.[51] Centrally mediated constrictor adjustments also occur in the vasculature of nonexercising tissues (skin, kidneys, splanchnic region, and inactive muscle). Constrictor action maintains adequate perfusion pressure within exercising muscle while simultaneously increasing blood supply to meet metabolic demands.

Factors that affect venous return are equally as important as factors that regulate arterial blood flow. Muscle and ventilatory pump actions and visceral vasoconstriction immediately return blood to the right ventricle when exercise begins and continue to facilitate venous return as cardiac output increases. These adjustments balance venous return with cardiac output. In upright exercise, venous blood flow regulation remains crucial because gravity impedes return of blood from the extremities.

INTEGRATIVE QUESTIONS

Discuss the following statement: "Task-specific, regular aerobic exercise not only trains the cardiovascular system, but also 'trains' the neuromuscular system to facilitate physiologic adjustments to the specific exercise mode."

EXERCISING AFTER CARDIAC TRANSPLANTATION

Patients with left ventricular dysfunction—ejection fraction less than 20%, referred to as end-stage heart disease—show poor long-term prognosis. Even though some asymptomatic and minimally symptomatic patients show near-normal function and survive for several years, most symptomatic patients die within 1 year of diagnosis. For these patients, cardiac transplantation becomes their only hope of survival. FIGURE 16.9A shows the number of transplants per calendar year reported to the registry of the International Society for Heart and Lung Transplantation (www.ishlt.org/), beginning with the first human transplant nearly 40 years ago. The steady decline in transplants after 1995 results from a reduction in donor availability. Prior to 1985, 1-year survival rate averaged 70% (Fig. 16.9B). With the introduction of the immunosuppressive drug cyclosporine in the early 1980s, overall 1-year survival rates increased to approximately 80%, with 4-year survival approaching 70%. In 1990, the 5-year survival rate for the 12,000 reported transplant patients averaged 72%.[33] Current postoperative therapy uses improved immunosuppressive drug combinations and applies the transvenous endomyocardial biopsy technique (first reported in the early 1970s) for early detection of tissue rejection.

Cardiac transplantation, also called **orthotopic transplantation**, illustrates the importance of extrinsic neural control of exercise heart rate. The procedure removes donor and recipient hearts by transection at the midatrial level—preserving pulmonary venous connections of the posterior wall of the left atrium of the recipient—and transection of the aorta just above the semilunar valves. Transplantation eliminates neural innervation of the myocardium, although hormonal feedback from circulating catecholamines, largely from the adrenal medulla, remains intact (FIG. 16.10A). Selected patients may receive a "piggyback" or **heterotropic transplant** that places the donor heart in the recipient's chest without removing the recipient's heart. Regardless of transplantation form, significant complications occur in recovery (e.g., donor heart rejection and infection), often requiring recurrent hospitalization and prolonged, costly medical care.

Improved Function but Altered Circulatory Dynamics

Following successful transplantation, patients generally report a favorable quality of life, and approximately 50% of individuals return to work. Successful pregnancy and vaginal delivery also have occurred, as well as completion of a full marathon in less than 6 hours. In general, a transplant patient demonstrates impaired exercise capacity and diminished physiologic and hemodynamic function that rarely exceeds 45 to 70% of normal.[2,9,15,20,41,45] For younger patients, this does not necessarily represent the rule; the 1998 United States' top-ranked junior golfer (an 18-year-old) received a heart transplant at age 12, when dilated congestive cardiomyopathy reduced his heart function below 30% of normal. Depressed levels of aerobic fitness and exercise tolerance magnify in heart transplant patients who also suffer from impaired pulmonary diffusion capacity.[64]

FIGURE 16.11 A–C illustrates peak oxygen consumption ($\dot{V}O_{2peak}$) for an initial pool of 140 patients evaluated prior to transplantation and up to 9 years after the procedure. Cardiac transplantation produced an average 50% improvement in $\dot{V}O_{2peak}$ (Fig. 16.11A) from 14.2 mL · kg^{-1}min^{-1} before to 21.4 mL · kg^{-1}min^{-1} 11.2 months after surgery. In comparing $\dot{V}O_{2peak}$ with a typical healthy population, 44% of the patients achieved 50 to 70% of the predicted value, 31% reached 70 to 90%, and several patients achieved more than 90%. The patients maintained improved aerobic capacity up to 9 years postsurgery (Fig. 16.11B). Figure 16.11C shows that the younger patients exhibited the greatest improvement following transplantation.

Sluggish Circulatory Response

An elevated resting heart rate characterizes the denervated heart because the intrinsic activity of the donor SA node governs heart rate. Without extrinsic neural control, the SA node generally depolarizes about 100 times each minute. The short-term exercise response for transplant patients classifies as abnormal. These patients demonstrate limited cardiac output and oxygen consumption during exercise, with accompanying reduced left ventricular ejection capacity. Figure 16.10B reveals that circulatory sluggishness results from the denervated heart's inability to accelerate significantly with increasing exercise demands (often by only 20

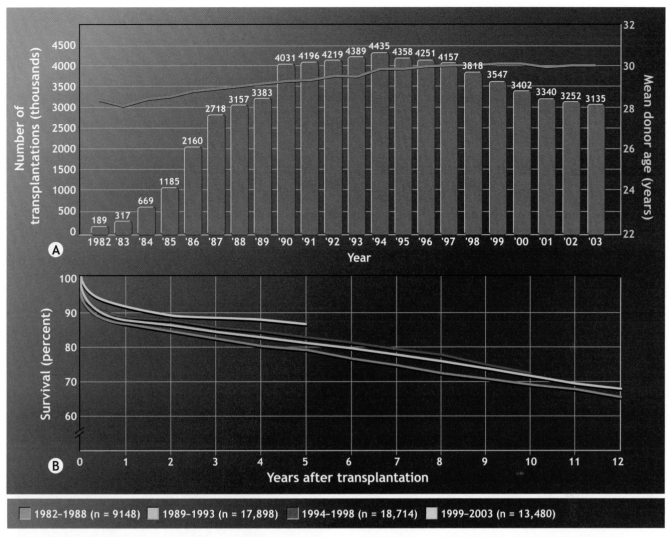

Figure 16.9   A. Number of hearts transplanted by year and mean donor age (*green line*) from 1982 to 2003 as reported by the International Society for Heart and Lung Transplantation. **B.** Survival of heart transplantation by era. Half-life survival (time when one half of those who underwent transplantation had died) was 9.4 years between 1994 and 1998 compared to 8.1 years between 1982–1988. Data based on results reported in J Heart Lung Transplant 2005;24:945.

to 40 b · min^{-1}).[4,38] The exercise response of the denervated transplanted heart does improve over the 12-month post-surgery period. However, the adaptations exert no meaningful effect on submaximal or peak exercise oxygen consumption.

In healthy individuals, stroke volume increases up to approximately 50% of $\dot{V}O_{2max}$ and then plateaus; further increases in cardiac output come mainly from increases in heart rate. Transplant patients, in contrast, have no stroke volume plateau during graded exercise; instead, stroke volume progressively increases by the Frank-Starling mechanism throughout the exercise range. Stroke volume increases represent the primary mechanism for these patients to increase cardiac output during more intense exercise.

Evidence indicates possible reinnervation of the donor heart with parasympathetic cardiac fibers.[65] Thirty-two months after transplantation, two P waves at somewhat different rates were recorded from the hearts of two young, fit transplant patients. These waves appeared to arise from donor *and* recipient SA nodes. They accompanied rapid heart rate

acceleration at the start of exercise for both patients. Chapter 32 discusses the effects of exercise training for the heart transplant patient.

INTEGRATIVE QUESTIONS

If heart transplantation surgically removes all nerves to the myocardium, explain why heart rate increases for these patients during physical activity.

Summary

1. The cardiovascular system provides rapid heart rate regulation and effective distribution of blood through the vascular circuit (while maintaining blood pressure) in response to overall metabolic and physiologic needs.

FOCUS On Research

AGE-RELATED CHANGES IN EXERCISE-INDUCED CARDIOVASCULAR FUNCTION

Robinson S. Experimental studies of physical fitness in relation to age. Arbeitsphysiologie 1938;10:18.

▲ Robinson's classic comprehensive cross-sectional study documents the relationship of aging to physiologic responses during rest and exercise in 93 healthy, nonathletic males aged 6 to 91 years. Measurement variables included resting and exercise oxygen consumption ($\dot{V}O_2$), lung volume, heart rate (HR), arterial blood pressure, submaximal treadmill walking performance at 5.6 km · h^{-1} at an 8.6% incline for 15 minutes, and a 2- to 5-minute treadmill run to exhaustion.

The *top figure* shows that HR$_{max}$ in older men is nearly 20% lower compared to young boys. The younger individuals also showed greater variability in HR response to exercise and more rapid HR acceleration at the start of exercise; their HRs returned to baseline more rapidly in recovery than older subjects. In the *middle figure*, $\dot{V}O_{2peak}$ increased from age 8 to 10 years, declined for the next few years, then increased further until about age 17, and decreased steadily thereafter. Interestingly, Robinson suggested that the $\dot{V}O_{2peak}$ decrease with age was probably related to a reduced level of general physical activity and was not necessarily true "aging." Thus, recognition of the deleterious effects of a sedentary lifestyle on cardiovascular function occurred as early as 1938. The *bottom figure* depicts pulmonary ventilation relative to body mass (BM; $\dot{V}_E$ · kg BM^{-1}), breathing rate (breaths · min^{-1}), and tidal air volume (TV) expressed as a percentage of forced vital capacity (TV × 100 ÷ FVC) during maximal exercise. Measures of ventilatory function declined with age, and older men used a greater fraction of FVC as TV than younger men. Boys increased ventilation over resting values principally by increasing breathing frequency; adults increased ventilation by increasing breathing rate and tidal volume.

This pioneering cross-sectional study demonstrated an age- and sedentary lifestyle-related decline in cardiovascular and pulmonary function variables during rest and throughout the full range of exercise intensity. Subsequent research verified Robinson's assertion that a significant component of the functional capacity decline with aging coincides more with lifestyle characteristics than chronologic age per se.

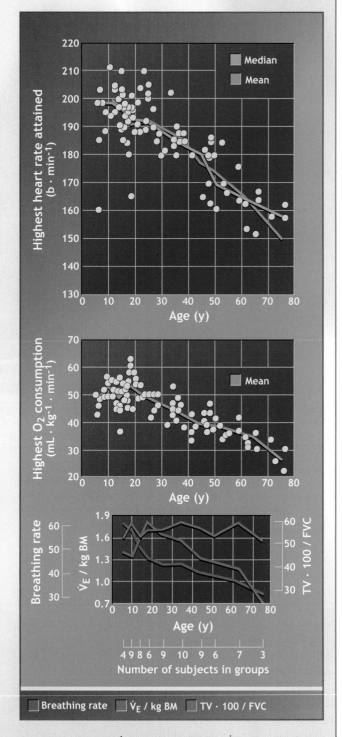

Top. HR$_{max}$ (b · min^{-1}) versus age. *Middle.* $\dot{V}O_{2peak}$ versus age. *Bottom.* Pulmonary minute ventilation ($\dot{V}_E$), breathing rate, and tidal volume (TV) versus age.

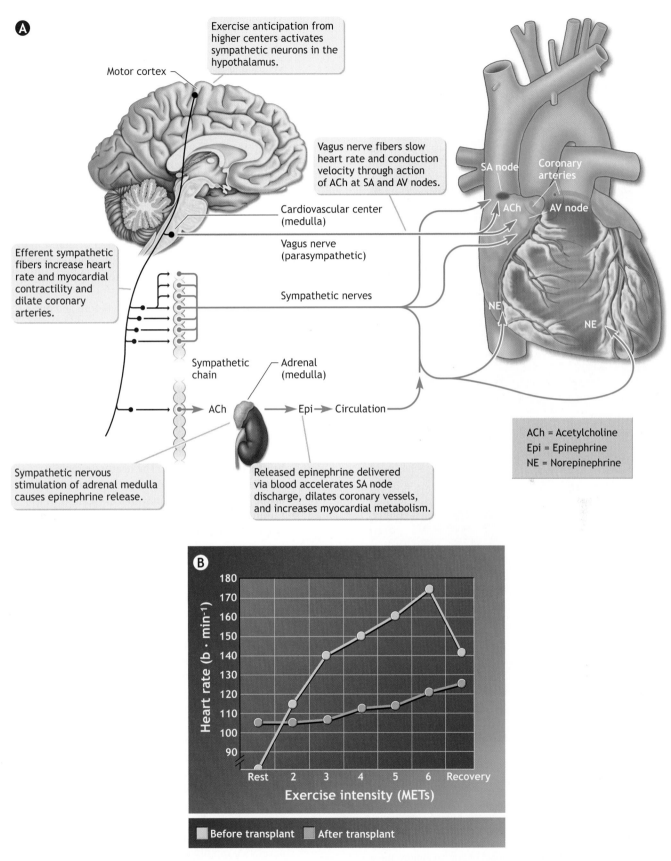

Figure 16.10 A. Regulation of heart rate under normal conditions. Heart transplantation produces cardiac denervation by removing vagal and sympathetic efferent stimulation to the myocardium. Consequently, circulating epinephrine from the adrenal medulla provides the primary mechanism to regulate exercise heart rate. **B.** Heart rate response of a patient during graded exercise before and after orthotopic cardiac transplantation. Note the elevated resting heart rate and delayed [and] depressed heart rate response after transplantation. (Figure B from Squirers RW. Exercise training after cardiac transplantation. Med Sci Sports Exerc 1991;23:686.)

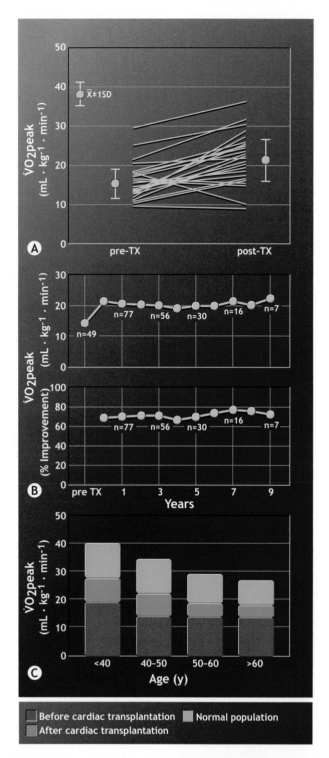

Figure 16.11 Long-term effects of heart transplantation (TX) on aerobic functional capacity. **A.** $\dot{V}O_{2peak}$ before and 11.2 months after cardiac transplantation in 43 patients who underwent testing at both intervals. Post-TX average is significantly higher than pre-TX. **B.** Significant improvements in peak oxygen consumption ($\dot{V}O_{2peak}$) and percentage improvement occurred as early as 6 months after transplantation and remained improved up to 9 years after the transplant procedure. **C.** Impact of age on improvement in $\dot{V}O_{2peak}$ in 43 patients who underwent exercise testing before and 1 year after cardiac transplantation. (From Osada N, et al. Long-term cardiopulmonary exercise performance after heart transplantation. Am J Cardiol 1997;79:451.)

2. The cardiac rhythm originates at the SA node. The impulse then travels across the atria to the AV node. After a brief delay, it spreads across the large ventricular mass. This normal conduction pattern initiates atrial and ventricular contractions to provide impetus for blood flow.

3. The electrocardiogram (ECG) records the sequence of the heart's electrical events during the cardiac cycle. The ECG detects various heart function abnormalities during rest and increasing exercise intensity.

4. Epinephrine and norepinephrine accelerate heart rate and increase myocardial contractility. Acetylcholine acts through the vagus nerve to slow heart rate.

5. The heart "turns on" in the transition from rest to exercise from increased sympathetic and decreased parasympathetic activity integrated with central command input.

6. Cortical influence in anticipation before and during the initial stage of physical activity governs a substantial part of the heart rate adjustment to exercise.

7. Reflex sensory input from peripheral receptors in blood vessels, joints, and muscles provides the cardiovascular center with continual feedback about the physical and chemical state of active muscles.

8. Neural and hormonal extrinsic factors modify the heart's inherent rhythm. The heart rate rapidly accelerates in anticipation of exercise and can reach about $200\ b \cdot min^{-1}$ in maximal exercise.

9. Carotid artery palpation accurately accesses heart rate during and immediately after exercise in healthy individuals.

10. Nerves, hormones, and local metabolic factors act on the smooth muscle bands in blood vessels to alter the vessels' internal diameter and regulate blood flow in response to metabolic demands.

11. Blood flow in the vascular circuit changes with the vessels' radius raised to the fourth power in accord with Poiseuille's law.

12. Nitric oxide, an extraordinarily important and potent endothelium-derived relaxing factor, facilitates blood vessel dilation and decreases vascular resistance.

13. The kidneys and splanchnic regions dramatically compromise their blood flow in exercise to augment delivery of blood to the muscles and maintain systemic blood pressure.

14. Patients who successfully undergo orthotopic transplantation have a depressed cardiovascular response to exercise; the denervated heart cannot accelerate rapidly to meet the increased demands of physical activity.

References are available on the Student CD and online at http://connection.lww.com/mkk6e.

Functional Capacity of the Cardiovascular System

17

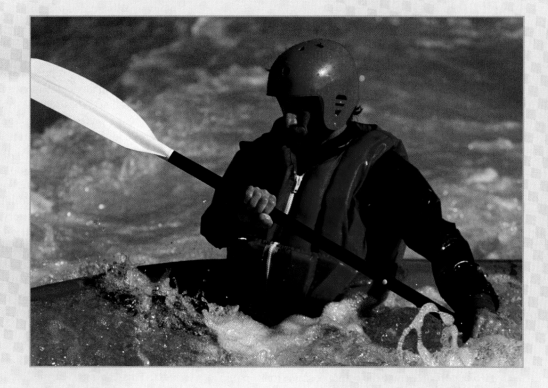

CHAPTER OBJECTIVES

- Describe the direct Fick, indicator dilution, and CO_2 rebreathing methods used to measure cardiac output, and discuss the advantages and disadvantages of each

- Compare cardiac output during rest and maximal exercise for an endurance-trained and sedentary person

- Explain the influence of each component of the Fick equation on $\dot{V}O_{2max}$

- Discuss two physiologic mechanisms that influence exercise stroke volume

- Contrast the components of cardiac output during rest and maximal exercise for sedentary and endurance-trained individuals

- Discuss the contribution of the Frank-Starling mechanism to augment cardiac output during different exercise modes

- Outline the dynamics and proposed mechanisms for cardiovascular drift

- Outline cardiac output distribution to body tissues during rest and intense aerobic exercise

- Describe the relationship between maximal cardiac output and $\dot{V}O_{2max}$ among individuals who vary in aerobic fitness

- Indicate factors that contribute to expanding the a-$\bar{v}O_2$ difference during graded exercise

- Contrast cardiovascular and metabolic dynamics during upper-body versus lower-body graded exercise

CARDIAC OUTPUT

Cardiac output ($\dot{Q}$) expresses the amount of blood pumped by the heart during a 1-minute period. The maximal value reflects the functional capacity of the cardiovascular system to meet physical activity demands. Output from the heart, as with any pump, depends on its rate of pumping (**heart rate; HR**) and quantity of blood ejected with each stroke (**stroke volume; SV**). Cardiac output computes as follows:

$$\text{Cardiac output} = \text{Heart rate} \times \text{Stroke volume}$$

Measuring Cardiac Output

The output from a hose, pump, or faucet is determined by opening the valve and collecting and measuring the volume of fluid ejected over a given time. In humans with a closed circulatory system, three common methods assess cardiac output: (1) direct Fick, (2) indicator dilution, and (3) CO_2 rebreathing.

Direct Fick Method

Two factors determine the output of fluid from a pump in a closed circuit: (1) change in concentration of a substance between the outflow and inflow ports of the pump and (2) total quantity of that substance taken up (or given off) by the fluid in a given time. For cardiovascular dynamics, calculating cardiac output requires knowledge of two factors: (1) average difference between the oxygen content of arterial and mixed-venous blood (**a-$\bar{v}O_2$ difference**) and (2) oxygen consumption during 1 minute ($\dot{V}O_2$). The question then becomes how much blood circulates during the minute to account for the observed oxygen consumption given the observed a-$\bar{v}O_2$ difference. The **Fick equation**, derived and published by influential German physiologist Adolph Fick (1829–1901) in 1870, expresses the relationships among cardiac output, oxygen consumption, and a-$\bar{v}O_2$ difference. These variables could not be determined in humans until the acceptance of cardiac catheterization as a clinical tool in 1940.

$$\begin{array}{c}\text{Cardiac output} \\ \text{(mL} \cdot \text{min}^{-1}\text{)}\end{array} = \frac{\dot{V}O_2 \text{ mL} \cdot \text{min}^{-1}}{\begin{array}{c}\text{a-}\bar{v}O_2 \text{ difference} \\ \text{(mL per 100 mL blood)}\end{array}} \times 100$$

FIGURE 17.1 illustrates the Fick principle for determining cardiac output. In this example, the person consumes 250 mL of oxygen during 1 minute at rest, and the a-$\bar{v}O_2$ difference

during this time averages 5 mL of oxygen per 100 mL (deciliter [dL]) of blood. Substituting these values in the Fick equation computes cardiac output as follows:

$$\begin{array}{c}\text{Cardiac output} \\ \text{(mL} \cdot \text{min}^{-1}\text{)}\end{array} = \frac{250 \text{ mL O}_2}{5 \text{ mL O}_2} \times 100 = 5000 \text{ mL blood}$$

Although straightforward in principle, the actual Fick method to determine cardiac output requires complex methodology usually limited to a clinical setting where the benefits of measurement exceed any potential risk. Measuring oxygen consumption involves open-circuit spirometry methods summarized in Chapter 8. The more difficult task is to determine a-$\bar{v}O_2$ difference. A representative sample of arterial blood can come from any convenient systemic artery (e.g., femoral, radial, brachial). These arteries are easily located, but the arterial puncture has some risk. Sampling mixed-venous blood presents additional difficulties because the blood in each vein only reflects the metabolic activity of the specific area it drains. An accurate estimate of the average oxygen content of all venous blood requires sampling from an anatomic "mixing chamber" such as the right atrium, right ventricle, or most accurately, the pulmonary artery. Such sampling requires threading a small flexible catheter through the antecubital vein in the arm into the superior vena cava that drains into the right heart. Arterial and mixed-venous blood are then sampled simultaneously with measurement of oxygen consumption.

Numerous studies of cardiovascular dynamics have applied the direct Fick method under various experimental conditions. The method generally serves as the criterion standard to validate other techniques for cardiac output measurement. The main criticism of the Fick method concerns its *invasiveness*. This can alter normal cardiovascular dynamics during the measurement period that may not reflect the person's usual cardiovascular response.

Indicator Dilution Method

The **indicator dilution method** involves venous and arterial punctures but does not require cardiac catheterization. A known quantity of an inert dye such as indocyanine green or a radioactive substance is injected into a large vein. The indicator material remains in the vascular stream, usually bound to plasma proteins or red blood cells. It then mixes in the blood as the blood travels to the lungs and returns to the heart before ejection throughout the systemic circuit. A radioactive counter or photosensitive device continually assesses arterial blood samples. The area under the dilution–concentration curve (obtained by repetitive sampling) reflects the average concentration of indicator material in blood leaving the heart. From the dilution of a known quantity of dye in an unknown quantity of blood, cardiac output computes as follows:

$$\begin{array}{c}\text{Cardiac} \\ \text{output}\end{array} = \frac{\text{Quantity of dye injected}}{\begin{array}{c}\text{Average dye concentration blood in for} \\ \text{duration of curve} \times \text{Duration of curve}\end{array}}$$

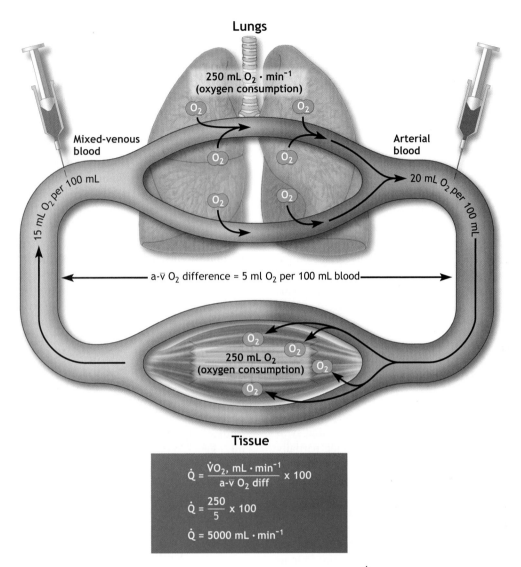

Lungs

250 mL $O_2 \cdot min^{-1}$
(oxygen consumption)

Mixed-venous blood

Arterial blood

15 mL O_2 per 100 mL

20 mL O_2 per 100 mL

a-v̄ O_2 difference = 5 ml O_2 per 100 mL blood

250 mL O_2
(oxygen consumption)

Tissue

$$\dot{Q} = \frac{\dot{V}O_2, mL \cdot min^{-1}}{\text{a-}\bar{v}\ O_2\ \text{diff}} \times 100$$

$$\dot{Q} = \frac{250}{5} \times 100$$

$$\dot{Q} = 5000\ mL \cdot min^{-1}$$

Figure 17.1   The Fick principle to measure cardiac output per minute (Q̇).

CO₂ Rebreathing Method

One can determine cardiac output by substituting CO_2 values for O_2 values in the Fick equation.[23,45] The same open-circuit spirometry method for determining oxygen consumption in the typical Fick technique determines CO_2 production in the rebreathing method. Using a rapid CO_2 gas analyzer and making certain reasonable assumptions concerning gas exchange provides valid estimates of mixed-venous and arterial CO_2 levels. This noninvasive or "bloodless" technique requires breath-by-breath CO_2 analysis. Values for CO_2 production and mixed-venous and arterial CO_2 concentrations (derived from expired CO_2 obtained during different times) provide the data to compute cardiac output in accordance with the Fick principle as follows:

$$\frac{\text{Cardiac output}}{(mL \cdot min^{-1})} = \frac{\dot{V}CO_2}{\bar{v}\text{-a } CO_2 \text{ difference}} \times 100$$

The **CO₂ rebreathing method** offers obvious advantages over the direct Fick and indicator dilution methods. It does not require blood sampling or close medical supervision and only minimally interferes with the subject during bicycle ergometer or treadmill exercise. This noninvasive method may provide more accurate estimates of the "real" cardiovascular dynamics during exercise than the invasive strategies. One limitation of CO_2 rebreathing requires that subjects exercise under steady-rate aerobic metabolism. This restricts the method's use during maximal and "supermaximal" exercise and in the transition from rest to exercise.

INTEGRATIVE QUESTION

How does the Fick equation fully explain the physiologic components that determine $\dot{V}O_{2max}$?

CARDIAC OUTPUT AT REST

Cardiac output varies considerably during rest. Influencing factors include emotional conditions that alter cortical outflow (central command) to the cardioaccelerator nerves and nerves that modulate arterial resistance vessels. Each minute, the left ventricle pumps the entire 5-L blood volume of a representative 70-kg adult male. A 5-L cardiac output at rest represents an average value for both trained and untrained males. Resting cardiac output for a representative 56-kg woman averages nearly 4.0 L $\cdot$ min^{-1} (see next section).

Untrained

For the average sedentary person at rest, an average heart rate of 70 b $\cdot$ min^{-1} usually sustains the 5-L cardiac output. Substituting this heart rate value in the cardiac output equation, the heart's calculated stroke volume equals 0.714 L or 71.4 mL (SV = $\dot{Q}$ ÷ HR). Stroke volume and cardiac output for women average about 25% below values for men; in women, the stroke volume at rest averages 50 to 60 mL. This "gender difference" generally relates to the average woman's smaller body size.

Endurance Athletes

Endurance training brings the heart's sinus node under greater influence of acetylcholine, the parasympathetic hormone that slows heart rate. At the same time, resting sympathetic activity decreases. This training adaptation partially explains the low resting heart rates of many elite endurance athletes. Relatively brief training periods exert only a minimal lowering effect on resting heart rate.[1,51]

Heart rates in healthy endurance athletes generally average 50 b $\cdot$ min^{-1} at rest, although heart rates below 30 b $\cdot$ min^{-1} have been reported but infrequently. Consequently, the endurance athlete's resting cardiac output of 5 L $\cdot$ min^{-1} circulates with the relatively large stroke volume of 100 mL. The following summarizes average values for cardiac output, heart rate, and stroke volume for endurance-trained and untrained men at rest:

Rest

	Cardiac output	=	Heart rate	×	Stroke volume
Untrained:	5000 mL $\cdot$ min^{-1}	=	70 b $\cdot$ min^{-1}	=	71 mL
Trained:	5000 mL $\cdot$ min^{-1}	=	50 b $\cdot$ min^{-1}	=	100 mL

These straightforward computations do not clarify the underlying physiologic mechanisms for the different response patterns of trained and untrained persons. Two factors probably explain the large stroke volume and low heart rate of endurance-trained athletes:

1. Increased vagal tone and decreased sympathetic drive, both of which slow the heart
2. Increased blood volume, myocardial contractility, and compliance of the left ventricle, all of which augment the heart's stroke volume

CARDIAC OUTPUT DURING EXERCISE

Systemic blood flow increases directly with exercise intensity. Cardiac output increases rapidly during the transition from rest to steady-rate exercise. Thereafter, cardiac output rises gradually until it plateaus when blood flow meets the exercise metabolic requirements.

In sedentary, college-aged males, cardiac output during maximal exercise increased four times above the resting level to 20 to 22 L $\cdot$ min^{-1}. Maximum heart rate for these young adults averaged 195 b $\cdot$ min^{-1}. Consequently, the stroke volume generally ranged between 103 and 113 mL (20,000 mL $\cdot$ min^{-1} ÷ 195 b $\cdot$ min^{-1} = 103 mL $\cdot$ b^{-1}; 22,000 mL $\cdot$ min^{-1} ÷ 195 b $\cdot$ min^{-1} = 113 mL). In contrast, world-class endurance athletes achieve maximum cardiac outputs of 35 to 40 L $\cdot$ min^{-1}. This high value assumes greater significance when one considers that the trained person generally achieves a slightly *lower* maximum heart rate than a sedentary person of similar age. *The endurance athlete achieves a large maximal cardiac output solely through a large stroke volume.* For example, the cardiac output of an Olympic medal winner in cross-country skiing increased to 40 L $\cdot$ min^{-1} in maximum exercise (almost 8 times above rest); the stroke volume was 210 mL. This nearly doubled the maximum volume of blood pumped per beat by a sedentary counterpart. As a point of comparison among species, thoroughbred racehorses achieve cardiac outputs of 600 L $\cdot$ min^{-1} (accompanying a 120 to 150 mL $\cdot$ kg^{-1} $\cdot$ min^{-1} $\dot{V}O_{2max}$).[9,30]

The following summarizes average values for cardiac output, heart rate, and stroke volume for endurance-trained and untrained men during maximal exercise:

Maximal Exercise

	Cardiac output	=	Heart rate	×	Stroke volume
Untrained:	22,000 mL	=	195 b $\cdot$ min^{-1}	=	113 mL
Trained:	35,000 mL	=	195 b $\cdot$ min^{-1}	=	179 mL

Stroke Volume: Diastolic Filling Versus Systolic Emptying

Three physiologic mechanisms increase the heart's stroke volume during exercise. The first, intrinsic to the myocardium, involves enhanced cardiac filling in diastole followed by a more forceful systolic contraction. Neurohormonal influence governs the second mechanism that involves normal ventricular filling with a subsequent forceful ejection and emptying during systole. The third mechanism comes from training adaptations that expand blood volume and reduce resistance to blood flow in peripheral tissues.[10,19,44,46]

Enhanced Diastolic Filling

Any factor that increases venous return or slows the heart produces greater ventricular filling (preload) during the cardiac cycle's diastolic phase. An increase in **end-diastolic**

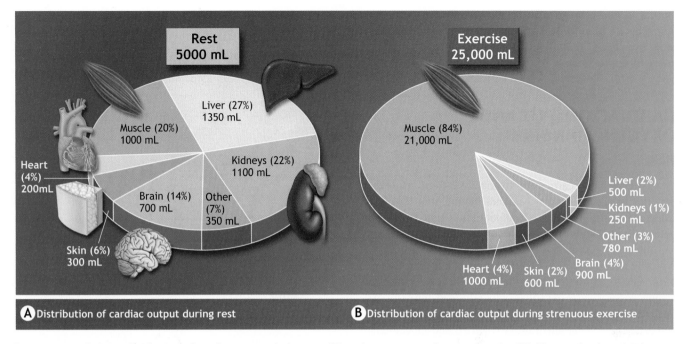

Figure 17.3 Relative distribution of cardiac output during rest (**A**) and strenuous endurance exercise (**B**). The number in parentheses indicates percentage of the total cardiac output. The large absolute mass of muscle tissue at rest receives about the same quantity of blood as the much smaller kidneys. In strenuous exercise, approximately 84% of the cardiac output diverts to the active muscles.

portion of the exercise cardiac output diverts to active muscles. Approximately 4 to 7 mL of blood flows each minute to each 100 g of muscle at rest. This flow increases steadily in graded exercise, with active muscle receiving up to 50 to 75 mL per 100 g of tissue each minute of maximal exertion.[36,37] Blood flow within active muscle is highly regulated. The greatest quantity of blood diverts to the oxidative portions of the muscle at the expense of those areas with high glycolytic capacity.[5,21] Thus, peak blood flow in a small portion of active quadriceps muscle achieve perfusion as high as 300 to 400 mL $\cdot 100$ g^{-1} $\cdot$ min^{-1}.[32,33] During "big muscle" activities such as running and cycling at maximum intensity, muscle blood flow accounts for 80 to 85% of the total cardiac output.[38]

Redistribution of Blood

Increases in cardiac output contribute greatly to increased muscle blood flow during exercise. In addition, blood flow to muscle increases disproportionately relative to flow to other tissues. For trained individuals, blood redistribution—from one organ to another by vasoconstriction in one and vasodilation in the other—begins in the anticipatory period just prior to exercise.[5] Two factors, hormonal vascular regulation and local metabolic conditions, cause blood to route through active muscles from areas that temporarily tolerate compromised blood flow.[25] Blood redistribution among specific tissues occurs primarily during high-intensity exercise. For example, blood flow to the skin, the primary heat-exchange organ, increases during light and moderate exercise in response to the rise in core temperature.[15,55] During near-

maximal effort, the skin restricts its blood flow redirecting it to active muscle, even in a hot environment.[34]

The kidneys and splanchnic tissues consume only 10 to 25% of the oxygen in their normal blood supply. These tissues tolerate a considerably reduced blood flow before oxygen demand exceeds supply and compromises function.[28] Renal blood flow can decrease up to four fifths of the blood supply at rest. Increased oxygen extraction from the available blood supply generally maintains the oxygen needs of tissues with reduced blood flow. The visceral organs sustain a substantially reduced blood supply for more than 1 hour during intense exercise. Redistribution of 2 to 3 L of blood away from these tissues "frees" up to 600 mL of oxygen each minute for use by active muscles. Sustained blood flow reduction to the liver and kidneys, however, may contribute to fatigue often experienced during prolonged submaximal exercise. Regular aerobic training diminishes the typical vasoconstrictor response to splanchnic and renal tissues with exercise.[25] An improved capacity to maintain blood flow to the liver and kidneys during sustained exercise probably contributes to improved endurance.

Blood Flow to the Heart and Brain

Some tissues cannot compromise their blood supply (Fig. 17.3). At rest, the myocardium normally uses approximately 75% of the oxygen in the blood flowing through the coronary circulation. With such a limited margin of reserve, increased coronary blood flow primarily supplies the increased myocardial oxygen needs with exercise. Thus, a four- to fivefold increase in coronary circulation accompanies a similar increase in myocardial work during exercise; this amounts to a blood flow of about 1 L · min⁻¹ during maximum exercise. Cerebral blood flow also increases during exercise by approximately 25 to 30% compared with the resting flow.[47]

CARDIAC OUTPUT AND OXYGEN TRANSPORT

Rest

Arterial blood carries approximately 200 mL of oxygen per liter in a person with a normal hemoglobin level (see Chapter 13). If resting cardiac output each minute equals 5 L, potentially 1000 mL of oxygen becomes available to the body (5 L blood × 200 mL O₂). The resting oxygen consumption typically averages 250 to 300 mL · min⁻¹, allowing 750 mL of oxygen to return unused to the heart. This does not reflect an unnecessary waste of cardiac output. Instead, the extra oxygen circulating above the resting requirement represents oxygen in reserve—a margin of safety when a tissue's metabolism increases dramatically.

Exercise

A healthy, young adult with a maximum heart rate of 200 b · min⁻¹ and stroke volume of 80 mL (0.08 L) generates a maximum cardiac output of 16 L · min⁻¹ (200 × 0.08 L). Even during maximal exercise, hemoglobin saturation with oxygen remains nearly complete, so each liter of arterial blood carries about 200 mL of oxygen. Consequently, 3200 mL of oxygen circulates each minute via a 16-L cardiac output (16 L × 200 mL O₂ · L⁻¹). Even if the tissues could extract all of the oxygen from all of the blood as it traveled throughout the body, the $\dot{V}O_{2max}$ could not exceed 3200 mL. This represents a purely theoretical value because the oxygen needs of some tissues such as the brain and skin do not increase markedly with exercise, yet they still require a substantial blood supply.

Based on the preceding example, increasing the heart's stroke volume from 80 to 200 mL while maintaining the maximum heart rate at 200 b · min⁻¹ dramatically increases maximum cardiac output to 40 L · min⁻¹. This represents a 2.5-fold increase in oxygen circulated during each minute of exercise (from 3200 to 8000 mL). *An increase in maximum cardiac output clearly produces a proportionate increase in capacity to circulate oxygen and profoundly affects an individual's maximal oxygen consumption.*

Close Association Between Maximum Cardiac Output and $\dot{V}O_{2max}$

FIGURE 17.4 depicts the close relationship between maximum cardiac output and capacity for a high level of aerobic exercise metabolism. $\dot{V}O_{2max}$ values represent averages for the sedentary person to the elite endurance athlete. An unmistakable association exists—a low maximal oxygen consumption corresponds closely with a low maximum cardiac output,

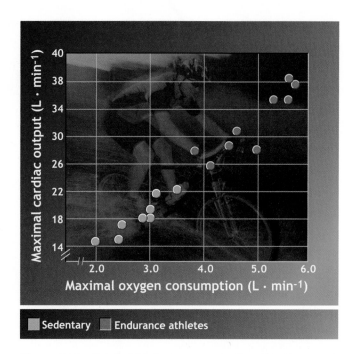

Figure 17.4 Relationship between maximal cardiac output and maximal oxygen consumption ($\dot{V}O_{2max}$) in endurance trained and untrained individuals. Maximal cardiac output relates to $\dot{V}O_{2max}$ in the ratio of about 6:1.

whereas a 5- or 6-L $\dot{V}O_{2max}$ invariably accompanies a 30- to 40-L cardiac output.

A 5- to 6-L increase in blood flow accompanies each 1-L increase in oxygen consumption above the resting value; this relationship remains essentially unchanged regardless of exercise mode over a broad range of dynamic exercises. *High levels of maximal oxygen consumption and cardiac output provide distinguishing characteristics for preadolescent and adult endurance athletes.* An almost proportionate increase in maximum cardiac output accompanies increases in $\dot{V}O_{2max}$ with endurance training (see Chapter 21).

Cardiac Output Differences Among Men and Women and Children

Cardiac output and oxygen consumption remain linearly related during graded exercise for boys and girls and men and women. However, teenage and adult females generally exercise at any level of *submaximal* oxygen consumption with a 5 to 10% *larger* cardiac output than males.[31] The 10% lower hemoglobin concentration in women than in men helps to explain any apparent gender difference in submaximal cardiac output. A proportionate increase in submaximal cardiac output compensates for this small decrease in the blood's oxygen-carrying capacity.

Higher heart rates in children than in adults during submaximal treadmill and cycle ergometer exercise do not fully compensate for their smaller stroke volume. This produces a smaller cardiac output for children at a given submaximal exercise oxygen consumption.[18,40,50] As such, the a-v̄O₂ difference expands to meet the oxygen requirements. The biologic significance remains unclear of this difference in central circulatory function between children and adults. Comparisons of cardiac responses (stroke volume, aortic peak blood flow velocity, systolic ejection time) between prepubertal children and adults fail to demonstrate any age-related exercise impairment.[39]

Oxygen Extraction: The a-$\bar{v}O_2$ Difference

If only blood flow increased a tissue's oxygen supply, then increasing cardiac output from 5 L · min^{-1} at rest to 100 L · min^{-1} during maximum exercise would achieve the 20-fold oxygen consumption increase common among endurance athletes. Fortunately, strenuous exercise does not require this large cardiac output. Instead, hemoglobin releases a considerable quantity of its "reserve" oxygen from blood that perfuses active tissues. Exercise oxygen consumption increases by two mechanisms:

1. Increased total quantity of blood pumped by the heart (i.e., increased cardiac output)
2. Greater use of the already existing relatively large quantity of oxygen carried by the blood (i.e., expanded a-$\bar{v}O_2$ difference)

Rearranging the Fick equation summarizes the important relationship among cardiac output, a-$\bar{v}O_2$ difference, and $\dot{V}O_2$ as follows:

$$\dot{V}O_2 = \dot{Q} \times \text{a-}\bar{v}O_2 \text{ difference}$$

a-$\bar{v}O_2$ Difference During Rest

Resting metabolism uses an average of 5 mL of oxygen from the 20 mL of oxygen in each deciliter of arterial blood (50 mL per liter) that passes through the tissue capillaries. This represents an a-$\bar{v}O_2$ difference of 5 mL of oxygen per deciliter of blood perfusing the tissue–capillary bed. Thus, 15 mL of oxygen or 75% of the blood's original oxygen load still remains bound to hemoglobin.

INTEGRATIVE QUESTION

How would factors that influence the a-$\bar{v}O_2$ difference in maximal exercise explain the specificity of $\dot{V}O_{2max}$ improvement with different modes of aerobic training?

a-$\bar{v}O_2$ Difference During Exercise

FIGURE 17.5 shows a progressive expansion of the a-$\bar{v}O_2$ difference from rest to maximal exercise for physically active men. A similar pattern emerges for women, except that the arterial oxygen content averages 5 to 10% lower because of lower hemoglobin concentrations. The figure includes values for the oxygen content of arterial and mixed-venous blood

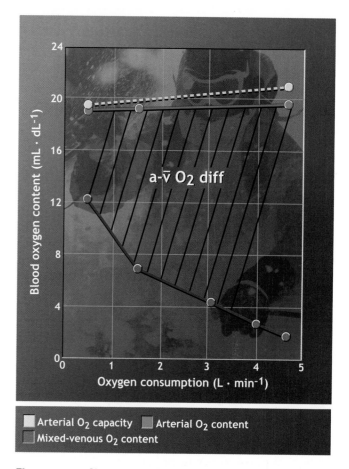

Figure 17.5 Changes in a-$\bar{v}O_2$ difference from rest to maximal exercise in physically active men.

during different exercise oxygen consumptions. Arterial blood oxygen content varies little from its value of 20 mL · dL^{-1} at rest throughout the full exercise intensity range. In contrast, mixed-venous oxygen content varies between 12 and 15 mL · dL^{-1} during rest to a low of 2 to 4 mL · dL^{-1} during maximal exercise. The difference between arterial and mixed-venous blood oxygen content at any discrete time (i.e., the a-$\bar{v}O_2$ difference) represents oxygen extraction from arterial blood as it circulates throughout the body.

The progressive expansion of the a-$\bar{v}O_2$ difference to at least three times resting value results from a reduced venous oxygen content, which in maximal exercise approaches 20 mL · dL^{-1} in active muscle (all oxygen extracted). The oxygen content of a true *mixed-venous sample* from the pulmonary artery rarely falls below 2 to 4 mL · dL^{-1} because blood returning from active tissues mixes with oxygen-rich venous blood from metabolically less active regions.

Figure 17.5 also shows that the capacity of each deciliter of arterial blood to carry oxygen increases during exercise from an increased concentration of red blood cells (hemoconcentration). Hemoconcentration results from the progressive movement of fluid from the plasma to the interstitial space with (1) increases in capillary hydrostatic pressure as blood pressure rises and (2) metabolic byproducts of exercise metabolism that osmotically draw fluid into tissue spaces from the plasma.

PREDICTING $\dot{V}O_{2MAX}$ USING RUNNING AND SWIMMING

■ The 1.5-mile run and the 12-minute swim provide reliable and valid tests to predict $\dot{V}O_{2max}$. The tests are effective for mass testing in schools and with recreational runners and swimmers. We do not recommend these tests for unconditioned beginners, men over age 40, and women over age 50 without proper medical clearance, symptomatic individuals, and those with known disease or coronary heart disease risk factors. The swim test assumes relatively high-level swimming skill.

THE TESTS
1.5-Mile Walk–Run Test

1. Testing site: a school track (each lap measures 1/4 mile) or premeasured 1.5-mile course.
2. Warm-up for at least 3 minutes (easy stretching, mild calisthenics, and jogging in place).
3. Walk, jog, and/or run the 1.5-mile distance as fast as possible.
4. Record run time in min:s.
5. Allow a 5-minute cool-down upon test completion.
6. Refer to Table 1 for predicting $\dot{V}O_{2max}$.

Cooper KH. A means of assessing maximal oxygen uptake. JAMA 1968;203:201.

12-Minute Swim Test

Individuals swim as far as possible in 12 minutes, with distance measured in yards. Differences in skill level, swim conditioning, and body composition greatly affect oxygen consumption (exercise economy), thus making $\dot{V}O_{2max}$ predictions less valid than those based on walking and running tests (with smaller variation in economy).

1. Warm up for at least 3 minutes with easy stretching and mild calisthenics followed by several laps of easy swimming.
2. Swim as many laps as possible in 12 minutes; paced swimming is preferred to intervals of fast and slow effort.
3. Determine total distance swam in yards; if the test ends in the middle of the pool, estimate distance; find swim fitness and $\dot{V}O_{2max}$ prediction in Table 2.

TABLE 1 ■ PREDICTED $\dot{V}O_{2MAX}$ $(ML \cdot KG^{-1} \cdot MIN^{-1})$ FOR 1.5-MILE WALK—RUN TEST (MIN:S)

TIME	$\dot{V}O_{2max}$	TIME	$\dot{V}O_{2max}$	TIME	$\dot{V}O_{2max}$
6:10	80.0	10:30	48.6	14:50	34.0
6:20	79.0	10:40	48.0	15:00	33.6
6:30	77.9	10:50	47.4	15:10	33.1
6:40	76.7	11:00	46.6	15:20	32.7
6:50	75.5	11:10	45.8	15:30	32.2
7:00	74.0	11:20	45.1	15:40	31.8
7:10	72.6	11:30	44.4	15:50	31.4
7:20	71.3	11:40	43.7	16:00	30.9
7:30	69.9	11:50	43.2	16:10	30.5
7:40	68.3	12:00	42.3	16:20	30.2
7:50	66.8	12:10	41.7	16:30	29.8
8:00	65.2	12:20	41.0	16:40	29.5
8:10	63.9	12:30	40.4	16:50	29.1
8:20	62.5	12:40	39.8	17:00	28.9
8:30	61.2	12:50	39.2	17:10	28.5
8:40	60.2	13:00	38.6	17:20	28.3
8:50	59.1	13:10	38.1	17:30	28.0
9:00	58.1	13:20	37.8	17:40	27.7
9:10	56.9	13:30	37.2	17:50	27.4
9:20	55.9	13:40	36.8	18:00	27.1
9:30	54.7	13:50	36.3	18:10	26.8
9:40	53.5	14:00	35.9	18:20	26.6
9:50	52.3	14:10	35.5	18:30	26.3
10:00	51.1	14:20	35.1	18:40	26.0
10:10	50.4	14:30	34.7	18:50	25.7
10:20	49.5	14:40	34.3	19:00	25.4

TABLE 2 ■ 12-MINUTE SWIM TEST FITNESS CATEGORIES (AGE 18–29 YEARS)

DISTANCE (YD)	FITNESS CATEGORY	ESTIMATED $\dot{V}O_{2MAX}$ $(ML \cdot KG^{-1} \cdot MIN^{-1})$ MALES	FEMALES
≥700	Excellent	>52.5	>41.0
500–700	Good	46.5–52.4	37.0–40.0
400–500	Average	42.5–46.4	33.0–36.9
200–400	Fair	36.5–42.4	29.0–32.9
≤200	Poor	33.0–36.4	23.6–28.9

Cooper KH. The aerobics program for total well-being. New York: Bantam Books, 1982.

Severe Heart Disease

The myocardium in advanced coronary artery disease shows impaired capacity to perform work or improve function with regular exercise. These individuals exhibit negligible training adaptations in maximal stroke volume and cardiac output. Nevertheless, patients can improve exercise tolerance and $\dot{V}O_{2max}$ because regular aerobic exercise increases how skeletal muscles' receive, extract, and metabolize oxygen. These adaptations expand the a-$\bar{v}O_2$ difference, allowing patients to exercise at higher intensities or at sub-maximal levels with a lower cardiac output. A reduced sub-maximal exercise cardiac output also decreases myocardial workload, which greatly benefits patients with exertional angina.

Factors Affecting the Exercise a-$\bar{v}O_2$ Difference

Central and peripheral factors interact to increase oxygen extraction in active tissue during exercise. Diverting a large portion of the cardiac output to the active musculature influ-

FOCUS On Research

CONSEQUENCES OF STOPPING REGULAR EXERCISE

Coyle EF, et al. Time course of loss of adaptations after stopping prolonged intense endurance training. J Appl Physiol 1984;57:1857.

▲ Considerable research frames the understanding of physiologic and metabolic adaptations to diverse types of exercise training. Much less attention has focused on what happens when training stops. A clearer picture of the dynamics of "detraining" would clarify the importance of regular physical activity and the consequences of adapting a sedentary lifestyle.

Coyle and colleagues studied cessation of exercise training in seven highly trained runners or cyclists. Subjects had trained for 10 to 12 months at least 5 days weekly for 60 minutes daily at 70 to 80% of $\dot{V}O_{2max}$. Fifty-seven sedentary subjects served as controls. Testing included muscle biopsies on the last day of training and on days 12, 21, 56, and 84 of detraining. Physiologic variables included oxygen consumption ($\dot{V}O_2$), cardiac output ($\dot{Q}$), heart rate (HR), stroke volume (SV), and arteriovenous oxygen difference (a-$\bar{v}O_2$ diff) during 15 minutes of exercise at 75% of $\dot{V}O_{2max}$ and at $\dot{V}O_{2max}$. Muscle biopsies included the left gastrocnemius for runners and vastus lateralis for cyclists.

Except for exercise during testing, the subjects limited their physical activity to the minimal level required in their sedentary jobs and walked less than 500 m daily at a slow pace. The inset figure shows average changes in physiologic variables at each testing session. $\dot{V}O_{2max}$ decreased in all subjects, declining 7% below training levels after 12 days, 14% after 56 days, and 16% by day 84. $\dot{Q}$, SV, and a-$\bar{v}O_2$ diff$_{max}$ each declined, while HR$_{max}$ increased during detraining. Stroke volume decreased by 11% during the first 12 days and stabilized at 86% of the trained value by day 56. No further decreases occurred in the final 4 weeks. The increase in HR$_{max}$ partially compensated for the decrease in SV$_{max}$. Thus, $\dot{Q}_{max}$ declined by only 8% during the initial 3 weeks of detraining, with an average total decrease of 10% over 84 days.

The muscle biopsy data also indicated impressive detraining changes. Citrate synthase and succinate dehydrogenase, key enzymes in aerobic respiration, declined in parallel to reach their lowest levels at day 56. Detraining did not affect myoglobin levels or muscle capillarization. Because capillary density did not change with detraining, the researchers attributed the decreased oxygen extraction (a-$\bar{v}O_2$ diff$_{max}$) to reduced mitochondrial oxidative capacity reflected in depressed respiratory enzyme levels.

This study confirmed that decreases in maximum SV (central factor) *and* a-$\bar{v}O_2$ diff (peripheral factor) contributed to reductions in $\dot{V}O_{2max}$ with detraining. The results thus support the age-old dictum, *"use it or lose it."*

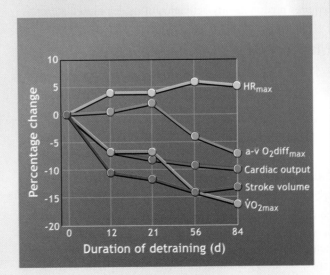

Average changes in maximum heart rate (HR$_{max}$), stroke volume, arteriovenous oxygen differences (a-$\bar{v}O_2$ diff$_{max}$), cardiac output, and $\dot{V}O_{2max}$ over 84 days of detraining.

ences the magnitude of the a-$\bar{v}O_2$ difference in maximal exercise. Some tissues temporarily compromise their blood supply during exercise by redistributing blood to make more oxygen available for muscle metabolism. Exercise training redirects a greater portion of the central circulation to active muscle.

Increases in skeletal muscle microcirculation also increase tissue oxygen extraction.[4,20] Muscle biopsy specimens from the quadriceps femoris show a relatively large ratio of capillaries to muscle fibers in individuals who exhibit large a-$\bar{v}O_2$ differences during intense exercise. An increased capillary-to-fiber ratio reflects a positive endurance training adaptation that enlarges the interface for nutrient and metabolic gas exchange during exercise. Individual muscle cells' ability to generate energy aerobically represents another important factor that governs oxygen extraction capacity.

Increasing the size and number of mitochondria and augmenting aerobic enzyme activity improve a muscle's metabolic capacity in exercise.[13,14] Local vascular and metabolic improvements within muscle ultimately enhance its capacity to produce ATP aerobically.[52] These local training adaptations translate to an increased oxygen extraction capacity.

INTEGRATIVE QUESTION

Present a physiologic rationale to support or refute the contention that either (1) central circulatory factors or (2) peripheral factors residing within the active muscle mass limit $\dot{V}O_{2max}$.

CARDIOVASCULAR ADJUSTMENTS TO UPPER-BODY EXERCISE

Exercise with the upper body creates different metabolic and cardiovascular responses than lower-body exercise that requires predominantly activation of the leg musculature.

Maximal Oxygen Consumption

The highest oxygen consumption during arm exercise averages 20 to 30% lower than leg exercise. Similarly, arm exercise produces lower maximal values for heart rate and pulmonary ventilation. In large part, these differences relate to the relatively smaller muscle mass activated in arm exercise.

Submaximal Oxygen Consumption

Submaximal exercise reverses the pattern for oxygen consumption between upper- and lower-body exercise observed in maximal effort.[8,17] FIGURE 17.6 shows higher oxygen consumption during arm exercise at all submaximal power outputs. The small differences during light exercise become progressively larger as intensity increases. This additional oxygen cost at higher intensities of arm exercise results from (1) lower mechanical efficiency in upper-body exercise from the additional cost of static muscle actions that do not

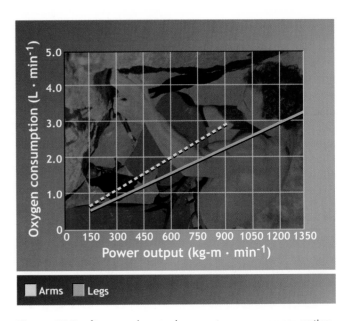

Figure 17.6 Arm exercise requires greater oxygen consumption than leg exercise at any submaximal power output throughout the comparison range. The largest differences occur during intense exercise. Data represent averages for men and women. (From Laboratory of Applied Physiology, Queens College, Flushing, NY.)

contribute to external work and (2) recruitment of additional musculature to stabilize the torso during arm exercise.

Physiologic Response

Any level of submaximal oxygen consumption (or percentage $\dot{V}O_{2max}$) or power output with upper-body exercise provides greater physiologic strain than lower-body exercise.[41,48,49] More specifically, submaximal arm exercise produces higher heart rates, pulmonary ventilations, and perceptions of effort than comparable intensities of leg exercise. This also applies to blood pressure during arm versus leg exercise (see Chapter 15).

The elevated heart rate response in submaximal arm exercise probably results from two factors: (1) greater feedforward stimulation from the brain's central command to the medullary control center and (2) increased feedback stimulation to the medulla from peripheral receptors in active tissue. Upper-body exercise places a greater strain (i.e., greater force per unit muscle, greater percentage of maximum capacity, and more metabolic byproducts) on the relatively smaller upper-body musculature for any submaximum exercise level. Added strain augments peripheral feedback to the medulla; this increases heart rate and blood pressure. More than likely, activating a smaller muscle mass as in arm exercise accounts for the lower maximum heart rate in upper-body exercise. This effect reduces input to the medullary cardiovascular control center from the motor cortex, with less peripheral feedback from the smaller upper-body muscle mass.

Implications. *A standard submaximal exercise load (power output or oxygen consumption) with the upper body produces greater metabolic and physiologic strain than leg exercise.*

For this reason, exercise prescriptions based on running and bicycling do *not* apply to arm exercise. Low correlations often emerge between $\dot{V}O_{2max}$ in arm versus leg exercise so one should not expect to accurately predict aerobic capacity for arm exercise from a test that uses the legs and vice versa.[7,22] This lack of strong association between the two exercise modes further amplifies the specificity concept applied to aerobic fitness.

Summary

1. Cardiac output reflects the functional capacity of the cardiovascular system. Heart rate and stroke volume determine the heart's output capacity expressed as follows: Cardiac output = Heart rate × Stroke volume.
2. Several invasive and noninvasive methods measure cardiac output in humans. Each has specific advantages and disadvantages during exercise.
3. Cardiac output increases proportionally with exercise intensity, starting from approximately $5 \text{ L} \cdot \text{min}^{-1}$ at rest to a maximum of 20 to 25 $\text{L} \cdot \text{min}^{-1}$ in untrained, college-aged men and 35 to $40 \text{ L} \cdot \text{min}^{-1}$ in elite male endurance athletes.
4. The large stroke volumes of endurance athletes explain the difference in maximum cardiac outputs compared with untrained persons.
5. Stroke volume increases during upright exercise from the interaction between greater ventricular filling during diastole and more complete emptying during systole.
6. Sympathetic hormones augment systolic ejection by increasing stroke power during systole.
7. Blood flows to specific tissues in proportion to their metabolic activity. The kidneys and splanchnic regions temporarily compromise blood supply to redistribute blood to exercising muscles; most of the cardiac output diverting to active muscles during exercise.
8. Maximum cardiac output and maximum $a\text{-}\bar{v}O_2$ difference determine maximal oxygen consumption. A large cardiac output clearly differentiates endurance athletes from untrained counterparts.
9. Arm exercise generates 25% lower $\dot{V}O_{2max}$ than leg exercise.
10. Any level of submaximal oxygen consumption (or $\%\dot{V}O_{2max}$) or power output with upper-body exercise provides greater physiologic strain than lower-body exercise.

References are available on the Student CD and online at http://connection.lww.com/mkk6e.

Skeletal Muscle: Structure and Function

18

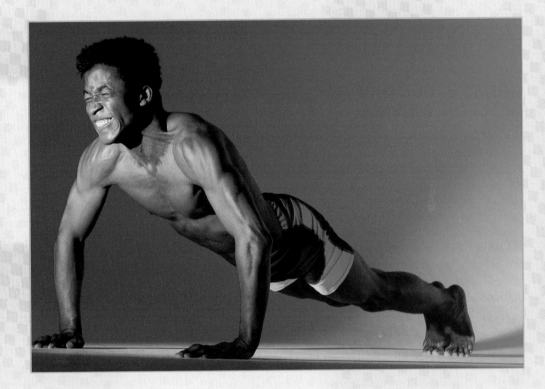

CHAPTER OBJECTIVES

- Outline the levels of organization in the gross structure of skeletal muscle

- List four major protein constituents of skeletal muscle and their functions

- Draw and label the structures that characterize a skeletal muscle fiber's striated appearance under the light microscope at low magnification

- Describe the different arrangements of individual muscle fibers along the long axis of skeletal muscle and explain the biomechanical advantage of each

- Draw and label a skeletal muscle fiber's ultrastructural components

- Summarize the salient features of the sliding filament model of muscle contraction

- Outline the sequence of chemical and mechanical events during skeletal muscle excitation–contraction coupling and relaxation

- Discuss the function of the triad and T-tubule system

- Contrast slow-twitch and fast-twitch (including subdivisions) muscle fiber characteristics

- Outline the distribution patterns of muscle fiber type among diverse groups of elite athletes

- Discuss modifications in muscle fibers and fiber types with specific exercise training

Human movement through the action of skeletal muscle, the body's most abundant tissue, requires conversion of the chemical energy in adenosine triphosphate (ATP) to mechanical energy. Muscle forces act on the body's bony lever system to move one or more bones about their joint axis to propel an object, move the body itself, or do both simultaneously. The following sections present the architectural organization of skeletal muscle with focus on its gross and microscopic structures. We also highlight the sequence of chemical and mechanical events in muscle action and relaxation, including differences in muscle fiber characteristics among sedentary and elite athletes in different sports.

GROSS STRUCTURE OF SKELETAL MUSCLE

Each of the body's more than 660 skeletal muscles contains various wrappings of fibrous connective tissue. FIGURE 18.1 illustrates the gross structural details of a skeletal muscle and its thousands of cylindrical cells called **fibers**. These long, slender, multinucleated fibers (whose number probably remains fixed by the second trimester of fetal development) lie parallel to each other, with the force of action directed along the fiber's long axis. Individual fiber length varies from a few millimeters in the eye muscles to nearly 30 cm in the large antigravity muscles of the leg (with width reaching 0.15 mm).

Levels of Organization

A fine layer of connective tissue, the endomysium, wraps each muscle fiber and separates it from neighboring fibers. Another layer of connective tissue, the **perimysium**, surrounds a bundle of up to 150 fibers called a **fasciculus**. A fascia of fibrous connective tissue, the **epimysium**, surrounds the entire muscle. This protective sheath tapers at its distal and proximal ends as it blends into and joins the intramuscular tissue sheaths to form the dense, strong connective tissue of the **tendons**. The tendons connect both ends of the muscle to the **periosteum**, the bone's outermost covering.

The tissues of the tendon intermesh with the collagenous fibers within the bone. This forms a powerful link between muscle and bone that remains inseparable except during severe stress when it can sever or literally pull away from the bone. When the tendon attaches to the end of a long bone, the bone adapts by enlarging at that end to create a more stable union. Depending on bone size, the term *tubercle, tuberosity,* or *trochanter* describes this overgrowth.

The force of muscle action transmits directly from the connective tissue harness to the tendons, which then pull on the bone at the point of attachment. The forces exerted on the tendinous attachments under muscular exertion range from 20 to 50 newtons (197 to 492 kg) per cm^2 of cross-sectional area—forces often much larger than the muscle fibers themselves can tolerate. The muscle's **origin** refers to the location

where the tendon joins a relatively stable skeletal part, generally the proximal or fixed end of the lever system or that nearest the body's midline; the point of distal attachment to the moving bone represents the **insertion**. Figure 18.1B illustrates the tendon's ultrastructural details. The protein collagen comprises about 70% of the tendon's dry mass.

Beneath the endomysium and surrounding each muscle fiber lies the **sarcolemma**, a thin, elastic membrane that encloses the fiber's cellular contents. It contains a plasma membrane (plasmalemma) and a basement membrane. The plasma membrane, a bilayer lipid structure, conducts the electrochemical wave of depolarization over the surface of the muscle fiber. The membrane also insulates one fiber from another during depolarization. The basement membrane contains proteins and strands of collagen fibrils that fuse with the collagenous fibers in the outer covering of the tendon. Between the basement and plasma membranes lie myogenic stem cells known as **satellite cells**, the normally quiescent myoblasts that function in regenerative cellular growth, possible adaptations to exercise training, and recovery from injury.[20,38,52] Incorporation of satellite cell nuclei into existing muscle fibers seems a likely explanation for exercise-induced muscle fiber hypertrophy.

The fiber's aqueous protoplasm (**sarcoplasm**) contains enzymes, fat and glycogen particles, nuclei (approximately 250 per mm of fiber length) that contain the genes, mitochondria, and other specialized organelles. Figure 18.1C details the **sarcoplasmic reticulum**, an extensive longitudinal latticelike network of tubular channels and vesicles. This highly specialized system provides structural integrity to the cell. It allows the wave of depolarization to spread rapidly from the fiber's outer surface to its inner environment through the T-tubule system to initiate muscle action. The sarcoplasmic reticulum that surrounds each myofibril contains biologic "pumps" that take up Ca^{2+} from the fiber's sarcoplasm. This produces a calcium concentration gradient between the sarcoplasmic reticulum (higher $[Ca^{2+}]$) and the sarcoplasm surrounding the filaments (lower $[Ca^{2+}]$).

Chemical Composition

Water makes up approximately 75% of skeletal muscle mass and protein composes 20%. The remaining 5% contains salts and other substances, including high-energy phosphates; urea; lactate; the minerals calcium, magnesium, and phosphorus; various enzymes; sodium, potassium, and chloride ions; amino acids, fats, and carbohydrates. **Myosin** (approximately 60% of muscle protein), **actin**, and **tropomyosin** are the most abundant muscle proteins. Each 100 g of muscle tissue contains about 700 mg of the oxygen-binding, conjugated protein **myoglobin**.

Blood Supply

Arteries and veins that lie parallel to individual muscle fibers provide a rich vascular supply. These vessels divide into numerous arterioles, capillaries, and venules to form a vast net-

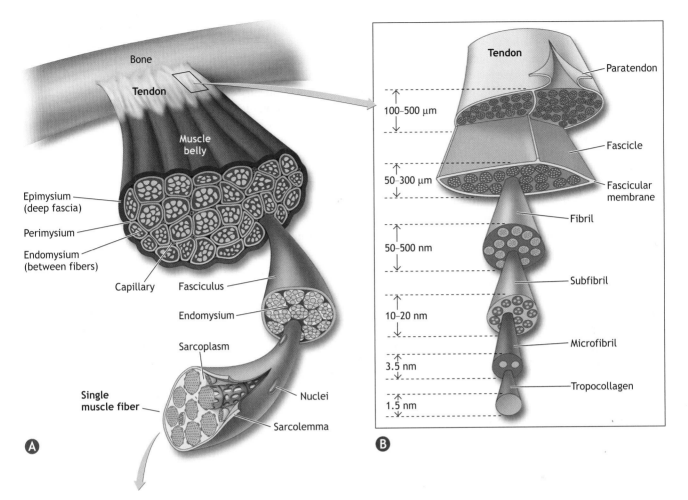

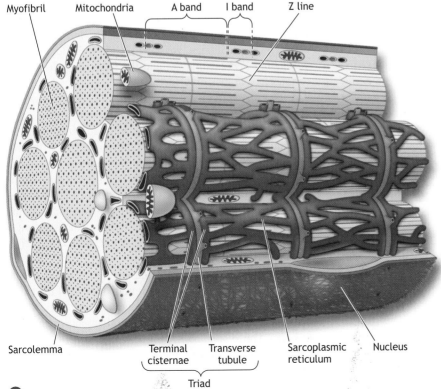

Figure 18.1 Cross section of skeletal muscle structures and arrangement of connective tissue wrappings.
A. Endomysium covers individual fibers. Perimysium surrounds groups of fibers called fasciculi, and epimysium wraps the entire muscle in a sheath of connective tissue. The sarcolemma, a thin, elastic membrane, covers the surface of each muscle fiber. **B.** Details of tendon structure. The microfibril forms from five parallel tropocollagen molecules that unite to form fibrils and then collagen fibers. An endotendon encloses a bundle of fibers, and an epitendon sheath, known as a fascicle, surrounds a group of endotendons. The fascicles combine into a tendon that becomes surrounded by its own sheath, the paratendon ($\mu m = 10^{-6}$ m; $nm = 10^{-9}$ m). **C.** Cross section of the sarcoplasmic reticulum and T-tubule system that surrounds the myofibrils. Note the close contact of the mitochondria and network of intracellular membranes and tubules.

work in and around the endomysium. Extensive branching of blood vessels ensures each muscle fiber an adequate supply of oxygenated blood from the arterial system and rapid removal of carbon dioxide in the venous circulation. During intense exercise, the muscle's oxygen uptake increases nearly 70 times to approximately 11 mL per 100 g per minute or a total muscle $\dot{V}O_2$ of 3400 mL · min^{-1} for an elite endurance athlete. The local vascular bed channels large quantities of blood through active tissues to accommodate this oxygen requirement. Blood flow distribution fluctuates in rhythmic activities such as running, swimming, or cycling. It decreases during the muscle's contraction phase and increases during relaxation to provide a "milking action" that moves blood through the muscles and propels it back to the heart. The rapid dilation of previously dormant capillaries complements the pulsatile blood flow. Between 200 and 500 capillaries deliver blood to each square millimeter of active muscle cross-section, with up to four capillaries directly contacting each fiber. In endurance athletes, five to seven capillaries surround each fiber; this adaptation ensures greater local blood flow when needed (see next section).

Physical activities that require straining present a somewhat different picture for muscle blood flow. When a muscle generates about 60% of its force-generating capacity for several seconds, elevated intramuscular pressure occludes local blood flow during the contraction. With a sustained contraction, the intramuscular high-energy phosphates and glycolytic anaerobic reactions provide the main energy source for muscular effort.

Capillarization

Trained muscles' increased capillary-to-muscle fiber ratio helps to explain improved exercise capacity with endurance training.[2,7] An enhanced capillary microcirculation expedites the removal of heat and metabolic byproducts from active tissues in addition to facilitating delivery of oxygen, nutrients, and hormones. Electron microscopy reveals the total number of capillaries per muscle (and capillaries per mm^2 of muscle tissue) averages about 40% higher in endurance-trained athletes than untrained counterparts. This almost equaled the 41% difference in $\dot{V}O_{2max}$ between the two groups. A positive association also exists between $\dot{V}O_{2max}$ and average number of muscle capillaries.[40] Enhanced vascularization on the capillary level proves particularly beneficial during exercise that requires a high level of steady-rate aerobic metabolism. Vascular stretch and shear stress on the vessel walls from increased blood flow during exercise stimulates capillary development with intense aerobic training.[31]

SKELETAL MUSCLE ULTRASTRUCTURE

Electron microscopy, x-ray diffraction, histochemical staining, helium–neon laser diffraction, in vitro motility assays, and optical tweezer technologies (see Chapter 33) reveal the microscopic anatomy (ultrastructure) of skeletal muscle. FIGURE 18.2 shows the different levels of gross and subcellular organization within a skeletal muscle fiber. A single multinucleated muscle fiber contains smaller functional units that lie parallel to the fiber's long axis. These **fibrils** or **myofibrils**, approximately 1 μm (1 μm = 1/1000 mm) in diameter, contain even smaller subunits called **filaments** or **myofilaments** that lie parallel to the long axis of the myofibril. The myofilaments chiefly consist of ordered assemblages of the proteins **actin** and **myosin** that account for about 85% of the myofibrillar complex. Twelve to 15 other proteins either serve a structural function or affect protein filament interaction during muscle action. Examples include (1) **tropomyosin**, located along the actin filaments (5%); (2) **troponin** (which consists of troponin-1, T, C), located in the actin filaments (3%); (3) **α-actinin**, distributed in the Z band region (7%); (4) **β-actinin**, found in the actin filaments (1%); (5) **M protein**, identified in the region of the M lines within the sarcomere (less than 1%); and (5) **C protein** (less than 1%), which contributes to the sarcomere's structural integrity.

The Sarcomere

At low magnification, the alternating light and dark bands along the length of the skeletal muscle fiber give it a characteristic **striated** appearance. FIGURE 18.3 *(top)* illustrates the structural details of this cross-striation pattern within a myofibril. The lighter area is the *I band,* and the darker zone, the *A band.* The *Z line* bisects the I band and adheres to the sarcolemma; it provides stability to the entire structure. Optical properties denote the specific bands. When polarized light passes through the I band, it moves at the same velocity in all directions (isotropic). Light passing through the A band does not scatter equally (anisotropic). The letter *Z* indicates between (from German, *zwischenscheibe*); the letter *M* (*mittelscheibe*) *denotes* middle; and the letter *H* (*hellerscheibe*) denotes a clear disk or zone.

*The **sarcomere** consists of the basic repeating unit between two Z lines. This structural entity makes up the functional unit of a muscle fiber.* The actin and bipolar myosin filaments within the sarcomere contribute primarily to the mechanics of muscle contraction. Sarcomeres lie in series, and their filaments have a parallel configuration within a given fiber. In the resting state, the length of each sarcomere averages 2.5 μm. Thus, a myofibril 15-mm long contains about 6000 sarcomeres joined end to end. The length of the sarcomere largely determines a muscle's functional properties.

The position of thin actin and thicker myosin proteins in the sarcomere creates an interdigitating overlap of the two filaments. The center of the A band contains the *H zone,* a region of lower optical density because actin filaments are absent in this area. The *M band* bisects the central portion of the H zone, which delineates the sarcomere's center. The M band consists of the protein structures that support the arrangement of the myosin filaments. Figure 18.3 *(bottom)* shows a detailed view of a sarcomere and TABLE 18.1 lists proposed functions of a sarcomere's proteins.

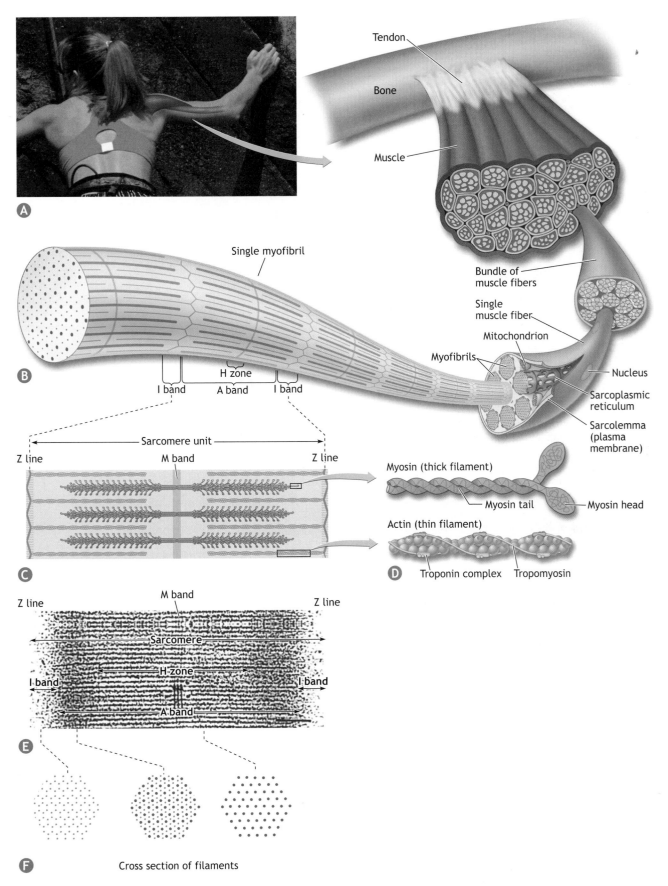

Figure 18.2 Gross and subcellular microscopic organization of skeletal muscle. **A.** Individual fibers constitute the whole muscle. **B.** Fibers consist of myofibrils with actin and myosin protein filament subdivisions. **C–F.** Details of a single sarcomere with the actin and myosin filaments, a microscopic view of the sarcomere (note the two Z lines), and a cross-sectional view of the filaments.

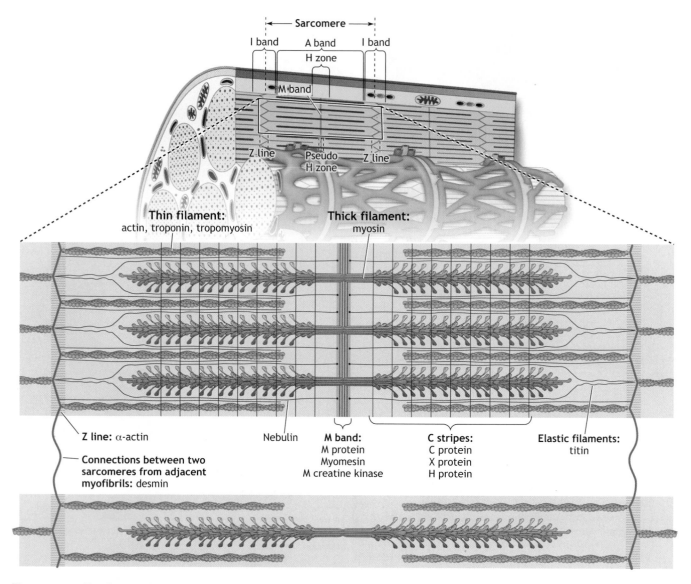

Figure 18.3 *Top.* Structural position of the filaments in a sarcomere. The Z line bounds a sarcomere at both ends. *Bottom.* Detailed view of a sarcomere, including the proteins listed in Table 18.1.

MUSCLE FIBER ALIGNMENT

The long axis of the muscle determines the arrangement of individual fibers from an imaginary line drawn through the origin and insertion, or the fiber angle relative to the force-generating axis. Differences in sarcomere alignment and length strongly affect a muscle's force- and power-generating capacity (FIG. 18.4). Fusiform or spindle-shaped fibers run parallel to the muscle's long axis (e.g., biceps brachii) and taper at the tendinous attachment. In contrast, pennate or fan-shaped fibers' fasciculi (bundles of fibers) lie at an oblique pennation angle that varies up to 30°. In the soleus muscle, for example, the pennation angle averages 25°, whereas for the vastus medialis it equals 5°; the sartorius muscle has no angle of pennation. Of functional significance, the degree of pennation directly affects the number of sarcomeres per cross-sectional muscle area (no fibers run full muscle length). In essence, pennation allows individual muscle fibers to remain short while the overall muscle may reach considerable length. A fusiform fiber has no pennation so the fiber's cross-sectional area represents the true anatomic cross section. In pennate muscle, the complex arrangement of connective tissue, tendons, and relatively short fibers creates a larger cross-sectional area than fusiform fibers because more sarcomeres "pack" into a given volume of muscle. The term **physiologic cross-sectional area** (**PCSA**) refers to the total cross-sectional areas of all fibers within a particular muscle. An unusually large pennation angle of 30° results in only a 13% loss in an individual fiber's force capacity; this makes for a huge increase in total fiber packing ability.[32,43] Thus, pennation per se allows packing of a large number of fibers into a smaller cross-sectional area. Pennate muscles tend to generate considerable power. The bottom of Figure 18.4 illustrates the effect of pennation on fiber packing and force-generating capacity.

TABLE 18.1 ■ TWELVE PROTEINS ASSOCIATED WITH A MUSCLE FIBER'S SARCOMERE AND THEIR PROPOSED FUNCTIONS

STRUCTURE	PROTEIN	FUNCTION
Thin filament	Actin	The main protein of actin that interacts with myosin during excitation–contraction coupling
	Tropomyosin	Transduces the conformational change of the troponin complex to actin
	Troponin	Binds Ca^{2+} and affects tropomyosin; represents the "switch" that transforms the Ca^{2+} signal into a molecular signal that induces crossbridge cycling
	Nebulin	Present next to actin and believed to control the number of actin monomers joined to each other in a thin filament
Thick filament	Myosin	Splits ATP and is responsible for the "power stroke" of the myosin head
C stripes	C protein	Holds the myosin thick filaments in a regular array; may hold the H protein of adjacent thick filaments at an even distance during force generation; may also control the number of myosin molecules in a thick filament
M line	M protein	Helps hold thick filaments in a regular array
	Myomesin	Provides a strong anchoring point for the protein titin
	M-CK	Provides ATP from phosphocreatine; located proximal to the myosin heads
Z line	α-actinin	Holds the thin filaments in place spatially
	Desmin	Forms the connection between adjacent Z lines from different myofibrils; helps to keep the sarcomeres in register so they maintain their striated appearance
Elastic filament	Titin	Helps keep the thick filament centered between two Z lines during contraction; believed to control the number of myosin molecules contained in the thick filament

The fibers in a fusiform muscle run parallel to the muscle's long axis. In this case, fiber length equals muscle length, and a fiber's force generation transmits directly to the tendon. *This arrangement facilitates rapid muscle shortening.* A unipennate fiber arrangement, where muscle fibers lie at an oblique angle to the tendon, produces a larger effective cross-sectional area than in fusiform muscle. *Muscles with greater pennation, although slower in contractile velocity, generate greater force and power than fusiform muscles (other factors being equal) because more sarcomeres contribute to the muscle action.* A bipennate muscle has two sets of fibers that lie obliquely on both sides of a common tendon (e.g., gastrocnemius and rectus femoris muscles). A multipennate muscle like the deltoid contains more than two sets of fibers that converge at different angles and insert directly into tendons at both their ends. Pennate muscles differ from fusiform fibers in three ways: (1) they generally contain shorter fibers, (2) they possess a greater number of individual fibers, and (3) they exhibit less range of motion.

Complex Fusiform Arrangement

The **complex parallel muscle (series-fibered muscle)** features individual fibers that run parallel to the muscle's line of pull. Unlike the simple fusiform arrangement where a fiber runs the entire muscle length, the complex parallel arrangement features muscle fibers that terminate in the muscle's midbelly and taper to interact with the connective tissue matrix and/or adjacent muscle fibers. This arrangement enables parallel packing of relatively short fibers within in a long muscle (e.g., the 50-cm long sartorius). This structural specialization with diverse intrafascicular terminations also creates lateral tension—either through connective tissue into tendon or through adjacent and series fibers into connective tissue—at various points along the fiber's surface.

INTEGRATIVE QUESTION

List the advantages of a skeletal muscle organ system composed of muscles whose fibers vary in architectural design.

Fiber Length–Muscle Length Ratio

The ratio of individual fiber length to a muscle's total length usually varies between 0.2 and 0.6. This means that individual fibers in the longest muscles such as the upper and lower limbs remain significantly shorter than the muscle's overall length. FIGURE 18.5 *(left)* illustrates the architectural properties of four lower limb muscles. On average, quadriceps muscle fibers maintain pennation angles that average 4.6°, a PCSA of approximately 21.7 cm^2, and a fiber length that averages 68 mm. This contrasts with the biceps femoris (hamstring) muscle with relatively long fibers (111 mm) and an intermediate PCSA (11.7 cm^2). Quadriceps muscles exhibit approximately 50% greater force capacity than the hamstrings, whose design provides rapid shortening. These design differences suggest susceptibility of the hamstrings to tearing should an abrupt force output imbalance occur during maximal activation between the quadriceps and hamstrings as often occurs in sprint running. Part of the imbalance may be from a strength deficit between the hamstrings and quadriceps, which predisposes individuals to recurrent hamstring injuries and discomfort.[12] The hamstring-to-quadriceps strength ratio typically computes by dividing the maximal knee flexor (hamstring) moment by the maximal

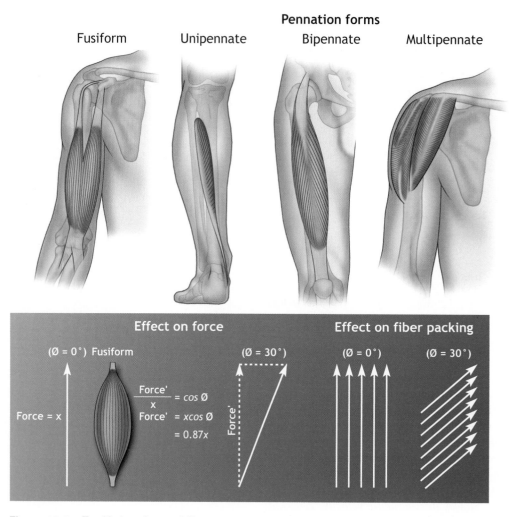

Figure 18.4   *Top.* Various forms of fiber arrangement in human skeletal muscle. *Bottom.* Force development in a fusiform muscle with no angle of pennation ($\varnothing = 0°$) and when $\varnothing = 30°$. A 30° angle of pennation results in a 13% loss of each fiber's maximum force on the tendon, solely a result of muscle mechanics. Pennation angle increases the number of fibers that pack into a given volume of muscle *(bottom right)*. Muscle mass and the contractile capacity relate proportionately for a given muscle in comparisons among individuals. Because of the effect of pennation angle, it does not necessarily follow that muscle mass per se relates to an equivalent tension output among different muscle groups. (Modified from Lieber RL. Skeletal muscle structure and function. 2nd ed. Baltimore: Lippincott Williams & Wilkins, 2002.)

knee extensor (quadriceps) moment.[1] Specific exercise training at preset velocities designed to improve this ratio is now an integral part of functional rehabilitation of hamstring-to-quadriceps deficits.[10,16,33]

Figure 18.5 (*right inset, A* and *B*) shows the generalized muscle force–muscle length and muscle force–muscle velocity relationships for fusiform and pennate muscles with the same amount of contractile protein and identical muscle fiber type. In this hypothetical example, the muscle force–muscle length curve for fusiform muscle shows a longer working range and lower maximum force output because of longer individual fibers and a smaller PCSA (Fig. 18.5C). The opposite occurs for pennate muscle with shorter fibers and larger PCSA—these fibers generate about double the force of fusiform muscles. For the muscle force–muscle velocity curve, the fusiform muscle

with longer fibers exhibits a higher contractile velocity but lower force–output capacity.

ACTIN–MYOSIN ORIENTATION

Thousands of myosin filaments lie along the line of actin filaments in a muscle fiber. FIGURE 18.6A illustrates the sarcomere's actin–myosin orientation at resting length; Figure 18.6B shows the hexagonal arrangement of myosin and actin filaments. Myosin filaments consist of bundles of molecules with polypeptide tails and globular heads. Actin filaments have two twisted chains of monomers bound by tropomyosin polypeptide chains. Six relatively thin actin filaments, each about 50 Å in diameter and 1 μm long, encircle the thicker myosin filament (150 Å in diameter and 1.5 μm long). This represents an extremely

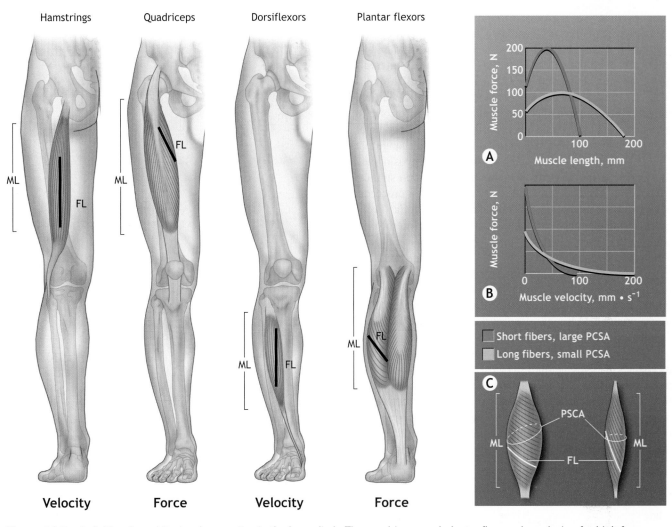

Figure 18.5 *Left.* Muscle architectural properties in the lower limb. The quadriceps and plantar flexors show design for high force production because of their low fiber length-to-muscle length (FL:ML) ratios and relatively large physiologic cross-sectional areas (PCSA). The hamstrings and dorsiflexor muscles, in contrast, show architecture designed for high contractile velocity because of their relatively high FL:ML and long FL. *Right.* Hypothetical pennate (short fibers) muscles and fusiform (long fibers) muscles of the same length and with the same amount of contractile machinery. The muscle force–muscle length curve (**A**) shows the fusiform muscle with a longer working range and lower maximum force output than the pennate muscle. Lower force capacity (dorsiflexors and hamstrings) occurs because for a given change in muscle length, the individual sarcomeres lengthen less, with the change in muscle length distributed over more sarcomeres. A greater force output (quadriceps and plantar flexors) results from a greater PCSA (**C**). The muscle force–muscle velocity curve (**B**) shows that the fusiform muscle with longer fibers exhibits higher contractile velocity but a lower maximum force output. (Modified from Lieber RL. Skeletal muscle structure and function. 2nd edition. Baltimore: Lippincott Williams & Wilkins, 2002.)

impressive substructural configuration. For example, a myofibril 1 μm in diameter contains approximately 450 thick filaments in the sarcomere's center and 900 thin filaments at each end. A muscle fiber 100 μm in diameter and 1 cm long contains approximately 8000 myofibrils; each myofibril consists of 4500 sarcomeres on average. In a single fiber, this arrangement consists of 16 billion thick filaments and 64 billion thin filaments.

FIGURE 18.7 illustrates the spatial orientation of various components of contractile filaments. Projections or "**crossbridges**" spiral around the myosin filament in the region of overlap of the actin and myosin filaments. The crossbridges repeat at intervals of approximately 450 Å along the filament.

Globular "lollipop-like" myosin heads extend perpendicularly to latch onto the thinner double-twisted actin strands to create structural and functional links between myofilaments. The unique feature of myosin's two heads concerns their opposite orientation at the ends of the thick filament. ATP hydrolysis activates the two heads, placing them in an optimal orientation to bind actin's active sites, thus pulling the thin filaments and Z lines of the sarcomere toward the middle.

Tropomyosin and troponin are two other important constituents of the actin helical structure. These proteins regulate the make-and-break contacts between the myofilaments during muscle action. Tropomyosin distributes along the length of the actin filament in a groove formed by the double helix. Tropomyosin inhibits actin and myosin interaction (coupling) and thus prevents their permanent bonding. Troponin and its three-subunit proteins embedded at fairly regular intervals along the actin strands exhibit a high affinity for calcium ions (Ca^{2+}), a mineral that plays a crucial role in muscle action and fatigue.[29] For example, Ca^{2+} and troponin trigger myofibrils to interact and slide past each other. During muscle fiber stimulation, troponin molecules undergo a conformational change that "tugs" on tropomyosin protein strands. Tropomyosin then moves deeper into the groove between the two actin strands, "uncovering" actin's active sites so muscle action proceeds. Muscle fatigue relates to considerable reductions in Ca^{2+} concentration in the transverse tubules during intense exercise, in addition to intrinsic alterations in the contractile apparatus and sarcoplasmic reticulum function.[8,51]

The M band consists of transversely and longitudinally oriented proteins that maintain myosin filament orientation within a sarcomere. As Figure 18.7 illustrates, the perpendicularly oriented M bridges connect with six adjacent myosin filaments in a hexagonal pattern.

An exciting area of muscle biochemistry, physiology, and mechanics involves the study of cytoskeletal proteins and structures that serve as an intermediate intracellular filament system.[35] The intracellular cytoskeleton provides (1) structural integrity in the inactive muscle cell, (2) lateral force transmission to adjacent sarcomeres through interaction with actomyosin during muscle action, and (3) connections to the cell's surface

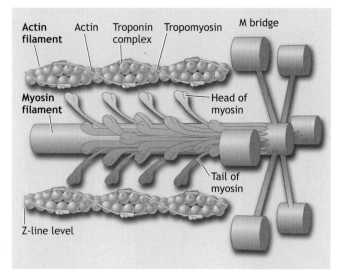

Figure 18.7   Details of the thick and thin protein filaments including tropomyosin, troponin complex, and M bridge. The globular heads of the myosin contain myosin ATPase; this "active" head frees the energy from ATP for muscle action.

membrane. A better understanding of the role of the cytoskeleton, its diverse proteins, and the myofibrillar lattice structure should enhance current understanding of muscle action, including processes in muscle injury, repair, and overload.

Intracellular Tubule Systems

Figure 18.8 illustrates the complex tubule system within a muscle fiber. The lateral end of each tubule channel terminates in a saclike vesicle that stores Ca^{2+}. Another network of tubules—the transverse tubule system or **T-tubule system**—runs perpendicular to the myofibril. T tubules lie between the most lateral part of two sarcoplasmic channels; vesicles of these structures abut the T tubule. The term **triad** describes this repeating pattern of two vesicles and a T tubule in each Z line region. Each sarcomere contains two triads, with the pattern repeated regularly along the myofibril's length.

The T tubules pass through the fiber and open externally from the inside of the muscle cell. *The triad and T-tubule system function as a microtransportation network by spreading the action potential (wave of depolarization) from the fiber's outer membrane inward to deeper cell regions.* Propagation of the action potential stimulates the triad sacs to release Ca^{2+}, which diffuses a short distance to "activate" the actin filaments. Muscle action begins when myosin filament crossbridges momentarily attach to active sites on the actin filaments. When electrical excitation ceases, Ca^{2+} concentration in cytoplasm decreases; this relates to muscle relaxation. To some extent, propagating an action potential (and countering fatigue in exercise) depends on maintaining continued steep gradients of Na^+ and K^+ across the sarcolemma. Decreased chemical gradients of these electrolytes (from a reduction in Na^+/K^+ pump activity) severely affect muscle fiber excitability and consequent contractile performance of active muscles.[34]

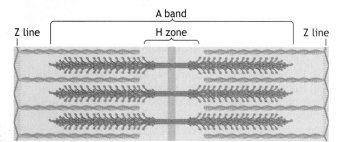

A Resting sarcomere

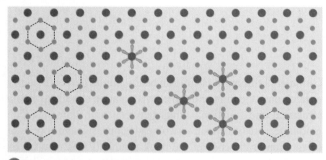

B Cross-section of myofibrils

Figure 18.6   A. Ultrastructure of actin–myosin orientation within a resting sarcomere. **B.** Representation of electron micrograph through a cross-section of myofibrils in a single muscle fiber. Note the hexagonal orientation of the smaller actin and larger myosin filaments, including crossbridges that extend from a thick to thin filament.

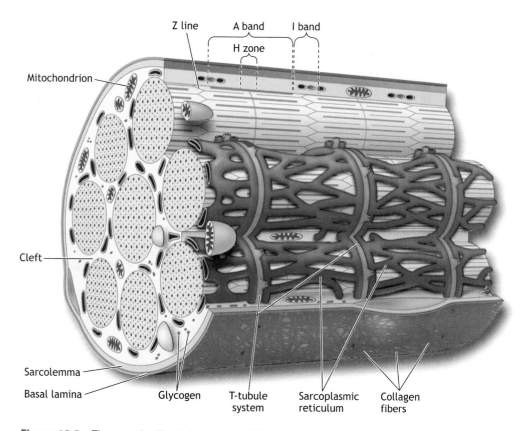

Z line
A band
I band
H zone
Mitochondrion
Cleft
Sarcolemma
Basal lamina
Glycogen
T-tubule system
Sarcoplasmic reticulum
Collagen fibers

Figure 18.8 The complex T-tubule system within a muscle fiber.

CHEMICAL AND MECHANICAL EVENTS DURING MUSCLE ACTION AND RELAXATION

Electron microscopy, x-ray diffraction, and biochemical methods have unraveled many secrets of cellular structure and kinetics, providing testable hypotheses about chemical and mechanical events during muscle activation and relaxation. Many pieces of the puzzle remain unanswered, but considerable evidence supports the **sliding-filament model** to explain muscle contraction. Proposed some 60 years ago to explain the molecular movements that underlie muscle action, the model still fits nicely with the ever-expanding details about muscle ultrastructure and function.[21]

Mechanism of Muscle Action: The Sliding-Filament Model

In the early 1950s, two British biologists, Hugh Huxley and Andrew Huxley (unrelated and working independently), proposed a sliding-filament model of muscle contraction. In 1957, A. Huxley extended the theory to include specifics of crossbridge behavior.[22,23] *The theory proposes that a muscle shortens or lengthens because the thick and thin filaments slide past each other without changing length. The myosin crossbridges, which cyclically attach, rotate, and detach from the actin filaments with energy from ATP hydrolysis, provide the **molecular motor** to drive fiber shortening.*[15,39] This pro-

duces a major conformational change in relative size within the sarcomere's zones and bands and produces a force at the Z bands. FIGURE 18.9 shows that the thin actin filaments move past the myosin myofilaments (translate over them by a preset amount) and into the A band region during shortening (and move out during the lengthening or relaxation phase).[5,6] Thus, the major structural rearrangement during shortening occurs in the region of the I band. This band decreases as the Z bands are pulled toward the center of each sarcomere. No change occurs in the width of the A band, although the H zone can disappear when the actin filaments make contact at the sarcomere center. A static (isometric) muscle action generates force, but the fiber's length remains unchanged, with the relative spacing of I band and A band remaining constant. In this case, the same molecular groups interact repeatedly. The A band widens in an eccentric action as the fiber lengthens during force generation.

Mechanical Action of Crossbridges

Myosin plays both an enzymatic and structural role in muscle action. The globular head of the myosin crossbridge, which contains an actin-activated ATPase in its actin-binding site, provides the mechanical power stroke for the actin and myosin filaments to slide past each other. The cyclic, oscillating to-and-fro motion of the crossbridges (powered by ATP hydrolysis) moves like oars slicing through water (FIG. 18.10). But unlike oars, crossbridges do not all move synchronously.

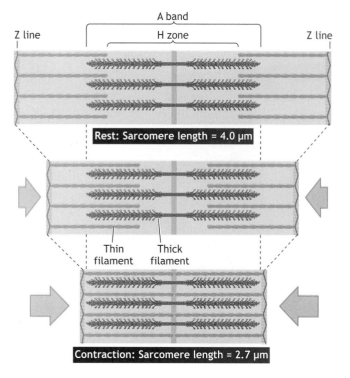

Figure 18.9 Structural rearrangement of actin and myosin filaments at rest (sarcomere length, 4.0 μm) and during muscle shortening (contracted sarcomere length, 2.7 μm).

If they did, the muscle action would produce a series of uneven actions instead of finely graded, smoothly modulated movements and force outputs. During shortening, each crossbridge undergoes many repeated but independent cycles of asynchronous movement.

At any one time, approximately 50% of the crossbridges make contact with the actin filaments to form the protein complex **actomyosin**, which exhibits contractile properties. The remaining crossbridges move through other positions in their vibrating cycle. Figure 18.10 shows that each crossbridge action contributes only a small longitudinal displacement to the filament's full sliding action. The process resembles the movement of a person climbing a rope. The arms and legs represent the crossbridges. Climbing progresses by first reaching with the arms; then grabbing, pulling, and breaking contact while the legs extend; and then repeating this procedure throughout the climb as the person traverses from one point to the next point and so on.

The biochemical technique of in vitro motility assays has played a key role in quantifying the behavior of actin and myosin molecules.[29] Careful experimentation has determined that myosin elicits a 1 to 10 piconewton (pN; 10^{-2} N) force, in which myosin movement ranges from 1 to 20 nanometers (nm; 10^{-9} m) over a brief period of about 5 ms. Researchers have devised four elegant tools to determine the chemical and mechanical properties of the actomyosin complex.

1. *Microneedles*. A glass needle placed in contact with myosin molecules and an actin filament records the mechanical movements of the molecules. Research-

ers then deduce the forces produced by the myosin heads as they slide along the actin strand.[24]

2. *Optical tweezers*. This technique interfaces powerful laser technology with a microscope to isolate individual molecules and measure molecular movement one molecule at a time.[14]

3. *Atomic force microscope*. The displacement and forces from a probe (with actin and myosin mole-

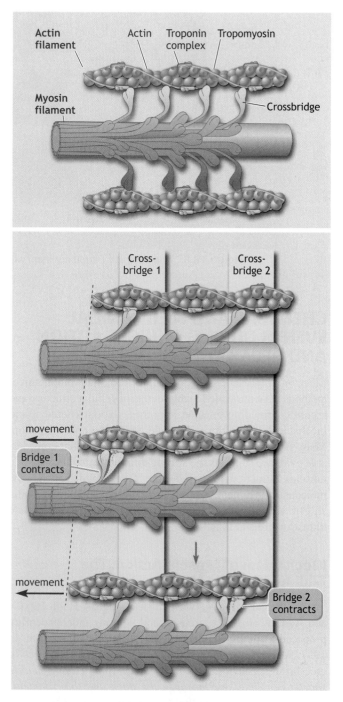

Figure 18.10 *Top.* Relative positioning of actin and myosin filaments during crossbridge oscillation. *Bottom.* The action of each crossbridge contributes a small displacement of movement. For clarity, we show only one actin strand.

cules attached) interfaced with a microscope yields quantitative data about actin–myosin interaction.[27]

4. *Fluorescent probes.* Light-emitting probes quantify the kinetics of molecular binding and release between myosin and actin and how ATP releases energy when degraded to ADP and inorganic phosphate.[17] The technique also has revealed how actin rotates slightly as it moves along myosin[41] and the behavior of the myosin heads during their power stroke.[49]

INTEGRATIVE QUESTION

Discuss the meaning of the term molecular motor to describe how the myofilament crossbridges contribute to muscle fiber action.

Sarcomere Length–Isometric Tension Curve in an Isolated Fiber

FIGURE 18.11 displays the interactions between actin and myosin during isometric tension development in an isolated skeletal muscle preparation. British and Swedish researchers developed this length–tension curve approximately 40 years ago by electrically stimulating a single frog muscle fiber (8 mm long and 75 μm in diameter) and plotting maximum tension output at selected muscle sarcomere lengths.[13,19] The length of the sarcomere along the horizontal axis ranged from 1.6 μm at maximum overlap of the actin filaments (approximately 70% of maximum tension) to 3.6 μm when fully relaxed. Note that the crest of the upward curve for tension occurred at a sarcomere length between 2.0 and 2.25 μm; this length for maximal

tension represents the region of maximum actin and myosin filament interaction. Interestingly, the difference of 0.2 μm at this part of the curve equals precisely the width of the region where no change takes place in actin–myosin interaction. The curve shifts downward when the sarcomere stretches beyond 2.2 μm, thus indicating a decline in peak tension. This decline occurs from reduced overlap between actin and myosin filaments; less overlap produces less crossbridge interaction and diminished active tension development. The fiber fails to develop tension at the maximum point of stretch of 3.65 μm (maximum actin filament length, 2.0 μm; maximum myosin filament length, 1.65 μm). Crossbridge interaction cannot take place at a sarcomere length of 3.65 μm and above.

Sarcomere Length–Isometric Tension Curve in Human Muscle Fibers in Vivo

An elegant procedure determines the range over which sarcomeres in intact human muscle operate on their length–tension curve. FIGURE 18.12 illustrates sarcomere action during different wrist position angles in patients who undergo surgery to correct chronic lateral epicondylitis ("tennis elbow"). The researchers compared the length–tension characteristics of an animal preparation (Fig. 18.11) with those of human muscle in vivo. Figure 18.12 *(top right)* depicts the intraoperative helium–neon laser to quantify sarcomere length. The laser, positioned beneath the lateral end of the extensor carpi radialis brevis muscle (ECRB), quantified sarcomere lengths at three different wrist positions: (1) full flexion to increase sarcomere length, (2) neutral, and (3) full extension to decrease sarcomere length. The *top left* of Figure 18.12 shows the laser diffraction pattern for computing

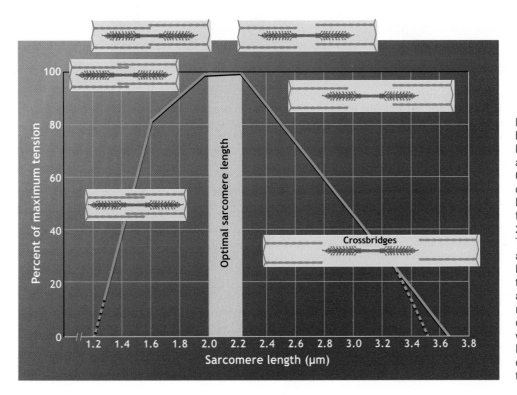

Figure 18.11 Relationship between tension and sarcomere length in skeletal muscle during an isometric muscle action. Optimal sarcomere length (i.e., the one with the greatest interaction between actin and myosin filaments) occurs between 2.0 and 2.25 μm (*light blue vertical band*). Tension output decreases steadily as sarcomere length increases beyond the optimal length. Note the amount of overlap in the actin and myosin filaments at various regions of the tension–length curve and how tension output varies at different sarcomere lengths. Thin filament thickness equals 1.0 μm; thick filament thickness, 1.6 μm.

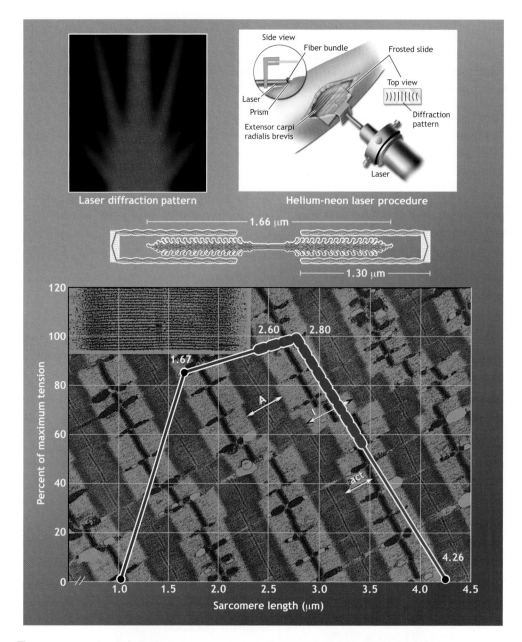

Figure 18.12 Changes in the length–tension curve for sarcomeres in vivo during human wrist flexion and extension. The *top insets* illustrate the helium–neon laser procedure (and view of the illumination prism) used during the surgery. The electron micrograph depicted behind the length–tension curve shows the actin and myosin filaments and the A and I bands from biopsy samples of the extensor carpi radialis brevis muscle to verify sarcomere lengths. The *thickened blue portion* of a hypothetical length–tension curve represents sarcomere length change during wrist flexion (causing sarcomere length increase) and wrist extension (causing sarcomere length decrease). The numbers over the curve represent the inflection points based on the measured filament lengths. (Modified from Lieber RL, et al. In vivo measurement of human wrist extensor muscle sarcomere length changes. J Neurophysiol 1994;71:874. Illustration of the experimental procedure, including the example of the laser diffraction pattern and electron micrograph courtesy of Dr. R. L. Lieber, Professor of Orthopaedics and Bioengineering, Muscle Physiology Laboratory, University of California and Veterans Administration Medical Centers, San Diego, CA.)

sarcomere length. Biopsy specimens from the same muscle verified the laser determinations. An electron micrograph displayed behind the length–tension curve shows the actin and myosin filaments and A and I bands from a muscle biopsy sample. In this experiment, actin filament length equaled 1.30 μm while the myosin filaments were 1.66 μm long. The

thicker blue portion for the plateau and downward parts of the curve show the operating range of the ECRB sarcomeres during both passive (2.6–3.4 μm) and active (2.44–3.33 μm) muscle actions. These data objectify the intrinsic relation between sarcomere length and muscle fiber force capacity (length–tension curve) measured in vivo in human muscle.

Link Between Actin, Myosin, and ATP

The interaction and movement of the protein filaments during muscle action require that myosin crossbridges continually undergo oscillatory movements by combining, detaching, and recombining with new sites along the actin strands (or the same sites in a static action). The myosin crossbridges detach from the actin filament when ATP molecules join the actomyosin complex. The myosin crossbridge in this chemical reaction returns to its original state ready to bind to a new active actin site. The dissociation of actomyosin occurs as follows:

$$\text{Actomyosin} + \text{ATP} \rightarrow \text{Actin} + \text{Myosin-ATP}$$

Energy from ATP hydrolysis transduces into mechanical force when ADP and inorganic phosphate end products form. One of the reacting sites on the globular head of the myosin crossbridge binds to an actin reactive site. The other myosin active site serves as the actin-activated enzyme **myofibrillar adenosine triphosphatase** (**myosin ATPase**). This enzyme splits ATP to yield energy for muscle action. The rate of ATP splitting is relatively slow if myosin and actin remain apart; when they join, myosin ATPase reaction rates increase substantially. Energy released from ATP splitting activates the crossbridges, causing them to oscillate. This course of energy transfer produces a conformational change in myosin's globular head so it interacts with the appropriate actin molecule. The actin filament slides forward from conformational change at multiple points of contact between myosin and actin.

Prior to muscle action, the elongated, pear-shaped, flexible myosin head literally bends around the energy-carrying ATP molecule and cocks like a spring. The myosin then interacts with the adjacent actin filament, splits a phosphate from ATP, and releases its stored mechanical energy as it straightens. This forces the sliding motion that generates muscle tension. The actin and myosin filaments slide past each other at speeds up to 15 μm · s⁻¹.³

Excitation–Contraction Coupling

Excitation–contraction coupling provides the physiologic mechanism whereby an electrical discharge at the muscle initiates chemical events at the cell surface, releasing intracellular Ca^{2+} and ultimately causing muscle action. Intracellular Ca^{2+} plays an intimate role in regulating a muscle fiber's contractile and metabolic activity. Ca^{2+} concentration within a nonactive muscle fiber remains relatively low compared with the extracellular fluid that bathes the cell. Muscle fiber stimulation causes an immediate, small increase in intracellular Ca^{2+}, which precedes contractile activity. Cellular Ca^{2+} increases when the action potential at the transverse tubules causes Ca^{2+} release from the lateral sacs of the sarcoplasmic reticulum. The inhibitory action of troponin (prevents actin–myosin interaction) rapidly dissipates when Ca^{2+} binds with this and other proteins in the actin filaments. In a sense, the muscle "turns on" for action.

$$\text{Actin} + \text{Myosin ATPase} \rightarrow \text{Actomyosin} + \text{ATPase}$$

Joining the active sites on actin and myosin activates myosin ATPase to split ATP. The energy generated causes myosin crossbridge movement to produce muscle tension.

$$\text{Actomyosin ATP} \rightarrow \text{Actomyosin} + \text{ADP} + \text{Pi} + \text{Energy}$$

The crossbridge uncouples from actin when ATP binds to the myosin crossbridge. Coupling and uncoupling continue when Ca^{2+} concentration remains high enough to inhibit the troponin–tropomyosin system. When neural stimulation ceases, Ca^{2+} moves back into the lateral sacs of the sarcoplasmic reticulum. This restores the inhibitory action of troponin–tropomyosin, and actin and myosin stay apart provided ATP concentration remains adequate. In rigor mortis, the muscles stiffen and become rigid soon after death because the cell no longer contains ATP. Without ATP, the myosin crossbridges and actin remain attached and do not separate. FIGURE 18.13 illustrates the interaction between actin and myosin filaments, Ca^{2+}, and ATP in both a relaxed and shortened muscle fiber.

Stimulation produces a threefold rise in Ca^{2+} concentration and accompanying increase in the action potential in type II (fast-twitch) muscle fibers compared with type I (slow-twitch) muscle fibers in isolated muscle preparations. Such differences reflect faster Ca^{2+} transport through the sarcoplasmic reticulum and ultimately to the contractile proteins in type II fibers. During excitation–contraction coupling, electrochemical events occur within the cell membrane at the site of excitation. The

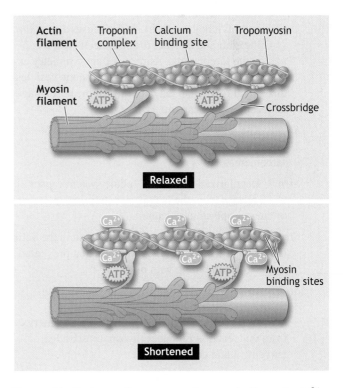

Figure 18.13 Interaction among actin–myosin filaments, Ca^{2+}, and ATP in relaxed and shortened muscle. In the relaxed state, troponin and tropomyosin interact with actin, preventing the myosin crossbridge from coupling to actin. During muscle action, the crossbridge couples with actin because of Ca^{2+} binding with troponin–tropomyosin.

common pathway for precisely targeting the chemical signal to the contractile proteins depends mostly on ion channel regulators. These structures serve as selective "gates" or "sensors" to modulate ion passage between the intracellular and extracellular fluids before myofilament activation.

Relaxation

When muscle stimulation ceases, Ca^{2+} flow stops and troponin frees up to inhibit actin–myosin interaction. Recovery involves active pumping of Ca^{2+} into the sarcoplasmic reticulum where it concentrates in the lateral vesicles. Retrieval of Ca^{2+} from the troponin–tropomyosin protein complex "turns off" the active sites on the actin filament. Deactivation serves two purposes: (1) prevents any mechanical link between the myosin crossbridges and actin filaments and (2) inhibits myosin ATPase activity, which curtails ATP splitting. Muscle relaxation occurs when the actin and myosin filaments return to their original states.

Sequence of Events in Muscle Action

FIGURE 18.14 summarizes the main events in muscle activation, contraction, and relaxation. The sequence begins with the initiation of an action potential by the motor nerve. The impulse then propagates over the entire fiber surface (sarcolemma) as it depolarizes. The following nine steps correspond to the numbered sequence in Figure 18.14:

Step 1: Small, saclike vesicles within the terminal axon release acetylcholine (ACh). ACh diffuses across the synaptic cleft and attaches to specialized ACh receptors on the sarcolemma. Almost perfect symmetry exists between the "imprint" of the presynaptic vesicles that contain ACh and the "imprint" of the postsynaptic receptors that capture ACh.

Step 2: The muscle action potential depolarizes the transverse tubules at the A–I junction of the sarcomere.

Step 3: Depolarization of the T-tubule system causes Ca^{2+} release from the lateral sacs (terminal cisternae) of the sarcoplasmic reticulum.

Step 4: Ca^{2+} binds to troponin–tropomyosin in the actin filaments. This releases the inhibition that prevented actin from combining with myosin.

Step 5: During muscle action, actin combines with myosin–ATP. Actin also activates the enzyme myosin ATPase, which then splits ATP. The energy from this reaction produces myosin crossbridge movement and creates tension.

Step 6: ATP binds to the myosin crossbridge; this breaks the actin–myosin bond and allows the crossbridge to dissociate from actin. The thick and thin filaments then slide past each other and the muscle shortens.

Step 7: Crossbridge activation continues when Ca^{2+} concentration remains high enough (from membrane depolarization) to inhibit the troponin–tropomyosin system.

Step 8: When muscle stimulation ceases, intracellular Ca^{2+} concentration rapidly decreases as Ca^{2+} moves back into the lateral sacs of the sarcoplasmic reticulum through active transport that requires ATP hydrolysis.

Step 9: Ca^{2+} removal restores the inhibitory action of troponin–tropomyosin. In the presence of ATP, actin and myosin remain in the dissociated, relaxed state.

MUSCLE FIBER TYPE

Skeletal muscle does not simply contain a homogeneous group of fibers with similar metabolic and contractile properties. Researchers have identified and classified *two* distinct fiber types by their *contractile* and *metabolic* characteristics. A common technique for establishing the specific muscle fiber type assesses the myosin molecule's heavy chain that exists in three different forms or isoforms. Assessment evaluates a fiber's differential sensitivity to altered pH of the enzyme myosin ATPase (a measure of myosin phenotype).[28,30,36,37] The different characteristics of this enzyme determine the rapidity of ATP hydrolysis in the myosin heavy chain region and thus the velocity of sarcomere shortening. More specifically, acid pH inactivates the activity of the specific myosin ATPase in fast-twitch fibers, but this enzyme remains fairly stable at an alkaline pH; these fibers stain *dark* for this enzyme. In contrast, specific myosin ATPase activity for slow-twitch fibers remains high at an acid pH but becomes inactive in an alkaline milieu; these fibers stain *light* for myosin ATPase. FIGURE 18.15 illustrates serial cross sections of the human vastus lateralis muscle with identification of type I and type II muscle fibers and subdivisions. TABLE 18.2 lists different classification schemes for skeletal muscle fiber types on the basis of morphology, histochemistry and biochemistry, function, and contractility.

Fast-Twitch Fibers

Fast-twitch muscle fibers exhibit the following four characteristics:

1. High capability for electrochemical transmission of action potentials
2. High myosin ATPase activity
3. Rapid Ca21 release and uptake by an efficient sarcoplasmic reticulum
4. High rate of crossbridge turnover

These four factors contribute to this fiber's rapid energy generation for quick, powerful actions. The fast-twitch fiber's intrinsic speed of shortening and tension development ranges three to five times faster than slow-twitch fibers (see following section). Fast-twitch fibers rely on a well-developed, short-term glycolytic system for energy transfer. *Fast-twitch fiber activation predominates in anaerobic-type sprint activities*

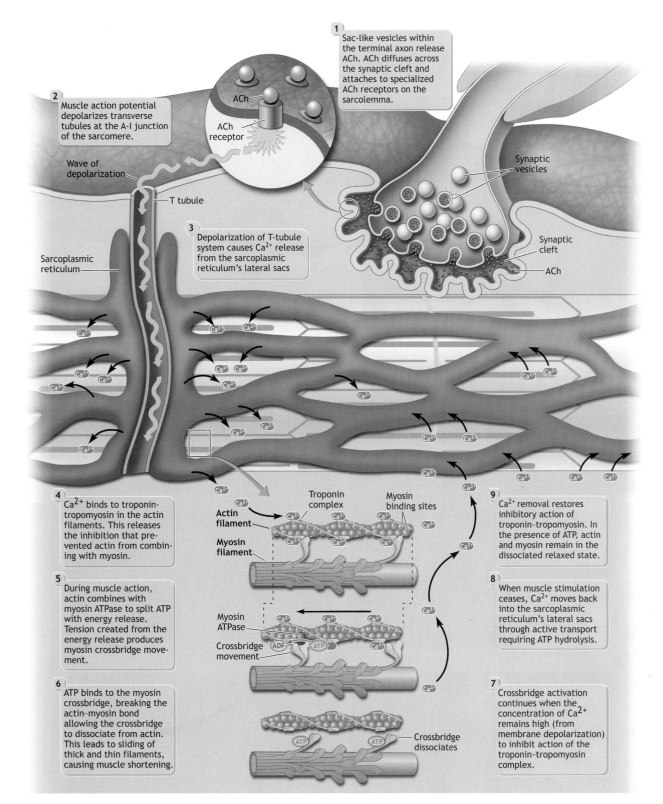

1 Sac-like vesicles within the terminal axon release ACh. ACh diffuses across the synaptic cleft and attaches to specialized ACh receptors on the sarcolemma.

2 Muscle action potential depolarizes transverse tubules at the A-I junction of the sarcomere.

ACh

ACh receptor

Synaptic vesicles

Wave of depolarization

T tubule

Synaptic cleft

ACh

3 Depolarization of T-tubule system causes Ca^{2+} release from the sarcoplasmic reticulum's lateral sacs

Sarcoplasmic reticulum

Ca^{2+}

Troponin complex

Myosin binding sites

9 Ca^{2+} removal restores inhibitory action of troponin-tropomyosin. In the presence of ATP, actin and myosin remain in the dissociated relaxed state.

4 Ca^{2+} binds to troponin-tropomyosin in the actin filaments. This releases the inhibition that prevented actin from combining with myosin.

Actin filament

Myosin filament

5 During muscle action, actin combines with myosin ATPase to split ATP with energy release. Tension created from the energy release produces myosin crossbridge movement.

Myosin ATPase

Crossbridge movement

ADP

ATP

8 When muscle stimulation ceases, Ca^{2+} moves back into the sarcoplasmic reticulum's lateral sacs through active transport requiring ATP hydrolysis.

6 ATP binds to the myosin crossbridge, breaking the actin-myosin bond allowing the crossbridge to dissociate from actin. This leads to sliding of thick and thin filaments, causing muscle shortening.

ATP

ATP

Crossbridge dissociates

7 Crossbridge activation continues when the concentration of Ca^{2+} remains high (from membrane depolarization) to inhibit action of the troponin-tropomyosin complex.

Figure 18.14 Schematic view of the nine main events in muscle contraction and relaxation. *Numbers* correspond to the sequence of nine steps outlined on p. 380. The neurotransmitter acetylcholine (ACh), released from saclike vesicles within the terminal axon, initiates transmission at the myoneural junction. Here, the electrochemical signal "jumps" across the 0.05-μm cleft between neuron and muscle fiber. The electrical impulse, traveling at a velocity of $1 \text{ m} \cdot \text{s}^{-1}$ or faster spreads through the fiber's tubule system to the inner contractile "machinery" of the myofibrils.

and other forceful muscle actions that rely almost entirely on anaerobic energy metabolism.[18,26] Activation of fast-twitch fibers plays an important role in the stop-and-go or change-of-pace sports such as basketball, soccer, lacrosse, or field hockey. These types of activities demand rapid energy that only anaerobic pathways generate. "In a Practical Sense" on p. 384 describes a popular jumping test to infer the immediate power output from ATP and PCr. Theoretically, individuals with a predominance of fast-twitch muscle fibers should achieve relatively high scores on such a test.

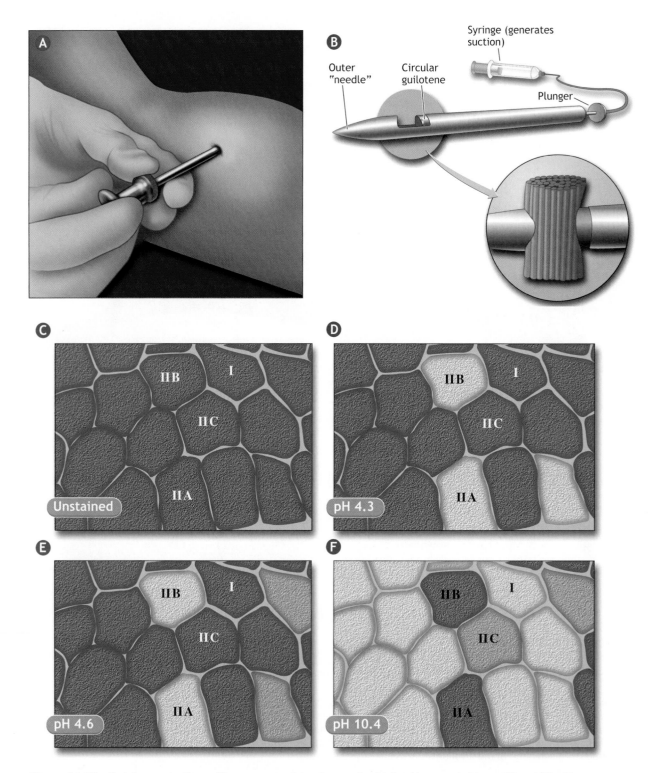

Figure 18.15   Serial cross sections of human vastus lateralis muscle obtained by muscle biopsy (**A** and **B**) with identification of type I and type IIA, B, and C fiber subdivisions. **C.** Thick unstained section (40–50 μm) where all fibers appear similar. Three other panels indicate same fibers stained for myosin–ATPase activity at a preincubation pH of (**D**) 4.3 (highly acidic), (**E**) 4.6 (intermediate acidity), and (**F**) 10.6 (alkaline).

TABLE 18.2 ■ CLASSIFICATION SCHEMES OF SKELETAL MUSCLE FIBER TYPES

	FIBER TYPES		
CHARACTERISTIC	**FAST-TWITCH TYPE IIB**	**TYPE IIA**	**SLOW-TWITCH TYPE I**
Electrical activity patterns	Phasic; high frequency		Tonic; low frequency
Morphology	**FTb**	**FTa**	**ST**
Color	White	White/red	Red
Fiber diameter	Large	Intermediate	Small
Capillaries/mm²	Low	Intermediate	High
Mitochondrial volume	Low	Intermediate	High
Histochemistry and biochemistry	**FG**	**FOG**	**SO**
Myosin ATPase	High	High	Low
Calcium capacity	High	Medium/high	Low
Glycolytic capacity	High	High	Low
Oxidative capacity	Low	Medium/high	High
Function and contractility	**FF**	**FR**	**S**
	FT	**FT**	**ST**
Speed of action	Fast	Fast	Slow
Speed of relaxation	Fast	Fast	Slow
Fatigue resistance	Low	Moderate/high	High
Force capacity	High	Intermediate	Low

From Kraus W. Skeletal muscle adaptation to chronic low-frequency motor nerve stimulation. Exerc Sport Sci Rev 1994;22:313.

FT, fast twitch; FG, fast, glycolytic; FOG, fast, oxidative, glycolytic; SO, slow, oxidative; FF, fast contracting, fast fatigue; FR, fast contracting, fatigue resistant; S, slow contracting.

Slow-Twitch Fibers

Slow-twitch fibers generate energy for ATP resynthesis predominantly through the aerobic system of energy transfer. Their four distinguishing characteristics include:

1. Low myosin ATPase activity
2. Slow calcium handling ability and shortening speed
3. Less well-developed glycolytic capacity than fast-twitch fibers
4. Large and numerous mitochondria

Slow-twitch fibers receive their characteristic red pigmentation from their rich mitochondria supply and accompanying iron-containing cytochromes combined with high myoglobin levels. A high concentration of mitochondrial enzymes links closely to a slow-twitch fiber's enhanced aerobic metabolic machinery. *These characteristics make slow-twitch fibers highly fatigue resistant and ideally suited for prolonged aerobic exercise.* The fibers have been labeled **SO (slow-oxidative) fibers** to describe their slow shortening speed and reliance on oxidative metabolism. Unlike fast-twitch fibers that fatigue readily, SO fibers (more precisely, motor units) are selectively recruited in aerobic activities.[25]

Muscle glycogen depletion patterns indicate that prolonged, high-intensity aerobic exercise demands almost exclusive reliance on slow-twitch muscle fibers. Even after exercising for 12 hours, the limited glycogen remaining in active muscle exists mostly in the relatively "unused" fast-twitch fibers. Differences in oxidative capacity of the two fiber types

also determine the magnitude of blood flow through muscle, with slow-twitch fibers receiving the largest quantity.[31,45]

Most researchers classify slow-twitch fibers as **type I**, and fast-twitch fibers (and proposed subdivisions) as **type II.** *Both fiber types contribute during near-maximum aerobic and anaerobic exercise as in middle-distance running or swimming or basketball, field hockey, or soccer, which combine high levels of aerobic and anaerobic energy transfer.*

INTEGRATIVE QUESTION

Present the pros and cons for muscle fiber typing of children to "guide" them into sports to increase their likelihood of future success.

Fast-Twitch Subdivisions

Several subdivisions characterize fast-twitch muscle fibers. The intermediate **type IIa fiber** exhibits fast shortening speed and a moderately well-developed capacity for energy transfer from both aerobic (high level of aerobic enzyme succinic dehydrogenase, or SDH) and anaerobic (high level of anaerobic enzyme phosphofructokinase, or PFK) sources. These fibers represent the **fast–oxidative–glycolytic (FOG) fibers**. Another subdivision, the **type IIb fiber** (also termed *type IIx*) possesses the greatest anaerobic potential and most rapid shortening velocity; it represents the "true" **fast–glycolytic (FG) fiber**. The **type IIc fiber**, normally rare and undifferentiated, may contribute to reinnervation and motor unit transformation.

IN A PRACTICAL SENSE

PREDICTING PEAK ANAEROBIC POWER OUTPUT USING A VERTICAL JUMP TEST

■ Peak anaerobic power output underlies success in many sports activities. The vertical jump test is often used to predict "explosive" peak anaerobic power output from the intramuscular high-energy phosphates.

VERTICAL JUMP TEST

The vertical jump test measures the highest distance jumped from a semicrouched position in the following protocol:

1. Establish standing reach height. The subject, standing with the preferred shoulder adjacent to a wall and feet flat on the floor, reaches as high as possible to touch the wall. The starting point (standing reach height) represents the distance from the wall mark (middle finger) to the floor, recorded in centimeters (cm) (Fig. *A*).
2. Bend the knees to about a 90° angle while moving the arms back in a winged position (Fig. *B*).
3. Thrust forward and upward, touching as high as possible on the wall (Fig. *C*).
4. Perform three trials of the jump test; use the highest score as the vertical height.
5. Compute vertical jump height (cm) as the difference between standing reach height and vertical height achieved in the jump.

PREDICTING IMMEDIATE ANAEROBIC POWER OUTPUT

The following equation for males and females predicts peak anaerobic power output in watts (PAP_w) from vertical jump height in cm (VJ_{cm}) and body mass in kilograms (BM_{kg}):

$$PAP_w = 60.7\ (VJ_{cm}) + 45.3\ (BM_{kg}) - 2055$$

EXAMPLE

A 21-year-old male who weighs 78 kg records a vertical jump of 43 cm (standing reach height, 185 cm; vertical height, 228 cm); predict peak anaerobic power output in watts.

COMPUTATIONS

$$
\begin{aligned}
PAP_w &= 60.7\ (VJ_{cm}) + 45.3\ (BM_{kg}) - 2055 \\
&= 60.7\ (43\ \text{cm}) + 45.3\ (78\ \text{kg}) - 2055 \\
&= 4088.5\ \text{W}
\end{aligned}
$$

COMPARISONS

The average peak power output measured with this vertical jump protocol averages 4620.2 (SD ± 822.5) W for males and 2993.7 (SD ± 542.9) W for females.

REFERENCE

Sayers S, et al. Cross-validation of three jump power equations. Med Sci Sports Exerc 1999;31:572.

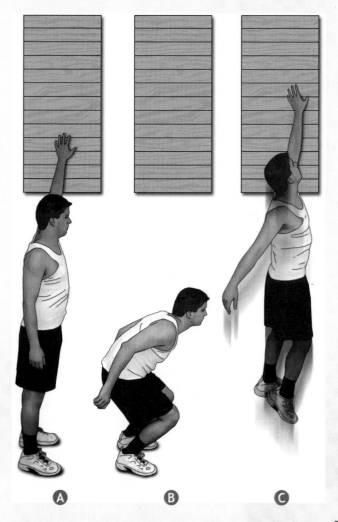

Ⓐ   Ⓑ   Ⓒ

(A) Starting point (standing reach height), *(B)* just prior to jumping, and *(C)* final point in determining vertical jump height.

SPECIES DIFFERENCES: A COMPARATIVE LOOK AT MUSCLE METABOLISM AND DYNAMICS

The study of comparative physiology provides an appreciation for the diversity of function and adaptation among species and insight into a better understanding of human physiology and muscle metabolism. Throughout the animal kingdom—from the elephant that weighs 100,000 times more than a mouse to the smallest shrew, about one-millionth the elephant's size—extraordinary examples of muscular strength, power, and endurance make the athletic feats of humans pale by comparison. For example, the world's fastest human runs 200 m at an average velocity of $10.4 \, m \cdot s^{-1}$ (23.2 mph; 1996 World Record), yet the greyhound dog covers the same distance at 60% greater velocity ($16.6 \, m \cdot s^{-1}$). For elite human endurance athletes, aerobic metabolism during sustained exercise exceeds the resting requirement by about 25 times. However, the muscle machines of other animal species have adapted over millions of years to perform extraordinary metabolic and performance feats. FIGURE 18.16 shows the maximal rates of oxygen consumption during treadmill running for 22 species of wild and domestic African mammals. On average,

a 10-fold difference occurs in the ratio of resting to maximal oxygen consumption. The ratio, termed the **factorial aerobic scope** or **metabolic scope**,[42] displays considerable intraspecies variation. For example, in four species of canids with different body masses (gray fox, 4.7 kg; coyote, 12.4 kg; timber wolf, 23.3 kg; dog, 25.3 kg) the metabolic scope ranged from 24 for the gray fox to 32 for the dog, a value about the same as for a champion human endurance athlete.

Contractile Dynamics

From the perspective of muscle fiber dynamics, consider the hummingbird, a super avian athlete that sustains a wing beat frequency of 80 Hz, with an ATP turnover rate of 500 mmol per gram of muscle per minute (500 times the value at rest). This represents the highest metabolic rate in the vertebrate world, accomplished from the resting state to full wing activity in less than 15 ms! Intuitively, one might expect the hummingbird to have an advanced chemical system to fuel a multifaceted network of different muscle fiber types. Some might argue that unique metabolic pathways would sustain high-intensity fiber activity without the negative, fatiguing consequences of anaerobic metabolism characteristic of the

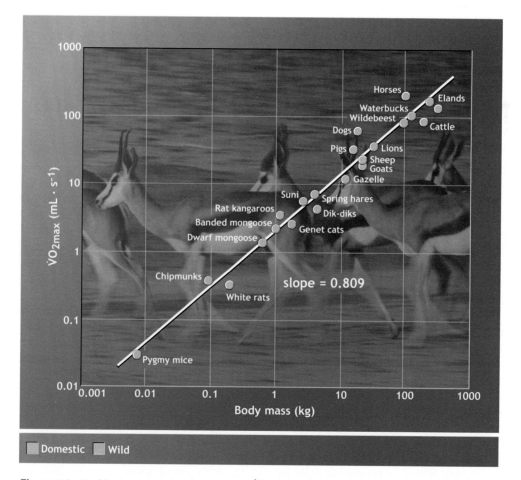

Figure 18.16 Maximal oxygen consumption ($\dot{V}O_{2max}$) during running for 22 species of African mammals, ranging in body mass from 0.007 kg (pygmy mouse) to 263 kg (horse). (From Taylor CR, et al. Design of the mammalian respiratory system. III. Scaling maximum aerobic capacity to body mass: wild and domestic mammals. Respir Physiol 1981;44:25.)

human response to all-out effort. In actuality, the hummingbird's flight muscles show a simple architecture of only FOG fibers. The homogeneity of the internal metabolic machinery of these fast-acting fibers shows tremendous upregulation of aerobic functions. Fibers have five to seven times the mitochondrial density of human muscle fibers. Capillaries literally wrap around each fiber. Fibers also contain a large sarcoplasmic reticulum volume, a larger than normal mitochondrial cristae surface area, reduced diameter of individual fibers (to facilitate diffusion), and high concentrations of key aerobic enzymes. Fat droplets lie against the mitochondria for immediate uptake as aerobic fuel along with glucose. To accentuate these remarkable aerobic adaptations, the fibers possess essentially no capacity for anaerobic metabolism. For most mammals, total muscle mass represents about 40 to 45% of body mass, regardless of body size. In flying birds, pectoral muscles average 15% of body mass, except in the hummingbird, where the value increases to nearly 30%. This makes sense from a standpoint of muscle because the power output requirement for hovering flight exceeds that for forward flight.[50]

Other species in the animal and insect world also show remarkable adaptation in muscle functions to support tasks required for survival.[9] The fast-twitch muscle fibers of "sprint-type" fish (e.g., pike and white tuna) demonstrate homogeneity in cellular architecture and function. Such tremendous upregulation emphasizes glycolytic and high-energy phosphate–driven power performance with a corresponding blunting of aerobic function. At a different extreme, the muscle machinery of the electric eel creates a 2000-fold increase in ATP production to generate a paralyzing electric charge within 300 ms.[4]

Force and Power

For generating muscle power, the limiting factor in humans and animals depends on the energy-producing capacity of the muscle's protein filaments. Maximal force of any muscle (roughly 3 to 4 kg · cm^{-2} cross section of muscle [300–400 kN · m^{-2}]) relates to its cross-sectional area, independent of total body size; this is about the same for a mouse, elephant, and human. The reason for the narrow intraspecies range relates to the similarity in dimensions of the actin and myosin filaments and quantitative similarity in crossbridge number. A microscopist would have difficulty distinguishing between the muscular ultrastructure of an elephant and a mouse, except for the larger number of mitochondria in the muscles of smaller animals and the relative length of individual fibers.[42] This gives smaller animals a tremendous advantage in endurance activities, whether they move horizontally or vertically.

Compared with a human, the small animal would easily win any speed and power contest by a large margin. Anyone who has run on a treadmill at 20% grade knows the difficulty in sustaining power output for a minute or two, even at a relatively slow speed of 6 mph. If it were possible to triple the treadmill elevation to 60%, how long could a human maintain the 6 mph velocity? Although the answer remains unknown, the task would clearly tax the cardiovascular, metabolic, and

muscular systems beyond limits. The small mammal, however, performs this task with relative ease. Mice trained to run on a treadmill at a 15° incline exhibited no difference in oxygen consumption between uphill and level running.[44] For chimpanzees and horses, the energy expenditure more than doubles as it does for humans when running up the same incline. Thus, the smaller animal "athlete" such as a squirrel runs up and down tall trees rapidly with relative ease for extended durations. The best-conditioned human endurance or strength athletes would offer no match in uphill climbing competition against a small, furry mammal.

The same would hold true for jumping events. The world's high-jump champion (Javier Sotomayor, Cuba; height, 2.45 m) exceeded his own length (stature) in jumping height by a relatively small amount. In contrast, the galago—a 1.3-m bush baby prosimian primate found in many regions south of the Sahara desert and characterized by a hopping gait similar to a kangaroo—can leap vertically (2.25 m) more than 70% of its stature![20] The galago's jumping ability relates to its large muscles for jumping (10% of body mass), nearly double that of humans. On a relative basis, the maximal vertical jumping ability of a human, properly scaled to body size (see Chapter 22, "Allometric Scaling"), falls far short of a flea (*Pulex;* body mass of 50 mg). The 2 mm-long flea leaps more than 100 times its body length or twice as far as its human "competition" when appropriately adjusted for the large body size differences. The flea, a remarkable "athlete" in its own right, has a muscular system perfectly adapted to its needs, as do most locomotor and flying members of the animal kingdom.

FIBER TYPE DIFFERENCES AMONG ATHLETIC GROUPS

Several observations concern muscle fiber type and the possible influence of specific training on fiber composition and metabolic capacity. Men, women, and children on average possess 45 to 55% slow-twitch fibers in their arm and leg muscles. The fast-twitch fibers probably distribute equally between type IIa and type IIb subdivisions. While no gender differences exist in fiber distribution, large interindividual variation occurs. Generally, the trend in one's muscle fiber type distribution remains consistent among the body's major muscle groups.

Certain patterns of muscle fiber distribution appear readily in comparisons among highly proficient athletes.[46] For example, successful endurance athletes have predominantly slow-twitch fibers in the major muscles activated in their specific sport. In contrast, fast-twitch fibers predominate for elite sprint athletes. FIGURE 18.17 illustrates fiber-type distribution for top Nordic competitors in different sports. Athletic groups with the highest aerobic and endurance capacities (e.g., distance runners and cross-country skiers) possess the highest percentage of slow-twitch fibers, often as high as 90 to 95% in the leg's gastrocnemius muscle. Weight lifters, ice hockey players, and sprinters have more fast-twitch fibers and relatively lower aerobic capacities. As might be expected, men and women who perform in middle-distance events display

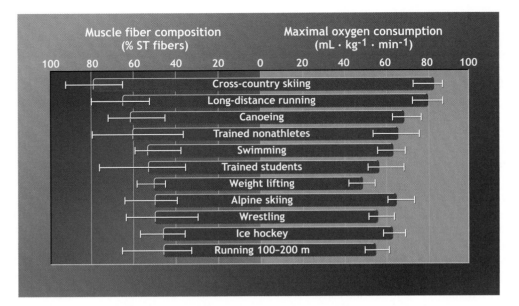

Figure 18.17 Muscle fiber composition (% slow-twitch fibers, *left side*) and maximal oxygen consumption *(right side)* in athletes representing different sports. The *outer white bars* denote the range. (From Bergh U, et al. Maximal oxygen uptake and muscle fiber types in trained and untrained humans. Med Sci Sports 1978;10:151.)

approximately equal percentages of the two fiber types. The same distribution also occurs in power athletes—throwers, jumpers, and high jumpers.[11]

The relatively clear-cut distinctions between exercise performance and muscle fiber composition pertain mainly to elite athletes with prominence in a sport category. Even among this group, muscle fiber composition does not solely determine performance success. This seems reasonable because successful performance reflects blending of many physiologic, biochemical, neurologic, and biomechanical "support systems," not simply the single factor of muscle fiber type.

Endurance athletes have relatively normal-sized muscle fibers, with a tendency toward enlargement of the slow twitch fibers. Conversely, weight lifters and other power athletes show definite enlargement in both fiber types, particularly fast-twitch fibers, which may exceed by 45% those of endurance athletes or sedentary persons of the same age.[47,48] Strength and power training induce enlargement of the fiber's contractile apparatus—specifically the actin and myosin filaments—and total glycogen content. *Larger muscle fibers in male athletes and a larger total muscle mass are the principal gender differences in muscle morphology.* Chapter 22 discusses the potential for exercise training to alter the metabolic and fiber-type characteristics and size of skeletal muscle.

Summary

1. Various connective tissue wrappings that encase skeletal muscle blend into and join the tendinous attachment to bone. This harness enables muscles to act on bony levers to transform chemical energy of ATP into mechanical energy of motion.

2. A skeletal muscle fiber by weight consists of 75% water, 20% protein, and the remainder inorganic salts, enzymes, pigments, fats, and carbohydrates.

3. The muscle's oxygen consumption during vigorous exercise increases up to 70 times the resting level. Immediate adjustments and longer term training adaptations that increase the size of the local vascular bed support this elevated metabolic requirement.

4. The sarcomere provides the functional unit of the muscle fiber. It contains the contractile proteins actin and myosin. An average muscle fiber contains 4500 sarcomeres and 16 billion thick (myosin) and 64 billion thin (actin) filaments.

5. Myosin projections or crossbridges serve as structural links between thick and thin contractile filaments. During muscle action, tropomyosin and troponin regulate the make-and-break contacts between the filaments.

6. Tropomyosin inhibits actin and myosin interaction; troponin plus Ca^{2+} trigger the myofibrils to interact and slide past each other.

7. The triad and T-tubule system function as a microtransportation network to spread the action potential from the fiber's outer membrane inward to deeper cell regions.

8. Muscle action takes place when Ca^{2+} activates actin, causing the myosin crossbridges to attach to active sites on the actin filaments. Relaxation occurs when Ca^{2+} concentration decreases.

9. The sliding filament model proposes that a muscle shortens or lengthens because protein filaments slide past each other without altering their length. The

FOCUS On Research

A TISSUE RESPONSIVE TO REGULAR EXERCISE

Tipton CM, et al. Influence of exercise on strength of medial collateral knee ligaments of dogs. Am J Physiol 1970;218:894.

▲ Prior to 1970, evidence showing that exercise improved connective tissue strength came from studies using laboratory mice and rats. The pioneering study by Tipton and colleagues provides direct experimental evidence of exercise training benefits on the strength of either intact or surgically repaired medial collateral ligaments of dogs. These data provide an important framework to justify the current commonly accepted therapeutic use of exercise—not immobilization—to rehabilitate soft tissue injury and surgical repair.

Tipton studied more than 100 male mongrel dogs (age >1 year) to answer several questions, including the effects of 6 weeks of increased or decreased physical activity (exercise training, immobilization, normal cage activity, and sham surgical procedures) on intact knee ligament strength. A second goal was to describe the effects of variations in exercise training, immobilization, and normal cage activity on the strength of surgically repaired ligaments, a question of primary interest in sports medicine.

In all evaluations of ligament strength, the plantaris, gastrocnemius, and extensor digitorum longus muscles were removed (along with the joint's surrounding soft tissue), leaving the capsule and ligaments intact. A testing apparatus held the bone–capsule–bone preparation as the tibia was pulled from the femur at a constant speed of $0.25 \text{ mm} \cdot \text{s}^{-1}$. The force (kg) necessary to separate the ligament from the bone—stress–strain measurement—represented the separation force (SF). The SF-to-body mass ratio (SFR) adjusted for the animals' differences in body mass. Exercise training included treadmill running at different speeds, grades, and durations for a maximum of 6 days weekly for 6 weeks; 3 days of endurance and 3 days of "wind sprint" training. By week 3, the animals were exercising 1 hour daily.

Immobilization involved fixing one of the hind legs with the knee flexed at 60 to 80° with pins placed through the femur and one through the tibia. A fast-drying plaster cast then secured the leg. Surgical repair of the left medial collateral ligament exposed the ligament by making an incision through its superficial and deep portions along the joint line while preserving the blood supply. Two steel-wire sutures reattached the ligament at

its original location. Sham operations (no ligament cut) included pin insertion, skin incision, ligament exposure, and wound closure.

FIGURE 1 shows that strength of the intact knee ligament relates to the animal's level of physical activity, with immobilization (group 2) producing the least strength (lowest SF) and 6 weeks of treadmill running (group 4) yielding the greatest strength. Strength of the surgically repaired ligaments (FIG. 2) depended on the time interval before sacrifice and the amount of activity performed by the experimental leg. Location of separation also varied between intact and repaired ligaments; intact ligaments separated from their tibial attachment, while surgically repaired ligaments invariably separated at the repair site.

The data indicated that physical activity markedly improves ligament strength. These important findings showed that connective tissue responds to the mechanical stress of exercise.

Tipton's innovative work provided the first experimental verification that ligaments from immobilized legs

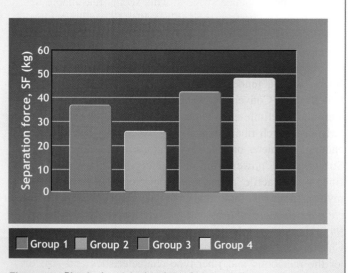

Figure 1 Physical activity levels and strength (separation force) of intact knee ligaments. Group 1, sham procedure on left leg; group 2, decreased physical activity by leg immobilization; group 3, normal cage activity; group 4, increased physical activity with exercise training. Group 2 data are significantly lower than other group means.

continued on page 389

Continued

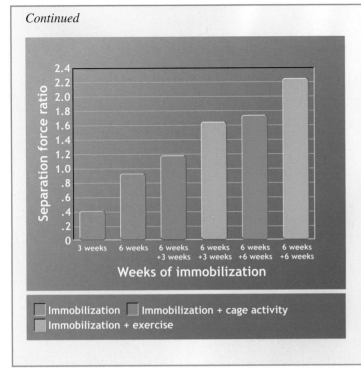

Separation force ratio vs Weeks of immobilization

■ Immobilization ■ Immobilization + cage activity
■ Immobilization + exercise

were weaker and weighed less than ligaments from normal control and exercised legs. The study also cast doubt on the efficacy of immobilization following ligament surgery. Instead, they support exercise training as a first line of rehabilitation following soft tissue surgery.

Figure 2 Strength of surgically repaired ligaments in relation to duration of immobilization and level of physical activity.

mechanism of excitation–contraction coupling links electrochemical and mechanical events to achieve muscle action.

10. Contractile and metabolic characteristics classify the two types of muscle fibers: (1) fast-twitch (FT) fibers that generate energy predominantly anaerobically for quick, powerful actions and (2) slow-twitch (ST) that shorten relatively slowly and generate energy predominantly by aerobic metabolism.

An intermediate, fast–oxidative–glycolytic (FOG) fiber also exists.

11. Significant interindividual differences exist in the percentage of fiber type distribution. Most likely, genetic factors explain the variation, yet specific exercise training may produce some modification.

References are available on the Student CD and online at http://connection.lww.com/mkk6e.

Neural Control of Human Movement

19

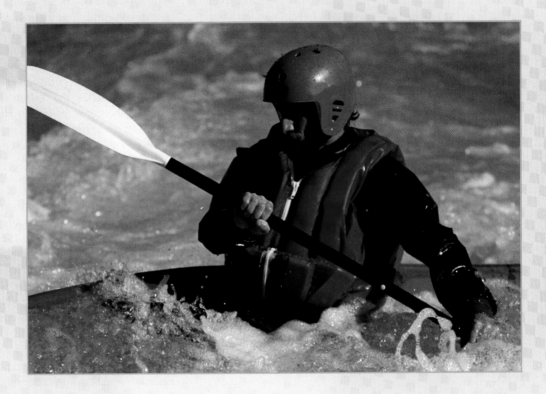

CHAPTER OBJECTIVES

- Draw the major structural components of the brain including the four lobes of the cerebral cortex

- Discuss specific pyramidal and extrapyramidal tract functions

- Diagram the anterior motor neuron and discuss its role in human movement

- Draw and label the basic components of a reflex arc

- Define the terms (1) *motor unit,* (2) *neuromuscular junction,* and (3) *autonomic nervous system*

- Summarize the events in motor unit excitation prior to muscle action

- Outline motor unit facilitation and inhibition and the contribution of each to exercise performance and responsiveness to resistance training

- Discuss variations in twitch characteristics, resistance to fatigue, and tension development in the different motor units

- Describe mechanisms that adjust force of muscle action along the continuum from slight to maximum

- Define fatigue and discuss factors that act and interact to induce neuromuscular fatigue

- List and describe functions of the specific proprioceptors within joints, muscles, and tendons

The effective application of force during complex learned movements (e.g., tennis serve, shot put, golf swing) depends on a series of coordinated neuromuscular patterns, not just on the strength of muscle groups recruited for the activity. Neural control mechanisms linked together by diverse pathways regulate such movements. The neural circuitry in the brain, spinal cord, and the periphery functions as a modern computer network, although today's most complex high-speed computer is no match for the exquisite integrative and organizational structure of the human nervous system. In response to changing internal and external stimuli, hundreds of millions of bits of sensory input automatically synchronize for near-instantaneous processing by central neural control mechanisms. The input becomes properly organized, routed, and transmitted with extreme efficiency to the effector organs, the skeletal muscles.[27]

The following sections present a general outline of the neural control of human movement:

- Structural organization for motor control
- Neuromuscular transmission
- Motor unit function and activation
- Sensory input from muscle activity

NEUROMOTOR SYSTEM ORGANIZATION

The human nervous system consists of two major parts: (1) **central nervous system** (**CNS**) consisting of the brain and spinal cord and (2) **peripheral nervous system** (**PNS**) that contains nerves that transmit information to and from the CNS. FIGURE 19.1 presents an overview of these two subdivisions.

Central Nervous System—The Brain

The human brain exhibits great complexity with selective growth of different anatomic areas. From a comparative perspective, mammalian brains share similarities in structure and function but differ in size and intricacy (FIG. 19.2). Notably, the size of the human brain exceeds that of most (but not all) mammals. A larger brain (Fig. 19.2A and B) permits more complexity, but factors other than size explain variations in functional differentiation. Figure 19.2C shows the lateral view of the cerebral cortex in the human, cat, and rat, with primary sensory and motor areas identified. Note the expansion of the human cortex that serves neither strict primary sensory nor motor functions. Evolution of the cortex, particularly the frontal and temporal lobes coincides with unique human functions like spoken and written language, reasoning, and abstract thinking. Such differentiation frames the hypothesis that larger, more complex brains allow greater neural circuitry within the cortex and hence increased intellectual functioning.

For decades, conventional wisdom maintained that the number of brain cells was fixed at birth, unlike the cells of other organ systems that continually renew themselves throughout life. Neurobiologists now believe that brain cells (and perhaps spinal neurons; German anatomist Heinrich Wilhelm Gottfried

Waldeyer-Hartz [1836–1921] coined the term "neurone" in 1891) and neural circuits are created throughout life with elimination of unneeded or redundant synapses in developing neural tissues. From birth through late adolescence, the brain probably adds billions of new cells, literally constructing new circuits from these newly formed cells.[14] After adolescence, the plasticity of neuronal addition and formation of new circuits slows but does not stop, even into old age. Regular physical activity appears to contribute to the development and maintenance of optimal neural circuitry in middle and older age.

FIGURE 19.3 categorizes the brain into six main areas: **medulla oblongata**, **pons**, **midbrain**, **cerebellum**, **diencephalon**, and **telencephalon**. Figure 19.3C depicts four lobes of the cerebral cortex and associated sensory areas. As a frame of reference, the body has roughly 10 million sensory (afferent) neurons, 50 billion central neurons, and 500,000 motor (efferent) neurons. This represents a ratio of about 20 to 1 between the sensory and motor circuits.

Brainstem

The medulla, pons, and midbrain compose the **brainstem**. The medulla, located immediately above the spinal cord, extends into the pons and serves as a bridge between the two hemispheres of the cerebellum. The midbrain, only 1.5 cm long, attaches to the cerebellum and forms a connection between the pons and cerebral hemispheres. The midbrain contains parts of the extrapyramidal motor system, specifically the red nucleus and substantia. The **reticular formation** integrates various incoming and outgoing signals that flow through it. These signals originate from the stretching of sensors in joints and muscles, from pain receptors in the skin, and as visual signals from the eye and auditory impulses from the ear. Once activated, the reticular system produces either inhibitory or facilitory effects on other neurons. Twelve pairs of cranial nerves innervate predominantly the head region. Each cranial nerve has a name and associated number (originally derived by Galen about 1800 years ago).

Cerebellum

The cerebellum consists of two peach-size mounds of folded tissue with lateral hemispheres and a central vermis. It functions by means of intricate feedback circuits to monitor and coordinate other areas of the brain and spinal cord involved in motor control. The cerebellum receives motor output signals from the central command in the cortex. This specialized brain tissue also obtains sensory information from peripheral receptors in muscles, tendons, joints, and skin and from visual, auditory, and vestibular end organs. *The cerebellum serves as the major comparing, evaluating, and integrating center for postural adjustments, locomotion, maintenance of equilibrium, perceptions of speed of body movement, and other diverse reflex functions related to movement.* Movement tasks first learned by trial and error, like riding a bicycle or swinging a golf club, remain coded as coordinated patterns in the cerebellar memory banks. In essence, this motor control center "fine tunes" all forms of muscular activity.[29]

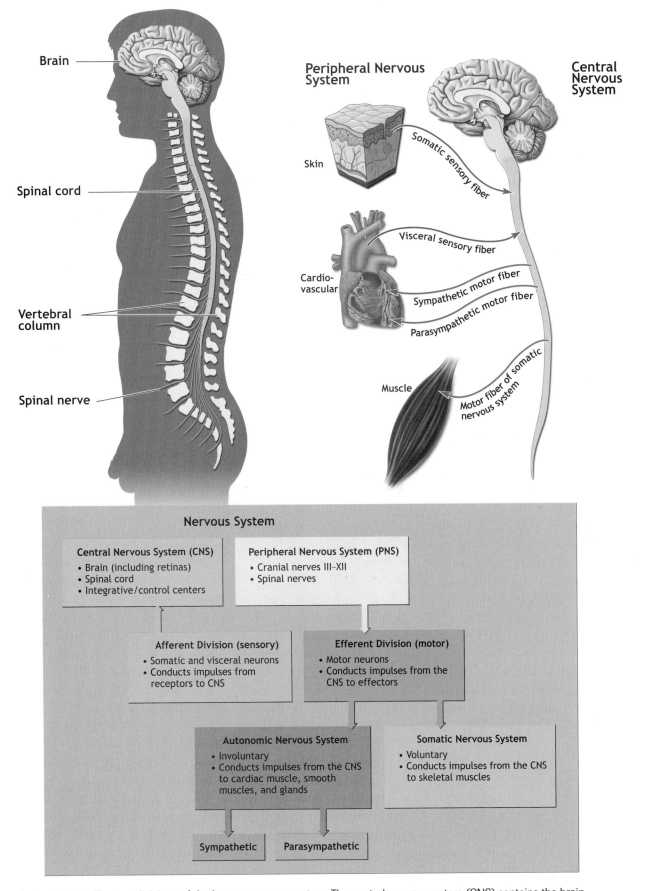

Figure 19.1 The two divisions of the human nervous system. The central nervous system (CNS) contains the brain (including retinas), spinal cord, and integrating and control centers; the cranial nerves and spinal nerves compose the peripheral nervous system (PNS). The PNS further subdivides into the afferent (sensory) and efferent (motor) divisions. The efferent division consists of the somatic nervous system and autonomic nervous system (sympathetic and parasympathetic divisions).

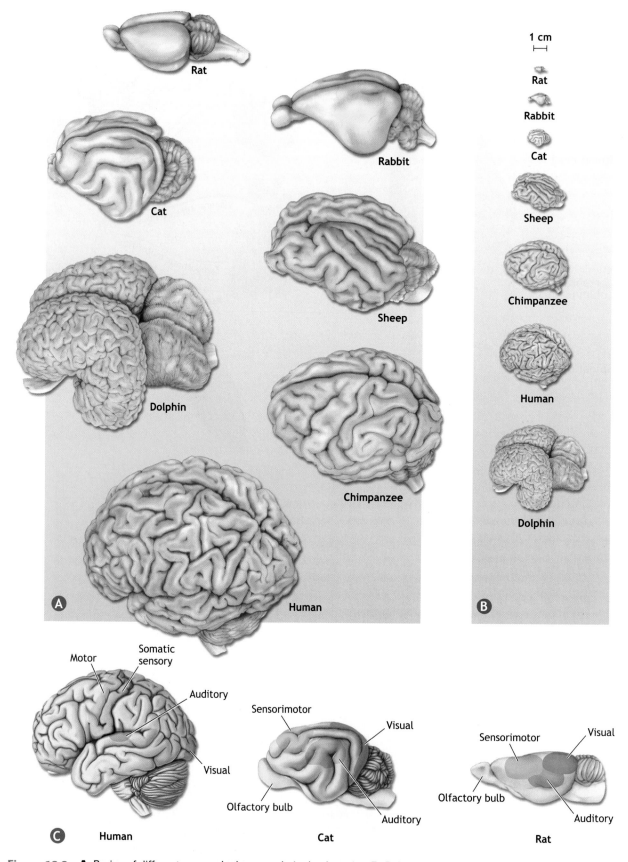

Figure 19.2   A. Brains of different mammals drawn to their absolute size. **B.** Relative brain sizes. **C.** Lateral view of the cerebral cortex in three species, showing expansion of the human cortex that is neither strictly primarily sensory nor strictly motor. (From Bear MF, et al. Neuroscience: exploring the brain. 2nd ed. Baltimore: Lippincott Williams & Wilkins, 2000.)

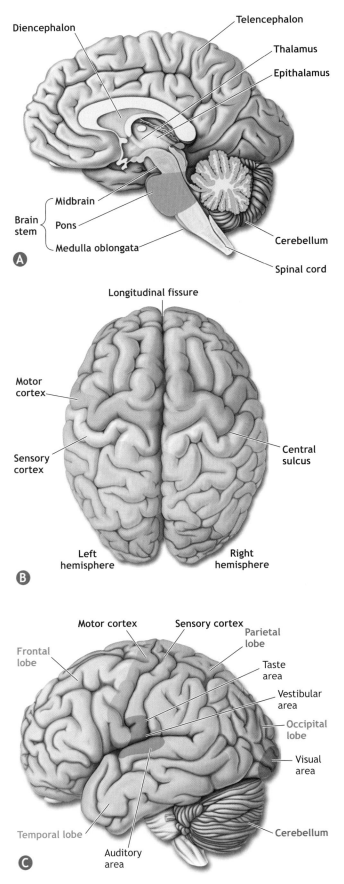

Figure 19.3 **A.** Side (medial) view of the brain and brainstem. **B.** Superior view of the brain. **C.** Four lobes of the cerebral cortex.

Diencephalon

The diencephalon, located immediately above the midbrain, forms part of the cerebral hemispheres. The thalamus, hypothalamus, epithalamus, and subthalamus compose the major structures of the diencephalon. The **hypothalamus**, situated below the thalamus, regulates functions that include metabolic rate and body temperature. The hypothalamus also influences activity of the autonomic nervous system (see p. 400); it receives regulatory input from the thalamus and limbic brain system and responds to the effects of diverse hormones (see Chapter 20). Changes in arterial blood pressure and blood gas tensions influence hypothalamic activity via peripheral receptors located in the aortic arch and carotid arteries. In essence, the hypothalamus regulates and maintains the body's internal milieu.

Telencephalon

The telencephalon contains the two hemispheres of the **cerebral cortex**, including the corpus striatum and medulla. The cerebral cortex makes up approximately 40% of the total brain weight. It divides into four lobes: frontal, temporal, parietal, and occipital. Neurons in the cortex provide specialized sensory and motor functions. Beneath each cerebral hemisphere and in close association with the thalamus lie the basal ganglia, which play an important role in the control of motor movements.

Limbic System

In 1878, French surgeon, neurologist, and anthropologist Paul Pierre Broca (1824–1880) described a group of areas on the medial surface of the cerebrum that were distinctly different from the surrounding cortex. Using the Latin word for "border" *(limbus),* Broca named the area the **limbic lobe** because its structures formed a ring or border around the brainstem and corpus callosum on the medial surface of the temporal lobe.[3] Broca also discovered the speech center now known as Broca's area, or the third circumvolution of the frontal lobe. He was the founder of modern brain surgery.

Central Nervous System— The Spinal Cord

FIGURE 19.4 illustrates the spinal cord, about 45 cm in length and 1 cm in diameter, encased by 33 vertebrae (7 cervical, 12 thoracic, 5 lumbar, 5 sacral, and 4 coccygeal). The bony vertebral column encases and protects the spinal cord, which attaches to the brainstem. The spinal cord provides the major conduit for the two-way flow of information from the skin, joints, and muscles to the brain. It provides for communication throughout the body via spinal nerves of the PNS (see p. 398). These nerves exit the cord through small openings or notches between the vertebrae. Each spinal nerve connects to the spinal cord by the dorsal root and ventral root branches. TABLE 19.1 lists common names that describe the collections of spinal cord neurons and axons.

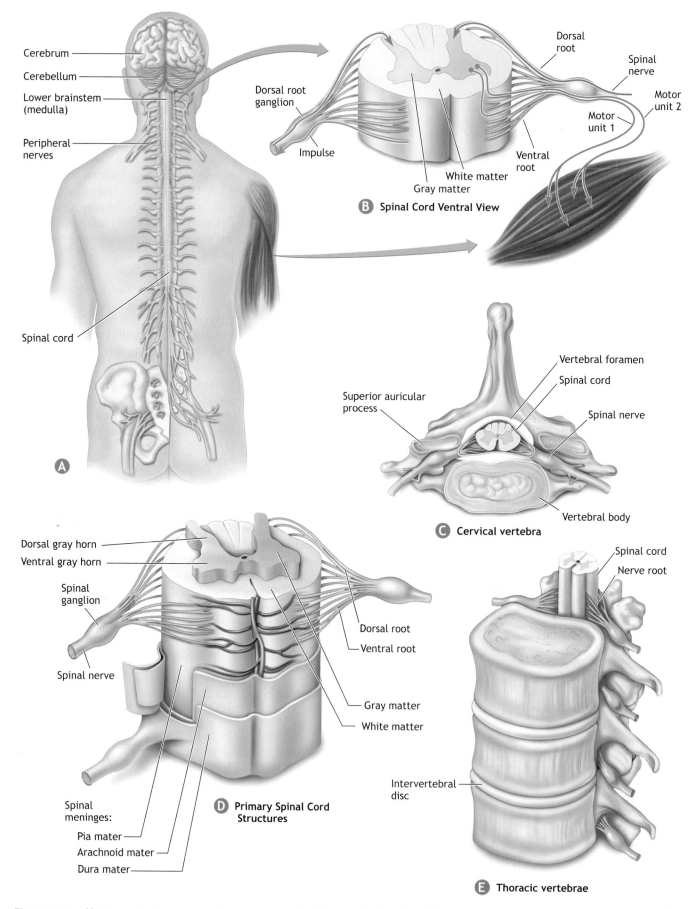

Figure 19.4 Human central nervous system anatomy. **A.** Spinal cord showing the peripheral nerves. **B.** Ventral view of spinal cord section illustrates dorsal and ventral root neural pathways and nerve impulse direction. **C.** Cross-section through one cervical vertebra. **D.** Primary spinal cord structures. **E.** Enlarged view of the junction of three thoracic vertebral bodies.

TABLE 19.1 ■ COMMON NAMES DESCRIBING NEURONS AND AXONS OF THE SPINAL CORD

NAME	DESCRIPTION/EXAMPLE
Neurons	
Gray matter	Generic term for a collection of neuronal cell bodies in the CNS (neurons appear gray in a freshly dissected brain)
Cortex	Collection of neurons forming a thin sheet, usually at the brain's surface; example: *cerebral cortex*, the sheet of neurons found just under the surface of the cerebrum
Nucleus	Distinguishable mass of neurons, usually deep in the brain (not to be confused with the nucleus of a cell); example: *lateral geniculate nucleus*, a cell group in the brainstem relaying information from the eye to the cerebral cortex
Substantia	Related neurons deep within the brain, but with less distinct borders than those of nuclei; example: *substantia nigra*, a brainstem cell group involved in voluntary movement control
Locus (plural—loci)	Small, well-defined group of cells; example: *locus coeruleus*, a brainstem group of cells involved in control of wakefulness and behavioral arousal
Ganglion (plural—ganglia)	From the Greek term for knot; collection of neurons in the peripheral nervous system; example: *dorsal root ganglia* that contain the cell bodies of sensory axons entering the spinal cord in the dorsal roots; only one cell grouping, the *basal ganglia*, in the CNS goes by this name; the basal ganglia that lie deep within the cerebrum control movement
Axons	
Nerve	A bundle of axons in the peripheral nervous system; the optic nerve is the only collection of CNS axons termed *nerve*
White matter	Generic term for a collection of CNS axons (neurons appear white in a freshly dissected brain)
Tract	Collection of CNS axons having a common site of origin and a common destination; example: *corticospinal tract that* originates in the cerebral cortex and ends in the spinal cord
Bundle	Collection of axons running together but not necessarily having the same origin and destination; example: *medial forebrain bundle* that connects the brainstem with the cerebral cortex
Capsule	Collection of axons that connect the cerebrum with the brainstem; example: *internal capsule* that connects the brainstem with the cerebral cortex
Commissure	Any collection of axons that connect one side of the brain to the other side
Lemniscus	A tract that meanders through the brain in ribbonlike fashion; example: *medial lemniscus* that brings tactile information from the spinal cord through the brainstem

From Bear MF, et al. Neuroscience: exploring the brain. 2nd ed. Baltimore: Lippincott Williams & Wilkins, 2000.

When viewed in cross section, the spinal cord shows an H-shaped core of gray matter (FIG. 19.5). The **ventral** (anterior) and **dorsal** (posterior) **horns** describe the limbs of this core. The spinal cord core contains principally three types of neurons: **motor neurons**, **sensory neurons**, and **interneurons**. The motor neurons (**efferent**) run through the ventral horn to supply the extrafusal and intrafusal skeletal muscle fibers (see p. 411). Sensory (**afferent**) nerve fibers enter the spinal cord from the periphery by way of the dorsal horn. The white matter, containing the ascending and descending nerve tracts, surrounds the gray matter within the cord.

Ascending Nerve Tracts

Ascending nerve tracts in the spinal cord forward sensory information from peripheral receptors to the brain for processing. Three neurons typically make up the sensory pathway. The dorsal root ganglion contains the cell body of the first neuron whose axon relays information into the spinal cord. The cell body of the second neuron lies within the spinal cord itself; its axon passes up the cord to the thalamus, which contains the third neuron's cell body. The axon of the third neuron passes up to the central command center in the cerebral cortex.

Sensory Receptors. *Peripheral sensory nerve endings serve as specialized receptors that detect conscious and subconscious sensory information.* The "conscious" receptors show sensitivity to body position (kinesthesia and proprioception), temperature, and sensations of light, sound, smell, taste, touch, and pain. Receptors also monitor subconscious changes in the body's internal environment; these include **chemoreceptors** that respond to changes in blood gas tension (Po_2,

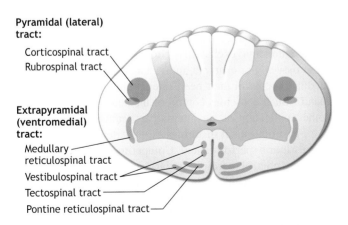

Pyramidal (lateral) tract:
- Corticospinal tract
- Rubrospinal tract

Extrapyramidal (ventromedial) tract:
- Medullary reticulospinal tract
- Vestibulospinal tract
- Tectospinal tract
- Pontine reticulospinal tract

Figure 19.5 Descending spinal cord tracts from the brain. (From Bear MF, et al. Neuroscience: exploring the brain. 2nd ed. Baltimore: Lippincott Williams & Wilkins, 2000.)

P_{CO_2}) and pH and **baroreceptors** that react rapidly to changes in arterial blood pressure.

Descending Nerve Tracts

Axons from the brain move downward through the spinal cord along two major pathways displayed in Figure 19.5. The lateral or **pyramidal tract** activates the skeletal musculature in voluntary movement under direct cortical control. The other pathway, the ventromedial or **extrapyramidal tract**, controls posture and muscle tone via the brainstem.

Pyramidal (Lateral) Tract. Neurons in the pyramidal tract (including the corticospinal and rubrospinal tracts) transmit impulses downward through the spinal cord. By means of direct routes and interconnecting neurons in the cord, these nerves eventually excite the **alpha (α) motor neurons** that control the activity of skeletal muscles. The corticospinal tract, the longest and one of the largest CNS tracts, has two thirds of its axons originating from the brain's frontal lobe, collectively called the **motor cortex**.

Extrapyramidal (Ventromedial) Tract. The extrapyramidal neurons (reticulospinal, vestibulospinal, and tectospinal tracts) originate in the brainstem and connect at all levels of the spinal cord. They control posture and provide a continual background level of neuromuscular tone.

Reticular Formation

James Papez (1883–1958), an American neuroanatomist, published a definitive work in 1926 that described the reticular formation's projections in the spinal cord of the rat. Further research in the 1950s revealed that the reticular formation provides an extensive and intricate neural network through the core of the brainstem that integrates the spinal cord, cerebral cortex, basal ganglia, and cerebellum. It receives a continuous flow of sensory data. Once activated, it either inhibits or facilitates other neurons. For example, the reticular formation helps to control posture by regulating the sensitivity of neurons to the antigravity muscles. Excitation of peripheral sensory neurons arouses the reticular nerve cells to excite the cerebral cortex. This initiates transmission of signals back to the reticular system to maintain appropriate cortical arousal and wakefulness. The reticular formation also exerts a powerful influence on cardiovascular and pulmonary regulation.

The modulating influences of other feedback networks superimpose on reticular formation activity. As an example, increased neural outflow to the postural muscles augments the tension of these muscles. An increase in neuromuscular tone also stimulates the muscle's own set of internal sensors, the spindles (see p. 411), to redirect impulses back to the CNS to maintain proper activation of the reticular formation. This level of integrated response exemplifies **multiple feedback control**, one of the most complex aspects of nervous system function.

Peripheral Nervous System

The peripheral nervous system contains 31 pairs of spinal nerves and 12 pairs of cranial nerves. FIGURE 19.6 shows the distribution of the 12 pairs of cranial nerves numbered I through XII. Cranial nerves I and II serve visual and olfactory functions and are part of the CNS. Cranial nerves emerge through foramina or fissures in the skull (cranium). Like their spinal counterparts, cranial nerves contain fibers that transmit sensory and/or motor information. Their neurons innervate muscles or glands or transmit impulses from sensory areas into the brain. The spinal nerves consist of 8 pairs of cervical nerves, 12 pairs of thoracic nerves, 5 pairs of lumbar nerves, 5 pairs of sacral nerves, and 1 pair of coccygeal nerves. A specific letter and number identifies these nerves (e.g., C-1, first nerve from the cervical region; T-4, fourth nerve in thoracic region). Careful research has traced the exact location of the spinal nerves by mapping the tissues they innervate. This is fortuitous because an injury to a specific area of the spinal cord produces predictable neurologic damage. For example, severe damage to the upper thoracic vertebra and corresponding descending nerve tract usually produces quadriplegia. FIGURE 19.7 maps the distribution of the different spinal nerves related to the sensory innervation of the skin. The term **dermatome** defines the skin area (delineated by a set of stripes on the body surface) innervated by the dorsal roots of a single spinal segment; one-to-one correspondence exists between dermatomes and spinal segments.

The peripheral nervous system includes afferent neurons that relay sensory information from receptors in the periphery *toward* the CNS and efferent neurons that transmit information *away from* the brain to peripheral tissues. **Somatic** and **autonomic** nerves are the two types of efferent neurons. Somatic nerve fibers (also called *motor neurons,* or *motoneurons*) innervate skeletal muscle. Their firing always produces an excitatory response to activate muscle. The autonomic nerves (also called *visceral, involuntary,* or *vegetative* nerves) activate cardiac muscle, sweat and salivary glands, some endocrine glands, and smooth muscle cells (also called *involuntary muscle*) in the intestines and walls of blood vessels. Autonomic activity produces either an excitatory or inhibitory effect depending on the specific neurons activated.

Whereas tissues of the heart and viscera display considerable autonomic excitability, conscious control also affects these tissues. For example, individuals who practice yoga or meditation control their heart rate and blood flow "on command." Such conscious control of the autonomic system has some application as an alternative treatment in medicine (e.g., gastrointestinal disturbances, hypertension) and to enhance sports performance. Competitors in archery and biathlon control cardiovascular activity and respiratory movements to temporarily halt the normal breathing cycle and slow heart rate during the crucial "steadiness" phase of the performance (i.e., immediately prior to releasing the bowstring or firing the rifle).

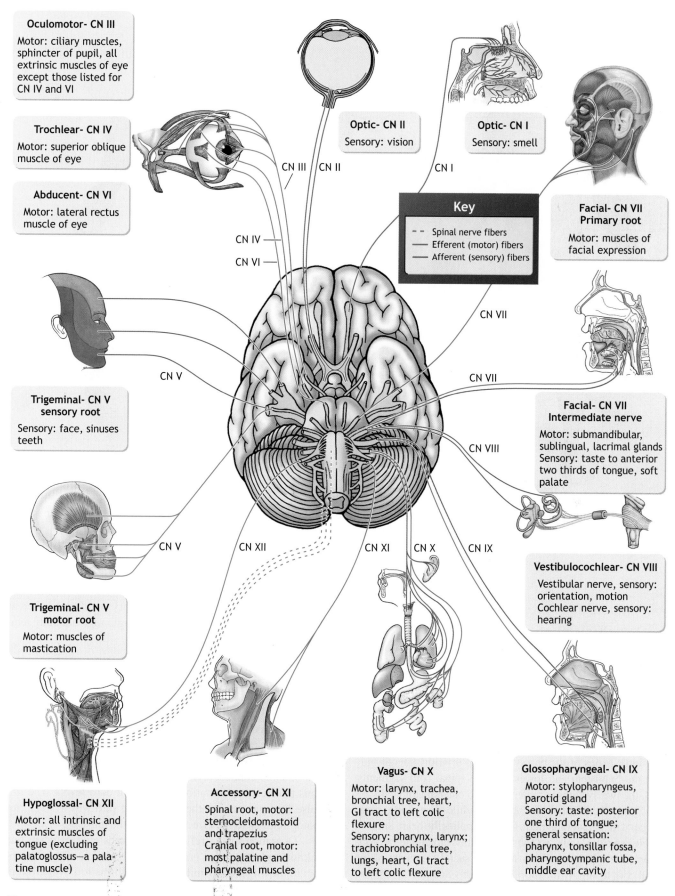

Oculomotor- CN III

Motor: ciliary muscles, sphincter of pupil, all extrinsic muscles of eye except those listed for CN IV and VI

Trochlear- CN IV

Motor: superior oblique muscle of eye

Abducent- CN VI

Motor: lateral rectus muscle of eye

Optic- CN II
Sensory: vision

Optic- CN I
Sensory: smell

Facial- CN VII Primary root

Motor: muscles of facial expression

Key
- - - Spinal nerve fibers
—— Efferent (motor) fibers
—— Afferent (sensory) fibers

Trigeminal- CN V sensory root

Sensory: face, sinuses teeth

Facial- CN VII Intermediate nerve

Motor: submandibular, sublingual, lacrimal glands
Sensory: taste to anterior two thirds of tongue, soft palate

Vestibulocochlear- CN VIII

Vestibular nerve, sensory: orientation, motion
Cochlear nerve, sensory: hearing

Trigeminal- CN V motor root

Motor: muscles of mastication

Hypoglossal- CN XII

Motor: all intrinsic and extrinsic muscles of tongue (excluding palatoglossus—a palatine muscle)

Accessory- CN XI

Spinal root, motor: sternocleidomastoid and trapezius
Cranial root, motor: most palatine and pharyngeal muscles

Vagus- CN X

Motor: larynx, trachea, bronchial tree, heart, GI tract to left colic flexure
Sensory: pharynx, larynx; trachiobronchial tree, lungs, heart, GI tract to left colic flexure

Glossopharyngeal- CN IX

Motor: stylopharyngeus, parotid gland
Sensory: taste: posterior one third of tongue; general sensation: pharynx, tonsillar fossa, pharyngotympanic tube, middle ear cavity

CN III CN II CN I
CN IV
CN VI
CN VII
CN V
CN VII
CN VIII
CN V CN XII CN XI CN X CN IX

Figure 19.6 Distribution of the 12 cranial nerves (CN). (From Moore KL, Dalley AF II, eds. Clinically oriented anatomy. 5th ed. Baltimore: Lippincott Williams & Wilkins, 2005.)

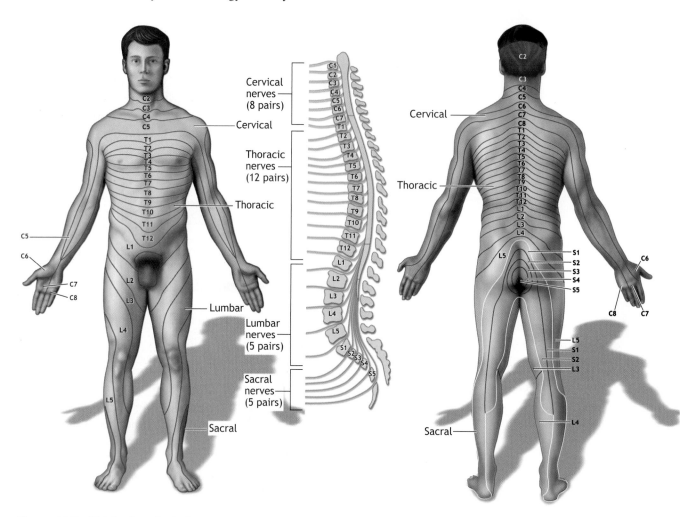

Figure 19.7 Distribution of spinal nerves related to sensory innervation of skin. *Center inset,* lateral view of vertebral column, spinal cord, spinal ganglia, and outflow of spinal nerves in the adult.

Sympathetic and Parasympathetic Nervous Systems

The **autonomic nervous system** subdivides into **sympathetic** and **parasympathetic** components. These neurons, based on anatomic and physiologic differences, operate in parallel but use structurally distinct pathways and differ in their transmitter systems. Figure 16.5 shows that axons of the sympathetic division emerge only from the middle one third of the spinal cord (thoracic and lumbar segments); in contrast, preganglionic axons of the parasympathetic division emerge only from the brainstem and lowest (sacral) spinal cord segments. Thus, the two systems complement each other anatomically.

Sympathetic fiber distribution, while displaying some overlap with parasympathetic fibers, supplies the heart, smooth muscle, sweat glands, and viscera. Parasympathetic nervous system fibers leave the brainstem and sacral segments of the spinal cord to supply the thorax, abdomen, and pelvic regions.

Regions of the medulla, pons, and diencephalon control the autonomic nervous system. For example, fibers that originate in the medullary region of the lower brainstem control blood pressure, heart rate, and pulmonary ventilation, whereas nerve fibers of upper hypothalamic origin regulate body temperature.

The Reflex Arc

FIGURE 19.8 diagrams the neural arrangement for a typical **reflex arc** in one of the 31 spinal cord segments. Afferent neurons that enter the spinal cord through the dorsal (sensory) root transmit sensory input from peripheral receptors. These neurons interconnect (**synapse**) in the cord through **interneurons** that relay information to different cord levels. The impulse then passes over the **motor root pathway** via anterior motor neurons to the effector organ—the muscles.

Operation of the reflex arc becomes evident when one unknowingly touches a hot object. Stimulation of pain receptors in the fingers transmits sensory information over afferent fibers to the spinal cord. This activates efferent motor fibers to elicit an appropriate muscular response (removing the hand rapidly). Concurrently, the signal transmits through

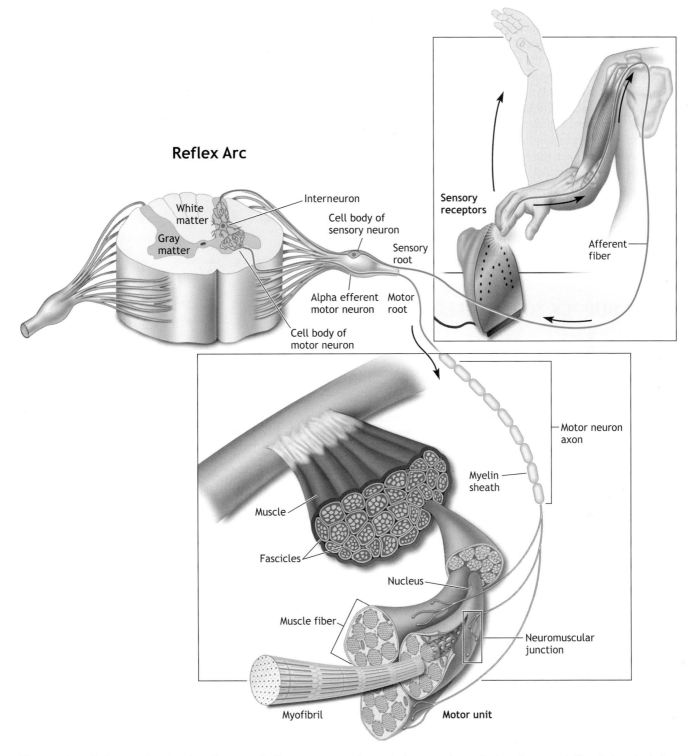

Figure 19.8 Reflex arc showing the afferent and efferent neurons plus an interneuron in a spinal cord segment. The *darker shaded* or gray matter contains the neuron cell bodies; longitudinal columns of nerve fibers make up the white matter. Stimulation of a single α-motor neuron activates up to 3000 muscle fibers. The motor neuron and the fibers it innervates collectively constitute the motor unit. The figure shows only one side of the spinal nerve complex.

interneuron activity up the cord to sensory areas in the brain, the area that actually "feels" the pain. These various levels of operation for sensory input, processing, and motor output, including the reflex action just described, cause removal of the hand from the hot object before the perception of pain. Reflex actions in the spinal cord and other subconscious areas of the CNS control many muscle functions. Hundreds of hours of practicing a particular skill "grooves" the neuromuscular movements to become automatic, requiring little or no conscious control. Unfortunately, improper practice also can automate a task to produce less than optimal neuromuscular actions. Most individuals who practice the golf swing do so by reinforcing poor habits. It starts with the grip and the first 6 inches of the takeaway in the backswing. Setting up with an improper grip, followed by a rapid cocking of the wrists at the start of the backswing, fuels a recipe for disaster (meaning that continual "poor" practice reinforces nonoptimal mechanics). Instead of hitting one ball after another, hours on end, the aspiring golfer must learn how to mimic or emulate the desirable swing mechanics. If not, the "groove" once learned to perfection tends to become more permanent. That is, the neural pathways responsible for the swing become established and automatic. Thus, trying to correct a wicked slice without changing the basic patterns of motion during purposeful practice just reinforces the movements required to produce the slice! The adage "practice makes perfect" should be amended to "perfect practice makes perfect."

NERVE SUPPLY TO MUSCLE

One nerve or its terminal branches innervate at least one of the body's approximately 250 million muscle fibers. The typical individual possesses only about 420,000 motor neurons; thus, a single nerve usually supplies many individual muscle fibers. *The number of muscle fibers per motor neuron generally relates to a muscle's particular movement function.* Delicate and precise work of the eye muscles, for example, requires that a neuron control fewer than 10 muscle fibers. For less complex movements of the large muscle groups, a motor neuron may innervate as many as 2000 or 3000 fibers. For muscular activity, the spinal cord is the major processing and distribution center for motor control. The ensuing sections take a closer look at how information processed in the CNS activates the muscles to trigger an appropriate motor response.

Motor Unit Anatomy

*The **motor unit** makes up the functional unit of movement; this anatomic unit consists of the anterior motor neuron and the specific muscle fibers it innervates.* Muscle action results from the individual and combined actions of motor units. Each muscle fiber generally receives input from only one neuron, yet a motor neuron may innervate many muscle fibers because the terminal end of an axon forms numerous branches. **Motor neuron pool** describes the collection of α-motor neurons that innervate a single muscle (e.g., triceps or biceps) (FIG.19.9). Diverse motor points exist within the muscle to allow neural stimulation throughout the muscle's length.[26] Some motor units contain up to 1000 or more muscle fibers, whereas motor units of the larynx, fingers, or eyeball contain relatively few. For example, the first dorsal interosseous muscle of the finger contains 120 motor units that control 41,000 fibers; the medial gastrocnemius (calf) muscle contains 580 motor units and 1,030,000 muscle fibers. The average ratio of muscle fibers to motor unit is 340 for the finger muscle and about 1800 for the gastrocnemius muscle.

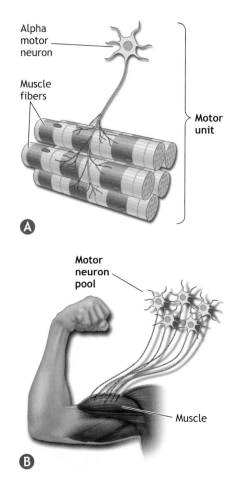

Figure 19.9   Motor unit and motor neuron pool. **A.** Motor unit represents an α-motor neuron and the fibers it innervates. **B.** Motor neuron pool represents all the α-motor neurons that innervate one muscle.

The Anterior Motor Neuron

The anterior motor neuron, illustrated in FIGURE 19.10, consists of a **cell body**, **axon**, and **dendrites**. Its unique design allows transmission of an electrochemical impulse from the spinal cord to the muscle. The cell body houses the neuron's control center—the structures involved in replication and transmission of the genetic code. The spinal cord's gray matter contains this part of the motor neuron. The axon extends from the cord to deliver the impulse to the muscle; the dendrites consist of the short neural branches that receive impulses through numerous connections and conduct them toward the cell body. Nerve cells conduct impulses in one direction only—down the axon, away from the point of stimulation.

The **myelin sheath**, a lipoprotein membrane that wraps around the axon over most of its length, encases the larger nerve fibers. A large part of this sheath acts as an electrical insulator that envelops the axon akin to the plastic coating around a copper electrical wire. A specialized cell known as a **Schwann cell** covers the bare axon and then spirals around it, sometimes up to 100 times in the biggest fibers. A thinner outermost membrane, the **neurilemma**, covers the myelin sheath. The **nodes of Ranvier** (named for Paris physician and histologist Louis Antoine Ranvier, 1835–1922) interrupt the Schwann cells and

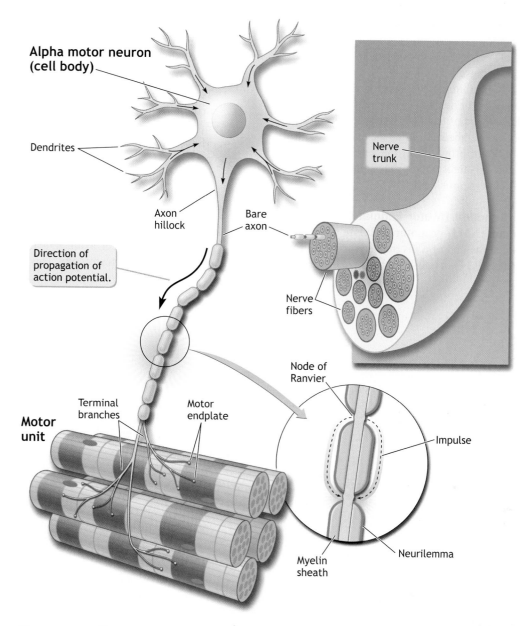

Alpha motor neuron (cell body)

Dendrites

Axon hillock

Bare axon

Direction of propagation of action potential.

Nerve trunk

Nerve fibers

Terminal branches

Motor endplate

Motor unit

Node of Ranvier

Impulse

Myelin sheath

Neurilemma

Figure 19.10 The anterior (α) motor neuron consists of a cell body, axon, and dendrites. *Top inset* shows a nerve trunk containing numerous individual nerve fibers, including a bare axon. *Bottom inset* shows a node of Ranvier on the bare axon, which permits impulses to jump from one node to another as the electrical current travels toward the terminal branches at the motor endplate.

myelin every 1 or 2 mm along the axon's length. Whereas the myelin sheath insulates the axon to the flow of ions, the nodes of Ranvier permit depolarization of the axon. This alternating sequence of myelin sheath and node of Ranvier at about 1-mm intervals allows impulses to "jump" from node to node (saltatory conduction) as the electrical current travels toward the terminal branches at the **motor endplate**. This means of conduction causes faster transmission velocities in myelinated than unmyelinated fibers. Conduction speed in a nerve fiber increases in direct proportion to a fiber's diameter and thickness of its myelin sheath. Large, myelinated neurons conduct impulses at speeds that exceed $100 \text{ m} \cdot \text{s}^{-1}$ (224 mph).

Four different nerve fiber groups exist based on size (and thus transmission velocity): (1) A-alpha (A-α [13–20 μm;

$80–120 \text{ m} \cdot \text{s}^{-1}$]), (2) A-beta (A-β [6–12 μm; $35–75 \text{ m} \cdot \text{s}^{-1}$]), (3) A-delta (A-δ [1–5 μm; $5–35 \text{ m} \cdot \text{s}^{-1}$]), and (4) C-nerve fibers (0.2–1.5 μm; $0.5–2.0 \text{ m} \cdot \text{s}^{-1}$). Myelin insulation covers the A-α, A-β, and A-δ nerve fibers, while C nerve fibers remain unmyelinated. The thickness of a nerve fiber dictates the speed of neural transmission within the fiber—the thickest A-α fibers have the fastest transmission speeds, while the smallest C fibers have the slowest transmission speed. These relatively tiny fibers relay information related to pain, temperature, and itch. To give some perspective about the speed of transmission, impulses in C nerve fibers travel about 2.2 mph, slower than most people walk. In contrast, the A-δ fibers conduct action potentials at the speed of the winning 100-m Olympic dash, while the A-β fibers that relay information related to touch travel at speeds close to that of most propellor-driver aircraft. As discussed in the section on proprioception, the γ-efferent fibers connect with special stretch sensors in skeletal muscle that detect minute changes in muscle fiber length.

All muscle action ultimately depends on three primary sources of input to α-motor neurons (motor units): (1) dorsal root ganglion cells with axons that innervate specialized muscle spindle sensory units embedded within the muscle, (2) motor neurons in the brain, primarily in the cerebral cortex's precentral gyrus, and (3) largest input from excitatory and inhibitory spinal cord interneurons.

Neuromuscular Junction (Motor Endplate). The **neuromuscular junction (NMJ)** or **motor endplate** represents the interface between the end of a myelinated motor neuron and muscle fiber (FIG. 19.11). It transmits the nerve impulse to initiate muscle action. Each skeletal muscle fiber usually contains one NMJ.

Five common features describe the NMJ[5]:

1. Presence of Schwann cells
2. Terminal section of the neuron contains the neurotransmitter substance acetylcholine (ACh)
3. Basement membrane that lines the synaptic space
4. Membrane across from the synaptic space (the postsynaptic membrane) contains ACh receptors
5. Connector microtubules at the postsynaptic membrane transmit the electrical signal deep within the muscle fiber

The terminal portion of the axon below the myelin sheath forms several smaller axon branches whose endings become the **presynaptic terminals**. This region possesses

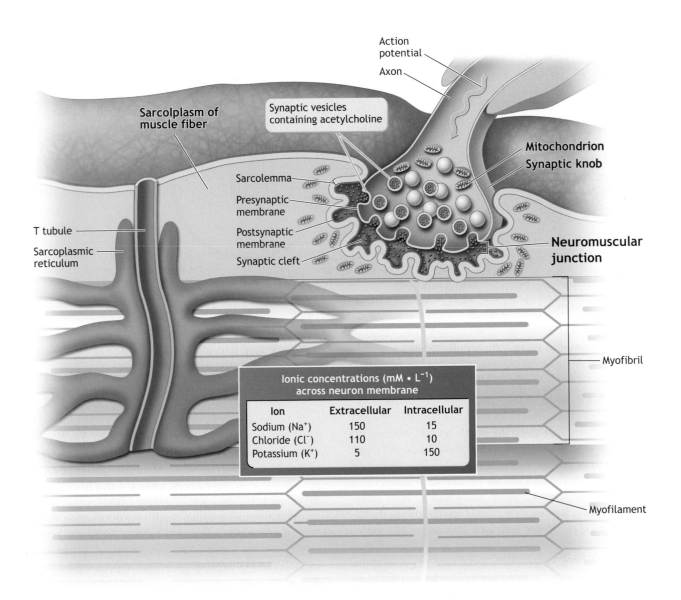

Ionic concentrations (mM · L⁻¹) across neuron membrane		
Ion	Extracellular	Intracellular
Sodium (Na⁺)	150	15
Chloride (Cl⁻)	110	10
Potassium (K⁺)	5	150

Figure 19.11 Microanatomy of the neuromuscular junction, including details of the presynaptic and postsynaptic contact area between the motor neuron and the muscle fiber it innervates. *Inset table* shows representative values for ionic concentrations across the motor neuron membrane.

approximately 50 to 70 ACh-containing vesicles per square micrometer. They lie close to (but do not come in contact with) the muscle fiber's sarcolemma. The invaginated region of the **postsynaptic membrane** (also called the *synaptic gutter*) has many infoldings that increase the membrane's surface area. The **synaptic cleft** between the synaptic gutter and the presynaptic terminal of the axon provides the region for neural impulse transmission between nerve and muscle fiber.

Excitation. *Excitation normally occurs only at the NMJ.* When an impulse arrives at the NMJ, ACh releases from saclike vesicles in the terminal axons into the synaptic cleft. ACh, which changes a basically electrical neural impulse into a chemical stimulus, then combines with a transmitter–receptor complex in the postsynaptic membrane. The resulting change in electrical properties of the postsynaptic membrane elicits an **endplate potential** that spreads from the motor endplate to the extrajunctional sarcolemma. This causes an **action potential** (wave of depolarization) to travel the length of the fiber, enter the T-tubule system, and spread to the inner structures of the muscle fiber to prime the contractile machinery.

The enzyme **cholinesterase** (concentrated at the borders of the junctional folds at the synaptic cleft) degrades ACh within 5 ms of its release from the synaptic vesicles. ACh hydrolysis by cholinesterase allows the postsynaptic membrane to repolarize rapidly. The axon resynthesizes the end products of cholinesterase action (acetic acid and choline) to ACh so the entire process can begin again when another neural impulse arrives.

Facilitation. ACh release from synaptic vesicles excites the postsynaptic membrane of its connecting neuron. This changes membrane permeability so sodium ions can diffuse into the stimulated neuron. An action potential generates if the change in transmembrane microvoltage (influx of extracellular sodium and/or efflux of intracellular potassium) reaches the **threshold for excitation**. The term **excitatory postsynaptic potential** (EPSP) describes this change in membrane potential at the junction between two neurons (FIG. 19.12A). The arrival of a subthreshold EPSP does not cause the neuron to discharge. Instead, the flow of positive charges into the cell increases to lower its **resting membrane potential** (usually an electrical potential of 65 mV between outside and inside the cell), temporarily increasing its tendency to "fire." The neuron fires when many subthreshold excitatory impulses arrive in rapid succession and the resting membrane potential lowers to about 50 mV. **Temporal summation** describes this condition of repeated subthreshold stimulation. Simultaneous stimulation of different presynaptic terminals of the same neuron produces **spatial summation**. This can induce an action potential from the "summing" of each individual effect.

INTEGRATIVE QUESTION

Describe neuromuscular factors that help to explain performance differences among individuals who devote equal time practicing a specific sports skill?

The phenomenon of neural facilitation (disinhibition) affects neurons within the CNS rather than electrochemical events at the NMJ because the NMJ does not release inhibitory neurotransmitters. Neuronal facilitation can result from (1) decreased sensitivity of the motor neuron to inhibitory neurotransmitters, (2) reduced quantity of inhibitory neurotransmitter substance transported to the motor neuron, or (3) combined effect of both mechanisms.

Neural facilitation exerts an important influence under certain exercise conditions. In all-out strength and power activities, for example, ability to disinhibit and maximally activate all motor neurons required for a movement becomes crucial to topflight performance.[14,16,24] *Enhanced facilitation (disinhibition) leads to full activation of muscle groups during all-out effort and largely accounts for the rapid and highly specific strength increases during the early stages of resistance training.*[9,10,25,28] Chapter 22 discusses the potential for augmenting maximal strength performance through CNS facilitation with intense concentration or "psyching."

Inhibition. Some presynaptic terminals produce inhibitory impulses. The inhibitory transmitter substance increases the postsynaptic membrane's permeability to the efflux of potassium and chloride ions. This increases the cell's resting membrane potential to create an **inhibitory postsynaptic potential** (**IPSP**; Fig. 19.12B). The IPSP hyperpolarizes the neuron, making it more difficult to fire. A large IPSP prevents initiation of an action potential when a motor neuron receives both excitatory and inhibitory stimulation. For example, one usually can override (inhibit) the reflex to pull the hand away when removing a splinter and so steady the hand to expedite this usually unpleasant but necessary task.

The precise neurochemical that provokes an IPSP remains unknown, although γ-aminobutyric acid (GABA) and the amino acid glycine exert inhibitory effects. Neural inhibition has protective functions and reduces the input of unwanted stimuli to produce a smooth, purposeful response.

INTEGRATIVE QUESTION

How can drugs that mimic neurotransmitters affect physiologic response and exercise performance?

MOTOR UNIT FUNCTIONAL CHARACTERISTICS

A motor unit contains only one specific muscle fiber type (type I or type II) or a subdivision of the type II fiber with the same metabolic profile. TABLE 19.2 classifies motor units based on physiologic and mechanical properties of the muscle fibers they innervate:

- Twitch characteristics
- Tension characteristics
- Fatigability

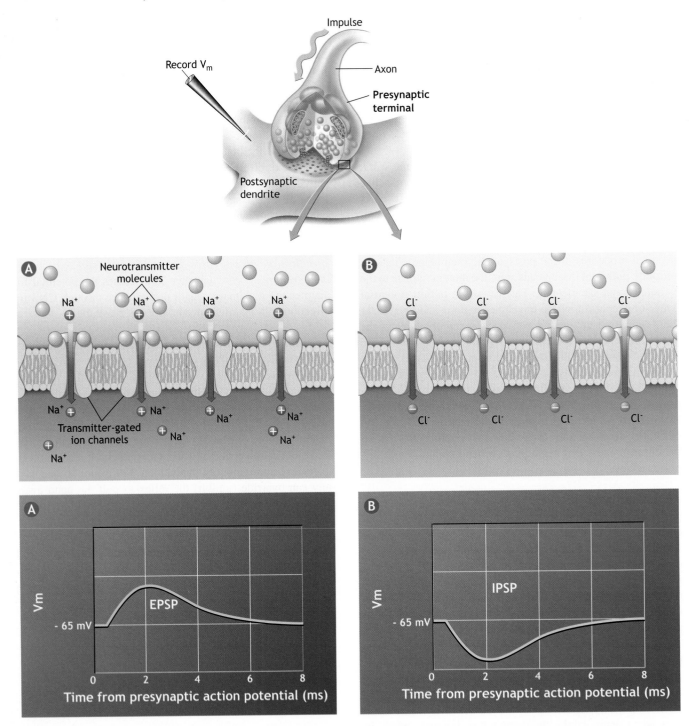

Figure 19.12   A. Generation of an excitatory postsynaptic potential (EPSP). An impulse arriving in the presynaptic terinal *(top inset)* causes neurotransmitter release. The molecules bind to transmitter-gated ion channels in the postsynaptic membrane. If Na$^+$ enters the postsynaptic cell through the open channels, the membrane becomes hypopolarized. The EPSP represents the resulting microvoltage change in membrane potential (V$_m$) recorded by a microelectrode in the cell. **B.** Generation of an inhibitory postsynaptic potential (IPSP). An impulse arriving in the presynaptic terminal *(top inset)* causes neurotransmitter release. The molecules bind to transmitter-gated ion channels in the postsynaptic membrane. If Cl$^-$ enters the postsynaptic cell through the open channels, the membrane becomes hyperpolarized. The IPSP represents the resulting change in V$_m$ recorded by a microelectrode in the cell. (From Bear MF, et al. Neuroscience: exploring the brain. 2nd ed. Baltimore: Lippincott Williams & Wilkins, 2000.)

TABLE 19.2 ■ CHARACTERISTICS AND CORRESPONDENCE BETWEEN MOTOR UNITS AND MUSCLE FIBER TYPES

MOTOR UNIT DESIGNATION	FORCE PRODUCTION	CONTRACTION SPEED	FATIGUE RESISTANCE	SAG[a]	MUSCLE FIBER TYPE IN THE MOTOR UNIT
Fast fatigable (FF)	High	Fast	Low	Yes	Fast glycolytic (FG)
Fast fatigue-resistant (FR)	Moderate	Fast	Moderate	Yes	Fast oxidative glycolytic (FOG)
Slow (S)	Low	Slow	High	No	Slow oxidative (SO)

Modified from Lieber RL. Skeletal muscle structure, function, & plasticity: the physiologic basis of rehabilitation. 2nd ed. Baltimore: Lippincott Williams & Wilkins, 2002.

[a]Under repetitive stimuli, some motor units respond smoothly with a systematic increase in tension, while others first increase tension and then decrease or "sag" in response to the same tetanic stimulus. These sag characteristics can classify the different motor units. Only the slow motor units do not exhibit sag. This probably relates more to their diminished force-generating capabilities than fatigue characteristics.

Twitch Characteristics

Early experiments in motor unit physiology revealed that motor units developed high, low, or intermediate tension in response to a single electrical stimulus. Additionally, motor units with low force capacity exhibited a slow shortening time (and time to peak force) but remained fatigue resistant, whereas units with higher force capacity shortened rapidly but fatigued earlier. FIGURE 19.13 illustrates the major characteristics for the three common motor unit categories:

1. Fast twitch, high force, and fast fatigue (type IIb)
2. Fast twitch, moderate force, and fatigue resistant (type IIa)
3. Slow twitch, low force, and fatigue resistant (type I)

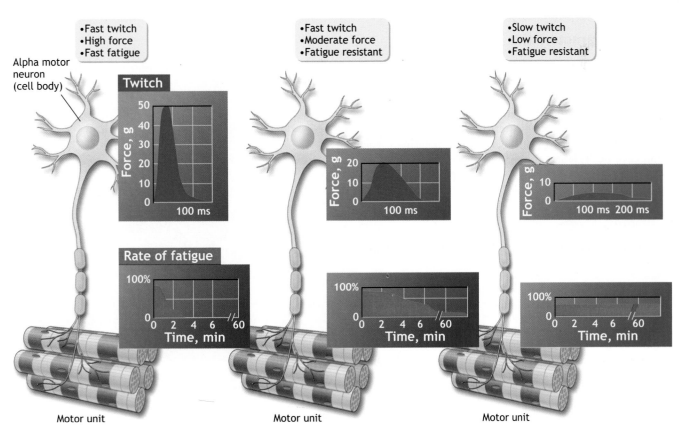

Figure 19.13 Speed, force, and fatigue characteristics of motor units. "Phasic" motor neurons fire rapidly with short bursts; "tonic" motor neurons fire slowly but continuously.

Relatively large motor neurons with fast conduction velocities innervate the two major subdivisions of fast-twitch muscle fibers. These motor units generally contain between 300 and 500 muscle fibers. The fast-fatigable (FF) and fast–fatigue-resistant (FR) units reach greater peak tension and develop it faster than slow-twitch (S) motor units that receive innervation from smaller motor neurons with slow conduction velocities. The slower contracting units, however, exhibit more fatigue resistance than the fast-twitch units. As discussed in Chapter 22, specific exercise training modifies the unique metabolic characteristics of each specific muscle fiber type. *With prolonged aerobic training, fast-twitch muscle fibers become almost as fatigue resistant as their slow-twitch counterparts.*

Motor neurons themselves have a trophic or stimulating effect on the muscle fibers they innervate in a way that modulates the fibers' properties and adaptive response to stimuli.[8] Surgically innervating fast-twitch muscle fibers with the neuron from a slow-twitch motor unit eventually alters the twitch characteristics of the fast-contracting fibers. Furthermore, application of long-term, low-frequency stimulation to intact fast-twitch motor units induces conversion of the muscle fibers to the slow-twitch type.[14,22] This neurotrophic effect suggests that the myoneural junction takes on much greater significance than just serving as the site of muscle fiber depolarization. It indicates a remarkable plasticity of skeletal muscle that may indeed be altered through long-term use.

Tension Characteristics

A stimulus strong enough to trigger an action potential in the motor neuron activates all of the accompanying muscle fibers in the motor unit to contract synchronously. A motor unit does not exert a force gradation—either the impulse elicits an action or it does not. After the neuron fires and the impulse reaches the NMJ, all fibers of the motor unit react simultaneously. This action embodies the principle of **"all-or-none"** that relates to the normal function of skeletal muscle.

Gradation of Force

The force of muscle action varies from slight to maximal via two mechanisms:

1. Increased *number* of motor units recruited
2. Increased *frequency* of motor unit discharge

A muscle generates considerable force when activated by all of its motor units. Repetitive stimuli that reach a muscle before it relaxes also increase the total tension. Blending recruitment of motor units and modification of their firing rate permits optimal patterns of neural discharge that allow a wide variety of graded muscle actions. These range from the delicate touch of the eye surgeon to the maximal effort in throwing a baseball from deep center field on a straight line to throw out a runner approaching home plate.

Motor Unit Activity. Low-force muscle actions activate only a few motor units; a higher force requirement progressively enlists more motor units. **Motor unit recruitment** describes adding motor units to increase muscle force. As muscle force requirements increase, motor neurons with progressively larger axons are recruited. This exemplifies the **size principle**—an anatomic basis for the orderly recruitment of specific motor units to produce a smooth muscle action.

All of the motor units in a muscle do not fire at the same time (FIG. 19.14). If they did, it would be virtually impossible to control muscle force output. Consider the tremendous gradation of forces and speeds that muscles generate. For example, when lifting a barbell, specific muscles act to move the limb at a particular speed under a set rate of tension development. One can lift a relatively light weight at a number of speeds. As weight increases, however, the speed options decrease accordingly. With a pencil, for example, one generates the proper force to lift the pencil regardless of how fast or slowly the arm moves. *From the standpoint of neural control, the selective recruitment and firing pattern of the fast-twitch and slow-twitch motor units provide the mechanism to produce the desired coordinated response.*

In accordance with the size principle, slow-twitch motor units with the lowest threshold for activation are selectively recruited during light to moderate effort. Activation of slow-twitch units occurs during sustained jogging or cycling on a level grade or during slow swimming or slowly lifting a relatively light weight. More rapid, powerful movements progressively activate fast-twitch fatigue-resistant (type IIa) units up

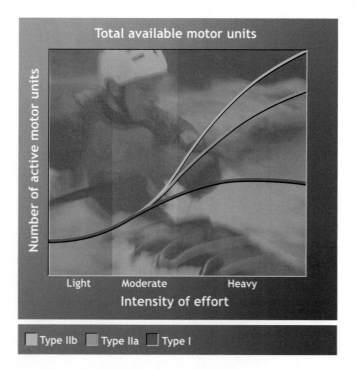

Figure 19.14 Recruitment of slow-twitch (type I) and fast-twitch (type IIa and b) muscle fibers (motor units) in relation to exercise intensity. More intense exercise progressively recruits more fast-twitch fibers.

through the fast-twitch fatigable (type IIb) units at peak force. As a runner or cyclist reaches a hill during a distance race, some fast-twitch units become activated to maintain a fairly constant pace over varying terrain. Large single muscles with broad origins and/or insertions (like the deltoid), contain smaller, independently controlled "muscles within muscles" that are activated depending on the segment's line of action and direction of the intended motion. Such an arrangement allows CNS flexibility to fine tune skeletal muscle activity to fit the demands of the imposed motor task.[30]

The differential control of motor unit firing patterns represents a major factor that distinguishes skilled from unskilled performances and specific athletic groups.[6] For example, weight lifters generally exhibit a synchronous pattern of motor unit firing (i.e., many motor units recruited simultaneously during lifting), whereas the firing pattern of endurance athletes is more asynchronous (i.e., some units fire, others recover). As discussed previously, a muscle's composition of specific motor units (muscle fibers) also contributes to an athlete's successful performance. The synchronous firing of fast-twitch motor units allows the weight lifter to generate force quickly for the desired lift. In contrast, for the endurance athlete the asynchronous firing of predominantly slow-twitch, fatigue-resistant units provides a built-in recuperative period so performance can continue with minimal fatigue. This occurs because motor units share the burden of multiple movements and intensities during exercise.

 INTEGRATIVE QUESTION

How can knowledge of neuromuscular exercise physiology help to enhance an athlete's (1) strength and power and (2) sports skill performance?

Neuromuscular Fatigue

Fatigue represents the decline in muscle tension or force capacity with repeated stimulation. This definition also encompasses perceptual alterations of increased difficulty to achieve a desired submaximal or maximal exercise outcome. Many complex factors produce motor unit fatigue, each relating to the specific exercise demands that produce it.[1,13,15,17,18]

Voluntary muscle actions exhibit four main components listed in the following order of nervous system hierarchy:

1. Central nervous system
2. Peripheral nervous system
3. Neuromuscular junction
4. Muscle fiber

Fatigue occurs from interrupting the chain of events between the CNS and muscle fiber, regardless of the reason. Examples include:

- Exercise-induced alterations in levels of CNS neurotransmitters serotonin, 5-hydroxytryptamine (5-HT), dopamine, and ACh in various brain regions, along with the neuromodulators ammonia and cytokines secreted by immune cells alter one's psychic or perceptual state to disrupt ability to exercise.[4,19]

- Reduced glycogen content of the active muscle fibers relates to fatigue during prolonged intense exercise.[2,7] This "nutrient fatigue" occurs even with sufficient oxygen available to generate energy through aerobic pathways. Depletion of phosphocreatine (PCr) and a decline in total adenine nucleotide pool (ATP + ADP + AMP) also accompanies the fatigue state in prolonged submaximal exercise.[2]

- Oxygen lack and increased level of blood and muscle lactate relate to muscle fatigue in short-term, maximal exercise. The dramatic increase in $[H^+]$ in the active muscle dramatically disrupts the intracellular environment.[12,23] Alterations in contractile function in anaerobic exercise also relate to five factors: (1) PCr depletion, (2) changes in myosin ATPase, (3) impaired glycolytic energy transfer capacity from reduced activity of the key enzymes phosphorylase and phosphofructokinase, (4) disturbance in the T-tubule system for transmitting the impulse throughout the cell, (5) and ionic imbalances.[11] Downregulation in muscle Na^+, K^+, and Ca^{2+} release, distribution, and uptake alters the myofilament activity and impairs muscular performance,[16] even though nerve impulses continue to bombard the muscle fiber.

- Fatigue occurs at the NMJ when an action potential fails to cross from the motor neuron to the muscle fiber. The precise mechanism for this aspect of "neural fatigue" remains unknown.

As muscle function deteriorates during prolonged submaximal exercise, additional motor-unit recruitment maintains the crucial force output required for activity. In all-out exercise that presumably activates all motor units, a decrease in neural activity (as measured by the electromyogram or EMG) accompanies fatigue. Reduced neural activity supports the contention that failure in neural or myoneural transmission produces fatigue in maximal effort.

 INTEGRATIVE QUESTION

In terms of neuromuscular physiology, discuss the validity of the adage "Perfect practice makes perfect."

RECEPTORS IN MUSCLES, JOINTS, AND TENDONS: THE PROPRIOCEPTORS

Muscles and tendons contain specialized sensory receptors sensitive to stretch, tension, and pressure. These end organs, known as **proprioceptors**, rapidly relay information about muscular dynamics and limb movement to conscious and subconscious portions of the CNS. Proprioception allows continual monitoring of the progress of any sequence of movements and serves to modify subsequent motor behavior.[20]

MUSCULAR FATIGUE: A COMPLEX PHENOMENON

Merton PA. Voluntary strength and fatigue. J Physiol (Lond) 1954;123:553.

▲ Since the turn of the 20th century, scientists have tried to explain why repeated maximal muscular activity produced decreased tension output in muscle (fatigue). The debate over the site of fatigue focuses on the existence of either a central or peripheral mechanism. *Central mechanism* refers to a location proximal to the motor neuron (i.e., mainly the brain); a *peripheral mechanism* involves the motor units (i.e., anterior motor neurons, motor endplates, and muscle fibers). Merton reasoned that he could distinguish central and peripheral mechanisms by inducing fatigue in a muscle group by maximal voluntary contractions (MVCs) and then stimulating the motor unit electrically. "Extra" localized electrical stimulation's failure to increase force production (i.e., no change in fatigue pattern) would indicate a purely peripheral fatigue site. In contrast, an increase in muscle tension (i.e., pattern of fatigue decreased) with electrical stimulation would support a central site hypothesis for muscular fatigue.

Merton experimented mainly on himself with an apparatus modified from one used to measure force recordings of excised muscle from animals *[left figure]* that measured muscle tension output of the isolated adductor pollicis that produces thumb adduction. The upper arm remained fixed in a flexed position with the hand rotated outward and stabilized in a grasping position. The arm and hand rested in a splint-type device that allowed only thumb abduction/adduction movement. This hand and arm position enabled isolation and recording of muscle tension by either voluntary muscle action or electrical stimulation via the ulnar nerve.

Subjects performed maximal isometric actions to fatigue. Merton then delivered a series of single twitches evoked by stimulation of the ulnar nerve at approximately 12-second intervals preceding and following fatigue. The *top tracing* in the *right figure below* shows the fatigue curve for the muscles during the sustained isometric MVC. Tension declined linearly over time, reaching one half its initial value in 1 minute. The *lower tracing* shows the corresponding action potentials in response to repeated nerve stimulation. Stimulating the motor nerve electrically did not alter the fatigue pattern. Merton reasoned that some part of the peripheral apparatus directly affected fatigue during MVC. Nerve stimulation did not diminish the amplitude of the action potential during fatigue *(lower tracing)*, so the site of fatigue must have been within the muscle fiber itself rather than at the neuromuscular junction. Merton's classic experiments provided the first strong support for the role of peripheral factors in muscular fatigue.

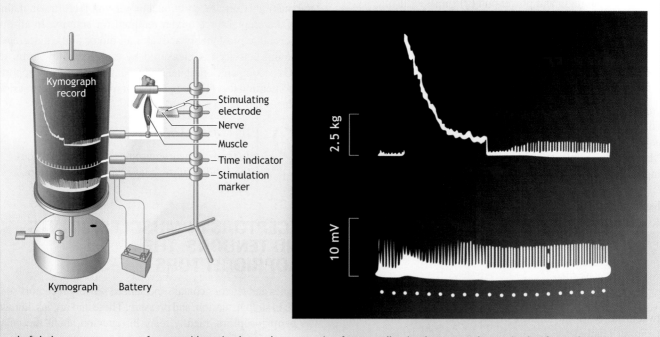

Left. Laboratory apparatus for use with excised muscle preparation from small animals to record magnitude of muscle action in response to repeated electrical nerve stimulation. *Right.* Results from modification by Merton of technique on left for use on intact muscle of humans to show fatigue curve during sustained isometric maximal voluntary muscle action *(top)* and corresponding action potentials in response to repeated electrical stimulation of the motor nerve *(bottom).*

Muscle Spindles

The **muscle spindles** provide sensory information about changes in muscle fiber length and tension. They primarily respond to any stretch of a muscle. Through reflex response, they initiate a stronger muscle action to counteract this stretch.

Structural Organization

FIGURE 19.15 shows a fusiform muscle spindle aligned in parallel to regular muscle fibers or **extrafusal fibers**. Consequently, when the muscle stretches, the spindle also stretches. The number of spindles within a quantity of muscle varies depending on the muscle group. On a relative basis, muscles involved in complex movements contain more spindles per gram than muscles that perform gross movement patterns. The spindle, covered by a sheath of connective tissue, contains two specialized types of muscle fiber called **intrafusal fibers**. One type of intrafusal fiber, the fairly large **nuclear bag fiber**, contains numerous nuclei packed centrally through its diameter. Each spindle usually contains two nuclear bag fibers. The other type of intrafusal fiber, the **nuclear chain fiber**, contains many nuclei along its length. These fibers attach to the surface of the longer nuclear bag fibers. Each spindle usually contains four to five chain fibers. The ends of the intrafusal fibers contain actin and myosin filaments and exhibit shortening capability.

Two sensory afferent fibers and one motor efferent fiber service the spindles. A primary afferent nerve fiber, the **annulospiral nerve fiber** (composed of a set of rings in spiral configuration), entwines about the midregion of the bag fiber. This fiber responds directly to the stretch of the spindle; its firing frequency or discharge rate increases in proportion to the stretch. A second group of smaller sensory nerve fibers, the **flower-spray endings**, makes connections mainly on the chain fibers but also attaches to the bag fibers. These endings show less sensitivity to stretch than annulospiral fibers. Activation of the annulospiral and flower-spray sensors relays impulses through the dorsal root into the cord to produce reflex activation of the motor neurons to the stretched muscle. This causes the muscle to act more forcefully and shorten, which reduces the stretch stimulus from the spindles.

The third type of spindle nerve fiber, the thin **γ-efferent fiber** that innervates the contractile, striated ends of the intrafusal fibers, serves a motor function. Higher centers in the brain activate these fibers to maintain optimal sensitivity of the spindle at all muscle lengths. γ-efferent stimulation activates the intrafusal fibers to regulate their length and sensitivity regardless of the muscle's overall length. This mechanism prepares the spindle for other lengthening actions, even if the muscle remains shortened. Adjustments in γ-efferent activation allow the spindle to continuously monitor the length of the muscles that contain them.

The Stretch Reflex

The muscle spindle detects, responds to, and modulates changes in the length of the extrafusal muscle fibers. This provides an important regulatory function for movement and maintenance of posture. Postural muscles continuously receive neural input to sustain their readiness to respond to conscious (voluntary) movements. These muscles require continual subconscious activity to adjust to the pull of gravity in upright posture. Without this monitoring and feedback mechanism, the body would literally fall down upon itself from the absence of tension in neck muscles, spinal muscles, hip flex-

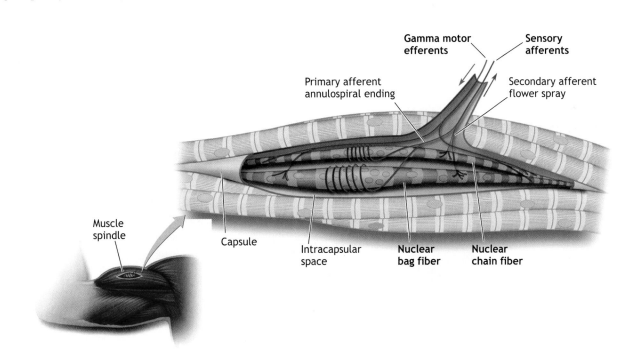

Figure 19.15 Structural organization of the muscle spindle with an enlarged view of the equatorial region of the spindle.

IN A PRACTICAL SENSE

HOW TO DETERMINE UPPER-ARM MUSCLE AND FAT

■ Girth measurements include bone surrounded by a mass of muscle tissue ringed by a layer of subcutaneous fat (Fig. A). Muscle represents the largest component of girth (except in obese and elderly persons), so girth indicates one's relative muscularity. The procedure for estimating limb muscle area assumes similarity between a limb and a cylinder, with subcutaneous fat evenly distributed around the cylinder (Fig. A).

MEASUREMENTS
Determine the following:
1. Upper-arm girth (relaxed triceps; G_{arm}): Measure with arm extended relaxed at the side (or parallel to the ground in an abducted position). Measure girth (cm) midway between the acromial and olecranon process (Fig. B).
2. Triceps skinfold (Sf_{tri}): Measure in decimeters (dm; mm ÷ 10) on the back of the arm over the triceps muscle as a vertical fold at the same level as the relaxed arm girth (Fig. C).

EXAMPLE
Data: Upper-arm girth (G_{arm}) in cm = 30.0; Sf_{tri} = 2.5 dm (25 mm).

COMPUTATIONS
1. Arm muscle girth, cm
   $= G_{arm} - (\pi Sf_{tri})$
   $= 30.0 \text{ cm} - (\pi 2.5 \text{ dm})$
   $= 30.0 - 7.854$
   $= 22.1 \text{ cm}$
2. Arm muscle area, cm^2
   $= [G_{arm} - (\pi Sf_{tri})] \div 4\pi$
   $= (30.0 \text{ cm}) - (\pi 2.5 \text{ dm})^2 \div 4\pi$
   $= 488.4 \div 12.566$
   $= 38.9 \text{ cm}^2$
3. Arm area (A), cm^2
   $= (G_{arm})^2 \div 4\pi$
   $= (30.0 \text{ cm})^2 \div 4\pi$
   $= 900 \div 12.566$
   $= 71.6 \text{ cm}^2$
4. Arm fat area, cm^2
   $= \text{arm area} - \text{arm muscle area}$
   $= 71.6 \text{ cm}^2 - 38.9 \text{ cm}^2$
   $= 32.7 \text{ cm}^2$
5. Arm fat index, % fat area
   $= (\text{arm fat area} \div \text{arm area}) \times 100$
   $= (32.7 \text{ cm}^2 \div 71.6) \times 100$
   $= 45.7\%$

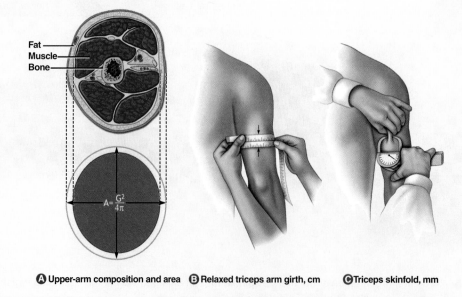

Fat
Muscle
Bone

$A = \dfrac{G^2}{4\pi}$

Ⓐ Upper-arm composition and area   Ⓑ Relaxed triceps arm girth, cm   Ⓒ Triceps skinfold, mm

ors, abdominal muscles, and large leg musculature. To this end, the stretch reflex provides a fundamental controlling mechanism.

Three main components make up the stretch reflex: (1) muscle spindle that responds to stretch, (2) afferent nerve fiber that carries the sensory impulse from the spindle to the spinal cord, and (3) efferent spinal cord motor neuron that activates the stretched muscle fibers.

FIGURE 19.16 illustrates the patellar tendon stretch reflex (knee-jerk reflex), the simplest autonomic reflex arc involving only one synapse (monosynaptic). Because the spindles lie parallel to the extrafusal fibers, they become stretched when these fibers elongate as the hammer strikes the patellar tendon. The spindle's sensory receptors fire when its intrafusal fibers stretch. This directs impulses through the dorsal root into the spinal cord to directly activate the anterior motor neurons. The gray matter contains neuron cell bodies; the white matter carries longitudinal columns of nerve fibers. Stimulation of a single α-motor neuron affects up to 3000 muscle fibers. The reflex also activates interneurons within the cord to facilitate the appropriate motor response. For example, excitatory impulses activate synergistic muscles that support the desired movement, while inhibitory impulses flow to motor units that normally counter the movement. In this way, the stretch reflex acts as a self-regulating, compensating mechanism. This salient feature allows the muscle to adjust automatically to differences in load (and length) without requiring immediate information processing through higher CNS centers.

Golgi Tendon Organs

In contrast to the muscle spindles that lie parallel to the extrafusal muscle fibers, the **Golgi tendon organs** connect to up to 25 extrafusal fibers near the tendon's junction to the muscle. These sensory receptors detect differences in the tension generated by active muscle rather than muscle length. FIGURE 19.17 shows that the Golgi tendon organs respond as a feedback monitor to discharge impulses under either of two conditions: (1) to tension created in the muscle when it shortens and (2) to tension when the muscle stretches passively.

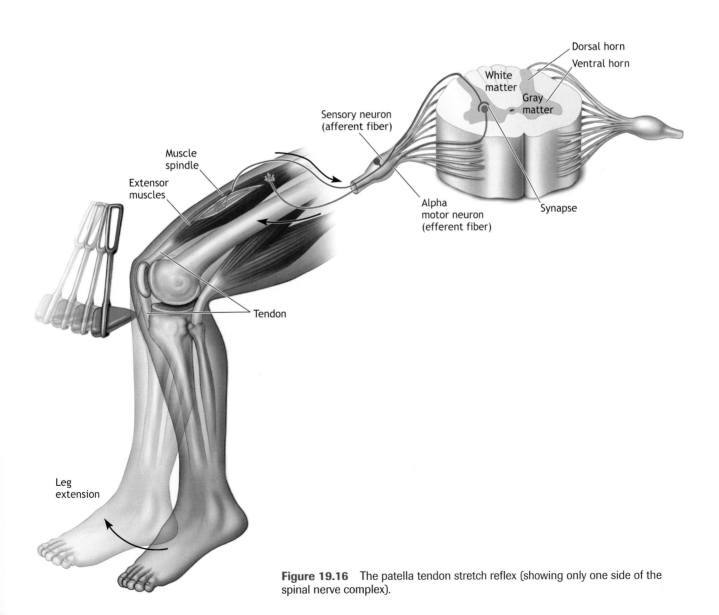

Figure 19.16 The patella tendon stretch reflex (showing only one side of the spinal nerve complex).

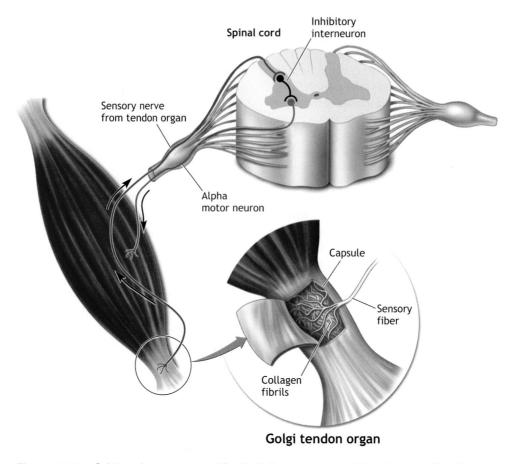

Golgi tendon organ

Figure 19.17 Golgi tendon organ named for the Italian anatomist and Nobel laureate Camillo Golgi (1843–1926) who first described these proprioceptors in the late 1800s. Excessive tension or stretch on a muscle activates the Golgi receptors to initiate a reflex inhibition of the muscles they supply. The Golgi tendon organ functions as a protective sensory mechanism that detects and subsequently inhibits undue strain within the muscle–tendon structure.

When stimulated by excessive tension, the Golgi receptors conduct signals rapidly to the spinal cord to elicit *reflex inhibition* of the muscles they supply. This occurs because of the overriding influence of the inhibitory spinal interneuron on the motor neurons supplying the muscle. Therefore, Golgi tendon organs functions as a *protective* sensory mechanism much like a "governor" mechanism that prevents motorized go-carts from moving too fast. Excessive change in muscle tension increases the Golgi sensor's discharge; this depresses motor neuron activity and reduces force output. If muscle action produces little tension, Golgi receptors remain relatively inactive and exert little influence. *Ultimately, the Golgi tendon organs protect the muscle and its connective tissue harness from injury from excessive load.*

Pacinian Corpuscles

Pacinian corpuscles are small, ellipsoidal bodies located close to the Golgi tendon organs and embedded in a single, unmyelinated nerve fiber. These sensory receptors are sensitive to quick movement and deep pressure. Deformation or compression of the onionlike capsule by a mechanical stimulus transmits pressure to the sensory nerve ending within its core.

This produces a change in the electric potential of the sensory nerve ending. If this generator potential reaches sufficient magnitude, a sensory signal propagates down the myelinated axon that leaves the corpuscle and enters the spinal cord.

Pacinian corpuscles are fast-adapting mechanical sensors because they discharge a few impulses at the onset of a steady stimulus and then remain electrically silent or may discharge a second volley of impulses when the stimulus ceases. They detect *changes* in movement or pressure rather than the magnitude of movement or the quantity of pressure applied.

Summary

1. Neural control mechanisms located in the central nervous system (CNS) finely regulate human movement. In response to internal and external stimuli, bits of sensory input automatically become coded, routed, organized, and transmitted to the effector organ—the skeletal muscles.

2. Tracts of neural tissue descend from the brain to influence spinal cord neurons. Neurons in the extrapyramidal tract control posture and provide a continual background level of neuromuscular tone;

the pyramidal tract neurons stimulate discrete muscular movements.

3. The cerebellum fine tunes muscle activity through its function as the major comparing, evaluating, and integrating center.

4. The spinal cord and other subconscious areas of the CNS control diverse muscle functions. The reflex arc provides the basic mechanism to process "automatic" muscle actions.

5. The motor unit makes up the functional unit of movement. The number of muscle fibers in a motor unit depends on a muscle's movement function. Intricate movement patterns require a small fiber-to-neuron ratio, whereas a single neuron may innervate a thousand muscle fibers for gross movements.

6. The anterior motor neuron (cell body, axon, and dendrites) transmits electrochemical nerve impulses from the spinal cord to the muscle. The dendrites receive impulses and conduct them toward the cell body, whereas the axon transmits the impulse in one direction only—down the axon to the muscle.

7. The neuromuscular junction (NMJ) establishes the interface between motor neuron and muscle fiber. Acetylcholine (ACh) release at the NMJ provides the chemical stimulus that activates the muscle fiber.

8. Stimulation of a muscle fiber progresses in the following six-step sequence: (1) action potential propagates down the motor neuron's axon; (2) calcium channels open at the end of the nerve terminal; (3) calcium moves into the nerve terminal; (4) ACh primes for release; (5) ACh traverses the synapse and binds to ACh receptors on the postsynaptic membrane at the sarcolemma; and (6) endplate potential generates and a depolarization wave spreads throughout the T-tubular network.

9. Excitatory and inhibitory impulses continually bombard the synaptic junctions between neurons. These impulses alter a neuron's threshold for excitation by either increasing or decreasing its tendency to fire.

10. During all-out power exercise, a high degree of neural facilitation (disinhibition) proves beneficial because it maximally activates a muscle's motor units.

11. Motor units classify into three types depending on speed of muscle action, force generated, and fatigability: (1) fast twitch, high force, fast fatigue; (2) fast twitch, moderate force, fatigue resistant; and (3) slow twitch, low force, fatigue resistant.

12. Muscle force gradation progresses through the interaction of factors that regulate the number and type of motor units recruited and their discharge frequency. Low-intensity exercise recruits slow-twitch motor units, followed by activation of fast-twitch units when requiring more powerful forces.

13. Alterations in motor unit recruitment and firing pattern help to explain the rapid strength improvement during the early stages of resistance training.

14. Special sensory receptors in muscles, tendons, and joints relay information about muscle dynamics and limb movement to specific portions of the CNS. This provides important sensory feedback during physical activity.

References are available on the Student CD and online at http://connection.lww.com/mkk6e.

The Endocrine System: Organization and Acute and Chronic Responses to Exercise

20

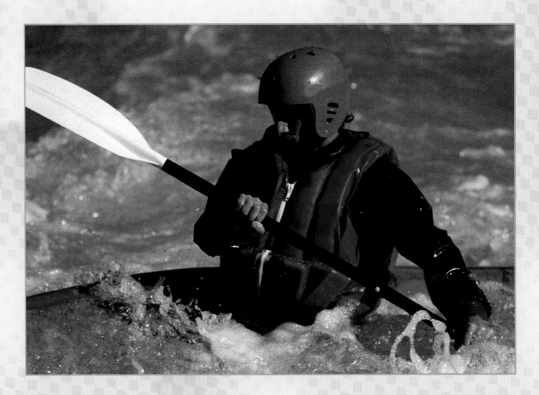

CHAPTER OBJECTIVES

- Draw the locations of the body's major endocrine glands

- List the sequence of events to show how hormones affect specific "target cell" functions

- Outline the role of the intracellular messenger cyclic 3′,5′-adenosine monophosphate (cyclic AMP)

- Discuss how hormones affect enzyme activity and enzyme-mediated membrane transport

- Describe the influence of hormonal, humoral, and neural stimulation on endocrine gland activity

- List the anterior and posterior pituitary gland hormones, their functions, and how acute and chronic exercise affect their release

- List the thyroid gland hormones, their functions, and how acute and chronic exercise affect their release

- List the adrenal medulla and adrenal cortex hormones, their functions, and how acute and chronic exercise affect their release

- List hormones of the α- and β-cells of the pancreas, their functions, and how acute and chronic exercise affect their release

- Define *type 1* and *type 2 diabetes* and the symptoms and effects of each disorder

- Describe three test options for diagnosing diabetes mellitus

- List the fasting blood glucose classification categories for type 2 diabetes

- List risk factors for type 2 diabetes and benefits of regular exercise to prevent and treat this disease

- Outline how exercise training affects endocrine function

- Describe the effect of resistance training on testosterone and growth hormone release

- Characterize the functions of opioid peptides, their response to exercise, and possible role in the "exercise high"

- Outline interactions among short-term, moderate, and exhaustive exercise, exercise training, susceptibility to illness, and immune function

The endocrine system integrates and regulates bodily functions and thus provides stability to the internal environment. Hormones produced by endocrine glands affect almost all aspects of human function; they activate enzyme systems, alter cell membrane permeability, cause muscular contraction and relaxation, stimulate protein and fat synthesis, initiate cellular secretion, and augment how the body responds to physical and psychologic stress. The following sections provide a general overview of the endocrine system, its functions during rest and physical activity, and responses to acute exercise and chronic training.

ENDOCRINE SYSTEM OVERVIEW

Relatively small compared with other organs, the combined weight of the endocrine organs averages 0.5 kg. FIGURE 20.1 shows the location of the major endocrine organs—the pituitary, thyroid, parathyroid, adrenal, pineal, and thymus glands. Several other organs contain discrete areas of endocrine tissue that also produce hormones. These include the pancreas, gonads (ovaries and testes), hypothalamus, and adipose (fat) cells. The hypothalamus also serves as a major

organ of the nervous system; thus it functions as a **neuroendocrine organ**. Pockets of hormone-producing cells also form in the walls of the small intestine, stomach, kidneys, and myocytes in the heart's atria, although these organs exert little influence on hormone production per se.

New discoveries in obesity research have identified the hormone adiponectin, which increases the body's sensitivity to insulin, and resistin, which increases insulin resistance (studied mostly in mice). These discoveries add further evidence that the nervous and endocrine systems act synchronously to regulate all aspects of human physiology from conception to death. Researchers who focus on endocrinology study the intimate workings of the body's chemical communication systems. In essence, endocrinologists examine the detailed workings of hormones and the receptors and signaling pathways they target.

ENDOCRINE SYSTEM ORGANIZATION

The endocrine system consists of a host organ (gland), minute quantities of chemical messengers (hormones), and a target or receptor organ. Glands classify as either **endocrine** or **exocrine**. Some glands serve both functions.

Endocrine glands possess no ducts (referred to as *ductless glands*), so they secrete substances directly into the extracellular spaces around the gland. FIGURE 20.2 shows that these hormones then diffuse into the blood for transport throughout the body to fulfill their intercellular communication functions. The term *endocrine* means *hormone secreting*. Exocrine glands, in contrast, contain secretory ducts that carry substances directly to a specific compartment or surface. The nervous system controls almost all exocrine glands. Examples of exocrine glands include sweat glands and glands of the upper digestive tract.

Types of Hormones

Hormones, *chemical substances synthesized by specific host glands, enter the bloodstream for transport throughout the body.* Hormones generally fit into one of two categories: **steroid-derived hormones** and **amine** and **polypeptide hormones** synthesized from amino acids. In contrast to steroid hormones, amine and peptide hormones are soluble in blood plasma. This allows easy uptake at target sites. The term **half-life** describes the time required to reduce a hormone's blood concentration by one half. For example, the half-life of epinephrine is slightly less than 3 minutes. Most orally consumed anabolic hormones such as testosterone have a half-life of approximately 3.5 hours. A hormone's half-life gives a good indication of how long its effect persists. TABLE 20.1 compares the storage, synthesis, release mechanism, transport medium, receptor location and receptor-ligand binding, and target organ response of the peptide, steroid, and amine hormones.

TABLE 20.2 lists eight different hormones produced by organs other than the major endocrine glands. Of these, **prostaglandins** constitute a third chemical class of hormones;

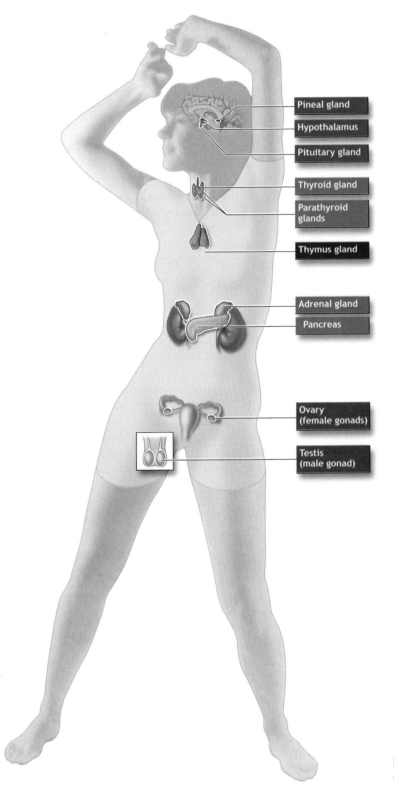

Figure 20.1 Location of the hormone-producing endocrine organs.

they represent biologically active lipids found in the plasma membrane of nearly all cells. **Erythropoietin**, a glycoprotein, stimulates the bone marrow's production of red blood cells.

Most hormones circulate in the blood as messengers that affect tissues a distance from the specific gland. Other hormones (e.g., prostaglandins and the gastrointestinal hormone **gastrin**) exert local effects in their region of synthesis.

Hormone–Target Cell Specificity

Hormones alter cellular reactions of specific "target cells" in four ways:

1. Modify rate of intracellular protein synthesis by stimulating DNA in the nucleus
2. Change rate of enzyme activity

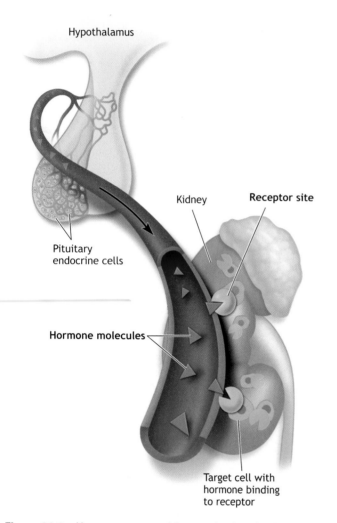

Hypothalamus

Pituitary
endocrine cells

Kidney

Receptor site

Hormone molecules

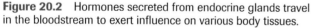

Target cell with
hormone binding
to receptor

Figure 20.2 Hormones secreted from endocrine glands travel in the bloodstream to exert influence on various body tissues.

3. Alter plasma membrane transport via a second-messenger system
4. Induce secretory activity

A target cell's response to a hormone depends largely on the presence of specific protein receptors that bind the hormone in a complementary way. Target cell receptors occur either on the plasma membrane (up to 10,000 receptors per cell) or in the cell's interior switch as occurs for fat-soluble steroid hormones that pass through the plasma membrane. Hormone receptors exist in specific local areas or more diffusely throughout the body. For example, adrenal cortex cells contain receptors for **adrenocorticotropic hormone (ACTH)**. In contrast, all cells contain receptors for **thyroxine**, the principal hormone that stimulates cellular metabolism.

Hormone–Receptor Binding

Hormone–receptor binding is the first step in initiating hormone action. The extent of a target cell's activation by a hormone depends on three factors: (1) hormone concentration in the blood, (2) number of target cell receptors for the

hormone, and (3) sensitivity or strength of the union between hormone and receptor. Consider cell hormone receptors as dynamic structures that continually adjust to physiologic demands. **Upregulation** describes the state whereby target cells form more receptors in response to increasing hormone levels. In contrast, prolonged exposure to high hormone concentrations desensitizes target cells to blunt hormonal stimulation. Such **downregulation** also involves a loss of receptors to prevent target cells from overresponding to persistently high hormone levels.

Cyclic AMP: The Intracellular Messenger. The binding of a hormone with its specific receptor in the plasma membrane alters the target cell's permeability to a particular chemical (e.g., insulin's effect on cellular glucose uptake) or modifies the target cell's manufacture of intracellular substances, primarily proteins. Such actions ultimately affect cellular function. FIGURE 20.3 shows that for the nonsteroid hormones epinephrine and glucagon, the binding hormone acts as **first messenger** to react with the enzyme **adenylate cyclase** in the plasma membrane. This forms the compound **cyclic 3′5′-adenosine monophosphate (cyclic AMP)** from an original ATP molecule. Cyclic AMP then acts as a ubiquitous **second messenger** to activate a specific protein kinase, which then activates a target enzyme to alter cellular function.

The sequence of reactions set into motion by cyclic AMP depends on three factors: (1) type of target cell, (2) specific enzymes contained in the target cell, and (3) specific hormone that acts as first messenger. In thyroid cells, for example, cyclic AMP generated from the binding of thyroid-stimulating hormone promotes thyroxine synthesis. In bone and muscle cells, the cyclic AMP produced via growth-hormone binding activates anabolic reactions to synthesize amino acids into tissue proteins.

Effects on Enzymes

Major hormone actions include altering enzyme activity and enzyme-mediated membrane transport. A hormone increases enzyme activity in one of three ways:

1. Stimulates enzyme production
2. Combines with the enzyme to alter its shape and ability to act, a chemical process known as **allosteric modulation**, which increases or decreases the enzyme's catalytic effectiveness
3. Activates inactive enzyme forms, thus increasing the total amount of active enzyme

In addition to altering enzyme activity, hormones either facilitate or inhibit uptake of substances by cells. Insulin, for example, facilitates glucose transport into the cell by combining with extracellular glucose and a glucose carrier within the plasma membrane. In contrast, epinephrine inhibits insulin release, thus slowing cellular glucose uptake.

Hormone action can exert potent, although often indirect, secondary effects. For instance, insulin release increases

TABLE 20.1 ■ STORAGE, SYNTHESIS, RELEASE MECHANISM, TRANSPORT MEDIUM, RECEPTOR LOCATION AND RECEPTOR-LIGAND BINDING, AND TARGET ORGAN RESPONSE OF THE PEPTIDE, STEROID, AND AMINE HORMONES

	PEPTIDE HORMONES	STEROID HORMONES	AMINE HORMONES	
			CATECHOLAMINES	THYROID HORMONES
Examples	Insulin, glucagon, leptin, IGF-1	Androgens, DHEA, cortisol	Epinephrine, norepinephrine	Thyroxine (T_4)
Synthesis and storage	Made in advance; stored in secretory vesicles	Synthesized on demand from precursors	Made in advance; stored in secretory vesicles	Made in advance; precursor stored in secretory vesicles
Release from parent cell	Exocytosis[a]	Simple diffusion	Exocytosis	Simple diffusion
Transport medium	Dissolved in plasma	Bound to carrier proteins	Dissolved in plasma	Bound to carrier proteins
Lifespan (half-life[b])	Short	Long	Short	Long
Receptor location	On cell membrane	Cytoplasm or nucleus; some have membrane receptors	On cell membrane	Nucleus
Response to receptor-ligand binding[c]	Activation of second messenger system; may activate genes	Activate genes for transcription and translation; may have nongenomic actions	Activation of second messenger systems	Activate genes for transcription and translation
General target response	Modification of existing proteins and induction of new protein synthesis	Induction of new protein synthesis	Modification of existing proteins	Induction of new protein synthesis

[a] Process in which intracellular vesicles fuse with the cell membrane and release their contents into the extracellular fluid.
[b] Amount of time required to reduce hormone concentration by one half.
[c] A ligand (the molecule that binds to a receptor) binds to a membrane protein, which triggers endocytosis (process of how a cell brings molecules into the cytoplasm in vesicles formed from the cell membrane).

glucose uptake by muscle fibers (primary effect), which increases synthesis of muscle glycogen (secondary effect). This effect of insulin on glucose uptake (and glycogen synthesis) maintains fuel homeostasis during exercise. In insulin-deficient individuals, depressed glucose metabolism impairs exercise performance. Inadequate cellular glucose uptake from chronic insulin deficiency abnormally increases blood glucose concentrations. In the extreme, glucose spills into the urine. We discuss the conditions of insulin insufficiency and/or insulin resistance in more detail on pp. 441–446.

Factors That Determine Hormone Levels

Hormone secretion rarely occurs at a constant rate. As with nervous system activity, hormone secretion usually adjusts rapidly to meet the demands of changing bodily conditions. For this reason, all protein hormones secrete in a pulsatile manner (see next section). Four factors determine plasma concentration of a particular hormone: (1) quantity synthesized in the host gland, (2) rate of either catabolism or

secretion into the blood, (3) quantity of transport proteins present (for some hormones), and (4) plasma volume changes.

The rate that endocrine glands secrete hormones depends on the magnitude of chemical stimulatory or inhibitory input from more than one source. For example, insulin secretion from the pancreas responds directly to plasma changes in glucose and amino acids, norepinephrine (from sympathetic neurons) and circulating epinephrine, and acetylcholine released from parasympathetic neurons. Each of these chemical messengers supplies inhibitory or excitatory input that determines whether insulin secretion increases or decreases. Over an extended time, hormone synthesis tends to equal hormone release. For a relatively short time, however, hormone release can exceed its synthesis. The term **secreted amount** describes the plasma concentration of a hormone. In reality, this represents the sum of hormone synthesis and release by the host gland, in addition to its uptake by receptor tissues and removal by liver and kidneys.

Hormone concentration depends on its rate of secretion into the blood and/or the rate of its metabolism (i.e., it becomes inactive). Hormone inactivation takes place at or near

TABLE 20.2 ■ HORMONES PRODUCED BY ORGANS OTHER THAN THE MAJOR ENDOCRINE ORGANS

HORMONE	COMPOSITION	SOURCE AND STIMULUS FOR SECRETION	TARGET AND OUTCOME
Prostaglandins	20-carbon fatty acid synthesized from arachidonic acid	*Source:* plasma membrane of different body cells *Stimulus:* local irritation, different hormones	*Target:* multiple sites *Outcome:* controls local hormone response; stimulates arterioles to increase blood pressure; increases uterine contractions, HCl and pepsin secretion in stomach, platelet aggregation, blood clotting, constriction of bronchioles, inflammation, pain, and fever
Gastrin	Peptide	*Source:* stomach *Stimulus:* food	*Target:* stomach *Outcome:* release of HCl
Enterogastrin	Peptide	*Source:* duodenum *Stimulus:* food (especially lipids)	*Target:* stomach *Outcome:* inhibits HCl secretion and gastro-intestinal motility
Secretin	Peptide	*Source:* duodenum *Stimulus:* food	*Target:* pancreas *Outcome:* release of bicarbonate-rich juice *Target:* liver *Outcome:* release of bile *Target:* stomach *Outcome:* inhibits secretion
Cholecystokinin	Peptide	*Source:* duodenum *Stimulus:* food	*Target:* pancreas *Outcome:* release of bicarbonate-rich juice *Target:* gallbladder *Outcome:* expulsion of bile *Target:* sphincter of Oddi *Outcome:* relaxes sphincter and allows bile to enter duodenum
Erythropoietin	Glycoprotein	*Source:* kidneys[a] *Stimulus:* hypoxia	*Target:* bone marrow *Outcome:* production of red blood cells
Active vitamin D_3	Steroid	*Source:* kidneys activate vitamin D from epidermal skin cells *Stimulus:* parathyroid hormone	*Target:* intestine *Outcome:* active transport of dietary Ca^+ across intestinal membranes
Atrial natriuretic hormone	Peptide	*Source:* atrium of heart *Stimulus:* atrial stretching	*Target:* kidneys *Outcome:* inhibits Na^+ reabsorption and renin release *Target:* adrenal cortex *Outcome:* inhibits secretion of aldosterone

[a] The kidneys release an enzyme that modifies a circulating blood protein to produce erythropoietin.

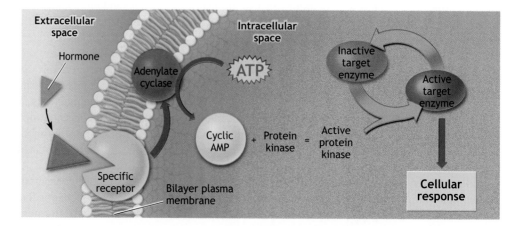

Figure 20.3 Action of non-steroid hormones. Circulating hormone (first messenger) binds to a specific receptor in the cell's plasma membrane to trigger production of cyclic AMP from ATP catalyzed by adenylate cyclase. Cyclic AMP then acts as second messenger to activate a protein kinase within the cell. This in turn activates a target enzyme to elicit the cellular response.

receptors or in the liver or kidneys. Because blood flow to splanchnic and renal areas decreases during exercise (blood distributes to active muscle), hormone inactivation rate decreases and plasma hormone concentration rises.

Steroid hormones must dissociate from their plasma protein carriers before exerting their influence. The quantity and affinity of the transport protein affects the amount of free hormone and its potential effect on tissue. Changes in plasma volume also alter hormone concentrations, independent of the host organ's secretion rate. For example, decreased plasma volume during prolonged exercise concurrently increases plasma hormone concentration, even without an absolute change in hormone amount.

FIGURE 20.4 shows that three factors—hormonal, humoral, and neural—stimulate endocrine gland activity.

- *Hormonal stimulation:* Hormones influence secretion of other hormones. For example, release-inhibiting hormones produced by the hypothalamus regulate the secretion of most anterior pituitary hormones. Anterior pituitary hormones, in turn, stimulate other endocrine organs to release their hormones into the bloodstream. The increased blood levels of a hormone produced by the final target gland provide feedback to *inhibit* release of anterior pituitary hormones and ultimately their own release.
- *Humoral stimulation:* Changing levels of ions and nutrients in blood, bile, and other body fluids stimulate hormone release. The term *humoral stimuli* describes these chemicals to distinguish them from hormonal stimuli, which also are fluid-borne

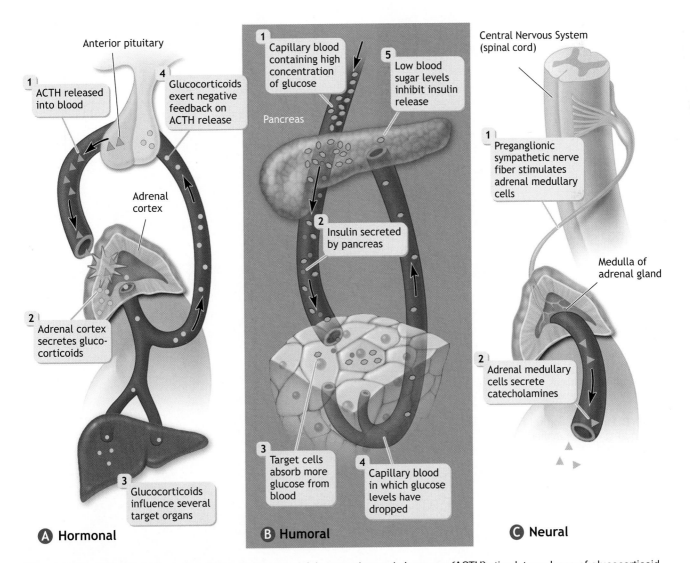

Figure 20.4 Endocrine gland stimulation. **A.** *Hormonal.* Adrenocorticotropic hormone (ACTH) stimulates release of glucocorticoid hormones by the adrenal cortex. **B.** *Humoral.* High blood glucose concentrations trigger insulin release, causing rapid cellular glucose uptake. The subsequent decrease in blood glucose removes the stimulus for insulin release. **C.** *Neural.* Sympathetic nervous system fibers trigger catecholamine release to blood. (From Marieb E. Anatomy and physiology. 6th edition, Redwood City, CA: Benjamin/Cummings, 2003.)

chemicals. For example, an increase in blood sugar concentration (the humoral agent) prompts the pancreas to release insulin. Insulin promotes glucose entry into cells, causing blood sugar levels to decline, thus ending the humoral stimulus for insulin release.

- *Neural stimulation:* Neural activity affects hormone release. For example, sympathetic neural activation of the adrenal medulla during stress releases epinephrine and norepinephrine. The nervous system can override normal endocrine control to maintain homeostasis. Insulin action normally maintains blood sugar levels between 80 and 120 mg per 100 mL (1 dL) of blood. During exercise, however, activation of the hypothalamus and sympathetic nervous system blunts insulin release. This attenuates a further decline in

blood sugar thus ensuring sufficient carbohydrate to fuel neural tissue and active muscle.

Patterns of Hormone Release

Most hormones respond to peripheral stimuli on an as-needed basis. Others release at regular intervals during a 24-hour cycle referred to as **diurnal variation**. Some secretory cycles span several weeks while others follow daily cycles. Cycling patterns are not confined to one category of hormones. FIGURE 20.5 shows the pulsatile release profiles during a normal day for the peptide luteinizing hormone (LH) and cortisol, a steroid hormone. Graph A illustrates two different LH pulsatile patterns: (1) during acute anorexia nervosa and (2) following clinical remission of anorexia nervosa

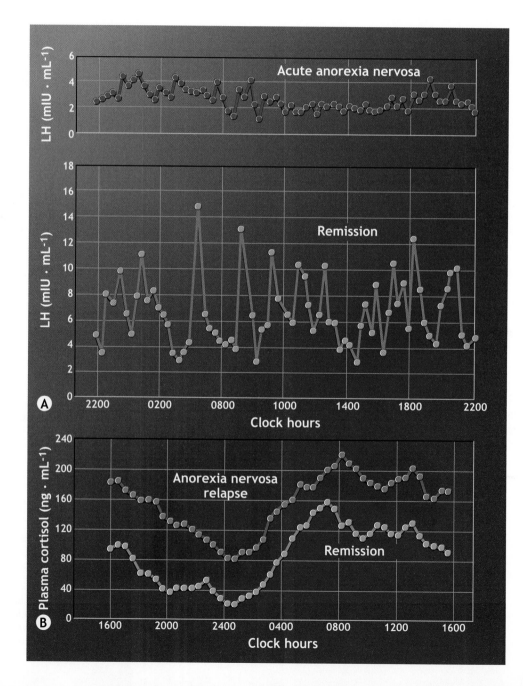

Figure 20.5   A. Cycling pattern of depressed LH release during acute episode of anorexia nervosa *(upper graphic)* and after clinical remission when body weight returns to normal *(lower graphic).* **B.** Pattern of cortisol release during relapse *(upper data points)* and after subsequent recovery *(lower data points)* in patients with anorexia nervosa. (From Boyar R, et al. Anorexia nervosa: immaturity of the 24-hour luteinizing hormone secretory pattern. N Engl J Med 1974; 291:861; Doerr P, et al. Relationship between weight gain and hypothalamic pituitary adrenal function in patients with anorexia nervosa. J Steroid Biochem 1980;13:529.)

with return of body weight to normal. The data points during anorexia resemble a prepubertal or early puberty pattern, while the remission data show a near-normal pulsatile pattern. The two sets of data points in part B of the figure show pulsatile patterns for plasma cortisol, an adrenocortical hormone, during relapse and after recovery in anorectic patients. Similar pulsatile patterns emerge under both conditions, but absolute hormone concentrations differ considerably between conditions.

Pulsatile hormone release patterns reveal information not available from a single blood sample that fails to show potentially significant variation in hormone levels during a daily cycle. Patterns of release and/or amplitude and frequency of discharge provide more meaningful information about hormone dynamics than simply examining mean concentration at any single time.

 INTEGRATIVE QUESTION

Discuss the meaning of the following statement: "Hormones act as silent messengers to integrate the body as a unit."

RESTING AND EXERCISE-INDUCED ENDOCRINE SECRETIONS

TABLE 20.3 lists the different endocrine host organs and nonglandular endocrine tissues, specific hormones secreted, hormone targets, and main effects. The following sections review these hormones, with special emphasis on their immediate response to exercise and adaptations to physical training.

Anterior Pituitary Hormones

Figure 20.6 illustrates the pituitary gland (also called the **hypophysis**), its secretions, and various target glands and their hormone secretions. Located beneath the base of the brain, the pituitary secretes at least six specialized polypeptide hormones. Because of its widespread influence, the anterior pituitary gland was often called the *master gland;* we now know, that the hypothalamus actually controls anterior pituitary activity; therefore, the hypothalamus should truly claim that title. Each of the primary pituitary hormones has its own hypothalamic releasing hormone, called a **releasing factor**. Neural input to the hypothalamus from anxiety, stress, and physical activity controls output of these releasing factors. In addition to the hormones displayed in FIGURE 20.6, the pituitary secretes **proopiomelanocortin (POMC)**, a large precursor molecule of other active molecules. POMC is the source of a number of neurotransmitters and hormones including ACTH, melanocortin peptides, and some of the naturally produced opiates such as β-endorphin (see p. 457). These hormones exert a remarkable range of influence, including effects on pigmentation, adrenocortical function, food intake and fat storage, and nervous and immune system functions.

Growth Hormone

Growth hormone–releasing factor from the hypothalamus influences resting **growth hormone** (**GH**) secretion by directly stimulating the anterior pituitary gland. GH (also called **somatotropin**) represents a family of related polypeptides (derived from one gene) that exert widespread physiologic activity because they promote cell division and cellular proliferation throughout the body. In adults, GH facilitates protein synthesis by (1) increasing amino acid transport through the plasma membrane, (2) stimulating RNA formation, or (3) activating cellular ribosomes that increase protein synthesis. GH also slows carbohydrate breakdown and initiates subsequent mobilization and use of fat as an energy source.

Growth Hormone, Exercise, and Tissue Synthesis. Short-term physical activity stimulates a sharp rise in GH pulse amplitude and the amount of hormone secreted per pulse.[14,102,148, 226] Perhaps more importantly, exercise stimulates release of GH isoforms with extended half-lives, thereby extending the action of this anabolic hormone on target tissues.[162] Augmented GH release benefits muscle, bone, and connective tissue growth and remodeling.[137] It also optimizes the fuel mixture during exercise, principally decreasing tissue glucose uptake, increasing free fatty acid mobilization, and enhancing liver gluconeogenesis. The net metabolic effect of increased exercise-induced GH production preserves plasma glucose concentration for central nervous system and muscle functions. Many of the growth-promoting effects of GH result from actions of intermediary chemical messengers on different target tissues, rather than a direct effect of GH itself. These peptide messengers, produced in the liver, are termed somatomedins or **insulin-like growth factors** (IGF-1 and IGF-II; see next section) because of their structural similarity to insulin. These factors exert potent peripheral effects on motor units and other tissues.

How exercise stimulates GH release to augment protein synthesis (and subsequent muscle hypertrophy), cartilage formation, skeletal growth, and cell proliferation remains unclear. Concurrent measurements of circulating lactate, alanine, and pyruvate; blood glucose; and body temperature reveal no association with GH secretory patterns during exercise.[106] One hypothesis suggests that exercise directly stimulates GH release (or release of somatomedins from the liver or kidneys), which in turn stimulates anabolic processes.[15] Exercise also may indirectly affect GH by stimulating cholinergic pathways to trigger GH release. Exercise stimulates endogenous opiate production that facilitates GH release by inhibiting the liver's production of somatostatin, a hormone that blunts GH release.[220]

FIGURE 20.7 outlines the overall metabolic actions of GH. GH modulates the metabolic mixture during exercise by stimulating fatty acid release from adipose tissue while simultaneously inhibiting cellular glucose uptake. This glucose-sparing action maintains blood glucose at relatively high levels to augment prolonged exercise performance.

Trained and sedentary individuals show similar increases in GH concentration when they exercise to exhaustion. In con-

TABLE 20.3 ■ ENDOCRINE ORGANS AND THEIR SECRETIONS, TARGETS, AND MAIN EFFECTS

LOCATION	GLAND OR CELL	CHEMICAL TYPE	HORMONE	TARGET	MAIN EFFECT
Adipose tissue	Cells	Peptide	Leptin; adiponectin (resistin)	Hypothalamus, other tissues	Food intake, metabolism, reproduction
Adrenal cortex	Gland	Steroid	Mineralocorticoids (aldosterone)	Kidney	Stimulates Na$^+$ reabsorption and K$^+$ secretion
			Glucocorticoids (cortisol; corticosterone)	Many tissues	Promotes protein and fat catabolism; raises blood glucose levels; adapts body to stress
			Androgens (androstenedione; dehydroepiandro-sterone [DHEA]; estrone)	Many tissues	Promotes sex drive
Adrenal medulla	Gland	Amine	Epinephrine, norepinephrine	Many tissues	Facilitates sympathetic activity; increases cardiac output; regulates blood vessels; increases glycogen catabolism and fatty acid release
Gastrointestinal tract (stomach and small intestine)	Cells	Peptide	Gastrin; cholecystokinin (CCK); secretin; glucose-dependent insulinotropic peptide (GIP)	GI tract and pancreas	Assist digestion and absorption of nutrients; regulates gastrointestinal motility
Heart	Cells	Peptide	Atrial natriuretic peptide (ANP)	Kidney tubules	Inhibits sodium reabsorption
Hypothalamus	Clusters of neurons	Peptide	Trophic hormones (releasing and release-inhibiting hormones: corticotropin-releasing hormone [CRH]; thyrotropin-releasing hormone [TRH]; growth hormone-releasing hormone [GHRH]; gonadrotropin-releasing hormone [GnRH])	Anterior pituitary	Release or inhibit anterior pituitary hormones
Kidney	Cells	Peptide Steroid	Erythropoietin (EPO) 1,25 Dihydroxy-vitamin D$_3$ (calciferol)	Bone marrow Intestine	Red blood cell production Increases calcium absorption
Liver	Cells	Peptide	Angiotensinogen	Adrenal cortex, blood vessels, brain	Aldosterone secretion; increases blood pressure
			Insulin-like growth factors (IGF-1)	Many tissues	Growth
Muscle	Cells	Peptide	Insulin-like growth factors (IGF-1, IGF-II); myogenic regulatory factors (MRFs)	Many tissues	Growth
Pancreas	Gland	Peptide	Insulin	Many tissues	Lowers blood glucose levels; promotes protein, lipid, and glycogen synthesis
			Glucagon	Many tissues	Raises blood glucose levels; promotes glycogenolysis and gluconeogenesis

TABLE 20.3 ■ *continued*

Location	Gland or Cell	Chemical Type	Hormone	Target	Main Effect
			Somatostatin (SS)	Many tissues	Inhibits secretion of pancreatic hormones; regulates digestion and absorption of nutrients by GI system
Parathyroid	Gland	Peptide	Parathyroid hormone (PTH)	Bone, kidney	Promotes Ca^{++} release from bone, Ca^{++} absorption by intestine, and Ca^{++} reabsorption by kidney; raises blood Ca^{++} levels; stimulates vitamin D_3 synthesis
Pineal gland	Gland	Amine	Melatonin	Unknown	Controls circadian rhythms
Pituitary-anterior	Gland	Peptides	Growth hormone (GH)	Many tissues	Growth; stimulates bone and soft tissue growth; regulates protein, lipid, and CHO metabolism
			Adrenocorticotropic hormone (ACTH)	Adrenal cortex	Stimulates glucocorticoid secretion
			Thyroid-stimulating hormone (TSH)	Thyroid gland	Stimulates secretion of thyroid hormones
			Prolactin	Breast	Milk secretion
			Follicle-stimulating hormone (FSH)	Gonads	Females: stimulates growth and development of ovarian follicles and estrogen secretion; Males: sperm production by testis
			Luteinizing hormone (LH)	Gonads	Females: stimulates ovulation, secretion of estrogen and progesterone; Males: testosterone secretion by testis
Pituitary-posterior	Extension of hypothalamic neurons	Peptide	Oxytocin (OT)	Breast and uterus	Females: stimulates uterine contractions and milk ejection by mammary glands; Males: unknown function
			Antidiuretic hormone (ADH or vasopressin)	Kidney	Decreases urine output by kidneys; promotes blood vessel (arteriole) constriction
Placenta (pregnant female)	Gland	Steroid	Estrogens and progesterone	Many tissues	Fetal and maternal development
		Peptide	Chorionic somatomammotropin (CS)		Metabolism
			Chorionic gonadotropin (CG)		Hormone secretion
Skin	Cells	Steroid	Vitamin D_3	Intermediate hormone form	Precursor of 1,25 dihydroxy-vitamin D_3
Ovaries (female)	Glands	Steroid	Estrogens (estradiol)	Many tissues	Egg production; secondary sex characteristics
			Progestins (progesterone)	Uterus	Promotes endometrial growth to prepare uterus for pregnancy
		Peptide	Ovarian inhibin	Anterior pituitary	Inhibits FSH secretion
Testes (male)	Glands	Steroid	Androgen	Many tissues	Sperm production; secondary sex characteristics
		Peptide	Inhibin	Anterior pituitary	Inhibits FSH secretion
Thymus	Gland	Peptide	Thymosin, thymopoietin	Lymphocytes	Stimulates proliferation and function of T lymphocytes
Thyroid	Gland	Iodinated amines	Triiodothyronine (T_3); thyroxine (T_4)	Many tissues	Increases metabolic rate; normal physical development
		Peptide	Calcitonin (CT)	Bone	Promotes calcium deposition in bone; lowers blood calcium levels

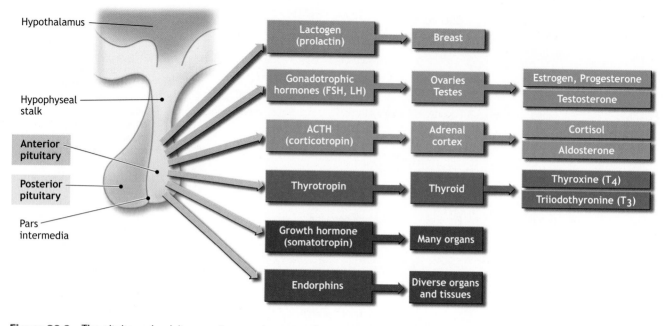

Figure 20.6 The pituitary gland, its secretions, and target options.

trast, the sedentary person maintains higher GH levels for several hours into recovery. During a standard bout of submaximal exercise, sedentary individuals have a greater GH response. Because this absolute submaximal exercise level represents greater stress for the less fit person, GH release generally relates more to the *relative* strenuousness of physical effort.

Insulin-Like Growth Factors

IGFs (or somatomedins) mediate many of GH's effects. In response to GH stimulation, liver cells synthesize **IGF-I** (a 70–amino acid polypeptide) and **IGF-II** (a 67–amino acid polypeptide), a process that requires between 8 and 30 hours. IGFs travel in the blood attached to one of five types of binding proteins for release as free hormones to interact with specific receptors. The factors that influence IGF transport include binding proteins within muscle, nutritional status, and plasma insulin levels.

The time required for IGF synthesis to GH stimulation affects any IGF appearance during or immediately following exercise. This suggests that its release results from disruption of cells already containing IGF. Also, GH-mediated release of IGF with exercise may reflect a different time course than typically observed in nonexercise conditions.[91]

Thyrotropin

Thyrotropin, also known as **thyroid-stimulating hormone (TSH)**, controls hormone secretion by the thyroid gland. TSH maintains growth and development of the thyroid gland and increases thyroid cell metabolism. Considering the important role of thyroid hormones in regulating overall body metabolism, one would expect TSH output from the pituitary

to increase during exercise, but this response does not occur consistently.

Adrenocorticotropic Hormone

ACTH, also known as **corticotropin**, functions as part of the **hypothalamic–pituitary–adrenal axis** to regulate adrenal cortex output of hormones in a manner similar to TSH control of thyroid gland secretion. ACTH acts directly to enhance fatty acid mobilization from adipose tissue, increase gluconeogenesis, and stimulate protein catabolism. Owing to difficulty in assay methods and rapid disappearance of this hormone from the blood, data remain scarce concerning ACTH response during exercise. ACTH concentrations may increase proportionately with exercise intensity and duration if intensity exceeds 25% of aerobic capacity.[46,85] Corticotropin-releasing hormone (CRH) and arginine vasopressin (AVP) mediate ACTH release. CRH exhibits a definite diurnal rhythm, with highest levels in early morning just after rising. As the day progresses, CRH levels decline, essentially blocking ACTH release. Factors that alter the normal ACTH rhythm by triggering CRH release include fever, hypoglycemia, and other forms of stress. Because CRH is both an ACTH regulator and a central nervous system neurotransmitter, it often is termed the *stress response integrator*. High-intensity exercise may favor AVP release while prolonged exercise favors CRH release, both resulting in ACTH inhibition.[88]

Prolactin

Prolactin (PRL) initiates and supports milk secretion from the mammary glands. PRL levels increase at high exercise intensities and return toward baseline within 45 minutes during recovery.[20] Owing to its important role in female sexual func-

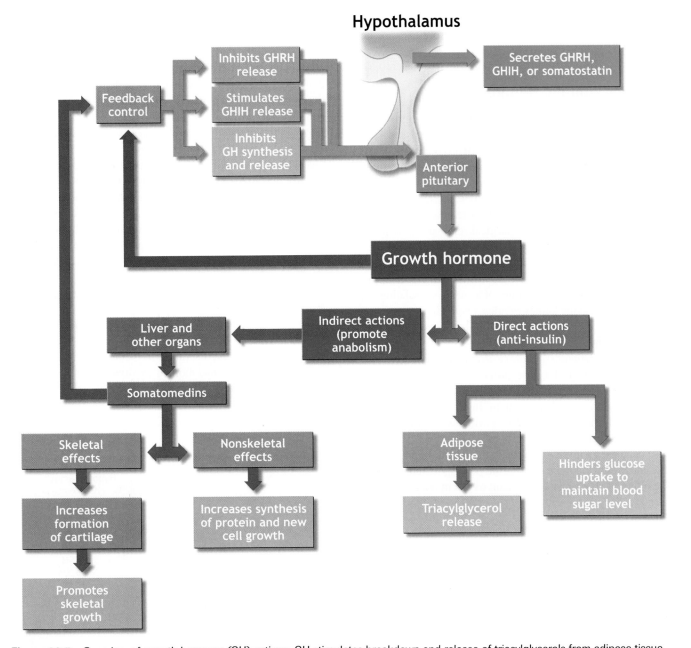

Figure 20.7 Overview of growth hormone (GH) actions. GH stimulates breakdown and release of triacylglycerols from adipose tissue and hinders cellular glucose uptake (antiinsulin effect) to maintain a relatively high blood glucose level. Somatomedins mediate the indirect anabolic effects of GH. Elevated GH levels and somatomedins provide feedback to promote GH-inhibiting hormone (GHIH) release and depress hypothalamic release of GH-releasing hormone (GHRH); this further inhibits GH release by the anterior pituitary gland.

tion, repeated exercise-induced PRL release may inhibit ovarian function and contribute to menstrual cycle alterations when females train intensely for athletic competition.[17,136] Greater increases in PRL occur in women who run without wearing an undergarment support;[172] either fasting or consuming a high-fat diet enhances release of this hormone.[95] PRL concentration increases in men following maximal exercise.[35]

Gonadotropic Hormones

Gonadotropic hormones stimulate the male and female sex organs to grow and secrete their hormones at a faster rate.

Follicle-stimulating hormone (FSH) and **luteinizing hormone (LH)** are the two gonadotropic hormones. FSH initiates follicle growth in the ovaries and stimulates these organs to secrete estrogen, one type of female sex hormone. LH complements FSH action to cause estrogen secretion and rupture of the follicle, which allows the ovum to pass through the fallopian tube for fertilization. In the male, FSH stimulates germinal epithelium growth in the testes to promote sperm development. LH also stimulates the testes to secrete testosterone.

Inconsistent reports describe short-term exercise–associated alterations in FSH and LH. LH release is normally pulsatile, making it difficult to separate any specific exercise-related change from the normal pulsatile pattern (see Fig. 20.5). Generally, LH concentration rises before exercise begins and peaks during recovery.

Posterior Pituitary Hormones

The posterior pituitary gland forms as an outgrowth of the hypothalamus and resembles true neural tissue (Fig. 20.6). This tissue, often called the **neurohypophysis**, stores **antidiuretic hormone** (**ADH** or **vasopressin**) and **oxytocin.** The posterior pituitary does not synthesize its hormones. Instead, the hypothalamus produces these hormones and secretes them to the neurohypophysis for release as needed via neural stimulation. Damage or surgical removal of the posterior pituitary does not dramatically affect ADH or oxytocin production.

ADH influences water excretion by the kidneys. Its action limits production of large volumes of urine by stimulating water reabsorption in the kidney tubules. Oxytocin initiates muscle contraction in the uterus and stimulates ejection of milk during lactation.

Exercise provides a potent stimulus for ADH secretion.[212] Increased ADH release, probably stimulated by sweating, helps to conserve body fluids, particularly during hot-weather exercise and accompanying dehydration. This water-conserving effect of ADH contributes to efficient modulation of the cardiovascular response to exercise.[141] ADH release decreases with fluid overload, thus increasing urine volume and producing more dilute urine (i.e., lighter color urine). The effect of short-term exercise on oxytocin release remains unknown.

Thyroid Hormones

The 15- to 20-g reddish brown thyroid gland, located nearer the first part of the trachea just below the larynx, comes under the influence of TSH produced by the anterior pituitary gland. In addition to secreting the calcium-regulating hormone calcitonin, the thyroid gland secretes two protein-iodine-bound hormones, **thyroxine** (T_4) and **triiodothyronine** (T_3, the active form of thyroid hormone). These two hormones are often referred to as the *major metabolic hormones*. More T_4 is secreted than T_3; although less abundant, T_3 acts several times faster than T_4. The majority of T_3 comes from the deiodination of T_4 in peripheral tissues, principally liver and kidney. Most receptor cells for T_4 metabolize it to T_3. T_3 and T_4 are not readily soluble in water, which means they bind to carrier proteins that circulate in blood. Thyroxine-binding globulin (glycoprotein synthesized in the liver) serves as the main transporter of thyroid hormones. This carrier protein (along with two others—transthyretin and albumin) permits a more consistent availability of thyroid hormones from which the active, free hormones release for target cell uptake.

Through its stimulating effect on enzyme activity, T_4 secretion raises metabolism of all cells except those in the brain, spleen, testes, uterus, and thyroid itself. For example, abnor-

mally high T_4 secretion raises basal metabolic rate (BMR) up to fourfold. This potent thermogenic effect produces large BMR deviations that often indicate thyroid gland abnormality (see Chapter 9). A person may lose weight rapidly with abnormally high thyroid activity. In contrast, depressed thyroid production blunts BMR, which usually leads to gains in body weight and body fat. *Fewer than 3% of obese persons show abnormal thyroid functions, so depressed thyroid activity cannot explain excessive body fat gain in most individuals.* For nervous system function, T_3 release facilitates neural reflex activity, whereas low T_4 levels cause sluggishness, often inducing people to sleep for up to 15 hours a day. Thyroid hormones provide important regulation for tissue growth and development, skeletal and nervous system formation, and maturation and reproductive capabilities. They also play a role in maintaining blood pressure by provoking an increase in adrenergic receptors in blood vessels.

Whole-body metabolism influences synthesis of thyroid hormones. Depressing the metabolic rate to some critical value directly stimulates hypothalamic release of TSH. This increases thyroid output and increases resting metabolism. Conversely, a chronic elevation in metabolism reduces TSH production, causing metabolism to slow. FIGURE 20.8 illustrates this exquisitely regulated feedback system.

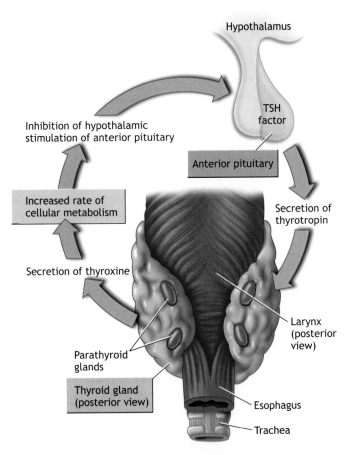

Hypothalamus

TSH factor

Inhibition of hypothalamic stimulation of anterior pituitary

Anterior pituitary

Secretion of thyrotropin

Increased rate of cellular metabolism

Secretion of thyroxine

Larynx (posterior view)

Parathyroid glands

Thyroid gland (posterior view)

Esophagus

Trachea

Figure 20.8   Feedback system that controls the release of thyroid hormone.

During exercise, blood levels of *free T_4* (thyroxine not bound to plasma proteins) increase by approximately 35%.[54] This increase could occur from an exercise-induced elevation in core temperature, which alters the protein binding of several hormones, including T_4. The importance of these transient exercise-induced alterations in thyroid hormone dynamics requires further study.[183]

Thyroid Hormones Affect Quality of Life

Thyroid hormones are not essential for life but they do affect its quality. In children, full expression of growth hormone requires thyroid activity. Thyroid hormones provide essential stimulation for normal growth and development, especially of nervous tissue. The actions of thyroid hormones become most noticeable in people who suffer from either hypersecretion or hyposecretion.

Hypersecretion of thyroid hormones (**hyperthyroidism**) produces the following four effects:

1. Increased oxygen consumption and metabolic heat production during rest (heat intolerance is a common complaint)
2. Increased protein catabolism and subsequent muscle weakness and weight loss
3. Heightened reflex activity and psychological disturbances that range from irritability and insomnia to psychosis
4. Rapid heart rate (tachycardia)

Hyposecretion of thyroid hormones (**hypothyroidism**) produces the following four effects:

1. Reduced metabolic rate and cold-intolerance from reduced internal heat production
2. Decreased protein synthesis produces brittle nails, thinning hair, and dry, thin skin
3. Depressed reflex activity, slow speech and thought processes, and feeling of fatigue (in infancy causes cretinism, marked by decreased mental capacity)
4. Slow heart rate (bradycardia)

Parathyroid Hormones

Normally, four parathyroid glands, measuring 6-mm long, 4-mm wide, and 2-mm deep embed in the posterior aspect of the thyroid gland (Fig. 20.8). As many as eight glands have been reported, and some have been found in other regions of the neck or in the thorax. The structure of the parathyroid glands differs considerably from thyroid tissues. The cells that synthesize and secrete parathyroid hormone are arranged in densely packed cords or nests surrounded by abundant capillaries. This contrasts with the cells responsible for thyroid hormone synthesis that arrange in spheres (*thyroid follicles*) filled with a proteinaceous colloid depot of thyroid hormone precursor. **Parathyroid hormone** (**PTH** or parathormone) controls blood calcium balance. A decrease in blood calcium levels triggers PTH release; increasing calcium concentrations inhibit its release. PTH's major effect increases ionic calcium levels by stimulating three target organs—bone, kidneys, and small intestine (FIG 20.9). PTH release results in the following three effects:

1. Activation of bone-reabsorbing cells (osteoclasts) to digest some of the bone matrix to release ionic calcium and phosphate to the blood
2. Enhancement of calcium ion reabsorption and decreased retention of phosphate by the kidneys
3. Increased calcium absorption by intestinal mucosa

Plasma calcium ion homeostasis modulates nerve impulse conduction, muscle contraction, and blood clotting. Limited evidence suggests that physical activity increases PTH release in young, middle-aged, and older individuals, an effect that contributes to the positive effects of exercise on bone mass accretion.[9,121,209] For example, one study exercised six subjects on bicycle ergometers at different intensities for 10 minutes.[19] Blood samples were analyzed for ionized calcium, total calcium, calcitonin, pH, and plasma PTH. Moderate exercise at 50% $\dot{V}O_{2max}$ initially depressed PTH levels, whereas near-maximal effort elevated hormone concentration during and in recovery from exercise. PTH release and calcium mobilization may provide the osteogenic raw material that allows mechanical forces from exercise to positively affect skeletal mass and density.

Adrenal Hormones

The adrenal glands appear as flattened, caplike tissues situated just above each kidney (FIG. 20.10). The glands have two distinct parts: **medulla** (inner portion) and **cortex** (outer portion). Each part secretes different types of hormones; consequently, the cortex and medulla are generally considered two distinct glands.

Adrenal Medulla Hormones

The adrenal medulla makes up part of the sympathetic nervous system. It acts to prolong and augment sympathetic effects by secreting two hormones, **epinephrine** and **norepinephrine**, collectively called **catecholamines**. FIGURE 20.11 shows the chemical structure of epinephrine and norepinephrine and the role of each in substrate mobilization. Norepinephrine, a hormone in its own right, serves as a precursor of epinephrine. It also acts as a neurotransmitter when released by sympathetic nerve endings. *Epinephrine represents 80% of adrenal medulla secretions, whereas norepinephrine provides the principle neurotransmitter released from the sympathetic nervous system.* An outflow of neural impulses from the hypothalamus stimulates the adrenal medulla to increase catecholamine release. These hormones then affect the heart, blood vessels, and glands in the same, albeit slower-acting way as direct sympathetic nervous system stimulation. Epinephrine's primary function in energy metabolism stimulates glycogenolysis (in the liver and active muscles) and lipolysis (in adipose tissue and active muscles); norepinephrine provides powerful lipolytic stimulation in adipose

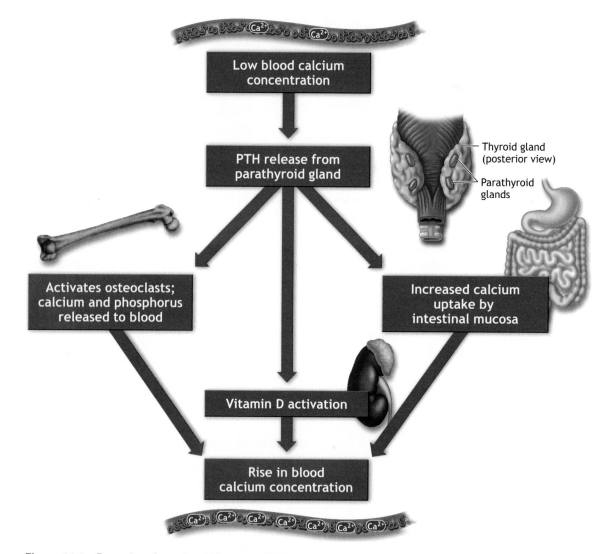

Figure 20.9 Dynamics of parathyroid hormone (PTH) release and its actions.

tissue.[48,202] Sympathetic nerve endings (including those to the adrenal gland) secrete both epinephrine and norepinephrine so it is more appropriate to discuss the "sympathoadrenal" response to exercise and training rather than simply the adrenal gland response. *The sympathoadrenal response to exercise most closely relates to relative rather than absolute exercise intensity.*

FIGURE 20.12 illustrates the catecholamine response at various exercise intensities (expressed as $\%\dot{V}O_{2max}$) in 10 male subjects. Norepinephrine increases markedly at intensities that exceed 50% $\dot{V}O_{2max}$, whereas epinephrine levels remain unchanged until exercise intensity exceeds about 60% $\dot{V}O_{2max}$. At maximum effort, an approximate two- to sixfold increase in norepinephrine release takes place. More than likely, increased secretion occurs from sympathetic postganglionic nerve endings and relates to cardiovascular and metabolic adjustments in active tissues. Exercise also increases epinephrine output from the adrenal medulla with the magnitude of increase directly related to intensity and duration of effort.[31,116,117,142] Athletes involved in sprint–power training show greater sympathoadrenergic activation during maximal

exercise than counterparts trained in aerobic exercise.[203] This difference relates to the higher anaerobic contribution to maximal exercise energy supply by the sprint–power athletes. Age does not affect the catecholamine response to exercise among individuals equal in aerobic fitness.[107,133] The effects of increased adrenal medulla activity on blood flow distribution, cardiac contractility, and substrate mobilization all benefit the exercise response.

Adrenocortical Hormones

The adrenal cortex, stimulated by corticotropin from the anterior pituitary, secretes **adrenocortical hormones**. These corticosteroid hormones fit functionally into one of three groups: (1) **mineralocorticoids**, (2) **glucocorticoids**, and (3) **androgens**—each produced in a different zone (layer) of the adrenal cortex.

Mineralocorticoids. As the name suggests, mineralocorticoids regulate the mineral salts sodium and potassium in the extracellular fluid. **Aldosterone**, the most physiologically im-

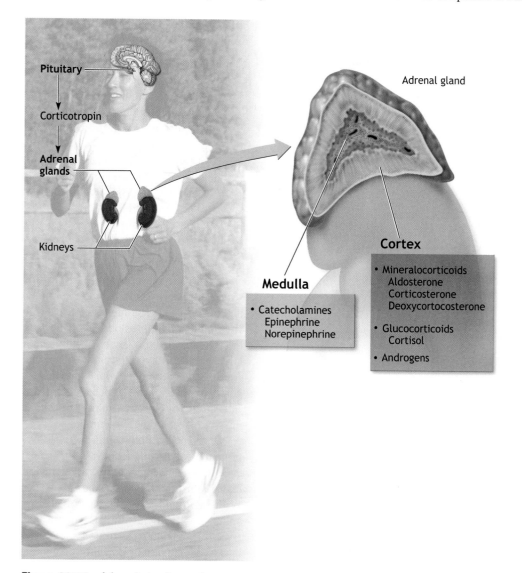

Figure 20.10 Adrenal gland secretions.

portant of the three mineralocorticoids, represents almost 95% of all mineralocorticoids produced.

FIGURE 20.13 shows four major controlling factors for aldosterone release from the adrenal cortex. *Aldosterone secretion controls total sodium concentration and extracellular fluid volume. It stimulates sodium ion reabsorption (along with fluid) in the distal tubules of the kidneys by increasing synthesis of sodium transporter proteins by the epithelial cells of the tubules and collecting duct.* Consequently, little sodium (and fluid) voids in the urine. Increases in cardiac output and arterial blood pressure also accompany increases in plasma volume with aldosterone secretion. In contrast, sodium and water literally flow into the urine when aldosterone secretion ceases. Aldosterone also helps to stabilize serum potassium and pH because the kidneys exchange either a K^+ or H^+ for each Na^+ reabsorbed. Proper mineral balance maintains nerve transmission and muscle function. Neuromuscular activity ceases without effective regulation of sodium and potassium exchange. As

with all steroid hormones, cellular response to increased aldosterone production is slow. It requires relatively prolonged exercise (>45 min) for aldosterone's effect to emerge; hence, its major effects occur during recovery.

Renin–Angiotensin Mechanism. Increased sympathetic nervous system activity during exercise constricts blood vessels to the kidneys. Reduced renal blood flow stimulates the kidneys to release the enzyme **renin** into the blood. Increased renin concentration activates production of two kidney hormones, **angiotensin II** and **angiotensin III**. These hormones stimulate arterial constriction and adrenocortical secretion of aldosterone, which causes the kidneys to retain sodium and excrete potassium. Renal absorption of sodium also conserves water, causing plasma volume to expand and blood pressure to increase.

Chronic reduction in renal blood flow at rest, perhaps from abnormal sympathetic stimulation, activates the **renin–angiotensin system**. Prolonged overresponse of this

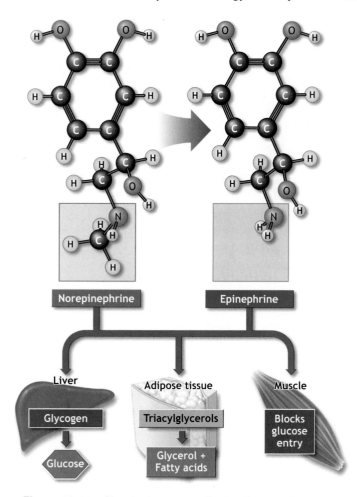

Figure 20.11 Chemical structure of epinephrine and norepinephrine and their role in mobilizing glucose from the liver and free fatty acids from adipose tissue and blunting glucose uptake by skeletal muscle. Norepinephrine serves both as a hormone and as a precursor of epinephrine. It also functions as a neurotransmitter when released by sympathetic nerve endings.

mechanism with resulting excess aldosterone output causes hypertension. High blood pressure associated with increased aldosterone production often occurs in teenage obesity.[178] Teenage hypertension relates to (1) decreased salt sensitivity (hence increased water retention), (2) increased sodium intake, and (3) decreased sensitivity to the effects of insulin (hyperinsulinemia). These interrelationships suggest a direct link between obesity as a disease and subsequent development of hypertension. Similar relationships have been reported for adults.[39,41,70]

Glucocorticoids. Emotionally charged situations or the stress of physical activity stimulate the hypothalamus to secrete **corticotropin-releasing factor** that causes the anterior pituitary to release ACTH. In turn, ACTH promotes glucocorticoid release by the adrenal cortex. **Cortisol** (hydrocortisone), the major glucocorticoid of the adrenal cortex,

affects glucose, protein, and free fatty acid metabolism as follows:

- Promotes breakdown of protein to amino acids in all cells except the liver; the circulation delivers these "liberated" amino acids to the liver for synthesis to glucose via gluconeogenesis
- Supports action of other hormones, primarily glucagon and GH in the gluconeogenic process
- Serves as an insulin antagonist by inhibiting cellular glucose uptake and oxidation
- Promotes triacylglycerol breakdown in adipose tissue to glycerol and fatty acids
- Suppresses immune system function
- Produces negative calcium balance

FIGURE 20.14 shows factors that affect cortisol secretion and its effects on target tissues. Cortisol is secreted with a strong diurnal rhythm; secretion normally peaks in the morning and diminishes at night. Cortisol secretion increases with stress; thus it is sometimes called the "stress" hormone. Even though considered a catabolic hormone, cortisol's important effect counters hypoglycemia and is thus essential for life. Animals whose adrenal glands have been removed die if exposed to severe environmental stress. Cortisol, required for full activity of glucagon and the catecholamines, exerts a permissive effect on these hormones.

Chronically high-serum cortisol levels initiate excessive protein breakdown, tissue wasting, and negative nitrogen balance. Cortisol secretion also accelerates fat mobilization for energy during starvation and intense, prolonged exercise. With rapid and large increases in cortisol output, the liver splits mobilized fat into its simple ketoacid components. Excess ketoacid concentrations in the extracellular fluid can lead to the potentially dangerous condition of **ketosis** (a form

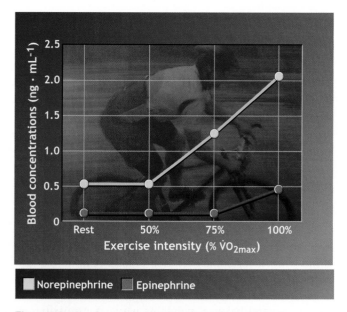

Figure 20.12 Catecholamine response to exercise of increasing intensity in 10 male subjects. (From Applied Physiology Laboratory, University of Michigan, Ann Arbor.)

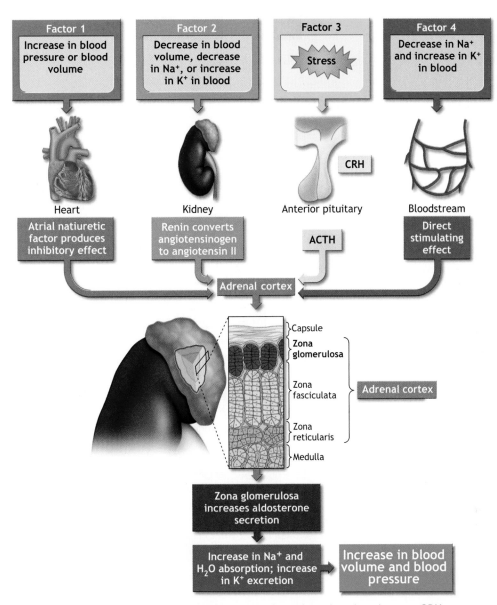

Figure 20.13   Four major factors control aldosterone release from the adrenal cortex. *CRH,* corticotropin-releasing hormone; *ACTH,* adrenocorticotropic hormone.

of acidosis). Individuals who subsist on very low carbohydrate, low-calorie weight-loss diets (termed *ketogenic diets*; see Chapter 30) can experience ketosis, augmented by elevated cortisol secretion.

Cortisol turnover, the difference between its production and removal, provides a convenient means to study cortisol response to exercise. Considerable variability exists in cortisol turnover with exercise, depending on intensity and duration, fitness level, nutritional status, and even circadian rhythm.[38,204] Most research indicates that cortisol output increases with exercise intensity; this accelerates lipolysis, ketogenesis, and proteolysis. In addition, extremely high cortisol levels occur following long-duration exercise such as marathon running or an intense bout of resistance training.[32,171] Even during more moderate exercise, plasma cortisol concentration rises with prolonged duration. Data for cortisol turnover indicate that highly trained runners maintain a state of hypercortisolism that height-

ens before competition or intense training.[72,128] Cortisol levels also remain elevated for up to 2 hours following exercise, suggesting that cortisol plays a role in tissue recovery and repair. Unlike the direct, active metabolic effect of epinephrine and glucagon on fuel homeostasis during exercise, cortisol exerts a more facilitating effect on substrate use.

Gonadocorticoids. The reproductive organs (gonads) provide the major source of the so-called sex steroids, but the adrenal cortex produces androgen hormones (gonadocorticoids) with similar actions. For example, the adrenal cortex produces **dehydroepiandrosterone**, which exerts effects similar to those of the dominant male hormone testosterone. Treatment with 50 mg of dehydroepiandrosterone in women with adrenal insufficiency over a four-month trial improved well being and sexual responsiveness as well as scores for depression and anxiety compared to placebo treatment.[227] The adrenal cortex also pro-

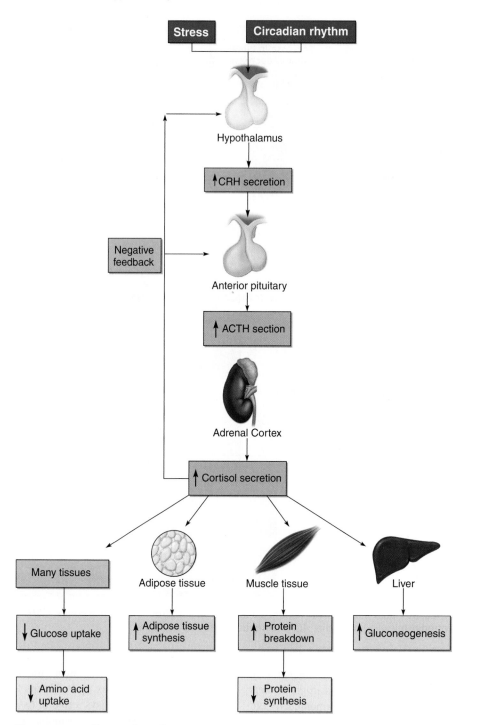

Figure 20.14   Factors that affect cortisol secretion and its actions on target tissues. CRH, corticotropic releasing hormone; ACTH, adrenocorticotropic hormone.

duces small amounts of the "female" hormones estrogen and progesterone.

GONADAL HORMONES

The testes in the male and ovaries in the female are the reproductive glands. These endocrine glands produce hormones that promote sex-specific physical characteristics and initiate and maintain reproductive function. No distinctly "male" or "female" hormones exist but rather general differences in hormone

concentrations between the sexes. **Testosterone** is the most important androgen secreted by the interstitial cells of the testes. FIGURE 20.15 shows that testosterone initiates sperm production and stimulates development of male secondary sex characteristics. In addition, testosterone's anabolic, tissue-building role contributes to the male–female differences in muscle mass and strength that emerge at the onset of puberty. As noted in Chapter 2, testosterone conversion to estrogen in peripheral tissues, under control of the enzyme aromatase, provides the male with protection in maintaining bone structure throughout life.

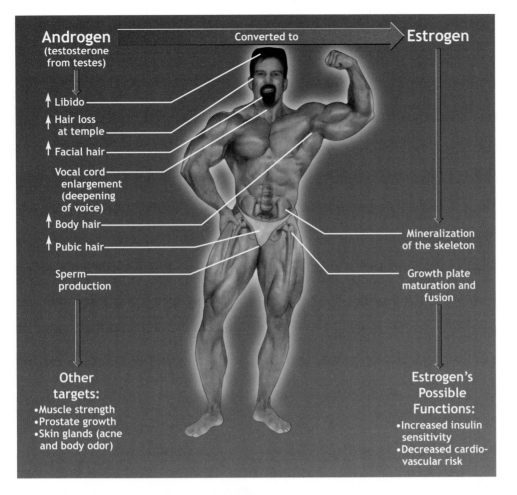

Androgen
(testosterone
from testes)

Converted to → **Estrogen**

↑ Libido
↑ Hair loss
   at temple
↑ Facial hair
   Vocal cord
   enlargement
   (deepening
   of voice)
↑ Body hair
↑ Pubic hair
   Sperm
   production

Mineralization
of the skeleton

Growth plate
maturation and
fusion

**Other
targets:**
• Muscle strength
• Prostate growth
• Skin glands (acne
  and body odor)

**Estrogen's
Possible
Functions:**
• Increased insulin
  sensitivity
• Decreased cardio-
  vascular risk

Figure 20.15 Androgen's effects in men. Binding with special receptor sites in muscle and various other tissues, androgen (testosterone) contributes to male secondary sex characteristics and sex differences in muscle mass and strength that develop at the onset of puberty. Some androgen converts to estrogen in peripheral tissues and gives males a considerable edge over females in maintaining bone mass throughout life.

The ovaries provide the primary source of estrogens, particularly **estradiol** and **progesterone**. Estrogens regulate ovulation, menstruation, and physiologic adjustments during pregnancy. Estrogen, both circulating in the bloodstream and generated locally in peripheral tissues, also exerts effects on blood vessels, bone, lungs, liver, intestine, prostate, and testes through action on α- and β-receptor proteins. Progesterone contributes specific regulatory input to the female reproductive cycle, uterine smooth muscle action, and lactation. Controversy exists concerning the role of estrogen and progesterone in substrate metabolism, particularly during exercise.[5,144] Estradiol-17β (biologically active estrogen synthesized from cholesterol) increases free fatty acid mobilization from adipose tissue and inhibits glucose uptake by peripheral tissues. In this way, the increases in estradiol-17β and GH during exercise exert similar metabolic effects.

Testosterone

Plasma testosterone concentration commonly serves as a physiologic marker of anabolic status. In addition to its direct effects on muscle tissue synthesis, testosterone indirectly affects a muscle fiber's protein content by promoting GH release, which leads to IGF synthesis and release from the liver. Testosterone also interacts with neural receptors to increase neurotransmitter release and initiate structural protein changes that alter the size

of the neuromuscular junction. These neural effects enhance the force-production capabilities of skeletal muscle.

Testosterone's effect on the cell nucleus remains controversial. More than likely, a transport protein (sex-hormone–binding globulin) delivers testosterone to target tissues, after which testosterone associates with a membrane-bound or cytosolic receptor. It subsequently migrates to the cell nucleus where it interacts with nuclear receptors to initiate protein synthesis.

Plasma testosterone concentration in females, although only one tenth that in males, increases with exercise. Exercise also elevates estradiol and progesterone levels. In untrained males, both resistance exercise and moderate aerobic exercise increase serum and free testosterone levels after 15 to 20 minutes. The mechanism for this increase remains unclear. Findings remain equivocal concerning the effect of intense endurance exercise on testosterone levels.[171,210]

FIGURE 20.16 shows the pattern of plasma cortisol and testosterone 48 hours before swimming, and immediately following 15 × 200-m freestyle at the swimmer's competitive velocity with a 20-second rest between swims, and 1 hour into recovery. Four 6-week periods formed the training program with careful monitoring of training volume. The bar graphs (right) show values for swim volume during the four training periods, including average performance during time trials. The results show clearly that cortisol and testosterone

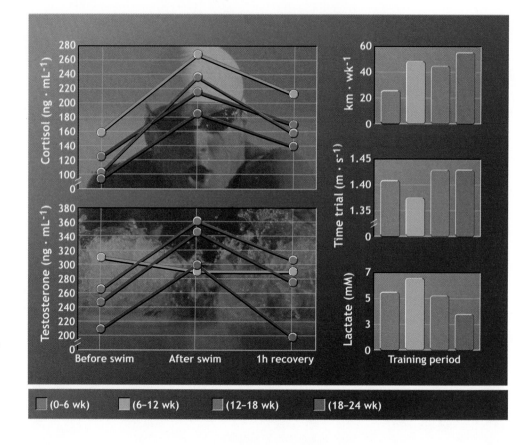

Figure 20.16 Pattern of plasma cortisol and testosterone concentrations measured at three time intervals (4 h before swimming, immediately after multiple sprint swims, and after 1-h recovery) over a 24-week swim-training season. *Bar graphs on right show* values for swim volume, time-trial performance, and blood lactate during the four 6-week training periods. (Modified from Bonifazi M, et al. Blood levels of exercise during the training season. In: Miyashita M. et al., eds. Medicine and science in aquatic sports. Basel: Karger, 1994.)

remain elevated post exercise. Values remained higher 1 hour after exercise except for testosterone levels in training weeks 6–12 and 18–24. The generalized decrease in cortisol and testosterone concentrations when the swimmers "peaked" for the championships (weeks 18–24) indicates long-term adaptation for these hormones, not the immediate result of excess stress induced by overtraining and subsequent poor performance. The depressed performance during weeks 18–24 might indicate overtraining; this period corresponded to a large increase in training volume. Chapter 21 provides an in-depth discussion of overtraining and its related syndrome.

 INTEGRATIVE QUESTION

Hormones play crucial roles in normal growth and development and the regulation of physiologic function. Give specific examples of why "more is not necessarily better" for these chemicals.

Pancreatic Hormones

The pancreas gland, approximately 14-cm long and weighing about 60 g, lies just below the stomach on the posterior abdominal wall. Two different types of tissues, **acini** and **islets of Langerhans**, named for German scientist Paul Langerhans who first described this cluster of cells (FIG. 20.17), compose the pancreas. The islets are comprised of about 20% **α-cells** that secrete glucagon and 75% **β-cells** that secrete insulin and a peptide called amylin. The remaining cells are somatostatin-secreting D cells and PP cells that produce pancreatic polypeptide. The acini serve an exocrine function and secrete digestive enzymes.

Insulin

Insulin regulates glucose entry into all tissues (primarily muscle and adipose cells) except the brain. Insulin's action mediates **facilitated diffusion**. In this process, glucose combines with a carrier protein on the cell's plasma membrane for transport into cells. In this way, insulin regulates glucose metabolism. Any glucose not immediately catabolized for energy either stores as glycogen for later use or synthesizes to triacylglycerol. Without insulin, only trace amounts of glucose enter the cells. FIGURE 20.18A illustrates that the anabolic functions of insulin promote glycogen, protein, and fat synthesis; Figure 20.18B outlines the target tissues and specific metabolic responses to insulin's action.

Insulin-mediated glucose uptake by cells (and correspondingly reduced hepatic glucose output) following a meal decreases blood glucose levels. In essence, insulin exerts a hypoglycemic effect by reducing blood glucose concentration. Conversely, with insufficient insulin secretion (or decreased insulin sensitivity), blood glucose concentration increases from a normal level of about 90 mg · dL^{-1} to a high of 350 mg · dL^{-1}. When blood glucose levels remain high, glucose ultimately

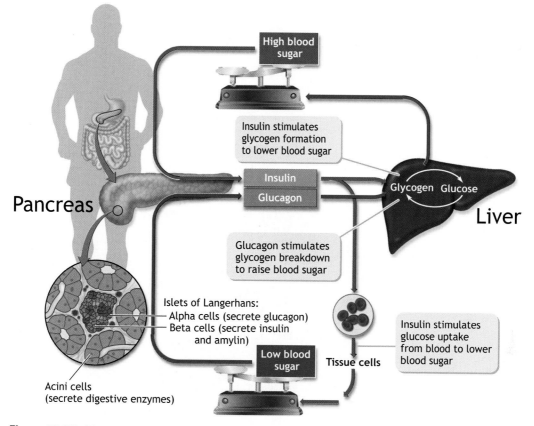

Figure 20.17 The pancreas, its secretions, and their actions.

spills into the urine. In the absence of insulin, fatty acids mobilize as the primary energy substrate.

Insulin also exerts a pronounced effect on fat synthesis. A rise in blood glucose levels (as normally occurs after a meal) stimulates insulin release. This causes some glucose uptake by fat cells for synthesis to triacylglycerol. Insulin's action also triggers intracellular enzyme activity that facilitates protein synthesis. This occurs by one or all of the following actions: (1) increasing amino acid transport through the plasma membrane, (2) increasing cellular levels of RNA, and (3) increasing protein formation by ribosomes.

Insulin Transport into Cells: Glucose Transporters. Cells possess different glucose transport proteins (termed **glucose transporters** or **GLUTs**), which vary in response to insulin and glucose concentrations.[131,181] Muscle fibers contain GLUT-1 and GLUT-4, with most glucose entering by the GLUT-1 carrier during rest. With high blood glucose or insulin concentrations, as occur after eating or during exercise, muscle cells receive glucose via the insulin-dependent GLUT-4 transporter. GLUT-4 action is mediated through a second messenger, perhaps stimulated by muscle action, which permits migration of the intracellular GLUT-4 protein to the surface to promote glucose uptake. The fact that GLUT-4 moves to the cell surface through a separate, *insulin-independent* mechanism coincides with observations that active muscles can take up glucose without insulin.

Glucose–Insulin Interaction. *Blood glucose levels within the pancreas directly control insulin secretion.* Elevated blood glucose levels cause insulin release. This, in turn, induces glucose entry into cells, lowers blood glucose, and removes the stimulus for insulin release. In contrast, a decrease in blood glucose concentration dramatically lowers blood insulin levels, thus providing a favorable milieu for increasing blood glucose. The interaction between glucose and insulin provides a feedback mechanism that normally maintains blood glucose concentration within narrow limits. Insulin secretion also increases in response to rising levels of plasma amino acids.

FIGURE 20.19 relates plasma insulin concentration to exercise duration for cycling at 70% $\dot{V}O_{2max}$. The inset graph shows insulin response as a function of exercise intensity (%$\dot{V}O_{2max}$). The decreased insulin concentration (below rest values) as exercise duration extends or intensity increases results from inhibitory effects of an exercise-induced catecholamine release on pancreatic β-cell activity. Catecholamine suppression of insulin relates directly to exercise intensity. *Exercise inhibition of insulin output explains why no excessive insulin release (and possible rebound hypoglycemia) occurs with a concentrated glucose feeding during exercise.* Prolonged exercise derives progressively more energy from free fatty acids mobilized from the adipocytes from reduced insulin output and decreased carbohydrate reserves. Blood glucose lowering with prolonged exercise directly enhances hepatic glucose output

A

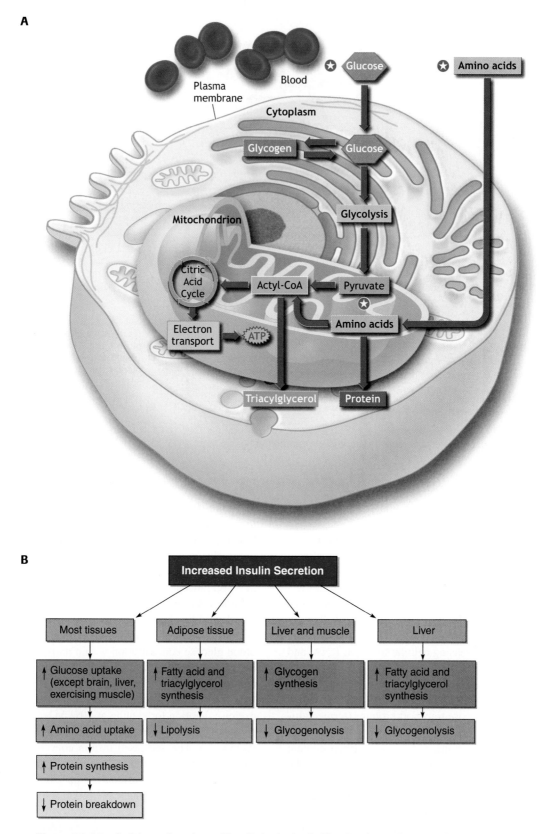

Figure 20.18   A. Primary functions of insulin in the body. The ⊛s show where insulin exerts its influence in metabolism. **B.** Target tissues and specific metabolic responses to insulin's action. The anabolic functions of increased insulin promote glycogen, protein, and fat synthesis.

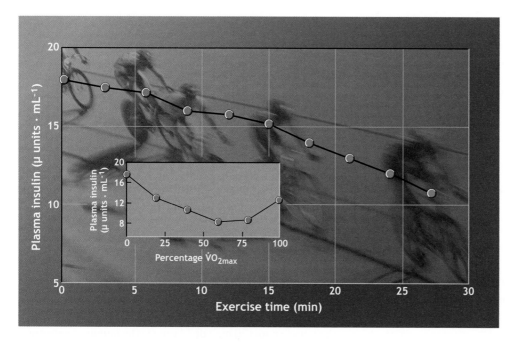

Figure 20.19 Plasma insulin levels during 30 minutes of cycle ergometer exercise at 70% $\dot{V}O_{2max}$. *Inset,* data show insulin concentrations related to exercise intensity (%$\dot{V}O_{2max}$). (From Applied Physiology Laboratory, University of Michigan, Ann Arbor.)

and sensitizes the liver to the glucose-releasing effects of glucagon and epinephrine, whose actions help to stabilize blood glucose levels.

Diabetes Mellitus. Diabetes mellitus consists of subgroups of disorders (with different pathophysiologies) that currently afflict 18.2 million Americans (6.3% of U.S. population in 2002), with the number expected to increase to 23 million by 2025 (FIG. 20.20). Above age 60, the disease afflicts 8.6 million people or 18.3% of all individuals in this age group. Each year, more than 1.3 million Americans age 20 years or older learn they have diabetes. Diabetes is the sixth leading cause of death by disease in the United States (213,000 diabetes-related deaths in 2000) and the leading cause of blindness, kidney failure, and limb amputations. Diabetes most likely represents an independent risk factor for cardiovascular disease.[66] The terms **type 1** and **type 2** identify the two largest diabetes subgroups. Terms *insulin-dependent diabetes mellitus* (type 1) and *non–insulin-dependent diabetes mellitus* (type 2), in addition to Roman numerals I and II for subgroup identification, respectively, have been discontinued because they imply specific and different treatments rather than reflecting an underlying etiology. For example, many persons with type 2 diabetes require exogenous insulin.

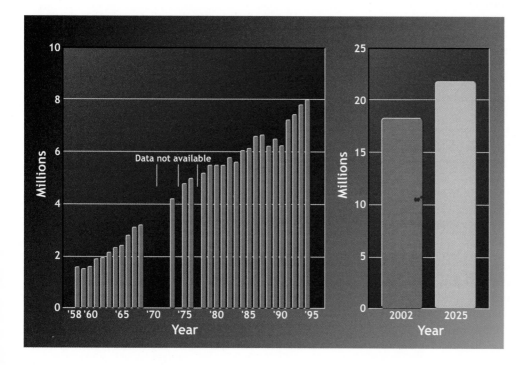

Figure 20.20 Rates of diagnosed cases of type 1 and type 2 diabetes between 1958 and 1995 and projected increases in new cases to the year 2025. Type 2 diabetes represents nearly 95% of all cases. (Source: National Institutes of Health.) Recent data and statistics from: diabetes. niddk.nih.gov/dm/pubs/statistics/.

Diabetes symptoms include:

- Presence of glucose in the urine (glycosuria)
- Frequent urination (polyuria)
- Excessive thirst (polydipsia)
- Extreme hunger (polyphagia)
- Unexplained weight loss
- Increased fatigue
- Irritability
- Blurry vision
- Numbness or tingling in the extremities (hands, feet)
- Slow-healing wounds or sores
- Abnormally high frequency of infection

Use the following Internet site to calculate your diabetes risk: www.diabetes.org/risk-test.jsp.

Tests for Diabetes Mellitus. Different tests diagnose diabetes, including the laboratory-based glucose and insulin clamp methodology, an oral glucose-tolerance test, and a simple 8-hour fasting plasma glucose test.

- The clamp procedure involves maintaining insulin at a constantly above-normal blood concentration using infusion technology (termed **hyperinsulinemic clamp**). Once insulin stabilizes at the higher level, the body's use of glucose is measured by infusing a known amount of glucose into the patient's blood. A **euglycemic clamp** maintains blood glucose at near-normal concentration with insulin production measured. A **euglycemic–hyperinsulinemic clamp** combines both clamp procedures. A large glucose uptake for a given insulin concentration reflects increased **insulin sensitivity**, while increased insulin release to a constant glucose condition relates to augmented **insulin responsiveness**. Decreased insulin sensitivity indicates inability of cells to respond adequately to insulin to increase glucose uptake. Type 2 diabetes commonly reflects inadequacies in either insulin receptors or cellular response to insulin binding. Decreased insulin responsiveness indicates impaired β-cell function evident in some type 2 diabetics and is the primary cause of type 1 diabetes.
- **Oral glucose-tolerance test** evaluates blood sugar levels 2 hours after drinking a concentrated glucose-containing solution. Delayed removal of ingested glucose indicates diabetes.
- **Fasting plasma glucose (FPG) test** measures plasma glucose following an 8-hour fast. The American Diabetes Association (www.diabetes.niddk.gov/) currently recommends the FPG test.

Considerable risks exist for impaired glucose homeostasis—probably a genetic trait that can manifest itself in adolescence—in which blood glucose remains elevated but not high enough for diabetic classification. Nondiabetic middle-aged men whose FPG falls in the upper range of normal show a higher risk of death from heart disease than those in the low-

CLASSIFICATION CATEGORIES FOR FASTING BLOOD GLUCOSE

CATEGORY	FASTING PLASMA GLUCOSE
Normal	<110 mg $\cdot$ dL^{-1}
Impaired range	$110–125$ mg $\cdot$ dL^{-1}
Suspected diabetes	>125 mg $\cdot$ dL^{-1}

normal range.[10] Men with fasting blood glucose levels above 85 mg $\cdot$ dL^{-1} have a 40% higher risk of cardiovascular death than men with lower values, even after adjusting for age, smoking habits, blood pressure, and fitness status. The current plasma glucose cutoff for suspected diabetes is an FPG of 126 mg $\cdot$ dL^{-1}, down from the previous standard of 140 mg $\cdot$ dL^{-1} set in 1979. This lower cutoff acknowledges that patients can remain asymptomatic despite microvascular complications (damaged small blood vessels) with FPG values in the low- to mid-120 mg $\cdot$ dL^{-1} range. The *impaired range* represents a transition between normal and overt diabetes. In this situation, the body no longer responds properly to insulin and/or secretes inadequate insulin to achieve a more healthful blood glucose concentration.

Metabolic Syndrome X

Metabolic syndrome X (or simply metabolic syndrome), first mentioned in the late 1980s,[52,105,173–175] represents a multifaceted grouping of coronary artery disease risks.[12,51,125] Diet-induced insulin resistance/hyperinsulinemia often occurs before manifestations of the metabolic syndrome of obesity, insulin resistance, glucose intolerance, dyslipidemia, and hypertension.[6,147,196] In essence, the syndrome reflects a concurrence of four factors:

1. Disturbed glucose and insulin metabolism (fasting glucose ≥ 110 mg $\cdot$ dL^{-1})
2. Overweight with abdominal fat distribution (waist circumference: men >102 cm [40 in]; women >88 cm [35 in])
3. Mild dyslipidemia (triacylglycerols ≥ 150 mg$\cdot$dL^{-1}; high-density lipoprotein cholesterol: men, <40 mg $\cdot$ dL^{-1}; women <50 mg $\cdot$ dL^{-1})
4. Hypertension ($\geq 130/\geq 85$ mm Hg)

These individuals exhibit high risk for cardiovascular disease, type 2 diabetes, Alzheimer's disease, and all-cause mortality.[124] Some researchers maintain that inappropriate diet consumption, sedentary lifestyle, and poor levels of muscular strength and cardiorespiratory fitness not only associate with the syndrome but represent features of it.[99,123,177] Estimates place the age-adjusted prevalence of the metabolic syndrome in the United States at nearly 25% or about 47 million men and women.[51] The age-adjusted prevalence is similar for men (24%) and women (23.4%). Mexican Americans have the highest age-adjusted prevalence of the syndrome (31.9%). The lowest prevalence occurs among whites (23.8%), African

METABOLIC SYNDROME X

- Insulin resistance
- Glucose intolerance
- Dyslipidemia (high triacylglycerols, low HDL, high LDL)
- Stroke
- Upper-body obesity
- Type 2 diabetes mellitus
- Hypertension
- Coronary artery disease
- Reduced ability to dissolve blood clots

Americans (21.6%), and people reporting "other" for race or ethnicity (20.3%). Among African Americans, women had about a 57% higher prevalence than men; Mexican American women had a 26% higher prevalence.

This "disease of modern civilization" afflicts a large number of adults (more common in men than women) in western industrialized countries. Disease occurrence relates to genetic, hormonal, and lifestyle factors of obesity, physical inactivity, and nutrient excesses, including high intakes of saturated and *trans*-fatty acids. Although characterized by the clustering of insulin resistance and hyperinsulinemia, dyslipidemia (atherogenic plasma lipid profile), essential hypertension, abdominal (visceral) obesity, and glucose intolerance, the syndrome also relates to abnormalities of blood coagulation, hyperuricemia, and microalbuminuria.

Psychosocial stress, socioeconomic disadvantage, and abnormal psychiatric traits also link to the syndrome's pathogenesis.[11,12] In all likelihood, such factors relate to a central neuroendocrine origin as enhanced activation of the hypothalamic–pituitary–adrenal axis, with endpoints of hyperinsulinemia, obesity, coronary artery disease, type 2 diabetes, stroke, and increased colorectal cancer risk.[188]

TABLE 20.4 provides percentage body fat ranges and associated risk equivalent to the traditional BMI cutoffs for the metabolic syndrome for black and white men and women. Lifestyle modifications that include increased regular physical activity represent the cornerstone of national recommendations to prevent the metabolic syndrome.[147]

Insulin Actions and Impaired Glucose Homeostasis

FIGURE 20.21 summarizes insulin's normal response and the response under insulin-resistant and type 2 diabetes conditions. The increase in blood glucose concentration following a meal induces insulin release from the β-cells in the islets of Langerhans. Insulin then migrates in the blood to target cells throughout the body where it binds to receptor molecules on the cell surface. Insulin–receptor interaction triggers a series of events within the cell that enhance glucose uptake and subsequent catabolism or storage as glycogen and/or fat. A defect anywhere along the pathway for glucose uptake signals diabetes. Possible causes include (1) destruction of β-cells, (2) abnormal insulin synthesis, (3) depressed insulin release, (4) inactivation of insulin in the blood by antibodies or other blocking agents, (5) altered insulin receptors or a decreased number of receptors on peripheral cells, (6) defective processing of the insulin message within the target cells, and (7) abnormal glucose metabolism.

Type 1 Diabetes. Type 1 diabetes, formerly called juvenile-onset diabetes, typically occurs in younger individuals and represents between 5 and 10% of all diabetes cases. This

TABLE 20.4 ■ THRESHOLDS OF PERCENTAGE BODY FAT (%BF) CORRESPONDING TO ESTABLISHED BODY MASS INDEX CUTOFFS ASSOCIATED WITH METABOLIC SYNDROME RISK

	%BF AND CORRESPONDING PERCENTILES									
	MEN					WOMEN				
	BLACK		WHITE			BLACK		WHITE		
BMI CUTOFFS (KG/M²)	CUTOFF	PERCENTILE	CUTOFF	PERCENTILE	MEAN[a]	CUTOFF	PERCENTILE	CUTOFF	PERCENTILE
18.5	12.7	8.9	11.0	3.9	12	25.4	11.7	22.5	24
25	21.7	43.5	21.2	41.0	21	32.0	29.3	30.8	31
30	28.3	80.9	29.1	87.6	29	37.1	52.5	37.2	37
35	35.0	97.6	37.0	99.4	36	42.1	75.9	43.5	43

[a]Values were rounded.

From Zhu S, et al. Percentage body fat ranges associated with metabolic syndrome risk: results based on the third National Health and Nutrition Examination Survey (1988–1994). Am J Clin Nutr 2003;78:228.

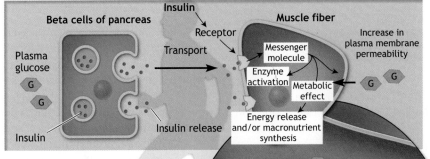

A Normal response

The rise in blood glucose G after eating stimulates insulin I release from the beta cells of the pancreas. Insulin mediates facilitated diffusion into the cell where glucose combines with a carrier on the plasma membrane of muscle and adipose tissue cells. Any glucose not immediately catabolized for energy stores as glycogen or synthesizes to fat for later use.

B Insulin-resistant response

The pancrease overproduces insulin (abnormal output) in response to a rise in blood glucose as occurs from the rapid digestion and absorption of some dietary starches and simple sugars. Excess insulin production maintains blood glucose at the upper level of the normal range. Thus, the person does not classify as a type 2 diabetic. However, a chronic high insulin output in response to elevations in blood glucose after eating strongly relates to the metabolic syndrome of dyslipidemia, hypertension, upper-body obesity, and increased risk for heart attack and stroke.

C Type 2 diabetes

The pancreas continues to secrete insulin. However, the severity of insulin resistance exceeds the pancreas' maximum insulin output to regulate blood glucose within the normal range. This results in the diagnosis of type 2 diabetes.

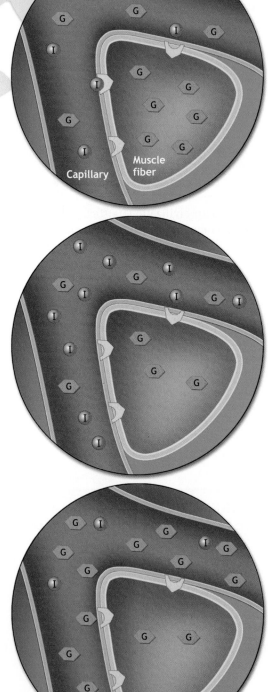

Figure 20.21 Normal insulin–glucose interaction (**A**), with insulin resistance (**B**), and type 2 diabetes (**C**).

diabetes form represents an autoimmune response, possibly from a single protein that renders the β-cells incapable of producing insulin and often other pancreatic hormones.[231] Type 1 diabetic patients present a more severe abnormality for glucose homeostasis than individuals in the type 2 subgroup. Exercise exerts more-pronounced effects on the metabolic state in type 1 individuals, and the management of exercise-related problems requires greater attention (see "In a Practical Sense," p. 456).

Type 2 Diabetes

So ingrained is the belief that type 2 diabetes occurs primarily in overweight, middle-aged men and women that it is frequently called adult-onset diabetes. Although type 2 diabetes tends to occur after age 40, a sharp increase has occurred in the number of children with type 2 diabetes, some younger than age 10. This alarming new health trend signals that type 2 diabetes may represent a "pediatric disease."[63] Recent estimates indicate that the disease has more than tripled in children over the last 3 to 5 years. Physicians consider the spiraling rate of childhood obesity—particularly among African Americans, Native Americans, and Hispanics (most notably children of Mexican descent)—as the predominant factor in the rising number of children with type 2 diabetes. Type 2 diabetes accounts for nearly 95% of all diabetes cases in the United States; it represents the leading cause of death from the disease. Treatment costs exceed $105 billion annually.

High blood glucose levels in type 2 diabetes can result from three factors: (1) inadequate insulin produced by the pancreas to control blood sugar (**relative insulin deficiency**), (2) decreased insulin effects on peripheral tissue (**insulin resistance**), particularly skeletal muscle, or (3) combined effect of factors 1 and 2. A dysregulation in glycolytic and oxidative capacities of skeletal muscle also relates to insulin resistance in type 2 diabetes.[195] The disease most likely results from the interaction of genes and lifestyle factors—physical inactivity, weight gain, (up to 80% of type 2 diabetes are obese) aging, and possibly a high-fat diet. No doubt, these lifestyle factors have contributed to the 70% increase in the disorder among persons in their 30s during the last decade of the 20th century, and a 33% overall increase nationally. Also, the form of insulin resistance in type 2 diabetes has a strong genetic component. Diabetic-prone individuals possess a gene that directs synthesis of a protein that inhibits insulin's action in cellular glucose transport.

Obesity, particularly upper-body fat distribution, and lack of regular physical activity represent major risks for type 2 diabetes in adults and children. An estimated 60 to 80 million Americans show insulin resistance but have not developed overt symptoms of type 2 diabetes. One-third of these individuals will eventually become full-blown diabetics, and many others are at heightened risk of cardiovascular disease. The term **insulin-resistant** means that the pancreas overproduces insulin (abnormal output) when blood glucose rises from the rapid digestion and absorption of dietary high-

glycemic carbohydrates (Fig. 20.21). Increased blood glucose levels of these individuals are not high enough for a type 2 diabetes classification. Failure of insulin to exert its normal effect increases glucose conversion to triacylglycerol and storage as body fat. For the insulin-resistant individual, a diet high in simple sugars and refined carbohydrates (with a relatively high glycemic index) facilitates body fat accumulation. Fat cell enlargement further exacerbates the situation, because these cells exhibit insulin resistance from their reduced insulin receptor density.

As with type 1 diabetes, adequate glucose fails to enter the cells of a person with type 2 diabetes. This triggers abnormally high levels of blood glucose that the kidney tubules filter and void in the urine (**glycosuria**). Excessive glucose particles in

AT RISK FOR TYPE 2 DIABETES

- Body mass exceeds 20% of ideal
- First-degree relative with diabetes (genetic influence)
- Member of a high-risk ethnic group (black, Hispanic American, Pacific Islander, American Indian, Asian)
- Delivered a baby weighing more than 9 pounds or developed gestational diabetes
- Blood pressure at or above 140/90 mm Hg
- HDL cholesterol level of 35 mg · dL^{-1} or below and/or a triacylglycerol level of 250 mg · dL^{-1} or above
- Impaired fasting plasma glucose or impaired glucose tolerance on previous testing

CHARACTERISTICS OF TYPE 1 AND TYPE 2 DIABETES

CHARACTERISTICS	TYPE 1 DIABETES	TYPE 2 DIABETES
Age of onset	Usually <20 y	Usually >40 y (but increasing in children)
Proportion of all diabetics	<10%	>90%
Appearance of symptoms	Acute or subacute	Slow
Metabolic ketoacidosis	Frequent	Rare
Obesity at onset	Uncommon	Common
ß-cells	Decreased	Variable
Insulin	Decreased	Variable
Inflammatory cells in islets	Present initially	Absent
Family history	Uncommon	Common

renal filtrate create an osmotic effect that diminishes water reabsorption, which results in loss of large amounts of fluid (**polyuria**). With decreased cellular glucose uptake, a diabetic person relies largely on fat catabolism for energy. This produces an excess of ketoacids and a tendency toward acidosis. In extreme situations, diabetic coma occurs as plasma pH falls as low as 7.0. Arteriosclerosis, small blood vessel and nerve disease, and susceptibility to infection occur at increased rates in type 2 diabetes. Obese diabetic women also face an almost three-fold greater risk of endometrial cancer than diabetic women of normal weight, perhaps from their persistently high insulin levels (insulin insensitivity).[189]

Since 1970, heart disease mortality has declined by 36% in nondiabetic males and 27% in nondiabetic females; unfortunately, it has decreased only 13% in diabetic males and increased by 23% in women with diabetes.[67] The observed discrepancies probably occur either from more limited reductions in risk factors over time among those with diabetes or a blunted response to risk factor reduction.

Diabetes and Exercise. Hypoglycemia is the most common disturbance in glucose homeostasis during exercise in diabetic persons who take exogenous insulin. Severe hypoglycemia occurs for patients that undergo intensive insulin therapy to normalize plasma glucose levels throughout the day. Under normal conditions, hypoglycemia occurs during prolonged, intense exercise when hepatic glucose release does not match increased glucose use by active muscle. In addition, persons with type 2 diabetes often demonstrate reduced exercise tolerance independent of glycemic control. Contributing factors include genetics, undesirable lifestyle characteristics, excessive body fat, and poor physical fitness.

INTEGRATIVE QUESTION

What would explain the sweet-smelling breath of individuals who suffer from poorly regulated diabetes mellitus or malnutrition from starvation?

Glucagon

The α-cells of the islets of Langerhans secrete **glucagon**, the "insulin antagonist" hormone. In contrast to insulin's effect in lowering blood sugar levels, glucagon primarily stimulates both glycogenolysis and gluconeogenesis by the liver and increases lipid catabolism. (FIG. 20.22). The glucose generated by glucagon action then moves into the blood. Glucagon exerts its effect by activating adenylate cyclase. This enzyme stimulates cyclic AMP in liver cells and causes hepatic glycogen breakdown to glucose (glycogenolysis). Glucagon also stimulates gluconeogenesis by promoting amino acid uptake by the liver.

As with insulin, plasma glucose concentration controls glucagon output by the pancreas. A decrease in blood glucose concentration from prolonged high-intensity exercise or food (or carbohydrate) restriction stimulates glucagon release.[206]

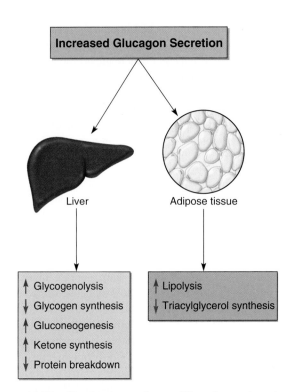

Figure 20.22   Glucogen secretion and its action on target tissues. The anabolic functions of glucagon promote liver glycogenolys and gluconeogenesis and lipid catabolism.

Unlike its effects on insulin secretion, autonomic nervous stimulation does not mediate glucagon release. Also, no gender differences exist in the glucagon response to exercise when individuals exercise at the same percentage of aerobic capacity.[37,207] Because glucagon release occurs later in exercise, this hormone exerts little influence in the early regulation of hepatic glycogenolysis. More than likely, it primarily contributes to blood glucose regulation as exercise progresses and glycogen reserves deplete.

Other Glands and Hormones

Other hormones also influence bodily functions. The liver secretes somatomedins, which affect growth of muscle, cartilage, and other tissues. The mucosal lining of the small intestine secretes **secretin**, **gastrin**, and **cholecystokinin**, to promote and coordinate digestive processes. The hypothalamus itself constitutes an important endocrine gland that secretes stimulating or releasing hormones that activate or release anterior pituitary hormones. The hypothalamus also releases **somatoliberin**, which stimulates somatotropin secretion from the anterior pituitary gland.

EXERCISE TRAINING AND ENDOCRINE FUNCTION

TABLE 20.5 lists the different hormones and their general response to exercise training. Because of the complex interactions between endocrine secretions and the nervous system, only lim-

TABLE 20.5 ■ **HORMONES AND THEIR RESPONSES TO ENDURANCE TRAINING**

HORMONE	TRAINING RESPONSE
Hypothalamus–pituitary hormones	
Growth hormone	No effect on resting values; less dramatic rise during exercise
Thyrotropin	No known training effect
ACTH	Increased exercise values
Prolactin	Some evidence that training lowers resting values
FSH, LH, and testosterone	Trained females have depressed values; reduced testosterone in males (testosterone levels may increase in males with long-term resistance training)
Posterior pituitary hormones	
Vasopressin (ADH)	Slightly reduced ADH at a given workload
Oxytocin	No research results available
Thyroid hormones	
Thyroxine (T_4)	Reduced concentration of total T_3 and increased free thyroxine at rest
Triiodothyronine (T_3)	Increased turnover of T_3 and T_4 during exercise
Adrenal hormones	
Aldosterone	No training adaptation
Cortisol	Slight elevation during exercise
Epinephrine and norepinephrine	Decreased secretion at rest and at the same absolute exercise intensity after training
Pancreatic hormones	
Insulin	Increased sensitivity to insulin; normal decrease in insulin during exercise greatly reduced with training
Glucagon	Smaller increase in glucose levels during exercise at absolute and relative workloads
Kidney enzyme and hormone	
Renin and angiotensin	No apparent training effect

ited research has evaluated multiple hormone secretions and changes consequent to exercise training. *The magnitude of hormonal response to a standard exercise load generally declines with endurance training.* For example, when highly trained athletes perform at the same absolute exercise level as sedentary subjects, hormonal responses remain lower in the athletes. Improved target tissue sensitivity and/or responsiveness to a given amount of hormone accounts for much of this "efficiency" in response.[33,55,83,179] A similar level of hormonal response occurs regardless of state of training when subjects exercise at the same relative exercise intensity (i.e., same percentage of maximum [lower absolute load for the untrained]). With maximal exercise, trained subjects have an identical or somewhat greater hormonal response than untrained subjects.

Anterior Pituitary Hormones

Growth Hormone

GH stimulates lipolysis and inhibits carbohydrate breakdown so one could hypothesize that training enhances GH secretion and conserves glycogen reserves. This does not occur. Compared with untrained counterparts, endurance-trained individuals show *less* rise in blood GH levels at a given exercise intensity—a response attributed to reduced exercise stress as training progresses and fitness improves.[15] Regardless of training status, women typically maintain higher GH levels at rest than men; this difference disappears during prolonged exer-

cise.[23] FIGURE 20.23A illustrates the training-induced depression of GH response of a representative subject from a group of six men during 20 minutes of constant-load, high-intensity exercise before and after 3 and 6 weeks of endurance training. Integrated GH concentrations (exercise plus recovery) for the group averaged 45% lower than pretraining values at both training measures. Responses for plasma catecholamines (Fig. 20.23B and C) and blood lactate (Fig. 20.23D) paralleled the decrease in GH. Because the constant-load exercise test represented less physiologic demand after training (reflected by lower catecholamine and lactate levels), a similar release of GH after training probably requires higher absolute exercise intensity. The effect of exercise training on GH release also may occur under nonexercise conditions. For example, aerobic training above the lactate threshold level amplifies the 24-hour pulsatile GH release during rest (see "Focus on Research," p. 449).

ACTH (Adrenocorticotropic Hormone)

ACTH, secreted by the posterior pituitary gland, provides potent stimulation to the adrenal cortex and thus increases free fatty acid mobilization for energy. Training increases ACTH release during exercise—a response that stimulates adrenal gland activity to promote fat catabolism and spare glycogen.[16,76] This effect would certainly benefit prolonged, high-intensity exercise performance.

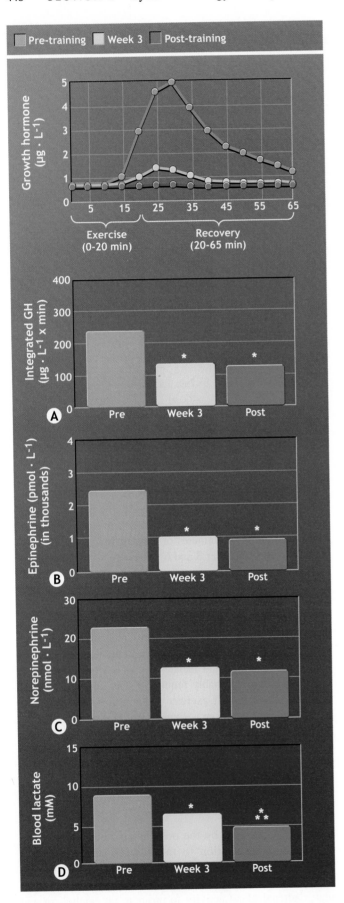

PRL (Prolactin)

Little information exists concerning exercise training changes in PRL. It does appear that resting PRL levels of male runners average below values for sedentary nonrunners.[69,222]

FSH (Follicle-Stimulating Hormone), LH (Leuteinizing Hormone), and Testosterone

Regular exercise depresses reproductive hormone responses in women and men.[34,42,223] Male endurance athletes generally maintain resting testosterone levels between 60 and 85% of values for sedentary men. The implications of these findings remain unclear.

Women. Women with a long history of exercise participation have altered FSH and LH levels at different times in their menstrual cycles, which may contribute to menstrual dysfunction.[17] For example, FSH levels remain depressed in trained females throughout an abbreviated anovulatory menstrual cycle, whereas LH and progesterone concentrations rise in the cycle's follicular phase. Several concomitant factors other than exercise per se alter reproductive function. These include energy drain, weight loss, dietary changes, alterations in the lean-to-fat ratio, the physical and emotional stress of strenuous training and competition, and altered clearance rates of gonadal steroid hormones. However, variations in the menstrual cycle do not affect metabolic and hormonal responses to acute bouts of physical activity.[56,101]

Men. Endurance training affects a man's pituitary–gonadal function, including levels of testosterone and PRL.[82] FIGURE 20.24 compares 46 male runners (average weekly running distance, 64 km) and 18 nonrunners matched for age, stature, and body mass. The runners showed lower testosterone than nonrunners, with no differences in LH and FSH levels. Reduced testosterone concentration (both increased clearance and lower production) in endurance-trained men parallels the sex-steroid reductions observed in women who undergo endurance training and associated reductions in body fat.[17,201] No difference exists in LH and FSH levels between trained and untrained men; thus, impaired gonadotropin release from the anterior pituitary does not cause the lower testosterone levels during standard exercise in the trained state.

Figure 20.23 *Top.* Serum growth hormone (GH) concentrations in a representative subject during 20 minutes of constant-load exercise and 45 minutes of recovery at pretraining, after 3 weeks of training, and after 6 weeks of training. *Bottom.* Effects of 6 weeks of training on integrated GH concentration (**A**), and end-exercise concentrations of epinephrine (**B**), norepinephrine (**C**), and blood lactate (**D**) in response to constant-load cycle ergometry exercise (*n* = 6, mean). Pre week 3, after 3 weeks of training; Post, after 6 weeks of training. * P < .05 versus pretraining; ** P < .05 versus week 3. (From Weltman A, et al. Exercise training decreases the growth hormone (GH) response to acute constant-load exercise. Med Sci Sports Exerc 1997;29:669.)

FOCUS On Research

TRAINING INTENSITY AFFECTS GROWTH HORMONE RELEASE

Weltman A, et al. Endurance training amplifies the pulsatile release of growth hormone: effects of training intensity. J Appl Physiol 1992;72:2188.

▲ Research has focused on growth hormone (GH) responses to a single session of exercise and long-term training. The dynamics of GH secretions during exercise training takes on clinical importance because of the causal relationship between GH availability and maintenance of lean body tissue during aging and weight loss.

Weltman and colleagues studied GH dynamics with 52 weeks of aerobic run training in two groups of 21 healthy, eumenorrheic women. One group ran at a speed corresponding to lactate threshold (@*LT*) and the other at a faster speed above the lactate threshold level (>*LT*). Nontraining women served as controls (*C*). Both training groups completed similar weekly mileage. The distance covered during the first week was 5 miles. Weekly mileage then gradually increased to 24 miles by week 20 and continued at 24 miles per week until week 40. Thereafter, weekly mileage increased by 1.25 miles for three of the weeks. Subjects ran between 35 and 40 miles per week by the end of the study.

Yearlong training increased $\dot{V}O_{2max}$ by 9.9% for the @LT group and 11.8% for the >LT group. In addition,

the @LT group increased exercise $\dot{V}O_2$ at LT ($\dot{V}O_{2\text{-LT}}$) by 21.5%, while the >LT group's $\dot{V}O_{2\text{-LT}}$ increased by 28%. The C group remained unchanged on all measures. No differences in body mass, fat mass, or percentage body fat emerged within or among groups, although the >LT group showed a trend toward body fat reduction. Both exercise groups increased fat-free body mass with training.

The figure illustrates the effects of the run training program on resting 24-hour integrated serum GH concentrations. Training induced a 50% increase in resting GH concentration for the >LT group. GH concentrations remained unchanged for the C and @LT groups. The investigators speculated that the release of endogenous opiates and catecholamines and inhibition of somatostatin release in more intense exercise performed by the >LT group facilitated GH release.

This research showed that exercise training augments resting pulsatile GH release by amplitude enhancement, but only with training intensity above LT. Training at intensities above the LT may provide a natural and healthful means to increase pulsatile GH secretion under conditions that depress GH release, as in aging. Increased GH release through regular physical activity can conserve the lean tissue mass during weight loss.

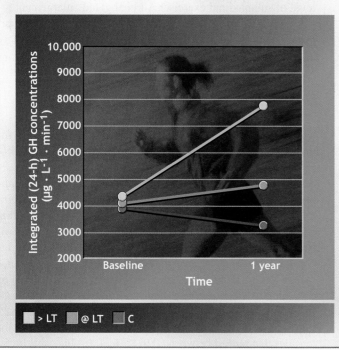

Integrated 24-hour resting GH concentrations for the control group *(C)* and groups that exercised either at an intensity equivalent to the lactate threshold *(@LT)* or greater than the lactate threshold *(>LT)*. Note the large (50%) increase in GH concentration for the >LT group compared with the @LT and C groups.

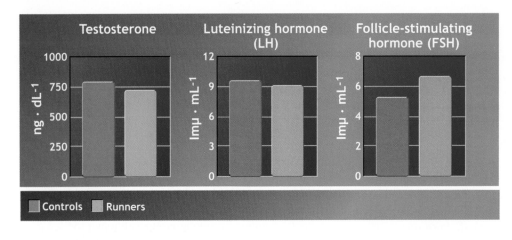

Figure 20.24 Comparison of testosterone, LH, and FSH levels in trained male runners and untrained controls. Runners show lower testosterone levels than controls and no significant difference in LH and FSH. (From Wheeler GD, et al. Reduced serum testosterone and prolactin levels in male distance runners. JAMA 1984;252:514.)

Posterior Pituitary Hormones

ADH (Antidiuretic Hormone)

High-intensity exercise to exhaustion or prolonged submaximal exercise at the same relative intensity produces no difference in ADH levels between trained and untrained individuals. ADH concentration decreases with training when exercising at the same absolute submaximal intensity.[212]

Oxytocin

We are unaware of research on training-induced changes in oxytocin.

PTH (Parathyroid Hormone)

Endurance training enhances exercise-related increases in PTH in young and elderly adults.[185,232] The significance of a training-induced augmented rise in PTH for preserving bone mass with aging awaits further study.

Thyroid Hormones

Exercise training produces a coordinated pituitary–thyroid response that reflects increased turnover of thyroid hormones. Increased thyroid turnover often reflects excessive hormonal action that ultimately leads to hyperthyroidism (i.e., overproduction of T_3 and T_4 hormones). However, no evidence indicates a higher incidence of hyperthyroidism in highly trained individuals. For example, inordinately high BMR levels and basal body temperatures rarely occur in the trained state. Consequently, the greater T_4 turnover that accompanies physical training occurs through a mechanism that differs from "normal" thyroid hormone dynamics.

Research on women who endurance train yields interesting results regarding thyroid turnover. Changing from a baseline of relatively sedentary living to running 48 km per week produced a mild thyroid impairment reflected by decreased T_3 and T_4 levels.[18] In contrast, nearly doubling the weekly distance increased plasma hormone levels. To explain these apparent conflicting effects of regular exercise, the researchers suggested that greater body fat loss with more intense training produced an exercise-induced increase in thyroid output. Six months of resistance training in men slightly reduced the concentrations of T_4 and plasma free T_4, without change in TSH. However, the magnitude of the change was of no clinical or physiologic significance.[164] The importance of any changes in thyroxine levels in adapting to training remains unclear.

Adrenal Hormones

Aldosterone

The renin–angiotensin–aldosterone system contributes to homeostatic control of body fluid volumes, electrolytes, and blood pressure, but exercise training does not affect resting levels of these compounds or their normal response to exercise.[57]

Cortisol

Plasma cortisol levels increase less in trained subjects than in sedentary subjects who perform the same absolute level of submaximal exercise. Adrenal gland enlargement results from both cellular hypertrophy and hyperplasia with repeated bouts of intense exercise training and correspondingly high cortisol output.

Epinephrine and Norepinephrine

Sympathoadrenal activity (principally norepinephrine release) in response to an *absolute* submaximum workload remains lower in trained than in untrained individuals.[45,71] Epinephrine and norepinephrine output in standard exercise falls dramatically during the first several weeks of training. *The appearance of bradycardia and a smaller rise in blood pressure during submaximal exercise represent the most familiar consequences of the sympathoadrenal training adaptation.* Reductions in exercise heart rate and blood pressure reflect favorable adaptations because they lower myocardial oxygen demands during exercise and possibly other forms of stress. For equivalent *relative* exercise intensities, a *higher* sympathoadrenal response occurs following aerobic training.[65] FIGURE 20.25 illustrates norepinephrine and epinephrine during exercise at intensities that ranged between 60 to 85% of aerobic capacity by

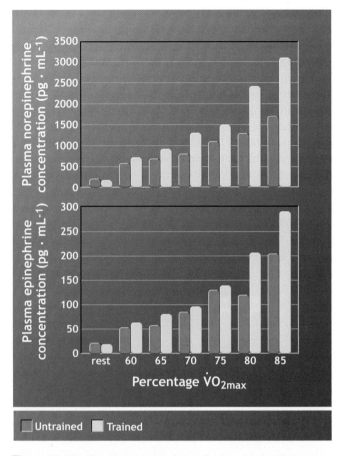

Figure 20.25 Plasma norepinephrine *(top)* and epinephrine concentrations *(bottom)* at rest and after 15 minutes of exercise at the same relative exercise intensity (%$\dot{V}O_{2max}$) before and after 10 weeks of endurance exercise training. (From Greiwe JS, et al. Norepinephrine response to exercise at the same relative intensity before and after endurance training. J Appl Physiol 1999;86:531.)

three adult men and six women prior to and following 10 weeks of aerobic training that increased $\dot{V}O_{2max}$ by 20%. Plasma norepinephrine levels (Fig. 20.25, *top*) increased progressively with exercise intensity before and after training. However, training produced higher plasma norepinephrine levels, particularly at the higher intensities of effort. Consistently higher epinephrine values also emerged following training (Fig. 20.25, *bottom*), but the differences did not reach statistical significance. More than likely, greater catecholamine output at the same relative exercise intensity following training reflects three factors requiring greater sympathetic nervous system activation: (1) greater absolute demand for substrate use via glycogenolysis and lipolysis, (2) increased overall cardiovascular response (e.g., cardiac output), and (3) larger muscle mass activation. Whether exercise training alters resting catecholamine levels remains unclear.

Pancreatic Hormones

Endurance training maintains blood levels of insulin and glucagon during exercise closer to resting values. *In essence, the trained state requires less insulin at any stage from rest through light to moderately intense exercise.* FIGURE 20.26

shows insulin and glucagon responses in 10 young males before and after 20 weeks of training at 60 to 80% $\dot{V}O_{2max}$. Aerobic training depressed the exercise response of both hormones, with glucagon showing the most pronounced reduction. These findings agree with previous reports for adults who trained for 10 weeks by running and cycling.[68]

Regular Physical Activity and Type 2 Diabetes Risk

Cross-sectional, retrospective, prospective, and interventional epidemiologic research, including studies of enforced inactivity, provide strong evidence that regular exercise reduces type 2 diabetes risk in adolescents and adults with or without concomitant body composition changes.[2,21,78,89,103,211,217,224] Refer to http://connection.lww.com/productores.asp?area =49 for the ACSM position stand on exercise and type 2 diabetes.) Those individuals at greatest risk for type 2 diabetes (obese, hypertensive, family history, sedentary lifestyle) gain the greatest benefit from regular exercise.[1,63,135,165] For adult men and women, low fitness levels coincide with increased

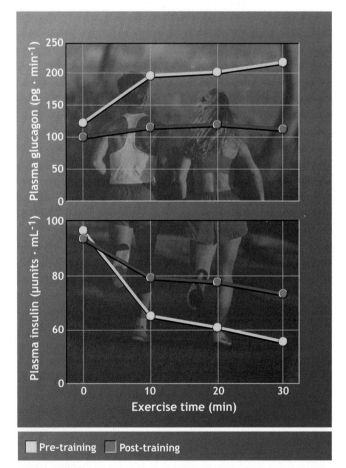

Figure 20.26 Pre–post differences in plasma glucagon and insulin responses to exercise before and after 20 weeks of an aerobic training program. (From Applied Physiology Laboratory, University of Michigan.)

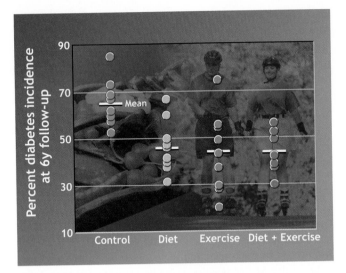

Figure 20.27 Effects of dietary and exercise lifestyle interventions on the occurrence of type 2 diabetes in individuals with impaired glucose tolerance. (From Xiao-ren P, et al. Effects of diet and exercise in preventing NIDDM in people with impaired glucose tolerance. Diabetes Care 1997;20:537.)

sponse relationship remained consistent in those at low or high risk for diabetes and stayed significant after BMI adjustment. Women who walked regularly achieved greater benefits with a brisker walking pace; the most vigorous exercise lowered diabetes risk by 46%. Equivalent energy expenditures from walking or other forms of physical activity produced comparable risk reduction.

Adult Native Americans of the Pima tribe in Arizona, a group with 10 to 15 times more type 2 diabetes than the typical U.S. population, retrospectively rated their participation in various sports and leisure activities at various life stages.[119]

clustering of the metabolic abnormalities associated with the **insulin-resistant syndrome** (see "Metabolic Syndrome X," p. 442), the "deadly quartet" of insulin resistance, glucose intolerance, upper-body obesity, and dyslipidemia.[43,221] For sedentary, middle-aged men, aerobic exercise plus weight loss lowers blood pressure and improves glucose and fat metabolism.[40] A 6-year clinical trial evaluated the effects of diet and exercise lifestyle interventions on the occurrence of type 2 diabetes in individuals with impaired glucose tolerance.[230] In one study, 577 men and women were randomly assigned to either control, diet-only, exercise-only, or diet-plus-exercise groups. Diet modification consisted of 25 to 30 kCal per kg of body mass (55–60% carbohydrate, 25–30% lipid, and 10–15% protein) for individuals with a BMI below 25. Those with a BMI above 25 maintained the same macronutrient mixture as the leaner group while gradually losing weight at a rate of 0.5 to 1.0 kg per month until their BMI decreased to 23. Exercise intervention required a progressive increase in the quantity of mild-to-moderate regular physical activity. The diet–exercise intervention combined the major components of both diet and exercise treatments. FIGURE 20.27 shows that diet, exercise, and combined diet–exercise interventions decreased incidence of diabetes after the 6-year intervention.

A large prospective study evaluated diabetes risk for a cohort of 70,102 female nurses aged 40 to 65 years without diabetes, cardiovascular disease, or cancer at baseline measurements in 1986.[87] In agreement with previous prospective research on men, an 8-year follow-up found increased physical activity correlated with a substantially reduced relative risk for type 2 diabetes. FIGURE 20.28 indicates that after adjustment for smoking, alcohol use, history of hypertension, and elevated cholesterol levels, relative risk across physical activity quintiles (20-percentile units) related inversely to diabetes risk in lean and overweight women. The dose–re-

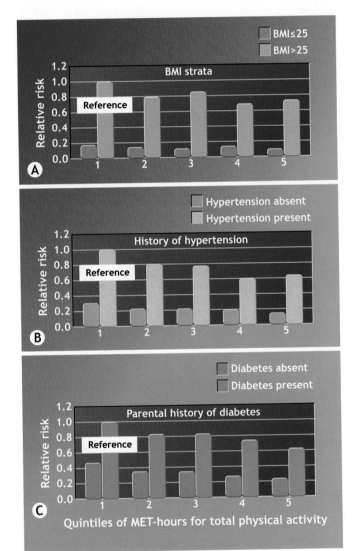

Figure 20.28 Multivariate relative risks of type 2 diabetes according to MET-hours for total physical activity quintile (ascending 20-percentile units) within strata of (**A**) body mass index (BMI), (**B**) history of hypertension, and (**C**) parental history of diabetes. *MET-hours for total physical activity* represents average time per week spent in each of eight physical activities multiplied by the MET value of each activity. The MET value equals energy need per kilogram of body mass per hour of activity divided by the energy need per kilogram of body mass per hour at rest. (From Hu GB, et al. Walking compared with vigorous physical activity and the risk of type 2 diabetes in women: a prospective study. JAMA 1999;282:1433.)

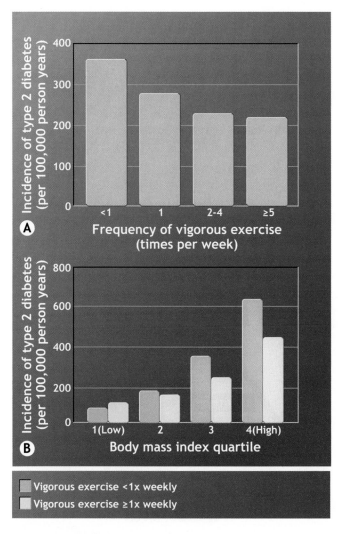

Figure 20.29   A. Age-adjusted incidence rates of type 2 diabetes in relation to frequency of vigorous exercise, and (**B**) for individuals with similar values for body size assessed by the body mass index. (From Manson JE, et al. A prospective study of exercise and incidence of diabetes among US male physicians. JAMA 1993;268:63.)

Individuals with diabetes, regardless of gender, consistently reported less physical activity over their lifetime than disease-free individuals. This relationship existed even after accounting for age, body mass, body fat distribution, family history, and current physical activity level. These retrospective data agree with prospective data obtained over a 5-year follow-up of more than 21,000 healthy U.S. male physicians aged 40 to 85 years (FIG. 20.29).[132] Physicians reporting more physical activity, regardless of body mass, experienced a lower incidence of type 2 diabetes. FIGURE 20.30 outlines the possible mechanisms by which exercise training—via its effects on skeletal muscle, adipose tissue, liver, and pancreatic hormone output—improves insulin action and blood glucose control in type 2 diabetes.

Exercise Benefits for Type 2 Diabetes. Exercise training provides considerable benefits for persons with type 2 diabetes.

Glycemic Control. Skeletal muscle consumes the major amount of the glucose transported in blood. Muscle, for example, generally clears between 70 and 90% of the glucose in an oral or intravenous glucose challenge. A single bout of moderate or intense exercise abruptly decreases plasma glucose levels, an effect that persists for up to several days.[104,109] Most likely, the immediate effects of each exercise session on increasing the active muscles' **insulin sensitivity** causes long-term improvement in glycemic control with regular exercise, not any exercise-induced chronic adaptations in tissue function. When resuming a sedentary lifestyle, the muscle's sensitivity to insulin decreases, thus requiring more insulin to clear a given quantity of blood glucose.[157] *Improved insulin sensitivity with regular exercise provides type 2 diabetics with important "therapy" that ultimately lowers the insulin requirement.* Improved insulin sensitivity for glucose transport in skeletal muscle and adipose tissue after a bout of exercise results from (1) translocation of the glucose transporter protein GLUT-4 from the endoplasmic reticulum to the cell surface, (2) increase in total quantity of GLUT-4, and (3) increase in glycogen synthase activity and subsequent glucose storage as glycogen (independent of any effect on insulin signaling).[30,49,75,81,90] For example, 4 days of vigorous training increased skeletal muscle GLUT-4 content and insulin-stimulated glucose transport by up to 100%.[176] The hyperinsulinemic patient who requires the largest insulin release for glucose regulation derives the greatest benefits from regular exercise.[109,214] This observation supports the theory that regular exercise acts by reversing insulin resistance (i.e., exercise increases insulin sensitivity). *Improved insulin sensitivity imparts one of the most important health benefits that regular physical activity confers to the diabetic.*

A wide range of intensity and volume of physical activity minimizes insulin resistance that develops with a sedentary lifestyle. Extending duration of weekly exercise from 115 minutes to 170 minutes produces the greatest increase in insulin sensitivity.[84] Combining resistance exercise *and* endurance training improves markers of insulin resistance and body composition for insulin-resistant individuals more than endurance training alone.[213] Benefits of resistance plus endurance training for hyperinsulinemia most likely come from the specific effects of activating a relatively larger muscle mass (than with endurance training alone) and additional caloric expenditure. Improvements in blood glucose homeostasis with regular exercise rapidly decrease once training ceases and completely dissipate within several weeks of inactivity.[3]

Cardiovascular Disease. Excess morbidity and mortality in type 2 diabetes results from coronary heart disease, stroke, and peripheral vascular disease from accelerated atherosclerosis. Disease risk factors that improve with regular exercise include hyperinsulinemia, hyperglycemia, abnormal plasma lipoproteins, some blood coagulation parameters, and hypertension.

Weight Loss. Weight loss and accompanying reduction in body fat and its distribution enhance glucose tolerance and insulin sensitivity.[8,118,120] The beneficial effects of exercise on fat loss

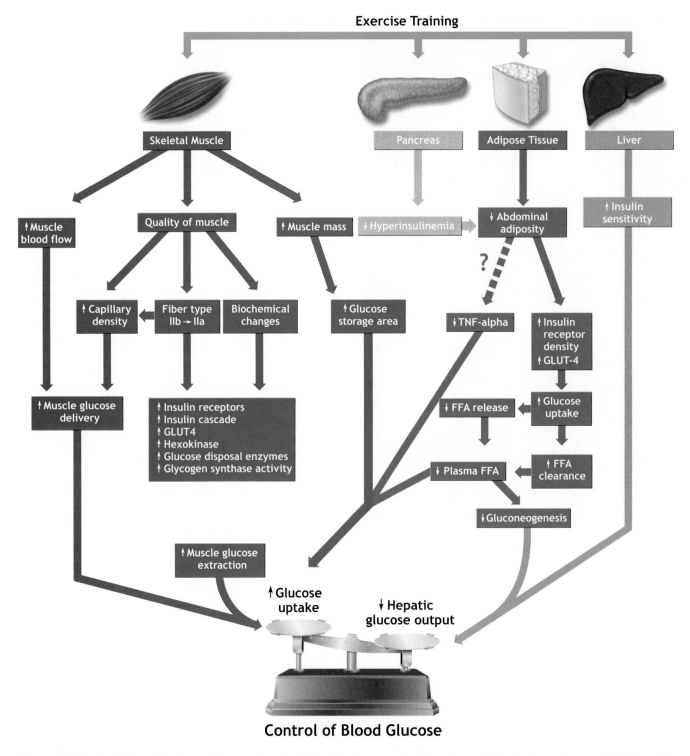

Figure 20.30   Possible mechanisms of how regular physical activity improves insulin action and blood glucose homeostasis in type 2 diabetes. *TNF-alpha,* tumor necrosis factor-alpha, a hormonelike substance released from active adipocytes in the abdominal region, which may depress insulin-regulated glucose transport. (Modified from Ivy JL, et al. Prevention and treatment of non-insulin-dependent diabetes mellitus. Exerc Sport Sci Rev 1999;27:1.)

often are underestimated because body weight changes with exercise do not necessarily reflect even more favorable, exercise-induced body composition changes (fat loss and muscle gain). Combining diet and regular exercise reduces body fat in diabetic persons more effectively than either treatment alone.

Psychologic Profile. Improved exercise capacity in diabetic persons relates to decreased anxiety, improved mood and self-esteem, increased sense of well-being and psychologic control, enhanced socialization, and improved quality of life.[143]

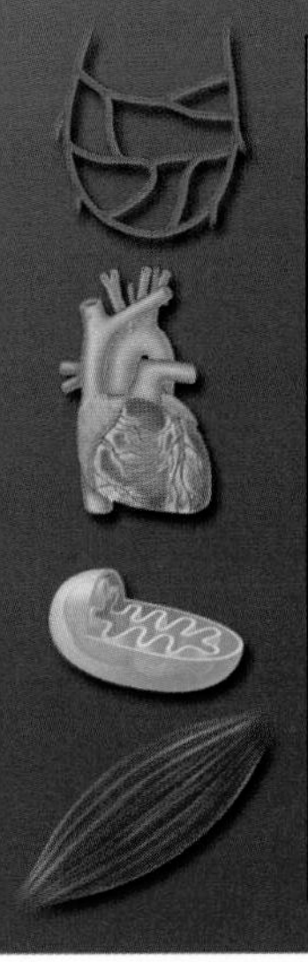

System	Potential Problem
Systemic	•Retinal hemorrhage •Increased proteinuria •Acceleration of microvascular lesions
Cardio-vascular	•Cardiac arrhythmias •Ischemic heart disease (often silent) •Excessive blood pressure during exercise •Postexercise orthostatic hypertension
Metabolic	•Increased hyperglycemia •Increased ketosis
Musculo-skeletal	•Foot ulcers (in presence of neuropathy) •Orthopedic injury related to neuropathy •Accelerated degenerative joint disease

Figure 20.31 Potential physical and physiologic problems and problem areas faced by type 2 diabetics who begin an exercise program.

Occurrence of Type 2 Diabetes. Regular exercise contributes to delaying and even preventing the onset of insulin resistance and type 2 diabetes in persons at high risk for developing this disease. Exercise benefits are particularly pronounced for obese individuals and perhaps all persons with increased abdominal fat deposition.[120,132]

Exercise Risks for Type 2 Diabetes. One must consider the possible complications from exercise for patients with diabetes. FIGURE 20.31 lists potential adverse effects of exercise in type 2 diabetics. One can minimize these risks by properly screening patients before they start an exercise program and carefully monitoring them during exercise when the program begins.

Exercise Guidelines for Type 1 Diabetes. The clinical usefulness of regular exercise to improve glucose control in type 1 diabetes remains uncertain. To complicate matters for type 1 diabetics, exercise can trigger a potentially dangerous dual response: (1) enhanced glucose uptake by active muscles and (2) greater-than-anticipated exogenous insulin distributed by more rapid circulation that accompanies exercise. These two factors could *worsen* the imbalance between glucose supply and use, increasing the risk of serious complications from hypoglycemia. The "In a Practical Sense" feature on p. 480 offers exercise guidelines for the diabetic patient. The guidelines also apply to patients with well-controlled type 1 diabetes who wish to perform prolonged and strenuous exercise while minimizing the principle risk of hypoglycemia.[63]

RESISTANCE TRAINING AND ENDOCRINE FUNCTION

Muscle remodeling in resistance training reflects a complex process of cell receptor interaction with different hormones and the DNA-mediated production of new contractile proteins. The specific exercise response to muscular overload initially links to configuration of the exercise stimulus—intensity, frequency, volume, sequence, mode, and recovery interval. FIGURE 20.32 proposes how resistance exercise training improves overall muscular size, strength, and power. Factors responsible for exercise-induced changes in muscle size and function include the following: (1) changes in hepatic and extrahepatic hormone clearance rates, (2) differential rates of hormone secretion (and accompanying fluid shifts around the receptor sites), and (3) altered receptor-site activation via neurohumoral control. In general, early-phase adaptations to resistance training reflect a response that mediates neuromuscular system adaptations that improve muscle strength.

Testosterone and GH are two primary hormones that affect adaptations to resistance training. Testosterone augments GH release and interacts with nervous system function to increase muscle force production. These roles may be more important than any direct anabolic effect of testosterone per se. A single session of resistance training generally elicits a short-term rise in serum testosterone and decrease in cortisol, with a greater response in men than women.[37,62,114,179] Concurrently, catecholamine release from the adrenal medulla increases with the acute stress of high-force and high-power exercise protocols.[24]

Resistance training in men increases frequency and amplitude of testosterone and GH secretion, thereby creating a favorable hormonal environment for muscular growth (hypertrophy). In contrast, most studies fail to demonstrate changes in testosterone and GH concentrations with training in females. Thus, gender differences in hormone output with long-term resistance training may ultimately explain variations in responsiveness of muscle strength and size to prolonged muscular overload.

Testosterone response to resistance exercise reveals several factors that increase its release. These include activation of large-muscle groups with dead lifts, power cleans and squats, and other forms of heavy resistance exercise (i.e., 85 to 95%

IN A PRACTICAL SENSE

DIABETES, HYPOGLYCEMIA, AND EXERCISE

■ Persons with type 1 or type 2 diabetes should exercise regularly as part of a comprehensive treatment regimen. Hypoglycemia represents the major risk of exercise for individuals who take insulin or oral hypoglycemic agents. A physically active diabetic person needs to pay particular attention to the following:

• Warning signs of hypoglycemia
• Immediate response to a hypoglycemia attack
• Treatment of late-onset hypoglycemia

HYPOGLYCEMIA WARNING SIGNS

Symptoms of moderate and severe hypoglycemia (see Table) result from inadequate glucose supply to the brain. In general, hypoglycemic symptoms appear only after blood glucose concentration drops below 60 mg · dL^{-1}.

Symptoms of low blood glucose vary considerably. Some diabetic persons with autonomic neuropathy who lose the ability to secrete adrenaline-like hormones in response to hypoglycemia experience *hypoglycemic unawareness*. They require regular blood glucose monitoring during and after exercise. Individuals who take β-blocker medication also have increased risk for hypoglycemic unawareness.

WARNING SIGNS OF HYPOGLYCEMIA

Mild hypoglycemic reaction

• Trembling or shakiness
• Nervousness
• Rapid heart rate
• Palpitations
• Increased sweating
• Excessive hunger

Moderate hypoglycemic reactions

• Headache
• Irritability and abrupt mood changes
• Impaired concentration and attentiveness
• Mental confusion
• Drowsiness

Severe hypoglycemic reactions

• Unresponsiveness
• Unconsciousness and coma
• Convulsions

HYPOGLYCEMIA ATTACK: WHAT TO DO

1. *Respond quickly:* Hypoglycemic reactions appear suddenly and progress rapidly.
2. *Stop exercising:* Test blood glucose to confirm hypoglycemia.
3. *Eat or drink carbohydrate:* Immediately consume 10 to 15 g of simple sugar. A diabetic person should always carry high-glycemic carbohydrate while exercising (e.g., hard candy, sugar cubes, raisins, juice). Consuming ice cream or chocolates is a poor choice; their high fat content depresses the glycemic index and impedes glucose absorption.
4. *Rest 10 to 15 minutes:* This allows for intestinal absorption of glucose. Test blood glucose levels before resuming exercise. If blood glucose registers below 100 mg · dL^{-1}, do not exercise but eat more sugar.
5. *Remonitor during exercise:* After resuming exercise, pay close attention to further signs of hypoglycemia. If possible, measure blood glucose within 30 to 45 minutes.
6. *Replenish carbohydrate immediately after exercise:* Consume complex carbohydrates. If carbohydrate intake does not increase blood glucose concentration, be prepared to administer glucagon subcutaneously to boost glucose levels.

LATE-ONSET HYPOGLYCEMIA

Late-onset hypoglycemia describes the condition of excessively low blood glucose more than 4 hours (and up to 48 h) after exercise. It occurs more frequently in new exercisers or after a strenuous workout. Insulin sensitivity remains high for 24 to 48 hours after exercise, so late-onset hypoglycemia poses a particular problem for many medicated diabetics. The following precautions can guard against late-onset hypoglycemia:

• Adjust insulin dosage or other medication before exercising. If needed, increase food intake before and during exercise.

continued on page 457

Continued

- If exercise lasts beyond 45 minutes, monitor blood glucose at 2-hour intervals for 12 hours into recovery or until sleep. Consider reducing insulin or oral hypoglycemic agents until bedtime. Before retiring, eat some low-glycemic food to increase blood glucose levels.
- Use caution when initiating an exercise program. Start slowly and gradually increase exercise intensity and duration over a 3- to 6-week period.
- If planning to exercise longer than 45 to 60 minutes, exercise with a friend who can assist in an emergency. Always carry snacks and important phone numbers (doctor, hospital, home) and wear a medical ID bracelet.

ADJUSTING INSULIN LEVELS

For intense exercise, consider the following:

- Intermediate-acting insulin: Decrease dose by 30 to 35% on the day of exercise.
- Intermediate- and short-acting insulin: Omit dose if it normally precedes exercise.
- Multiple doses of short-acting insulin: Reduce dose before exercise by 30% and supplement with carbohydrate-rich food.
- Continuous subcutaneous insulin infusion: Eliminate mealtime bolus or insulin increment that precedes or follows exercise.
- Avoid exercising for 1 hour the muscles that receive the short-acting insulin injection.
- Avoid exercising in late evening.

1-RM) or moderate- to high-volume (total quantity) training with multiple sets and/or exercises with less than 1-minute rest intervals.[115] Long-term resistance training in men increases resting testosterone levels, which correlates with the pattern of strength improvement over time.[72]

OPIOID PEPTIDES AND EXERCISE

Scientists who studied the pain-relieving effects of opioid peptides (e.g., morphine) on brain function in the 1970s reported that these substances exhibited neurotransmitter effects that reflected activation of specific opioid brain receptor sites.

With this finding came the realization that perhaps the brain itself produced endogenous opioid, mood-altering substances. Evidence for the existence of endogenous substances with opiate-like behavior first emerged with the isolation and purification of two opioid pentapeptides, methionine and leucine enkephalin (Greek, meaning *in the brain*). These opioids form part of a larger propiocortin precursor molecule produced in the anterior pituitary. Other opioid substances include β-lipotropin, β-endorphin, and dynorphin, (the most potent of the opioid peptides).

The various endogenous opioids exert widespread effects with a range in function from neurohormones to neurotransmit-

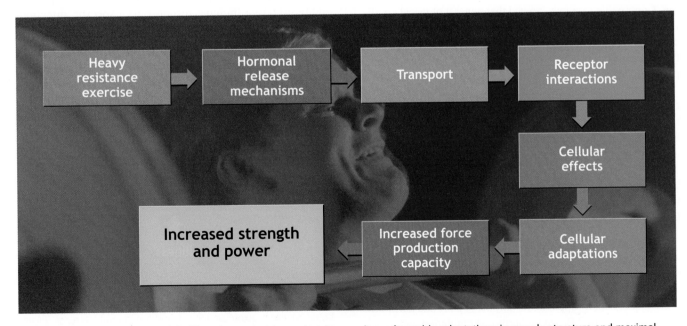

Figure 20.32 Schematic model of how heavy resistance training produces favorable adaptations in muscle structure and maximal strength performance. (Modified from Kraemer WJ. Endocrine responses and adaptations to strength training. In: Komi PV, ed. Strength and power in sport. London: Blackwell Scientific, 1992.)

ters. Endogenous opiates strongly inhibit hormonal release from the anterior pituitary, principally LH and FSH release. This inhibition may play a key role in menstrual cycle disturbances—delay in menarche, dysfunctional uterine bleeding, secondary amenorrhea, and inadequacy of the luteal phase—observed among many physically active women. In contrast to their inhibitory role, the opioid peptides stimulate release of GH and PRL.

Endorphins also regulate other hormones, including ACTH, the catecholamines, and cortisol.[136] Serum concentrations of endogenous opioids, primarily β-endorphin and/or β-lipotropin, generally increase with exercise similarly in men and women, although the response varies among individuals and varies inversely with exercise intensity.[44,61,112] Exercise increases β-endorphin up to five times the resting level and probably even more in the brain itself.[60,76,96] With resistance exercise, β-endorphin release varies with the exercise protocol; longer duration (lighter resistance) and longer interset rest intervals elicit the greatest response.[113]

The precise physiologic significance of the response of the various endogenous opioid peptides to exercise remains unclear, but several noteworthy effects emerge. These include the postulated opioid effect in triggering the so-called **exercise high**, a state described as euphoria and exhilaration as the duration of moderate to intense aerobic exercise increases. Endorphin secretion also may increase pain tolerance, improve appetite control, and reduce anxiety, tension, anger, and confusion. Interestingly, these effects generally reflect the documented psychologic benefits of regular exercise.

The effect of exercise training on endorphin response remains controversial, partly because of limited data and partly from variations in training and testing protocols.[76,86] One study reported no significant change in β-endorphin response to prolonged exercise following 8 weeks of endurance training. Contrasting research showed that general physical conditioning augmented β-endorphin and β-lipotropin release in exercise.[26] Greater endorphin release also occurs with sprint-type training, suggesting that anaerobic factors affect endorphin dynamics.[112]

Exercise training can also increase an individual's sensitivity to opioid effects, thus reducing the amount of hormone required to induce a specific effect. Regular exercise causes the opioids produced during exercise to degrade more slowly than in the pretraining condition.[92] A slower rate of hormone disposal facilitates and prolongs an opioid response and possibly augments one's tolerance for extended exercise. Taken in total, one could view the endogenous opioid response to regular exercise as a form of "positive addiction."

INTEGRATIVE QUESTION

List supplements at your local health food store that claim to enhance exercise performance. Which supplements purport to simulate hormone release? Based on hormonal regulation and function, can any of these products deliver on their claims?

EXERCISE, INFECTIOUS ILLNESS, CANCER, AND IMMUNE RESPONSE

"Don't exercise when fatigued or you'll get sick" reflects the common perception of parents, athletes, and coaches that excessive intense exercise increases susceptibility to certain illnesses. In contrast, some also believe that regular, more moderate exercise improves health and reduces susceptibility to infectious illnesses as the common cold.

Studies as early as 1918 reported that most cases of pneumonia in boys in boarding school occurred among athletes, and respiratory infections seemed to progress toward pneumonia after intense sports training. Anecdotal reports also related the severity of poliomyelitis to participation in intense physical activity at the critical time of infection. Current epidemiologic and clinical findings from the field of **exercise immunology**—the study of the interactions of physical, environmental, and psychologic factors on immune function—support the contention that short-term, unusually strenuous physical activity affects immune function to increase susceptibility to illness, particularly upper respiratory tract infection (URTI). Repeated URTI may signal a state of overtraining (see Chapter 21).[167]

The immune system comprises a highly complex and self-regulating grouping of cells, hormones, and interactive modulators that defend the body from invasion from outside microbes (bacterial, viral, and fungal), foreign macromolecules, and abnormal cancerous cell growth. This system has two functional divisions: (1) **innate immunity** and (2) **acquired immunity**. The innate immune system includes anatomic and physiologic components (skin, mucous membranes, body temperature, and specialized defenses such as natural killer cells, diverse phagocytes, and inflammatory barriers). The acquired immune system consists of specialized B- and T-lymphocyte cells. When activated these cells regulate a highly effective immune response to a specific infectious

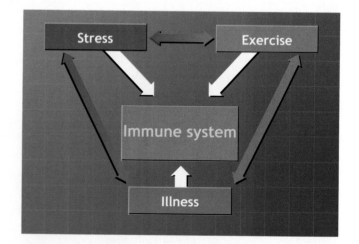

Figure 20.33   Theoretical model of the interrelationships between stress, exercise, illness, and the immune system. (From MacKinnon LT. Current challenges and future expectations in exercise immunology: back to the future. Med Sci Sports Exerc 1994;26:191.)

agent. If infection does occur, an optimal immune system diminishes the severity of illness and speeds recovery.

FIGURE 20.33 shows a proposed model for the interactions of exercise, stress, illness, and the immune system. Within this framework, exercise, stress, and illness interact, each exerting its separate effect on immunity. For example, exercise affects susceptibility to illness, while certain illnesses clearly affect exercise capacity. Likewise, psychologic factors (via links between the hypothalamus and immune function) and other forms of stress, including nutritional deficiencies and acute alterations in normal sleep schedule, influence resistance to illness. Concurrently, exercise can either positively or negatively modulate the response to stress. Each factor—stress, illness, and short- and long-term exercise—exerts an independent effect on immune status, immune function, and resistance to disease.

Upper Respiratory Tract Infections

FIGURE 20.34 describes the general J-shaped curve of the relationship between exercise volume and/or intensity and susceptibility to URTI. Diverse markers of immune function generally follow an *inverted* J-shaped curve.[163,229] Implications drawn from this relationship may be simplistic, but light to moderate physical activity offers more protection against URTI and possibly diverse cancers than a sedentary life-

style.[98,129,130,134,192] In addition, moderate exercise does not exacerbate the severity and duration of illness when an infection occurs.[218] In contrast, a marathon run or intense training session provides an "open window" (3 to 72 h) that decreases antiviral and antibacterial resistance and increases risk of URTI that manifests itself within 1 to 2 weeks.[36,151,169] For example, approximately 13% of the participants in a Los Angeles marathon reported an episode of infectious URTI during the week following the race. For runners of comparable ability who did not compete for reasons other than illness, the infection rate approximated just 2%.[152]

Short-Term Exercise Effects

- **Moderate exercise:** *A moderate exercise bout boosts natural immune functions and host defenses for up to several hours.*[108] Noteworthy effects include an increase in **natural killer (NK) cell** activity. These phagocytic lymphocyte subpopulations enhance the blood's cytotoxic capacity and provide the first line of defense against pathogens. The NK cell does not require prior or specific sensitization to foreign bodies or neoplastic cells. Rather, these cells demonstrate spontaneous cytolytic activity that ultimately ruptures and/or inactivates viruses and depresses the metastatic potential of tumor cells.[67,225]

- **Exhaustive exercise:** Prolonged exhaustive exercise (and other forms of extreme stress or increased training) severely depresses the body's first line of defense against infection.[22,100,110,111,126,150,166,193,219] Repeated cycles of unusually intense exercise and sports participation further compound the risk. For example, impaired immune function from strenuous exercise "carries over" to a second bout of exercise on the same day to augment negative changes in neutrophils, lymphocytes, and select CD cells.[182] Elevated temperature, cytokines, and various stress-related hormones (epinephrine, GH, cortisol, β-endorphins) in exhaustive exercise may mediate the transient depression of innate (NK cell and neutrophil cytotoxicity) and depress adaptive immune defenses (T- and B-cell function).[7,153,200,205] Reduced immunity following strenuous exercise remains in the mucosal immune system of the upper respiratory tract.[59,146,215] This negative effect on immune response clearly supports the wisdom of advising individuals with URTI symptoms to refrain from physical activity (or at least "go easy") to optimize normal immune mechanisms that combat infection. TABLE 20.6 summarizes components of the immune system that exhibit transient changes after prolonged intense exertion.

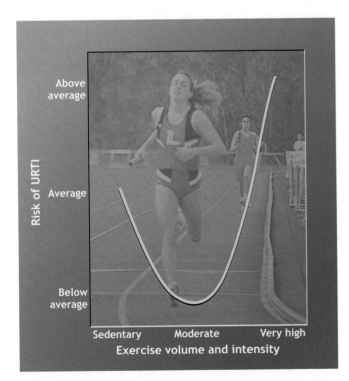

Figure 20.34 General model for the relationship between intensity of physical activity and susceptibility to upper respiratory tract infection *(URTI)*. Moderate exercise reduces risk of URTI, whereas exhaustive competition or training places the participant at increased risk. (From Nieman DC. Exercise, upper respiratory tract infection, and the immune system. Med Sci Sports Exerc 1994;26:128.)

Long-Term Exercise Effects

Aerobic training positively affects natural immune functions in young and old individuals and in obese persons during weight loss.[47,50,186,191,198] Areas of improvement include

TABLE 20.6 ■ IMMUNE SYSTEM COMPONENTS THAT EXHIBIT CHANGE FOLLOWING PROLONGED, INTENSE EXERCISE

- High neutrophil and low lymphocyte blood counts, induced by high concentrations of plasma cortisol
- Increase in blood granulocyte and monocyte phagocytosis (engulfing of infectious agents and of breakdown products of muscle fiber); decrease in nasal neutrophil phagocytosis
- Decrease in granulocyte oxidative-burst activity (killing activity)
- Decrease in nasal mucociliary clearance (sweeping movement of cilia)
- Decrease in NK-cell cytotoxic activity (the ability to kill infected cells or cancer cells)
- Decrease in mitogen-induced lymphocyte proliferation (a measure of T-cell function)
- Decrease in the delayed-type hypersensitivity skin response (the ability of the immune system to produce hard red lumps after the skin is pricked with antigens)
- Increase in plasma concentrations of pro- and antiinflammatory cytokines (e.g., interleukin-6 and interleukin-1 receptor antagonist)
- Decrease in ex vivo production of cytokines (interferon-8, interleukin-1, and interleukin-6) to mitogens and endotoxin
- Decrease in nasal and salivary IgA concentration (an important antibody)
- Blunted expression of major histocompatibility complex (MHC) II in macrophages (an important step in recognition of foreign agents by the immune system)

From Nieman DC. Immunity in athletes: current issues. Sports Sci Exchange, Gatorade Sports Science Institute 1998;11(2).

enhanced functional capacity of natural cytotoxic immune mechanisms (e.g., antitumor actions of NK cell activity) and diminished age-related decrease in T-cell function and associated cytokine production.[96,155] The cytotoxic T cells defend directly against viral and fungal infections and help to regulate other immune mechanisms.

If exercise training enhances immune function, one might ask why trained individuals show increased susceptibility to URTI after intense competition. The **open window hypothesis** maintains that an inordinate increase in training or competition exposes the highly conditioned athlete to nonnormal stress that transiently but severely depresses NK cell function. This period of immunodepression (open window) decreases natural resistance to infection. The inhibitory effect of strenuous exercise on ACTH and cortisol's maintenance of optimal blood glucose concentrations may negatively affect the immune process. For individuals who exercise regularly but only at moderate levels, the window of opportunity for infection remains "closed," thus maintaining the protective benefits of regular exercise on immune function.

Resistance Training. In contrast to the beneficial effect of regular aerobic exercise on immune function, nine years of prior resistance exercise training did not affect resting NK cell activity or number compared to sedentary controls.[156] Comparisons

also indicated that resistance training activated monocytes more than typically observed for aerobic training. Monocyte activation releases prostaglandins that downregulate NK cells following exercise, thus blunting the long-term positive effect of exercise on NK cells. These researchers had previously shown a substantial 225% increase in NK cells following a short-term bout of resistance exercise,[157] a response similar to the short-term effect of moderate aerobic exercise.[53,74]

Perhaps a Role for Nutritional Supplements.
Macronutrients. Nutrition may optimize immune system function with strenuous exercise and training.[29,58,79,138,187] For example, consuming a fat-rich diet (62% energy from lipids) negatively affected the immune system compared to a carbohydrate-rich diet (65% energy from carbohydrates).[168] In general, endurance athletes who ingest carbohydrate during a race experience lower disruption in hormonal and immune measures (indicating a diminished level of physiologic stress) than athletes not consuming carbohydrate. Supplementing with a 6% carbohydrate beverage (0.7l L before; 0.25 L every 15 min during; 500 mL every h throughout a 4.5-h recovery) depressed cytokine levels in the inflammatory cascade after 2.5 hours of running at 77% $\dot{V}O_{2max}$.[149] Consuming carbohydrates (4 mL per kg of body mass) every 15 minutes during 2.5 hours of high-intensity running or cycling maintained higher plasma glucose levels in 10 triathletes during exercise than a placebo.[159] A blunted cortisol response and diminished pro- and anti-inflammatory cytokine responses accompanied the higher plasma glucose levels with supplementation in both forms of exercise. Similar benefits from carbohydrate ingestion for cortisol and select anti-inflammatory cytokines occur following marathon competition, regardless of age or gender.[160] *This suggests a carbohydrate-induced reduction in overall physiologic stress in prolonged high-intensity exercise.* In contrast, carbohydrate ingestion during two hours of intense resistance training produced no effect on immune changes compared to similar training with placebo ingestion.[161]

Micronutrients. Combined supplementation with the antioxidant vitamins C and E produces more prominent immunopotentiating effects (enhanced cytokine production) in young, healthy adults than supplementation with either vitamin alone.[93] Also, a 200-mg daily vitamin E supplement enhanced several clinically relevant indices of T-cell–mediated function in healthy elderly subjects.[139] However, long-term daily supplementation with a physiologic dose of vitamins and minerals or with 200 mg of vitamin E *did not lower* the incidence and severity of acute respiratory tract infections in noninstitutionalized persons aged 60 and older. For individuals with infections, those receiving vitamin E had *longer* total illness duration and restriction of activity.[64]

Daily supplementation with vitamin C benefits individuals engaged in intense exercise, particularly those predisposed to frequent URTI.[77,170] Runners who received a 600-mg daily vitamin C supplement before and for 3 weeks following a 90-km ultramarathon competition experienced fewer symptoms of URTI—running nose, sneezing, sore throat, coughing, fever—than runners given a placebo.[169] Interestingly, infection risk inversely related to race performance; those with the fastest times suffered more symptoms. URTI also appeared most frequently in runners with strenuous training regimens. For these individuals, additional vitamin C and E and perhaps carbohydrate ingestion before, during, and after prolonged stressful exercise may boost immune mechanisms for combating this type of infection.[153,158] More than likely, other stressors—sleep deficit, mental stress, poor nutrition, or weight loss—magnify stress on the immune system from a single or repeated bout of exhaustive exercise.[29,153]

Glutamine and the Immune Response. The nonessential amino acid glutamine plays an important role in normal immune function. One protective aspect concerns glutamine's role as an energy fuel for nucleotide synthesis by disease fighting cells, particularly lymphocytes and macrophages that defend against infection.[4,25,194] In humans, sepsis, injury, burns, surgery, and endurance exercise lower plasma and skeletal muscle glutamine levels. Lowered plasma glutamine levels most likely occur because glutamine demand by the liver, kidneys, gut, and immune system exceeds its supply from the diet and skeletal muscle. The lowered plasma glutamine concentration contributes in part to the immunosuppression that accompanies extreme physical stress.[13,80,184,197] Thus, glutamine supplementation might reduce susceptibility to URTI following prolonged competition or a bout of exhaustive training.[190]

Marathoners who ingested a glutamine drink (5 g L-glutamine in 330 mL mineral water) at the end of a race and then 2 hours later reported fewer URTI symptoms than unsupplemented athletes.[27] In subsequent studies by the same researchers to determine a possible protective mechanism, glutamine's effect on postexercise infection risk did not relate to any change in blood lymphocyte distribution.[28] Appearance of URTI in athletes during intense training does not fluctuate with changes in plasma glutamine concentration. Furthermore, preexercise glutamine supplementation does not affect the immune response following repeated bouts of intense exercise.[124] Glutamine supplements taken 0, 30, 60, and 90 minutes after a marathon race prevented the drop in glutamine concentrations following the race but *did not influence* lymphokine-activated killer cell activity, proliferative responses, or exercise-induced changes in leukocyte subpopulations.[180] Based on current evidence, we cannot recommend glutamine supplements to reliably blunt immunosuppression from exhaustive exercise.

A General Recommendation

A lifestyle that emphasizes regular physical activity, maintenance of a well-balanced diet, reducing stress to a minimum, and obtaining adequate sleep generally optimizes immune function. For weight loss, we recommend a gradual approach because more rapid weight loss with accompanying severe caloric restriction suppresses immune function.[154] With prolonged intense exercise, ingesting about 1 L · h⁻¹ of a typical carbohydrate-rich sports drink lessens negative changes in immune function from the stress of exercise and accompanying carbohydrate depletion. In general, endurance athletes who consume carbohydrate during a race experience a lower disruption in hormonal and immune measures than athletes who do not consume carbohydrate.

The Exercise–Cancer Connection

Epidemiologic studies generally demonstrate a protective association between regular physical activity and risk of cancers of the breast, colon, lung, and prostate (see Chapter 31).[127,140] Long-term enhancement of other natural immune functions may contribute to the cancer-protective effect of regular exercise in addition to exercise's beneficial effect on NK cell activity. Upgraded defenses include augmented phagocytic capacity of the monocyte–macrophage lineage combined with more robust cytotoxic and intracellular killing capacities (T-cell activity) that inhibit tumor growth and destroy cancer cells.[225,228] Other potential effects of regular exercise on aspects of cancer development include beneficial changes in the body's antioxidant functions, endocrine profiles, prostaglandin metabolism, body composition, and, in the case of colon cancer, a beneficial increase in intestinal transit time. In Chapter 31, we review the role of exercise in the prevention and treatment of different cancers.

Summary

1. The endocrine system consists of a host organ, a transmitted substance (hormone), and a target or receptor organ. Hormones consist of steroids or amino acid (polypeptide) derivatives.
2. Hormones alter rates of cellular reactions by acting at specific receptor sites to enhance or inhibit enzyme function.
3. The amount of hormone synthesized, the amount released or taken up by the target organ, and the removal rate from the blood influence blood hormone concentration.
4. Most hormones respond to peripheral stimulus on an as-needed basis; others release at regular intervals. Some secretory cycles span several weeks; others pattern on a 24-hour cycle.
5. The anterior pituitary secretes at least six hormones: PRL, the gonadotropic hormones FSH and LH, corticotropin, TSH, and GH.
6. GH promotes cell division and cellular proliferation. IGFs (or somatomedins) mediate many of GH's effects.
7. TSH controls the amount of hormone secreted by the thyroid gland; ACTH regulates output of hormones from the adrenal cortex; PRL affects reproduction and development of secondary sex

characteristics of females; FSH and LH stimulate the ovaries to secrete estrogen in females and the testes to secrete testosterone in males.

8. The posterior pituitary secretes ADH, which controls water excretion by the kidneys. It also secretes oxytocin, an important hormone in birthing and lactation.

9. PTH controls blood calcium balance; a decrease in blood calcium concentration triggers its release. It increases ionic (free) calcium levels by stimulating three target organs: bone, kidneys, and the small intestine.

10. TSH stimulates metabolism of all cells and increases carbohydrate and fat breakdown in energy metabolism.

11. The inner (medulla) and outer (cortex) regions of the adrenal gland secrete two different types of hormones. The medulla secretes epinephrine and norepinephrine. The adrenal cortex secretes mineralocorticoids (regulate extracellular sodium and potassium levels), glucocorticoids (stimulate gluconeogenesis and serve as insulin antagonists), and androgens (control male secondary sex characteristics).

12. Testes in the male produce testosterone and ovaries in the female produce the estrogens estradiol and progesterone.

13. Moderate aerobic and resistance exercise increases testosterone in untrained males. For females, plasma testosterone and estrogen levels increase during moderate exercise.

14. Secreted by the β-cells of the pancreas' islets of Langerhans, insulin increases glucose transport into cells to control blood glucose levels and carbohydrate metabolism.

15. Total lack of insulin or decreased sensitivity or increased resistance to this hormone produces diabetes mellitus.

16. The β-cells of the pancreas secrete glucagon, an insulin antagonist that raises blood sugar levels.

17. Exercise training exerts differential effects on resting and exercise-induced hormone production and release. Trained persons have elevated hormone response during exercise for ACTH and cortisol, and depressed values for GH, PRL, FSH, LH, testosterone, ADH, thyroxine, catecholamines, and insulin. No training response occurs for aldosterone, renin, and angiotensin.

18. Exercise-induced elevation of β-endorphins and other opioid-like hormones contributes to euphoria, increased pain tolerance, "exercise high," and altered menstrual function.

19. Unusually intense physical activity affects immune function in a manner that increases susceptibility to URTI. Moderate exercise upgrades immune responses to protect against URTI.

20. Regular exercise training positively affects natural immune functions. An enhanced immune profile protects against URTI and various cancers.

References are available on the Student CD and online at http://connection.lww.com/mkk6e.

two

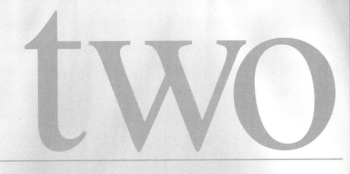

Applied
Exercise
Physiology

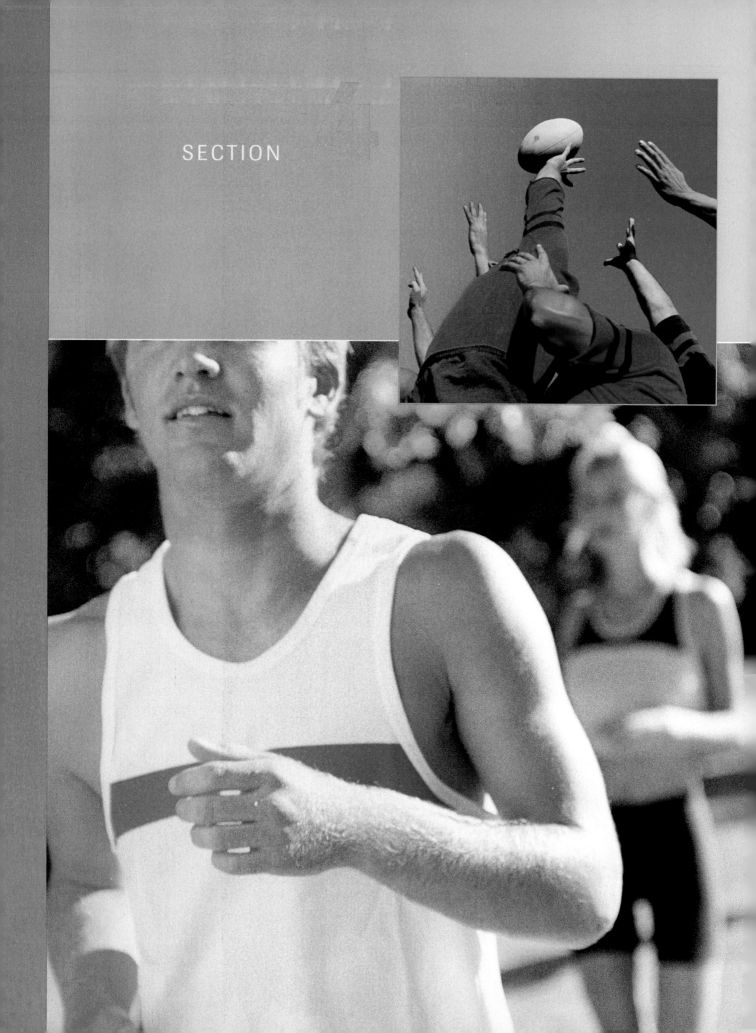

SECTION 4

Enhancement of Energy Transfer Capacity

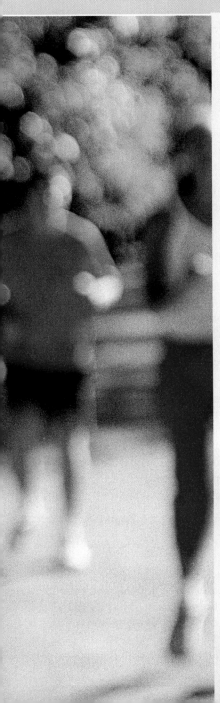

Interview *with* **Bengt Saltin**

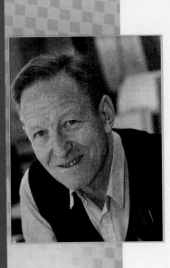

Name: Bengt Saltin

Education: Södertälje Gymnasium (1955); Medical School, Karolinska Institute, Stockholm (1956–62); Thesis in physiology, Karolinksa Institute, Stockholm (1964).

Current Affiliation: Director, Copenhagen Muscle Research Centre at Rigshospitalet and the University of Copenhagen; Adjunct professor, August Krogh Institute, University of Copenhagen.

Honors and Awards: See Appendix E, which is available on the Student CD and online at http://connection.lww.com/mkk6e.

Research Focus: Exploration of integrative cardiovascular and metabolic response to physical exercise, including studies on skeletal muscle in humans by direct needle biopsy.

Memorable Publication: Saltin B, et al. Response to exercise after bed rest and after training: a longitudinal study of adaptive changes in oxygen transport and body composition. Circulation 1968;38(Suppl 7):79.

Statement of Contributions: ACSM Honor Award

In recognition of his studies which provide a better understanding of maximal oxygen uptake in human subjects under different physiological and patho-physiological conditions, particularly thermal stress and dehydration.

His classic study on exercise after bed rest and after training was the scientific foundation for the current early ambulation and exercise treatment of patients with coronary heart disease and the understanding of deconditioning that occurs in space travel.

In the late 1960s, he began his seminal studies on skeletal muscle in humans obtained by direct needle biopsy. This pioneering work has had a profound influence on our understanding of the anatomical, physiological, and biochemical behavior of skeletal muscle and its interactions with the cardiovascular system. His recent work has determined the maximal flow capacity in active skeletal muscle, and shows that the limiting factor in maximal oxygen uptake is the pumping capacity of the heart.

Dr. Saltin has provided training for many of the current leaders in exercise and sports science and they have greatly benefited from his unique ability to acquire new knowledge by studying at all levels of integration.

What first inspired you to enter the exercise science field? What made you decide to pursue your advanced degree and/or line of research?

■ In January of 1958, I had my oral examination in physiology as part of my medical studies. The examiner was Professor Ulf von Euler (later the 1970 Nobel Prize winner in physiology or medicine for discoveries concerning humoral transmitters in the nerve terminal and the mechanisms for their storage, release, and inactivation). At the end of the examination I was asked whether I would be interested in staying on as a student instructor. My answer was yes. As I had an interest in orienteering (a common sport in Scandinavia), I wanted to be associated with exercise-related research. Professor Euler called Erik Hohwü-Christensen, who was the professor of physiology at the Royal School of Gymnastics. The week after I met with Professor Hohwü-Christensen in the summer of 1958, I started to work with him on a project that evaluated energy demands in intermittent exercise. During the semesters, I helped with teaching while at the same time continuing my medical studies. In the fall of 1961, I decided to go for a doctoral thesis in physiology, which I defended in May 1964.

Who were the most influential people in your career, and why?

■ Two people played a very important role in my scientific career. I would like to acknowledge Professor Erik Hohwü-Christensen and Professor Per-Olof Åstrand. Professor Hohwü-Christensen had been a student of Johannes Lindhard, the first Docent of the equivalent of an endowed Chair in Anatomy, Physiology, and Theory of Gymnastics at the University of Copenhagen, and had also done cooperative research with 1920 Nobel Prize winner August Krogh. Professor Per-Olof Åstrand at the Karolinska Institute was the equivalent of my PhD dissertation research advisor. My projects were concerned with trying to better understand maximal oxygen uptake in human subjects and its determinants under different physiological and pathophysiological conditions, particularly thermal stress and dehydration. The knowledge and passion of these two pioneer scientists encouraged a younger generation of researchers-to-be to focus on human integrative physiology.

What has been the most interesting/enjoyable aspect of your involvement in science? What was the least interesting/enjoyable aspect?

■ This is a difficult question to answer. I have been very fortunate to work with many scientists from all over the world. For example, in 1965, I spent 1 year in the Department of Medicine at the University of Texas in Dallas. Later, I worked for 5 months at the John B. Pierce Institute and Department of Physiology at Yale University in New Haven, Connecticut. In 1972, I spent 2 months in the Department of Medicine at the University of California, San Francisco, and

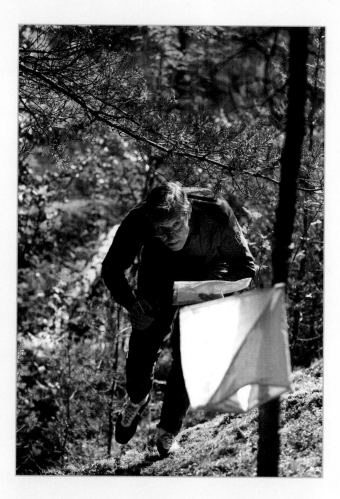

then in 1976, I spent 3 months working with David Costill in The Human Performance Laboratory at Ball State University in Muncie, Indiana. I also spent 4 months at Cumberland College and the Department of Physiology at New South Wales University in Sydney, Australia. For my interest in high-altitude physiology and temperature regulation, I was fortunate to spend from 1 to 5 months between the years of 1960 and 1989 in laboratories in Northern Norway studying the physical profile and health of Nomadic Lapps, and at the following locations studying high-altitude physiology: Mt. Evans (Colorado), Mexico City, the Andes and Himalayan mountains, and Kenya. I also had a wonderful experience studying the physiological responses to exercise in racing camels in the Arabian desert.

What is your most meaningful contribution to the field of exercise science, and why is it so important?

■ To try to better understand, not only to describe, basic phenomena concerned with physiological responses to exercise under various environmental conditions. Exercise science was a key area in science in the latter part of the 19th century and in the first three decades of the 20th century. There are many reasons for the lack of major contributions since then. One reason could be that the majority of exercise scientists describe a phenomenon, but they do not try hard enough to penetrate the mechanisms and thereby contribute to the fundamental understanding of the phenomenon.

What advice would you give to students who express an interest in pursuing a career in exercise science research?

■ Become very focused and learn basic techniques. Today, exercise science is to a large extent the study of acute and chronic adaptations. Thus, one route I would highlight is to identify the exercise stimulus and the intracellular signalling of genes of importance for muscle adaptation. In an article in *Scientific American* (September 2000), we pointed out that Olympic athletes depend on how well their muscles adapt to the stress of high-intensity aerobic, anaerobic, and resistance training. However, recent research suggests that the ratio of fast-to-slow-twitch muscle fibers depends on inherited characteristics. Unfortunately, future genetic technologies could change even that as athletes experiment with methods to enhance muscle performance.

What interests have you pursued outside your professional career?

■ I have been heavily involved in the sport of orienteering, both as a runner and administrator. From 1982 to 1988, I served as a Board Member and President of the International Orienteering Federation. I am a theater freak and have an interest in literature. Ibsen and Strindberg are my favorites, but

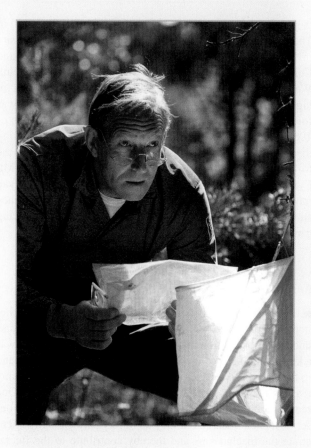

most classical plays from antique Greece onwards will bring me to the theater. Throughout life my "reading companions" have been Katherine Mansfield, Albert Camus, Joseph Brodsky, and to name a Dane, J. P. Jacobsen.

You have the opportunity to give a last lecture. Describe its primary focus.

■ I have given my "last" lecture. It focused on how young exercise physiologists could best serve an area in research and also make a major contribution to science. A major point was to identify an important phenomenon. If there are ample methods to study it, then stay with it until it has been solved. In other words, be mechanistic, carefully explain the phenomena, and then do whatever you can to understand it.

Training for Anaerobic and Aerobic Power

21

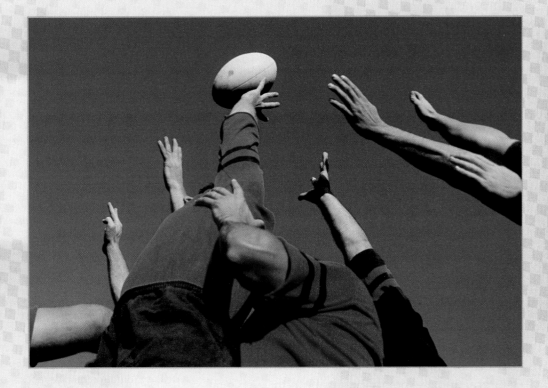

CHAPTER OBJECTIVES

- Discuss and provide examples of the exercise training principles of (1) overload, (2) specificity, (3) individual differences, and (4) reversibility

- Outline the metabolic adaptations to anaerobic exercise training

- Outline the metabolic, cardiovascular, and pulmonary adaptations to aerobic exercise training

- Discuss factors that expand the a-v̄O$_2$ difference during graded exercise, and how endurance training affects each component

- Explain the effects of endurance training on regional blood flow

- Explain the term *athlete's heart;* contrast structural and functional characteristics of an endurance athlete's heart and a resistance-trained athlete's heart

- Describe the influence of (1) initial fitness level, (2) genetics, (3) training frequency, (4) training duration, and (5) training intensity on the aerobic training response

- Discuss the rationale for using heart rate to establish exercise intensity for aerobic training

- Discuss the term *training-sensitive zone,* including its rationale, advantages, limitations, and use for men and women of different ages

- Give the reason for adjusting the training-sensitive zone for swimming and other forms of upper-body exercise

- Justify the "rating of perceived exertion" to establish exercise intensity for aerobic training

- Outline advantages of training at the lactate threshold

- Contrast continuous and intermittent aerobic exercise training and advantages and disadvantages of each

- Summarize current recommendations by the American College of Sports Medicine concerning the quantity and quality of exercise to develop and maintain cardiorespiratory and muscular fitness and joint flexibility in healthy adults

- Outline the application of the overload principle to train the (1) intramuscular high-energy phosphates and (2) glycolytic energy system

- Summarize important factors about the exercise prescription for interval training

- Describe the most common form of overtraining syndrome and summarize interacting factors that contribute to overtraining in endurance athletes

- Summarize current recommendations for regular physical activity during pregnancy

Throughout this book we emphasize that different physical activities, depending on duration and intensity, activate highly specific energy transfer systems. FIGURE 21.1 illustrates examples of sport and physical activities broadly classified for duration and predominant energy pathways. We realize the difficulty in placing certain activities into one category. For example, as a person increases aerobic fitness, an activity previously classified as anaerobic may become aerobic. In many cases, all three energy-transfer systems—adenosine triphosphate–phosphocreatine (ATP–PCr) system, lactic acid system, and aerobic system—operate predominantly at different times during exercise. Their relative contributions to the energy continuum directly relate to the duration and intensity (power output) of a specific activity.

Brief power activities lasting up to 6 seconds in duration rely almost exclusively on "immediate" energy generated from breakdown of the stored intramuscular high-energy phosphates, ATP and PCr. Consequently, power athletes (e.g., sprinters, football players, shot putters, pole vaulters) must gear training toward improving this energy-transfer capacity. As all-out exercise progresses to 60 seconds in duration and power output decreases, most of the energy for exercise still arises through anaerobic pathways. These metabolic reactions also involve the glycolytic short-term energy system with subsequent lactate accumulation. As exercise intensity diminishes and duration extends to 2 to 4 minutes, reliance on energy from the intramuscular phosphagens and anaerobic glycolysis decreases, and aerobic ATP production becomes increasingly important. Prolonged exercise progresses on a "pay-as-you-go" basis, with aerobic metabolism generating more than 99% of the energy requirement. Clearly, an efficient training program allocates a proportionate commitment to targeted training of specific energy and physiologic systems activated in the activity. In the sections that follow, we discuss anaerobic and aerobic conditioning with emphasis on principles, methods, and short-term responses and longer term training adaptations. *The basic approach to physiologic conditioning applies similarly to men and women within a broad age range: both respond and adapt to training in essentially the same way.*

TRAINING PRINCIPLES

Stimulating structural and functional adaptations to improve performance in specific physical tasks remains the major objective of exercise training. These adaptations require adherence to carefully planned programs, with attention focused on frequency and length of workouts, type of training, speed, intensity, duration, and repetition of the activity, rest intervals, and appropriate competition. Application of these factors varies depending on the performance and fitness goals. Several principles of physiologic conditioning are common to improving performance in the diverse physical activity classifications illustrated in Figure 21.1.

Overload Principle

*Regular application of a specific exercise **overload** enhances physiologic function to induce a training response.* Exercising at intensities greater than normal stimulates highly specific adaptations so the body functions more efficiently. Achieving the appropriate overload requires manipulating training *frequency, intensity,* and *duration,* with focus on exercise *mode.*

The concept of individualized and progressive overload applies to athletes, sedentary persons, disabled persons, and even cardiac patients. An increasing number in this latter group have applied appropriate exercise rehabilitation to walk, jog, and eventually run and compete in marathons and triathlons. As we discuss in Chapter 31, achieving health-related benefits of regular exercise requires lower exercise intensity (but greater volume) than required to improve aerobic fitness.[7,46,47,113,133,135,217,220]

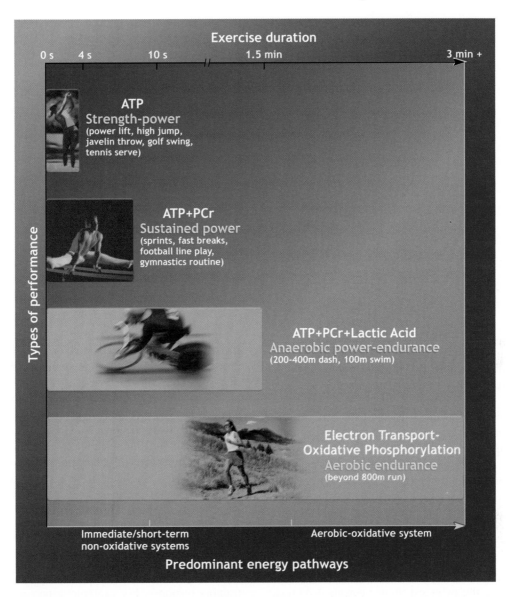

Figure 21.1 Classification of physical activity based on duration of all-out exercise and the corresponding predominant intracellular energy pathways.

Specificity Principle

Exercise training specificity refers to adaptations in metabolic and physiologic functions that depend upon the type and mode of overload imposed. A specific anaerobic exercise stress (e.g., strength–power training) induces specific strength–power adaptations; specific endurance exercise stress elicits specific aerobic system adaptations—with only a limited interchange of benefits between strength–power training and aerobic training. Nonetheless, the specificity principle extends beyond this broad demarcation. Aerobic training, for example, does not represent a singular entity requiring *only* cardiovascular overload. Aerobic training that relies on the specific muscles in the desired performance most effectively improves aerobic fitness for swimming,[132] bicycling,[158] running,[137] or upper-body exercise.[118] Some evidence even suggests a temporal specificity in training response such that indicators of training improvement peak

when measured at the time of day when training regularly occurred.[84] The most effective evaluation of sport-specific performance occurs when the laboratory measurement most closely simulates the actual sport activity and/or uses the muscle mass and movement patterns required by the sport.[14,62,117,190] *Simply stated, specific exercise elicits specific adaptations to create specific training effects.*

Specificity of $\dot{V}O_{2max}$

TABLE 21.1 presents evidence for the specificity of endurance swim training on aerobic capacity improvements. Fifteen men trained 1 hour daily, 3 days a week, for 10 weeks. For all subjects, treadmill running and tethered swimming tests measured $\dot{V}O_{2max}$ before and after training. Vigorous swimming elicits a general circulatory overload, so the researchers expected at least minimal improvement (or "transfer") in aerobic power from swimming to running. This did

TABLE 21.1 ■ EFFECTS OF 10 WEEKS OF INTERVAL SWIM TRAINING ON CHANGES IN $\dot{V}O_{2MAX}$ AND ENDURANCE PERFORMANCE DURING RUNNING AND SWIMMING

SUBJECTS	MEASURE	RUNNING TEST			SWIMMING TEST		
		Pretraining	Posttraining	% Change	Pretraining	Posttraining	% Change
Swim Training	$\dot{V}O_{2max}$						
	$L \cdot min^{-1}$	4.05	4.11	1.5	3.44	3.82	11.0
	$mL \cdot kg^{-1} \cdot min^{-1}$	54.9	55.7	1.5	46.6	51.8	11.0
	Max work time						
	min	19.6	20.5	4.6	11.9	15.9	34.0
Nontraining Controls							
	$\dot{V}O_{2max}$						
	$L \cdot min^{-1}$	4.12	4.18	1.5	3.51	3.40	3.1
	$mL \cdot kg^{-1} \cdot min^{-1}$	55.1	55.5	0.7	46.8	45.0	−3.8
	Max work time						
	min	20.7	19.7	−4.8	11.5	11.5	0

From Magel JR, et al. Specificity of swim training on maximum oxygen uptake. J Appl Physiol 1975;38:151.

not occur. Almost total specificity accompanied the $\dot{V}O_{2max}$ improvement with swim training. Treadmill running alone to assess swim training effects would have mistakenly concluded no swim training effect!

When training for specific aerobic activities such as cycling, swimming, rowing, or running, the overload must (1) engage the appropriate muscles required by the activity and (2) provide exercise at a level sufficient to stress the cardiovascular system. Little improvement occurs when measuring aerobic capacity with dissimilar exercise, yet the greatest improvement occurs when the test exercise duplicates the training exercise. These results also apply in exercise rehabilitation of patients with coronary artery disease.[153] The data in Table 21.1 also indicate that while swimming $\dot{V}O_{2max}$ improved 11% with swim training, maximum exercise time increased 34% during the swim test. Improvements in $\dot{V}O_{2max}$ probably reach a peak in training. Thereafter, other mechanisms (only partly related to the capacity of the oxygen transport system) support performance improvements. These adaptations most likely take place within the active musculature rather than the central circulatory system (see "Focus on Research," p. 473).

General improvements take place in cardiac function, whereas aerobic exercise training induces a highly specific $\dot{V}O_{2max}$ improvement. For example, ventricular contractility that improves with one mode of exercise training also improves when exercising the untrained limbs.[222] This finding indicates that individuals can train the myocardium per se with diverse "big-muscle" exercise modes.

Specificity of Local Changes

Overloading specific muscle groups with endurance training enhances exercise performance and aerobic power by facilitating oxygen transport *and* use at the local level of the trained muscles.[85,128,185] For example, the vastus lateralis muscle of well-trained cyclists has greater oxidative capacity than that of endurance runners; oxidative capacity in this muscle improves considerably following training on a bicycle ergometer. Such local adaptations increase the capacity of the trained muscles to generate ATP aerobically before the onset of lactate accumulation. The specificity of aerobic improvement may also result from greater regional blood flow in active tissues from (1) increased microcirculation, (2) more effective distribution of cardiac output, or (3) the combined effect of both factors. Regardless of the mechanism, these adaptations take place *only* in the specifically trained muscles and *only* become apparent in exercise that activates this musculature.

Individual Differences Principle

Many factors contribute to individual variation in the training response. For example, a person's relative fitness level at the start of training exerts an influence. This subprinciple of **initial values** states that individuals with lower fitness show the greatest improvement with training. This principle operates for healthy individuals and older adults with cardiovascular disease or at high risk for the disease.[19,177,239] When a relatively homogenous group starts exercise training, one cannot expect each person to reach the same state of fitness (or exercise performance) after 10 or 12 weeks. A coach should not insist that all athletes on the same team (or even in the same event) train the same way or at the same relative or absolute exercise intensity. All individuals do not respond similarly to a given training stimulus.

FIGURE 21.2 shows the heart rate curves of two college varsity forwards (same age) during warm-up and four consecutive 15-minute quarters of a basketball game. The heart rate for player A (*yellow line*) averaged 174 $b \cdot min^{-1}$ during each of the four quarters. Player B (*red line*) showed a similar heart rate response pattern, except heart rate averaged 163 $b \cdot min^{-1}$ during the game, with relatively small heart rate variation for both players. This difference in the magnitude of heart rate response during the hour-long game illustrates that two

HIGHLY SPECIFIC NATURE OF THE TRAINING RESPONSE

Saltin B, et al. The nature of the training response: peripheral and central adaptations to one-legged exercise. Acta Physiol Scand 1976;96:289.

▲ In 1976, Saltin and colleagues performed one of the first studies to document that regular exercise induces marked local adaptations in trained muscle. Importantly, these adjustments enhance local blood flow and metabolism in response to physical activity and also contribute to general cardiovascular function during exercise.

An elegant series of experiments separated local and general training effects. They applied different combinations of one-legged bicycle exercise to study simultaneously adaptations of skeletal muscles and central circulatory functions with training. Healthy but otherwise sedentary males with pretraining $\dot{V}O_{2max}$ of 46 mL $\cdot$ kg^{-1} $\cdot$ min^{-1} (range, 37 to 54) were placed into three training groups: group A—one-legged endurance training (E) and the other leg sprint training (S); group B—one-legged S and the other leg no training (NT); group C—one-legged E and the other leg NT. Exercise training performed on a bicycle ergometer with intensity adjusted to heart rate lasted 4 weeks with an average of 5 workouts per leg each week. The exercise intensity throughout training represented 75% for E and 150% for S of the one-legged $\dot{V}O_{2max}$ assessed pretraining and at week 3 to ensure proper training progression. Intensity and duration of each type of training produced similar total work output for each training bout. Total weekly energy output averaged 12,558 kCal per trained leg, with all groups achieving within 5 to 10% of this value; group A, however, performed 90 to 95% more work than group B because their training required both legs.

Pre- and posttraining measurements included needle biopsy samples from the quadriceps femoris for histochemical identification of muscle fiber type and area, glycogen concentration, and succinate dehydrogenase (SDH) and ATPase activity. Subjects performed submaximal and maximal exercise for each leg and during two-legged maximal cycling (8 of 13 subjects provided data to evaluate local metabolic adaptations to training). Measures included oxygen consumption, heart rate, arteriovenous oxygen difference (a-vO$_2$ diff) in muscle blood flow (catheters inserted in the two femoral arteries and veins to measure each leg's blood flow), and glucose and lactate. The major findings were:

- Exercise training improved $\dot{V}O_{2max}$ (particularly for the E-trained leg) and lowered heart rate and blood lactate in submaximal exercise *only* when exercising with a trained leg.

- Training induced no change in muscle fiber composition but produced pronounced metabolic adaptations reflected by enhanced SDH activity of the S- and E-trained legs, with no change in the NT leg. These changes generally paralleled increases in $\dot{V}O_{2max}$.

- Glycogen use during two-legged exercise remained lowest in the trained leg. Moreover, only the untrained leg continuously released lactate during submaximal exercise.

1. **One-legged exercise**
   Figure 1 shows that $\dot{V}O_{2max}$ increased nearly 20% with training in the E-trained leg, 11% in the S-trained leg, and 8% when exercising both legs (group A). S training of one leg only (group B) increased $\dot{V}O_{2max}$ by 15%, whereas $\dot{V}O_{2max}$ of the nontrained leg increased less than 2%. One-legged endurance training for group C increased $\dot{V}O_{2max}$ by 24% in the trained leg while $\dot{V}O_{2max}$ with the NT leg increased just 6%. These results confirmed that training only one leg exerts little effect on the nontrained leg, thus indicating considerable *training specificity*.

2. **Two-legged exercise**
   Analysis of pre- and posttraining two-legged $\dot{V}O_{2max}$ revealed mean increases for groups A (9%), B (10%), and C (8%). Figure 2 shows similar leg blood flow *(left panel)* in trained and untrained legs and in E-trained leg compared with S-trained legs. In addition, similarity existed for a-vO$_2$ difference *(middle panel)* for S- and E-trained legs during exercise. In the four subjects with one trained and one untrained leg, the slightly higher a-vO$_2$ differences in the trained leg resulted from a lower oxygen content in the femoral blood draining the trained leg (greater O$_2$ extraction). Endurance- and sprint-trained legs showed similar calculated oxygen consumptions during exercise *(right panel);* some subjects, however, showed higher values in the trained leg than in the untrained leg.

The study's major impact was demonstrating that an exercise training regimen elicits a distinct pattern of local adaptations *only* in the trained muscles. These specific local changes provide essential stimulation for the central cardiovascular response to exercise. Saltin and coworkers concluded that peripheral adaptations to training probably contribute as much to the training response as the well-documented improvement in central circulatory function.

continued on page 474

Continued

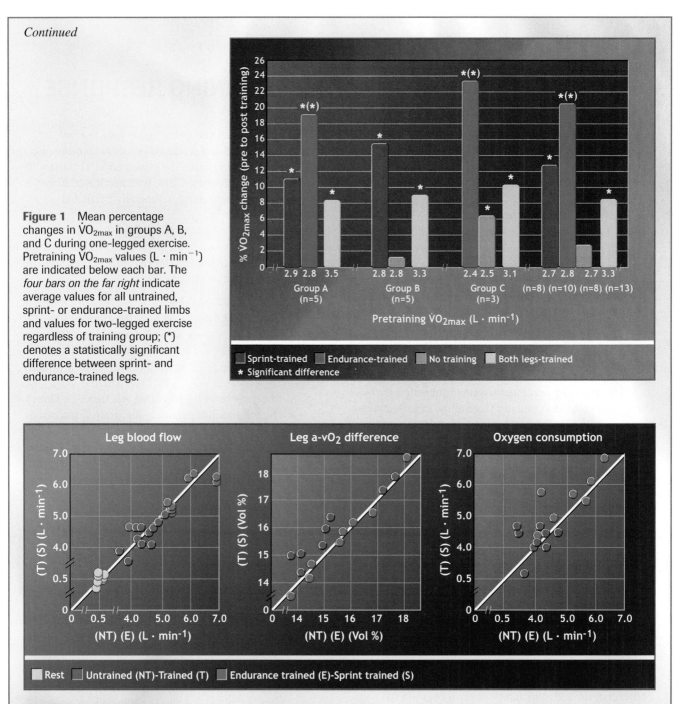

Figure 1   Mean percentage changes in $\dot{V}O_{2max}$ in groups A, B, and C during one-legged exercise. Pretraining $\dot{V}O_{2max}$ values (L · min^{-1}) are indicated below each bar. The *four bars on the far right* indicate average values for all untrained, sprint- or endurance-trained limbs and values for two-legged exercise regardless of training group; (*) denotes a statistically significant difference between sprint- and endurance-trained legs.

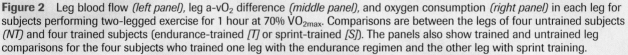

Figure 2   Leg blood flow *(left panel)*, leg a-vO₂ difference *(middle panel)*, and oxygen consumption *(right panel)* in each leg for subjects performing two-legged exercise for 1 hour at 70% $\dot{V}O_{2max}$. Comparisons are between the legs of four untrained subjects *(NT)* and four trained subjects (endurance-trained *[T]* or sprint-trained *[S]*). The panels also show trained and untrained leg comparisons for the four subjects who trained one leg with the endurance regimen and the other leg with sprint training.

individuals can perform at approximately equivalent intensity but at a 6.3% different level of cardiovascular strain as reflected by average exercise heart rate. *Optimal training benefits occur when exercise programs focus on the individual needs and capacities of the participants.* Chapter 11 and p. 495 of this chapter emphasize that genetic factors clearly interact to influence the training response.

Reversibility Principle

Loss of physiologic and performance training adaptations (**detraining**) occurs rapidly when a person terminates participation in regular exercise. Only 1 or 2 weeks of detraining reduces both metabolic and exercise capacity, with many training improvements lost within several months.[149] TABLE 21.2

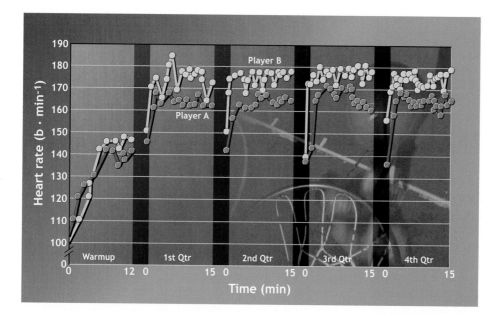

Figure 21.2 Individual differences in heart rate response in two forwards (same age) during a 60-minute basketball game. For player A *(yellow line)*, heart rate averaged 174 b · min⁻¹, and for player B *(red line)*, 163 b · min⁻¹. A miniature telemetry transmitter taped to each player's lower back monitored heart rate continuously throughout the game. (Data from F. Katch, Department of Exercise Science, University of Massachusetts, Amherst.)

TABLE 21.2 ■ CHANGES IN MEASURES OF PHYSIOLOGIC AND METABOLIC FUNCTION WITH VARIOUS DURATIONS OF DETRAINING[a]

VARIABLE	TRAINED	DETRAINED	CHANGE, % SHORT-TERM DETRAINING[b]	CHANGE, % LONGER-TERM DETRAINING[c]
$\dot{V}O_{2max}$, mL · min⁻¹ · kg⁻¹	62.2	57.3	−8	
	62.1	50.8		−18
$\dot{V}O_{2max}$, L · min⁻¹	4.45	4.16	−7	
Cardiac output, L · min⁻¹	27.8	25.5	−8	
	27.8	25.2		−10
Stroke volume, mL	155	139	−10	
	148	129		−13
Heart rate, b · min⁻¹	186	193	4	
	187	197		5
Oxygen pulse, mL · b⁻¹	12.7	10.9		−14
Sum 3-min recovery HR	190	237		25
Plasma volume, L	2.91	2.56	−12	
a-v̄ O₂ diff, mL · 100 mL⁻¹	15.1	15.4	−2 (NS)	
	15.1	14.1		−7
PCr, mM · (g wet wt)⁻¹	17.9	13.0		−27
ATP, mM · (g wet wt)⁻¹	5.97	5.08		−15
Glycogen, mM · (g wet wt)⁻¹	113.9	57.4		−50
Capillary density, cap · mm⁻²	511	476	−7	
	464	476		−2 (NS)
Oxidative enzyme capacity			−29	−32
Myoglobin, mg (g protein)⁻¹	43.3	41.0	−5 (NS)	
	43.3	40.7		−6
Insulin (rest)			17–120	
Norepinephrine/epinephrine (rest)			No change	
Norepinephrine/epinephrine (exercise)				65–100
Blood lactate			88	
Lactate threshold			−7	−18
Exercise lipolysis			−52	
Muscle glycogen synthesis			−29	−40
Time to fatigue, min			−10	
Swim power, W				−14
Elbow extension strength, ft-lb	39.0	25.5		−35

[a] Data represent an average computed from individual studies as cited in the following sources: McArdle WD, et al. Essentials of exercise physiology. 3rd ed. Lippincott Williams & Wilkins, 2006, and Wilber RL, Moffatt RJ. Physiological and biochemical consequences of detraining in aerobically trained individuals. J Strength Cond Res 1994;8:110. Note that a change for heart rate represents a decline in functional capacity. Omitted values for trained and detrained excluded in original sources.

[b] Short term, 3 weeks or less in primarily aerobically trained individuals.

[c] Longer term, 3 to 12 weeks in primarily aerobically trained individuals. NS, not statistically significant.

shows the biologic consequences of various durations of short-term (<3 weeks) and longer-term (3 to 12 weeks) detraining in endurance-trained individuals. The data represent average responses reported in the literature. One research group confined five subjects to bed for 20 consecutive days.[194] $\dot{V}O_{2max}$ decreased by 25%. This decrease accompanied a similar decrement in maximal stroke volume and cardiac output, which decreased aerobic capacity an average of 1% each day. Additionally, the number of capillaries within trained muscle decreased between 14 and 25% within 3 weeks after training ceased.[193] For elderly subjects, 4 months of detraining caused complete loss of endurance training adaptations on cardiovascular functions and body water distribution.[163]

Even among highly trained athletes, the beneficial effects of many years of prior exercise training remain transient and reversible. For this reason, most athletes begin a reconditioning program several months prior to the start of the competitive season or maintain some moderate level of off-season, sport-specific exercise to blunt the decline in physiologic functions from deconditioning.

PHYSIOLOGIC CONSEQUENCES OF TRAINING

The following sections present a more detailed listing of the diverse adaptations to anaerobic and aerobic exercise training outlined in TABLE 21.3. We also present many of the biologic changes that accompany training in other sections throughout the text.

ANAEROBIC SYSTEM CHANGES WITH TRAINING

FIGURE 21.3 summarizes the metabolic adaptations in anaerobic function that accompany strenuous physical training that overloads the anaerobic energy transfer systems. Consistent with the concept of training specificity, activities that demand a high level of anaerobic metabolism induce specific changes in the immediate and short-term energy systems without concomitant increases in aerobic functions.

TABLE 21.3 ■ TYPICAL METABOLIC AND PHYSIOLOGIC VALUES FOR HEALTHY, ENDURANCE-TRAINED AND UNTRAINED MEN[a]

VARIABLE	UNTRAINED	TRAINED	PERCENTAGE DIFFERENCE[b]
Glycogen, mM · (g wet muscle)$^{-1}$	85.0	120	41
Number of mitochondria, mmol^3	0.59	1.20	103
Mitochondrial volume, % muscle cell	2.15	8.00	272
Resting ATP, mM · (g wet muscle)$^{-1}$	3.0	6.0	100
Resting PCr, mM · (g wet muscle)$^{-1}$	11.0	18.0	64
Resting creatine, mM · (g wet muscle)$^{-1}$	10.7	14.5	35
Glycolytic enzymes			
Phosphofructokinase, mM · (g wet muscle)$^{-1}$	50.0	50.0	0
Phosphorylase, mM · (g wet muscle)$^{-1}$	4–6	6–9	60
Aerobic enzymes			
Succinate dehydrogenase, mM · (kg wet muscle)$^{-1}$	5–10	15–20	133
Max lactate, mM · (kg wet muscle)$^{-1}$	110	150	36
Muscle fibers			
Fast twitch, %	50	20–30	−50
Slow twitch, %	50	60	20
Max stroke volume, mL	120	180	50
Max cardiac output, L · min^{-1}	20	30–40	75
Resting heart rate, b · min^{-1}	70	40	−43
Max heart rate, bmin^{-1}	190	180	−5
Max a-$\bar{v}O_2$ diff, mL · dL^{-1}	14.5	16.0	10
$\dot{V}O_{2max}$, mL · kg^{-1} · min^{-1}	30–40	65–80	107
Heart volume, L	7.5	9.5	27
Blood volume, L	4.7	6.0	28
V_{Emax}, L · min^{-1}	110	190	73
Percentage body fat	15	11	−27

[a] In some cases, approximate values are used. In all cases, the trained values represent data from endurance athletes. Caution is advised in assuming that the percentage differences between trained and untrained necessarily results from training because genetic factors exert a strong influence on many of these factors.
[b] Percentage by which the value for the trained differs from the corresponding value for the untrained.

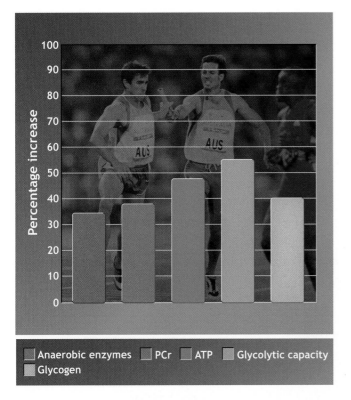

Figure 21.3 Generalized potential for increases in anaerobic energy metabolism of skeletal muscle with heavy training.

Important changes that occur with sprint–power training include:

- *Increased levels of anaerobic substrates.* Muscle biopsy specimens taken before and after resistance training (TABLE 21.4) show significant increases in the trained muscle's resting levels of ATP, PCr, free creatine, and glycogen, accompanied by a 28%

improvement in muscular strength. Other studies have shown higher levels of ATP and total creatine content in the trained muscles of sprint runners and track speed cyclists than in distance runners and road racers.[152] Speed–power training also increases PCr content of the trained skeletal muscle.

- *Increased quantity and activity of key enzymes that control the anaerobic (glycolytic) phase of glucose catabolism.* These changes do not reach the magnitude observed for oxidative enzymes with aerobic training. The most dramatic increases in anaerobic enzyme function and fiber size occur in fast-twitch muscle fibers.
- *Increased capacity to generate high levels of blood lactate during all-out exercise.* This adaptation probably results from (1) increased levels of glycogen and glycolytic enzymes and (2) improved motivation and "pain" tolerance to fatiguing exercise. Research has yet to demonstrate that exercise training augments buffering capacity. Motivational factors probably improve training-induced tolerance to elevated plasma acidity.

AEROBIC SYSTEM CHANGES WITH TRAINING

FIGURE 21.4 shows the diverse physiologic and metabolic factors related to oxygen transport and use. *With an adequate training stimulus, adaptations in many of these factors remain independent of race, gender, age and, to some extent, health status.*[33,69,95,200,232,238]

Metabolic Adaptations

Aerobic training improves the capacity for respiratory control in skeletal muscle.

VARIABLE[a]	CONTROL	POSTTRAINING	PERCENTAGE DIFFERENCE[b]
PCr	17.07	17.94	+5.1
Creatine	10.74	14.52	+35.2
ATP	5.07	5.97	+17.8
Glycogen	86.28	113.90	+32.0

TABLE 21.4 ■ CHANGES IN RESTING CONCENTRATIONS OF PCR, CREATINE, ATP, AND GLYCOGEN FOLLOWING 5 MONTHS OF HEAVY RESISTANCE TRAINING IN 9 MALE SUBJECTS

From MacDougall JD, et al. Biochemical adaptation of human skeletal muscle to heavy resistance training and immobilization. J Appl Physiol 1977;43:700.
[a]All values are averages expressed in mM per gram of wet muscle.
[b]All percentage differences are statistically significant.

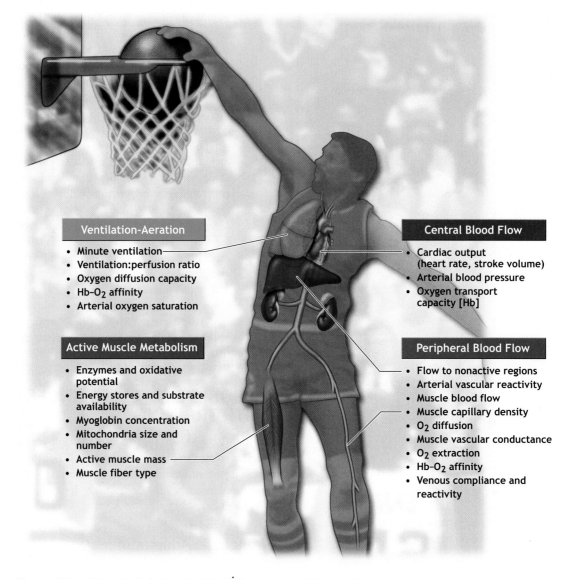

Figure 21.4   Physiologic factors that limit $\dot{V}O_{2max}$ and aerobic exercise performance.

Metabolic Machinery

To some extent, mitochondrial potential and not oxygen supply limits the muscle oxidative capacity of untrained individuals.[77] Endurance-trained skeletal muscle contains *larger* and *more numerous* mitochondria than less active muscle fibers. The enlarged mitochondrial structural machinery and enzyme activity adaptations with training (up to 50% increase in a few weeks) greatly *increases* capacity of subsarcolemmal and intermyofibrillar muscle mitochondria to generate ATP aerobically.[68,87,212] A nearly twofold increase in aerobic system enzymes within 5 to 10 days of training coincides with increased mitochondrial capacity to generate ATP aerobically.

Enzyme changes result from increases in total mitochondrial material rather than increased enzymatic activity per unit of mitochondrial protein. The increase in mitochondrial protein by a factor of two exceeds the typical 10 to 20% increases in $\dot{V}O_{2max}$ with endurance training. More than likely, the en-

zymatic changes allow a person to sustain a higher percentage of aerobic capacity during prolonged exercise without blood lactate accumulation.

Fat Metabolism. FIGURE 21.5 shows that endurance training increases the oxidation of fatty acids for energy during submaximal exercise.[34,57,88] Enhanced fat catabolism becomes particularly apparent at the same absolute submaximal exercise workload without regard to fuel input (fed or fasted).[9,13,35] Impressive increases also occur in the trained muscle's capacity to use intramuscular triacylglycerols as the primary source for fatty acid oxidation.[134] Four factors contribute to a more lively, training-induced lipolysis:

1. Greater blood flow within trained muscle
2. More fat-mobilizing and fat-metabolizing enzymes
3. Enhanced muscle mitochondrial respiratory capacity
4. Decreased catecholamine release for the same absolute power output

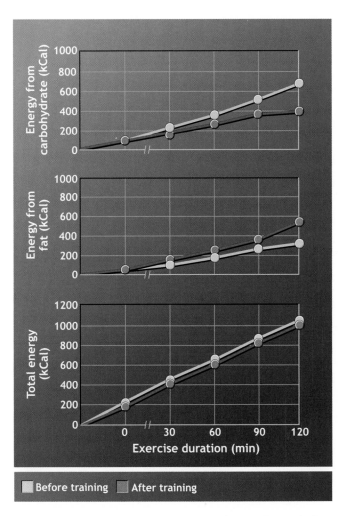

Before training ■ After training

Figure 21.5 Aerobic exercise training enhances fat catabolism in submaximal exercise. During constant-load, prolonged exercise, total energy derived from fat oxidation increases considerably following training. The carbohydrate-sparing adaptation results from facilitated release of fatty acids from adipose tissue depots (augmented by a reduced blood lactate level) and an increased amount of triacylglycerol within the endurance-trained muscle fibers. (From Hurley BF, et al. Muscle triglyceride utilization during exercise: effect of training. J Appl Physiol 1986;5:62.)

Enhanced fat catabolism in submaximal exercise benefits endurance athletes because it conserves the glycogen stores so important during high-intensity prolonged exercise. Improved fatty acid β-oxidation and respiratory ATP production contributes to a cell's integrity and high level of function. This enhances endurance capacity independent of increases in glycogen reserves or aerobic capacity.

Carbohydrate Metabolism. *Trained muscle exhibits enhanced capacity to oxidize carbohydrate during maximal exercise.* Consequently, large quantities of pyruvate flow through the aerobic energy pathways in intense exercise; an effect consistent with increased mitochondrial oxidative capacity and enhanced glycogen storage within muscles. Reduced carbohydrate as fuel and increased fatty acid combustion in submaximal exercise with endurance training results from the

combined effects of (1) decreased muscle glycogen use and (2) reduced glucose production (decreased hepatic glycogenolysis and gluconeogenesis) and use of plasma-borne glucose.[32] Training-enhanced hepatic gluconeogenic capacity provides further resistance to hypoglycemia during prolonged exercise.[45]

Muscle Fiber Type and Size

Aerobic training elicits metabolic adaptations in each type of muscle fiber. The basic fiber type probably does not "change" to any great extent; rather, all fibers maximize their already-existing aerobic potential.

Selective hypertrophy occurs in the different muscle fiber types with specific overload training. Highly trained endurance athletes have larger slow-twitch fibers than fast-twitch fibers in the same muscle. Conversely, the fast-twitch fibers of athletes trained in anaerobic power activities occupy a greater portion of the muscle's cross-sectional area.

Myoglobin. As might be expected, slow-twitch muscle fibers with high capacity to generate ATP aerobically contain relatively large quantities of myoglobin. Among animals, a muscle's myoglobin content relates to their level of physical activity. The leg muscles of hunting dogs, for example, contain more myoglobin than the muscles of sedentary house pets; similar findings exist for grazing cattle compared with penned animals. Whether regular exercise exerts any effect on myoglobin levels in humans remains undetermined.

Cardiovascular Adaptations

FIGURE 21.6 summarizes important adaptations in cardiovascular function with aerobic exercise training that increase oxygen delivery to active muscle. Because of the intimate linkage of the cardiovascular system to aerobic processes, endurance training produces dimensional and functional cardiovascular adaptations.

Cardiac Hypertrophy: The "Athlete's Heart"

Long-term aerobic training generally *increases* the heart's mass and volume with greater left-ventricular end-diastolic volumes noted during rest and exercise. Moderate cardiac hypertrophy secondary to longitudinal myocardial cell enlargement reflects a fundamental and normal training adaptation of muscle to an increased workload independent of age.[145,146] This enlargement, characterized by increased size of the left ventricular cavity (**eccentric hypertrophy**) and modest thickening of its walls (**concentric hypertrophy**), returns to control levels when training ceases.

Long-term exercise alters the contractile properties of cardiac muscle fibers that include increased sensitivity to activation by Ca^{2+}, changes in force–length relationship, and increased power output.[42] Myocardial overload stimulates greater cellular protein synthesis with concomitant reductions in protein breakdown. Increasing the trained muscle's RNA content accelerates protein synthesis. Individual myofibrils

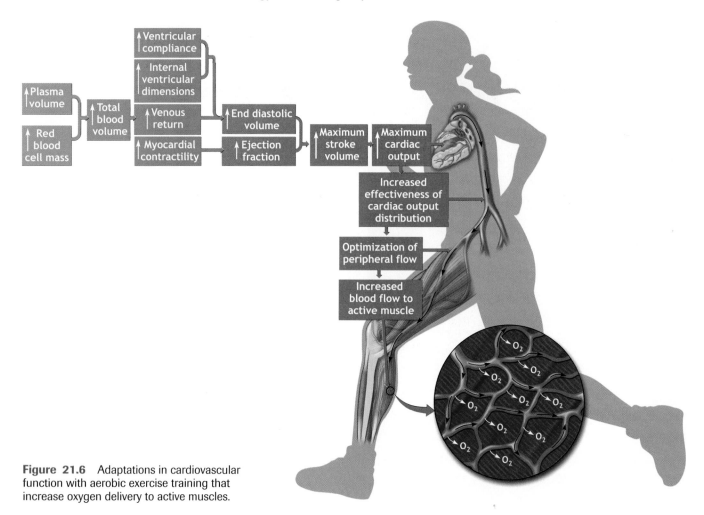

Figure 21.6 Adaptations in cardiovascular function with aerobic exercise training that increase oxygen delivery to active muscles.

thicken, while the number of contractile filaments increases. The heart volume of sedentary men averages 800 mL. In athletes, increases in heart volume relate to the aerobic nature of the sport—endurance athletes average a 25% larger heart volume than sedentary counterparts. The degree to which the large heart volumes of endurance athletes reflect genetic endowment, training adaptations, or combined effect of both factors remains unanswered. Training duration affects cardiac size and structure. Several studies report no changes in cardiac dimensions with short-term training despite improvements in $\dot{V}O_{2max}$ and submaximal-exercise heart response.[178,222] When endurance training increases left ventricular size, the enlargement does not reflect a permanent adaptation. Instead, heart size decreases to pretraining levels—with apparently no deleterious effects—as training intensity decreases.[41,83] FIGURE 21.7 depicts the general trend for cardiac enlargement (reflected by left-ventricular mass) in untrained and trained athletic groups.

Disease also induces considerable cardiac enlargement. In hypertension, for example, the heart *chronically* works against excessive resistance to blood flow (afterload). This stretches the heart muscle, which, in accord with the Frank-Starling mechanism, generates compensatory force to overcome the added resistance to systolic ejection. In addition to ventricular dilation, individual muscle cells enlarge to adjust

to the increased myocardial work imposed by a hypertensive state. In untreated hypertension, myocardial fibers stretch beyond their optimal length so the dilated heart weakens and eventually fails. To the pathologist, a "hypertrophied" heart represents an enlarged, distended, and functionally inadequate organ unable to deliver enough blood to satisfy minimal resting requirements.

Specific Nature of Cardiac Hypertrophy. The ultrasonic technique of **echocardiography** incorporates sound waves to "map" myocardial dimensions and heart chamber volume (see Chapter 32). Echocardiography has evaluated the structural characteristics of the hearts of male and female athletes (and other species of mammals) to determine how various modes of exercise training differentially affect cardiac enlargement.[159,214]

Cardiac dimensions of male swimmers, water polo players, long-distance runners, wrestlers, and shot putters were compared during their competitive seasons with those of untrained college men. The swimmers and runners represented athletes in "isotonic" or endurance events; the wrestlers and shot putters represented "isometric" or resistance-trained power athletes. TABLE 21.5 shows clear distinctions in the structural characteristics of the hearts of apparently healthy athletes and healthy untrained individuals. Heart structure differences

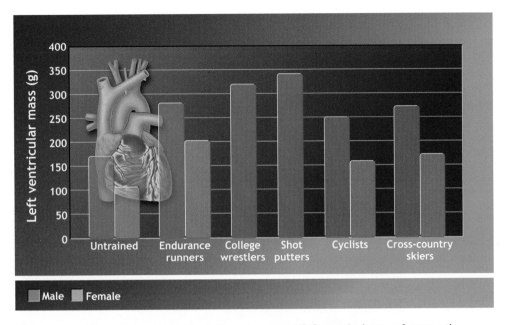

Figure 21.7 General trend toward cardiac enlargement (left-ventricular mass) among the untrained and various groups of male and (where applicable) female athletes.

among athletes also relate to the nature of exercise training. In swimmers, left-ventricular volume averaged 181 mL and mass equaled 308 g. In wrestlers, left-ventricular volume averaged 110 mL and mass averaged 330 g; the nonathletic controls averaged 101 mL for ventricular volume and 211 g for ventricular mass. The resistance-trained athletes had thicker ventricular walls, while the walls of endurance athletes remained within the normal range. Cardiac morphologic and functional adaptations, including resting bradycardia, increased stroke volume, and enlarged ventricular internal dimensions also occur in prepubertal children who undergo intense endurance training.[154]

FIGURE 21.8 shows the distribution of left-ventricular end-diastolic dimensions in 1309 elite Italian athletes aged 13 to 59 years. These dimensions ranged from 38 to 66 mm (average, 48.4 mm) in women and 43 to 70 mm (average, 55.5

mm) in men. Ventricular cavity size of the majority of athletes remained within normal range, but 14% showed substantially enlarged dimensions. A large body surface area and participation in endurance cycling, cross-country skiing, and canoeing represented the major determinants of enlarged cavity dimension. The subjects remained free of heart problems over the 12-year study. Other athletic groups also show an enlarged ventricular cavity (increased end-diastolic volume) with normal wall thickness,[141,181] with the effect less pronounced among females.[159]

Possible Explanation. *Myocardial structural and dimensional adaptations to regular exercise generally reflect specific training demands.*[48,157,166,187] As discussed in the section titled "Plasma Volume," a plasma volume increase

TABLE 21.5 ■ COMPARATIVE AVERAGE CARDIAC DIMENSIONS IN COLLEGE ATHLETES, WORLD-CLASS ATHLETES, AND NORMAL SUBJECTS

DIMENSION[a]	COLLEGE RUNNERS (N = 15)	COLLEGE SWIMMERS (N = 15)	WORLD-CLASS RUNNERS (N = 10)	COLLEGE WRESTLERS (N = 12)	WORLD-CLASS SHOT PUTTERS (N = 4)	NORMALS (N = 16)
LVID	54	51	48–59[b]	48	43–52[b]	46
LVV, mL	160	181	154	110	122	101
SV, mL	116	NR	113	75	68	NR
LV wall, mm	11.3	10.6	10.8	13.7	13.8	10.3
Septum, mm	10.9	10.7	10.9	13.0	13.5	10.3
LV mass, g	302	308	283	330	348	211

From Morganroth J, et al. Comparative left-ventricular dimensions in trained athletes. Ann Intern Med 1975;82:521.
[a] LVID, left-ventricular internal dimension at end diastole; LVV, left-ventricular volume; SV, stroke volume; LV wall, posterobasal left-ventricular wall thickness; Septum, ventricular septal thickness; LV mass, left-ventricular mass.
[b] Range.
NR, Values not reported.

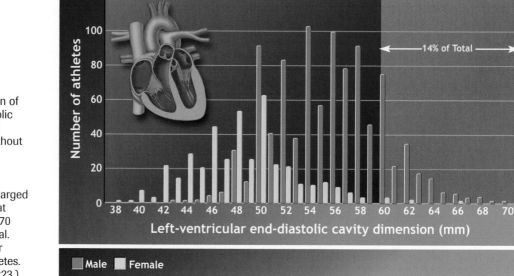

Figure 21.8 Distribution of left-ventricular end-diastolic cavity dimensions in 1309 highly trained athletes without evidence of structural cardiovascular disease. Fourteen percent of the athletes had markedly enlarged left ventricular cavities that ranged in size from 60 to 70 mm. (From Pelliccia A, et al. Physiologic left ventricular cavity dilation in elite athletes. Ann Intern Med 1999;130:23.)

within a day or two of the onset of endurance training contributes to intraventricular enlargement or eccentric hypertrophy.[204,243] Increased plasma volume, coupled with a decreased heart rate and increased myocardial compliance, dilates the left-ventricular cavity like the way added water stretches a rubber balloon.

In contrast, male and female resistance-trained athletes possess the largest intraventricular septum, ventricular wall thickness, and ventricular mass with little enlargement in the left ventricle's internal cavity.[61,116] These athletes do not experience volume overload with training. Instead, their training produces short-term episodes of elevated arterial blood pressure (see Chapter 15) from high forces generated by a limited mass of skeletal muscle. An increase in ventricular wall thickness (that generally falls within the normal range when expressed as ventricular mass per unit body size, particularly fat-free body mass)[51,159,160] compensates for the additional afterload on the left ventricle without affecting ventricular cavity size. More than likely, considerable intraindividual variability exists for the heart's structural response to different forms of training. When changes do occur, the implications for myocardial blood supply and long-term cardiovascular health remain unknown. *No compelling scientific evidence indicates that specific forms of arduous exercise and training can damage a healthy heart.*[99] The same also is true for cardiac patients who undergo a proper exercise-based cardiac rehabilitation program.[23]

Functional Versus Pathologic Hypertrophy. Cardiac hypertrophy to chronic hypertension is sometimes confused with moderate compensatory myocardial growth and left ventricular cavity enlargement with endurance training. Exercise stress requires that myocardial fibers generate increased tension, a critical requirement to initiate compensatory hypertrophy. This form of overload application differs considerably

from the *chronic* pressure overload from vascular disease. Exercise training imposes only a *temporary* myocardial stress so nonexercise periods provide time for "recuperation." Also, dilation and weakening of the left ventricle, a frequent response to chronic hypertension, does not accompany the compensatory myocardial adaptations with exercise training. The heart size of elite athletes usually exceeds that of untrained individuals, but it generally falls within the upper range of normal limits for either body size or increased end-diastolic volume. One possible exception concerns resistance-trained athletes who abuse anabolic steroids. A considerable increase in both systolic and diastolic blood pressure as well as exacerbation of the normal cardiac hypertrophy occurs with steroid use.[66,75,97] *The "athlete's heart" does not represent a dysfunctional organ. Rather, it demonstrates normal systolic and diastolic functions and superior functional capacity for stroke volume and cardiac output.*

INTEGRATIVE QUESTION

In what way might cardiac hypertrophy with pressure overload training (e.g., resistance training) affect oxygenation of myocardial tissues?

Plasma Volume

A 12 to 20% *increase* in plasma volume, in the absence of changes in red blood cell mass, occurs after three to six aerobic training sessions. In fact, a measurable change takes place within 24 hours of the first exercise bout with expansion of the extracellular fluid volume requiring several weeks.[195] Intravascular volume expansion directly relates to increased synthesis and retention of plasma albumin.[143,151,243] A plasma volume increase enhances circulatory reserve and increases end-diastolic volume, stroke volume, oxygen transport,

$\dot{V}O_{2max}$, and temperature-regulating ability during exercise.[65,70] The expanded plasma volume returns to pretraining levels within 1 week after training stops.[204,233] For endurance athletes in different sports, hemoglobin mass and blood volume averaged 35% higher than in untrained subjects with no difference in hemoglobin concentration among groups.[79]

Heart Rate

Endurance training creates an imbalance between the tonic activity of sympathetic accelerator and parasympathetic depressor neurons in favor of greater vagal dominance—a response mediated primarily by increased parasympathetic activity and a small decrease in sympathetic discharge.[64,112,203] Training also decreases the intrinsic firing rate of sinoatrial (SA) nodal pacemaker tissue.[196] These adaptations contribute to the resting and submaximal exercise bradycardia in highly conditioned endurance athletes or previously sedentary individuals who train aerobically. Submaximal exercise heart rate reductions reflect the magnitude of training improvement because they generally coincide with increased maximum stroke volume and cardiac output.

Exercise Heart Rate: Training Effects. Submaximal heart rate for a standard exercise task frequently decreases by 12 to 15 b · min^{-1} with endurance training, while a much smaller decrease occurs for resting heart rate. FIGURE 21.9 illustrates the relationship between heart rate and oxygen consumption during graded exercise for athletes and sedentary students.[192] The group of six endurance athletes had trained for several years; the other group consisted of three sedentary college students. The researchers evaluated the students' exercise responses before and after a 55-day training program to improve aerobic fitness. The lines relating heart rate and oxygen consumption remain essentially linear for both groups throughout the major portion of the exercise range. Whereas the untrained students' heart rates accelerate rapidly as exercise intensity (oxygen consumption) increases, the athletes' heart rates rise much less; that is, the slope or rate of change of the HR–$\dot{V}O_2$ lines differs considerably. Consequently, an athlete (or trained student) performs more intense exercise and achieves a higher oxygen consumption before reaching a specific submaximal heart rate than does a sedentary student. At an oxygen consumption of 2.0 L · min^{-1}, the athletes' heart rate averaged 70 b · min^{-1} less than for sedentary students. After 55 days of training, the difference in submaximal heart rate decreased to about 40 b · min^{-1}. In each instance, cardiac output remained essentially unchanged—an increase in stroke volume compensated for the lower heart rate.

Stroke Volume

Endurance training causes the heart's stroke volume to *increase* during rest and exercise regardless of age or gender. This change results from four factors:[52,102,139,240]

1. Increased internal left ventricular volume (consequent to the training-induced plasma volume expansion) and mass

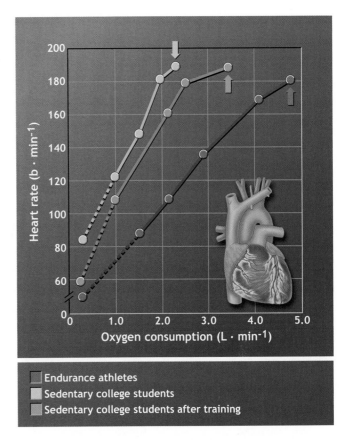

Figure 21.9 Heart rate and oxygen consumption during upright exercise in endurance athletes (■) and sedentary college students before (□) and after (■) 55 days of aerobic training (⬆ maximal values).

2. Reduced cardiac and arterial stiffness
3. Increased diastolic filling time (from training-induced bradycardia)
4. Possibly, improved intrinsic cardiac contractile function

Exercise Stroke Volume: Trained Versus Untrained. FIGURE 21.10 shows the stroke volume response during exercise for the men depicted in Figure 21.9. Several important training-related observations emerge from these data:

- The endurance athlete's heart exhibits a considerably larger stroke volume during rest and exercise than an untrained person of similar age.
- The greatest stroke volume increase during upright exercise for trained and untrained persons occurs in transition from rest to moderate exercise. Only small increases in stroke volume accompany further increases in exercise intensity.
- Maximum stroke volume generally occurs between 40 and 50% of $\dot{V}O_{2max}$ (untrained persons); this takes place at a heart rate of 110 to 120 b · min^{-1} in young adults. Debate currently focuses on whether the stroke volume of endurance athletes actually plateaus during graded exercise (as it does in the untrained) or

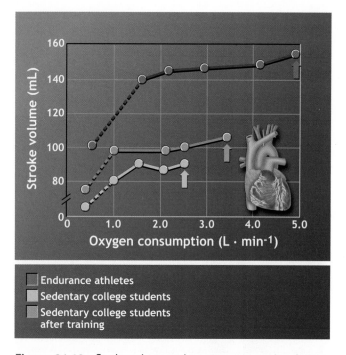

Figure 21.10 Stroke volume and oxygen consumption during upright exercise in endurance athletes (■) and sedentary college students before (□) and after (■) 55 days of aerobic training (⬆ maximal values).

continues to gradually increase from an enlarged plasma volume. More than likely, endurance training minimizes the small decrease in stroke volume often observed during intense exercise. Even at near-maximal heart rates, sufficient time exists for the trained heart's ventricles to fill during diastole without diminution in stroke volume.[63,211,245]

- For untrained persons, only a small increase in stroke volume occurs during transition from rest to exercise. Consequently, a cardiac output increase occurs from acceleration in heart rate. For endurance athletes, heart rate and stroke volume *both* increase to increase cardiac output; the athlete's stroke volume generally expands 60% above resting values. Relatively large stroke volume increases in transition from rest to exercise also take place in endurance-trained children

and older men compared with healthy but untrained counterparts.[70,189]
- Eight weeks of aerobic training by previously sedentary individuals substantially increases stroke volume, but these values remain well below values for elite athletes.

Stroke Volume and V̇O$_{2max}$. The data in TABLE 21.6 amplify the importance of stroke volume in differentiating persons with high and low V̇O$_{2max}$ values. These data represent three groups: (1) athletes, (2) healthy but sedentary men, and (3) patients with mitral stenosis, a valvular heart disease that causes inadequate emptying of the left ventricle.[187] The differences in V̇O$_{2max}$ among groups relate closely to differences in maximal stroke volume. Patients with mitral stenosis achieved an aerobic capacity and maximum stroke volume one half that of sedentary subjects. The importance of stroke volume also emerges in comparisons among healthy groups. Athletes achieved an average 62% larger V̇O$_{2max}$ than sedentary subjects, almost entirely from the athletes' 60% larger stroke volume and cardiac output.

Cardiac Output

An increase in maximum cardiac output represents the most significant adaptation in cardiovascular function with aerobic training. Maximal heart rate decreases slightly with training, so increased cardiac output capacity results directly from improved stroke volume. A large maximum cardiac output (stroke volume) distinguishes champion endurance athletes from other well-trained athletes and from untrained counterparts.

FIGURE 21.11 illustrates the important role of cardiac output in achieving a high level of aerobic metabolism. In trained athletes and students, cardiac output increases *linearly* with oxygen consumption throughout the major portion of the exercise intensity range with the athletes achieving the highest values for both variables. A linear relationship between cardiac output and oxygen consumption in graded exercise also occurs in children and adolescents. For these young persons, increased stroke volume (and proportionate increase in cardiac output) closely matches the added cost of exercise during growth.[37]

TABLE 21.6 ■ **MAXIMAL VALUES FOR OXYGEN CONSUMPTION, HEART RATE, STROKE VOLUME, AND CARDIAC OUTPUT IN THREE GROUPS WITH LOW, NORMAL, AND HIGH AEROBIC CAPACITIES**

GROUP	V̇O$_{2MAX}$ (L · MIN^{-1})	MAX HEART RATE (B · MIN^{-1})	MAX STROKE VOLUME (ML · B^{-1})	MAX CARDIAC OUTPUT (L · MIN^{-1})
Mitral stenosis	1.6	190	50	9.5
Sedentary	3.2	200	100	20.0
Athlete	5.2	190	160	30.4

Modified from Rowell LB. Circulation. Med Sci Sports 1969;1:15.

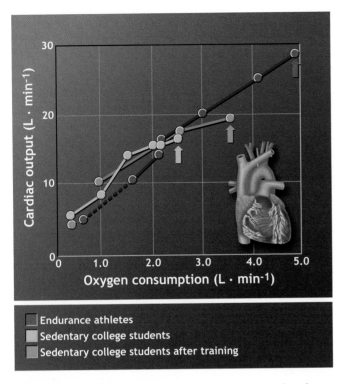

Figure 21.11 Cardiac output and oxygen consumption during upright exercise in endurance athletes (■) and sedentary college students before (□) and after (■) 55 days of aerobic training (⬆ maximal values).

Training and Submaximal Cardiac Output. Early reports showed that training, while improving maximal cardiac output, reduced the heart's minute volume during moderate exercise. In one study, average cardiac output of young men after 16 weeks of aerobic training decreased by 1.1 and 1.5 $L \cdot min^{-1}$ at a specific submaximal oxygen consumption.[49] As expected, maximal cardiac output increased 8% from 22.4 to 24.2 $L \cdot min^{-1}$. With reduced submaximal cardiac output, a corresponding increase in oxygen extraction in the active muscles matches the exercise oxygen requirement. A training-induced reduction in submaximal cardiac output presumably reflects two factors: (1) more effective distribution of blood flow and (2) trained muscles' enhanced capacity to generate ATP aerobically at a lower tissue P_{O_2}.

Oxygen Extraction (a-v̄O₂ Difference)

Aerobic training *increases* the quantity of oxygen extracted from circulating blood.[197] An increase in the maximum arteriovenous oxygen (a-v̄O₂) difference results from more effective cardiac output distribution to active muscles combined with enhanced capacity of trained muscle fibers to extract and process the available oxygen. The a-v̄O₂ difference takes on even greater importance in contributing to improved aerobic capacity with training in older men and women.[105,199]

FIGURE 21.12 compares the relationship between oxygen extraction (a-v̄O₂ difference) and exercise intensity for the trained athletes and untrained students depicted in Figure 21.9. The a-v̄O₂ difference for the students increases steadily during graded exercise to a maximum of 15 mL per deciliter of blood. Following 55 days of training, the students' maximum oxygen extraction increased 13% to 17 mL of oxygen. This means that during intense exercise, arterial blood released approximately 85% of its oxygen content. Actually, the active muscles extract even more oxygen because the a-v̄O₂ difference reflects an *average* based on sampling of mixed-venous blood. This sample contains blood returning from tissues that use less oxygen during exercise than active muscle. The posttraining value for maximal a-v̄O₂ difference for the students equals the value of the endurance athletes. Obviously, the students' lower cardiac output capacity explains the rather large difference in $\dot{V}O_{2max}$ that clearly differentiates athletes from students.

Blood Flow and Distribution

Submaximal Exercise. Trained persons perform submaximal exercise with *lower* cardiac output (and unchanged or slightly lower muscle blood flow) than untrained persons. A relatively larger portion of the submaximal cardiac output flows to the high oxidative skeletal muscles (composed primarily of type I fibers) at the expense of blood flow to muscles with a large percentage of type IIB fibers with low oxidative capacity.[38] Two factors contribute to reduced muscle blood flow in submaximal exercise:

1. Relatively rapid training-induced changes in the vasoactive properties of large arteries and local resistance vessels within skeletal and cardiac muscle, mediated by the dilation effects of endothelium-derived nitric oxide[21,39,67,110,221,231,241]

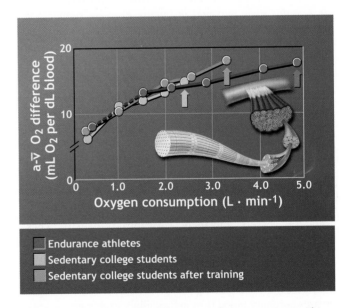

Figure 21.12 The a-v̄O₂ difference and oxygen consumption during upright exercise in endurance athletes (■) and sedentary college students before (□) and after (■) 55 days of aerobic training (⬆ maximal values).

2. Changes within the muscle cells that enhance oxidative capacity

Both adaptations support the principle of training specificity. As the muscle's ability to deliver, extract, and use oxygen increases, the active tissue's oxygen needs require proportionally less regional blood flow.

Maximal Exercise. Three factors affect how aerobic training increases total skeletal muscle blood flow during *maximal* exercise:

1. Larger maximal cardiac output
2. Distribution of blood to muscle from nonactive areas that temporarily compromise blood flow during all-out effort
3. Enlargement of the cross-sectional areas of the large and small arteries (arteriogenesis) and veins, and 10 to 20% increase in capillarization per gram of muscle (angiogenesis)[80,107,173,180]; this effect begins rapidly from increased vascular endothelial growth factors—produced by skeletal muscle cells to induce angiogenesis—after a single bout of exercise in trained and untrained persons[60,101]

Training-induced *decreases* in splanchnic and renal blood flow in exercise occur from reduced sympathetic nervous system outflow to these tissues.[136] This frees a relatively large quantity of blood for distribution to active muscles. Concurrently, exercise training and accompanying frequent exposure to elevated core temperatures produces heat loss adaptations via enhanced endothelium-dependent increases in blood flow to the skin for a given internal temperature.[93,104] Augmented cutaneous blood flow facilitates the endurance-trained person's capacity to dissipate metabolic heat generated in exercise.

The observation that oxygen extraction in skeletal muscle remains near maximal in intense exercise supports the hypothesis that oxygen supply (blood flow), not oxygen use (extraction), limits the maximal respiratory rate of muscle tissue.[12,148,179]

Myocardial Blood Flow. For both normal persons and cardiac patients, structural and functional changes in the heart's vasculature, including modifications in mechanisms that regulate myocardial perfusion, parallel a modest training-induced myocardial hypertrophy.[73,109,237] Structural vascular modifications include an increase in the cross-sectional area of the proximal coronary arteries, possible arteriolar proliferation and longitudinal growth, recruitment of collateral vessels, and increased capillary density. These adaptations provide adequate perfusion to support blood flow and energy demands of the functionally improved myocardium.

Two mechanisms help to explain how aerobic training increases coronary blood flow and capillary exchange capacity:

1. Ordered progression of structural remodeling that improves myocardial vascularization when new

capillaries form and develop into small arterioles[108,237]
2. More effective control of vascular resistance and blood distribution within the myocardium[226,231]

The significance of vascular and cellular adaptations to the heart's functional capacity during exercise remains unclear—mainly because the healthy, untrained heart does not suffer from oxygen lack during maximum exercise. Training adaptations may provide some cardioprotection by enabling myocardial tissue to better tolerate and recover from transient episodes of ischemia (i.e., become more resistant to ischemic injury). The trained tissue also functions at a lower percentage of its total oxidative capacity during exercise. Vascular adaptations do not accompany the myocardial hypertrophy that occurs with chronic resistance training.[146]

Blood Pressure

Regular aerobic training *reduces* systolic and diastolic blood pressure during rest and submaximal exercise. The largest reduction occurs in systolic pressure, particularly in hypertensive subjects (see Chapter 32 for a more complete discussion).

Pulmonary Adaptations with Training

Aerobic training stimulates adaptations in pulmonary ventilation during submaximal and maximal exercise. The adaptations generally reflect a breathing strategy that minimizes respiratory work at a given exercise intensity. This frees oxygen for use by the nonrespiratory active musculature.

Maximal Exercise

Maximal exercise ventilation *increases* from increased tidal volume and breathing rate as maximal oxygen consumption increases. This makes sense physiologically because any increase in $\dot{V}O_{2max}$ raises the oxygen requirement and corresponding need to eliminate additional carbon dioxide via alveolar ventilation.

Submaximal Exercise

Several weeks of aerobic training *reduce* the ventilatory equivalent for oxygen ($\dot{V}_E/\dot{V}O_2$) during submaximal exercise and lowers the percentage of the total exercise oxygen cost attributable to breathing. Reduced oxygen consumption by the ventilatory musculature enhances exercise endurance for two reasons: (1) it reduces the fatiguing effects of exercise on the ventilatory musculature and (2) any oxygen freed from use by the respiratory musculature becomes available to the active locomotor muscles.[74,91]

Healthy adolescents and young and older adults consistently show positive training adaptations in pulmonary ventilation during submaximal exercise. In general, tidal volume increases and breathing frequency decreases. Consequently, air remains in the lungs for a longer time between breaths; this increases oxygen extraction from inspired air. For example, the exhaled air of trained individuals during submaximal exercise contains only 14 to 15% oxygen, whereas the expired air of untrained persons averages 18% at the same exercise intensity. This translates to the common observation that untrained persons ventilate proportionately more air to achieve the same submaximal oxygen consumption.

Substantial specificity exists for ventilatory responses relative to the type of exercise and training adaptations. When subjects performed arm-only and leg-only exercise, consistently higher ventilatory equivalents occurred with the arms (FIG. 21.13). As expected, the ventilatory equivalent decreased with each mode of exercise training. However, the reduction occurred *only* with exercise that used the specifically trained muscles. For the group trained by arm-crank ergometry, the ventilation equivalent decreased only during arm exercise and vice versa for the leg-trained group. The ventilatory training adaptation linked closely to a less pronounced rise in blood lactate and heart rate during the specific training exercise. This suggests that local adaptations in specifically trained muscles affect the ventilatory adjustment to training.

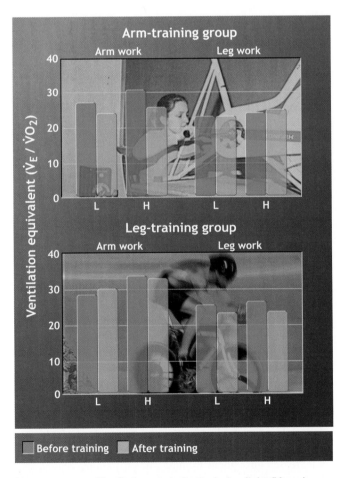

Figure 21.13 Ventilation equivalents during light (L) and intense (H) submaximal arm and leg exercise before and after arm training *(top)* and leg training *(bottom)*. (From Rasmussen B, et al. Pulmonary ventilation, blood gases, and blood pH after training of the arms and the legs. J Appl Physiol 1975;38:250.)

Lower lactate levels with training remove the drive to ventilation from any additional carbon dioxide produced in lactate buffering.

Training May Benefit Ventilatory Endurance

Inspiratory muscle fatigue occurs during prolonged, intense exercise.[10,89,91] Such exercise also reduces the abdominal muscles' capacity to generate maximal expiratory pressure.[58]

Exercise training enhances the ability to sustain exceptionally high levels of submaximum ventilation.[20,92,208] Endurance training stabilizes the body's internal milieu during submaximal exercise. Consequently, exercise causes less disruption in whole-body hormonal and acid–base balance that could negatively affect inspiratory muscle function. The ventilatory muscles also benefit directly from exercise training. For example, 20 weeks of run training by healthy men and women improved ventilatory muscle endurance by approximately 16% (less lactate accumulation during standard breathing exercise). The documented training-induced increase in aerobic enzyme levels and oxidative capacity of the respiratory musculature contribute to enhanced ventilatory muscle function.[171,172,210,229] Exercise training increases inspiratory muscle capacity to generate force and sustain a given level of inspiratory pressure.[27] These training adaptations benefit exercise performance in three ways:

1. Reduces overall exercise energy demands because of less respiratory work
2. Reduces lactate production by the ventilatory muscles during high-intensity, prolonged exercise
3. Enhances how ventilatory muscles metabolize circulating lactate as metabolic fuel

Blood Lactate Concentration

FIGURE 21.14 illustrates the generalized effect of endurance training in lowering blood lactate levels and extending exercise before the onset of blood lactate accumulation (OBLA) during exercise of progressively increasing intensity. The explanation underlying this effect centers on three possibilities related to central and peripheral adaptations to training discussed in this chapter: (1) decreased rate of lactate formation during exercise, (2) increased rate of lactate clearance (removal) during exercise, and (3) combined effects of decreased lactate formation and increased lactate removal. More than likely, the combination of the first and second factors exerts the influence.

Other Aerobic Training Adaptations

- *Body composition changes:* For the obese or borderline obese person, regular aerobic exercise reduces body mass and body fat. Small increases in fat-free body mass also accompany training. Exercise only or combined with calorie restriction reduces

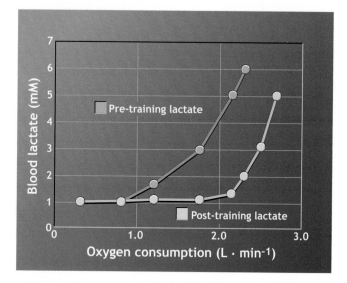

Figure 21.14   Generalized response for pre- and posttraining lactate accumulation during graded exercise. (Plots based on data from the Applied Physiology Laboratory, University of Michigan, Ann Arbor, MI.)

body fat more than weight lost with dieting only because exercise promotes conservation of the body's lean tissue.

- *Body heat transfer:* Well-hydrated, trained individuals exercise more comfortably in hot environments because of a larger plasma volume and more responsive thermoregulatory mechanisms. (They dissipate heat faster and more economically than sedentary

individuals.) As a result, metabolic heat generated by exercise poses less potential detriment to exercise performance and overall safety.

- *Performance changes:* Enhanced endurance performance accompanies the physiologic adaptations with training. FIGURE 21.15 depicts the results of cycling exercise following training performed for 40 to 60 minutes, 4 days per week for 10 weeks at an intensity of 85% $\dot{V}O_{2max}$. In the performance test, subjects attempted to maintain a constant work rate of 265 watts for 8 minutes. Training produced significantly less drop-off in power output during the prescribed 8-minute exercise test.
- *Psychologic benefits:* Important potential benefits on psychologic state result from regular exercise regardless of age.[53,106,223] Adaptations often occur to a degree equal to that achieved with other therapeutic interventions including pharmacologic therapy.

POTENTIAL PSYCHOLOGIC BENEFITS FROM REGULAR EXERCISE

- Reduction in state of anxiety (i.e., the level of anxiety at the time of measurement)
- Decrease in mild-to-moderate depression
- Reduction in neuroticism (long-term exercise)
- Adjunct to professional treatment of severe depression
- Improvement in mood, self-esteem, and self-concept
- Reduction in the various indices of stress

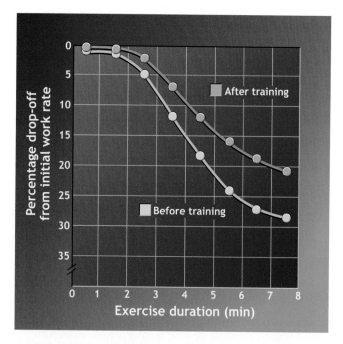

Figure 21.15   Percentage drop-off from initial exercise intensity before and after 10 weeks of endurance cycling training. (From the Applied Physiology Laboratory, University of Michigan, Ann Arbor, MI.)

Summary View

FIGURE 21.16 summarizes adaptive changes in active muscle that accompany $\dot{V}O_{2max}$ improvements with endurance training. Aerobic capacity generally increases 15 to 25% over the first 3 months of intensive training and may improve by 50% over a 2-year period. When training stops, $\dot{V}O_{2max}$ decreases toward the pretraining level. Even more impressive training effects occur for aerobic enzymes of the citric acid cycle and electron-transport chain within the mitochondria of trained muscles. These enzymes increase rapidly and substantially throughout training in both fiber types and subdivisions. Conversely, a few weeks of detraining cause loss of a large portion of enzymatic adaptations. The number of muscle capillaries increases throughout training. When training ceases, this adaptation in blood supply probably decreases relatively slowly.

Local metabolic improvement greatly exceeds improvements in the capacity to circulate, deliver, and use oxygen (reflected by $\dot{V}O_{2max}$ and cardiac output) during intense

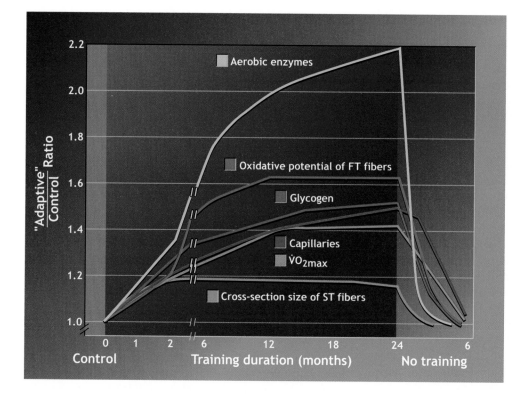

Figure 21.16 Generalized summary of increase in aerobic capacity and muscle adaptations with endurance training. (Modified from Saltin B, et al. Fiber types and metabolic potentials of skeletal muscles in sedentary man and endurance runners. Ann NY Acad Sci 1977;301:3.)

exercise. With local training adaptations, a muscle's lactate remains at lower levels (lower production and/or greater removal rate) than similar submaximal exercise before training. *These cellular adjustments account for how a trained person performs steady-rate exercise at a greater percentage of $\dot{V}O_{2max}$.*

INTEGRATIVE QUESTION

Respond to the question "How long must I exercise to 'get in shape'?"

FACTORS THAT AFFECT THE AEROBIC TRAINING RESPONSE

Four factors influence the aerobic training response:

1. Initial level of aerobic fitness
2. Training intensity
3. Training frequency
4. Training duration

Initial Level of Aerobic Fitness

The magnitude of the training response depends upon initial fitness level. Someone who rates low at the start has considerable room for improvement. If capacity already rates high, the magnitude of improvement remains relatively small. Studies of sedentary, middle-aged men with heart disease showed that $\dot{V}O_{2max}$ improved by 50%, while similar training in normally active, healthy adults improved 10 to 15%.[179] Of course, a 5% improvement in aerobic capacity represents as crucial a change for an elite athlete as a 40% increase for a

sedentary person. *As a general guideline, aerobic fitness improvements with endurance training range between 5 and 25%.* Some of this improvement occurs within the first week of training.

Training Intensity

Training-induced physiologic adaptations depend primarily on the intensity of overload. There are at least seven different ways to express exercise intensity:

1. Energy expended per unit time (e.g., 9 kCal $\cdot$ min^{-1} or 37.8 kJ $\cdot$ min^{-1})
2. Absolute exercise level or power output (e.g., cycle at 900 kg-m $\cdot$ min^{-1} or 147 W)
3. Relative metabolic level expressed as percentage of $\dot{V}O_{2max}$ (e.g., 85% $\dot{V}O_{2max}$)
4. Exercise below, at, or above the lactate threshold or OBLA (e.g., 4 mM lactate)
5. Exercise heart rate or percentage of maximum heart rate (e.g., 180 b $\cdot$ min^{-1} or 80% HR$_{max}$)
6. Multiples of resting metabolic rate (e.g., 6 METs)
7. Rating of perceived exertion (e.g., RPE = 14)

An example of absolute training intensity involves having all individuals exercise at the same power output or energy expenditure (e.g., 9.0 kCal $\cdot$ min^{-1}) for 30 minutes. When everyone performs at the same intensity, the task can elicit considerable stress for one person yet fall short of the training threshold for another more fit person. For this reason, the *relative stress* on a person's physiologic systems more properly establishes exercise intensity. The assigned exercise intensity usually relates to some breakpoint for steady-rate exercise (e.g., lactate threshold, OBLA) or some percentage of maximum physiologic capacity (e.g., $\%\dot{V}O_{2max}$, $\%HR_{max}$) or maximum exercise capacity. General practice establishes aerobic training intensity via direct measurement (or estimation) of $\dot{V}O_{2max}$ (or HR_{max}) and then assigns an exercise level to correspond to some percentage of these maximums.

Establishing training intensity from measures of oxygen consumption provides a high degree of accuracy, but its use requires sophisticated equipment that renders this method impractical for the general population. An effective alternative uses *heart rate* to classify exercise for relative intensity when individualizing the training protocol. Exercise heart rate is convenient because $\%\dot{V}O_{2max}$ and $\%HR_{max}$ relate in a predictable way regardless of gender, race, fitness level, exercise mode, or age. Exercise training does not affect a particular individual's heart rate at a given $\%\dot{V}O_{2max}$, so there is no need to frequently test to adjust the exercise prescription relative to training-induced changes in aerobic capacity.[207]

TABLE 21.7 presents selected values for $\%\dot{V}O_{2max}$ and corresponding $\%HR_{max}$ obtained from several sources.[4,134] The error in estimating $\%\dot{V}O_{2max}$ from $\%HR_{max}$, or vice versa, equals about 8%. Thus, one need only monitor heart rate to estimate the relative exercise stress or $\%\dot{V}O_{2max}$ within the given error range. The relationship between $\%HR_{max}$ and $\%\dot{V}O_{2max}$ remains essentially the same for arm or leg exercises among healthy subjects, normal-weight and obese persons, cardiac patients, and persons with spinal cord injuries.[56,86,140] *Importantly, arm (upper-body) exercise produces lower HR_{max} than leg exercises. One must consider this difference when formulating the exercise prescription for different exercise modes* (see p. 491).

Train at a Percentage of HR_{max}

Aerobic capacity improves if exercise intensity regularly maintains heart rate between 55 and 70% of maximum. During lower-body exercise such as cycling, walking, or running, this heart rate increase equals about 40 to 55% of the $\dot{V}O_{2max}$; for college-aged men and women, the training heart rate ranges from 120 to 140 b $\cdot$ min^{-1}.

An alternative and equally effective method to establish the training threshold, termed the **Karvonen method**, requires that subjects exercise at a heart rate equal to 60% of the difference between resting and maximum.[98] With the Karvonen method, one computes the training heart rate as follows:

$$HR_{threshold} = HR_{rest} + 0.60\,(HR_{max} - HR_{rest})$$

This approach to determining heart rate training threshold gives a somewhat *higher* value than computing the threshold heart rate simply as 70% of HR_{max}.

Clearly, positive training adaptations do not require strenuous exercise. For most healthy persons, an exercise heart rate of 70% maximum represents moderate exercise with little or no discomfort. This training level, frequently referred to as "**conversational exercise**," reaches sufficient intensity to stimulate a training effect yet does not produce a level of discomfort (e.g., lactate accumulation and associated hyperpnea) that prevents talking during the workout. *A previously sedentary person need not exercise above this heart rate to improve physiologic capacity.*

FIGURE 21.17 shows that as aerobic fitness improves, submaximal exercise heart rate decreases 10 to 20 b $\cdot$ min^{-1} for a given level of exercise or oxygen consumption. To keep pace with physiologic improvement, the exercise level then increases periodically to achieve the desired exercise heart rate. A person who begins training by walking then walks more briskly; jogging then replaces walking for periods of the workout, and eventually continuous running elicits the desired exercise heart rate. In each progression, exercise remains at the *same* relative intensity or strenuousness. If exercise intensity progression does not adjust to training improvements, the exercise program essentially becomes a maintenance program for aerobic fitness without further improvement.

Is Strenuous Training More Effective?

Generally, the higher the training intensity above threshold, the greater the training improvement, particularly for $\dot{V}O_{2max}$. Some minimal threshold intensity exists below which no training effect occurs, yet a "ceiling" may exist above which no further gains accrue. More fit men and women generally require higher threshold levels to stimulate a training response than less fit persons. The ceiling for training intensity remains unknown, although about 85% $\dot{V}O_{2max}$ (corresponding to 90% HR_{max}) probably represents an upper limit. Importantly, regardless of the exercise level selected, more does not necessarily produce greater results. Excessive training intensity and abrupt increases in training volume increase the risk for injury to bones, joints, and muscles.[3,94,212] For men and women, the number of miles run per week was the only variable consistently associated with running injuries. In preadolescent children, running excessive distances strains the articular cartilage. This type of strain could injure the bone's growth plate (epiphysis) to adversely affect normal growth.

The "Training-Sensitive Zone"

One can determine maximum exercise heart rate immediately after several minutes of all-out effort in a specific form of exercise. This exercise intensity requires considerable

TABLE 21.7 ■ RELATIONSHIP BETWEEN PERCENTAGE MAXIMAL HEART RATE AND PERCENTAGE $\dot{V}O_{2MAX}$	
PERCENTAGE HR_{MAX}	**PERCENTAGE $\dot{V}O_{2MAX}$**
50	28
60	40
70	58
80	70
90	83
100	100

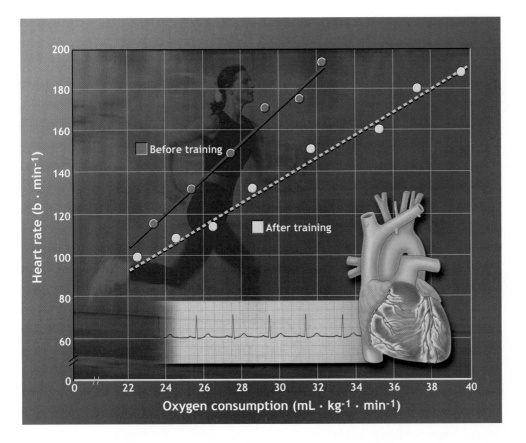

Figure 21.17 Improvement in exercise heart rate response with aerobic training in relation to oxygen consumption. A reduction in exercise heart rate with training usually reflects enhanced stroke volume.

motivation and stress—a requirement inadvisable for adults without medical clearance, particularly those predisposed to coronary heart disease. Persons should consider themselves average and use the **age-predicted maximum heart rates** presented in FIGURE 21.18.

Individuals of a given age have varying HR_{max} values, but the inaccuracy from individual variation (± 10 b · min^{-1} standard deviation for any age-predicted HR_{max}) has little influence in establishing effective training for healthy persons. *Maximum heart rate has commonly been estimated as 220 minus the person's age in years, with values independent of race or gender in children and adults.*[90,120,121]

$$HR_{max} = 220 - age\ (y)$$

An alternative formula for estimating HR_{max} that has high accuracy for non-fit males and females is as follows:[219]

$$HR_{max} = 208 - 0.7 \times age\ (y)$$

For example, the estimated maximum heart rate for a 20-year-old man or woman predicts as:

$$HR_{max} = 208 - (0.7 \times 20)$$
$$= 208 - 14$$
$$= 194\ b \cdot min^{-1}$$

Reduced sympathetic output from the medulla and age-related changes in the inherent characteristics of the SA node decrease maximum heart rate with age.[188] This formula represents a convenient rule of thumb, but it does not determine a specific person's maximum heart rate. Within normal variation, the maximum heart rate of 95% (± 2 standard deviations) of 40-year-old men and women ranges between 160 and 200 b · min^{-1}. Figure 21.18 also depicts the "training-sensitive zone" related to age. Aerobic system conditioning occurs when exercise heart rate remains within this zone.

A 40-year-old woman or man who wants to train at moderate intensity but still achieve the threshold level would select a training heart rate equal to 70% of age-predicted HR_{max}, or a target exercise heart rate of 126 b · min^{-1} (0.70 × 180). Applying progressive increments of light-to-moderate exercise, the person achieves a walking, jogging, or cycling intensity that produces this heart rate. To increase training to 85% of maximum, exercise intensity must increase to produce a heart rate of 153 b · min^{-1} (0.85 × 180).

Running Versus Swimming and Other Forms of Upper-Body Exercise. Estimation of HR_{max} requires an adjustment when swimming or performing other upper-body exercises for training. Maximum heart rate during these exercise modes averages about 13 b · min^{-1} lower for trained and untrained men and women than while running.[56,62,132,137] This difference probably results from less feed-forward stimulation from the motor cortex to the medulla, in addition to less feedback stimulation from the smaller, active upper-body muscle mass. In swimming, the horizontal body position and cooling effect of the water may also contribute to a lower HR_{max}.

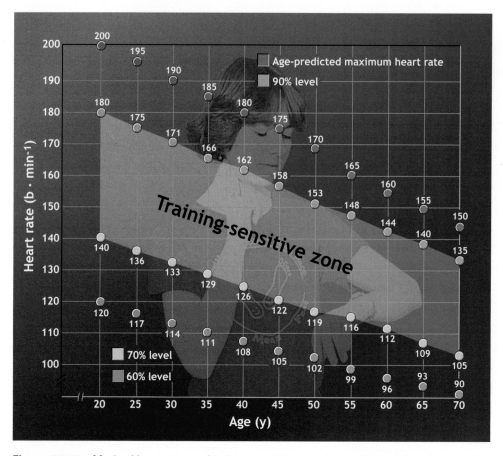

Figure 21.18 Maximal heart rates and training-sensitive zone for aerobic training of men and women of different ages.

Establishing the appropriate exercise intensity for swimming and upper-body exercise requires subtracting 13 b · min^{-1} from the age-predicted HR$_{max}$ in Figure 21.18. A 30-year-old person who swims at 70% HR$_{max}$ should select a swimming speed that produces a heart rate of 124 b · min^{-1} (0.70 × [190 − 13]). This more accurately represents the proper threshold training heart rate for swimming. Without this heart rate adjustment, a prescription of upper-body exercise based on %HR$_{max}$ in leg exercise *overestimates* the appropriate threshold training heart rate.

Is Less Intense Training Effective?

The often-cited recommendation of 70% HR$_{max}$ as a training threshold for aerobic improvement represents a *general guideline* for effective yet comfortable exercise. The lower limit may depend on the participant's initial exercise capacity and current state of training. In addition, older and less fit, and sedentary, overweight men and women have training thresholds closer to 60% HR$_{max}$ (about 45% $\dot{V}O_{2max}$). Twenty to 30 minutes of continuous exercise at 70% HR$_{max}$ stimulates a training effect; exercise at the lower intensity of 60% HR$_{max}$ for 45 minutes also proves beneficial. *Generally, the longer exercise duration offsets the lower exercise intensity.*

Train at a Perception of Effort

The **rating of perceived exertion** (**RPE**) can be used in addition to oxygen consumption, heart rate, and blood lactate to indicate exercise intensity.[17,184] With this psychophysiologic approach, the exerciser rates on a numerical scale perceived feelings relative to exertion level. Monitoring and adjusting RPE during exercise provides an effective means to prescribe exercise from an individual's perception of effort that coincides with objective measures of physiologic/metabolic strain (%HR$_{max}$, %$\dot{V}O_{2max}$, blood lactate concentration).

Exercise that corresponds to higher levels of energy expenditure and physiologic strain produces higher RPE ratings. For example, an RPE of 13 or 14 (exercise that feels "somewhat hard;" FIG. 21.19) coincides with about 70% HR$_{max}$ during cycle ergometer and treadmill exercise; an RPE between 11 and 12 corresponds to exercise at the lactate threshold for trained and untrained individuals. The RPE establishes an exercise prescription for exercise intensities that correspond to blood lactate concentrations of 2.5 mM (RPE ∼ 15) and 4.0 mM (RPE ∼ 18) during a 30-minute treadmill run where subjects self-regulated exercise intensity.[218] Individuals learn quickly to exercise at a specific RPE. In similar fashion, a simple "talk test" that

	RPE Scale	Equivalent % HR_{max}	Equivalent % $\dot{V}O_{2max}$
6			
7	Very, very light		
8			
9	Very light		
10			
11	Fairly light	52–66	31–50
12			
13	Somewhat hard	61–85	51–75
14			
15	Hard	86–91	76–85
16		92	85
17	Very hard		
18			
19	Very, very hard		

Figure 21.19 The Borg scale (and accompanying estimates of relative exercise intensity) for obtaining the RPE during exercise. (Modified from Borg GA. Psychological basis of physical exertion. Med Sci Sports Exerc 1982;14:377.)

asks whether comfortable speech is possible produces exercise intensities within accepted guidelines for exercise prescription for both treadmill and cycle ergometer exercise.[161]

Train at the Lactate Threshold

Exercising at or slightly above the lactate threshold provides effective aerobic training, with the higher exercise levels producing the greatest benefits, particularly for fit individuals.[119,234] FIGURE 21.20 illustrates how to determine the appropriate exercise level by plotting exercise intensity (e.g., running speed) in relation to blood lactate level. In this example, the running speed that produced a blood lactate concentration at the 4-mM level (OBLA) represented the recommended training intensity. Many coaches use the 4-mM blood lactate level as the optimal aerobic training intensity, yet no convincing evidence exists to justify this particular blood lactate level as "ideal." Regardless of the specific blood lactate level chosen for endurance training, the blood lactate–exercise intensity relationship should be evaluated periodically and the exercise intensity adjusted as aerobic fitness improves. If regular blood lactate measurement proves impractical, the exercise heart rate at the initial lactate determination remains a convenient and relatively stable marker to set an appropriate predetermined exercise intensity. This is because no systematic training-induced change occurs in the heart rate–blood lactate relationship during incremental exercise.[54]

The RPE can be an effective tool to estimate blood lactate threshold when setting training intensity for continuous exercise. However, a change in the blood lactate concentration–RPE relationship occurs with repeated exercise bouts. The relationship remains altered from a single exercise bout, even after 3.5 hours of recovery.[235] This limits the use of RPE to gauge exercise intensity for a specific blood lactate concentration if repeated bouts of exercise occur during the same training session (e.g., during interval training; see p. 498).

One important distinction between %HR_{max} and lactate threshold for setting training intensity lies in the physiologic dynamics each method reflects. The %HR_{max} method establishes a level of exercise stress to overload the central circulation (e.g., stroke volume, cardiac output), whereas the capability of the peripheral vasculature and active muscles to sustain steady-rate aerobic metabolism dictates exercise intensity adjustments based on lactate threshold.

Training Duration

No threshold duration per workout exists for optimal aerobic improvement. If a threshold exists, it probably depends on the interaction of total work accomplished (duration or training volume), exercise intensity, training frequency, and initial fitness level. Whereas 3- to 5-minute daily exercise periods produce training effects in some poorly conditioned people, 20- to 30-minute sessions achieve more optimal results (within practicality for time) if intensity reaches at least 70% HR_{max}. With higher intensity training, improvement occurs with only a 10-minute workout. Conversely, it requires at least 60 minutes of continuous exercise to produce a training effect when exercise intensity remains below 70% HR_{max}.

As for training volume, more does not necessarily produce greater improvements. For collegiate swimmers, one group trained for 1.5 hours daily while another group per-

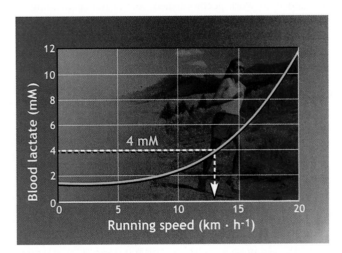

Figure 21.20 Blood lactate concentration in relation to running speed for one subject. At a lactate level of 4.0 mM, the corresponding running speed was approximately 13 km · h⁻¹. This speed establishes the subject's initial training intensity.

formed two 1.5-hour exercise sessions each day.[36] Even when one group exercised at twice the daily volume, *no differences* in swimming power, endurance, or performance time improvements emerged between groups.

Training Frequency

Do 2- or 5-day-a-week training produce different effects if exercise duration and intensity remain constant for each training session? Unfortunately, the precise answer remains elusive. Some investigators report that training frequency influences cardiovascular improvements, while others maintain this factor contributes considerably less than either exercise intensity or duration.[168] Studies using interval training show that training 2 days per week produced $\dot{V}O_{2max}$ changes similar to training 5 days weekly.[55] In other studies that held total exercise volume constant, no differences emerged in $\dot{V}O_{2max}$ improvement between training frequencies of 2 and 4 or 3 and 5 days a week. As with training duration, more frequent training is beneficial when training occurs at a lower intensity.

While the extra time invested to increase training frequency may not prove profitable for improving physiologic function, the extra quantity of exercise (e.g., 3 vs. 6 days per week) often represents a considerable caloric expenditure. *To effect meaningful weight loss through exercise, each exercise session should last at least 60 minutes at sufficient intensity to expend 300 kCal or more.* Training only 1 day a week generally does not meaningfully change anaerobic or aerobic capacity, body composition, or body weight.[5]

Typical aerobic exercise training programs take place 3 days per week, usually with a rest day spaced between workout days. One could reasonably ask whether training on consecutive days would produce equally effective results. In an experiment concerned with this question, nearly identical improvements in $\dot{V}O_{2max}$ occurred regardless of sequencing of the 3-days-per-week training schedule.[144] Thus, the stimulus for aerobic training probably links closely to exercise intensity and total work accomplished, *not* to the sequencing of training days.

Exercise Mode

Holding exercise intensity, duration, and frequency constant produces a similar training response regardless of training mode—provided exercise involves relatively large muscle groups. Bicycling, walking, running, rowing, swimming, in-line skating, rope skipping, bench-stepping, stair climbing, and simulated arm–leg climbing all provide excellent overload for the aerobic system.[22,127,167,230] Based on the specificity concept, the magnitude of training improvement varies considerably depending on testing mode. Individuals trained on a bicycle show greater improvement when tested on a bicycle than on a treadmill.[158] Likewise, individuals who train by swimming or arm–cranking show the greatest improvement when measured during upper-body exercise.[62,132]

AMERICAN COLLEGE OF SPORTS MEDICINE'S UPDATED FITNESS GUIDELINES AND RECOMMENDATIONS

The American College of Sports Medicine (ACSM) has published guidelines for a "well-rounded training program" that include flexibility exercises and modifications in previous recommendations for aerobic and resistance training and joint flexibility in light of current knowledge.[6] For example, a combined program of aerobic training and resistance training increases muscular strength and aerobic power, decreases body fat, and increases basal metabolic rate. In contrast, singular-focus programs of either resistance *only* or aerobic training *only* produce singularly larger but more limited overall effects.[44]

- *Cardiovascular function.* Recommended changes focus on helping the average person—more gradual approach with older and unfit individuals—adhere to a fitness program that improves the full range of physical fitness components. Professionals now view exercise as exerting an additive effect; cardiovascular and health benefits derived from three 10-minute daily exercise bouts throughout the day almost equal the effects of one continuous 30-minute session. This enables individuals to benefit from daily lifestyle exercise without formally exercising for a distinct period in a structured gymnasium setting.[7,47] Clarifications also have delimited the dose of exercise required for aerobic fitness improvement. Persons should exercise at an intensity of 40–50 to 85% $\dot{V}O_{2max}$ or 55–65 to 90% HR_{max} (lower number for unfit, elderly, or sedentary persons) at least 20 to 60 minutes more than twice weekly. Previously sedentary or unfit individuals should exercise more than 2 days a week for at least 10 minutes. From a health perspective, further good news indicates that just moderate exercise (e.g., gardening or walking >60 min per week) performed regularly reduces the risk of a first heart attack to the same extent as higher intensity workouts.[115] These findings support current exercise recommendations of the American Heart Association and the Centers for Disease Control and Prevention to strive for at least 30 minutes of moderate-intensity physical activity on most days.

- *Muscular strength.* The guidelines acknowledge the positive contributions of resistance training to fat-free body mass, particularly muscle and bone mass. Single-set exercise produces only slightly less strength improvement than multiple-set exercise. This means men and women under age 50 should exercise major muscle groups with one set of 8 to 10 different exercises 2 to 3 days a week; weight loads should allow completion of 8 to 12 repetitions. Older and previously sedentary persons perform one set of 10 to 15 repetitions. Also recognized are the potential cardiovascular benefits of regular, moderate resistance exercise—specifically, reductions in heart rate and blood pressure.[169]

- *Joint flexibility*. A balanced fitness program incorporates static and dynamic range-of-motion (flexibility) exercises of the body's major muscle/tendon groups (four repetitions per group) performed 2 to 3 days a week.

INTEGRATIVE QUESTION

What factors account for differences in responsiveness of individuals to the same exercise-training program?

HOW LONG BEFORE IMPROVEMENTS OCCUR?

Aerobic fitness adaptations occur rapidly with improvement noted within several weeks. FIGURE 21.21 shows absolute and percentage improvements in $\dot{V}O_{2max}$ for subjects who trained

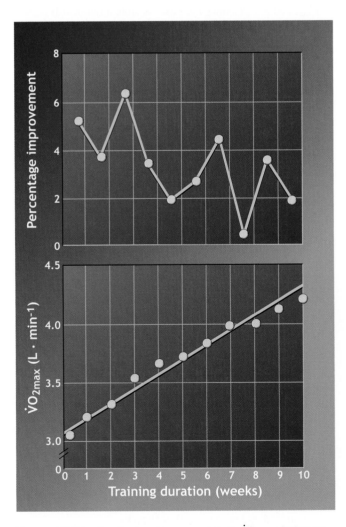

Figure 21.21 Continuous improvements in $\dot{V}O_{2max}$ during 10 weeks of high-intensity aerobic training. (From Hickson RC, et al. Linear increases in aerobic power induced by a program of endurance exercise. J Appl Physiol 1977;42:373.)

6 days a week for 10 weeks. Training consisted of stationary cycling for 30 minutes 3 days per week combined with running for up to 40 minutes on alternate days. The continuous week-to-week improvement in aerobic capacity indicates that training improvement in previously sedentary persons occurs rapidly and progresses in relatively steady fashion. Adaptive responses eventually level off as subjects approach their "genetically predisposed" maximums. The exact time for this leveling off remains unknown, particularly for high-intensity training. The data presented in Figure 21.16 indicate that each physiologic and metabolic system responds differently.

The data in TABLE 21.8 complement those in FIGURE 21.21; they show the rapidity of maximum cardiovascular adaptations to aerobic exercise training. Five young adult men and five women trained daily for 10 consecutive days. Exercise consisted of 1 hour of cycling—10 minutes at 65% $\dot{V}O_{2peak}$, 25 minutes at 75% $\dot{V}O_{2peak}$ and the last 25 minutes of repeat 5, 3-minute intervals at 95% $\dot{V}O_{2peak}$ followed by a 2-minute recovery. This relatively brief 10-day training period induced a 10% increase in $\dot{V}O_{2peak}$ and a 12% increase in cardiac output, 15% increase in stroke volume, and a slight decrease in heart rate during peak exercise. Resting plasma volume increased nearly 9% during the 10 days of training and correlated with the increases in exercise cardiac output and stroke volume. Exercise training augmented the contractile (inotropic) response of the heart to β-adrenergic stimulation. These results indicate that cardiovascular adaptations occur with short-term exercise training in young men and women. The stroke volume increases during exercise reflect the *combined effects* of increased left ventricular end-diastolic dimension (preload in accordance with the Frank-Starling mechanism) and increased systolic ejection.

Trainability and Genes

A vigorous exercise program enhances a person's level of fitness regardless of genetic background, with the limits for developing fitness capacity linked closely to natural endowment. Of two individuals in the same exercise program, one might show 10 times more improvement than the other. A genotype dependency exists for much of one's sensitivity in responding to maximal aerobic and anaerobic power training, including adaptations of most muscle enzymes.[18,43,71,174] Stated differently, both identical twins in a pair generally show a training response of similar magnitude. FIGURE 21.22 (A and B) indicates a clear similarity in the response of $\dot{V}O_{2max}$ (both mL · kg^{-1} · min^{-1} and % improvement) among 10 pairs of male identical twins participating in the same 20-week aerobic exercise training program. If one twin showed high responsiveness to training, a high likelihood existed that the other twin would also be a **responder**; similarly, the brother of a **nonresponder** to exercise training generally showed little improvement. Presence of the muscle-specific creatine kinase gene provides one example of the possible contribution of genetic makeup to individual differences in responsiveness of $\dot{V}O_{2max}$ to endurance training.[182,183]

TABLE 21.8 ■ **MAXIMUM PHYSIOLOGIC RESPONSES DURING PEAK CYCLE ERGOMETER EXERCISE BEFORE AND AFTER 10 CONSECUTIVE DAYS OF AEROBIC TRAINING**

VARIABLE	PRETRAINING	POSTTRAINING
$\dot{V}O_{2peak}$, $L \cdot min^{-1}$	2.54 ± 0.29	2.80 ± 0.32^{a}
Cardiac output, $L \cdot min^{-1}$	18.3 ± 1.3	20.5 ± 1.7^{a}
Heart rate, $b \cdot min^{-1}$	189 ± 2	184 ± 2^{a}
Stroke volume, mL	97 ± 7	112 ± 9^{a}
$a\text{-}\bar{v}O_2$ diff, $mL \cdot dL^{-1}$	13.6 ± 0.8	13.4 ± 0.6
Plasma volume (rest), mL	2896 ± 175	3152 ± 220^{a}

From Mier CM, et al. Cardiovascular adaptations to 10 days of cycle exercise. J Appl Physiol 1997; 83:1900.
^{a}Statistically significant at the .05 level from pretraining value.

MAINTENANCE OF AEROBIC FITNESS GAINS

An important question concerns optimal exercise frequency, duration, and intensity to maintain aerobic improvements with training. In one study, healthy young adults increased $\dot{V}O_{2max}$ 25% with 10 weeks of interval training by bicycling and running for 40 minutes, 6 days a week.[81] They then joined one of two groups that continued to exercise an additional 15 weeks at the same intensity and duration but at reduced *frequency* to either 4 or 2 days a week. Both groups maintained their gains in aerobic capacity despite up to two-thirds reduction in training frequency.

A similar study evaluated reduced training duration on maintenance of improved aerobic fitness.[82] Upon completion of the same protocol outlined previously for the initial 10 weeks of training, subjects continued to maintain intensity and frequency of training for an additional 15 weeks, but at reduced training *duration* from the original 40-minute sessions to either 26 or 13 minutes per day. They maintained almost all $\dot{V}O_{2max}$ and performance increases despite a two-thirds reduction in training duration. Importantly, if training *intensity* decreased and frequency and duration remained constant, even a one-third reduction in exercise intensity reduced the $\dot{V}O_{2max}$.[83]

It appears that aerobic capacity improvement involves somewhat different training requirements than its maintenance. *With intensity held constant, the frequency and duration of exercise required to maintain a certain level of aerobic fitness remain considerably lower than required for its improvement.* In contrast, a small drop-off in exercise intensity reduces $\dot{V}O_{2max}$. This indicates that exercise intensity plays a principal role in maintaining the increase in aerobic capacity achieved through training.

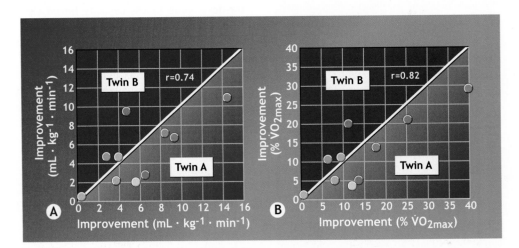

Figure 21.22 Responsiveness of $\dot{V}O_{2max}$ (**A**, $mL \cdot kg^{-1} \cdot min^{-1}$; **B**, % improvement) of 10 pairs of identical twins to a 20-week program of aerobic exercise training. *r*, Pearson product-moment correlation coefficient. Each of the 10 colored data points represents a twin pair. (From Bouchard C. Heredity, fitness, and health. In: Bouchard C, et al., eds. Physical activity, fitness, and health, Champaign, IL: Human Kinetics, 1990.)

Components Other Than $\dot{V}O_{2max}$

Fitness components other than $\dot{V}O_{2max}$ more readily suffer adverse effects of reduced exercise training volume. Well-trained endurance athletes who normally trained 6 to 10 hours a week reduced weekly training to one 35-minute session over a 4-week period.[131] $\dot{V}O_{2max}$ remained constant during this period of reduced training volume. However, endurance capacity at 75% $\dot{V}O_{2max}$ *decreased*; this performance decrement related to reduced preexercise glycogen stores and a diminished level of fat oxidation during exercise. *A single measure such as $\dot{V}O_{2max}$ cannot adequately evaluate all of the factors that affect training and detraining adaptations.*

Tapering for Peak Performance

In most instances, little improvement occurs in the aerobic systems *during* the competitive season. At best, athletes strive to prevent physiologic and performance deterioration as the season progresses. Before major competition, athletes often **taper** training intensity and/or volume believing such adjustments reduce physiologic and psychologic stress of daily training and optimize exercise performance. The taper period and exact alterations in training vary by sport.

No clear answers exist about optimum taper duration or training modification. From a physiologic perspective, probably 4 to 7 days provide sufficient time for maximum muscle and liver glycogen replenishment, optimal nutritional support and restoration, alleviation of residual muscle soreness, and healing of minor injuries. In one study of competitive runners, a 1-week taper period applied either no training (rest), low-intensity running (2 to 10 km daily at 60% $\dot{V}O_{2max}$), or high-intensity running while reducing training volume (five 500-m repeats on day 1, decreasing one repeat each day).[202] Measurements during the taper period included blood volume, red blood cell mass, muscle glycogen content, muscle mitochondrial activity, and 1500-m race performance. Compared with rest and low-intensity exercise taper conditions, high-intensity exercise taper produced the most benefit. This finding suggests that an optimal taper should include progressive reductions in training volume while maintaining a high level of training intensity. With proper tapering, expected performance improvement usually ranges between 0.5 and 6.0%.[150]

METHODS OF TRAINING

Each year, performance improvements occur in almost all athletic competitions. These advances generally relate to increased opportunities for participation: individuals with "natural endowment" have opportunities to participate in different sports. Improved nutrition and health care, better equipment, and more systematic and scientific approaches to athletic training also contribute to superior performance. The following sections present general guidelines for effective anaerobic and aerobic exercise training.

Anaerobic Training

Figure 21.1 shows that the capacity to perform all-out exercise for up to 60 seconds largely depends on ATP generated by the immediate and short-term anaerobic systems for energy transfer.

INTEGRATIVE QUESTION

In what specific ways would anaerobic exercise training improve performance in all-out physical activity?

The Intramuscular High-Energy Phosphates

American football, weight lifting, and other brief sprint–power sport activities rely almost exclusively on energy derived from ATP and PCr, the intramuscular high-energy phosphates. Engaging specific muscles in repeated 5- to 10-second maximum bursts of effort overloads energy transfer from this phosphagen pool. Consequently, only small amounts of lactate accumulate and recovery progresses rapidly. Exercise can begin again after a 30-second rest period. The use of brief, all-out exercise interspersed with recovery represents a specific application of interval training to anaerobic conditioning (see p. 498).

Activities selected to enhance ATP–PCr energy transfer capacity must engage the specific muscles at the movement speed and power output for which the athlete desires improved anaerobic power. This enhances metabolic capacity of specifically trained muscle fibers; it also facilitates recruitment and modulation of the firing sequence of appropriate motor units activated in the particular movement.

Lactate-Generating Capacity

Dependence on anaerobic energy from the intramuscular high-energy phosphates decreases as duration of all-out effort extends beyond 10 seconds. This coincides with a proportionate increase in anaerobic energy transfer from glycolysis. To improve energy transfer capacity by the short-term lactic acid energy system, training must overload this aspect of energy metabolism.

Training of the short-term energy system requires extreme physiologic and psychologic demands. An exercise bout of up to 1-minute maximum exercise stopped 30 seconds before subjective feelings of exhaustion raises blood lactate to near-maximum levels. The individual repeats the exercise bout after 3 to 5 minutes of recovery. Repetition of exercise causes "lactate stacking," which produces a higher blood lactate level than just one all-out exhaustive effort. Of course, as with all training, one must exercise the specific muscle groups that require enhanced anaerobic capacity. A backstroke swimmer trains by swimming the backstroke, a cyclist should bicycle, and basketball, hockey, or soccer players rapidly perform various movements and direction changes similar to those requirements in their sport.

As discussed in Chapter 7, recovery requires considerable time when exercise involves a large anaerobic component. For this reason, anaerobic power training should occur at the end of the conditioning session. Otherwise, fatigue can hinder ability to perform subsequent aerobic training.

Aerobic Training

FIGURE 21.23 indicates two important factors in formulating an aerobic training program:

1. Cardiovascular overload must be sufficiently intense to increase stroke volume and cardiac output.
2. Cardiovascular overload must occur from activation of sport-specific muscle groups to enhance local circulation and the muscle's "metabolic machinery."

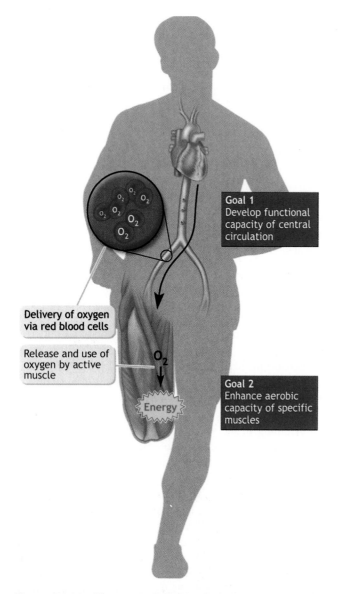

Goal 1
Develop functional capacity of central circulation

Delivery of oxygen via red blood cells

Release and use of oxygen by active muscle

O₂

Energy

Goal 2
Enhance aerobic capacity of specific muscles

Figure 21.23 The two major goals of aerobic training: *Goal 1*, develop the capacity of the central circulation to deliver oxygen; *Goal 2*, enhance the capacity of the active musculature to supply and process oxygen.

In essence, proper endurance training overloads all components of oxygen transport and use. This consideration embodies the specificity principle as applied to aerobic training. Simply stated, runners must run, cyclists must bicycle, rowers must row, and swimmers must swim.

Relatively brief bouts of repeated exercise, as well as continuous, long-duration efforts, enhance aerobic capacity, provided exercise reaches sufficient intensity to overload the aerobic system. **Interval training**, **continuous training**, and **fartlek training** represent three common methods to improve aerobic fitness.

INTEGRATIVE QUESTION

What information would you need to effectively improve aerobic capacity for the specific physical job performance requirements for (1) firefighters, (2) police officers, and (3) oil field workers?

Interval Training

With correct spacing of exercise and rest, one can perform extraordinary amounts of high-intensity exercise, normally not possible if exercise progressed continuously. Repeated exercise bouts (with rest periods or relief intervals) vary from a few seconds to several minutes or longer, depending on the desired training outcome.[110,111,215,216,229] The interval training prescription evolves from the following considerations:

- Intensity of exercise interval
- Duration of exercise interval
- Length of recovery (relief) interval
- Number of repetitions of the exercise–relief interval

Consider the following example of performing a large volume of high-intensity exercise during an interval-training workout. Few people can maintain a 4-minute-mile pace for longer than 1 minute, let alone complete a mile within 4 minutes. Suppose we limited running intervals to only 10 seconds followed by 30 seconds recovery. This scenario makes it reasonably easy to maintain the exercise–relief intervals and complete the mile in 4 minutes of actual running. This does not parallel a world-class performance, but the example indicates that a person can accomplish a considerable quantity of normally exhausting exercise given proper spacing of rest and exercise intervals.

Rationale for Interval Training. Interval training has a sound basis in physiology and energy metabolism. In the example of a continuous run at a 4-minute-mile pace, anaerobic glycolysis provides a large portion of energy. Within a minute or two, the lactate level rises precipitously and the runner fatigues. For interval training, repeated 10-second exercise bouts permit completion of intense exercise without appreciable lactate buildup because intramuscular high-energy phosphates provide the primary energy source. Minimal fatigue

TABLE 21.9 ■ GUIDELINES FOR DETERMINING INTERVAL-TRAINING EXERCISE RATES FOR RUNNING AND SWIMMING DIFFERENT DISTANCES

INTERVAL TRAINING DISTANCES (YARDS)		WORK RATE FOR EACH EXERCISE INTERVAL OR REPEAT
RUN	**SWIM**	
55	15	1.5 ⎧ seconds *slower* than best
110	25	3.0 ⎨ times from a running (or swimming) start
220	55	5.0 ⎩ for each distance
440	110	1 to 4 seconds *faster* than the average 440-yard run or 110-yard swim times recorded during a mile run or 440-yard swim
660–1320	165–320	3 to 4 seconds *slower* than the average 440-yard run or 100-yard swim times recorded during a mile run or 440-yard swim

From Fox EL, Mathews DK. Interval training. Philadelphia: WB Saunders, 1974.

develops during the predominantly "alactic" exercise interval and recovery progresses rapidly. The exercise interval can then begin following only a brief rest.

In interval training, exercise intensity must activate the particular energy systems that require improvement. TABLE 21.9 provides practical guidelines to determine the appropriate exercise and recovery intervals for running and swimming different distances.

- *Exercise interval*: Generally *add* 1.5 to 5.0 seconds to the exerciser's "best time" for training distances between 55 and 220 yards for running and 15 and 55 yards for swimming.[55] If a person can run 60 yards from a running start in 8 seconds, the training time for each repeat equals 8 + 1.5, or 9.5 seconds. For an interval-training distance of 110 yards add 3 seconds, and for a distance of 220 yards add 5 seconds to the best running times. This particular type of interval training applies to training the intramuscular ATP–PCr energy system.

- Training distances of 440 yards running or 110 yards swimming: determine the exercise rate by *subtracting* 1 to 4 seconds from the best 440-yard part of a mile run or 110-yard part of a 440-yard swim. If a person runs a mile in 7 minutes (averaging 105 s per 440 yd), the interval time for each 440-yard repeat range is 104 seconds (105 − 1) to 101 seconds (105 − 4). For training intervals beyond 440 yards, *add* 3 to 4 seconds for each 440-yard portion of the interval distance. In running an interval of 880 yards, the 7-minute miler runs each interval at about 216 seconds [(105 + 3) × 2 = 216].

- *Relief interval*: The relief interval is either passive (rest–relief) or active (work–relief). A ratio of exercise duration to recovery duration usually formulates the duration of the relief interval. *The ratio 1:3 generally applies to training the immediate energy system.* Thus, for a sprinter who runs 10-second intervals, the relief interval equals about 30 seconds (3 × 10 s). *For*

training the short-term glycolytic energy system, the relief interval averages twice the exercise interval or a ratio of 1:2. These specific work–relief ratios for anaerobic training supposedly ensure sufficient restoration of intramuscular phosphates and/or sufficient lactate removal so the next exercise bout can continue with minimal fatigue.

- *To train the long-term aerobic energy system, the exercise–relief interval ratio usually is 1:1 or 1:1.5.* During a 60- to 90-second high-intensity exercise interval, oxygen consumption increases rapidly to a high level but remains insufficient to meet exercise energy requirements. The recommended relief interval causes the succeeding exercise interval to begin before complete recovery (before return to baseline oxygen consumption). This ensures that cardiovascular and aerobic metabolic stress reach near peak levels with repeated but relatively short exercise intervals. The duration of the rest interval takes on less importance with longer periods of intermittent exercise because sufficient time exists for adjustments in metabolic and circulatory parameters during exercise.

 INTEGRATIVE QUESTION

A coach insists that a single exercise mode improves aerobic capacity for all physical activities requiring a high level of aerobic fitness. Give your opinion regarding the potential effectiveness of single-mode exercise to produce generalized cross-training effects?

Sprint-Type Interval Training Affects Anaerobic and Aerobic Physiologic Systems. FIGURE 21.24 shows that relatively brief but intense sprint-type interval training increases parameters of both anaerobic and aerobic metabolic capacity. The 7-week training program for 12 young, adult men consisted of 30 seconds of maximum sprint effort

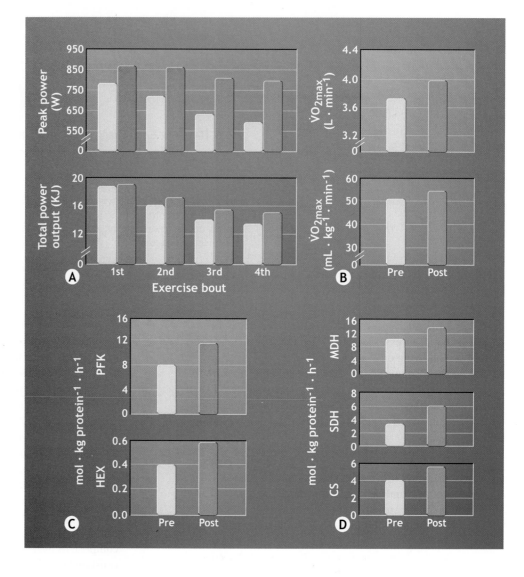

Figure 21.24 Peak power output and total power output during four successive maximum 30-second efforts (**A**), V̇O₂max (**B**), maximal enzyme activity for phosphofructokinase *(PFK)* and hexokinase *(HEX)* (**C**), and maximal enzyme activity for malate dehydrogenase *(MDH)*, succinate dehydrogenase *(SDH)*, and citrate synthase *(CS)* (**D**) before *(yellow bars)* and after *(red bars)* 7 weeks of sprint interval training. (From MacDougall JD, et al. Muscle performance and enzymatic adaptations to sprint interval training. J Appl Physiol 1998;84:2138.)

(Wingate protocol) interspersed with 2 to 4 minutes of recovery performed three times a week. Week 1 began with four exercise intervals with 4 minutes recovery per interval and progressed to 10 exercise intervals with a 2.5-minute recovery per exercise bout by week 7. Despite this relatively brief training stimulus in which exercise duration reached only 5 minutes per session during week 7, improvements occurred in V̇O₂max, short-term power output, and maximal activity of key marker enzymes in the aerobic and anaerobic energy pathways. Positive clinical and cardiovascular adaptations to interval training also emerge among healthy elderly persons.[2]

Continuous Training

Continuous or long, slow, distance (LSD) training involves steady-paced, prolonged exercise at either moderate or high aerobic intensity, usually 60 to 80% V̇O₂max. The exact pace can vary, but it must at least meet a threshold intensity to ensure aerobic physiologic adaptations. Previously, we outlined the method to establish the training-sensitive zone (pp. 490–491). Continuous training for an hour or longer has become popular among fitness enthusiasts, including competi-

tive endurance athletes such as triathletes and cross-country skiers. For example, some elite distance runners train twice a day and run between 100 and 150 miles each week to prepare for competition.

Because of its submaximal nature, continuous exercise training progresses in relative comfort. This contrasts with the potential hazards of high-intensity interval training for coronary-prone individuals and the high level of motivation required for such strenuous exercise. Continuous training ideally suits those beginning an exercise program or wishing to accumulate a large caloric expenditure for weight loss. When applied in athletic training, continuous training truly represents "overdistance" training, with most athletes training two to five times the actual distances of competitive events.

Continuous training allows endurance athletes to exercise at nearly the same intensity as actual competition. Specific motor unit recruitment depends on exercise intensity, so continuous training may best apply to endurance athletes in terms of adaptations at the cellular level. In contrast, interval training often places disproportionate stress on the fast-twitch motor units, *not* slow-twitch units predominantly recruited in endurance competition.

Fartlek Training

Fartlek, a Swedish word meaning "speed play," represents a training method introduced to the United States in the 1940s. This relatively unscientific blending of interval and continuous training has particular application to exercise out-of-doors over natural terrain. The system uses alternate running at fast and slow speeds over level and hilly terrain.

In contrast to the precise exercise-interval training prescription, fartlek training does not require systematic manipulation of exercise and relief intervals. Instead, the performer determines the training schema based on "how it feels" at the time, similar to gauging exercise intensity based on one's rating of perceived exertion (RPE). If used properly, this method can overload one or all of the energy systems. Fartlek training provides an ideal means of general conditioning and off-season training, although it lacks the systematic and quantified approaches of interval and continuous training. It also adds freedom and variety in workouts.

Insufficient evidence prevents proclaiming superiority of any specific training method to improve aerobic capacity and associated physiologic variables, provided equality exists in absolute training intensity and total amount of work completed.[147] Each form of training produces success. One can probably use the various methods interchangeably, particularly to modify training and achieve a more psychologically pleasing exercise or training regimen.

OVERTRAINING: TOO MUCH OF A GOOD THING

Ten to 20% of athletes experience the syndrome of **overtraining** or "staleness." The overtrained condition represents more than just a short-term inability to train hard or a slight dip in competition-level performance. Based on complex interactions among biologic and psychologic influences, an athlete can fail to endure and adapt to training so that normal exercise performance deteriorates, and the individual encounters increasing difficulty fully recovering from a workout.[24,26,176,227] This takes on crucial importance for elite athletes for whom performance decrements of 1 to 3% can cause a gold medalist to fail to qualify for competition. Overtraining also relates to increased incidence of infections, persistent muscle soreness, and general malaise and loss of interest in sustaining high-level training. Injuries occur more frequently in the overtrained state.[228]

Two clinical forms of overtraining have been described:

1. The less common **sympathetic form** (*basedowian* for thyroid hyperfunction patterns), characterized by increased sympathetic activity during rest; generally typified by hyperexcitability, restlessness, and impaired exercise performance. This form of overtraining may reflect excessive psychologic/emotional stress that accompanies the interaction among training, competition, and responsibilities of normal living.[114]

2. The more common **parasympathetic form** (*addisonoid* for adrenal insufficiency patterns) characterized by predominance of vagal activity during rest and exercise. More properly termed **overreaching** in the early stages (within as few as 10 days), the syndrome is qualitatively similar in symptoms to the full-blown parasympathetic overtraining syndrome but of shorter duration. Excessive and protracted exercise overload with inadequate recovery and rest leads to overreaching. Initially, maintaining exercise performance requires greater effort; this eventually leads to performance deterioration in training and competition. Short-term rest intervention of a few days up to several weeks usually restores full function. Untreated overreaching eventually leads to the overtraining syndrome.

Parasympathetic overtraining syndrome involves chronic fatigue during exercise workouts and recovery periods. Associated symptoms include sustained poor exercise performance, altered sleep patterns and appetite, frequent infections, persistently high fatigue ratings, altered immune and reproductive functions, acute and chronic alterations in systemic inflammatory responses, mood disturbances (anger, depression, anxiety), and general malaise and loss of interest in high-level training. Complex interactions and effects of short- and long-term alterations in systemic inflammatory responses also produce the syndrome.[209]

DEFINITIONS OF TERMS RELATED TO THE OVERTRAINING SYNDROME[175]

- Overload: A planned, systematic, and progressive increase in training to improve performance.
- Overreaching: Unplanned, excessive overload with inadequate rest. Poor performance is observed in training and competition. Successful recovery should result from short-term (i.e., a few days up to 1 or 2 weeks) interventions.
- Overtraining syndrome: Untreated overreaching that produces long-term decreased performance and impaired ability to train. Other problems may require medical attention.

FIGURE 21.25 illustrates possible factors that interact to initiate the parasympathetic-type overtraining syndrome. Interactions among chronic neuromuscular, neuroendocrine, psychologic, immunologic, and metabolic overload during long-term, high-volume training (with insufficient recuperation) eventually alter physiologic function and the stress response to produce the overtrained state.[72,129,186] Preexisting medical conditions, poor diet (e.g., inadequate carbohydrate or dehydration), environmental stress (e.g., heat, humidity,

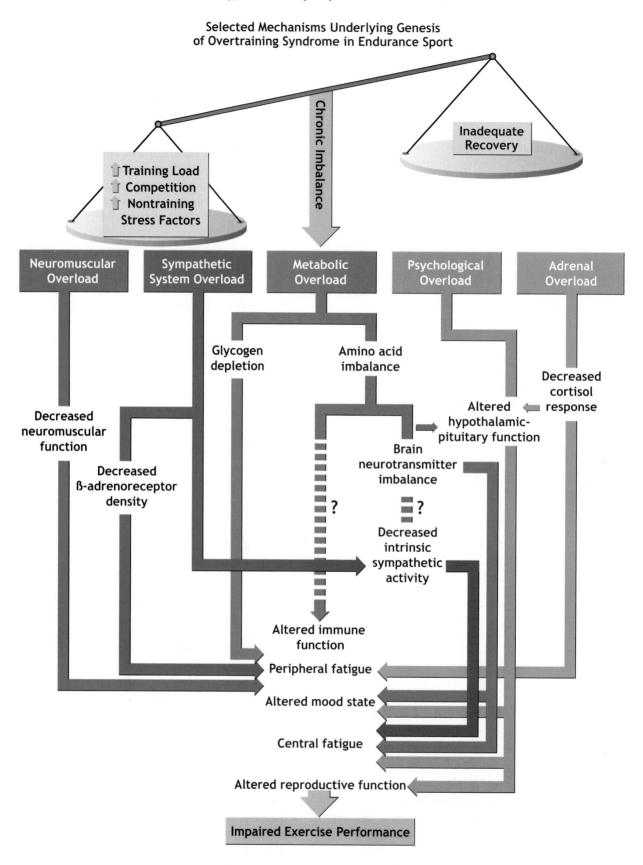

Figure 21.25 Schematic overview of the genesis of the overtraining syndrome in endurance sports requiring prolonged high-volume training. (Modified from Lehmann M, et al. Autonomic imbalance hypothesis and overtraining syndrome. Med Sci Sports Exerc 1998;30:1140.)

TABLE 21.10 ■ THE OVERTRAINING SYNDROME: SYMPTOMS OF STALENESS
• Unexplained and persistently poor performance and high fatigue ratings • Prolonged recovery from typical training sessions or competitive events • Disturbed mood states characterized by general fatigue, apathy, depression, irritability, and loss of competitive drive • Persistent feelings of soreness and stiffness in muscles and joints • Elevated resting pulse and increased susceptibility to upper respiratory infections (altered immune function) and gastrointestinal disturbances • Insomnia • Loss of appetite, weight loss, and inability to maintain proper body weight for competition • Overuse injuries

altitude), and psychosocial pressures (e.g., monotonous training, frequent competition, personal conflicts) often exacerbate training demands and increase the risk of developing the overtraining syndrome.

Significant effects of overtraining include (1) functional impairments in the hypothalamo–pituitary–gonadal and adrenal axes and sympathetic neuroendocrine system as reflected by depressed urinary excretion of norepinephrine[114,224] and (2) exercise-induced increases in adrenocorticotropic hormone and growth hormone and decreases in cortisol and insulin levels.[227] In some ways the syndrome reflects the body's attempt to enforce upon the athlete an appropriate recuperative period from the sustained arousal levels from intense training and competition. Despite the highly individualized specific symptoms of the overtraining syndrome, those outlined in TABLE 21.10 are most common. No simple method can diagnose overtraining in its earliest stages.[59,76,103] Deterioration in physical performance, alterations in mood, a relatively high cortisol/cortisone ratio, and possibly decreased nocturnal heart rate variability provide the best indications.[8,155,162,201] Conditions that cause some athletes to thrive in training initiate an overtraining response in others. Generally, when symptoms emerge they persist unless the athlete rests, with complete recovery requiring weeks or even months. No reliable method currently exists to determine the point of complete recovery from the overtraining syndrome.

Proper periodization of training contributes to preventing the overtraining syndrome. Coaches must provide for adequate recuperation during the most intense training cycles or when an athlete attempts to regain peak form following a layoff. Nutrition becomes particularly important during intense training;[205] special emphasis placed on glycogen replenishment (sufficient recovery time plus high levels of dietary carbohydrate[1]) and rehydration reduce symptoms but cannot prevent the syndrome's development.[175]

EXERCISING DURING PREGNANCY

Estimates indicate that 40% or more of women in the United States exercise during pregnancy.[78,244] FIGURE 21.26 illustrates the prevalence and pattern of exercise during pregnancy among 9953 randomly selected pregnant women from 48 states, including the District of Columbia and New York City, who gave birth to live infants. Forty-two percent of all women reported exercising, one half of whom exercised longer than 6 months. Walking was the leading activity (43% of all reported), followed by swimming (12%) and aerobic dancing (12%). Older mothers and women who had multiple gestations, previous children, or an unfavorable reproductive history were less likely to exercise during pregnancy.

Exercise Effects on the Mother

Maternal cardiovascular dynamics follow normal response patterns; moderate exercise offers no greater physiologic stress to the mother other than the additional weight gain and possible encumbrance of fetal tissue. Pregnant women showed the same capacity as postpartum women to perform 40 minutes of cycling at 70 to 75% $\dot{V}O_{2max}$. The physiologic responses to this weight-supported exercise remained largely independent of gestation.[123] Pregnancy does not compromise the absolute value for aerobic capacity ($L \cdot min^{-1}$).[124,191] As pregnancy progresses, the increase in maternal body mass and changes in coordination and balance adversely affect exercise economy; this adds to exercise effort with weight-bearing exercise. Pregnancy, particularly in the last trimester, also increases pulmonary ventilation at a given submaximal exercise level.[123]

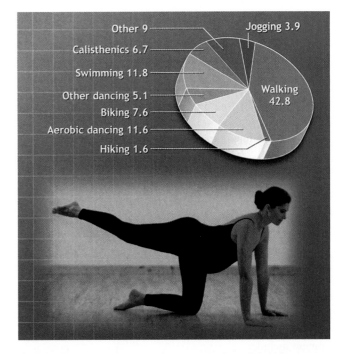

Figure 21.26 Pattern of exercising (% of total) in U.S. women during pregnancy. (From Zhang J, Savitz DA. Exercise during pregnancy among US women. Ann Epidemiol 1996;6:53.)

TABLE 21.11 ■ IMPORTANT METABOLIC AND CARDIORESPIRATORY ADAPTATIONS DURING PREGNANCY
• Blood volume increases 40 to 50%; hemodilution reduces hemoglobin concentration • Increase in blood volume dilates the left ventricle • Slight increase in oxygen consumption during rest and submaximal, weight-supported exercise such as stationary cycling • Substantial increase in oxygen consumption during weight-bearing exercise such as walking and running • Increased heart rate during rest and submaximal exercise • No change in $\dot{V}O_{2max}$ (L · min^{-1}) • Increased ventilatory response—largely progesterone induced—during rest and submaximal exercise • Possible magnified hypoglycemic response during exercise, especially late in pregnancy • Possible depressed sympathetic nervous system response to exercise in late gestation
Modified from Wolfe LA, et al. Maternal exercise, fetal well-being and pregnancy outcome. Exerc Sport Sci Rev 1994;22:145.

The direct stimulating effects of progesterone and increased chemoreceptor sensitivity to carbon dioxide contribute to maternal exercise "hyperventilation."[242] Regular, moderate exercise during the second and third trimesters reduces submaximal ventilatory demands and RPE.[156] This training adaptation increases the mother's ventilatory reserve and possibly inhibits exertional dyspnea. TABLE 21.11 summarizes the important maternal metabolic and cardiorespiratory adaptations during pregnancy.

Exercise Effects on the Fetus

Prudent guidelines and recommendations are required for exercise during pregnancy.[4] Epidemiologic evidence indicates that exercise during pregnancy does not relate to increased risk of fetal deaths or low birth weights.[198] In fact, beginning a moderate program of weight-bearing exercise early in pregnancy and continuing to exercise until term enhances fetoplacental growth.[31] A study of middle-class women evaluated the effects of daily low–moderate exercise (<1000 kCal · wk^{-1}), more intense exercise (>1000 kCal · wk^{-1}), or no exercise on timely delivery and the safety and potential benefits of regular exercise during pregnancy.[78] No association emerged between low–moderate exercise and gestation length. A positive finding indicated that higher volume weekly exercise lowered rather than raised the risk of preterm birth; among births after the projected term, women who exercised more heavily delivered faster than nonexercisers.

Potential exercise risks of intense maternal exercise for which repeated exposures could alter fetal growth and development include:

- Reduced placental blood flow and accompanying fetal hypoxia

- Fetal hyperthermia
- Reduced fetal glucose supply

Any factor that might temporarily compromise fetal blood supply raises concern in counseling pregnant women about exercise. Research on humans in this area remains sparse, but other species of mammals have been studied. In one investigation, treadmill exercise to exhaustion caused uterine blood flow and arterial oxygen pressure to decline in near-term pregnant ewes.[28] Despite this potentially negative response, facilitated unloading of oxygen from the available blood supply maintained oxygen consumption by the uteroplacental tissues and fetus. However, animals with one umbilical artery tied off to restrict placental circulation displayed a reduction in fetal oxygen supply during exercise.[50] The researchers concluded that the fetus tolerated vigorous maternal exercise without adverse effects under normal conditions. In contrast, intense exercise posed a potentially harmful reduction in oxygen supply to a fetus with some limitation in umbilical circulation.

Neonates born to exercising mothers exhibit a neurobehavioral profile as early as the fifth day after birth, earlier than neonates from more sedentary counterparts.[30] Exercising mothers either ran, performed aerobics, swam, or used stair-climbing exercise at least three times weekly for more than 20 minutes at 55% of aerobic capacity or above. The women in the control group led active lives that did not include regular, sustained exercise bouts. FIGURE 21.27 shows data for five behavioral clusters of the Brazelton Neonatal Assessment Scales for the offspring of 34 women who exercised regularly and 31 sedentary women. No significant differences emerged between neonates born to exercising women and sedentary controls for clusters of factors that assessed motor organization, autonomic stability, and range of state behaviors. Neonates born to exercising women scored higher in orientation behavior and ability to regulate state (i.e., more alert and interested in the surroundings and less demanding of their mothers). The inset table indicates that axial length and head circumference remained similar between groups. The offspring of the exercising women were lighter and leaner than offspring from the control group. The findings support the concept that continuing regular exercise throughout pregnancy modifies neonatal behavior by positively affecting early neurodevelopment.

 INTEGRATIVE QUESTION

What weight control advantage during pregnancy would a daily walking program offer compared with stationary cycling if each program remained at the same initial exercise level (i.e., constant walking speed or cycling power output), frequency, and duration?

Current Opinion

Reports document extreme levels of physical activity nearly to term for highly conditioned pregnant women without adverse effects on mother or fetus. Exercise protocols for these athletes included resistance training, endurance training,

■ **IN A PRACTICAL SENSE**

THE EXERCISE PRESCRIPTION DURING PREGNANCY

■ Pregnancy alters normal physiology, necessitating some modification in exercise prescription. Pregnant women should consult their physician before initiating an exercise program (or modifying an existing program) to rule out possible complications. This pertains particularly to women of low fitness status and little exercise experience prior to pregnancy.

Exercise during pregnancy should heighten awareness about heat dissipation, adequate caloric and nutrient intake, and knowing when to reduce exercise intensity. For a normal, uncomplicated pregnancy, light-to-moderate exercise does not negatively affect fetal development; the benefits of properly prescribed regular exercise during pregnancy generally outweigh potential risks.

EXERCISE GUIDELINES

Exercise mode: Avoid exercise in the supine position, particularly after the first trimester. Supine exercise impairs venous return (mass of the fetus compresses inferior vena cava), which could affect cardiac output and uterine blood flow. Non–weight-bearing exercise (e.g., cycling, swimming) minimizes the effect of gravity and the added weight associated with fetal development. Low-impact, weight-bearing exercise in moderation should not pose a risk.

Exercise frequency: Exercise 3 days a week, emphasizing continuous, steady-rate effort. Reduce the intensity of more frequent exercise.

Exercise duration: Exercise 30 to 40 minutes, depending on how the person feels.

Exercise intensity: Pregnancy alters the relationship between heart rate and oxygen consumption, making it difficult to establish guidelines from heart rate. An effective alternative establishes exercise intensity based on RPE, which should range between 11 ("fairly light") to 13 ("somewhat hard").

Rate of progression: Perform exercise on a regular basis; moderate aerobic exercise maintains cardiovascular fitness and often produces a small

training effect. Most women should not strive to induce training effects, but, rather maintain cardiorespiratory fitness, muscle mass, and physician-recommended weight gain. The combined effects of pregnancy per se and regular exercise often produce improved fitness after delivery.

WHEN TO STOP EXERCISE AND SEEK MEDICAL ADVICE

Discontinue exercise immediately under the following conditions:
- Any signs of vaginal bleeding
- Any gush of fluid from the vagina (premature rupture of membranes)
- Sudden swelling of ankles, hands, or face
- Persistent, severe headaches and/or disturbances in vision; unexplained lightheadedness or dizziness
- Elevated pulse rate or blood pressure that does not rapidly return to normal following exercise
- Excessive fatigue, palpitations, or chest pain
- Persistent uterine contractions (more than 6 to 8 per h)
- Unexplained or unusual abdominal pain
- Insufficient weight gain (<1.0 kg per month during the last two trimesters)

Contraindications to exercise during pregnancy:
- Pregnancy-induced hypertension
- History of two or more spontaneous abortions
- Preterm rupture of membranes
- Preterm labor during the prior or current pregnancy
- Incompetent cervix
- Excessive alcohol intake
- Persistent second to third trimester bleeding
- History of premature labor
- Intrauterine growth retardation
- Anemia
- Type 1 diabetes
- Significant obesity
- Multiple pregnancy
- Smoking

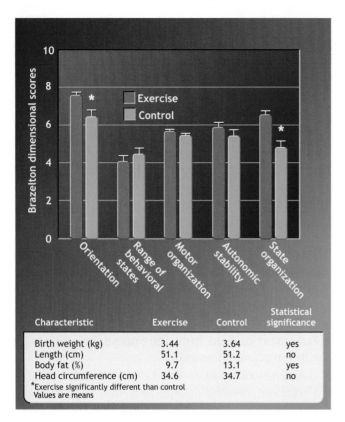

Characteristic	Exercise	Control	Statistical significance
Birth weight (kg)	3.44	3.64	yes
Length (cm)	51.1	51.2	no
Body fat (%)	9.7	13.1	yes
Head circumference (cm)	34.6	34.7	no

*Exercise significantly different than control
Values are means

Figure 21.27 Behavioral constellation scores of neonates in exercise and nonexercise control groups on Brazelton Neonatal Behavioral Assessment Scales. *Numbers* preceding each set of vertical bars represent an optimum score for each constellation; *asterisks* indicate statistical significance at the .01 level. *Insert table* presents neonatal morphometric values. (From Clapp JF III, et al. Neonatal behavioral profile of the offspring of women who continue to exercise regularly throughout pregnancy. Am J Obstet Gynecol 1999;180:91.

and interval training 6 days a week to within 4 days of labor.[96] For an elite marathoner pregnant with twins, regular exercise consisted of training an average of 107 km (66.5 mi) weekly up to 3 days before giving birth.[11] For active women with uncomplicated pregnancies, maximal exercise testing produced no untoward responses in fetal heart rate (minimal changes) or abnormal neonatal outcomes.[130] Despite these examples of extreme physical activity for well-trained women without apparent negative affect on maternal or fetal health, more conservative, prudent recommendations apply to most healthy, pregnant women. *Thirty to 40 minutes of moderate aerobic exercise for a previously active, healthy, low-risk woman during an uncomplicated pregnancy does not compromise fetal oxygen supply or acid–base status, induce heart rate signs of fetal distress, or produce other adverse effects to mother or fetus.*[40,123] Performed on a regular basis, such exercise maintains cardiovascular fitness and generates a training effect.[164,170] Hormonal action via the sympathetic nervous system during strenuous exercise probably diverts some blood from the uterus and visceral organs for preferential distribution to active muscles. This could pose a hazard to a fetus with restricted placental blood flow. The accompanying "In a

Practical Sense" on p. 505 outlines guidelines for formulating the exercise prescription in pregnancy. The prudent approach dictates that a pregnant woman (in consultation with her health care provider) should exercise in moderation, especially if the pregnancy is at all compromised. In addition, exercise late in pregnancy can magnify the normal maternal hypoglycemic response by increasing glucose consumption by maternal skeletal muscle; in the extreme, this response could adversely affect fetal glucose supply.[16,29]

Pregnant women should avoid supine exercise, contact sports, high-altitude exertion, hot tub immersion, and scuba diving. A decrease in uterine blood flow or elevation in maternal core temperature with extended-duration exercise during environmental heat stress could compromise heat dissipation from the fetus through the placenta.[138] Hyperthermia negatively affects fetal development (e.g., increased risk of neural tube defect), particularly in the first trimester,[142] so pregnant women should exercise during warm weather in the cool part of the day for shorter intervals while maintaining regular fluid intake. Within this framework, aquatic exercise serves as an ideal form of maternal exercise.

Current fitness level and previous physical activity patterns should guide a woman's exercise behavior throughout an uncomplicated pregnancy and postpartum. Regular aerobic exercise plays an important role to maintain functional capacity and general well-being during pregnancy. It also optimizes overall weight gain during the later stages of pregnancy[29] and may reduce risk for cesarean delivery in women who have never borne children.[25] Controversy remains about whether (1) extremes of maternal exercise benefit either mother or fetus or (2) exercise during pregnancy benefits labor, delivery, birth weight, and general outcome.[15,165] Beginning regular exercise 6 to 8 weeks postpartum produces no deleterious effect on volume or composition of lactation and improves aerobic fitness without impairing immune function.[40,122,126] Combining moderate exercise with a reduced energy intake of about 500 kCal a day allows overweight lactating women to safely lose 0.5 kg per week without adversely affecting infant growth.[125]

Summary

1. Physical activities generally classify by the specific energy transfer system predominantly activated. An effective exercise program trains the appropriate energy system(s) to improve a desired physiologic function or performance goal.

2. Physical conditioning based on sound principles optimizes improvements. The four primary training principles are overload, specificity, individual differences, and reversibility.

3. Exercise training initiates cellular adaptations and gross physiologic changes that enhance functional capacity and exercise performance.

4. Anaerobic training increases resting levels of intramuscular anaerobic substrates and key glycolytic enzymes. Adaptations usually accompany concomitant increases in maximal exercise performance.

5. Aerobic training adaptations increase mitochondrial size and number, quantity of aerobic enzymes, muscle capillarization, and fat and carbohydrate oxidation. These improvements contribute to enhanced aerobic ATP production.

6. A linear relationship exists between heart rate and oxygen consumption from light to moderately intense exercise in trained and untrained individuals. Improved stroke volume with aerobic training shifts this line to the right, thereby decreasing heart rate at any submaximal exercise level.

7. Aerobic training induces functional and dimensional changes in the cardiovascular system. These changes decrease resting and submaximal exercise heart rate, enhance stroke volume and cardiac output, and expand the a-$\bar{v}O_2$ difference.

8. Cardiac hypertrophy represents a fundamental biologic adaptation to increased myocardial workload imposed by exercise training. Cardiac enlargement with endurance training increases left ventricular volume and enhances stroke volume.

9. Structural and dimensional changes in the left ventricle vary with exercise training modes. No scientific evidence shows that regular exercise harms normal cardiac function.

10. Factors that affect the magnitude of training improvements include initial fitness level; frequency, intensity, and duration of exercise; and training type (mode). Of these, exercise intensity is the most crucial.

11. Training intensity can be applied on either an absolute basis for exercise load or relative to a person's physiologic response. The most practical approach sets exercise intensity to a percentage of HR_{max}. Training levels between 60 and 90% HR_{max} induce meaningful changes in aerobic fitness.

12. Training duration and intensity interact in affecting the training response. Generally, 30-minute exercise sessions are practical and effective. Extending duration compensates for reduced exercise intensity.

13. Two to 3 days a week is probably the minimum frequency for aerobic training. Optimal training frequency remains undetermined.

14. Similar improvements occur with intensity, duration, and frequency held constant, regardless of exercise mode when training involves large muscle groups and training evaluation remains mode specific.

15. The frequency and duration of training to maintain improved aerobic fitness are lower than required to improve it. Even small decreases in exercise intensity reduce $\dot{V}O_{2max}$.

16. Interval, continuous, and fartlek training improve the capacity of the different energy transfer systems. Interval training most effectively improves the immediate and short-term anaerobic energy systems.

17. Aerobic training must overload both cardiovascular function and metabolic capacity of specific muscles. Peripheral adaptations in trained muscle profoundly enhance endurance performance.

18. Prolonged and intense endurance training can cause the syndrome of overtraining or staleness, with associated alterations in neuroendocrine and immune functions. The syndrome includes chronic fatigue, poor exercise performance, frequent infections, and general loss of interest in training. Symptoms generally persist until the athlete relinquishes training, possibly for several days to months.

19. At least 40% of American women exercise during pregnancy. Walking is the most common form of exercise (42%) followed by swimming (12%) and aerobics (12%).

20. Reduced placental blood flow and accompanying fetal hypoxia, fetal hyperthermia, and reduced fetal glucose supply pose the most serious potential exercise risks during pregnancy.

21. For previously active, healthy women, moderate aerobic exercise does not compromise fetal oxygen supply.

References are available on the Student CD and online at *http://connection.lww.com/ mkk6e.*

Muscular Strength: Training Muscles to Become Stronger

22

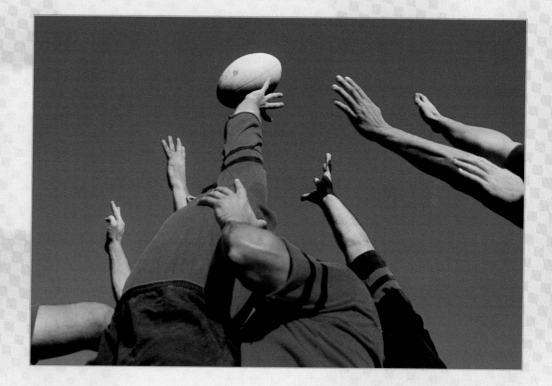

CHAPTER OBJECTIVES

- Describe the following four methods to assess muscular strength: (1) cable tensiometry, (2) dynamometry, (3) one-repetition maximum (I-RM), and (4) computer-assisted isokinetic dynamometry

- Outline a procedure to assess 1-RM for trained and untrained individuals

- Describe how to ensure test standardization and fairness to evaluate muscular strength

- Compare absolute and relative upper- and lower-body muscular strength in men and women

- Describe allometric scaling to "equalize" individuals when comparing physical and exercise performance characteristics

- Define concentric, eccentric, and isometric muscle actions, and give examples of each

- Discuss the advisability of resistance training for children and adolescents

- Summarize the main research findings on optimal number of sets and repetitions, and frequency and relative intensity of progressive-resistance training

- Outline the model for strength-training periodization

- Discuss specificity of the strength-training response related to sports and occupational tasks

- Differentiate between resistance training goals of competitive athletes and untrained middle-aged and elderly persons

- Respond to the question: "Which is better for strength improvement: progressive resistance weight training, isometric training, or isokinetic training?"

- Describe advantages and disadvantages of plyometric training for power athletes

- Describe how "psychologic" factors and "muscular" factors influence maximum strength capacity and training responsiveness

- List physiologic adaptations with chronic resistance training

- Summarize current opinion concerning resistance training's effect on muscle fiber type and number

- Outline a circuit resistance training program for middle-aged men and women to improve muscular strength and aerobic fitness

- Discuss whether specific resistance training can "shape" a muscle's appearance

- Review (1) the type of exercise most frequently associated with delayed-onset muscle soreness (DOMS), (2) the best way to minimize DOMS when initiating training, and (3) significant cellular alterations with DOMS

PART 1 • *Strength Measurement and Resistance Training*

Weight lifting began in America in the early 1840s as a spectator sport practiced by "strongmen" who showcased their prowess in traveling carnivals and sideshows. By the mid-1880s, measuring muscular strength became more commonplace. As pointed out in the text's "Introduction: A View of the Past," the military evaluated the strength of conscripts during the Civil War; strength measurements also provided

the basis for routine fitness assessments in college and university physical education programs. An 1897 meeting of College Gymnasium Directors (Dr. D. A. Sargent, committee chair from Harvard University) established strength contests for college undergraduates to determine overall body strength and the college's "strongest man." Measures included back, leg, arm, and chest strength evaluated with several of the devices depicted in Figure 9 of the "Introduction." Harvard, Columbia, Amherst, University of Minnesota, and Dickinson were the first five colleges to rank in the 1898–1899 competitions.

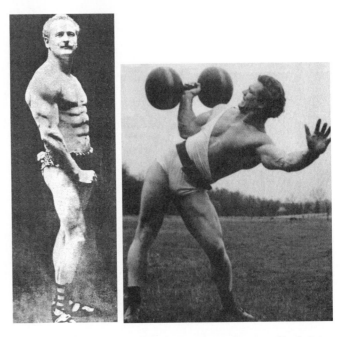

Left. Early 1890s pose of strongman Eugene Sandow (Frederick Mueller), billed by showman Florenz Ziegfeld as "The Most Perfect Man." Sandow helped to design a physical fitness training program for the British military, inspiring a future generation of body builders. *Right.* John Grimek, member of the United States 1936 Olympic weight lifting team, two-time Mr. America (1940, 1941), 1948 Mr. Universe, and undefeated in body-building competition. Recognized as the "best-built human" of the first half of the 20th century.

Strength assessment became commonplace after the turn of the century, and by the mid-1900s, physical culture specialists, circus performers, body builders, competitive weight lifters, field event athletes, and wrestlers trained predominantly using "weight-lifting" exercises. Most other athletes refrained from lifting weights for fear such training would slow them and increase muscle size to the point where they would lose joint flexibility and become *musclebound*. Subsequent research in the late 1950s and early 1960s dispelled this myth when experiments revealed that muscle-strengthening exercises did not reduce speed or range of joint motion. Instead, the opposite usually occurred; elite weight lifters, body builders, and "muscle men" had exceptional joint flexibility without limitations in general limb movement speed. For untrained healthy individuals, heavy-resistance exercises increased speed and power of muscular effort. Certainly, these effects would not impair subsequent sports performance.

In the sections that follow, we explore the rationale that underlies resistance training and physiologic adaptations when training muscles to become stronger. The discussion centers on different methods to measure muscular strength, gender differences in strength, and resistance-training programs to increase muscle strength and power.

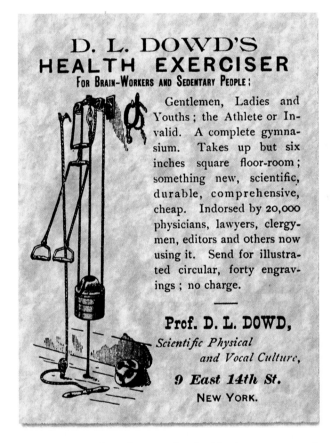

Late 1890s strength equipment advertised for home gym use. By the mid-1850s, rowing machines and strengthening devices became commonplace, eventually leading to studies of their effectiveness in American colleges (Harvard and Amherst) in the 1890s.

MEASUREMENT OF MUSCLE STRENGTH

One of the following four methods commonly measures muscle strength or, more precisely, maximum force or tension generated by a single muscle or related muscle groups:

1. Tensiometry
2. Dynamometry
3. One-repetition maximum
4. Computer-assisted force and power output determinations

Cable Tensiometry

FIGURE 22.1A shows a **cable tensiometer** for measuring knee extension muscle force. Increasing the force on the cable depresses the riser over which the cable passes. This deflects the pointer and indicates the subject's strength score. The instrument measures muscle force in a static (isometric) muscle action that elicits little or no change in the muscle's external length. This application of the tensiometer differs considerably from its original use in the early 1900s for measuring the tension on steel cables linking the upper and lower wings of biplane aircraft. The tensiometer (lightweight, portable, and easy to use) provides the advantage of versatility for recording force measurements at virtually all angles about a specific joint's range of motion (ROM). Standardized cable-tension strength-test batteries assess static force capacity of all major muscle groups.[31] The tests document strength impairment in muscles weakened from disease or injury. Muscle evaluation takes place at a specific joint angle, and repeated measurements determine strength status prior to and following resistance training. A particular movement activates more than one muscle group, so the clinician or researcher applies the tensiometer at multiple angles in the full ROM. This approach often gives a clearer picture of muscular strength (or weakness) than solely standard weight-lifting tests.

Dynamometry

Figure 22.1B and C illustrate hand-grip and leg and back-lift **dynamometers** for static strength measurement based on the compression principle. An external force applied to the dynamometer compresses a steel spring and moves a pointer. The force required to move the pointer a given distance determines the external force applied to the dynamometer.

One-Repetition Maximum

A dynamic procedure for measuring muscular strength applies the **one-repetition maximum (1-RM) method**. 1-RM refers to the maximum amount of weight lifted *one time* using proper form during a standard weight-lifting exercise. To assess 1-RM for any muscle group, the tester makes a reasonable guess at an initial weight close to, but below, the person's maximum lifting capacity. Weight is progressively added to the exercise device on subsequent attempts until the person reaches maximum lift capacity. The weight increments usually range between 1 and 5 kg depending on the muscle group evaluated. Rest intervals of 1 to 5 minutes usually provide sufficient recuperation before attempting a lift at the next heavier weight.

Estimate the 1-RM

Impracticality and/or potential risk in performing 1-RM with preadolescents, the elderly, hypertensives, cardiac patients, and other special populations requires that equations estimate 1-RM from submaximal effort. We present equations (next page) for untrained and resistance-trained young adults because resistance training alters the relationship between a

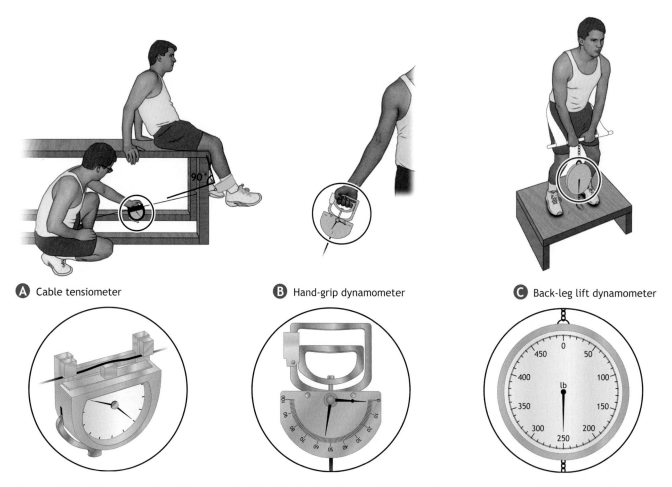

Figure 22.1 Measurement of static strength with (**A**) cable tensiometer, (**B**) hand-grip dynamometer, and (**C**) back-leg lift dynamometer.

submaximal performance (7- to 10-RM) and maximal lift (1-RM). Generally, the weight that one lifts for 7- to 10-RM represents about 68% of the 1-RM score for the untrained person and 79% of the new 1-RM after training.[20]

Untrained:

1-RM (kg) = 1.554 × 7- to 10-RM weight (kg) − 5.181

Trained:

1-RM (kg) = 1.172 × 7- to 10-RM weight (kg) + 7.704

For example, estimate 1-RM bench press score for a trained person whose 10-RM bench press equals 70 kg, as follows:

1-RM (kg) = 1.172 × 70 kg + 7.704
= 89.7 kg

Computer-Assisted, Electromechanical, and Isokinetic Methods

Microprocessor technology rapidly quantifies forces, torques, accelerations, and velocities of body segments in numerous movement patterns. Force platforms measure the external application of muscle force by a limb as in jumping.

Other electromechanical devices assess forces generated during all phases of an exercise movement (e.g., cycling) or during movements that primarily use the arms (supine bench press) or legs (leg press).

An electromechanical accommodating resistance instrument, termed an **isokinetic dynamometer**, contains a speed-controlling mechanism that accelerates to a preset, constant velocity with force application. Once attaining this speed, the isokinetic loading mechanism adjusts automatically to provide a counterforce to variations in force generated by the muscle as movement continues throughout the "strength curve." *Thus, maximum force (or any percentage of maximum effort) generates throughout the full ROM at a preestablished velocity of limb movement.* This allows training under either high-velocity (low-force) or low-velocity (high-force) conditions. A microprocessor within the dynamometer continuously monitors the immediate level of applied force. An electronic integrator in series with a monitor displays the average or peak force generated during any period. The integrator's voltage output interfaces directly with a computer for almost instantaneous feedback about performance (e.g., force, torque, work).

The interface of microprocessor technology with mechanical devices provides the exercise scientist with valuable data to evaluate, test, and train muscles. This technology,

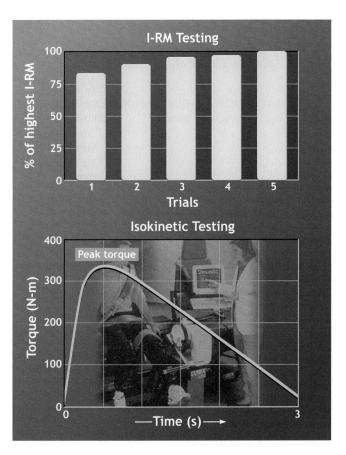

Figure 22.2 *Top.* Conventional 1-RM testing. The heaviest weight lifted constitutes the 1-RM. If 150 kg (100%) is the maximum lifted, then 150 kg equals the 1-RM. *Bottom.* Force curve obtained during an isokinetic test performed at an angular velocity of 30° · s^{-1} over a 3-second interval. Peak torque in this example equals 342 N-m. Average torque is the force-time integral, or impulse divided by time. Impulse equals 602 N-m · s^{-1}, and average torque equals 200.7 N-m (602 N-m ÷ 3). Work equals the product of average torque × distance moved (90°, or 1.57 radians). Using the data for average torque and distance, work equals 174 N-m × 157 radians = 273 N-m, or 273 joules (J). Power is work per unit time, or 273 J ÷ 3.0 s = 91 W.

however, lacks universal acceptance because many still consider a maximum lift (1-RM) the best criterion of overall muscular strength. The argument for isokinetic strength measurement maintains that muscle strength dynamics involve considerably more than *just* the final outcome of 1-RM. For example, two individuals with identical 1-RM scores could exhibit dissimilar force curves throughout the movement. Individual differences in force dynamics (e.g., time to peak tension) throughout the full ROM may reflect an entirely different underlying neuromuscular physiology that 1-RM does not assess. FIGURE 22.2 illustrates the differences between conventional 1-RM knee extension (*top;* highest force score during five lifts represents *only* total weight lifted) and a microprocessor-controlled, isokinetic resistance device that produces a force curve throughout the ROM (*bottom;* force related to movement duration). Note that peak torque occurred in the early phase of movement at the most advantageous angle in the ROM; the lowest torque occurred at full knee extension. TABLE 22.1 lists measurement units for various expressions of muscular performance during linear and angular movements.

INTEGRATIVE QUESTION

Explain why many resistance-trained athletes have their spotters during a free-weight bench press apply external force (to make the lift more difficult) in the early phase of the lift and provide assistance toward its completion.

Resistance-Training Equipment Categories

Resistance training typically uses one of three categories of exercise equipment to manipulate movement speed and/or resistance on the muscle throughout the ROM. The first category includes common weight-lifting with free weights and barbells. This equipment does not control for

TABLE 22.1 ■ INTERNATIONAL SYSTEM (SI) OF UNITS FOR EXPRESSING MUSCULAR STRENGTH AND POWER DURING LINEAR AND ANGULAR MOTIONS[a]

	LINEAR MOTION	ANGULAR MOTION	
QUANTITY	**UNIT**	**QUANTITY**	**UNIT**
Force	Newton, N	Torque, T	Newton meter, N-m
Velocity, v	Meters per second, m · s^{-1}	Velocity, v	Radians per second, rad · s^{-1}
Mass	Kilogram, kg	Moment of inertia, I or J	Kilogram meters squared, kg-m^2
Acceleration, a	Meters per second squared, m · s^{-2}	Acceleration, a	Radians per second squared, rad · s^{-2}
Displacement, d	Meter, m	Displacement, θ	Radian, rad
Time, t	Second, s	Time, t	Second, s

[a]Appendix A, available on the Student CD and online at http://connection.lww.com/mkk6e, provides additional information about SI units, including interconversions.

(or measure) speed of movement or resistance through a full ROM. Two subdivisions exist within the second category. One subdivision provides constant speed—controlled by true isokinetic equipment—and variable resistance. The other subdivision provides constant speed and variable resistance with a hydraulic device but the individual controls movement speed. In the third category, movement speed varies and resistance remains constant; this category includes some cam devices and concentric–eccentric apparatus. No machine currently allows muscles to exert force under conditions of true constant speed and constant resistance.

Strength-Testing Considerations

Important considerations exist for muscle strength testing, regardless of measurement method:

- Standardize instructions prior to testing.
- Ensure uniformity in duration and intensity of the warm up.
- Provide adequate practice prior to testing to minimize "learning" that could compromise initial results (see next section).
- Ensure consistency among subjects in the angle of limb measurement and/or body position on the test device.
- Predetermine a minimum number of trials (repetitions) to establish a criterion strength score. For example, if administering five repetitions of a test, what score represents the individual's strength score? Is the highest score best, or should one use the average? In most cases, an average of several trials provides a more representative (reliable) strength or power score than a single measure. High test–retest reliability exists for repeated measurements of maximal-effort muscle actions when administering multiple repetitions of bench press and squat 1-RM and bidirectional hydraulic exercise on the same and different days.
- Select test measures with high test score reproducibility. This crucial but often overlooked aspect of testing evaluates the variability of the subject's responses on repeated efforts. Lack of test score consistency (unreliability) often masks an individual's representative performance on the measure (or change in performance when evaluating strength improvement).
- Recognize individual differences in body size and composition when evaluating strength scores among individuals and groups. For example, consider the "fairness" of comparing absolute muscular strength of a 120-kg football lineman with the strength of a 62-kg distance runner. No clear-cut answer resolves this dilemma; in the section on Allometric Scaling on p. 517 we present alternatives for comparing strength scores relative to body size.

EXERCISE EQUIPMENT TO OVERLOAD SKELETAL MUSCLE

CATEGORY	SPEED	RESISTANCE	EQUIPMENT EXAMPLE
(I)	Variable	Variable	Barbells (resistance varies through ROM even though absolute weight remains constant)
(II)	Constant	Variable	Hydraulic (person controls speed)
	Constant	Variable	Computer-regulated (movement speed controlled by computer)
(III)	Variable	Constant	CAM-adjusted equipment and concentric-eccentric apparatus
(IV)	Constant	Constant	None available

Learning Factors That Affect Strength Measurements

In Chapter 19, we emphasized that initial gains in muscular strength with resistance training result largely from neural factors instead of structural changes within muscle fibers. FIGURE 22.3 presents data for repetition-by-repetition performance improvements in maximal effort movement at an angular velocity of $5° \cdot s^{-1}$ during a supine bench press with a 5-second interval between maximal effort repetitions. The dynamometer also assessed static 1-RM at a 100° angle in the ROM. This measurement differs from the conventional 1-RM determination that adds small increments of free weights on repeated lifts. The amount of improvement averaged 11.4% between maximal force on attempt 1 and attempt 5 and 2.1% between the last two attempts. Strength "improvement" with repeated testing indicates the necessity for *at least* three attempts before maximum force scores begin to stabilize or plateau. The scores remained unchanged with 3-, 4-, or 5-minute rest intervals between maximal attempts. Only 1-minute intervals between trials prove satisfactory for achieving the maximum lift.[198] Importantly, use of only one or two 1-RM attempts underestimates the "true" 1-RM by as much as 11%. If a single 1-RM trial preceded a 15-week strength training program, then any strength gains attributable to training would include the 11% "learning" improvement simply from exercise familiarization, regardless of the training effect!

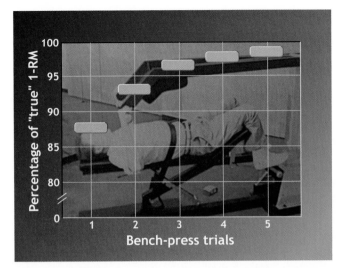

Figure 22.3 Five repeated determinations of 1-RM for the supine bench press with an electromechanical dynamometer. Strong verbal encouragement was provided on each attempt. A rest interval of 5 seconds occurred between maximal-effort trials. (From F. Katch, Human Performance Laboratory, University of Massachusetts, Amherst, MA.)

GENDER DIFFERENCES IN MUSCLE STRENGTH

Several approaches determine if a true gender difference exists in muscle strength. These evaluations relate to (1) the muscle's cross-sectional area, (2) an absolute basis as total force exerted, (3) architectural characteristics (e.g., fiber pennation angle), and (4) relative strength indexed to body mass or fat-free body mass (FFM).

Strength Related to Muscle Cross-Sectional Area

Human skeletal muscle, regardless of gender, generates a maximum of between 16 and 30 newtons (N) of force per square centimeter of muscle cross section. *In the body, force-output capacity varies depending on the arrangement of the bony levers and muscle architecture* (see Chapter 18). Applying the value of 30 N as a representative force capacity per cm^2 of muscle tissue indicates that a muscle with a cross-sectional area of 5.0 cm^2 develops maximal force of 150 N. If all of the body's muscles became maximally activated simultaneously (with force applied in the same direction), the resulting force would equal 168 kN. This estimation assumes a muscle total cross section of 0.56 m^2.

FIGURE 22.4A compares the absolute arm flexor strength of men and women related to the flexor muscle's total cross-sectional area. Clearly, individuals with the largest muscle cross sections generate the greatest absolute force. The near-linear relation between strength and muscle size indicates little difference in arm flexor strength for the same size muscle in men and women. Figure 22.4B further demonstrates this point when expressing the strength of the men and women per unit area of muscle cross section. In addition, women and men

matched for absolute muscular strength show similar fatigability of the elbow flexor muscles during sustained low level isometric contraction.[86]

Absolute Muscle Strength

Comparisons of muscular strength on an *absolute* score basis (i.e., total force in lb or kg) indicate that men possess considerably greater strength than women for all muscle groups tested. Women score about 50% lower than men for upper-body strength and about 30% lower for leg strength.

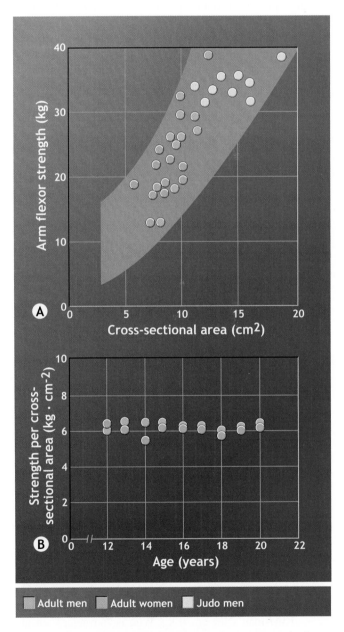

Figure 22.4 **A.** Variability of upper-arm flexion strength of men and women related to the flexor muscle's total cross-sectional area. **B.** Strength per unit muscle cross-sectional area in males and females aged 12 to 20 years. (From Ikai M, Fukunaga T. Calculation of muscle strength per unit cross-sectional area of human muscle by means of ultrasonic measurements. Arbeitsphysiologie 1968;26:26.)

This gender disparity exists independent of the measuring device and generally coincides with gender-related difference in muscle mass distribution. Exceptions usually emerge for strength-trained female track-and-field athletes and body builders who have trained for years with progressive resistance exercise to develop the strength and size of specific muscle groups.

Gender Differences in Weight-Lifting Championships

A unique set of data exists on gender differences in weight-lifting competitions in which men and women participate in the same categories on the basis of identical body mass. FIGURE 22.5 displays the percentage differences in maximum weight lifted in the combined snatch and clean-and-jerk lifts during national championship competitions. These comparisons do not "equate" or "adjust" performance scores on the basis of the well-documented gender difference in body composition. The six body weight categories range from 52 to 82.5 kg. The lighter-weight categories usually produce the smallest gender difference, with the effect most pronounced in the heavier lifters. Women of 75- and 82.5-kg body mass lift only about 60% of the maximal weight lifted by male counterparts. This represents a more pronounced gender difference than other comparisons that matched competitors for body composition, not just body mass.

INTEGRATIVE QUESTION

What performance would you expect in maximum weight-lifting tests comparing (1) an average-size man and average-size woman, (2) a man and woman of equivalent training history and identical body mass, and (3) a man and woman of equivalent training history and identical fat-free body mass?

Relative Muscle Strength

Traditionally, strength performance comparisons among individuals required creating a ratio by dividing the strength score by a reference measurement such as body mass, FFM, muscle cross section, or limb volume or girth. For example, comparing men and women for strength using a ratio score based on body mass or FFM considerably reduces (if not eliminates) the large absolute strength differences between genders.[28]

Consider the following example. A male who weighs 95 kg bench presses 114 kg; a 60-kg woman presses only 62% of the man's lift or 70 kg. Who is "stronger?" In absolute terms the male is clearly stronger. However, the bench press score divided by body mass creates a different situation. For the man, strength divided by body mass equals 1.20; the ratio for the woman is 1.17. In the first comparison, the male was "stronger" by 61.3%. Using the ratio

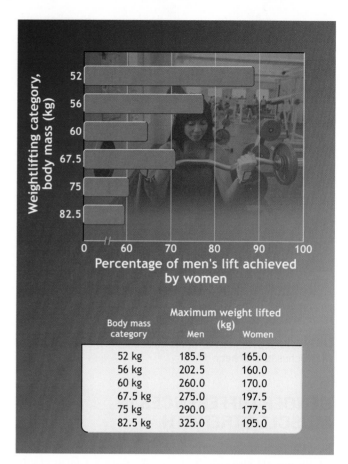

Body mass category	Maximum weight lifted (kg)	
	Men	Women
52 kg	185.5	165.0
56 kg	202.5	160.0
60 kg	260.0	170.0
67.5 kg	275.0	197.5
75 kg	290.0	177.5
82.5 kg	325.0	195.0

Figure 22.5 Difference in maximum weight lifted between men and women in the same body mass categories during a national weight-lifting competition. The *inset* shows the absolute weight lifted for each body mass category.

score reduced the percentage difference in bench press strength to only 2.5%! Such findings support the argument that no differences exist in muscle "quality" of men and women; the observed gender difference in absolute muscle strength merely reflects differences in muscle quantity (cross-sectional area) rather than muscle fiber architectural characteristics (e.g., fiber-pennation angle) or metabolic functions. Men and women generally do not differ significantly in either upper- or lower-body strength when comparisons are made applying ratios with FFM (or cross section of muscle) as the divisor.

We must point out that this traditional ratio adjustment may not equalize women and men on the basis of the underlying physiology. As with aerobic capacity (discussed in Chapter 11), a fair way to evaluate a potential gender difference in a criterion trait such as muscular strength or aerobic capacity either (1) compares men and women who do not differ in body size variables such as body mass or FFM and who exhibit similar training status or (2) adjusts for these variables through appropriate statistical control. These methods preclude the need to create a ratio score because men and women become equalized for body size and/or body composition. With this approach, researchers assessed five measures of muscular strength for men and women using 1-RM concentric (shortening) muscle actions for the bench press and squat and isokinetic dynamometry to assess maximum force during knee flexion and extension and seated shoulder press. FIGURE 22.6 shows that matching men and women for body mass produced larger gender differences in the sedentary group (44.0% for the shoulders and 25.1% for knee flexion) than in the trained group (33.0% for the bench press and 10.7% for knee flexion). The percentage differences decreased (but were not eliminated) for both groups by matching subjects for FFM. The shoulder press (39.4%) and bench press (31.2%) produced the largest gender differences in the sedentary group, while the corresponding differences for the trained group were 30.6% (shoulder press) and 35.4% (bench press).

These results differ from prior studies that used the traditional ratio score approach to express the strength of women and men. Without doubt, ratio scoring supports the argument that few gender differences exist in muscle quality, at least reflected by force output capacity. In contrast, matching men and women for body size, body composition, and training status before testing yields higher upper- and lower-body strength scores for men.[142] In a latter study of military personnel (2061 men, 1301 women), mean lift capacity averaged 51% greater in men, despite a regression, ratio, or exponential mathematical adjustment in the strength score based on interindividual differences in FFM.

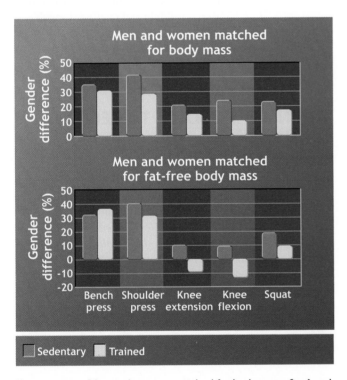

Figure 22.6 Men and women matched for body mass *(top)* and fat-free body mass *(bottom)* for five measures of muscle strength. Above the zero line indicates the percentage by which values for men exceed values for women. (Data courtesy of Keller B. The influence of body size variables on gender differences in strength and maximum aerobic capacity. Unpublished doctoral dissertation, University of Massachusetts, Amherst, 1989.)

INTEGRATIVE QUESTION

Based on gender-related differences in physical fitness components, devise a physical test that (1) minimizes and (2) maximizes performance differences between men and women.

Allometric Scaling

Allometric scaling represents a mathematical procedure to establish a proper relationship between a body size variable (usually stature, body mass, or FFM) and some factor of interest such as muscular strength, aerobic capacity, jumping height, or running speed.[17,96,189] The technique provides proper statistical adjustment to evaluate the relative contribution of diverse independent variables (e.g., gender, maturation, habitual physical activity) on the dependent measure of interest (e.g., muscular strength, $\dot{V}O_{2max}$, pulmonary function).

Allometric scaling requires three assumptions: (1) a curvilinear relationship exists between the two variables in question (e.g., body mass and muscular strength), (2) the slope of the relationship passes through the origin (i.e., someone with zero body mass exhibits no muscular strength), and (3) the equation $Y = bX^a$ best describes the form of the relationship, where Y represents the outcome variable (muscular strength); X, the scaling variable (body mass); b is a constant multiplier representing the line's slope; and a is a constant based on the slope. Solving the scaling equation for the exponent a eliminates the influence of individual differences in the scaling factor (in this case, body mass) on the outcome variable muscular strength. Stated another way, allometric scaling permits a variable of interest to remain free of confounding effects that inherently relate to it. Transforming the basic allometric scaling equation in assumption (3) above into a log–linear model enables one to solve for exponent a. This is done by taking the log of both sides of the equation in (3) and substituting values for the outcome variable (muscular strength) and the scaling variable (body mass). The equation becomes log strength = a log body mass + log b. Linear regression then solves for a by entering the log of strength and the log of body mass into the regression. For muscular strength, slope b usually equals 0.67, but the value may vary somewhat depending on the particular data set. Data for grip strength of college-age men and women reported a body mass exponent of 0.51 as the appropriate scaling factor. However, this study did not scale to FFM, which might have provided a scaling value closer to a body mass exponent to the 0.67 power. *If a linear relationship existed between muscular strength and body mass, b would equal 1.0; this would justify expressing strength per unit body mass without a correction. Since this does not* occur, one must express muscular strength per unit body mass raised to an appropriate power determined for the particular data set.

Is Scaling Fair? Applying allometry to an outcome variable such as muscular strength permits comparison of individuals who exhibit large individual differences in a body-size variable. The comparison becomes free of confounding effects that inherently relate in a nonlinear manner to the variable in question. For example, how can one best compare the maximum strengths of two individuals who vary widely in body size? If one competitor weighs 100 kg (190 cm tall) and the other 70 kg (178 cm tall)—with strength scores of 125 kg for the taller, heavier person and 110 kg for the shorter, lighter person—how can we "equate" both individuals for their "expected" muscular strength? Because body mass relates to muscular strength, the traditional approach simply divides the strength score by body mass to produce a proportionate ratio score of 1.250 for the heavier person (125 kg lifted 100 kg body mass) and 1.571 for the lighter competitor. This system deems the lighter person "stronger." In effect, the approach penalizes the heavier person because of the disproportionately large divisor in the ratio. But is this procedure fair? The answer becomes complicated from failure to consider differences in stature (stature also relates strongly to body mass) or total muscle mass (by FFM or lean body mass) related to body mass. To identify the strongest person (considering factors that normally affect muscular strength), one must properly scale the muscular strength outcome variable to remove the confounding influence of the body size variable(s).

Should strength be expressed per unit cross-sectional area of the active muscles? Unfortunately, no simple answer emerges to this question or to questions raised previously. Additional complications arise when physical size characteristics between males and females and between individuals of different ages (particularly during growth and aging) potentially affect exercise performance scores. Anthropologists, biologists, and other scientists since the mid-1600s have raised and debated questions of body size scaling and outcome variables.[179,185] Ample discussion exists among today's exercise scientists concerning proper scaling of variables commonly measured in exercise physiology.[98,188]

Strength and Allometric Scaling Using Body Mass.

FIGURE 22.7 illustrates the relationship between body mass and several different expressions of muscular strength. The *top left graph* (A) plots the total weight lifted versus body mass for Olympic weight lifters. Each point represents body mass of the top weight lifters in each body mass category. Importantly, total weight lifted and body mass do not relate linearly but curvilinearly, thus supporting the belief that weight-lifting strength relates proportionally to body mass raised to the exponent 0.7 (slope of line). The *bottom six curves* (B) depict the relationship between maximal grip strength and body mass in college-age men (*purple*) and women (*green*). The *top graphs* illustrate the simple relationship between body mass and grip strength without adjustment for body size. A positive relationship emerges ($r = 0.51$ for males and $r = 0.33$ for females). The *middle graphs* depict

the relationship with grip strength indexed to body mass (i.e., strength divided by body mass in kg). In this case, dividing strength by body mass penalized heavier males and females ($r = -0.43$ for males and -0.38 for females). If body mass does not represent a confounding variable, the ratio score should have approximately zero correlation ($r = 0.00$) with muscular strength. This represents an ideal situation that levies no penalty on heavier persons (who may also possess a higher percentage body fat). The bottom graphs illustrate the relationship between strength and allometric scaling of body mass. The body mass exponent is a $= 0.54$ for males and 0.475 for females; the resulting correlations between strength and strength raised to the appropriate exponent fall essentially to zero ($r = 0.013$ for males and 0.030 for females). This satisfies one of the basic tenets of allometry—the correlation between the scaled variable (muscular strength) and the scaling factor (body mass) must equal zero. The *inset table* (C) presents percentile norms for grip strength adjusted to body mass exponent 0.51 (grip strength per $kg^{0.51}$) for college-age men and women.

INTEGRATIVE QUESTION

You have a list of the names of young adults with the body weight of each. Justify your selection of two people: one must push a vehicle stuck in the mud while the other must move hand-over-hand on a rope strung across a ravine. *Hint:* Consider absolute and relative strength requirements of each task and association between body mass and absolute and relative muscular strength.

TRAINING MUSCLES TO BECOME STRONGER

A muscle strengthens when trained close to its current force-generating capacity. Standard weight-lifting equipment, pulleys or springs, immovable bars, or a variety of isokinetic and hydraulic devices provide effective muscle overload. *Importantly, overload intensity (level of tension placed on muscle), not the type of exercise that applies the overload, generally governs strength improvements.* Certain exercise methods lend themselves to precise and systematic overload applications. **Progressive-resistance weight training**, **isometric training**, and **isokinetic training** are three common exercise systems to train muscles to become stronger. These systems rely on the types of muscle actions illustrated in FIGURE 22.8, A–C.

Different Muscle Action Forms

Neural stimulation of a muscle causes the contractile elements of its fibers to attempt to shorten along the longitudinal axis. The terms *isometric* and *static* describe muscle activation without observable change in muscle fiber length. A **dynamic** muscle action produces movement of the skele-

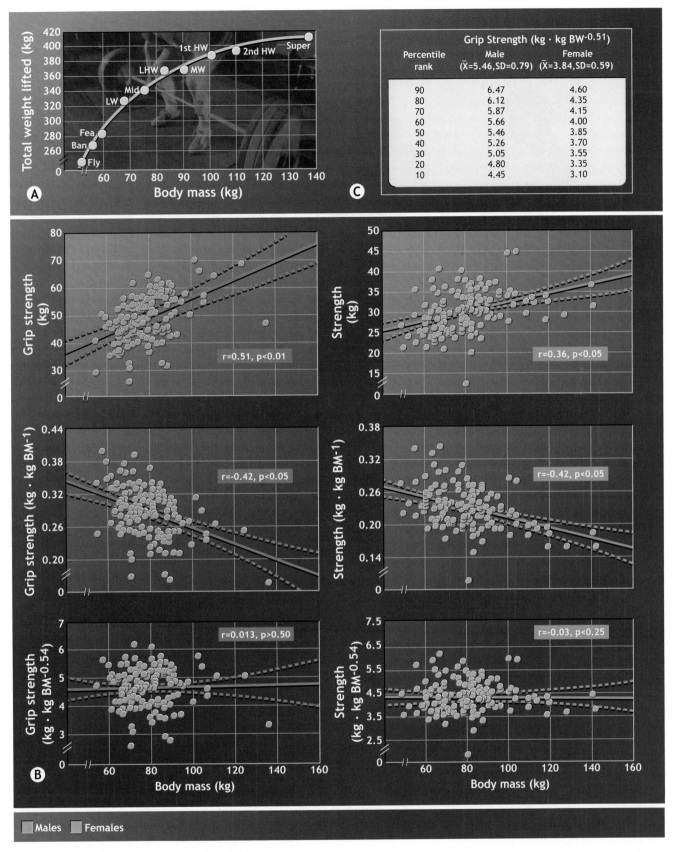

Figure 22.7 Relationship between body mass and different expressions of muscular strength. **A.** Total weight lifted in two events as a function of body mass of Olympic weight lifters (1980 Olympic games). Each point represents the body mass of the top six male weight lifters in each of the following weight categories: *Fly,* flyweight; *Ban,* bantamweight; *Fea,* featherweight; *LW,* lightweight; *Mid,* middleweight; *LHW,* light-heavyweight; *MW,* middle-heavyweight; *1st HW,* 1st heavyweight; *2nd HW,* 2nd heavyweight; and *Super,* superheavyweight. (Modified from data of Lathan and cited by Titel K, Wutscherk H. In: Komi PV, ed. Strength and power in sport. Oxford: Blackwell Scientific Publications, 1993.) **B.** Maximal absolute grip strength, relative grip strength, and strength scaled allometrically to body mass of 100 men and 105 women of college age. **C.** Percentile norms for grip strength scaled to body mass. (Data courtesy of Dr. Paul Vanderburgh.)

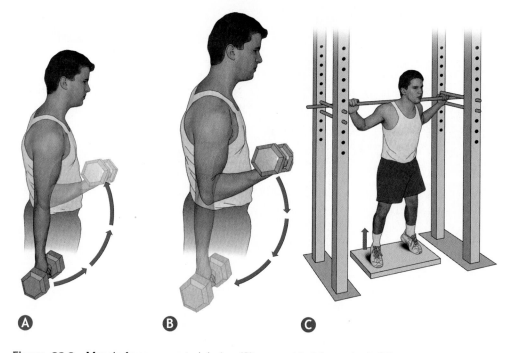

Figure 22.8   Muscle force generated during (**A**) concentric (shortening), (**B**) eccentric (lengthening), and (**C**) isometric (static) muscle actions.

ton. Concentric and eccentric actions represent the two types of dynamic muscle actions.

- **Concentric action** occurs when the muscle shortens and joint movement occurs as tension develops. Figure 22.8A illustrates a concentric action when raising a dumbbell from the extended to the flexed elbow position. Similarly, lifting a fork to deliver food from the plate to the mouth requires a concentric biceps muscle action.
- **Eccentric action** occurs when external resistance exceeds muscle force and the muscle lengthens while developing tension (Fig. 22.8B). The weight slowly lowers against the force of gravity. As with the food analogy for a concentric muscle action, returning the fork to the plate involves an eccentric biceps muscle action. The muscle fibers (more specifically the sarcomeres) of the upper-arm muscles lengthen in an eccentric action to prevent the weight (or fork) from crashing to the surface. In weight lifting, muscles frequently act eccentrically as the weight slowly returns to the starting position to begin the next concentric (shortening) action. Eccentric muscle action during this "recovery" phase adds to the total work and effectiveness of the exercise repetition.
- **Isometric action** occurs when a muscle generates force and attempts to shorten but cannot overcome the external resistance (Fig. 22.8C). From a physics standpoint, this type of muscle action does not produce external work. An isometric (static) action can generate considerable force despite the lack of

noticeable lengthening or shortening of muscle sarcomeres and subsequent joint movement.

The term *isotonic,* derived from the Greek word *isotonos* (*iso* meaning the same or equal, *tonos* meaning tension or strain), commonly refers to concentric and eccentric muscle actions because movement occurs in both cases. This term lacks precision when applied to most dynamic muscle actions that involve movement; the muscle's effective force-generating capacity continually varies as the joint angle changes throughout the ROM.

Resistance Training for Children

Exercise physiologists know relatively little concerning the benefits and possible risks of resistance training for preadolescents. Obvious concern arises regarding the potential for injury from excessive musculoskeletal loading (epiphyseal fractures, ruptured intervertebral disks, lower-back bony disruptions, acute low-back trauma). In addition, a child's hormonal profile lacks full development—particularly the tissue-building hormone testosterone. One might question whether resistance training in children could even induce significant strength improvements.

Supervised resistance training using concentric-only muscle actions with relatively high repetitions and low resistance improves muscular strength of children and adolescents without adverse effect on bone, muscle, or connective tissue.[52,147,200] More than likely, learning and enhanced neuromuscular activation rather than substantial increases in muscle size account for children's strength gains.[145] Studies must determine the benefit-to-risk ratio and long-term effects on growth and development of regular and more stressful muscle overload on children. The guidelines presented in TABLE 22.2 provide prudent recommendations for initiating resistance exercise training for children and adolescents.

Resistance Training

The most popular form of resistance training involves weight lifting. Through appropriate and progressive manipulation of training volume, intensity, and frequency to optimize dose response, this method selectively strengthens specific muscles by causing them to overcome a fixed initial resistance.[105,156] This resistance typically takes the form of a barbell, dumbbell, or weight plates on a pulley- or cam-type machine. For some individuals, intensive resistance training produces a two- to three-fold increase in muscle size. As with cardiovascular training, muscular strength improvements vary inversely on a continuum with initial training status. Generally, improvements average 40% for the untrained, 20% in the moderately trained, 15% in the trained, 10% in the advanced, and 2% in elite athletes who achieve a high level of competition.[3]

Progressive Resistance Exercise

Progressive resistance exercise (PRE) provides a practical application of the overload principle and forms the basis of most resistance-training programs. In a rehabilitation setting after World War II, researchers devised weight-training regimens to improve the strength of previously injured limbs (see "Focus on Research," p. 522). The procedure involved three sets of exercises, each set consisting of 10 repetitions done consecutively without resting. The first set required one half the maximum weight that could be lifted 10 times or 1/2 10-RM; the second set used 3/4 10-RM, and the final 10-RM required maximum weight. As patients trained, the muscles of the exercised limbs became stronger so the 10-RM resistance increased periodically to maintain continued strength improvements. Similar improvements occurred even when reversing the exercise intensity progression so patients performed the 10-RM as the first set.

Variations of PRE. Research has studied the optimal number of sets and repetitions, including frequency and relative intensity of PRE training, for optimal strength improvement. General findings are as follows:

- Eight- to twelve-RM proves effective in novice training, whereas 1- to 12-RM effectively loads for intermediate training. This can then increase to heavy loading using 1- to 6-RM
- Rest 3 minutes between sets of an exercise at moderate movement velocity (1 to 2 s concentric; 1 to 2 s eccentric)
- For PRE at a specific RM load, increase load 2 to 10% when the individual performs 1 to 2 repetitions above the current workload
- Performing one exercise set induces only slightly less strength improvement in recreational weight lifters than performing two or three sets.[26,73] For those who desire to maximize muscle strength and size gains, higher volume, multiple-set paradigms emphasizing 6- to 12-RM at moderate velocity with 1- to 2-minute rests between sets prove most effective.
- Single-set programs, although less effective for optimal strength improvement, generally produce most of the health and fitness benefits of multiple-set

TABLE 22.2 ■ GUIDELINES FOR RESISTANCE-EXERCISE TRAINING AND PROGRESSION IN CHILDREN AND ADOLESCENTS

AGE (Y)	CONSIDERATIONS
7 or younger	Introduce child to basic exercises with little or no weight; develop the concept of a training session; teach exercise techniques; progress from body weight calisthenics, partner exercises, and lightly resisted exercises; keep volume low
8–10	Gradually increase the number of exercises; practice exercise technique in all lifts; start gradual progressive loading of exercises; keep exercises simple; gradually increase training volume; carefully monitor toleration to the exercise stress
11–13	Teach all basic exercise techniques; continue progressive loading of each exercise; emphasize exercise techniques; introduce more advanced exercises with little or no resistance
14–15	Progress to more advanced youth programs in resistance exercise; add sport-specific components; emphasize exercise techniques; increase volume
16 or older	Move child to entry-level adult programs after all background knowledge has been mastered and a basic level of training experience has been gained

From Kraemer WJ, Fleck SJ. Strength training for young athletes. Champaign, IL: Human Kinetics, 1993.
Note: If a child of any age begins a program without previous experience, start the child at previous levels and move to more advanced levels as exercise toleration, skill, amount of training time, and understanding permit.

FOCUS On Research

DEVELOP STRENGTH BY INCREASING LOAD, NOT REPETITIONS

DeLorme TL. Restoration of muscle power by heavy-resistance exercises. J Bone Joint Surg 1945;27:645.

▲ The accepted principle for muscle rehabilitation from injury prior to DeLorme's classic research involved low-resistance, high-repetition exercises called *endurance-building exercises*. Examples include stationary cycling, stair climbing, and repetitively lifting light sandbags or weights with the aid of pulleys. The prevailing approach to restoring atrophied, weak, or "neglected" muscles relied on developing muscular endurance, not muscular strength and power. DeLorme challenged conventional wisdom by advocating heavy-resistance exercise. He reasoned that proportionality existed between the load resisting the muscle action and the rate and extent of muscle hypertrophy. DeLorme predicted that an inactive or injured person's strength would return to normal levels faster with heavier resistance exercise than lighter resistance exercise.

Based on observations of 300 patients, most of whom required lower-extremity rehabilitation, DeLorme developed a new training system named *progressive resistance exercise* (PRE). Within the PRE system, he introduced the concepts of one-repetition maximum (1-RM) strength and 10-RM strength for (1) setting initial overload and adjusting increasing resistance, (2) establishing maximal sets and repetitions, and (3) applying the concept of muscle-training specificity. For muscle rehabilitation, DeLorme recommended that patients accumulate 70 to 100 repetitions of an exercise using 7 to 10 sets with a *maximum* of 10 repetitions per set. Initially, workouts began with a weight considerably lighter than the maximum weight lifted for 10 repetitions (10-RM) so subjects could complete 10-RM in the final set. When the person achieved 10-RM, total repetitions equaled 70 to 100. For example, if 10-RM for the first week equaled 20 pounds, then beginning the first set with 2.5 pounds and increasing 1.5 pounds after each 10-repetition set accumulated 80 repetitions when performing the final 20-pound 10-RM.

DeLorme advocated exercising once daily, 5 days weekly, with workouts not exceeding 30 minutes. The patient performed one maximal lift (1-RM) only once each week. DeLorme believed that a person should exercise "smoothly, rhythmically, and without haste, but not

so slowly that the mere holding of the weight would tire the patient. Sudden motions should be avoided, and a momentary pause at the end of each repetition was advocated." Weekly 1-RM measurement provided the basis for progressively adjusting the load to maintain the 10-RM training level. The figure illustrates strength improvement in one patient undergoing rehabilitation from a femur fracture. After 36 days, note the 8% gain in thigh girth (1.8 in) and the 40-pound (200%) increase in quadriceps muscle strength.

The DeLorme paper represented the first in the modern strength-training literature to advocate the concept of *training specificity*. DeLorme argued that power-building and endurance exercises "were two entirely different types, each one producing its own results, and each being incapable of producing the results obtained by the other." More than 60 years of subsequent research has validated the specificity concept for strength improvement, including almost every claim made by DeLorme about PRE's beneficial effects.

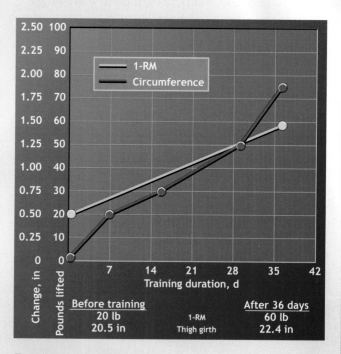

Time course of 1-RM *(yellow line)* and changes in thigh girth *(red line)* for a representative subject during 35 days of progressive resistance exercise.

programs. These "lower volume" programs also produce greater compliance and reduce financial cost and time commitment.

- Novices and intermediates should train 2 to 3 days a week, whereas the advanced can train 3 to 4 days per week.
- Training twice every second day produces overall superior results compared with training daily.[70] This may occur from the effects of low muscle glycogen content (with training twice every second day) on enhanced transcription of genes involved in training adaptations.
- If training includes multiple exercises, 4 or 5 days per week may produce less improvement than training 2 or 3 times per week, because near-daily training of the same muscles impairs muscle recuperation between training sessions. Inadequate recovery retards progress in neuromuscular and structural adaptations and strength development.
- A fast rate of moving a given resistance generates more strength improvement than moving at a slower rate. Neither free weights (barbells, weight plates, dumbbells) nor an array of exercise machines shows inherent superiority for developing muscle strength
- Exercise should sequence to optimize workout quality by engaging large before small muscle groups, multiple-joint exercises before single-joint exercises, and higher intensity exercise before lower intensity exercise.
- Combined resistance-training concentric and eccentric muscle actions augment effectiveness; include both single-joint and multiple-joint exercises to enhance muscle strength and fiber size.[3,75,144]
- Overload training that includes eccentric muscle actions preserves strength gains better during a maintenance phase than concentric-only training.[33]
- Power training should apply the strategy to improve muscular strength plus include lighter loads (30–60% of 1 RM) performed at fast contraction velocity. Use 2- to 3-minute rest periods between sets. Emphasize multiple-joint exercises that activate large muscle groups.

Table 22.3 summarizes the major recommendations of the American College of Sports Medicine in their position stand on progression models in resistance training for healthy adults.

Periodization. In 1972, Russian scientist Leonid Matveyev introduced the concept of strength-training periodization or periodized training;[124] it has since become incorporated into the training regimens of novice and champion athletes involved in long-term resistance training.[60,123] Conceptually, periodization varies training intensity and volume to ensure that peak performance coincides with major competition. It also proves effective for achieving recreational and rehabilitative goals. Periodization subdivides a specific resistance-training period such as 1 year (macrocycle) into smaller periods or phases (mesocycles), with each mesocycle again separated into weekly microcycles. In essence, the training model progressively decreases training volume (develops hypertrophy) and increases intensity (develops strength) as duration of the program progresses to maximize gains in muscular strength and power. Fractionating the macrocycle into components allows manipulation of training intensity, volume, frequency, sets, repetitions, and rest periods (to prevent overtraining). It also provides a way to alter workout variety. Periodization variation can reduce negative overtraining or "staleness" effects so the athlete achieves peak performance at competition. FIGURE 22.9 (*top*) depicts the generalized design for periodization and a typical macrocycle's four distinct phases. As competition approaches, training volume gradually decreases while training intensity concurrently increases.

- **Preparation phase** emphasizes modest strength development with *high-volume* (3–5 sets, 8–12 reps), *low-intensity* workouts (50 to 80% 1-RM plus flexibility and aerobic and anaerobic training).
- **First transition phase** emphasizes strength development with workouts of *moderate volume* (3–5 sets, 5–6 reps) and *moderate intensity* (80 to 90% 1-RM plus flexibility and interval aerobic training).
- **Competition phase** lets the participant peak for competition. Selective strength development is emphasized with *low-volume, high-intensity* workouts (3–5 sets, 2–4 reps at 90 to 95% 1-RM) plus short periods of interval training that emphasize sport-specific exercises.
- **Second transition phase** (**active recovery**) emphasizes recreational activities and low-intensity workouts that incorporate different exercise modes. For the next competition, the athlete repeats the periodization cycle.

Periodization structures an inverse relation between training volume and training intensity through the competition phase; it then decreases both aspects during the second transition or recuperation period. Note the increase in time devoted to technique training as competition approaches, with training volume at the cycle's lowest point. The *bottom part* of Figure 22.9 shows how training volume and intensity interact within a mesocycle for an athlete in a specific sport.

Sport-specific training principles usually apply in periodization to design a training regimen based on a sport's distinct strength, power, and endurance requirements. A detailed analysis of metabolic and technical requirements of the sport also frames the training paradigm. The concept of periodization makes intuitive sense, yet limited data exist for the superiority of this training approach from difficulties in controlling training intensity, training volume, the participants' general fitness level, and composite integration of strength and rate of force development.[104,123] Periodized resistance training has produced greater improvements in upper- and lower-body muscular strength

TABLE 22.3 ■ SUMMARY OF RESISTANCE TRAINING RECOMMENDATIONS: AN OVERVIEW OF DIFFERENT PROGRAM VARIABLES NEEDED FOR PROGRESSION WITH DIFFERENT FITNESS LEVELS

	Muscle Action	Selection	Order	Loading	Volume	Rest Intervals	Velocity	Frequency
Strength								
Nov.	ECC & CON	SJ & MJ ex.	*For Nov, Int, Adv:* Large < small MJ < SJ HI < LI	60–70% of 1RM	1–3 sets, 8–12 reps	*For Nov, Int, Adv:* 2–3 min for core 1–2 min for others	S, M	2–3×/week
Int.	ECC & CON	SJ & MJ ex.		70–80% of 1RM	Mult. sets, 6–12 reps		M	2–4×/week
Adv.	ECC & CON	SJ & MJ ex.—emphasis: MJ		1RM–PER	Mult. sets 1–12 reps–PER		US-F	4–6×/week
Hypertrophy								
Nov.	ECC & CON	SJ & MJ ex.	*For Nov, Int, Adv:* Large < small MJ < SJ HI < LI	60–70% of 1RM	1–3 sets, 8–12 reps	1–2 min	S, M	2–3×/week
Int.	ECC & CON	SJ & MJ ex.		70–80% of 1RM	Mult. sets, 6–12	1–2 min	S, M	2–4×/week
Adv.	ECC & CON	SJ & MJ		70–100% of 1RM with emphasis on 70–85%–PER	Mult. sets 1–12 reps with emphasis on 6–12 reps–PER	2–3 min–VH; 1–2 min–L–MH	S, M, F	4–6×/week
Power								
Nov.	ECC & CON	*For Nov, Int, Adv:* Mostly MJ	*For Nov, Int, Adv:* Large < small	*For Nov, Int, Adv:* Heavy loads (>80%)–strength; Light (30–60%) –velocity–PER	Train for strength	*For Nov, Int, Adv:* 2–3 min for core	M	2–3×/week
Int.	ECC & CON		Most complex < least complex		1–3 sets, 3–6 reps	1–2 min for others	F	2–4×/week
Adv.	ECC & CON		HI < LI		3–6 sets, 1–6 reps–PER		F	4–6×/week
Endurance								
Nov.	ECC & CON	SJ & MJ ex.	*For Nov, Int, Adv:* Variety in sequencing is recommended	50–70% of 1RM	1–3 sets, 10–15 reps	*For Nov, Int, Adv:* 1–2 min for high rep sets	S–MR	2–3×/week
Int.	ECC & CON	SJ & MJ ex.		50–70% of 1RM	Mult. sets, 10–15 reps or more	<1 min for 10–15 reps	M–HR	2–4×/week
Adv.	ECC & CON	SJ & MJ		30–80% of 1RM–PER	Mult. sets, 10–25 reps or more–PER			4–6×/week

ECC, eccentric; CON, concentric; Nov., novice; Int, Intermediate; Adv. advanced; SJ, single-joint; MJ, multiple-joint; ex., exercises; HI, high intensity; LI, low intensity; 1RM, 1-repetition maximum; PER, periodized; VH, very heavy; L-MH, light-to-moderately heavy; S, slow; M, moderate; US, unintentionally slow; F, fast; MR, moderate repetitions; HR, high repetitions. From ACSM position stand on: Progression models in resistance training for healthy adults. Med Sci Sports Exerc 2002;34:364.

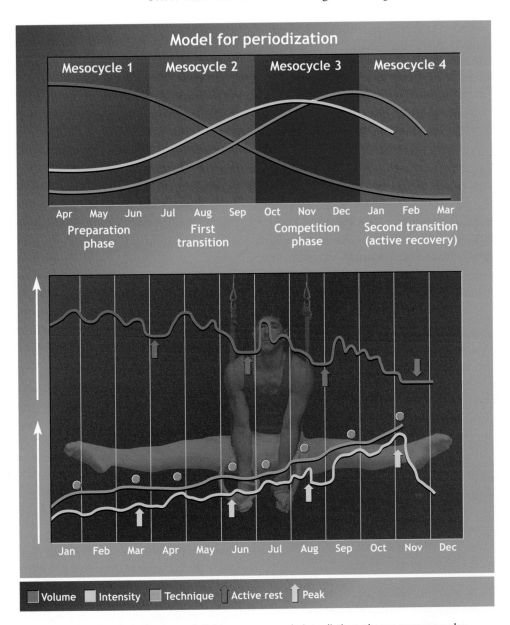

Figure 22.9 *Top.* Periodization subdivides a macrocycle into distinct phases or mesocycles. These in turn separate into weekly microcycles. The general plan provides modifications, but mesocycles typically include a preparation phase, a first transition phase, a competition phase, and a second transition or active recovery phase. *Bottom.* Example of periodization for an elite athlete (gymnast) preparing for competition. Competitions took place throughout the yearly training program so periodization focused on achieving peak performance at the end of each macrocycle. Periodization structures intensity, duration, and frequency of strength–power workouts, attempting to avoid overtraining (staleness), minimize injury potential, and reduce training monotony, while progressing toward peak competition performance *(filled circles)*.

and sport-specific motor performance than a traditional resistance-training program in collegiate women tennis players.[107]

Researchers have studied shorter mesocycles to determine what combination of factors optimizes performance improvements. One study that equated training volume and intensity among three approaches to periodization (linear periodization, undulating periodization, and a nonperiodized time interval) found each training method equally effec-

tive.[10] The training groups made similar gains in muscular strength (25% squat, 13.1% bench press) and muscular power (7.6% vertical jump). Without equating training volume and intensity, it is impossible to evaluate differences in training effects reported previously.[202] A critical review of the few studies of periodized strength training concluded that this approach produced greater improvements in muscular strength, body mass, lean body mass, and percentage body fat than nonperiodized multiset and single-set training programs.[56] Research must evaluate how periodization interacts with fitness status, age, gender, and specific sports (motor) performance. Studies must equate participants on various fitness parameters and then manipulate different training protocols, accounting for factors that affect training response. Program evaluation must consider the following four factors: (1) biomechanical and motor control sequences in the targeted sport skill, (2) changes in segmental and whole-body composition, (3) biochemical and ultrastructural tissue adaptations, and (4) transfer of newly acquired strength to subsequent sport performance measures.

Combining Resistance Training and Periodization: Application in HIV-Infected Men.

Weight loss during HIV infection adversely affects disease outcome and increases mortality. Testosterone therapy and exercise offer relatively inexpensive and safe therapeutic modalities. In HIV-infected men, weight loss accompanies low testosterone levels and deficits in muscle mass and strength.[36,66,158,165] Combining resistance exercise with pharmacologic therapy potentially offers alternative methods to improve physical function and health outcomes by increasing muscle mass and muscle strength (via either resistance training, resistance training with testosterone treatments, or either separately).

To test these possibilities, a placebo-controlled, double-blind, randomized clinical trial evaluated the effects of testosterone replacement with and without resistance-exercise training on muscle strength and body composition in HIV-infected men with low testosterone levels and existing weight loss.[18] Resistance training for 16 weeks included five standard free-weight exercises using periodization procedures and testing with the same equipment and exercises as in training in accordance with the specificity-of-training principle. Changes in strength, thigh muscle volume, and lean body mass were compared among the four treatment modalities (placebo, no exercise; intramuscular testosterone injections, [100 mg per wk], no exercise; placebo and exercise; testosterone and exercise).

Men treated with testosterone alone, exercise alone, or both increased muscular strength in the leg press (+22 to 30%), leg curls (+18 to 36%), and latissimus pulls (+17 to 33%). Body mass, strength, and MRI-measured thigh muscle volume improved more in men in the testosterone-exercise group or exercise-alone group than in the placebo-alone group. Also, average lean mass increased by 2.3 kg in the testosterone-alone group and 2.6 kg in the testosterone-plus-exercise group but remained unchanged in the placebo-alone group. The results convincingly demonstrate that progressive resistance exercise training incorporating periodization plus testosterone treatments promoted significant gains in body mass, muscle strength, and lean body mass in HIV-infected men with weight loss and low testosterone levels. Muscle strength per unit of muscle mass increased more in men who resistance trained than in men who only received testosterone, implying that without resistance training, testosterone-only treatments failed to improve the contractile quality of skeletal muscle. Incorporating resistance-exercise training to evaluate

clinical outcomes during disease progression offers great promise as a clinical intervention for HIV-infected patients.[119,178]

INTEGRATIVE QUESTION

Discuss the statement "There is no one *best* system of resistance training."

Resistance Training Guidelines for Sedentary Adults, the Elderly, and Cardiac Patients: Benefits in Health and Disease

Currently, the American College of Sports Medicine, American Heart Association, Centers for Disease Control and Prevention, American Association of Cardiovascular and Pulmonary Rehabilitation, and the U.S. Surgeon General's Office consider regular resistance exercise an important component of a comprehensive, health-related physical fitness program.[2,6,7,57,151,187] Resistance training goals for competitive athletes focus on optimizing muscular strength, power, and hypertrophy ("high-intensity" with 1-RM to 6-RM training loads). *In contrast, goals for most middle-aged and older adults focus on maintenance (and possible increase) of muscle and bone mass and muscular strength and muscular endurance to enhance the overall health and physical-fitness profile.*[51,53,87,112,113,201] Adequate muscular strength in midlife maintains a margin of safety above the necessary threshold to prevent injury in later life. Among 45- to 68-year-old men, hand-grip strength accurately predicted functional limitations and disability 25 years later (FIG. 22.10). Men in the lowest one third for grip strength showed the greatest risk; those in the middle one third showed intermediate risk, and men in the top one third experienced the least disability risk at the 25-year follow-up. The resistance training program recommended for middle-aged and older men and women classifies as "moderate intensity." In contrast to the multiple-set, heavy-resistance approach of younger athletes, the program uses single sets of diverse exercises performed between 8- and 15-RM a minimum of twice a week. TABLE 22.4 presents guidelines from different groups and health organizations for prudent resistance training of older men and women and cardiac patients.

Does Resistance Training Plus Aerobic Training Equal Less Strength Improvement?

Debate concerns whether concurrent resistance and aerobic training yields less muscular strength and power improvement than training for strength only.[15,63,80,106,131] This has caused many power athletes and body builders to refrain from endurance activities while they participate in resistance training. Advocates for abstaining from aerobic training when attempting to optimize gains in muscle size and strength maintain that the added energy (and perhaps

IN A PRACTICAL SENSE

THE LOWER BACK

■ According to the Bone and Joint Decade Monitor Project and the World Health Organization (WHO) (www.ota.org/downloads/bjdExecSum.pdf), the total costs in the United States related to musculoskeletal conditions amount to more than $250 billion per year. Of this amount, direct costs account for $88.7 billion. Thirty-eight percent was spent on hospital admissions, 21% on nursing home admissions, 17% on physician visits, and 5% on administrative costs. Indirect costs account for 58% of the total ($126.2 billion), which include lost wages through morbidity or premature mortality. Musculoskeletal diseases include approximately 150 different diseases and syndromes typically associated with pain or inflammation. Back injuries account for one fourth of all work-related injuries and one third of all compensation costs. Most cases result from on-the-job injuries, particularly in men in lumber and building retailing (highest risk) and construction (most cases); major-risk industries for women include nursing and personal care centers (highest risk) and hospitals (most cases). Grocery stores and agricultural production of crops rank among the top 10 occupations for lower-back injury for men and women. Estimates indicate that more than 32 million adult Americans frequently experience lower-back pain, the primary cause for workplace disability.[111] Workplace disability from lower back injuries also occurs in common tasks like refuse collection and other manual handling and lifting tasks.[42,45,102]

Muscular weakness, particularly in the abdominal and lower lumbar back regions, lumbar spine instability, and poor joint flexibility in the back and legs represent primary external factors related to low-back pain syndrome. Prevention of and rehabilitation from chronic low-back strain commonly use muscle-strengthening and joint-flexibility exercises.[16,132,161,192] Continuing normal activities of daily living (within limits dictated by pain tolerance) yields more rapid recovery from acute back pain than bed rest. Maintaining normal physical activity facilitates greater recovery than specific back-mobilizing exercises performed after pain onset.[122] Prudent use of resistance training isolates and strengthens the abdomen and lower lumbar extensor muscles that support and protect the spine through its full range of motion.[151] Patients with low back pain who strengthen the lumbar extensors with the pelvis stabilized experience less pain, fewer chronic symptoms, and improved muscular strength, endurance, and range of motion.[25]

Improper performance of a resistance-exercise movement (with a relatively heavy load and hips thrust forward with arched back) creates considerable compressive force on the lower spine. For example, pressing and curling exercises with back hyperextension create unusually high shearing stress on the lumbar vertebrae, often triggering low-back pain. Compressive forces with heavy lifting also can cause physiologic changes that hasten damage to the disks that cushion the vertebrae. Performing half squats with barbell loads from 0.8 to 1.6 times body mass produces compressive loads on the L3-L4 segment of the spine equivalent to 6 to 10 times body mass.[24,30] A person who weighs 90 kg and squats with 144 kg can create peak compressive forces in excess of 1367 kg (13,334 N)! A sudden amplification of compressive force can produce anterior disk prolapse; a lower-intensity but sustained compressive force that produces fatigue can increase posterior bulging of the lamellas in the posterior annulus.[5] In national-level male and female powerlifters, average compressive loads on L4–L5 reached 1757 kg (17,192 N).

Experiments with mice indicate that chronic disk compression in their tails—an extension of its spine, with disks similar to those in the human back—killed disk cells, eventually causing them to dehydrate outward and bulge. One should not sacrifice proper execution of an exercise to lift a heavier load or "squeeze out" additional repetitions. The extra weight lifted through improper technique does not facilitate muscle strengthening; instead, improper body alignment or unwarranted muscle substitution during force production can precipitate debilitating injury.

Wearing a weight-lifting belt during heavy lifts (squats, dead lifts, clean-and-jerk maneuvers) reduces intraabdominal pressure, compared with lifting without a belt.[71] The belt reduces potentially injurious compressive forces on

continued on page 528

Continued

spinal disks during near-maximal lifting, including most Olympic and power-lifting events and associated training. A person who normally trains wearing a belt should generally refrain from lifting without one. Further recommendations include performing at least some submaximal resistance training without a belt to strengthen the deep abdominal muscles. This also develops the proper pattern of muscle recruitment to generate high intra-abdominal pressures when not wearing a belt. Wearing a back belt to increase intra-abdominal pressure to ameliorate low-back injuries in the workplace does not provide a clear-cut biomechanical advantage.[148] A 2-year prospective study of nearly 14,000 material-handling employees in 30 states evaluated the effectiveness of using back belts to reduce back injury worker's compensation claims and reports of low-back pain.[196] Neither frequent back belt use (usually once a day and once or twice a week) nor a store policy that required the use of these belts reduced injury or reports of low-back pain. Researchers continue to probe for answers about the etiology of low-back pain syndrome and how to minimize its severity and reduce its occurrence. Studies have focused on numerous contributing factors that include intradisk pressure;[133] facet loads and disk fiber strains;[166] lumbar disk height and cross-sectional area;[138] compressive follower loads;[146] spinal joint force distribution;[29] ligament strain, disk shear, and facet impingement;[78] and prediction models to estimate spinal compression and shear forces.[67,99]

The following summary statement comes from *The Global Economic and Healthcare Burden of Musculoskeletal Disease.* 2005.

In the developed world, musculoskeletal disorders are the most frequent causes of physical disability. As the aging global population increases, the prevalence of many musculoskeletal disorders will increase in both the developed and developing parts of the world with the likely result being an increase in the number of people with chronic disabling disorders. This will have a definite negative impact on healthcare provision and the economies of countries in the coming years.

The following 12 exercises provide general strengthening of the abdomen and lower back and improve hamstring and lower-back flexibility for individuals with no apparent lower-back and spinal injuries. Symptomatic individuals require specific back exercises prescribed by a health care professional.

I. Lower-back stretches (hold each exercise for 30 to 60 s)
  1. *Knees-to-chest stretch:* Lie supine and pull the knees into the chest while keeping the lower back flat on the surface.

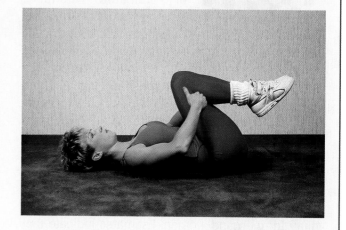

  2. *Cross-leg stretch:* Cross the legs and pull one 90°-flexed knee toward the chest.

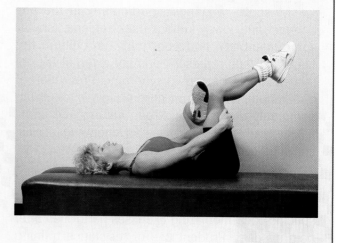

continued on page 529

Continued

3. *Hamstring stretch:* Wrap a strap over the foot, keeping lower back flat; pull leg upward toward the head.

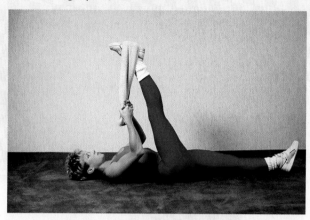

4. *Allah stretch:* Sit, buttocks on bilateral heels; move hands as far as possible forward along the surface.

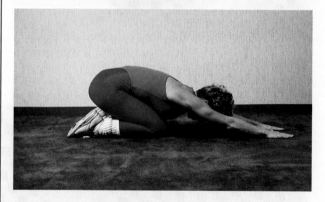

II. Abdominal exercises

5. *Bent-knee sit-up:* Keep hands low on neck (or across chest) with the head positioned over the shoulders. Roll up slowly, engaging one row of the abdominals at a time. Raise shoulders 4 to 6 inches off the surface.

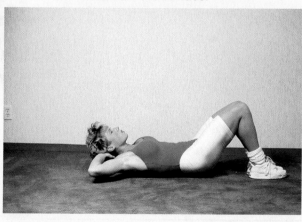

6. *Dying bug:* Flex the pelvis to flatten lower back against the surface. Over one side bring an extended arm and flexed knee together. On opposing side, extend arm straight overhead and leg straight backward. Maintain pelvic flexion while exchanging opposing arms and legs in this position.

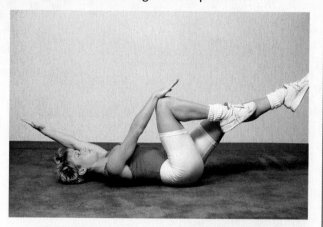

III. Prone lumbar extension exercises

7. *Dry-land swimming:* Lying prone with pelvic flexion, alternately lift opposite arm and leg.

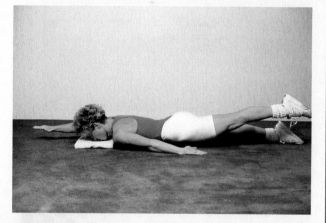

continued on page 530

Continued

8. *Both legs up:* Lie prone with pelvic flexion, and lift both legs simultaneously while keeping the head on the floor.

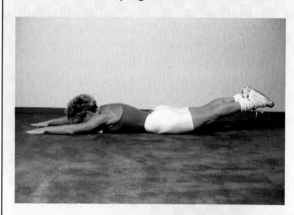

9. *Upper-body up:* Lying prone with pelvic flexion and arms outstretched or behind the back, lift upper torso while keeping legs on the floor.

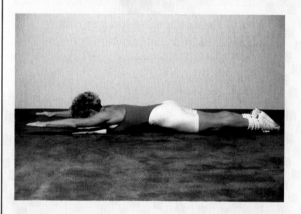

10. *Pointer (bird dog):* Start with hands and knees on the floor. Flex pelvis into a counter position. Exchange by pointing opposite arm and leg while keeping torso level.

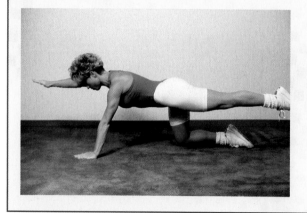

IV. Supine pelvic-flexion exercises

11. *Leg pointer:* Lie supine on the floor and flex pelvis with lower abdominals to flatten the lower back into the surface. Extend one arm upward and one leg outward while keeping quadriceps level.

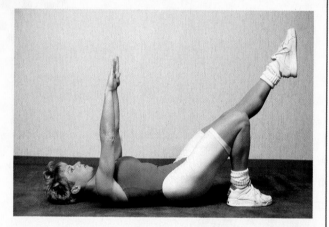

12. *Prone cobra push-up:* Keep pelvis on the floor while pressing up with arms to produce lower-back extension.

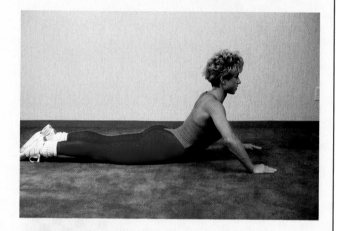

(Photos courtesy of Dr. Bob Swanson, Santa Barbara Back and Neck Care Center. Santa Barbara, CA 93108.)

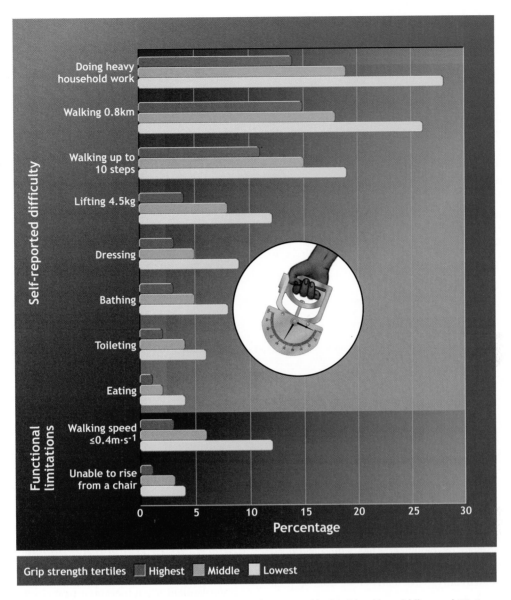

Figure 22.10 Relationship between grip strength assessed in 3218 healthy middle-aged 45- to 68-year-old men and functional limitations and difficulties 25 years later. (From Rantanen T, et al. Midlife hand grip strength as a predictor of old age disability. JAMA 1999;281:558.)

protein) demands of intense endurance training limit a muscle's growth and metabolic responsiveness to resistance training. Also, a short-term bout of high-intensity endurance exercise inhibits performance in subsequent muscular strength activities.[115] Further research must determine whether this acute effect on maximal force output limits the ability to overload skeletal muscle optimally to a degree that impairs strength development with concurrent strength and endurance training. If it does, then a 20- to 30-minute recovery between aerobic and strength training components might enhance the quality of the subsequent strength workout. These considerations should not deter those who desire a well-rounded conditioning program that offers the specific fitness and health benefits from *both* training modes.[46,87]

Isometric Strength Training

Research in Germany during the mid-1950s showed that isometric strength could increase about 5% weekly by performing a daily single, maximum isometric muscle action of only 1-second duration, or a 6-second action at two-thirds maximum.[81] Repeating this action 5 to 10 times daily produced greater gains in isometric strength.

Isometric Exercise Limitations

Isometric exercise provides muscle overload and improves strength yet offers limited benefits for sports training. Without movement, one cannot readily evaluate the overload level and/or training progress. Also, a high degree of *specificity*

TABLE 22.4 ■ STRENGTH TRAINING GUIDELINES FOR SEDENTARY ADULTS, ELDERLY PERSONS, AND CARDIAC PATIENTS

GUIDELINE	SETS	REPETITIONS[a]	NUMBER OF EXERCISES	FREQUENCY (DAYS/WEEK)
Healthy sedentary adults				
1990 ACSM Position Stand[b]	1	8–12	8–10[c]	2
1995 ACSM Guidelines[d]	1	8–12	8–10	2
1996 Surgeon General's Report[e]	1–2	8–12	8–10	2
Elderly persons				
Pollock et al,[f] 1994	1	10–15	8–10	2
Cardiac patients				
1995 AHA Exercise Standards[g]	1	10–15	8–10	2–3
1995 AACVPR Guidelines[h]	1	10–15	8–10	2–3

From ACSM, American College of Sports Medicine; AHA, American Heart Association; AACVPR, American Association of Cardiovascular and Pulmonary Rehabilitation.
[a] For healthy persons under age 50, weight should be sufficient to induce volitional fatigue with the number of repetitions listed. For older persons, lighter loads may be used.
[b] American College of Sports Medicine. The recommended quantity and quality of exercise for developing and maintaining cardiorespiratory and muscular fitness in healthy adults. Med Sci Sports Exerc 1990;22:265.
[c] Minimum one exercise per major muscle group (e.g., chest press, shoulder press, triceps extension, biceps curl, pull-down [upper back], lower-back extension, abdominal crunch/curl-up, quadriceps extension, leg curls [hamstrings], calf-raise).
[d] American College of Sports Medicine. Guidelines for exercise testing and prescription. 5th ed. Baltimore: Williams & Wilkins, 1995; also included low-risk diseased populations.
[e] U.S. Department of Health and Human Services. Physical activity and health: a report of the surgeon general. Atlanta: US Dept. of Health and Human Services, Centers for Disease Control and Prevention, National Center for Chronic Disease Prevention and Health Promotion, 1996.
[f] Pollock ML, et al. Exercise training and prescription for the elderly. South Med J 1994;87:S88.
[g] Fletcher GF, et al. Exercise standards: a statement for health care professionals from the American Heart Association. Circulation 1995;91:580.
[h] American Association of Cardiovascular and Pulmonary Rehabilitation. Guidelines for cardiac rehabilitation programs. 2nd ed. Champaign, IL: Human Kinetics, 1995.

affects isometric strength development. Thus, a muscle trained isometrically demonstrates improved strength primarily when the muscle acts isometrically, particularly at the training joint angle and body position.

Isometric training to develop "strengths" for a particular movement probably necessitates training at many points through the ROM. This becomes time consuming, particularly given the availability of conventional dynamic weight training and isokinetic and other resistance activities.

Isometric Exercise Benefits

The isometric method benefits muscle testing and rehabilitation. Isometric techniques detect specific muscle weakness, thus forming a basis for optimizing muscle overload at the appropriate joint angle.

Which Are Better, Static or Dynamic Methods?

Static and dynamic resistance training methods each increase muscle "strengths." An individual's specific needs determine the optimal resistance training method governed by the specificity of the training response.[135,210]

Specificity of Training Response

An isometrically trained muscle shows greatest strength improvement when measured isometrically; similarly, a dynamically trained muscle tests best when evaluated in resistance activities that require movement. Isometric strength developed at or near one joint angle does not readily transfer to other angles or body positions that demand use of the same muscles.[197] In dynamic exercise, muscles trained through movement over a limited ROM show the greatest strength improvement when measured in that ROM.[14,65] Even body position specificity exists; muscular strength of ankle plantar and dorsiflexors developed in the standing position with concentric and eccentric muscle actions showed no transfer with the same muscles evaluated in the supine position.[152] Resistance training specificity makes sense because strength improvement blends adaptations in two factors: (1) muscle fiber and connective tissue harness itself and (2) neural organization and excitability of motor units that power discrete patterns of voluntary movement.[117,137,153,176] Likewise, a muscle's maximal force output depends on neural factors that effectively recruit and synchronize firing of motor units, not *just* local factors such as muscle fiber type and cross-sectional area.[34,101,144,170]

A 3-month study of young adult men and women emphasized the highly specific nature of resistance-training adaptations.[48] One group trained the adductor pollicis muscle isometrically with 10 daily actions of 5-seconds duration at a frequency of 1 per minute. The other group trained the same muscle dynamically with 10 daily 10-repetition bouts of weight movement at one-third maximal strength. The untrained muscle served as the control. To eliminate any training influence from psychologic factors and central nervous system adaptations, a supermaximal electrical stimulation applied to the motor nerve evaluated the force capacity of the trained muscle. The results were clear—both training groups improved maximal force capacity and peak rate of force development. The improvement in maximal force for the isometrically trained group nearly doubled the improvement for the dynamically trained group. Conversely, improvement in speed of force development averaged about 70% greater in the group trained with dynamic muscle actions. Such findings provide strong evidence that resistance training per se does not induce all-inclusive (general) adaptations in muscle structure and function. Rather, a muscle's contractile properties (maximal force, velocity of shortening, rate of tension development) improve in a manner highly specific to the muscle action in training. Both static and dynamic training methods produce strength increases, yet no one system rates consistently superior to the other in evaluations of muscle function. The crucial consideration concerns the intended purpose of the newly acquired strength.

Practical Implications. The complex interaction between the nervous and muscular systems helps to explain why leg muscles strengthened in squats or deep knee bends fail to show equivalent improved force capability in other leg movements such as jumping or leg extension.[139] Low relationships emerge between dynamic measures of leg extension force at any speed and vertical jumping height. A muscle group strengthened and enlarged by dynamic resistance training does not demonstrate equal improvement in force capacity when measured isometrically or isokinetically.[170] Consequently, strengthening muscles for a specific athletic or occupational activity (e.g., golf, tennis, rowing, swimming, football, firefighting, package handling) demands more than just identifying and overloading the muscles in the movement. It requires training specifically in the important movements that necessitate improved strength. Increasing leg muscle "strength" through general weight lifting will not improve performance in a variety of subsequent leg movements.[128] *Newly acquired strength seldom transfers fully to other types of movements, even those that activate the same trained muscles.* A standard program of weight training for leg extension increased leg extension strength by 227%. However, evaluating leg extension peak torque of the same leg with an isokinetic dynamometer detected only a 10 to 17% improvement![59] *To improve a specific physical performance through resistance training, one must train the muscle(s) in movements that mimic the movement requiring* *force–capacity improvement, with focus on force, velocity, and power requirements.*

Physical Testing in the Occupational Setting: The Role of Specificity

A comprehensive review outlines the development of physical tests and professionally and legally defensible validation strategies for preemployment occupational testing requiring diverse physical abilities or specific fitness characteristics.[93] The high specificity of components of physical performance and physiologic function (e.g., muscular strength and power, joint flexibility, aerobic fitness) combined with the specific nature of the training response casts serious doubt that broad *constructs* of physical fitness exist to any important extent. Clearly, no single measure of overall muscular strength or aerobic fitness exists. *Instead, an individual expresses an array of muscular strengths and powers and aerobic "fitnesses."* These expressions of muscle function and performance often relate poorly to each other, if at all. Likewise, testing a person for aerobic fitness produces different fitness scores depending on the activity. For example, it would be undesirable to administer the 12-minute run test in the occupational setting to infer aerobic capacity for firefighting or lumbering (both requiring considerable upper-body aerobic function) or measuring static-grip or leg-strength tests to evaluate diverse dynamic strengths and powers required in these occupations.

Measurements applied in the occupational setting should most closely resemble the actual requirements of the job, not only for specific tasks but also in a manner that faithfully reflects the intensity, duration, and pace (i.e., physiologic demands) of the job. If such "content testing" remains impractical, one must substantiate alternative testing based on carefully conducted validation studies.

INTEGRATIVE QUESTION

Advise a candidate for a firefighter's job about the most effective way to train for a physical test that requires 7 minutes of a series of job-related tasks (e.g., stair climb with equipment, hose drag, ladder raise, forcible entry with sledge hammer, simulated rescue dummy drag).

Isokinetic Resistance Training

Isokinetic resistance training combines the positive features of isometric exercise and dynamic weight lifting. It provides muscle overload at a preset constant speed while the muscle mobilizes its force-generating capacity *throughout* the full ROM. Any effort during the exercise movement encounters an opposing force to that applied to the mechanical device; this represents **accommodating-resistance exercise**. Theoretically, isokinetic-type training activates the largest number of motor units to overload muscles consistently—even at the relatively "weaker" joint angles—as the bone–muscle–lever mechanics produce variations in force capacity throughout the ROM.

Isokinetics Versus Standard Weight Lifting

An important distinction exists between a muscle overloaded isokinetically and one overloaded with a standard weight-lifting exercise. FIGURE 22.11 shows that the force capacity of a muscle (or muscle group) varies with the bony lever configuration (joint angle) as the joint moves through its ROM. During weight training, the external weight lifted usually remains fixed at the greatest load that allows completion of the movement for the desired number of repetitions.

Resistance cannot exceed the maximum force generated at the weakest point in the ROM. If it did not, then one could not complete the movement. The term *sticking point* describes this point in the ROM.

The fact that muscles do not generate the same maximum force through all movement phases represents a major limitation of weight lifting. To help alleviate this problem, manufacturers have devised **variable-resistance training equipment** that adjusts resistance in accord with the generalized lever characteristics of a particular joint movement. This equipment still represents a classic mode of weight lifting except the *relative resistance* offered to the muscle theoretically remains fairly constant throughout the ROM. The machine

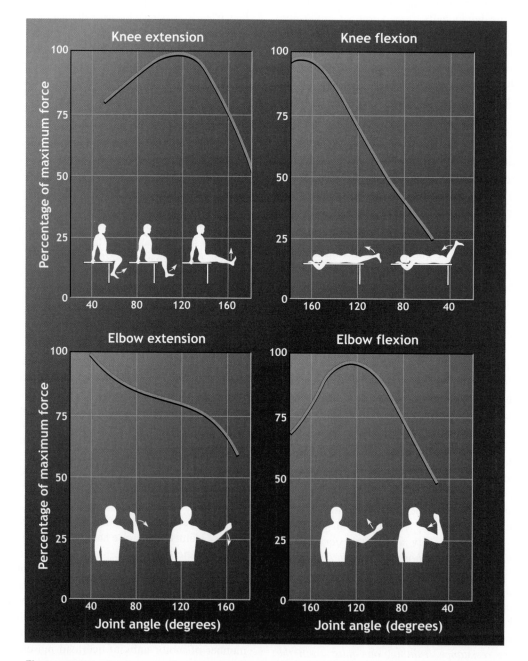

Figure 22.11 Force-generating capacity of a muscle or muscle group varies with joint angle in flexion and extension throughout the ROM.

does not control the speed of movement, and the design of the mechanical device uses the average physical dimensions of a population to achieve a variable resistance. Consequently, one cannot adjust for individual variations in body structure. With an isokinetically loaded muscle, the desired movement speed occurs almost instantaneously with force application, and the muscle generates peak power output throughout the ROM at a controlled shortening velocity.

Isokinetic Exercise and Training Experiments

Experiments with isokinetic exercise have explored the force–velocity patterns in various movements related to muscle fiber type composition. FIGURE 22.12 shows the progressive decline in peak torque output with increasing angular velocity of knee extensor muscles in two groups who differed in sports training and predominant muscle fiber type. For movement at $180° \cdot s^{-1}$, maximal torque decrement averaged about 55% of maximal isometric ($0° \cdot s^{-1}$) force. The two curves in Figure 22.12 differ in peak torque, depending on the group's muscle fiber composition. Peak force at zero velocity (isometric force) remained similar for athletes with relatively high (power athletes) or low (endurance athletes) percentages of fast-twitch muscle fibers; this indicated activation of *both* fast- and slow-twitch motor units in maximal isometric knee extension. As movement velocity increased, individuals with higher percentages of fast-twitch fibers exerted greater torque per unit body mass. This indicates the desirability of activating a high percentage of fast-twitch fibers for power activities where success largely depends on capacity to generate torque at rapid movement velocities.

Fast- Versus Slow-Speed Isokinetic Training

Studies of strength and power improvement with isokinetic training at slow and fast limb speeds further support the specificity of exercise performance and training response. For example, several studies show that strength and power gains from slow-speed isokinetic training relate specifically to the angular velocity of the movement in training. In contrast, exercising at fast speeds facilitates more general improvement; power output increased at fast *and* slow movement speeds, although measurement at the fast angular velocity in training improved the most.[149] Muscle hypertrophy generally occurs only from fast-speed training and only in the fast-contracting type II muscle fibers.[37] Muscle fiber hypertrophy may account for the more general strength improvement with fast-speed training. Concentric muscle actions produce greater power increases and type II fiber hypertrophy from training than eccentric training at equivalent relative power levels.[125]

The attractiveness of isokinetic training allows muscular overload through a full ROM at many shortening velocities. However, applications remain limited because the most rapid speed of movement of the current isokinetic dynamometers approximates $400° \cdot s^{-1}$. Even this relatively "fast" movement speed does not approach limb speeds during sports activities. In baseball pitching, where upper-limb extension velocity exceeds $2000° \cdot s^{-1}$ in professional pitchers, even the relatively "slow" hip rotators move at $600° \cdot s^{-1}$ during a pitch.[23] Also, the present generation of isokinetic dynamometers cannot overload eccentric muscle actions that serve important functions in limb deceleration and "braking" control in normal movements.

Plyometric Training

For sports that require powerful, propulsive movements—football, volleyball, sprinting, high jump, long jump, and basketball—athletes apply a special form of exercise training termed **plyometrics** or explosive jump training. Plyometric exercise requires various jumps in place or rebound jumping (drop jumping from a height) to mobilize the inherent stretch–recoil characteristics of skeletal muscle and its modulation via the stretch (myotatic) reflex. Stated somewhat differently, plyometric exercise involves the rapid stretching followed by shortening of a muscle group during a dynamic movement. Stretching produces a stretch reflex and elastic recoil within the muscle. When combined with a vigorous muscle contraction, plyometric actions should greatly increase the force that overloads the muscles, thereby facilitating increases in strength and power. Plyometric exercises range in difficulty from calf jumps off the ground to multiple one-leg jumps to and from boxes of different heights. The basic principle for all jumping and plyometric exercises is to absorb the shock with the arms or legs and then immediately contract the muscles. For example, when doing a series of squat jumps, jump again as quickly as possible as soon as you land. Quicker jumps provide greater overload to the muscles.

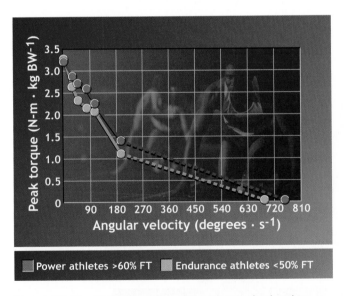

Figure 22.12 Peak torque (per unit body mass) related to angular velocity of joint movement in two groups of athletes with different predominance of muscle-fiber type. The torque–velocity curves were extrapolated *(dashed line)* to the approximated maximal velocity for knee extension. (From Thorstensson A. Muscle strength, fiber types, and enzyme activities in man. Acta Physiol Scand Suppl 1976:443.)

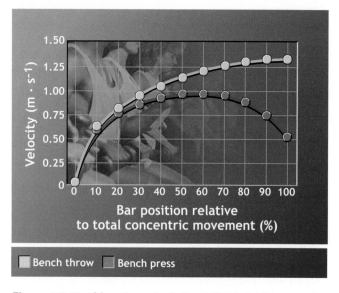

Figure 22.13 Mean bar velocity in relation to total concentric bar movement for bench throw and traditional bench press performed as rapidly as possible. (Data from Newton RU, et al. Kinematics, kinetics, and muscle activation during explosive upper body movements. J Appl Biomech 1996;12:31.)

In essence, "fast" plyometric exercise "trains" the nervous system to react quickly in order to activate muscles rapidly.

Plyometric maneuvers avoid the disadvantage of having to decelerate a mass in the latter part of the joint ROM during a fast movement; this provides for maximal power production. FIGURE 22.13 compares the traditional bench press movement to achieve maximal power output with a ballistic bench throw that attempts to maximize power output by projecting the barbell from the hands. The results were unequivocal. During the traditional bench press, deceleration begins at about 60% of the bar position relative to the total concentric movement distance *(purple line)*. In contrast, velocity during the bench throw *(yellow line)* continues to increase throughout the ROM and remains higher at all bar positions after the movement begins. This translates into greater average force, average power, and peak power outputs. Simultaneous monitoring of electromyographic (EMG) activity during the two conditions also showed greater muscle activity for the pectoralis major (+19%), anterior deltoid (+34%), triceps brachii (+44%), and biceps brachii (+27%) during the throw condition. Achieving a faster average and peak velocity throughout the ROM produces greater power output and muscle activation (assessed by EMG) than the traditional weight-lifting exercise movement.

Allowing the athlete to develop greater power at the end of the movement more closely simulates the projection phase of throwing an object (ball or implement), maximal effort jumping movements, or impact in striking movements. In this form of training, called **ballistic resistance training**,[104] the person moves the weight or projectile as fast as possible while trying to produce maximal force before releasing it. Sports performance examples include shot put, overhead soccer throw, javelin and discuss throws, push off in the pole vault, takeoff jump for a volleyball spike, jumping for a basketball rebound, punching in boxing, and takeoff in the high jump.

Plyometric exercise overloads a muscle to provide forcible and rapid stretch (eccentric, or stretch, phase) immediately before the concentric or shortening phase of action. Like many sports situations, the rapid lengthening phase in the **stretch-shortening cycle** produces a more powerful subsequent movement from two main factors:[38,92,186]

1. Attainment of a higher active muscle state (greater potential energy) before the concentric, shortening action
2. Stretch-induced evoking of segmental reflexes that potentiate subsequent muscle activation

These two effects form the basis for the speed–power benefits of this training mode.[139,195,205,208] FIGURE 22.14

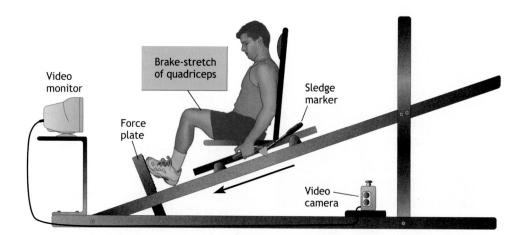

Figure 22.14 The sledge ergometer for plyometric (stretch-shortening cycle) exercise, training, and research protocols. Illustration shows braking phase (and subsequent muscle stretch) just prior to maximal activation of leg and foot extensor muscles. (Modified from Strojnik V, Komi PV. Fatigue after submaximal intensive stretch-shortening cycle exercise. Med Sci Sports Exerc 2000;32:1314.)

shows the sledge ergometer to (1) quantify force-generating capacity when affected by the stretch-shortening cycle, (2) train under such conditions, and (3) evaluate stretch reflex sensitivity and muscle stiffness under fatiguing exercise.

Practical Application of Plyometrics

A plyometric drill uses body mass and gravity for the important rapid prestretch or "cocking" phase to activate the muscle's natural elastic recoil elements. Prior stretch augments the subsequent concentric muscle action in the opposite direction. Forcibly dropping the arms to the side before vertical jumping produces an eccentric prestretch of the quadriceps muscle group and exemplifies a natural plyometric movement. Lower-body plyometric drills include a standing jump, multiple jumps, repetitive jumping in place, depth jumps or drop jumping from a height of about 1 m, single- and double-leg jumps, and various modifications. Proponents believe that repetitive plyometric actions provide neuromuscular training to enhance power output of specific muscles and sport-specific power performances as in jumping.[77,110,139,209]

Testimonials tout the benefits of plyometric training, but such pronouncements cannot substitute for the absence of carefully controlled evaluation of both benefits and possible orthopedic risks of such workouts. Concern for musculoskeletal injury stems partly from the estimation that drop jumping generates external skeletal loads equal to up to 10 times body mass. Research must quantify the appropriate role of plyometric drills in a complete strength–power training program, particularly for children and older recreational athletes. A position paper from the National Strength and Conditioning Association suggests that athletes first achieve lifts of 1.5 times body weight in the squat exercise before initiating high-intensity plyometric training.[204] This practical guideline requires validation. FIGURE 22.15 shows the rebound jumping technique in plyometric training along with four examples of plyometric exercise drills.

Window for Explosive Power Development

FIGURE 22.16 lists five components that contribute to the **window of explosive power development**. In this model, each component makes important neuromuscular contributions to maximal power training. The window of adaptation opportunity shrinks for an athlete with already well-developed components and expands for components in need of considerable improvement. As an athlete approaches his or her high-velocity strength potential, that component's contribution to overall maximal power development diminishes. Athletes must focus on training their least-developed components. Stated somewhat differently, maximal power performance improves more readily when targeting specific training routines to improve the weakest links because these have the largest adaptation window to develop explosive power.

ELECTROMYOGRAPHY DURING MAXIMAL BALLISTIC MUSCLE ACTIONS

The EMG signal provides a convenient way to study intricacies of neuromuscular physiology during different muscle actions. EMG reflects both the quality and quantity of electrical activity generated by muscle. In isometric actions, the EMG signal changes in proportion to muscle force generated. Dynamic actions reflect greater complexity from the changing force–torque characteristics during the ROM. Rapid, ballistic movements produce an EMG characterized by alternating bursts of electrical activity in agonistic and antagonistic muscles. This produces a triphasic EMG pattern: the first burst of electrical activity occurs in the agonist, followed by signals from the antagonist (when the agonist remains electrically silent) and then another burst of agonist activity. Each phase of EMG activity relates to certain aspects of the movement pattern. The first agonist burst creates the propulsive force that initiates limb motion; the antagonist's first burst stops the limb, and the agonist's second burst produces the final limb positioning.

Our studies of professional baseball pitchers (Boston Red Sox) and champion body builders (Mr. Universe contestants) showed striking between-group differences in triphasic EMG patterns during maximal-speed, unloaded arm flexion. FIGURE 22.17 compares the integrated EMG signal in baseball pitchers and body builders during rapid arm flexion. For the 19 pitchers, the second burst of muscle electrical activity occurs sooner (probably a protective mechanism to slow the extremely fast limb speed), with less amplitude than for the body builders. For the 11 body builders, the first agonistic burst occurs rapidly, followed by a distinct delay before the antagonist fires. The difference in timing of electrical activity probably relates to training adaptations to distinct differences in limb acceleration patterns (baseball pitching vs. weight lifting) over many years of specific limb movement training.

Summary

1. Tensiometry, dynamometry, 1-RM testing with weights, and computer-assisted force and work-output determinations including isokinetic-type measurements provide the most common methods to measure muscular performance.
2. Human skeletal muscle generates a maximum force of about 30 N per cm^2 of muscle cross section, regardless of gender. On an absolute basis, men generally exert greater maximal force than women.
3. The traditional method to evaluate gender differences in muscle strength creates a ratio score for strength (i.e., strength per unit body size [body mass, FFM, limb volume, girth]). When considering body size and/or composition in this manner, the large strength differences between men and women decrease considerably.

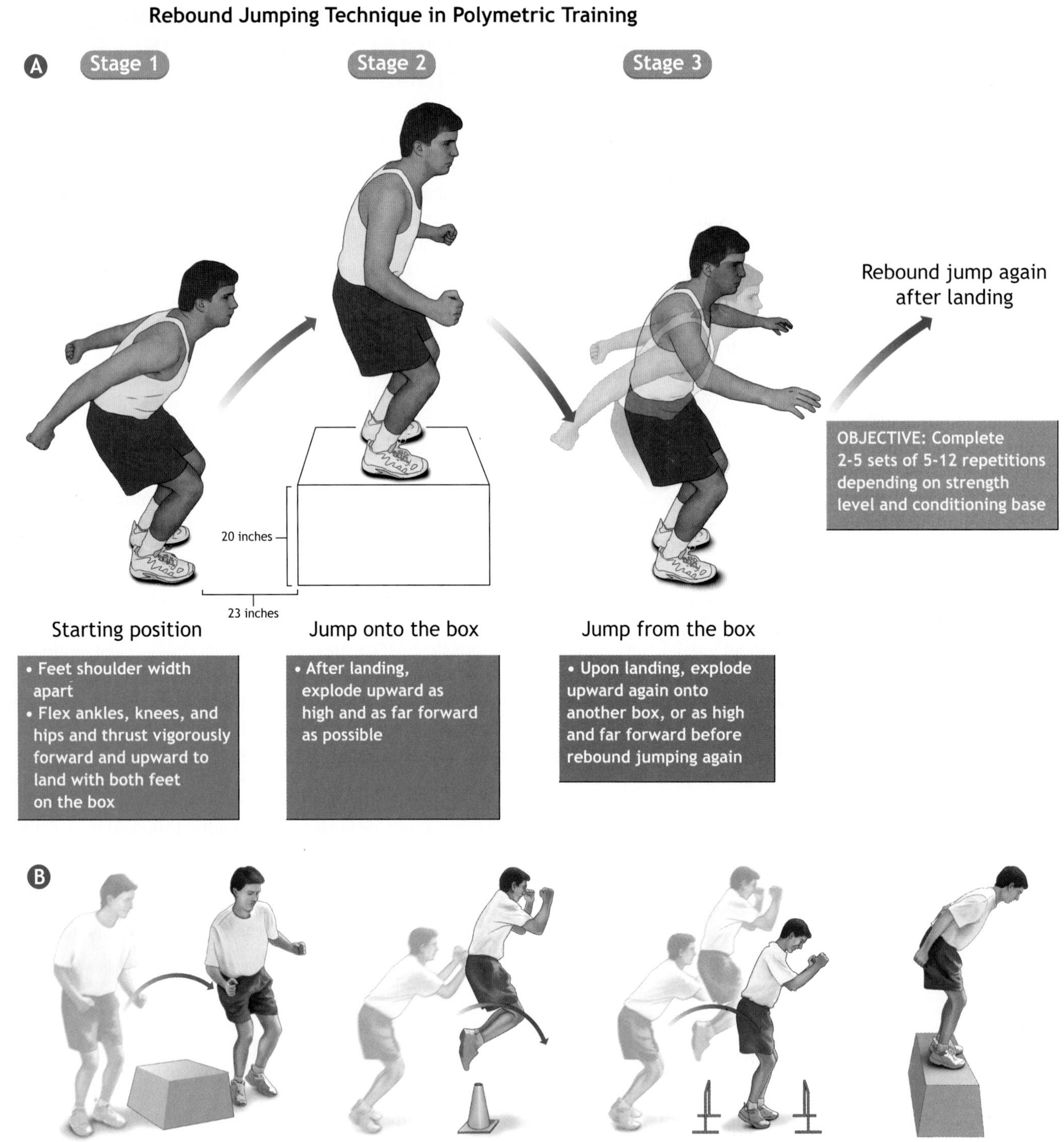

Rebound Jumping Technique in Polymetric Training

Figure 22.15 (**A**) Rebound jumping technique in plyometric training. (**B**) Four examples of plyometric exercise drills. 1. Box jump. 2. Cone hop. 3. Hurdle hop. 4. Long jump from box. (Examples courtesy of Dr. Thomas D. Fahey, California State University at Chico, Chico, CA.)

4. Allometric scaling mathematically establishes a "proper" relationship between a body size variable (e.g., stature, body mass, FFM) and some other variable of interest such as muscular strength or aerobic capacity. Allometry eliminates the confounding effects of factors inherently and non-linearly related to the variable in question.

5. Optimal overload training to strengthen muscles involves three factors: (1) increasing resistance (load) to muscle action, (2) increasing speed of muscle action, or (3) combining increased load and speed.

6. An overload between 60 and 80% of a muscle's force-generating capacity induces strength gains.

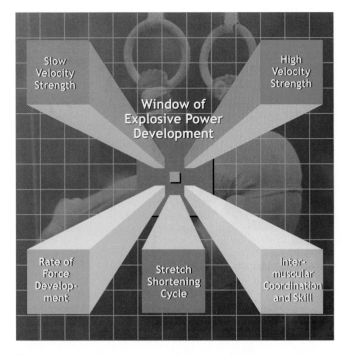

Figure 22.16 Five components that contribute to explosive power development. Adapted with permission from Dr. William J. Kraemer, Human Performance Laboratory, Ball State University, Muncie, IN. (From Kraemer WJ, Newton RU. Training for muscular power. Phys Med Rehabil Clin 2000;11:341.)

7. Three major strength-training systems include progressive resistance weight training, isometrics, and isokinetic training. Each produces strength gains highly specific to the type of training. Isokinetic training offers potential to generate maximum force throughout the full ROM at different angular velocities of limb movement.

8. Closely supervised resistance training programs using relatively moderate concentric muscle actions improve children's strength without adverse effects on bone, muscle, or connective tissue.

9. Periodization divides a distinct period of resistance training (macrocycle) into smaller training mesocycles; these subdivide into weekly microcycles. Compartmentalization of training minimizes staleness and overtraining effects to maximize peak performance that coincides with competition.

10. Resistance training for competitive athletes optimizes muscular strength, power, and hypertrophy. Training goals for middle-aged and older adults aim to modestly improve muscular strength and endurance, maintain muscle and bone mass, and enhance overall health and fitness.

11. Concurrent training for muscular strength and aerobic capacity inhibits the magnitude of strength improvement compared with training only for muscular strength.

12. Plyometric training emphasizes the inherent stretch–recoil characteristics of the neuromuscular system to facilitate muscle power development.

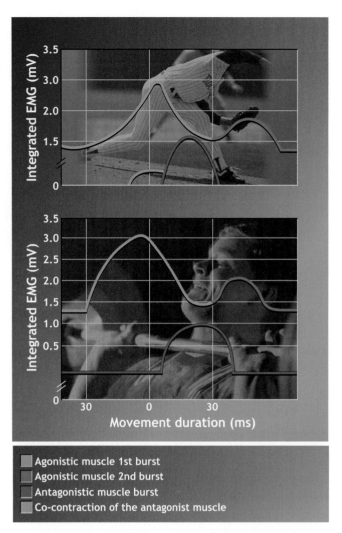

☐ Agonistic muscle 1st burst
☐ Agonistic muscle 2nd burst
☐ Antagonistic muscle burst
☐ Co-contraction of the antagonist muscle

Figure 22.17 The triphasic EMG pattern during rapid elbow flexion in professional baseball pitchers and champion body builders. (Data courtesy of Dr. Pierre Lagasse, Human Motor Performance Research Laboratory, Laval University, Quebec City, Quebec, Canada.)

13. Specificity of physiologic and performance measures and their response to training casts doubt on the efficacy of general fitness measures to predict ability to perform specific tasks or occupations.

14. A triphasic EMG activity pattern characterizes rapid, ballistic limb movements. EMG patterns often differ among individuals depending on prior athletic training and methods of strength acquisition.

PART 2 • *Structural and Functional Adaptations to Resistance Training*

Muscle tissue exists in a dynamic state where proteins are alternately synthesized (net deposition of amino acids) and degraded (net release of amino acids). FIGURE 22.18 lists six

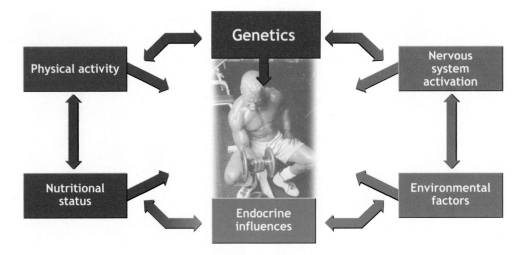

Figure 22.18   Six factors that act and interact to develop and maintain muscle mass.

factors that develop and maintain muscle mass. Without a doubt, genetic factors provide the governing frame of reference that modulates each of the other factors that increase muscle mass and strength.[155] Muscular activity contributes little to tissue growth without appropriate nutrition, particularly amino acid availability, to provide essential building blocks. Similarly, specific hormones (e.g., testosterone, growth hormone, cortisol, and, most importantly, insulin and systemic and local insulin-like growth factors) and nervous system innervation provide crucial input for patterning the appropriate training response. Without tension overload, each of the other factors cannot effectively produce the desired training response.

FACTORS THAT MODIFY THE EXPRESSION OF HUMAN STRENGTH

FIGURE 22.19 shows that factors broadly characterized as psychologic (neural) and muscular influence the expression of human strength. A resistance-training program modifies many components of these factors; other factors remain training resistant, probably determined by natural endowment or established early in life.

Psychologic–Neural Factors

Adaptive alterations in nervous system function that elevate motor neuron output largely account for the rapid and large strength increases early in training, often without an increase in muscle size and cross-sectional area.[1,109,137,160,176] Neural adaptations play a particularly important role in the dramatic muscular strength and power improvements of the elderly with resistance training compared with training-induced alterations in muscular hypertrophy.[68]

FIGURE 22.20 shows the general response for neural facilitation and muscle size increases with resistance training. Neural adaptations rather than changes inherent to muscle account for almost all of the relatively large strength improvements in the early phase of resistance training.

NEURAL ADAPTATIONS WITH RESISTANCE TRAINING THAT INCREASE MUSCULAR STRENGTH

- Greater efficiency in neural recruitment patterns
- Increased motor neuron excitability
- Increased central nervous system activation
- Improved motor unit synchronization and increased firing rates
- Lowering of neural inhibitory reflexes
- Inhibition of Golgi tendon organs

Research has considered the effects of exercise training on structural changes associated with the neuromuscular junction (NMJ). In one study with rats, endurance training improved the ratio of nerve terminal area to muscle fiber size by reducing fiber diameter without altering nerve terminal size.[193] In humans, high- and low-intensity training differentially affected the size of the NMJ.[44] Less intense, prolonged workouts produced a more expansive NMJ area, whereas intense exercise produced greater dispersion of synapses. Further research must clarify the compensatory effects of exercise training on NMJ structure and function.

A unique series of classic experiments illustrates the importance of psychologic factors in expressing muscular strength in humans.[90] The researchers measured arm strength in college-age men under (1) normal conditions, (2) immediately after a loud noise, (3) while the subject screamed loudly at the time of exertion, (4) under the influence of alcohol and amphetamines ("pep pills"), (5) and under hypnosis (told they possessed considerable strength and should not fear injury). Each of the alterations generally increased strength above normal levels; hypnosis, the most "mental" of all treatments, produced the greatest increments.

The investigators theorized that temporary modifications in central nervous system function accounted for strength im-

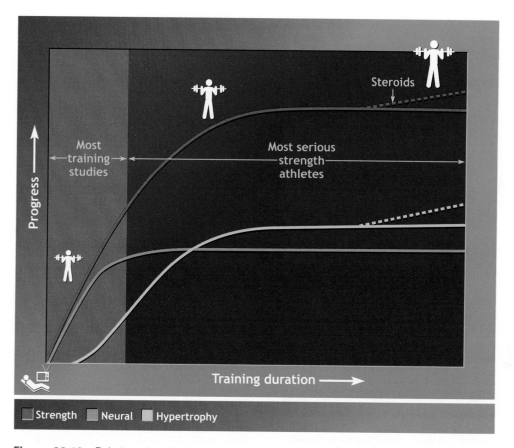

Figure 22.19 Relative roles of neural and muscular adaptations in strength improvement with resistance training. Note that neural adaptations predominate in the early phase of training (this phase encompasses the duration of most research studies). Hypertrophy-induced adaptations place the upper limit on longer term training improvements. This tempts many athletes to use anabolic steroids and/or human growth hormone *(dashed line)* to induce continual hypertrophy if training alone fails. (From Sale DG. Neural adaptation to resistance training. Med Sci Sports Exerc 1988;20:135.)

provements under the various experimental treatments. They argued that most persons normally operate at a level of neural inhibition, perhaps via protective reflex mechanisms that constrain the expression of strength capacity. Three factors, muscle cross section, fiber type, and mechanical arrangement of bone and muscle, explain strength capacity. Neuromuscular inhibition can come from unpleasant past experiences with exercise, an overly protective home environment, or fear of injury. Regardless of the reason, the person usually cannot express maximum strength capacity. The excitement of intense competition or influence of disinhibitory drugs or hypnotic suggestion often induces a "supermaximal" performance from greatly reduced neural inhibition and optimal motor neuron recruitment.

Highly trained athletes often create an almost self-hypnotic state by concentrating intensely, or "psyching," before competition. It sometimes takes years of training to perfect the "block out" of extraneous stimuli (e.g., crowd noise) so the muscle action relates directly to the performance. This occurs in power-lifting competition where success depends on precise, coordinated movements *with* maximal muscle tension output. Enhanced arousal level and accompanying neural disinhibition (or facilitation) fully activate muscle groups. Increased neurologic arousal also may account for "unex-

plainable" feats of strength and power during highly charged emergency situations.

Muscular Factors

Psychologic disinhibition and learning factors greatly modify muscle strength in the early phase of training. Ultimately, however, anatomic and physiologic factors within the joint–muscle unit determine strength capacity. TABLE 22.5 lists the physiologic and performance changes associated with long-term resistance training. Most of these components adapt to training, with some modifications occurring within several weeks. Resistance training's effects on muscle fibers generally relate to adaptations in the contractile structures; these usually accompany substantial increases in muscular force and power through a given ROM.

Muscle Hypertrophy

An increase in muscular tension (force) with exercise training provides the primary stimulus to initiate the relatively slow process of skeletal muscle growth, or hypertrophy. Mechanical stress on the components of the muscular system

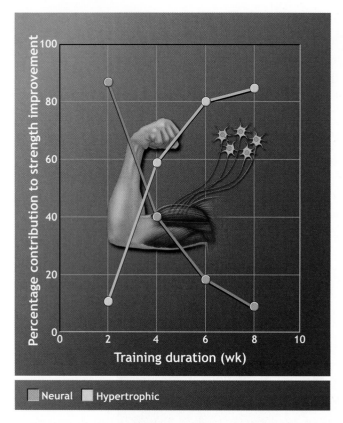

Figure 22.20 Generalized response curve for gains in muscle strength with resistance training from neural *(orange)* or muscular *(yellow)* factors. During a typical 8-week training period, neural factors account for approximately 90% of the strength gained over the first 2 weeks. In the subsequent 2 weeks, between 40 and 50% of the strength improvement still relates to nervous system adaptation. Thereafter, muscle fiber adaptations become progressively more important to strength improvement. Experiments of this type generally evaluate neural factors from integrated EMG recordings of the muscle groups trained.

TABLE 22.5 ■ PHYSIOLOGIC ADAPTATIONS TO RESISTANCE TRAINING

SYSTEM/VARIABLE	RESPONSE
Muscle fibers	
Number	Equivocal
Size	Increase
Type	Unknown
Strength	Increase
Capillary density	
In body builders	No change
In power lifters	Decrease
Mitochondria	
Volume	Decrease
Density	Decrease
Twitch contraction time	Decrease
Enzymes	
Creatine phosphokinase	Increase
Myokinase	Increase
Enzymes of glycolysis	
Phosphofructokinase	Increase
Lactate dehydrogenase	No change
Aerobic metabolism enzymes	
Carbohydrate	Increase
Triglyceride	Not known
Basal metabolism	Increase
Intramuscular fuel stores	
Adenosine triphosphate	Increase
Phosphocreatine	Increase
Glycogen	Increase
Triglycerides	Not known
$\dot{V}O_{2max}$	
Circuit resistance training	Increase
Heavy resistance training	No change
Connective tissue	
Ligament strength	Increase
Tendon strength	Increase
Collagen content of muscle	No change
Body composition	
% fat	Decrease
Lean body mass	Increase
Bone	
Mineral content and density	Increase
Cross-sectional area	No change

Modified from Fleck SJ, Kramer WJ. Resistance training: physiological responses and adaptations (part 2 of 4). Phys Sportsmed 1988;16:108.

triggers signaling proteins to activate the genes that activate translation of messenger RNA and stimulate protein synthesis in excess of protein breakdown. Accelerated protein synthesis, particularly when combined with the effects of insulin and adequate amino acid availability, increases muscle size during resistance training.[100] Hypertrophy reflects a fundamental biologic adaptation to increased workload independent of gender and age.[27] As mentioned earlier, improving muscular strength and power does not necessarily require muscle fiber hypertrophy because important neurologic factors initially affect the expression of human strength. The later, slower occurring strength improvements generally coincide with noticeable alterations in a muscle's subcellular molecular architecture.

Overload training enlarges individual muscle fibers with subsequent muscle growth. The fast-twitch fibers of weight lifters average about 45% larger than fibers of healthy sedentary persons and endurance athletes. The hypertrophic process couples directly to increased mononuclear number and synthesis of cellular components, particularly protein filaments

(myosin heavy chain and actin) that constitute the contractile elements.[11,74,129] Resistance exercise creates more efficient translation of mRNA that mediates stimulation of myofibrillar protein synthesis.[199] Muscle growth results from repeated muscle fiber injury (particularly with eccentric actions) followed by overcompensation of protein synthesis to produce a net anabolic effect. The cell's myofibrils thicken and increase in number, and additional sarcomeres form from accelerated protein synthesis and corresponding decreased protein breakdown. Intramuscular ATP, PCr, and glycogen also increase considerably. These anaerobic energy stores contribute to the rapid energy transfer required in resistance training. Body build characteristics also help to explain individual differences in responsiveness to resistance training. The greatest increases in muscle mass occur for individuals with the largest relative FFM corrected for stature and body fat before training begins.[191]

FIGURE 22.21 shows the change in muscle fiber size that accompanies exercise-induced hypertrophy. Figure 22.21A (*left*) compares exercised and nonexercised rat soleus muscle. The hypertrophied exercised muscle appears on the right. Figure 22.21B represents a typical cross section of untrained and hypertrophied muscles. Hypertrophied muscle diameter averages 30% larger and the fibers contain 45% more nuclei, which increase relative to fiber size. These compensatory changes relate to marked increases in DNA synthesis and proliferation of connective tissue cells and small, mononucleated satellite cells located beneath the basement membrane adjacent to the muscle fibers. These satellite cells, rich among type II

muscle fibers, facilitate growth, maintenance, and repair of damaged muscle tissue.[69,76] Connective tissue cellular proliferation thickens and strengthens the muscle's connective tissue harness to improve the structural and functional integrity of tendons and ligaments (cartilage lacks sufficient circulation to stimulate growth).[103] Such adaptations protect joints and muscles from injury. These adaptations justify including resistance exercise in preventive and rehabilitative orthopedic programs (see "Focus on Research"; Chapter 18).

Resistance-trained muscle fibers have increased total contractile protein and energy-generating compounds *without* parallel increases in capillarization, total volume of mitochondria, or mitochondrial enzymes. Thus, the ratio of mitochondrial volume and/or enzyme concentration to myofibrillar (contractile protein) volume decreases. This training response does not hinder performance in strength and power activities because of the anaerobic nature of such efforts. It does, however, impede endurance in prolonged exercise by reducing the fiber's aerobic capacity per unit of muscle mass.

Significant Metabolic Adaptations Occur

Undoubtedly, success at elite levels of sport performance requires optimization of muscle fiber distribution. The relatively fixed nature of muscle fiber type suggests an obvious genetic predisposition for exceptional performance. Considerable plasticity exists for metabolic potential because specific training enhances the anaerobic and aerobic energy transfer capacity of both fiber types.

The heightened oxidative capacity of fast-twitch fibers with endurance training brings them to a level nearly equal to the aerobic capacity of the slow-twitch fibers of untrained counterparts. Endurance training induces some conversion of type IIb fibers to the more aerobic type IIa fibers.[32,206] The well-documented increase in mitochondrial size and number and corresponding increase in total quantity of citric acid cycle and electron transport enzymes accompany these fiber subdivision changes.[82] Only the specifically trained muscle fibers adapt to regular exercise; this explains why trained athletes who change to a sport that requires different muscle groups (or different portions of the same muscle) often feel untrained for the new activity. Within this framework, swimmers or canoeists (with well-trained upper-body musculature) do not necessarily transfer upper body fitness to a running sport that relies predominantly on a highly conditioned lower-body musculature.

Metabolic characteristics of specific fibers and fiber subdivisions undergo modification within 4 to 8 weeks of resistance training. This occurs despite the lack of dramatic changes in inherent muscle fiber type. A decrease in the percentage of type IIb and corresponding increase in type IIa fibers denotes one of the more prominent and rapid training adaptations.[4,75,176] Furthermore, the volume of the trained fast-twitch fibers increases. FIGURE 22.22 clearly illustrates this increase for the relative areas of the fast- and slow-twitch muscle fibers before and after training. Considerable hypertrophy,

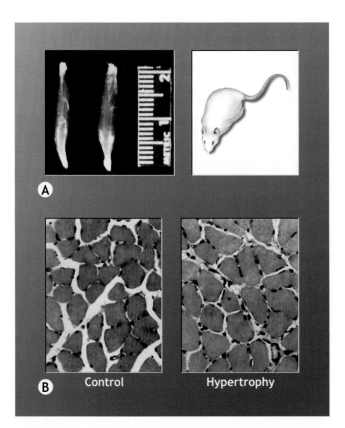

Figure 22.21 **A.** Control *(left)* and hypertrophied *(right)* rat soleus muscle. **B.** Cross sections of control and hypertrophied muscles shown in A. The average diameter for 50 fibers of the hypertrophied muscle was 24 to 34% greater than for controls; the average number of nuclei in hypertrophied muscle averaged 40 to 52% greater than controls. (From Goldberg AL, et al. Mechanism of work-induced hypertrophy of skeletal muscle. Med Sci Sports 1975;3:185.)

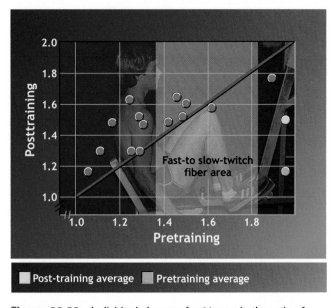

Figure 22.22 Individual changes for 14 men in the ratio of fast- to slow-twitch muscle fiber area after 8 weeks of resistance training. *Orange circle on right* indicates average pretraining FT:ST area ratio; *yellow circle* represents the posttraining average. (From Thorstensson A. Muscle strength, fiber types, and enzyme activities in man. Acta Physiol Scand Suppl 1976:443.)

predominantly of the fast-twitch fibers, occurs in power and Olympic-type lifters who train diligently over many years with progressive resistance training.[181,183] This makes sense within the framework of exercise specificity because near-maximal, high-resistance exercise requiring high levels of anaerobic power primarily recruits fast-twitch motor units.

TABLE 22.6 summarizes changes in skeletal muscle with specific training modalities. Generally, physical activity recruits both fiber types; however, certain activities require activation of a much greater proportion of one fiber type than another.

Muscle Cell Remodeling: Current Thinking

Skeletal muscle represents dynamic tissue whose cells do not remain as fixed populations throughout life. Rather, muscle fibers undergo regeneration and remodeling in response to diverse functional demands (e.g., resistance or endurance training) to alter their phenotypic profile.[206] Activation of muscle via specific types and intensities of long-term use stimulates otherwise dormant myogenic stem cells (satellite cells) situated under a muscle fiber's basement membrane to proliferate and differentiate to form new fibers. Fusion of satellite cell nuclei and incorporation into existing muscle fibers allows the fiber to synthesize more protein to form additional myofibril contractile elements. While this process does not create new muscle fibers per se, it does contribute directly to muscular hypertrophy and may stimulate transformation of existing fibers from one type to another.

A variety of extracellular signal molecules, primarily peptide growth factors (e.g., insulin-like growth factor [IGF], fibroblast growth factors, transforming growth factors, and hepatocyte growth factor) govern satellite cell activity and possibly exercise-induced muscle fiber proliferation and differentiation. FIGURE 22.23 proposes a model for muscle cell remodeling that involves satellite cell incorporation into an existing muscle fiber. A specific set of genes (gene A in the figure) is expressed in the fiber's preexisting nuclei. Chronic activation from physical activity stimulates satellite cell proliferation, with some cells differentiating and fusing with preexisting muscle fibers. The new muscle nuclei alter gene expression (gene B in the figure) in the adapting muscle.

Some fiber-type transformation may occur with specific exercise training. Studies with humans and animals support the concept that skeletal muscle adapts to functional demands. For example, arduous training may induce some transformation in fiber type. In one study, four athletes trained anaerobically for 11 weeks followed by 18 weeks of aerobic training. Anaerobic training increased the percentage of type IIc fibers and de-

TABLE 22.6 ■ EFFECTS OF SPECIFIC FORMS OF TRAINING ON SKELETAL MUSCLE

	SLOW-TWITCH FIBERS		FAST-TWITCH FIBERS	
	TYPE OF TRAINING			
MUSCLE FACTOR	**STRENGTH**	**ENDURANCE**	**STRENGTH**	**ENDURANCE**
Percentage composition	0 or ?	0 or ?	0 or ?	0 or ?
Size	+	0 or +	++	0
Contractile property	0	0	0	0
Oxidative capacity	0	++	0	+
Anaerobic capacity	? or +	0	? or +	0
Glycogen content	0	++	0	++
Fat oxidation	0	++	0	+
Capillary density	?	+	?	? or +
Blood flow during exercise	?	? or +	?	?

0, no change; ?, unknown; +, moderate increase; ++, large increase.

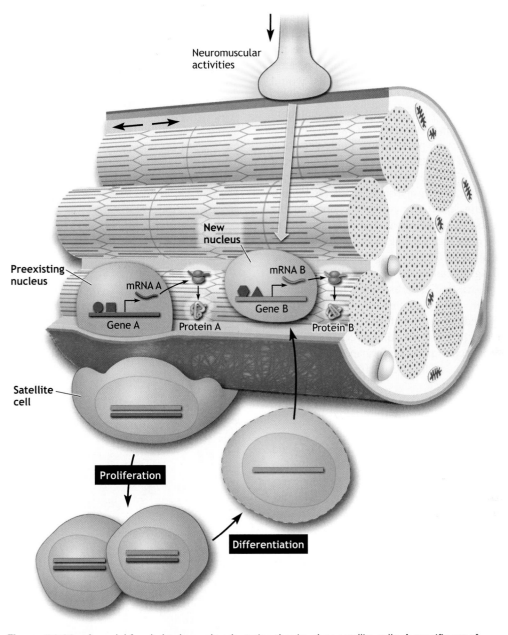

Figure 22.23 A model for skeletal muscle adaptation that involves satellite cells. A specific set of genes *(gene A)* is expressed in the preexisting myonuclei. Upon stimulation from increased neuromuscular activity, the satellite cells proliferate, and some of them differentiate and fuse with the preexisting myofibers. These myonuclei may alter gene expression *(gene B)* in the adapting muscle because they undergo altered differentiation from increased neuromuscular activities. (From Yan Z. Skeletal muscle adaptation and cell cycle regulation. Exerc Sport Sci Rev 2000;1:24.)

creased the percentage of type I fibers; the opposite occurred during the aerobic training phase.[95] Similarly, 4 to 6 weeks of sprint training increased the percentage of fast-twitch fibers with a commensurate decrease in slow-twitch fiber percentage.[41] Increasing daily training duration also increases the fast- to slow-twitch shift in myosin heavy-chain phenotype in rat hind limb muscles.[43] Specific training (and perhaps inactivity) may convert type I to type II fibers (and vice versa).[167,181] Available evidence does not permit definitive statements concerning the fixed nature of a muscle's fiber composition. *The genetic code more than likely exerts the greatest influence on fiber-type distribution.* The major direction of a muscle's fiber

composition probably becomes fixed before birth or during the first few years of life.

Myostatin: Perhaps a Governing Role in Muscle Growth. Studies with mice have indicated that when both copies of a gene for a protein called myostatin were inactivated the animals grew lean and extremely muscular. Years earlier, cattle breeders made the same observation and developed a strain of cattle with inactive myostatin genes. These cattle, known as Belgian Blue, were heavy, muscular, and lean. The precise role of myostatin in muscle growth is unclear, but it may normally function to limit muscle growth by keeping satellite cells quiescent. These immature cells surround muscle fibers and lie dormant until a muscle is injured. They then migrate into the muscle to replace the injured cells. Without myostatin, the normal brake on satellite cells would be removed and muscle cells would proliferate.

DNA testing has recently uncovered a genetic mutation, the first documented case in a human, in an extremely muscular young German boy who possessed a double dose of a mutation that inactivates myostatin similar to that produced in mice and cattle.[163] In essence, the boy produced no myostatin at all. Natural variation in myostatin levels (and genes that activate myostatin) may help researchers explain the considerable variation in responsiveness among humans to similar programs of resistance training. Ways exist to deactivate myostatin, deplete myostatin, or apply antibodies that block its action. Drugs are under development that may help persons with muscle-wasting diseases such a muscular dystrophy, AIDS, cancer, and other illnesses, including those with normal age-related muscle loss. From an ergogenic perspective, amateur and professional athletes could use myostatin blockers to enhance exercise performance and training responsiveness. Currently, the long-term effects of inhibiting this molecule remain unknown.

Benefits Regardless of Gender or Age

Women and men experience important physiologic and performance adaptations to resistance training independent of age.[32,74,108,154,168,207] A study of five older healthy men (average age 68 y) demonstrates the remarkable plasticity of human skeletal muscle (FIG. 22.24). The men trained for 12 weeks using heavy-resistance isokinetic and free-weight exercises. Training increased muscle volume and cross-sectional area of the biceps brachii (13.9%) and brachialis (26.0%), while hypertrophy increased by 37.2% in the type II muscle fibers. Increases of 46.0% in peak torque and 28.6% in total work output accompanied cellular adaptations. Similarly, older men experience percentage improvements in these variables similar to younger counterparts in response to a rapid, high-power periodized resistance-training program.[140]

Equally impressive training responses occur for elderly persons. One hundred nursing home residents (average age 87.1 y) trained for 10 weeks with high-intensity resistance exercise.[54] For the 63 women and 37 men who participated, muscle strength increased an average of 113%. Strength increases also paralleled improved function reflected by an 11.8% increase in normal gait velocity and 28.4% increase in stair-climbing speed; thigh muscle cross-sectional area increased by 2.7%.

Muscle Hyperplasia: Are New Muscle Fibers Made?

A common question concerns whether training increases the number of muscle cells (**hyperplasia**). If this does occur, to what extent does it contribute to muscle en-

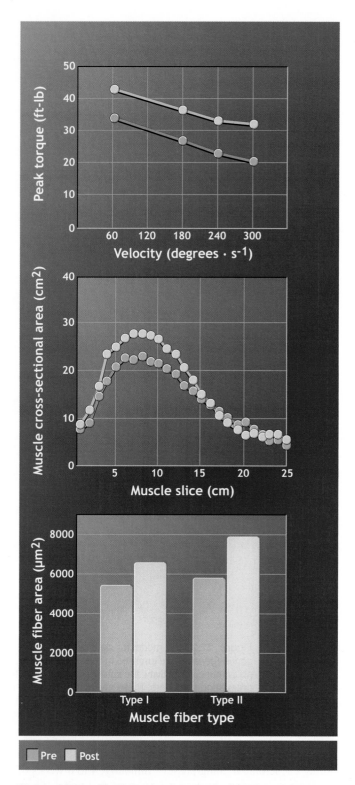

Figure 22.24 Plasticity of aging muscle. Data from five men, 68 years of age, before *(orange)* and after *(yellow)* 12 weeks of heavy-resistance training. *Top.* Peak torque of elbow flexors. *Middle.* Plot of flexor cross-sectional area computed from MRI scans from proximal *(right)* to distal *(left)* end of muscle. *Bottom.* Average for type I and type II fiber areas. (From Roman WJ, et al. Adaptations in the elbow flexors of elderly males after heavy-resistance training. J Appl Physiol 1993;74:750.)

largement in humans? Chronic overload of skeletal muscle in various animal species develops new muscle fibers from satellite cells or by longitudinal splitting.[8] Under conditions of stress, neuromuscular disease, and muscle injury, the normally dormant satellite cells develop into new muscle fibers (see Fig. 22.23). With **longitudinal splitting**, a relatively large muscle fiber splits into two or more smaller, individual daughter cells through lateral budding. These fibers function more efficiently than the large single fiber from which they originated.[9]

Generalizing findings from research on animals to humans poses a problem. The massive cellular hypertrophy observed in humans with resistance training does not occur in many animal species. In cats, for example, muscle fiber proliferation (hyperplasia) often reflects the primary compensatory adjustment to overload. Some evidence supporting hyperplasia in humans does exist. For example, autopsy data from young, healthy men who died accidentally show that muscle fiber counts of the larger and stronger leg (leg opposite the dominant hand) contained 10% more muscle fibers than the smaller leg.[169] Cross-sectional studies of body builders with relatively large limb circumferences and muscle masses failed to show they possessed above-normal size individual muscle fibers.[120,121,182] Some of the body builders may have inherited an initially large number of small muscle fibers (that "hypertrophied" to normal size with resistance training), yet the findings suggest hyperplasia with certain modes of resistance training. Muscle fibers probably adapt differently to the high-volume, high-intensity training practiced by body builders than the typical low-repetition, heavy-load system favored by strength and power athletes. *Even if other human studies replicate a training-induced hyperplasia (and even if the response reflects a positive adjustment), enlargement of existing individual muscle fibers represents the greatest contribution to increased muscle size from overload training.*

Changes in Muscle Fiber Type with Resistance Training

Research has evaluated the effects of 8 weeks of resistance exercise on muscle fiber size and fiber composition for the leg extensor muscles of 14 men who performed three sets of 6-RM leg squats three times weekly.[184] Biopsy specimens from the vastus lateralis muscle before and after training showed *no change* with resistance training in percentage distribution of fast- and slow-twitch muscle fibers. This finding agreed with previous short-term resistance and endurance-type training studies and indicates that several months of resistance training in adults does not alter the basic fiber composition of skeletal muscle. It remains unclear whether specific training early in life or for prolonged durations practiced by Olympic-caliber athletes alters a muscle fiber's inherent twitch (speed of shortening) characteristics. Some progressive fiber-type transformation may occur with longer duration, specific training (see Chapter 18). Current thinking posits that genetic factors largely determine one's predominant muscle fiber type distribution.

COMPARATIVE TRAINING RESPONSES IN MEN AND WOMEN

In today's society, women participate successfully in all sports and physical activities. Women had generally not used resistance training to avoid developing overly enlarged muscles similar to men. This hesitation was unfortunate because specific strength acquisition enhances performance in tennis, golf, skiing, dance, gymnastics, and most other sports including physically demanding occupations such as firefighting and construction work. The question often arises whether muscular strength acquisition differs between men and women, and if so, what factors might be responsible?

INTEGRATIVE QUESTION

If women respond to resistance training essentially the same way as men, explain the disparity between the upper-arm girth of male and female body builders.

Muscular Strength and Hypertrophy

The amount of absolute muscle hypertrophy with resistance training represents a primary gender difference. Computed axial tomography (CAT) scans for direct evaluation of muscle cross-sectional area show that men and women respond similarly in hypertrophic response to resistance training. Without doubt, men experience a greater absolute change in muscle size because of their larger initial muscle mass, but muscular enlargement on a percentage basis remains similar between genders.[39,145] Comparisons between elite male and female body builders also indicate substantial muscular hypertrophy in females with many years of resistance training.[174,175]

The limited data from relatively short-duration training studies suggest that women safely can use conventional resistance training exercise without developing overly large muscles. Gender-related differences in hormonal response to resistance exercise (e.g., increased testosterone and decreased cortisol for men) may determine any ultimate gender differences in muscle size and strength adaptations with prolonged training.[207] This intriguing area requires longitudinal research for a richer description of gender differences in how skeletal muscle responds to resistance training.

Does Muscle Strength Relate to Bone Density?

Men and women who participate in strength and power activities have as much or more bone mass as endurance athletes.[157] The lumbar spine and proximal femur bone mass of elite teenage weightlifters exceeds representative values for fully mature bone of reference adults.[35] A linear relation exists between increases in bone mineral density (BMD) and total and exercise-specific weight lifted during a 1-year strength-training program.[40] Such findings have raised speculation about the possible relationship between muscular strength and bone mass. Laboratory experiments have documented greater maximum flexion and extension dynamic strength in postmenopausal women without osteoporosis than in osteoporetic counterparts.[94,177] For female gymnasts, BMD correlated moderately with maximal muscle strength and serum progesterone.[79] For adolescent female athletes, absolute knee extension strength moderately associated with total body, lumbar spine, femoral neck, and leg BMD.[49] FIGURE 22.25 shows chest flexion and extension strength in normal and osteoporotic women. Women with normal BMD (measured by dual-photon absorptiometry in the lumbar spine and femur neck) exhibited 20% greater strength in 11 of 12 test comparisons for flexion; 4 of 12 comparisons for extension showed 13% higher strength values for women with normal bone density. Subsequent data complement these findings; they indicate that regional lean tissue mass (often an indication of muscular strength) accurately predicts bone mineral density.[141] Differences in maximum dynamic strength among postmenopausal women may serve a clinically useful role in osteoporosis screening.

Women at risk for osteoporosis or with osteoporosis can attenuate their *factor of risk* (ratio of the load on bone to the bone's failure load) for fracture in one of two ways: (1) strengthen bone by increasing bone density and (2) avoid risky activities that increase bone load or spinal compression (e.g., heavy lifting activities).[136]

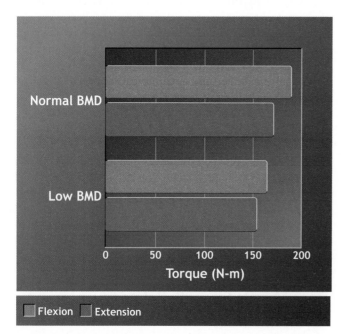

Figure 22.25 Comparison of chest press extension and flexion strength in age- and weight-matched postmenopausal women with normal and low bone mineral density (BMD). Women with low BMD scored significantly lower on each measure of muscular strength than a reference group. (From Stock JL, et al. Dynamic muscle strength is decreased in postmenopausal women with low bone density. J Bone Miner Res 1987;2:338; Janey C, et al. Maximum muscular strength differs in postmenopausal women with and without osteoporosis. Med Sci Sports Exerc 1987;19:S61.)

DETRAINING

Limited data document muscle strength decrements and associated factors with cessation of resistance training. Discontinuing training for 2 weeks caused male power lifters to lose 12% of their isokinetic eccentric muscle strength and 6.4% of their type II muscle fiber area, without loss in type I fiber area.[84] Abstaining for a short period of resistance training in previously sedentary men caused loss of strength gains within several weeks, most likely from reversal of training-induced neuromuscular and hormonal adaptations.[33] Reducing training frequency to only one or two weekly sessions provides sufficient stimulus to *maintain* training-induced strength gains.[64]

METABOLIC STRESS OF RESISTANCE TRAINING

High-intensity, variable-resistance strength training produces no improvement in $\dot{V}O_{2max}$ or submaximal exercise heart rate and stroke volume,[88] although intense resistance-exercise training may slightly increase blood volume.[130] Lack of cardiovascular improvement probably results from the relatively low "whole body" metabolic and circulatory demands and high anaerobic metabolic requirements of standard resistance training. This is reflected by the potent stimulation of glucose uptake and lactate release by the active muscle.[50] Data from young men during maximal isometric and 8- to 10-RM weight-lifting exercises indicate that such activity elicits only light-to-moderate heart rate response (generally less than 130 $b \cdot min^{-1}$) and oxygen consumption (3 to 4 METs).[126]

Undoubtedly, resistance training places considerable localized stress on specific muscles. The brief activation period and typically small muscle mass activated in such exercise creates lower heart rates and aerobic metabolic demands than dynamic big-muscle running, hiking, climbing, swimming, or cycling. A person may devote an hour or more completing a strength-training workout, yet the total time devoted to exercising does not usually exceed 8 minutes per hour. Clearly, traditional resistance-training workouts should not constitute the major portion of a program designed for cardiovascular improvement and weight control.

CIRCUIT RESISTANCE TRAINING

Modifying the traditional approach to resistance training increases the caloric cost of exercise to improve several important fitness aspects. **Circuit resistance training (CRT)**, deemphasizes the brief intervals of heavy, local-muscle overload in standard resistance training. It provides more-general conditioning that improves body composition, muscular strength and endurance, and cardiovascular fitness.[12,97] With CRT, a person lifts a weight between 40 and 55% of 1-RM as many times as possible with good form for 30 seconds. After a 15-second rest, the participant moves to the next resistance exercise station and so on to complete the circuit, usually composed of 8 to 15 different exercises. A modification that produces similar CRT energy expenditure uses exercise-to-rest ratios of 1:1, with either 15- or 30-second exercise periods.[13] The circuit, repeated several times, allows for 30 to 50 minutes of continuous exercise, not just the 6 to 8 minutes of the traditional resistance-training workout. As strength increases, a new 1-RM determined for each exercise provides the basis for increasing resistance.

The CRT modification of standard resistance training offers an attractive alternative to those who desire a more general conditioning program. Medically supervised CRT programs effectively train coronary-prone, cardiac, and spinal cord-injured patients for a well-rounded fitness program.[172] CRT supplements off-season conditioning for sports that require high levels of strength, power, and muscular endurance.

Specificity of Aerobic Improvement

Some research indicates that CRT produces nearly 50% less aerobic fitness improvement than bicycle or run training.[61] Importantly, CRT usually involves substantial upper-body exercise, but assessment of aerobic benefits from this training relied on treadmill or bicycle tests that predominantly activate lower-body musculature. To compensate for this limitation, one study assessed CRT effects on aerobic capacity with treadmill running and arm-crank ergometry tests.[72] Aerobic capacity increased 7.8% with treadmill testing *and* 21.1% with arm-crank testing, thus confirming the training specificity principle. These findings take on added significance because they occurred without negative effects in a group of borderline hypertensives. The program also increased muscular strength, decreased blood pressure, and modestly improved body composition.

Energy Cost of Different Resistance-Exercise Methods

TABLE 22.7 displays energy expenditures for exercise performed using free weights, Nautilus (eccentric), Universal Gym (concentric/eccentric), Cybex (isokinetic), and Hydra-Fitness (hydraulic-concentric). Energy expenditure for hydraulic exercises averaged 9.0 kCal · min^{-1}; this averaged 35% higher than exercise with free weights, 29.4% higher than Nautilus exercise, and 11.5% more than CRT using Universal Gym equipment. The energy expenditure values for hydraulic exercise averaged about 6.4% less than slow- and fast-speed isokinetic circuit exercise. For comparison, the last line lists the energy expenditure for walking at a normal pace on a level surface.

Specificity of Hypertrophic Response

One should not assume that a single resistance exercise creates uniform strength improvement or hypertrophic response in the muscle(s) activated.[8] For example, biceps curls performed at close to 1-RM do *not* produce equal strength gains from the muscle's origin to its insertion. If they did, then the maximal force-generating capacity of the muscle would show similar percentage improvements throughout its

TABLE 22.7 ■ **ENERGY EXPENDITURE FOR DIFFERENT MODES OF RESISTANCE EXERCISE COMPARED WITH WALKING**^{a}

MODE	SEX	kJ · MIN^{-1}	kCAL · MIN^{-1}
Nautilus, circuit	M	29.7	7.1
	F	24.3	5.8
Nautilus, circuit	M	22.6	5.4
Universal, circuit	M	33.1	7.9
	F	28.5	6.8
Isokinetic, slow	M	40.2	9.6
Isokinetic, fast	M	41.4	9.9
Isometric and free-weight	M	25.1	6.0
Hydra-Fitness, circuit	M	37.7	9.0
Walking on level	M	22.6	5.4

Data from Katch FI, et al. Evaluation of acute cardiorespiratory responses to hydraulic resistance exercise. Med Sci Sports Exerc 1985;17:168.
^{a} Based on a body weight of 68 kg.

ROM. This does not occur. Similarly, electrical activity measured by surface or needle EMG or MRI to assess a muscle's cross-sectional area does not produce a homogeneous response within the entire muscle during maximal activation.[21,134,162] A single muscle compartmentalizes into distinct regions, indicating that the muscle's different areas respond differentially to the imposed stress. In essence, skeletal muscle remodels its internal architecture, potentially reconfiguring external orientation and hence its shape. The overall lack of homogeneity in skeletal muscle's response to overload, coupled with intramuscular differences in fiber type and composition, governs the training adaptation to specific resistance exercise. The nonuniformity in skeletal muscle response to overload training also occurs in animal models with considerable molecular differentiation.[83,159,173]

MUSCLE SORENESS AND STIFFNESS

Following an extended layoff from exercise, most persons experience soreness and stiffness in the exercised joints and muscles. Temporary soreness may persist for several hours immediately after unaccustomed exercise, whereas residual **delayed-onset muscle soreness** (**DOMS**) appears later and can last for 3 or 4 days. Any one of the following factors may produce DOMS:

- Minute tears in muscle tissue or damage to its contractile components with accompanying release of creatine kinase (CK), myoglobin (Mb), and troponin I, the muscle-specific marker of muscle fiber damage
- Osmotic pressure changes that produce fluid retention in the surrounding tissues
- Muscle spasms

- Overstretching and tearing of portions of the muscle's connective tissue harness
- Acute inflammation
- Alteration in the cell's mechanism for calcium regulation
- Combination of the above factors

Eccentric Actions Produce Muscle Soreness

The precise cause of muscle soreness remains unknown, although the degree of discomfort and muscle disturbance depends largely on the intensity and duration of effort and type of exercise performed.[47,89,150] The magnitude of active strain imposed on a muscle fiber (rather than absolute force) precipitates muscle damage and soreness.[116] *Eccentric muscle actions trigger the greatest postexercise discomfort, particularly magnified in older individuals.*[171,180,194] Existing muscle damage or soreness from previous exercise does not exacerbate subsequent muscle damage or impair the repair process.[143]

In one study, subjects rated muscle soreness immediately after exercise and 24, 48, and 72 hours later. Greater soreness occurred from exercise that involved repeated intense strain during active lengthening in eccentric actions than from concentric and isometric actions. Soreness did not relate to lactate buildup because high-intensity, level running (concentric actions) produced no residual soreness despite significant elevations in blood lactate. In contrast, downhill running (eccentric actions) caused moderate-to-severe DOMS without lactate elevation during exercise.

TABLE 22.8 highlights muscle soreness and CK activity following an exercise circuit of either concentric-only or concentric and eccentric muscle actions. Group 1 performed three sets of eight exercises (concentric–eccentric) at 60% of 1-RM on Universal Gym equipment: one set equaled 20 seconds of exercise followed by 40 seconds of rest; total exercise time was 24 minutes. Group 2 followed the same exercise protocol, but they exercised maximally for each repetition on hydraulic resistance devices (Hydra-Fitness) that used concentric-only actions. Blood samples and ratings of perceived muscle soreness took place before exercise and 5, 10, and 25 hours after exercise. The major difference in soreness ratings between exercise groups occurred 25 hours postexercise; the concentric–eccentric workout produced higher perceived ratings of soreness for the major muscle groups exercised. The magnitude of increase in serum CK remained the same between groups from 5 to 25 hours postexercise. Both exercise modes elevated serum CK, but the concentric-only muscle actions did not cause DOMS.

Cell Damage

Running downhill at a 10° slope for 30 minutes produced considerable DOMS 42 hours after exercise.[22] Corresponding increases also occurred in serum levels of Mb and the muscle-specific enzyme CK, both common markers

---

TABLE 22.8 ■ ACUTE EFFECTS OF CONCENTRIC-ONLY AND CONCENTRIC–ECCENTRIC EXERCISE ON DOMS 25 HOURS AFTER EXERCISE[a]

	SORENESS RATINGS			SORENESS RATINGS	
SITE	CONCENTRIC $\overline{X}$	CONCENTRIC–ECCENTRIC $\overline{X}$	SITE	CONCENTRIC $\overline{X}$	CONCENTRIC–ECCENTRIC $\overline{X}$
Chest	2.3	5.1	Forearm (front)	1.7	3.4
Back (upper)	2.6	2.8	Forearm (back)	1.7	2.9
Shoulders (front)	2.2	3.6	Back (lower)	1.7	2.9
Shoulders (back)	1.9	3.6	Buttocks	1.8	2.5
Biceps (mid)	1.9	4.3	Quadricep (mid)	2.0	4.1
Biceps (lower)	1.8	3.5	Quadricep (lower)	2.1	3.8
Triceps (mid)	1.9	3.4	Hamstrings (mid)	2.1	3.5
Triceps (lower)	1.9	3.0	Hamstrings (lower)	2.1	3.0

	CK ACTIVITY (mU · mL^{-1})	
SAMPLE TIME	CONCENTRIC $\overline{X}$	CONCENTRIC–ECCENTRIC $\overline{X}$
Pre	86.7	126.9
5 h post	344.8	232.0
10 h post	394.3	368.5
25 h post	288.0	482.2

From Byrnes WC. Muscle soreness following resistance exercise with and without eccentric muscle actions. Res Q Exerc Sport 1985;56:283.
[a]All differences between groups were statistically significant.
$\overline{X}$ = mean

of muscle injury. Acute inflammation also augments greater mobilization of leukocytes and neutrophils. Subject testing also took place after 3, 6, and 9 weeks. FIGURE 22.26 shows the perceived soreness rating for the leg muscles related to elapsed postexercise time for the three study durations. For the 3- and 6-week comparisons, differences between exercise bouts reached statistical significance, with diminished DOMS noted in the second trial *(orange)*. Similar patterns emerged for perception of muscle soreness and CK and Mb levels. Interestingly, peak soreness ratings at 48 hours did not relate to absolute or relative CK or Mb changes. Individuals who reported the greatest DOMS did not necessarily have the highest CK and Mb values. The first bout of repetitive, high-force exercise probably disrupts the integrity of the sarcolemma to produce mitochondrial swelling and temporary ultrastructural muscle damage in a pool of stress-susceptible or degenerating muscle fibers. This response occurs with an increase in blood markers such as protein carbonyls that reflect oxidative stress.[58]

The early mechanical damage to the myocytes (reflected by increased CK release) 24 hours postexercise does coincide with acute inflammatory cell infiltration within the muscle.[19] The subsequent decrease in muscle performance for several days following eccentric injury primarily stems from failure in excitation–contraction coupling and increased myofibrillar proteolysis.[91,203] The fast-twitch fibers with low oxidative capacities show particular vulnerability, with more extensive damage several days after exercise than in the immediate postexercise period. Changes in plasma CK activity, soreness ratings, and skeletal muscle injury with eccentric exercise do not differ between young adult Caucasian and African-American men.[164]

A single exercise bout protects against muscle soreness and decrements in muscle strength in subsequent exercise, with the effect lasting up to 6 weeks. Resistance to muscle damage in succeeding exercise may result from an eccentric exercise–induced increase in muscle fiber sarcomeres connected in series.[118] Such adaptations support the wisdom of initiating a training program with light exercise to protect against the muscle soreness that almost always follows an initial intense exercise bout that includes an eccentric component. Intense concentric exercise performed just prior to strenuous eccentric exercise does not magnify muscle damage. It may prepare the muscle to respond more effectively to the next eccentric exercise stress. Even prior lower intensity exercise of specific muscles does not fully protect from DOMS with more intense exercise.

Altered Sarcoplasmic Reticulum

Four factors produce major alterations in sarcoplasmic reticulum structure and function with unaccustomed exercise: (1) changes in pH, (2) changes in intramuscular high-energy phosphates, (3) changes in ionic balance, and (4) changes in temperature. These effects depress the rates of Ca^{2+} uptake and release and increase free Ca^{2+} concentration as the mineral rapidly moves into the cytosol of the

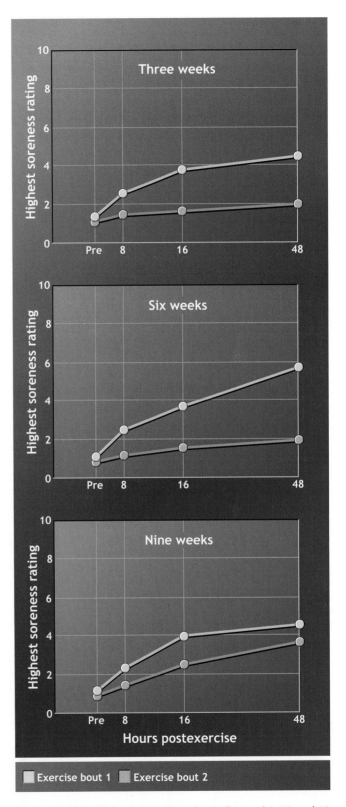

Figure 22.26 Highest soreness rating before and 6, 18, and 48 hours after exercise bout 1 *(yellow)* and a subsequent exercise bout (bout 2, *orange*) performed either 3, 6, or 9 weeks later. CK and Mb showed similar results. (From Byrnes WC, et al. Delayed onset muscle soreness following repeated bouts of downhill running. J Appl Physiol 1985;59:710.)

damaged fibers. Intracellular Ca^{2+} overload contributes to the autolytic process within damaged muscle fibers that degrades the contractile and noncontractile structures. Such changes lead to reduced force capacity and eventual muscle soreness. Vitamin E supplementation, and perhaps vitamin C and selenium, protects against cellular membrane disruption and enzyme loss following muscle damage from resistance exercise (see Chapter 2).[62,127,190] Postexercise protein supplementation also may protect against muscle soreness in severely exercise-stressed individuals.[55] In contrast, supplementing daily with either fish oil (high in omega-3 and omega-6 fatty acids) or isoflavones (soy isolate) for 30 days prior to and during the week of testing to reduce the inflammatory response produced no benefit to DOMS (strength, pain ratings, limb girth, and blood measures related to muscle damage, inflammation, and lipid peroxidation) compared with placebo treatment.[114]

Current DOMS Model

FIGURE 22.27 diagrams the probable steps in the development of DOMS and subsequent recuperation.

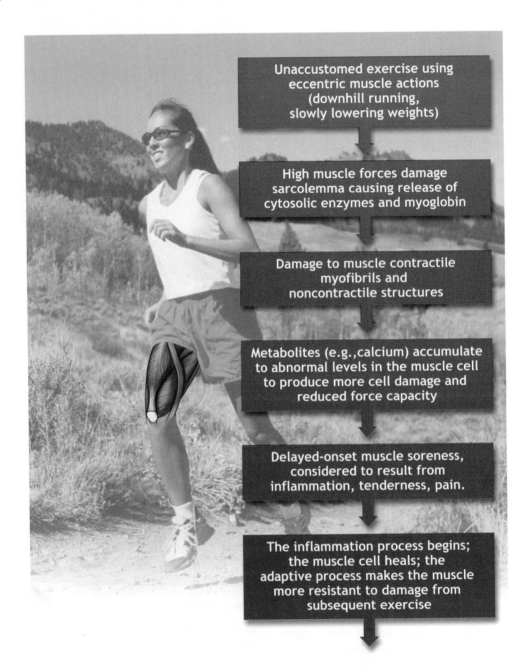

Figure 22.27 Proposed sequence for delayed-onset muscle soreness following unaccustomed exercise. Cellular adaptations to short-term exercise provide enhanced resistance to subsequent damage and pain.

INTEGRATIVE QUESTION

Respond to the following: "I run and work out with free weights regularly, yet every spring my muscles are sore a day or two after a few hours of yard work."

Summary

1. The size and type of muscle fibers and the anatomic lever arrangement of bone and muscle (physiologic factors) largely govern the upper limit to human muscular strength.
2. Central nervous system influences activate the prime movers in a specific action to affect maximal force capacity.
3. Six factors, genetic, exercise, nutritional, hormonal, environmental, and neural, interact to regulate skeletal muscle mass and corresponding strength development with resistance training.
4. Three factors contribute to increased muscle strength with resistance training: (1) improved capacity for motor unit recruitment, (2) changes in motor neuron firing pattern efficiency, and (3) alterations within the muscle fibers' contractile elements.
5. Muscular overload increases strength and selectively stimulates muscle fiber hypertrophy. Muscle hypertrophy includes increased protein synthesis with myofibrillar thickening, connective tissue cell proliferation, and an increase in the number of satellite cells around each fiber.
6. Muscle hypertrophy entails structural changes within the contractile apparatus of individual fibers, particularly fast-twitch fibers, and increased anaerobic energy stores.
7. The genetic code exerts the greatest influence on muscle fiber-type distribution; a muscle's fiber composition is largely fixed before birth or during the first few years of life.
8. Human muscle fibers adapt to increased functional demands via action of myogenic stem cells (satellite cells) that proliferate and differentiate to remodel the muscle.
9. Relatively brief periods of resistance training generates similar strength improvements (on a percentage basis) for women and men.
10. Muscle weakness in the abdominal and lower lumbar back regions (core) and poor flexibility in back and legs represent primary factors related to low-back syndrome. Core muscle-strengthening and flexibility exercises effectively protect against and rehabilitate this condition.
11. Women at risk for osteoporosis (or with the disease) reduce fracture risk by increasing bone density and avoiding activities that increase spinal compression and bone stress.
12. Conventional resistance training does not improve aerobic fitness. These workouts do not affect weight loss because of their relatively low caloric cost.
13. Circuit resistance training, by using lower resistance and higher repetitions, effectively combines the muscle-training benefits of resistance exercise with the cardiovascular, calorie-burning benefits of continuous dynamic exercise.
14. Eccentric muscle actions induce greater DOMS than concentric-only or isometric actions. Serum markers of muscle damage (CK and Mb) increase with each form of muscle action.
15. A single exercise bout protects against DOMS and muscle damage from subsequent exercise. The protection mechanism supports the wisdom of progressing gradually (lower intensity; minimize eccentric actions) when beginning an exercise program that requires application of considerable muscular force.
16. The body initiates a series of adaptive cellular events (basically an inflammation response) to unaccustomed exercise that produces DOMS.

References are available on the Student CD and online at *http://connection.lww.com/mkk6e.*

Special Aids to Exercise Training and Performance

23

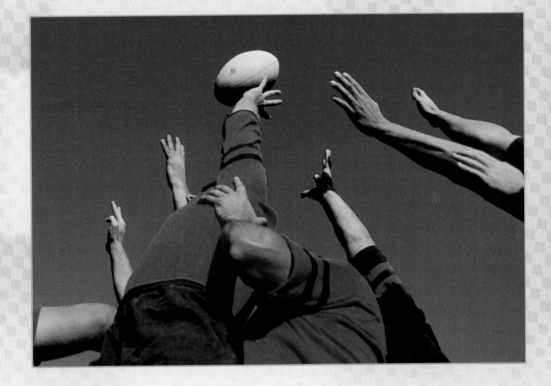

CHAPTER OBJECTIVES

- Define *ergogenic aids* and outline possible mechanisms for their purported effects

- List the categories of substances currently banned by the International Olympic Committee

- Give examples of substances and procedures with alleged ergogenic benefits

- Discuss the mode of action of anabolic steroids, their effectiveness, and risks when used by males and females

- Summarize ACSM's "Position Stand on Use of Anabolic Steroids"

- Give positive and negative findings from research on animals of the effect of β_2-adrenergic agonists

- Discuss the medical use of human growth hormone and potential dangers for healthy athletes

- Outline the general trend for endogenous dehydroepiandrosterone (DHEA) production during a lifetime

- Discuss the rationale for DHEA as an ergogenic aid and its potential risks

- Summarize the controversy about androstenedione as a benign nutritional supplement or a harmful drug

- Discuss the effects of oral supplements of amino acids, carbohydrate–protein, or carbohydrate on hormone secretion, training responsiveness, and exercise performance

- Summarize the research findings about ergogenic benefits and risks of amphetamines, caffeine, buffering solutions, chromium picolinate, L-carnitine, glutamine, and β-hydroxy-β-methylbutyrate

- Describe the typical time course for red blood cell reinfusion and the mechanism for ergogenic effects on endurance performance and $\dot{V}O_{2max}$

- Discuss the medical use of erythropoietin and potential dangers for healthy athletes

- Define *general warm-up* and *specific warm-up* and the potential benefits of each

- Describe possible cardiovascular benefits of moderate warm-up prior to extreme physical effort

- Provide a rationale for breathing hyperoxic gas mixtures to enhance exercise performance; quantify its potential to increase tissue oxygen availability

- Outline the classic carbohydrate-loading procedure and modified-loading procedure to augment glycogen storage

- Describe the theoretical role for an ergogenic effect of creatine supplements, and indicate physical activities that benefit from supplementation

- Summarize the research and rationale for consuming medium-chain triacylglycerols to enhance endurance performance

- Discuss the effects of pyruvate supplementation on endurance and body fat loss

Considerable literature exists about **ergogenic aids** and athletic performance—*ergogenic* referring to the application of a nutritional, physical, mechanical, psychologic, or pharmacologic procedure or aid to improve physical work capacity or athletic performance. This literature includes studies of potential performance benefits of alcohol, amphetamines, ephedrine, hormones, carbohydrates, amino acids, fatty acids, additional red blood cells, caffeine, carnitine, creatine, phosphates, oxygen-rich breathing mixtures, massage, wheat-germ oil, vitamins, minerals, ionized air, music, hypnosis, and even marijuana and cocaine! Athletes routinely use only a few of these aids, and only a few evoke real controversy. Specific concern focuses on the use of anabolic steroids, dehydroepiandrosterone (DHEA), and other exogenous hormones and prohormones, nutritional components, amphetamines, and "blood doping." Warm-up and breathing hyperoxic gas are common procedures, so we include these in our discussion of the effectiveness and practicality of ergogenic aids for exercise training and performance.

We discuss nutritional requirements for macro- and micronutrients for active individuals in the specific chapters dealing with these nutrients. The increasing use of herbs of undocumented quality by fitness enthusiasts and athletes raises concern about efficacy and possible toxicity. The "In a Practical Sense" feature on p. 560 summarizes ingredients, purported benefits, and possible side effects of commonly used herbal compounds.

Several explanations account for heightened interest in factors that might enhance exercise capacity and training responsiveness other than one's innate physical ability and commitment to training. First, more persons participate in high-level amateur and professional athletics. Second, success in competition brings considerable personal recognition and approval but also more tangible rewards ranging from valuable college scholarships to lucrative professional contracts and commercial endorsements. For many individuals, athletic success paves the way to riches, a route that sometimes spells personal misfortune. Concurrently, exercise science continues to research how pharmacologic agents and nutritional modification and supplementation affect energy supply, muscle metabolism, physiologic function, and overall growth and development.

AN INCREASING CHALLENGE TO FAIR COMPETITION

The indiscriminate use of alleged ergogenic substances increases the likelihood of adverse side effects that range from benign physical discomfort to life-threatening episodes.[8] Many of these compounds fail to conform to labeling requirements to correctly identify the strength of the product's ingredients.[130,170] A study at the Institute of Biochemistry at the German Sports University of Cologne (www.dopinginfo.de) supported by the Medical Commission of the International Olympic Committee (IOC) revealed that up to 20% of nutritional supplements contain substances that produce a positive result for doping. These included nandrolone, testosterone, and other steroids not declared on the label. The supplements analyzed included vitamins and minerals, amino acid mixtures, and creatine. These findings raise the likelihood that cross contamination occurs in laboratories that produce both prohormone products and nutrient supplements. Use of a dietary supplement contaminated with the prohibited anabolic substance 19-norandrostendine was the explanation offered by a member of the United States Olympic bobsled team for his disqualification just prior to the start of the 2002 Salt Lake City Winter Games.

Examples of illegal drug use by athletes abound. On July 16, 1998, the international governing body of bicycle racing suspended the coach of the top-ranked Festina team of France in a drug scandal that threatened to overwhelm the 85th Tour de France, bicycle racing's most prestigious and financially rewarding competition. The suspension resulted after large quantities of prohibited drugs were found in the team car. These included amphetamines, steroids, masking drugs (usually diuretics to prevent steroid detection or the chemical probenecid, which inhibits substances from reaching the urine), and the blood-boosting epoetin, a genetically engineered copy of the kidney hormone erythropoietin, linked to more than a dozen heart attacks among competitive cyclists. The following day, after the sixth stage of the Tour, the governing body suspended all nine members of Festina after its coach admitted supplying illegal drugs to his riders.

One week later during its world championships, the International Swimming Federation (FINA; www.fina.org), the swimming world's governing body, suspended four Chinese swimmers for 2 years for using triamterene, a banned diuretic that masks anabolic steroid use. On August 6, 1998, the organization banned from competition for 4 years the Irish swimmer who won three gold medals at the 1996 Summer Olympics, accusing her of manipulating a drug test by spiking her urine sample with alcohol to mask forbidden performance-enhancing drugs. Germany's leading Paralympian became the first athlete ejected from a Winter Paralympics for a doping scandal. He was stripped of two gold medals (biathlon and 5-km cross-country skiing) on March 12, 2002, and ejected from the Salt Lake Winter Games after testing positive for methenolone, a muscle-building steroid. In January 2003, a member of the United States Pan American Games swim team tested positive for 19-norandrosterone (a prohibited steroid), for which the swimmer received a 4-year ban from competition by the United States Anti-Doping Agency (USDA). The

USADA now offers online (www.usantidoping.org/) information for medical professionals, trainers, athletes, and others involved in sports medicine on whether specific U.S. pharmaceutical products and some over-the-counter medicinal products are permitted for use by athletes.

Researchers worldwide were gratified following the 2004 Athens Olympics because improvements in doping control apparently had a major impact on sports performance. FIGURE 23.1 shows the lack of improvement in new world records, mainly in track and field, as evidence that the drug-tainted past has temporarily been put on hold. Twenty-three athletes were barred from the 2004 games and only one world record was tied (12.92 s in the 110-m men's hurdles). Note particularly the decline in men and women's performances in the shot put, discus, javelin, and long jump.

ON THE HORIZON

The day may be near when individuals born lacking certain "lucky" genes that augment growth and development and exercise performance will simply add them, doping undetectably with DNA not drugs. In these instances, the use of "gene doping" misappropriates the medical applications of gene therapy that treats atherosclerosis, cystic fibrosis, and other diseases. Gene doping offers the promise to increase the size, speed, and strength of healthy humans. Genes that cause muscles to enlarge would be ideal for sprinters, weight lifters, and other power athletes. Endurance athletes would benefit from genes that boost red blood cell production (e.g., gene for erythropoietin) or stimulate blood vessel development (e.g., gene for vascular endothelial growth factor). The world of sports doping has changed dramatically in the past 10 years, and it seems that thrust will continue, but this time with a new arsenal of "magic bullet" genetically engineered drugs.

The following chart presents six mechanisms by which diverse agents might induce ergogenic effects.[151]

MECHANISM FOR HOW PURPORTED ERGOGENIC AIDS MIGHT WORK

- Act as a central or peripheral nervous system stimulant (e.g., caffeine, choline, amphetamines, alcohol)
- Increase storage and/or availability of a limiting substrate (e.g., carbohydrate, creatine, carnitine, chromium)
- Act as a supplemental fuel source (e.g., glucose, medium-chain triacylglycerols)
- Reduce or neutralize performance-inhibiting metabolic byproducts (e.g., sodium bicarbonate or sodium citrate, pangamic acid, phosphate)
- Facilitate recovery (e.g., high-glycemic carbohydrates, water)

Men	World Record (Year)	2004 Winning Time/Distance	Percentage Difference from World Record
100M	9.78 (2002)	9.85	- 0.7
200M	19.32 (1996)	19.79	- 2.4
400M	43.18 (1999)	44.00	- 1.9
800M	1:41.11 (1997)	1:44.45	- 3.3
1500M	3:26.00 (1998)	3:34.20	- 4.0
5000M	12:37.35 (2004)	13.14.39	- 4.9
10,000M	26:20.31 (2004)	27:05.10	- 2.8
Steeplechase	7:55.28 (2001)	8:05.80	- 2.2
110M Hurdles	12.91 (1993)	12.91	Tied World Record
400M Hurdles	46.78 (1992)	47.63	- 1.8
Shot-put	75.10 1/4 (1990)	69-5 1/4	- 8.5
Discus	243 (1986)	229-3 1/2	- 5.7
Hammer	284-7 (1986)	272-11 1/4	- 4.1
Javelin	323-1 (1996)	283-9 1/2	- 12.2
Long Jump	29-4 1/2 (1991)	28-2 1/4	- 4.0
Triple Jump	60- 1/4 (1995)	58-4 1/2	- 2.7
High Jump	8- 1/2 (1993)	7-8 3/4	- 3.7
Pole Vault	20- 1 3/4 (1994)	19-6 1/4	- 3.1
Decathlon	9026 (2001)	8893	- 1.5

Women	World Record (Year)	2004 Winning Time/Distance	Percentage Difference from World Record
100M	10.49 (1988)	10.93	- 4.2
200M	21.34 (1988)	22.05	- 3.2
400M	47.60 (1985)	49.41	- 3.8
800M	1:53.28 (1983)	1:56.38	- 2.7
1500M	3:50.46 (1993)	3:57.90	- 3.2
5000M	14:24.68 (2004)	14.45.65	- 2.4
10,000M	29:31.78 (2004)	30:24.36	- 3.0
110M Hurdles	12.21 (2001)	12.37	- 1.3
400M Hurdles	52.34 (1993)	52.82	- 0.9
Shot-put	74-3 (1987)	64- 3 1/4	- 13.4
Discus	252 (1988)	219- 10 1/2	- 12.7
Hammer	249-7 (1999)	246-1 1/2	- 1.4
Javelin	234-8 1/2 (2001)	234-8 1/4	- 0.01
Long Jump	24-8 (1988)	23-2 1/2	- 6.0
Triple Jump	50-10 1/4 (1995)	50-2 1/2	- 1.3
High Jump	6- 10 1/4 (1987)	6-9	- 1.4
Pole Vault	16- 3/4 (2004)	16-11/4	+ 0.20
Heptathlon	7291 (1988)	6952	- 4.7

Figure 23.1 Track and field world records compared with 2004 Athens Olympic performances. Negative values *(red)* reflect poorer performances in Athens for men *(top)* and women *(bottom)*. Note the *gold-colored area* for the shot-put, discus, hammer, and javelin events that emphasize muscular strength and power.

PHARMACOLOGIC AGENTS

Many athletes use pharmacologic agents, believing that a specific drug can improve skill, strength, power, or endurance. Athletes go to great lengths to promote all aspects of their health; they train hard, eat well-balanced meals, and seek and receive medical advice for various injuries (no matter how minor). Yet ironically, they will ingest synthetic agents, many of which precipitate adverse effects ranging from nausea, hair loss, itching, and nervous irritability to severe consequences such as sterility, liver disease, drug addiction, and even death caused by liver and blood cancer.

The IOC currently bans the following seven categories of substances:

1. Stimulants
2. Narcotic analgesics
3. Androgenic–anabolic steroids
4. β-Blockers
5. Diuretics
6. Peptide hormones and analogues
7. Substances that alter urine sample integrity

The competitive athlete should contact the United States Anti-Doping Agency (USADA: www.usantidoping.org/) for the latest information about doping. Another organization, the World Anti-Doping Agency or WADA (www.wada-ama.org) publishes a 31-page guide to prohibited substances and the intricacies of the comprehensive doping control process. In 2003, the World Anti-Doping Code (**the Code**) was unanimously approved by sports organizations and governments and entered into force on 1 January 2004. The downloadable Code ensures uniformity concerning rules and regulations governing antidoping for all athletes in all sports and in all countries.

Anabolic Steroids

Anabolic steroids gained prominence in the early 1950s for medical purposes to treat patients deficient in natural androgens or with muscle-wasting diseases. Other legitimate steroid uses include treatment of osteoporosis and severe breast cancer in women and countering the excessive decline in lean body mass and increase in body fat often observed in elderly men, HIV patients, and individuals who undergo kidney dialysis.[71]

Prescription use of steroids is legal in the United States. However, the Anabolic Steroid Control Act of 1990 criminalizes the sale and possession of any anabolic steroid intended for nonmedical use. It also is a felony to buy a known counterfeit steroid or one not approved by the Food and Drug Administration (FDA). Screening for anabolic steroid use among competitive athletes includes measuring the ratio of testosterone to luteinizing hormone (T:LH) in urine or testosterone to epitestosterone (T:E). A urinary T:LH ratio ≥ 30 provides a more sensitive marker of anabolic steroid use than the urinary T:E ratio ≥ 6.0, currently the prohibited level set by the IOC.

INTEGRATIVE QUESTION

A student maintains that a chemical compound added to his diet produced profound improvements in weight-lifting performance. Your review of the research literature indicates no ergogenic benefits for this compound. How would you reconcile the discrepancy?

Up to 4 million athletes (90% of male and 80% of female professional bodybuilders) currently use androgens, often combined with stimulants, hormones, and diuretics, believing their use augments training effectiveness. Even in the sport of baseball, *estimates* based on interviews of strength trainers and current players indicate that up to 30% of professionals use anabolic steroids in their quest to enhance performance.

Structure and Action

Anabolic steroids function in a manner similar to testosterone, the chief male hormone. By binding with receptor sites on muscle and other tissues, testosterone contributes to male secondary sex characteristics. This includes gender differences in muscle mass and strength that develop at puberty onset. Testosterone production takes place mainly in the testes (95%), with the adrenal glands producing the remainder. Synthetically manipulating the steroid's chemical structure to increase muscle growth (from anabolic tissue building and nitrogen retention) reduces the hormone's androgenic or masculinizing effects. A masculinizing effect of synthetically derived steroids still exists, particularly in females.

Athletes typically combine multiple steroid preparations in oral and injectable form, a practice called **stacking**, because they believe that the various androgens differ in physiologic action. They also progressively increase drug dosage—a practice called **pyramiding**—usually in 6- to 12-week cycles. The drug quantity far exceeds the recommended medical dose, often by 40-fold. The athlete then progressively reduces drug dosage in the months before competition to lower the chance of detection during drug testing. The difference between dosages used in research studies and those used by athletes contributes to the credibility gap between scientific findings (often, no effect of steroids) and what most in the athletic community believe to be true. TABLE 23.1 lists examples of oral and injectable anabolic steroids, including typical retail cost and black market prices. Black market prices vary considerably in different domestic regions and internationally: conservative estimates suggest at least twice the retail cost up to 100 times retail!

Designer Drug Unmasked. Researchers in the Department of Molecular and Medical Pharmacology at UCLA's Olympic Analytical Laboratory have recently unmasked an illegal "designer" compound that mimics the chemical structure of the banned steroids gestrinome and trenbolone. Discovery of this new stand-alone steroid chemical entity, not a "pro-steroid" or "precursor steroid" like many performance-boosting substances on the market, introduced a drug with no prior

IN A PRACTICAL SENSE

COMMONLY USED HERBAL COMPOUNDS FOR EXERCISE AND TRAINING: USER BEWARE

■ Aside from the influence of genetics and proper training, nutrition often exerts an important influence on athletic performance. In seeking the competitive edge, exercise enthusiasts and athletes fall prey to fad diets and unnecessary supplements whose potency, quality, and effectiveness lack scientific validation. Athletes often eat a suboptimal diet, particularly when attempting to reduce body weight while training strenuously. This leads to the use of a diverse array of "nutritional" supplements, including herbal compounds (used by 23% of U.S. adults), in the hope of overcoming nutritional inadequacies and ensuring optimal performance and training responsiveness.

Intake of a broad range of herbal compounds as supplements for ergogenic purposes has expanded considerably during the last decade. Aside from the lack of documentation concerning the efficacy of these chemicals, many carry the potential for health risk. The prudent coach and exercise specialist should know the common herbs used by athletes and their purported effects, contraindications, and possible adverse side effects. The table lists the more popular herbs with uses, active ingredients, common dosage, and precautionary information.

HERBS FREQUENTLY USED TO IMPROVE HEALTH, REDUCES STRESS, ELEVATE EMOTIONAL AND COGNITIVE RESPONSES, ENHANCE MUSCULAR DEVELOPMENT AND EXERCISE PERFORMANCE, AND SPEED RECOVERY

HERB	OTHER NAME	PURPORTED USE/BENEFIT	ACTIVE INGREDIENTS	DOSAGE	SIDE EFFECTS/ INTERACTIONS/ COMMENTS
Astragulus	*Huang qi*	Supports immune system; benefits cardiovascular system; increases energy level; promotes tissue repair	Flavonoids, polssaccharides, triterpene glycosides, amino acids, and trace minerals	$9–15\ g \cdot d^{-1}$	None
Bilberry	*Vaccinium myrtillus*	Diabetes; macular degeneration; retinopathy	Anthocyanosides (bioflavonoid)	$240–600\ mg \cdot d^{-1}$ as herbal extract or $20–60\ g \cdot d^{-1}$ fruit	None
Bee pollen	*Buckwheat pollen; puhuang*	Allergies; asthma; cholesterol and triacylglycerol lowering	Protein, carbohydrates, minerals, and essential fatty acids	$500–1000\ mg \cdot d^{-1}$	Allergic reactions; avoid with hypoglycemic agents
Chamomile	*Camomile, roman camomile*	Stress reduction; supports immune function; assists sleep; promotes tissue repair	α-Bisabol; bioflavonoids	Taken as tea 3 to 4 times per day	Avoid if allergic to plants
Echinacea	*Echinacea purpurea; echinacea angustifolia*	Common cold/sore throat; immune function; infection; influenza	Alkylamides, polyacetylenes; increases interferon production	At onset of cold or flu; $3–4\ mL \cdot 2h^{-1}$ or $300\ mg$ powder $\cdot d^{-10}$	Avoid if allergic to sunflower plant family
Ephedra	*Ephedra sinica; Ephedra equisetina*	Asthma; cough; weight loss; increases energy level	Alkaloids ephedrine and pseudo-ephedrine	$1.5–6\ g \cdot d^{-1}$ in tea form; $12.5–25$ $mg \cdot 4\ h^{-1}$ as over-the-counter drug	Banned substance; amphetamine-like side effects; avoid with hypertension or pregnancy

continued on page 561

Continued

Herb	Other Name	Purported Use/Benefit	Active ingredients	Dosage	Side Effects/ Interactions/ Comments
Garlic	*Allium sativum*	High blood pressure; high triacylglycerols; intermittent claudication	Sulfer compound allicin	600–900 mg · d^{-1}	Avoid with stomach problems; heartburn, gastritis, or ulcers
Ginseng, Asian	*Pannax*	Mental alertness; memory; physical endurance; type 2 diabetes; hyperlipidemia; congestive heart failure	Eleutherosides	200–600 mg · d^{-1}	Avoid with hypertension, heart disease; pregnancy and lactation; nervousness; fever or sleep disorders
Ginseng, Siberian	*Eleuthero root*	Physical endurance; fatigue prevention; immune function; motion sickness	Eleutherosides	200–600 mg · d^{-1}	Avoid with hypertension, heart disease, pregnancy, and lactation; nervousness; fever or sleep disorders
Ginkgo biloba	*Maidenhair tree*	Age-related cognitive decline; Alzheimer's disease; intermittent claudication; depression; atheroscleroisis; impotence (of vascular origin)	Gingko flavone glycosides (bioflavonoid), terpene (lactones)	120–240 mg · d^{-1}	Mild headaches lasting 1 or 2 days; mild upset stomach
Guarana	*Paullinia cupana*	Fatigue prevention; weight loss	Guaranine (identical to caffeine)	200–800 mg · d^{-1}	Avoid with pregnancy, glucoma, heart disease, high blood pressure, history of stroke
Kava Kava	*Piper methysticum*	Anxiety; restlessness; stress, muscle relaxing	Kava-lactones	200–250 mg · d^{-1}	Avoid with pregnancy or if lactating; can cause drowsiness
Milk thistle	*Silybum marianum*	Alcohol-related liver disease; hepatitis; liver support	Bioflavonoid complex-silymarin	200–400 mg · d^{-1}	None
Glucosamine sulfate[a]		Osteoarthritis; joint inflammation; joint stiffness		1500 mg · d^{-1}	Avoid with diabetes
Grape seed extract		Circulatory disorders; varicose veins; atherosclerosis		75–300 mg · d^{-1}	None
Saw palmetto	*Serenoa repens, sabal serrulata*	Benign prostatic hyperplasia; urination problems in males	Liposterolic extract of saw palmetto provides fatty acids, sterols, and esters	200–300 mg · d^{-1}	None
St. John's wort	*Hypericum perforatum*	Depression; anxiety or nervous unrest; mood disturbance of menopause	Hypericin, flavonoids	900 mg · d^{-1}	Heightens sun sensitivity; interferes with iron absorption
Witch hazel	*Hamamelis virginiana*	Eczema; hemorrhoids; varicose veins	Tannins and volatile oils	As ointment or cream 3–4 times · d^{-1}	Not for internal use; causes stomach irritation
Yohimbe	*Pausinystalia ohimbe*	Impotence; depression	Yohimbine (alkaloid)	15–30 mg · d^{-1}	Use only under medical supervision
Valerian	*Heliotrope; setwall; vandal root*	Stress reduction; improves sleep; benefits cardiovascular system	Essential oils	300–500 mg before sleep	None

[a]Not truly listed as an herb; usually listed as a supplement.
From Fetrow C, Avila JR. Professionals handbook of complementary & alternative medicines. Springhouse, PA: Springhouse Corporation, 1999; and Schuyler W, et al. The natural pharmacy. 2nd ed. Rocklin, CA: Healthnotes, 1999.

TABLE 23.1 ■ EXAMPLES OF ORAL AND INJECTABLE ANABOLIC STEROIDS, INCLUDING TYPICAL RETAIL COST AND BLACK MARKET PRICES

GENERIC NAME	COMMERCIAL NAME	FORM[a]	RETAIL COST[b]	BLACK MARKET[b] COST
Oxymetholone	Anadrol-50	Oral; 50 mg	$115/100 tabs	$300–700
Oxandrolone	Oxandrin	Oral; 2.5 mg	$420/100 tabs	$850–2200
Stanazolol	Winstrol V	Oral; 2 mg	$100/100 tabs	$300–700
Nandrolone phenpropionate	Durabolin Nandrobolic	Injectable; 25 mg · mL^{-1}	$27/5 mL vial	$300–700
Nandrolone deconate	Deca-Durabolin Neo-Durabolic Androlone-D 200	Injectable; 50 mg · mL^{-1}	$12/2 mL vial	$500–900

[a] Anabolic steroids are taken by mouth or injected into a muscle. Tablets or capsules taken by mouth are often called "orals." Oral androgens do not metabolize into testosterone but act directly on androgen receptors. The injectable forms, known as "oils" or "waters," usually have longer lasting effects than orals. Injectables release slowly into the body once the injection enters a muscle (usually the buttocks). One injection (at normal concentrations prescribed medically) can maintain normal serum testosterone levels for 10–14 days. Oral androgens are not as biologically active as injectable forms.
[b] 2005 typical retail prices in the Amherst/Boston area. Prices vary depending on country and local conditions. The black market price reflects a range of prices from various sources, 2005.

record of manufacture or existence. The USADA, which oversees drug testing for all sports federations under the U.S. Olympic umbrella, said that an anonymous tipster provided a syringe sample of the steroid identified as tetrahydrogestrinone, or THG. The researchers developed a new test to detect THG, apparently taken not by injection but in droplets under the tongue. They then reanalyzed 350 urine samples from participants at the U.S. track and field championships in June 2003 and 100 samples from random out-of-competition tests. A remarkably high half-dozen athletes tested positive. On October 17, 2003, the National Football League began testing players for THG to avoid the scandal that has embarrassed track and field. The USADA specifically states: "The use of dietary/nutritional supplements is completely at the athlete's own risk, even if the supplements are 'approved' or 'verified'."

In subsequent events, scientists with WADA announced on February 1, 2005, the discovery of a designer steroid of considerable more complexity than THG. The drug was uncovered after an anonymous e-mail tip directed the agency to investigate a substance seized by Canadian customs officials in June 2004. The drug desoxymethyltestosterone, dubbed DMT, is a clear, oily substance modified from methyltestosterone. Although no evidence exists of use of the drug by athletes, scientists with the antidoping agency, Canadian customs, and the University of Laval in Quebec are working to uncover the structure of the compound and its metabolic pathways and developing a test for it in the urine.

On October 23, 2003, the **American College of Sports Medicine (ACSM)**, the largest sports medicine and exercise science organization in the world (www.acsm-msse.org), issued a statement that called for increased vigilance in identifying and eradicating steroid use. They condemned the development and use of new "designer" steroids such as THG that are cloaked to avoid detection. ACSM considers the use of these chemicals "serious threats to the health and safety of athletes, as well as detriments to the principle of fair play in sports. Any effort to veil or disguise steroid use in sports through stealth, designer, or precursor means, puts elite, amateur and even recreational athletes at risk."

A Drug with a Considerable Following

One often pictures steroid abusers as extremely muscular bodybuilders, but abuse is also frequent among competitive athletes in road cycling, tennis, track and field, American collegiate and professional football, and swimming. Surveys of United States Powerlifting Team members indicate that up to two thirds used androgenic–anabolic steroids.[74] Many competitive and recreational athletes obtain steroids on the black market. Thus, misinformed individuals may take massive and prolonged dosages without medical monitoring and suffer harmful alterations in physiologic function.

Steroid abuse among adolescents and its accompanying risks, including extreme virilization and premature cessation of bone growth, remains particularly worrisome. Boys and girls as young as 11 years of age use anabolic–androgenic steroids.[100] Teenagers cite improved athletic performance as the most common reason for taking steroids, although 25% acknowledge enhanced appearance as a main reason. In this regard, a body image disturbance may contribute to anabolic steroid abuse among teenagers and young men.[366] The National Institutes of Drug Abuse, an arm of the National Institutes of Health, claims that steroid use among high school sophomores more than doubled nationwide between 1992 and 2000. A Blue Cross/Blue Shield national survey noted a 25% increase in steroid and similar drug use from 1999 to 2000 among boys ages 12 to 17. These findings run counter to the Healthy People 2010 report that indicates a decline in steroid use of 2.8% for male and 0.3% for female high school seniors based on 1998 data.[324] Abuse of doping agents appears to be a new public health problem, not just confined to athletes, which requires detection, medical care, and prevention.[93]

Effectiveness Questioned

For five decades, researchers and athletes have debated the true effect of anabolic steroids on human body composition and exercise performance. Much of the confusion about the ergogenic effectiveness of anabolic steroids stems from variations in experimental design, lack of control groups, specific drugs and dosages, treatment duration, accompanying nutritional supplementation, training intensity, evaluation techniques, previous experience of subjects, and individual differences in responsiveness to a drug's effectiveness.[138,139] The relatively small residual androgenic effect of the steroid facilitates central nervous system activation to make the athlete more aggressive (so-called *roid rage*), competitive, and fatigue resistant. Such facilitatory effects allow the person to train harder for a longer time or to believe that augmented training effects have actually occurred. Abnormal mood alterations and psychiatric dysfunction sometimes accompany androgen use.[60,111,311,314]

Research with animals suggests that anabolic steroid treatment combined with exercise and adequate protein intake stimulates protein synthesis and increases muscle protein content (myosin, myofibrillar, sarcoplasmic factors).[276] In contrast, other research revealed that steroid treatment did not benefit leg muscle weight of rats subjected to functional overload by surgical removal of the synergistic muscle.[211] Treatment with anabolic steroids did not complement functional overload to stimulate additional muscular development.

The situation with humans is difficult to interpret. Some studies show that steroid use by men who train augments body mass gains and reduces body fat, while other studies show no effect on strength and power or body composition, even with sufficient energy and protein intake to support an anabolic effect.[106,188,361] When steroid use produces body weight gains, the compositional nature of the gains (water, muscle, fat) remains unclear. Patients receiving dialysis and those infected with the HIV virus commonly experience malnutrition, a decrease in muscle mass, and chronic fatigue. Dialysis patients given 6 months of supplementation with the anabolic steroid nandrolone decanoate increased lean body mass and level of daily function.[165] Similarly, in men with HIV, a moderately supraphysiologic androgen regimen that included the anabolic steroid oxandrolone increased lean tissue accrual and strength gains from resistance training substantially more than physiologic testosterone replacement alone.[310]

Dosage Is an Important Factor

In many instances, dosage variations contribute to the confusion and create a credibility gap between scientist and steroid user regarding effectiveness. One study focused on 43 healthy men with some resistance-training experience. Experimental controls accounted for diet (energy and protein intake) and exercise (standard weight lifting, 3 times weekly) with steroid dosage (600 mg of testosterone enanthate injected weekly or placebo) exceeding values in previous studies with humans. FIGURE 23.2 illustrates changes from baseline values for fat-free body mass (FFM; hydrostatic weighing), triceps and quadriceps cross-sectional muscle areas (magnetic resonance imaging),

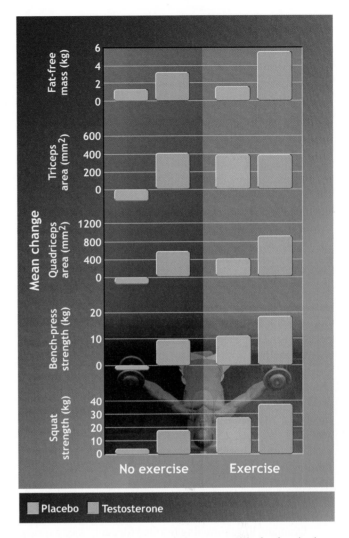

Figure 23.2 Changes from baseline in average fat-free body mass, tricep and quadricep cross-sectional areas, and muscle strength in bench press and squatting exercises over 10 weeks of testosterone treatment. (From Bhasin S, et al. The effects of supraphysiological doses of testosterone on muscle size and strength in normal men. N Engl J Med 1996;335:1.)

and muscle strength (1-RM) after 10 weeks of treatment. The men who received the hormone while continuing to train gained about 0.5 kg of lean tissue weekly with no increase in body fat. Even the group receiving the drug without training increased muscle mass and strength compared with men receiving the placebo. However, their increases averaged less than men who trained while taking testosterone. The researchers emphasized that that they did not design the study to justify or endorse steroid use for athletic purposes because of the health risks (see below). These data indicated the potential for medically supervised anabolic steroid treatment to restore and enhance muscle mass in individuals suffering from tissue-wasting diseases.

Risks Do Exist

Whether anabolic steroid use by athletes carries health risks remains controversial because research on risk has involved medical observations of hospitalized patients treated for anemia, renal insufficiency, impotence, or pituitary gland dysfunction. [*In our opinion, the infrequent but distinct possibility of harmful side effects from anabolic steroids, particularly orally administered steroids, greatly outweighs any potential ergogenic effect.*] Prolonged high dosages of steroids (often at levels 10 to 200 times therapeutic recommendations) can lead to long-lasting impairment of normal testosterone endocrine function. In male power athletes, for example, 26 weeks of steroid administration reduced serum testosterone to less than one half the level when the study began, with the effect lasting throughout a 12- to 16-week follow-up.[106] Infertility, reduced sperm concentrations (azoospermia), and decreased testicular volume pose additional problems for the steroid user.[114] Gonadal function usually returns to normal within several months. Other hormonal alterations during steroid use by males include a sevenfold increase in estradiol concentration, the major female hormone. The higher estradiol level represented the average value for normal females; this possibly explains the **gynecomastia** (usually irreversible, excessive development of the male mammary glands, sometimes secreting milk) often reported when taking anabolic steroids.

Steroid use with exercise training may damage connective tissue to decrease tendon tensile strength and elastic compliance.[198] Steroids also cause (1) chronic stimulation of the prostate gland (with possible size increase), (2) injury and functional alterations in cardiovascular function and myocardial cell cultures, (3) decreased diastolic relaxation and exacerbation of normal cardiac hypertrophy with resistance training, and (4) increased blood platelet aggregation.[3,82,83,121,140,172,313] The latter effect could compromise cardiovascular system health and function and possibly increase risk of stroke and myocardial infarction.

Dramatic life shortening resulted for adult mice exposed for 6 months to the type and relative levels of steroids used by athletes. One year after termination of steroid exposure, 52% of mice given a high steroid dose died compared with 35% given a low steroid dosage and only 12% of the control animals given no exogenous hormones (FIG. 23.3). Autopsy of steroid-treated mice revealed a broad array of pathologic effects that did not appear until long after steroid use ceased— liver and kidney tumors, lymphosarcomas, and heart damage, frequently in combination. A 6-month exposure represents about one fifth of a male mouse's life expectancy, a relative duration considerably longer than exposure of most humans to steroid use. Liver damage, represents a typical effect in athletes who take steroids. If such findings prove applicable to humans, several decades may elapse before the true negative effects of anabolic steroid use emerge.

Steroid Use and Life-Threatening Disease. TABLE 23.2 lists adverse effects and medical risks of anabolic steroid use. Concern centers on possible links between androgen abuse and abnormal liver function.[220] Because the liver almost exclusively metabolizes androgens, it becomes susceptible to damage from long-term steroid use and toxic excess. The development of localized blood-filled lesions, a condition called **peliosis hepatitis,** is one of the serious effects of

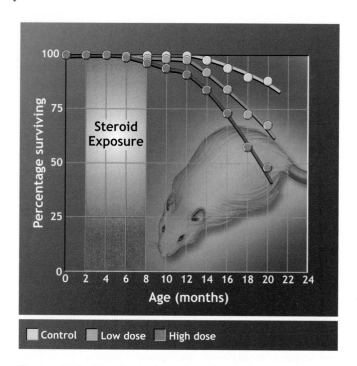

Figure 23.3 Life-shortening effects of exogenous anabolic steroid use in mice. (Modified from Bronson FH, Matherne CM. Exposure to anabolic–androgenic steroids shortens life span of male mice. Med Sci Sports Exerc 1997;29:615.)

androgens on the liver. In the extreme case, the liver eventually fails and the patient dies. We present these data not as a scare tactic but to emphasize the potentially serious adverse effects, even when a physician prescribes the drug in the recommended dosage. Patients often take steroids for a longer duration than do athletes, yet some athletes take steroids on and off for years at dosages exceeding typical therapeutic levels (50–200 mg · d^{-1} versus the usual therapeutic dosage of 5–20 mg · d^{-1}).

Steroid and Plasma Lipoproteins. Anabolic steroid use (particularly the orally active 17-alkylated androgens) by healthy men and women reduces high-density lipoprotein cholesterol (HDL-C) levels, elevates both low-density lipoprotein cholesterol (LDL-C) and total cholesterol levels, and reduces the HDL-C:LDL-C ratio.[63] Weight lifters who take anabolic steroids averaged an HDL-C level of 26 mg · dL^{-1} compared with 50 mg · dL^{-1} for weight lifters not taking this drug![171] Reducing HDL-C to this level increases a steroid user's risk of coronary artery disease. The dramatically low HDL-C levels among weight lifters remain low, even after they abstain for at least 8 weeks between consecutive steroid cycles.[283] The long-term effects of steroid use on cardiovascular morbidity and mortality remain unknown.

ACSM Position Statement on Anabolic Steroids. As part of their long-range educational program, the ACSM has taken a stand on the use of anabolic–androgenic steroids. We endorse their position, which follows.[7]

AMERICAN COLLEGE OF SPORTS MEDICINE: POSITION STAND ON USE OF ANABOLIC STEROIDS

Based on a comprehensive survey of the world literature and a careful analysis of the claims made for and against the efficacy of anabolic–androgenic steroids in improving human physical performance, it is the position of the American College of Sports Medicine that:

- Anabolic–androgenic steroids in the presence of an adequate diet and training can contribute to increases in body weight, often in the lean mass compartment.
- The gains in muscular strength achieved through high-intensity exercise and proper diet can occur by the increased use of anabolic–androgenic steroids in some individuals.
- Anabolic–androgenic steroids *do not* increase aerobic power or capacity for muscular exercise.
- Anabolic–androgenic steroids have been associated with adverse effects on the liver, cardiovascular system, reproductive system, and psychologic status in therapeutic trials and in limited research on athletes. Until further research is completed, the potential hazards of the use of the anabolic–androgenic steroids in athletes must include those found in therapeutic trials.
- The use of anabolic–androgenic steroids by athletes is contrary to the rules and ethical principles of athletic competition as set forth by many of the sports governing bodies. The American College of Sports Medicine supports these ethical principles and deplores the use of anabolic–androgenic steroids by athletes.

Additional Risks for Females. Females have additional concerns about dangers from anabolic steroids. These include virilization (more apparent than in men), disruption of normal growth pattern by premature closure of the plates for bone growth (also for boys), altered menstrual function, dramatic increase in sebaceous gland size, acne, hirsutism (excessive body and facial hair), and generally irreversible deepening of the voice, decreased breast size, enlarged clitoris, and hair loss. Serum levels of LH, FSH, progesterone, and estrogens also decline. These may negatively affect follicle formation, ovulation, and menstrual function. The long-term effects on reproductive function, including possible sterility, require further clarification.

Clenbuterol and Other β_2-Adrenergic Agonists: Anabolic Steroid Substitutes?

Gas chromatography coupled to high-resolution mass spectrometry introduced in the 1996 Atlanta Olympic Games detects most anabolic steroid use as far back as 18 months. Extensive, random testing of competitive athletes for steroid use has ushered in a number of steroid "substitutes." These have appeared on the illicit health food, mail order, and "black market" drug network as competitors try to circumvent detection. One such drug, the sympathomimetic amine **clenbuterol** (brand names Clenasma, Monores, Novegan, Prontovent, and Spiropent) has become popular among athletes because of its purported tissue-building, fat-reducing benefits. When a body builder discontinues steroid use before competition to avoid detection and possible disqualification, the athlete substitutes clenbuterol to retard loss of muscle mass and facilitate fat burning to achieve the desirable "cut" look. Clenbuterol has particular appeal to female athletes because it does not produce the androgenic side effects of anabolic steroids.

TABLE 23.2 ■ **SIDE EFFECTS AND MEDICAL RISKS OF ANABOLIC STEROID USE**

MALES		FEMALES	
INCREASE	**DECREASE**	**INCREASE**	**DECREASE**
Testicular atrophy	Sperm count	Voice change (deepening)	Breast tissue
Gynecomastia	Testosterone levels	Facial hair	
		Menstrual irregularities	
		Clitoral enlargement	

MALES AND FEMALES		
INCREASE	**DECREASE**	**POSSIBLE**
LDL-C	HDL-C	Hypertension
LDL-C/HDL-C		Connective tissue damage
Potential for neoplastic liver disease		Myocardial damage
Aggressiveness, hyperactivity, irritability		Myocardial infarction
Withdrawal and depression when steroid use stops		Impaired thyroid function
Acne		Altered myocardial structure
Peliosis hepatitis		

Clenbuterol, one of a group of chemical compounds (albuterol, clenbuterol, salbutamol, salmeterol, terbutaline, formoterol) classified as β_2-adrenergic agonists, facilitates responsiveness of adrenergic receptors to circulating epinephrine, norepinephrine, and other adrenergic amines. A review of the available studies of animals (to our knowledge no human exercise studies have been conducted) indicates that when fed to sedentary, growing livestock in dosages in excess of those prescribed in Europe for human use for bronchial asthma, clenbuterol increases skeletal and cardiac muscle protein deposition and slows fat gain (enhanced lipolysis). It also increases FFM and decreases fat mass when administered long term at therapeutic levels to thoroughbred racehorses.[174] Clenbuterol has been used experimentally in animals to counter the effects on muscle of aging, immobilization, malnutrition, and pathologic tissue-wasting conditions. In these situations, the β_2-agonists show specific growth-promoting actions on skeletal muscle.[87,368,370] For rats, clenbuterol altered muscle fiber type distribution, inducing enlargement and increased proportion of type II muscle fibers.[73] A decrease in protein breakdown and increase in protein synthesis accounted for the animals' increased muscle size.[2,25,202]

Potential Negative Effects on Muscle, Bone, and Cardiovascular Function

Female rats treated with clenbuterol ($2 \text{ mg} \cdot \text{kg}^{-1}$) injected subcutaneously versus controls sham-injected with the same volume of fluid carrier each day for 14 days increased muscle mass, absolute maximal force-generating capacity, and hypertrophy of fast- and slow-twitch muscle fibers.[85] A negative finding was hastened fatigue during short-term, intense muscle actions. In contrast, regular exercise combined with clenbuterol decreased muscular dystrophy progression in mice, reflected by increased muscle force-generating capacity.[370] The group receiving clenbuterol experienced increased muscle fatigability and cellular deformities not noted in the exercise-only group. This negative effect on muscle structure and function may explain findings that clenbuterol treatment negated the beneficial effects of exercise training on endurance performance, despite increased muscle protein content.[150] Clenbuterol treatment induced muscular hypertrophy in young male rats but concomitantly inhibited longitudinal bone growth.[179] The negative effect on bone may relate to clenbuterol's acceleration of epiphyseal closure in the bones of growing animals and certainly would contraindicate its use for prepubescent and adolescent humans.

Echocardiographic evaluations of Standard bred mares showed that chronic clenbuterol administration, even at low therapeutic levels, alters the heart's structural dimensions, which negatively affects cardiac function.[296] Effects occurred whether the animals exercised or remained inactive. Clenbuterol also caused aortic enlargement after exercise to a degree that indicated increased risk of aortic rupture and sudden death. Clenbuterol treatment when combined with aerobic training blunts the normal training-induced increase in plasma volume in Standard bred mares; this effect accompanied decreased aerobic exercise performance and ability to recover.[173]

Clenbuterol, not approved for human use in the United States, is commonly prescribed abroad as an inhaled bronchodilator to treat obstructive pulmonary disorders. Reported short-term side effects in humans who accidentally "overdosed" from eating clenbuterol-tainted meat include: skeletal muscle tremor, agitation, palpitations, dizziness, nausea, muscle cramps, rapid heart rate, and headache. Despite such negative side effects, clenbuterol use may benefit humans in treating muscle wasting in disease, forced immobilization, and aging. Unfortunately, no data exist for potential toxicity level or its efficacy and long-term safety. Clearly, clenbuterol can not be justified or recommended as an ergogenic aid.

Other Adrenergic Agonists

Research has focused on possible strength-enhancing effects of sympathomimetic β_2-adrenergic agonists other than clenbuterol. Men with cervical spinal-cord injuries took 80 mg of metaproterenol daily for 4 weeks in conjunction with physical therapy. Increases occurred in estimated muscle cross-sectional area and elbow flexor and wrist extensor strength compared with a placebo condition.[293] Albuterol administration (16 mg $\cdot$ d^{-1} for 3 wk) without exercise training improved muscular strength 10 to 15%.[205] Therapeutic doses of albuterol also facilitated isokinetic strength gains from slow-speed concentric/eccentric isokinetic training.[51]

Training State Makes a Difference

Animals. Untrained skeletal muscle of animals responds to the effects of β_2-adrenergic agonists. The increase in muscle mass with clenbuterol treatment plus exercise training is more pronounced in animals without prior training experience than in trained animals that continue training and then receive this drug. [226]

Humans. Some research with humans shows augmented muscle power output with albuterol administration.[292] No ergogenic effect occurred from salbutamol on short-term performance in two 10-minute cycling trials.[64] Similarly, no effect occurred in power output during a 30-second Wingate test in nonasthmatic trained cyclists who received 360 μg (twice the normal dose administered by inhaler in 4 measured doses of 90 μg each) 20 minutes before testing.[192] In other research, twice the recommended dose of salbutamol (albuterol; 400 mg administered in four inhalations 20 minutes before exercising) did not enhance anaerobic power output, endurance performance, ventilatory threshold, or dynamic lung function of trained endurance cyclists.[231] The researchers maintained that competitive athletes should not be prohibited from these compounds because they provide no ergogenic benefit, yet "normalize" individuals with obstructive pulmonary disorders. Differences in training status may explain discrepancies among studies concerning albuterol's effect on short-term power output.

Albuterol's ergogenic benefit supposedly comes from its stimulating effects on skeletal muscle β_2-receptors to increase muscle force and power. With exercise training, the muscle β_2-receptors undergo downregulation (become less sensitive to a given stimulus) from chronic exposure to training-induced elevations in blood catecholamine levels. This makes the trained athlete *less responsive* to a sympathomimetic drug than an untrained counterpart. Additional research must verify any ergogenic benefit of exogenous β_2-adrenergic agonists, elucidate possible mechanisms for action, and determine their influence on muscle mass.

Growth Hormone: Genetic Engineering Comes to Sports

Human growth hormone (**GH** or **hGH**), also known as **somatotropin**, currently competes with anabolic steroids in the illicit market of alleged tissue-building, performance-enhancing drugs (the Atlanta Olympics were dubbed by many the "Growth Hormone Games"). The adenohypophysis of the pituitary gland produces GH, which serves as a potent anabolic and lipolytic agent in tissue-building processes and growth. Specifically, GH stimulates bone and cartilage growth, enhances fatty acid oxidation, and reduces glucose and amino acid breakdown. Reduced GH secretion accounts for some of the decrease in FFM and increase in fat mass that accompanies aging. This condition reverses somewhat with exogenous recombinant GH supplements produced by genetically engineered bacteria. Healthy elderly men who received GH supplements increased FFM (4.3%) and decreased fat mass (13.1%).[240] *Supplementation did not reverse the negative effects of aging on functional measures of muscular strength and aerobic capacity.* Men receiving the supplement also experienced hand stiffness, malaise, arthralgias, and lower-extremity edema. One of the largest studies to date determined the effects of exogenous GH over a 6-month period on changes in body composition and functional capacity of healthy men and women aged mid-60s to late 80s.[31] Men who took GH gained 7 pounds of lean body mass and reduced a similar amount of fat mass. Women gained about 3 pounds of lean body mass and lost 5 pounds of body fat compared with counterparts receiving a placebo. Unfortunately, serious side effects afflicted between 24 and 46% of the subjects. These included swollen feet and ankles, joint pain, carpal tunnel syndrome (swelling of tendon sheath over a nerve in the wrist), and development of a diabetic or prediabetic condition. As in previous research, no effects were noted for GH treatment on measures of muscular strength or endurance capacity despite increases in lean body mass.

Excessive GH production during skeletal growth produces **gigantism**, an endocrine and metabolic disorder characterized by abnormal size or overgrowth of the entire body or any of its parts. Excessive hormone production following growth cessation produces the irreversible disorder **acromegaly** that presents as enlarged hands, feet, and facial features. Medically, children who suffer from kidney failure or who produce insufficient GH receive thrice-weekly biosynthetic GH injections until adolescence to help them achieve near-normal size. In young adults with hypopituitarism, GH replacement therapy improves muscle volume, isometric strength, and exercise capacity.

No Unanimity Among Researchers

At first glance, GH use seems appealing to strength and power athletes because at physiologic levels, this hormone stimulates amino acid uptake and muscle protein synthesis while enhancing fat breakdown and conserving glycogen reserves. Unfortunately, few well-controlled studies have examined how GH supplements affect healthy subjects who undertake exercise training. In one study, six well-trained men maintained a high-protein diet while taking either biosynthetic GH or a placebo.[72] During 6 weeks of standard resistance training with GH, percentage body fat decreased and FFM increased. No changes in body composition occurred for the group training with the placebo. Subsequent investigations failed to replicate these findings. For example, 16 previously sedentary young men who participated in a 12-week resistance training program received recombinant human GH supplements ($40 \, \mu g \cdot kg^{-1} \cdot d^{-1}$) or a placebo.[369] FFM, total body water, and whole-body protein synthesis increased more in the GH recipients. No significant differences emerged between groups in fractional rate of protein synthesis in skeletal muscle, torso and limb circumferences, or muscle function in dynamic and static strength measures (TABLE 23.3). The authors attributed the greater increase in whole-body protein synthesis in the GH group to a possible increase in nitrogen retention in lean tissue other than skeletal muscle—for example, connective tissue, fluid, and noncontractile protein.

GH occurs naturally in the body, making ready detection as an ergogenic substance difficult. Blood markers are currently available for screening. Such testing requires a change in current Olympic policy that permits only urine testing. Nonprescription GH can only be obtained on the black market and often in an adulterated form. Human cadaver-derived GH (used until May 1985 by U.S. physicians to treat children of short stature) greatly increases risk for contracting Creutzfeldt-Jakob disease, an infectious, incurable, and fatal brain-deteriorating disorder. A synthetic form of GH (Protoropin and Humantrope), produced by genetic engineering, currently treats GH-deficient children (cost $20,000 to $40,000 per year). Undoubtedly, child athletes who receive GH believing they gain a competitive edge will suffer increased incidence of gigantism, while adults will develop acromegalic syndrome. Additional, less obvious side effects include insulin resistance that leads to type 2 diabetes, water retention, and carpal tunnel compression syndrome.

DHEA: A Worrisome Trend?

Dehydroepiandrosterone (**DHEA** and its sulfated ester, DHEA sulfate, or DHEAS, the most common hormone in the body) is a weak steroid hormone synthesized primarily from cholesterol by the adrenal cortex of primates. The body produces more DHEA than all other known steroids. This

TABLE 23.3 ■ MAXIMAL FORCE PRODUCTION OF KNEE EXTENSOR AND FLEXOR MUSCLE GROUPS BEFORE AND AFTER TRAINING WITH OR WITHOUT GROWTH HORMONE SUPPLEMENTS

	EXERCISE PLUS PLACEBO			EXERCISE PLUS GH		
	INITIAL	FINAL	% CHANGE	INITIAL	FINAL	% CHANGE
Concentric						
Knee extensors	212 ± 13^a	248 ± 10	17	191 ± 11	214 ± 9	12
Knee flexors	137 ± 11^a	158 ± 7	15	122 ± 12	143 ± 6	17
Isometric						
Knee extensors	220 ± 13^a	252 ± 13	14	198 ± 15	207 ± 7	5
Knee flexors	131 ± 8^a	158 ± 8	20	127 ± 13	140 ± 16	10

From Yarasheski KF, et al. Effect of growth hormone and resistance exercise on muscle growth in young men. Am J Physiol 1992;262:E261.
[a] Values are mean $\pm$ SE. Maximum force (N · m) determined using a Cybex dynamometer. Concentric force measured at $60° · s^{-1}$ angular velocity. Isometric force measured at $135°$ of knee extension. The maximum concentric force production of knee flexor and extensor muscles increased significantly in both groups ($P < .05$), but these increments and the increments in maximum isometric force production were not greater in the exercise plus GH group.

"mother hormone" has a chemical structure that closely resembles testosterone and estrogen; a small amount of DHEA and related prohormone compounds are naturally derived precursors to testosterone or other anabolic steroids. FIGURE 23.4 outlines the major pathways for synthesizing DHEA, androstenedione, and related compounds.

Because DHEA occurs naturally, the FDA exerts no control over its distribution or claims for its action and effectiveness. The Drug Enforcement Administration does not consider DHEA an anabolic steroid as defined in section 102(6) of the Controlled Substances Act. Instead, DHEA fits the definition of a dietary supplement.

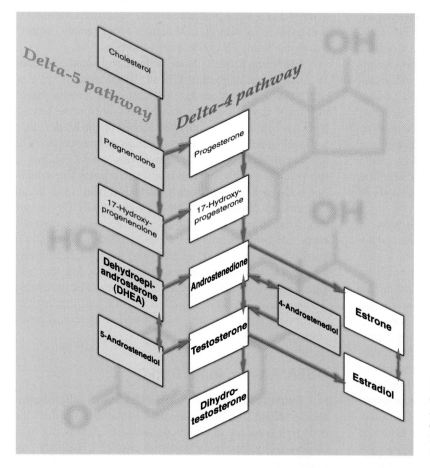

Figure 23.4 Outline of metabolic pathways for dehydroepiandrosterone (DHEA), androstenedione, and related compounds. *Directional arrows* signify one-way and two-way conversions. Compounds in *bold print* are products currently available on the market.

The lay press, mail order, and health food industry and advertisements tout DHEA as a "superhormone"—a Holy Grail that increases testosterone production; protects against cancer, heart disease, diabetes, and osteoporosis; bolsters the immune system; preserves youth; invigorates sex life; decreases joint pain and fatigue; facilitates lean tissue gain and body fat loss; enhances mood and memory and generally counters the debilitating effects of aging; and extends life. The hormone's detractors consider it the "snake oil" of the 21st century. The IOC and USOC have placed DHEA on their banned substance list at zero-tolerance levels.

FIGURE 23.5 illustrates the generalized trend for plasma DHEA levels during a lifetime, with six common claims by manufacturers of supplements. Boys and girls have substantial levels of DHEA at birth, which then decline sharply. DHEA production increases steadily from age 6 to 10 years (may contribute to the beginning of puberty and sexuality), with peak production (higher in males than females) between ages 20 and 25 years. In contrast to the glucocorticoid and mineralocorticoid adrenal steroids, whose plasma levels remain relatively high with aging, DHEA levels undergo a steady decline after age 30. By age 75, the plasma level averages only about 20% of that in young adults. This has led to speculation that plasma DHEA levels might serve as a biochemical marker of biologic aging and disease susceptibility.

Popular reasoning concludes that supplementing with DHEA blunts the negative effects of aging by raising plasma levels to more "youthful" concentrations. Many persons supplement with this "natural" hormone just in case it proves beneficial—typically without considering the potential for biologic harm.

An Unregulated Compound with Uncertain Safety

In 1994, the FDA reclassified DHEA (along with many other "natural" chemicals under the Dietary Supplement and Education Act) from the category of unapproved new drug (prescription required) to a dietary supplement for over-the-counter sale without prescription. Pharmaceutical companies synthesize DHEA from chemical ingredients or extract it from wild yams. Many consider the current unregulated and unmonitored use of DHEA (daily dosage varies from 5–10 mg to as much as 2000 mg) a disaster waiting to happen. Despite its quantitative significance as a hormone, researchers know little about DHEA with respect to the following:

- Health and aging
- Cellular or molecular mechanism(s) of action
- Possible receptor site interaction (although its sulfate interacts with brain receptors for the neurotransmitter γ-aminobutyric acid [GABA])
- Potential for adverse effects from exogenous dosage among young adults with normal DHEA levels

Appropriate DHEA dosage for humans remains uncertain. Concern exists about possible harmful effects on blood lipids, glucose tolerance, and prostate gland health, particularly because medical problems associated with hormone supplementation often do not appear until years after initiation of drug use.

Early support for DHEA comes from studies of rodents fed daily supplements. Beneficial effects included preventing cancer, atherosclerosis, viral infections, obesity, and diabetes; enhancing immune function; and even extending life span. Scientists have argued that research findings on rats and mice—who produce little if any DHEA—do not necessarily apply to healthy humans. With humans, cross-sectional observations relating DHEA levels to risk of death from heart disease provided early indirect evidence for a beneficial effect. A high DHEA level conferred protection in men; for women, elevated DHEA increased heart disease risk. Subsequent research showed only a moderate protective association for men and no association for women. Studies suggest that DHEA supplements may provide cardioprotection during aging (more beneficial in men than in

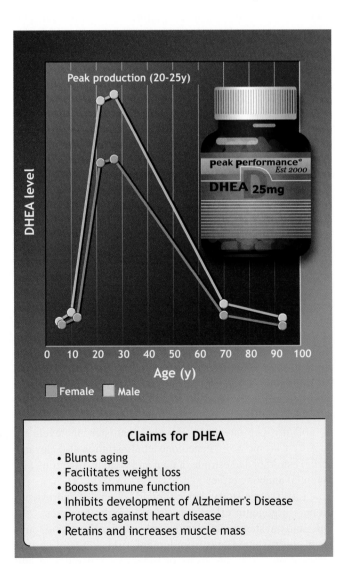

Peak production (20-25y)

peak performance® *Est 2000*

DHEA 25mg

DHEA level

0 10 20 30 40 50 60 70 80 90 100

Age (y)

☐ Female ☐ Male

Claims for DHEA

- Blunts aging
- Facilitates weight loss
- Boosts immune function
- Inhibits development of Alzheimer's Disease
- Protects against heart disease
- Retains and increases muscle mass

Figure 23.5 Generalized trend for plasma levels of DHEA for men and women over a lifetime.

women),[158] decrease abdominal fat and improve insulin sensitivity among the elderly, which could play a role in the prevention and treatment of the metabolic syndrome,[340] boost immune function in disease,[335] and provide antioxidant protection.[10]

In additional research on humans, eight men and eight women (ages 50 to 65 y) received either 100 mg of DHEA or a placebo daily for 3 months and the other treatment for the next 3 months.[224] All subjects showed a 1.2% increase in lean body mass during DHEA supplementation. Fat mass decreased in men but increased slightly in women. Chemical markers indicated improved immune function. These findings suggest some positive effects of exogenous DHEA on muscle mass and immune function in middle-aged men and women. Subsequent research evaluated short-term ingestion of 50 mg of DHEA daily on serum steroid hormones and 8 weeks supplementation (150 mg daily) on resistance-training adaptations in young men.[39] Short-term supplementation rapidly increased serum androstenedione (see next section) concentrations but exerted *no effect* on serum testosterone and estrogen concentrations. Furthermore, long-term DHEA supplementation elevated serum androstenedione levels but did not affect anabolic hormones, serum lipids, liver enzymes, muscular strength, and lean body mass, compared with a placebo for men undergoing similar training. These and similar results verify that relatively low dosages of DHEA do not increase serum testosterone levels, enhance muscular strength, change muscle and fat cross-sectional areas, or facilitate adaptations to resistance training.[245,352]

Concern exists about the effect of unregulated long-term DHEA supplementation (particularly at or above 50-mg daily) on bodily function and overall health. Converting DHEA into potent androgens such as testosterone promotes facial hair growth in females and alters normal menstrual function. Like exogenous anabolic steroids, DHEA lowers HDL-C levels to increase heart disease risk. Conflicting data concern its effects on breast cancer risk. Clinicians have expressed fear that elevating plasma DHEA by supplementation might stimulate the growth of otherwise dormant prostate gland tumors or cause benign hypertrophy of the prostate gland. If cancer exists, DHEA may accelerate its growth. *Despite its popularity among exercise enthusiasts, no data support an ergogenic effect of exogenous DHEA on young adult men and women.*

Androstenedione: Benign Prohormone Nutritional Supplement or Potentially Harmful Drug?

The over-the-counter supplement **androstenedione** (in addition to norandrostenediol and norandrostenedione, which convert to the steroid nandrolone) supposedly (1) stimulates production of endogenous testosterone or forms androgen-like derivatives (as shown in Fig 23.4), (2) enables more intense training, (3) builds muscle mass, and (4) rapidly repairs tissue injury. Found naturally in meat and some plant extracts, the World Wide Web touts androstenedione as "a prohormone, a

metabolite only one step away from the biosynthesis of testosterone." The National Football League, NCAA, Men's Tennis Association, and the IOC ban its use because they believe it provides unfair competitive advantage and may endanger health. The IOC banned the1996 Olympic shot-put gold medalist for life because he used androstenedione. Presently, Major League Baseball, the National Basketball Association, and the National Hockey League have not taken a stand against using the substance and have not banned it.

INTEGRATIVE QUESTION

Respond to the question "If testosterone, growth hormone, and DHEA occur naturally in the body, what harm could exist in supplementing with these 'natural' compounds?"

Researchers first synthesized androstenedione in the 1930s. By the late 1960s and early 1970s, sports physicians in East Germany administered androstenedione in addition to other testosterone-based steroids as part of a government-sanctioned program to enhance performance of their elite athletes. In the United States in 1994, the FDA developed rules for marketing androstenedione as a food not as a drug. By calling the substance a supplement and avoiding any claims of medical benefit, savvy marketers and distributors have created a lucrative business for androstenedione, mostly via Internet sales and over-the-counter at health food stores. Because many countries consider androstenedione a controlled substance, international athletes travel to the United States to purchase the compound, further contributing to the supplement industry's more than $15 billion yearly sales. Currently available are an androstenedione-containing chewing gum and a steroid lozenge that dissolves under the tongue.

Androstenedione is an intermediate (precursor) hormone between DHEA and testosterone; it therefore aids the liver in synthesizing other biologically active steroid hormones. Androstenedione is normally produced by the adrenal glands and gonads and converted to testosterone enzymatically by 17β-hydroxysteroid dehydrogenase found in the body's diverse tissues. It is also an estrogen precursor.

Research has demonstrated the effectiveness of exogenous androstenedione for raising testosterone levels. For example, daily oral treatment with 200 mg of 4-androstene-3,17-dione or 200 mg of 4-androstene-3β,17β-diol increased peripheral plasma total and free testosterone concentrations compared with a placebo.[89] Androstenedione dosages as high as 300 mg per day have elevated testosterone levels by 34%.[191] Chronic androstenedione administration also elevates serum estradiol and estrone in men and women, offsetting any potential anabolic effect.

Little scientific evidence supports claims of androstenedione's ergogenic effectiveness or anabolic qualities.[78,260] One study systematically evaluated whether short- and long-term androstenedione supplementation elevates blood testosterone concentrations or enhances muscle size and strength gains during resistance training. In one phase of the investigation, young-adult men received either a single 100-

mg dose of androstenedione or a placebo containing 250 mg of rice flour.[10] FIGURE 23.6A shows that serum androstenedione rose 175% during the first 60 minutes following ingestion and then increased further to about 350% above baseline values between minutes 90 and 270. However, short-term supplementation did *not* affect serum concentrations of either free or total testosterone.

In the experiment's second phase, 20 young, untrained men received 300 mg of androstenedione daily ($N = 10$) or 250 mg of a rice flour placebo during weeks 1, 2, 4, 5, 7, and 8 of an 8-week total-body resistance-training program. Serum androstenedione levels increased 100% in the androstenedione-supplemented group and remained elevated throughout training. Serum testosterone levels (Fig. 23.6B) remained higher in the androstenedione-supplemented group than the placebo group before and following supplementation. Free and total testosterone levels remained unaltered for

both groups. Serum estradiol and estrone concentrations only increased during training for the supplemented group, suggesting increased aromatization of the ingested androstenedione to estrogens (Fig. 23.6C). While resistance training increased muscle strength and lean body mass and reduced body fat for both groups, *no* synergistic effect emerged for the group supplemented with androstenedione. The supplement produced a 12% HDL-C *reduction* after only 2 weeks, which remained lower for the 8 weeks of training and supplementation. Serum liver enzyme concentrations stayed within normal limits for both groups throughout the experiment.

Taken together, these findings indicate *no effect* of androstenedione supplementation on basal serum concentrations of testosterone or training response for muscle size and strength and body composition. The potential negative effects of the HDL-C reduction on overall heart disease risk and the

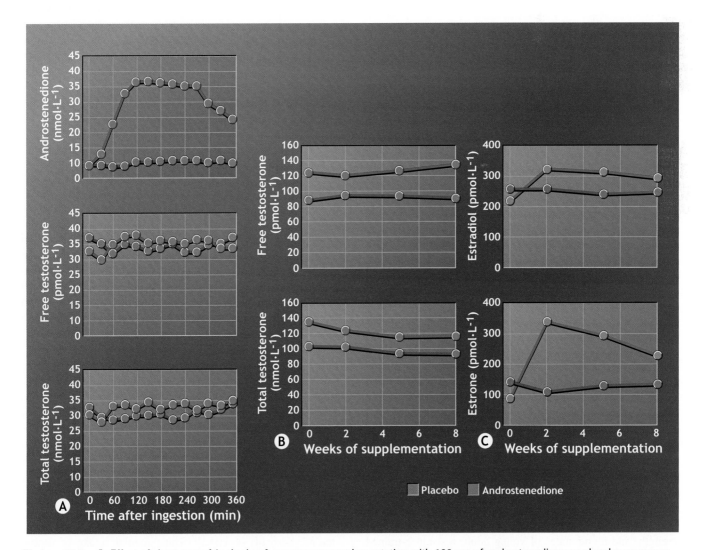

Figure 23.6   A. Effect of short-term (single dose) exogenous supplementation with 100 mg of androstenedione or placebo on serum concentrations of androstenedione and free and total testosterone. **B.** Serum free and total testosterone, and (**C**) serum estradiol and estrone with 300-mg daily supplementation of androstenedione ($N = 9$) and placebo ($N = 10$) during 8 weeks of resistance training. (From King DS, et al. Effect of oral androstenedione on serum testosterone and adaptations to resistance training in young men. JAMA 1999;281:2020.)

elevated serum estrogen levels on risk of gynecomastia and possibly pancreatic and other cancers cause concern. In addition, findings must be viewed within the context of this specific study, because subjects took smaller amounts of an-

---

RESEARCH FINDINGS CONCERNING ANDROSTENEDIONE

- Conflicting findings concerning elevation of plasma testosterone concentrations
- No favorable effect on muscle mass
- No favorable effect on muscular performance
- No favorable alterations in body composition
- Elevates a variety of estrogen subfractions
- No favorable effect on muscle protein synthesis or tissue anabolism
- Impairs blood lipid profile in healthy men
- Increases likelihood of a positive steroid test result

---

drostenedione than routinely consumed for ergogenic purposes (500 to 1200 mg per day).

Questions have concerned the legal use of androstenedione by professional baseball players during the 1998 season in their attempt to break the home run records of Babe Ruth and Roger Maris. The sport-related issues focus on whether supplementation increases muscular strength and power and whether any fitness increases transfer to improved performance in the precise motor skills required in baseball, basketball, ice and field hockey, soccer, and golf. If positive effects occur, then scientists can objectively assess any improvements in such tasks. As far as we know, no reliable evidence demonstrates such sport-specific enhancements. Longer term studies in larger groups of men and women must determine what dosage, if any, raises testosterone to high enough levels for a long enough time to provide ergogenic effects and whether such a practice is safe.

A Modified Version

Norandrostenedione and norandrostenediol are norsteroid compounds available over the counter in the United States. They are chemically similar to androstenedione and androstenediol, respectively, except with slight chemical modification that supposedly enhances anabolic properties without converting to testosterone but to the steroid nandrolone. These modifications should theoretically confer anabolic effects via the compounds' direct activation of the androgen receptors in skeletal muscle. To test this hypothesis, research evaluated 8 weeks of low-dose norsteroid supplementation on body composition, girth measures, muscular strength, and mood states of young adult, resistance-trained men.[329] The men received 100 mg of 19-nor-4-androstene-3,17-dione plus 56 mg of 19-nor-4-androstene-3,17-diol (156 mg total norsteroid per day) or a multivitamin placebo. Each subject resistance trained 4 days weekly for the duration of the

study. Norsteroid supplementation provided *no additional effect* on any of the body composition or exercise performance variables.

Competitive Athletes Beware

Elite athletes who take androstenedione can fail a urine test for the banned anabolic steroid nandrolone. This occurs because the supplement often contains contaminates with trace amounts (as low as 10 μg) of 19-norandrosterone, the standard marker for nandrolone use. Many androstenedione preparations are grossly mislabeled. Analysis of nine different brands of 100-mg doses indicate wide fluctuations in overall content ranging from zero to 103 mg of androstenedione, with one brand contaminated with testosterone.[54]

INTEGRATIVE QUESTION

Outline the points you would make in a talk to a high school football team concerning whether or not they should consider using performance-enhancing chemicals and hormones.

Regular Intake of Amino Acid Supplements for an Anabolic Effect

An emerging trend involves using nutrition as a "legal" alternative to activate the body's normal anabolic mechanisms. Highly specific dietary changes supposedly create a hormonal milieu that facilitates protein synthesis in skeletal muscle. More than 100 companies in the United States promote such alleged ergogenic stimulants. Weight lifters, bodybuilders, and fitness enthusiasts regularly use amino acid supplements, believing they boost the body's natural production of testosterone, GH, insulin, or insulin-like growth factor I (IGF-I) and so improve muscle size and strength and decrease body fat. The rationale for nutritional ergogenic stimulants comes from the clinical use of amino acid infusion or ingestion to regulate anabolic hormones in deficient patients.

Research on healthy subjects does not provide convincing evidence for an ergogenic effect of regular intake of amino acid supplements on hormone secretion, training responsiveness, or exercise performance. In studies with appropriate design and statistical analysis, oral supplements of arginine, lysine, ornithine, tyrosine, and other amino acids, either singly or in combination, produced no effect on GH levels,[104,189] insulin secretion,[43,104] diverse measures of anaerobic power,[103] or all-out running performance at $\dot{V}O_{2max}$.[307] Elite junior weight lifters who regularly supplemented with all 20 amino acids did not improve physical performance or change resting or exercise levels of testosterone, cortisol, or GH.[110] Thus, regular intake of amino acids in the quantities recommended in commercial supplements does not benefit the hormonal profile, body composition and muscle size, and exercise performance. Additionally, indiscriminate consumption of amino acid supplements at dosages considered pharmacologic rather than nutritional raises the possibility of direct toxic effects or the creation of an amino acid imbalance.[203]

Stimulating an Anabolic Effect

Manipulation and timing of intake of nutritional variables in the immediate pre- and postexercise periods can affect the responsiveness to resistance training via mechanisms that alter nutrient availability, enzyme activity, circulating metabolites and hormonal secretions, interactions with receptors on target tissues, and gene translation and transcription.[178,319,343] Resistance training stimulates protein synthesis and protein degradation in exercised muscle fibers. Muscle hypertrophy occurs when a *net increase* in protein synthesis results from a shift in the body's normal dynamic state of synthesis and degradation. The normal hormonal milieu (e.g., insulin and GH levels) in the period following resistance exercise stimulates the muscle fiber's anabolic processes while inhibiting muscle protein degradation. Dietary modifications that increase amino acid transport into muscles, raise energy availability, or increase anabolic hormones, particularly insulin, should theoretically increase the rate of anabolism and/or depress catabolism. Either effect would create a positive body protein balance to improve muscle growth and strength.

Carbohydrate–Protein Supplementation Immediately in Recovery Augments Hormonal Response to Resistance Exercise.
Studies of hormonal dynamics and protein anabolism indicate a transient but potential ergogenic effect (up to 4-fold increase in protein synthesis[259]) of carbohydrate and/or protein supplements consumed *prior to*[318,365] or *immediately following* a resistance exercise workout.[29,30,96,154,217,259,264,280,358] Supplementation in the immediate postexercise period may also enhance repair and synthesis of muscle proteins following aerobic exercise.[193,194]

Drug-free male weight lifters with at least 2 years of training experience consumed carbohydrate and protein supplements immediately after a standard workout.[55] Treatment included either (1) placebo of pure water or a supplement of (2) carbohydrate (1.5 g per kg body mass), (3) protein (1.38 g per kg body mass), or (4) carbohydrate/protein (1.06 g carbohydrate plus 0.41 g protein per kg body mass) consumed immediately following and then 2 hours following the training session. Each nutritive supplement produced a hormonal environment (elevated plasma insulin and GH concentrations) during recovery more conducive to protein synthesis and muscle tissue growth than the placebo condition. Subsequent research showed that protein–carbohydrate supplementation before and immediately following resistance training altered the metabolic and hormonal responses to 3 consecutive days of heavy resistance training.[181] Changes in the immediate recovery period included increased concentrations of glucose, insulin, GH, and IGF-I and decreased blood lactate concentration. Such data provide indirect evidence for a possible training benefit (e.g., enhanced glycogen and protein synthesis in recovery) from increasing carbohydrate or protein intake immediately after a workout. However, long-term augmented muscle growth and muscle strength from these dietary manipulations awaits documentation.

Postexercise Glucose Augments Protein Balance After Resistance-Training Workouts.
Research with postexercise glucose ingestion complements the previously described studies of carbohydrate/protein supplementation following resistance training.[279] Healthy men familiar with resistance training performed eight sets of 10 repetitions of unilateral knee extensor exercise at 85% of maximum strength in a placebo-controlled, randomized, double-blind trial. Immediately after the exercise session and 1 hour later, subjects received either a glucose supplement (1.0 g per kg body mass) or a placebo (Nutrasweet). Measurements consisted of (1) urinary 3-methylhistidine excretion (3-MH) as a marker of muscle protein degradation, (2) vastus lateralis muscle incorporation rate for the amino acid leucine (L-[I-^{13}C]leucine) to indicate protein synthesis, and (3) urinary nitrogen excretion to reflect protein breakdown. FIGURE 23.7A and B shows that glucose supplementation reduced myofibrillar protein breakdown, as reflected by decreased excretion of 3-MH and urinary nitrogen. Although not statistically significant, glucose supplementation also increased the rate of leucine incorporation into the vastus lateralis over the 10-hour postexercise period (Fig. 23.7C). These alterations all indicated a more positive body protein balance after exercise in the supplemented condition. The beneficial effect of postexercise glucose supplementation most likely occurred from increased insulin release with intake of glucose, a high-glycemic carbohydrate. Higher plasma insulin concentrations should enhance muscle protein balance in recovery.

One should view the effects of immediate postexercise carbohydrate and/or protein supplementation in perspective. The question awaiting answer concerns the degree that any transient (albeit positive) change in hormonal milieu favoring anabolism and net protein synthesis caused by postexercise dietary maneuvers contributes to long-term muscle growth and strength enhancement. In this regard, recent research failed to show any effect of immediate postexercise ingestion of an amino acid–carbohydrate mixture on muscular strength or size gains of older men undergoing 12-weeks of knee extensor resistance training.[117] Differences in study population, criterion variables, specific amino acid mixtures, overall diet composition, and subjects' age may account for future discrepancies in research findings.

Dietary Lipid May Affect Hormonal Milieu.
The diet's lipid content may modulate resting neuroendocrine homeostasis to modify tissue synthesis and training responsiveness. Research evaluated the effects of an intense resistance-exercise bout on postexercise plasma testosterone.[345] In agreement with prior research, testosterone levels increased 5 minutes postexercise. A more impressive finding was a close association between the macronutrient composition of the individual's regular diet and resting testosterone levels. TABLE 23.4 shows that the quantity and percentage of dietary macronutrients

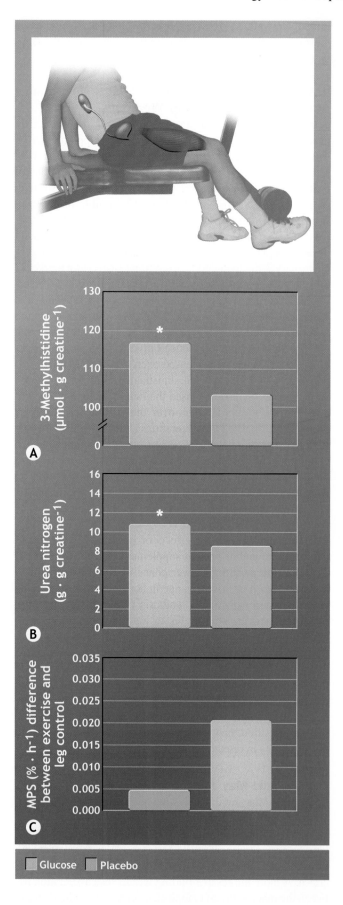

NUTRIENT	CORRELATION WITH TESTOSTERONE[a]
Energy, kJ	−0.18
Protein, %[b]	−0.71*
CHO, %[b]	−0.30
Lipid, %[b]	0.72*
SFA, g 1000 kCal^{-1} · d^{-1}	0.77†
MUFA, g 1000 kCal^{-1} · d^{-1}	0.79‡
PUFA, g 1000 kCal^{-1} · d^{-1}	0.25
Cholesterol, g 1000 kCal^{-1} · d^{-1}	0.53
PUFA/SFA	−0.63‡
Dietary fiber, g 1000 kCal^{-1} · d^{-1}	−0.19
Protein/CHO	−0.59‡
Protein/lipid	0.16
CHO/lipid	0.16

TABLE 23.4 ■ RELATIONSHIPS BETWEEN PREEXERCISE TESTOSTERONE CONCENTRATION AND SELECTED NUTRITIONAL VARIABLES

[a] Correlation coefficients are Pearson product-moment correlations.
[b] Nutrient percentage values expressed as percentage of total energy per day.
*P ≤ .01; †P ≤ .005; ‡P ≤ .05.
SFA, saturated fatty acids; MUFA, monounsaturated fatty acids; PUFA, polyunsaturated fatty acids; CHO, carbohydrate.
From Volek JS, et al. Testosterone and cortisol in relationship to dietary nutrients and resistance exercise. J Appl Physiol 1997;82:49.

correlated with preexercise testosterone concentrations. Dietary lipid and saturated and monounsaturated fatty acid levels best predicted testosterone concentrations at rest—lower levels of each of these dietary components accompanied lower resting levels of testosterone. These findings support prior studies that showed that a low-fat diet (~20% fat) produced lower testosterone levels than a diet with higher lipid content (~40% fat).[256,317] The data in Table 23.4 also show that the diet's protein percentage correlated inversely with resting testosterone levels—*higher* dietary protein related to *lower* testosterone levels. Many resistance-trained athletes consume considerable dietary protein, so the implications of this association for the training response remain unresolved. If a low dietary lipid intake decreases resting testosterone levels, then in-

Figure 23.7　Effects of glucose (1.0 g per kg body mass) versus Nutrasweet placebo, ingested immediately after exercise and 1 hour later, on protein degradation reflected by 24-hour urinary output of (**A**) 3-methylhistidine, (**B**) urinary urea nitrogen, and (**C**) rate of muscle protein synthesis (MPS) measured by vastus lateralis muscle incorporation of leucine (L-[l-^{13}C]). *Bars* for MPS indicate difference between exercise and control leg for glucose and placebo conditions. * Significantly different from placebo condition. (From Roy BD, et al. Effect of glucose supplement timing on protein metabolism after resistance training. J Appl Physiol 1997;82:1882.)

dividuals who consume low-fat diets (e.g., vegetarians, dancers, gymnasts, wrestlers) may experience a diminished training response. Furthermore, athletes who show low plasma testosterone levels from overtraining may benefit from changing their diet's macronutrient composition to lower protein and higher fat.

Nutrient Timing to Optimize Muscle Response to Resistance Training

An evidence-based nutritional approach has been proposed to enhance the quality of resistance training and facilitate muscle growth and strength development.[153] This easy-to-follow new dimension to sports nutrition emphasizes not only the specific type and mixture of nutrients but also the timing of nutrient intake. Its goal is to blunt the catabolic state (release of hormones glucagon, epinephrine, norepinephrine, cortisol) and activate the natural muscle-building hormones (testosterone, growth hormone, IGF-1, insulin) to facilitate recovery from exercise and maximize muscle growth. Three phases for optimizing specific nutrient intake are proposed:

1. The *energy phase* enhances nutrient intake to spare muscle glycogen and protein, enhance muscular endurance, limit immune system suppression, reduce muscle damage, and facilitate recovery in the postexercise period. Consuming a carbohydrate/protein supplement in the immediate preexercise period and during exercise extends muscular endurance; the ingested protein promotes protein metabolism thus reducing demand for amino acid release from muscle. The carbohydrates consumed during exercise suppress release of cortisol. This blunts the suppressive effects of exercise on immune system function and lessens the use of branched-chain amino acids generated by protein breakdown for energy.

   The recommended *energy phase* supplement contains the following nutrients: 20–26 g of high-glycemic carbohydrates (glucose, sucrose, maltodextrin), 5–6 g of whey protein (rapidly digested, high-quality protein separated from milk in the cheese-making process), 1 g of leucine; 30–120 mg of vitamin C, 20–60 IU of vitamin E, 100–250 mg of sodium, 60–100 mg of potassium, and 60–220 mg magnesium. Ingestion of the more slowly digested whole protein casein after exercise produces similar increases in muscle protein net balance, resulting in a short-term net muscle protein synthesis compared with whey protein.[319]

2. The *anabolic phase* consists of the 45-minute postexercise metabolic window—a period of enhanced insulin sensitivity for muscle glycogen replenishment and repair and synthesis of muscle tissue. This shift from catabolic to anabolic state occurs largely by blunting the action of the catabolic hormone cortisol and increasing the anabolic, muscle-building effects of the hormone insulin by consuming a standard high-glycemic carbohydrate/protein supplement in liquid form (e.g., whey protein and high-glycemic carbohydrates). In essence, the high-glycemic carbohydrate consumed postexercise serves as a nutrient activator to stimulate insulin release, which, in the presence of amino acids, increases muscle tissue synthesis and decreases protein degradation.

   The recommended *anabolic phase* supplement profile contains the following nutrients: 40–50 g of high-glycemic carbohydrates (glucose, sucrose, maltodextrin), 13–15 g of whey protein, 1–2 g of leucine; 1–2 g of glutamine, 60–120 mg of vitamin C, and 80–400 IU of vitamin E.

3. The *growth phase* extends from the end of the anabolic phase to the beginning of the next workout. It represents the time period to maximize insulin sensitivity and maintain an anabolic state to accentuate gains in muscle mass and muscle strength. The first several hours *(rapid segment)* of this phase is geared to maintaining increased insulin sensitivity and glucose uptake to maximize glycogen replenishment. It also speeds elimination of metabolic wastes via increased blood flow and stimulates tissue repair and muscle growth. The next 16 to 18 hours *(sustained segment)* maintains a positive nitrogen balance. This occurs with a relatively high daily protein intake (between 0.91 and 1.2 g of protein per pound of body weight) that fosters sustained but slower muscle tissue synthesis. An adequate carbohydrate intake emphasizes glycogen replenishment.

   The recommended *growth phase* supplement contains the following nutrients: 14 g of whey protein, 2 g of casein, 3 g of leucine, 1 g of glutamine, and 2–4 g of high-glycemic carbohydrates.

Amphetamines

Amphetamines, or "pep pills," comprise a group of pharmacologic compounds that exert powerful stimulating effects on central nervous system function. Amphetamine (Benzedrine) and dextroamphetamine sulfate (Dexedrine) are used most frequently by athletes. Amphetamines exert sympathomimetic effects—their action mimics epinephrine and norepinephrine. These sympathetic hormones increase blood pressure, heart rate, cardiac output, breathing rate, metabolism, and blood glucose. Five to 20 mg of amphetamine usually exerts its effect for 30 to 90 minutes after ingestion, although its influence often persists for much longer. Amphetamines supposedly increase alertness, wakefulness, and capacity to perform work by depressing the sensation of muscle fatigue. The deaths of two famed cyclists in the 1960s during competitive road racing were attributed to amphetamine use. In one of these deaths in 1967, British Tour de France rider Tom Simpson overheated and suffered a fatal heart attack during the ascent of Mont Ventoux in Provence.

Dangers of Amphetamines

Amphetamine use in athletics makes little sense for the following reasons:

- Regular use can lead to either physiologic or emotional drug dependency. This causes a cyclical reliance on "uppers" (amphetamines) or "downers" (barbiturates)—the barbiturates reduce or tranquilize the "hyper" state brought on by amphetamines.
- General side effects include headache, tremulousness, agitation, fever, dizziness, and confusion, all of which negatively affect sports performance that requires rapid reaction and judgment and a high level of steadiness and mental concentration.
- Larger doses are required to achieve the same effect because drug tolerance increases with prolonged use; this can aggravate and precipitate cardiovascular disorders.
- Inhibition or suppression of the body's normal mechanisms for perceiving and responding to pain, fatigue, or heat stress jeopardizes health and safety.
- Effects of prolonged intake of high doses remain unknown.

Amphetamine Use and Athletic Performance

TABLE 23.5 summarizes the results of seven experiments on amphetamines and physical performance. In general, amphetamines did not affect exercise capacity or performance of simple psychomotor tasks.

Athletes take amphetamines to "get up" for the event and keep psychologically ready to compete. The day or evening before a contest, competitors often become nervous and irritable and have difficulty relaxing. Under these circumstances, a barbiturate induces sleep. The athlete then regains the hyper condition by popping an "upper" prior to competition. Individuals knowledgeable about these drugs urge banning them from sport competition. The IOC, American Medical Association, and international sport-governing groups disqualify athletes for amphetamine use. Ironically, most research indicates that amphetamines do *not* enhance physical performance. Perhaps their greatest influence lies in the psychologic realm; athletes are easily convinced that any supplement augments performance. A placebo containing an inert substance often produces similar results!

Caffeine

Caffeine represents a possible exception to the general rule against taking stimulants. Caffeine's classification and prior regulatory status depends on its use as either a drug (over-the-counter migraine products), food (in coffee and soft drinks), or dietary supplement (alertness products).[105] The most widely consumed behaviorally active substance in the world, caffeine belongs to a group of lipid-soluble purines (proper chemical name, 1,3,7-trimethylxanthine), found naturally in coffee beans, tea leaves, chocolate, cocoa beans, and cola nuts and

TABLE 23.5 ■ EFFECTS OF AMPHETAMINES ON ATHLETIC PERFORMANCE

STUDY	DOSE (MG)	EXPERIMENT	EFFECT OF AMPHETAMINES
(1)	10–20	Two all-out treadmill runs with 10-min rest between runs	None
		Consecutive 100-yd swims with 10-min rest intervals	None
		220–440-yd swims for time	None
		220-yd track runs for time	None
		100-yd to 2-mile track runs for time	None
(2)	10	Bench stepping to fatigue carrying weights equal to one-third body mass, 3 times with 3-min rest intervals	None
(3)	5	100-yd swim for speed	None
(4)	15	All-out treadmill runs	None
(5)	10	Stationary cycling at work rates of 275–2215 kg-m · min^{-1} for 25–35 min followed by a treadmill run to exhaustion	None on submaximal or maximal $\dot{V}O_2$, heart rate, ventilation volume, or blood lactate; time on the bicycle and treadmill increased significantly
(6)	20	Reaction and movement time to a visual stimulus	None; subjective feelings of alertness or lethargy unrelated to reaction or movement time
(7)	5	Psychomotor performance during a simulated airplane flight	Enhanced performance and lessened fatigue; if preceded by secobarbital (barbiturate), performance decreased

1. Karpovich PV. Effect of amphetamine sulfate on athletic performance. JAMA 1959;170:558.
2. Foltz EE, et al. The influence of amphetamine (Benzedrine) sulfate and caffeine on the performance of rapidly exhausting work by untrained subjects. J Lab Clin Med 1943;28:601.
3. Haldi J, Wynn, W. Action of drugs on efficiency of swimmers. Res Q 1959;17:96.
4. Golding LA, Barnard RJ. The effects of d-amphetamine sulfate on physical performance. J Sports Med Phys Fitness 1963;3:221.
5. Wyndham CH, et al. Physiological effects of the amphetamines during exercise. S Afr Med J 1971;45:247.
6. Pierson WR, et al. Some psychological effects of the administration of amphetamine sulfate and meprobamate on speed of movement and reaction time. Med Sci Sports 1961;12:61.
7. McKenzie RE, Elliot LL. Effects of secobarbital and D-amphetamine on performance during a simulated air mission. Aerospace Med 1965;36:774.

often added to carbonated beverages and nonprescription medicines (see TABLE 23.6). For coffee consumption, this translates to a total of over 500 million cups of coffee consumed daily! Sixty-three plant species contain caffeine in their leaves, seeds, or fruits. In the United States, 75% (14 million kg) of caffeine intake (per capita, 150 mg · d^{-1}) comes from coffee (3.5 kg per person per year), 15% from tea, and the remainder from the items listed in Table 23.6. Depending on preparation, one cup of brewed coffee contains between 60 and 150 mg of caffeine, instant coffee about 100 mg, brewed tea between 20 and 50 mg, and caffeinated soft drinks about 50 mg. For comparison, 2.5 cups of percolated coffee contain 250 to 400 mg or generally between 3 and 6 mg per kg of body mass. In January 2004 the IOC removed caffeine from its list of restricted substances.

The intestinal tract absorbs caffeine rapidly; peak plasma concentration is reached within 1 hour. It also clears from the

---

TABLE 23.6 ■ CAFFEINE CONTENT OF COMMON FOODS, BEVERAGES, AND OVER-THE-COUNTER MEDICATIONS

BEVERAGES AND FOOD		OVER-THE-COUNTER PRODUCTS	
SUBSTANCE	**CAFFEINE CONTENT (MG)**	**SUBSTANCE**	**CAFFEINE CONTENT (MG)**
Coffee		**Cold remedies**	
Coffee, Starbucks, grande, 16 oz	550	Dristan Coryban-D, Triaminicin, Sinarest	30–31
Coffee, Starbucks, tall, 12 oz	375	Excedrin	65
Coffee, Starbucks, short, 8 oz	250	Actifed, Contac, Comtrex, Sudafed	0
Coffee, Starbucks, Americano, tall, 12 oz	70		0
Coffee, Starbucks, Latte or		**Diuretics**	
Cappuccino, grande, 16 oz	70	Aqua-ban	200
Brewed, drip method	110–150	Pre-Mens Forte	100
Brewed, percolator	64–124		
Instant	40–108	**Pain remedies**	
Expresso	100	Vanquish	33
Decaffeinated, brewed or instant; Sanka	2–5	Anacin; Midol	32
		Aspirin, any brand; Bufferin, Tylenol,	0
		Excedrin P.M.	
Tea 5 oz cup[a]			
Brewed, 1 min	9–33	**Stimulants**	
Brewed, 3 min	20–46	Vivarin tablet, NoDoz maximum-strength	200
Brewed, 5 min	20–50	caplet, Caffedrine	
Iced tea, 12 oz; instant tea	12–36	NoDoz tablet	100
		Energets Lozenges	75
Chocolate			
Baker's semi-sweet, 1 oz; Baker's		**Weight control aids**	
chocolate chips, 1/4 cup	13	Dexatrim, Dietac	200
Cocoa, 5 oz cup, made from mix	6–10	Prolamine	140
Milk chocolate candy, 1 oz	6		
Sweet/dark chocolate, 1 oz	20	**Pain drugs**[b]	
Baking chocolate, 1 oz	35	Cafergot	100
Chocolate bar, 3.5 oz	12–15	Migrol	50
Jello chocolate fudge mousse	12	Fiornal	40
Ovaltine	0	Darvon compound	32
Soft drinks			
Jolt	100		
Sugar-Free Mr. Pibb	59		
Mellow Yellow, Mountain Dew	53–54		
Tab	47		
Coca Cola, Diet Coke, 7-Up Gold	46		
Shasta-Cola, Cherry Cola, Diet Cola	44		
Dr. Pepper, Mr. Pibb	40–41		
Dr. Pepper, sugar free	40		
Pepsi Cola	38		
Diet Pepsi, Pepsi Light, Diet RC,	36		
RC Cola, Diet Rite			

Data from product labels and manufacturers and National Soft Drink Association, 1997.
[a] Brewing tea or coffee for longer periods slightly increases the caffeine content.
[b] Prescription, 1 oz or 30 mL.

body relatively quickly, taking about 3 to 6 hours for blood caffeine concentrations to decrease by one half, compared with about 10 hours for the stimulant methamphetamine.

Ergogenic Effects

Drinking 2.5 cups of regularly percolated coffee up to 1 hour before exercising extends endurance in strenuous aerobic exercise under laboratory conditions; it also improves higher intensity, shorter duration exercise performance.[41,86,294] Elite distance runners who consumed 10 mg of caffeine per kg of body mass immediately before a treadmill run to exhaustion improved performance time compared with placebo or control conditions.[108] Ergogenic effects during exhaustive exercise at 80% $\dot{V}O_{2max}$ that follows a 5-mg · kg^{-1} caffeine dose are maintained 5 hours later in a subsequent exercise challenge.[20] Thus, no need exists to ingest an additional dose to maintain high blood caffeine levels and ergogenic effects during subsequent exercise within 5 hours. Furthermore, caffeine ingestion does not impede glycogen resynthesis with carbohydrate supplementation after extreme depletion of muscle glycogen.[18]

Data presented in "Focus on Research," p. 579, show that subjects performed 90.2 minutes of exercise with caffeine and 75.5 minutes without it. Consuming caffeine before exercise increased fat catabolism and reduced carbohydrate oxidation. The ergogenic effect of caffeine also applies to exercise performed at high ambient temperatures.[62]

Caffeine benefits maximal swimming performance. In a double-blind, cross-over research design, seven male and four female competent distance swimmers (<25 min for 1500 m) consumed caffeine (6 mg · kg body mass^{-1}) 2.5 hours before

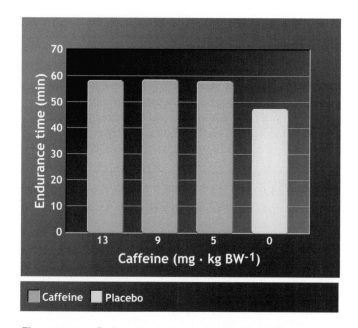

Figure 23.9 Endurance performance (time to fatigue) following preexercise doses of caffeine in different concentrations. Cycling time (min) represents the average for nine male cyclists. All caffeine trials produced significantly better performance than the placebo condition. No dose–response relationship emerged between caffeine concentration and endurance performance. (From Pasman WJ, et al. The effect of different dosages of caffeine on endurance performance time. Int J Sports Med 1995;16:225.)

swimming 1500 m. FIGURE 23.8 shows that split times improved with caffeine for each 500-m of the swim. Swim time averaged 1.9% faster with caffeine than without it (20:58.6 vs. 21:21.8). Enhanced performance with caffeine associated with a lower plasma potassium concentration before exercise and higher blood glucose levels at the end of the trial. These responses suggest a possible caffeine effect on electrolyte balance and glucose availability.

No Dose–Response Relationship. FIGURE 23.9 illustrates the effects of preexercise caffeine intake on endurance time of nine trained male cyclists. Subjects received a placebo or a capsule containing 5, 9, or 13 mg of caffeine per kg of body mass 1 hour before cycling at 80% of maximal power output on a $\dot{V}O_{2max}$ test. All caffeine trials showed a 24% improvement in performance with no additional benefit from caffeine quantities above 5 mg · kg body mass^{-1}.

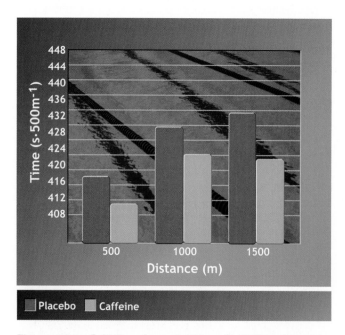

Figure 23.8 Split times for each 500 m of a 1500-m time trial with caffeine and placebo. Caffeine produced significantly faster split times. (From MacIntosh BR, Wright BM. Caffeine ingestion and performance of a 1,500-metre swim. Can J Appl Physiol 1995;20:168.)

Proposed Mechanism for Ergogenic Effect

A precise explanation for the ergogenic boost from caffeine remains elusive. The ergogenic effect of caffeine (or related methylxanthine compounds) in intense endurance exercise has generally been attributed to facilitated fat use as an exercise fuel, thus sparing carbohydrate reserves. In the quantities usually administered to humans, caffeine probably affects

ERGOGENIC BENEFITS OF CAFFEINE

Costill DL, et al. Effects of caffeine ingestion on metabolism and exercise performance. Med Sci Sports Exerc 1978;10:155.

▲ The potential ergogenic benefits of various substances and procedures have always interested sports competitors and exercise physiologists. Costill and colleagues tested the hypothesis that ingesting caffeine stimulated free fatty acid (FFA) mobilization, retarded depletion of muscle glycogen, and consequently enhanced endurance exercise performance. Previous research with animals and humans demonstrated that elevating plasma FFA spared muscle glycogen and extended exercise capacity. FFA concentration typically rose after injection of heparin, a substance that stimulates increased FFA mobilization and subsequent oxidation. Because caffeine also mobilizes FFA, Costill tested its effects on muscle glycogen levels, the metabolic mixture in exercise, and endurance performance in humans.

Two female and seven male competitive cyclists (average $\dot{V}O_{2max} = 60$ mL $\cdot$ kg^{-1} $\cdot$ min^{-1}), consuming the same diet, performed a cycle ergometer $\dot{V}O_{2max}$ test and two additional endurance exercise trials separated by 3 days. In one trial, they consumed 200 mL of hot water containing 5 g of decaffeinated coffee (D), 60 minutes before the exercise trial. The cycling test continued for as long as possible at a work intensity of 80% $\dot{V}O_{2max}$. In the second trial, subjects consumed a hot drink containing 5 g of D plus 330 mg of caffeine (C) 60 minutes before the exercise test. Subjects remained unaware of the experiment's purpose, with test order randomized for C and D trials. Blood samples, taken before and during each trial, provided information on plasma lactate, FFA, glycerol, glucose, and triacylglycerols. In addition, respiratory gas exchange throughout exercise allowed computation of RQ and estimation of the nonprotein metabolic mixture.

The accompanying figure shows that total exercise time to exhaustion increased 19.5% during trial C (90.2 min) compared with trial D (75.5 min). FFAs did not differ significantly between conditions (although consistently higher in C trial), but the caffeinated drink produced significantly higher plasma glycerol levels and significantly lower RQ values. The RQ allowed the researchers to estimate carbohydrate oxidation during exercise (about 240 g in both trials). In contrast, fat oxidation with caffeine (118 g) exceeded oxidation without caffeine (57 g). Subjects also perceived the exercise as easier in the C condition.

This study demonstrated that caffeine ingestion before exercise increased the lipolysis rate during sustained exercise. Increased lipolysis could spare liver and muscle glycogen early in exercise for later use. Subsequent research has confirmed caffeine's ergogenic role in endurance exercise performance.

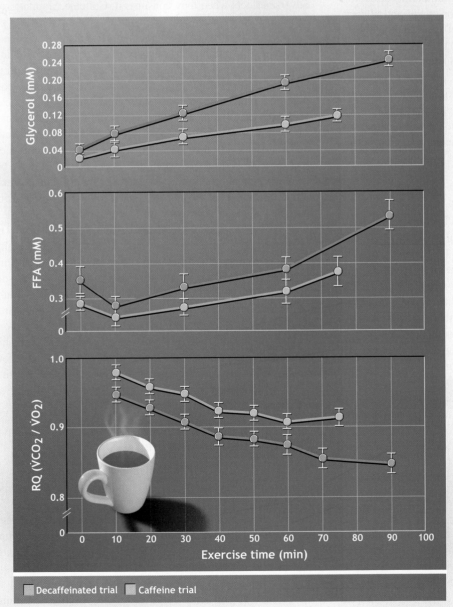

Decaffeinated trial   Caffeine trial

Average values for plasma glycerol, free fatty acid (FFA), and respiratory quotient (RQ) during endurance exercise after consuming either a caffeinated or decaffeinated liquid. *Vertical bars* (I) represent standard error of the mean.

metabolism in either of two ways: (1) directly on adipose and peripheral vascular tissues[123,334] or (2) indirectly by stimulating epinephrine release from the adrenal medulla. Epinephrine then acts as an antagonist of the adenosine receptors on adipocyte cells,[122,229] which normally repress lipolysis. Caffeine's inhibition of adenosine receptors increases cellular levels of the second messenger cyclic $3',5'$-adenosine monophosphate or cyclic AMP. Cyclic AMP then activates hormone-sensitive lipases to promote lipolysis; this effect causes the release of free fatty acids (FFAs) into the plasma. Elevated FFA levels increase fat oxidation, thus conserving liver and muscle glycogen to benefit high-intensity endurance exercise.

Caffeine's ergogenic effects also appear unrelated to hormonal or metabolic changes.[323] This suggests a possible action of caffeine on specific tissues including the nervous system. Caffeine and its metabolites readily cross the blood–brain barrier to produce analgesic effects on the central nervous system, potentially reducing the perception of effort during exercise. Caffeine enhances motoneuronal excitability to facilitate motor unit recruitment. The stimulating effects of caffeine do not occur from its direct action on the central nervous system. Instead, caffeine acts indirectly by blocking the receptors for adenosine (discussed earlier) that also serve a neuromodulator function to calm brain and spinal cord neurons. The following four factors probably interact to produce caffeine's facilitating effect on neuromuscular activity: (1) lower threshold for motor unit recruitment, (2) alter excitation/contraction coupling, (3) facilitate nerve transmission, and (4) increase ion transport within the muscle. Conflicting evidence exists concerning the effect of preexercise caffeine on $\dot{V}O_{2max}$.[84,320]

Inconsistent Effects. Prior nutrition partly accounts for why individuals vary in response to exercise after consuming caffeine. Those who normally consume a high-carbohydrate diet show a depressed effect for caffeine on FFA mobilization.[354] Individual differences in caffeine sensitivity, tolerance, and hormonal response from short- and long-term patterns of caffeine consumption also affect this drug's ergogenic qualities. Interestingly, the ergogenic effects of caffeine are less for caffeine in coffee than for an equivalent dose in capsule form.[124] Apparently, components in coffee antagonize caffeine's actions. Beneficial effects do not occur consistently in habitual caffeine users. This indicates that an athlete should consider "caffeine tolerance" rather than assume that caffeine provides a consistent benefit to all people. From a practical standpoint, the athlete should omit caffeine-containing foods and beverages 4 to 6 days before competition to optimize caffeine's potential for ergogenic effects.[333]

Effects on Muscle

Caffeine acts directly on muscle to enhance exercise capacity, particularly repeated submaximum muscle actions.[219,281] A double-blind research design evaluated voluntary and electrically stimulated muscle actions under "caffeine-free" conditions and following oral administration

of 500 mg of caffeine.[199] Electrically stimulating the motor nerve allowed the researchers to remove central nervous system control and quantify caffeine's direct effects on skeletal muscle. Caffeine produced no effect on maximal muscle force during voluntary or electrically stimulated muscle actions. For submaximal effort, caffeine increased force output for low-frequency electrical stimulation before and after muscle fatigue. Preexercise caffeine administration also increased by 17% repeated submaximum isometric muscular endurance.[247] Caffeine exerts no ergogenic effect on anaerobic metabolic capacity (glycolysis) as measured during repeated high-intensity Wingate exercise tests.[132] Page 604 of this chapter discusses how caffeine dramatically lessens the ergogenic effect of creatine supplementation on short-term muscular power.

Warning About Caffeine

Individuals who normally avoid caffeine may experience adverse effects when they consume it. Caffeine stimulates the central nervous system and in quantities greater than 1.5 g per day can produce typical symptoms of caffeinism: restlessness, headaches, insomnia, nervous irritability, muscle twitching, tremulousness, psychomotor agitation, and elevated heart rate and blood pressure and trigger premature left-ventricular contractions. From the standpoint of temperature regulation, caffeine acts as a diuretic. In extreme cases, this causes unnecessary preexercise fluid loss, negatively affecting thermal balance and exercise performance in hot environments. Caffeine's effect on fluid loss lessens when consumed during exercise because catecholamine release in exercise greatly reduces renal blood flow and exercise enhances renal solute reabsorption and consequently water conservation (osmotic effect).

While the effects of excess caffeine generally pose no health risk, a caffeine overdose can be lethal. The LD_{50} (lethal oral dose required to kill 50% of the population) for caffeine is about 10 g (150 mg · kg body mass^{-1}) for a 70-kg person. A 50-kg woman has an acute health risk with a caffeine intake of 7.5 g. Moderate caffeine toxicity exists for small children who consume 35 mg per kg of body mass. Such observations provide clear indication of the inverted U-shaped relationship between certain exogenous chemicals and health and safety (and probably exercise performance). With caffeine, ingesting small quantities produces desirable effects—consuming an excess can wreak havoc.

Ginseng and Ephedrine

The popularity of herbal and botanical remedies to improve health, control body weight, and improve exercise performance has soared. In 2005, Americans spent over $5 billion on such products. Ginseng and ephedrine have been commonly marketed as nutritional supplements to "reduce tension," "revitalize," "burn calories," and "optimize mental and physical performance," particularly during fatigue and stress. Ginseng also plays a role as an alternative therapy to treat diabetes and male impotence and stimulate immune function. Clinically, 1 to 3 g of ginseng administered 40 minutes before an oral glucose challenge reduces postprandial glycemia in nondiabetic subjects.[349]

Ginseng

The ginseng root (*Panax ginseng* C. A. Meyer), often sold as Panax or Chinese or Korean ginseng, serves no recognized medical use in the United States except as a soothing agent in skin ointments. Commercial ginseng root preparations generally take the form of powder, liquid, tablets, or capsules; widely marketed foods and beverages also contain various types and amounts of ginsenosides. Dietary supplements need not meet the same quality control for purity and potency as pharmaceuticals. Considerable variation exists in the concentrations of marker compounds for ginseng, including potentially harmful levels of impurities and toxins such as pesticides and heavy metals.[136]

A common claim for ginseng in the Western world is as an energy booster and to diminish the negative effects of overall stress and to reduce the severity of cold symptoms. Reports of an ergogenic effect often appear in nontraditional journals.[42] Little objective evidence exists to support the effectiveness of ginseng as an ergogenic aid.[4,12] For example, volunteers consumed either 200 or 400 mg of the standardized ginseng concentrate daily for 8 weeks in a double-blind research protocol.[94] Neither treatment affected submaximal or maximal exercise performance, ratings of perceived exertion, or physiologic parameters of heart rate, oxygen consumption, or blood lactate concentrations. Similarly, no ergogenic effects occurred for many physiologic and performance variables following a 1 week treatment with a ginseng saponin extract administered in doses of either 8 or 16 mg per kg of body mass.[223] Similarly, 8 weeks of ginseng supplementation failed to affect physical performance or recovery from 30-second Wingate tests.[86] Supplementation had no effect on mucosal immunity indicated by changes in secretory IgA at rest or following intense exercise.[95] When effectiveness has been demonstrated, the research failed to use adequate controls, placebos, or double-blind testing protocols.[107] At present, no compelling scientific evidence exists that ginseng supplementation offers ergogenic effects for physiologic function or exercise performance.[195,342]

Ephedrine

Unlike ginseng, Western medicine recognizes the potent amphetamine-like alkaloid compound ephedrine (with sympathomimetic physiologic effects) present in several species of the plant ephedra (dried plant stem called ma huang [ma wong; *Ephedra sinica*]). The ephedra plant contains two major active components first isolated in 1928, ephedrine and pseudoephedrine. The medicinal role includes treatment of asthma, symptoms of the common cold, hypotension, and urinary incontinence and as a central stimulant to treat depression. Physicians in the United States discontinued ephedrine as a decongestant and asthma treatment in the 1930s in favor of safer medications. The milder pseudoephedrine remains common in nonprescription cold and flu medications and

clinically treats mucosal congestion that accompanies hay fever, allergic rhinitis, sinusitis, and other respiratory conditions. Labeling that indicates ephedra compounds includes ephedra, ma huang, ephedrine, Ephedra sinica, sida cordifolia, epitonin, pseudoephedrine, and methyl ephedrine.

Ephedrine exerts central and peripheral effects, with the latter reflected in increased heart rate, cardiac output, and blood pressure. Ephedrine produces bronchodilation in the lungs owing to its β-adrenergic effect. High ephedrine dosages produce hypertension, insomnia, hyperthermia, and cardiac arrhythmias. Other side effects include dizziness, restlessness, anxiety, irritability, personality changes, gastrointestinal symptoms, and difficulty concentrating.

Despite the legal and scientific categorizations of ephedrine as a potent drug, one could legally sell it as a dietary supplement. Its claim for accelerated metabolism and enhanced exercise performance greatly increased ephedrine's popularity as a nutritional supplement. Supplements containing ephedra accounted for nearly $1.4 billion in 2002, or about 7% of dietary supplement sales, and included an array of products in capsule, drink, and chewing gum form. The botanical source of ephedra alkaloids also had popularity as a weight-loss dietary supplement.[367] Many commercial weight-loss products have contained combinations of ephedrine and caffeine designed to speed up metabolism. No credible evidence exists that the initial weight loss with high doses of ephedrine plus caffeine lasts beyond 6 months.[289]

The potent physiologic effects of ephedrine have led researchers to investigate its potential as an ergogenic aid—sold commercially as Ripped Fuel, Metabolift, Xenadrine RFA-1, Hyrocut, and ThermoSpeed. No effect of a 40-mg dose of ephedrine occurred on indirect indicators of exercise performance or ratings of perceived exertion (RPE).[79] The less concentrated pseudoephedrine also produce no effect on $\dot{V}O_{2max}$, RPE, aerobic cycling efficiency,[146,312] anaerobic power output (Wingate test), time to exhaustion on a bicycle and a 40-km cycling trial,[116] or physiologic and performance measures during 20 minutes of running at 70% of $\dot{V}O_{2max}$ followed by a 5000-m time trial.[57]

In contrast, a series of double-blind, placebo-controlled studies by the Canadian Defense and Civil Institute of Environmental Medicine using a relatively high preexercise ephedrine dosage (0.8 to 1.0 mg per kg body mass), either alone or combined with caffeine, produced small but statistically significant effects on endurance performance[19,21,23] and anaerobic power output during the early phase of the Wingate test.[22] Ephedrine supplementation also increased muscular endurance during the first set of traditional resistance-training exercise.[157] Whether central mechanisms that increase arousal and tolerance to discomfort, peripheral mechanisms that influence substrate metabolism and muscle function, or the combined effect of both account for any ergogenic effect remains undetermined.

Not Without Risk

Nearly 1400 adverse effects from ephedra use have been reported to the FDA (www.fda.gov) from January 1993 to February 2000. Incidents included 81 deaths, 32 heart attacks,

62 cases of cardiac arrhythmia, 91 cases of increased blood pressure, 69 strokes, and 70 seizures. An evaluation of more than 16,000 adverse reactions showed "five deaths, five heart attacks, 11 cerebrovascular accidents, four seizures, and eight psychiatric cases as 'sentinel events' associated with prior consumption of ephedra or ephedrine.[289] During 2001, 1178 adverse reactions were reported to American poison control centers. In general, the cardiovascular toxic effects of ephedra (increased heart rate and blood vessel constriction) are not limited to massive doses but rather to the amount recommended by the manufacturer. In 2002, an Alabama jury awarded $4.1 million to four persons who suffered strokes or heart attacks after taking an ephedra-based appetite suppressant produced by Metabolite International. In addition, the supplement maker Twin Laboratories Inc. has been sued by the families of a 28-year-old bodybuilder and a 27-year-old Marine Corps officer, blaming the men's deaths on the ephedra supplement called Ripped Fuel. For additional information on the untoward effects of ephedra, visit the web site of the Centers for Disease Control and Prevention (www.cdc.gov).

The IOC and NCAA currently ban ephedrine, and the National Football League (NFL) represents the first professional sports league to do so. Professional baseball discourages ephedrine use, but it does not ban it. On July 1, 2002, the NFL tested for this stimulant under the league's Policy on Anabolic Steroids and Related Substances. Any player that tests positive for ephedra may receive a four- game suspension. Many players acknowledge using this herbal stimulant seeking to lose weight or get a "quick burst of energy." The rationale for testing put forth by the NFL and the NFL Players Association was the growing evidence linking ephedrine-containing products to life-threatening strokes, seizures, thermoregulatory disorders that predispose to heat stroke, and heart arrhythmia. In spring training of 2003, ephedrine use was implicated in the death from organ failure complications in heat stroke of Baltimore Orioles pitcher Steve Bechler. He allegedly used the ephedrine-containing supplement Xenadrine RFA-1 to facilitate weight loss.

Risk-benefit assessments have caused physicians to declare ephedra use unsafe, even when taken in recommended doses. Products containing ephedra represent less than 1% of sales of all herbal supplements, yet they account for 64% of the adverse reactions. Consequently, ephedra poses a 200-fold greater risk than all other herbal supplements combined. Based on analysis of existing data, including commissioning a safety study by independent research group (the Rand Corporation), the FDA banned ephedra on December 31, 2003, the first time this federal agency banned a dietary supplement.

Buffering Solutions

Maximal exercise for 30 to 120 seconds dramatically alters the chemical balance between intra- and extracellular fluids because the active muscle fibers rely predominantly on anaerobic energy transfer. Lactate accumulates with a concurrent fall in intracellular pH. Increased acidity ultimately inhibits energy transfer and contractile dynamics in the active muscle fibers, and exercise performance deteriorates.[167]

The bicarbonate aspect of the body's buffering system (see Chapter 14) provides a rapid first line of defense against intracellular increases in H^+ concentration. Maintaining extracellular bicarbonate at a high level facilitates H^+ efflux from the cell, which reduces intracellular acidosis. Increasing the bicarbonate reserve before short-term anaerobic exercise might enhance performance by delaying the fall in intracellular pH associated with exhaustive effort. Variations in preexercise dosage of sodium bicarbonate and type of exercise to evaluate preexercise alkalosis have produced conflicting results about the ergogenic effectiveness of buffering agents.[126,253,286,308,332]

To improve experimental design, one study investigated the effects of acute metabolic alkalosis on exhaustive exercise that increased anaerobic metabolites.[357] Six trained middle-distance runners ran an 880-m race under control conditions and following alkalosis induced by ingesting a sodium bicarbonate solution (300 mg per kg body mass) or a calcium carbonate placebo of similar concentration. TABLE 23.7 shows that the alkaline drink raised pH and standard bicarbonate level before exercise. Subjects ran on average 2.9 seconds faster under alkalosis and exhibited higher postexercise blood lactate, pH, and extracellular H^+ concentration than in the placebo condition. Augmented anaerobic energy transfer and/or delayed onset of intracellular acidification during intense exercise most likely explains the ergogenic effect of preexercise alkalosis.[147,254,263] Increased extracellular buffering from preexercise sodium bicarbonate ingestion facilitates H^+ efflux from active muscle fibers during exercise. This delays the fall in intracellular pH and its subsequent negative effects on muscle function. An improvement of 2.9 seconds in 800-m race time represents a dramatic performance improvement—a distance of 19 m at race pace brings a last-place finisher to first place in most 800-m races!

The ergogenic effect of **preexercise alkalosis** (use not banned by the IOC) also occurs for women (FIG. 23.10).[214] Physically active women performed one bout of maximal cycle ergometer exercise for 60 seconds on separate days under three conditions in a double-blind research design: (1) control, no treatment; (2) sodium bicarbonate dose of 300 mg · kg body mass^{-1} in 400 mL of low-calorie flavored water 90 minutes before testing; and (3) placebo of equimolar dose of sodium chloride (to maintain intravascular fluid status similar to bicarbonate condition) administered like the bicarbonate treatment. Exercise capacity represented total work accomplished in the 60-second ride. The figure's *inset box* shows that total work and peak power output reached higher levels with preexercise bicarbonate treatment than under either control or placebo conditions. The bicarbonate treatment produced a higher blood lactate level in the immediate and 1-minute postexercise period; the effect explains the greater work capacity attained in the short-term, anaerobic exercise trial. Similar ergogenic benefits occur with exogenous sodium citrate as the preexercise alkalinizing agent.[142,212]

TABLE 23.7 ■ **PERFORMANCE TIME AND ACID–BASE PROFILES FOR SUBJECTS UNDER CONTROL (PLACEBO) AND INDUCED PREEXERCISE ALKALOSIS CONDITIONS BEFORE AND AFTER AN 800-M RACE**

VARIABLE	CONDITION	PRETREATMENT	PREEXERCISE	POSTEXERCISE
pH	Control	7.40	7.39	7.07
	Placebo	7.39	7.40	7.09
	Alkalosis	7.40	7.49[a]	7.18[b]
Lactate	Control	1.21	1.15	12.62
(mmol · L^{-1})	Placebo	1.38	1.23	13.62
	Alkalosis	1.29	1.31	14.29[b]
Standard HCO$_3$$^{-1}$	Control	25.8	24.5	9.90
(mEq · L^{-1})	Placebo	25.6	26.2	11.00
	Alkalosis	25.2	33.5[a]	14.30[b]

	CONTROL	PLACEBO	ALKALOSIS
Performance time (min:s)	2:05.8	2:05.1	2:02.9[c]

From Wilkes D. et al. Effects of induced metabolic alkalosis on 800-m racing time. Med Sci Sports Exerc 1983;15:277.
[a] Preexercise values significantly higher than pretreatment values.
[b] Alkalosis values significantly higher than placebo and control values after exercise.
[c] Alkalosis time significantly faster than control and placebo times.

Effect Related to Dosage and Degree of Anaerobiosis

Bicarbonate dosage and the cumulative anaerobic nature of exercise interact to influence the potential ergogenic effect of preexercise bicarbonate loading. Doses of at least 0.3 g per kg body mass facilitate H$^+$ efflux from the cell and enhance a single 1- to 2-minute maximal effort[208,214] and longer-term arm or leg exercise that exhausts within 6 to 8 minutes.[272] No ergogenic effect emerges for performance typical of heavy resistance training, perhaps because of the lower absolute anaerobic metabolic load than in supramaximal whole-body running or cycling.[251] Bicarbonate loading with all-out effort of less than 1 minute exerts an ergogenic effect with repetitive

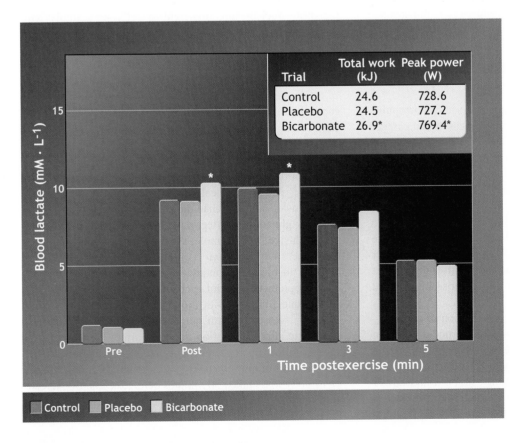

Trial	Total work (kJ)	Peak power (W)
Control	24.6	728.6
Placebo	24.5	727.2
Bicarbonate	26.9*	769.4*

Figure 23.10 Effects of bicarbonate loading on total work, peak power output, and post-exercise blood lactate levels in moderately trained women. *Significantly higher than either control or placebo. (From McNaughton LR, et al. Effect of sodium bicarbonate ingestion on high intensity exercise in moderately trained women. J Strength Cond Res 1997;11:98.)

(intermittent) exercise.[69] Species differences also influence the ergogenic effects of bicarbonate loading; improvements occur for racehorses but not for racing greyhounds.[176,190]

INTEGRATIVE QUESTION

Advise an Olympic-calibre weight lifter who plans to bicarbonate load because the competitive event requires all-out effort of an anaerobic nature.

High-Intensity Endurance Performance

Preexercise-induced alkalosis does not benefit low-intensity, aerobic exercise because pH and lactate remain at near-resting levels, but it may enhance aerobic exercise of higher intensity. High-intensity endurance exercise, while predominantly aerobic, increases blood lactate and decreases pH, which negatively affects performance. Eight trained male cyclists consumed sodium citrate (0.5 g per kg body mass) before a 30-km time trial.[252] Race times were faster and plasma pH and lactate concentrations higher after sodium citrate ingestion than with the placebo. Despite the relatively small anaerobic component in high-intensity aerobic exercise (compared with short-term, maximal exercise), ingesting a buffer before such exercise facilitates lactate and hydrogen ion efflux and improves muscle function.[213]

Individuals who bicarbonate load often experience abdominal cramps and diarrhea about 1 hour after ingestion. This adverse effect would surely minimize any potential ergogenic effect. Substituting sodium citrate (0.4 to 0.5 g per kg body mass) for sodium bicarbonate reduces or eliminates adverse gastrointestinal effects.[197,212]

Anticortisol Compounds: Glutamine and Phosphatidylserine

The hypothalamus normally secretes corticotrophin-releasing factor in response to emotional stress, trauma, infection, surgery, and physical exertion. This releasing factor stimulates the anterior pituitary gland to release adrenocorticotropic hormone (ACTH), which induces the adrenal cortex to discharge the glucocorticoid hormone **cortisol** (hydrocortisone). Cortisol decreases amino acid transport into the cell; this depresses anabolism and stimulates protein breakdown to its building-block amino acids in all cells except the liver. The circulation delivers these "liberated" amino acids to the liver for glucose synthesis (gluconeogenesis). Cortisol also serves as an insulin antagonist by inhibiting glucose uptake and oxidation.

A prolonged, elevated serum concentration of cortisol—usually from therapeutic exogenous glucocorticoid intake in drug form—leads to excessive protein breakdown, tissue wasting, and negative nitrogen balance. The potential catabolic effect of cortisol has convinced many strength and power athletes to use supplements thought to inhibit normal cortisol release. They believe that depressing cortisol's normal rise

following exercise augments muscular development by attenuating catabolism. In this way, muscle tissue synthesis progresses unimpeded in recovery. Glutamine and phosphatidylserine are two supplements used to produce an anticortisol effect.

Glutamine

Glutamine, a nonessential amino acid, is the most abundant amino acid in plasma and skeletal muscle. It accounts for more than one half of the muscles' free amino acid pool. Glutamine exerts many regulatory functions, one of which provides an anticatabolic effect that augments protein synthesis.[160,210,356] From a clinical perspective, glutamine supplementation effectively counteracts the decline in protein synthesis and muscle wasting from repeated glucocorticoid use.[145] Infusing glutamine following exercise promotes muscle glycogen accumulation, perhaps by serving as a gluconeogenic substrate in the liver.[337]

The potential anticatabolic and glycogen synthesizing effects of exogenous glutamine have promoted speculation that supplementation might benefit responses to resistance training.[9] Daily glutamine supplementation (0.9 g per kg lean tissue mass) during 6 weeks of resistance training in healthy young adults did not affect muscle performance, body composition, or muscle protein degradation compared with a placebo.[50]

Glutamine and the Immune Response

Glutamine plays an important role in normal immune function. One protective aspect concerns glutamine's use as metabolic fuel by infection-fighting cells, particularly lymphocytes and macrophages. Glutamine plasma concentration decreases following prolonged intense exercise, so glutamine deficiency has been linked to the immunosuppression from strenuous exercise (see Chapter 7).[32,278]

Glutamine supplementation might lessen increased susceptibility to upper respiratory tract infection (URTI) following prolonged competition or a bout of strenuous training. Marathoners who ingested a glutamine drink (5 g L-glutamine in 330 mL mineral water) at the end of a race and then 2 hours later reported fewer URTI symptoms than unsupplemented athletes.[52] More specifically, 65% more athletes reported no symptoms of infection than did a placebo group. The mechanism for glutamine's effect on postexercise infection risk remains elusive. For example, subsequent studies by the same researchers showed *no effect* of glutamine supplementation on changes in blood lymphocyte distribution.[53] Dietary glutamine supplementation did *not* benefit lymphocyte metabolism or immune function with more moderate exercise training in rats.[290] Research with humans indicates that preexercise glutamine supplementation does *not* affect the immune response following repeated bouts of intense exercise.[266,353] Supplements of nine equal doses of 100 mg of L-glutamine per kg of body mass taken 30 minutes before the end of exercise, at the end of exercise, and 30-minutes into recovery abolished the postexercise decline in glutamine following a race but did *not effect* immune function.[265] Insufficient data exist to recommend glutamine supplements to reliably blunt immunosuppression and infection risk from exhaustive exercise.

Phosphatidylserine

Phosphatidylserine (PS) is a glycerophospholipid typical of a class of natural lipids that compose the structural components of the internal layer of the plasma membrane that surrounds all cells. Through its potential for modulating functional events in the plasma membrane (e.g., number and affinity of membrane receptor sites), PS might modify the neuroendocrine response to stress. In one study, healthy men consumed 800 mg of PS derived from bovine cerebral cortex daily for 10 days.[222] Three 6-minute intervals of cycle ergometer exercise of increasing intensity induced physical stress. Compared with the placebo condition, PS treatment diminished ACTH and cortisol release without affecting growth hormone release. These results confirmed earlier findings by the same researchers that a single intravenous PS injection counteracted hypothalamic-pituitary–adrenal axis activation with exercise.[221] Soybean lecithin provides most PS for supplementation, yet research showing physiologic effects have used bovine-derived PS. Subtle differences in the chemical structure of these two forms of PS may create differences in physiologic action, including the potential for ergogenic effects.

β-Hydroxy-β-methylbutyrate

β-Hydroxy-β-methylbutyrate (HMB), a bioactive metabolite generated in the breakdown of the essential branched-chain amino acid leucine, decreases protein loss during stress by inhibiting protein catabolism. In rats and chicks, less protein breakdown and slight increase in protein synthesis occurred in muscle tissue (in vitro) exposed to HMB.[181] An HMB-induced increase occurred in fatty acid oxidation in vitro in mammalian muscle cells exposed to HMB.[56] Depending on the quantity of HMB in food (relatively rich sources include catfish, grapefruit, and breast milk), humans synthesize between 0.3 and 1.0 g of HMB daily, about 5% from dietary leucine catabolism. Because of its potential nitrogen-retaining effects, HMB supplements are taken to prevent or slow muscle damage and inhibit muscle breakdown (proteolysis) with intense physical effort.

Research has studied the effects of exogenous HMB on skeletal muscle's response to resistance training.[112,166,183,239,295] Young-adult men participated in two randomized trials.[230] In study #1, 41 subjects received either 0, 1.5, or 3.0 g of HMB daily at two protein levels, either 117 g or 175 g daily, for 3 weeks. The men resistance trained during this time for 1.5 hours, 3 days a week. In study #2, 28 subjects consumed either 0 or 3.0 g of HMB daily and resistance trained for 2 to 3 hours, 6 days a week, for 7 weeks. In the first study, HMB supplementation depressed the exercise-induced rise in muscle proteolysis (reflected by urinary 3-methylhistidine and plasma creatine phosphokinase [CPK] levels) during the first 2 weeks of exercise training. These biochemical indices of muscle damage were 20 to 60% lower in the HMB-supplemented group. In addition, the supplemented group lifted more total weight during each training week (FIG. 23.11A), with the greatest effect in the group receiving the largest HMB supplement. Muscular strength increased 8% in the unsupplemented group and more in the HMB-supplemented groups (13% for the 1.5-g group and 18.4% for the 3.0-g group). Added protein (not indicated in graph) did not affect any of the measurements, but one should view this lack of effect in proper context—the "lower" protein quantity (115 g · d^{-1}) equaled twice the RDA.

In the second study, individuals who received HMB supplementation had higher FFM than the unsupplemented group at 2 and 4–6 weeks of training (Fig. 23.11B). At the last measurement during training, the difference between groups decreased and did not differ significantly from the difference between pretraining baseline values.

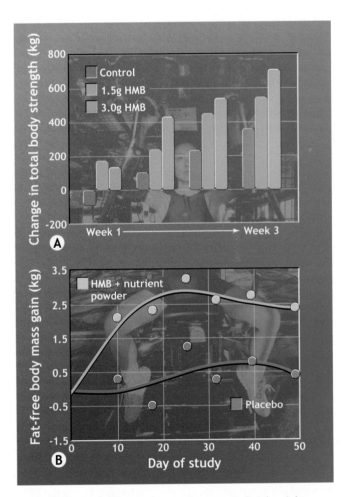

Figure 23.11 **A.** Change in muscle strength (total weight lifted in upper- and lower-body exercises) during study 1 (week 1 to week 3) in subjects who supplemented with HMB. Each *group of bars* represents one complete set of upper- and lower-body workouts. **B.** Total body electrical conductivity–assessed change in FFM during study 2 for a control group that received a carbohydrate drink *(placebo)* and a group that received 3 g of Ca-HMB each day mixed in a nutrient powder *(HMB + nutrient powder)*. (From Nissen S, et al. Effect of leucine metabolite β-hydroxy-β-methylbutyrate on muscle metabolism during resistance-exercise training. J Appl Physiol 1996;81:2095.)

The mechanism for HMB's effect on muscle metabolism, strength improvement, and body composition remains unknown. Perhaps this metabolite inhibits normal proteolytic processes that accompany intense muscular overload. While the results demonstrate an ergogenic effect for HMB supplementation, it remains unclear just what component of the FFM (protein, bone, water) HMB affects. Furthermore, the data in Figure 23.11B indicate potentially transient body composition benefits of supplementation that tend to revert toward the un-supplemented state as training progresses.

Not all research shows beneficial effects of HMB supplementation with resistance training.[112,258,295] One study evaluated the effects of variations in HMB supplementation (approximately 3 vs. 6 g · d^{-1}) on muscular strength during 8 weeks of whole-body resistance training in untrained, young adult men.[112] The study's primary finding indicated that HMB supplementation, regardless of dosage, produced *no difference* in most of the strength data (including 1-RM strength) compared with the placebo group. In contrast to the findings presented in Figure 23.11A, increases in training volume remained similar among groups. In both HMB-supplemented groups, lower CPK levels in recovery indicated some potential effect of HMB to inhibit muscle breakdown. The group that consumed the lower HMB dosage increased more in FFM than the other two groups. Inferences from these findings are limited because skinfolds assessed body composition changes. HMB supplementation with a daily dosage as high as 6 g · d^{-1} during 8 weeks of resistance training does not adversely affect hepatic enzyme function, blood lipid profile, renal function, or immune function.[113] Additional studies must assess the long-term effects of HMB supplements on body composition, training response, and overall health and safety. Age does not affect responsiveness to HMB supplementation.[348]

NONPHARMACOLOGIC APPROACHES

Besides pharmacologic procedures, athletes often use physical, mechanical, physiologic, and nutritional means to potentiate ergogenic effects.

Red Blood Cell Reinfusion—Blood Doping

Red blood cell reinfusion, often called *induced erythrocythemia, blood boosting,* or *blood doping,* gained public prominence as a possible ergogenic technique during the 1972 Munich Olympics when an athlete allegedly used this procedure prior to his two gold medal–winning endurance runs.

How It Works

Red blood cell reinfusion involves withdrawing 1 to 4 units (1 unit = 450 mL of whole blood) of a person's blood, immediately reinfusing the plasma, and placing the packed red cells in frozen storage for later infusion (**autologous transfusion**). **Homologous transfusion** infuses a type-matched donor's blood. To prevent dramatic reductions in blood-cell concentration, each unit of blood withdrawal takes place at 3- to 8-week intervals because it takes this time to reestablish normal red blood cell levels. Stored blood cells are then infused 1 to 7 days before an endurance event; this increases red blood cell count and hemoglobin levels from 8 to 20%. Hemoconcentration translates to an average hemoglobin increase for men from a normal 15 g per dL of blood to 19 g per dL (hematocrit increases 40 to 60%). Hematologic parameters remain elevated for at least 14 days. Theoretically, the added blood volume contributes to a larger maximal cardiac output, while red blood cell packing increases the blood's oxygen-carrying capacity. Enhanced oxygen transport and delivery to active tissues provides meaningful performance benefits to endurance athletes.[37]

An ergogenic effect occurs with infusion of 900 to 1800 mL of freeze-preserved autologous blood. Each 500-mL infusion of whole blood (equivalent to 275 mL of packed red cells) adds about 100 mL of oxygen to the blood's total oxygen-carrying capacity—each 100 mL of whole blood carries about 20 mL of oxygen. An elite endurance athlete's total blood volume circulates 5 to 6 times each minute in intense exercise, so the potential "extra" oxygen available to the tissues from red cell reinfusion averages 500 mL (0.5 L).

Blood doping might also produce effects opposite to those intended. For example, a large red blood cell infusion (and increase in blood cell concentration) could increase blood viscosity, or "thickness," and thus *decrease* cardiac output, blood flow velocity, and peripheral oxygen supply—important factors that reduce aerobic capacity and endurance performance. Any increase in blood viscosity might also compromise blood flow through the narrowed, atherosclerotic vessels of individuals with artery disease, thereby increasing risk for heart attack or stroke.

Does It Work?

A theoretical basis for blood doping exists and experimental evidence justifies its use for physiologic reasons.[285] Much of the early conflict concerning ergogenic benefits came from poor experimental design, inconsistent criteria for exercise performance, diverse blood storage techniques, and variations in timing and quantity of blood withdrawn and replaced. Early research in this area noted a rapid increase in $\dot{V}O_{2max}$ following infusion of whole blood.[90] One study reported a 23% overnight increase in exercise performance and a 9% increase in $\dot{V}O_{2max}$ with blood doping.[92] Subsequent investigations (including a study by a past critic of the technique) support previous findings and show physiologic and performance improvements with red blood cell reinfusion.[271,299]

Differences in results among various studies of exercise performance following red blood cell reinfusion largely result from variations in blood storage methods. Freezing red blood cells permits storage for more than 6 weeks without significant loss of cells. With storage at 4°C (used in some earlier

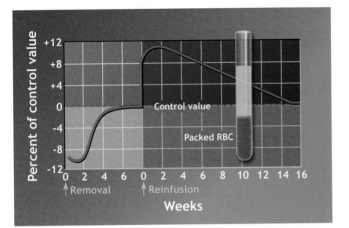

Figure 23.12 Time course of hematologic changes after removal and reinfusion of 900 mL of freeze-preserved blood. (From Gledhill N. Blood doping and related issues: a brief review. Med Sci Sports Exerc 1982;14:183.)

studies), substantial hemolysis occurs after only 3 weeks. This represents an important difference because it usually takes a person 5 to 6 weeks to reestablish blood cells lost after withdrawal of two units of whole blood (FIG. 23.12).

With appropriate blood storage methods, red blood cell reinfusion elevates hematologic parameters of men and women. This in turn translates to a 5 to 13% increase in aerobic capacity, decreased heart rate and blood lactate during submaximal exercise, and augmented endurance at sea level and altitude. In addition, thermoregulatory benefits during exercise in the heat (reduced body heat storage and improved sweating response) result from red blood cell reinfusion. Increased oxygen content in arterial blood in the infused state likely "frees" blood for delivery to the skin for heat dissipation during exercise heat stress. TABLE 23.8 illustrates hematologic, physiologic, and performance responses for five adult men during submaximal and maximal exercise before and 24 hours after infusion of 750 mL of packed red blood cells. These response patterns generally represent the more recent research findings in this area.

A New Twist: Hormonal Blood Boosting

To eliminate the cumbersome and lengthy process of blood doping, endurance athletes now use epoetin, a synthetic form of **erythropoietin** (**EPO**). This hormone, produced by the kidneys, regulates red blood cell production within the marrow of the long bones, but also is essential in the synthesis and proper functioning of several erythrocyte membrane proteins, particularly those facilitating lactate exchange.[66] Medically, exogenous recombinant human EPO, commercially available since 1988, has proved useful in combating anemia in patients undergoing chemotherapy or with severe renal disease. Normally, a decrease in red blood cell concentration or decline in the pressure of oxygen in arterial blood—as in severe pulmonary disease or on ascent to high altitude—releases this hormone to stimulate erythrocyte production. The 12% increase in hemoglobin and hematocrit that typically follows a 6-week EPO treatment greatly improves endurance exercise performance.[91,282] Unfortunately, self-administration in an unregulated and unmonitored manner—simply injecting the hormone requires much less sophistication than procedures for blood doping—can increase hematocrit more than 60%. This dangerously high hemoconcentration (and corresponding increase in blood viscosity) increases the likelihood for stroke, heart attack, heart failure, and pulmonary edema.

EPO use has become particularly prevalent in cycling competition and allegedly contributed to at least 18 deaths (mainly from heart attack) among competitive cyclists. Because EPO cannot be detected in urine, the blood hematocrit serves as a surrogate marker. During the 1997 and 1998 competitive seasons, Tour de France officials spot checked hematocrits, suspending for 2 weeks any rider with an abnormally high level. This resulted in suspension of 12 riders during 1997 and 6 midway through the 1998 competitive season. The International Cycling Union has set a hematocrit threshold of 50% for males and 47% for females; the International Skiing Federation uses a hemoglobin concentration of 18.5 g · dL^{-1} as the threshold for disqualification. Hematocrit cutoff values of 52% for men and 48% for women (roughly 3 standard deviations above the mean)

TABLE 23.8 ■ PHYSIOLOGIC, PERFORMANCE, AND HEMATOLOGIC CHARACTERISTICS BEFORE AND 24 HOURS AFTER REINFUSION OF 750 ML OF PACKED RED BLOOD CELLS

VARIABLE	PREINFUSION	POSTINFUSION	DIFFERENCE	DIFFERENCE, %
Hemoglobin, g · dL blood^{-1}	13.8	17.6	3.8[b]	+27.5[b]
Hematocrit[a], %	43.3	54.8	11.5[b]	+26.5[b]
Submaximal $\dot{V}O_2$, L · min^{-1}	1.60	1.59	−0.01	−0.6
Submaximal HR, b · min^{-1}	127.4	109.2	18.2	−14.3[b]
$\dot{V}O_{2max}$, L · min^{-1}	3.28	3.70	0.42[b]	+12.8[b]
HR$_{max}$, b · min^{-1}	181.6	180.0	−1.6	−0.9
Treadmill run time, s	793	918	125[b]	15.8

From Roberston RJ, et al. Effect of induced erythrocythemia on hypoxia tolerance during exercise. J Appl Physiol 1982;53:490.
[a] Hematocrit expressed as the percentage (%) of 100 mL (1 dL) of whole blood occupied by red blood cells.
[b] Difference statistically significant.

represent "abnormally high" or extreme values in triathletes.[236] Use of hematocrit level cutoff raises the unanswered question of the number of disqualified "clean" cyclists. Estimates place this number between 3 and 5% because of factors that affect normal variation in hematocrit such as genetics, posture, altitude training, and hydration level.[11,40]

The 2002 Olympics did not escape controversy; the Russian Olympic Committee threatened to withdraw from the Salt Lake City Winter Games. One of four incidents cited as the basis of their complaint concerned disqualification of the 20-km cross-country ski relay team because of elevated hemoglobin concentration of one of its members, a nine-time Olympic medalist. The Russians claimed a false-positive test result. Additionally, the IOC stripped two cross-country skiers from Spain and Russia of gold medals (and banished them from future Olympic competition) after they tested positive for darbepoietin, a blood-boosting analog of EPO.

Current concern centers on an anomaly in iron metabolism frequently observed among high-level international cyclists. Many of these athletes show serum iron levels above $500 \, ng \cdot L^{-1}$ (normal, $100 \, ng \cdot L^{-1}$), with some values as high as $1000 \, ng \cdot L^{-1}$. The elevated iron level results from their regular injections of supplemental iron to support increased synthesis of red blood cells induced by repeated EPO use. Chronic iron overload increases the risk of liver dysfunction among these athletes.

The enhancement of oxygen availability to muscles by EPO analog and mimetics constitutes one of the main challenges to doping control. In 2004, the concern shifted from simple red blood cell reinfusion to concern about transfection to an athlete's genes that code for erythropoietin and its subsequent impact on exercise performance.[242] Sports authorities have now incorporated such "gene doping" among the prohibited practices.

Other Means to Enhance Oxygen Transport

New classes of substances may emerge to enhance aerobic exercise performance.[288] These doping threats include perfluorocarbon emulsions and solutions formulated from either bovine or human hemoglobin that improve oxygen transport and delivery to muscle. Despite their potential benefits in clinical use, these substances exhibit potentially lethal side effects that include increased systemic and pulmonary blood pressure, renal toxicity, and impaired immune function.

Warm-Up (Preliminary Exercise)

Coaches, trainers, and athletes at all levels of competition generally recommend engaging in some type of physical activity or warm-up prior to vigorous exercise. Conventional wisdom maintains that preliminary exercise helps the performer prepare physiologically or psychologically and reduces the likelihood of joint and muscle injury. With animals, injuring a "warmed-up" muscle requires more force and greater muscle length than injuring a muscle in the "cold" condition.[284] The warming-up process stretches the muscle-tendon unit to allow greater length and less tension on exposure to a given external load.

Warm-up generally fits into one of two categories (although overlap exists):

- **General warm-up** uses body movements or "loosening-up" exercises unrelated to the specific neuromuscular actions of the anticipated performance. Examples include calisthenics and stretching.
- **Specific warm-up** applies big-muscle, rhythmic movements that provide skill rehearsal in the activity. Examples include swinging a golf club, throwing a baseball or football, tennis practice, basketball shooting and movements, and preliminary lead-up in the high jump or pole vault.

Psychologic Considerations

Competitors at all levels generally believe that performing some prior skill-related activity prepares them mentally for their event so they can focus on the upcoming performance. A specific warm-up related to the intended activity also may improve the necessary skill and coordination requirements. Consequently, sports that require accuracy, timing, and precise movements generally benefit from some type of specific or "formal" preliminary practice.

The notion also exists that prior exercise before strenuous effort gradually prepares a person to go "all out" without fear of injury. The ritual warm-up of baseball pitchers exemplifies this belief. Is it conceivable that a pitcher would enter a game, throwing at competitive speeds, without previously warming up? Would any athlete begin competition without first stretching and engaging in a particular form, intensity, or duration of warm-up? Most performers would respond with a definite no, yet objective support for this response remains elusive. One reason is the difficulty designing a well-controlled experiment with topflight athletes to determine the necessity of warming up and whether it improves subsequent performance with reduced injury risk. For preexercise stretching, research with army recruits indicates that a typical muscle-stretching protocol in the preexercise warm-up produces *no* clinically meaningful reductions in risk of exercise-related injury compared with subsequent exercise without warm-up.[249] In addition, strength loss, loss of motion, soreness, or markers of muscle damage from eccentric exercise were no different between groups that received preexercise passive warm-up with short-wave diathermy, active warm-up with concentric muscle actions, or no warm-up.[98]

Certain sport-related situations require peak performance with little time for warming up. For example, a reserve player entering the last few minutes of a game has no time for stretching, vigorous calisthenics, or taking practice shots; the player must go all out and achieve optimal performance without warm-up, except that done before the game or at intermission. Do more injuries occur in such cases? Does physical performance (e.g., shooting, rebounding, or basketball defense) deteriorate during the first few minutes of this "unwarmed" condition from that proceeded by a warm-up? Future research must address such questions.

Psychologic factors, including an athlete's ingrained belief in the importance of warming up, establish a definite bias when comparing maximum performance with and without warm-up. It is difficult if not impossible to obtain a maximum effort without warm-up if a subject believes in the importance of preliminary exercise. In this regard, some researchers have hypnotized subjects to neutralize preconceived notions about warm-up.

Physiologic Considerations

One study evaluated the effect of warm-up on 2-minute sprint-cycling performance at 120% of the power output at $\dot{V}O_{2max}$. Warm-up produced a higher muscle temperature, lower blood lactate level, and higher oxygen consumption during the first minute of exercise than the no-warm-up condition.[269] Warm-up augments local blood flow at the onset of exercise, thus increasing the aerobic contribution to muscle energy metabolism early in exercise.[133] However, increased muscle temperature per se does not contribute to the slow component (after several minutes) of oxygen-consumption kinetics during intense exercise. Any oxygen delivery–use benefits early in exercise from increased muscle temperature with warm-up may not carry over as exercise progresses. An active warm-up 5 minutes prior to a 30-second maximal sprint on a bicycle ergometer produced less blood and muscle lactate than equivalent effort without a physical warm-up.[127] Differences in muscle temperature with an active warm-up could not account for the ergogenic effect because exercise in the control condition also involved passively heating the muscle to the same temperature. These findings suggest a decreased reliance on anaerobic sources of energy during the exercise period preceded by a physical warm-up.

Five mechanisms explain why warm-up "should" improve physical performance and exercise capacity because of subsequent increases in blood flow and muscle and core temperature:

1. Faster muscle contraction and relaxation
2. Greater economy of movement from lowered viscous resistance within active muscles
3. Facilitated oxygen delivery and use by muscles because hemoglobin releases oxygen more readily at higher temperatures (Bohr effect)
4. Facilitated nerve transmission and muscle metabolism because increased temperature accelerates bodily processes; a specific warm-up may also facilitate recruitment of required motor units
5. Increased blood flow through active tissues as the local vascular bed dilates from increased metabolism and higher muscle temperature

Effects on Performance

Because of the strong psychologic component and possible physiologic benefits of warming-up, whether passive (massage, heat applications, and diathermy), general (calisthenics, jogging), or specific (practicing the actual movements), allied health and fitness professionals typically recommend continuing such procedures until evidence justifies its elimination. A warm-up provides a comfortable lead-in to more vigorous exercise. *The warm-up should progress gradually at sufficient intensity to increase muscle and core temperatures without fatigue or reducing energy stores.* These considerations become highly individualized; a warm-up for an Olympic swimmer would exhaust the recreational swimmer. To gain the possible benefits from increased body temperature, the competition or activity should begin within several minutes following the warm-up. When possible, the warm-up should activate specific muscles in a way that mimics the anticipated activity and brings about full range of joint motion.

Sudden Strenuous Exercise

Sudden exertion can trigger the onset of myocardial infarction, particularly in sedentary persons and those with latent coronary artery disease.[44,218] With this in mind, consideration of possible benefits from warming up takes on clinical significance. Several studies have evaluated the effects of preliminary exercise on the cardiovascular response to sudden, strenuous exercise. The findings provide an essentially different physiologic framework to justify warm-up that relates importantly to adult fitness and cardiac rehabilitation programs and occupations and sports that require sudden bursts of physical effort.

In one study, 44 men free of overt symptoms of coronary artery disease ran on a treadmill at high intensity for 10 to 15 seconds without prior warm-up.[16] Evaluation of postexercise ECGs revealed that 70% of the subjects displayed abnormal changes attributable to inadequate myocardial oxygen supply. The altered ECG did not relate to age or fitness level. To evaluate the effect of a warm-up, 22 of the men with an abnormal ECG from the treadmill run jogged in place at moderate intensity (heart rate, 145 b · min⁻¹) for 2 minutes before treadmill running. With this warm-up, 10 men now showed normal tracings during sudden exertion, while another 10 men displayed improved ECG responses; only two subjects showed significant abnormalities. In a subsequent study, the exercise blood pressure response also improved with prior warm-up.[17] For seven men with no warm-up, systolic blood pressure averaged 168 mm Hg immediately after the 15-second treadmill run. This decreased to 140 mm Hg when the 2-minute jog-in-place warm-up preceded exercise.

Coronary blood flow does not adjust instantaneously to a sudden increase in myocardial work; transient myocardial ischemia (poor oxygen supply) can occur in apparently healthy and fit individuals. *Prior warm-up (at least 2 min of easy jogging) benefits the subsequent ECG and blood pressure responses to vigorous exercise in a manner that indicates a more favorable relationship between myocardial oxygen supply and demand.* A prudent practice for all persons, warming up before strenuous exercise is particularly important for individuals with limited myocardial blood flow from coronary artery disease. A brief warm-up provides more optimal blood pressure and hormonal adjustments at the onset of subsequent strenuous exercise. The warm-up serves two beneficial purposes under these conditions: (1) it reduces myocardial workload and thus the myocardial oxygen requirement and (2) it augments blood flow through the coronary arteries.

Oxygen Inhalation (Hyperoxia)

Athletes breathe oxygen-enriched or **hyperoxic gas mixtures** during time-outs, at half-time, or following strenuous exercise. They believe this procedure enhances the blood's oxygen-carrying capacity to facilitate oxygen transport to active or recovering muscles. The fact remains that when healthy persons breathe ambient air at sea level, hemoglobin in blood leaving the lungs normally remains 95 to 98% saturated with oxygen (see Chapter 13). In physiologic terms consider the following:

- Breathing air with a higher-than-normal oxygen concentration increases oxygen transport by hemoglobin to only a small extent—by about 1 mL of extra oxygen for every deciliter of blood (10 mL O_2 per liter).
- Oxygen that dissolves in plasma when breathing a hyperoxic mixture also increases by about 0.4 mL per deciliter of blood (4.0 mL O_2 per liter), or from the normal 0.3 mL per deciliter (3.0 mL per liter) to about 0.7 mL per deciliter (7.0 mL per liter) of blood.

The blood's oxygen-carrying capacity under hyperoxic conditions potentially increases by about 14 mL of oxygen for every liter of blood—10 mL "extra" attached to hemoglobin and 4 mL "extra" dissolved in plasma.

Preexercise Oxygen Breathing

Blood volume for a 70-kg person averages about 5000 mL (5.0 L). Breathing hyperoxic gas adds about 70 mL of oxygen to the total blood volume (5.0 L of blood $\times$ 14 mL "extra" O_2 per liter of blood). Despite any potential psychologic benefit for the athlete who believes that preexercise oxygen breathing helps subsequent performance, this procedure confers only a trivial physiologic advantage from any additional oxygen per se. This small benefit emerges only if subsequent exercise takes place without breathing ambient air in the interval between hyperoxic breathing and exercise. This is because ambient air's lower oxygen pressure causes any additional oxygen in the blood to exit the body.

The football player who breathes an oxygen-rich mixture on the sideline before returning to the game or the swimmer who takes a few breaths of oxygen before moving to the blocks for the starting instructions does not gain a competitive edge from physiologic benefits. This is particularly ironic in football, because metabolic reactions without oxygen generate almost all of the energy to power each play.

Oxygen Breathing During Exercise

Breathing hyperoxic gas during submaximal and maximal aerobic exercise enhances endurance performance. Oxygen breathing during vigorous exercise accelerates oxygen consumption at the onset of exercise (smaller oxygen deficit in repeated bouts of intense effort); reduces blood lactate, heart rate, and pulmonary ventilation in submaximal exercise; and increases $\dot{V}O_{2max}$ and the exercise training intensity.[201,243,267] In one study, subjects performed a 6.5-minute endurance ride on a bicycle ergometer at an exercise level equal to 115% of $\dot{V}O_{2max}$ while breathing either room air or 100% oxygen.[355] Tanks of compressed gas supplied both air and oxygen to mask a subject's knowledge of the breathing mixture. FIGURE 23.13A

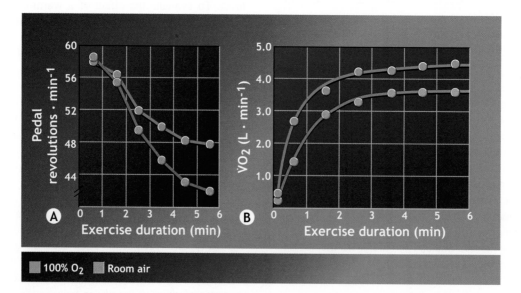

■ 100% O_2 ■ Room air

Figure 23.13   A. Endurance (measured by pedal revolutions each minute) while breathing 100% oxygen or ambient air. **B.** Oxygen consumption curves during the endurance rides show enhanced oxygen consumption while breathing oxygen. (Data from Weltman A, et al. Effects of increasing oxygen availability on bicycle ergometer endurance performance. Ergonomics 1978;21:427.)

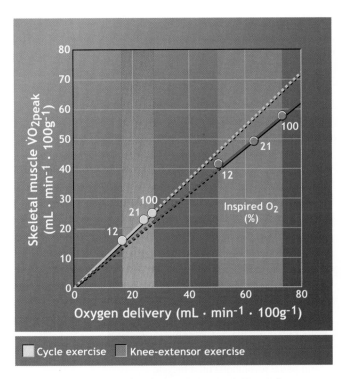

Figure 23.14 Relationship between skeletal muscle $\dot{V}O_{2peak}$ and oxygen delivery per 100 g of muscle during conventional maximal cycle ergometry exercise *(yellow)* and knee-extension exercise *(purple)* under hypoxia, normoxia, and hyperoxia. (From Richardson RS, et al. Evidence of O_2 supply–dependent $\dot{V}O_{2max}$ in exercise-trained human quadriceps. J Appl Physiol 1999;86:1048.)

shows superior endurance (less drop-off in pedal revolutions) while breathing oxygen during exercise. Figure 23.13B shows that the hyperoxic condition produced higher oxygen consumptions throughout exercise.

FIGURE 23.14 shows that oxygen consumption of the quadriceps muscle of seven trained subjects during maximum knee-extension exercise varied with the level of inspired oxygen, averaging lower in hypoxia (12% O_2) than in normoxia (21% O_2) and higher in hyperoxia (100% O_2) than normoxia. The figure also includes confirmatory results *(dotted yellow line)* from a previous study of cycle ergometry under comparable conditions.[180] Cycle ergometry produced lower muscle-specific $\dot{V}O_{2peak}$ values than knee-extension exercise. However, the slopes of the lines relating oxygen delivery to peak muscle oxidative metabolism were remarkably similar for both exercise modes. For maximal knee-extension exercise, oxygen content of venous blood leaving the active muscles remained essentially equal among conditions averaging 4 mL · dL^{-1}. Oxygen delivery in arterial blood increased from 17.3 to 19.5 to 21.8 mL · dL^{-1} with increasing levels of oxygen inhalation. Consequently, the hyperoxic condition during maximal exercise produced the largest skeletal muscle a-vO_2 difference and $\dot{V}O_{2peak}$. Similarly, maximal exercise intensity decreased 25% when breathing 12% inspired oxygen and increased 14% under 100% inspired oxygen compared with normoxic conditions. *Such findings support the contention that oxygen delivery to active muscles in the circulation, not use via mitochondrial metabolism, limits aerobic exercise.*

Breathing hyperoxic gas does not increase maximal cardiac output; thus, an expanded a-$\bar{v}O_2$ difference must account for the increased exercise oxygen consumption. The small increases in arterial hemoglobin saturation and dissolved plasma oxygen with hyperoxic breathing increase *total* oxygen availability as blood volume circulates 4 to 7 times each minute in strenuous exercise. The additional 14 mL of oxygen in each 1 L of blood from breathing hyperoxic gas represents considerable extra oxygen when exercising at a 20- to 30-L cardiac output. If the muscles metabolized the added oxygen during exercise, $\dot{V}O_{2max}$ would increase by 5 to 10%. The increased partial pressure of oxygen in solution from breathing hyperoxic gas also facilitates its diffusion across the tissue–capillary membrane into the mitochondria. More rapid oxygen diffusion may account for the higher oxygen consumption early in exercise under hyperoxic conditions. Reduced pulmonary ventilation under hyperoxic conditions lowers the oxygen cost of breathing. Theoretically, this liberates oxygen for use by the active, nonventilatory skeletal muscles. Hyperoxia also increases sustained muscle performance in intense static and dynamic movements not affected by central circulatory factors. The high oxygen pressure in blood and fluids within the active muscle environment may explain this ergogenic effect.

Breathing hyperoxic mixtures offers positive ergogenic benefits *during* endurance exercise, but offers limited practical sports application. The "legality" of using an appropriate breathing system during actual competition seems unlikely.

Oxygen Breathing During Recovery

Breathing hyperoxic mixtures does not facilitate recovery from exercise or improve performance in a subsequent exercise bout. FIGURE 23.15 illustrates the effects of breathing hyperoxic gas in recovery from strenuous exercise on subsequent exercise performance. Following 1 minute of all-out bicycle ergometer exercise, subjects recovered while breathing either room air or 100% oxygen for 10 or 20 minutes. They then repeated the all-out bicycle ride. No significant differences emerged in cumulative revolutions (graph A) and 6-second-by-6-second revolutions (graph B) for the 1-minute ride after breathing room air or 100% oxygen during recovery from previous exercise. Also, breathing either room air or oxygen yielded similar blood lactate levels in the 10- or 20-minute recovery periods. This indicated that breathing oxygen in recovery did not facilitate lactate removal. Subsequent research supports these findings; breathing oxygen after short intervals of submaximal and maximal exercise did not affect recovery kinetics for minute ventilation, heart rate, or serum lactate or the level of ensuing exercise performance.[268,363]

Modification of Carbohydrate Intake

Increased carbohydrate intake before and during high-intensity aerobic exercise, including periods of intense training, is a sound macronutrient manipulation that benefits exercise performance, lowers ratings of perceived exertion, and improves psychologic state.[1,325] Vigilance and mood also

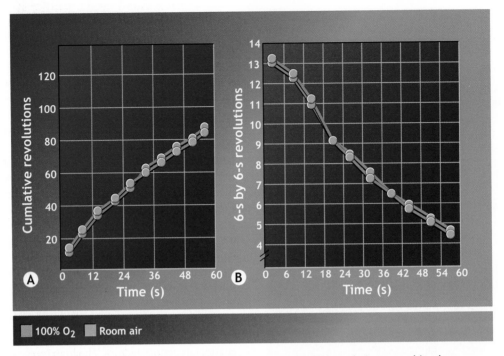

Figure 23.15 Cumulative (**A**) and absolute (**B**) 6-second pedal revolutions on a bicycle ergometer during 1 minute of maximal exercise after breathing either 100% oxygen or ambient air during recovery from a previous maximal exercise bout. (From Weltman A, et al. Exercise recovery, lactate removal, and subsequent high intensity exercise performance. Res Q 1977;48:786.)

improve with a carbohydrate beverage administered during a day of sustained aerobic activity interspersed with rest periods.[196] One of the more popular nutritional exercise modifications used by endurance athletes to augment glycogen reserves involves **carbohydrate loading** or **glycogen supercompensation**. The procedure produces considerably higher "packing" of muscle glycogen than simply maintaining a high-carbohydrate diet. Normally, each 100 g of muscle contains about 1.7 g of glycogen; carbohydrate loading packs up to 4 to 5 g of glycogen.

Nutrient-Related Fatigue in Prolonged Exercise

Glycogen stored in the liver and active muscle supplies most of the energy for intense aerobic exercise. Prolonging such exercise reduces the body's glycogen reserves. This allows fat catabolism—from adipose tissue and liver fatty acid mobilization and intramuscular fat stores—to supply a progressively greater percentage of energy. A substantially lowered muscle glycogen level precipitates fatigue even though active muscle maintains sufficient oxygen with an almost unlimited potential energy from fat. Consuming a glucose and water solution near the point of fatigue allows exercise to continue, but for all practical purposes, "the muscles' fuel tank reads empty." Reliance on fat catabolism decreases power output from the considerably slower mobilization and breakdown of fat than carbohydrate. Marathon runners use the term **hitting the wall** (endurance cyclists use *bonking*) to describe sensations of fatigue and muscle pain associated when exercising with severe glycogen depletion.

In the late 1930s, Nordic scientists reported enhanced endurance performance when athletes consumed carbohydrate-rich diets. Conversely, switching to high-fat diets drastically reduced endurance capacity. Modifying the diet's macronutrient composition alters carbohydrate stores and profoundly affects subsequent prolonged high-intensity exercise performance. In a classic series of experiments, endurance capacity for subjects fed a high-carbohydrate diet was triple that when the same subjects consumed a high-fat diet of similar energy content.[27] Carbohydrate represents the important energy substrate during 1 to 2 hours of high-intensity exercise, so researchers searched for additional ways to increase preexercise glycogen reserves.

Classic Loading Procedure

TABLE 23.9 presents the classic procedure for achieving the supercompensation effect. The first phase involves reducing the muscle's glycogen content with prolonged exercise about 6 days before competition. Glycogen supercompensation occurs *only* in the specific muscles depleted by exercise, so athletes must engage the muscles activated in their sport. Preparing for marathon running, endurance swimming, or bicycling requires 90 minutes of moderately intense submaximal exercise in the specific activity. The athlete then maintains a low-carbohydrate diet (about 60 to 100 $g \cdot d^{-1}$) for several days to further deplete glycogen stores. (*Note:* Glycogen depletion increases intermediate forms of the glycogen-storing enzyme **glycogen synthase** within the depleted muscle fibers.) Moderate training continues during this time. Then, 3 days before competing, the athlete switches to

---

TABLE 23.9 ■ TWO-STAGE DIETARY PLAN TO INCREASE MUSCLE GLYCOGEN STORAGE

Stage 1—Depletion
Day 1: Exhausting exercise to deplete muscle glycogen in specific muscles
Days 2, 3, 4: Low-carbohydrate intake (60–100 g · d^{-1}; high percentage of protein and lipid in daily diet)

Stage 2—Carbohydrate loading
Days 5, 6, 7: High-carbohydrate intake (400–700 g · d^{-1}; normal percentage of protein in daily diet)

Competition day
High-carbohydrate precompetition meal

---

a high-carbohydrate diet (400 to 700 g · d^{-1}) and maintains this intake up to the precompetition meal. The supercompensation diet should also contain adequate daily protein, minerals, and vitamins and abundant water. Supercompensated muscle glycogen levels remain stable for at least 3 days during a maintenance phase (in a nonexercising individual) if the diet contains 60% of calories as carbohydrate.[118]

Athletes should learn all they can about carbohydrate loading before manipulating dietary and exercise habits to achieve a supercompensation effect. If an athlete decides to supercompensate after weighing the pros and cons (see pp. 594–595), the new food regimen should proceed in stages during training, not for the first time before competition. For example, the athlete should start with a long run followed by a high-carbohydrate diet. A detailed log should record how the dietary manipulation affects performance. A record of subjective feelings should include exercise depletion and replenishment phases. With positive results, the athlete can try the entire series—depletion, low-carbohydrate diet, and high-carbohydrate diet—but maintain the low-carbohydrate diet for only 1 day. With no adverse effects, the low-carbohydrate diet can gradually extend to a maximum of 4 days.

Sample Diets to Achieve the Supercompensation Effect. TABLE 23.10 provides a sample meal plan for carbohydrate depletion (stage 1) and carbohydrate loading (stage 2) preceding an endurance event.

Limited Applicability. *Carbohydrate loading's benefits to exercise performance apply only to intense aerobic activities longer than 60 minutes. Exercise lasting less than 60 minutes requires only normal carbohydrate intake and glycogen reserves.* For example, carbohydrate loading did not benefit trained runners in a 20.9-km (13-mile) run compared with a run following a low-carbohydrate diet. Similarly, no ergogenic effect emerged for time trial performance, heart rate, and rating of perceived exertion (RPE) for endurance-trained cyclists in a 100-km trial that simulated continuous changes in exercise intensity typical of competition.[47] Ingesting 40 g of carbohydrate immediately before exercise had no effect on 30-minute maximal cycling performance of well-trained cyclists.[238] Varying the carbohydrate percentage between 40 and 70% in an isocaloric diet produced no effect on intense exercise lasting either 10 or 30 minutes.[246] Anaerobic

---

TABLE 23.10 ■ SAMPLE MEAL PLAN FOR CARBOHYDRATE DEPLETION AND CARBOHYDRATE LOADING PRECEDING AN ENDURANCE EVENT

MEAL	STAGE 1 DEPLETION	STAGE 2 CARBOHYDRATE LOADING
Breakfast	0.5 cup fruit juice 2 eggs 1 slice whole-wheat toast 1 glass whole milk	1 cup fruit juice 1 bowl hot or cold cereal 1 to 2 muffins 1 Tbsp butter
Lunch	6 oz hamburger 2 slices bread salad (normal size) 1 Tbsp mayonnaise and salad dressing 1 glass whole milk	2–3 oz hamburger with bun 1 cup juice 1 orange 1 Tbsp mayonnaise 1 Tbsp mayonnaise pie or cake (one 8-in slice)
Snack	1 cup yogurt	1 cup yogurt, fruit, or cookies
Dinner	2–3 pieces of chicken, fried 1 baked potato with sour cream 0.5 cup vegetables iced tea (no sugar) 2 Tbsp butter	1–1.5 pieces of chicken, baked 1 cup vegetables 0.5 cup sweetened pineapple iced tea (sugar) 1 Tbsp butter
Snack	1 glass whole milk	1 glass chocolate milk with 4 cookies

During stage 1, the intake of carbohydrate approaches 60 g or 240 kCal; in stage 2, the carbohydrate intake increases to 400–700 g or about 1600–2800 kCal.

power output of 75 seconds' duration did not improve when preexercise dietary manipulation increased muscle glycogen availability above normal levels.[135] A 2-day maintenance of a high-carbohydrate diet (61% carbohydrate) or a low-to-moderate carbohydrate diet (31% carbohydrate) produced no effect on intermittent anaerobic exercise of five 20-second bouts interspersed with a 100-second recovery period followed by a sixth 30-second bout to exhaustion.[200] In contrast, ergogenic benefits did emerge for high-carbohydrate versus low-carbohydrate intakes when performing *multiple bouts* of short-term, sprints.[15]

Endurance training increases the rate and magnitude of glycogen replenishment.[227] For sports competition and exercise training, a daily diet that contains about 60 to 70% of calories as carbohydrates provides adequate muscle and liver glycogen reserves. This diet ensures about twice as much muscle glycogen as a typical diet of 45 to 50% carbohydrate. For well-nourished athletes, the supercompensation effect remains relatively small. During intense training, athletes who do not upgrade daily calorie and carbohydrate intakes to meet energy demands can experience chronic muscle fatigue and staleness.[70]

Gender Differences in Glycogen Storage and Catabolism in Exercise

Gender-related differences in muscle glycogen supercompensation remain controversial. One study reported a relatively small 13% increase in the muscle glycogen content of women when they switched from a mixed diet to a high-carbohydrate diet.[350] Other research indicated that women do not increase glycogen storage when dietary carbohydrate increases from 60 to 75% of total caloric intake.[315] Importantly, this increase in carbohydrate intake as a percentage of total calories represents *significantly less total carbohydrate intake* relative to lean body mass for women than for men. FIGURE 23.16 illustrates that equalizing daily carbohydrate intake for endurance-trained men and women at 12 g per kg of lean body mass for 3 consecutive days produced no gender differences in glycogen loading. These and other findings show that men and women possess an equal capacity to accumulate muscle glycogen when fed comparable amounts of carbohydrate relative to lean body mass.[316]

Gender differences do exist in carbohydrate metabolism in exercise before and after endurance training. During submaximal exercise at equivalent percentages of $\dot{V}O_{2max}$ (same relative workload), women derive a *smaller* proportion of total energy from carbohydrate oxidation than men. This gender difference in substrate oxidation during exercise does not persist into recovery.[148]

With similar endurance-training protocols, women and men display a decrease in glucose flux for a given submaximal power output.[61,109] At the same relative workload after training, women show an exaggerated shift toward fat catabolism whereas men do not. This suggests that endurance training induces greater glycogen-sparing at a given relative submaximal exercise intensity for women. Gender differences in

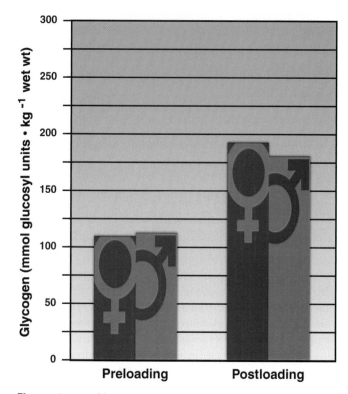

Figure 23.16 Muscle glycogen concentrations pre- and post-carbohydrate loading (12 g carbohydrate per kg lean body mass) in exercise-trained men and women. (From James AP, et al. Muscle glycogen supercompensation: absence of a gender-related difference. Eur J Appl Physiol 2001;85:533.)

exercise substrate metabolism may reflect differences in sympathetic nervous system adaptation to training (i.e., more blunted catecholamine response for women). A glycogen-sparing metabolic adaptation to training could benefit women's performance during high-intensity endurance competition.

Glycogen Supercompensation Enhanced by Prior Creatine Supplementation

A synergy exists between glycogen storage and creatine supplementation. For example, preceding glycogen loading with a 5-day creatine loading protocol (20 g per day) produced 10% greater glycogen packing in the vastus lateralis muscle than achieved with only glycogen loading.[274] More than likely, increases in creatine and cellular volume with creatine supplementation facilitate subsequent storage of muscle glycogen.

Negative Aspects of Carbohydrate Loading

The addition of 2.7 g of water with each gram of glycogen makes this a heavy fuel compared with equivalent energy stored as fat. The athlete often feels "heavy" and uncomfortable with this added water weight; any extra load also directly adds to the energy cost of running, racewalking, cross-country skiing, and other weight-bearing activities. The extra weight may negate any potential benefits from increased glycogen storage. On the positive side, water liberated during glycogen breakdown aids in temperature regulation, which benefits exercise in hot environments.

The classic model for supercompensation may pose potential hazards for individuals with specific health problems. A severe, chronic carbohydrate overload, interspersed with periods of high lipid and/or high protein intake, can increase blood cholesterol and urea nitrogen levels. High lipid intake often causes gastrointestinal distress plus poor recovery from the exercise-depletion sequence of the loading procedure. During the low-carbohydrate phase of loading, marked ketosis can occur in individuals who exercise while carbohydrate depleted. Failure to eat a balanced diet also produces mineral and vitamin deficiencies, particularly of the water-soluble vitamins. The glycogen-depleted state reduces the ability to train, possibly leading to a detraining effect during portions of the loading sequence. Dramatically reducing dietary carbohydrate for 3 or 4 days could set the stage for lean tissue loss because muscle protein serves as gluconeogenic substrate to maintain blood glucose levels in the glycogen-depleted state.

Modified Loading Procedure

The less-stringent **modified loading procedure** outlined in FIGURE 23.17 eliminates many potential negative aspects of the classic glycogen-loading sequence. The protocol increases glycogen synthase without requiring dramatic glycogen depletion with exercise as with the classic loading procedure; it increases glycogen storage to nearly the *same* level. The 6-day

protocol does not require prior exercise to exhaustion. Rather, the athlete trains at about 75% of $\dot{V}O_{2max}$ (85% HR_{max}) for 1.5 hours and then, on successive days, gradually reduces (tapers) exercise duration. During the first 3 days, carbohydrates represent about 50% of total calories. Three days before competition, the diet's carbohydrate content increases to 70% of total energy intake.

INTEGRATIVE QUESTION

What advice would you give to a sprint athlete who plans to carbohydrate load for competition?

Rapid Loading Procedure: A One-Day Requirement. The 2–6 days required to achieve supranormal muscle glycogen levels represents a limitation of typical carbohydrate loading procedures. A shortened time period that combines a relatively brief bout of high-intensity exercise with only 1 day of high-carbohydrate intake achieves the desired loading effect.[101] Endurance-trained athletes cycled for 150 seconds at an exercise intensity of 130% $\dot{V}O_{2max}$ followed by 30 seconds of all-out cycling. In the recovery period, the men consumed 10.3 g · kg body mass^{-1} of high glycemic carbohydrate foods. Biopsy data presented in FIGURE 23.18 indicated that glycogen in the vastus lateralis muscle increased from a 109.1 mmol · kg^{-1} preloading average to 198.3 mmol · kg^{-1} after only 24 hours. This 82% increase in glycogen storage equaled or exceeded values reported by others using a 2- to 6-day regimen. The short-duration loading procedure benefits individuals who do not wish to disrupt normal training with the time required and potential negative aspects of longer loading protocols.

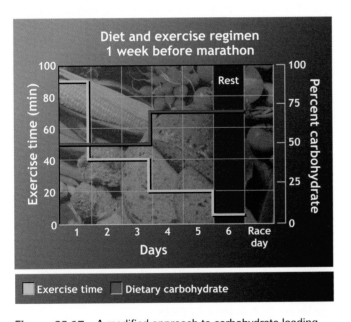

Figure 23.17 A modified approach to carbohydrate loading. Recommended combination of diet and exercise for overloading muscle glycogen stores in the week before an endurance contest. Exercise time is gradually reduced during the week, while the diet's carbohydrate content increases for the last 3 days. (From Sherman WM, et al. Effect of exercise-diet manipulation on muscle glycogen and its subsequent utilization during performance. Int J Sports Med 1981;2:114.)

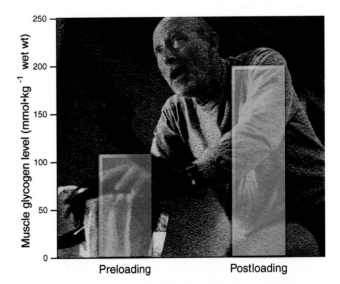

Figure 23.18 Muscle glycogen concentration of the vastus lateralis before (preloading) and after 180 seconds of near-maximal intensity cycling exercise followed by 1 day of high-carbohydrate intake (postloading). (From Fairchild TJ, et al. Rapid carbohydrate loading after short bout of near maximal-intensity exercise. Med Sci Sports Exerc 2002;34:980.)

L-Carnitine

L-Carnitine (L-3-hydroxytrimethylaminobutanoate), a short-chain carboxylic acid that contains nitrogen, is a vitamin-like compound found mostly in meat and dairy products. The liver and kidneys synthesize L-carnitine from methionine and lysine, with about 95% of the body's carnitine located in muscle cells. Carnitine facilitates influx of long-chain fatty acids into the mitochondrial matrix (as part of the carnitine acyltransferase enzyme system) where they enter β-oxidation during energy metabolism as follows:

$$Carnitine + acyl\text{-}CoA \Leftrightarrow acylcarnitine + CoA$$

The reaction enables the acyl components of long-chain fatty acyl-CoA (carbon chain lengths $\geq$ 10) to cross the mitochondrial membrane as substrate for oxidation. This carnitine-dependent process represents an important rate-limiting step in fatty acid oxidation.[35] Intracellular carnitine contributes to the maintenance of the acetyl-CoA:CoA ratio within the cell. Optimizing this ratio augments skeletal muscle energy metabolism by reducing inhibition of the pyruvate dehydrogenase enzyme; this facilitates conversion of pyruvate (and lactate) to acetyl-CoA, particularly in type I, slow-twitch muscle fibers. Theoretically, enhanced carnitine function could inhibit lactate accumulation and enhance exercise performance.[67,321] TABLE 23.11 outlines the potential mechanisms for carnitine supplementation to enhance exercise performance.

Rate of Fatty Acid Oxidation Affects Aerobic Exercise Intensity

During prolonged exercise, plasma FFAs often increase more than required by the energy expenditure. Plasma FFA elevation could result from inadequate mitochondrial fatty acid uptake and oxidation because of insufficient L-carnitine. Hence, increasing intracellular L-carnitine by dietary supplementation should promote fatty acid oxidation during exercise. This effect would increase aerobic energy transfer from fat breakdown while conserving limited glycogen reserves. Supplementation should provide the most benefit under glycogen depletion, which places the greatest demands on fatty acid oxidation. L-carnitine marketing targets endurance athletes who believe this "metabolic stimulator" enhances fat burning and spares glycogen. The alleged fat-burning benefits of L-carnitine appeal to bodybuilders as a practical way to reduce body fat. Unfortunately, *research does not support ergogenic benefits, positive metabolic alterations (aerobic or anaerobic), or body fat–reducing effects from L-carnitine supplementation.*[143,257]

Muscle carnitine levels do not differ between young and middle-aged men who consume a normal carnitine intake of 100 to 200 mg daily. For them, typical variations in muscle carnitine levels do not reflect capacity for aerobic metabolism.[305] Furthermore, no L-carnitine deficit occurs during long-term exercise or intense training.[76]

Consuming up to 2000 mg of L-carnitine either orally or intravenously during aerobic exercise does not affect the fuel mixture metabolized, endurance performance, aerobic capacity, or the exercise level for the onset of blood lactate accumulation (OBLA).[347] Short-term administration of 2000 mg of L-carnitine to endurance athletes either 2 hours before a marathon or 20-km into an endurance run increased plasma concentrations of all carnitine fractions but did not affect running performance, alter the metabolic mixture during the run, or enhance recovery.[65] Even with exercise prolonged and intense enough to deplete glycogen reserves, individuals receiving L-carnitine supplements did not alter substrate metabolism to indicate enhanced fat oxidation.[77] Carnitine supplementation also exerts no effect on repetitive short-term anaerobic exercise. Lactate accumulation, acid–base balance, or performance in five 100-yard swims with 2-minute rest intervals did not differ between male swimmers who consumed 2000 mg of L-carnitine in a citrus drink twice daily for 7 days and those who consumed only the citrus drink.[321]

Perhaps of Some Benefit

L-Carnitine acts as a vasodilator in peripheral tissues to possibly enhance regional blood flow and oxygen delivery.[143] In one study, subjects consumed either L-carnitine supplements (3000 mg · d^{-1} for 3 weeks) or an inert placebo to evaluate effects on delayed-onset muscle soreness (DOMS) after eccentric muscle actions.[115] Compared with placebo conditions, subjects receiving L-carnitine experienced less postexercise muscle pain and tissue damage, reflected by lower plasma levels of the muscle enzyme creatine kinase. The vasodilation property of L-carnitine might improve oxygen supply to damaged tissue and promote clearance of muscle damage by-products to reduce DOMS.

Chromium

The trace mineral chromium serves as a cofactor (as trivalent chromium) for a low-molecular-weight protein that potentiates insulin function, yet its precise mechanism of ac-

---

TABLE 23.11 ■ POTENTIAL MECHANISMS FOR A BENEFICIAL EFFECT OF CARNITINE SUPPLEMENTATION ON EXERCISE PERFORMANCE IN HEALTHY HUMANS

- Enhance muscle fatty acid oxidation
- Decrease muscle glycogen depletion rates
- Shift substrate use in muscle from fatty acid to glucose
- Replace muscle carnitine redistribution into acylcarnitine
- Activate pyruvate dehydrogenase via lowering of acetyl-CoA content
- Improve muscle fatigue resistance
- Replace carnitine lost during training

From Brass EP. Supplemental carnitine and exercise. Am J Clin Nutr 2000;72 (suppl):618S.

tion remains unclear. Insulin promotes carbohydrate transport into cells, augments fatty acid catabolism, and triggers cellular enzyme activity that facilitates protein synthesis. Chronic chromium deficiency can increase blood cholesterol and decrease the body's sensitivity to insulin, thus raising the risk for type 2 diabetes. Some adult Americans consume less than the 50 to 200 µg of chromium considered the estimated safe and adequate daily dietary intake (ESADDI). This occurs largely because chromium-rich foods—brewer's yeast, broccoli, wheat germ, nuts, liver, prunes, egg yolks, apples with skins, asparagus, mushrooms, wine, and cheese—do not usually form part of the regular diet. Food processing also removes substantial chromium from foods. In addition, strenuous exercise and associated high-carbohydrate intake promote urinary chromium losses, thus increasing the potential for chromium deficiency. For athletes with chromium-deficient diets, dietary modification to increase chromium intake or prudent use of chromium supplements seems appropriate.

Numerous Alleged Benefits

Touted as a "fat burner" and "muscle builder," chromium is one of the most hyped minerals in the health food/fitness literature. Supplemental intake of chromium, usually as **chromium picolinate**, often reaches 600 µg daily. This chelated picolinic acid combination supposedly yields better chromium absorption than the inorganic salt chromium chloride. Millions of Americans believe the unsubstantiated claims of health food faddists, television infomercials, and exercise zealots that additional chromium promotes muscle growth, curbs appetite, fosters body fat loss, and even lengthens life. Advertising targets chromium to bodybuilders and other resistance-trained athletes as a safe alternative to anabolic steroids to favorably change body composition. Chromium supplements supposedly potentiate insulin action to increase amino acid anabolism in skeletal muscle. This belief persists despite data that chromium supplements exert no effect on glucose or insulin concentrations in nondiabetic individuals.[6]

Generally, studies suggesting beneficial effects of chromium supplements on body fat and muscle mass infer body composition changes from changes in body weight (or unvalidated anthropometric measurements). One study observed that supplementing daily with 200 µg (3.85 µmol) of chromium picolinate for 40 days produced a small increase in FFM (estimated from skinfold thickness) and decrease in body fat in young men who resistance trained for 6 weeks.[97] The researchers provided no data to show increased muscular strength. Another study reported increases in body mass without changes in strength or body composition in previously untrained female college students (no change in males) who received a daily 200-µg chromium supplement during 12 weeks of resistance training compared with unsupplemented controls.[141]

Other research evaluated the effects of a chromium supplement of 200-µg daily on muscle strength, body composition, and chromium excretion in 16 untrained males during 12 weeks of resistance training.[134] Muscular strength improved

24% for the supplemented group and 33% for the placebo group during training. No changes occurred in any of the body composition variables. The group receiving the supplement did show higher chromium excretion than controls after 6 weeks of training. The researchers concluded that chromium supplements provided *no ergogenic effect* on any measured variable. Furthermore, supplementing with 800 µg of chromium picolinate (plus 6 mg of boron) proved no more effective than a maltodextrin placebo to enhance lean tissue gain or promote fat loss during resistance training.[5] Daily supplementation with 400 µg of chromium picolinate for 9 weeks did not promote weight loss in sedentary obese women; it actually caused weight gain during the treatment period.[125]

In support of chromium supplementation, greater body fat loss (no increase in FFM) occurred in subjects "recruited from a variety of fitness and athletic clubs" who consumed 400 µg of chromium daily over 90 days than in subjects who received a placebo.[169] Hydrostatic weighing and DEXA techniques assessed body composition. However, body compositional data from hydrostatic weighing do not appear in the report, and the DEXA-derived analysis indicated average body fat values of 42% for both control and experimental subjects, an extraordinary level of obesity for members of fitness clubs. Collegiate football players who received daily 200-µg supplements of chromium picolinate for 9 weeks showed no changes in body composition and muscular strength from intense weight training compared with controls receiving a placebo.[59] Similar findings of no benefit on body composition and exercise performance emerged from a 14-week study of NCAA Division I wrestlers that compared combined chromium picolinate supplementation with a typical preseason training program with identical training without supplementation.[351]

Loss of muscle mass commonly affects older individuals, so any potential ergogenic effect on muscle from chromium supplementation should emerge readily in this age group. This did not occur for older men involved in high-intensity resistance training; a high chromium picolinate dosage (924 µg · d^{-1}) did not augment muscle size, strength, or power or FFM accretion above the unsupplemented condition.[49] Obese personnel enrolled in the United States Navy's mandatory remedial physical-conditioning program who consumed an additional 400 µg of chromium picolinate daily showed no greater loss in body weight or percentage body fat or increase in FFM than a group receiving a placebo.[322]

A comprehensive double-blind study examined the effects of a daily chromium supplement (3.3 to 3.5 µmol as either chromium chloride or chromium picolinate) or a placebo for 8 weeks during resistance training in 36 young men. For each group, dietary intakes of protein, magnesium, zinc, copper, and iron equaled or exceeded recommended levels during training; subjects also maintained adequate baseline dietary chromium intakes. Supplementation increased serum chromium concentration and urinary chromium excretion equally regardless of its ingested form. TABLE 23.12 shows that compared with placebo treatment, chromium supplementation did not affect training-related changes in muscular strength, FFM, or muscle mass.

TABLE 23.12 ■ **EFFECTS OF TWO DIFFERENT FORMS OF CHROMIUM SUPPLEMENTATION ON AVERAGE VALUES FOR ANTHROPOMETRIC, BONE, AND SOFT-TISSUE COMPOSITION MEASUREMENTS BEFORE AND AFTER WEIGHT TRAINING**

	PLACEBO		CHROMIUM CHLORIDE		CHROMIUM PICOLINATE	
	PRE	POST	PRE	POST	PRE	POST
Age (y)	21.1	21.5	23.3	23.5	22.3	22.5
Stature (cm)	179.3	179.2	177.3	177.3	178.0	178.2
Weight (kg)	79.9	80.5[a]	79.3	81.1[a]	79.2	80.5
$\sum$4 skinfold thickness (mm)[b]	42.0	41.5	42.6	42.2	43.3	43.1
Upper-arm girth (cm)	30.9	31.6[a]	31.3	32.0[a]	31.1	31.4
Lower-leg girth (cm)	38.2	37.9	37.4	37.5	37.1	37.0
FFMFM (kg)[c]	62.9	64.3[a]	61.1	63.1[a]	61.3	62.7[a]
Bone mineral (g)	2952	2968	2860	2878	2918	2940
Fat-free body mass (kg)	65.9	67.3[a]	64.0	65.9[a]	64.2	66.1[a]
Fat (kg)	13.4	13.1	14.7	15.1	14.7	14.5
Body fat (%)	16.4	15.7	18.4	18.2	18.4	17.9

From Lukaski HC, et al. Chromium supplementation and resistance training: effects on body composition, strength, and trace element status of men. Am J Clin Nutr 1996;63:954.
[a] Significantly different from pretraining value.
[b] Measured at biceps, triceps, subscapular, and suprailiac sites.
[c] Fat-free, mineral-free mass.

Not Without a Potential Downside

Chromium competes with iron for binding to transferrin, the plasma protein that transports iron from ingested food and damaged red blood cells for delivery to tissues in need. The chromium picolinate supplement for the group whose data appear in Table 23.12 reduced serum transferrin (a measure of adequacy of current iron intake) compared with chromium chloride or placebo treatments. Conversely, other researchers observed that giving middle-aged men 924 µg of supplemental chromium daily as chromium picolinate for 12 weeks did not affect hematologic measures or indices of iron metabolism or status.[48] More research must determine whether chromium picolinate intake above recommended values adversely affects iron transport and distribution in the body. No studies have evaluated the safety of long-term chromium supplementation or the ergogenic efficacy of supplementing in individuals with suboptimal chromium status. Concerning the bioavailability of trace minerals in the diet, excessive dietary chromium inhibits zinc and iron absorption. At the extreme, this could induce iron-deficiency anemia, blunt the ability to train intensely, and negatively affect exercise performance requiring high-level aerobic metabolism.

Further potential bad news emerges from studies in which human tissue cultures that received extreme doses of chromium picolinate showed eventual chromosomal damage. Critics contend that such high laboratory dosages would not occur with supplement use in humans. Nonetheless, one could argue that cells continually exposed to excessive chromium (e.g., long-term supplementation) accumulate this mineral and retain it for years.

Coenzyme Q_{10} (Ubiquinone)

Coenzyme Q_{10} (CoQ_{10}, ubiquinone in oxidized form and ubiquinol when reduced), found primarily in meats, peanuts, and soybean oil, functions as an integral component of the mitochondrion's electron transport system of oxidative phosphorylation. This lipid-soluble component of all cells exists in high concentrations within myocardial tissue. CoQ_{10} has been used therapeutically to treat cardiovascular disease because of its role in oxidative metabolism and antioxidant properties that promote scavenging of free radicals that damage cellular components.[159,338] Owing to positive effect on oxygen uptake and exercise performance in cardiac patients, some consider CoQ_{10} a potential ergogenic nutrient for endurance performance. Based on the belief that supplementation increases electron flux through the respiratory chain to augment aerobic resynthesis of ATP, the popular literature touts CoQ_{10} supplements to improve "stamina" and enhance cardiovascular function.

CoQ_{10} supplementation increases serum CoQ_{10} levels, but it does not improve aerobic capacity, endurance performance, plasma glucose or lactate levels in submaximal exercise, or cardiovascular dynamics when compared with a placebo.[36,270,371] One study evaluated oral supplements of CoQ_{10} on exercise tolerance and peripheral muscle function of healthy, middle-aged men. Measurements included $\dot{V}O_{2max}$, lactate threshold, heart rate response, and upper-extremity exercise blood flow and metabolism.[250] For 2 months, subjects received either CoQ_{10} (150 mg per day) or placebo. Blood levels of CoQ_{10} increased during the treatment period and remained unchanged in the controls. No differences occurred between groups for any of the physiologic or metabolic variables. Similarly, for trained young and older men, CoQ_{10} supplementation of 120 mg per day for 6 weeks did not benefit aerobic capacity or lipid peroxidation, a marker of oxidative stress.[187] CoQ$_{1010}$ supplements (60 mg daily combined with vitamins E and C) did not affect lipid peroxidation during exercise in endurance athletes.[338] In contrast, rats supplemented with CoQ$_{10}$ (10 mg per day for 4 days), showed marked suppression of exercise-induced lipid peroxidation in liver, heart, and gastrocnemius muscle tissues.[99]

Future research must elucidate potential benefits from exogenous CoQ$_{10}$ supplementation. If benefits result, do they depend on the health status of one's cardiovascular system? On a negative note, CoQ$_{10}$ supplementation may induce harmful effects. Increased cell damage (increased plasma creatine kinase) occurred during intense exercise in subjects who received 60 mg of CoQ$_{10}$ twice daily for 20 days.[204] Researchers speculate that under conditions of high proton concentrations as occur in high-intensity aerobic exercise, CoQ$_{10}$ supplementation augments free radical production.[80,204] If this proves true, supplementation could trigger plasma membrane lipid peroxidation and eventual cellular damage. This is indeed paradoxical in light of CoQ$_{10}$'s wide use as an antioxidant supplement.

Creatine

Meat, poultry, and fish provide a rich source of creatine, containing 4 to 5 g of creatine per kg of food. The body synthesizes only about 1 g of this nitrogen-containing organic compound daily from the nonessential amino acids arginine, glycine, and methionine in the kidneys, liver, and pancreas. The animal kingdom contains the richest creatine-containing foods, placing vegetarians at a distinct disadvantage for ready sources of exogenous creatine. Skeletal muscle contains approximately 95% of the body's total 120 to 140 g of creatine.

Creatine sold in supplemental form as **creatine monohydrate (CrH$_2$O)** comes as a powder, tablet, capsule, and stabilized liquid. Adding phosphate salts to the CrH$_2$O molecule creates phosphocreatine (PCr), a less frequently used form of creatine supplementation. Supplements in this form produce the same training effects on body mass, muscular strength, and FFM (estimated from skinfolds) as creatine ingested in monohydrate form.[244] Creatine can be purchased over-the-counter or mail order as a nutritional supplement (but without guarantee of purity). Ingesting a liquid suspension of creatine monohydrate at the relatively high dosage of 20 to 30 g per day for 2 weeks increases intramuscular concentrations of free creatine and PCr up to 30%. These levels remain high for weeks after only a few days of supplementation.[149,209] Sports' governing bodies do not consider creatine an illegal substance.

Important Component of High-Energy Phosphates

Creatine passes through the digestive tract unaltered and is absorbed into the bloodstream by the intestinal mucosa. Just about all ingested creatine incorporates into skeletal muscle (average concentration, 125 mM [range 90 to 160 mM] per kg dry muscle). About 40% exists as free creatine; the remainder combines readily with phosphate (in the creatine kinase reaction shown below) to form PCr. Type II, fast-twitch muscle fibers store about 4 to 6 times more PCr than ATP. As emphasized in Chapter 5, PCr serves as the cells' "energy reservoir" to provide rapid phosphate-bond energy to resynthesize ATP (more rapid than ATP regenerated in glycogenolysis[131]) in the reversible reaction:

$$PCr + ADP \xrightarrow{\text{creatine kinase}} C + ATP$$

PCr also shuttles intramuscular high-energy phosphate between the mitochondria and muscle filament cross-bridge sites that initiate muscle action. Maintaining a high sarcoplasmic ATP:ADP ratio by energy transfer from PCr is important in maximum effort lasting up to 10 seconds. This exercise duration places high demands on ATP resynthesis that exceed energy transfer from intracellular macronutrient breakdown.[33,107] Improved energy transfer capacity from PCr also lessens reliance on energy from anaerobic glycolysis with associated increase in intramuscular H$^+$ and decrease in pH from lactate accumulation.[14] Because of limited intramuscular PCr, it seems reasonable that any PCr increase should accomplish the following:

- Accelerate ATP turnover to maintain power output during short-term muscular effort
- Delay PCr depletion
- Diminish dependence on anaerobic glycolysis and decrease subsequent lactate formation
- Facilitate muscle relaxation and recovery from repeated bouts of intense, brief effort via faster ATP and PCr resynthesis; rapid recovery allows continued higher level power output

Documented Benefits in Humans

Creatine supplementation received notoriety as an ergogenic aid when British sprinters and hurdlers used it in the 1992 Barcelona Olympic Games. Creatine supplementation at recommended levels exerts the following three effects:

1. Improves performance in muscular strength and power activities
2. Augments short bursts of muscular endurance
3. Provides for greater muscular overload to augment training effectiveness

No serious adverse effects from creatine supplementation for up to 4 years have been reported.[287] Studies with animals suggest that creatine or creatine analogs exert beneficial effects on a number of diseases, although some data suggest an increased potential for renal dysfunction.[119] The typical use of creatine for ergogenic purposes does not alter insulin action in healthy, active untrained men.[228] Anecdotes indicate a possible association between creatine supplementation and cramping in multiple muscle areas during competition or lengthy practice in American football players. This effect may result from (1) altered intracellular dynamics because of increased levels of free creatine and PCr or (2) osmotically induced enlarged cell volume (greater cellular hydration) from the muscle fibers' increased creatine content. Gastrointestinal tract disturbances (nausea, indigestion, and difficulty absorbing food) have been linked to exogenous creatine ingestion.

FIGURE 23.19 illustrates the ergogenic effects of creatine supplementation on total work accomplished during repetitive sprint cycling performance. Physically active but untrained males performed sets of maximal 6-second bicycle sprints interspersed with various recovery periods (24, 54, or 84 s) to simulate sport conditions. Performance evaluations took place under creatine-loaded (20 g per day for 5 days) or placebo conditions. Supplementation increased muscle creatine (48.9%) and PCr (12.5%), which produced a 6% increase in total work accomplished (251.7 kJ presupplement vs. 266.9 kJ creatine loaded) compared to the placebo group (254.0 kJ pretest vs. 252.3 kJ placebo). Creatine supplements have benefited an on-court "ghosting" routine of simulated positional play of competitive squash players.[277] Supplementation also augments repeated sprint cycle performance after 30 minutes of constant load, submaximal exercise in the heat, without adversely affecting thermoregulatory dynamics.[346]

FIGURE 23.20 outlines possible mechanisms for enhancement of exercise performance and training response by elevating intramuscular free creatine and PCr. Taking a high dose of creatine helps replenish muscle creatine following intense exercise. This metabolic "reloading" promotes recovery of muscle contractile capacity, enabling athletes to maintain repeated efforts of high-intensity exercise and training. A facilitated rate of muscle relaxation may also contribute to the ergogenic action of creatine supplementation.[330] Besides benefiting weight

lifting and bodybuilding, improved immediate anaerobic power output capacity aids sprint running, swimming, kayaking, cycling, jumping, football, and volleyball. Oral creatine supplementation combined with heavy resistance training affects cellular processes in a manner that increase protein deposition within the muscle's contractile mechanism.[360] This response could explain any increase in muscle size and strength associated with creatine supplementation in vivo.

Creatine monohydrate supplements substantially increase muscle creatine content and performance in high-intensity exercise, particularly repeated intense muscular effort (TABLE 23.13).[34,215,233,261,262,275,297,328,344] It remains unclear whether the ergogenic effect differs in vegetarians and meat eaters.[291] One research study evaluated a creatine dose of 30 g daily for 6 days in trained runners under two conditions: (1) four repeated 300-m runs with a 4-minute recovery and (2) four 1000-m runs with a 3-minute recovery.[137] Compared with placebo treatment, creatine supplementation improved performance under both conditions with the most impressive gains in repeated 1000-m runs. Supplementing with 20 g of creatine daily for 4 days also benefited anaerobic capacity in three 30-second Wingate tests with a 5-minute rest between trials. For Division I football players, creatine supplementation with resistance training increased body mass, lean body mass, cellular hydration, and muscular strength and performance.[24] Similarly, supplementation augmented muscular strength and size increases during 12-weeks of resistance training.[360] The enhanced hypertrophic response with supplementation and resistance training possibly results from accelerated myosin heavy-chain synthesis. For resistance-trained men classified as "responders" to creatine supplementation (i.e., a creatine increase ≥ 32 mmol · kg dry wt muscle^{-1}), 5 days of supplementation increased body weight and FFM, and peak force and total force during repeated maximal isometric bench-presses.[177] For men classified as "nonresponders" to supplementation (i.e., creatine increase ≤ 21 mmol · kg dry wt muscle^{-1}), no ergogenic effect occurred.

Creatine supplementation does not improve cardiovascular and metabolic responses during continuous incremental treadmill running,[104,128] or performance that requires a high level of aerobic energy transfer.[13,93]

Are There Risks?

Potential dangers of short-term creatine supplementation have been studied in healthy individuals, particularly the effects on cardiac muscle and kidney function (creatine degrades to creatinine before excretion in urine). Creatine consumed 20 g per day for 5 consecutive days produced no detrimental effect on blood pressure, plasma creatine, plasma CK activity, or renal function, measured by glomerular filtration rate and total protein and albumin excretion rates.[168,185,216] Only limited information exists about the effects of long-term, high-dose supplementation with creatine. For healthy subjects, no differences in plasma contents and urinary excretion rates for creatinine, urea, and albumin emerged between control sub-

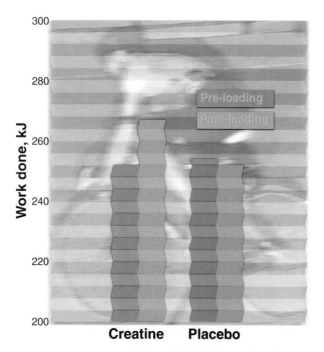

Figure 23.19 Effects of creatine loading versus placebo on total work accomplished during repetitive sprint-cycling performance. (From Preen CD, et al. Effect of creatine loading on long-term sprint exercise performance and metabolism. Med Sci Sports Exerc 2001;33:814.)

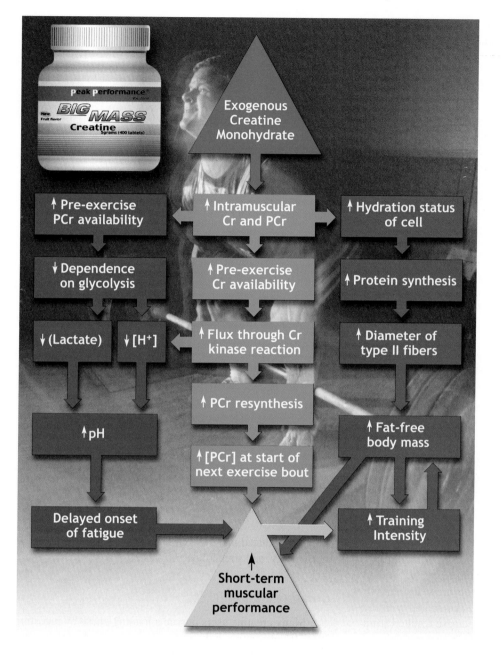

Figure 23.20 Mechanisms to explain why increased intracellular creatine *(Cr)* and phosphocreatine *(PCr)* might enhance intense, short-term exercise performance and the exercise-training response. (Modified from Volek JS, Kraemer WJ. Creatine supplementation: its effect on human muscular performance and body composition. J Strength Cond Res 1996;10:200.)

jects and individuals who consumed creatine for up to 5 years.[248] Glomerular filtration rate, tubular reabsorption, and glomerular membrane permeability also remained normal with long-term creatine use. Individuals with suspected renal malfunction should refrain from creatine supplementation because of the potential for exacerbating the disorder.[255]

Age Effects Uncertain. Whether or not creatine supplementation augments the training response in older individuals remains equivocal. For 70-year old men, a creatine supplementation loading phase (0.3 g per kg body mass for 5 days) followed by a daily maintenance phase (0.07 g per kg body mass) increased lean tissue mass, leg strength, muscular endurance, and average power of the legs during resistance training to a greater extent than a placebo.[58] Similarly, creatine supplements benefit muscular performance in normally active older men.[120] In con-

trast, no enhancement in resistance training response to creatine ingestion occurred among sedentary and weight-trained older adults.[28] These results were attributed to an age-related decline in creatine transport efficiency. Short-term creatine supplementation per se, without resistance training, does not increase muscle protein synthesis or FFM.[241]

Effects on Body Mass and Body Composition. Body mass increases between 0.5 and 5.2 kg often accompany creatine supplementation,[88,155,166,346] independent of changes in testosterone or cortisol concentrations.[345] Short-term creatine supplementation exerts no effect on the hormonal response to resistance training.[234] It is unclear how much of the weight gain occurs from the anabolic effect of creatine on muscle tissue synthesis, retention of intracellular water from increased creatine stores, or other factors.

TABLE 23.13 ■ SELECTED STUDIES SHOWING INCREASES IN EXERCISE PERFORMANCE FOLLOWING CREATINE MONOHYDRATE SUPPLEMENTATION

REFERENCE	EXERCISE	PROTOCOL	EXERCISE PERFORMANCE
d	Isokinetic, unilat, knee extensions ($180°·s^{-1}$)	5 bouts of 30 ext, w/1-min rest periods	Less decline in peak torque production during bouts 2, 3, and 4
e	Running	4–300 m w/4-min rest periods	Improved time for final 300- and 1000-m runs
		4–1000 m w/3-min rest periods	Improved total time for 4–1000-m runs; reduction in best time for 300- and 1000-m runs
a	Cycle ergometry (140 rev·min^{-1})	Ten 6-s bouts w/1-min rest periods	Better able to maintain pedal frequency during second 4–6 of each bout
f	Cycle ergometry (140 rev·min^{-1})	Five 6-s bouts w/30-s recovery followed by one 10-s bout	Better able to maintain pedal frequency near end of 10-s bout
b	Cycle ergometry (80 rev·min^{-1})	Three 30-s bouts w/4-min rest periods	Increase in peak power during bout 1 and increase in mean power and total work during bouts 1 and 2
c	Bench press	1-RM bench press and total reps at 70% 1-RM	Increase in 1-RM; increase in reps at 70% of 1-RM
g	Bench press	5 sets bench press w/2-min rest periods	Increase in reps completed during all 5 sets
g	Jump squat	5 sets jump squat w/2-min rest periods	Increase in peak power during all 5 sets

[a] Balsom PD, et al. Creatine supplementation and dynamic high-intensity intermittent exercise. Scand J Med Sci Sports 1995;3:143.
[b] Birch R, et al. The influence of dietary creatine supplementation on performance during repeated bouts of maximal isokinetic cycling in man. Eur J Appl Physiol 1994;69:268.
[c] Earnest CP, et al. The effect of creatine monohydrate ingestion in anaerobic power indices, muscular strength and body composition. Acta Physiol Scand 1995;153:207.
[d] Greenhaff PL, et al. Influence of oral creatine supplementation on muscle torque during repeated bouts of maximal voluntary exercise in man. Clin Sci 1993;84:565.
[e] Harris RC, et al. The effect of oral creatine supplementation on running performance during maximal short-term exercise in man. J Physiol 1993;467:74P.
[f] Soderlund K, et al. Creatine supplementation and high-intensity exercise: influence on performance and muscle metabolism. Clin Sci 1994;87(suppl):120.
[g] Volek JS, et al. Creatine supplementation enhances muscular performance during high-intensity resistance exercise. J Am Diet Assoc 1997;97:765.
From Volek JS, Kraemer WJ, Creatine supplementation: its effect on human muscular performance and body composition. J Strength Cond Res 1996;10:200.

Creatine intake during resistance training (4-d pretraining dosage, 20 g · d^{-1}, followed by 5 g · d^{-1} during training) by young adult females increased maximal strength of trained muscles (20–25%), maximal intermi ttent exercise capacity of the arm flexors (10–25%), and FFM (6%) compared with the placebo condition.[327] Part of the FFM increase resulted from additional muscle water content. A 2.42-kg body mass gain associated with creatine supplementation and resistance/agility training resulted partly from increases in fat/bone-free body mass unrelated to an increase in total body water.[182]

Resistance-trained men matched for physical characteristics and maximal strength randomly received a placebo or creatine supplement. Supplementation consisted of 25 g daily followed by maintenance at 5 g daily. Both groups engaged in heavy resistance training for 12 weeks. FIGURE 23.21A shows the greater training-induced increase in body mass and FFM for the creatine-supplemented group compared with controls. Greater maximum bench press and squat strength increases occurred in the creatine group than in controls Fig. 23.21B). Creatine supplementation induced greater muscle fiber hypertrophy with resistance training, indicated by greater enlargement in types I (35 vs. 11%), IIA (36 vs. 15%), and IIAB muscle fiber cross-sectional areas (35 vs. 6%; Fig. 23.21C). The larger volume of weight lifted during weeks 5 to 8 by the creatine supplement group suggests that higher quality training

sessions mediated more favorable adaptations in FFM, muscle morphology, and strength performance.

Creatine Loading

Many creatine users pursue a loading phase by ingesting 20 to 30 g of creatine daily for 5 to 7 days. Individuals who consume vegetarian-type diets show the greatest increase in muscle creatine levels because of their low dietary creatine content. Particularly large increases characterize individuals with normally low basal levels of intramuscular creatine.[45] A maintenance phase follows the loading phase. During this time, the athlete supplements with as little as 2 to 5 g of creatine daily.

Practical questions for the athlete desiring to elevate intramuscular creatine levels concern the magnitude and time course of intramuscular creatine increase with supplementation, dosage needed to maintain creatine increase, and rate of creatine loss, or "washout," when supplementation ceases. To provide insight into these questions, researchers studied two groups of men. In one experiment, six men ingested 20 g of creatine monohydrate (approximately 0.3 g per kg of body mass) for 6 consecutive days and then stopped the supplementation. Biopsies assessed muscle creatine levels before supplement ingestion and at days 7, 21, and 35. Similarly, nine men took 20 g of creatine monohydrate daily for 6 consecutive days. Instead

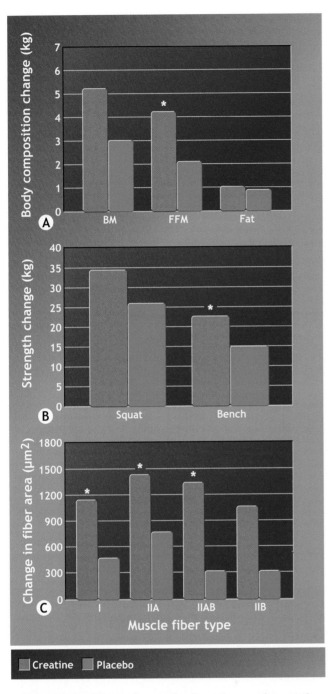

Figure 23.21 Effects of 12 weeks of creatine supplementation plus heavy resistance training on changes in (**A**) body mass *(BM)* fat-free body mass *(FFM)*, and body fat, (**B**) muscular strength in the squat and bench press, and (**C**) cross-sectional areas of specific muscle fiber types. The placebo group underwent identical training and received an equivalent quantity of powdered cellulose in capsule form. * Change significantly greater than in placebo group. (From Volek JS, et al. Performance and muscle fiber adaptations to creatine supplementation and heavy resistance training. Med Sci Sports Exerc 1999;31:1147.)

declined to near baseline in 35 days. The group that continued to supplement with reduced creatine intake for an additional 28 days maintained muscle creatine at the higher level (Fig. 23.22B).

For both groups, the increase in total muscle creatine content during the initial 6-day supplementation period averaged about 23 mmol per kg of dry muscle; this represented about 20 g (17%) of total creatine ingested. A similar 20% increase in total muscle creatine concentration occurred with only a 3-g daily supplement. The increase occurred more gradually and required 28 days rather than 6 days with the 6-g supplement.

A rapid way to creatine-load skeletal muscle requires ingesting 20 g of creatine monohydrate daily for 6 days; switching to a reduced 2-g per day dosage keeps these levels

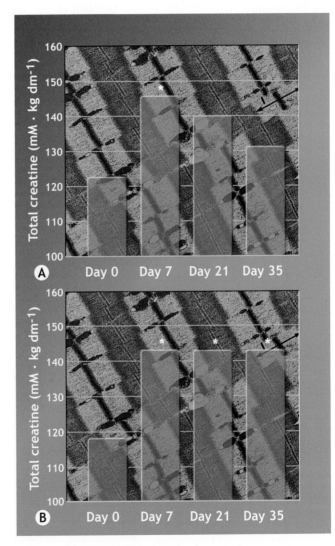

Figure 23.22 **A.** Total muscle creatine concentration in six men who ingested 20 g of creatine for 6 consecutive days and then stopped the supplement. Muscle biopsies done before ingestion (day 0) and on days 7, 21, and 35. **B.** Total muscle creatine concentration in nine men who ingested 20 g of creatine for 6 consecutive days and then ingested 2 g of creatine daily for the next 28 days. Muscle biopsies done before ingestion (day 0) and on days 7, 21, and 35. Values refer to averages per dry mass *(dm)*. * Significantly different from day 0. (From Hultman E, et al. Muscle creatine loading in men. J Appl Physiol 1996;81:232.)

of discontinuing supplementation, they reduced dosage to 2 g daily (approximately 0.03 g per kg body mass) for an additional 28 days. FIGURE 23.22A shows that total muscle creatine concentration increased approximately 20% after 6 days. Without continued supplementation, muscle creatine content gradually

elevated for up to 28 days. If rapidity of loading does not matter, supplementing with 3 g daily for 28 days achieves the same high levels.

Carbohydrate Ingestion Augments Creatine Loading.

Consuming creatine with a sugar-containing drink increases creatine uptake and storage in skeletal muscle (FIG. 23.23).[129,298] For 5 days, subjects received either 5 g of creatine four times daily or a 5-g supplement followed 30 minutes later by 93 g of a high-glycemic simple sugar four times daily. The creatine-only group increased muscle PCr (7.2%), free creatine (13.5%), and total creatine (20.7%). Much larger increases occurred for the creatine plus sugar-supplemented group (14.7% for PCr, 18.1% for free creatine, and 33.0% for total creatine). Creatine supplementation alone did not affect insulin secretion, whereas adding sugar elevated plasma insulin levels. More than likely, augmented creatine storage with a creatine-plus-sugar supplement resulted from insulin-mediated glucose transport into skeletal muscle, which facilitated creatine transport into muscle fibers.

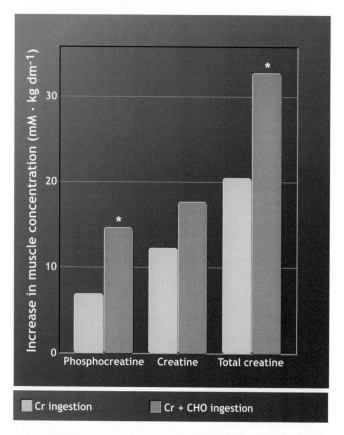

Figure 23.23 Increases in dry muscle (dm) concentrations of phosphocreatine (PCr), creatine (Cr), and total creatine in one group after 5 days of Cr supplementation and in another group after 5 days of Cr and carbohydrate (CHO) supplementation. Values represent averages. * Significantly greater than creatine-only supplementation. (From Green AL, et al. Carbohydrate ingestion augments skeletal muscle creatine accumulation during creatine supplementation in humans. Am J Physiol 1996;271:E821.)

Stop Caffeine When Using Creatine. *Caffeine negates the ergogenic effect of creatine supplementation.* To evaluate the effect of preexercise caffeine ingestion on intramuscular creatine stores and high-intensity exercise performance, subjects consumed either a placebo, a daily creatine supplement ($0.5 \ g \cdot kg^{-1}$ body mass), or the same daily creatine supplement plus caffeine ($5 \ mg \cdot kg^{-1}$ body mass) for 6 days.[326] Under each condition, subjects performed maximal intermittent knee-extension exercise to fatigue on an isokinetic dynamometer. Creatine supplementation, with or without caffeine, increased intramuscular PCr (evaluated by nuclear magnetic resonance spectroscopy) between 4 and 6%. Dynamic torque production also increased 10 to 23% with creatine compared with the placebo. Consuming caffeine *totally negated* creatine's ergogenic effect. *Athletes who load creatine should abstain from caffeine-containing foods and beverages for several days before competition.*

Some Research Shows No Benefit

Not all research confirms positive effects of creatine supplementation. Ergogenic effects may not emerge under the following conditions:

- In untrained subjects performing a single 15-second bout of sprint cycling[68]
- In trained subjects performing bouts of sport-specific physical activities such as swimming, cycling, and running[46,102,264]
- In trained and untrained older adults[156,364]
- In resistance-trained individuals[309]
- In trained rowers[81]
- During rapid weight loss[232]
- When short-term supplementation does not increase muscle PCr[102,225]

The reason for the discrepancies remains unknown.

Ribose: The Next Creatine on the Supplement Scene?

Ribose has emerged as a competitor to creatine as a supplement to increase power and replenish high-energy compounds following intense exercise. The body readily synthesizes ribose, and the diet provides small amounts through ripe fruits and vegetables. Metabolically, this 5-carbon sugar serves as an energy substrate for ATP resynthesis. Because of this role in energy metabolism, exogenous ribose ingestion is promoted to quickly restore the body's limited amount of ATP. To maintain optimal ATP levels, recommended ribose doses range from 10 g to 20 g per day. Clearly, any compound that either increases ATP levels or facilitates its resynthesis would benefit short-term, high-power physical activities. Only limited experimentation exists to assess this potential for ribose. A double-blind randomized study evaluated the effect of oral ribose supplementation (4 doses per day at 4 g per dose) on repeated bouts of maximal exercise and ATP replenishment after intermittent maximal muscle contractions.[235] No significant difference in any measure (e.g., intermittent isokinetic knee-extension force, blood lactate, and plasma ammonia concentration) emerged between ribose and placebo trials. The exercise did decrease intramuscular ATP and total adenine nucleotide content immediately after exercise and 24 hours later, yet ribose supplementation proved ineffective in facilitating recovery of these compounds. Other researchers have also shown no ergogenic effects of ribose supplementation in healthy untrained or trained groups.[26,184]

Inosine and Choline

Inosine

Many popular articles and advertisements tout inosine as an amino acid, when in fact it is a nucleic acid derivative found naturally in brewer's yeast and organ meats. Inosine (and choline) are not considered essential nutrients. The body synthesizes inosine from precursor amino acids and glucose. Metabolically, inosine participates in forming purines such as adenine, one of the structural components of ATP. Strength and power athletes supplement with inosine believing that it increases ATP stores to improve training quality and competitive performance. Some also theorize that inosine supplementation augments synthesis of red blood cell 2,3-diphosphoglycerate, thus facilitating oxygen release from hemoglobin at the tissue level. Others suggest that inosine plays an ergogenic role by stimulating insulin release to speed glucose delivery to the myocardium, augmenting cardiac contractility, or acting as a vasodilating agent. These theoretical considerations, plus anecdotal claims, provide the basis for popular marketing themes that extol inosine as a supplement to boost anaerobic and aerobic exercise performance. *Objective data do not support an ergogenic role for inosine supplementation.*

Highly trained young and older men and women who supplemented daily with 6000 mg of inosine for 2 days failed to improve 3-mile treadmill run time, peak oxygen uptake, blood lactate level, heart rate, or RPE.[359] Interestingly, subjects could not exercise as long on a test for aerobic capacity when supplemented with inosine as in the unsupplemented state. In another study, male competitive cyclists received either a placebo or a 5000-mg per day oral inosine supplement for 5 days.[306] They then performed a Wingate bicycle test, a 30-minute self-paced bicycle endurance test, and a constant load, supramaximal cycling sprint to fatigue. FIGURE 23.24 shows the results for maximal anaerobic power output on the 30-second Wingate test (A) and heart rate (B), RPE (C), and total work accomplished (D) during segments of the 30-minute endurance ride. No significant differences occurred in any of the criterion variables between placebo and supplemented conditions. In agreement with the ergolytic effect of inosine noted above,[359] cyclists fatigued nearly 10% more rapidly on the supramaximal sprint test when they consumed inosine than without it. Additionally, serum uric acid levels nearly doubled following 5 days of inosine supplementation—a level normally associated with gout, an inherited metabolic disorder characterized by recurrent acute arthritis and deposition of crystalline urate in connective tissues and articular cartilage. *These findings alone contraindicate any use of inosine supplements for possible ergogenic effects.*

Choline

All animal tissues contain choline, an important compound for normal cellular functioning. Although humans synthesize choline, it (like inosine) also must be obtained in the diet. Lecithin, a structural component of lipoproteins and the cells' phospholipid plasma membrane, and the neurotransmitter acetylcholine (which controls skeletal muscle activation at the myoneural junction) incorporate choline into their chemical structures. Choline functions as a lipotrophic agent as part of the lecithin molecule either to depress accumulation of fat in the liver or to increase fatty acid uptake by the liver. Very low density lipoproteins (the major transporting vehicle of triacylglycerols synthesized in the liver) also contain choline. A subpar choline intake increases the liver's triacylglycerol content. Many foods contain ample choline; top food sources include eggs (yolk), brewer's yeast, liver (beef, pork, lamb), wheat germ, soybeans, dehydrated potatoes, oatmeal, and vegetables in the cabbage family.

Inositol and choline supplements depress fat accumulation in the liver when given to animals deficient in these compounds. However, supplements did not affect percentage carcass fat of aerobically trained rats, although the supplemented animals gained less weight during the training period.[175] Body builders frequently take choline- and inositol-containing "metabolic optimizing powders" and "fat-burning tablets" prior to competition, hoping to increase muscle mass/fat mass ratio to achieve the "cut" look. We are unaware of research on humans that supports supplementation with inositol–choline products for such purposes.

Lipid Supplementation with Medium-Chain Triacylglycerols

Do high-fat foods or lipid supplements elevate plasma fatty acid levels to increase energy availability from fat during prolonged aerobic exercise? Several factors affect the answer to this question. First, consuming triacylglycerols composed of predominantly long-chain fatty acids (12 to 18 carbons) delays gastric emptying. This negatively affects the rapidity of fat availability and slows fluid and carbohydrate replenishment, both crucial factors in intense endurance exercise. Second, after digestion and intestinal absorption (normally 3 to 4 h), long-chain triacylglycerols reassemble with phospholipids, fatty acids, and a cholesterol shell to form fatty droplets called *chylomicrons*. These substances travel slowly to the systemic circulation via the lymphatic system. They eventually empty into the systemic venous blood in the neck region by way of the thoracic duct. Through the action of the enzyme lipoprotein lipase that lines capillary walls, chylomicrons in the bloodstream readily hydrolyze to provide free fatty acids and glycerol for use by peripheral tissues. The relatively slow rate of gastric emptying and subsequent digestion, absorption, and assimilation of long-chain triacylglycerols makes this energy source an undesirable supplement to augment energy metabolism during exercise.

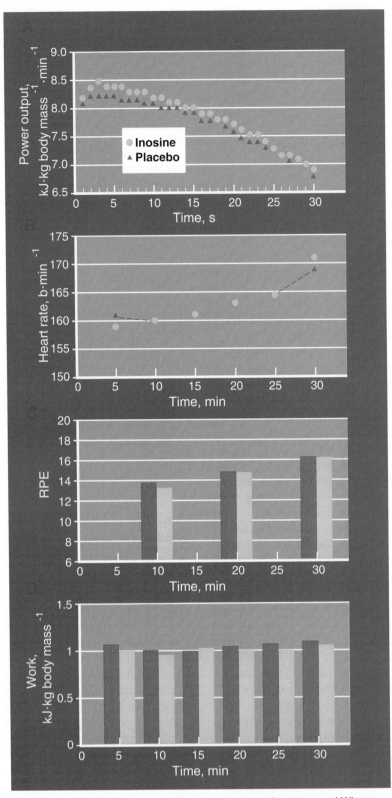

Figure 23.24   Maximal anaerobic power output on the 30-second Wingate test (**A**) and for heart rate (**B**), ratings of perceived exertion (RPE) (**C**), and total work accomplished (**D**) during segments of the 30-minute endurance ride for inosine and placebo trials for 10 male competitive cyclists. (From Starling RD, et al. Effect of inosine supplementation on aerobic and anaerobic cycling performance. Med Sci Sports Exerc 1996;28:1193.)

Medium-chain triacylglycerols (MCTs) provide a more rapid source of fatty acid fuel. MCTs are processed oils, frequently produced for patients with intestinal malabsorption and tissue-wasting diseases. Marketing for the sports enthusiast hypes MCTs as "fat burners," "energy sources," "glycogen sparers," and "muscle builders." Unlike longer-chain triacylglycerols, MCTs contain saturated fatty acids with 8 to 10 carbon atoms along the fatty acid chain. During digestion, lipase in the mouth, stomach, and intestinal duodenum hydrolyzes MCTs to glycerol and medium-chain fatty acids (MCFAs). Their water solubility allows MCFAs to move rapidly across the intestinal mucosa directly into the bloodstream (portal vein) without first being transported as chylomicrons by the lymphatic system, as long-chain triacylglycerols require. Once at the tissues, MCFAs move readily through the plasma membrane where they diffuse across the inner mitochondrial membrane for oxidation—they enter the mitochondria largely independent of the carnitine–acyl-CoA transferase system. The speed of cellular uptake and mitochondrial oxidation contrasts with the relatively slower transfer and oxidation rate of long-chain fatty acids. MCTs do not usually store as body fat because of their relative ease of oxidation. Because ingesting MCTs rapidly elevates plasma FFAs, some speculate that these lipids might spare liver and muscle glycogen during aerobic exercise.[206,207]

Exercise Benefits Inconclusive

Consuming MCTs does not inhibit gastric emptying, as does common fat, but conflicting research supports their use in exercise.[163,164,336,341] In early studies, subjects consumed 380 mg of MCT oil per kg of body mass 1 hour before exercising at 60 to 70% of $\dot{V}O_{2max}$ for 1 hour.[75] Plasma ketone levels generally increased, but the exercise metabolic mixture did not change compared with a placebo trial or a trial after subjects consumed a glucose polymer. Catabolism of 30 g of MCTs (estimated maximal amount tolerated in the gastrointestinal tract) consumed before exercising contributed only 3 to 7% to the total exercise energy requirement.[161]

 INTEGRATIVE QUESTION

Discuss the importance of the psychologic or "placebo" effect to evaluate claims for the effectiveness of particular nutrients, chemicals, or procedures as ergogenic aids.

Subsequent research investigated possible metabolic and ergogenic effects of consuming 86 g of MCT (surprisingly well tolerated by subjects). Six endurance-trained cyclists rode for 2 hours at 60% of $\dot{V}O_{2peak}$ while ingesting 2 L of either 4.3% MCT emulsion, 10% glucose plus 4.3% MCT emulsion, or a 10% glucose solution during exercise. They then performed a simulated 40-km cycling time trial. FIGURE 23.25 shows the effects of the different beverages on average speed in the time trials. Replacing the carbohydrate beverage with only MCTs produced an 8% decrement in performance (in agreement with another study[163]), but the combined carbohydrate plus MCT solution consumed throughout exercise

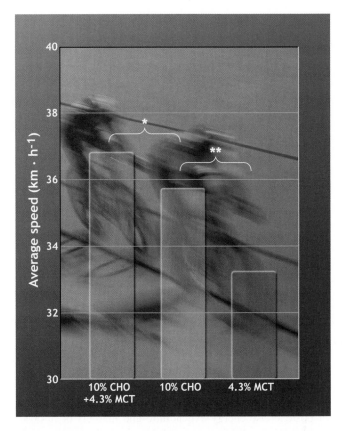

Figure 23.25 Effects of carbohydrate (CHO; 10% solution), medium-chain triacylglycerol (MCT; 4.3% emulsion), and carbohydrate + MCT (10% CHO + 4.3% MCT) ingestion during exercise on simulated 40-km time-trial cycling speeds after 2 hours of exercise at 60% of $\dot{V}O_{2peak}$. * Significantly faster than 10% CHO trials; ** Significantly faster than 4.3% MCT trials. (From Van Zyl CG, et al. Effects of medium-chain triglyceride ingestion on fuel metabolism and cycling performance. J Appl Physiol 1996;80:2217.)

produced a 2.5% improvement in cycling speed compared with the two other conditions. This ergogenic effect occurred with reduced total carbohydrate oxidation at a given level of oxygen consumption, higher final circulating FFA and ketone levels, and lower final glucose and lactate concentrations.

The small ergogenic enhancement by MCT supplementation probably occurred because this exogenous source of fatty acids contributes relatively little to the total energy expenditure (and total fat oxidation) during sustained exercise.[162] MCT ingestion does not stimulate release of bile, the gall bladder's fat-emulsifying agent. Thus, cramping and diarrhea often accompany excess intake of this lipid. It provides little ergogenic effect.

(−)-Hydroxycitrate: A Potential Fat Burner?

(—)-hydroxycitrate (HCA), a principal constituent of the rind of the fruit of *Garcinia cambogia* used in Asian cuisine, is a compound promoted as a "natural fat burner" to facilitate weight loss and enhance endurance performance. Metabolically, HCA operates as a competitive inhibitor of citrate lyase that catalyzes the breakdown of citrate to oxaloacetate and acetyl-CoA in the cytosol. Inhibition of this enzyme limits the pool of two-carbon acetyl compounds and thus reduces cellular ability to synthesize fat. Because inhibition of citrate catabolism also slows carbohydrate breakdown, HCA supplementation should also conserve glycogen and increase lipolysis during exercise.[237]

Research has evaluated short-term effects of HCA ingestion on HCA availability in the plasma and fat oxidation rates during rest and moderate-intensity exercise.[331] Endurance-trained cyclists received either a 3.1 mL per kg of body mass HCA solution (19 g · L^{-1}; 6 to 30 times the dosage in weight-loss studies) or a placebo at 45 and 15 minutes before starting exercise (resting measure) and at 30 and 60 minutes during a 2-hour exercise bout at 50% maximal exercise capacity. Plasma concentrations of HCA increased at rest and during exercise after supplementation, but no difference occurred between trials in energy expenditure or in fat and carbohydrate oxidation. These findings indicate that increasing plasma HCA availability with supplementation exerts no effect on skeletal muscle fat oxidation during rest or exercise, at least in endurance-trained humans. In addition, no effects of HCA supplementation occurred for resting or postexercise energy expenditure and markers of lipolysis in healthy men[186] or on weight or fat loss in obese subjects.[144] Collectively, these findings seriously question the usefulness of large quantities of HCA as an antiobesity agent or ergogenic aid—claims frequently made by supplement purveyors.

Pyruvate

Ergogenic effects have been extolled for pyruvate, the three-carbon end product of the cytoplasmic breakdown of glucose in glycolysis. Exogenous pyruvate, as a partial replacement for dietary carbohydrate, allegedly augments endurance performance and promotes fat loss. Pyruvic acid, a relatively unstable chemical, causes intestinal distress. Consequently, various forms of the salt of this acid (sodium, potassium, calcium, or magnesium pyruvate) are provided in capsule, tablet, or powder form.

Dosage recommendations range between a total of 2 and 5 g of pyruvate spread throughout the day and taken with meals. One capsule usually contains 600 mg pyruvate. The calcium form of pyruvate also contains approximately 80 mg of calcium with 600 mg of pyruvate. Some advertisements recommend dosage of one capsule per 20 pounds of body weight. Manufacturers also combine creatine monohydrate and pyruvate; 1 g of creatine pyruvate provides about 80 mg of creatine and 400 mg of pyruvate. Recommended pyruvate dosages range from 5 to 20 g per day. Pyruvate content in the normal diet ranges from 100 to 2000 mg daily. The largest dietary amounts occur in fruits and vegetables, particularly red apples (500 mg each), with smaller quantities in dark beer (80 mg per 12 oz) and red wine (75 mg per 6 oz).

Effects on Endurance Performance

Several reports indicate beneficial effects of exogenous pyruvate on endurance performance. Two double-blind, crossover studies by the same laboratory showed that 7 days of daily supplementation of a 100-g mixture of pyruvate (25 g) plus 75 g of dihydroxyacetone (DHA; another three-carbon compound of glycolysis) increased upper- and lower-body aerobic endurance by 20% compared with exercise with a 100-g supplement of an isocaloric glucose polymer.[301,302] The pyruvate–DHA mixture increased cycle ergometer time to exhaustion of the legs by 13 minutes (66 vs. 79 min) while upper-body arm-cranking exercise time increased by 27 minutes (133 vs. 160 min). Exercising with the pyruvate–DHA mixture reduced local muscle and overall body ratings of perceived exertion compared with the placebo condition.[273]

Proponents of pyruvate supplementation maintain that elevated extracellular pyruvate augments glucose transport into active muscle. Enhanced "glucose extraction" from the blood provides the important energy source to sustain high-intensity aerobic exercise while conserving intramuscular glycogen stores.[152] When the individual's diet contains a normal level of carbohydrate (approximately 55% of total energy intake), pyruvate supplementation also increases preexercise muscle glycogen levels.[302] Both of these effects, higher pre-exercise glycogen levels and facilitated glucose uptake and oxidation by active muscle, benefit endurance exercise in much the same way as preexercise carbohydrate loading and glucose feedings during exercise exert ergogenic effects.

Body Fat Loss

Subsequent research by the same investigators who showed ergogenic effects of pyruvate supplementation indicates that exogenous pyruvate intake augments body fat loss when accompanied by a low-energy diet. Obese women in a metabolic ward maintained a liquid 1000-kCal daily energy intake (68% carbohydrate, 22% protein, 10% lipid). Adding 20 g of sodium pyruvate plus 16 g of calcium pyruvate (13% of energy intake) daily for 3 weeks induced greater weight loss (13.0 vs. 9.5 lb) and fat loss (8.8 vs. 5.9 lb) than a control group on the same diet who received an equivalent amount of extra energy as glucose.[303] These findings complement the researchers' previous study with obese subjects that showed that adding DHA and pyruvate (substituted as equivalent energy for glucose) to a severely restricted low-energy diet facilitated body weight and fat loss (without increased nitrogen loss).[304] The precise role of pyruvate in facilitating weight loss remains unknown. Consuming pyruvate may stimulate small increases in futile metabolic activity (metabolism not coupled to ATP production) with a subsequent wasting of energy.

Adverse side effects of a 30- to 100-g daily pyruvate intake include diarrhea and gastrointestinal gurgling and discomfort. *Until studies from independent laboratories reproduce existing findings for exercise performance and body fat loss, one should view the effectiveness of pyruvate supplementation with caution.*

Summary

1. The term *ergogenic aid* describes substances or procedures that improve physical work capacity, physiologic function, or athletic performance.

2. Anabolic steroids compose a group of pharmacologic agents frequently used for ergogenic purposes. These drugs function like the hormone testosterone; they increase muscle size, strength, and power with resistance training in some individuals.

3. The β_2-adrenergic agonists clenbuterol and albuterol increase skeletal muscle mass and slow fat gain in animals to counter aging, immobilization, malnutrition, and tissue-wasting pathology. A negative finding showed hastened fatigue during short-term, intense muscle actions.

4. Debate exists about whether administration of growth hormone to healthy individuals augments muscular hypertrophy when combined with resistance training. Health risks exist for those who abuse this chemical.

5. Dehydroepiandersterone (DHEA), a relatively weak steroid hormone synthesized from cholesterol by the adrenal cortex, steadily decreases throughout adulthood, prompting individuals to supplement, hoping to counteract the effects of aging. DHEA does not produce an ergogenic effect.

6. Research indicates no effect of androstenedione supplementation on basal serum concentrations of testosterone or training response for muscle size and strength and body composition. Worrisome are the potentially negative effects of lowered HDL-C on heart disease risk and elevated serum estrogen levels on risk of gynecomastia and certain cancers.

7. No ergogenic effects exist for healthy subjects from chronic oral amino acid supplements on hormone secretion, training responsiveness, or exercise performance.

8. Hormonal dynamics from carbohydrate and/or protein supplementation immediately following a resistance-exercise workout suggests an ergogenic effect on training responsiveness.

9. Amphetamines, or pep pills, do not aid exercise performance or psychomotor skills, other than a placebo effect. Adverse effects include drug dependency, headache, dizziness, confusion, and gastrointestinal distress.

10. Caffeine ingestion exerts an ergogenic effect in some individuals by extending endurance in aerobic exercise from increased fat use for energy and conservation of glycogen reserves.

11. No compelling evidence supports ginseng supplementation to benefit physiologic function or exercise performance. Significant health risks accompany ephedrine use.

12. Concentrated buffering solutions consumed before exercise improve anaerobic exercise performance.

13. Further research must determine the benefits and risks of glutamine, phosphatidylserine, and β-hydroxyl-β-methylbutyrate to provide a "natural" anabolic boost with resistance training.

14. The additional blood volume and increased red cell mass and concentration from red blood cell reinfusion contribute to a larger maximum cardiac output and an increase in the blood's oxygen-carrying capacity and $\dot{V}O_{2max}$.

15. A physiologic rationale for why warm-up should enhance exercise performance includes benefits on muscle-shortening velocity and efficiency, enhanced oxygen delivery and use, and facilitated transmission of nerve impulses. Limited research supports the benefits of warm-up beyond a positive psychologic component.

16. Moderate warm-up proves beneficial immediately before sudden, strenuous exercise by reducing myocardial work and augmenting coronary blood flow when exercise begins.

17. Breathing hyperoxic gas during exercise extends endurance by increasing oxygen consumption, reducing blood lactate, and lowering pulmonary ventilation. Using this procedure before or after exercise provides no ergogenic effect.

18. Carbohydrate loading augments endurance in prolonged submaximal exercise. Athletes should be well informed about this procedure because of potential negative effects.

19. A modification of the classic loading procedure provides the same high level of glycogen storage without dramatic alterations in the diet and exercise routine.

20. No ergogenic benefits occur from carnitine supplementation.

21. No benefits emerge from chromium supplements on training-related changes in muscular strength, physique, or muscle mass for individuals with adequate dietary chromium intake.

22. CoQ_{10} supplements in healthy individuals provide no ergogenic effect on aerobic capacity, endurance, submaximal exercise lactate levels, or cardiovascular dynamics.

23. Creatine supplements increase intramuscular creatine and PCr, enhance brief anaerobic power output capacity, and facilitate recovery from repeated bouts of intense effort.

24. No effect of inosine supplements occurs on physiologic or performance measures during aerobic or anaerobic exercise. A decidedly negative effect includes an increase in serum uric acid levels.

25. Body builders frequently supplement with choline to enhance fat metabolism and achieve the "cut look," but research does not support such effects.

26. Owing to relatively rapid digestion, assimilation, and catabolism for energy, athletes consume medium-chain triacylglycerols (MCTs) to enhance

fat oxidation and conserve glycogen during endurance exercise. This procedure does enhance performance by an additional 2.5%.

27. Increasing plasma (—)-hydroxycitrate (HCA) availability via supplementation exerts no effect on skeletal muscle fat oxidation at rest or during exercise.

28. Pyruvate supplementation purportedly augments endurance performance and promotes fat loss. A definitive conclusion concerning its effectiveness requires verification.

References are available on the Student CD and online at http://connection.lww.com/mkk6e.

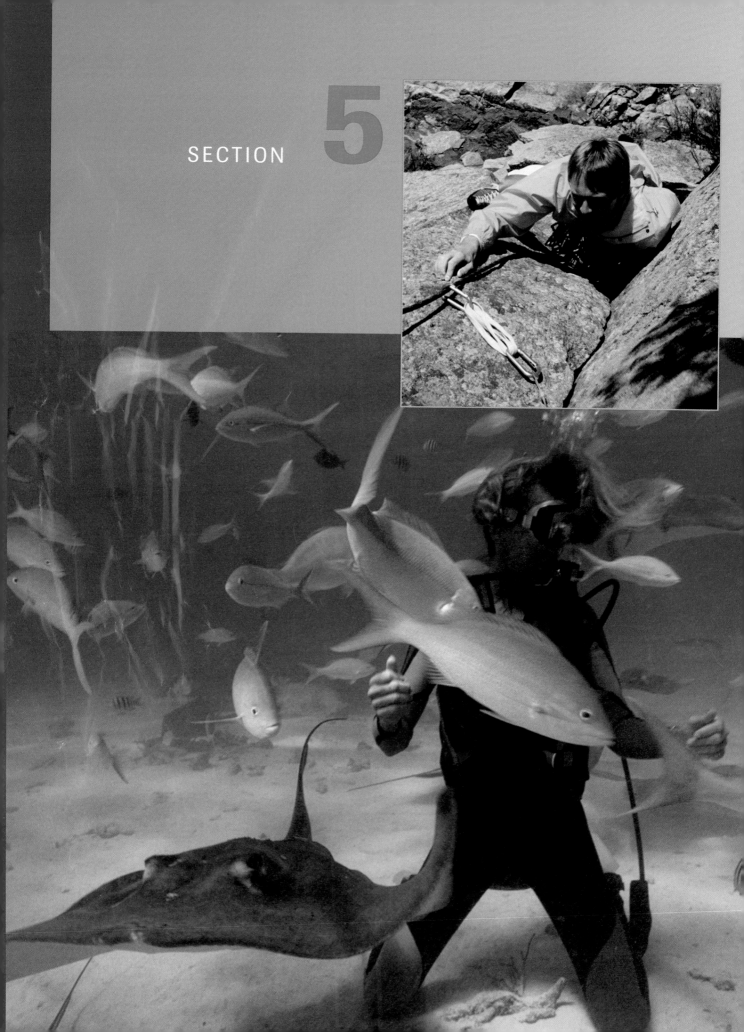

SECTION 5

Exercise Performance and Environmental Stress

"The true explorer does his work not for any hopes of reward or honor, but because the thing he has set for himself to do is a part of his being, and must be accomplished for the sake of the accomplishment. And he counts lightly hardships, risks, obstacles, if only they do not bar him from his goal."

Admiral Robert E. Peary, Polar Explorer

Sport activities often take place at terrestrial elevations that impair oxygenation of blood flowing through the lungs and severely limit aerobic energy metabolism for exercise. At the other extreme, exploration beneath the water's surface poses a different challenge. Divers must transport their sea-level environment as a gas mixture compressed in a scuba tank carried on the back. Some diving enthusiasts use no external assistance, and the length of an underwater excursion becomes limited by two factors: (1) the quantity of air inhaled into the lungs just before the dive and (2) the buildup of arterial carbon dioxide during the dive. In both breath-hold diving and scuba diving, the environment provides unique challenges and dangers for the participant, often independent of the stress of exercise. Consideration also must focus on the thermal quality of the environment. On land, exercising in a hot, humid environment or extreme cold imposes severe stress. These environmental demands impair exercise capacity and pose a severe threat to health and safety.

Space exploration and accompanying short- and long-term exposures to near-zero gravity present a unique set of environmental stressors that impinge on physiologic function, structural mass, and exercise capacity both during flight and upon return to Earth.

The extent that each environmental stressor deviates from neutral conditions and the duration of the exposure determine the total impact on the body. In addition, the effect of several simultaneous environmental stressors (e.g., extreme cold exposure at high altitude) may exceed the simple additive consequence of each stressor imposed separately.

In the four chapters that follow, we explore the specific problems encountered at altitude, during exercise in hot and cold environments, and prolonged exposure to microgravity. We also discuss the immediate physiologic adjustments and long-term adaptations as the body strives to maintain internal consistency despite an environmental challenge. The chapter on sport diving considers the unique problems associated with this increasingly popular form of sport and recreation.

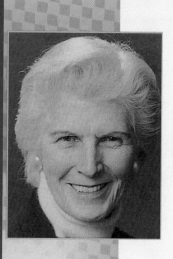

Interview *with* **Barbara Drinkwater**

Education: BS (Douglass College, Rutgers University, New Brunswick, NJ); MEd (University of North Carolina, Greensboro, NC); PhD (Purdue University, West Lafayette, IN).

Current Affiliation: Retired May 1, 2000. Previously, Research Physiologist, Department of Medicine, Pacific Medical Center, Seattle, WA.

Honors and Awards: See Appendix E, which is available on the Student CD and online at http://connection.lww.com/mkk6e.

Research Focus: The response of women to exercise as mediated by environmental factors and aging. Special areas of interest have been the female athlete, her physical performance under environmental stressors such as heat and altitude, the effect of exercise-associated amenorrhea on bone health, and the role of exercise, calcium, and exercise in preventing osteoporosis.

Memorable Publication: Drinkwater BL. Bone mineral content of amenorrheic and eumenorrheic athletes. N Engl J Med 1984;311:277.

Statement of Contributions: ACSM Honor Award

In recognition of her distinguished scientific contributions as one of the foremost investigators of exercise and physiological issues pertaining to women, particularly with, respect to the study of bone mineral content relative to menstrual function, pregnancy, physical activity, and calcium intake, and for her distinguished international leadership and professional contributions to exercise science and sports medicine.

Dr. Drinkwater began her well-known scientific work with a series of landmark studies, first on the aerobic capacity, training, and detraining characteristics of young women track athletes, and then on the influence of air pollutants and thermal stress on the working capacity of humans. She has demonstrated a continuing interest in gender differences and aging on aerobic capacity, body composition, and thermal responses. Indeed, an anthology of the woman in sport would be incomplete without reference to her data-based studies and scholarly reviews of the physiological responses of women to exercise, particularly in reference to age, fitness, and heat stress.

Dr. Drinkwater has earned the respect of the international scientific community for her primary scientific contribution, the interactions of menstrual function, estrogen and exercise on bone mineral content. Her work has clarified the importance of adequate menstrual function on bone mineral density in young athletic women, the long term consequences of bone mineral losses following athletic amenorrhea, and the role of estrogen relative to physical activity for the prevention of bone mineral loss in menopause.

Second only to her scientific contributions, Dr. Drinkwater has demonstrated an exemplary commitment to professional leadership and development of beginning

scholars and clinicians. She has served or chaired many of the vital committees of ACSM, and was elected as Trustee, Vice President, and President. She remains a strong voice that brings an important message to the American College of Sports Medicine Foundation, where she serves on the Board of Directors. Dr. Drinkwater is an icon that represents unfailing support, nurturing, and challenging of beginning investigators and clinicians in exercise science and sports medicine.

Dr. Drinkwater's highly regarded contributions to the international scientific community, her professional leadership, and her commitment to the development of beginning scientists and clinicians form the basis of recognizing her with ACSM's highest distinction.

What first inspired you to enter the exercise science field? What made you decide to pursue your advanced degree and/or line of research?

■ In 1965, I was teaching a methods course in track and field to physical education majors. One of them asked me why women weren't allowed to compete in the marathon and were restricted to running twice around the track. I decide to investigate the scientific rationale and found instead that myths and prejudice, not science, limited women's participation in sports. Several years later I had the opportunity to join the Institute of Environmental Stress at the University of California, Santa Barbara. With the encouragement of the director, Steven M. Horvath, PhD, I began the series of studies that would demonstrate clearly that women of all ages could attain high levels of aerobic power and that cardiovascular fitness, not gender, accounted for the previous notion that women could not tolerate exercise in the heat.

What influence did your undergraduate education have on your final career choice?

■ My undergraduate degree was in Physical Education. I had an excellent program that emphasized science as well as sports skills and teaching methods. However, none of the female faculty members had a doctorate degree, and graduate education was never mentioned. The assumption in those days was that we "majors" would go directly into teaching. However, I'm sure it was my love for sport and the excellent courses I had in physiology and kinesiology that later led me into the exercise science field.

Who were the most influential people in your career, and why?

■ Oddly enough, the most influential individual in my career was Ben Winer, PhD, who taught the statistics courses I took in the doctoral program at Purdue. He was an outstanding teacher, and the skills and knowledge of experimental design that I gained in his classes led to my unofficial role of statistician and advisor on study designs at Institute of Environmental Stress. Obviously, I owe a great deal to Steve Horvath as well, who gave me the opportunity to work at the Institute. A career encompasses not only your research and teaching, but your professional contributions as well. Individuals such as Charles Tipton, John Sutton, Carl Gilsolfi, Peter Raven, Chris Wells, Toby Tate, and a multitude of others all enhanced that aspect of my career. Their support and encouragement had a tremendous impact on my career and me.

What has been the most interesting/enjoyable aspect of your involvement in science? What was the least interesting/enjoyable aspect?

■ The most enjoyable aspect of my scientific career has been the opportunity to encourage and "open some doors" for younger women on the road toward their own careers. That, plus the opportunity to speak to a wide variety of audiences about topics of importance to their health and well being, have given me a great deal of satisfaction. The least enjoyable aspect has been the constant need to search for funds to keep the research program going.

What is your most meaningful contribution to the field of exercise science, and why is it so important?

■ I would like to think that my most meaningful contribution to the field of exercise science has been to stimulate interest of other investigators in evaluating women's response to exercise, environmental stress, and aging. In terms of a specific area of research, I would have to select the area of the Female Athlete Triad, which demonstrates that the amenorrhea experienced by many female athletes can lead to irreversible bone loss. Until our 1984 paper in the

New England Journal of Medicine, amenorrhea was assumed to be a benign—and welcome—condition by the athletes. When additional studies confirmed our results, athletes and those responsible for their health began to take the Triad seriously.

What advice would you give to students who express an interest in pursuing a career in exercise science research?

■ My advice to an undergraduate student would be to select as many science courses as possible in areas related to exercise science and work hard to get good grades. Your selection to the better graduate programs will depend largely on your grade point average and the recommendations of your professors. If you are not a serious student, you are not going to have a successful career in research. In selecting a doctoral program, investigate thoroughly before applying. Not only will you be spending 4 to 5 years of your life in that department, but you will be depending on the reputation of that program and the faculty to secure a postdoctoral position. Among the factors to consider are the publications of the faculty and graduate students, ongoing research in your area of interest, laboratory facilities and equipment, success of graduates in obtaining postdoctoral positions, and the requirements for the PhD. If possible, talk with some recent graduates of the program and get their honest appraisal of their experience.

What interests have you pursued outside of your professional career?

■ Sports, aviation, and animals. I've been active in a number of sports, but am now totally involved with golf—playing several times a week and even taking my clubs over to Australia to play when not at an Olympic venue. When I was in Santa Barbara, I found time to get a commercial pilot's license, an instrument rating, and an instrument instructor's rating. I spent many hours in the air on trips throughout California and the Southwest. When I moved to Vashon in 1982, I had two dogs and one cat. Within 6 months, a puppy found at the dump and another 6 cats that had come out of the woods joined the family. At that point, I decided the island needed a humane society so I started one. Sixteen years later, the program is going strong and now includes a low-cost spay neuter program, a lost-and-found hotline, an adoption service, education programs in the schools, and medical–surgical help as well.

Where do you see the exercise science field (particularly your area of greatest interest) heading in the next 20 years?

■ The exercise science field is so diverse that it may be impossible to make a general statement regarding future directions. I do believe there will be increasing interest in the

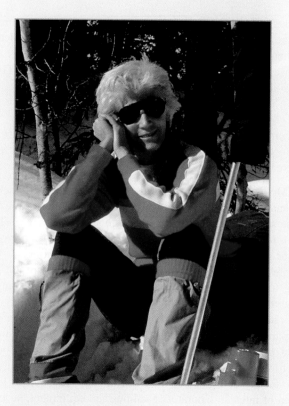

interaction of exercise and health. As our population continues to age, the rising cost of medical care will force an emphasis on lifestyle and other preventive measures. The Surgeon General's Healthy People 2000 Report has made physical activity and fitness the number one priority for health promotion and disease prevention. The responsibility for providing data-based evidence that physical activity does indeed prevent or ameliorate disease states, as well as defining the optimum exercise program for each segment of the population, will be the responsibility of the exercise scientist who is challenged by studying integrated physiological systems.

You have the opportunity to give a "last lecture." Describe its primary focus.

■ I can't even conceive of accepting an invitation to give a "last lecture"! The actual final lecture I give will be one that I probably accepted to give six months earlier, and in the interim I've decided I've said enough, I have nothing new to say, and it's time to leave the stage to younger professionals with new and exciting data and insights. I hope I have the good sense to recognize that time when it comes.

Exercise at Medium and High Altitude

24

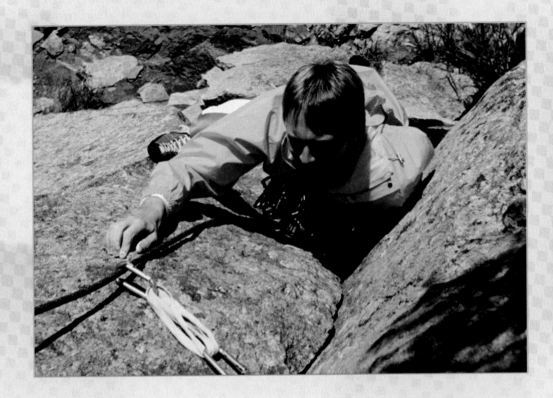

CHAPTER OBJECTIVES

- Outline the effects of increasingly higher altitudes on (1) partial pressure of oxygen in ambient air, (2) oxygen saturation of hemoglobin in pulmonary capillaries, and (3) $\dot{V}O_{2max}$

- Describe and quantify the oxygen transport cascade at sea level and 4300 m

- Discuss immediate and longer term physiologic adjustments to altitude exposure

- Give symptoms, possible causes, and treatment for acute mountain sickness, high-altitude pulmonary edema, and high-altitude cerebral edema

- Describe the "lactate paradox" and possible causes for its occurrence

- Summarize factors that affect the time course for altitude acclimatization

- Graph the relation between the decrease in $\dot{V}O_{2max}$ (% sea-level value) with increasing altitude exposure

- Discuss alterations in circulatory function that offset the benefits of altitude acclimatization on oxygen transport capacity

- Discuss whether altitude training produces greater improvement than sea-level training on sea-level exercise performance

- Describe the training concept of "living high, training low"

More than 40 million people live, work, and recreate at terrestrial elevations between 3048 m (10,000 ft) and 5486 m (18,000 ft) above sea level. In terms of the Earth's topography, these elevations encompass the range generally considered **high altitude**. High-altitude natives inhabit permanent settlements up to 5486 m in the Andes and Himalayas. Prolonged exposure of an unacclimatized person to this altitude causes death from the ambient air's subnormal oxygen pressure (**hypoxia**), even if the person remains physically inactive. The physiologic challenge of even medium-altitude exposure becomes readily apparent during physical activity. In the United States, close to 1 million people a year ascend Pikes Peak, Colorado (4300 m) by train, car, or railroad, and thousands of others do so by climbing, cycling, and running. Millions more throughout the world ascend to high altitudes for mountaineering, trekking, tourism, business, and scientific and military excursions. Many newcomers to altitude do not take sufficient time to acclimatize to the physiologic challenge of the reduced partial pressure of oxygen (P_{O_2}) in ambient air.

THE STRESS OF ALTITUDE

Altitude's physiologic challenge comes directly from decreased ambient P_{O_2}, not from reduced total barometric pressure per se or any change in the relative concentrations (percentages) of gases in inspired (ambient) air. FIGURE 24.1 illustrates the barometric pressure, pressures of the respired gases, and percentage saturation of hemoglobin at various terrestrial elevations. FIGURE 24.2 shows changes that occur in oxygen availability (reflected by P_{O_2}) in ambient air, alveolar air, and arterial and mixed-venous blood as one ascends from sea level to Pikes Peak. The progressive change in the environment's oxygen pressure and in various body areas is termed the **oxygen transport cascade.**

Air density decreases progressively as one ascends above sea level. For example, barometric pressure at sea level averages 760 mm Hg; at 3048 m, the barometer reads 510 mm Hg. At an elevation of 5486 m, the pressure of a column of air at the Earth's surface equals about one half of its sea-level pressure.

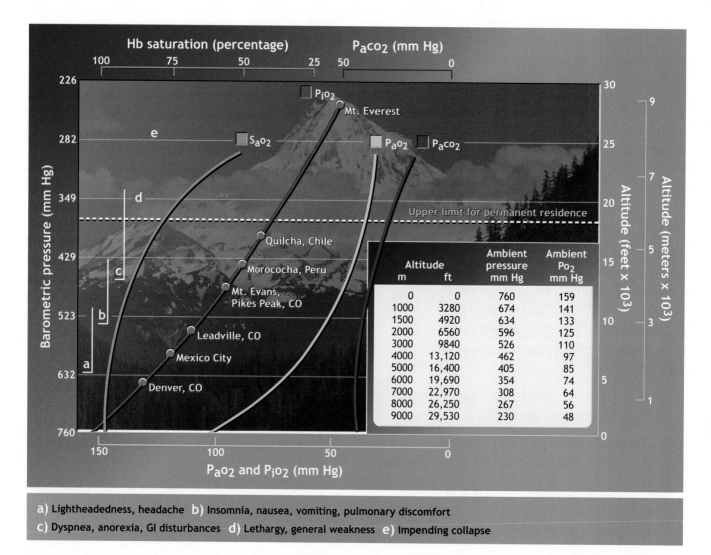

a) **Lightheadedness, headache**   b) **Insomnia, nausea, vomiting, pulmonary discomfort**
c) **Dyspnea, anorexia, GI disturbances**   d) **Lethargy, general weakness**   e) **Impending collapse**

| Altitude | | Ambient pressure | Ambient P_{O_2} |
m	ft	mm Hg	mm Hg
0	0	760	159
1000	3280	674	141
1500	4920	634	133
2000	6560	596	125
3000	9840	526	110
4000	13,120	462	97
5000	16,400	405	85
6000	19,690	354	74
7000	22,970	308	64
8000	26,250	267	56
9000	29,530	230	48

Figure 24.1   Changes in environmental and physiologic variables with progressive elevations in altitude ($P_{a}O_2$, partial pressure of arterial oxygen; $P_{a}CO_2$, partial pressure of arterial carbon dioxide; $P_{i}O_2$, partial pressure of oxygen in inspired air; $S_{a}O_2$; oxygen saturation of hemoglobin.).

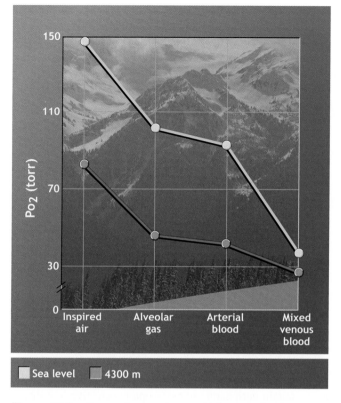

Figure 24.2 Oxygen transport cascade from sea level to 4300 m (14,108 ft).

Dry ambient air at sea level and altitude contains 20.93% oxygen, while the P_{O_2} (density of the oxygen molecules) of air decreases directly with the fall in barometric pressure upon ascending to higher elevations (P_{O_2} = 0.2093 × barometric pressure). Thus, ambient P_{O_2} at sea level averages 150 mm Hg, but only 107 mm Hg at 3048 m. At the summit of Mt. Everest (8848 m; 29,028 ft) ambient air pressure usually ranges between 251 and 253 mm Hg with a concomitant alveolar P_{O_2} of about 25 mm Hg (ambient air P_{O_2} between 42 and 43 mm Hg).[100] This equals only about 30% of the oxygen available in air at sea level. *Arterial hypoxia that accompanies the reduction in P_{O_2} precipitates both the immediate physiologic adjustments to altitude and longer term process of acclimatization.* **Acclimatization** refers to adaptations produced by changes in the natural environment, whether through a change in season or place of residence. In contrast, **acclimation** concerns adaptations produced in a controlled laboratory environment as in chambers that simulate high altitude or microgravity, hypoxic environments, and extremes of thermal stress.

Oxygen Loading at Altitude

The S-shaped nature of the oxyhemoglobin dissociation curve (see Chapter 13, Fig. 13.4) indicates that only a small change occurs in hemoglobin's percentage saturation with oxygen until an altitude of about 3048 m. At 1981 m (6500 ft), for example, alveolar P_{O_2} decreases from its sea-level value of 100 mm Hg to 78 mm Hg, yet hemoglobin remains 90% saturated with oxygen. This relatively small arterial desaturation

exerts little effect on a person during rest or even mild exercise but severely curtails performance in vigorous aerobic activities. The poorer performances of men and women in middle-distance and distance running and swimming during the 1968 Olympics in Mexico City (altitude 2300 m; 7546 ft) resulted from the small reduction in oxygen transport at this altitude. No new world records were established in events lasting longer than 2.5 minutes. Altitude does not impair the short-term anaerobic energy system at moderate altitude (e.g., glycogen storage, pathways of glycolysis and corresponding phosphorylase and phosphofructokinase enzyme activity) or success in sprint–power activities such as sprint running, speed skating, track cycling, jumping, and discus.[26,29] Performance in single bouts of such activities often improves because of lower air density (air resistance or drag force) at altitude than at sea level. The lessened air resistance from a 24% reduction in air density at 2300 m should also improve performance in the shot put, hammer throw, and javelin.[21] Impaired performance has been reported for *repeated intervals* of short-term power output (15-s training intervals) in elite athletes.[12]

In the transition from moderate altitude to higher elevations, values for alveolar (arterial) P_{O_2} position on the steep part of the oxyhemoglobin dissociation curve. This dramatically reduces hemoglobin oxygenation and oxygen transport capacity and negatively affects even mild-intensity aerobic activities. At high elevations in the Andes and Himalayas, oxygen loading of hemoglobin decreases dramatically, and physical activity becomes difficult to sustain. A small change in inspired P_{O_2} (i.e., barometric pressure) greatly affects aerobic capacity at the summit of Mt. Everest. For well-acclimatized mountain climbers, breathing ambient air with a P_{O_2} of 48.5 mm Hg produces a $\dot{V}O_{2max}$ of 1450 mL · min^{-1}. This declines to 1070 mL · min^{-1} with only a 6-mm Hg decrease in inspired P_{O_2}—a decrease of 63 mL · min^{-1} in $\dot{V}O_{2max}$ for each 1-mm Hg drop in inspired P_{O_2}.[98–100]

Sudden exposure to an altitude of 4300 m reduces aerobic capacity by 32% compared with sea-level values.[107] At altitudes above 5182 m (17,000 ft), permanent living becomes nearly impossible, and mountain climbing frequently requires the aid of hyperoxic breathing mixtures. At 5486 m (18,000 ft), arterial P_{O_2} averages 38 mm Hg, and hemoglobin maintains only 73% oxygen saturation. Amazingly, reports describe acclimatized mountaineers who lived for weeks at 6706 m (22,000 ft) breathing only ambient air.[41] In fact, members of two Swiss expeditions to Mt. Everest remained at the summit for 2 hours without breathing equipment![69] This represents an impressive feat considering that arterial P_{O_2} averaged only 25 mm Hg with a corresponding arterial blood oxygen saturation of 58%. An unacclimatized person becomes unconscious within 30 seconds under these conditions. For acclimatized men at simulated extreme altitudes that approach the summit of Mt. Everest, $\dot{V}O_{2max}$ decreases by 70% from 4.13 to 1.17 L · min^{-1}, or from 49.1 to 15.3 mL · kg^{-1} · min^{-1}.[32] These low values reflect the sea-level aerobic capacity of a sedentary 80-year-old man. Despite the considerable physiologic strain imposed by high altitude, mountaineer Tom Whittaker, age 50, became the first amputee to reach Mt. Everest's summit on his third attempt on May 27, 1998. Although remarkable performances at high altitude reflect exceptions and not the rule, they demonstrate the enormous adaptive capability of humans to survive and even work without external support at extreme terrestrial elevations (see "Focus on Research," p. 621).

 INTEGRATIVE QUESTION

Respond to this question: "If altitude has such negative effects on the body, why are certain track and field records broken during competition at higher elevations?"

ACCLIMATIZATION

During the many years that mountaineers attempted to climb the world's highest peaks, they knew it required weeks to adjust to successively higher elevations. *The term* **altitude acclimatization** *broadly describes adaptive responses in physiology and metabolism that improve tolerance to altitude hypoxia.* Each adjustment to a higher elevation proceeds progressively, and full acclimatization requires time. Successful adjustment to medium altitude affords only partial adjustment to a higher elevation. Residents of moderate altitudes, however, show less decrement in physiologic capacity and exercise performance than lowlanders when both groups travel to a higher altitude.[59]

TABLE 24.1 reveals that compensatory responses to altitude occur almost immediately, while other adaptations take weeks or even months. The rapidity of the body's response remains largely altitude dependent, yet considerable individual variability exists for both the rate and success of acclimatization. A person can retain many of the beneficial submaximal

exercise responses with 16 days of acclimatization at 4300 m despite intermittent 8-day sojourns to sea level.[8] This suggests that certain aspects of acclimatization regress more slowly than their acquisition.

Immediate Responses to Altitude

Arrival at elevations of 2300 m and higher initiates rapid physiologic adjustments to compensate for the thinner air and accompanying reduction in alveolar P_{O_2}. The two more important responses include:

1. Increase in the respiratory drive to produce hyperventilation
2. Increase in blood flow during rest and submaximal exercise

Hyperventilation

Hyperventilation from reduced arterial P_{O_2} reflects the most important and clear-cut immediate response of the native lowlander to altitude exposure. Once initiated, this "hypoxic drive" increases during the first few weeks and can remain elevated for a year or longer during prolonged altitude residence.[50]

The aortic arch and branching of the carotid arteries in the neck contain peripheral chemoreceptors sensitive to reduced oxygen pressure. Reduced arterial P_{O_2} that occurs at altitudes above 2000 m progressively stimulates these receptors. This modifies inspiratory activity to increase alveolar ventilation and cause alveolar P_{O_2} to rise toward the level in ambient air. Even small increases in alveolar P_{O_2} with hyperventilation facilitate oxygen loading in the lungs and provide the rapid first line of defense against reduced ambient P_{O_2}. For females, variations in menstrual cycle phase do not affect ventilatory responses and exercise performance decrements during short-

TABLE **24.1** ■ **IMMEDIATE AND LONGER TERM ADJUSTMENTS TO ALTITUDE HYPOXIA**

SYSTEM	IMMEDIATE	LONGER TERM
Pulmonary acid-base	Hyperventilation Bodily fluids become more alkaline due to reduction in carbon dioxide (H_2CO_3) with hyperventilation	Hyperventilation Excretion of base (HCO_3^-) via the kidneys and concomitant reduction in alkaline reserve
Cardiovascular	Increase in submaximal heart rate Increase in submaximal cardiac output Stroke volume remains the same or decreases slightly Maximum cardiac output remains the same or decreases slightly	Submaximal heart rate remains elevated Submaximal cardiac output falls to or below sea-level values Stroke volume decreases Maximum cardiac output decreases
Hematologic		Decreased plasma volume Increased hematocrit Increased hemoglobin concentration Increased total number of red blood cells
Local		Possible increased capillarization of skeletal muscle Increased red blood cell 2,3-DPG Increased mitochondrial density Increased aerobic enzymes in muscle Loss of body weight and lean body mass

FOCUS On Research

HIGH ALTITUDE: A HOSTILE ENVIRONMENT

Pugh LGCE, et al. Muscular exercise at great altitudes. J Appl Physiol 1964;19:431.

▲ Since the first ascent of Mt. Everest (8848 m; 29,028 ft) in 1953 by Sir Edmund Hillary and Tenzig Norgay, scientists have studied relationships among terrestrial elevation, partial pressure of oxygen in ambient air, arterial hemoglobin oxygen loading, and cardiovascular function to explain reduced exercise capacity at altitude. Early experiments at high altitude posed enormous scientific challenges owing to equipment limitations and lack of trained personnel with mountaineering experience. The experiments, carried out by the Himalayan Scientific and Mountaineering Expedition of 1960–1961 (sponsored by the publishers of *World Book Encyclopedia,* Chicago, and Medical Research Council, London, England), represent "classic" experiments in environmental physiology. Discoveries from this legendary scientific expedition provided the underpinnings to current understanding about physical work at high altitude. The research by L. G. C. E. Pugh and coworkers was part of the first series of studies to demonstrate that lung diffusion capacity, cardiac output, and the oxygen cost of extreme pulmonary ventilation limit exercise capacity at altitudes above 5800 m (19,000 ft).

The researchers used bicycle ergometer exercise to assess physical working capacity at sea level and at altitudes ranging from 4650 m to 7440 m (barometric pressure of 440 to 300 mm Hg). They established a base station at 4650 m but used a prefabricated laboratory hut at 5800 m (barometric pressure of 380 mm Hg) to conduct most of the research.

Subjects included eight men: six experienced mountaineers and one "sportsman,"—all acclimatized to high altitude—and one high-altitude Sherpa guide. The scientists with the Himalayan Scientific Expedition were five of the seven "lowland" subjects. The Sherpa guide carried the bicycle ergometer (20 kg) to the laboratory hut. Subjects pedaled at 50 RPM, with expired air collected by the Douglas bag method. A dry-gas meter measured expired air volumes with respiratory gas concentrations analyzed with a Lloyd-Haldane chemical analyzer. The exercise protocol (preceded by a 10-min warm-up) included 6 minutes of exercise (12 min at sea level) starting at 300 kg-m · min^{-1} with increments of 300 kg-m · min^{-1}. The test terminated when the subject would not exercise for at least 2 minutes at a given intensity. Oxygen consumption, pulmonary ventilation, heart rate, respiratory exchange ratio, and venous blood samples (not secured from all subjects) were obtained during the last 2 minutes at each exercise level.

Figure 1 presents the researchers' original plot of $\dot{V}O_{2max}$ in relation to terrestrial elevation. Clearly, $\dot{V}O_{2max}$ decreased from sea level upward and declined steeply above 6000 m, to reach an average of 1.42 L · min^{-1} at 7440 m.

Figure 2 shows pulmonary ventilation (STPD and BTPS) and heart rate in response to $\dot{V}O_2$ during exercise at different altitudes. The curves for pulmonary ventilation shift to the left and increase in slope during exercise at higher elevations, with submaximal effort requiring the greatest ventilation at the highest altitude. This altitude-related hyperventilation reflects the experience of mountain climbers at great altitude; any slight increase in mountain slope or snow conditions brings them to a halt with breathlessness. Only the highest altitude produced apparent impairment of maximum exercise ventilation. Heart rates remained elevated during submaximal exercise at altitude.

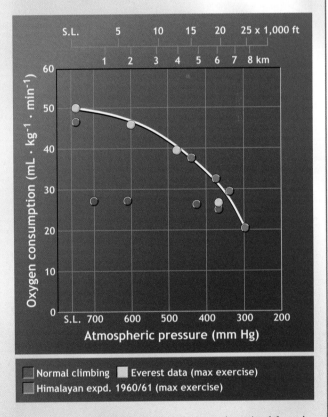

Figure 1 Oxygen consumption during submaximal (*purple symbols;* men climbing at their typical pace) and maximal (*yellow and orange symbols*) exercise in relation to ambient barometric pressure and terrestrial elevation. S.L., sea level.

continued on page 622

Continued

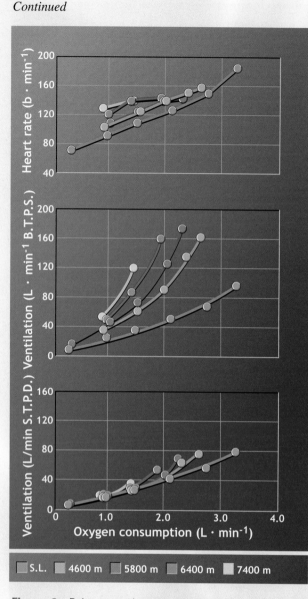

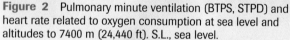

Figure 2   Pulmonary minute ventilation (BTPS, STPD) and heart rate related to oxygen consumption at sea level and altitudes to 7400 m (24,440 ft). S.L., sea level.

Figure 3 shows a tendency for a higher respiratory exchange ratio (R) at all exercise levels at 5800 m than at sea level. At $\dot{V}O_2$s above 2.0 L · min^{-1}, R increased nearly vertically, a response consistent with the extreme hyperventilation at high altitude. Altitude exposure increased

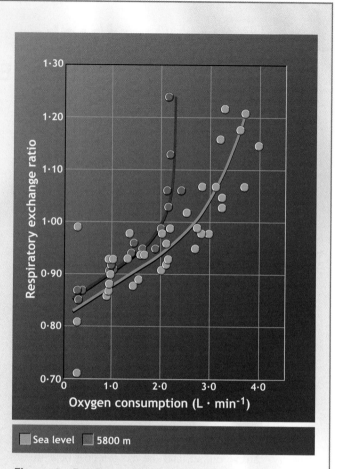

Figure 3   Respiratory exchange ratio during graded exercise at sea level and 5800 m (19,000 ft).

exercise blood lactate (not shown), which also contributed to hyperventilation. Finally, comparisons of data for the Sherpa guide with those from other subjects showed his superior work capacity, attributable to economy of ventilation with preservation of a normal blood pH and maintenance of a relatively higher arterial Po2. The guide also maintained a high pulmonary diffusing capacity for oxygen and high cardiac output relative to work intensity (measured in a separate experiment).

These pioneering studies demonstrated physiologic links to exercise limitations at high altitude and formed the foundation for expanding knowledge of human physical working capacity at extreme terrestrial elevations.

term altitude exposure compared with at sea level.[9] Mountaineers who respond with a strong, hypoxic ventilatory drive to sudden but extreme altitude exposure perform exercise tasks more effectively (and reach higher altitude) than climbers with a depressed hypoxic ventilatory response.[90]

INTEGRATIVE QUESTION

From a physiologic perspective, what represents a safe altitude for flight in an airplane with a nonpressurized cabin?

Increased Cardiovascular Response

Resting systemic blood pressure increases in the early stages of altitude adaptation.[42] In addition, submaximal exercise heart rate and cardiac output can rise to 50% above sea level values, while the heart's stroke volume remains unchanged. The increased submaximal exercise blood flow at altitude largely compensates for arterial desaturation. For example, a 10% increase in cardiac output during rest or moderate exercise offsets a 10% reduction in arterial oxygen saturation in terms of total oxygen transported through the body. FIGURE 24.3 shows that the oxygen cost of submaximal exercise at 100 watts on a bicycle ergometer at sea level and high altitude remains unchanged at about 2.0 L · min^{-1}, but the relative strenuousness of the effort increases dramatically at altitude. In this example, submaximal exercise representing 50% of sea-level $\dot{V}O_{2max}$ equals 70% of $\dot{V}O_{2max}$ at 4300 m.

Catecholamine Response

Sympathoadrenal activity progressively increases over time during rest and exercise with altitude exposure.[60,64,65] Increased blood pressure and heart rate at altitude coincide with the steady rise in plasma levels and excretion rates of epinephrine. Norepinephrine levels peak in women and men after 6 days of high-altitude exposure and then remain stable.[62,63,105] Increased sympathoadrenal activity also contributes to regulation of blood pressure, vascular resistance, and substrate mixture (enhanced carbohydrate use) during short- and long-term hypobaric exposures. FIGURE 24.4 shows the 24-hour urinary excretion of norepinephrine and epinephrine during control (sea level) measurements and following 7-days exposure to

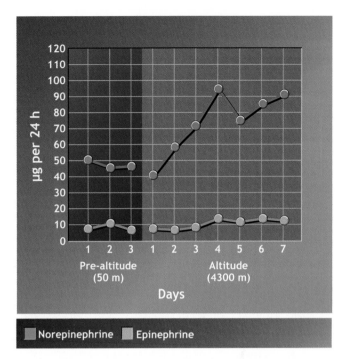

Figure 24.4 Effects of a 7-day stay at 4300 m (14,108 ft) on urinary norepinephrine and epinephrine in eight male sea-level residents. (Modified from Surks MJ, et al. Changes in plasma thyroxine concentration and metabolism, catecholamine excretion and basal oxygen uptake during acute exposure to high altitude [14,100 ft]. J Clin Invest 1966;45:1442.)

4300-m altitude. Epinephrine changed little but norepinephrine excretion increased by the fourth day. Urinary norepinephrine levels remain elevated for approximately 1 week following return to sea level.

TABLE 24.2 shows metabolic and cardiorespiratory responses to moderate and maximal cycling exercise in young men at sea level and during brief exposure to simulated altitude of 4000 m. Despite the increase in pulmonary ventilation during submaximal exercise at "altitude," arterial oxygen saturation decreased from 96% at sea level to 70% during all exercise intensities. In submaximal exercise, increased cardiac output entirely compensated for the blood's reduced oxygen content. Greater blood flow occurred from a higher heart rate (stroke volume remained unchanged). With an increase in cardiac output, submaximal exercise oxygen consumption remained essentially identical at sea level and altitude. The greatest altitude effect on aerobic metabolism emerged during maximal exercise when $\dot{V}O_{2max}$ decreased to 72% of the sea level value.

With maximal exercise during short-term altitude exposure (≤7 d), ventilatory and circulatory adjustments fail to compensate for the depressed arterial oxygen content. FIGURE 24.5 illustrates the relationship between pulmonary ventilation and oxygen consumption up to maximum during bicycle exercise at sea level and simulated altitudes from 1000 to 4000 m. Each 1000-m increase in altitude proportionately increased exercise ventilation volume. When exercise oxygen consumption exceeded 2.0 L · min^{-1}, pulmonary ventilation increased disproportionately at progressively higher elevations.

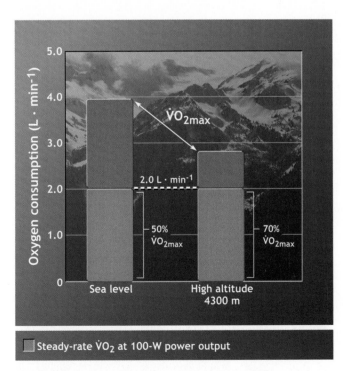

Figure 24.3 Comparison of oxygen cost and relative strenuousness of submaximal exercise at sea level and high altitude.

TABLE 24.2 ■ **CARDIORESPIRATORY AND METABOLIC RESPONSE DURING SUBMAXIMAL AND MAXIMAL EXERCISE AT SEA LEVEL AND SIMULATED ALTITUDE OF 4000 M (13,115 FT)**

EXERCISE LEVEL	$\dot{V}O_2$ (L · MIN^{-1})		$\dot{V}E$ (L · MIN^{-1} BTPS)		ARTERIAL SATURATION (%)	
Altitude, m	0	4000	0	4000	0	4000
600 kg-m · min^{-1}	1.50	1.56	39.6	53.7	96	71
900 kg-m · min^{-1}	2.17	2.23	59.0	93.7	95	69
Maximum	3.46	2.50	123.5	118.0	94	70

EXERCISE LEVEL	$\dot{Q}$ (L · MIN^{-1})		HR (B · MIN^{-1})		SV (ML)		A-$\bar{V}O_2$ DIFF (ML O$_2$ · dL^{-1})	
Altitude, m	0	4000	0	4000	0	4000	0	4000
600 kg-m · min^{-1}	13.0	16.7	115	148	122	113	10.8	9.4
900 kg-m · min^{-1}	19.2	21.6	154	176	125	123	11.4	10.4
Maximum	23.7	23.2	186	184	127	126	14.6	10.8

From Sternberg J, et al. Hemodynamic response to work at simulated altitude 4000 m. J Appl Physiol 1966;21:1589.
$\dot{Q}$, cardiac output; HR, heart rate; SV, stroke volume; A-$\bar{V}O_2$ Diff, arteriovenous oxygen difference.

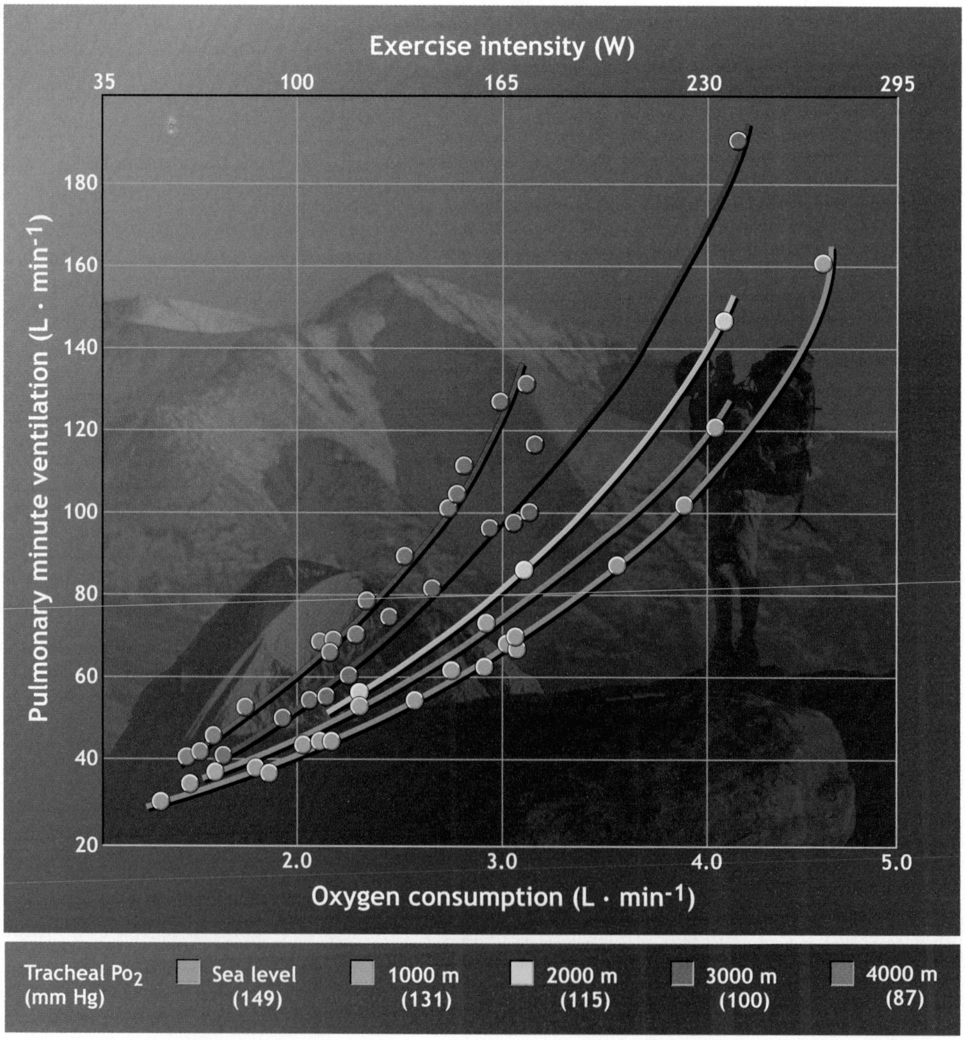

Figure 24.5 Effects of a progressive increase in simulated altitude from sea level (tracheal PO$_2$ = 149 mm Hg) to 4000 m (tracheal PO$_2$ = 87 mm Hg) on the relationship between pulmonary ventilation and oxygen consumption during cycle ergometry. (Modified from Åstrand PO. The respiratory activity in man exposed to prolonged hypoxia. Acta Physiol Scand 1954;30:343.)

Fluid Loss

Because ambient air in mountainous regions remains cool and dry, considerable body water evaporates as inspired air becomes warmed and moistened in the respiratory passages. This fluid loss often leads to moderate dehydration and accompanying dryness of the lips, mouth, and throat. Fluid loss becomes pronounced for physically active people because of their large daily total sweat loss and exercise pulmonary ventilation volumes (and hence water loss). These individuals should have access to water at all times.

Sensory Functions. FIGURE 24.6 shows deterioration in a variety of sensory and mental functions with decreases in arterial oxygen saturation at altitude. Neurologic alterations range from a 5% decrease in sensitivity to light at 1524 m to a further 25% decrease in light sensitivity and 30% decrease in visual acuity when elevation doubles to 3048 m; at 6096 m, a 25% deterioration occurs in coding task performance and simple reaction time.

Myocardial Function. Individuals with normal electrocardiograms at sea level including patients with stable chronic heart failure generally show no adverse changes to indicate myocardial ischemia (e.g., arrythmias, angina, ECG abnormalities) at simulated high altitudes, even during maximal exercise.[2,79,92] On Mt. Everest, the heart's contractile function remains stable despite considerable arterial hypoxia.[73] Little information exists about the effects of altitude on individuals with coronary artery disease, so such patients should avoid high-altitude exposure altogether.

Longer-Term Adjustments to Altitude

Hyperventilation and increased submaximal exercise cardiac output provide a rapid and relatively effective counter to the short-term challenge of altitude exposure. Concurrently, other slower acting adjustments occur during a prolonged al-titude stay. Three important longer term adjustments improve tolerance to the relative hypoxia of medium and high altitudes:

1. Regulation of acid–base balance of body fluids altered by hyperventilation
2. Synthesis of hemoglobin and red blood cells and accompanying changes in local circulation and aerobic cellular function
3. Elevated sympathetic neurohumoral activity reflected by increased norepinephrine that peaks within 1 week

Acid–Base Readjustment

The beneficial effect of hyperventilation at altitude to increase alveolar P_{O_2} produces the opposite effect on the body's carbon dioxide level. Ambient air contains essentially no carbon dioxide, so the increased breathing volumes at altitude dilute normal alveolar carbon dioxide concentrations. This creates a larger-than-normal gradient for diffusion ("wash out") of carbon dioxide from the blood to the lungs, causing a considerable decrease in arterial P_{CO_2}. For example, exposure to 3048 m decreases alveolar P_{CO_2} to about 24 mm Hg, in contrast to its usual 40 mm Hg sea-level value. Alveolar P_{CO_2} decreases to 10 mm Hg during a prolonged high-altitude stay.

Carbon dioxide loss from body fluids in a hypoxic environment creates a physiologic disequilibrium. In Chapter 13 we point out that carbonic acid (H_2CO_3) normally carries the largest quantity of carbon dioxide in the body. This relatively weak acid readily dissociates into H^+ and HCO_3^- that move to the lungs in the venous circulation. The H^+ and HCO_3^- recombine in the pulmonary capillaries to form H_2CO_3, which in turn forms carbon dioxide and water; carbon dioxide diffuses from the blood into the alveoli and leaves the body. A decrease in carbon dioxide level with hyperventilation increases the pH from loss of carbonic acid; thus, bodily fluids become more alkaline.

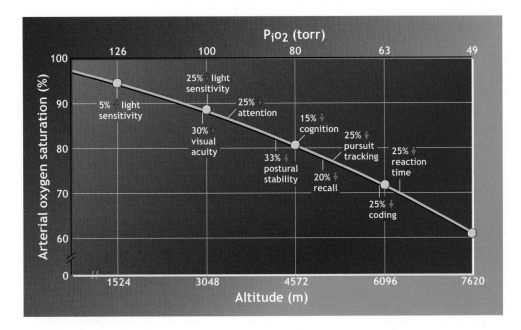

Figure 24.6 Arterial desaturation as a function of increasing altitude and corresponding impairment (↓) in diverse sensory and mental functions. (Modified from Fulco CS, Cymerman A. Human performance and acute hypoxia. In: Pandolf KB, et al., eds. Human performance physiology and environmental medicine at terrestrial extremes. Carmel, IN: Cooper Publishing Group, 1988.)

IDENTIFICATION AND TREATMENT OF ALTITUDE-RELATED MEDICAL PROBLEMS

Natives who live and work at high altitudes as well as newcomers risk a variety of medical problems associated with reduced arterial P_{O_2}. These problems usually remain mild and dissipate within several days depending on the rapidity of the ascent and degree of exposure. Other medical complications compromise overall health and safety. Three medical conditions threaten those who ascend to high altitude:

1. **Acute mountain sickness (AMS),** the most common malady
2. **High-altitude pulmonary edema (HAPE),** which reverses if the person returns quickly to a lower altitude
3. **High-altitude cerebral edema (HACE),** a potentially fatal condition if not diagnosed and treated immediately

ACUTE MOUNTAIN SICKNESS

Most people experience the discomfort of AMS during the first few days at altitudes of 2500 m and above. Factors that predispose to AMS include individual susceptibility, rapid rate of ascent, and lack of prealtitude exposure.[89] Nonspecific symptoms include headache, nausea, dizziness, fatigue, insomnia, and peripheral edema. This relatively benign condition, which becomes exacerbated by exercise in the first few hours of exposure,[77] possibly results from acute reduction in cerebral oxygen saturation.[82] It occurs most frequently in those who ascend rapidly to a high altitude without benefiting from gradual and progressive acclimatization to lower altitudes. Symptoms (Table 1) usually begin within 4 to 12 hours and dissipate within the first week.[34,38,52] Headache, the most frequent symptom, probably results from increased cerebral hemodynamics from short-term hyperventilation.[43] Most symptoms become prevalent above 3000 m. Rapid ascent to 4200 m almost guarantees some form of AMS.

Decreased thirst sensation and severe appetite suppression occurs during the early stages, often resulting in a 40% reduction in energy intake and consequent body mass loss. Diets low in salt and high in carbohydrates are well tolerated during the early stay at high altitude. A potential benefit of maintaining carbohydrate reserves through dietary intake lies in the liberation of more energy per unit oxygen with carbohydrate oxidation than with fat (5.0 kCal vs. 4.7 kCal per L of oxygen). Also, high blood lipid levels following a high-fat meal may reduce arterial oxygen saturation. Benefits of maintaining a high-carbohydrate diet include:

1. Enhanced altitude tolerance
2. Reduced severity of mountain sickness
3. Lessened physical performance decrements during the early stages of altitude exposure

Even moderate exercise becomes intolerable for persons who suffer the effects of AMS. Symptoms subside and often disappear as acclimatization progresses. Acclimatizing slowly to moderate altitudes below 3048 m followed by a gradual progression to higher elevations (termed *staged ascent*) usually prevents AMS. Climbers should spend several nights at 2500 to 3000 m before going higher, and an extra night should be added for each additional 600 to 900 m climbed. Abrupt increases of more than 600 m in the altitude for sleeping should be avoided at 2500 m or above ("climb high – sleep low"). If acclimatization proves ineffective, a 300-m descent usually alleviates symptoms; supplemental oxygen and the drug acetazolamide (Diamox) facilitate recovery.

HIGH-ALTITUDE PULMONARY EDEMA

For unknown reasons, about 2% of sojourners to altitudes above 3000 m experience HAPE. Symptoms (Table 1) usually manifest within 12 to 96 hours following rapid ascent. Major predisposing factors for HAPE include level of altitude, rate of ascent, and individual susceptibility.[6,7] Fluid accumulates in the brain and lungs in this life-threatening condition.[3,76] At first, symptoms do not seem severe, but the syndrome progresses to pulmonary edema and fluid retention by the kidneys. Chest examination reveals wheezy, raspy sounds known as *rales*. Even in well-acclimatized individuals, HAPE can develop with severe exertion at elevations above 5486 m (18,000 ft), probably the result of increased pulmonary artery pressure with damage to the blood–gas barrier.[101]

continued on page 627

Continued

TABLE 1 ■ IMPORTANT ALTITUDE-RELATED MEDICAL CONDITIONS

CONDITION	SYMPTOMS
Acute mountain sickness (AMS)	Severe headache, fatigue, irritability, nausea, vomiting, loss of appetite, indigestion, flatulence, generalized weakness, constipation, decreased urine output with normal hydration, sleep disturbance
High-altitude pulmonary edema (HAPE)	Debilitating headache and severe fatigue; excessively rapid breathing and heart rate; rales;[a] cough producing pink frothy sputum; bluish skin color (from low blood Po₂); disruption of vision, bladder, and bowel functions; poor reflexes; loss of coordination of trunk muscles; paralysis on one side of the body
High-altitude cerebral edema (HACE)	Staggered gait, dyspnea upon exertion, severe weakness/fatigue, persistent cough with pulmonary infection, pain or pressure in substernal area, confusion, impaired mental processing, drowsiness, ashen skin color, loss of consciousness

[a] Excess mucus in the lungs diagnosed as clicking sounds heard through a stethoscope.

Table 2 lists appropriate methods to avoid and treat HAPE. Treatment to prevent severe disability or even death requires immediate descent to lower altitude on a stretcher (or flown to safety) because physical activity from walking potentiates complications. With proper treatment, symptoms subside within hours, with complete clinical recovery within days. HAPE poses no problem for healthy individuals who journey to and recreate without acclimatization at altitudes below 1676 m.

HIGH-ALTITUDE CEREBRAL EDEMA

HACE is a potentially fatal neurologic syndrome that develops within hours or days in individuals with AMS. HACE occurs in about 1% of persons exposed to altitudes above 2700 m; it involves increased intracranial pressure that causes coma and death if left untreated. The early symptoms (Table 1), similar to those of AMS and HAPE, progressively worsen as the altitude stay progresses. Cerebral edema probably results from cerebral vasodilation and elevations in capillary hydrostatic pressure that moves fluid and protein from the vascular compartment across the blood–brain barrier.[35] An enlarged cerebral fluid volume eventually distorts brain structures, particularly the white matter, which exacerbates symptoms and increases sympathetic nervous system activity. Tissue hypoxia caused by high-altitude exposure also initiates a series of local events that stimulate angiogenesis (new capillary vessel growth) in brain tissue.[106] Immediate decent to a lower elevation is mandatory because of the difficulty in adequately diagnosing HACE at high altitude.

Other Conditions

Chronic mountain sickness (CMS), prevalent in a small number of altitude natives, can develop after months and years at altitude. CMS relates to excessive polycythemia, perhaps from a genetically linked variation in the EPO response to hypoxic stress.[68] CMS symptoms include lethargy, weakness, sleep disturbance, bluish skin coloring (cyanosis), and change in mental status. **High-altitude retinal hemorrhage (HARH)** affects virtually all climbers at altitudes above 6700 m (21,982 ft). HARH usually progresses unnoticed with no specific treatment or means for prevention. Hemorrhage in the macula of the eye—the oval "yellow spot" region in the back of the eyeball close to the optic disc—produces irreversible visual defects. Retinal bleeding probably results from surges in blood pressure with exercise that cause blood vessels in the eye to dilate and rupture from increased cerebral blood flow.

TABLE 2 ■ PREVENTION AND TREATMENT OF HIGH-ALTITUDE PULMONARY EDEMA

Prevention
1. Slow ascent for susceptible individuals (average increase in sleeping altitude of 300–350 m · d⁻¹ above 2500 m)
2. No ascent to higher altitude with symptoms of AMS
3. Descent when AMS symptoms do not improve after a day of rest
4. Under circumstances of high risk: avoid vigorous exercise when not acclimatized
5. Nifedipine: 20 mg slow-release formulation every 6 hours (or 30–60 mg sustained-release formulation once daily) for susceptible individuals when slow ascent is impossible

Treatment
1. Descent by at least 1000 m (primary choice in mountaineering)
2. Supplemental oxygen: 2–4 L · min⁻¹ (primary choice in areas with medical facilities)
3. When 1 and/or 2 are not possible:
   - Administer 20 mg nifedipine slow-release formulation every 6 hours
   - Use a portable hyperbaric chamber (see Fig. 26.9)
   - Descend to low altitude immediately

Because hyperventilation represents a sustained and beneficial response to altitude exposure, adjustments proceed during acclimatization to minimize the accompanying negative disruption in acid−base balance. Control of ventilatory-induced alkalosis advances slowly as the kidneys excrete base (HCO_3^-) through the renal tubules. In turn, restoration of normal pH increases the respiratory center's responsiveness, thus enabling even greater hyperventilation with altitude hypoxia.

Reduced Buffering Capacity and the "Lactate Paradox."

Establishing acid–base equilibrium with acclimatization occurs at the expense of a loss of absolute alkaline reserve. The pathways of anaerobic metabolism remain unaffected at altitude, yet the blood's capacity for buffering acid gradually decreases, lowering the critical level for acid metabolite accumulation.

On immediate ascent to high altitude, a given submaximal exercise load increases blood lactate concentration compared with sea level values. Greater reliance on anaerobic glycolysis with altitude hypoxia presumably increases lactate accumulation. Surprisingly, after several weeks of hypoxic exposure the same submaximal and maximal exercise with large muscle groups produces *lower lactate levels*. This occurs despite a lack of increase in either $\dot{V}O_{2max}$ or regional blood flow in active tissues. A general depression in maximum lactate concentrations becomes apparent in maximal exercise above 4000 m. A question arises concerning this apparent physiologic contradiction, termed the **lactate paradox**: "How is lactate accumulation reduced without a concomitant increase in tissue oxygenation, when the hypoxemia associated with high altitude should promote lactate accumulation?"

Research to resolve the lactate paradox points to reduced output of the glucose-mobilizing hormone epinephrine during chronic high-altitude exposure.[10] Because glucose and glycogen provide the only macronutrient sources for anaerobic energy (and lactate formation), reduced glucose mobilization from the liver reduces capacity for lactate formation. Reduced intracellular ADP during long-term altitude exposure may also inhibit activation of the glycolytic pathway. In addition, depressed lactate formation during maximal exercise may partly reflect an overall reduced central nervous system drive, which would diminish capacity for all-out physical effort.[61] Reduced blood lactate accumulation at high altitude does not relate to decreased buffering capacity with high-altitude acclimatization.[47]

Hematologic Changes

An increase in the blood's oxygen-carrying capacity provides the most important longer term adjustment to altitude exposure. Two factors account for this adaptation: (1) initial decrease in plasma volume followed by (2) increase in erythrocytes and hemoglobin synthesis.

Initial Plasma Volume Decrease. During the first several days of altitude exposure, the body's fluid shifts from the intravascular space to the interstitial and intracellular spaces. The decrease in plasma volume within several hours of altitude exposure increases red blood cell concentration.[87] After a week at 2300 m, for example, plasma volume declines by about 8%, whereas red blood cell concentration (hematocrit) increases 4% and hemoglobin 10%. A 1-week stay at 4300 m decreases plasma volume 16 to 25% with concomitant increases in hematocrit (6%) and hemoglobin (20%) concentration.[36] The rapid plasma volume reduction (and accompanying hemoconcentration) increases the oxygen content of arterial blood above values observed on arrival at altitude. Diuresis (increased urine output) accompanies the fluid shift from plasma during acclimatization; this maintains balance in the fluid compartments despite a lower total body water content.

Red Blood Cell Mass Increases. Reduced arterial P_{O_2} at altitude stimulates an increase in total number of red blood cells, a condition termed **polycythemia**. The erythrocyte-stimulating hormone **erythropoietin** (EPO), synthesized and released primarily from the kidneys in response to localized arterial hypoxia, initiates red blood cell formation within 15 hours after altitude ascent. In the weeks that follow, erythrocyte production in the marrow of the long bones increases and remains elevated throughout the altitude stay.[33] The blood of a typical miner in the Andes contains 38% more erythrocytes than a lowlander. In some apparently healthy high-altitude natives, red cell count may reach levels 50% above normal—8 million cells per mm^3 compared with 5.3 million for the native lowlander![58] Climbers acclimatized at 6500 m during a 1973 Mt. Everest expedition showed a 40% increase in hemoglobin concentration and a 66% increase in hematocrit.[16] Debate concerns the precise benefits of increased hematopoiesis with altitude exposure, and whether an optimum exists for hemoglobin concentration at high altitude.[74,97] Clearly, extreme erythrocyte packing increases blood viscosity and restricts blood flow and oxygen diffusion to the tissues.

INTEGRATIVE QUESTION

For their assault on Mt. Everest, elite mountaineers spend 3 months at camps at 4877 m (16,600 ft), 5944 m (19,500 ft), 6492 m (21,300 ft), 7315 m (24,000 ft), and 7925 m (26,000 ft) before the final ascent. Explain the physiologic rationale for this "stage ascent" approach to mountaineering.

Polycythemia translates directly to an increase in the blood's capacity to transport oxygen. For example, the oxygen-carrying capacity of blood in high-altitude residents of Peru averages 28% above sea-level values. The blood of well-acclimatized mountaineers carries 25 to 31 mL of oxygen per deciliter of blood compared with 20 mL for lowland residents.[70] Despite reduced hemoglobin oxygen saturation at altitude, the *quantity* of oxygen in arterial blood may approach or even equal sea-level values.

FIGURE 24.7A illustrates the general trend for increased hemoglobin and hematocrit during acclimatization for eight young women who lived and worked for 10 weeks at the 4267-m summit of Pikes Peak. Because the researchers' previous work showed fewer hematologic changes during acclimatization in women than in men (possibly from inadequate iron intake), each woman received iron supplementation prior to, during, and on return from altitude. Red blood cell concentration increased rapidly upon reaching Pikes Peak. A reduced plasma volume within the first 24 hours at altitude produced hemoconcentration. Hemoglobin concentration and hematocrit continued to rise in the month that followed and then stabilized for the remainder of the stay. Prealtitude values reestablished within 2 weeks after return to Missouri.

Figure 24.7B shows that iron supplementation increased the prealtitude values for hematocrit and hemoglobin. One might anticipate this finding because young women frequently suffer from mild dietary iron insufficiency with depressed iron reserves (see Chapter 2). Comparison of the acclimatization curves for the iron-supplemented women and another group of women not given additional iron showed greater hematocrit increase in the supplemented group. Iron supplementation enhanced hematocrit increases at altitude to a level equivalent to men at the same location. Athletes with borderline iron stores may not respond to acclimatization as effectively as individuals who arrive at altitude with iron reserves adequate to sustain increased erythrocyte production.

Cellular Adaptations

Debate concerns whether extreme terrestrial hypoxia stimulates vascular and cellular adaptations in humans that improve local oxygen extraction and maximize oxidative functions.[29,30,39,66,94] Animals born and raised at high altitude show more concentrated capillarization of skeletal muscle (number per mm^2) than sea-level counterparts.[96] Chronic hypoxia can initiate remodeling of capillary diameter and length, with formation of new capillaries to increase oxygen conductance to neural tissues.[11]

Human residents of sea level also increase tissue capillarization during an altitude stay.[67] A more prolific microcirculation reduces the oxygen diffusion distance between the blood and tissues to optimize tissue oxygenation at altitude when arterial PO_2 decreases. Muscle biopsy specimens from humans living at altitude indicate that myoglobin increases up to 16% after acclimatization.[75] Additional myoglobin augments oxygen "storage" in specific fibers and facilitates intracellular oxygen release and delivery at a low tissue PO_2. Researchers are unclear whether the small increase in mitochondrial number and concentration of aerobic energy transfer enzymes with prolonged exposure[56] (or when training under normobaric hypoxic versus normoxic conditions[66]) reflects exercise training effects or the hypoxic environment.[40,84]

High-altitude natives benefit from the slight shift to the right of the oxyhemoglobin dissociation curve at altitude. This effect decreases hemoglobin's affinity for oxygen to favor more oxygen release to tissues for a given cellular PO_2. Increased concentration of red blood cell 2,3-diphosphoglycerate (2,3-DPG; see Chapter 13) facilitates oxygen release from hemoglobin with long-term altitude exposure. Increased 2,3-DPG coupled with more circulating hemoglobin (and red blood cells) favorably affects the long-term resident's capacity to supply oxygen to active tissue during physical activity.

Body Mass and Body Composition

Prolonged high-altitude exposure reduces lean body mass (muscle fibers atrophy by 20%) and body fat, with the magnitude of weight loss directly related to terrestrial elevation. Six men

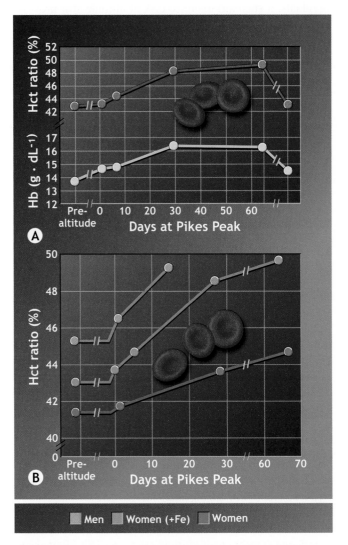

Figure 24.7 **A.** Effects of altitude on hemoglobin (Hb; *yellow line*) and hematocrit (Hct; *red line*) levels of 8 young women from the University of Missouri (213 m) prior to, during, and 2 weeks after exposure to 4267 m at Pikes Peak, Colorado. (From Hannon JP, et al. Effects of altitude acclimatization on blood composition of women. J Appl Physiol 1968;26:540.) **B.** Hematocrit response of young women receiving supplemental iron [+Fe] prior to and during altitude exposure compared with male and female subjects receiving no supplemental iron. (Courtesy of Dr. J. P. Hannon.)

participated in a 40-day progressive decompression to an ambient pressure of 249 mm Hg in a hypobaric chamber to simulate ascent of Mt. Everest.[81] Daily caloric intake from depressed appetite decreased by 43% during the exposure period. Reduced energy intake reduced body mass 7.4 kg, predominantly from the muscle component of the fat-free body mass. In addition to depressed appetite and food intake during high-altitude exposure, efficiency of intestinal absorption decreases to compound the difficulty in maintaining body weight.[13,22,102] Basal metabolic rate increases upon arrival at altitude to further affect the tendency to lose weight. To some extent, one can override an accelerated metabolic rate and minimize weight loss by consciously increasing energy intake while at altitude.[14]

Time Required for Acclimatization

The time required to acclimatize to altitude depends on terrestrial elevation. Acclimation to one altitude ensures only partial adjustment to a higher elevation. As a broad guideline, it takes about 2 weeks to adapt to altitudes up to 2300 m. Thereafter, each 610-m altitude increase requires an additional week to fully acclimatize up to 4600 m. Athletes who desire to compete at altitude should begin intense training immediately during acclimatization. Rapid initiation of training minimizes detraining effects induced by the normal tendency to reduce physical activity in the first few days at altitude. Acclimatization adaptations dissipate within 2 or 3 weeks after returning to sea level.

METABOLIC, PHYSIOLOGIC, AND EXERCISE CAPACITIES AT ALTITUDE

The stress of high altitude considerably restricts exercise capacity and physiologic function. Even at lower altitudes, the physiologic and metabolic adjustments do not fully compensate for the reduced ambient oxygen pressure, and exercise performance deteriorates. Certain circulatory parameters, particularly stroke volume and maximum heart rate, acclimatize in a direction that *reduces* oxygen transport capacity and $\dot{V}O_{2max}$.[25,28,83]

Maximal Oxygen Consumption

FIGURE 24.8A depicts the relationship between the decrease in $\dot{V}O_{2max}$ (% of sea-level value) and increasing altitude or simulated exposures (i.e., hypobaric chambers or normobaric hypoxic gas breathing) reported in diverse civilian and military studies. Disparities in experimental design and procedures and physiologic differences among subjects help to explain the variation in the points about the orange line that depict the relationship. Small declines in $\dot{V}O_{2max}$ become noticeable at an altitude of 589 m. *Thereafter, arterial desaturation decreases $\dot{V}O_{2max}$ by 7 to 9% per 1000-m altitude increase to 6300 m, where aerobic capacity declines at a more rapid, nonlinear rate.*[19,71] For example, aerobic capacity at 4000 m averages 75% of the sea-level value. At 7000 m, $\dot{V}O_{2max}$ averages one half that at sea level. The $\dot{V}O_{2max}$ of relatively fit men atop Mt. Everest averages about 1000 mL · min^{-1}; this corresponds to an exercise power output of only 50 watts on a bicycle ergometer.[69]

Physical conditioning prior to altitude exposure offers little protection because the endurance athlete experiences a slightly greater percentage reduction in $\dot{V}O_{2max}$ than an untrained person. In addition, large variability exists among individuals in the decrement in $\dot{V}O_{2max}$ with altitude exposure. Men experience the largest decrease, particularly those with (1) large lean body mass, (2) large sea-level aerobic capacity, and (3) low sea-level lactate threshold.[78] To some extent, arterial desaturation and decrease in $\dot{V}O_{2max}$ become more pronounced in individuals with a depressed hyperventilation response to exercise in a hypoxic environment.[27] Despite any unique effects of altitude exposure on aerobically fit individuals, a standard exercise task at altitude still provides relatively less stress for well-conditioned women and men because they perform it at a lower percentage of their $\dot{V}O_{2max}$.

Circulatory Factors

After several months of acclimatization to hypoxia, $\dot{V}O_{2max}$ remains below sea-level values, even with relatively rapid and pronounced increases in hemoglobin concentration. This occurs because reduced circulatory capacity—combined effect of lowered maximum heart and stroke volume—offsets the hematologic benefits of acclimatization.

Submaximal Exercise

The immediate altitude response to exercise increases submaximal cardiac output (Table 24.2), but this adjustment diminishes as acclimatization progresses and does not improve with prolonged exposure.[48] A progressive decrease in the heart's stroke volume (associated with diminished plasma volume) during the altitude stay reduces exercise cardiac output. With a lower cardiac output, submaximal oxygen consumption remains stable through an expanded a-$\bar{v}O_2$ difference. To some extent, an increased submaximal heart rate offsets the decrease in stroke volume during submaximal exercise.

Maximal Exercise

Maximum cardiac output decreases after about one week above 3048 m and remains lower throughout one's stay. *Reduced blood flow during maximal exercise results from the combined effect of decreases in maximum heart rate and stroke volume, both of which continue to decrease with the length and magnitude of altitude exposure.* This blunted cardiac response does not result from myocardial hypoxia as reflected by electrocardiographic and coronary blood flow measurements during vigorous exercise at high altitudes.[37,83] Decreased plasma volume and increased total peripheral vascular resistance contribute to the reduced maximum stroke volume. Enhanced parasympathetic tone induced by prolonged altitude exposure reduces maximum heart rate.[86]

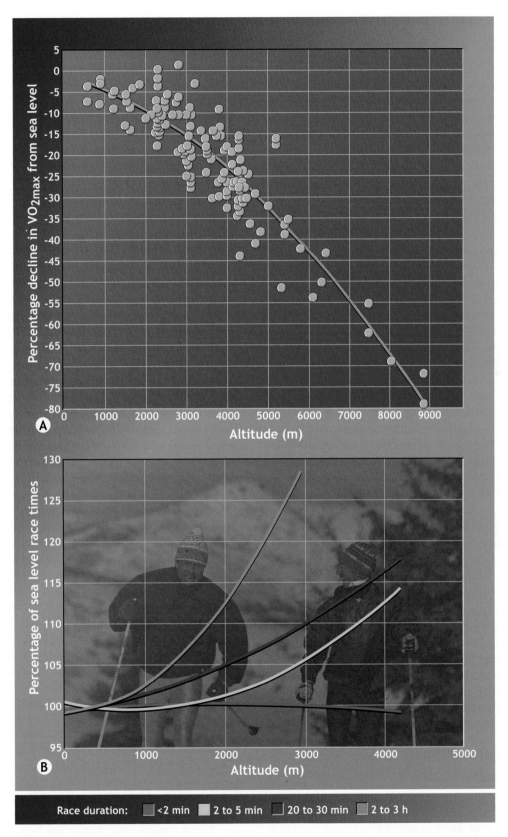

Figure 24.8 **A.** Reduction in $\dot{V}O_{2max}$ as a percentage of the sea-level value related to altitude exposure derived from 146 average data points from 67 different civilian and military investigations conducted at altitudes from 580 m (1902 ft) to 8848 m (29,021 ft). "Altitude" represents data from actual terrestrial elevations or simulated elevations with hypoxic chambers or hypoxic gas breathing. The *orange curvilinear line* is a database regression line drawn using the 146 points.
B. Generalized trend in performance decrements related to altitude exposure for runners and swimmers, primarily during competition. (Modified from Fulco CS, et al. Maximal and submaximal exercise performance at altitude. Aviat Space Environ Med 1998;69:793.)

INTEGRATIVE QUESTION

If altitude acclimatization improves endurance performance at altitude, why doesn't it improve similar performance immediately upon return to sea level?

Performance Measures

Figure 24.8B illustrates the generalized trend in exercise performance decrements primarily during competition for athletes at different altitude exposures. Altitude exerts *no* adverse effect on events lasting less than 2 minutes. For longer duration events, poorer performance occurs at higher elevations than at sea level. The threshold for decrements appears at about 1600 m for events of 2 to 5 minutes, while only a 600- to 700-m altitude induces poorer performance in events longer than 20 minutes. For the 1- and 3-mile runs, medium altitude (2300 m) decreases performance by 2 to 13% for fit subjects.[24] This coincides with the 7.2% increase in 2-mile run times for highly trained middle-distance runners at the same altitude.[1] After 29 days of acclimatization, high-altitude exposure still increases 3-mile run time, compared with sea-level runs.[72] The small improvement in endurance during acclimatization, despite lack of concomitant increase in $\dot{V}O_{2max}$, relates to three factors: (1) increased minute pulmonary ventilation (ventilatory acclimatization), (2) increased arterial oxygen saturation and cellular aerobic functions, and (3) blunting of the blood lactate response in exercise (see "lactate paradox," p. 628).

Aerobic Capacity on Return to Sea Level

Sea-level exercise performance does not improve after living at altitude when $\dot{V}O_{2max}$ serves as the improvement criterion.[44,54,67] An 18-day stay at 3100 m produced no change in the altitude-induced 25% reduction in aerobic capacity in young runners.[33] Also, $\dot{V}O_{2max}$ remained at the same prealtitude value on return to sea level. Even in studies that reported small improvements in $\dot{V}O_{2max}$ or exercise performance at altitude and on return to sea level, the change often relates to increased physical activity (i.e., effects of training and/or repeated testing) during altitude exposure.[20,49]

Possible Negative Effects

Several physiologic changes during prolonged altitude exposure negate adaptations that could improve exercise performance on return to sea level. For example, the residual effects of muscle mass loss and reduced maximum heart rate and stroke volume do not enhance sea-level performance. Any reduction in maximum cardiac output at altitude offsets benefits from an increase in the blood's oxygen-carrying capacity. A depressed circulatory capacity returns to normal after a few weeks at sea level, but so also do potentially positive hematologic adaptations. Within a physiologic context, the controversial use of blood doping (see Chapter 23) mimics the hematologic benefits of altitude exposure without the negative effects on maximum cardiovascular dynamics and body composition.

ALTITUDE TRAINING AND SEA-LEVEL PERFORMANCE

Endurance training at altitude does not improve subsequent sea-level exercise performance. Altitude acclimatization improves capacity for exercise at altitude, particularly high altitude. The effect of altitude training on aerobic capacity and endurance performance immediately on return to sea level remains unclear. As discussed previously, altitude adaptations in local circulation and cellular metabolism, combined with compensatory increases in the blood's oxygen-carrying capacity, should improve subsequent sea-level performance. Also, positive pulmonary adaptations and responses during prolonged hypoxic exposure do not regress immediately upon descent from altitude. If tissue hypoxia provides an important training stimulus, altitude plus training should act synergistically, making the total effect exceed similar training only at sea level. Unfortunately, much of the exercise training–altitude exposure research contains experimental design flaws that limit assessment of this possibility. Poor control over subjects' physical activity at altitude makes it difficult to discern whether improved $\dot{V}O_{2max}$ or performance score on return to sea level represents a training effect, an altitude effect, or synergism between the two effects.

Researchers used equivalent groups to compare effectiveness of altitude training (2300 m) and equivalent training at sea level. Six middle-distance runners trained at sea level for 3 weeks at 75% of sea-level $\dot{V}O_{2max}$. Another group of six runners trained an equivalent distance at the same percentage $\dot{V}O_{2max}$ at 2300 m. The groups then exchanged training sites and continued to train for 3 weeks at the same relative intensity as the preceding group. Initially, 2-mile run times averaged 7.2% slower at altitude than at sea level. Run times improved 2.0% for both groups during altitude training, but postaltitude performance at sea level remained the same as the prealtitude sea-level runs. FIGURE 24.9 shows that short-term altitude exposure decreased $\dot{V}O_{2max}$ 17.4% for both groups; it improved only slightly after 20 days of altitude training. When the runners returned to sea level after altitude training, aerobic capacity remained 2.8% *below* prealtitude sea-level values. Clearly, for these well-conditioned middle-distance runners, no synergistic effect emerged from combining aerobic training at medium altitude compared with equivalent sea-level training.

Other studies have duplicated these observations for $\dot{V}O_{2max}$ and endurance performance at moderate and higher altitudes in athletes from sea level.[23,51] Highly trained male track athletes flew to Nunoa, Peru (altitude 4000 m), where they continued to train and acclimatize for 40 to 57 days. $\dot{V}O_{2max}$ decreased 29% below sea-level values after the initial 3 days at altitude; after 48 days it still remained 26% lower.

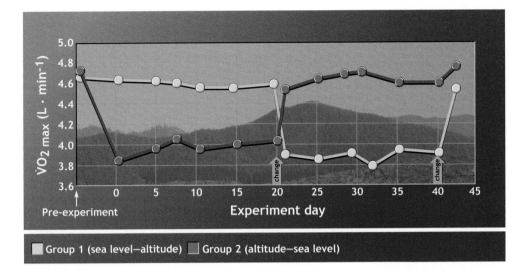

Figure 24.9 Maximal oxygen consumption of two equivalent groups during training for 3 weeks at altitude and 3 weeks at sea level. Group 1 trained first at sea level and continued training for 3 weeks at altitude. For group 2, the procedure reversed; they trained first at altitude and then at sea level. *Green arrows* indicate change in training site. (From Adams WC, et al. Effects of equivalent sea-level and altitude training on $\dot{V}O_{2max}$ and running performance. J Appl Physiol 1975;39:262.)

The 440-yard, 880-yard, and 1- and 2-mile runs during a "track meet" with the altitude natives measured running performance after acclimatization. The times after acclimatization remained considerably slower than prealtitude, sea-level times, particularly for the longer runs. When the athletes returned to sea level, $\dot{V}O_{2max}$ and running performance did not differ from prealtitude measures. On no occasion did a runner improve his previous prealtitude run time. Running times in the longer events averaged 5% *below* prealtitude trials. In other studies, training in a hypobaric chamber provided no additional benefit to sea-level performance compared with similar training (albeit at a higher absolute exercise level) at sea level. As expected, the "altitude-trained" group eventually showed better exercise performance at simulated altitude than sea-level residents.[93]

Altitude Natives May Respond Differently

For endurance athletes native to moderate altitude, total hemoglobin and blood volume synergistically increase by exercise training and altitude exposure compared to endurance athletes from sea level.[88] This adaptive response, unique to athletes born and living at altitude (e.g., Kenyan runners, Colombian cyclists, Mexican walkers) may contribute to their extraordinary endurance performance.

INTEGRATIVE QUESTION

Give your opinion (and rationale) about what effects a 2-week exposure to 3000 m would have on maximal exercise performance of 60-second duration.

Decrement in Absolute Training Level at Altitude

One must lower the absolute workload to perform aerobic exercise at the same relative intensity at altitude as at sea level. If not, anaerobic metabolism provides a larger portion of the energy for exercise at altitude (see Fig. 24.3) and fatigue develops. Exposure to 2300 m and above makes it nearly impossible to train at the same absolute exercise intensity as at sea level. TABLE 24.3 shows the reduction in exercise intensity for training relative to sea-level standards for six college athletes. At 4000 m, the runners could train only at the intensity equivalent to 39% of sea-level $\dot{V}O_{2max}$ compared with an intensity of 78% when training at sea level. The absolute exercise training level at altitude may become so reduced that an athlete cannot maintain peak condition for sea-level competition. In this regard, elite athletes benefit from periodically returning from altitude to sea level for intense training to offset "detraining" during a prolonged altitude stay (see next

TABLE 24.3 ■ **EFFECT OF ALTITUDE ON TRAINING EXERCISE INTENSITY FOR SIX COLLEGIATE ATHLETES**

	ALTITUDE (M)			
	300	**2300**	**3100**	**4000**
Intensity of workout (%$\dot{V}O_{2max}$ at 200 m)	78	60	56	39

From Kollias J, Buskirk ER. Exercise and altitude. In: Johnson WR, Buskirk ER, eds. Science and medicine of exercise and sports. 2nd ed. New York: Harper & Row, 1974.

section). Returning to a lower altitude intermittently does not interfere with acclimatization and might benefit altitude performance.[8,20,91] Regardless of the training model, athletes who train at altitude should include high-intensity speed work to maintain muscle power.

COMBINE ALTITUDE STAY WITH LOW-ALTITUDE TRAINING

Research has focused on the optimal combination of high-altitude stay plus low-altitude training in competitive runners. Athletes who lived at 2500 m but returned regularly to 1250 m to train at near–sea-level intensity (i.e., **live high–train low**) showed greater average increases in $\dot{V}O_{2max}$ and 5000-m run performance than athletes who lived and trained only at 2500 m or those who lived and trained only at sea level.[53] Strategies that combine altitude acclimatization and maintenance of sea-level training intensity provide *synergistic benefits* to sea-level endurance performance. Regular training exposure to a near–sea-level environment prevents the impaired systolic function (i.e., reduced maximum stroke volume and cardiac output) typically observed during altitude training. Such an approach to training also improves running economy and the hypoxic ventilatory drive of elite distance runners.[31,46,85,95] To remove the inconvenience and cost of the live high-train low strategy, a modification applies supplemental oxygen during training at altitude.[103] Compared with control trials, supplemental oxygen increases (1) arterial oxyhemoglobin saturation, (2) exercise oxygen consumption, and (3) average power output during high-intensity workouts at moderate altitude. This form of training allows athletes to live at altitude yet effectively "train low" with minimal travel expense and inconvenience, and without inducing additional free radical oxidative stress.[104] Researchers have not confirmed whether intermittent altitude exposure increases red blood cell mass and hemoglobin concentration.[4,55]

Not all individuals benefit to the same degree from the living high, training low strategy. Within the group that showed physiologic and performance increases with this protocol, certain individuals were "responders" while others showed little positive adjustment.[17] The "nonresponders" displayed a smaller increase in plasma concentration of the erythrocyte-producing hormone EPO after 30 hours at altitude than the responders. Such individuals experience a depressed increase in hematocrit during acclimatization to altitude exposure. There are three prerequisites to benefit from combining altitude living and lower altitude training:

1. The elevation must be high enough to raise EPO concentrations to increase total red blood cell volume and $\dot{V}O_{2max}$.
2. The athlete must respond positively with increased EPO output.
3. Training must take place at an elevation low enough to maintain training intensity and exercise oxygen consumption at near–sea-level values.

INTEGRATIVE QUESTION

Respond to a person who suggests that periodic breath-holding while exercising at sea level should produce physiologic adaptations similar to training at altitude.

At-Home Acclimatization

Application of the live high–train low training model poses significant practical and financial hurdles. Unfortunately, some endurance athletes use the banned (and dangerous) practices of either blood doping or EPO injections to increase hematocrit and hemoglobin concentration, without the potential negative effects of an altitude stay.

A more prudent approach makes use of the observation that altitude's beneficial effects on erythropoiesis and aerobic capacity may require relatively short-term exposures to hypoxia. For example, daily intermittent exposures of 3 to 5 hours for 9 days to simulated altitudes of 4000 to 5500 m in a hypobaric chamber increased endurance performance, red blood cell count, and hemoglobin concentration in elite mountain climbers.[15,80] This approach also decreases the rate of lactate appearance during intense exercise.[18] These effects may be time and protocol dependent because a 4-week regimen of intermittent normobaric hypoxia at rest (5:5 min hypoxia-to-normoxia ratio for 70 min, 5 days a week) did not improve endurance or augment erythropoietic markers in trained runners.[45] Intermittent hypoxic training under normobaric conditions provides an added bonus with clinical and cardioprotective implications—it augments training's effect on selected metabolic and cardiovascular risk factors.[5]

In the absence of a hypobaric chamber, three approaches create an "altitude" environment where an athlete, mountaineer, or hot-air balloonist living at sea level spends a large enough portion of the day to stimulate an altitude acclimatization response.

1. **Gamow Hypobaric Chamber**. A person rests and sleeps for about 10 hours each day. The chamber's total air pressure decreases to simulate the barometric pressure of a preselected altitude. Reduced barometric pressure proportionately reduces the inspired air's PO_2 to simulate altitude exposure and induce physiologic adaptations.
2. To eliminate the necessity of constructing an enclosure to withstand differentials between sea-level ambient air pressure and reduced hypobaric chamber pressure, one can simulate altitude at sea level by increasing the nitrogen percentage of the air within an enclosure. Increased nitrogen percentage correspondingly reduces the air's oxygen percentage, thus decreasing inspired air PO_2. Nordic skiers have applied this technique by living for 3 to 4 weeks in a house that provides "air" with only 15.3% oxygen rather than its normal concentration of 20.9%. The system requires mixing nitrogen gas and carefully

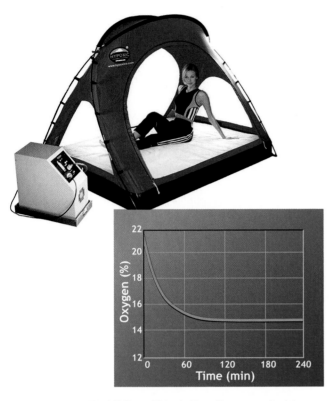

Figure 24.10 The Wallace Altitude Tent fits over a double or queen-size bed or can be constructed for in-home use as a semipermanent cubicle. Patches of "breathable" nylon allow ambient oxygen (at higher P_{O_2}) to diffuse into the tent (at lower P_{O_2}) to maintain the percentage of oxygen within the tent at about 15%. A hypoxic generator *(left of tent)* continuously supplies air with oxygen content that equilibrates within the tent to near 15%. The *bottom inset* shows the time course for equilibration of air within the tent to reach the 15% oxygen level. (Photo courtesy of Hypoxico Inc., www.hypoxico.com, and Shaun Wallace, Cardiff, CA.)

monitoring the breathing mixture. Interestingly, the Norwegian Olympic Organization has banned these "altitude houses" for its own athletes because they consider this practice "grey-zone" doping.

3. **Wallace Altitude Tent** (FIG. 24.10). A suitcase-sized unit developed by two-time British Olympic cyclist Shaun Wallace continuously supplies air with an oxygen content of approximately 15% to simulate an altitude of 2500 m. The 70-lb unit consists of a portable tent that fits over a normal bed. A "hypoxic generator" (housed in an airline suitcase) continually feeds altitude-simulating hypoxic air into the tent. The porosity of the tent's material limits the rate of diffusion of outside oxygen into the tent and maintains the 15% oxygen concentration. Equilibration of the tent's environment at the 15% oxygen level requires about 90 minutes.

Summary

1. The progressive reduction in ambient P_{O_2} with increasing altitude produces inadequate hemoglobin oxygenation in arterial blood. Arterial desaturation impairs aerobic physical activities at altitudes of 2000 m and above.

2. Altitude exposure does not adversely affect short-term (anaerobic) sprint and power performances that depend on energy from intramuscular high-energy phosphates and glycolytic reactions.

3. Reduced P_{O_2} and accompanying hypoxia at altitude stimulate physiologic responses and adjustments that improve altitude tolerance during rest and exercise. Hyperventilation and increased submaximal cardiac output via elevated heart rate provide the primary immediate responses.

4. Medical problems ranging from mild to life-threatening—AMS, HAPE, and HACE—often emerge during altitude exposure. The potentially lethal conditions of HAPE and HACE require immediate removal to a lower altitude.

5. Acclimatization entails physiologic and metabolic adjustments that improve tolerance to altitude hypoxia. The main adjustments involve (1) reestablishment of acid–base balance of the bodily fluids, (2) increased synthesis of hemoglobin and red blood cells, and (3) improved local circulation and cellular metabolism.

6. The rate of altitude acclimatization depends on the terrestrial elevation. Noticeable improvements occur within several days. The major adjustments require about 2 weeks, but acclimatization to high altitudes requires 4 to 6 weeks.

7. Alveolar P_{O_2} averages 25 mm Hg at the summit of Mt. Everest. For acclimatized men, this reduces $\dot{V}O_{2max}$ by 70% to about 15 mL $O_2 \cdot kg^{-1} \cdot min^{-1}$. An unacclimatized individual loses consciousness within 30 seconds at this altitude.

8. Despite acclimatization, $\dot{V}O_{2max}$ decreases about 2% for every 300 m above 1500 m. A decrement in endurance-related exercise performance parallels reduced aerobic capacity.

9. Altitude-related declines in maximum heart rate and stroke volume offset any beneficial effects of acclimatization. This partly explains the inability to achieve sea-level $\dot{V}O_{2max}$ values at altitude, even after acclimatization.

10. Training at altitude provides no greater benefit to sea-level exercise performance than equivalent training at sea level.

11. Athletes benefit from periodically returning from altitude to sea level for intense training to offset any "detraining" from lower levels of exercise during a prolonged altitude stay.

12. The Gammow hyperbaric chamber and Wallace tent system represent two approaches to creating an "altitude" environment under sea-level conditions.

References are available on the Student CD and online at http://connection.lww.com/mkk6e.

Exercise and Thermal Stress

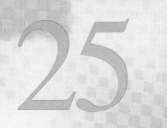

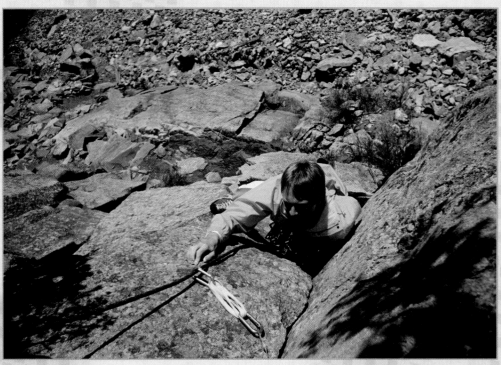

CHAPTER OBJECTIVES

- Explain how the hypothalamus maintains thermal balance

- Explain the four physical factors that contribute to heat gain and heat loss

- Discuss how the circulatory system serves as a "workhorse" for thermoregulation

- List desirable clothing characteristics for exercising in cold and warm weather

- Indicate how football equipment and the cycling helmet affect heat dissipation and thermoregulation in exercise

- Discuss factors that maintain cutaneous and muscle blood flow and blood pressure during exercise in the heat

- Describe cardiac-output, heart-rate, and stroke-volume response during exercise in the heat

- Graph the relationship between core temperature and exercise intensity (% $\dot{V}O_{2max}$)

- Quantify fluid loss during hot-weather exercise, and indicate the consequences of dehydration on physiology and performance

- Describe the purposes of fluid replacement and proposed benefits of preexercise hyperhydration and glycerol supplementation when exercising in a hot environment

- Explain how acclimatization, training, age, gender, and body fat modify heat tolerance during exercise

- Give symptoms, possible causes, and treatment for heat cramps, heat exhaustion, and exertional heat stroke

- Describe factors that constitute the WB-GT index and the relative importance of each factor

- List six factors that reduce the insulation properties of clothing

- Summarize the American College of Sports Medicine WB-GT recommendations for endurance running and cycling

- Discuss immediate and possible longer term physiologic adjustments to cold stress

- Explain the purpose of the wind chill index and factors that comprise it

Humans can tolerate a decline in deep body temperature of 10°C but only an increase of 5°C. **Temperature** technically represents the mean kinetic energy of a substance's molecules. The potential for heat exchange between substances (e.g., blood to capillary walls) or objects (e.g., playing surface to participant's body) reflects a functional definition of this term. Over the past 20 years, more than 100 football players have died from excessive heat stress during practice or competition. Hyperthermia and dehydration also contributed to the deaths of three apparently healthy collegiate wrestlers just before the 1997 competitive season.[134] A proper understanding of thermoregulation and the best ways to support these mechanisms should prevent such tragedies. Most of the responsibility for combating heat injuries rests with the people who organize and guide athletic events and physical activity programs.

PART 1 • *Mechanisms of Thermoregulation*

THERMAL BALANCE

FIGURE 25.1 shows that the temperature of the deeper tissues (**core**) represents a dynamic equilibrium between factors that add and subtract body heat. Integration of mechanisms that alter heat transfer to the periphery (**shell**) regulates evaporative cooling and varies the body's heat production to sustain thermal balance. Core temperature rises if heat gain exceeds heat loss as readily occurs with vigorous exercise in a warm, humid environment; in contrast, core temperature falls in the cold when heat loss exceeds heat production.

TABLE 25.1 presents thermal data for heat production and heat loss via sweating during rest and maximal exercise. The chemical reactions of energy metabolism produce body heat gains that can reach considerable levels during muscular activity. From shivering alone, whole body metabolism increases 3- to 5-fold.[54,133] Metabolism often rises 20 to 25 times above the resting level to about 20 kCal · min^{-1} during intense aerobic exercise by elite athletes; this theoretically can increase core temperature by 1°C (1.8°F) every 5 to 7 minutes. The body also absorbs heat from solar radiation and objects warmer than the body. Heat leaves the body via the physical mechanisms of radiation, conduction, and convection, and most importantly by water vaporization from the skin and respiratory passages. Under optimal conditions, evaporative cooling with maximal sweating accounts for a heat loss of about 18 kCal · min^{-1}.

Circulatory adjustments provide the "fine tuning" for temperature regulation. Heat conservation occurs when blood shunts rapidly to the deep cranial, thoracic, and abdominal cavities and portions of the muscle mass. This optimizes insulation from subcutaneous fat and other components of the body's shell. Conversely, when internal heat increases, peripheral vessels dilate and warm blood flows to the cooler periphery. The drive to maintain thermal balance remains so strong that it readily triggers a sweat rate of 2.0 L · h^{-1} in exercise in the heat, or an oxygen consumption of 1200 mL · min^{-1} from shivering in severe cold.

HYPOTHALAMIC REGULATION OF TEMPERATURE

*The **hypothalamus** contains the central coordinating center for temperature regulation.* This group of specialized neurons at the floor of the brain acts as a "thermostat"—usually set and carefully regulated at 37°C ± 1°C—that continually makes thermoregulatory adjustments to deviations from a temperature norm. Unlike the home thermostat, the hypothalamus cannot "turn off" the heat; it can only initiate responses to protect the body from either a buildup or loss of heat.

Two ways activate the body's heat-regulating mechanisms:

1. Thermal receptors in the skin provide input to the central control center.
2. Changes in the temperature of blood that perfuses the hypothalamus directly stimulate this area.

FIGURE 25.2 shows the diverse structures embedded within the skin and subcutaneous tissue. The *inset* on the right depicts the dynamics of sweat evaporation from the skin surface. Peripheral thermal receptors responsive to rapid changes in heat and cold exist predominantly as free nerve endings in the skin. The more numerous cutaneous cold receptors generally exist near the skin surface. Cold receptors play an important role in initiating regulatory responses to a cold environment. The cutaneous thermal receptors act as an "early warning system" that relays sensory information to the hypothalamus and cortex. This direct line of communication evokes appropriate heat-conserving or heat-dissipating physiologic adjustments, and the individual consciously seeks relief from the thermal challenge.

The central hypothalamic regulatory center plays the primary role in maintaining thermal balance. In addition to receiving peripheral input, cells in the anterior portion of the

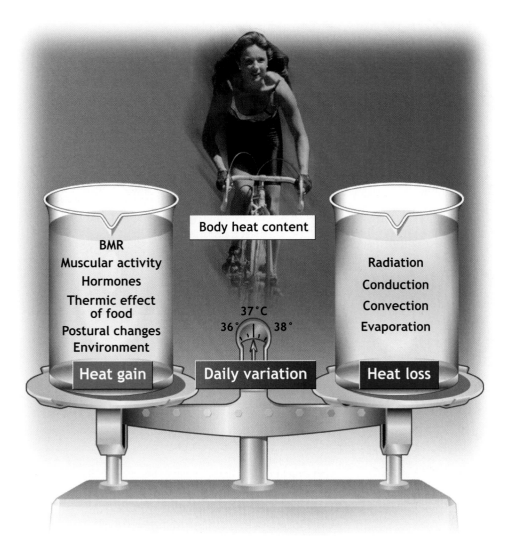

Figure 25.1 Contributing factors to heat gain and heat loss to regulate core temperature at about 37°C.

hypothalamus detect slight changes in blood temperature. These cells' heightened activity stimulates other hypothalamic regions to initiate coordinated responses for heat conservation (posterior hypothalamus) or heat loss (anterior hypothalamus). In contrast to the importance of peripheral receptors in detecting cold, the temperature of the blood that perfuses the hypothalamus provides the primary monitoring system to assess body warmth.

THERMOREGULATION IN COLD STRESS: HEAT CONSERVATION AND HEAT PRODUCTION

The normal heat transfer gradient flows from the body to the environment. Generally core temperature regulation involves no physiologic strain. However, excessive heat loss can occur in extreme cold, particularly at rest. In this case, the body's

TABLE 25.1 ■ THERMODYNAMICS DURING REST AND EXERCISE

CONDITION	REST	MAXIMAL EXERCISE
Body's heat production (1 L O_2 consumption = 4.82 kCal)	$\sim$0.25 L $O_2 \cdot min^{-1}$ $\sim$1.2 kCal $\cdot min^{-1}$	$\sim$4.0 L $O_2 \cdot min^{-1}$ $\sim$20.0 kCal $\cdot min^{-1}$
Body's capacity for evaporative cooling (Each 1 mL sweat evaporation = $\sim$0.6 kCal body heat loss)	**Maximal sweating** $\sim$30 mL $\cdot min^{-1}$ = 18 kCal $\cdot min^{-1}$	
Core temperature increase	No increase	$\sim$1°C every 5 to 7 minutes

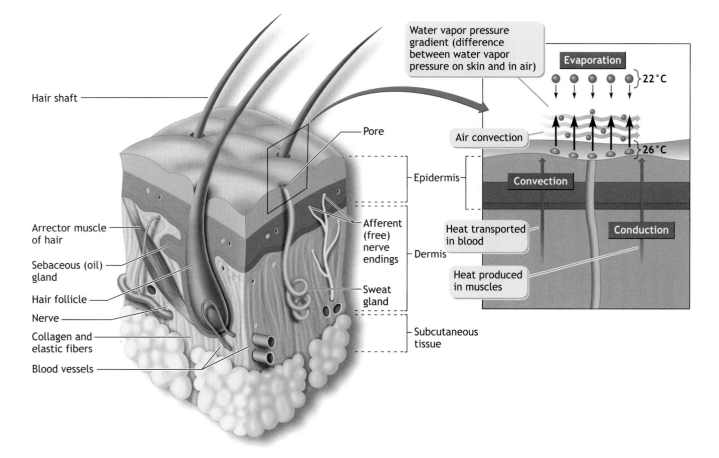

Figure 25.2 *Right inset.* Schematic illustration of the skin and underlying structures. The enlargement of the skin surface shows the dynamics of conduction, convection, and sweat evaporation for heat dissipation from the body. Each 1 L of water evaporated from the skin transfers 580 kCal of heat energy to the environment.

heat production increases while heat loss slows to minimize any core temperature decline.

Vascular Adjustments

Stimulation of cutaneous cold receptors constricts peripheral blood vessels, which immediately reduces the flow of warm blood to the body's cooler surface and redirects it to the warmer core. For example, cutaneous blood flow averages 250 mL · min^{-1} in a thermoneutral environment, yet with severe cold stress this flow approaches zero.[56] Consequently, skin temperature declines toward ambient temperature to maximize the insulatory benefits of skin, muscle, and subcutaneous fat. A person with excessive body fat exposed to cold stress greatly benefits from this heat-conserving mechanism. For a thinly clad person with normal body fat content, cutaneous blood flow regulation generally provides effective thermoregulation at ambient temperatures between 25 and 29°C (77–84°F).

Muscular Activity

Shivering generates metabolic heat, but physical activity provides the greatest contribution in defending against cold.

Exercise energy metabolism sustains a constant core temperature in air as cold as −30°C (−22°F) without reliance on a heavy, restrictive clothing barrier. Internal temperature, not the body's heat production per se, mediates the thermoregulatory response to cold. Shivering still occurs during vigorous exercise if the core temperature remains low. As a result, cold stress often induces higher exercise oxygen consumption from shivering than occurs performing the same exercise in a warmer environment.

When exercise metabolism decreases (e.g., from fatigue), shivering alone may not prevent a decline in core temperature.[133] To some extent, the variability among individuals in shivering response dictates the diverse outcomes for those caught unprepared for accidental wet–cold exposures. General muscle fatigue induced by prior heavy exercise does not depress the shivering response.[131]

Hormonal Output

Two "calorigenic" adrenal medulla hormones, epinephrine and norepinephrine, increase heat production during cold exposure. Prolonged cold stress also stimulates release of thyroxine, the thyroid hormone that increases resting metabolism.

THERMOREGULATION IN HEAT STRESS: HEAT LOSS

The body's thermoregulatory mechanisms primarily protect against overheating. Dissipating heat efficiently becomes crucial during exercise in hot weather when inherent competition exists between mechanisms that maintain a large muscle blood flow and thermoregulatory mechanisms. FIGURE 25.3 illustrates the potential avenues for heat exchange during exercise. Body heat loss occurs by four physical processes:

1. **Radiation**
2. **Conduction**
3. **Convection**
4. **Evaporation**

Heat Loss by Radiation

Objects continually emit electromagnetic heat waves. Our bodies usually remain warmer than the environment, making the net exchange of radiant heat energy move through the air to solid, cooler objects in the environment. This form of heat transfer does not require molecular contact between objects; it provides the means for the sun's warming effect on the Earth. A person can remain warm by absorbing radiant heat energy from direct sunlight or by reflection from snow, sand, or water, even in subfreezing air temperatures. The body absorbs radiant heat energy from the surroundings when an object's temperature exceeds skin temperature. This makes evaporative cooling the only avenue for heat loss.

Heat Loss by Conduction

Heat exchange by conduction involves direct heat transfer from one molecule to another through a liquid, solid, or gas. The circulation transports most body heat to the shell, but a small amount continually moves by conduction directly through the deep tissues to the cooler surface. Heat loss by conduction then involves warming air molecules and cooler surfaces that contact the skin.

The rate of conductive heat loss depends on two factors: (1) the temperature gradient between the skin and surrounding surfaces and (2) their thermal qualities. For example, immersing the body in cool water can produce considerable heat loss. Placing one hand in room-temperature water clearly illustrates this phenomenon. Why does the hand in water feel much colder than the hand in air, even though the water and air have identical temperatures? The answer is straightforward: water absorbs several thousand times more heat than air and conducts it away from the warmer body part. Sitting in an indoor swimming pool with water at 83°F provides more discomfort than sitting on the pool deck at the same temperature. Warm-weather hikers often gain considerable body heat when exercising in a warm environment. Lying on a rock shielded from the sun facilitates some body heat loss by conductance between the rock's cool surface and the hiker's warmer surface.

Heat Loss by Convection

The effectiveness of heat loss by conduction depends on how rapidly the air (or water) adjacent to the body exchanges once it warms. If air movement or convection proceeds slowly, the air next to the skin warms and acts as a "zone of insulation" that minimizes further conductive heat loss. Conversely, if cooler air continually replaces warmer air about the body on a breezy day, in a room with a fan, or when running, heat loss increases because convection continually replaces the zone of insulation. For example, air currents at 4 miles per hour are about twice as effective for body cooling as air currents at 1 mile per

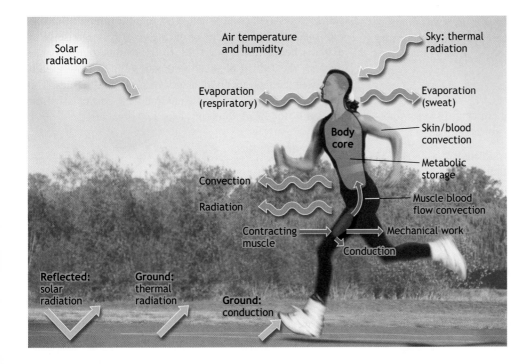

Figure 25.3 Heat production within active muscle and its transfer from the core to the skin. Under appropriate environmental conditions, excess body heat dissipates to the environment; this regulates core temperature within a narrow range. (From Gisolfi CV, Wenger CB. Temperature regulation during exercise: old concepts, new ideas. Exerc Sport Sci Rev 1984;12:339.)

hour. The cooling effect of airflow forms the basis of the wind chill temperature index (see p. 664). This index indicates the equivalent still-air temperature for a particular ambient temperature at different wind velocities. Convection also exerts an effect on thermal balance in water because the body loses heat more rapidly when swimming than when remaining motionless.

Heat Loss by Evaporation

Evaporation provides the major defense against overheating. Water vaporizing from the respiratory passages and skin surface continually transfers heat to the environment. Each vaporized liter of water extracts 580 kCal from the body and transfers it to the environment.

The body's surface contains approximately 2 to 4 million sweat glands. During heat stress, these eccrine glands—controlled by cholinergic sympathetic nerve fibers—secrete large quantities of hypotonic saline solution (0.2–0.4% NaCl). Evaporation of sweat from the skin exerts a cooling effect. The cooled skin in turn cools the blood diverted from interior tissues to the surface. In addition to heat loss through sweat evaporation, about 350 mL of insensible perspiration seeps through the skin each day and evaporates to the environment. Also, about 300 mL of water vaporizes daily from the moist mucous membranes of the respiratory passages. This is seen as "foggy breath" in cold weather.

Evaporative Heat Loss at High Ambient Temperatures

As ambient temperature increases, conduction, convection, and radiation decrease in their effectiveness to facilitate body heat loss. When ambient temperature exceeds body temperature, the body *gains* heat by these three thermal transfer mechanisms. In such environments (or when conduction, convection, and radiation are inadequate to dissipate a large metabolic heat load), sweat evaporation from the skin and respiratory tract provide the *only* means for heat dissipation. Increases in ambient temperature generally induce proportionate increases in sweating rate.

Heat Loss in High Humidity

Three factors influence the total amount of sweat vaporized from the skin and/or pulmonary surfaces:

1. Surface exposed to the environment
2. Temperature and relative humidity of the ambient air
3. Convective air currents about the body

Relative humidity represents the most important factor in determining the effectiveness of evaporative heat loss. Relative humidity refers to the ratio of water in ambient air at a particular temperature to the total quantity of moisture that air could contain, expressed as a percentage. For example, 40% relative humidity means that ambient air contains only 40% of the air's moisture-carrying capacity at that specific temperature. With high humidity, the ambient vapor pressure approaches that of moist skin (about 40 mm Hg). In this case, evaporation greatly diminishes even though large quantities of sweat bead on the skin and eventually roll off. This form of sweating represents useless water loss that can produce dehydration and overheating. A dangerous rise in core temperature can occur in athletes who compete in moderate- to high-intensity sports that exceed 30 minutes duration in environments above 35°C and 60% relative humidity. "In a Practical Sense," p. 644, describes how to assess the heat quality of the environment, with accompanying recommendations concerning physical activity related to ambient temperature, radiant heat, and relative humidity.

Continually drying the skin with a towel while sweating, as some tennis players do between games and sets, thwarts evaporative cooling. *Sweat per se does not cool the skin; evaporation cools the skin.* Individuals can tolerate relatively high environmental temperatures provided relative humidity remains low. Most persons find hot, dry desert climates more comfortable than cooler but more humid tropical climates.

 INTEGRATIVE QUESTION

In deciding on the starting time for an upcoming summer marathon, what prior meteorologic information would be most valuable and why?

Integration of Heat-Dissipating Mechanisms

The mechanisms for heat loss remain the same whether the heat load originates internally (metabolic heat) or externally (environmental heat).

Circulation

The circulatory system represents the "workhorse" to maintain thermal balance (see "Focus on Research," p. 650). At rest in the heat, heart rate and cardiac output increase while superficial arterial and venous blood vessels dilate to divert warm blood to the body shell. This manifests as a flushed or reddened face on a hot day or during vigorous exercise. With extreme heat stress, 15 to 25% of the cardiac output passes through the skin. Enhanced cutaneous blood flow greatly increases the thermal conductance of peripheral tissues. This favors radiative heat loss to the environment, particularly from the hands, forehead, forearms, ears, and tibial areas.

Evaporation

Sweating begins within several seconds of the start of vigorous exercise. After about 30 minutes, it achieves equilibrium in direct relation to the exercise load. An effective thermal defense exists when evaporative cooling combines with a large cutaneous blood flow. The cooled peripheral blood then flows to the deeper tissues to absorb additional heat on its return to the heart.

Hormonal Adjustments

Sweating produces loss of water and electrolytes; this initiates hormonal adjustments to conserve salts and fluid.

Fluid conservation makes urine more concentrated during heat stress. Concurrently, repeated days of exercise in the heat or just a single exercise bout stimulates adrenocortical release of the sodium-conserving hormone **aldosterone**. This hormone acts on the renal tubules to increase sodium reabsorption. Aldosterone also reduces sweat's osmolality. Thus, sweat sodium concentration decreases during repeated heat exposure to further conserve electrolytes. At the same time, exercise and/or hypohydration stimulates **vasopressin** (also called *antidiuretic hormone*) release from the neurohypophysis of the hypothalamus. Vasopressin increases permeability of the collecting tubules of the kidneys to facilitate fluid retention. The magnitude of aldosterone and vasopressin release depends on hypohydration severity and physical activity intensity.[88]

EFFECTS OF CLOTHING ON THERMOREGULATION

Clothing insulates the body from its surroundings. It can reduce radiant heat gain in a hot environment or retard conductive and convective heat loss in the cold.

Clothing Insulation (CLO Units)

Research by the military has established standards for the insulatory properties of clothing to meet environmental challenges. The **clo unit** represents an index of thermal resistance. It indicates the insulatory capacity provided by any layer of trapped air between the skin and clothing, including the clothing's insulation value. Assuming an environment with negligible air movement and body movement to disturb the insulatory layer of air about the body, a clo unit of 1 maintains a sedentary person at 1 MET indefinitely in an environment of 21°C (68.8°F), and 50% relative humidity.

An individual's metabolic rate at a given environmental temperature also affects the clo unit requirement. Data in the inset table on this page show six conditions of metabolic intensity from sleeping to heavy work (expressed in MET units) and three environmental temperatures (0°C, −20°C, −50°C). Note that for each activity condition, the clo unit requirement increases almost proportionally from sleeping to heavy work at the three temperature extremes. Stated somewhat differently, a close inverse relationship exists between metabolic intensity and the insulation requirement (more clothing required for less work). At rest (1 MET) at 0°C, the clo requirement is 5.4, but when temperature drops to −50°C, the clo requirement increases by 130% to 12.4.

Six factors affect the insulation (clo) value of clothing:

1. *Wind speed*—increased speed disturbs the zone of insulation
2. *Body movements*—pumping actions of arms and legs disturb the zone of insulation
3. *Chimney effect*—loosely hanging clothing ventilates the trapped air layers away from body
4. *Bellows effect*—vigorous body movements increase ventilation of air layers that conserve body heat

CLO VALUES REQUIRED TO MAINTAIN CORE TEMPERATURE RELATED TO PHYSICAL ACTIVITY LEVEL AND AMBIENT TEMPERATURE

ACTIVITY	TEMPERATURE, °C		
	0	−20	−50
Heavy work, 6.0 METs	1.0	1.6	2.2
Moderate work, 3.0 METs	1.6	2.8	4.2
Light work, 2.0 METs	2.6	4.0	6.2
Very light work, 1.5 METs	3.4	5.6	8.2
Rest, 1.0 MET	5.4	8.3	12.4
Sleep, 0.8 METs	6.7	10.6	15.5

5. *Water vapor transfer*—clothing resists the passage of water vapor and thus decreases heat loss by evaporative cooling
6. *Permeation efficiency factor*—how well clothing absorbs liquid (sweat) by capillary action (wicking); wicking sweat away from the body surface reduces the cooling effect of evaporation, thus improving clothing's effectiveness for conserving body heat

TABLE 25.2 presents clo values for common garments. To determine the total insulatory value of what a person wears, add the individual clo values for each garment. Without wind penetration or air movement around the clothing, the clo value for a given weight of clothes equals 0.15 times the clothing weight in pounds. For example, wearing 10 pounds of clothes produces a clo value of 1.5 (0.15 × 10 lb).

Cold-Weather Clothing

In providing insulation from the cold, the mesh of the cloth fibers traps air that then warms. This establishes a barrier to heat loss because the cloth and air conduct heat poorly; insulation becomes more effective with a thicker zone of trapped air above the skin. For this reason, several layers of light clothing, or garments lined with animal fur, feathers, or synthetic fabrics (with numerous layers of trapped air) provide better insulation than a single bulky layer. The clothing layer against the skin should also wick moisture from the body's surface to the next insulating clothing layer for subsequent evaporation. Wool or synthetics (e.g., polypropylene) that insulate well and dry quickly serve this purpose. A wool cap contributes considerably to heat conservation; nearly 30 to 40% of body heat dissipates through the highly vascularized head region that represents only about 8% of the body's total surface area. Conversely, cooling the head during exercise in hot weather reduces symptoms of thermal discomfort. When clothing becomes wet, through either external moisture or condensation from sweating, it loses almost 90% of its insulating properties. This facilitates heat loss from the body because water conducts heat 25 times faster than air.

The thermoregulatory challenge when exercising in cold air arises not from inadequate insulation, but from metabolic

IN A PRACTICAL SENSE

ASSESSING HEAT QUALITY OF THE ENVIRONMENT: HOW HOT IS TOO HOT?

■ A variety of factors determine the physiologic strain imposed by environmental heat. These include:

- Air temperature and relative humidity
- Individual differences in body size and fatness
- State of training
- Degree of acclimatization
- Environmental influences such as convective air currents and radiant heat gain
- Exercise intensity
- Amount, type, and color of clothing

Several football deaths from heat injury occurred with air temperature below 75°F (23.9°C) but with relative humidity above 95%. *Prevention is the most effective control of heat stress injuries.*[30] Most importantly, acclimatization mini-mizes the likelihood of heat injury. Another consideration requires evaluating the environment for its potential thermal challenge using the **wet bulb–globe temperature (WB-GT)** index. This index of environmental heat stress developed by the military provides important information to the National Collegiate Athletic Association to establish thresholds for increased risk of heat injury and exercise performance decrements. The WB-GT index depends on ambient temperature, relative humidity, and radiant heat as related in the following equation:

$$WB\text{-}GT = 0.1 \times DBT + 0.7 \times WBT + 0.2 \times GT$$

where DBT represents the dry-bulb temperature (air temperature) recorded by an ordinary mercury

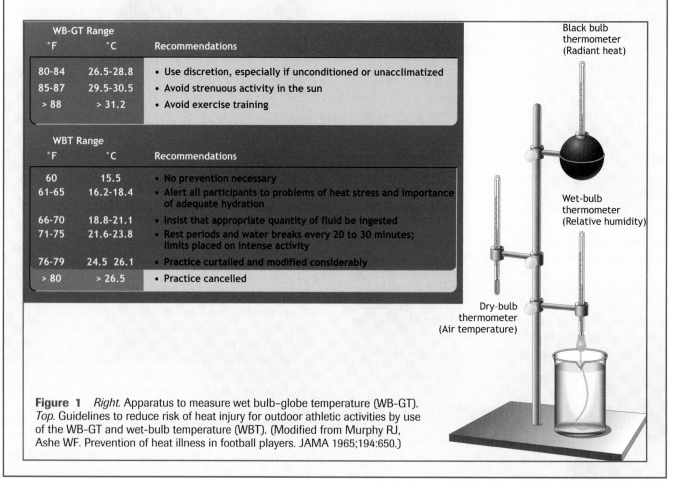

WB-GT Range		Recommendations
°F	°C	
80-84	26.5-28.8	• Use discretion, especially if unconditioned or unacclimatized
85-87	29.5-30.5	• Avoid strenuous activity in the sun
> 88	> 31.2	• Avoid exercise training

WBT Range		Recommendations
°F	°C	
60	15.5	• No prevention necessary
61-65	16.2-18.4	• Alert all participants to problems of heat stress and importance of adequate hydration
66-70	18.8-21.1	• Insist that appropriate quantity of fluid be ingested
71-75	21.6-23.8	• Rest periods and water breaks every 20 to 30 minutes; limits placed on intense activity
76-79	24.5 26.1	• Practice curtailed and modified considerably
> 80	> 26.5	• Practice cancelled

Black bulb thermometer (Radiant heat)

Wet-bulb thermometer (Relative humidity)

Dry-bulb thermometer (Air temperature)

Figure 1   *Right.* Apparatus to measure wet bulb–globe temperature (WB-GT). *Top.* Guidelines to reduce risk of heat injury for outdoor athletic activities by use of the WB-GT and wet-bulb temperature (WBT). (Modified from Murphy RJ, Ashe WF. Prevention of heat illness in football players. JAMA 1965;194:650.)

continued on page 645

Continued

thermometer, and WBT equals the wet-bulb temperature recorded by a similar thermometer except that a wet wick surrounds the mercury bulb (Fig. 1). With high relative humidity, little evaporative cooling occurs from the wetted bulb so this thermometer's temperature remains similar to the dry bulb. On a dry day, however, considerable evaporation occurs from the wetted bulb to maximize the difference between the two thermometer readings. A small difference between thermometer readings indicates high relative humidity, whereas a large difference indicates little air moisture and rapid evaporation. GT represents the globe temperature recorded by a thermometer with a black metal sphere enclosing its bulb. The black globe absorbs radiant energy from the surroundings to measure this source of heat gain. Most industrial supply companies sell this relatively inexpensive thermometer.

The *top* portion of the inset table in Figure 1 presents WB-GT guidelines to reduce the chance of heat injury in athletic activities. These standards apply to lightly clothed humans but do *not* consider the specific heat load imposed by uniforms or equipment. For American football, the lower end of each temperature range serves as the more prudent guide. One can assess ambient heat load from wet-bulb thermometer (WBT) because this reading reflects both air temperature and relative humidity. The *bottom* portion of the table presents heat stress recommendations based on WBT.

The American College of Sports Medicine proposes the following recommendations concerning risk for heat injury with continuous exercise based on the WB-GT:

AMERICAN COLLEGE OF SPORTS MEDICINE WB-GT RECOMMENDATIONS FOR CONTINUOUS ACTIVITIES SUCH AS ENDURANCE RUNNING AND CYCLING[2]
- *Very high risk:* Above 28°C (82°F)—postpone race

- *High risk:* 23 to 28°C (73–82°F)—heat-sensitive individuals (e.g., obese, low physical fitness, unacclimatized, dehydrated, previous history of heat injury) should not compete
- *Moderate risk:* 18 to 23°C (65–73°F)
- *Low risk:* Below 18°C (65°F)

Without the WBT, but knowing relative humidity (local meteorologic stations or media reports), the **heat-stress index** (Fig. 2) evaluates the relative heat stress. The index should rely on data close to the actual sport site to eliminate potential error from meteorologic data some distance from the event.

Relative humidity	Air temperature (°F)										
	70	75	80	85	90	95	100	105	110	115	120
	Heat sensation (°F)										
0%	64	69	73	78	83	87	91	95	99	103	107
10%	65	70	75	80	85	90	95	100	105	111	116
20%	66	72	77	82	87	93	99	105	112	120	130
30%	67	73	78	84	90	96	104	113	123	135	148
40%	68	74	79	86	93	101	110	123	137	151	
50%	69	75	81	88	96	107	120	135	150		
60%	70	76	82	90	100	114	132	149			
70%	70	77	85	93	106	124	144				
80%	71	78	86	97	113	136					
90%	71	79	88	102	122						
100%	72	80	91	108							

■	90°–105°F	Possibility of heat cramps
■	105°–130°F	Heat cramps or heat exhaustion likely, heat stroke possible
■	130°+	Heat stroke a definite risk

Figure 2 The heat-stress index.

heat dissipation through a thick air–clothing barrier. Cross-country skiers alleviate this problem by removing layers of clothing as the body warms. This practice maintains core temperature without reliance on evaporative cooling. *The ideal winter garment in cold, dry weather blocks air movement but also allows water vapor from sweating to escape through the clothing.*

Warm-Weather Clothing

Dry clothing, no matter how lightweight, retards heat exchange more than the same clothing fully wet. Switching to a dry tennis, basketball, or football uniform in hot weather makes little sense for temperature regulation. Evaporative heat loss occurs only when the clothing becomes wet throughout. A dry

TABLE 25.2 ■ CLO VALUES FOR SOME COMMON GARMENTS[a]

GARMENT DESCRIPTION	CLO	GARMENT DESCRIPTION	CLO
Underwear, pants		**Jacket**	
Pantyhose	0.02	Vest	0.13
Panties	0.03	Light summer jacket	0.25
Briefs	0.04	Jacket	0.35
Pants, long legs	0.1	**Coats, jacket, and overtrousers**	
Underwear, shirts		Coat	0.6
Bra	0.01	Down jacket	0.55
Shirt, sleeveless	0.06	Parka	0.7
T-shirt	0.09	**Accessories**	
Shirt with long sleeves	0.12	Socks	0.02
Half-slip, nylon	0.14	Thick, ankle socks	0.05
Shirts		Thick, long socks	0.1
Tube top	0.06	Slippers, quilted fleece	0.03
Short sleeve	0.09	Shoes (thin soled)	0.02
Light-weight blouse, long sleeves	0.15	Shoes (thick soled)	0.04
Light-weight blouse, long sleeves	0.20	Boots, gloves	0.05
Normal, long sleeves	0.25	**Skirts, dresses**	
Flannel shirt, long sleeves	0.3	Light skirt, 15 cm above knee	0.10
Trousers		Light skirt, 15 cm below knee	0.18
Shorts	0.06	Heavy skirt, knee-length	0.25
Walking shorts	0.11	Light dress, sleeveless	0.25
Light-weight trousers	0.20	Winter dress, long sleeves	0.4
Normal trousers	0.25	**Sleepwear**	
Flannel trousers	0.28	Long-sleeve, long gown	0.3
Overalls	0.28	Thin-strap, short gown	0.15
Sweaters		Hospital gown	0.31
Sleeveless vest	0.12	Long-sleeve, long pajamas	0.50
Thin sweater	0.2	**Robes**	
Long sleeves, turtleneck (thin)	0.26	Long-sleeve, wrap, long	0.53
Sweater	0.28	Long-sleeve, wrap, short	0.41
Thick sweater	0.35	**Coveralls**	
Long sleeves, turtleneck (thick)	0.37	Daily wear, belted, work	0.49
		Highly insulating multicomponent, filling coveralls	1.03
		Fibre-pelt	1.13

[a] Higher numbers indicate greater insulatory capacity.

uniform simply prolongs the time lag between sweating and evaporative cooling.

Different materials absorb water at different rates. Cottons and linens readily absorb moisture. In contrast, heavy sweatshirts and rubber or plastic clothing produce high relative humidity close to the skin. This retards vaporization of moisture from its surface, blunting or even preventing evaporative cooling. Warm-weather clothing should fit loosely to permit free circulation of air between the skin and environment to promote convection and evaporation from the skin. Moisture-wicking fabrics (e.g., polypropylene, coolmax, drylite) worn close to the skin optimally transfers heat and moisture from the skin to the environment, particularly during intense exercise in hot weather. They also benefit the individual during exercise in cold environments because dry clothing (in contrast to sweat-drenched clothing) reduces the risk for hypothermia. Color exerts an influence; dark colors absorb light rays and add to radiant heat gain, whereas lighter color clothing reflects heat rays.

Football Uniforms

Football uniforms and equipment present a considerable barrier to heat dissipation during environmental heat exposure.[83] Even with loose-fitting porous jerseys, the wrappings, padding (with its plastic covering), helmet, and other objects of "armor" effectively seal off 50% of the body's surface from the benefits of evaporative cooling. The 6 or 7 kg of equipment, frequently transported over a hot artificial playing surface adds to the player's total metabolic load. The large size of many of the athletes further magnifies heat stress, particularly for offensive and defensive linemen with relatively small surface

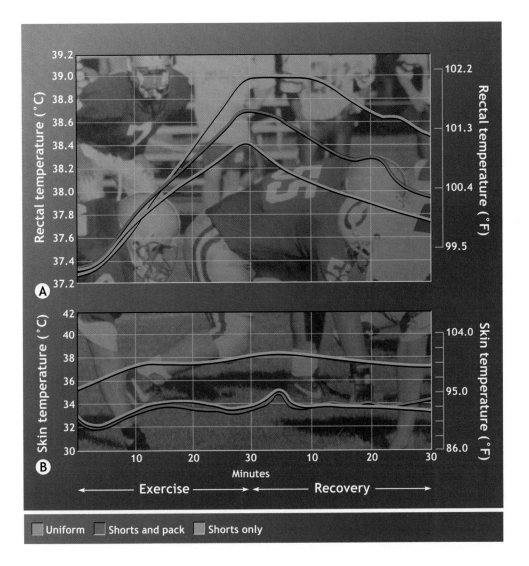

Figure 25.4 Effects of full football uniform and its equivalent weight on (**A**) rectal temperature and (**B**) skin temperature during exercise. Subjects ran at 9.6 km · h⁻¹ for 30 minutes at 25.6°C and 35% relative humidity. The uniform caused the largest heat stress, because of its effect in retarding evaporative cooling. This significantly elevated rectal and skin temperatures. (From Mathews DK, et al. Physiological responses during exercise and recovery in a football uniform. J Appl Physiol 1969;26:611.)

area : body mass ratio and higher body fat percentage than smaller teammates at the other skill positions.

FIGURE 25.4 shows the metabolic and thermal stress provided by the football uniform. The experiment tested nine men who ran for 30 minutes at 25.6°C (78°F) and 35% relative humidity. In one test, the men wore only shorts; in another, they wore the complete football uniform including helmet and plastic padding. In a third series, they wore shorts and carried a backpack that contained 6.2 kg, the exact weight of the uniform and equipment.

Wearing football gear while exercising produced higher rectal and skin temperatures during exercise and recovery than the other exercise conditions. Skin temperature directly beneath the padding averaged only 1°C less than rectal temperature. This indicates that subcutaneous blood in these areas cooled by only about one fifth as much as blood near the skin surface directly exposed to the environment. Rectal temperature remained elevated in recovery with uniforms, so a rest period offers limited value in normalizing thermal status unless the athlete removes the uniform. The dark green line shows that the weight of the uniform accounts for a large portion of the heat load. Not wearing the uniform (light green line) produced cooler skin temperatures and lower sweat rates.

Without the uniform, evaporation from the skin progressed freely, whereas the uniform insulated the athlete and reduced the effective evaporative surface.

The Modern Cycling Helmet Does Not Thwart Heat Dissipation

Wearing a commercially available cycling helmet provides vital protection against possible head trauma, but does the helmet impede thermoregulatory processes in a hot–dry or hot–humid environment? Because the head provides an important avenue for heat loss during exercise-induced hyperthermia, many competitive cyclists believe riding without a helmet reduces thermal strain and physical discomfort. This belief persists even though the design of the current commercial protective helmet retains aerodynamic and lightweight features with ventilation ports for convective and evaporative cooling. To evaluate physiologic and perceptual responses of wearing a helmet, 10 male and 4 female competitive cyclists pedaled for 90 minutes at 60% of $\dot{V}O_{2peak}$ in both hot–dry (35°C, 20% relative humidity) and hot–humid (35°C, 70% relative humidity) environments, with and without a protective helmet.[117] The results for oxygen consumption, heart rate, core, skin, and head skin temperatures, rating of perceived exertion, and perceived thermal sensations of the head and body revealed that exercising in a hot–humid environment produced greater thermal stress than exercising under thermoneutral conditions. Wearing the helmet did *not* increase the riders' heat strain or perceived heat sensation from the head or body.

Summary

1. Humans tolerate relatively small variations in internal (core) temperature. Exposure to heat or cold stress initiates thermoregulatory mechanisms that generate and conserve heat at low ambient temperatures and dissipate heat at high temperatures.

2. The "thermostat" for temperature regulation resides in the brain's hypothalamus. This coordinating center initiates adjustments in response to input from thermal receptors in the skin and changes in the temperature of the blood that perfuses the hypothalamic region.

3. Heat conservation in cold stress results from vascular adjustments that shunt blood from the cooler periphery to the warmer deep tissues of the body's core. If this mechanism proves ineffective, shivering provides input of metabolic heat. Prolonged cold stress stimulates release of hormones that elevate resting metabolism.

4. Heat stress diverts warm blood from the body's core to the shell. Four factors—radiation, conduction, convection, and evaporation—contribute to heat dissipation. Evaporation provides the major physiologic defense against overheating at high ambient temperatures and intense exercise.

5. Effectiveness of evaporative heat loss diminishes dramatically in warm, humid environments, making a person vulnerable to dehydration and spiraling core temperature.

6. Practical heat-stress indices (e.g., wet bulb–globe temperature index, heat-stress index) use ambient temperature, radiant heat, and relative humidity to evaluate the environment's potential heat challenge.

7. Three factors influence sweat vaporization from the skin or pulmonary surfaces: surface exposure, ambient air temperature and relative humidity, and convective air currents.

8. Vigorous exercise generates metabolic heat to maintain core temperature in cold air environments, even if the person wears little clothing.

9. The clo index reflects thermal resistance from clothing—the insulatory capacity of air trapped between skin and clothing including the clothing's insulation value. A clo value of 1.0 maintains thermal balance indefinitely at 1 MET at 68.8°F, and 50% relative humidity in still air.

10. Wearing several layers of light clothing traps a zone of air against the skin; this provides more effective insulation from cold than a single thick layer of clothing. Wet clothing loses its insulating properties; this greatly facilitates heat flow from the body.

11. Ideal warm-weather clothing is lightweight, loose fitting, and light colored. Even with these characteristics, heat loss slows until the clothing becomes wet and allows evaporative cooling.

12. Football uniforms impose a barrier to heat dissipation because they effectively shield about 50% of the body's surface from the beneficial effects of evaporative cooling.

PART 2 • *Thermoregulation and Environmental Stress During Exercise*

EXERCISE IN THE HEAT

The refrigerating mechanism of evaporative cooling dissipates metabolic heat during exercise, particularly in hot weather. This places a demand on the body's fluid reserves and often produces relative hypohydration. Excessive sweating leads to more serious fluid loss and reduced plasma volume. This causes circulatory failure in the extreme, and core temperature rises to lethal levels.

Circulatory Adjustments

The body faces two competitive cardiovascular demands when exercising in the heat:

1. The muscles require delivery of arterial blood (oxygen) to sustain energy metabolism.
2. Arterial blood diverts to the periphery to transport metabolic heat for cooling at the skin surface; this blood cannot deliver its oxygen to active muscle.

Submaximal exercise produces similar cardiac outputs in hot and cold environments.[110] However, the heart's stroke volume usually remains lower in the heat in proportion to the fluid deficit and reduced blood volume created in exercise.[41,91] This translates to *higher heart rates* at all submaximal levels of exercise in the heat. In contrast, the reflex compensatory increase in heart rate in maximal exercise cannot offset the stroke volume decrease so maximal cardiac output decreases.

Vascular Constriction and Dilation

Maintaining adequate cutaneous and muscle blood flow during exercise under heat stress requires that other tissues temporarily compromise their blood supply. For example, during environmental heat stress, compensatory constriction of the splanchnic vascular bed and renal tissues rapidly counteracts active vasodilation of the subcutaneous vessels responsible for 80 to 95% of elevated skin blood flow.[55,80,141] A prolonged reduction in renal and visceral tissue blood flow probably contributes to the relatively large number of liver and renal complications during exertional heat stress.

Maintenance of Blood Pressure

Vasoconstriction in the viscera increases total vascular resistance. A balance between dilation and constriction maintains arterial blood pressure during exercise in the heat. In intense exercise (with accompanying dehydration), relatively less blood diverts to peripheral areas for heat dissipation. Reduced peripheral blood flow reflects the body's attempt to maintain cardiac output in the face of diminishing plasma volume caused by sweating. *Circulatory regulation and muscle blood flow take precedence over temperature regulation during exercise in the heat.* When submaximal exercise progresses without excessive physiologic strain, a greater dependence still exists on anaerobic metabolism than in cooler conditions.[142] This produces earlier accumulation of lactate, encroachment on glycogen reserves, and premature fatigue during prolonged moderate exercise. Two factors increase blood lactate accumulation: (1) decreased lactate uptake by the liver from reduced hepatic blood flow and (2) reduced muscle catabolism of circulating lactate because heat dissipation diverts a large portion of the cardiac output to the periphery.

Core Temperature During Exercise

The heat generated by active muscles can raise core temperature to fever levels that would incapacitate a person if caused by external heat stress alone. Champion runners show no ill effects from rectal temperatures as high as 41°C (105.8°F) at the end of a 3-mile race. Aerobically fit subjects perform longer in uncompensably hot environments (thermoregulatory mechanisms inadequate) and tolerate higher levels of hyperthermia than less fit subjects.[14] An abnormally high core temperature for trained and untrained subjects impairs exercise performance. Fatigue generally coincides with core temperatures between 38 and 40°C. This temperature range reflects a "critical" high body temperature that impairs muscle activation directly from a high brain temperature that decreases the central drive to exercise. In addition to the fatiguing effects of altered cerebral blood flow and depressed neuromuscular drive, a thermally induced exercise impairment may also result from reduced blood flow to specific regions of the gastrointestinal tract to produce gastrointestinal barrier dysfunction and increased permeability. This effect allows endotoxins to enter the internal environment and contribute to fatigue.[15,65,98]

Temperature Regulated at a Higher Level

Within limits, the increase in core temperature with exercise does not reflect a failure of the heat-dissipating mechanisms or contribute to early fatigue. To the contrary, it represents a well-regulated response even during exercise in the cold. FIGURE 25.5A illustrates the relationship between esophageal (core) temperature and power output (oxygen consumption) for five men and two women of varying fitness levels during progressively more intense exercise. Core temperature increases to a higher level for all subjects as exercise intensity increases, although considerable intersubject variation occurs in temperature response. Note that the lines move closer together in Figure 25.5B, which plots core temperature related to exercise oxygen consumption expressed as a percentage of each person's $\dot{V}O_{2max}$. This indicates that relative workload (i.e., the percentage of exercise capacity) determines the change in core temperature with exercise. *More than likely, a modest rise in core temperature represents a favorable adjustment that optimizes physiologic and metabolic functions.*

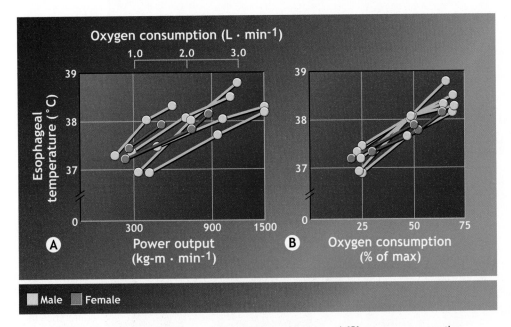

Figure 25.5 Relationship between esophageal temperature and **(A)** oxygen consumption (absolute exercise intensity expressed as power output) and **(B)** oxygen consumption as a percentage of $\dot{V}O_{2max}$. (From Saltin B, Hermansen L. Esophageal, rectal, and muscle temperature during exercise. J Appl Physiol 1966;21:1757.)

FOCUS On Research

HEAT STRESS AND CARDIOVASCULAR DYNAMICS IN EXERCISE

Rowell LB, et al. Reductions in cardiac output, central blood volume, and stroke volume with thermal stress in normal men during exercise. J Clin Invest 1966;45:1801.

▲ The 1966 research by Rowell and colleagues constituted the first study of cardiac output (CO) of unacclimatized men during heat stress and exercise. The data showed reduced CO at high ambient temperatures and exercise intensities, and helped explain an unacclimatized man's limited exercise capacity during environmental heat stress.

The researchers tested the hypothesis that maximum blood flow decreased during strenuous exercise in the heat in unacclimatized subjects (six men; mean age, 23 y; mean body surface area, 1.97 m^2; mean $\dot{V}O_{2max}$ at 23.6°C, 3.80 L · min^{-1}) by measuring CO seven times during each of four exercise intensities at 25.6°C and 43.3°C in the same subjects (56 CO determinations per subject). The men

walked for 15 minutes on a motor-driven treadmill at 3.5 mph at 7.5, 10, 12.5, and 15% grades. They rested for 15 to 20 minutes between walks.

The care given to accuracy of CO measurements represented a unique aspect of this research. Open-circuit spirometry measured oxygen consumption ($\dot{V}O_2$). The indicator dilution method assessed CO by indocyanine green dye injected into the right atrium and sampled from the aortic arch. Detailed repeat measurements reduced within-subject variability. Stroke volume (SV), arteriovenous oxygen differences (a-$\bar{v}O_2$ diff), heart rate (HR), and central blood volume (CBV) were also determined.

Figure 1 presents data for $\dot{V}O_2$, SV, a-$\bar{v}O_2$ diff, CBV, and HR at each work load at the two different temperatures. Exercise $\dot{V}O_2$ remained unaffected by ambient temperature, while HR increased markedly at 43.3°C. At the two lowest exercise intensities, CBV at 43.3°C remained 16% below control values at 25.6°C. Decrements in CBV

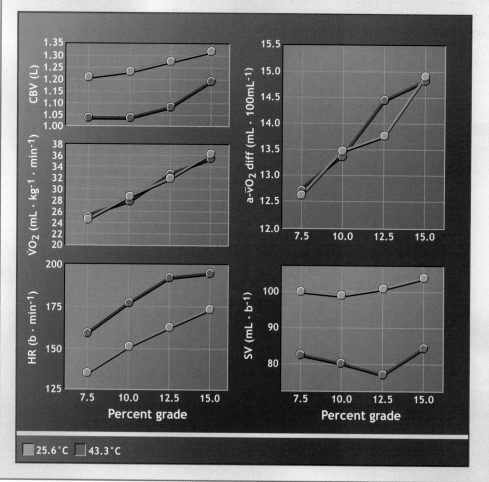

Figure 1 Central blood volume (CBV), oxygen consumption ($\dot{V}O_2$), heart rate (HR), arteriovenous oxygen difference (a-$\bar{v}O_2$ diff), and stroke volume (SV) during exercise of increasing intensity at 25.6°C and 43.3°C.

continued on page 651

Continued

paralleled the percentage decrease in SV (also 16%). CVC and SV remained reduced at the two higher exercise intensities, but SV showed more pronounced reductions.

Figure 2 presents the average CO responses to exercise at 25.6°C and 43.3°C at each of the four intensities (indicated as *percent grade* on the *right*). Ambient air temperature exerted only a small effect on CO during the first two exercise intensities. With further increases in intensity (12.5 and 15% grades), CO decreased more markedly during heat stress. For example, CO averaged $1.1 \text{ L} \cdot \text{min}^{-1}$ lower at 12.5% grade at 43.3°C than in the cooler environment. Three subjects attained near-maximal HRs at 12.5% grade. However, CO failed to increase at the most intense exercise level, although $\dot{V}O_2$ increased the expected amount via a widened a-$\bar{v}O_2$ difference.

This important experiment demonstrated that heat dissipation during moderate-to-severe exercise at a high ambient temperature occurs by repartitioning of CO rather than by increasing it. The decrease in CBV and SV during exercise in heat stress suggests a redistribution of blood from the core to the periphery coincident with a more rapid circulation time. The study showed for the first time that failure of cardiac output to increase adequately during heat stress constituted an important contributory factor that limited unacclimatized man's capacity to exercise in the heat.

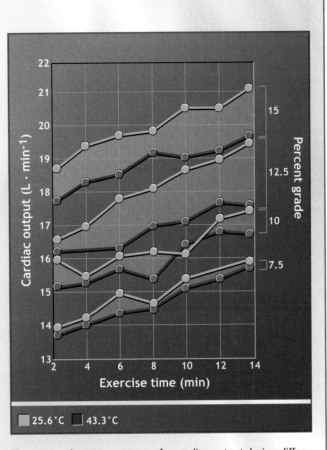

Figure 2 Average responses for cardiac output during different intensities (percent grade) of exercise at 25.6°C and 43.3°C.

In general, exercise at 50% $\dot{V}O_{2max}$ in a comfortable environment increases core temperature to a new steady level of about 37.3°C (99°F), whereas work at 75% of maximum elevates temperature to 38.5°C (101°F), regardless of the absolute exercise oxygen consumption. This means that a fit person generates more total energy (heat) in exercise than a less fit person at the same percentage of $\dot{V}O_{2max}$, yet both maintain about the same core temperature. The extra metabolic heat for the trained person dissipates via a larger sweat output. However, the trained person exercises with a lower core temperature than the untrained person at identical exercise levels.

INTEGRATIVE QUESTION

What mechanisms explain how improved aerobic fitness increases exercise tolerance in a warm, humid environment?

Water Loss in the Heat: Dehydration

Dehydration refers to body water loss from a hyperhydrated state to euhydration or from euhydration downward to hypohydration. A moderate exercise workout over 1 hour generally produces a sweat loss of 0.5 to 1.0 L. Greater water loss occurs from several hours of intense exercise in a hot environment. Exercise performed in less challenging thermal environments (e.g., cross-country skiing or swimming) still produce sweating. For swimmers and divers, water immersion also stimulates fluid loss through increased urine production. Non-exercise-induced water loss occurs when power athletes (wrestlers, boxers, weight lifters, and rowers) aggressively attempt to "make weight" through rapid weight loss induced by common dehydration techniques—external heat exposure via sauna, steam room, hot whirlpool or shower, fluid and food restriction, diuretic and laxative use, and vomiting. Athletes often combine these techniques, hoping to accelerate weight loss. *The risk of heat illness greatly increases when a person begins to exercise in a dehydrated state.*

Fluid deficits *(hypovolemia)* in the intracellular and extracellular compartments with hypohydration can rapidly reach levels that reduce the body's ability to dissipate heat and increase the rate of heat storage and cardiovascular strain owing to reductions in sweating rate and skin blood flow for a given core temperature. Reduced heat tolerance severely compromises cardiovascular function and exercise capacity with intense exercise in hot environments.[90,115] Sweat remains hypotonic to other body fluids, so the hypovolemia from sweating correspondingly increases plasma osmolality.

In terms of exercise performance, rapid weight loss through dehydration does not impair muscular strength (effects on muscular endurance remain equivocal) or a single bout of power performance up to 60-seconds duration.[42,89] Losing body water rapidly before exercising even improves muscular power and strength on a relative basis (per kg body mass).[53] When intense exercise lasts longer than 1 minute, dehydration profoundly impairs physiologic function and optimal ability to train and compete. For wrestlers, moderate hypohydration equivalent to 1.5% body mass produced poorer intermittent all-out exercise performance than similar exercise in the euhydrated state.[79] Dehydration associated with a 3% decrease in body weight also slows gastric emptying rate thus increasing epigastric cramps and feelings of nausea.

Magnitude of Fluid Loss

For an acclimatized person, water loss by sweating reaches a peak of about $3 \text{ L} \cdot \text{h}^{-1}$ an hour during intense exercise in the heat and totals nearly 12 L on a daily basis. Several hours of intense sweating can produce sweat-gland fatigue that ultimately interferes with core temperature regulation. Elite marathon runners frequently experience fluid loss in excess of 5 L during competition, a loss equivalent to 6 to 10% of body mass. For a slower paced ultramarathon, the average fluid loss rarely exceeds 500 mL per hour. Even in a temperate climate of 10°C (50°F), soccer players lose an average of 2 L during a 90-minute game.[75] *Acclimatized humans sustain their exceptional potential for evaporative cooling only with adequate fluid replacement.*

Sports other than distance running induce a large sweat output and accompanying fluid loss. Football, basketball, and hockey players lose large quantities of fluid during competition. Prior to a change in certification standards, high school wrestlers often lost 9 to 13% of preseason body weight prior to certification; the greatest portion of this weight loss came from voluntarily reducing water intake and excessive sweating just prior to the weigh-in. Collegiate wrestlers, excluding heavyweights, regained an average of 3.7 kg during the 20 hours between weigh in and competition.[116] In their desire to "make weight," high school and collegiate wrestlers usually competed in a dehydrated state, with reduced blood and plasma volumes.[1,140,144] Transient, reversible mood alterations and impaired short-term memory also accompanied rapid weight loss in collegiate wrestlers.[16]

Significant Consequences

Almost any dehydration impairs physiologic function and thermoregulation. As dehydration progresses and plasma volume decreases, peripheral blood flow and sweating rate diminish, making thermoregulation progressively more difficult. Preexercise dehydration equivalent to 5% of body mass increases rectal temperature and heart rate and decreases

sweating rate, $\dot{V}O_{2max}$, and exercise capacity, compared with exercise under normal hydration.[114,120] Reduced central blood volume lowers ventricular filling pressure and helps to explain the elevated heart rate and 25 to 30% stroke volume reduction in the dehydrated state. An increase in heart rate does not offset the reduced stroke volume; consequently, cardiac output and arterial blood pressure decline.[19,39] Elevation in core temperature relates directly to reduced sweating rate and cutaneous blood flow.

Fluid loss becomes most apparent during exercise in hot, humid environments because the high vapor pressure of ambient air thwarts evaporative cooling. FIGURE 25.6 shows the linear dependency between sweating rate during rest and exercise) and the air's moisture content reflected by wet-bulb temperature (see "In a Practical Sense," p. 644). Ironically, excessive sweat output in high humidity contributes little to cooling because of minimal evaporation.

Physiologic and Performance Decrements

Reduced peripheral blood flow and increased core temperature in exercise relate closely to dehydration level. A fluid loss equivalent to only 1% of body mass increases rectal temperature compared with the same exercise and normal hydration. For each liter of sweat-loss dehydration, exercise heart rate increases $8 \text{ b} \cdot \text{min}^{-1}$, with a corresponding $1.0 \text{ L} \cdot \text{min}^{-1}$ decrease in cardiac output.[19] A water loss of 4 to 5% of body mass impairs physical work capacity and physiologic function.[12] A large portion of water lost through sweating comes from blood plasma, so circulatory capacity progressively decreases as sweat loss progresses. Fluid loss coincides with the following: (1) decreased plasma volume, (2) reduced skin blood flow for a given core temperature, (3) reduced stroke volume, (4) increased near-compensatory heart rate, and

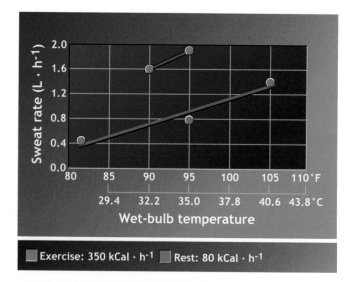

Figure 25.6 Effect of humidity (wet-bulb temperature) on sweat rate during rest and exercise in the heat. Ambient dry-bulb temperature was 43.4°C (110°F). (From Iampietro PF. Exercise in hot environments. In: Shephard RJ, ed. Frontiers of fitness. Springfield, IL: Charles C Thomas, 1971.)

(5) general deterioration in circulatory and thermoregulatory efficiency in exercise. For exercise performance, dehydration equal to 4.3% of body mass reduced walking endurance by 48%; concurrently, $\dot{V}O_{2max}$ decreased by 22%.[20] These same experiments showed decreased endurance performance (−22%) and $\dot{V}O_{2max}$ (−10%) when dehydration averaged only 1.9% of body mass. Clearly, even modest dehydration imposes adverse thermoregulatory effects during exercise.

Diuretics

Diuretic-induced dehydration draws a greater percentage of water from the plasma than body water lost through sweating. In addition, drugs that cause diuresis markedly impair neuromuscular function; this does not occur with comparable fluid loss through exercise. Chemicals that induce vomiting and diarrhea for sudden weight loss trigger dehydration and promote excessive mineral loss with accompanying muscle weakness and impaired neuromuscular function.

MAINTAINING FLUID BALANCE: REHYDRATION AND HYPERHYDRATION

Fluid replacement must focus on maintaining plasma volume so circulation and sweating progress at optimal levels. Ingesting fluid during exercise increases blood flow to the skin for more effective cooling, independent of any change in plasma volume. Prevention of dehydration and its consequences, especially hyperthermia, occurs *only* with an adequate and strictly observed water replacement schedule. Meeting this requirement often presents difficulties, because some coaches and athletes believe that ingesting water hinders performance. Left on their own, most individuals voluntarily replace only about one half of the water lost in exercise (<500 mL $\cdot$ h^{-1}).[99]

Adequate hydration provides the most effective defense against heat stress. The ideal hydration protocol balances water loss with water intake, not pouring water over the head or body. No evidence indicates that restricting fluid intake during training in some way makes an athlete better able to adjust to subsequent work in the heat. *A well-hydrated athlete always functions at a higher level than one who exercises in a dehydrated state.* Chapters 2 and 3 discuss the body's fluid compartments and factors that influence gastric emptying and intestinal fluid absorption. These chapters also provide practical recommendations for oral rehydration beverages and possible complications from hyponatremia—(excessive water intake that disrupts electrolyte balance).

Ingesting "extra" water (termed **hyperhydration**) before exercising in the heat offers thermoregulatory protection. Hyperhydration delays hypohydration from inadequate fluid replacement during exercise, increases sweating during exercise, and produces a smaller rise in core temperature in **uncompensable heat stress**, where evaporative cooling is inadequate to maintain thermal balance.[66] A practical way to promote acute preexercise hyperhydration involves consuming (1) at least 500 mL of water before sleeping the night before ex-

ercising in the heat, (2) another 500 mL upon awakening, and (3) an additional 400 to 600 mL of cold water 20 minutes before exercise. An extended, systematic regimen of hyperhydration (4.5 L $\cdot$ d^{-1}) 1 week before soccer competition by elite young soccer players in Puerto Rico increased body water reserves (despite greater urine output) and improved temperature regulation during a soccer match in warm weather.[104] The structured sequence of preexercise hyperhydration produced a 1.1 L greater total body fluid volume than with the athletes' normal daily 2.5-L fluid intake.

Preexercise hyperhydration does not replace the need for continual fluid replacement during exercise. The benefits of hyperhydration usually subside if the individual remains euhydrated during exercise. In distance running, for example, matching fluid loss with fluid intake becomes virtually impossible because only 800 to 1000 mL of fluid empty from the stomach each hour. This rate of stomach emptying does not match a water loss that can average nearly 2000 mL per hour. Under these conditions, preexercise hyperhydration proves beneficial.

Does Exogenous Glycerol Provide a Benefit?

The United States Olympic Committee (USOC) has banned the use of the diuretic glycerol. The three-carbon glycerol molecule achieved clinical notoriety (along with mannitol, sorbitol, and urea) for its role in producing an osmotic diuresis. The capacity to influence water movement within the body makes glycerol effective in reducing excess fluid accumulation (edema) in the brain and eye. An osmotic effect occurs because concentrated extracellular glycerol enters brain tissues, cerebrospinal fluid, and the eye's aqueous humor at a slow rate, thus drawing fluid from these tissues.

When consumed with 1 to 2 L of water, glycerol facilitates intestinal water absorption[135] and extracellular fluid retention, mainly in the plasma and interstitial fluid compartments.[35,105] An expanded body fluid volume potentially sets the stage for fluid excretion from increased renal filtrate and urine flow. Because proximal and distal kidney tubules reabsorb large amounts of glycerol, much of the fluid portion of the increased renal filtrate is also reabsorbed; this averts marked diuresis and promotes hyperhydration.

The normal plasma glycerol concentration at rest averages 0.05 mM; it may rise tenfold to 0.5 mM during prolonged exercise with accompanying carbohydrate depletion and elevated fat catabolism. The kidneys generally reabsorb from the renal filtrate almost all of the glycerol from food and metabolism. Thus, an exaggerated increase in urine glycerol concentration most likely indicates glycerol supplementation.

Proponents of glycerol supplementation maintain that its hyperhydration effect reduces overall heat stress in exercise as reflected by increased sweating rate; this leads to a lower exercise heart rate and body temperature and enhanced endurance performance. Reducing heat stress with augmented hyperhydration before exercise using glycerol plus water supplementation increases the safety of the participant. One gram of glycerol per kilogram of body mass with 1 to

2 L of water is the typical recommended preexercise glycerol dose; its hyperhydration effect lasts up to 6 hours.

Not all research demonstrates meaningful thermoregulatory benefits from glycerol hyperhydration over preexercise hyperhydration with plain water.[66] For example, exogenous glycerol diluted in 500 mL of water consumed 4 hours before exercise failed to promote fluid retention or ergogenic effects.[50] Also, no cardiovascular or thermoregulatory advantages result from consuming glycerol with small volumes of water during exercise.[93] Side effects of exogenous glycerol ingestion include headache, nausea, dizziness, bloating, and light-headedness. Those favoring glycerol supplementation argue that failure to reverse the USOC's glycerol ban only increases the exposure of elite athletes to risk of heat injury, including potentially fatal heat stroke. A definitive conclusion about thermoregulatory benefits of exogenous glycerol awaits further research.

Adequacy of Rehydration

Changes in body weight indicate water loss and adequacy of rehydration during and following exercise participation. Voiding small volumes of dark yellow urine with a strong odor qualitatively indicates inadequate hydration. Well-hydrated individuals typically produce large volumes of light-colored urine without a strong smell. TABLE 25.3 presents recommendations for fluid intake with short-term weight loss during exercise. These standards initially applied to a 90-minute football practice, but they easily adapt to most exercise situations.

The ideal condition replaces water losses from sweating during exercise at a rate close to or equal to sweating rate.

Athletes can be weighed before and after practice. Each pound of weight lost represents 450 mL (15 fl oz) of dehydration. Periodic water breaks during activity deter fluid depletion. Coaches and trainers must urge athletes to rehydrate because the thirst mechanism imprecisely monitors dehydration or the body's fluid needs (see American College of Sports Medicine Clarifies Indicators for Fluid Replacement [http://www.acsm-msse.org/]). The elderly generally require longer time to rehydrate after dehydration.[59] If a person relied entirely on thirst for rehydration, it could take several days to reestablish fluid balance following severe dehydration. Alcohol-containing beverages generally impede restoration of fluid balance, particularly if the rehydration fluid contains 4% or more alcohol.[122–124]

OPTIMIZING HYDRATION

PREEXERCISE
- Approximately 17 to 20 ounces 2 to 3 hours before activity
- Consume another 7 to 10 ounces after the warm-up (10 to 15 minutes before exercise)

DURING EXERCISE
- Approximately 28 to 40 ounces every hour of exercise (7 to 10 ounces every 10 to 15 minutes)
- Rapidly replace lost fluids (sweat and urine) within 2 hours after activity to enhance recovery by drinking 20 to 24 ounces for every pound of body weight lost through sweating

TABLE 25.3 ■ RECOMMENDED FLUID AVAILABILITY AND INTAKE FOR A STRENUOUS 90-MINUTE ATHLETIC PRACTICE[a]

WEIGHT LOSS		MINUTES BETWEEN WATER BREAKS	FLUID PER BREAK		FLUID AVAILABILITY FOR AN 11-MEMBER SQUAD	
LB	KG		OZ	ML	GAL	L
8	3.6	No practice recommended	—	—	—	
7.5	3.4		—	—	—	
7	3.2	10	8–10	266	6.5–8	27.4
6.5	3.0	10	8–9	251	6.5–7	25.5
6	2.7	10	8–9	251	6.5–7	25.5
5.5	2.5	15	10–12	325	5.5–6.5	22.7
5	2.3	15	10–11	311	5.5–6	21.8
4.5	2.1	15	9–10	281	5–5.5	19.9
4	1.8	15	8–9	251	4.5–5	18.0
3.5	1.6	20	10–11	311	4–4.5	16.1
3	1.4	20	9–10	281	3.5–4	14.2
2.5	1.1	20	7–8	222	3	11.4
2	0.9	30	8	237	2.5	9.5
1.5	0.7	30	6	177	1.5	5.7
1	0.5	45	6	177	1	3.8
0.5	0.2	60	6	177	0.5	1.9

[a] Based on an 80% replacement of weight loss.

Electrolyte Replacement

Sweat remains hypotonic to bodily fluids. This makes water replacement the immediate concern during exercise rather than mineral replenishment. For a fluid loss of less than 2.7 kg in adults, adding a slight amount of salt to food readily replenishes the sodium lost in sweat. Adding sodium and potassium chloride to the drinking water provided little benefit to men and women who became sweat-loss dehydrated by 3% of body mass on 5 successive days but received food and water ad libitum during each daily recovery period.[18] During prolonged exercise, the kidneys' sodium-conserving mechanisms generally balance sodium losses.

Added Sodium May Benefit Rehydration

Chapter 3 points out that electrolytes and glucose added to the rehydration beverage bring about a more complete rehydration than plain water.[103,118,138] Restoration of water and electrolyte balance in recovery occurs more rapidly by adding moderate-to-high amounts of sodium (between 20 and 60 mmol · L^{-1}) to the rehydration drink or combining solid food with appropriate sodium content with plain water.[76,77,111] Adding a small amount of potassium (2–5 mmol · L^{-1}) may en-

hance water retention in the intracellular space and reestablish any extra potassium excretion that accompanies sodium retention by the kidneys.[21] The ACSM recommends that sports drinks contain 0.5 to 0.7 g of sodium per liter of fluid consumed during exercise lasting more than 1 hour. A beverage that tastes good to the individual also contributes to voluntary rehydration during exercise and recovery.[107,139]

To restore fluid balance, the volume of ingested fluid following exercise must exceed by 25 to 50% the exercise sweat loss because the kidneys continually form some urine regardless of hydration status. Pure water absorbed from the gut rapidly dilutes plasma sodium. In turn, decreased plasma osmolality stimulates urine production and blunts the normal sodium-dependent stimulation of the thirst mechanism. These responses are counter to the goal of rehydration. Without sufficient sodium in the beverage, excess fluid intake merely increases urine output without fully benefiting rehydration.[125] *Maintaining a relatively high plasma sodium concentration by adding sodium to ingested fluid sustains the thirst drive, promotes retention of ingested fluids (lower urine output), and restores lost plasma volume more rapidly.*

FIGURE 25.7 illustrates the effect of a rehydration beverage with added sodium on ingested fluid retention in recovery.

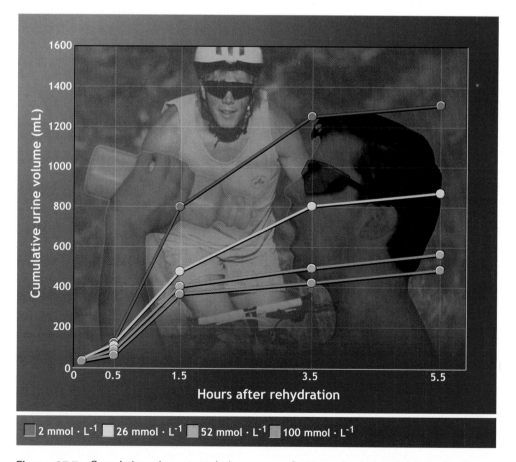

Figure 25.7 Cumulative urine output during recovery from exercise-induced dehydration. The oral rehydration beverages were four test drinks (equivalent to 1.5 times body weight loss, or 2045 mL) containing sodium (and matching anion) in a concentration of either 2, 26, 52, or 100 mmol · L^{-1}. (From Maughan RJ, Leiper JB. Sodium intake and post-exercise rehydration in man. Eur J Appl Physiol 1995;71:311.)

Six healthy men exercised in a warm, humid environment until sweating produced a 1.9% weight loss. They then ingested one of four test drinks (2045 mL) with sodium concentrations of either 2, 26, 52, or 100 mmol · L^{-1} (typical "sports drinks" contain 10–25 mM sodium; normal plasma sodium concentration ranges between 138 and 142 mM) over a 30-minute period beginning 30 minutes after stopping exercise. From the 1.5-hour urine sample onward, urine volume inversely related to the rehydration beverage's sodium content. At completion of the study period, a difference in total body water content of 787 mL existed between trials using drinks with the lowest and highest sodium content. The drink containing 100 mM sodium contributed to the greatest fluid retention.

With prolonged exercise in the heat, sweat loss can deplete the body of 13 to 17 g of salt (2.3–3.4 g · L^{-1} of sweat) daily, about 8 g more than typically consumed. It seems prudent in this deficit situation to replace the lost sodium by adding about one-third teaspoon of table salt to 1 L of water. Moderate exercise generally produces a negligible potassium loss in sweat. Even at competitive physical activity levels, potassium loss in sweat ranges between 5 and 18 mEq, which poses little or no immediate danger.[21] With heavy sweating, increasing the intake of potassium-rich citrus fruits and bananas replaces most potassium losses. *Except in unusual cases, minor adjustments in food intake and electrolyte conservation by the kidneys adequately compensate for mineral loss through sweating.*

Whole-Body Precooling

"Cold treatments" that periodically apply cold towels to the forehead and abdomen during exercise or a cold shower before exercising in the heat improve heat transfer at the body's surface only slightly above the same exercise without skin wetting.[6] However, whole-body precooling (core temperature decrease of 0.7°C) with up to 60 minutes immersion in water at 23.5°C increased subsequent exercise endurance in a hot, humid environment. Time to exhaustion inversely related to initial body temperature (lowered via precooling) and directly related to the rate of heat storage.[40] Precooling with cold-water immersion enhanced the rate of heat storage and caused less thermoregulatory strain—attenuated rise in skin and rectal temperatures and heart rates—during exercise.[9,137] In addition, whole-body precooling of the skin by 5 to 6°C without reduction in core temperature reduced thermal strain and increased distance cycled in 30 minutes under warm, humid conditions.[57] In contrast, whole-body precooling provided no thermoregulatory benefit during a simulated triathlon[8] or on the physiologic responses to a 90-minute soccer-specific exercise protocol under normal environmental conditions.[28]

Capitalizing on the potential beneficial effects of precooling, sporting goods manufacturers have developed specialized garments that circulate cold air through the garment with the intent of reducing central core temperature. For example, specially designed football shoulder pads now under evaluation have a port built into the back of the pads. When a player comes off the field, an assistant or teammate plugs in a hose to circulate cold air through ventilation channels that run up and down the pad's interior. The system includes a portable air compressor and cooler/dryer unit that adjusts cool air up to 40°F below skin temperature.

FACTORS THAT MODIFY HEAT TOLERANCE

Five factors interact to improve physiologic adjustments and exercise tolerance during environmental heat stress:

1. Acclimatization
2. Training status
3. Age
4. Gender
5. Body composition

Acclimatization

Relatively easy tasks performed in cool weather become taxing if attempted on the first hot day of spring. The early stages of preseason training for warm-weather sports often pose the greatest hazards for heat injury because thermoregulatory mechanisms have not adjusted to the dual challenge of exercise and environmental heat. Repeated exposure to hot environments when combined with exercise improves exercise capacity with less discomfort upon subsequent heat exposure.[97,114,]

The term **heat acclimatization** *describes the collective physiologic adaptive changes that improve heat tolerance.* Data from a classic study in the early 1960s show that major acclimatization occurs during the first week of heat exposure, with full acclimatization thereafter (FIG. 25.8). The process requires only 2 to 4 hours of daily heat exposure. The first several sessions in the heat should include 15 to 20 minutes of light-intensity physical activity. Thereafter, exercise sessions increase in duration and intensity.

INTEGRATIVE QUESTION

Your Maine, USA–based soccer team competes in Hawaii in early spring. Discuss how you would prepare the team to compete in this hot–humid environment making all precompetition preparations (1) at your school or (2) elsewhere, if time, money, and travel were not considerations.

TABLE 25.4 summarizes the main physiologic adjustments during heat acclimatization. *Optimal acclimatization requires adequate hydration.* During exercise, larger quantities of blood flow to cutaneous vessels to facilitate heat transfer from the core to periphery. A more effective cardiac output distribution also helps stabilize blood pressure during exercise. A lowered threshold for sweating complements these "circulatory acclimatizations." Consequently, cooling begins before core temperature increases appreciably. Sweating capacity, the most significant factor for heat acclimatization, increases early and nearly doubles after 10 days of heat exposure; sweat also

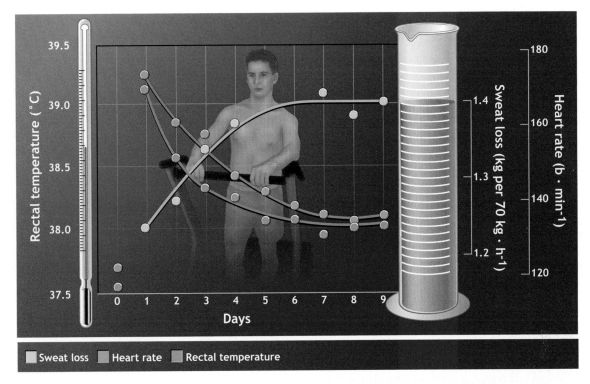

Figure 25.8 Average rectal temperature, heart rate, and sweat loss during 100 minutes of daily heat-exercise exposure for 9 days. On day 0, the men walked on a treadmill at an exercise intensity of 300 kCal · h⁻¹ in a cool climate. Thereafter, they performed the same daily exercise in the heat at 48.9°C (26.7°F wet bulb). (From Lind AR, Bass DE. Optimal exposure time for development of acclimatization to heat. Fed Proc 1963;22:704.)

becomes more dilute (less salt lost) and distributes more evenly over the skin surface. Concurrently, heat acclimatization reduces sodium loss from the kidneys. Adjustments in circulation and evaporative cooling enable the heat-acclimatized person to exercise with lower skin and core temperatures and heart rates. A lower exercise core temperature requires diversion of less blood to the skin, thus freeing a larger percentage of the cardiac output for active muscles. Acclimatization also reduces carbohydrate use in exercise, a response consistent with acclimatization-induced plasma epinephrine reduction.[34] The major benefits of acclimatization dissipate within 2 to 3 weeks after returning to a more temperate environment.

TABLE 25.4 ■ PHYSIOLOGIC ADJUSTMENTS DURING HEAT ACCLIMATIZATION

ACCLIMATIZATION RESPONSE	EFFECT
• Improved cutaneous blood flow	• Transports metabolic heat from deep tissues (core) to shell
• Effective distribution of cardiac output	• Appropriate circulation to skin and muscles to meet demands of metabolism and thermoregulation; greater blood pressure stability during exercise
• Lowered threshold for start of sweating	• Evaporative cooling begins early in exercise
• More effective distribution of sweat over skin surface	• Optimum use of effective body surface for evaporative cooling
• Increased sweat output	• Maximizes evaporative cooling
• Lowered salt concentration of sweat	• Dilute sweat preserves electrolytes in extracellular fluid
• Lower skin and core temperatures and heart rate for standard exercise	• Frees greater proportion of cardiac output to the active muscles
• Less reliance on carbohydrate catabolism during exercise	• Carbohydrate sparing

Training Status

Exercise-induced "internal" heat stress with training in a cool environment induces adjustments in peripheral circulation and evaporative cooling qualitatively similar to training in hot ambient temperatures. These training adaptations facilitate elimination of metabolic heat generated by exercise. They generally occur with an 8- to 12-week training period at an exercise intensity above 50% of aerobic capacity. This makes well-conditioned men and women living in a temperate climate respond effectively to sudden, severe heat stress than sedentary counterparts.[3] Exercise training increases the sensitivity and capacity of the sweating response so that sweating begins at a lower core temperature, thus producing larger volumes of more-dilute sweat. This results partly from intrinsic adaptations in the sweat glands.[11] Concurrently, a training-induced adjustment in cutaneous circulation provides greater skin blood flow at a given internal temperature or percentage of $\dot{V}O_{2max}$, independent of age.[55] Enhanced physical fitness sustains better blood flow to the gastrointestinal tract. This maintains the normal barrier to endotoxin movement from the gut lumen into the plasma, blunting the potential for endotoxin-induced fever that could aggravate exercise hyperthermia.[113] Plasma and extravascular fluid volumes also increase during the initial stages of aerobic training.[17,70,73,78] Controversy exists as to whether an expanded plasma volume enhances the sweating response or provides added thermoregulatory benefit during physical activity in hot weather (e.g., lower submaximal heart rate and increased stroke volume and cardiac output). The thermoregulatory benefit for exercise training occurs provided the individual remains fully hydrated during exercise.[114]

Exercise "heat conditioning" in cool weather offers fewer benefits than acclimatization from similar hot weather exercise training. *A physically active person cannot achieve full heat acclimatization without exposure to environmental heat stress.* Athletes who train and compete in hot weather have a distinct thermoregulatory advantage over athletes who train in cool climates and only periodically compete in hot weather.

Age

Debate concerns the effects of aging on tolerance and acclimatization to moderate heat stress. An early study exposed men and women aged 60 to 93 years to 70 minutes of heat stress during exercise at intensities that ranged from 2 to 5 METs. FIGURE 25.9 shows the relationship between heart rate and exercise intensity in the heat for these older subjects and young men and women. The less fit elderly subjects exercised at higher heart rates than young adults of the same gender. However, environmental heat imposed no greater physiologic strain for the older groups because their body temperature increased an average of only 0.3°C, compared with 0.2°C for the younger group. Testing the elderly subjects in the spring and fall evaluated their extent of natural heat acclimatization during the summer months. After the summer, all subjects had lower heart rates during the standard thermal–exercise stress.

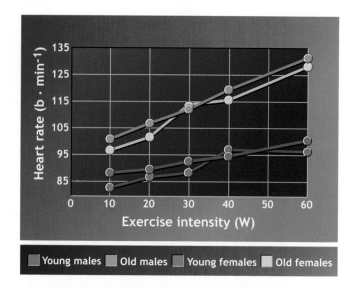

Figure 25.9   Heart rate during moderate exercise in the heat in young and older men and women. Dry-bulb ambient temperature was 33.5°C and wet-bulb was 28.5°C. (Modified from Henshel A. The environment and performance. In: Simonsen E, ed. Physiology of work capacity and fatigue. Springfield, IL: Charles C Thomas, 1971.)

Comparisons between young and middle-aged competitive runners indicate no age-related decrements in thermoregulation during marathon running.[108] Thermoregulatory function was not impaired in trained 50-year-old men compared with younger men.[101] Likewise, sweating capacity for men aged 58 to 84 years adequately regulated body temperature during prolonged desert walks.[24] *Research that controls for body size and composition, aerobic fitness, hydration, degree of acclimatization, and chronological age shows little or no age-related decrements on thermoregulatory capacity or heat-stress acclimatization.*[60,130]

Age-Related Differences

Some age-related factors affect thermoregulatory dynamics despite equivalence between young and older adults in capacity to regulate core temperature during heat stress. Aging delays the onset of sweating and blunts the magnitude of the sweating response in one of three ways: (1) modified sensitivity of thermoreceptors, (2) limited sweat gland output per se, or (3) dehydration-limited sweat output with insufficient fluid replacement.[52,58] Aging also alters the intrinsic structure and function of the skin and its vasculature.[51,62,74,109] Vascular changes include depressed peripheral sensitivity that impairs cutaneous vasodilation from two factors: (1) smaller release of vasomotor tone and (2) less active vasodilation once sweating begins. For example, older athletes show a 25 to 40% lower skin blood flow with increased core temperature than younger athletes.[61] Contributing factors include the combined effects of a lower cardiac output and reduced blood distribution from the splanchnic and renal circulations.[86] Older adults do not recover from dehydration as effectively as younger counterparts because of a reduced thirst drive.[60] This places these elderly individuals in a chronic state of hypohydration (with a less than optimal plasma volume), which could impair thermoregulatory dynamics. An altered thirst mechanism and shift in the operating point for control of body fluid volume and composition also decrease total blood volume.[22,72]

Children

Children sweat less and maintain higher core temperatures during heat stress than adolescents and adults, even though children possess a larger number of heat-activated sweat glands per unit skin area.[5,32] A reduced sweating response likely results from underdeveloped peripheral mechanisms, including the sweat glands and their surrounding tissues, rather than a depressed central drive for sweating.[119] The age difference in thermoregulation lasts through puberty; it generally does not limit exercise capacity except during extreme environmental heat stress.[31] Sweat composition differs between children and adults; children's sweat shows higher sodium and chlorine concentrations and lower concentrations of lactate, H^+, and potassium.[32,85] *From a practical standpoint, exercise intensity should decrease for children exposed to a hot environment; they also require more time to acclimatize than more mature competitors.*

Gender

Early comparisons of thermoregulation in men and women indicated that men exhibited greater tolerance to environmental heat stress during a standard bout of exercise. A major flaw in this research required that women exercise at a higher percentage of aerobic capacity than men. When researchers controlled for this factor and compared men and women of equal fitness (or exercised both at the same $\%\dot{V}O_{2max}$), thermoregulatory gender differences became less pronounced.[27,49] In essence, women tolerate the thermal stress of exercise at least as well as men of comparable aerobic fitness and level of acclimatization; both genders also acclimatize to the same degree.

Sweating

Sweating represents the distinct gender difference in thermoregulation. Women sweat less prolifically than men, despite possessing more heat-activated sweat glands per unit skin area.[11] Women start to sweat at higher skin and core temperatures and produce less sweat than men for a comparable heat-exercise load, even after equivalent acclimatization.[25]

Evaporative Cooling Versus Circulatory Cooling. Women tolerate heat similar to men of equal aerobic fitness at the same exercise level, despite a lower sweat output. Women probably use circulatory mechanisms for heat dissipation, whereas men make greater use of evaporative cooling. Clearly, producing less sweat to maintain thermal balance protects women from dehydration during exercise at high ambient temperatures.

Ratio of Body Surface Area to Body Mass. The typically smaller female has a relatively large external surface per unit of body mass exposed to the environment. This factor conveys favorable dimensional characteristic for heat dissipation. Under identical conditions of heat exposure, women tend to cool faster than men. Children possess a similar "geometric" advantage during heat stress from their larger ratio of surface area-to-mass than adults.

Menstruation. Phases of the menstrual cycle influence cutaneous vascular control in a manner that alters skin blood flow and sweating response during rest and physical activity.[13,128] For example, a higher core temperature threshold initiates sweating during the luteal phase at both 60% and 80% of aerobic capacity.[64] An upward resetting of the thermoregulatory setpoint for sweating occurs during the luteal phase and probably reflects a unique feature of hormone dynamics throughout the cycle.[47,128] An upward shift of approximately 0.4°C in oral temperature persists for about 6 days during the luteal phase. *The change in thermoregulatory sensitivity during this phase does not impair ability to exercise intensely.[71]*

Body Fat Level

Excess body fat is a liability when exercising in the heat. Because the specific heat of fat exceeds muscle tissue, fat increases the insulatory quality of the body shell and retards heat conduction to the periphery. The large, overly fat person also has a smaller ratio of body surface area-to-body mass for effective sweat evaporation than a leaner, smaller person with less body fat.

Excess body fat directly adds to the metabolic cost of weight-bearing activities. Compounding this effect by adding the weight of sports equipment (e.g., American football or lacrosse gear), intense competition, and a hot, humid environment places the overly fat person at a distinct disadvantage for temperature regulation and exercise performance. Fatal heat stroke (see next section) occurs 3.5 times more frequently in excessively overweight young adults than in individuals of average body size.

 INTEGRATIVE QUESTION

Describe the ideal physical and physiologic characteristics that minimize heat injury risk while exercising in the heat.

COMPLICATIONS FROM EXCESSIVE HEAT STRESS

Nearly 400 people die each year in the United States from excessive heat stress, and about one half of these were men and women age 65 and older. If the normal signs of heat stress go unheeded—thirst, tiredness, grogginess, and visual disturbances— cardiovascular compensation begins to fail. This initiates a cascade of disabling complications collectively termed **heat illness**. Heat cramps, heat exhaustion, and heat stroke constitute the major heat illnesses in order of increasing severity. Heat-related disabilities are more apparent among overweight, unacclimatized, and poorly conditioned individuals, including those who exercise when dehydrated.[29,36,44,102] No clear-cut demarcation exists between maladies because symptoms often overlap; exercise-induced heat injury frequently results from the cumulative effects of multiple adverse interacting stimuli.[127] TABLE 25.5 summarizes the salient features of the cardiovascular response patterns during three distinct stages of exercise hyperthermia. These stages—compensation, crisis, and failure—apply to heat exhaustion and heat stroke. The response patterns are broadly classified as either central circulatory, peripheral, or central nervous system effects. When serious heat illness occurs, only immediate corrective action reduces heat stress until medical help arrives.[26]

Heat Cramps

Heat cramps (involuntary muscle spasms) occur during or after intense physical activity, usually in the specifically exercised muscles. Core temperature often remains within normal range. An imbalance in the body's fluid level and electrolyte concentrations produces this form of heat illness. Crampers tend to have high sweat rates and/or high sweat sodium concentrations. With heat cramps, body temperature does not necessarily increase. Prevention involves two factors: (1) providing plentiful water that contains salt and

(2) increasing daily salt intake (e.g., adding salt to foods at mealtime) several days before heat stress. Sweating causes electrolyte loss during prolonged heat exposure. Failure to replenish these minerals often leads to muscle pain and spasm, most commonly in the abdomen and extremities. Drinking copious amounts of water and increasing daily salt intake several days before heat stress generally prevents this heat-related malady.

Heat Exhaustion

Heat exhaustion usually develops in unacclimatized persons during the first summer heat wave or with the first hard training session on a hot day. Exercise-induced heat exhaustion occurs from ineffective circulatory adjustments compounded by depletion of extracellular fluid, principally plasma volume from excessive sweating. Blood usually pools in the dilated peripheral vessels; this drastically reduces the central blood volume necessary to maintain cardiac output. Characteristics of heat exhaustion include a weak and rapid pulse, low blood pressure in the upright position, headache, dizziness, and general weakness. Sweating may decrease somewhat, but core temperature does not rise to dangerous levels (i.e., >40°C or 104°F). A person who experiences symptoms of heat exhaustion should stop exercising and move to a cooler environment. Intravenous therapy replenishes fluid most effectively.

TABLE 25.5 ■ CARDIOVASCULAR RESPONSES DURING THE THREE STAGES OF EXERCISE HYPERTHERMIA

	CENTRAL CIRCULATION		PERIPHERAL CIRCULATION	RECTAL TEMPERATURE	CENTRAL NERVOUS SYSTEM STATUS
Compensation	↑ CO ↑ SV, ↑ HR ↓ PV Respiratory alkalosis	↓ Low SPBF ↓ PV	↓ Low TPVR ↑ Skin BF ↑ Muscle BF	37.0°C to 39.5°C	Premonitory signs Dizziness Headache Euphoria Psychoses
Crises	↑↓ CO ↑ MABP ↓ SV ↑↑ HR Tachycardia (180 b · min⁻¹) Metabolic acidosis	↑↓ SPBF ↓ PV Moderate CVP	↓ TPVR ↑↓ Skin BF	39.5°C 41.5°C	↓ Cerebral congestion ↓ Cerebral edema Intracranial hypertension
Failure	↓↓ CO ↓↓ MABP ↑ HR Tachycardia Metabolic acidosis	↑↑ SPBF (autoregulatory escape); high CVP but low if hypovolemic	↓ TPVR ↓ Low skin BF	41.5°C	↓Coma, decreased cerebral perfusion ↓Cerebral ischemia Neurologic damage, seizures

Data from Hubbard RW, Armstrong LE. The heat illnesses: biochemical, ultrastructural, and fluid-electrolyte considerations. In: Pandolf K et al., eds. Human performance physiology and environmental medicine at terrestrial extremes. Carmel, IN: Cooper Publishing Group, 1994; original data of Kielblock AJ, et al. Cardiovascular origins of heatstroke pathophysiology: an anesthetized rat model. Aviat Space Environ Med 1982;53:171.

Abbreviations: CO, cardiac output; SV, stroke volume; HR, heart rate; SPBF, splanchnic blood flow; PV, plasma volume; TPVR, total peripheral vascular resistance; BF, blood flow; MABP, mean arterial blood pressure; CVP, central venous pressure. ↑ = moderate increase; ↑↑ = strong increase; ↓ = moderate decrease; ↓↓ = strong decrease; ↑↓ = increase then decrease; ↓ = progressing to.

Heat Stroke

Heat stroke, the most serious and complex of the heat-stress maladies, requires immediate medical attention. Heat stroke reflects failure of the heat-regulating mechanisms from an excessively high core temperature. The *classic form* of heat stroke—core temperature >105°F, altered mental status, absence of sweating—usually occurs during heat waves. It affects young children, the elderly, and those with chronic diseases. In classic heat stroke, environmental heat overloads the body's heat-dissipating mechanisms. Severe heat stress also produces a continuum of potentially negative alterations in the immune system and in leukocyte adhesion and activation processes (unrelated to elevated catecholamine levels).[45] One in every three individuals who survive a near-fatal case of classic heat stroke remains permanently disabled with multisystem organ dysfunction.[23]

Exertional heat stroke is a state of extreme hyperthermia from the interactive effects of two factors:

1. Metabolic heat load in exercise
2. Challenge for heat dissipation from a hot–humid environment

When thermoregulation fails, sweating diminishes, the skin becomes dry and hot, and body temperature rises to 41.5°C and above; this places an inordinate strain on cardiovascular function. The often subtle symptoms compound the complexity of emergency hyperthermia. With intense exercise, usually by young, highly motivated individuals, sweating may progress but body heat gain overpowers the avenues for heat loss. Other predisposing factors for exertional heat stroke include poor fitness status, obesity, inadequate acclimatization, sweat gland dysfunction, dehydration, and infectious disease. If left untreated, the disability progresses rapidly and death ensues from circulatory collapse and damage to the central nervous system and other organ systems. While awaiting medical treatment, aggressive steps must be taken to lower core temperature because mortality relates to the magnitude and duration of hyperthermia. Immediate treatment includes fluid replacement and body cooling with alcohol rubs, application of ice packs to the neck area, and whole-body immersion in cold or even ice water.[4,92,94] No attempt should be made to slow the respiratory rate because a rapid rate of breathing compensates for metabolic acidosis. Prudent treatment also includes specific drug therapy to counter possible endotoxin effects precipitated by heat stroke pathology.[43]

Oral Temperature Unreliable

Oral temperature inaccurately measures core temperature after strenuous exercise. Rectal temperature following a 14-mile race in a tropical climate averaged 103.5°F while oral temperature surprisingly remained normal at 98°F![112] Part of the discrepancy lies in the effects on oral temperature of evaporative cooling of the mouth and airways during high levels of exercise pulmonary ventilation.

Summary

1. Core temperature normally increases during exercise; the relative stress of exercise determines the magnitude of the increase. A well-regulated temperature increase creates a more favorable environment for physiologic and metabolic functions.
2. Excessive sweating compromises fluid reserves to create a relative state of dehydration. Sweating without fluid replacement decreases plasma volume, which leads to circulatory dysfunction and a precipitous rise in core temperature.
3. Exercise in a hot, humid environment poses a considerable thermoregulatory challenge because the large sweat loss in high humidity contributes little to evaporative cooling.
4. Fluid loss of more than 4% of body weight impedes heat dissipation, compromises cardiovascular function, and diminishes exercise capacity.
5. Adequate fluid replacement maintains plasma volume so circulation and sweating progress optimally. The ideal replacement schedule during exercise matches fluid intake to fluid loss, a process effectively monitored by changes in body weight.
6. The small intestine can absorb about 1000 mL of water each hour. A small amount of electrolytes in the rehydration beverage facilitates fluid replacement more than drinking plain water.
7. The diet generally replaces minerals lost through sweating. With prolonged exercise in the heat, adding a small amount of salt to the replacement fluid (1 tsp · L^{-1}) facilitates sodium and fluid replenishment.
8. Repeated heat stress initiates thermoregulatory adjustments that improve exercise capacity and reduce discomfort on heat exposure. Such heat acclimatization triggers favorable cardiac output distribution while increasing sweating capacity. Ten days of heat exposure promotes full acclimatization.
9. Aging affects thermoregulatory functions but does not appreciably alter temperature regulation during exercise or acclimatization to moderate heat stress.
10. Women and men show equivalent thermoregulation during exercise when controlled for levels of fitness and acclimatization. Women produce less sweat than men when exercising at the same core temperature.
11. Heat cramps, heat exhaustion, and heat stroke constitute the major heat illnesses. Heat stroke, a medical emergency, is the most serious and complex of these maladies.
12. Oral temperature after exercising inaccurately measures core temperature. This discrepancy results from evaporative cooling of the mouth and airways with high levels of pulmonary ventilation during exercise and recovery.

EXERCISE IN THE COLD

Human exposure to extreme cold produces significant physiologic and psychologic challenges. Cold ranks high among the differing terrestrial environmental stressors for its potentially lethal consequences. Core temperature becomes further compromised during chronic exertional fatigue and sleep loss, inadequate nourishment, reduced tissue insulation, and a depressed shivering heat production.[143]

Water provides an excellent medium to study physiologic adjustment to cold because it conducts heat about 25 times faster than air at the same temperature. Consequently, immersion in cool water of only 28° to 30°C imposes a thermal stress that rapidly initiates an array of thermoregulatory adjustments. Persons frequently shiver if they remain inactive in a pool or ocean environment because of a large conductive heat loss to the water. Even when exercising at moderate intensity in cold water, exercise metabolism often generates insufficient heat to counter the large thermal drain. This becomes most notable during swimming because heat transfer by convection increases when water moves past the skin surface.

Light and moderate exercise in cold water produces higher oxygen consumptions and lower body temperatures than identical exercise in warmer water.[81,129,132] For example, swimming at a submaximal pace in a flume at 18°C (64°F) requires 500 mL of oxygen more per minute than swimming at the same speed in 26°C (79°F) water.[95] The additional oxygen consumption directly relates to the energy cost of shivering as the body combats heat loss in colder water. Shivering also serves an important role in recovering from hypothermia; it attenuates the typical postexercise decline in core temperature and facilitates core rewarming.[38] While the body shows remarkable flexibility in oxidative fuel selection during sustained cold exposure, a shift from lipid to carbohydrate metabolism occurs in shivering substrate with intense cold stress.[46]

Body Fat, Exercise, and Cold Stress

Differences in body fat content among individuals influence physiologic function in the cold during rest and exercise.[82,100,121] Successful ocean swimmers, usually possess a larger amount of subcutaneous fat than highly trained non-ocean swimmers. The additional fat increases the effective insulation in cold water when peripheral blood diverts from the body's shell to the core. With this advantage, athletes with greater thermal insulation from fat accretion swim in cool ocean water with almost no decline in core temperature. For leaner swimmers, exercise does not generate sufficient heat to offset heat drain to the water, and the body's core cools.

To a large extent, consider the stress from "cold" as highly relative. The physiologic strain from cold-water and cold-land environments depends not only on environmental temperature, but also on one's level of metabolism and body fat's resistance to heat flow. A person with excess body fat who rests comfortably immersed to the neck in 26°C water may sweat about the forehead during vigorous exercise. For this person, 18°C provides a more favorable water temperature for high-intensity exercise. For a lean person, on the

other hand, water at 18°C proves debilitating during rest and exercise. An optimum water temperature exists for each person and for each physical activity. For most persons, water temperatures between 26°C (78.8°F) and 30°C (86.0°F) allow effective heat dissipation in sustained exercise without compromising exercise capacity from large deviations in core temperature. Even colder water may optimize performance in shorter term, near-maximal exercise, particularly for fatter people. For some as yet unexplained reason, older adults do not withstand the challenge of cold during rest and low-intensity exercise as effectively as younger counterparts with similar aerobic capacities.[33] Age-related variations in body composition or hormonal functions may provide part of the explanation.

Children and Cold Stress

Cold water provides an exceptionally stressful thermoregulatory environment for children. A child's distinctly large ratio of body surface area-to-mass facilitates heat loss in a warm environment but becomes a liability during cold stress because body heat dissipates rapidly. During exercise in the less stressful cold-air environment, children rely on two mechanisms to compensate for their relatively large body surface: (1) augmented energy metabolism and (2) more effective peripheral vasoconstriction in the limbs.[126]

ACCLIMATIZATION TO COLD

Humans possess much less capacity for adaptation to long-term cold exposure than to prolonged heat exposure. Indeed, the basic response of Eskimos and Lapps involves avoiding the cold or minimizing its effects. To this end, their clothing provides a near-tropical microclimate; the temperature inside an igloo typically averages 21°C (70°F).

The Ama

Studies of the **Ama**, the women divers of Korea and southern Japan, indicate some human cold adaptation.[48] These women tolerate daily prolonged exposure to diving for food in cold water that in winter averages 10°C (50°F). During the summer when water temperature rises to 25°C, the Ama perform three bouts of diving, each 45 minutes long. In winter, they perform only one 15-minute dive daily. The women generally remain in the water until oral temperature declines to about 34°C (93.2°F). FIGURE 25.10A shows skin and core temperature responses of the Ama relative to time in the water. Mean skin and mean body temperatures always remained lower during the winter dives. Figure 25.10B shows the relationship between water temperature and coldest water temperatures when at least 50% of the Ama and nondiving Korean women and men started shivering. The response curve for the Ama (light blue) shifted to the right, clearly indicating a blunted thermogenic response (higher shivering threshold) until water temperature reached about 28°C. An elevated resting metabolism may contribute to how the Ama tolerate extreme cold. In winter, resting metabolic rate increased by about 25%

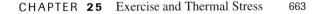

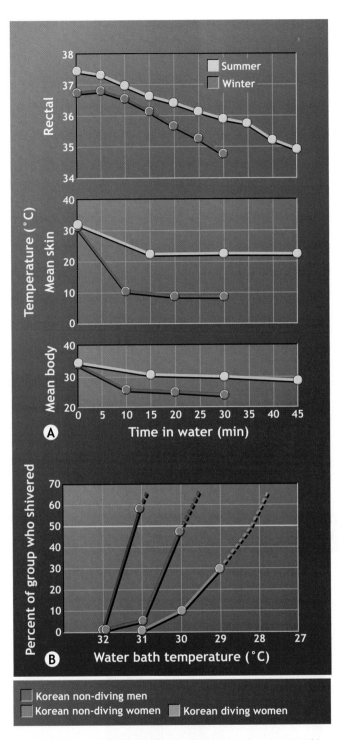

Figure 25.10 **A.** Differences in rectal temperature, mean skin temperature, and mean body temperature related to water temperature during summer and winter in Ama divers upon resurfacing from a dive. (Modified from Kang DH, et al. Energy metabolism and body temperature of the Ama. J Appl Physiol 1965;18:483.) **B.** Shivering response in professional Ama divers compared with nondiving Korean men and women at different immersion temperatures. The point where the lines cross the horizontal yellow line at 50 indicates the water temperature when 50% of a group began to shiver (Modified from Hong SK. Comparison of diving and nondiving women of Korea. Fed Proc 1963;22:831.)

compared with nondiving women from the same country. Interestingly, the Ama and nondiving female counterparts had equivalent body fat percentages. This suggests that circulatory adaptations aid the Ama by retarding heat transfer from the core to the skin during cold-water immersion.

Other Examples of Cold Adaptation

A type of general cold adaptation occurs with regular and prolonged cold-air exposure. As a result, heat production does not balance heat loss, and the person regulates at a lower core temperature during cold stress.[68,79] Some peripheral circulatory adaptations also reflect a form of acclimation with severe local cold exposure.[67,69] Repeated cold exposure of the hands or feet increases blood flow through these tissues during cold stress. This commonly occurs in fishermen who routinely handle nets and fish in cold water.[96] Local adaptations actually facilitate heat loss from the periphery but provide a self-defense because a vigorous circulation of warm blood in exposed tissue thwarts tissue damage from localized hypothermia. Long-term cold exposure may also blunt the typical depression of immune responses with acute cold stress.[63] Improved physical fitness as reflected by a high aerobic capacity and relatively large muscle mass enhances thermoregulatory defense against cold stress. This manifests itself in a larger shivering response and earlier (more sensitive) onset of shivering with cold exposure.[7]

INTEGRATIVE QUESTION

What information contributes to predicting an individual's survival time during extreme cold exposure?

HOW COLD IS TOO COLD?

Cold injuries from overexposure continue to rise because of increased participation by the general population in ice skating, ice fishing, cross-country skiing, snowboarding, snowmobiling, and all-season walking, hiking, jogging, and cycling. Pronounced peripheral vasoconstriction during severe cold exposure causes dangerously low skin and extremity temperatures, particularly when compounded by marked increases in convective and conductive heat loss. Predisposing factors to frostbite include alcohol use, low physical fitness, fatigue, dehydration, and poor peripheral circulation.[106] Early warning signs of cold injury include tingling and numbness in the fingers and toes or a burning sensation in the nose and ears. Overexposure from failure to heed these warning signs leads to frostbite; in the extreme, irreversible damage occurs that requires surgical removal of the damaged tissue. From military operations and occupational perspectives, application of external heat to the torso *during* cold exposure can overcome the local effects of environmental cold and maintain fingers and toes at a comfortable temperature for up to 3 hours with exposure to −15°C.[10]

In severe cold stress (e.g., near drowning in prolonged cold-water submersion), the brain experiences significant decrements in temperature, which reduce its oxygen needs. The central nervous system also benefits from a redistribution of blood from tissues that compromise their supply for relatively long periods. Other responses include potential benefits from the mammalian dive reflex (see Chapter 26, p. 676) and possibly cold-induced changes in neurotransmitter release.[37]

INTEGRATIVE QUESTION

Explain the greater likelihood for resuscitation and survival from cold-water drowning than from drowning in warmer water.

The Wind-Chill Temperature Index

One dilemma in evaluating the thermal quality of an environment relates to the inadequacy of ambient temperature alone to assess coldness. Many of us have experienced the chilling winds of a spring day even though air temperature remained well above freezing. In contrast, a calm subfreezing day may feel comfortable. *Wind creates the difference—air currents on a windy day magnify heat loss because the warmer insulating air layer surrounding the body continually exchanges with cooler ambient air.*

The **wind-chill temperature index**, presented in FIGURE 25.11 and used by the National Weather Service since 1973, was modified November 1, 2001. Based on advances in science, technology, and computer modeling, the revised for-

mula provides a more accurate, understandable, and useful way to understand the dangers from winter winds and freezing temperatures and provides frostbite threshold values.[87] For example, a 30°F ambient air reading is equivalent to 9°F with a wind speed of 25 mph, while a 10°F reading equals −11°F at the same wind velocity. If a person runs, skis, or skates into the wind the effective cooling increases directly with forward velocity. Thus, running at 8 mph into a 12-mph headwind creates the equivalent of a 20-mph wind speed. Conversely, running at 8 mph with a 12-mph wind at one's back creates a relative wind speed of only 4 mph. The *white zone in the left of the figure* denotes relatively little danger from cold injury for a properly clothed person. In contrast, the *yellow-, orange-, and red-shaded zones* indicate frostbite threshold values; the danger to exposed flesh increases, especially for the ears, nose, and fingers, when moving to the right of the chart. In the *red-shaded zone,* the equivalent wind-chill temperatures pose serious risk of exposed flesh freezing within minutes.

Respiratory Tract During Cold-Weather Exercise

Cold ambient air generally poses no special danger of damaging respiratory passages. Even in extreme cold, incoming air warms to between 26°C and 32°C as it reaches the bronchi, although values as low as 20°C have been observed with breathing large volumes of cold, dry air.[84] Warming an incoming breath of cold air greatly increases its capacity to hold moisture. Thus, humidification of inspired cold air

Temperature (°F)

Wind (mph) \ Calm	40	35	30	25	20	15	10	5	0	-5	-10	-15	-20	-25	-30	-35	-40	-45
5	36	31	25	19	13	7	1	-5	-11	-16	-22	-28	-34	-40	-46	-52	-57	-63
10	34	27	21	15	9	3	-4	-10	-16	-22	-28	-35	-41	-47	-53	-59	-66	-72
15	32	25	19	13	6	0	-7	-13	-19	-26	-32	-39	-45	-51	-58	-64	-71	-77
20	30	24	17	11	4	-2	-9	-15	-22	-29	-35	-42	-48	-55	-61	-68	-74	-81
25	29	23	16	9	3	-4	-11	-17	-24	-31	-37	-44	-51	-58	-64	-71	-78	-84
30	28	22	15	8	1	-5	-12	-19	-26	-33	-39	-46	-53	-60	-67	-73	-80	-87
35	28	21	14	7	0	-7	-14	-21	-27	-34	-41	-48	-55	-62	-69	-76	-82	-89
40	27	20	13	6	-1	-8	-15	-22	-29	-36	-43	-50	-57	-64	-71	-78	-84	-91
45	26	19	12	5	-2	-9	-16	-23	-30	-37	-44	-51	-58	-65	-72	-79	-86	-93
50	26	19	12	4	-3	-10	-17	-24	-31	-38	-45	-52	-60	-67	-74	-81	-88	-95
55	25	18	11	4	-3	-11	-18	-25	-32	39	-46	-54	-61	-68	-75	-82	-89	-97
60	25	17	10	3	-4	-11	-19	26	-33	-40	-48	-55	-62	-69	-76	-84	-91	-98

Wind Chill (°F) = 35.74 + 0.6215 T - 35.75 (V$^{0.16}$) + 0.4275 T (V$^{0.16}$)
Where, T = Air Temperature (°F); V = Wind Speed (mph)

■ Little Danger   Frostbite Times: ■ 30 minutes   ■ 10 minutes   ■ 5 minutes

Figure 25.11 The wind-chill temperature index.

causes considerable water and heat loss from the respiratory tract with large ventilatory volumes during exercise. Airway moisture loss during cold-weather exercise contributes to mouth dryness, a burning sensation in the throat, irritation of the respiratory passages, and general dehydration. Wearing a scarf or cellulose mask-type baklava that covers the nose and mouth and traps the water in exhaled air (and warms and moistens the next incoming breath) helps minimize uncomfortable respiratory symptoms.

Summary

1. Water conducts heat about 25 times faster than air; immersion in water of only 28 to 30°C provides considerable thermal stress that initiates rapid thermoregulatory adjustments.
2. Heat production from shivering and physical activity offsets heat flux to a cold environment. Shivering increases the metabolic rate by 3 to 6 METs.
3. Subcutaneous fat provides excellent insulation against cold stress. It greatly enhances the effectiveness of vasomotor adjustments so individuals with excess body fat to retain a large percentage of metabolic heat.
4. Individuals exhibit much less physiologic adaptation to chronic cold stress than to prolonged heat exposure. Wearing appropriate clothing enables humans to tolerate some of the coldest climates on Earth.
5. Ambient temperature and wind influence the coldness of an environment. The wind-chill index determines the wind's cooling effect on exposed tissue.
6. Considerable water loss occurs from the respiratory passages during exercise on a cold day, but inspired air temperature generally does not pose a danger to respiratory tract tissues.

References are available on the Student CD and online at http://connection.lww.com/mkk6e.

Sport Diving

26

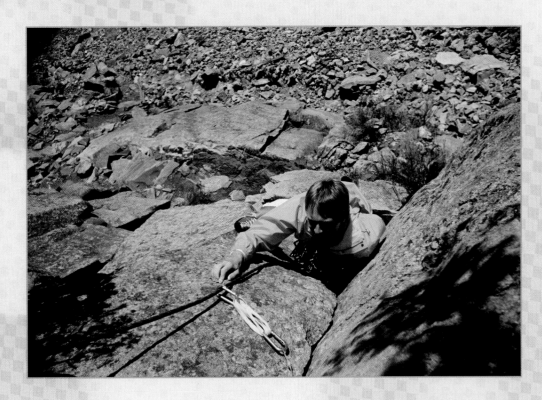

CHAPTER OBJECTIVES

- Outline the chronology of historical milestones in diving from antiquity to present

- Quantify, with examples, the relationship between depth under water and gas pressure and volume

- Discuss the rationale for snorkel size and underwater breathing depth

- Describe factors that limit the depth of a breath-hold dive

- Describe the effects of hyperventilation on breath-hold duration and potential risks before diving

- Outline evidence that supports a "diving reflex" in humans

- Describe open-circuit and closed-circuit scuba systems

- List causes, symptoms, and treatment of air embolism, lung burst, pneumothorax, mask squeeze, aerotitis, nitrogen narcosis, decompression sickness, and oxygen poisoning

- Discuss the decompression schedule for diving with compressed air in terms of its purpose and factors that influence it

- Outline the rationale for saturation diving, and describe the environment where the diver lives for prolonged dives to exceptional depths

- Give reasons for breathing helium–oxygen mixtures and discuss limitations to deep diving with these mixtures

- Describe the closed-circuit, mixed-gas system used by the U.S. Navy in technical diving

An estimated 5 million scuba divers work and recreate in the United States, with an additional 500,000 divers trained each year. Unquestionably, safe diving requires thorough knowledge of diving physics and physiology. We emphasize the relationships among diving depth, pressure, and gas volume and the potentially toxic effects of various gases breathed in diving.[4,21,22]

DIVING HISTORY—ANTIQUITY TO THE PRESENT

Men and women have practiced breath-hold diving for centuries as they hunted for sponges and food, salvaged artifacts and treasures, repaired ships, observed marine life, and participated in military maneuvers. The 5th century historian Herodotus tells of the underwater exploits of the Greek patriot Scyllias against the Persians. When Scyllias, taken as prisoner aboard ship, learned that Xerxes planned to attack a Greek flotilla, he escaped by jumping overboard. The Persians presumed he had drowned. To the contrary, Scyllias used a hollow reed as a snorkel and remained undiscovered, surfacing at night to cut each enemy ship loose from its moorings—saving the Greek Navy from sure disaster. Understandably, each dive could last only a few minutes until the discovery of how to remain underwater for longer durations. Using longer "snorkels" did not work because the diver could not inhale against water pressure at depths greater than several feet (see p. 673). Rebreathing from an air-filled bag submerged under water also failed because the buildup of exhaled carbon dioxide caused the diver to lose consciousness.

The first solutions to these problems took place in the 1530s with the invention of diving bells supplied with surface air. The bell, positioned a few feet from the surface, had its bottom open to water with its top portion containing air compressed by water pressure. A diver in the bell with his head surrounded by air could then hold his breath, swim from the bell for a minute or two and return for a short while, repeating the process until the air remaining in the bell became toxic.

In England and France in the 16th century, diving suits made of leather allowed descent to depths of 60 feet. Manual pumps delivered fresh air from the surface to the diver. Soon metal helmets could withstand greater water pressures, and divers could descend still further. By the 1830s, perfection of the surface-supplied air helmet allowed extensive underwater salvage work.

Starting in the 19th century, two main avenues of investigation—one scientific and the other technologic—accelerated underwater exploration. Two scientists, Paul Bert and John Scott Haldane, explained the physiologic effects of water pressure on body tissues and also defined safe limits for compressed air diving. Technologic improvements with compressed air pumps, carbon dioxide scrubbers, and demand-valve regulators allowed prolonged underwater explorations.

Chronology of Selected Events in Diving History

4500 BC: Archeologists unearth shells in Mesopotamia dated to this period that must have originated from the sea floor.

3200 BC: Archeologists discover mother-of-pearl (abalone) shell ornaments dated to this period from the Egyptian Theban VI dynasty.

2500 BC: Greek divers make sponges widely available in commerce; *The Iliad* and *The Odyssey* mention diving and sponges.

550 BC: Pearl diving documented in India and Ceylon.

500 BC: Scyllias demonstrates the practical use of breath-hold diving in military exploits against the Persian Navy.

100 BC: The Ama, Japan's women breath-hold divers of antiquity and modern times gather pearl oysters, shellfish, and edible seaweed.

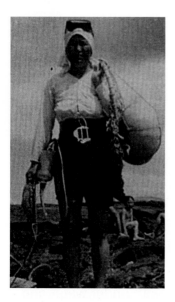

Ama diver.

1500: Da Vinci designs the first "snorkel" device and dive fins for the hands and feet.

1530: Invention of the first diving bell.

1650: First effective air pump developed by Von Guericke, which physicist Robert Boyle makes use of in compression and decompression experiments with animals.

1667: Robert Boyle makes first recorded observation of decompression sickness or "the bends" by documenting a gas bubble in the eye of a viper that had been compressed and then decompressed.

1690: Sir Edmund Halley (of comet fame) patents a practical diving bell (lead-coated wood with glass top to allow light to enter), 60 cubic feet (1.7 m^3) in volume and connected by a pipe to weighted barrels of air replenished from the surface, which permits dives to 60 feet for 90 minutes.

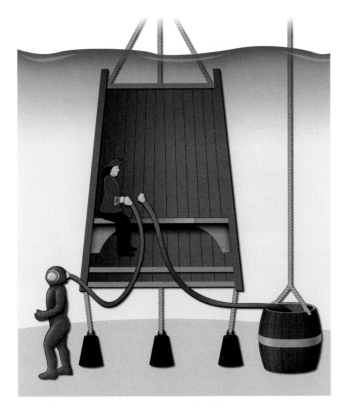

Halley's diving bell used weighted barrels of air to replenish the bell's atmosphere (late 17th century).

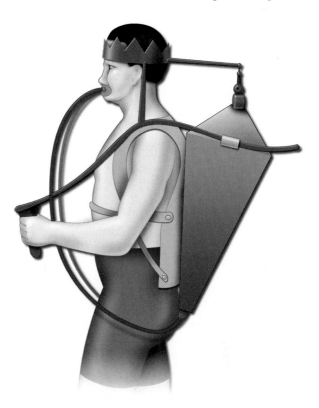

Triton diving apparatus invented by von Drieberg.

1715: John Lethbridge's constructs his "diving engine" built from an oak cylinder and supplied with compressed surface air. The diver remained submerged for 30 minutes at 60 feet while protruding his arms (sealed by greased leather cuffs) into the water for salvage work.

1776: First confirmed submarine battle; David Bushnell's American *Turtle* against the HMS *Eagle* (British) in New York harbor.

1788: John Smeaton's popular diving bell uses a hand pump to supply fresh surface air and a one-way valve to prevent air from returning to the pump when it stops.

1808: Freiderich von Drieberg invents a bellows-in-a-box device (named Triton) worn on the diver's back that delivers compressed air from the surface. The device never worked successfully, but nonetheless suggested compressed air could be used in diving, an idea conceived by Halley in the late 1690s.

1823: "Smoke helmet" patented by Charles Anthony Deane for fighting structural fires. Later modified for diving, the helmet fastened over the head with weights and received surface air through a hose. In 1828, Charles and his brother John market the helmet with a loosely attached "diving suit" so the diver could perform salvage work but only in the full vertical position to prevent water from entering the suit.

1825: First prototype for scuba invented by William James incorporates a cylindrical belt (air reservoir) around the diver's trunk that supplies air at 450 psi to a helmet by a

hand-operated valve and rubber tube. The diver inhales through the nose and exhales through a mouthpiece connected by a short tube to an escape valve in the helmets' crown. With the reservoir charged to 30 atmospheres, James believed a diver would have enough air to last 60 minutes.

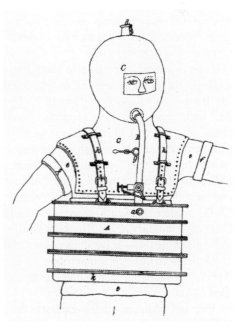

James's first practical self-contained diving apparatus, composed of a copper or leather helmet with a glass plate window attached to a waterproof tunic sealed at the waist and wrists by "elastic bandages."

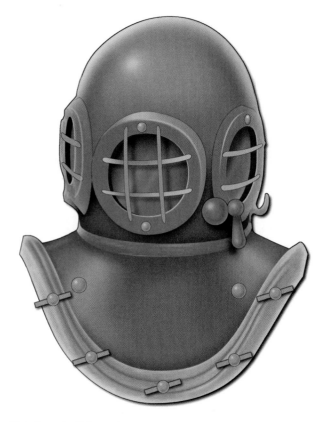

Siebe's early diving suit.

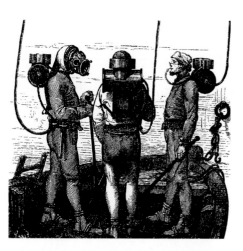

Aerophore SCUBA apparatus patented in 1865 by Benoit Rouquayrol and Auguste Denayrouse.

1837: Augustus Siebe, the father of diving, seals the Deane brothers' diving helmet to the waist-length jacket to create a full, watertight rubber suit that received surface air. This suit served as the forerunner for modern hardhat diving gear.

1839: Seibe's diving suit used during salvage of the British warship HMS *Royal George* sunk in 1782 to a depth of 65 feet; divers reported the first symptoms of decompression sickness.

1843: From experience salvaging the HMS *Royal George*, the British Royal Navy establishes the first diving school.

1865: Benoit Rouquayrol and Auguste Denayrouse patent their underwater breathing apparatus ("aerophore") that consisted of a steel tank of compressed air (250–350 psi) worn on the back connected through an automatic demand valve to a mouthpiece. This forerunner of modern scuba enabled the diver to disconnect from a tether that supplied surface air and swim freely with the tank for several minutes.

1873: Dr. Andrew H. Smith, surgeon to the New York Bridge Company (builders of the Brooklyn Bridge), reports about bends in workers who leave their pressurized caisson. Smith recommends chamber recompression for future projects but does not mention nitrogen bubbles as the cause of decompression sickness.

1878: First self-contained diving apparatus developed by Henry A. Fleuss uses compressed oxygen (not compressed air). Rope soaked in caustic potash absorbs carbon dioxide so the diver can rebreathe exhaled air without bubbles entering the water. The apparatus provides divers up to 3 hours of "bottom time."

1878: Paul Bert publishes *La Pression Barometrique,* which describes physiologic studies of pressure changes. Bert proves that nitrogen gas bubbles cause decompression sickness (the "bends" or caisson disease), gradual ascent prevents the problem, and recompression relieves pain.

1908: John Haldane, Arthur Boycott, and Guybon Damant publish "The Prevention of Compressed-Air Illness," a landmark paper that describes staged decompression to combat decompression sickness. Based on this work, the British Royal Navy and United States Navy develop diving tables for compressed air diving up to 200 feet deep.

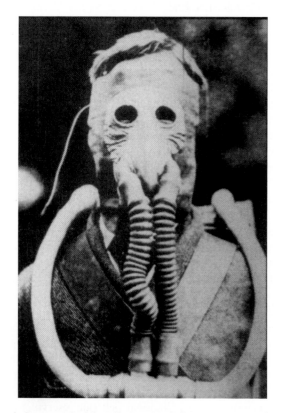

Fleuss's first practicable self-contained diving apparatus that employs the closed circuit principle.

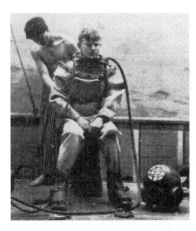

Deep sea pearl diver (circa 1896).

1912: Sir Robert Davis designs the first pressurized submersible decompression chamber.

1917: The U.S. Bureau of Construction and Repair first introduces the Mark V diving helmet, which revolutionizes salvage operations in World War II.

1920s: U.S. researchers experiment with helium–oxygen mixtures for deep dives.

1924: The U.S. Navy and Bureau of Mines conduct the first experiments with helium–oxygen mixtures.

1930: William Beebe and Otis Barton descend 1426 feet in a 4′9″ bathysphere attached to a barge by a steel cable.

1930s: Guy Gilpatric pioneers use of rubber goggles with glass lenses for skin diving. By the mid-1930s, face masks, fins, and snorkels are in common use.

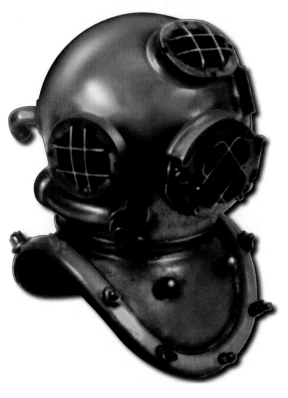

U.S. Navy Mark V diving helmet.

1933: French Navy captain Yves Le Prieur modifies the Rouquayrol-Denayrouse "aerophore" by combining a new demand valve with a 1500 psi high-pressure air tank without a regulator to eliminate restricting effects of hoses and lines. The diver breathes fresh air by opening a tap, while exhaled air escapes under the edge of the diver's mask.

1934: William Beebe and Otis Barton descend 3028 feet in a bathysphere near Bermuda, setting a depth record that remained until 1948.

1935: French navy adopts Le Prieur's scuba.

1936: Le Prieur establishes the world's first scuba diving club called the "Club of Divers and Underwater Life."

1938: Edgar End and Max Nohl make the first intentional saturation "dive" in a Milwaukee hospital hyperbaric chamber (27 h at a 101-ft depth). Decompression takes 5 hours, and Nohl suffers the bends.

1939: A new diving bell, the McCann-Erickson Rescue Chamber, makes the first successful rescue of men aboard the submarine USS *Squalus*, a new 310-foot submarine sunk in 243 feet of water in the North Atlantic. The chamber fits over the submarine's escape hatch, which four men at a time entered under one atmosphere of pressure.

1941–1944: Italian divers, working out of midget submarines during World War II, use closed-circuit scuba to place explosives under British naval and merchant marine vessels. The British adopt this technology to sink the German battleship *Tirpitz* on November 12, 1944 (www.bismarck-class.dk/tirpitz/tirpitz_menu.html).

1942–1943: Jacques-Yves Cousteau (French naval lieutenant) and Emile Gagnan (engineer for a Parisian natural gas company) redesign a car regulator to supply compressed air to a diver on initiation of a breathing cycle. They attach their new demand valve regulator to hoses, a mouthpiece, and a pair of compressed air tanks, which they patent as the AquaLung. Frederic Dumas descends to 210 feet in the Mediterranean Sea and experiences *l'ivresse des grandes profondeurs*—the rapture of the great depths. Cousteau achieves worldwide acclaim for his underwater explorations, movies, books, and dedication to environmental causes (www.cousteau.org/).

1947: Frederic Dumas uses the AquaLung and dives to 94 m (307 ft) in the Mediterranean Sea.

1948: Otis Barton descends in a modified bathysphere to 1370 m (4500 feet) off the coast of California.

1950s: Augus and Jaquet Picard develop the bathyscaphe (deep boat), a completely self-contained vessel. In 1954, the bathyscaphe sets a diving record of 4050 m (13,287 ft).

1959: The YMCA begins the first nationally organized course for scuba certification.

1960: Jacques Picard and Don Walsh descend to approximately 35,820 ft (10,916 m, 6.78 miles; water pressure 16,883 psi, temperature 37.4°F) in the August Picard-designed, Swiss-built, U.S. Navy-owned bathyscaphe *Trieste* to the bottom of the Mariana Trench (deepest known seafloor depression on Earth) in the Pacific Ocean.

1960s: As accident rates for scuba divers climb, the first national agencies form to train and certify divers; NAUI (National Association of Underwater Instructors) forms in

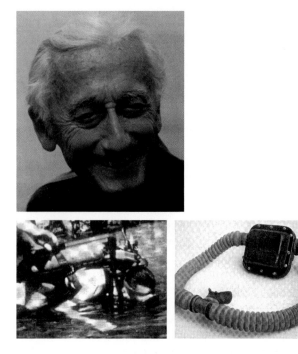

Top left. Captain Jacques Cousteau (1910–1997). *Bottom left.* First AquaLung dive in the Marne River. *Bottom right.* 1943 Cousteau-Gagnan regulator.

1960, and PADI (Professional Association of Diving Instructors) forms in 1966.

1962: Albert Falco and Claude Wesley spend 7 days under 10 m (33 ft) of water near Marseilles in an underwater-living habitat named *Diogenes*.

1963–1965: Divers live and work in underwater habitats for a month at a time at 60 m.

1968: John J. Gruener and R. Neal Watson dive to 133 m breathing compressed air.

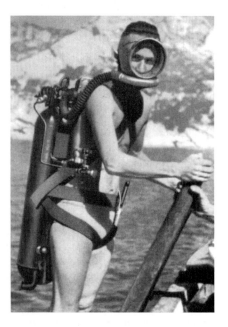

Dumas with the 1943 AquaLung Costeau-Gagnan unit. Note the waist level control valve.

1970s: Implementation of diving safety standards including the following: certification cards to indicate a minimum training level and as a requirement for tank refills, change from J-valve reserve systems to nonreserve K valves, adoption of submersible pressure gauges, and use of the buoyancy compensator and single-hose regulators.

1980: Divers Alert Network founded at Duke University as a nonprofit organization to promote safe diving.

1981: Record 686-m (2250-ft) "dive" is made in a Duke Medical Center chamber. Stephen Porter, Len Whitlock, and Erik Kramer live in the 8-foot chamber for 43 days, breathing a nitrogen, oxygen, and helium mixture.

1983: Introduction of the first commercially available dive computer (Orca Edge).

1985: Robert Ballard (*www.ife.org*) and Ralph White use a remote controlled camera to explore the wreck of the *Titanic* (12,500-ft or 3810-m depth).

1990s: Estimated 500,000 new scuba divers certified yearly in the United States as this activity's popularity increases for recreational and commercial purposes. Numerous scientific experiments using submersibles explore worldwide deep-diving sites in the Atlantic and Pacific oceans. The journeys include probing deep sea vulcanism, deep geology, and searching for artifacts from sunken vessels including the *Titanic* and two thousand-year-old shipwrecks in the Mediterranean Sea.

2003: Tanya Streeter, a world champion freediver, shattered the men's and women's variable ballast freediving world records by descending 400 feet (122 m in 3 min 38 s) to capture the variable ballast record (she becomes the first person to break all four deep freediving world records).

2004–2005: Expansion of technical diving by nonprofessionals who use mixed gases, new propulsion systems, full face masks, underwater voice communication, and digital cameras.

Loic Lefeme (France) sets the "no limits" free-diving record (maximum depth reached by a diver on a weighted sled before being pulled to the surface by a lift bag that the diver inflates at depth) of 171 m on October 30, 2004.

World records for the static apnea event (maximum time holding breath while submerged under water, usually face down) established by Tom Sietas (Germany; 8 min 58 s; December 12, 2004) and female Lotta Ericson (Sweden; 6 min 32 s; August 19, 2004).

PRESSURE–VOLUME RELATIONSHIPS AND DIVING DEPTH

Diving Depth and Pressure

Water remains essentially noncompressible owing to its high density. Consequently, its pressure against a diver's body increases directly with the depth of the dive. Two forces produce increased external pressure (**hyperbaria**) in diving: (1) weight of the column of water directly above the diver (hydrostatic pressure) and (2) weight of the atmosphere (*ata*, or *bar*) at the water's surface. TABLE 26.1 shows that a column of seawater exerts a force of 1 sea-level ata (760 mm Hg, or 14.7 lb per in² [*psi*]) for

TABLE 26.1 ■ RELATIONSHIP OF DEPTH IN WATER TO PRESSURE AND GAS VOLUME

DEPTH		PRESSURE		HYPOTHETICAL LUNG VOLUME	INSPIRED AIR (MM HG)	
FT	M	ATM	MM HG	ML	PO₂	PN₂
	Sea level	1	760	6000	159	600
33	10	2	1520	3000	318	1201
66	20	3	2280	2000	477	1802
99	30	4	3040	1500	636	2402
133	40	5	3800	1200	795	3003
166	50	6	4560	1000	954	3604
200	60	7	5320	857	1113	4204
300	90	10	7600	600	1590	6006
400	120	13	9880	461	2068	7808
500	150	16	12,160	375	2545	9610
600	180	19	14,440	316	3022	11,412

each 33-foot (10-m) descent below the water's surface. Because fresh water is less dense than sea water, a depth of approximately 34 feet corresponds to 1 ata in fresh-water diving. Thus, a dive to 33 feet in seawater exposes the diver to a pressure of 2 ata—1 ata from the weight of ambient air at the surface and the other from the weight of the column of water itself. Diving from sea level to 66 feet (20 m) exposes a diver to an absolute external pressure of 3 ata; the pressure is 4 ata at 99 feet (30 m), and so on. Clearly, considerable external pressure builds up when diving relatively short distances below the surface.

Water constitutes a large portion of the body's tissues so they too remain noncompressible and not particularly susceptible to increased external pressure during diving. The body also contains air-filled cavities—notably the lungs, respiratory passages, and sinus and middle ear spaces. Volume and pressure in these cavities change considerably with any increase or decrease in diving depth. Pain, injury, and even death occur unless adjustments *equalize* the rapid and large changes in pressure that occur in a hyperbaric environment.

Diving Depth and Gas Volume

Boyle's law states that at constant temperature, the volume of a given mass of gas varies inversely with its pressure. When pressure doubles, volume halves; conversely, reducing pressure by one half expands any gas volume to twice its previous size. FIGURE 26.1 (and Table 26.1) shows that if divers fill their lungs with 6 L of air at the surface and then descend to 10 m, the lung volume compresses to 3 L. Diving an additional 10 m to a depth of 20 m (external pressure now 3 ata) reduces the original 6-L lung volume by two thirds, to 2 L. At 91 m (300 ft), the lung volume compresses to 0.6 L, simply from the compressive force of water against the air-filled thoracic cavity. For most individuals, further increases in diving depth reduce the pulmonary air volume and seriously damage the chest wall and lung tissue. As the diver returns to the surface, the air volume reexpands to its *original*

6-L volume. For the scuba diver who breathes pressurized air beneath the water, a 6-L lung volume at a 10-m depth expands to 12 L at the water's surface; this 6-L volume at 50-m depth occupies 36 L at sea-level pressure. Failure to permit the "extra" air volume to escape through the nose or mouth during ascent ruptures lung tissue from the powerful force of expanding gases.

SNORKELING AND BREATH-HOLD DIVING

Swimming at the water's surface with fins, mask, and snorkel provides a common form of recreation and sport for spear fishing and exploring shallow areas of clear water. A J-shaped tube, or **snorkel**, allows the swimmer to breathe continually with the face immersed in water. The swimmer periodically takes a full breath of air and dives to explore beneath the water's surface. After about 30 seconds, the carbon dioxide level in arterial blood increases causing the diver to sense the need to breathe and surface quickly. Snorkeling is essentially an extension of swimming, limited entirely by the swimmer's breath-holding ability.

Limits to Snorkel Size

Novice skin divers often speculate that if only the snorkel were longer they could swim deeper in the water and still breathe ambient air through the top of the snorkel. Some neophytes believe they can sit at a pool bottom and breathe through a garden hose extending to the pool deck! The idea of a longer snorkel seems intriguing, but two factors limit snorkel length and volume:

1. Increased hydrostatic pressure on the chest cavity as one descends beneath the water
2. Increased pulmonary dead space by enlarging the snorkel's volume

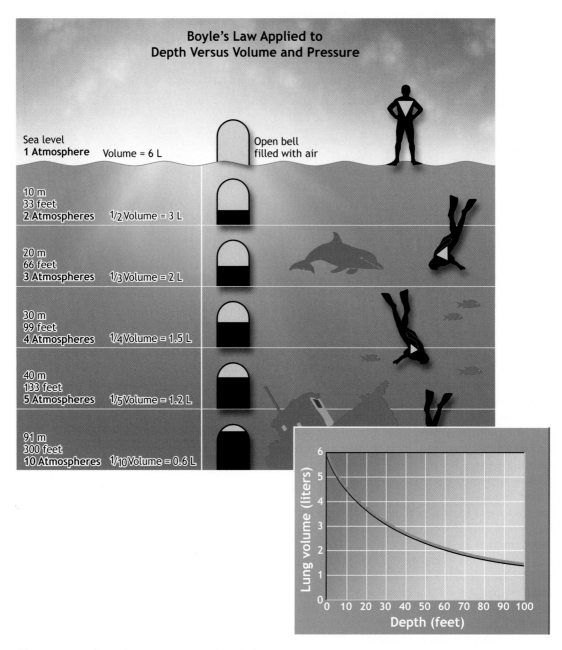

Figure 26.1 Gas volume varies inversely with the pressure acting upon it. A 6-L volume, whether in an open bell or in the flexible thoracic cavity, compresses to 3 L in 33 feet (10 m) of seawater (fsw) because of a doubling of the external water pressure. At 99 fsw, or 4 ata, the gas decreases to 25% of original volume, or 1.5 L. The *inset figure* graphically illustrates the curvilinear relation between lung volume at the surface and depth in seawater. The volume change per unit depth change is greatest nearest the water's surface.

Inspiratory Capacity and Diving Depth

When breathing through a snorkel, the diver inspires air at atmospheric pressure. At a depth of about 3 ft (1 m), the compressive force of water against the chest cavity becomes so large that the inspiratory muscles cannot overcome external pressure and expand thoracic dimensions. This makes inspiration impossible without external air at sufficient pressure to counter the compressive force of water at the particular depth. This reality forms the basis for scuba discussed on p. 676 of this chapter.

Snorkel Size and Pulmonary Dead Space

In Chapter 12 we explain that not all inspired air enters the alveoli. Approximately 150 mL of each breath fills the nose, mouth, and other nondiffusible portions of the respiratory tract. The snorkel, an extension of the airways, adds to the volume of the anatomic dead space. Consequently, the ideal snorkel averages about 15 inches (38 cm) in length, with an inside diameter of five-eighths to three-quarters of an inch to minimize the effects of added dead space and resistance to breathing.[24] Any further increase in snorkel size (volume) increases anatomic dead space volume, thus encroaching on alveolar ventilation.

Breath-Hold Diving

The duration of a breath-hold dive depends on two factors:

1. Breath-hold duration until arterial carbon dioxide pressure reaches the breath-hold breakpoint
2. Relationship between a diver's total lung capacity (TLC) and residual lung volume (RLV)

A full inspiration of ambient air causes 1 L of oxygen to move into the respiratory passages and lungs. Upon breath-hold, 650 mL of oxygen sustains metabolism before partial pressures of arterial oxygen (P_{O_2}) and carbon dioxide (P_{CO_2}) signal the need to renew breathing.[6] With some practice, most persons can breath-hold for up to 1 minute, and 2 minutes represents a typical upper limit. During this time, arterial P_{O_2} drops to 60 mm Hg, whereas P_{CO_2}, the most important factor controlling breath-holding, rises to 50 mm Hg, signaling an urgency to breathe. Physical activity greatly reduces breath-holding time because oxygen consumption and carbon dioxide production increase with exercise intensity.

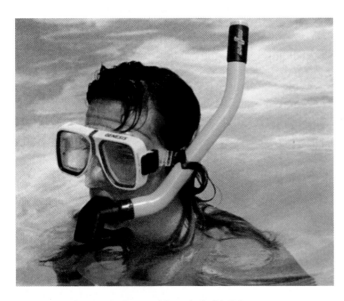

Basic tools for snorkeling and breath-hold diving.

Hyperventilation and Breath-Hold Diving: Blackout

Hyperventilation before breath-hold diving extends the breath-hold period; at the same time, the risk to the diver greatly increases. **Blackout**, a sudden loss of consciousness, poses a serious danger in skin diving; it usually afflicts divers who try to extend the dive's duration beyond reasonable limits. A critical reduction in arterial P_{O_2} causes blackout, a condition that contributes to a total relaxation of respiratory muscles.

The breakpoint for breath-holding corresponds to an increase in arterial P_{CO_2} to 50 mm Hg. Some persons can ignore this stimulus and continue breath-holding until arterial carbon dioxide reaches levels that cause severe disorientation and even blackout. When hyperventilation precedes breath-hold, arterial P_{CO_2} decreases from its normal value of 40 mm Hg to 15 mm Hg. Lowering the body's carbon dioxide content before the dive extends the breath-hold duration until arterial P_{CO_2} increases to a level that stimulates ventilation. For example, 313 seconds is the longest breath-hold recorded while breathing air without prior hyperventilation. Breath-holds of 15 to 20 minutes occur with hyperventilation followed by several deep breaths of pure oxygen.[13]

Combining hyperventilation, breath-holding, and exercise in the underwater environment poses serious risks. Consider the following scenario: A skin diver hyperventilates at the surface before a dive to reduce arterial P_{CO_2} to augment breath-hold duration. The diver now takes a full inhalation and descends beneath the water. Alveolar oxygen continually moves into the blood for delivery to active muscles. Owing to previous hyperventilation, arterial carbon dioxide levels remain low, freeing the diver from the urge to breathe. Concurrently, as the diver swims deeper, external water pressure compresses the thorax, increasing gas pressure within this cavity. Increased intrathoracic pressure maintains a relatively high alveolar P_{O_2}. Consequently, even though absolute alveolar oxygen quantity decreases as oxygen moves into the blood during the dive, P_{O_2} continually loads hemoglobin as the dive progresses. When the diver senses the need to breathe from carbon dioxide buildup and begins to ascend, reversals occur in intrathoracic pressure. As water pressure on the thorax decreases with ascent, lung volume expands and alveolar P_{O_2} decreases to a level where no gradient exists for oxygen diffusion into arterial blood. This places the diver in a hypoxic state. Near the surface, alveolar P_{O_2} reaches levels so low that dissolved oxygen diffuses *from* venous blood returning to the lungs and flows into the alveoli; this causes the diver to suddenly lose consciousness before surfacing.

Additional Considerations. Two responses provide additional risks from hyperventilation preceding a breath-hold dive.

1. A normal quantity of arterial carbon dioxide maintains the blood's acid–base balance, mediated by H^+ release as carbonic acid forms from the union of carbon dioxide and water. By reducing the blood's carbon dioxide content through hyperventilation, H^+ concentration decreases, thus increasing pH and alkalinity.
2. Normal arterial P_{CO_2} stimulates dilation of arterioles in the brain.[19] A decrease in arterial carbon dioxide with hyperventilation can reduce cerebral blood flow to produce dizziness or loss of consciousness.

Depth Limits with Breath-Hold Diving: Thoracic Squeeze

Progressing deeper beneath the water subjects the body's air cavities to tremendous compressive forces.

Generally, when the lung volume compresses below 1.5 to 1.0 L (i.e., to RLV), internal and external pressures fail to equalize and **lung squeeze** occurs. (The "In a Practical Sense" feature on p. 677 provides equations to estimate RLV from age, body mass, and stature.) Excessive hydrostatic pressure on pulmonary air volume causes extensive damage to pulmonary tissues.

Commercial breath-hold diving generally does not exceed depths of 100 fsw, and lung squeeze generally occurs at depths between 150 and 200 fsw. However, individuals show considerable variability in the safe depth for breath-hold diving without danger of lung squeeze. The world record for "no limits" breath-hold diving depth following a single breath of air is 492 fsw (150 m), a level about 20 yards above the typical cruising depth of nuclear submarines. Umberto Pelizzari (height 1.89 m; weight 84 kg; total lung capacity 7.9 L) achieved this remarkable physiologic feat in 1999. Estimates indicate that external water pressure against the diver's thoracic cavity at this depth would compress his chest girth from 50 inches to 20 inches. Wearing fins and a hooded wet suit, Pelizzari was lowered down a cable anchored to the ocean floor. At the desired depth, a balloonlike bag inflated that facilitated his ascent to the surface. The total round trip took about 2.5 minutes. Tanya Streeter redefined the limits of achievement in 2003 by setting the world accord for free breath-hold diving at 400 feet (122 m).

The ratio of the diver's TLC to RLV at the surface generally determines the critical diving depth before lung squeeze; this ratio typically averages 4:1 at the surface. For example, for a diver with a 6.0-L TLC and a 1.5-L RLV, Boyle's law predicts that TLC would compress to RLV at 30 m, or 4 ata external pressure. *No danger from lung squeeze exists if lung volume remains greater than RLV because sufficient air remains in the lungs and rigid respiratory passages to equalize pressure and prevent damage from compression.* If TLC during a dive decreases below RLV (i.e., if TLV:RLV falls below 1.00), pulmonary air pressure becomes less than the external water pressure. The unequalized pressure creates a relative vacuum within the lungs. In severe cases of lung squeeze, blood literally spurts from the pulmonary capillaries through the alveoli and into the lungs. In this situation, divers drown in their own blood. Further increases in depth cause compression fractures of the ribs as the chest cavity collapses from excessive external pressure.

In many instances, the ratio TLV:RLV at the surface considerably *underestimates* the actual impressive depths achieved by trained breath-hold divers. Part of the explanation may relate to a reduced RLV as immersion progresses because of a shift toward greater intrathoracic blood volume. Consequently, a smaller RLV underwater increases the TLV:RLV, allowing the individual to increase maximal depth before reaching the critical ratio.

Other Problems. If pressures within the internal air spaces do not continually equalize with external hydrostatic pressures, problems other than lung squeeze limit the depth of a breath-hold dive. For example, if air at ambient pressure remains trapped within the middle ear (from inflamed tissue or a mucous plug) and cannot equilibrate with air in the lungs, external hydrostatic pressure forces the eardrum inward and it ruptures. A ruptured eardrum frequently occurs at relatively shallow depths.

The sinus cavities also provide difficulty for skin divers. Air compressed in the lungs by the external force of water attempts to move into the paranasal sinuses. However, sinuses inflamed and irritated from infection provide extremely narrow openings that hinder sinus space equilibration with pressure changes in the respiratory tract. Failure to equilibrate creates a relative vacuum in the sinus cavities that distorts their tissues' shape and causes intense sinus pain. With severe disequilibrium, fluid and blood move into the sinuses to fill the vacuum.

A Diving Reflex in Humans?

Physiologic responses to immersion, collectively termed the **diving reflex**, enable diving mammals to spend considerable time under water. These responses include (1) bradycardia, (2) decreased cardiac output, (3) increased peripheral vasoconstriction, and (4) lactate accumulation in underperfused muscle. A modified diving response also has been described for humans during face immersion, breath-hold face immersion, and dives to modest depths.[1,8,10,15] The research has primarily documented increased vagal activity that induces bradycardia in humans during face immersion and diving, particularly in cool and cold water. Elevated blood lactate concentration during breath-hold dives to 65 m at energy expenditures only slightly above rest also suggests a diving-mediated peripheral vasoconstriction that decreases blood flow (oxygen supply) to skeletal muscles.[7]

More recent data have expanded the findings on blood lactate concentration to include hemodynamic aspects of breath-hold diving in thermoneutral and cool water by elite divers to depths of 40 to 55 m. FIGURE 26.2A illustrates the responses for one diver during descent to 40 m, bottom stay, and ascent (depth indicated by *green line*) in water at 25°C and 35°C. The electrocardiographic tracing (Fig. 26.2B) shows the longest R–R interval recorded during the cool-water dive. After an initial tachycardia, bradycardia rapidly ensued and became most pronounced in cool water where heart rate decreased to 16 b · min^{-1} near the bottom. Because stroke volume did not change appreciably during the dive, lower heart rates reduced cardiac output (*yellow line*). Output decreased to a low of 3 L · min^{-1} (25°C) compared with the value of 6.4 L · min^{-1} at the surface. A large number of diverse arrhythmic beats, often more frequent than true sinus beats, accompanied bradycardia, mainly in the cool-water dives. Arterial blood pressure increased suddenly and dramatically, reaching 280/200 and 290/150 mm Hg in two divers. This hypertensive response reflected overall peripheral vasoconstriction; the large increase in blood lactate concentrations reflected increased anaerobic metabolism.

Overall, the intense cardiovascular responses to breath-hold diving in elite divers resembles response patterns of diving mammals. The occurrence of arrhythmias and large increases in blood pressure probably reflects species differences and less perfect adaptation by humans.

SCUBA DIVING

The discussion of snorkeling emphasized that at depths below 1 m, inspiratory muscle power cannot overcome the compressive force of water against the thoracic cavity. Air under pressure from an external source to promote inspiratory action counteracts the external hydrostatic force. The **self-contained underwater breathing apparatus (scuba)**, principally developed in 1943 by French oceanographer Jacques-Yves Costeau (1910–1997) and Emile Gagnon (1915–2003),

---

IN A PRACTICAL SENSE

ESTIMATING RESIDUAL LUNG VOLUME FROM AGE, STATURE, AND BODY MASS

■ In breath-hold diving, RLV plays a significant role by affecting the depth a diver can achieve without danger of lung squeeze. In fact, the diver's TLC:RLV ratio at the surface generally determines the critical diving depth before lung squeeze.

Laboratory techniques of helium dilution, nitrogen washout, or oxygen dilution routinely measure RLV (see Chapter 12). Each procedure requires complicated and expensive laboratory equipment. An alternative but less valid approach estimates RLV with gender-specific prediction equations based on age, stature, and body mass. The standard error of estimate for predicting RLV ranges between 325 and 500 mL.

RLV PREDICTION EQUATIONS

Variables: age (y); St, stature (cm); BM, body mass (kg).

Normal-weight males

RLV (L) = (0.022 × Age) + (0.0198 × St)
          − (0.015 × BM) − 1.54

Normal-weight females (only age and stature used)

RLV (L) = (0.007 × Age) + (0.0268 × St) − 3.42

Overweight males (%fat 25) *and females* (%fat 30)

RLV (L) = (0.0167 × Age) + (0.0130 × BM)
          + (0.0185 × St) − 3.3413

EXAMPLES

1. Male: age, 21.0 y; body mass, 80 kg; stature, 182.9 cm
   RLV (L) = (0.022 × 21) + (0.0198 × 182.9)
             − (0.015 × 80) − 1.54

   = 0.462 + 3.621 − 1.2 − 1.54
   = 1.34 L

2. Female: age, 19 y; stature, 160.0 cm
   RLV (L) = (0.007 × 19) + (0.0268
             × 160.0) − 3.42
   = 0.133 + 4.288 − 3.42
   = 1.00 L

3. Overweight male: age, 35 y; body mass, 104 kg; stature, 179.5 cm
   RLV (L) = (0.0167 × 35) + (0.0130 × 104)
             + (0.0185 × 179.5) − 3.3413
   = 0.5845 + 1.352 + 3.321 − 3.3413
   = 1.39 L

Grimby G, Söderholm B. Spirometric studies in normal subjects, III: static lung volumes and maximum ventilatory ventilation in adults with a note on physical fitness. Acta Med Scand 1963;2:199.

Miller WCT, et al. Derivation of prediction equations for RV in overweight men and women. Med Sci Sports Exerc 1998;30:322.

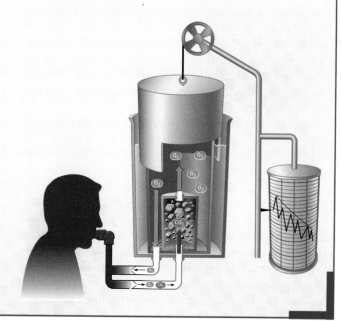

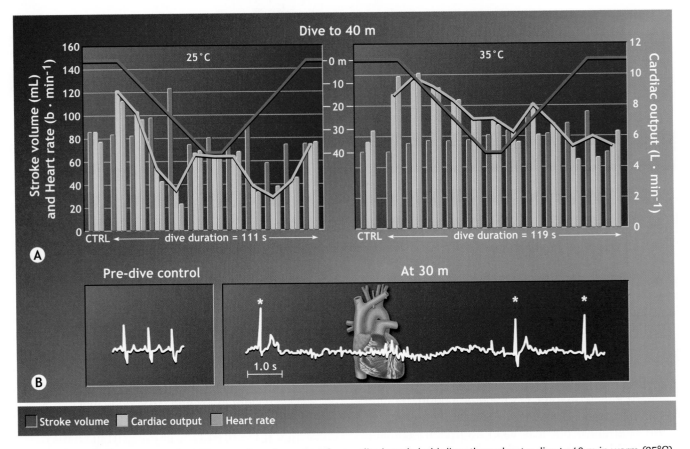

Figure 26.2   A. Heart rate, stroke volume, and cardiac output for an elite breath-hold diver throughout a dive to 40 m in warm (35°C) and cool (25°C) water. *Green line,* diving depth in relation to time; *yellow line,* cardiac output throughout the dive; *CTRL,* control measures prior to dive. **B.** Electrocardiographic tracing showing longest R-R interval during the dive in 25°C water. (*), QRS complex during the dive. (From Ferrigno M, et al. Cardiovascular changes during deep breath-hold dives in a pressure chamber. J Appl Physiol 1997;83:1282.)

is the most common apparatus to supply air under pressure for complete independence from the surface. *Sport divers should use only this form of scuba.* The scuba system, strapped to the diver's chest or back, includes a tank of compressed air and a demand regulator valve that delivers air the diver needs at a particular depth with hose and mouthpiece or full face mask. Two basic scuba designs exist: (1) the common **open-circuit system** and (2) the **closed-circuit system**, used primarily for clandestine military operations and special applications that require mixed gases.

Underwater commercial operations frequently apply surface-demand diving techniques in operations below a 50-m depth. This approach supplies air directly from a compressor at the surface to the diver via a direct reinforced hose. German inventor Augustus Siebe (1788–1872) provided the original design for this system in 1819; it consisted of a copper helmet (hard hat) riveted to a leather jacket, with air delivered continuously from the surface. The excess supplied air and the diver's expired air bubbled out from the bottom of the jacket. If the diver moved substantially from the vertical position, water would rush in through the bottom of the jacket and fill the headpiece. Siebe modified this design in 1840; he constructed a full waterproof diving suit bolted

to a breastplate and helmet that allowed a diver to work in any position because the suit encapsulated the entire body. Valves admitted air through the diver's helmet as needed, and expired air exited the helmet also through valves.[12] Siebe's "closed" diving helmet allowed divers to dive safely to depths previously impossible to attain.

Open-Circuit Scuba

FIGURE 26.3 illustrates the typical open-circuit scuba system for submerged swimming with neutral buoyancy in relatively shallow water. For most diving purposes, the steel or aluminum tanks (lightweight titanium that withstands high pressures also are used) contain 2000 L (70–80 ft³) of air compressed to about 3000 psi; deeper and longer exposures require 3500 L (120 ft³) of compressed air. One tank supplies enough air for a 0.5- to 1-hour dive to moderate depths. The start of inspiration creates a slight negative pressure. This opens the demand valve and releases air to the diver at a pressure nearly equal to the water's external pressure. The positive pressure created with exhalation closes the inspiratory valves and discharges the exhaled air into the water. The scuba gear contains gauges that continually monitor tank pressure and diving depth.

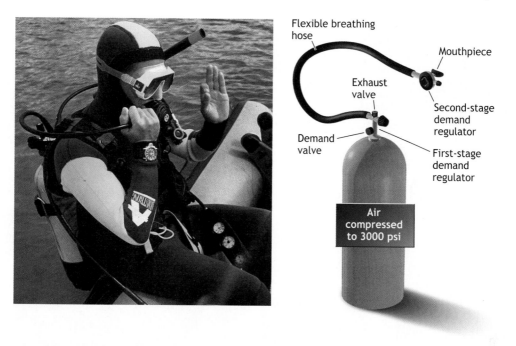

Figure 26.3 General design of an open-circuit scuba unit. Compressed air flows through a two-stage regulator valve that reduces tank pressure to a near-breathable pressure at a specific depth and releases air to the diver on demand at pressure equal to "ambient" so the diver breathes without difficulty.

Open-circuit scuba presents several drawbacks. The air exhaled into the water generally contains approximately 17% oxygen so the open-circuit system "wastes" about 75% of the total oxygen in the tank. In addition, the diver requires a considerable mass of air at increased depths to provide tidal volume for adequate pulmonary ventilation. As an extreme example, inhalation of a 5-L volume at 300 fsw (90 m) requires the equivalent of 50 L of air at sea level! This dramatic effect of pressure on air volume greatly limits the time one can remain at great depth before depleting the scuba tank's air. Factors that influence the energy cost of swimming under water (and thus pulmonary ventilation) include gender (lower in women than men), gear and number of tanks (25% higher with two tanks), fin type (flexible fin lower than rigid fin), and diver's experience (lower in advanced divers).[18] Diving tanks contain moisture-free compressed air, making each breath produce heat and moisture loss as the inspired air warms and humidifies on its passage down the respiratory tract. This causes substantial body heat loss during prolonged diving. To counter heat loss, the diver breathes a *heated* gas mixture of compressed helium-oxygen to avoid hypothermia during deep diving (see p. 687).

FIGURE 26.4 shows the theoretical air time limits for a diver who performs similar work at various underwater depths. These time limits assume a completely filled standard compressed air tank and ascent and descent at 60 feet per minute. For example, a single aluminum tank that contains 80 ft³ of air compressed to 3000 psi normally sustains an 80-minute dive near the surface. At a depth of 10 m, this tank supplies enough

air for about 40 minutes, whereas at 3 ata or 20 m, dive duration decreases by one third to 27 minutes. These time limits vary with the diver's body size, type and intensity of physical activity, fitness level, and diving experience, all of which affect exercise energy cost and ventilatory volumes.

The **wet suit**, the most common protective garment worn by recreational scuba divers and surfers, counters cold stress during

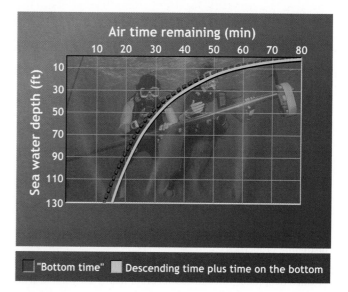

Figure 26.4 Theoretical air time for a single tank containing 80 ft³ of air. The *yellow line* includes the time spent descending (at a rate of 60 ft · min⁻¹) plus time on the bottom; *dashed line,* indicates only "bottom time."

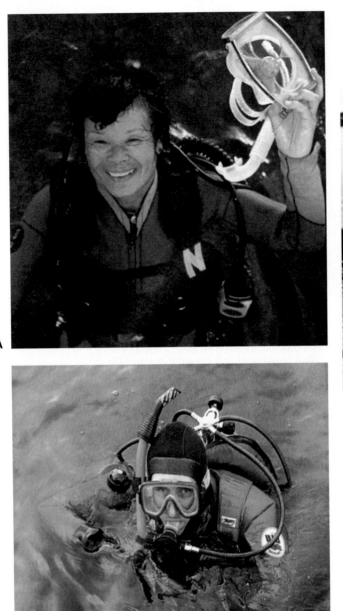

A

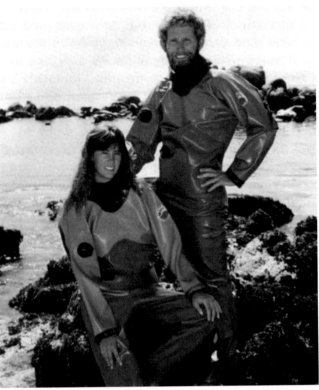

B

C

A. Wet suits are available in 3- to 9-mm thickness and a variety of styles. **B.** Dry suits are preferred for diving in colder water. **C.** A hood is important for cold-water diving because up to 50% of body heat escapes through the head.

diving. This garment, constructed of air-impregnated rubber (usually foam neoprene), traps water against the diver's skin, which warms to body temperature to provide the insulatory boundary. The suit, filled with thousands of tiny gas bubbles, provides insulation. Wet suits generally furnish sufficient thermal protection for relatively short dives, even in ice water. For longer dives in moderately cold water (17–18.5°C), a full wet suit offers insufficient thermal protection.[3] Compression of the wet suit as the diver descends progressively diminishes the suit's insulating properties.

The modern **dry suit**—made from foam neoprene, crushed neoprene, vulcanized rubber, or heavy-duty nylon with laminated waterproof materials, and often worn over insulating garments—maximizes protection from cold stress. This protective clothing ensemble keeps the diver dry, has seals at the neck, wrists, and ankles and a waterproof zipper to prevent water

from entering the suit. Dry-suit underwear traps a layer of air between the diver and the water for additional insulation. Layering of underwear adjusts insulation to water temperature.

Closed-Circuit Scuba

The need for shallow diving maneuvers during World War II produced a new diving form that used rebreathing of pure oxygen and absorption of carbon dioxide within a closed system. The closed-circuit underwater breathing apparatus operates similarly to the closed-circuit spirometer described in Chapter 8. A small cylinder feeds pure oxygen into a bellows or bag from which the diver breathes. The breathing bag acts as a pressure regulator. Valves in the breathing mask direct the exhaled gas through a carbon dioxide–absorbing canister that contains soda lime; the carbon dioxide–free gas then passes back to the diver. The oxygen cylinder replenishes the oxygen consumed in energy metabolism, allowing the diver to continually rebreathe oxygen, the only gas removed from the tank. Thus, only a small oxygen cylinder sustains the submerged diver for 3 hours or longer. Because no expired air releases into the water, the system provides a near-silent and bubble-free operation for clandestine activities. FIGURE 26.5 illustrates a closed-circuit scuba design currently used by the U.S. Navy that requires only a single bottle of compressed oxygen. The other type of closed-circuit system uses mixed gas: one bottle of pure oxygen and a second bottle of a mixed gas containing helium and oxygen (**Heliox**) or nitrogen and oxygen (**Nitrox**; see pp. 687–688).

The closed-circuit system requires a high level of proficiency for safe use. Two main problems exist with closed-circuit scuba. First, a serious medical emergency occurs if carbon dioxide output exceeds its rate of absorption or if absorption fails altogether. With a faulty rebreathing system, the diver may not receive warning symptoms and can drown from becoming anesthetized by arterial carbon dioxide buildup. Second, high concentrations of inspired oxygen, particularly when breathed under high pressures beneath the water, produce a variety of adverse effects on physiologic functions, particularly those related to the central nervous system. These problems remain minimal if the depth–time limits do not exceed the recommendations in TABLE 26.2 . Closed-circuit oxygen breathing generally should not exceed a maximum depth of 25 fsw and definitely should not exceed 50 fsw because oxygen poisoning produces high risk of central nervous system seizures. Minimal risk usually exists in military diving because most clandestine operations require swimming underwater in relatively shallow depths to avoid detection at night. Decompression sickness does not pose a problem because no inert gas absorption occurs when rebreathing pure oxygen. The increased resistance to breathing and the generally large dead space common with the closed-circuit system limit intense physical work.

TABLE 26.2 ■ U.S. NAVY–RECOMMENDED DEPTH–TIME LIMITS BREATHING PURE OXYGEN DURING WORKING DIVES[a]		
NORMAL OPERATIONS		
DEPTH		
(FT)	(M)	TIME (MIN)
10	3.0	240
15	4.6	150
20	6.1	150
25	7.6	75
EXCEPTIONAL OPERATIONS		
DEPTH		
(FT)	(M)	TIME (MIN)
30	9.2	45
35	10.7	20
40	12.2	10

[a]No symptoms of oxygen poisoning were noted at these depths and durations.

SPECIAL PROBLEMS WITH BREATHING GASES AT HIGH PRESSURES

Henry's law states that the quantity of gas dissolved in a liquid at a given temperature varies directly with the (1) pressure differential between the gas and the liquid and (2) gas solubility in the liquid. Underwater breathing systems must supply air, oxygen, or other gas mixtures at sufficient pressure to overcome the force of water against the diver's thorax. For example, at 3 ata (20-m depth) the respired gas requires delivery at approximately 2280 mm Hg (3×760 mm Hg), whereas gas delivery at 60 m requires a pressure of 5320 mm Hg. The following sections consider the specific dynamics of breathing gases at high pressures and their effects on physiologic functions. We also examine the physical responses of a gas to abrupt changes in pressure. FIGURE 26.6 summarizes the main hazards of scuba diving posed by improper equalization of pressure within the body's air spaces (and diving mask) to changes in external pressure.

Air Embolism

An air volume breathed underwater expands in direct proportion to the reduction in external pressure as the diver ascends to the surface. Air breathed at a depth of 10 m doubles in volume if brought to the surface. If normal breathing continues during ascent, the expanding air vents freely

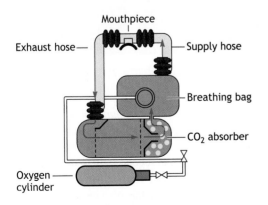

Figure 26.5 General design of a closed-circuit scuba system used by the U.S. Navy. A small cylinder of pure oxygen feeds into a bellows or bag from which the diver breathes. The breathing bag acts as a pressure regulator. Valves in the breathing mask direct the exhaled gas through a CO_2-absorbing canister containing soda lime; the CO_2-free gas then passes back to the diver. The oxygen cylinder replenishes oxygen consumed in metabolism. *Arrows* indicate direction of airflow.

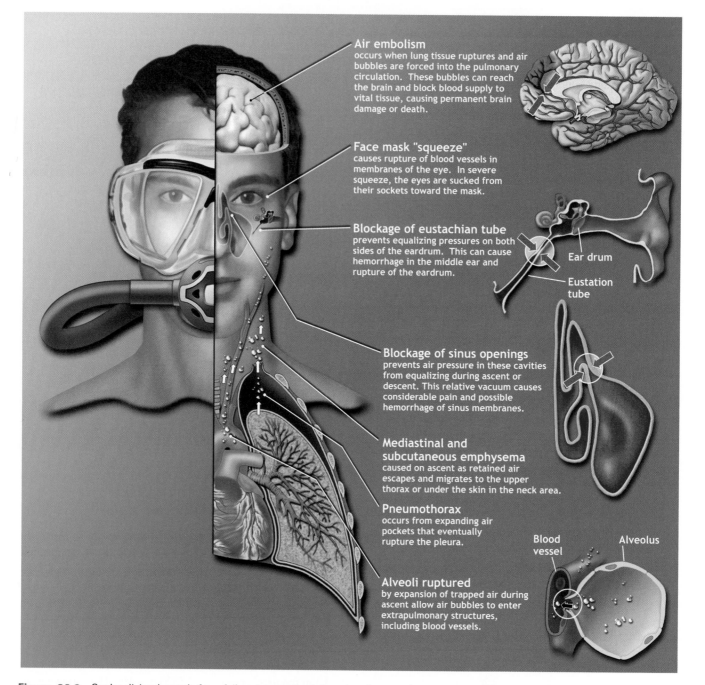

Figure 26.6 Scuba diving hazards from failure to equalize internal and external gas pressures.

through the nose and mouth. However, if a diver takes a full breath at 10 m but fails to exhale while ascending, the rapidly expanding gas eventually ruptures the lungs before the diver reaches the surface. **Lung burst** becomes a real possibility in scuba diving. Many inexperienced divers react to a perceived underwater danger by filling their lungs and then holding their breath while swimming rapidly to the surface. This particular diving hazard does not necessarily require a deep dive. Accidents caused by breath-hold ascent with scuba frequently occur in shallow dives; changes in pressure exert the greatest effect on the expanding lung volume near the water surface (see *inset box* in Fig. 26.1). *Inhaling a full breath of compressed air in 6 feet of water causes serious overdistension of lung tissue if the diver fails to exhale during ascent.* Fatal air embolism can occur in swimming pools as shallow as 8 feet for an inexperienced scuba diver. Air embolism from pulmonary barotrauma ranks second only to drowning as a cause of death among recreational scuba divers.

If expansion of air in the respiratory tract causes lung tissue to rupture during ascent from under water—from either breath-holding or pulmonary obstruction (bronchospasm, excessive pulmonary secretions, or bronchial inflammation)—air bubbles (**emboli**) enter the pulmonary venous system. Emboli then flow to the heart and enter the systemic circulation. Because the diver usually maintains a head-up, vertical position on ascent, the bubbles move upward in the body. Eventually, they lodge in the small arterioles or capillaries and restrict blood supply to vital tissue. General symptoms of air embolism include confusion, weakness, dizziness, and blurred vision. Severe blockage of pulmonary, coronary, and cerebral circulation causes collapse, unconsciousness, and frequently death. Effective treatment for air embolism requires rapid decompression to reduce bubble size and force them into solution to open the plugged vessels. Even with rapid, expert treatment, 16% of air embolism victims die.

Pneumothorax: Lung Collapse

Air forced through the alveoli when lung tissue ruptures sometimes migrates laterally to burst through the pleural sac that covers the lungs. In about 10% of cases of this form of pulmonary barotrauma, an air pocket forms in the chest cavity outside the lungs, between the chest wall and lung itself. Continued expansion of trapped air during ascent collapses the ruptured lung (**pneumothorax**). Pneumothorax treatment often requires surgical intervention with a syringe to extract the air pocket.

To eliminate the danger of air embolism and pneumothorax, instructors teach divers to ascend slowly and breathe normally when using scuba gear. The diver's lungs must remain free from any disease that could lead to air trapping (e.g., chronic obstructive pulmonary disease). Air trapping creates difficulty equalizing alveolar pressure and external pressure during ascent.

Mask Squeeze

Air in a facemask or goggles before a dive equals ambient air pressure at the surface. As the diver progresses deeper, a considerable pressure differential develops between the inside and outside of the mask to create a relative vacuum within the mask. For example, wearing swimming goggles to improve vision and protect the eyes from irritants during a dive beneath the water can cause the eyes to bulge or squeeze from their sockets. This leads to capillary rupture and hemorrhage of the eyes and surrounding soft tissue. The squeeze effect occurs because most goggles are constructed from rigid materials. Consequently, displacement of the eye and surrounding soft tissue into the air space between the eye and the goggles provides the only means to equalize the difference in air pressure between the goggle space and external water pressure during breath-hold diving. As newer pools with separate diving areas reach depths of 14 feet (4.3 m), goggles pose a distinct risk to swimmers who dive to this depth.

Breath-hold diving with a facemask that covers the eyes and nose represents a somewhat different situation than diving with only swim goggles. Air pressure within the mask that covers the eyes and nose readily equalizes to external water pressure as air flows freely between the nasal passages and the lungs' relatively large air volume. In breath-hold diving, air in the lungs compresses and passes through the nose to equalize mask pressure. With scuba, inspired air automatically adjusts to the external water pressure. Therefore, periodically exhaling through the nose into the mask balances pressures on both sides of the face mask.

Aerotitis: Middle-Ear Squeeze

Divers often encounter problems equalizing pressure within the air space of the eustachian tubes, the passages that connect the middle ear with the back of the throat.[26] These relatively narrow, mucus-lined channels generally resist air flow. In healthy individuals, the tubes remain clear enough so that changes in external pressure against the eardrum equalize by pressure changes transmitted from the lungs through the eustachian tubes. In skin and scuba diving (and air travel in nonpressurized aircraft), middle-ear pressure equalizes with external pressure by blowing gently against closed nostrils. Swallowing, yawning, or moving the jaws from side to side also helps to "pop" the ears.

In upper-respiratory tract infection, the eustachian tube membranes swell and produce mucus that can plug cranial air passages. The greatest difficulty involves equalizing middle-ear pressure during descent because an equal force from the ear canal does not readily match the pressure change against the eardrum's outer surface. The magnitude of pressure changes in diving considerably exceed those experienced in air travel. Divers can suffer severe pain only a few feet under water because the eardrum stretches and moves inward toward the plugged canal. Further pressure disequilibrium creates a relative vacuum in the middle ear that hemorrhages tissues. Complete blockage of the eustachian tubes can rupture the eardrum, forcing water into the middle ear as pressure equalizes.

Never Use Earplugs. *Never wear earplugs while diving.* During a dive, the external water pressure pushes the earplug deep into the external ear canal. A pocket of ambient air trapped between the plug and eardrum can rupture the eardrum outward during descent.

Aerosinusitis

Inflamed, congested sinuses prevent air pressure in these cavities from equalizing during diving. Sinus air pressure that does not equalize during descent remains at atmospheric pressure while external pressure increases. This relative vacuum creates "sinus squeeze," causing sinus membranes to bleed as blood occupies the space to equalize the pressure differential.[17]

Nitrogen Narcosis: Rapture of the Deep

The total pressure of the respired gas during diving increases in direct proportion to diving depth. Likewise, the partial pressure of each gas in the breathing mixture increases so at 10 m the nitrogen partial pressure doubles the sea-level value to 1200 mm Hg. With each additional 10-m depth, nitrogen partial pressure increases by 600 mm Hg—inspired P_{N_2}

equals 4200 mm Hg at a 60-m depth. At each successive depth, the gradient increases for the net flow of nitrogen across the alveolar membrane into the blood and eventually into all tissue fluids for equilibration. At 20 m, all tissues eventually contain three times as much nitrogen as before the dive. Tissue perfusion, tissue solubility coefficients, body composition, and temperature all influence nitrogen uptake at the tissue level.

Three-hundred fsw generally sets the limit for compressed air diving because dissolved nitrogen accumulation in the body's fluids and tissues renders all but the most experienced divers incapable of accomplishing meaningful work. The U.S. Navy sets the maximum operating depth at 190 fsw for breathing compressed air. In 1935, Dr. Albert Behnke (see Chapter 28) and coworkers demonstrated that the increase in inspired nitrogen pressure while breathing compressed air during diving produced the narcotic effect. An increase in the pressure and quantity of dissolved nitrogen causes physical and mental changes characterized by a general state of euphoria similar to alcohol intoxication termed **rapture of the deep**. Dissolved nitrogen at a depth of 30 m produces effects similar to those felt after consuming alcohol on an empty stomach. Divers often speak of "Martini's Law." This well-known dictum states that every 50 feet of seawater produces effects equal to 1 dry martini on an empty stomach. As a rough estimate, this would mean a diver at 200 feet experiences intoxication from pressurized nitrogen equal to 4 martinis! Eventually, high nitrogen levels produce a numbing, anesthetic effect on the central nervous system. The term **nitrogen narcosis** or "inert gas narcosis" collectively describes these mimicking effects of intoxication. The term was first coined in Jacques Cousteau's 1940s book, *The Silent World*. Cousteau's partner Frederic Dumas was diving to about 240 feet in the Mediterranean Sea. The following quote from Dumas was the first widely read description of the intoxicating effect of breathing nitrogen under pressure.

> I'm anxious about that line, but I really feel wonderful. I have a queer feeling of the beatitude. I am drunk and carefree. My ears buzz and my mouth tastes bitter. The current staggers me as though I had to many drinks. I [have] forgotten Jacques and the people in the boats. My eyes are tired. I lower on down, trying to think about the bottom, but I can't. I'm going to sleep, but I can't fall asleep in such dizziness.

At the extreme, mental processes deteriorate so that a diver may feel that the scuba serves little purpose and remove it and swim deeper instead of toward the surface.

Nitrogen diffuses slowly into body tissues so the narcosis effect depends on dive depth and duration. Considerable individual variation exists for nitrogen sensitivity, but a mild narcosis usually appears after an hour or more at 30 to 40 m—the maximum recommended depth for recreational scuba divers. Treatment requires that the diver ascend to a shallower depth, where complete recovery usually occurs rapidly.[24] The precise role of body fatness in nitrogen narcosis remains controversial.

Decompression Sickness

With rapid ascent, the external pressure against the diver's body decreases dramatically. Excess dissolved nitrogen in the body tissues begins to separate from the dissolved state; it eventually forms bubbles in the tissues, an effect not unlike the appearance of carbon dioxide bubbles when removing the cap from a carbonated beverage bottle. With the cap in place, the gas remains dissolved under pressure. Removing the cap suddenly reduces pressure above the fluid, causing bubbles to form. **Decompression sickness** *occurs when dissolved nitrogen moves out of solution and forms bubbles in body tissues and fluids.* It results from ascending to the surface too rapidly following a deep, prolonged dive, often made possible with double and triple air tanks. Nitrogen reaches equilibrium slowly in many tissues, particularly fatty tissues, so it leaves the body slowly.[11,28] This means that women (with a greater average percentage body fat than men) and obese men face greater risk for decompression sickness. FIGURE 26.7 compares nitrogen elimination after a simulated "dive" by two dogs that differed in fat content. The relatively fat dog eliminated considerably more nitrogen over the 4-hour decompression than the leaner dog.

The term *bends,* a synonym for decompression sickness, was coined during construction of piers for the Brooklyn Bridge (1869–1883) to reflect the bent-over position of limping workers who emerged from the caisson. The following poignantly describes the time course and fatal consequences of decompression sickness in an early history of this malady:[27]

> In 1900, for example, a Royal Navy diver descended to 150 fsw in 40 minutes, spent 40 minutes at depth searching for a torpedo, and ascended to the surface in 20 minutes without apparent difficulty. Ten minutes later, he complained of

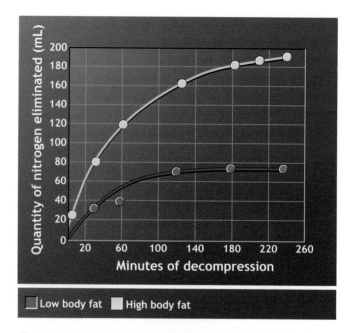

Low body fat   High body fat

Figure 26.7 Nitrogen elimination from body tissues of a relatively lean dog and one higher in body fat during decompression in a chamber. (Courtesy of Dr. A. R. Behnke.)

abdominal pain and fainted. His breathing was labored, he was cyanotic, and he died after 7 minutes. An autopsy the next day revealed the organs to be healthy, but gas was present in the liver, spleen, heart, cardiac veins, venous, subcutaneous, and cerebral veins and ventricles.

Nitrogen Elimination: Zero Decompression Limits

Diving at a depth of 30 m for up to 30 minutes represents the time limit before sufficient nitrogen dissolves to pose danger from decompression sickness. About 18 minutes is the limit at 40 m, and one can spend almost an hour at 20 m without danger from decompression sickness. If a diver exceeds the depth–duration recommendations for compressed air diving shown in FIGURE 26.8, the ascent to the surface must progress in a preestablished manner. With this approach, a recreational or commercial diver ascends at a prescribed, relatively slow rate designed not to require stops. This rate of ascent enables all excess dissolved nitrogen to diffuse from the tissues into the blood and escape through the lungs without bubbles forming.[24,28] **Stage decompression** requires the diver to make one or more stops on ascent to the surface. The time required for the slowest tissue compartment to lose sufficient nitrogen to allow ascent to the next depth determines the duration of such pauses (termed *stage-decompression stops*). For example, a dive to 30 m for 50 minutes requires one 2-minute decompression stop at 6 m (20 ft) and a 24-minute stop at 3 m (10 ft). Surface stage decompression involves transfer of the diver from the water (after several in-water stops) to a decompression chamber at the surface. The judicious use of a hyperoxic breathing mixture facilitates recompression.

A conservative approach recommends that the sport diver not exceed a 20- to 25-m depth (30-m maximum). During single or repetitive dives the diver should never approach the time limits indicated by the decompression tables. The recommendations in Figure 26.8 assume a *single* dive, with a minimum of 12 hours between dives. For repeated dives within 12 hours, the diver must consult the appropriate repetitive dive decompression schedules.[24] These recommendations account for the residual nitrogen remaining in the body at the start of the next dive if it occurs within the 12-hour period. Interestingly, air travel within 24 hours of scuba diving increases risk of decompression sickness because commercial airlines usually pressurize cabins to an equivalent altitude of 7000 feet. This further reduction in ambient atmospheric pressure may initiate bubble formation from excess nitrogen dissolved in body tissues during the prior preflight dive(s).

Consequences of Inadequate Decompression

Bubbles within the vascular circuit initiate complications from decompression injury. With the exception of bubbles in central nervous tissue that cause lesions in the brain and spinal cord and damage intravertebral disks, the primary bubbles form in the venous and arterial vascular bed. Symptoms of decompression sickness usually appear within 4 to 6 hours following a dive. Severe violation of decompression procedures (e.g., diver runs out of air and ascends too rapidly) initiates symptoms immediately; these symptoms progress to paralysis within minutes. Indications of inadequate decompression include dizziness, itchy skin, and aching pain in the legs and arms, particularly in tight tissues such as ligaments and tendons (the classic and most common characteristic). The degree of injury depends on the size of the bubbles and where they form. Bubbles in the lungs cause choking and asphyxia, whereas bubbles in the brain and coronary arteries block blood flow and deprive these vital tissues of oxygen and nutrients to produce cellular damage and death. Central nervous system bends occurs with some frequency; failure to provide immediate treatment leads to permanent neural damage.

Treatment for the bends involves lengthy recompression in a **hyperbaric chamber**. This specialized device elevates external pressure to force nitrogen gas back into solution. Gradual decompression then follows to provide time for the expanding gas to leave the body as the diver returns to the "surface." Immediate recompression offers the best chance for success; any delay decreases the prognosis for complete recovery. FIGURE 26.9 shows a collapsible, lightweight, transportable chamber for rapid deployment during transport of the diver to an appropriate facility to treat decompression accidents. The chances are slim for a sport diver to have ready access to such a recompression chamber. This makes it imperative that divers adhere strictly to recommendations for diving depth and duration.

Higher Prevalence with a Patent Foramen Ovale.

Decompression sickness sometimes occurs after uneventful dives, without any reported errors in recommended decompression procedures. Divers with lesions localized in the high cervical spinal cord and brain areas show a higher prevalence

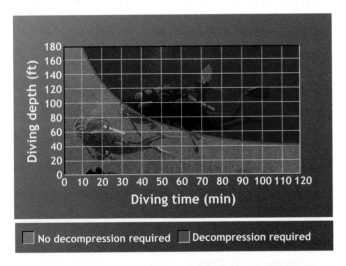

■ No decompression required ■ Decompression required

Figure 26.8 Zero decompression limits. Any single dive that falls on the left side of the curve requires no decompression provided the rate of ascent does not exceed 60 ft per minute (m = ft × 0.34048). Dives on the right side of the line require the decompression period specified in standard decompression tables.[25]

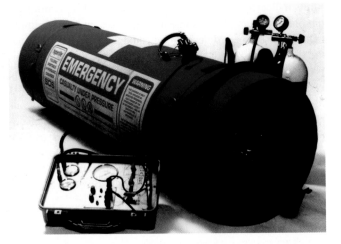

Figure 26.9   Portable, collapsible recompression chamber (50 kg) for diving in remote locations. A compressed air cylinder provides a working pressure differential of 2.1 ata (bars), or 70 fsw, between the chamber environment and ambient conditions; the diver receives oxygen via a breathing mask. The tube is constructed from para-aramid fiber (like Kevlar) in a matrix of silicone rubber. This provides flexibility (can fold when not in use) and considerable strength under pressure (burst pressure approximately 14 ata differential pressure). (Manufactured by SOS Limited, London, England; photo courtesy of John Selby.)

of patent foramen ovale (PFO) of the myocardium than divers who experience decompression sickness that localizes in the lower spinal cord.[9] PFO consists of an interatrial septum channel that forms a functional valve between the right and left atria. This channel could cause localized decompression sickness because nitrogen bubbles that the pulmonary vasculature normally filters pass through the PFO into the arterial circulation. The bubbles then migrate preferentially into the carotid and/or vertebral arteries. Divers with unexplained decompression sickness but with symptoms suggesting cerebral or high spinal localization should receive evaluation for PFO.

Oxygen Poisoning

Inspiring a gas with a P_{O_2} above 2 ata (1520 mm Hg) greatly increases a diver's susceptibility to **oxygen poisoning**, particularly at elevated metabolic rates during physical activity.[2] For this reason, closed-circuit scuba that uses pure oxygen severely restricts both diving depth and duration (TABLE 26.3). At depths greater than 25 fsw (7.6 m), the diver should *not* rebreathe pure oxygen except in extraordinary circumstances. A decreased vital capacity strongly indicates impaired pulmonary function under hyperoxic conditions.[5]

Breathing high pressures of oxygen negatively affects bodily functions in three ways:

1. Irritates respiratory passages and eventually induces bronchopneumonia if exposure persists
2. Constricts cerebral blood vessels at pressures above 2 ata and alters central nervous system function
3. Depresses carbon dioxide elimination

DEPTH (FSW)	MAXIMUM TIME (MIN)
25	240
30	80
35	25
40	15
50	10

TABLE 26.3 ■ REPRESENTATIVE DEPTH–TIME LIMITS FOR CLOSED-CIRCUIT DIVING WITH 100% OXYGEN

Adapted from United States Navy diving manual, vol 2. Mixed gas diving, rev 3. NAVSEA publ 0994 LP-001-9020. May 1991.

For carbon dioxide elimination, an elevated inspired P_{O_2} may force sufficient oxygen into solution in the plasma to supply the diver's metabolic needs. As such, oxygen remains combined with hemoglobin (oxyhemoglobin) as blood returns to the pulmonary capillaries. This causes carbon dioxide buildup because deoxygenated hemoglobin normally transports considerable carbon dioxide as carboaminohemoglobin from the tissues (see Chapter 13). Treatment for oxygen poisoning consists of breathing air at sea-level pressure.

Carbon Monoxide Poisoning

Potentially lethal carbon monoxide gas combines some 200 times more readily with hemoglobin than does oxygen. Consequently, only a small quantity of carbon monoxide in the inspired mixture induces tissue hypoxia. Carbon monoxide poisoning is of concern during deep dives because the partial pressures of all gases in the breathing mixture (including impurities) increase greatly.

Urban areas are likely candidates for high levels of contaminants from automotive and industrial exhausts, including carbon monoxide and oxides of sulfur. One should never fill a scuba tank during air pollution or "unhealthy air" alerts. Aside from the contaminants present in ambient air, operating gasoline or diesel engine compressors contributes additional carbon monoxide and oil impurities. Placing the compressor's engine exhaust downstream from the air intake eliminates this potential source of contamination. The antidote for carbon monoxide poisoning requires immediate breathing of hyperbaric oxygen. High pressures of inspired oxygen hasten dissociation of carbon monoxide from the hemoglobin molecule.

Are Women at Risk?

About 35% of recreational scuba divers in the United States are women. They do not experience a greater risk than men of equivalent physical fitness for decompression sickness, nitrogen narcosis, oxygen toxicity, air embolism, or diving accidents. Little research has assessed the risks of open-circuit scuba diving to the fetus during pregnancy. Prudent guidelines recommend that pregnant women *refrain* from scuba diving during pregnancy to eliminate risk of fetal injury from maternal breathing of compressed air at elevated pressures.[23]

DIVES TO EXCEPTIONAL DEPTHS: MIXED-GAS DIVING

Commercial, military, scientific, rescue, and technical divers often descend to depths in excess of 160 fsw. Recall that at depths greater than 60 fsw, diving with compressed air and saturation diving (see p. 685) increase risk of oxygen toxicity. Diving lower than this depth requires breathing compressed mixed gases (nonair) with a lower P_{O_2} (FIG. 26.10). Oxygen always exists in the breathing mixture in mixed-gas diving, but it represents only a small fraction of the mix in dives to extreme depths. Precise management of oxygen concentrations becomes a primary consideration in **mixed-gas diving**.

Helium–Oxygen Mixtures

Helium, the second lightest known element, is the most common inert gas substituted for nitrogen in deep diving. Helium is colorless, odorless, tasteless, nonexplosive, and relatively nontoxic and does not induce narcosis at any inspired pressure.[20]

Helium in the breathing mixture in diving came into its own during the 1939 rescue of remaining crew members and salvage of the submarine *Squalus* that sank in 75 m of water off Portsmouth, New Hampshire. For these purposes, a compressor at the water's surface continually supplied the divers with a helium-oxygen (**Heliox**) mixture. Because of helium's low density, breathing Heliox mixtures reduces the typically increased breathing resistance imposed by nitrogen.

During rapid descent to depths in excess of 300 fsw up to 2280 fsw, divers can experience potentially incapacitating nausea, muscle tremors, and other central nervous effects. This phenomenon was first noted in the 1960s and termed **high-pressure nervous syndrome** (**HPNS**) or initially as helium tremors. The condition probably results from the direct effects

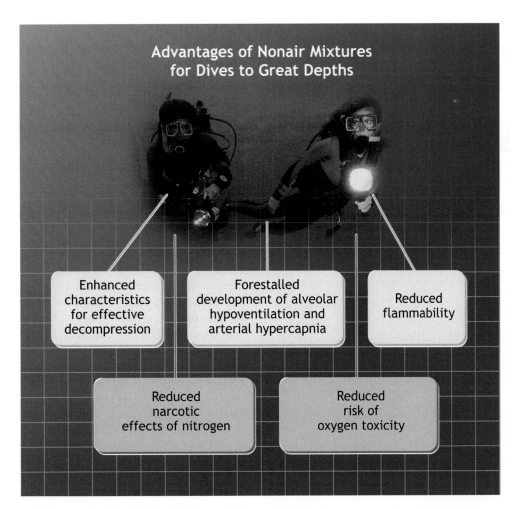

Figure 26.10 Rationale for breathing gas mixtures other than compressed air when diving to great depths. Avoidance of nitrogen narcosis and oxygen poisoning are the *overwhelming* reasons for breathing nonair mixtures.

of extremes of hydrostatic pressure on excitable nerve cells. Slowing the rate of descent (compression) and adding a small amount of narcotic gas (e.g., 5% N_2) to the Heliox breathing mixture relieves the tremor associated with HPNS. The term **Trimix** describes the helium–nitrogen–oxygen combination.

Other negative effects of breathing helium include:

- Changes in voice characteristics (high-pitched, cartoonlike quality), which interfere with voice communication among divers. Electronic voice unscramblers remedy this effect.
- Considerable heat loss for divers living in a Heliox environment from helium's high thermal conductivity (6 × air).[16] The thermal challenge contributes to weight loss, common among saturation divers.

Increased risk for central nervous system oxygen toxicity when breathing surface-supplied Heliox gas makes it crucial that the diver not exceed the oxygen exposure limits put forth in TABLE 26.4.

NATIONAL OCEANIC AND ATMOSPHERIC ADMINISTRATION (NOAA; http://www.dive. noaa.gov/): Recommendations to Avoid HPNS

- Do not dive Heliox (O_2/He) deeper than 400 fsw.
- Do not dive Trimix (O_2/He/N_2) deeper than 600 fsw. Adding 10% nitrogen to He/O_2 mix buffers mix so it can be used to 600 fsw without experiencing HPNS.
- Use slow descent rates. Descending slower than one fsw per minute beyond 400 fsw on Heliox and 600 fsw on Trimix keeps HPNS at bay. Unfortunately, this slow rate of decent is only practical in commercial diving and is of no use in technical diving.

TABLE 26.4 ■ REPRESENTATIVE NORMAL OXYGEN PARTIAL PRESSURE LIMITS FOR SURFACE-SUPPLIED HELIOX DIVING

EXPOSURE TIME (MIN)	MAXIMUM OXYGEN PARTIAL PRESSURE (ATA)
13	1.8
20	1.7
30	1.6
40	1.5
80	1.4
Unlimited	**1.3**

Adapted from United States Navy diving manual, vol 2. Mixed gas diving, rev 3. NAVSEA publ 0994 LP-001-9020. May 1991.

Saturation Diving

Breathing a Heliox mixture supports a safe dive to depths greater than 300 fsw, but the time the diver must remain "in-water" for decompression becomes prohibitive. Thus, dives below 300 fsw generally take place with **saturation diving** in a deep-diving system using a helium–oxygen–nitrogen breathing mixture that maintains oxygen pressure between 0.4 and 0.6 ata (Po_2, 300 to 450 mm Hg). In saturation diving, each inert gas in a mixture begins to concentrate in body tissues as depth and duration progress. Within 24 to 30 hours, the gases equilibrate and *saturate* body tissues to equal the pressures of the inspired gases. Once the tissues saturate, the decompression procedure remains identical regardless of the dive's duration.

The deep-diving system consists of a chamber where the divers live under pressure for up to 4 weeks. The system also contains a deck decompression chamber and transfer capsule or diving bell for transport of personnel under pressure to and from the worksite. Once at the worksite, the divers exit, tethered to an umbilicus-supplied breathing apparatus. Saturation diving provides benefits in offshore oil-field work with dives up to 30 days at depths of 1500 fsw. Successful dives to depths of 2300 fsw in a dry chamber apply principles of saturation diving with a breathing mixture of hydrogen, helium, and oxygen. Decompression from a saturation dive takes 8 to 24 hours per 10-m ascent.

A critical consideration in saturation diving with Heliox mixtures is to maintain normoxic Po_2. Breathing the wrong mixture or the correct mixture at the wrong pressure creates the potential for a tragic fatality. Oxygen percentages must remain within ±0.10% of the desired value to avoid either hypoxia or oxygen toxicity. FIGURE 26.11 shows the typical recommended percentage of oxygen in Heliox for various diving depths. For example, the oxygen concentration to obtain a desired Po_2 of 0.35 ata (Po_2, 270 mm Hg) at a depth of 1200 fsw requires a breathing mixture with approximately 0.7% oxygen.

Technical Diving

The term **technical diving** defines untethered dives (scuba or closed-circuit rebreathing) beyond the traditional compressed air range for military operations, science, salvage, and recreational pursuits. Many recreational scuba divers now consider the typical depth limit of 130 fsw imposed by diving with compressed air too restrictive. They wish to expand diving depths for personal achievement, recreation, and exploration (e.g., cave diving). Technical diving requires special equipment, expertise, and vigilant management of gas mixtures. Technical divers routinely use various mixtures of Trimix compressed gas to dive below 300 fsw. Blending a depth-specific gas mixture allows the diver to control the risk of hyperoxia and the narcotic potential of nitrogen.

Closed-circuit nitrogen-oxygen and helium-oxygen scuba originally developed for military operations now appear in the recreational technical diving community. These highly sophisticated systems maintain a constant partial pressure of oxygen in the inhaled mixture regardless of depth. FIGURE 26.12 illustrates a closed-circuit mixed-gas system

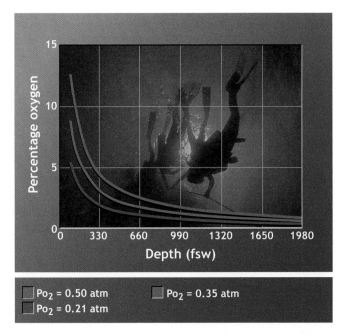

Figure 26.11   Range of oxygen concentrations for saturation diving. The *green line* represents the oxygen concentration that maintains oxygen at 0.35 atm ($P_{O_2} = 266$ mm Hg), a common choice for P_{O_2}. The *purple line* shows the oxygen needed to provide the normoxic level of 0.21 atm. The *red line* represents 0.5 atm ($P_{O_2} = 380$ mm Hg), the upper limit of continuous exposure to avoid whole-body oxygen toxicity. The low oxygen concentrations needed at great depths become difficult to mix and analyze within acceptable tolerance limits; thus, they are usually mixed as the diving chamber becomes pressurized. (From Hamilton RW. Mixed-gas diving. In: Bove AA, ed. Diving medicine. 4th ed. Philadelphia: WB Saunders, 2003.)

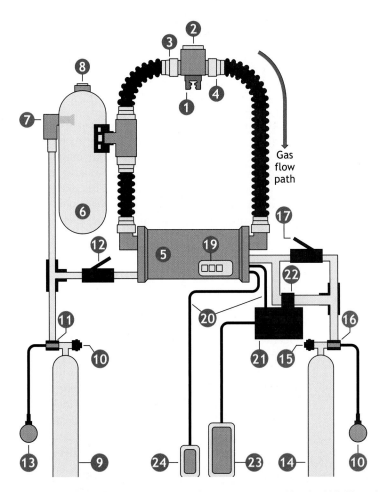

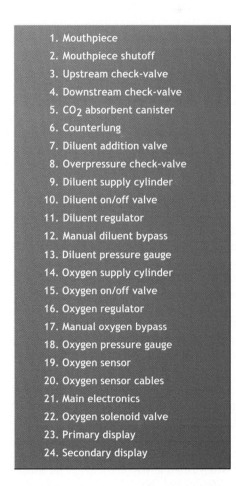

1. Mouthpiece
2. Mouthpiece shutoff
3. Upstream check-valve
4. Downstream check-valve
5. CO_2 absorbent canister
6. Counterlung
7. Diluent addition valve
8. Overpressure check-valve
9. Diluent supply cylinder
10. Diluent on/off valve
11. Diluent regulator
12. Manual diluent bypass
13. Diluent pressure gauge
14. Oxygen supply cylinder
15. Oxygen on/off valve
16. Oxygen regulator
17. Manual oxygen bypass
18. Oxygen pressure gauge
19. Oxygen sensor
20. Oxygen sensor cables
21. Main electronics
22. Oxygen solenoid valve
23. Primary display
24. Secondary display

Figure 26.12   Closed-circuit mixed-gas system used by the U.S. Navy for diving to great depths. A microprocessor and oxygen sensors in the breathing loop continually detect falling P_{O_2} and activate valves that add the precise amount of 100% oxygen to regulate the partial pressure of inspired oxygen. A single high-pressure gas bottle supplies pure oxygen, and a second provides either air or a Heliox mixture as a diluent. A chemical bed continually absorbs the carbon dioxide produced in metabolism (approximate cost, $35,000 to $45,000).

FOCUS On Research

THE OXYGEN COST OF SWIMMING UNDERWATER

Donald KW, Davidson WM. Oxygen uptake of "booted" and "fin swimming" divers. J Appl Physiol 1954;7:31.

▲ Scuba allows thousands of individuals to enjoy underwater diving. The duration of independence under water depends on the depth of the dive and the physiologic/metabolic demands of physical activity before the tank empties of compressed air. Minute pulmonary ventilation increases with increasing muscular effort under water, thus decreasing the duration of the stay.

Early research on underwater diving, particularly with closed-circuit scuba, attempted to establish the interactions among energy expenditure, pulmonary airflow, quantity of oxygen available in the tank, and the diver's rate of return to the surface, to avoid complications such as oxygen poisoning, anoxia, and nitrogen narcosis. Fundamental data required detailed measurements of oxygen consumption ($\dot{V}O_2$) and carbon dioxide production ($\dot{V}CO_2$) to determine the amount of oxygen supplied in the tank and the carbon dioxide absorbent required. The study by Donald and Davidson, completed in 1944 but not published until 1954, was among the first to quantify $\dot{V}O_2$ of divers and underwater swimmers during different forms of physical effort. This research demanded considerable technical expertise to permit accurate $\dot{V}O_2$ measurements in the underwater environment.

Subjects included 13 British military divers and 13 military "commando" frogmen, each in top physical condition. Subjects underwent multiple measurements under diverse exercise conditions. The researchers used a modified closed-circuit breathing system. Divers breathed pure oxygen under all conditions, which included work in a tank (12-ft depth) and open seawater. Divers wore either (1) a full rubber diving suit with leather or rubber boots (5–7 lb in the sole) that allowed them to assume the vertical position with ease or (2) the familiar frogman well-fitting rubber suit with rubber swim fins.

Measurements were taken during rest at the surface, sitting under water (12-ft depth), standing under water, with minimum movement (moving along the bottom as slowly and gently as possible without stopping and avoiding any marked postural changes), and with maximum movement (moving as fast as possible to cover the greatest distance).

Additional $\dot{V}O_2$ measurements were made during underwater cycle ergometer leg exercise with paddles attached to the pedals to increase resistance. Pedal revolutions per minute (rpm) controlled exercise intensity. A metronome placed in the diver's line of vision maintained

pedaling rate. Thirty rpm represented light exercise maintained easily for 15 minutes, 40 rpm provided intense exercise for 15 minutes, and 45 rpm caused fatigue within 10 minutes. For heavy arm exercise, the diver stood underwater while alternately lifting a 21-pound weight by means of a pulley system. The frogmen swam 2 to 3 feet below the surface at (1) a medium speed of 1.3 to 1.7 ft · s^{-1} for 20 minutes and (2) a fast speed of 1.7 to 2.3 ft · s^{-1} for 10 minutes.

TANK SERIES: BOOTED DIVERS

$\dot{V}O_2$ with subjects seated and standing still underwater remained low and remarkably near the divers' calculated resting values. These men experienced near-neutral buoyancy under water, so it is likely that lying and standing quietly required less postural effort than in air, hence the low underwater energy expenditure. While these resting data have little application to practical diving conditions, they do help to explain the prolonged periods that trained divers can remain under water with limited oxygen supply if they remain inactive.

$\dot{V}O_2$ during the minimum-movement experiments reached the same magnitude as for walking about 2.0 mph on the level in air; the underwater maximum-movement $\dot{V}O_2$ equaled the out-of-water $\dot{V}O_2$ for walking at 4 mph. Even though the energy expenditure values during underwater effort were relatively low, the divers complained of fatigue, possibly owing to the minimal involvement of the total leg musculature during work under water.

UNDERWATER SWIMMING WITH FINS

Eight of the 13 swimmers had $\dot{V}O_2$s of 2.3 L · min^{-1} or above during a 20-minute swim at the slower speed. At the faster speed, sustained for 10 minutes, 4 of 8 swimmers achieved $\dot{V}O_2$s over 3.0 L · min^{-1}, with one swimmer exceeding 4.0 L · min^{-1}, just slightly below his maximum level in air. The $\dot{V}O_2$s during underwater swimming are similar to those reported for athletes during different sustained sport activities out of water and considerably higher than previously calculated for underwater activities. The results indicated a need to reconsider the maximum size of carbon dioxide absorbent canisters used in most closed-circuit diving systems.

The figure shows the marked differences in $\dot{V}O_2$ under the different exercise conditions. These carefully designed experiments formed the foundation for further research on underwater energy expenditure. The data contributed to the growing understanding of diving physiology and construction of safer diving systems.

continued on page 691

Continued

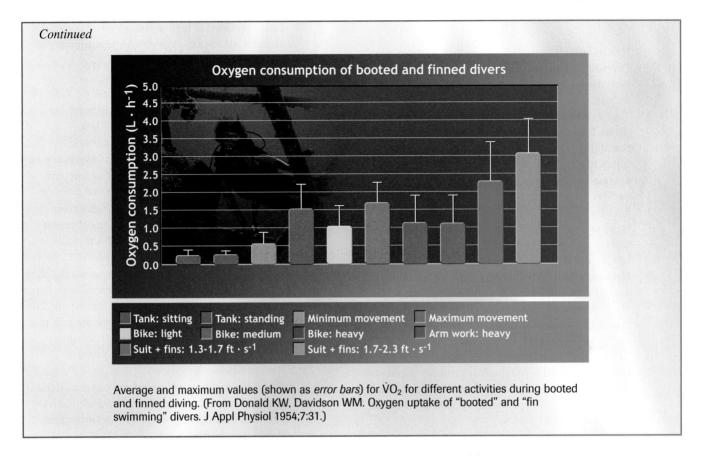

Average and maximum values (shown as *error bars*) for $\dot{V}O_2$ for different activities during booted and finned diving. (From Donald KW, Davidson WM. Oxygen uptake of "booted" and "fin swimming" divers. J Appl Physiol 1954;7:31.)

used by the U.S. Navy. An oxygen sensor *(19)* and microprocessor *(21)* in the breathing loop continually detect and regulate falling PO_2. The sensors activate valves that add the precise quantity of 100% oxygen to regulate inspired PO_2 at 0.75 ata (427 mm Hg). One of two high-pressure gas bottles *(9 and 14)* supplies pure oxygen, and the other provides either air or a Heliox mixture as the diluent gas. As with the typical closed-circuit system, a chemical bed absorbs carbon dioxide produced in metabolism. Monitors within the facemask provide continual feedback about PO_2 and diving depth. A fiberglass casing worn on the diver's back contains the microprocessor, gas bottles, breathing bag, and insulated carbon dioxide absorbent canister (cold decreases CO_2 absorbent life).

ENERGY COST OF UNDERWATER SWIMMING

As with surface swimming, drag forces impede the diver's forward movement and greatly increase the energy cost of swimming underwater. FIGURE 26.13 shows the curvilinear relationship between oxygen consumption and underwater swimming speed. For example, a swimmer with a $\dot{V}O_{2max}$ of $35 \text{ mL} \cdot \text{kg}^{-1} \cdot \text{min}^{-1}$ could swim underwater at a speed of 1.2 knots (1.4 mph) for only several minutes. This speed creates minimal stress for a diver with a $\dot{V}O_{2max}$ of $65 \text{ mL} \cdot \text{kg}^{-1} \cdot$

min^{-1}. The location and density of the gear can alter the diver's positioning in the water and increase the energy cost of swimming by as much as 30% at slow speeds. The type of fin used has an effect on the depth and frequency of the kick, thus influencing drag and swimming economy.[18]

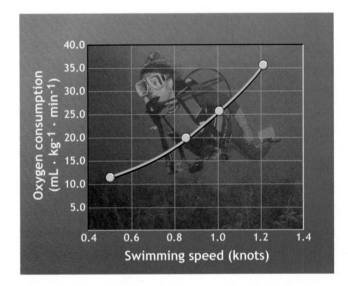

Figure 26.13 Generalized curvilinear relationship between oxygen consumption ($\text{mL} \cdot \text{kg}^{-1} \cdot \text{min}^{-1}$) and underwater swimming speed (1.0 knot = 1.15 mph).

Summary

1. Breath-hold diving has been practiced for centuries. Deep-sea diving had its origins in the 14th century with the invention of diving bells supplied with surface air.

2. The underwater environment routinely exposes divers to high pressures (hyperbaria) and the possibility of rapidly changing pressures. Severe injury and even death ensue unless divers adjust to equalize pressures in the body's air-filled cavities.

3. Two factors limit snorkel size: (1) increased hydrostatic pressure on the chest cavity during descent and (2) increased pulmonary dead space from enlarging the snorkel's internal volume.

4. Duration of a breath-hold dive depends on time until arterial P_{CO_2} reaches the breath-holding breakpoint.

5. Hyperventilation considerably lowers arterial P_{CO_2} increases breath-holding time; it also increases the likelihood of underwater blackout.

6. The point at which the diver's lung volume compresses to RLV generally determines maximum depth for breath-hold diving. Lung squeeze occurs below this critical depth when internal and external pressures cannot equalize.

7. Breath-hold diving by elite divers produces intense cardiovascular changes that resemble response patterns of diving mammals.

8. Scuba supplies breathing mixtures at great depths and pressures. Specific hazards result from improper equalization of pressures in the lungs, sinus, and middle-ear spaces with the external water pressure. Important dangers include air embolism, pneumothorax, mask and middle-ear squeeze, and aerosinusitis.

9. Gases breathed at high pressures move across the alveolar membrane to dissolve and equilibrate in the fluids of all tissues.

10. High tissue oxygen and nitrogen pressures exert profound negative effects on physiologic function. The maximum recommended diving depth for breathing compressed air is about 30 m.

11. Prolonged breathing of a gas with a P_{O_2} above 2 ata increases a diver's susceptibility to oxygen poisoning. Closed-circuit scuba systems that use pure oxygen severely restrict dive depth and duration.

12. Nitrogen bubbles form in tissues when excess nitrogen fails to exit through the lungs if ascent progresses too rapidly. Decompression sickness or bends describe this painful condition.

13. Diving to depths below 60 fsw requires inhalation of compressed mixed gases. Oxygen always exists in the breathing mixture in mixed-gas diving, but it represents only a small fraction of the mix in dives to extreme depths. Precisely managing oxygen concentrations becomes a primary consideration.

14. Breathing mixtures of helium and oxygen (Heliox) allows dives to depths of 2000 fsw. Heliox diving eliminates nitrogen narcosis risk and minimizes risk of oxygen poisoning.

15. Rapid descent to depths from 300 fsw to 2800 fsw breathing Heliox mixtures produces nausea, muscle tremors, and other central nervous system effects termed high-pressure nervous syndrome (HPNS).

16. Drag forces that impede a diver's forward movement increase the energy cost of swimming under water.

References are available on the Student CD and online at http://connection.lww.com/mkk6e.

Microgravity: The Last Frontier

27

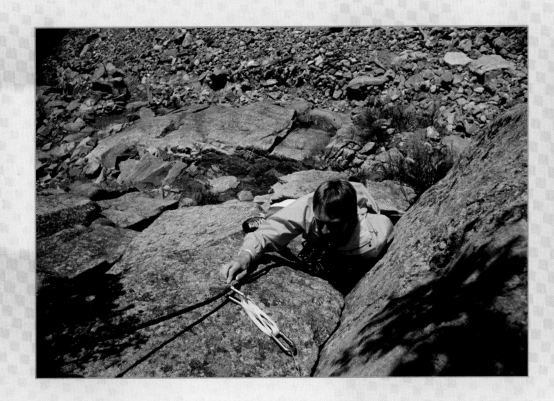

CHAPTER OBJECTIVES

- Define the term gravity and list factors that affect the magnitude of gravitational force

- Differentiate between zero-g and weightlessness

- Outline factors that contribute to a sense of "free fall" in a falling elevator

- Describe four strategies to simulate microgravity with inanimate objects and animals and humans

- Describe how the KC-135 airplane creates brief durations of microgravity during astronaut training

- List five physiologic/anatomic responses to microgravity exposure; differentiate between short-term and long-term responses

- Give reasons for denitrogenation prior to extravehicular activity and procedures to achieve this effect

- Discuss the role of hindlimb unloading to study mammalian responses to microgravity

- Outline the goals of exercise countermeasures to ensure astronaut health and safety during missions and return to Earth

- Describe the rational for applying lower-body negative pressure and its role as a countermeasure during space flight

- Outline interactions among energy balance, nutrition, and protein dynamics during current space missions

- Describe the time course for postflight recovery for physiologic systems from two-week and one-year space missions

- List 10 significant spin-off technologies from space biology research

THE WEIGHTLESS ENVIRONMENT

The pioneering efforts of mainly German, Russian, and American scientists and engineers advanced aerospace medicine from the early test flights of rocket-propelled jet aircraft to the technologic innovations of today's **International Space Station** (**ISS**) that orbits 220 nautical miles above Earth. The remarkable successes of man's escape from Earth's atmosphere and subsequent return originated in antiquity, when prophets and philosophers could only dream of contacting celestial bodies. From flying machine designs of da Vinci's Renaissance drawings five centuries ago at the dawn of modern science to successful hot-air balloon ascents during the mid-1700s, the obsession to explore the universe has not waned. The reliability of powerful rocketry now makes commercial space adventure possible, creating new challenges about how best to tame the short- and long-term physiologic stress imposed by escaping Earth's gravitational field.

The early jet flights could not test human responses to changing gravitational forces because that era's test aircraft could not accommodate specialized laboratory equipment. Nevertheless, knowing how to cope with the unique environmental stressors (and health challenges) of high-altitude exposure still required new understanding unavailable from conventional medicine. The field of **aerospace medicine** emerged from a need to deal with unconventional situations not encountered in normal gravity. Few in the medical establishment could predict the response of mice, cats, dogs, monkeys, or humans to space flight. Primates and eventually humans in more powerful rocket tests followed the earliest "space-travelers," lower life forms carried aloft by test aircraft. Concurrently, research progressed by use of space cabin simulators on Earth. Scientists focused on psychophysiologic responses to changing gravitational forces and prolonged isolation while performing complex motor and mental tasks. The experience from simulations and manned flights provided new understanding about space flights' impact on human structure, function, and response.

Gravity

On the Earth's surface, **gravity** provides an invisible attraction that makes any mass exert downward force or have weight. Gravity behaves in the same fundamental way between the Earth and any object on it, between any of

the planets that revolve about the sun in our solar system, or between a planet and its moons. The universality of the gravitational law, first proposed in 1687 by **Sir Isaac Newton** (1642–1727), can be stated as follows and depicted in the top of FIGURE 27.1.

> Every particle in matter in the universe attracts every other particle with a force directly proportional to the product of the masses of the particles and inversely proportional to the square of the distance separating them.

When a person sits in a chair on Earth, the force of gravity pulls the person into the seat because the chair provides an equal and opposite force (Newton's third law). Every mass (m) on Earth requires support from a force (F) equal to its weight (w) such that w (or F) $= mg$. Stated differently, the

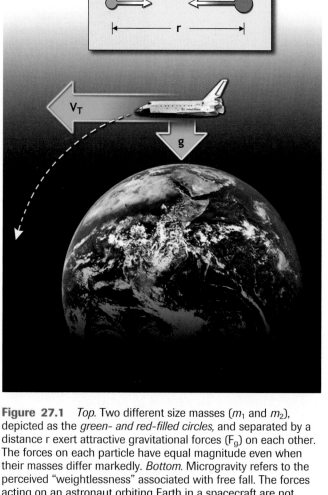

Figure 27.1 *Top.* Two different size masses (m_1 and m_2), depicted as the *green- and red-filled circles,* and separated by a distance r exert attractive gravitational forces (F_g) on each other. The forces on each particle have equal magnitude even when their masses differ markedly. *Bottom.* Microgravity refers to the perceived "weightlessness" associated with free fall. The forces acting on an astronaut orbiting Earth in a spacecraft are not balanced—both astronaut and spacecraft accelerate toward the Earth's center. They do not "fall" to the Earth because its surface is curved and they are moving at a tangential velocity (V_T) high enough to "balance" gravity's downward force on the spacecraft. No perceived force (i.e., weight) exists because nothing counteracts the force of gravity.

constant acceleration force per second (s) of descent on a freely falling body at or near Earth's surface has a value of 1g (acceleration due to gravity), or the equivalent magnitude of 9.80665 or 9.80 m $\cdot$ s^{-2}, 980 cm $\cdot$ s^{-2}, or 32 ft $\cdot$ s^{-2}. On the moon's surface, the attractive force of the moon rather than Earth causes the acceleration of gravity, where g = 1.6 m $\cdot$ s^{-2}. Near the sun's surface, the g value increases tremendously by a factor of nearly 169 to 270 m $\cdot$ s^{-2}.

Microgravity and Weightlessness

To achieve an orbit around Earth or move away from it, the velocity of a rocket must exceed the downward pull of Earth's gravity. The gravitational pull on the rocket decreases as the rocket moves farther from Earth. When the rocket reaches a specified distance from Earth sufficient for orbit, a traveler experiences a weightless feeling because *nearly* all of the forces acting on the body remain in balance. To reach a point in space where the gravitational pull from Earth equals one-millionth the force at Earth's surface requires traveling 6.37 million kilometers or 16.6 times the distance from Earth to the moon, or 1400 times the highway distance between New York City and San Francisco. In a practical sense, a rock dropped from a window 5 m above the ground requires 1 second to touch ground. In an environment with only 1% of Earth's gravitational pull, the same drop takes 10 seconds. In a microgravity environment equal to one-millionth of the gravity on Earth, the same 5-m drop would take 1000 seconds, or approximately 17 minutes.

The issue of gravitational force also applies to **escape velocity** (V_{esc}) required to evade gravity's pull, which depends on the mass (M) and radius (r) of the celestial body a spacecraft attempts to leave. V_{esc} from the Earth computes at 11.2 km $\cdot$ s^{-2}; on the moon, with considerably less gravity than Earth, a spacecraft must achieve approximately one-fifth the escape velocity or 2.38 km $\cdot$ s^{-2}. Leaving the planet Jupiter requires an extremely large escape velocity (59.5 km $\cdot$ s^{-2}) compared with leaving the Earth or moon because of Jupiter's huge mass, radius, and distance from Earth.

Spacecraft orbit Earth at a relatively close distance (typically 200 to 450 km), so astronauts experience only an *apparent* sense of weightlessness. In essence, the force of gravity never truly reaches an absolute value of zero (called **zero-g**), because a gravitational force still exists. Consequently, the term **microgravity**, not weightlessness (or zero-g), correctly describes what astronauts feel during space flight in Earth orbit when the rocket's altitude exceeds approximately 160 km (100 mi) at a velocity of approximately 17,500 mph. In a microgravity environment, an object's apparent weight is small compared with its weight on Earth because of the different gravitational effects. On the space shuttle or the ISS, the microgravity environment at 220-km altitude is qualitatively the same as in a spacecraft orbiting a thousand Earth radii away (6,370,000 km); here, g equals one-millionth the force of Earth's gravity.

The 121-ft space shuttle orbiting laboratory can carry a payload of 29,479 kg into orbit, with each main engine producing a thrust of 170,068 kg at sea level while burning a mixture of liquid oxygen and hydrogen. After achieving orbital velocity, the astronaut and spacecraft continually accelerate toward a single point at the Earth's center. However, they do not fall to Earth because of the planet's curved surface and because both craft and crew move at a high enough tangential velocity (V_T) to the Earth (see *bottom* of Fig. 27.1). The spacecraft's speed creates an outward centrifugal force that "balances" the downward gravitational force on the spacecraft. When spacecraft velocity decreases (reduced V_T)—a planned maneuver during reentry—the craft "plunges" toward Earth under gravity's pull.

The orbit essentially creates a state of continuous **free-fall** so the astronaut does not perceive any force (i.e., weight) because nothing counteracts gravity and the astronaut experiences a feeling of floating. During this time, astronaut and spacecraft accelerate at the same rate in orbit without buoyancy effects. No pressure gradient pushes the astronaut against the vehicle's floor or walls. In fact, the vehicle and its inhabitants maintain a state of continuous free-fall around the Earth in a microgravity environment as the vehicle's falling path remains parallel to the Earth's surface. The spacecraft and any unfixed object within it fall *around* the Earth, not toward it. All objects in a state of free-fall experience the same acceleration regardless of their mass. Interestingly, springboard divers launch themselves into the air when performing dives and then experience the free-fall of microgravity (at a rate independent of the diver's mass).

Spacecraft that maintain Earth orbit at an established velocity produce high-quality microgravity. The United States reusable launch vehicles (space shuttles) stay in orbit for no longer than 18 days (16-day planned mission plus a 2-day contingency capability). Before the Russian Mir Space Station deorbited on March 21, 2001, it had remained in orbit for 15 years (launched Feb. 20, 1986), maintaining continuous free-fall as it circled Earth. Currently, the 454-metric ton (356 × 290-ft wing span) ISS orbits Earth every 90 minutes.

Passenger in a Falling Elevator

When an elevator descends quickly, one feels a lessening of weight because of reduced force between the feet and elevator floor. If the elevator cable suddenly snaps and the elevator plummets downward, the force against the feet equals zero until the elevator strikes bottom. Consider the example of a 60-kg woman riding in the elevator. If she could lift her feet off the floor before hitting the ground, she would float within the elevator compartment. No force pushes her up because she and the elevator fall together at the same speed and acceleration. This applies equally to any other objects in the elevator. If a scale were present in the elevator, the woman's weight would not register because the scale too would be falling. *During free-fall, everything in the elevator remains weightless because the person and elevator car (including a scale) accelerate downward at the same rate from gravity alone.*

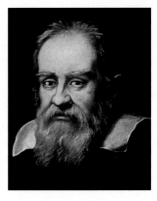

Galileo Galilei (1564–1642)

Galileo, in his classic *Two New Sciences* published in 1638, makes the case of a similar "falling" experiment in which, legend has it, he simultaneously dropped a cannonball and musket ball of different masses from the Leaning Tower of Pisa. Galileo observed that both objects fell downward at approximately the same rate and consequently touched the ground at the same time. In his demonstration of the two falling masses, *F* and *g* both equaled zero because both objects hit the ground at precisely the same time, similar to the situation of the person and elevator striking the ground simultaneously. The term *zero-g* correctly applies to these temporary weightless conditions.

Examples of Near–Zero-G During Space Flight

Space flight provides the ubiquitous condition of near–zero-g. Liquids fail to remain in open cups or glasses, so drinks must be squeezed into the mouth from special con-tainers. No "up" or "down" exists inside the space vehicle (FIG. 27.2); to keep from floating freely, astronauts must anchor or tether themselves to a fixed object within the cabin (e.g., a wall or other attached object). Astronauts aboard the 1973–1974 Skylab missions wore shoes with a triangle-shaped cleat on the sole. The floors, made of aluminum alloy webbing with triangular openings, provided a contact surface for the shoe, which when twisted, locked the foot in place. The cleated shoes provided a stable base to apply leverage for movement. The contact surface provides reaction forces to gravitational or inertial and accelerational forces. These enable the body's musculoskeletal-neural internal "sensors" to maintain control over posture and locomotion.

In microgravity, blood and fluid volumes shift upward and move into the thoracocephalic region. This causes a puffy-face appearance as fluid relocates from extracellular to intracellular spaces.[91] Correspondingly, a 2- to 5-cm decrease occurs in waist girth (a legitimate way in space to wear otherwise tight-fitting pants!). The initial net shift of fluid also produces eye redness, "bird-type" (skinny) legs, nasal congestion, headaches, and nausea. Concomitant reductions in blood volume affect cardiovascular function, manifested by decreased plasma and red blood cell volume, increased venous pooling, blunted baroreceptor reflex, and **orthostatic intolerance**, defined as compromised venous return to the heart during upright posture in a gravity environment.

On Earth, the constant downward pressure of 1 g compresses intervertebral disks. In microgravity, removal of gravitational force causes disks to expand making stature increase up to 5 cm (FIG. 27.3, *top*). The bottom of Figure 27.3 illustrates that posture also changes during microgravity exposure. Compared with preflight, joints move toward the midpoint in their range of motion so that hips and knees flex

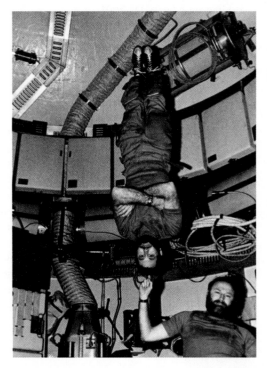

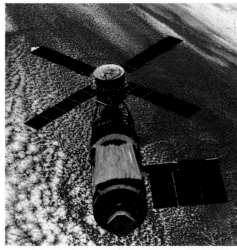

Figure 27.2 *Left.* Demonstration of microgravity aboard Spacelab where no "up" or "down" exists. *Above.* The entire vehicle in orbit; note the solar panels.

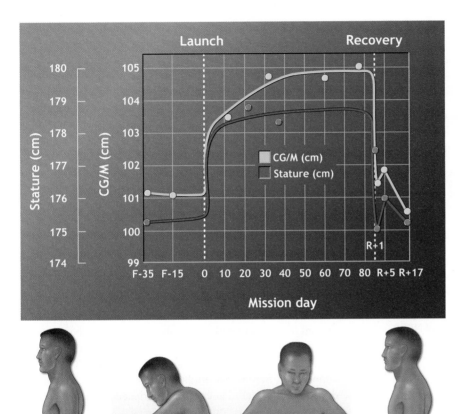

Figure 27.3 *Top.* Change in the center of gravity/mass (CG ÷ M) and stature before (F), during an 84-day Skylab 4 mission, and 17 days postflight (R). *Bottom.* General changes in posture under conditions of Earth's gravity (1g) and microgravity. (From Thornton WE, et al. Anthropometric changes and fluid shifts. In: Johnson RS, Dietlein LF, eds. Biomedical results from Skylab. NASA SP-377. Washington, DC: Government Printing Office, 1977.)

slightly causing the body to crouch. Arms tend to float in front of the body unless consciously forced downward. Note the postural sway with head protruding forward with accompanying lordosis immediately upon return to Earth.

New technology and techniques to offset the effects of microgravity often replace the most ordinary tasks on Earth. Anchoring eating utensils becomes essential or else they float freely away. The same holds true for food; crumbs fall downward to one's plate or napkin on Earth, while in a microgravity environment, they disperse in all directions to pose a menace if inhaled or if they migrate to clog a sensitive instrument. Similarly, sprinkled salt or pepper fails to reach the intended food. Spilled water does not drip downward but drifts

upward to form mostly stationary, suspended particles within the cabin. When these globules contact a solid object, they spread like pancake batter and cling to surfaces making them difficult to remove. Without the reacting force of friction, simple chores such as showering require new strategies and unique skills. FIGURE 27.4 shows the shower facility aboard the 1973 *Skylab 3* vehicle. Shower facilities were not included on subsequent shuttle flights because of the cumbersome equipment and the time required to shower. Astronauts now take a sponge bath with a sprayable hand washer. The sponge absorbs the sprayed water, which the astronaut then squeezes into an airflow system that carries the fluid into a waste collection tank.

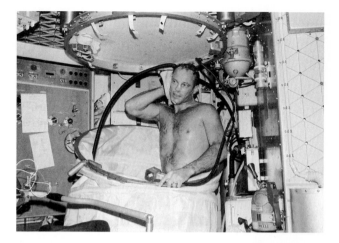

Figure 27.4 Astronaut Jack Lousma, Skylab 3 pilot, takes a hot bath in the crew quarters of the Orbital Workshop (OWS). In deploying the shower facility, the shower curtain pulled up from the floor and attached to the ceiling. The water came through a push-button showerhead connected to a flexible hose, and a vacuum system drew off the water. (Photo courtesy of NASA, Lyndon B. Johnson Space Center, Houston, TX.)

Strategies to Simulate Microgravity

Different strategies have simulated space flight's microgravity environment. This allows researchers to manipulate various experimental conditions before deciding on the best procedure(s) for a particular mission. One strategy uses sophisticated test equipment that creates zero-g conditions for relatively brief times with nonhuman objects dropped from towers and into tubes or within sounding rockets as they fall to Earth after achieving a maximum altitude. Another tactic uses parabolic airplane flights with living and nonliving objects, and a third strategy simulates microgravity conditions with animals and humans using head-down bed rest, confinement, water immersion, or immobilization.

Nonhuman Testing

The Microgravity Research Division of the **National Aeronautics and Space Administration** (**NASA**) Office of Life and Microgravity Sciences and Applications (microgravity.grc.nasa.gov/) directs a basic and applied research program from the Marshall Space Flight Center that supports ground-based and flight experiments that require microgravity conditions of varying duration and quality. In microgravity, researchers study the fundamental states of matter—solids, liquids, and gases—and the forces acting upon them. In addition to the space shuttles and ISS, NASA researchers use other methods to achieve microgravity or simulate it effects (FIG. 27.5). These include (1) two drop towers, one tower from which objects fall 24 m, and one in-ground shaft 132-m deep and 6.1-m in diameter, and one drop tube 105-m high for achieving 2.2 to 5.2 seconds of zero-g conditions; (2) sounding rockets that fly suborbital parabolic trajectories with a payload that produces several minutes of high-quality

microgravity during the rocket's coast and before atmospheric reentry; (3) bioreactor (rotating wall cylinder to randomize the gravity vector in cell culture samples. This reduces shear forces and simulates microgravity exposure (science.nasa.gov/newhome/br/bioreactor.htm) by rotation perpendicular to the gravity vector that intersects the center of the cell (which alters cytoplasmic viscosity and disrupts normal particle distribution, causing particle "suspension"); and (4) reduced-gravity aircraft that achieve microgravity conditions for 25 to 30 seconds.

The longest zero-g drop time currently available (approximately 10 s) occurs in Japan in a 490-m deep vertical mine shaft converted to a drop facility (spaceinfo.jaxa.jp/note/kankyo/e/kan9812_rakkasetubi_e.html). The Bremen Drop Tower at Bremen University, Germany consists of a 146-m tall concrete shaft that produces one-millionth of Earth's gravity (1.0 micro-g or 1.0×10^{-6}g; www.zarm.uni-bremen.de/6zarm_fab/fallturm/index.htm). In all of the drop facilities, polystyrene pellets decelerate the payload as it hits the ground from its fall within the tube whose air has been evacuated to minimize drag. The 105-m drop tube at Marshall Space Flight Center can create a vacuum of less than a billionth of an atmosphere. Sensations similar to those from a drop in the reduced gravity facilities can be experienced on most amusement park roller coaster rides.

Human Testing

Researchers have devised five basic strategies to simulate a microgravity environment and study its effects on humans: (1) head-down bed rest, (2) wheelchair confinement of paraplegics, (3) water immersion, (4) immobilization and confinement, and (5) parabolic flights.

Head-Down Bed Rest. Head-down bed rest has yielded the most information about human physiologic dynamics in simulated microgravity. These studies confirmed experimental findings in space about physiologic responses and adaptations including psychologic stress, hormonal changes, and immune function[24,98]; this makes the head-down bed rest strategy a useful space flight analogue. Subjects remain confined to bed for an extended time (weeks, months, or a year) in a horizontal or head-down tilt position (-3 to $-12°$), often followed by physiologic measurements to positive acceleration at forces up to 3g in a centrifuge.

Wheelchair Confinement of Paraplegics. Prolonged wheelchair confinement produces postural hypotension in paraplegics who seldom experience full erect posture following their disability.[28] As in longer space flight missions (>21 days), years of sitting constrain fluctuations in hydrostatic gradients normally experienced by nonparaplegics during routine daily activities. Short-term exercise stress (e.g., graded, arm-crank exercise to maximum[113]) evaluates paraplegics' responses for heart rate, systolic and diastolic blood pressure, forearm vascular resistance (FVR), and vasoactive hormones.[49] In general, exercise eliminated orthostatic hypotension and increased FVR and baroreflex sensitivity independ-

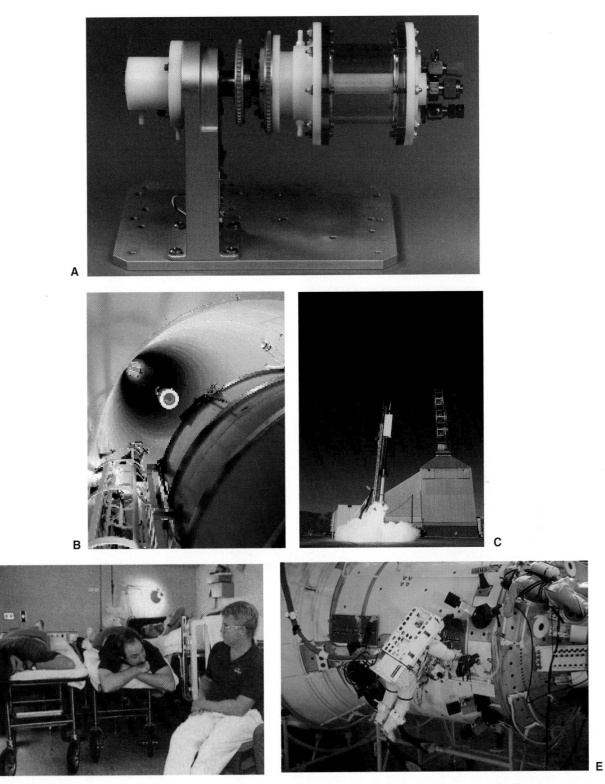

Figure 27.5   Methods to achieve microgravity or simulate its effects. **A.** Bioreactor apparatus. **B.** Drop tower facility. Note object in midflight within the tower. **C.** Launch of sounding rocket. **D.** Bed rest, head-down experimental strategy to study postural hypotension and associated cardiovascular functions. **E.** An astronaut with the assistance of scuba divers performs a simulated EVA maneuver to the space shuttle in the Weightless Environment Training Facility. (Photos courtesy of NASA, Lyndon B. Johnson Space Center, Houston, TX.)

ent of blood volume changes. The positive cardiovascular adjustments in paraplegics to less frequent but relatively intense exercise have relevance as a postflight countermeasure to the potentially debilitating effects of prolonged missions on orthostatic stability and baroreflex functions following return to Earth's gravitational environment. The intriguing possibility of immediate benefit from short-term, intense postflight exercise would maximize overall mission efficiency by reducing time devoted to in-flight exercise and concomitant demands for additional food and water associated with daily exercise.[50]

Water Immersion. Subjects lie supine in a water tank for up to 24 hours (wet immersion technique) or lie on a thin sheet to prevent the skin from touching the water (dry immersion technique). Figure 27.5E illustrates maneuvers under water in a space suit as a simulation modality of near–zero-g conditions. The astronaut performs complex hand–eye coordination tasks to mimic skills required in extravehicular activity (EVA) during orbital missions.

Immobilization and Confinement

- Whole-body or segmental casts restrict limb and body movements in humans and animals. One approach immobilizes the nondominant arm in a sling, except during sleep and bathing, for 4 weeks.[113] This procedure produces an effective analogue for simulating the effects of "weightlessness" on human skeletal muscle loading. Changes in muscle structure and function (e.g., torque production, cross-sectional area, histochemical muscle fiber analysis, and integrated electromyography or IEMG) produce results similar in magnitude and direction to data obtained from humans following exposure to real and simulated microgravity environments.
- Confining animals to a small cage severely restricts their movement.
- A harness provides partial body support by suspending an animal in a head-down position with gravitational loading removed from the hind limbs (see figure on p. 737).

Parabolic Flights. FIGURE 27.6 *(top)* illustrates the strategy to evaluate physiologic responses to microgravity produced when NASA's KC-135 aircraft climbs rapidly at a 45° angle and then follows a path called a parabola (jsc-aircraft-ops.jsc.nasa.gov/kc135/). The four-engine turbojet aircraft produces a near–zero-g effect (1×10^{-3}g) for about 30 seconds (*center purple area* in the figure) just as the aircraft achieves 9500 m of the 10,000-m ascent (termed *pull-up*) before it slows. The plane then traces a parabola (pushover), descending rapidly at a 45° angle (termed *pull-out*) to 7300 m. The forces of acceleration and deceleration produce 2 to 2.5 times normal gravity during the pull-up and pull-out phases of the flight; the brief pushover at the apogee generates an environment with less than 1% of Earth's gravity. The nickname "vomit comet" aptly describes the gut-wrenching sensations produced during KC-135 training flights.

During repeated brief parabolic roller coaster-like maneuvers, scientists evaluate how humans and equipment function during intermittent forces that range from 1.8g to near–zero-g, similar to those experienced during liftoff and reentry of space vehicles. Depending on the mission, astronaut training can include up to 60 **parabolic flights** daily for a week, providing about 3 hours of cumulative weightlessness. Some career astronaut–researchers have accumulated 4000 and 5000 parabolas during a decade of KC-135 flight experiments, equivalent to 28 to 36 hours of simulated weightlessness. In addition to astronauts and mission specialists, more than 2000 students and 460 college teams have conducted experiments on board the KC-135. The final flight of the KC-135 occurred on October 29, 2004; its replacement, a C-9 aircraft, is the military version of the DC-9 used by commercial airlines and military for medical evacuation, passenger transportation, and special missions.

The *bottom left* of Figure 27.6 shows scientists measuring shock-absorption parameters from vibrations during motorized treadmill exercise on KC-135 parabolic flights. Adding 245 kg to the base of the treadmill blunted the impact forces (and vibration effects) of the exercising subject. The *bottom right* photo shows astronauts testing aerobic (rowing) and resistance-training equipment during the flights. Scientific information gleaned from the reduced-gravity aircraft flights has translated into on-board exercise regimens as countermeasures to the lack of gravity's deleterious effects during space shuttle and ISS missions. The new field of **bioastronautics** focuses on biologic and medical effects of space flight on human systems. The National Space Biomedical Research Institute (NSBRI; www.nsbri.org) discussed below has developed long-range plans to implement research to prevent and reduce the known risks to astronaut health, safety, and mission performance.

National Space Biomedical Research Institute. A consortium of 12 institutions that study physiologic and medical solutions to health problems related to long-duration space travel and prolonged exposure to microgravity compose the NSBRI research program. The Institute's 95 research and education projects take place at 75 institutions in 22 states and involve almost 300 investigators. The NSBRI's primary mission objective is to ensure safe and productive human space flight. Established in 1997, the NSBRI actively researches microgravity's effects on bone loss, cardiovascular alterations, human performance factors, sleep and chronobiology, immunology, infection, and hematology, muscle alterations and atrophy, neurobehavioral and psychosocial factors, neurovestibular adaptation, nutrition, physical fitness, and rehabilitation, radiation effects, smart medical systems, technology development, and space medicine.[102]

Mathematical Modeling and Computer Simulations

Researchers generally consider an entire physiologic system (e.g., cardiovascular, thermoregulatory, hormonal, respiratory, muscular) or subdivide it into its component parts. For

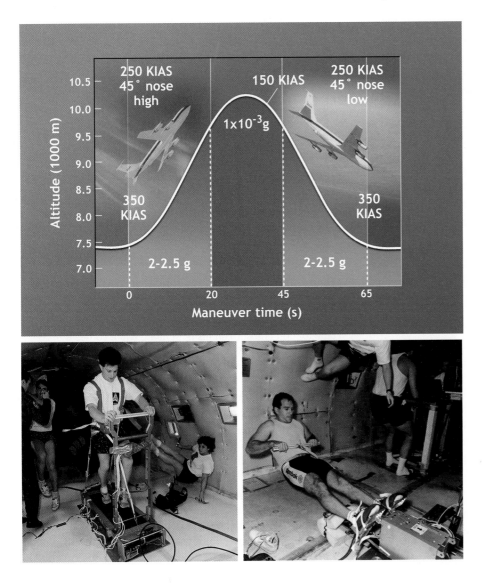

Figure 27.6 *Top.* Parabolic (Keplerian trajectory) flight profile of NASA's KC-135 aircraft to achieve brief periods of weightlessness. *KIAS,* knots indicating air speed. (From Nicogossian AE, et al. Space physiology and medicine. 3rd ed. Philadelphia: Lea & Febiger, 1994.) *Bottom left.* Evaluating the shock absorption qualities caused by vibrations while running on a motorized treadmill during KC-135 flights. *Bottom right.* Evaluating exercise equipment (aerobic and strength) during KC-135 flights. (Photos courtesy of NASA, Lyndon B. Johnson Space Center, Houston, TX.)

example, elements of the cardiovascular system include the heart, lungs, blood vessels, and blood. Each constituent can further subdivide into parts and factors such as wall compliance, wall thickness, and blood flow within the heart's chambers or through its valves and specific vasculature. Researchers mathematically model each component on the basis of known values for a particular function (e.g., HR_{max} in young adults averages 200 b · min^{-1}).

Armed with facts about the entire physiologic system, a computer-based model recreates how the system would respond to weightlessness when changes affect single or multiple components. Researchers have applied mathematical models of the thermoregulatory and cardiovascular systems to establish design criteria for the astronaut's space suit. For example, the model predicts the range of energy expenditures an astronaut might encounter with EVA (from 180 to 200 kCal · kg^{-1} · h^{-1} assessed during different space missions[112]; spacesuit design details are discussed in the following section).

On the shuttle *Atlantis* STS-98 flight of 12 days and 21 hours (Feb. 7, 2001–Feb. 20, 2001), astronauts conducted 3 space walks over a period of 19 hours and 49 minutes. They used hand and power tools to bolt the U.S. Laboratory Module *Destiny* to the station. By 2006, about 160 space walks were completed that totaled 960 clock-hours or 1920 man-hours to assemble and maintain the station. Knowing the limits of sustained energy expenditure based on prior laboratory research establishes a reasonable completion time for the EVA and provides parameters for garment design to effectively dissipate the work-induced heat load. Simulating different aspects of the EVA (speed of movement, intensity of effort, duration of task) and how different physiologic systems respond and adapt allows researchers the luxury of predicting outcomes under specified conditions. Well-designed mathematical models should ultimately predict with high accuracy physiologic responses in microgravity, especially on long-duration flights to Mars and eventually beyond.

Extravehicular Mobility Unit. An important aspect of the prediction models involves protective suits astronauts wear, called extravehicular mobility units or EMUs, as they perform building and repair tasks outside the space vehicle. From 1965 to 1996, astronauts' averaged 20 hours per year performing EVA. The current ISS assembly target will require 135 hours of EVA per year, and 138 hours per year for postconstruction maintenance. Thus, exercise and repeated exposure to hypobaric conditions in EMU protective gear, with its low pressure of 4.3 psi, increases astronauts' risk of decompression sickness (DCS). Changes in EVA support systems and training require more research into the physiologic responses to exercise in the EVA environment to ensure the health, safety, and efficiency of working astronauts.[39]

The EMU worm by Astronaut Edward White II in FIGURE 27.7 combines soft and hard components to provide support, mobility, and comfort compared with the early spacesuits made entirely of soft fabrics. The 127-kg suit (weight on Earth) consists of 13 layers of different materials, including an inner cooling garment (two layers), pressure garment (two layers), thermal micrometeroid garment (eight layers) and outer cover (one layer). The materials include Kevlar, the material used in bulletproof vests. The layers are sewn and cemented together to form the suit. In contrast to early spacesuits individually tailored for each astronaut, the EMU consists of component pieces to fit astronauts of any size. In effect, the EMU is a spacecraft in and of itself, independent of the shuttle vehicle or space station. There are many interesting aspects about the $12 million spacesuit; we highlight two of them.

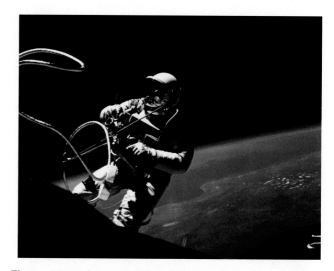

Figure 27.7 Astronaut Edward H. White II performed an EVA during the third revolution of the *Gemini 4* spacecraft (June 9, 1965). White remained secured to the spacecraft by a 25-foot umbilical line and a 23-foot tether line, both wrapped in gold tape to form one cord. In his right hand, White carries a handheld, self-maneuvering unit. His gold-plated helmet visor protected him from unfiltered sun rays.

1. **In-Suit Drink Bag**. Astronaut performance and health require access to water during up to 7 hours of EVA. The spacesuit includes an in-suit drink bag (IDB), a plastic pouch in the shape of a vest mounted inside the hard fiberglass shell. The IDB supports structures that include the arms, lower torso, helmet, life-support backpack, mini-tool carrier, and control module. It holds 32 ounces (1.9 L) of water, including a small tube and straw positioned next to the astronaut's mouth. A slot in the helmet accommodates a rice paper-covered fruit and cereal bar the astronaut can consume during an EVA. An astronaut must consume the entire bar to prevent crumbs from floating within the helmet. Most astronauts eat prior to the spacewalk and prefer not to eat the bar.

2. **Primary Life-Support Subsystem**. The primary life-support subsystem (PLSS), the backpack astronauts wear during EVA, contains the oxygen tanks (1.2 lb [0.54 kg] at 518 atm tank pressure), carbon dioxide scrubbers/filters, cooling water (10 lb [4.6 kg] total), radio, electrical power, ventilating fans, and warning systems. Oxygen flows into the suit behind the astronaut's head and out of the suit at the feet and elbows. The air first flows through a charcoal cartridge to remove odors and then into the carbon dioxide scrubber cartridge. The gas then flows through a fan to a sublimator that removes water vapor for return to the cooling-water supply. Airflow temperature is maintained at 55°F (12.8°C). The PLSS provides up to 7 hours of oxygen supply and carbon dioxide removal. A complementary secondary oxygen pack (SOP) provides an emergency oxygen supply that fits below the PLSS on the backpack frame. Its two oxygen tanks contain 2.6 pounds (1.2 kg) at 408-atm tank pressure; this provides enough oxygen for 30 minutes, sufficient time for a crewmember to reenter the spacecraft. The system automatically turns on if the oxygen pressure in the suit drops below 0.23 atm.

HISTORICAL OVERVIEW OF AEROSPACE PHYSIOLOGY AND MEDICINE

This section highlights the early history of aerospace medicine, paying tribute to pioneers and their accomplishments that ushered in the modern space age. Today's astronauts must overcome numerous challenges as they prepare to live in space for prolonged periods. Perhaps during the middle of this century, thousands of individuals will routinely travel into space, some establishing permanent space colonies relatively near Earth orbit, while others participate in exploration-class missions to Mars and beyond.

In addition to experiencing varied gravitational forces, astronauts on Mars must contend with a hostile environment that includes viscous windstorms of several hundred miles per hour that can last for weeks, not to mention temperature extremes from −220°F to +81°F. The thin atmosphere consists mostly of carbon dioxide (93.5%), so living on Mars requires

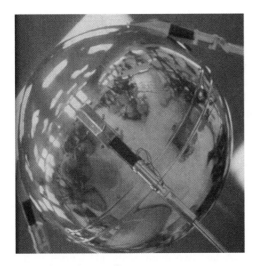

Figure 27.9 *Sputnik 1* satellite.

propulsion systems, physiologic requirements and adaptations to manned space flight, and more than 30,000 practical "technology-transfer" payoffs (discussed on p. 762) from interdisciplinary experiments in physical chemistry, microbiology, genetics, medicine, and exercise physiology.

National Aeronautics and Space Administration

Reacting swiftly to the perceived Soviet threat of technologic superiority, the United States Congress passed the National Aeronautics and Space Act signed into law on July 29, 1958 by President Dwight D. Eisenhower (1890–1969). As a new federal agency, NASA began operation on October 1, 1958, less than a year after the successful Sputnik-1 launch. For the first time in United States history, a single government agency had responsibility for conquering a new frontier only dreamt about by the early aeronaut explorers. These pioneers included Scottish meteorologists Drs. Alexander Wilson (1714–1786) and Thomas Melville from the University of Glasgow. These scientists, the first to record temperatures above the Earth's surface, in 1749 hoisted thermometers on six kites (balloons) to heights up to 3000 feet; thermometers were then dropped from different altitudes. Pilâtre de Rozier and Marquis d'Arlandes made the first manned hydrogen balloon free ascent to 85 m on November 21, 1783 (FIG. 27.10). The Montgolfier brothers Joseph and Etienne, in 1783 ascended in large-capacity hot air balloons that they designed. Their balloon, made of cloth and lined with paper and coated with alum as fireproofing, with about 2000 buttons holding its segments together, rose to 1000 m and traveled 2 km. The balloon was 75 feet tall, 49 feet wide, and contained 77,000 cubic feet of hot air heated by burning straw and wool. French physicist Jacques Alexandre César Charles (1746–1823; Charles' Law—at a fixed pressure, gas volume is proportional to its temperature) made one of the first untethered ascents with Professor M. N. Robert (1758–1820) in a hydrogen-filled, rubberized silk balloon Charles designed that covered about 44 km from liftoff in the Tuileries Gardens in Paris to Nesle. Upon landing, Robert departed and Charles soared alone in the wicker gondola with netting and valve-and-ballast system to a height of 9000 ft in about 10 minutes, making temperature and pressure measurements during the ascent; this was the first solo balloon flight (1783). Grey, Piccard, Anderson, and Steven flew in high-altitude balloons (1920s–1930s). Aida de Costa was the first woman to pilot a powered gasoline aircraft (dirigible) solo, in Paris on June 29, 1903, months before Orville (1871–1948) and Wilbur Wright's (1867–1912) flight. Scientists emerged such as Johannes Kepler (1571–1630), who penned an imaginary moon visit *(Somnium, sive Astronomia Lunaris)* and a cadre of science writers (e.g., Jules Verne, 1865, *De la Terre a la Lune;* Hale, *Brick Moon,* serialized in *Atlantic Monthly* magazine in 1869–1870; Eyraud, *Voyage a Venus,* 1875).

At its inception, NASA inherited 8000 employees and a $100 million budget; it supervised three major research laboratories (Langley Aeronautical Laboratory, established in 1918; Ames Aeronautical Laboratory, founded in 1940; and Lewis Flight Propulsion Laboratory, created in 1941).

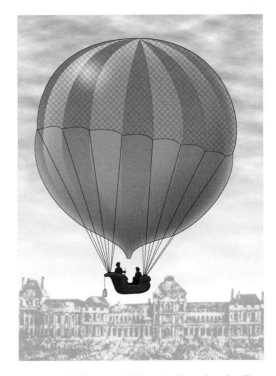

Figure 27.10 A physician (Pilâtre de Rozier) and military officer (Marquis d' Arlandes) made the first manned, sustained hydrogen balloon free ascent to 85 m, which lasted 25 minutes and covered 8 km over Paris, France, on November 21, 1783. The two men carried a pail of water and sponge to arrest sparks that often ignited small fires and threatened the 23-by-15-m balloon, which was made of painted cloth fabric and paper. The balloon weighed 725 kg (including a fire basket made of wrought iron wire) with an estimated lift (payload) of 770 kg. In 1785, de Rozier became the first fatality when his balloon exploded at about 1000 m.

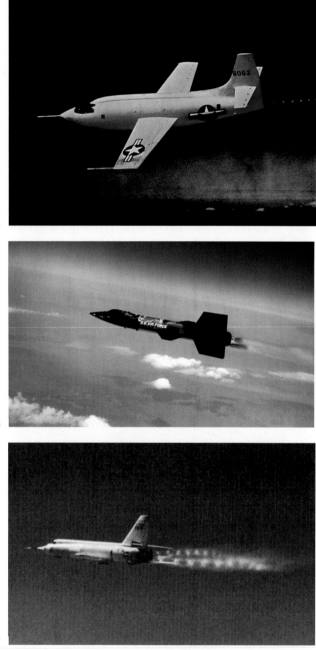

Figure 27.11 *Top.* The X-1 made the world's first supersonic flight (Mach 1.45) by breaking the sound barrier on October 14, 1947. The Douglas D-558-2 skyrocket (not shown) flew to Mach 2 on November 20, 1953. *Middle.* The X-2 achieved Mach 3 on September 27, 1956. *Bottom.* Top view of the X-15 during high altitude and speed trials. Test pilot Joe Walker flew the X-15 to a world-record altitude of 354,200 feet (67.1 mi) on August 22, 1963. Three years later on October 3, 1967, Peter Knight piloted the X-15 to Mach 6.7. His vehicle's launch weight (rocket plus fuel) was approximately 33,000 pounds (landing weight, 14,700 lb). The X-15 had a fuel capacity of 1003 gallons of liquid oxygen and 1445 gallons of anhydrous ammonia. (Photos from Stillwell WH. X-15. Research results with a selected bibliography. www.hq.nasa.gov/office/pao/History/SP-60/cover.html.)

NASA also supervised two smaller facilities at Monroc Dry Lake in the California desert for high-speed flight research and Wallops Island, Virginia, for testing rockets. NASA absorbed the Jet Propulsion Laboratory (www.jpl.nasa.gov)—managed by the California Institute of Technology and Army Ballistic Missile Agency—whose engineers were developing the massive rocket engines required for space flight. NASA assimilated the technical resources obtained from 13 prior years of jet aircraft research with the X-1 (that achieved Mach 1) and X-2 (that achieved Mach 3) rocket airplanes, including engineering information gleaned from hundreds of other rocket and jet airplane flights. FIGURE 27.11 shows the X-1, X-2, and X-15 rocket aircraft, the predecessors of NASA's successful but now aging shuttle aircraft.

NASA had two main goals: (1) launching a man into space and returning him safely to Earth and (2) developing the capability of humans to endure space missions.[109] Achieving this second goal had been a Herculean task because the current knowledge of microgravity's effects remained restricted to laboratory simulations. Scientists knew little about how humans would respond to the rigors of microgravity and what might happen during extended sojourns beyond Earth's gravitational field. Experts publicly expressed concern about possible deleterious effects of space flight on human function and overall health. In 1958, the National Academy of Sciences National Research Council Committee on Bioastronautics listed 30 potential ill effects from human exposure to the space environment during launch and reentry (TABLE 27.1). Some concerns proved justified and are discussed in subsequent sections.

In the race to become first in space, scientists could not afford the luxury of years to conduct systematic research. Instead, a test pilot's prior flight experience provided "seat-of-the pants" solutions to important aeronautical questions. The fully pressurized flight suits Navy test pilots used during high-altitude reconnaissance became the first "space suits" during the early rocket missions. This allowed NASA to proceed on a fast track toward eventually putting a human into space.

United States Races into Space

NASA's top priority besides initiating human space flight centered on a plan to allow humans to work for extended periods during prolonged space missions. These two goals required advanced technologies in rocket design and effective approaches to prepare test pilots for missions never attempted previously. To put a human into Earth orbit required new ways of looking at the man–machine interface. On the human side, engineers had to design a fail–safe life-support system, provide for food and water, integrate an efficient method to remove metabolic byproducts, and implement temperature control to ensure crew safety during liftoff, flight, and reentry. Research had to determine physiologic responses to extremes of acceleration and reduced gravity, including short- and long-term adjustments to prolonged weightlessness. Could a human function competently

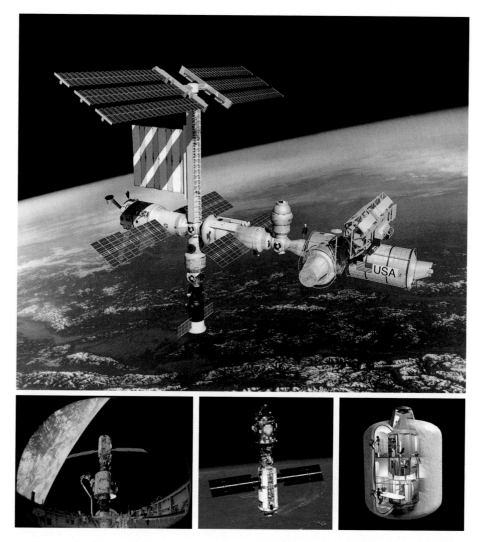

Figure 27.12 *Top.* The International Space Station (ISS), the most complex (and expensive) construction project ever undertaken, involves 16 nations. The program uses more than 100,000 people at space agencies and hundreds of contractors and subcontractors worldwide. The 460-ton ISS necessitates 45 United States and Russian rocket missions to launch and assemble the more than 100 major components. When completed, the ISS will have a mass of about 1,040,000 pounds and measure 356 feet across and 290 feet long. Construction will require 160 spacewalks (approximately 1800 h) by pairs of astronauts. A shuttle mission to visit the ISS during 2002 delivered the Expedition 6 crew and P1 (P-One) Truss. The space shuttle fleet was grounded following the loss of Space Shuttle *Columbia* on Feb. 1, 2003. Mission LF1 on July 26, 2005, the return-to-flight mission, restocked the station with supplies and equipment. The next mission in March 2006 will deliver cargo and supplies and test new equipment and safety procedures. Three crew exchanges have occurred since that time using Soyuz spacecraft instead of shuttles. *Bottom left.* A robot arm from the Space Shuttle *Endeavor* lifts *Unity*, the first of the ISS modules, to join the Russian control module *Zayra. Bottom middle.* ISS view from STS-96 *Discovery* during a fly-around following separation of the American and Russian spacecraft. *Bottom right.* Computer-generated cutaway view of the Translab Module, ISS's large-volume (12,000 ft^3) habitation module.

TABLE 27.1 ■ POTENTIAL DELETERIOUS EFFECTS OF WEIGHTLESSNESS FOR LAUNCH, TRAVEL, AND REENTRY

• Anorexia	• Bone demineralization
• Nausea	• Renal calculi
• Disorientation	• Motion sickness
• Sleeplessness	• Pulmonary atelectasis
• Fatigue	• Tachycardia
• Restlessness	• Hypertension
• Euphoria	• Hypotension
• Hallucinations	• Cardiac arrhythmia
• Decreased g tolerance	• Postflight syncope
• Gastrointestinal disturbance	• Decreased work capacity
• Urine retention	• Reduced blood volume
• Diuresis	• Reduced plasma volume
• Muscular incoordination	• Dehydration
• Muscle atrophy	• Weight loss
• Sleepiness	• Infectious illnesses

Modified from Dietlein LF. Skylab: a beginning. In: Johnston RS, Dietlein LF, eds. Biomedical results from Skylab (NASA SP-377). Washington, DC: U.S. Government Printing Office, 1977.

during liftoff, propelled upward at thousands of miles per hour and then perform flawlessly in maneuvering the space vehicle and returning it to Earth safely? Engineers needed to develop rocket engines with sufficient thrust to achieve escape velocity. The pilot's capsule required intricate communication and navigation controls. The capsule's weight and size had to dovetail with rocket design and launch requirements. In addition, a capsule recovery system required development for safe reentry. The human and engineering requirements facing NASA provided considerable challenges to say the least, but the race into space was on with no turning back.

The current human space program owes a debt of gratitude to thousands of men and women from many countries whose imaginations and careers spearheaded possibilities of space exploration. The following sections review key achievements of the United States and Russian space programs related to advances in space medicine and physiology. These superpowers played the dominant role in the space effort, but not without significant contributions from European, Japanese, and Canadian human space programs. Their remarkable successes culminated in the launches (Nov. and Dec. 1998) of Russian and United States rockets to initiate assembly of the ISS (FIG. 27.12). On October 30, 2000, the Soyuz *Expedition 1* crew began its rendezvous with the ISS for a 4-month stay to prepare the ISS for future missions to continue the on-orbit assembly. This included installation of solar arrays and batteries, thermal control systems, communications equipment, and the 8.5-m long, 4.3-m diameter U.S. Laboratory Module *Destiny*, the centerpiece of the ISS for conducting fundamental scientific experiments. The *Destiny* focused on basic and applied research in biotechnology, fluid physics, combustion, and the life sciences.

Following the *Columbia* STS-107 Shuttle catastrophe in February 2003, NASA scuttled future missions to complete the ISS until mission-critical recommendations could be made. The shuttle disaster was caused by a chunk of insulating foam that broke away from the external fuel tank during liftoff and damaged the left wing. The *Columbia*, with a crew of seven astronauts, disintegrated during reentry into the Earth's atmosphere following a successful 16-day science mission. Shuttle *Discovery* resumed the ambitious NASA schedule on July 26, 2005 (see timeline, p. 711) to work on construction of the ISS. NASA plans 28 shuttle flights to finish building the ISS by 2010.

United States Human Space Program

TABLE 27.2 summarizes the salient accomplishments of NASA's human space program beginning with Project Mercury and continuing with Gemini, Apollo, Skylab, Apollo-Soyuz, and Space Shuttle. Voluminous medical data exist from the initial six Mercury flights (1961–1963) to the present extended-duration flights of the United States and Soviet cooperative endeavors. NASA currently oversees 15 flight and research facilities in the United States (www.nasa.gov/about/highlights/index.html).

Perhaps the most significant technologic achievement of the 20th century took place on July 20, 1969, when *Apollo 11* astronauts Edwin "Buzz" Aldrin (1930–; www.buzzaldrin.com/) and Neil Armstrong (1930–; www.grc.nasa.gov/www/pao/html/neilabio.htm) landed on the moon's surface in the lunar module *Eagle* after it separated from the main spacecraft at 50,000 feet (FIG. 27.13). With these words, "Houston, Tranquility Base here. The *Eagle* has landed," the world knew a momentous accomplishment had taken place. Seven hours later, Armstrong's hopeful words as he set foot on the lunar

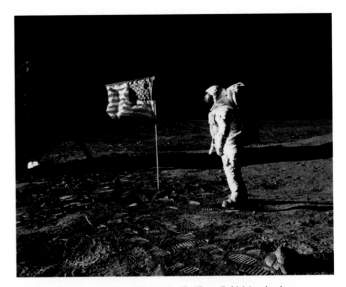

Figure 27.13 Astronaut Edwin E. "Buzz" Aldrin, Jr., lunar module pilot of the first lunar landing mission, poses beside the deployed United States flag (stiffened by inserts) during *Apollo 11* EVA on the lunar surface (July 20, 1969). The lunar module is darkly outlined on the left, and the astronaut's footprints are visible in the soil (foreground).

TABLE 27.2 ■ ACCOMPLISHMENTS OF THE UNITED STATES AND SOVIET HUMAN SPACE PROGRAMS: FROM PROJECT MERCURY TO THE INTERNATIONAL SPACE STATION

PROGRAM	YEARS	ACCOMPLISHMENTS
Project Mercury	May 1961 to May 1963 Feb 12, 1962 May 15–16, 1963	Twenty unmanned missions; two suborbital, four orbital manned missions. Longest flight 34 h, 19 min, 49 s; 22 Earth orbits. Alan Shepard, (1923–1998) first U.S. astronaut makes suborbital flight of 15 min, 28 s on May 5, 1961 (5 astronauts completed successful missions) John Glenn became the first American to orbit Earth (3 times), in spacecraft *Friendship 7* Astronaut L. Gordon Cooper piloted *Faith 7* during a 22-orbit mission, becoming the first astronaut to launch a satellite (beacon) while in orbital flight and first American to reentry in manual mode (maximum orbital speed achieved was 17,546.6 mph at a perigee of 100.2 and apogee of 165.9 statute mi). His flight suit temperature reached 92°F and 109°F cabin temperature
Project Gemini	May 1961 to Nov 1966	Two unmanned missions; 10 human space missions; first U.S. extra-vehicular activity (EVA; 22 min on *Gemini IV*); first rendezvous and docking (*Gemini VIII*; 6 h, 33 min after liftoff); first use of fuel cells for electrical power; evaluation of guidance and naviga-tion systems for future rendezvous missions; bio-medical experiments successfully conducted on *Gemini IV, V, VII*. Longest EVA on last *Gemini XII* (5 h, 30 min) The Kennedy Space Center (KSC) at Cape Canaveral, FL, serves as the primary launch facility for the U.S. Space Program. Over a 20-month period (Mar 1965 to Nov 1966), the 10 Project Gemini human missions built a bridge between the relatively "simple" Mercury flights and the technologically challenging Apollo moon program. They accomplished rendezvous between two spacecraft in orbit, mastered space docking, and made the first controlled re-entries to Earth
Apollo Program	Oct 1961 to Dec 1972	Six unmanned Apollo-Saturn missions; 12 manned missions achieved significant biomedical results concerning physiologic responses: • Vestibular disturbances • Suboptimal food consumption (1260–2903 kCal · d^{-1}) • Postflight dehydration and weight loss • Decreased postflight orthostatic tolerance from tilt tests • Reduced postflight orthostatic tolerance first 3 days • Cardiac arrhythmias (*Apollo 15*) • Decreased red cell mass (2–10%) and plasma volume (4–9%) **Moon Flights:** *Apollo 10* launched from KSC on May 18, 1969, on a 9-day mission. The spacecraft orbited the moon and the lunar module (LM) descended to an altitude of 15 km over the planned site for the first lunar landing. Color TV was transmitted to Earth. The command module (CM) landed safely in the Pacific May 26, 1969 *Apollo 11* orbits the moon; Apollo astronauts Neil Armstrong and Edwin Aldrin Jr. became the first men to walk on the moon. The spacecraft returned and landed in the Pacific on July 24, 1969, fulfilling the space goal set by President Kennedy on May 25, 1961

continued on page 710

TABLE 27.2 ■ *continued*

PROGRAM	YEARS	ACCOMPLISHMENTS

Apollo Program, *continued*

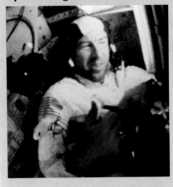

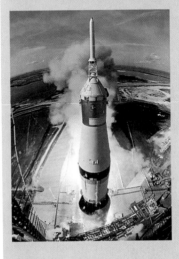

Apollo 12 launched on Nov. 14, 1969, and landed on the moon 163 m from the *Surveyor III* spacecraft. The two astronauts performed two EVAs on the lunar surface; retrieved samples and pans of *Surveyor III*; left the lunar surface after a stay of 31 h, 31 min; redocked and landed in the Pacific on Nov. 24, 1969

Apollo 13 launched on a lunar landing mission on April 11, 1970, but 7 h, 55 min into the flight an explosion in an oxygen tank required an abort. The astronauts powered up the LM and used the LM propellant for a free-return trajectory around the moon. They returned safely to Earth and landed in the mid-Pacific on April 17

Apollo 14 launched from KSC on Jan. 31, 1971, and the LM landed on the Fra Mauro area of the moon on February 5. Two EVAs were performed, the second using a mobile equipment transporter to permit a longer traverse. The LM lifted off from the moon February 6 and the CM splashed down in the Pacific on Feb. 9, 1970

Apollo 15 launched July 26, 1971, and on July 30 the LM landed in the Hadley-Apennine region of the moon. Three EVAs were completed with a total EVA time of 18 h, 35 min. The LM ascent stage liftoff on August 2 was the first televised, and the lunar roving vehicle was used for the first time. *Apollo 15's* CM landed in the Pacific on August 7, 1971

Apollo 16 launched from KSC on April 16, 1972, and landed in the moon's Descartes region April 20. Three EVAs were completed using the lunar roving vehicle for a distance of 26.7 km. The LM lifted off April 23 and docked with the command service module (CSM) to transfer astronauts and samples. The CM landed in the Pacific April 27

Apollo 17, the final manned lunar landing mission, launched from KSC on Dec. 7, 1972. The astronauts in the LM landed in the Taurus-Littrow region of the moon on Dec. 11 and explored the area on the lunar roving vehicle during three 22-h EVAs. Lift-off occurred on Dec. 14, and the CM landed in the Pacific Dec. 19

Project Skylab Program

May 1973 to Feb 1974

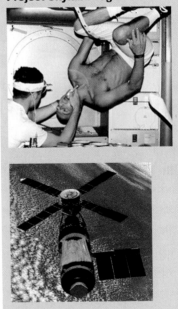

One unmanned and three manned missions

Skylab 1 (unmanned) launched into orbit May 14, 1973, by a Saturn V booster. Almost immediately, technical problems developed due to vibrations during lift-off. A critical meteoroid shield ripped off, taking one of the craft's two solar panels with it; a piece of the shield wrapped around the other panel, keeping it from deploying. *Skylab 1* maneuvered so its Apollo Telescope Mount (ATM) solar panels faced the sun to maximize electricity. Because of the loss of the meteoroid shield, workshop temperatures increased to 52°C (126° F). The *Skylab 2* launch was postponed while NASA engineers trained (10 d) the crew to make the workshop habitable. The engineers "rolled" *Skylab 1* to lower workshop temperature. Extensive scientific studies on 28-, 59-, and 85-day missions showed humans could live and work in space for extended periods using countermeasures against deleterious adaptations

Skylab 2, first manned mission, launched May 25, 1973, for 28 d, 50 min. The crew rendezvoused with *Skylab 1* on the fifth orbit. After making substantial repairs, including deployment of a parasol sunshade that cooled the inside temperature to 23.8°C (75°F), by June 4 the workshop became fully operational. The crew conducted solar astronomy and Earth resources experiments, medical studies, and five student experiments; 404 orbits and 392 experiment-hours completed; three EVAs totaled 6 h, 20 min

continued on page 711

TABLE 27.2 ■ *continued*

PROGRAM	YEARS	ACCOMPLISHMENTS
Project Skylab Program, *continued*		*Skylab 3* (July 28–Sep. 25, 1973; 59 d, 11 h). Continued maintenance of the space station and extensive scientific and medical experiments completed. Completed 858 Earth orbits and 1081 hours of solar and Earth experiments; three EVAs totaled 13 h, 43 min *Skylab 4* (Nov. 16, 1973–Feb. 8, 1974; 84 d, 1 h). Last of the Skylab missions; included observation of the comet *Kohoutek* among numerous experiments. Completed 1214 Earth orbits and four EVAs totaling 22 h, 13 min
Apollo-Soyuz Test Project (ASTP) 	July 1975 (9 d)	First U.S. and Soviet project that successfully tested rendezvous and docking systems and medical and technical cooperation from July 15–24, 1975 (9 d, 7 h, 28 min). The *Soyuz* launched just over 7 hours before launch of the *Apollo* CSM. *Apollo* then maneuvered to rendezvous and docked 52 h after the *Soyuz* launch. The *Apollo* and *Soyuz* crews conducted diverse exper-iments for 2 d. After separation, *Apollo* remained in space an additional 6 d. *Soyuz* returned to Earth approx-imately 43 h after separation
Space Shuttle Program 	Mar 1979	First reusable spacecraft that operated under sea-level atmospheric pressure while in orbit. The pressurized Spacelab module provides a sophisticated scientific laboratory to study physiologic and medical aspects of extended flight, including extended EVA
	Mar 8, 2001 to Aug 2001	The crew worked with 18 different experiments. Shuttle Flight STS-104 (July 12, 2001) consisted of five assembly and resupply flights, including the Joint Airlock. STS-105 launched August 9, 2001. The mission rotated the ISS crew, bringing water, equipment, and supplies to the station and completed a series of spacewalks and robotics tasks
	Mar 2002 to Dec 2002	Shuttle flights STS-109–STS-113 provided pay-loads to the ISS, including the successful serv-icing of the Hubble Space Telescope (STS-109)
	Jan 16, 2003 to Feb 1, 2003	Shuttle *Columbia* (STS-107) with a crew of seven astronauts disintegrated during reentry into the Earth's atmosphere following a successful 16-day science mission dedicated to research in physical, life, and space sciences. The mission conducted approx-imately 80 separate exper-iments, comprising hun-dreds of samples and test points. The photo (*left*) is a tribute to the memory of the crew of Space Shuttle *Columbia*
	Jul 26, 2005 to Aug 21, 2005	The launch of Space Shuttle *Discovery* (STS 114) ended a 2½-year wait for the historic return-to-flight mission. NASA accomplished many goals while learning important lessons. At liftoff, a large piece of insulating foam broke off the External Tank. Using the new Orbiter Boom Sensor System, *Discovery* crewmembers took an unprecedented up-close look at the orbiter's thermal protection system. This also included the first-ever "rendezvous pitch maneuver" as the orbiter approached the ISS for docking. During the first of three spacewalks, the astronauts tested new repair techniques for the outer skin of the space shuttle's heat shield and installed equipment outside the station. They also repaired a failed Control Moment Gyro. Two thermal protection tile gap-fillers were spotted jutting from *Discovery*'s underside, protrusions that could have caused above-normal temperatures on the shuttle during atmospheric reentry. An astronaut rode the station's robotic arm and retrieved the gap-fillers without incident.

continued on page 712

TABLE 27.2 ■ *continued*

PROGRAM	YEARS	ACCOMPLISHMENTS
International Space Station 		The International Space Station (ISS), an international coop-erative research platform, provides a state-of-the-art research facility; studies gravity's effects on physical, chemical, and biologic systems; and serves as an advanced facility for technology and human exploration and a commercial platform for space research and development. The ISS is designed to accomplish three main goals: (1) advance scientific knowledge; (2) live, explore, and work productively in space; and (3) use attributes of space to improve products and processes on Earth. Major research areas include fundamental biology, physical science (materials science, biotechnology, fundamental physics, fluid physics, combustion), biomedical research and coun-termeasures, advanced human support technology, space science, and Earth observation
	Nov 1998 to Feb 2002	Dec 7, 1998, Shuttle *Endeavor* mated *Unity* module with Russian control module *Zayra*
	Nov 2000 to Feb 2001	Four modules on-orbit (*Unity* node; *Zarya* functional cargo block; *Zvezda* service module, U.S. Lab *Destiny*). Five assembly and resupply flights. Expedition I crew arrived November 2, 2000 on *Soyuz*
	Feb 2001 to Jun 2001	Six assembly and resupply flights (lab outfitting and remote manipulator); major focus on radiation research, bone and muscle studies, psychosocial studies, fluids science, protein crystallization. Expedition 2 crew arrived February 2001 on shuttle
	Jun 2001 to Oct 2001	Studies of subregional bone and muscle structure and function; effects of prolonged space flight on human skeletal muscle (pre/postflight measurements); crystal growth, cell biology, pulmonary function, susceptibility to renal stone formation
	Oct 2001 to Feb 2002	Studies of multiple plant experiments in space, biomass production, astroculture, commercial generic bioprocessing, biologic habitats, centrifuge, physical sciences apparatus (fluids, laser cooling, low temperature, materials science, alpha magnetic spectrometry)
	Mar 8, 2001 to Aug 2001	Expedition 2 arrived on Space Shuttle *Discovery* (STS-102) March 8, 2001, with the Multi-Purpose Logistics Module (unpiloted, reusable cargo cylindrical carrier 6.4 m long and 4.5 m diameter, 4.5 tons, that provides equipment and supplies for the *Destiny* module. This new module also included components that provide life support, fire detection and suppression, electrical distribution, and computer functions. The crew worked with 18 different experiments. Shuttle Flight STS-104 (July 12, 2001) consisted of five assembly and resupply flights, including the Joint Airlock. STS-105 launched August 9, 2001. The mission rotated the ISS crew, bringing water, equipment and supplies to the station and completed a series of spacewalks and robotics tasks
	Dec 2001 to Apr 2005	The next flight, STS-108, arrived at the station in early December 2001 and delivered the *Expedition* 4 crew. The first shuttle mission to visit the station in 2002 was STS-110. The seven-member crew installed the S0 (S-Zero) Truss onto the station. The S0 was the second piece of the 11-piece Integrated Truss Structure delivered to the station. The second shuttle mission of 2002 to visit the station was STS-111 in mid-June. STS-111 delivered the Expedition 5 crew and the Mobile Base System to the orbital outpost. Also, STS-111 returned the Expedition 4 crew to Earth. Carl Walz and Dan Bursch set the record for the longest U.S. space flight with 196 days in space during Expedition 4. Outward expansion of the station occurred during STS-112 with the delivery of the S1 Truss that was attached to the starboard side of the S0 Truss. STS-113, the last shuttle mission to visit the ISS during 2002, delivered the Expedition 6 crew and P1 Truss. The STS-113 crew performed three spacewalks to activate and outfit P1 after it was attached to the port side of the S0 Truss. Expedition 5 returned to Earth on Shuttle *Endeavour,* wrapping up a 6-month space stay. Five crew exchanges occurred since the loss of Space Shuttle *Columbia* using Soyuz spacecraft instead of shuttles.

continued on page 713

TABLE 27.2 ■ *continued*

PROGRAM	ACCOMPLISHMENTS
International Space Station, *continued* 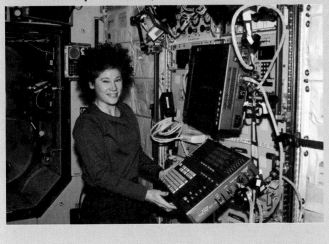	The STS-114 mission delivered a new control moment gyroscope (External Stowage Platform-2) and tons of much-needed supplies to the station. During three spacewalks, the crew installed the platform on the Quest airlock, replaced one gyroscope and repaired another. The ISS *Soyuz 6* spacecraft delivered the Expedition 7 crew to the ISS on April 28, 2003 to replace Expedition 6, which returned to Earth aboard the ISS *Soyuz 5* spacecraft. Expedition 7 was the station's first two-person crew. Expedition 8 arrived at the ISS on Oct. 20, 2003. Commander Michael Foale and Flight Engineer Alexander Kaleri became the first Expedition crew to perform a spacewalk without a crewmember inside the station. The ISS *Soyuz 8* spacecraft delivered the Expedition 9 crew to the station on April 21, 2004. The Expedition 11 crew arrived aboard a Soyuz spacecraft in April 2005.

Resources:
Johnston RS. Introduction. In: Biomedical results of Apollo (NASA SP-368). Johnson RS, et al., eds. Washington, DC: U.S. Government Printing Office, pp. 3–7, 1975.
Link MM. Space medicine in Project Mercury (NASA SP-4003). Washington, DC: U.S. Government Printing Office, 1965.
Nicogossian AE, et. al. Space physiology and medicine. 3rd ed. Philadelphia: Lea & Febiger, 1994. www.spaceflight.NASA.gov.

surface—"One small step for man, one giant leap for mankind"—resonated worldwide to demonstrate that humans could travel to the moon, explore its surface, and return safely to Earth. Aldrin joined him on the surface several minutes later, and for 2 hours they collected rocks, planted the American flag on lunar soil in the Sea of Tranquility, and took photographs. Thus, it had taken almost a decade and $25.4 billion to achieve the goal President John F. Kennedy (1917–1963) first stated on May 25, 1961:

> I believe that this nation should commit itself to achieving the goal, before this decade is out, of landing a man on the Moon and returning him safely to the Earth. No single space project in this period will be more impressive to mankind, or more important for the long-range exploration of space; and none will be so difficult or expensive to accomplish.

Indeed, the Apollo program achieved its three main objectives: (1) ensuring the safety and health of crew members, (2) preventing contamination of Earth by extraterrestrial organisms, and (3) studying specific effects of space exposure on the human body. During the Apollo program, 12 astronauts walked on the moon during six lunar landings. TABLE 27.3 summarizes this program's significant medical findings.

Soviet Space Program

The Soviet human space program began in 1957 when *Sputnik 1* crystallized the United States' efforts to join the race into space. The first Soviet cosmonaut in space, Lt. Colonel Yuri Gagarin (FIGURE 27.14; 1934–1968; killed in plane

crash), prepared for manned space flight as a test pilot in the Vostok program. On April 12, 1961, Gagarin completed a single Earth orbit in 108 minutes and ejected from the Vostok spacecraft at 7000 m in a parachute landing. The Soviets withheld the news that Gagarin might have perished when the Vostok spacecraft malfunctioned on reentry. His return unharmed scored another key space victory for the Soviet Union in their quest for supremacy in space. Longer duration missions for up to 5 days in space followed this historic flight. The

TABLE 27.3 ■ SIGNIFICANT BIOMEDICAL FINDINGS FROM APOLLO SPACE MISSIONS

- Vestibular disturbances
- In-flight cardiac arrhythmia
- Reduced postflight orthostatic tolerance
- Reduced postflight exercise tolerance
- Postflight dehydration and weight loss
- Flight diet adequate; food consumption suboptimal
- Decreased red cell mass, plasma volume
- Negative in-flight balance trend for nitrogen, calcium, other electrolytes
- Increased in-flight adrenal hormone secretion
- No in-flight diuresis

Dietlein LF. Summary and conclusions. In: Biomedical results from Skylab (NASA SP-377). Johnston RS, Dietlein LF, eds. Washington, DC: U.S. Government Printing Office 1977:579.

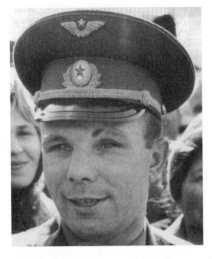

Figure 27.14 Pioneer cosmonaut Yuri A. Gagarin ("Columbus of the Cosmos"; 1934–1968), the first human to orbit the Earth, in the *Vostok I* spacecraft.

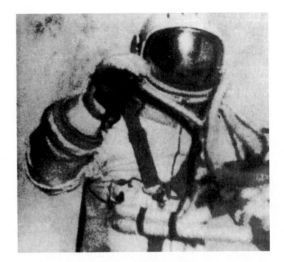

Figure 27.16 Cosmonaut Aleksei Leonov (1934–), copilot of *Voskhod 2*, performed the first EVA for 10 minutes during the second orbit of a 1-day flight before returning safely to the spacecraft through an inflatable airlock, but not without first releasing air from his spacesuit as a desperate measure when he had difficulty reentering the narrow passageway (March 18, 1964). The Soviets did not disclose this brush with disaster, so Leonov returned a hero, once again demonstrating Soviet supremacy in space. Leonov also served as command pilot for *Soyuz 19* in the Apollo-Soyuz Test Project (July 15–21, 1975).

first woman in space, Valentina Tereshkova (FIG. 27.15), flew in *Vostok 6* in 1963, the last mission of this series. The two succeeding Soviet missions, named Voskhad, advanced space science by completing the first EVA that lasted 8 minutes (manned by cosmonaut Aleksei Leonov [FIG. 27.16], who exited the spacecraft through a canvas tube attached to the *Voskhod 2*) and medical studies of lung function, middle-ear (vestibular) function, blood pressure, muscular strength (hand grip), and blood composition from the first blood sample taken during weightlessness by Dr. Boris Yegorov, the first space physician.

The next period of Soviet exploration included manned flight aboard the advanced *Soyuz 1* spacecraft, but a tragic accident stalled several planned rendezvous and docking missions. In January 1969, Soyuz flights 4 and 5 completed

mission-critical maneuvers (rendezvous, docking, EVA transfer) for a future moon landing. Unfortunately, four unmanned spacecraft designed to test a powerful booster rocket needed to achieve moon orbit exploded on launch, canceling that phase of the program. One year later, the 18-day Soyuz mission included extensive experiments to evaluate microgravity's effects on heart function, vision, muscular strength, and hematologic variables. Unfortunately, an in-flight exercise countermeasures effort did *not* reduce problems experienced with balance (one aspect of orthostatic intolerance) and muscle weakness.

April 19, 1971 marked the launch of the world's first space station, *Salyut 1* (FIG. 27.17). Forty-nine days later, three cosmonauts from *Soyuz 11* boarded *Salyut 1* to become the space station's first crew. Over the next 6 years, the Soviets launched four additional Salyut space stations, the cosmonauts performing biomedical experiments involving humans on 24 missions,[10] but only 5 experiments considered successful. The longest mission (*Soyuz 18*) lasted 63 days. Subsequent missions on advanced *Salyut 6* and *Salyut 7* space stations lengthened flight duration and increased the number of crewmembers. Between 1977 and 1981, five two-man crews completed flights of 96, 140, 175, 185, and 74 days. Thirteen other crews completed shorter flights. During the Salyut-6 program, the Soviets accumulated about 3 years of flight experience and 5 hours of EVA. In 1982, two cosmonauts accumulated 211 days in orbit. American and Soviet cooperation in space commenced during July 15–24, 1975 with the first docking of an Apollo spacecraft with a Soyuz spacecraft (Apollo–Soyuz Test Project or ASTP). This mission established the basis for future American–

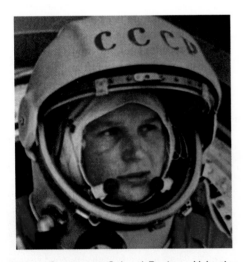

Figure 27.15 Cosmonaut Colonel-Engineer Valentina Tereshkova (1937–) the first woman in space, orbited Earth 48 times during a 3-day flight (June 17–19, 1963). Nineteen years later, Svetlana Savitskaya became the second Russian woman in space (1982, 1984).

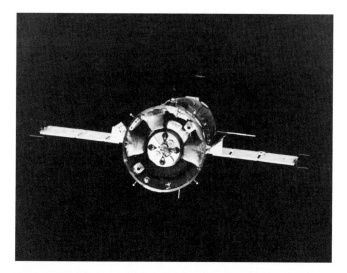

Figure 27.17 *Salyut 1*, the first scientific space station, launched from the Baikonur launch cosmodrome (Kazakhstan, Russia) on June 6,1971 and stayed in orbit for 23.8 days. The 6790-kg station included a telescope, spectrometer, electrophotometer, and television. The crew conducted medical-biologic experiments.

Russian cooperation between the American Space Shuttle and Mir Space Station. The 143-ton Mir, almost twice as heavy as Skylab (76 tons) and the largest manufactured object in space ($4.2 billion to build and maintain), was purposely deorbited after 15 years of unprecedented scientific achievements (46 expeditions and 23,000 experiments, including the longest continuous space mission [438 d] and 16 spacewalks totaling 77 h). Mir plunged in fiery descent from the Earth's atmosphere into the Pacific Ocean on March 22, 2001. Twenty-two years earlier, the first U.S. space station Skylab, despite three repair attempts to save this science space station from failure after only 6 years in orbit, also met a fiery reentry from Earth's atmosphere in the southeastern Indian Ocean on July 11, 1979.

EVA Medical Support on the Mir Space Station. Thirty-six male crewmembers participated in 78 two-person EVAs conducted during the Mir Space Program since its inception in 1986.[74] The maximum length of a space walk was 7 h:14 min, total duration of all space walks was 717.1 man-hours, and maximum frequency of EVAs was 10 per year. Sixty-seven EVAs were performed at mission elapsed time that ranged from 31 to 180 days. The Orlan space suit (FIG. 27.18) oxygen atmosphere of 40 kPa (kPa refers to spacesuit pressure; multiply kPa by 0.1451 to convert kPA vacuum pressure units to psi), combined with a normobaric cabin environment and a 30-minute oxygen prebreathe protocol produced no incidence of decompression sickness. At peak EVA activity, metabolic rate ranged from 9.9 to 13 kCal $\cdot$ min^{-1}, and heart rate ranged from 150 to 174 b $\cdot$ min^{-1}. All of the EVAs were completed safely. Minor medical problems included feelings of moderate overcooling during a rest period in a shadow outside of the capsule following a difficult work period, some tachycardia accompanied by cardiac rhythm disorders at moments of emotional

stress, minor muscle soreness, and general tiredness following a high-workload EVA. Interestingly, Skylab crews went from a ground-based, sea-level launch environment to the 34.5 kPa (5.0 psi) environment of the Skylab cabin, which contained 70% oxygen and 30% nitrogen, and did not experience any difference in energy expenditure and alertness. During prolonged Russian flights of up to 1 year, cabin pressure is maintained at 101.4 kPa (14.71 psi at 21% oxygen), while spacesuit pressure for the Orlan-M is 38 kPa (5.52 psi) using 100% oxygen. On typical 10-day shuttle missions, the cabin pressure is the same as in the Russian spacecraft, but spacesuit pressure is lower at 29.6 kPa (4.29 psi).

Chinese Space Program

On October 15, 2003, China launched its first manned space flight mission, *Shenzhou 5* (*Shenzhou* means divine vessel) from the 2000 square mile Jiuquan Satellite Launch Center (JSLC) in northwest China's Gansu Province. The rocket, a CZ-2F launch vehicle, is a 2-stage, 50-m tall core vehicle with four strap-on stages. The rocket is powered by UDMH (unsymmetrical dimethylhydrazine [$(CH_3)_2NHH_2$]),

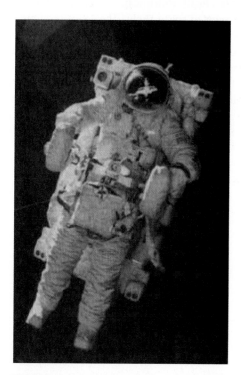

Figure 27.18 The Russian Orlan spacesuit consists of flexible limbs attached to a one-piece rigid body/helmet unit. Cosmonauts entered the suit through a hatch in the rear of the torso. The exterior of the hatch housed the life support equipment established as a 9-hour EVA. No external hoses are required as in American space suits. Electrical power and communications occur via an umbilical cord to the space vehicle. The suit was operated via a chest panel with the markings in mirror image, which the cosmonaut viewed using a wrist-worn reflective mirror on the suit. The following web site provides an in-depth review (including audio and animations) of the life support systems used by the Russian and American space programs: paperairplane.mit.edu/16.423J/ Space/SBE/projects/LSSWEBSITE/Pages/physiology.htm.

a hypergolic liquid rocket fuel derived from hydrazine and nitrogen tetroxide. Ten minutes after liftoff, the modified Russian Soyuz capsule module entered an initial 200-km × 343-km orbit piloted by 38-year-old Lt. Col. Yang Liwei, China's first man in space. FIGURE 27.19 shows the location of the JSLC with the rocket used in the launch, and the reentry, kettle-shaped capsule that touched down only 4.8 km from the anticipated grasslands landing site in Inner Mongolia. The single-pilot flight circled the globe 14 times in the 21 h:31 min-long mission. Ground stations in China, Namibia, and the South Pacific-island of Kiribati with ship-based tracking in the Indian, Atlantic, and Pacific Oceans tracked the spacecraft. The mission catapulted China into an elite group of nations capable of independent human space flight.

The reentry module that remained in orbit was outfitted with solar power panels and rocket motors to perform subsequent scientific experiments to prepare for future space ventures. These included launching *Shenzhou 6* and *Shenzhou 7* in a late 2005 and 2007 timeframe to conduct two-man space walks and docking and eventual three-man missions around the moon and return to earth by 2010.

Shenzhou Flight Planning. China has a long history of planning manned space flight. The space program known as Project 921 officially began in 1992, but preparations for manned orbital flight had begun in 1968 with the founding of the Spaceflight Medical Research Center and launches of China's first DFH-1 satellite. During the 1970s and 1980s, China launched test rockets, developed strategies for satellite recovery, and began human studies to assess physiologic responses to microgravity. The Chinese joined with Russian counterparts in cooperative space ventures that included astronaut training at the Yuri Gagarin Cosmonaut Training Center. This cooperation included development of a new launch vehicle patterned after the successful Soyuz space vehicle.

The inaugural unmanned Shenzhou flight took place on November 20, 1999 from the Jiuquan Satellite Launch Center. The first test flight lasted 21 h:11 min, and made 14 Earth orbits. The spacecraft performed without life support and emergency escape systems, and no experimental payloads were onboard. In January 2001, *Shenzhou 2*, the next vehicle in the series, stayed aloft for 7 d:10 h:22 min and made 117 orbits. The flight carried 64 experimental payloads that included 15 in the reentry module, 12 in the orbital module, and 37 on the forward external pallet. The experiments included a microgravity crystal-growing device, life sciences experiments with 19 species of animals and plants, cosmic ray and particle detectors, and China's first gamma ray burst detectors. *Shenzhou 3*, a precursor flight to a planned mission, was launched in March 2002. The flight included life support and emergency escape systems, and a dummy astronaut to test reliability of the required life-support system in a space environment. The flight lasted 6 d:18 h:51 min during 107 orbits. Nine months later on December 30, 2002, the *Shenzhou 4* launched carrying a fully functioning crew module with two dummy astronauts to assess viability for the planned *Shenzhou 5* manned launch. The spaceship carried 52 science payloads for Earth observation, space environment monitoring, microgravity fluid physics, and biotechnology research. The spacecraft remained in Earth orbit for 7 days and made 107 orbits.

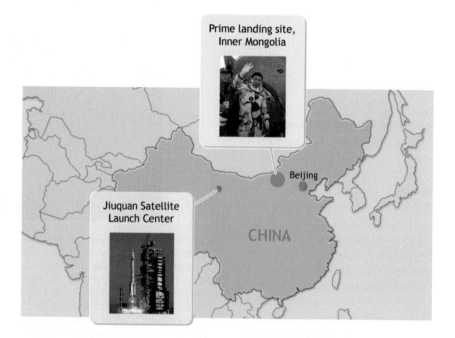

Figure 27.19 China's entry into human space flight puts that nation into an exclusive club—the third country to launch humans into space. The first Chinese astronaut, Yang Liwei, piloted *Shenzhou 5* in Earth orbit 14 times during the inaugural 21-hour mission. On October 12, 2005, the *Shenzhou 6* space capsule carried astronauts Fei Junlong and Nie Haisheng on a 5-day flight 210 miles above Earth. The newest space travelers—called "yuhangyuans" or "taikonauts," the Chinese term for space navigator—successfully landed 5 days later on October 17, 2005 at the Inner Mongolian landing site. The *Shenzhou 7* flight will involve an EVA and an unmanned probe to the moon by 2010.

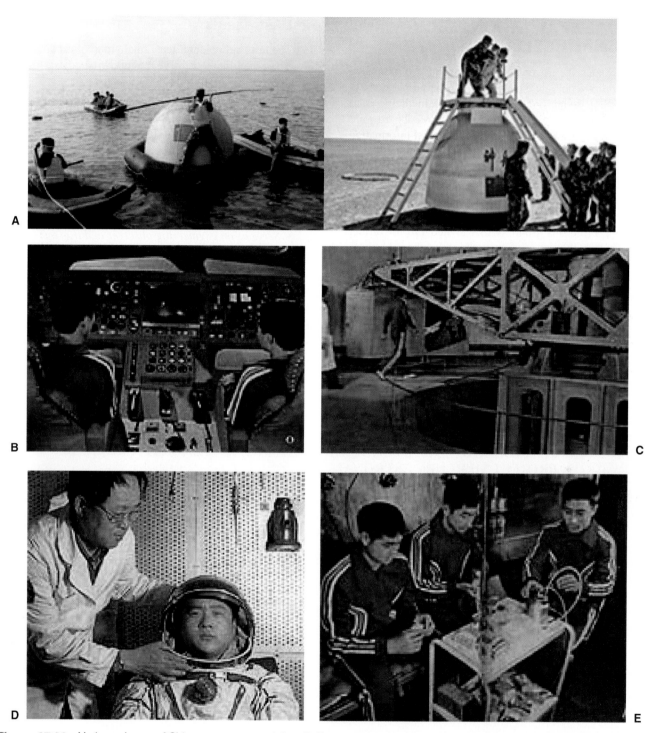

Figure 27.20 Various phases of Chinese astronaut training. **A.** Emergency escape procedures. **B.** Pilots receive flight training in a space module simulator. **C.** The first Chinese astronauts trained on a centrifuge to monitor physiologic responses to increasing g-forces. **D.** Testing of Chinese-developed spacesuits. **E.** Chinese astronauts test specially prepared foods for on-board flights.

Astronaut Training. Training of Chinese astronauts began in 1968 at the Space Flight Medical Research Institute to investigate physiologic responses to the space environment. The once secret program named Project 714 began with 80 candidates from a pool of 1800 fighter pilots. A final group of 20 astronaut trainees continued to train until the program was cancelled in 1975 because of poor funding and lack of political support. In 1995, China and Russia signed a cooperative agreement to share aerospace technologies that included the design of the spacecraft capsule, spacesuit, and life support system. A total of 20 astronauts currently comprise the Chinese Astronaut Corp. The astronauts, all air force pilots with at least 800 hours of flight experience, are university-educated with advanced knowledge of physics, fluid dynamics, electronics, and psychology. Aspects of their training shown in FIGURE 27.20 include landing procedures, emergency escape procedures, and zero-g instruction.

MEDICAL EVALUATION FOR ASTRONAUT SELECTION

Candidates for astronaut currently undergo extensive medical and psychologic evaluation;[66,119] the primary objective of U.S.–Russian cooperation in space medicine is to maintain the health and fitness of space crews aboard joint missions to the ISS.[58,106] However, little factual information existed about what to expect during space flight or the personal characteristics necessary for mission success when NASA devised the first medical evaluation in 1959. Approximately 600 active military test pilots from the Navy, Air Force, Army, and Marine Corps served as the initial candidate pool. From this group, NASA invited 110 for further testing. Thirty-two pilot finalists qualified for the next phase of testing, which included the exhaustive 23-item test battery listed in TABLE 27.4. The final evaluative criteria for the Mercury astronaut selection included (1) younger than age 40 years, (2) less than 71 inches tall (no weight requirement), (3) excellent physical condition, (4) college degree in engineering or equivalent, (5) minimum of 1500 hours flying time, (6) graduation from test pilot school, and (7) qualified test pilot.

First Astronauts

The test battery identified a final group of candidates believed best qualified to achieve the following goals:

- *Survive*—demonstrate ability to fly in space and return safely
- *Perform*—demonstrate ability to perform effectively under the conditions of space flight
- *Serve as a backup for automatic controls and instrumentation*—increase the reliability of flight systems
- *Serve as a scientific observer*—go beyond what the instruments and satellites can observe and report
- *Serve as an engineering observer and true test pilot*—to improve the flight system and its components

In April 1959, NASA selected the final seven astronauts. This elite group, survivors of an extraordinarily elaborate search and selection process, would train to enter an unknown environment with a life-support system previously tested only during high-altitude balloon flights.

TABLE 27.4 ■ **PHYSIOLOGIC AND PSYCHOLOGIC TESTING OF THE FIRST AMERICAN PROJECT MERCURY ASTRONAUTS**

PHYSIOLOGIC TESTS	PSYCHOLOGIC TESTS
1. *Harvard step test:* Subject steps up 20 inches to platform and down once every 2 s for 5 min to measure physical fitness 2. *Treadmill maximum workload:* Subject walks at constant rate on moving platform elevated 1° each min; test continues until heart rate reaches 180 b · min^{-1}; test of physical fitness 3. *Cold pressor:* Subject plunges feet into tub of ice water; pulse and blood pressure measured before and during test 4. *Complex behavior simulator:* A panel with 12 signals, each requiring a different response, measures ability to react reliably in confusing situations 5. *Tilt table:* Subject lies on steeply inclined table for 25 min to measure heart's ability to compensate for unusual body position for extended duration 6. *Partial pressure suit:* Subject taken to simulated altitude of 65,000 ft for 1 h in MC-1 partial pressure suit; measure of cardiovascular efficiency and breathing at low ambient pressures 7. *Isolation:* Subject enters a dark, soundproof room for 3 h to assess adaptation to unusual circumstances and coping without external stimuli 8. *Acceleration:* Subject placed in centrifuge with seat inclined at various angles; assesses near–multiple gravity forces 9. *Heat:* Subject spends 2 h in chamber at 130°F; measures reactions of heart and body functions to this stress 10. *Equilibrium and vibration:* Subject seated on chair that rotates simultaneously on two axes; subject required to maintain chair on even keel using control stick with and without vibration; subject tested with and without blindfold 11. *Noise:* Subject exposed to different sound frequencies to determine susceptibility to high-frequency tones	1. Extensive interviews (psychiatrists) 2. Rorschach (ink blot) 3. Thematic apperception (stories suggested by pictures) 4. Draw-a-person 5. Sentence completion 6. Self-inventory from 566-item questionnaire 7. Officer effectiveness inventory 8. Personal-preference schedule from 225 pairs of self-descriptive statements 9. Preference evaluation from 52 statements 10. Determination of authoritarian attitudes 11. Peer ratings 12. Interpretation of the question, "Who am I?" 13. Wechsler Adult Scale 14. Miller Analogies Test 15. Raven Progressive Matrices 16. Doppelt Mathematical Reasoning Scale 17. Engineering analogies 18. Mechanical comprehension 19. Air Force Officer Qualification Test 20. Aviation qualification test (USN) space memory 21. Spatial orientation 22. Gottschaldt Hidden Figures 23. Guilford-Zimmerman Spatial Visualization

Unknown at that time, NASA had identified, conducted, and completed similar tests with female test pilots with extensive flight experience. However, an executive decision had been made that the new astronauts would only be males with commissions in the armed services with prior fighter pilot training and experience.

Beginning in 1977, NASA adopted medical evaluation criteria for astronaut selection, relying on some test procedures gleaned from exercise physiology research that assessed maximal physiologic responses during treadmill and cycle-ergometer tests. The standards, modified in 1991, reflect changes in NASA's objectives for space exploration; personnel now include pilots, mission specialists, payload specialists, and space flight participants. The strictest standards for vision and hearing apply to pilots and mission specialists, with less stringent requirements in these two areas for the two other personnel categories. Soviet selection and training program standards for cosmonauts clearly resemble the United States model.

In addition to medical screening and testing, NASA conducts retrospective and longitudinal studies of astronauts matched against a large control group of Johnson Space Center employees. Until about age 40, astronauts score better on health and fitness variables than controls. The comparative data provide an important baseline for future studies of the possible effects of short- and long-term microgravity exposure on parameters concerned with long-term health and aging. NASA sponsors three types of studies:[66]

1. *Data analysis from single flights*. Research involves on-going data collection about space motion sickness symptoms experienced before, during, and after flights. Experiments aim to validate ground-based predictive tests of an individual's susceptibility to this malady and to define operationally acceptable countermeasures.
2. *Longitudinal studies spanning several missions*. Such studies quantify the cumulative effects of repeated exposure to the space environment, particularly radiation effects on cancer risk and bone mineral loss.
3. *Longitudinal studies throughout careers*. Long-term medical surveillance documents occupational injuries and maladies during or following space missions. The longest-duration study of physiologic responses after microgravity exposure involves studies of astronaut John Glenn, Jr. (1921–), the first American to orbit Earth, who piloted the 1962 *Friendship 7* Earth-orbital space mission. Thirty-six years later on October 29, 1998 at age 77, Glenn served as a Payload Specialist 2 on Shuttle *Discovery* STS-95 for an 8-day mission. The experiments involved studies of bone and muscle loss, balance, and sleep disorders (www.spaceflight. nasa.gov/shuttle/archives/sts-95/index.html).

Occupational Health Program

In addition to NASA's exercise physiology laboratory, the Occupational Health Program (OHP) (ohp.nasa.gov/) consists of approximately 400 occupational medicine and environmental health professionals distributed across 10 primary NASA centers. This team provides comprehensive medical support to a diverse, highly technologic workforce of more than 60,000 civil servant and contractor employees involved in human exploration and development of space, aeronautics research, and Earth and space science activities. The traditional occupational health program elements include medical surveillance, industrial hygiene, health physics, emergency medical response, employee assistance programs, physical fitness programs, and overall health and wellness programs. Astronauts in training for a mission participate at the Johnson Space Center in developmental fitness regimens in modern facilities similar to most university and commercial gymnasia.

Radiation Effects. *For astronauts living in low-Earth orbit for extended periods, including exploratory Mars missions and beyond, radiation exposure poses potentially serious health concerns.*[136,172] Current preflight requirements include projecting a mission radiation dosage, assessing the probability of solar flares during the mission, and quantifying the radiation exposure history of flight crewmembers. Each crewmember carries a passive dosimeter (radiation-measuring device), and highly sensitive dosimeters located throughout the spacecraft continually monitor radiation in case of solar flares or other radiation contingencies.

Future research must resolve the short- and long-term biologic impact on cellular microarchitecture of galactic cosmic ray particles (nuclei of high atomic number) with high energies (HZE) and high linear energy transfer (LET). Different kinds of radiation during liftoff and aboard the spacecraft on short-duration missions at nominal orbit generally pose an "acceptable" level of hazard to astronaut health (e.g., blood-forming organs, lens of eyes, skin).[9,108,171]

PHYSIOLOGIC ADAPTATIONS TO MICROGRAVITY

Space flight has produced considerable biomedical information about human physiology in microgravity, beginning in 1961 with astronaut Alan Shepard's brief solo flight aboard *Freedom 7* (see Table 27.2 and FIG. 27.21). In the ensuing 50 years, researchers have quantified physiologic adaptations to relatively brief space missions (1–14 d) and flights lasting longer than 2 weeks, including postflight adaptations.

FIGURE 27.22 displays a generalized schema of the dynamics of physiologic functions with microgravity exposure. These include the effects of two major factors: reduced hydrostatic gradients and reduced loading and disuse of weight-bearing tissues. The graphic reveals how these two factors influence the following six systems: (1) cardiovascular

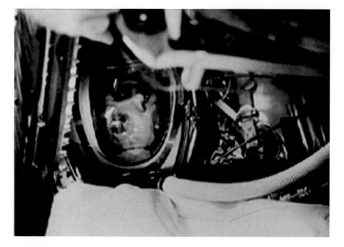

Figure 27.21   Astronaut Alan Shepard's (1923–1998) historic 15-min, 28-s solo flight on May 5, 1961, on Mercury 3 rocket *Freedom 7,* achieved 116.5 statute mi-altitude and traveled 303 statute mi at a maximum velocity of 5134 mph. Shepard logged 216 cumulative hours of space flight, including 9 hours of cumulative EVA on Apollo 14.

and cardiopulmonary, (2) hematologic, (3) fluid, electrolyte, and hormonal, (4) muscle, (5) bone, and (6) neurosensory and vestibular. Each system has been color coded, with *arrows* indicating how one system might influence another. For example, trace the pathways between a decrease in hydrostatic gradients *(top left)* and reduced total blood volume *(bottom center)*. How many different pathways interact to reduce total blood volume? Similarly, trace how altered sensory and balance information also affects blood volume and maximal exercise capacity. Two of the current NASA research efforts focus on the impact of reduced bone density on risk of bone fractures and functional impact of skeletal muscle atrophy (reduced strength) on performing mission-related tasks. These physiologic responses to microgravity, in addition to reduced stroke volume related to orthostatic hypotension and possible syncope, have implications for developing and testing effective countermeasure strategies (see pp. 741–742).

In addition to the flow chart of physiologic events, we present separate tables with detailed information about the cardiovascular, pulmonary, body fluid, sensory, and musculoskeletal responses to microgravity. The information comes from almost four decades of cumulative research from Mercury, Gemini, Apollo, ASTP, Vostok, Voskhod, Soyuz, Shuttle Spacelab, Skylab, Salyut, and Mir missions. Excellent summary resource materials exist about these responses.[14,20,30,31,40,42,44–47,52,55,65,69,81,110,135, 152,157,166,168]

Cardiovascular Adaptations

The decrease in total fluid volume during the first few days in microgravity reduces the heart's total work effort. With continued microgravity exposure, overall heart size decreases mainly from reduced left ventricular volume, particularly left ventricular end-diastolic volume. Such adaptations represent an

appropriate response to microgravity without compromising "normal" cardiovascular function during a mission.

TABLE 27.5 summarizes adaptations in 15 cardiovascular variables for space missions through 1992, while FIGURE 27.23 displays pre- to postflight changes in stroke volume during upright exercise expressed as a percentage of preflight baseline. Also shown are changes in aerobic capacity (not listed in Table 27.5) as a function of intensity and frequency of 20-minute in-flight cycle ergometer exercise bouts during four different missions. Maximal oxygen consumption declined significantly regardless of training regimen, except for group 1, which maintained heart rate above $130 \text{ b} \cdot \text{min}^{-1}$ and exercised longer than 20 minutes more than three times weekly. In contrast to these studies, some in-flight ergometer and treadmill studies have reported astronauts maintained their level of aerobic capacity during relatively brief missions.

A recent experiment measured changes in cardiac function (left and right ventricular mass and left ventricular end-diastolic volume) assessed by magnetic resonance imaging to isolate whether microgravity per se or frank atrophy from physical inactivity produced changes in cardiac loading functions. In four astronauts on a 10-day mission and in controls on ground measured at 2, 6, and 12 weeks of bed rest and 6 weeks of routine daily activities, left ventricular mass declined by 12% (±7.9%). Thus, cardiac atrophy occurs both during relatively long 6 weeks of horizontal bed rest (inactivity) and after short-term space flight (microgravity). The authors postulated that physiologic adaptation to reduced myocardial load and work in real or simulated microgravity produces the cardiac atrophy, demonstrating the plasticity of cardiac muscle under different loading conditions.[116]

INTEGRATIVE QUESTION

Contrast the hemodynamic responses when a person moves from the upright to the upside-down position on Earth and in a microgravity environment.

Pulmonary Adaptations

Tight linkage exists between the cardiovascular, pulmonary, and metabolic systems. The cells' demand for oxygen during rest and exercise remains invariant regardless of environment. Any change in external work above a resting baseline triggers immediate ventilatory responses that increase breathing rate and tidal volume. Augmented alveolar ventilation maintains an adequate pressure differential for oxygen diffusion across lung tissues for delivery to the site of increased energy metabolism.

TABLE 27.6 summarizes changes in pulmonary variables during two Spacelab missions. FIGURE 27.24 depicts changes in pulmonary diffusing capacity for carbon monoxide measured preflight on days 2, 4, and 9 during the mission and within 6 hours before or after landing and then at days 1, 2, 4,

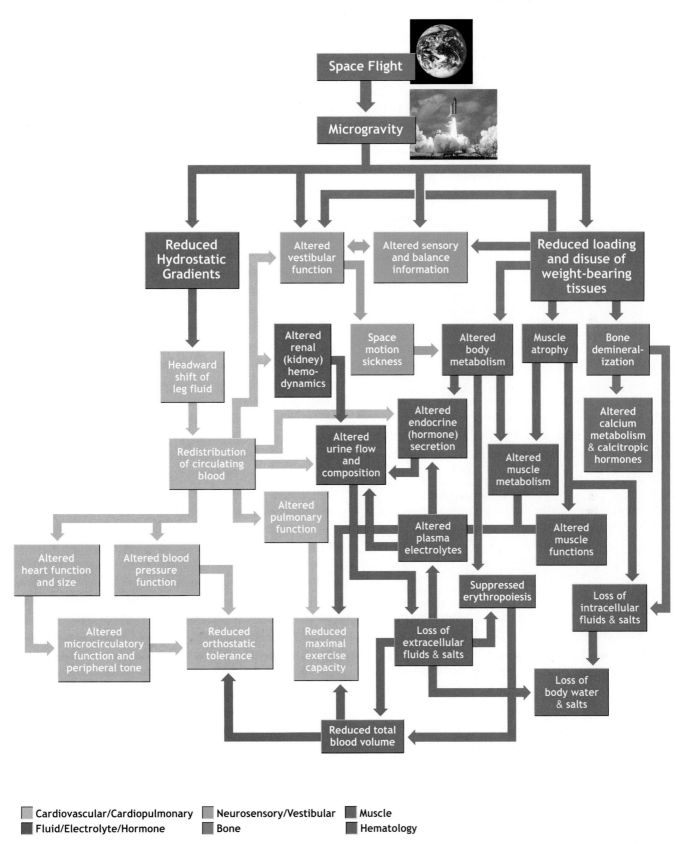

Figure 27.22 General schema of microgravity's effects on physiologic alterations from (1) reduced hydrostatic gradients and (2) reduced loading and disuse of weight-bearing tissues. (Modified from Lujan BF, White RJ. Human physiology in space. [www.nsbri.org/humanphysiologyspace/].)

TABLE 27.5 ■ CHANGES IN CARDIOVASCULAR VARIABLES ASSOCIATED WITH MICROGRAVITY

PHYSIOLOGIC MEASURE	SHORT SPACE FLIGHTS (1–14 D)	LONG SPACE FLIGHTS (>2 WK)	
		PREFLIGHT VS. IN-FLIGHT	PREFLIGHT VS. POSTFLIGHT
Heart rate (resting)	Variable in flight; increased after flight; peaks during launch and reentry; RPB up to 1 w	Normal or slightly increased	Increased; RPB 3 w
Blood pressure (resting)	Normal; decreased after flight	Diastolic blood pressure reduced or unchanged	Decreased mean arterial pressure
Orthostatic tolerance	Decreased after flights longer than 5 h; exaggerated cardiovascular responses to tilt test, stand test, and LBNP after flight; RPB 3–14 d	Exaggerated cardiovascular responses to in-flight LBNP (especially during first 2 w); last in flight test comparable to recovery-day test	Exaggerated cardiovascular responses to LBNP; RPB up to 3 w
Total peripheral resistance	Decreased in flight; no increase at landing despite drop in stroke volume and increase in HR	Tendency toward decrease	Increased after landing
Cardiac size	Normal or slightly decreased C/T ratio after flight	C/T ratio decreased after flight	
Stroke volume	Increased in flight by as much as 60% (SLS-1); compensated by decreased HR	Increased early in flight then decreased	12% decrease on average
Left end-diastolic volume	Same as stroke volume	Same as in short-duration missions	16% decrease on average
Cardiac output	Elevated 30–40% in flight (SLS-1); reduced immediately after flight	Unchanged	Variable; RPB 3–4 weeks
Central venous pressure	Elevated above resting supine level before launch; transient increase followed by levels below preflight upon attaining orbit	Not measured	Not measured
Left cardiac muscle mass thickness	Unchanged	Unchanged	11% decrease; return to normal after 3 w
Cardiac electrical activity (ECG/VCG)	Moderate rightward shift in QRS and T waves after flight	Increased P-R interval, QT interval, and QRS vector magnitude	Slight increase in QRS duration and magnitude; increase in P-R interval duration
Arrhythmia	Usually PABs and PVBs; isolated cases of nodal tachycardia, ectopic beats, and supraventricular bigeminy in flights	PVBs and occasional PABs; sinus or nodal arrhythmia at release of LBNP in flight	Occasional unifocal PABs and PVBs
Systolic time intervals	Not measured	Not measured; PEP/ET ratio RPB 2 w	Increase in resting and LBNP-stressed
Exercise capacity	No change or decreased ≤12% after flight; increased HR for same VO_2; no change in efficiency; RPB 3–8 d	Submaximal exercise capacity unchanged	Decreased after flight; recovery time inversely related to amount of in-flight exercise rather than mission duration
Venous compliance in legs	Not measured	Increased: continues to increase for 10 d or more; slow decrease later in flight	Normal or slightly increased

Data from Nicogossian AE, et al. Space physiology and medicine, 3rd ed. Philadelphia: Lea & Febiger, 1994:216.
RPB, return to preflight baseline; LBNP, lower-body negative pressure; C/T, cardiothoracic; ECG, electrocardiogram; VCG, vectorcardiogram; PAB, premature atrial beat; PVB, premature ventricular beat; HR, heart rate; SLS-1, Spacelab Life Sciences 1.

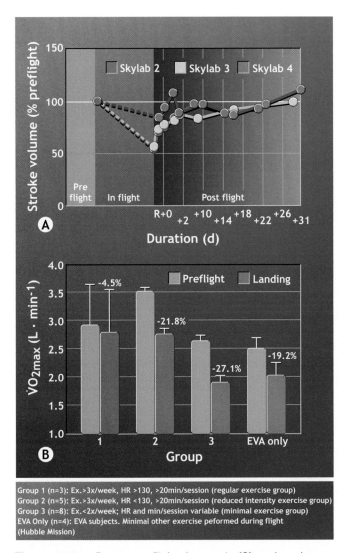

Group 1 (n=3): Ex.>3x/week, HR >130, >20min/session (regular exercise group)
Group 2 (n=5): Ex.>3x/week, HR <130, >20min/session (reduced intensity exercise group)
Group 3 (n=8): Ex.<2x/week; HR and min/session variable (minimal exercise group)
EVA Only (n=4): EVA subjects. Minimal other exercise peformed during flight
(Hubble Mission)

Figure 27.23 Pre- to postflight changes in (**A**) stroke volume during upright exercise (*Skylab 2–4*). *R,* return to Earth, and (**B**) aerobic capacity related to intensity and frequency of 20-minute in-flight cycle ergometry. (Data for A from Michel EL, et al. Results of Skylab medical experiment M171-metabolic activity. In: Johnson RS, Dietlein LF, eds. Biomedical results from Skylab. NASA SP-377. Washington, DC: Government Printing Office, 1977. Data for B from Sawin CF. Biomedical investigations conducted in support of the extended duration orbiter medical project. Aviat Space Environ Med 1999;70:169.)

and 6 postflight. Note that diffusing capacity increases in the sitting and standing positions during 3 days in microgravity and then returns to preflight baseline values.

Denitrogenation and EVA

Before astronauts perform EVA maneuvers, they must "washout" the nitrogen from their fluids and tissues to prevent decompression sickness (DCS or bends) from differentials in gas pressures within the cabin and EVA garment. They do this by using a 10.2 lb per square inch atmosphere (psia) staged decompression of the shuttle for at least 12 hours. This also includes 100 minutes of **preoxygenation**

breathing 100% O_2 at 14.7 psia prior to decompression and before decompression to the suit pressure of 4.3 psia (equivalent to 9144-m altitude). Even a slight incapacitation from DCS during EVA could hinder safe return to the spacecraft and provoke a medical emergency. Scientists have proposed several ways to induce **denitrogenation**. First, reduce the total pressure inside the spacecraft from 760 to 630 torr (approximate barometric pressure of Denver, CO) to shorten overall time for denitrogenation prior to EVA. Second, have astronauts sleep in a special low-pressure compartment prior to EVA. Thus, the several hours devoted to denitrogenation during sleep would not encroach upon valuable work time. A seemingly simple solution would increase the pressure within the space suit to keep N_2 in solution to avoid bubble formation. Unfortunately, this would cause the suit to stiffen considerably, rendering limb maneuverability nearly impossible.

The rate of denitrogenation depends on at least two factors: (1) tissue nitrogen capacity, which increases with body fat content (N_2 elimination takes longer in fatter people) and (2) the tissues' oxygenation, which ultimately depends on cardiac output, which decreases during flight in the supine position.[120] In prolonged missions, as lower limb muscles begin to atrophy in the weightless environment, the time for denitrogenation also may change.

Exercise-Enhanced Preoxygenation. Recent experiments with exercise-enhanced preoxygenation (10 min of upper- and lower-body exercise at 75% estimated $\dot{V}O_{2max}$ breathing 100% O_2) eliminated DCS during 36 U-2 reconnaissance flights at altitudes of 29,000 to 30,000 feet in a pilot who previously experienced 25 episodes of DCS.[64] Another experiment investigated the efficiency of either a 1- or a 15-minute preoxygenation period, each beginning with 10 minutes of dual-cycle ergometry performed at 75% of $\dot{V}O_{2peak}$ for enhancing preoxygenation efficiency by increasing perfusion gradients and minute ventilation.[167] Male subjects accomplished a 1-hour preoxygenation with exercise, a 15-minute preoxygenation with exercise, or a 1-hour resting preoxygenation before exposure to 4.3 psia for 4 hours while performing light-to-moderate exercise. The incidence of DCS following the 1-hour preoxygenation with exercise was significantly lower (42%; $n = 26$) than following the 1-hour resting preoxygenation (77%; $n = 26$). The incidence and onset of DCS following the 15-minute preoxygenation with exercise (64%; $n = 22$) did not differ from the 1-hour resting control. *Thus, 1-hour of preoxygenation with exercise improves resistance to DCS, illustrating the potentially positive exercise effect on ameliorating DCS during critical mission EVA maneuvers.*

Body Fluid Adaptations

TABLE 27.7 summarizes preflight to postflight adaptations in 24 body fluid variables. FIGURE 27.25 reports data for three variables: (1) percentage change in plasma volume and red cell mass during *Spacelab 1* and three Skylab missions, (2)

TABLE 27.6 ■ PULMONARY SYSTEM CHANGES ASSOCIATED WITH MICROGRAVITY DURING SPACELAB LIFE SCIENCES-1 (FLIGHT STS-40, JUNE 5, 1991) AND GERMAN SPACELAB MISSION D-2 ABOARD STS-55 (APRIL 26, 1993)

PHYSIOLOGIC RESPONSE TO MICROGRAVITY (1–14 D)	REFERENCE LETTER	NUMBER OF SUBJECTS	CHANGES IN MICROGRAVITY (IN-FLIGHT VS. PREFLIGHT STANDING MEASUREMENTS)
Pulmonary blood flow			
Total pulmonary blood flow (cardiac output)	A	4	18% increase
Cardiac stroke volume	A	4	4% increase
Diffusing capacity (carbon monoxide)	A	4	28% increase
Pulmonary capillary blood volume	A	4	28% increase
Diffusing capacity of alveolar membrane	A	4	27% increase
Pulmonary blood flow distribution	C	7	More uniform but some inequality remained
Pulmonary ventilation			
Respiration frequency	E	8	9% increase
Tidal volume	E	8	15% decrease
Alveolar ventilation	E	8	Unchanged
Total ventilation	E	8	Small decrease
Ventilatory distribution	B	7	More uniform but some inequality remained
Maximal peak expiratory flow rate	E	7	Decreased by ≤12.5% early in flight, then returned to normal
Pulmonary gas exchange			
O_2 uptake	E	8	Unchanged
CO_2 output	E	8	Unchanged
End-tidal P_{O_2}	E	8	Unchanged
End-tidal P_{CO_2}	E	8	Small increase when CO_2 concentration in spacecraft increased
Lung volumes			
Functional residual capacity	D	4	15% decrease
Residual lung volume	D	4	18% decrease
Closing volume	B	7	Unchanged as measured by argon bolus

Modified from West JB, et al. Pulmonary function in space. JAMA 1997;277:1957.

Note: Pulmonary blood flow in normal subjects equals cardiac output. How well carbon monoxide diffuses into the blood is a standard clinical test of the integrity of the alveolar membrane and its surrounding capillary blood supply. The data indicate that more alveoli are expanded and ventilated in space than on Earth. Closing volume refers to the volume in the lung where the alveoli close in significant numbers.

A. Prisk OK, et al. Pulmonary diffusing capacity, capillary blood volume and cardiac output during sustained microgravity. J Appl Physiol 1993;75:15.
B. Guy HJB, et al. Inhomogeneity of pulmonary ventilation during sustained microgravity as determined by single-breath washouts. J Appl Physiol 1994;76:1719.
C. Prisk OK, et al. Inhomogeneity of pulmonary ventilation during sustained microgravity on Spacelab SLS-1. J Appl Physiol 1994;76:1730.
D. Elliott AR, et al. Lung volumes during sustained microgravity on Spacelab SLS-1. J Appl Physiol 1994;77:2005.
E. Prisk OK, et al. Pulmonary gas exchange and its determinants during sustained microgravity on Spacelab SLS-1. J Appl Physiol 1995;76:1290.

percentage change in total hemoglobin during four Salyut (Russian) missions, and (3) blood volume related to orthostatically stressed heart rate response during Apollo, SMEAT (Skylab Medical Experiments Altitude Tests), and Skylab missions.

Sensory System Adaptations

TABLE 27.8 summarizes space flight adaptations in the sensory system categories of audition, gustation and olfaction, somatosensory, and vision for relatively short (<14 d) and longer (>14 d) space missions. The *bottom* of the table lists general vestibular system changes. Part A of FIGURE 27.26 schematically shows multisensory interactions that readjust the sensory responses disturbed by micrograv-

ity. Sensorimotor integration plays a pivotal role in posture and movement control, ambulation, and manipulating objects at 1g, which necessitate proper adjustment in body orientation. In essence, the sensorimotor control system consists of a highly complex, tightly integrated neural complex that modulates vestibular, visual, somatosensory, tactile, and proprioceptive input within a central command-processing center. Disturbance in one aspect of the system usually initiates an override, readjustment, or temporary substitution by other system components to maintain the system's functional integrity.[53,79,89,99,100,117,162] Considerable research has assessed how microgravity affects spatial orientation, postural control,[88] vestibuloocular reflexes, and vestibular processing. Studies have also focused on mechanisms related to space motion sickness and perceptual motor per-

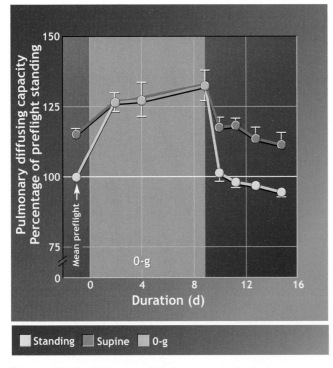

Figure 27.24 Pulmonary diffusing capacity for carbon monoxide preflight on flight days 2, 4, and 9 and 6 hours following landing and on days 1, 2, 4, and 6 postflight. Data are referenced to the preflight standing value. (From Prisk GK, et al. Pulmonary diffusing capacity, capillary blood volume, and cardiac output during sustained microgravity. J Appl Physiol 1993;75:15,1993.)

formance.[111,112] The unnumbered figure below shows an inflight experiment on 1993 Spacelab Life Sciences 2 shuttle flight STS-58 using a rotating chair to study vestibular function.

Part B of Figure 27.26 displays the immediate effects of space flight on postural reflexes in crewmembers from eight missions that lasted 4 to 10 days. Immediate postflight measurements were made within 1 to 5 hours in 10 of the 13 subjects. The greatest postural instability occurred in tests that required vestibular information. These experiments demonstrated a two-stage readaptation process that followed microgravity exposure. The first stage occurred quickly, within a few hours after landing; in a second, slower stage, stability returned to near normal in approximately 4 days. On longer Russian Mir missions (140 and 175 d), recovery of postural parameters to preflight levels required approximately 6 weeks. Apparently, readaptation of postural control upon return from space coincides with mission duration, with a prominent role played by visual cues.[40]

Musculoskeletal Adaptations

TABLE 27.9 examines musculoskeletal adaptations during exposure to microgravity. *NASA's greatest biomedical concern involves the 1% per month loss in weight-bearing bone mass during space missions.*

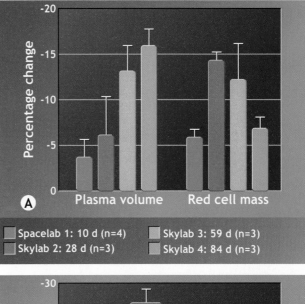

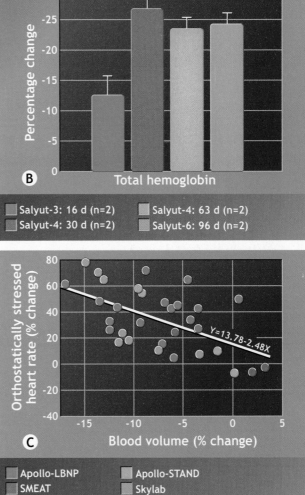

Figure 27.25 Pre- to postflight changes in (**A**) plasma volume and red blood cell mass (*Spacelab 1; Skylab 2–4*), (**B**) total hemoglobin (*Salyut 3–4; 6*), and (**C**) blood volume in relation to orthostatically stressed heart rate (Apollo, Skylab, and SMEAT [Skylab Medical Experiments Altitude Tests]). *Error bars* in A and B represent standard errors of measurement. (Data for A and B redrawn from Convertino VA. Physiological adaptations to weightlessness: effects on exercise and work performance. Exerc Sports Sci Rev 1990;18:119.)

TABLE 27.7 ■ BODY FLUID CHANGES ASSOCIATED WITH MICROGRAVITY

PHYSIOLOGIC MEASURE	SHORT SPACE FLIGHTS (1–14 D)[a]	LONG SPACE FLIGHTS (>2 W)[b]	
		PREFLIGHT VS. IN-FLIGHT	PREFLIGHT VS. POSTFLIGHT
Total body water	3% decrease by flight day 4 or 5		Decreased after flight
Plasma volume	Decreased after flight (except Gemini 7 and 8); decreased in flight (SLS-1)		Markedly decreased after flight. RPB 2 w increased at R + 0; decreased R + 2 (hydration effect)
Hematocrit	Slightly increased after flight		Decreased after flight; RPB 2–4 w after landing
Hemoglobin	Normal or slightly increased after flight	Increased in first in-flight sample; slowly declines later in flight	Decreased from near-preflight values on landing day; RPB 1–2 months
Red blood cell (RBC) mass	Decreased after flight (approx. 9% on SLS-1); RPB at least 2 w	Decreased ~15% during first 2–3 w in flight; begins to recover after about 60 d; recovery of RBC mass independent of time spent in space	Decreased after flight; RPB 2 w to 3 months after landing
Red blood cell morphology	No significant changesafter flight	Increased percentage of echinocytes; decrease in discocytes	Rapid reversal of in-flight changes in distribution of red blood cell shapes; significantly increased potassium influx; RPB 3 d
Red blood cell half-life (^{51}Cr)	No change; verified on SLS-1		No change
Reticulocytes	Decreased after flight; RPB 1 w		Decreases at landing, then shifts to increases over preflight values by 7 d after landing; greatest changes seen after longer flights
Iron turnover	No change		No change
Mean corpuscular volume	Increased after flight; RPB at least 2 w		Variable, but within normal limits
White blood cells	Increased after flight, especially neutrophils; lymphocytes decreased; RPB 1–2 d; no significant change in T/B lymphocyte ratio		Increased, especially neutrophils; postflight reduction in number of T cells and T-cell function as measured by PHA responsiveness, RPB 3–7 d; transient postflight elevation in B cells, RPB 3 d
Plasma lipids	Decreased cholesterol and triacylglcerols in flight		
Plasma glucose	Decreased during and immediately after flight	Decreased for the first 2 months then leveled off	Postflight hyperglycemia with increased lactate and pyruvate
Plasma proteins	Occasional postflight elevations in α_2-globulin from increases of haptoglobin, ceruloplasmin, and α_2-macroglobulin; elevated IgA and C_3		No significant changes
Red blood cell enzymes	No consistent postflight changes	Decreased phosphofructo-kinase; no evidence of lipid peroxidation or red blood cell damage	No consistent postflight changes
Serum/plasma electrolytes	Increased K and Ca in flight (SLS-1); decreased Na in flight; decreased K and Mg after flight	Decreased Na, Cl, and osmolality; slight increase in K and PO$_4$	Postflight decreases in Na, K, Cl, Mg; increase in PO$_4$ and osmolality
Serum/plasma hormones	Decreased ANF, aldosterone, and ADH in flight (SLS-1); increased cortisol and angiotensin 1 in flight (SLS-1)	Increased cortisol; decreased ACTH, insulin	Postflight increases in angiotensin, aldosterone, thyroxine, TSH and GH; decrease in ACTH
Insulin		Decreased during long missions	Decreased after flight

continued on page 727

TABLE 27.7 ■ *continued*

PHYSIOLOGIC MEASURE	SHORT SPACE FLIGHTS (1–14 D)[a]	LONG SPACE FLIGHTS (>2 W)[b]	
		PREFLIGHT VS. IN-FLIGHT	PREFLIGHT VS. POSTFLIGHT
Serum/plasma metabolites and enzymes	Postflight increases in blood urea nitrogen, creatinine, and glucose; decreases in lactic acid dehydrogenase, creatinine phosphokinase, albumin, triacylglycerols, cholesterol, and uric acid		Postflight decrease in cholesterol, uric acid
Urine volume	Decreased after flight	Decreased early in flight	Decreased after flight
Urine electrolytes	Postflight increases in Ca, creatinine, PO$_4$, and osmolality; decreases in Na, K, Cl, Mg	Increased osmolality, Na, K, Cl, Mg, Ca, PO$_4$; decrease in uric acid excreation	Increased Ca excretion; initial postflight decreases in Na, K, Cl, Mg, PO$_4$, uric acid; Na and Cl excretion increased in second and third week after flight
Urinary hormones	In-flight decreases in 17-OH-corticosteroids, increase in aldosterone; postflight increases in cortisol, aldosterone, ADH, and pregnanediol; decreases in epinephrine, 17-OH-corticosteroids, androsterone, and etiocholanolone	In-flight increases in cortisol, aldosterone, and total 17-ketosteroids; decrease in ADH	Increased cortisol, aldosterone, norepinephrine; decreases in total 17-OH-corticosteroids, ADH
Urinary amino acids	Postflight increases in taurine and β-alanine; decreases in glycine, alanine, and tyrosine	Increased in flight	Increased after flight

[a] Biomedical data from Mercury, Gemini, Apollo, ASTP, Vostok, Voskhod, Soyuz, Shuttle, Spacelab.
[b] Biomedical data from Skylab, Salyut, Mir missions.
Data from Nicogossian AE, et al. Space physiology and medicine. 3rd ed. Philadelphia: Lea & Febiger, 1994:217.
SLS, Spacelab Life Sciences; RPB, return to preflight baseline; R, return to Earth.

Increased Calcium Loss

TABLE 27.10 summarizes data from 18 male crewmembers aboard Russian Mir station missions lasting between 4 and 14.4 months. Bone mineral density (BMD) declined at all seven sites measured, with spine, neck of femur, trochanter, and pelvis decreasing more than 1% per month. On the shorter 4- to 14-day Gemini flights, BMD decreased 3 to 9% in the os calcis (heel bone).[164] Loss of BMD at the os calcis and radius occurred during Apollo Skylab missions and showed no recovery, even 97 days postflight.[151,163] During the Skylab 2 28-day orbital mission, crewmembers experienced a daily negative 50-mg calcium imbalance;[169] daily calcium loss averaged 140 mg on the 84-day mission. Increased bone calcium loss, if coupled with a high fluid and salt intake, could alter plasma filtrate composition and pH to favor supersaturation of kidney stone-forming salts.[170]

FIGURE 27.27 illustrates how reduced mechanical stress in microgravity affects calcium balance. The *top panel* shows how three skeletal loading factors—reduced gravity (microgravity), normal gravity, and above-normal gravity—adjust calcium distribution in the digestive (intestine), cardiovascular, renal (kidney), and skeletal (bone) systems. Under normal gravity conditions, the small intestine absorbs approximately 250 to 500 mg of calcium for every 1000 mg consumed, with the remainder excreted in feces (▼▼). In a microgravity environment, reduced calcium intestinal absorption exacerbates calcium fecal loss (▼▼▼). Abnormal calcium excretion from bone resorption disrupts calcium homeostasis, which in turn decreases total body calcium and bone mass. With increased gravitational loading, calcium absorption by bone increases to spare overall calcium loss (▼). In the *bottom panel*, the flow diagram shows proposed parallel dynamics of the calcium/endocrine response and skeletal structure and composition to altered gravitational loading with adequate diet and endocrine balance.[70]

Without suitable countermeasures, progressive calcium losses during future missions of several years duration will compromise astronaut well-being, increasing bone fracture risk upon return to Earth. On-board, multimode exercise training and lower-limb exercise has *not* prevented BMD loss, despite United States and Soviet crewmembers' commitment to intense workouts. Hopefully, future research using valid animal and bed rest models will reveal the basic mechanism of bone remodeling during prolonged microgravity exposure.[107,133,153,155] These studies must consider hormonal and cellular factors as affected by alterations in mechanical stimulation that alter bone sensors to subsequently affect the structural integrity of bones.[57] Biochemical markers of bone

TABLE 27.8 ■ SENSORY SYSTEM CHANGES ASSOCIATED WITH MICROGRAVITY

PHYSIOLOGIC MEASURE	SHORT SPACE FLIGHTS (1–14 D)	LONG SPACE FLIGHTS (>2 W)	
		PREFLIGHT VS. IN-FLIGHT	PREFLIGHT VS. POSTFLIGHT
Audition	No change in thresholds after flight	One report of lowered thresholds during a 1-year flight	No change in thresholds after flight
Gustation and olfaction	Subjective and varied human experience; no impairments noted	Same as shorter missions	Same as shorter missions
Somatosensory	Subjective and varied human experience; no impairments noted	Subjective experiences (e.g., tingling in feet)	
Vision	Intraocular tension tends to increase during flight and decrease at landing; postflight decreases in visual field; retinal blood vessels constricted after flight; dark-adapted crews reported light flashes with eyes open or closed; decrease in visual motor task performance and contrast discrimination; no change in in-flight contrast discrimination or distant and near visual acuity	Light flashes reported by dark-adapted subjects; frequency related to latitude (highest in South Atlantic, lowest over poles)	No significant changes except transient decreases in intraocular pressure
Vestibular system	40–70% of astronauts/cosmonauts exhibit in-flight neurovestibular effects including immediate reflex motor responses (postural illusions, sensations of tumbling or rotation, nystagmus, dizziness, vertigo) and space motion sickness (pallor, cold sweating, nausea, vomiting); motion sickness symptoms appear early in flight and subside or disappear in 2–7 days; postflight difficulties in postural equilibrium with eyes closed or other vestibular disturbances	In-flight vestibular disturbances are the same as for shorter missions; markedly decreased susceptibility to provocative motion stimuli (cross-coupled angular acceleration) after adaptation period of 2–7 days; cosmonauts reported occasional reappearance of illusions during long missions	Immunity to provocative motion continues for several days after flight; marked postflight disturbances in postural equilibrium with eyes closed; some cosmonauts exhibit additional vestibular disturbances after flight, including dizziness, nausea, and vomiting

Data used by permission from Nicogossian AE, et al. Space physiology and medicine. 3rd ed. Philadelphia: Lea & Febiger, 1994:219.

turnover during 120 days of bed rest (skeletal unloading) showed the combined effects of accelerated bone resorption and retarded bone formation accounted for bone loss.[71] BMD measurements at the distal radius and tibia in 15 cosmonauts on the MIR space station on missions of 1, 2, and 6 months revealed the following:[160]

1. Cancellous and cortical bone of the radius decreased progressively at each of the time points.
2. For the weight-bearing tibial site, cancellous BMD appeared normal after 1 month and deteriorated thereafter. After 2 months, bone loss became noticeable in the tibial cortices.
3. At 6 months, cortical bone loss was less evident than cancellous bone loss; cumulative time in microgravity did not relate to BMD changes.
4. Tibial bone loss still persisted after return to Earth for durations similar to time in space (1–6 months).

Even with on-board, dedicated physical exercise intervention, bone loss persists and can remain pathologic for a prolonged period following a mission. Alterations in circulation to bone during microgravity exposure can alter the balance between bone resorption and bone formation. Thus, bone blood flow may play an important role in bone remodeling in microgravity.[25]

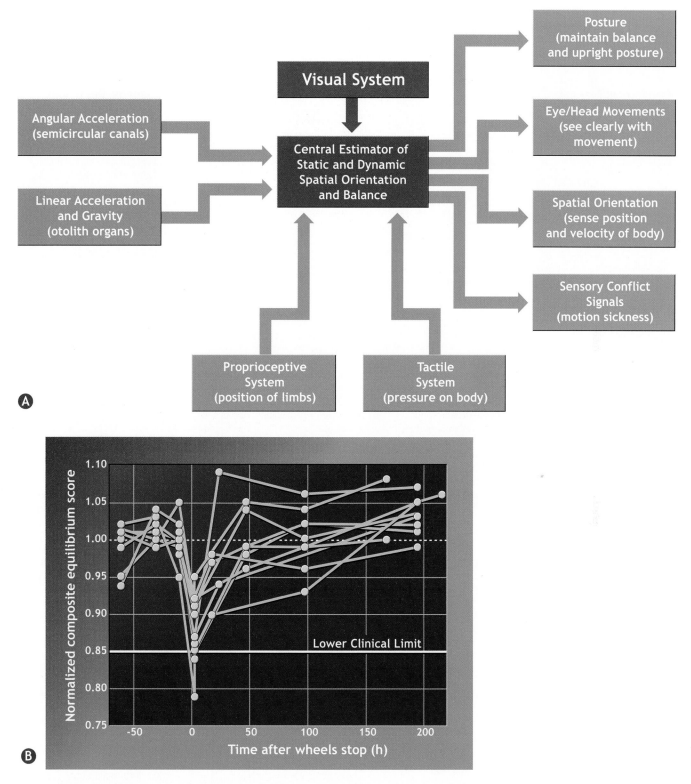

Figure 27.26   A. Schematic representation of sensory motor system that controls eye movements and posture, and perception of orientation and motion. **B.** Changes in anterior–posterior sway (composite equilibrium score) in 10 astronauts at various times after the space shuttle returned to Earth *(wheels stop)*. The tests involved perturbation of a posture platform under different conditions of visual, vestibular, and proprioceptive input. *Dashed horizontal line* at 1.00 represents normal response. (Data reported in Daunton NG. Adaptation of the vestibular system to microgravity. In: Fregly MJ, Blatteis CM, eds. Handbook of physiology. Section 4, Environmental physiology, vol 2. American Physiological Society. New York: Oxford University Press, 1996:765. Data for A modified from Young LR, et al. M.I.T./Canadian vestibular experiments on the Spacelab 1 mission: 2. Visual vestibular tilt interaction in weightlessness. Exp Brain Res 1986;64:299. Data for B modified from Paloski WH, et al. Recovery of postural equilibrium control following space flight. Ann NY Acad Sci 1992;656:747.)

TABLE 27.9 ■ MUSCULOSKELETAL CHANGES ASSOCIATED WITH MICROGRAVITY

PHYSIOLOGIC MEASURE	SHORT SPACE FLIGHTS (1–14 D)	LONG SPACE FLIGHTS (>2 W)	
		PREFLIGHT VS. IN-FLIGHT	PREFLIGHT VS. POSTFLIGHT
Stature	Slight increase during first week in flight (~1.3 cm); RPB 1 d	Increased during first 2 w in flight (maximum 3–6 cm); stabilizes thereafter	Height returns to normal on R + 0
Body mass	Postflight weight losses average about 3.4%; about 2/3 of the loss from water loss, the remainder from loss of lean body mass and fat	In-flight weight losses average 3–4% during first 5 d; thereafter, weight either declines or increases for the remainder of mission; early in-flight losses probably from fluid loss; later losses are metabolic	Rapid weight gain during first 5 d after flight, mainly replenishment from fluid; slower weight gain from R + 5 days to R + 2 or 3 w; amount of postflight weight loss inversely related to in-flight caloric intake
Protein synthesis	Elevated 40% on flight day 8 (SLS-1), suggesting a "stress response"		
Body composition		Fat is probably replacing muscle tissue; muscle mass is partially preserved depending on exercise regimen	
Total body volume	Decreased after flight	Center of mass shifts headward	Decreased after flight
Limb volume	In-flight leg volume decreases exponentially during the first flight day; thereafter, rate of decrease declines and plateaus within 3–5 d; postflight decrements in leg volume up to 3%; rapid increase immediately after flight, followed by slower RPB	Same as short missions early in flight; leg volume continues to decrease slightly throughout mission; arm volume decreases slightly	Rapid increase in leg volume immediately after flight followed by slow RPB
Muscle strength	Decreased during and after flight; RPB 1–2 w		Postflight decrease in leg muscle strength, particularly extensors; increased use of in-flight exercise reduces postflight losses in strength regardless of mission duration; arm strength normal or slightly decreased after flight
EMG analysis	Postflight EMGs from gastrocnemius suggest increased susceptibility to fatigue and reduced muscular efficiency; EMGs from arm muscles show no change		Postflight EMGs from gastrocnemius show shift to higher frequencies, suggesting deterioration of muscle tissue; EMGs indicate increased susceptibility to fatigue; RPB in about 4 d
Reflexes (Achilles tendon)	Reflex duration decreased after flight		Reflex duration decreased after flight by 30% or more; reflex magnitude increased; compensatory increase in reflex duration about 2 w after flight; RPB about 1 month
Nitrogen and phosphorus balance		Negative balances early in flight shift to less negative or slightly positive balances later	Rapid return to markedly positive balances after flight

continued on page 731

TABLE 27.9 ■ *continued*

Physiologic Measure	Short Space Flights (1–14 d)	Long Space Flights (>2 w)	
		Preflight vs. In-Flight	Preflight vs. Postflight
Bone density	Os calcis density decreased after flight; radius and ulna show variable changes depending on measurement method		Os calcis density decreased after flight; amount of loss correlated with mission duration; little or no loss from non–weight-bearing bones; RPB is gradual; time course undetermined
Calcium balance	Progressive negative calcium balance in flight	Ca excretion in urine increases during first month in flight, then plateaus; fecal Ca excretion declines until day 10, then increases continually throughout flight; Ca balance becomes increasingly negative throughout flight	Urine Ca content drops below preflight baselines by day 10; fecal Ca content declines but does not reach preflight baseline by day 20; markedly negative Ca balance after flight, becomes less negative by day 10; Ca balance remains slightly negative on day 20; RPB at least several weeks

Data used by permission from Nicogossian AE, et al. Space physiology and medicine. 3rd ed. Philadelphia: Lea & Febiger, 1994:220.
RPB, return to preflight baseline; SLS, Spacelab Life Sciences; R, return to Earth; EMG, electromyography.

Part of the solution to the problem of bone loss in prolonged microgravity lies in selecting crewmembers with the greatest resistance to bone loss, including applying targeted prevention and/or treatment strategies.[154] Individual differences in the rate of bone loss during space flight relates to genetic factors. Identifying the genetic basis of osteoporosis may exclude susceptible individuals from prolonged missions. One hopes that effective combinations of pharmacologic, nutritional, and exercise countermeasures together with screening procedures can attenuate bone loss during space missions. Studying female crewmembers should offer a wealth of new information to compare with terrestrial research on gender-related bone loss including how reduced gravity affects hormone status. Carefully controlled, longitudinal studies in a microgravity environment (i.e., long-term studies on the ISS) become crucial to better understand skeletal biology.[154] Altering the ratio of animal protein intake to potassium intake can affect bone metabolism in ambulatory and bed-rest subjects. Changing this ratio may help attenuate bone loss on Earth and during space flight.[174]

Skeletal Muscle Adaptations

Bone loss during prolonged microgravity exposure coincides with considerable decrements in muscle mass and strength. Deterioration in muscle structure and function (see

TABLE 27.10 ■ BONE LOSS ON MIR SPACE STATION EXPRESSED AS PERCENTAGE OF BONE MINERAL DENSITY LOST PER MONTH

Variable	Crew Members (N)	Mean Loss (%)	SD[a]
Spine	18	1.07[b]	0.63
Neck of femur	18	1.16[b]	0.85
Trochanter	18	1.58[b]	0.98
Total body	17	0.35[b]	0.25
Pelvis	17	1.35[b]	0.54
Arm	17	0.04	0.88
Leg	16	0.34[b]	0.33

From LeBlanc A, et al. Bone mineral and lean tissue loss after long duration space flight. Am Soc Bone Miner Res 1996;11:S323.
[a]Standard deviation.
[b]$p < 0.01$.

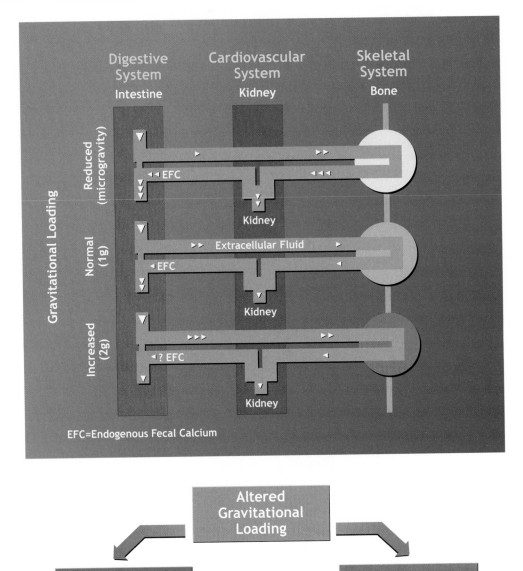

Figure 27.27 Influence of gravitational loading on calcium balance. *Top.* How the digestive system (intestine), cardiovascular system (kidney), and skeletal system (bone) adjust calcium distribution in response to (1) reduced (microgravity), (2) normal (1g), and (3) increased (2g) gravitational skeletal loading. The *shading within the circle in the right panel* represents the adaptation in whole-body bone mineral (*darker shading*, greater Ca accretion) to the different loading conditions. *Bottom.* Flow diagram proposing parallel calcium/endocrine and skeletal adaptive responses to changing gravitational loading, assuming adequate diet and endocrine balance. (Adapted from Morey-Holton ER, et al. The skeleton and its adaptation to gravity. In: Fregly MJ, Blatteis CM, eds. Handbook of physiology. Section 4, Environmental physiology, vol 2. American Physiological Society. New York: Oxford University Press, 1996.)

"Focus on Research," p. 734) could compromise crew health and safety during an exploration-class mission, including performance of critical EVA tasks, landing maneuvers, and procedures for leaving orbit on return to Earth. The absence of gravity virtually eliminates the load-bearing effects on antigravity muscles, rendering them susceptible to impaired performance in emergencies.

Such exigencies also apply to low-orbit missions. For example, egress from an orbiting spacecraft, even under normal conditions, taxes major muscle groups of the arms, legs, and torso. The current launch and entry suit (LES) that must be worn during all landing and exiting procedures weighs 23 kg, including a 12-kg parachute pack in the event of an emergency bailout. The additional weight could impair operational performance during an emergency that requires lifting, pushing and pulling, climbing, and jumping. In an expedited contingency landing, a crewmember deploys a 20-kg flight package that includes an inflatable slide that must be lifted up against the side hatch and locked into designated slots before inflation. Another scenario involves escape through the top window of the flight deck. This requires climbing out of the spacecraft's top window using a ground descent device to rappel to the surface.

Concentric and Eccentric Strength

The important role of concentric and eccentric muscle actions in space missions has focused experiments on pre- and postflight assessment of submaximal and maximal-muscle functions.[3,18,23,26,27,29,32,38,48,61] The preponderance of research in exercise countermeasures supports the use of resistance exercise training on various modes of exercise equipment to hypertrophy "space-bound" muscle to improve its force-generating capacity and produce positive ultrastructural changes and complimentary neural components.[1,2,7,8,43,68,75,130,147] Standard concentric and eccentric methods, including isokinetic loading devices and newer on-board equipment,[4,5,6,11,13,118,129,132,146] produce such improvements. For example, concentric strength of Skylab crews tested isokinetically before and 5 days after the 28-day flight showed decrements of approximately 25% in leg extensor strength.[150] Greater losses would probably have occurred had testing been conducted immediately upon landing. Subsequently, longer Skylab missions (59, 84, and 59 d) provided preflight fitness and conditioning that emphasized strengthening exercises for the lower extremities. This emphasis on preflight fitness produced smaller strength decrements during flight than during Skylab 2. On longer (110–237 d) and short (7 d) Russian missions, isokinetic concentric strength declined up to 28%.[63] The 7-day Salyut 6 mission decreased torque/velocity relationships in the gastrocnemius/soleus, anterior tibialis, and ankle extensor musculature. On longer 110- to 237-day missions, cosmonauts' average triceps strength loss ranged between 20 and 50%. Considerable losses in peak torque occurred for isokinetic ankle flexion and extension at all measured angular velocities of movement (Fig. 27.28). Studies of cosmonauts investigated the use of

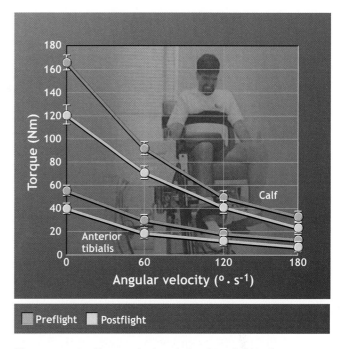

Figure 27.28 Force–velocity relationship of ankle flexors (anterior tibialis) and extensor calf muscles measured by isokinetic dynamometry at four angular velocities in six cosmonauts before and after 110 to 237 days in microgravity on *Salyut 7*. (Data summarized from Convertino VA. Effects of microgravity on exercise performance. In: Garrett WE, Kirkendall DT, eds. Exercise and sport science. Philadelphia: Lippincott Williams & Wilkins, 2000.)

functional electrostimulation (FES) to minimize atrophy, morphologic changes, and neuromuscular coordination patterns of skeletal muscles during prolonged space missions.[101] FES trains lower-extremity muscle groups using 1-second tetanic muscle actions followed by 2 seconds of relaxation continuously at 20 to 30% of maximum tetanic muscle force up to 6 hours daily.

Extended-Duration Orbiter Medical Project. TABLE 27.11 displays changes between 17 astronauts' preflight and landing (postflight) concentric and eccentric abdominal strength, eccentric strength of the quadriceps/soleus, and concentric quadriceps strength assessed at $30° \cdot s^{-1}$. Note that for each muscle group tested, a greater strength loss occurred in concentric than eccentric modes, with the greatest losses in the back (−23%) and quadriceps (−12%) muscles within 5 hours postflight. The three *inset figures* display the percentage strength changes in upper- and lower-leg and trunk flexor muscles. The unique aspect of these data compares space "exercisers" with "nonexercisers."[127,128] The exercisers trained by running on the treadmill (see p. 740) at intensities from 60 to 85% of preflight $\dot{V}O_{2peak}$ estimated from heart rate. Interestingly, testing conducted 7 days postflight revealed that on-board treadmill exercise did *not* ameliorate strength loss in all muscle groups. Preservation of muscle integrity even after only 9 to 11 days of space flight may target those muscles exercised—in accord with the principle of specificity of exercise training.

FOCUS On Research

MICROGRAVITY'S EFFECTS ON MUSCLE FIBERS

Edgerton VR, et al. Human fiber size and enzymatic properties after 5 and 11 days of space flight. J Appl Physiol 1995;78:1733.

▲ From the beginning of manned space flight, it has been assumed that prolonged exposure to near–zero-g would negatively affect neuromuscular function. Early experiments by the Soviet Union showed that space flight impaired a number of neuromotor components. Some neural adaptations persisted for days and weeks after space flight. A principal issue not addressed by the Soviets was the degree that neuromotor changes related to muscular components. This study by Edgerton and colleagues was the first to objectify space flight's effects on human muscle fibers. The researchers measured size and capillarization of single muscle fibers and activities of myofibrillar adenosine triphosphatase (ATPase), succinate dehydrogenase (SDH), and α-glycerophosphate dehydrogenase (GPD) of astronauts who flew either one 11-day or one of two 5-day missions.

Five male (age 40 y; range 33–46 y) and three female (age 38 y, range 36–40 y) astronauts served as subjects.

jects. Five subjects participated in a 261–hour flight; two subjects flew for 120 hour; and one subject flew for 128 hours. Preflight (3–16 weeks before the mission) and postflight (2–3 h after landing), a 6-mm needle was used to obtain muscle biopsies from the midportion of the vastus lateralis muscle. For postflight measures, all subjects minimized their walking and standing between landing and the biopsy. Tissue was quick-frozen in liquid nitrogen for subsequent analyses according to standard procedures.

Figures 1 and 2 present results for muscle fiber type and cross-sectional area (CSA), respectively, for type I and type II muscle fibers. The percentage of fibers classified as type I averaged 6 to 8% less after the mission. This reduction seemed to be compensated for by an increase in the percentage of type IIA fibers, with no change in type IIB fibers. A similar pre- to postflight difference was noted for the three subjects who flew for 5 days, but this difference was not statistically significant.

After the 11-day flight, CSA averaged 16 to 36% smaller than preflight values. Relative atrophy among fiber types was greatest for type IIB and least for

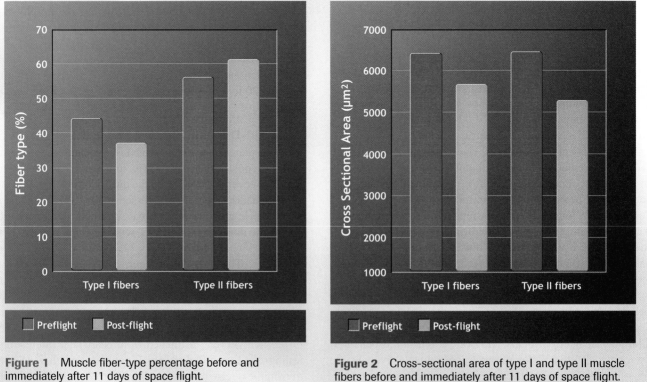

Figure 1   Muscle fiber-type percentage before and immediately after 11 days of space flight.

Figure 2   Cross-sectional area of type I and type II muscle fibers before and immediately after 11 days of space flight.

continued on page 735

Continued

type I fibers, yet mean fiber size decreased for all fibers. Crew members of 5-day missions also exhibited evidence of muscle atrophy.

The table presents results for fiber enzyme activities, enzyme ratios, total enzyme activities per fiber, and number of capillaries per fiber for all subjects on 5- and 11-day missions. A 32% decrease in total SDH activity in type II fibers was the only significant difference in enzyme activity during space flight. SDH activity per unit mass of the fibers did not change for either type I or type II fibers, but SDH activity per fiber decreased from muscle atrophy. No loss of total activity occurred for ATPase or GPD because the increase in activity per unit mass countered any atrophy effect.

The absolute number of capillaries supplying each type of muscle fiber decreased significantly from space flight. Mean fiber size also decreased (Fig. 2), so capillary number per unit muscle CSA remained unchanged.

Because of the close association between the CSA of single fibers, motor units, and whole muscle and the muscle's force-generating capacity, the present results suggest a loss in strength of the vastus lateralis within 11 days of space flight. The loss in CSA within 11 (and perhaps even 5) days of microgravity exposure agrees with previous data on rats and supports the usefulness of animal models to study human responses to space travel. Astronauts showed considerable variation in preflight and in-flight physical activity levels. More than likely, some of the between-subject variation in muscle atrophy related to physical activities during flight. For example, two of the three subjects who exercised four or more times during the flight showed little or no atrophy, while an astronaut with a high level of preflight physical fitness exhibited the greatest atrophy.

The work of Edgerton and colleagues demonstrated that skeletal muscle adapts rapidly to microgravity exposure, with a significant loss in CSA, selected enzyme activity, and fiber capillarization. These highly variable responses may partly relate to physical fitness level before launch and the extent of in-flight exercise.

■ **EFFECTS OF 5 TO 11 DAYS OF SPACE FLIGHT ON MUSCLE FIBER CAPILLARIZATION AND SELECTED ENZYME LEVELS**

Variable	TYPE I FIBERS			TYPE II FIBERS		
	Preflight	Postflight	%Diff	Preflight	Postflight	%Diff
ATPase activity	383.0	376.0	−2	471.0	513.0	−9[a]
SDH activity	232.0	203.0	−13	184.0	158.0	−14
ATP/SDH	1.8	2.1	17*	2.9	4.0	38[a]
GPD activity	5.9	10.6	80	25.0	23.0	−8
Total ATPase	212.0	177.0	−17	258.0	211.0	−18
Total SDH	133.0	97.0	−27	105.0	71.0	−32[a]
Capillaries per fiber	4.7	3.8	−19*	4.8	3.6	26[a]

[a] Significantly different at the 0.05 level.

Muscle Ultrastructural Changes

Permanent neuromuscular dysfunction has not yet been demonstrated during prolonged space missions. Nevertheless, in-flight and postflight changes during missions of nearly 1 year reveal altered muscular coordination patterns, some delayed-onset muscle soreness (DOMS), and generalized muscular fatigue and weakness. Many unanswered questions remain about human muscle physiology and biochemical adaptations related to microgravity exposure in humans. Animal models using head-down, tail-suspended, non–weight-bearing rodents (see FIG. 27.29) rely on reduced gravity's effects on skeletal muscle contractile morphology and physiology. Placing rodents in a harness that elevates the hindquarters eliminates the normal loading of weight-bearing hindlimb muscles (Fig. 27.29). The model mimics the fluid shifts of microgravity; it produces reduced sensory input to the motor centers and less mechanical stimulation of connective, muscular, and osseous tissues. Specifically, both space flight and non–weight-bearing confinement atrophies rat skeletal muscles, mainly the slow twitch (type 1) leg-extensor fibers.[10,15,48,76,123,125] Also, non–weight bearing in microgravity reduces contractile activity assessed by EMG of male rat hindlimb soleus muscle by 75%.[30,49]

Maximal Explosive Leg Power Before and After Space Missions

FIGURE 27.30 shows different duration space flight effects on maximal explosive power (MEP) and maximal cycling power (MCP) assessed preflight and 26 days postflight for astronauts exposed to microgravity for up to 180 days. The *inset illustration at bottom left* shows the ergometer–dynamometer to assess MEP. Subjects made six maximal pushes with both

TABLE 27.11 ■ *TOP LEFT.* CHANGES IN SKELETAL MUSCLE STRENGTH PERFORMANCE ON LANDING VERSUS PREFLIGHT. *BOTTOM LEFT.* PERCENTAGE CHANGES IN UPPER-LEG, LOWER-LEG *(TOP RIGHT),* AND TRUNK STRENGTH *(BOTTOM RIGHT)* FOLLOWING SPACE FLIGHT IN "SPACE EXERCISERS" VS. NONEXERCISERS

	TEST MODE	
MUSCLE GROUP	**CONCENTRIC**	**ECCENTRIC**
Back	−23 (±4)*	−14 (±4)*
Abdomen	−10 (±2)*	−8 (±2)*
Quadriceps	−12 (±3)*	−7 (±3)
Hamstrings	−6 (±3)	−1 (±0)
Tibialis anterior	−8 (±4)	−1 (±2)
Gastroc/soleus	1 (±3)	2 (±4)
Deltoids	1 (±5)	−2 (±2)
Pecs/lats	0 (±5)	−6 (±2)
Biceps	6 (±6)	1 (±2)
Triceps	0 (±2)	8 (±6)

*Significantly lower than preflight value.

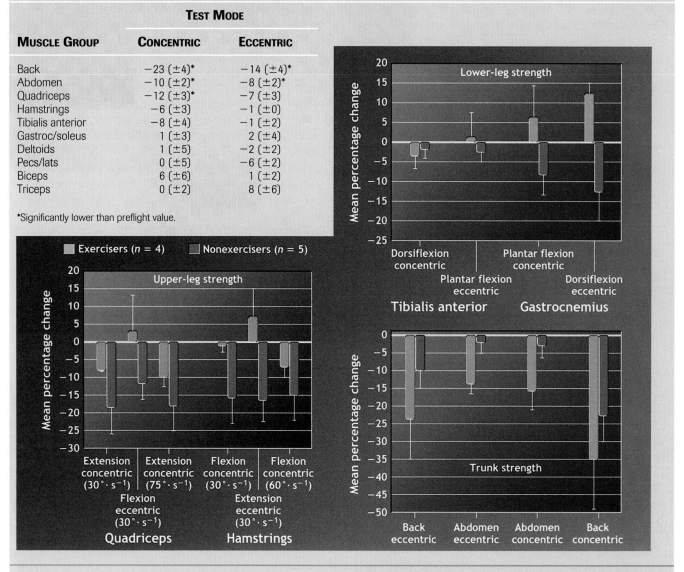

Data from Extended Duration Orbiter Medical Project. 1989–1995. Final report NASA/SP-1999-534. NASA. Lyndon B. Johnson Space Center. Houston, TX, 1999.

feet against the force platform for approximately 250 ms at a knee angle of 110° with a 2-minute rest between pushes. MCP involved five to seven "all-out" pedal revolutions for 5 to 6 seconds on a bicycle ergometer following either 5 to 7 minutes of mild aerobic exercise or free-wheel pedaling. The *top figure* shows the percentage of premission scores for MEP and MCP for four astronauts at four periods after mission completion. Astronaut 1, who spent 31 days in orbit, recovered nearly all MEP by 11 days postflight. For the other three astronauts, whose missions lasted 169 to 180 days, MEP recovery approached only 77% of the preflight value. For the two astro-

nauts tested 26 days postflight, MEP for astronaut 3 was 80% of his premission score, while astronaut 4 achieved only 57%. In contrast, each astronaut's MCP, a measure of more sustained power output, recovered more rapidly throughout the postflight measurement period, with final scores within 10% of premission values.

The *bottom figure (right)* compares all values for MCP plotted relative to the corresponding MEP scores expressed as a percentage of premission values. On average, MCP deterioration exceeded MEP loss. The researchers attributed the differential deterioration in the two forms of maximal exercise to

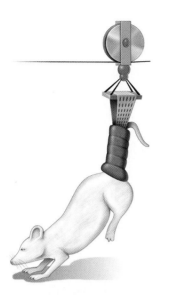

Figure 27.29 Hind limb suspension (uploading).

muscular and neurologic factors involved in each form of effort. In essence, the absence of gravity appears to rearrange postural muscle tone and locomotor coordination substantially. This adversely affects the motor control system; in one astronaut it negatively affected the normal pattern of motor unit recruitment. Changes in neural drive during long-term missions of 90 to 180 days could impact the contractile and elastic characteristics of lower limb musculature.[80]

COUNTERMEASURE STRATEGIES

Countermeasures systematically attempt to neutralize (or minimize) space flight's potentially harmful deconditioning effects on crew physiologic function, performance, and overall health during mission-critical maneuvers, particularly reentry and landing. In the absence of gravity, no linear, downward head-to-foot acceleration forces (referred to as +Gz) act on the body. This makes normal biologic functions more susceptible to short- and longer term maladaptations such as **space motion sickness (SMS)**. This syndrome usually manifests within the first 72 hours of a mission and often is characterized by clumsiness, difficulty concentrating, disorientation, persisting sensation after-effects, nausea, pallor, drowsiness, vomiting, vertigo while walking and standing, difficulty walking a straight line, blurred vision, and dry heaves. Some symptoms resemble those of terrestrial motion sickness. SMS symptoms often dissipate on their own or with medication during the first few days of space flight. On reentry after short-duration missions, SMS can manifest as a general reentry syndrome (GRS) that imposes potentially deleterious effects on astronaut performance. GRS symptoms include vertigo, nausea, instability, and fatigue induced by reimposition of increased +Gz during reentry and landing. In contrast to the relatively acute emergence of SMS, weeks and months of prolonged absence of normal gravitational loading

adversely affect bone and muscular structure and function. Concurrently, fluid shifts within the vascular system produce considerable loss of electrolytes and bone minerals. Cumulative negative effects during sustained missions could trigger more severe medical complications that include increased risk for developing renal stones, orthostatic intolerance, neurosensory and motor dysfunctions, and musculoskeletal injuries (including bone fracture) in the weeks and months following return to Earth.

Without appropriate countermeasures, microgravity's deleterious effects mimic the adverse changes with prolonged bed rest. For example, 30-days of bed rest dramatically impairs skeletal muscle function; knee extensor strength declines nearly 23%, while knee flexor strength and leg volume decrease 10 to 12%. Reductions in limb volume result from decreased muscular cross-sectional area from muscle fiber protein loss. The 28-day Skylab 2 mission decreased muscular function and leg volume to an extent comparable with bed rest.[30] The protein loss has been attributed in part to a normal adaptive response to decreased workload on weight-bearing muscles.[142] Decrements in cardiovascular function generally parallel losses in muscle strength and size.[148,149]

Projected travel time for an exploration-class mission to Mars requires approximately 6 months of isolation in microgravity, more than a year of planetary habitation at 0.38g, followed by a 6-month return trip to Earth (in microgravity). Thus, on-board countermeasures play a critical role in minimizing pathology or impaired motor task performance to preserve crew health and safety.[126] More than likely, gender-related factors affect these health and performance goals.[54] In-flight resistance and endurance exercises show the greatest overall potential as exercise countermeasures to combat microgravity's sustained deleterious effects. TABLE 27.12 lists examples of adverse effects and clinical consequences of prolonged microgravity exposure in four functional body areas and possible countermeasure strategies. A recent review assesses countermeasures strategies (fluid loading, G-suit inflation, pharmacologic agents, artificial gravity, short-term physical exercise to elicit maximal effort) to minimize microgravity-induced orthostatic intolerance.[35] A compelling argument posits that combining multiple countermeasures could afford astronaut's optimal protection against potential adverse effects of long-duration space missions.

In-Flight Exercise

Four exercise modes have played predominant roles during in-flight workouts aboard space missions: (1) treadmill walking and running, (2) cycle ergometry, including maximal exercise performed 24 hours before landing,[105] (3) leg rowing, and (4) upper- and lower-body multijoint dynamic resistance exercise. The latest resistance exercise training equipment aboard the ISS, the interim Resistance Exercise Device (iRED) allows astronauts to exercise dynamically with increasing resistance throughout a full range of motion (ROM) for three basic exercise movements that stress the hip, back, and spine. Peak

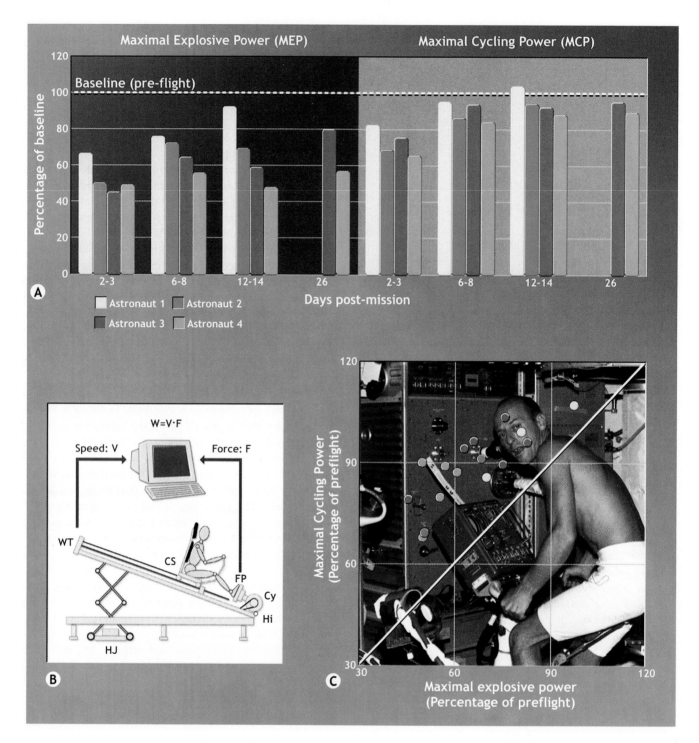

Figure 27.30   **A.** Effects of up to 180 days in microgravity on changes in maximal explosive power (MEP) and maximal cycling power (MCP). **B.** The ergometer–dynamometer assessed MEP of the lower limbs by varying either force or velocity. *HJ,* hydraulic jack; *WT,* wire tachometer; *CS,* carriage seat; *FP,* force platform; *Cy,* isokinetic cycle ergometer; *Hi,* hinge. MEP was assessed within less than 0.3 s, and MCP was determined during all-out pedaling on a cycle ergometer for 5 to 6 s. **C.** Plot of MCP versus MEP scores expressed as a percentage of premission values. (Data modified from Antonutto G, et al. Effects of microgravity on maximal power of lower limbs during very short efforts in humans. J Appl Physiol 1999;86:85.)

TABLE 27.12 ■ **ADVERSE EFFECTS OF SPACE FLIGHT AND PROPOSED COUNTERMEASURES**

AREA	MAJOR FINDINGS	CLINICAL/OPERATIONAL CONSEQUENCES	COUNTERMEASURES UNDER EVALUATION
Cardiovascular	Fluid loss Electrolyte changes Electrical activity disturbances Neuroreflex readjustments Electrolyte changes Electrical activity disturbances Neuroreflex readjustments	Orthostatic intolerance	Fluid/electrolyte replenishment Exercise
Neurovestibular	Motion sickness Gait disturbances Motor performance degradation	Decreased productivity	Palliative treatments (intramuscular promethazine) Adaptation trainers
Musculoskeletal	Bone mass loss Muscle mass loss	Renal stone formation Muscle/joint injuries Bone fractures	Diet Exercise; lower-body negative pressure Drugs (biphosphonates, etc.)
Immunologic endocrinologic	Changes in immune response in vitro Inappropriate hormonal secretion or metabolism	Susceptibility to infection (?) Synergistic radiation effects Allergic reactions and disorders	Growth factors (?)

From Nicogossian AE, et al. Countermeasures to space deconditioning. In: Nicogossian AE, et al., eds. Space physiology and medicine. 3rd ed. Philadelphia: Lea & Febiger, 1994:447.
Note: Third column lists factors (renal stone formation, muscle/joint injuries, bone fractures) undocumented in NASA reports.

force, average force, and ROM are recorded for each repetition.[129] FIGURE 27.31 shows different exercise modes during KC-135 flights and space missions, including the iRED in row D. At the end of this section, we discuss unique exercise countermeasures devices, human-powered centrifuges.

Lunar–Mars Life Support Test Experiment

NASA conducts research to examine the efficacy of exercise testing and prescription protocols for onboard countermeasures on future space flights. The experiments provide insights into potentially useful training methodologies for application to space missions, particularly targeted resistance exercise for lower-extremity muscles—those most likely to suffer impairment. The trial studied men and women before, during, and after a 60-day confined-chamber experiment at 1g in the Life Support Systems Integration Unit, a component scheduled for a future ISS mission. A combined exercise countermeasure protocol quantified the following:

• Training effects from exercise countermeasures
• Tolerance to combined aerobic and resistance training countermeasures
• Methods to quantify the performance of exercise countermeasures for valid monitoring of exercise compliance

Measurements included:

1. $\dot{V}O_{2peak}$. Subjects pedaled an electronically braked cycle ergometer in the upright position at 75 rpm at increasing workloads of 50, 100, and 150 W for men and 50, 75, and 100 W for women. Exercise then continued in 25-W increments to volitional termination.
2. *Submaximal and maximal sustained aerobic exercise.* Subjects cycled for three 5-minute periods at 75 rpm at exercise intensities of 25, 50, 75, and 100% $\dot{V}O_{2peak}$.
3. *Resistance exercise.* Subjects performed maximal-effort bench press, seated shoulder press, latissimus dorsi pull, squat, and heel raise on a multifunction exercise station preprogrammed for fast- and slow-speed movement velocities.

In the chamber, subjects exercised 6 days per week, alternating between preprogrammed 32-minute cycle ergometer aerobic workouts at 40 to 80% of $\dot{V}O_{2peak}$ and the five resistance exercises in the pretest assessment. They performed three sets of 6- to 12-RM of each exercise beginning with a warm-up at 50% 1-RM. Movement speed varied from $10° \cdot s^{-1}$ at the slow speed to $20° \cdot s^{-1}$ at the fastest speed. Submaximal ergometer tests were administered on days 15, 30, and 58 in lieu of the aerobic workout. Subject compliance averaged 91% with the exercise program.

FIGURE 27.32 shows peak torque developed at low, medium, and high movement speeds with resistance exercises during training weeks 2, 5, and 8. Within-subject evaluation revealed that all subjects improved in strength measures (peak torque, average peak torque, total work) at each speed over the 8-week period. The pre- to post-chamber exercise oxygen consumptions shown in the *top left panel* of FIGURE 27.33 reveal that average $\dot{V}O_{2peak}$ increased 7% during chamber confinement, ranging between 1 and 20%; the initially high-fit subjects improved the least. Peak posttraining workload also

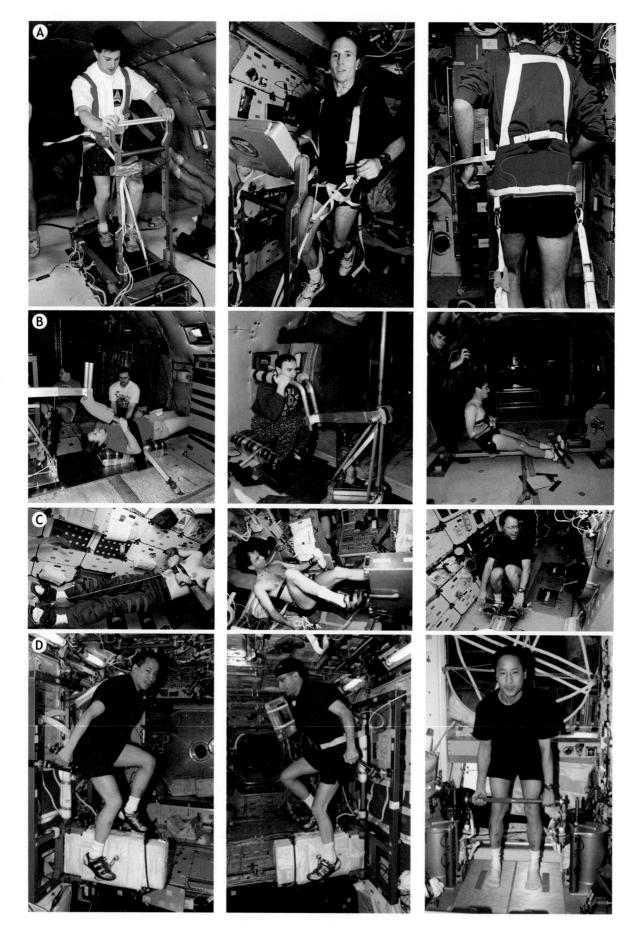

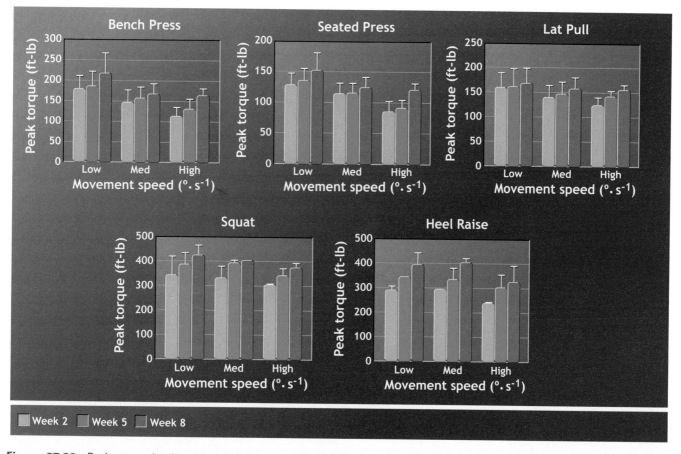

Figure 27.32 Peak torque developed at low, medium, and high movement during bench press, seated press, lat pull, squat, and heel raise during weeks 2, 5, and 8. (Adapted from Lee SL, et al. Exercise Countermeasures Demonstration Project during the Lunar-Mars Life Support Test Project. Phase IIA. NASA. NASA/TP-98-206537. Lyndon B. Johnson Space Center, Houston, TX. 1998.)

increased (13%), as did exercise duration (7%). Submaximal exercise heart rate *(bottom left panel)* declined 6% during the last test session ("submax 3") compared with pretraining values. Ratings of perceived exertion and systolic blood pressure during the three training sessions did not change. In contrast, diastolic blood pressure declined by 19% after 30 days ("submax 2") and 13% at 58 days ("submax 3").

Countermeasures on Long-Duration Missions

The prolonged Russian Mir missions made extensive use of exercise countermeasures based on considerable prior experience with extended space missions. Like their American counterparts, cosmonauts did not exercise during the flight's first 48

Figure 27.31 Examples of exercise training and measurement for different exercise modes during microgravity conditions. **A.** Tethered treadmill exercise during KC-135 training *(left)* and space shuttle mission *(middle and right)*. Note the strap arrangement around the upper body and straps anchored to the hips to keep the astronaut tethered to the treadmill. **B.** KC-135 training for upper-arm bench press exercise *(left)*, squat exercise *(middle)*, and upper-arm rowing exercise *(right)*. **C.** Exercise training aboard different space shuttle missions showing upper-arm, cycling, and rowing modes. **D.** The *left* and *middle* photos show astronauts exercising on the Cycle Ergometer with Vibration Isolation System (CEVIS) in the Destiny laboratory on the ISS. The *right photo* shows the astronaut using the short bar for the Interim Resistive Exercise Device (IRED) to perform upper-body strengthening pull-ups in the Unity node on ISS. (Photos courtesy of NASA, Lyndon B. Johnson Space Center, Houston, TX.)

Alkner BA, et al. Effects of strength training, using a gravity-independent exercise system, performed during 110 days of simulated space station confinement. Eur J Appl Physiol 2003;90:44.

Convertino VA. Planning strategies for development of effective exercise and nutrition countermeasures for long-duration space flight. Nutrition 2002;18:880.

Cowell SA, et al. The exercise and environmental physiology of extravehicular activity. Aviat Space Environ Med 2002;73:54.

Lee SM, et al. Foot-ground reaction force during resistive exercise in parabolic flight. Aviat Space Environ Med 2004 75: 405.

McCrory JL, et al. Locomotion in simulated zero gravity: ground reaction forces. Aviat Space Environ Med 2004 75: 203.

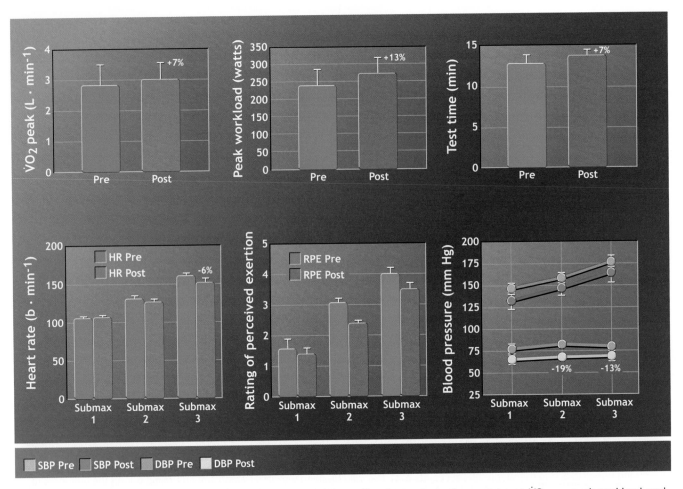

Figure 27.33 The 60-day Lunar–Mars countermeasures experiment. *Top,* Comparison of pre- and post-$\dot{V}O_{2peak}$, peak workload, and test duration on the bicycle ergometer. *Bottom,* Heart rate, rating of perceived exertion *(RPE),* and blood pressure during three submaximal test sessions. *SBP,* systolic blood pressure; *DBP,* diastolic blood pressure. (Adapted from Lee SL, et al. Exercise Countermeasures Demonstration Project during the Lunar-Mars Life Support Test Project. Phase IIA. NASA. NASA/TP-98-206537. Lyndon B. Johnson Space Center, Houston, TX. 1998.)

to 72 hours to provide sufficient recovery from SMS that affects nearly 70% of astronauts and cosmonauts on their first flight. The Soviet cosmonaut Titov deserves credit as the first person to experience SMS—refractory dizziness when making head movements and subsequent nausea and illness after 6 hours during the 1961 Vostok-2 mission.[59] On current space shuttle missions, an intramuscular injection of Phenergan relieves SMS, replacing Dexedrine and other drug combinations that evoke strong negative central nervous system responses.

Toward the end of the flight's first week and over the next 24 days, cosmonauts exercised twice daily, progressing to 1 hour of continuous ergometer cycling at an initial workload of 900 kg-m · min^{-1}. Exercise intensity progressively increased to maintain heart rate between 80 and 90% of age-predicted maximum. They added 5 to 15 minutes of daily strengthening exercise (hamstrings, trunk extensors) using bungee-cord devices. On missions exceeding 1 month, cosmonauts exercise twice daily for 1 hour on a passive (subject-driven) treadmill with a restraint system similar to that used by space shuttle astronauts (see FIG. 27.34 for schematic of U.S. Space Shuttle passive treadmill in which a rapid-onset centrifugal brake provides seven braking levels to control drag

forces on the running track). To simulate gravitational forces, straps from their side—called subject load devices—secure the cosmonaut to the treadmill. Treadmill exercise, using a harness and bungee tether system, generates the effects of 0.5 to 0.7g, while exercise on Salyut and Mir treadmills generated a "gravitational" pull of 0.62g. The nonmotorized treadmill requires running at a positive percentage grade to overcome frictional resistance. At present, the treadmill provides the only mode of on-board exercise. Astronauts wear a monitor secured to the ear (ear oximeter) to record heart rate continuously by an infrared sensor that detects pulsating blood flow in the earlobe. A mechanical sensor wire on the side of the treadmill displays distance run from the number of treadmill revolutions completed.

FIGURE 27.35 compares heart rate response during continuous *(top)* and intermittent *(bottom)* treadmill exercise during two shuttle missions. Astronauts did not attain assigned target heart rates (representing 60, 70, or 80% VO_{2max}) when exercising continuously for 30 minutes during an 11-day mission. More than likely, altered running mechanics while wearing the bungee apparatus reduced target heart rates.

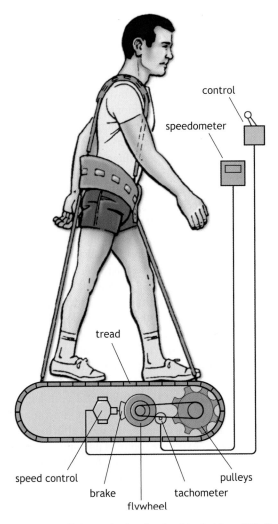

Figure 27.34 Schematic details of subject-driven U.S. Space Shuttle treadmill.

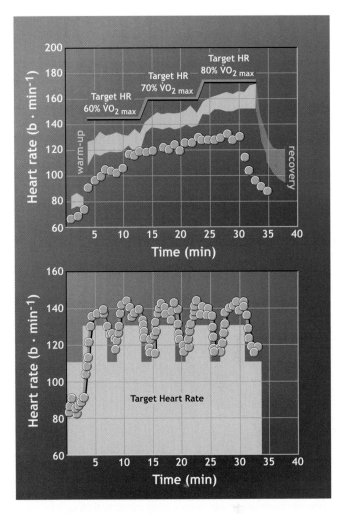

Figure 27.35 *Top.* Heart rate during continuous treadmill exercise at 60, 70, and 80% of $\dot{V}O_{2max}$ on an 11-day shuttle mission. The *light green shaded area* shows the exercise heart rate range during workout days 3 to 11. *Green circles* represent heart rate during a familiarization run on flight day 2. The intense workouts helped to minimize orthostatic dysfunction upon landing. *Bottom.* Heart rate during five intervals of a treadmill exercise routine using the shuttle treadmill. (Adapted from Lee SL, et al. Exercise Countermeasures Demonstration Project during the Lunar–Mars Life Support Test Project. Phase IIA. NASA. NASA/TP-98-206537. Lyndon B. Johnson Space Center, Houston, TX. 1998.)

INTEGRATIVE QUESTION

What type of exercise training program would you advise an astronaut to undertake 6 months prior to a Mars mission and during the mission?

New Approach: Human-Powered Centrifuges Simulate Gravitational Loading

NASA currently supports new countermeasures that use unique exercise devices to combat the deleterious effects of space flight deconditioning.

Self-Powered Human Centrifuge. Force and acceleration represent two distinct entities ($F = m \times a$), so simply applying force to an object (e.g., bungee cord or lower-body negative-pressure device) in microgravity does not mean that it regulates a beneficial "loading" of the skeleton similar to exercise on Earth. An animal or human placed in a rotating centrifuge experiences the force benefits produced by a sustained-acceleration "gravity" field. In this regard, a self-powered human centrifuge displayed schematically in FIGURE 27.36, offers promise for counteracting adverse physiologic effects of extended-duration space missions.[77]

Pedaling the **Space Cycle** propels the centrifuge in a curvilinear motion about a fixed central shaft rigidly fixed within the spacecraft. A centrifuge effect produces artificial gravity as the rider rotates about the shaft while pedaling. Irregularly shaped cams fixed to the foot crankshaft allow an adjustable spring-loaded device to trace a path around the cam and provide resistance to pedaling. Altering cam configuration generates foot force profiles to simulate walking, jogging, and cycling. Combining artificial gravity with impact-loading

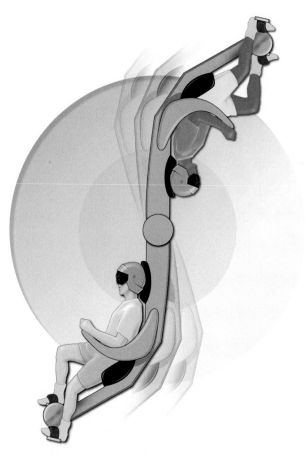

Figure 27.36 Pedaling the self-powered human centrifuge (Space Cycle) creates artificial gravity by producing head-to-foot acceleration (+Gz). Added instrumentation can monitor extremity strength, power output, body mass, and other parameters for ongoing functional and medical research. Restricting head movements by wearing a harness attached to the frame, combined with virtual reality headgear to maintain a horizontal visual experience, could minimize sensory input conflict during cycling, dramatically reducing space motion sickness. (From Kreitenberg A, et al. The "Space Cycle"™ self powered human centrifuge: a proposed countermeasure for prolonged human space flight. Aviat Space Environ Med 1998;69:66.)

exercise offers the potential for an effective countermeasures strategy against orthostatic intolerance, macro- and microscopic skeletal muscle deterioration, and loss of bone mass.

The Space Cycle designed for the ISS simulates gravitational acceleration (+Gz) experienced while standing on Earth and provides axial loading on the rider's long bones. The added "stress" in microgravity should provide similar 1g stresses on the musculoskeletal system. Thus, missions lasting a year or more should benefit from artificially induced gravity produced by human powered, in-flight centrifugation. A recent experiment comparing Gz (upright cycle ergometry) and 2 Gz conditions (Space Cycle) at the same work rate on hemodynamic measures (heart rate, systolic and diastolic blood pressure, oxygen uptake) revealed few differences between the two experimental conditions. The authors concluded that the subject's hemodynamic responses were well tolerated under the Space Cycle's low hypergravity conditions.[21]

In addition to the Space Cycle, NASA's Ames Research Center has developed its own self-powered human centrifuge to evaluate the countermeasure potential of this exercise mode with and without the effect of +Gz acceleration (FIG. 27.37).[60] The Ames centrifuge consists of a short-arm, dual-couch device powered by a chain-linked cycle foot drive. Approximately two pedal revolutions produce a 360° rotation of the centrifuge to generate a maximum of 5g. Research with this device required subjects to perform exercise under two conditions: (1) pedaling the centrifuge for 2 minutes at 25, 50, and 75% of maximum cycling rpm, defined as all-out until volitional fatigue and (2) exercising at the same three intensities without centrifuge acceleration. Changes in heart rate under the two conditions assessed the effects of only exercise and exercise coupled with +Gz acceleration. Subjects remained blindfolded during exercise to prevent nausea or vertigo. They achieved 3.9 Gz (43.7 rpm) for maximal-acceleration exercise, 0.2 Gz at 25% (11.0 rpm), 1.0 Gz at 50% (21.8 rpm), and 2.2 Gz (32.8 rpm) at 75% maximum Gz. The *bottom* of Figure 27.21 compares the effects of the two conditions (exercise acceleration and passive acceleration) on heart rate response at different percentages of maximal acceleration. The numbers at the end of each trial (shown at the *right*) represent heart rate at the end of exercise minus heart rate at the start. Pedaling the Ames centrifuge produced its intended effect—it augmented heart rate response to exercise at 75% maximum Gz. Additional research must quantify the most effective exercise and artificial gravity exposure (optimal magnitude, frequency, and duration) during space missions for full adaptation of head, arm, and leg movement equilibrium.[78]

Space Pharmacology

SMS remains the most persistent short-term problem during space flight. Approximately 50% of cosmonauts, 60% of Apollo astronauts, and 71% of first-time shuttle astronauts encountered mild-to-severe SMS. TABLE 27.13 lists the incidence and severity of SMS during 36 space shuttle flights through 1991. Note the decline in prevalence from 77 episodes to 34 episodes for crewmembers on their second shuttle flight. On the 1993 Space Shuttle Life Sciences mission (SLS-2), only one astronaut experienced nausea but without sickness during the mission's first few days.[137]

SMS is not confined to orbital flight; nearly 10% of astronauts experience it during reentry or immediately upon landing, including training during parabolic flights.[128] Ninety-two percent of cosmonauts report SMS upon return from missions that last several months or longer.[73] To date, no single pharmacologic treatment prevents or cures SMS. On shuttle missions, the disorder shows no preference for commanders, pilots, or mission specialists, gender or age, career versus noncareer astronauts, or first-time versus repeat flyers. Incomplete understanding of the cause(s) of SMS hampers its treatment, but pharmacologic treatment usually relieves most symptoms within the first 3 days in the space environment. Additional countermeasure strategies to minimize SMS effects include mechanical and electrical stimulation and biofeedback techniques. Despite these efforts,

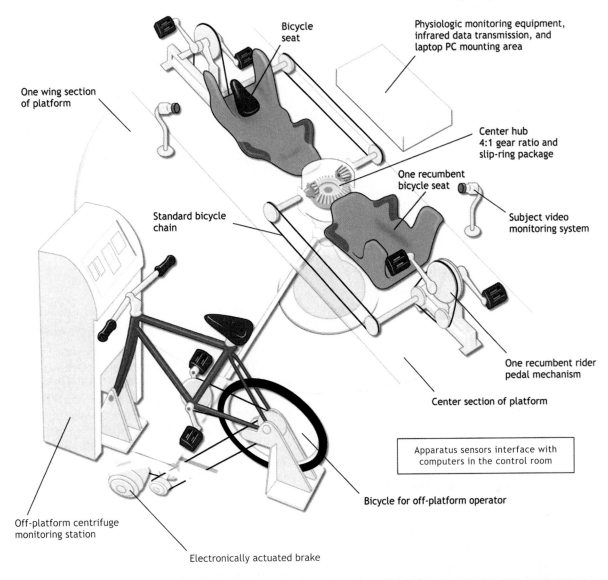

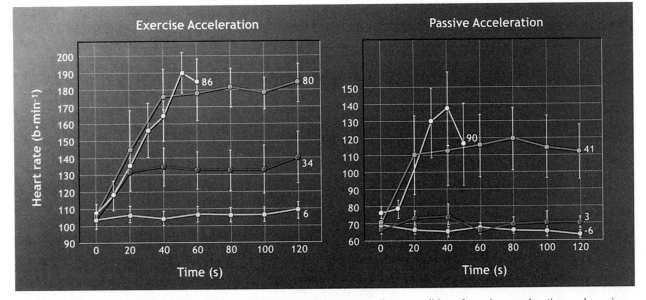

Figure 27.37   *Top.* The Ames centrifuge. *Bottom.* Comparison of the effects of two conditions (exercise acceleration and passive acceleration) on heart rate response at different percentages of maximal acceleration. Numbers at the *end of lines* represent final HR increase above rest. (Modified from Greenleaf JE, et al. Cycle-powered short radius [1.9 m] centrifuge: effect of exercise versus passive acceleration on heart rate in humans. NASA technical memorandum 110433. 1997. NASA. Ames Research Center. Moffett Field, CA, 1997.)

TABLE 27.13 ■ INCIDENCE AND SEVERITY OF SPACE MOTION SICKNESS DURING 36 SPACE SHUTTLE FLIGHTS

MOTION SICKNESS RATING	NUMBER OF CREWMEMBERS		
	FIRST SHUTTLE FLIGHT	LATER SHUTTLE FLIGHT	TOTALS
None	32 (29%)	28 (45%)	60 (35%)
Mild	36 (33%)	24 (39%)	60 (35%)
Moderate	29 (27%)	10 (16%)	39 (23%)
Severe	12 (11%)	0 (0%)	12 (7%)
Totals	109 (64%)	62 (36%)	171 (100%)

From Nicogossian AE, et al. Countermeasures to space deconditioning. In: Nicogossian AE, et al., eds. Space physiology and medicine. 3rd ed. Philadelphia: Lea & Febiger, 1994:230.

medication provides the most effective pharmacologic therapy against SMS.

Medications

The following classes of drugs help to minimize SMS effects:

1. *Anticholinergics (parasympatholytics)* blunt parasympathetic nervous system effects. Scopolamine in a dose of 0.6 to 1.0 mg proves most effective to eradicate approximately 90% of symptoms. Researchers believe that scopolamine blocks neural communication between the nerves of the vestibule and the brain's vomiting center (located in the reticular formation of the medulla) to retard the action of acetylcholine. Scopolamine also may work directly on the vomiting center.
2. *Antihistamines* (action antagonistic to histamine) offer some protection but are not as effective as scopolamine.
3. *Sympathomimetics* mimic sympathetic nervous system effects. Amphetamine with scopolamine confers beneficial effects.
4. *Sympatholytics* inhibit sympathetic nervous system effects.

"Scope-dex," a combination of scopolamine (parasympatholytic) and amphetamine (sympathomimetic) exhibits the best overall success in minimizing SMS. Meclazine, a promising medication in land-based trials to maintain optimal cognitive functioning (histamine receptor blocker medication), also may blunt SMS's deleterious effects.[114]

Lower-Body Negative Pressure

FIGURE 27.38 shows the in-flight lower-body negative pressure (LBNP) apparatus aboard Skylab (A, B) and Shuttle (C) missions. This device serves two functions:

1. Assesses orthostatic deconditioning during space flight and postlanding.

2. As a countermeasure against adverse orthostatic changes with short- and long-term missions.

The LBNP device applies negative pressure to the lower limbs. This forces fluid in the vascular system to migrate downward from the upper torso to the lower body—an effect that counters the in-flight response to microgravity. During three 6-month Mir missions, cosmonauts wore thigh cuffs (rather than rely on an LBNP device) at 1, 3 to 4, and 5 to 5.5 months and assessed cardiovascular parameters with echocardiography. Data were contrasted with control sessions 30 days preflight and 3 and 7 days postflight.[67] In all cosmonauts, a reduced vasoconstrictive response and a less efficient blood flow redistribution toward the brain coincided with orthostatic intolerance during postflight stand tests.[131] The vascular response to LBNP tests remained depressed during the flights. Thus, the thigh cuffs compensated partially for the cardiovascular changes induced by microgravity but not for microgravity deconditioning. Upregulation of nitric oxide (NO; a potent vasodilator and natriuretic) may explain orthostatic intolerance in microgravity.[158] If this mechanism proves correct, administration of an inducible nitric oxide synthase inhibitor (iNOS) may attenuate orthostatic intolerance when astronauts return to Earth following a mission; it also may benefit patients following extended bed rest.

Assessing Orthostatic Deconditioning Effects

Disruptions in cardiovascular dynamics—heart rate, blood pressure, and leg volume changes during space missions—could compromise crew performance and mission success.[17,34] For example, orthostatic testing conducted after Gemini (14 days) and during Skylab (80 days) missions documented the degree of orthostatic deconditioning effects. The Gemini vehicles (including Mercury and Apollo) barely had enough room for the astronauts, so the mission could not accommodate an on-board LBNP chamber. Thus, testing on Gemini took place only before and after flights. Also, Gemini flights used a tilt table rather than LBNP (FIG. 27.39, *top panel*). A 15-minute, 70° vertical LBNP tilt test produced dra-

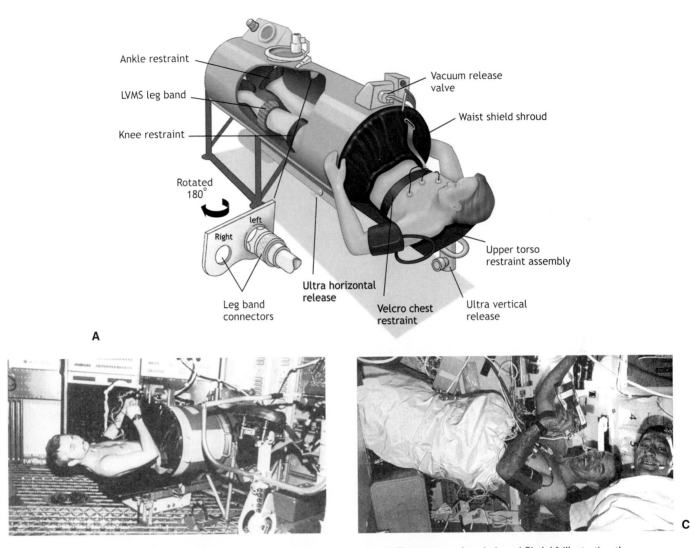

Figure 27.38   A. Schematic diagram of the lower-body negative pressure (LBNP) apparatus (used aboard Skylab) illustrating the upper- and lower-body restraint assembly, including the leg volume measuring system (LVMS) leg band. The waist seal shroud maintains controlled and regulated negative pressure from 0 to 50 mm Hg below ambient pressure. During ground tests, a vacuum provides negative pressure; during flight, negative pressure occurs from the space vacuum. **B.** LBNP device beginning with the 28-day Skylab 2 mission (1973). The 20-inch diameter, 48-inch long cylindrical chamber separates longitudinally to provide access to the legs, beginning at the subject's waist at the iliac crests, and ease of securing leg bands to measure change in lower-limb (calf) volume.[133] Lower-leg volume changes on exposure to negative pressure because of caudal displacement of blood and other fluids. **C.** LBNP assessment aboard an early shuttle mission. (From Nicogossian AE, et al., eds. Space physiology and medicine. 3rd ed. Philadelphia: Lea & Febiger, 1994.)

matic changes in heart rate, systolic and diastolic blood pressure, and leg volume during the prolonged Skylab mission compared with the same variables assessed 3 weeks prior to liftoff. Heart rate increased 100% from 70 b · min^{-1} at rest at the start of the LBNP tilt test to 140 b · min^{-1} at the end of the procedure. Systolic blood pressure declined more (30%) than diastolic blood pressure (<10%) during the tilt, whereas leg volume increased 10-fold during the test.

The *bottom* of Figure 27.39 shows the pattern of resting heart rate in a −50-mm Hg LBNP test in one crewmember during the 80-day Skylab 4 mission and 2 months postflight. While not as dramatic as the shorter duration Gemini experiments, the resting heart rate increase in response to LBNP during Skylab confirmed the relative instability (and variability)

of heart rate, particularly during the first month of space flight compared with the end of the mission. Heart rate with LBNP during preflight never exceeded 75 b · min^{-1}, but it always exceeded this value throughout the mission. On Skylab missions 2 and 3, resting heart rate averaged 109 b · min^{-1}, a 55% increase over preflight values.

LBNP Combined Countermeasures

A countermeasure combination of LBNP and increased fluid ingestion during space flight improves performance on an upright standing posture test postflight.[19,159] For example, two groups of 26 male astronauts consumed either no fluid or a loading volume of 32 oz of water or juice plus eight salt

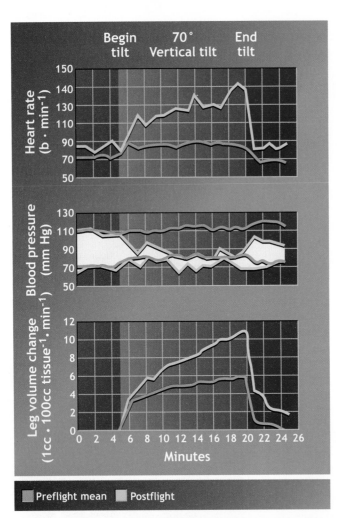

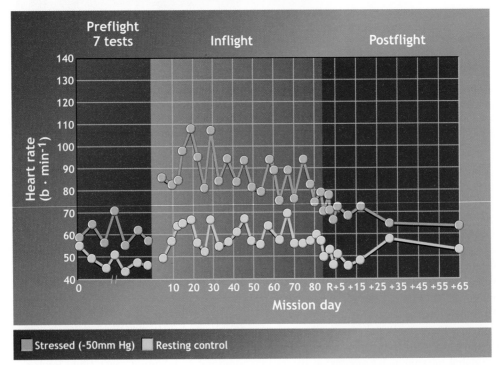

Figure 27.39 LBNP evaluation of cardiovascular dynamics during space missions: *Top.* Gemini 14-day pre–postflight changes in heart rate, blood pressure, and leg volume. *Bottom.* Resting heart rate in a −50-mm Hg LBNP test in one crew member during an 80-day Skylab mission. (From Charles JB, et al. Cardiopulmonary function. In: Nicogossian AE, et al., eds. Space physiology and medicine. 3rd ed. Philadelphia: Lea & Febiger, 1994.)

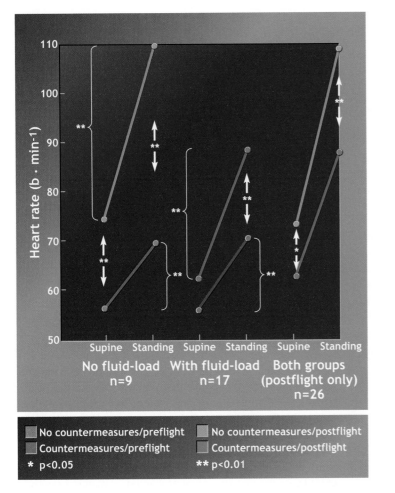

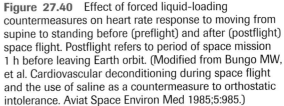

Figure 27.40 Effect of forced liquid-loading countermeasures on heart rate response to moving from supine to standing before (preflight) and after (postflight) space flight. Postflight refers to period of space mission 1 h before leaving Earth orbit. (Modified from Bungo MW, et al. Cardiovascular deconditioning during space flight and the use of saline as a countermeasure to orthostatic intolerance. Aviat Space Environ Med 1985;5:985.)

tablets (to facilitate fluid retention) 1 hour before leaving Earth orbit during shuttle missions 1 through 8.[22] FIGURE 27.40 shows the fluid-loading countermeasure effects on postflight heart rate responses in the supine and standing positions. All crewmembers showed similar preflight heart rates. Crew members who used the liquid countermeasures did not experience syncope after landing mainly because about 40% of the ingested fluid increased plasma volume for nearly 4 hours. Astronauts who loaded fluid before reentry also had lower heart rates and maintained a more stable mean blood pressure. Overall, the hyperhydration countermeasures were more effective during short 3- to 7-day missions than during longer 10-day ones.

The protective benefits of *combined* countermeasures reduce the incidence of orthostatic intolerance assessed by postural tests postflight to only 5%.[127] In contrast, fluid loading alone prior to reentry loses its effectiveness after 7 days in microgravity[33] or during a 7-day, 6° head-down bed rest[36] because the vascular space cannot maintain enough fluid to restore plasma volume to a level that exerts benefits. Another countermeasure tactic reduces air temperature inside the space cabin the night before landing. Keeping the cabin "as cold as tolerable" helps to dissipate heat in the cabin (and ultimately in the space garments) during reentry and postlanding, when cabin air temperature can reach 26.7 to 32°C. The astronaut's

liquid cooling garment uses a thermoelectric cooler to keep the precirculated water cool before it circulates through the full-torso garment. Reducing sweating response during reentry and landing minimizes fluid loss.

NASA Guidelines. The flight rule requiring astronauts to *load isotonic fluid* (hyperhydrate) prior to reentry with 8 g of NaCl in 1 L of water (referred to as the "soak") sometimes produced nausea and vomiting, causing some astronauts to ignore the rule. Adding natural sugars to sweeten the fluid and increase palatability also triggered undesirable fluid loss through copious urine flow (diuresis). More than likely, this discontinued fluid countermeasure application may itself have contributed negatively to postflight evaluation of physiologic parameters.

Current NASA guidelines concerning combined countermeasures for reentry now require (1) preinflation of anti-g suit, (2) a liquid cooling garment that circulates chilled water through tubes in the flight suit, and (3) consumption of 15 mL per kg of preflight body mass of an isotonic fluid, consommé, or potassium citrate (Astroade) 2 hours before landing. Determining the efficacy of these combined procedures requires additional research with appropriate control conditions during reentry and landing. Nevertheless, incorporation of the liquid cooling garment decreased the frequency of orthostatic symptoms to approximately 5%, with a corresponding 50% decrease in postflight nausea.[127]

Nutrition

An optimal diet for space flight should theoretically provide energy (calorie) intake equal to the energy required for the mission. Dietary management may also counter the diverse, adverse effects of physiologic adaptation to microgravity.[50] This goal, seemingly straightforward, has not been reached successfully on most missions. *Almost every space journey produces weight loss compared with similar-duration ground-based activities on Earth.*[121,122,137,161] Disruption in energy balance results from combined effects of two factors: (1) increased energy demands of the physical requirements of space flight and (2) decreased food intake during microgravity exposure. Both factors negatively affect the space traveler's energy balance. The effects of a negative energy balance became manifested not only in weight loss but in impaired fluid, electrolyte, and mineral balance. Each of these factors influences cardiovascular, musculoskeletal, immunologic, and endocrinologic functions. Cosmonauts in the Russian space program also have reported weight loss during extended missions.

Adequacy of Food Intake

During the relatively brief 1961–1963 Mercury missions of up to 34 hours, astronauts ate pureed foods and bite-sized cubes through their helmet faceplates. John Glenn, the first American space diner, consumed 270 kCal of pureed applesauce and beef and gravy with vegetables during the flight. Before this mission, there was no knowledge that humans could swallow and hence, consume food in weightlessness. On the longer Gemini flights, astronauts were supposed to consume 2800 kCal daily but ate only 30 to 50% of this amount. Their rations consisted of bite-sized cubes of meat, dessert, and bread, in addition to rehydratable fruits, salads, meats, soups, desserts, and beverages. The meals were designed to supply a macronutrient mixture of 16% protein, 31% lipid, and 53% carbohydrate.

To improve taste, the meals on Apollo flights contained greater variety—astronauts could preselect from 70 foods—with the foods thermostablized to withstand temperature extremes and with relatively normal moisture content to improve taste. Bread made from irradiated flour could be preserved for at least 1 month; this enabled astronauts to consume sandwiches throughout their mission. They were supposed to consume their individualized diets for 21 days preflight, throughout the flight, and 18 days postflight. The spacecraft's galley area contained a freezer, food chiller, and hot and cold outlets to provide drinking water and to rehydrate foods. During EVA and moon missions, astronauts consumed calorie-dense fruit bars and fruit-flavored beverages from a delivery system within their space suit. Crewmembers were encouraged to consume an additional 800 to 1000 kCal as food bars every third day. Protein intake varied between 52 and 126 g daily, averaging 76 g.

Physiology experiments on subsequent Skylab missions required more stringent guidelines and control of food intake to maintain validity of on-board studies of mineral balance, body fluid characteristics, bone mineral composition, body mass, and other biomedical parameters. The Skylab contains freezers and refrigerators to give astronauts and cosmonauts more varied food choices. Experience in planning nutritious meals in space has carryover to human health, particularly because the tools for space-based nutrition research must meet stringent design criteria for flight. New technologies developed in space have positive heath potential in studies of normal and abnormal nutritional states on Earth, such as those involving malnutrition in special populations from infants to the elderly.[82,83] Currently, astronauts on the ISS consume a wide variety of foods similar to those consumed on Earth. On extended planetary journeys, growing plants will help to recycle air and water and provide the crew with a source of food nutrients for preparation into palatable but nutritious menu items.[115]

Effects on Body Weight

The graphs in FIGURE 27.41 summarize the large individual variation in body weight changes for the commander, scientist–pilot, and pilot crew members during three Skylab missions lasting 24, 56, and 84 days. On each mission, all crewmembers lost weight and did not regain it except for the commander (Skylab 4), whose weight returned to prelaunch values by mission's end. The most dramatic weight loss (3–4%) generally occurred over the first 10 days of each mission, mainly from fluid loss. Weight loss reversed within 5 days after the crew returned to Earth. This same weight loss pattern during space flight and weight regain postflight occurred during the 1996 Life Sciences and Microgravity (LSM) mission.[138]

INTEGRATIVE QUESTION

How would you measure an astronaut's body weight in microgravity?

Food Intake on Skylab

The relatively large Skylab vehicle with its own food galley changed the way astronauts dined in space. The crew preselected commercially available foods, preassembled into complete meals. Flexible aluminum and plastic pouches contained beverages and natural food items, and cans contained the thermostabilized foods (www.neurolab.jsc.nasa.gov/eatdrink.htm). Estimated basal energy expenditure using the Harris-Benedict equation to predict BMR multiplied by 1.7 for men and 1.6 for women established the total energy content of daily meals. A basal requirement of 1752 kCal for a male allowed an additional 1226 kCal for nonbasal activities (1752 kCal $\times$ 1.7 = 2978 kCal [1752 + 1226]). With these conservative computations, astronauts still fail to balance energy intake with energy expenditure and thus lose weight. For example, on Columbia shuttle flight STS-40 (June 5–14,

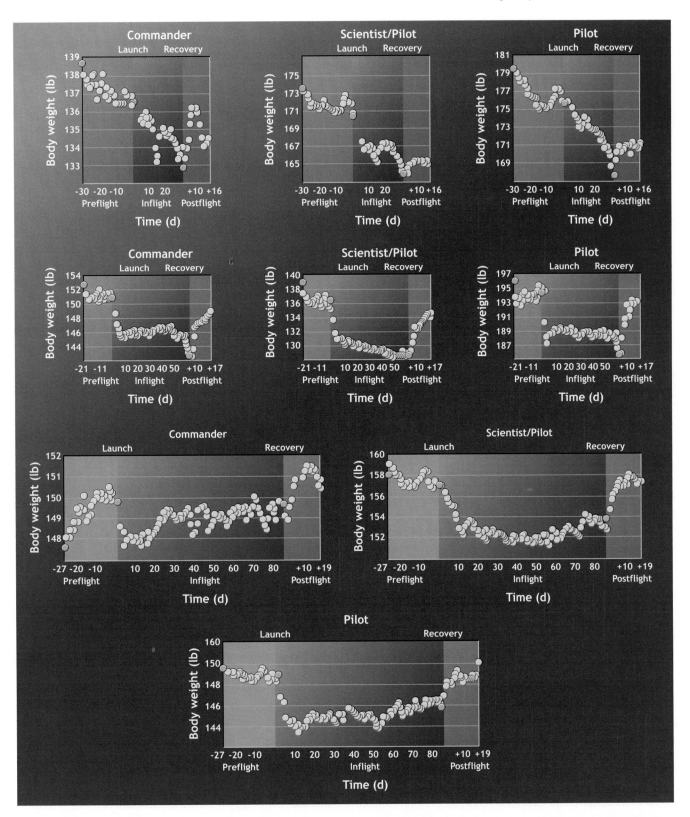

Figure 27.41 Changes in body weight of crew personnel during three Skylab missions. Top, Skylab 2, 24 days. *Middle,* Skylab 3, 56 days. *Bottom three,* Skylab 4, 84 days. *Orange circles* denote body weight at transitions at various phases in mission sequence. Note that each astronaut's body weight decreases dramatically during microgravity exposure. (From Thornton WE, Ord J. Physiological mass measurements in Skylab. In: Johnson RS, Dietlein LF, eds. Biomedical results from Skylab. NASA SP-377. Washington, DC: Government Printing Office, 1977.)

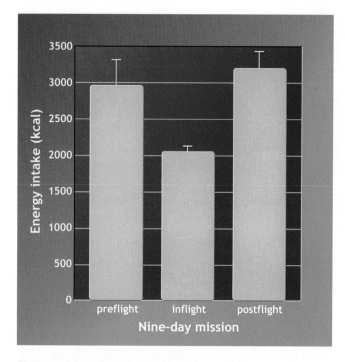

Figure 27.42 Daily energy intake during the shuttle STS-40 flight before, during, and postflight. (From Lane HW, Rambaut PC. Nutrition. In: Nicogossian AE, et al., eds. Space physiology and medicine. 3rd ed. Philadelphia: Lea & Febiger, 1994.)

1991), the fifth dedicated SLS-1 mission, four payload crewmembers weighed and recorded all food consumed before, during, and after flight. FIGURE 27.42 shows clearly that the astronauts under-consumed recommended energy intake by 33% during the 9-day mission, with considerable individual variation in macronutrient intake. Daily protein intake varied between 34 and 149 g; lipid intake ranged between 11 and 42% of total calories ingested, and carbohydrate ranged between 37 and 72%.

Comparison of Energy and Macronutrient Intake for Apollo, Skylab, and Space Shuttle Missions

TABLE 27.14 *(top)* summarizes the dietary intakes for Apollo, Skylab, and Space Shuttle astronauts during space flight; the *bottom* of the table lists macronutrient proportions, expressed as a percentage of total energy intake.[138] For comparison, the space flight intakes are contrasted with World Health Organization equations that predict daily requirements. Three salient findings emerge. First, for each mission, energy intake never achieved the predicted optimum. It came closest on Skylab (99.1% predicted), but achieved only 64.2% of predicted on Apollo and 67.5% on the space shuttle. Second, astronauts consumed a relatively higher percentage of carbohydrate (58%) and lower percentage of lipid (28%) during flight than in preflight; preflight calories from carbohydrate averaged 52%; those from lipid averaged 33%. Third, considerable individual variation exists in energy expenditure during space flight, ranging from 28 to 47 kCal $\cdot$ kg^{-1} $\cdot$ d^{-1}.

Perhaps the relative ease of preparing foods of high carbohydrate content explains the shift in macronutrient preference during space flight.[84,87] Of nutritional significance, daily calcium intake averaged 25% lower than recommended values. The reduced total water consumption during flight[84] occurs from food intake and reduced fluid consumption, possibly from depressed sensitivity of the thirst mechanism.[93]

Daily Nutritional Recommendations for 90- to 360-Day Space Missions. TABLE 27.15 lists recommended daily macro- and micronutrient intake proposed by the Biomedical Operations Research Branch of NASA charged with nutritional optimization of space missions. The reference values for space travelers frequently exceed the Dietary Reference Intakes for an average American man and woman. Nevertheless, because of large variations among individuals in energy expenditure, it will not be possible for a single recommended nutrient intake to apply to all astronauts on their missions. Instead, astronauts receive individually customized meal plans to meet the mission's nutrient and energy requirements. The astronauts' total energy expenditure consists of their BMR, energy cost of planned inflight exercise, and any EVA activity.

During future stays on Space Station Freedom, the iron requirement (see Table 27.15) changes from the current daily standard of 15 mg $\cdot$ d^{-1} for women to 10 mg $\cdot$ d^{-1} from decreased red blood cell mass and turnover and altered iron metabolism in space.[92,156] Researchers now must identify ways to ensure that astronauts have a total food intake adequate to balance energy requirements and achieve optimal macro- and micronutrient intake to sustain "good" health throughout a mission regardless of duration. This will pose a challenge for future interplanetary travel with respect to whether pregnancy and birth can be sustained successfully without gravity.[124]

Altered Protein Dynamics. *Atrophy of skeletal muscles that support posture and locomotion represents a characteristic maladaptation to microgravity during short- and long-duration exposures*[51] Decreases in lean body mass, muscle volume, and muscle strength, and changes in muscle fiber microarchitecture[173] accompany space-induced muscle atrophy. Such changes suggest poor adaptation in whole-body protein (nitrogen) balance.[95,137,139] Isotopic methods that assess tissue protein turnover show that astronauts increase protein breakdown rate by approximately 30% on mission days 2 to 8, thereby producing negative nitrogen balance. In addition, increases occur in urinary cortisol, fibrinogen, and interleukin-2 (IL-2). These changes suggest that space flight triggers a stress response similar to response patterns from physical injury.[137] In both of these stressful situations, tissue protein serves as a substrate for energy metabolism that fosters a negative nitrogen balance (protein catabolism). This supports the recommendation of a daily protein intake of 1.5 g per kg of body mass during space travel.[86] In addition, long space missions (4 to 9 months on the Russian Mir Space Station) and shorter duration space shuttle flights (up to 15 d) are associated with decreased oxidative damage owing to reduced oxygen radical production (in the electron transport chain) from reduced energy intake. Increased oxidative damage occurs postflight from combined

TABLE 27.14 ■ *TOP.* DIETARY INTAKES FOR APOLLO, SKYLAB, AND SPACE SHUTTLE ASTRONAUTS DURING SPACE FLIGHT. *BOTTOM.* MACRONUTRIENT PROPORTIONS AS A PERCENTAGE OF ENERGY INTAKE (%kJ) IN APOLLO, SKYLAB, AND SPACE SHUTTLE DIETS BEFORE AND DURING SPACE FLIGHT

	APOLLO	SKYLAB	SPACE SHUTTLE
Energy			
$kJ \cdot d^{-1}$	7864 ± 1734[a]	11,906 ± 1300	8346 ± 1364
WHO predicted requirements (%)	64.2 ± 13.6	99.1 ± 8.2	67.5 ± 19.3
Protein			
$g \cdot d^{-1}$	76.1 ± 18.7	111.0 ± 18.4	75.7 ± 20.2
% of kJ intake	16.2 ± 2.1	15.5 ± 1.2	15.0 ± 2.8
Carbohydrate intake			
$g \cdot d^{-1}$	268.8 ± 49.1	413.3 ± 59.3	282.9 ± 49.5
% of kJ intake	58.1 ± 7.1	58.1 ± 4.4	57.0 ± 5.1
Lipid			
$g \cdot d^{-1}$	61.4 ± 21.4	83.2 ± 13.8	62.7 ± 13.8
% of kJ intake	28.8 ± 5.4	26.4 ± 3.8	28.2 ± 4.1
Water ($mL \cdot d^{-1}$)	1647 ± 188[b]	2829 ± 529	1923 ± 376
Calcium ($mg \cdot d^{-1}$)	774 ± 212	902 ± 152	853 ± 226
Before flight			
Carbohydrate	NA[c]	50.5 ± 3.5	53.1 ± 6.2
Lipid	NA	33.4 ± 3.2	31.7 ± 5.0
Protein	NA	16.1 ± 0.9	14.7 ± 2.1
During flight			
Carbohydrate	58.1 ± 7.1	58.1 ± 4.4	57.0 ± 5.1
Lipid	28.8 ± 5.4	26.4 ± 3.8	28.2 ± 4.1
Protein	16.2 ± 2.1	15.5 ± 4.1	15.0 ± 2.8

Modified from Lane HW, et al. Nutrition in space: lessons from the past applied to the future. Am J Clin Nutr 1994;60:801S.
To convert kJ to kCal, divide by 4.186.
[a] Values are means ± standard deviations.
[b] $n = 3$.
[c] Not available.

increases in metabolic rate and possible loss of in-flight host antioxidant defenses.[141] The potential beneficial effects of postflight antioxidant supplementation remain unknown.

FIGURE 27.43 plots daily energy intake and urine-based nitrogen balance assessment during three Skylab missions and two SLS missions. Note the in-flight negative nitrogen balance on Skylab compared with a preflight baseline despite near-normal energy intake. On the two shuttle missions, daily calorie intake and nitrogen balance were affected negatively compared with preflight values. Based on Russian data aboard the Salyut-7 space mission, the estimated energy cost of twice-daily in-flight exercise sessions was approximately 20 kCal per kg of body mass. Adding this energy requirement to an already inadequate daily energy intake would provoke further protein loss to absorb the energy deficit.[72] Research must determine effective combinations of exercise and nutritional supplementation to stabilize energy and protein balance during space missions.

INTEGRATIVE QUESTION

Explain whether consuming additional protein during a space mission would help to restore fat-free body mass.

Energy Expenditure and Balance Dynamics on the Space Shuttle

The 1996 LMS shuttle mission measured energy expenditure and energy balance in four crew members for 12 days before liftoff, during the 17-day flight, and 15 days postflight.[138] In addition, a complementary bed-rest study with 6° head-down tilt to simulate microgravity evaluated energy expenditure and energy balance in eight subjects. The bed-rest study had three phases: (1) 15-day pre–bed rest ambulatory period, (2) 17 days of bed rest (except when subjects exercised to match the in-flight exercise routines), and (3) a 15-day recovery period. Subjects in both experiments performed submaximal and maximal bicycle ergometer exercise tests on days 13 and 8 before launch and on days 4 and 8 postflight. During space flight days 2, 8, and 13, crewmembers performed an additional ergometer test to assess cardiorespiratory responses to exercise at 85% $\dot{V}O_{2max}$.

Measurements included doubly labeled water (DLW; $^2H_2^{18}O$) and body composition by dual-energy x-ray absorptiometry (DXA) before and after space flight/bed rest to quantify positive energy balance (fat stored) or negative energy balance (fat catabolized). Subjects quantified each food item

TABLE 27.15 ■ DAILY MACRO- AND MICRONUTRIENT NASA RECOMMENDATIONS FOR 90- TO 360-DAY SPACE MISSIONS

NUTRIENT	RECOMMENDATIONS[a]
Energy	WHO (moderate activity level)
Protein	12–15% of total energy consumed
Carbohydrate	50% of total energy consumed
Lipid	30–35% of total energy consumed
Fluid	238–357 mL per MJ consumed
Fiber	10–25 g
Vitamin A	1000 μg retinol equiv
Vitamin D	10 μg
Vitamin E	20 mg α-tocopherol equiv
Vitamin K	80 μg for men; 65 μg for women
Vitamin C	100 mg
Vitamin B_{12}	2.0 μg
Vitamin B_6	2.0 mg
Thiamin	1.5 mg
Riboflavin	2.0 mg
Folate	400 μg
Niacin	20 mg
Biotin	100 μg
Pantothenic acid	5.0 mg
Calcium	1000–1200 mg
Phosphorus	1000–1200 mg
Magnesium	350 mg for men; 280 mg for women
Sodium	<3500 mg
Potassium	3500 mg
Iron	10 mg
Copper	1.5–3.0 mg
Manganese	2.0–5.0 mg
Fluoride	4.0 mg
Zinc	15 mg
Selenium	70 μg
Iodine	150 μg
Chromium	100–200 μg

[a]Recommendations generated by two nutritional advisory committees to NASA. Courtesy of Dr. Helen Lane, NASA Chief Nutritionist. Biomedical Research Branch at the NASA Houston Space Center, Houston, TX. WHO, World Health Organization.

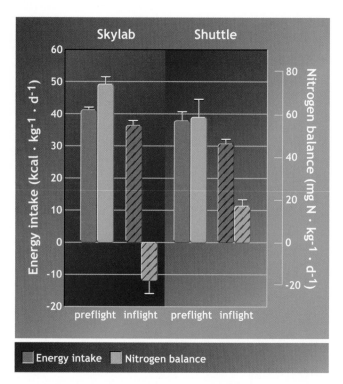

Figure 27.43 Daily energy intake *(left axis)* and daily urine-based nitrogen balance *(right axis)* during space flight on three Skylab missions and two Life Sciences Space Shuttle missions (SLS-1 and SLS-2). Values are means ±SE. (Modified from Stein TP, et al. Diet and nitrogen metabolism during space flight on the shuttle. J Appl Physiol 1996;81:82.)

consumed and not consumed with a bar code reader and verbal description (using a cassette recorder) to estimate the contents remaining in the individual food package. During pre- and postflight periods, subjects consumed prepared meals of known nutrient content. The Spacelab contained a system to collect, measure, and save a 20-mL daily urine sample to estimate nitrogen balance from nitrogen and creatinine excretion.

The top of FIGURE 27.44 displays three energy intake periods expressed as kCal · kg^{-1} · d^{-1} during preflight, flight, and postflight. Note that within each period, a relative stabilization (adaptation) takes place for energy intake. This probably occurs from resetting of setpoint mechanisms that regulate energy balance. The *histogram inset* expresses average energy intake in kCal daily to highlight the dramatic 45% lower in-flight energy intake (1708 kCal · kg^{-1} · d^{-1}) compared with

the remarkably similar values preflight (3025 kCal · kg^{-1} · d^{-1}) and postflight (3151 kCal · kg^{-1} · d^{-1}) intakes.

The *bottom* graphic compares the energy intake during the first 2 weeks of space flight for Skylab missions 2, 3, and 4 and the two shuttle LMS missions. Astronauts on the shuttle LMS *(bottom red curve)* remained in substantial negative energy balance throughout the flight. Astronauts on the previous three Skylab missions participated in a metabolic balance study so daily energy intakes remained fairly stable during the different-duration missions. In contrast, astronauts on shuttle LMS consumed food ad libitum. At the same time, they performed vigorous daily exercise that contributed to their relatively high average total daily energy expenditure of 40.8 kCal · kg^{-1} · d^{-1} (3238 kCal). No differences occurred among the three methods of estimating energy balance. This result supported the validity of the methodology and the main two research conclusions:

1. Severe negative energy balance and corresponding loss of body mass, body fat, and protein could compromise a mission and adversely affect an astronaut's health in a manner resembling prolonged malnutrition.
2. High levels of physical activity during space flight may disrupt mechanisms that maintain energy balance.

Persistent, severe 1400-kCal negative daily energy balance on future extended-duration flights would ultimately

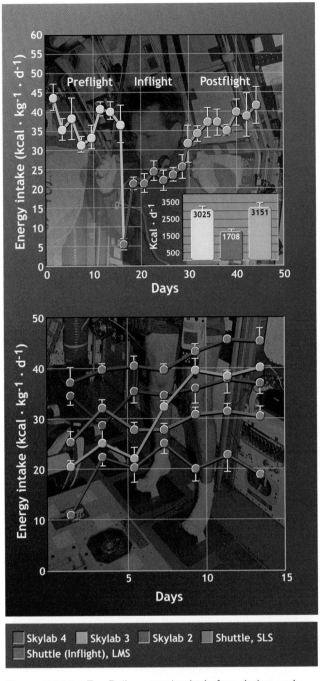

Figure 27.44 *Top.* Daily energy intake before, during, and after space flight on shuttle LMS. The *histogram inset* expresses the data as average kCal · d⁻¹ during each mission phase. *Bottom.* Daily energy intake during the first 2 weeks of space flight for Skylab missions 2 (28 d), 3 (56 d), and 4 (84 d); two shuttle missions (SLS-1 and SLS-2 combined); and shuttle LMS. (Data modified from Stein TP, et al. Energy expenditure and balance during space flight on the space shuttle. Am J Physiol 1999;45:R1739.)

mobilize an astronaut's entire fat energy reserves (approximately 160,000 kCal) within 120 days and produce terminal starvation. Researchers obviously must determine how best to ensure that astronauts consume adequate daily nutrition to counterbalance (1) the energy requirements of space flight, (2) the demands of exercise countermeasures and

normal work tasks, and (3) the decreased efficiency in removing the metabolic byproducts of exercise (e.g., CO_2, heat).[143] Cosmonauts on the Mir mission partially resolved their inflight energy deficits by curtailing physical activity. Theoretically, they could remain in orbit for 660 days before severe undernutrition compromised physiology, performance, and health.

Nutritionally Related Effects of Space Flight on Physiologic Functions

Since the first space missions, researchers have tracked adaptations in physiologic function during microgravity exposure. A prevailing theory about such changes concerns the interactions among nutritional variables and endocrine functions and their combined effects on cardiopulmonary, hormonal, skeletal, and body fluid functions and body mass and composition.[37,56,62,92,96,134,144,145] FIGURE 27.45 shows the triad of nutritionally related effects of space flight on physiologic systems. The interrelated triad components—fluid shifts, physical unloading of weight-bearing structures, and metabolic changes—in many ways link to shifts in endocrine function. The *inset table* shows endocrine changes during stress, simulated microgravity (bed rest), and space flight. Note that the responses to bed rest do not generally mirror endocrine changes in space flight, but instead mimic the stress-mediated responses. An attractive hypothesis posits that the endocrine effects of space flight relate more to nutritional changes characterized by stress-related models, not a model that includes bed rest.[85] The similarity between the catabolic effects of the increased demands on energy metabolism (and negative energy balance) and catabolic effects of space flight "stress" help to explain space-induced decreases in body mass, lean body mass, and bone density. This includes shifts in extracellular and intracellular water compartments.

Body Composition Changes. FIGURE 27.46 shows percentage changes in body composition variables of 10 astronauts assessed by densitometry and bioelectrical impedance analysis before and 2 days following 7- to 16-day missions. No changes occurred in body fat or extracellular water, with the 2.3% decline in body mass attributable to a loss in fat-free body mass (FFM). Note that all three components of FFM (water, protein, and mineral) declined from 3 to 4% in the postflight measures. The 3% loss of intracellular water—attributable to decreased protein and mineral levels within other tissues including muscle—explains the decrease in total-body water.[140] Whether such alterations in body composition parameters affect in-flight performance awaits further study. However, body composition variables did not explain the 12% postflight reduction in $\dot{V}O_{2max}$. An integrative approach assesses regional body composition (calf muscle volume[165]) and MRI-derived characteristics of muscle (transverse relaxation of calf muscles) following multiple shuttle/Mir missions lasting 16 to 28 weeks.[94] The newer technique of bioelectrical impedance spectroscopy (BIS) has

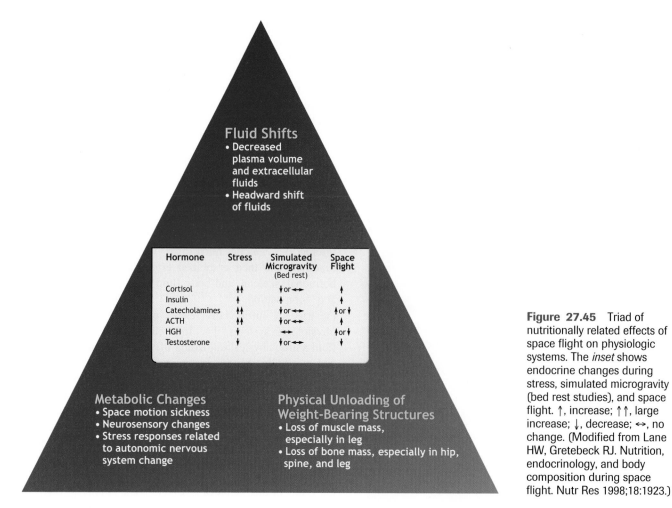

Hormone	Stress	Simulated Microgravity (Bed rest)	Space Flight
Cortisol	↑↑	↓or↔	↑
Insulin	↑	↑	↑
Catecholamines	↑↑	↓or↔	↑or↓
ACTH	↑↑	↓or↔	↑
HGH	↓	↔	↑or↓
Testosterone	↓	↓or↔	↓

Fluid Shifts
- Decreased plasma volume and extracellular fluids
- Headward shift of fluids

Metabolic Changes
- Space motion sickness
- Neurosensory changes
- Stress responses related to autonomic nervous system change

Physical Unloading of Weight-Bearing Structures
- Loss of muscle mass, especially in leg
- Loss of bone mass, especially in hip, spine, and leg

Figure 27.45 Triad of nutritionally related effects of space flight on physiologic systems. The *inset* shows endocrine changes during stress, simulated microgravity (bed rest studies), and space flight. ↑, increase; ↑↑, large increase; ↓, decrease; ↔, no change. (Modified from Lane HW, Gretebeck RJ. Nutrition, endocrinology, and body composition during space flight. Nutr Res 1998;18:1923.)

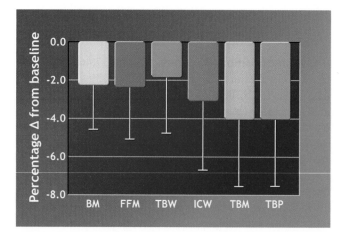

Figure 27.46 Percentage changes (Δ) in body composition variables of 10 astronauts assessed by densitometry and multifrequency bioelectrical impedance analysis before and 2 days after 7- to 16-day missions. *BM,* body mass; *FFM,* fat-free body mass; *TBW,* total body water; *ICW,* intracellular water; *TBM,* total body mineral; *TBP,* total body protein. (Data from Greenisen MC, et al. Functional performance evaluation. In: Extended Duration Orbiter Medical Project. NASA Johnson Space Center final report. 1989–1995. [NASA/SP-1999-534] NASA. Lyndon B. Johnson Space Center. Houston, TX. 1999.)

assessed nutritional status during space flight, but its limitations in precision and insensitivity to short-term intracellular water changes require further validation.[12]

 INTEGRATIVE QUESTION

What role should diet and exercise play in prolonged-duration space missions?

OVERVIEW OF PHYSIOLOGIC RESPONSES TO SPACE FLIGHT

Numerous research reports discuss short- and long-term consequences of space flight on human physiology.[10,16,19,30,36,65,90] From the first single-pilot flights of Project Mercury in the early 1960s to the extended Soviet Soyuz missions of the 1990s and now the manned Chinese missions, scientists have pondered how best to minimize the deleterious effects of microgravity during flight and upon return to Earth. FIGURE 27.47 diagrams the two main physical stressors from space travel: (1) decreased hydrostatic pressure gradients within the cardiovascular system (displayed

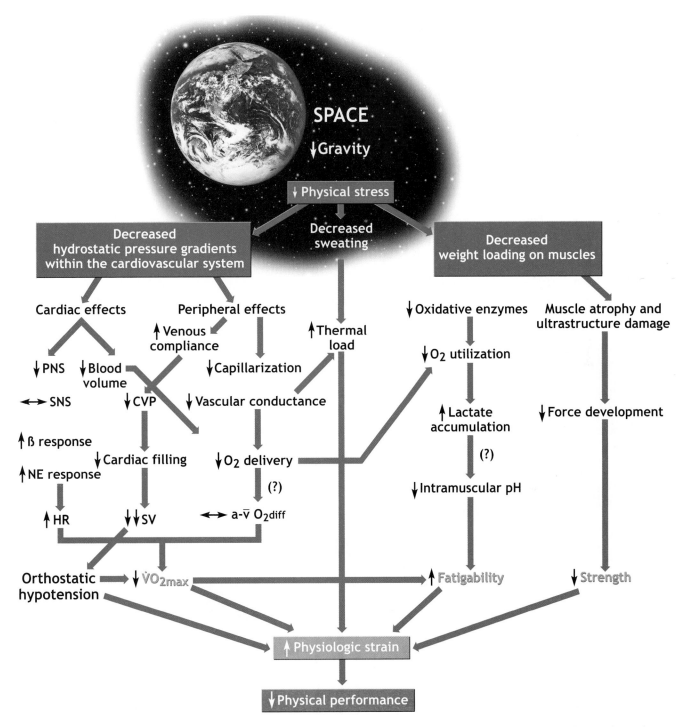

Figure 27.47 Model of the relationship between physical stress of the space environment and adaptation of cardiovascular and muscular systems with resulting increased physiologic strain and decreased physical performance. *SNS,* sympathetic nervous system; *CVP,* central venous pressure; β, beta-adrenergic; *NE,* norepinephrine; *HR,* heart rate; *SV,* stroke volume; *a-v̄O₂diff,* arteriovenous oxygen difference; ↑, increase; ↓, decrease; ↓↓, large decrease; ↔, no change. (From Convertino VA. Effects of microgravity on exercise performance. In: Garrett WE, Kirkendall DT, eds. Exercise and sport science. Philadelphia: Lippincott Williams & Wilkins, 2000.)

on the *left*), and (2) decreased weight loading on muscles (displayed on the *right*), both of which ultimately increase physiologic strain (*orange box* at the *bottom*) and negatively affect an astronaut's physical performance (*red box* at the *bottom*).[30] Note that the three effects (decreased $\dot{V}O_{2max}$ and muscular strength and increased fatigability), combined with an increased thermal load, add substantially to the total phys-

iologic strain. Exercise countermeasures (specifically site-specific lower-body eccentric and concentric resistance exercise) coupled with relatively intense cardiovascular workouts on a cycle ergometer and treadmill can mitigate deleterious effects from prolonged microgravity sojourns. This is particularly germane when astronauts return to a 1g Earth environment.

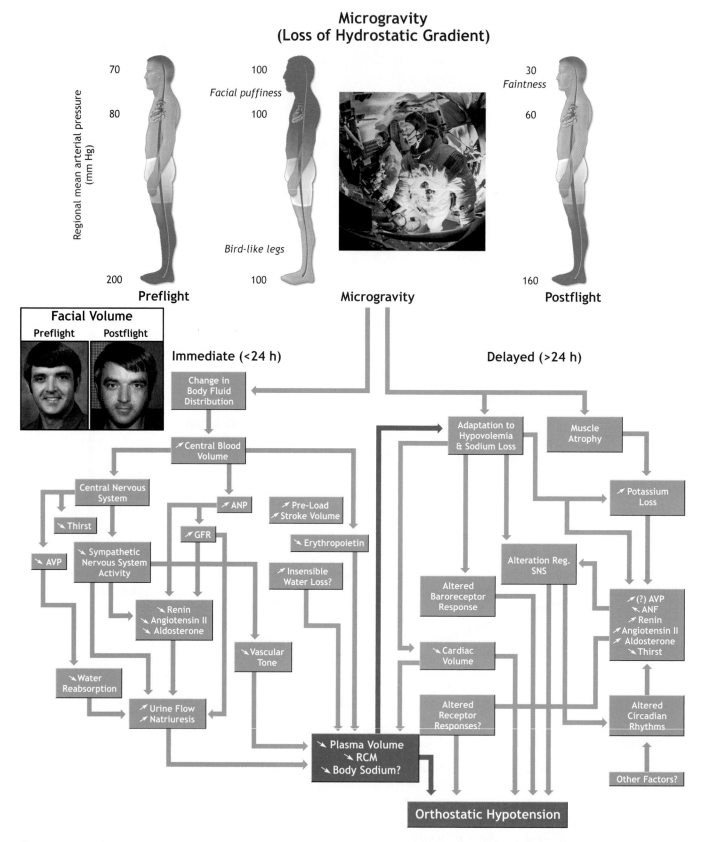

Figure 27.48 Proposed immediate (<24 h) and delayed (>24 h) responses to microgravity compared with those under preflight (1g) and postflight (1g) conditions. *AVP,* arginine vasopressin; *ANP,* atrial natriuretic peptide; *GFR,* glomerular filtration rate; *RCM,* red cell mass; *SNS,* sympathetic nervous system; ↗ increase; ↘ decrease, ?, possible. (Photos courtesy of NASA, Lyndon B. Johnson Space Center, Houston, TX. Figures denoting changes in mean arterial pressure modified from Hargens AR, et al. Control of circulatory function in altered gravitational fields. Physiologist 1992;35:S80. Additional graphic information modified from Maillet A, et al. Cardiovascular and hormonal changes induced by isolation and confinement. Med Sci Sports Exerc 1996;28:S53.)

Short- and Long-Term Responses

Two categories, short- and long-term, describe the time course of physiologic response and adaptation in the transitions from Earth's 1g environment to microgravity in low-Earth orbit and then return to 1g following a mission. Short-term responses occur within 24 hours or the first few days of a mission. The second category describes longer term changes following a mission. FIGURE 27.48 presents a generalized flow diagram of the immediate or short-term (<24 h) and delayed or long-term (>24 h) responses. Both immediate and delayed responses eventually contribute to orthostatic hypotension *(bottom purple box),* the most common malady following space flight.

In space, body fluids no longer move "downward" from gravity's pull, so fluids redistribute toward the chest and upper body (note facial puffiness from cranial edema). Lower-body fluid loss gives the legs a birdlike appearance. Excess fluid buildup in the torso triggers fluid elimination by the kidneys. Mean arterial pressure increases in the cranial region from a preflight normal of 70 mm Hg to 100 mm Hg in space (Fig. 27.48, *top*), while mean pressure at the feet declines 50% from its normal 200 mm Hg; heart volume also decreases slightly. The immediate change in body fluid distribution activates a plethora of additional responses and lower sympathetic nervous system activity. Restricted stimulation environments such as space flight and other stress-inducing situations from prolonged confinement and isolation share many of the same responses and adaptations.[97]

Time Course of In-Flight Adaptations

FIGURE 27.49 depicts the time course for shifts in four main categories of physiologic function during 1 year of sustained microgravity. The *green horizontal line* represents baseline function on Earth (denoted as 0% change). Within the first 3 weeks, up to a 10% change in cardiovascular function reflects a deconditioning response; within 14 days, a 10% change occurs in body fluid redistribution, and within 3 months, bone mass declines by 5%. Bone mass declines farther to 15% between months 5 and 6 when it stabilizes for several months before decreasing farther to 17% after 1 year. Like bone mass, muscle structure and function deteriorate at a slower rate than do cardiac deconditioning and fluid redistribution, but the magnitude of the decrement reaches higher values.

Time Course of Postflight Readaptations

FIGURE 27.50 shows how 3 months of recovery (readaptation) affects neurovestibular and cardiovascular functions, fluid and electrolyte balance, red blood cell mass, and lean body mass. For reference, the *lower horizontal line,* indicated by the *arrow* at *bottom left (1g set point),* represents baseline measures expected under normal 1g conditions. The *colored lines* for each variable indicate average trends, but considerable inter- and intraindividual differences exist.

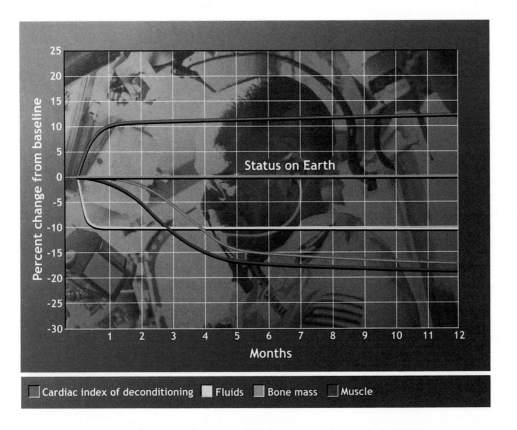

Figure 27.49 Time course of four main shifts in physiologic function during 1 year in microgravity. The *horizontal green line* represents baseline function on Earth at 1g (denoted as zero percent change). The cardiac index of deconditioning *(red line)* reflects severity of orthostatic intolerance to gravitational stress. (Modified from: Nicogossian A, et al. Overall physiologic response to space flight. In: Nicogossian AE, et al., eds. Space physiology and medicine. 3rd ed. Philadelphia: Lea & Febiger, 1994.)

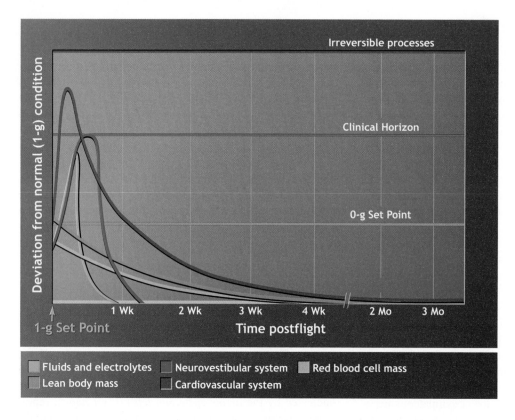

Figure 27.50 Time course of physiologic shifts during readaptation to 1g, in which flight duration only minimally affects the readaptations. (Modified from Nicogossian AE, et al., eds. Space physiology and medicine. 3rd ed. Philadelphia: Lea & Febiger, 1994.)

Analysis of the recovery curves reveals two characteristics: (1) the response rate is nonlinear, with some processes appearing bimodal with relatively high rate constants and (2) recovery time varies depending on the variable evaluated. For example, the rapid change in fluid distribution during the first few weeks of microgravity exposure shown previously in Figure 27.33 recovers to baseline within the first week of return to 1g (*yellow curve*). In contrast, the *light green curve* for lean body mass and *purple curve* for cardiovascular deconditioning require approximately 6 weeks to approach baseline.

FUTURE RESEARCH PRIORITIES

Before NASA attempts an interplanetary Mars mission, a host of questions remain concerning astronaut health and safety, including priorities for the most-productive research strategies in gravitational biology.[47,104] The Office of Biological and Physical Research (www.spaceresearch.nasa.gov/general_info/priorities.html) is developing a comprehensive research strategy that includes a 10-year plan based around five organizing questions to propel NASA into the next realm of exploration (www.exploration.nasa.gov/).

1. How can we ensure the survival of humans traveling far from Earth?
2. How does life respond to gravity and space environments?
3. What new opportunities can research bring to expand understanding of the laws of nature and enrich lives on Earth?

4. What technology must we create to enable the next explorers to go beyond where we have been?
5. How can we educate and inspire the next generation to take the journey?

NASA's cooperative efforts with the scientific and industrial sector continue to develop advanced instrumentation and methodologies for space-based studies at the cellular level. The new generation of space vehicles now under development for interplanetary-class explorations will integrate cutting-edge research in the physical sciences to make endeavors to tame the space environment a success.

VISION FOR THE FUTURE OF SPACE EXPLORATION

On January 4, 2004, President George W. Bush announced a new vision for the United States space exploration program. The president committed the United States to a long-term human and robotic program to explore the solar system, starting with a return to the moon to ultimately enable future exploration of Mars and other destinations. The president's plan for human and robotic space exploration is based on the following goals:

1. America will complete its work on the ISS by 2010, fulfilling the United States commitment to the 15 partner countries involved in the space program. The United States will launch a refocused research effort on board the ISS to better understand and overcome the effects of human space flight on astronaut health, increasing the safety of future space missions. To

accomplish this goal, NASA will return the Space Shuttle to flight consistent with safety concerns and the recommendations of the *Columbia* Accident Investigation Board. The shuttle's chief purpose is to help finish assembly of the ISS before it will be retired by the end of this decade following 30 years of service.

2. The United States will develop a new manned exploration vehicle to explore beyond our orbit to other worlds—the first of its kind since the Apollo Command Module. The new spacecraft, the Crew Exploration Vehicle (CEV), will be developed and tested by 2008 and conduct its first manned mission no later than 2014. The CEV will transport astronauts and scientists to the ISS after the shuttle retires.

3. America will return to the moon as early as 2015 and no later than 2020 (twice-yearly lunar missions from lunar orbit to the moon's surface), including it as a stage for more ambitious missions that will ferry groups of six astronauts to Mars. A series of robotic missions to the moon, similar to the *Spirit* Rover that currently transmits remarkable images back to Earth from Mars (www.marsrovers.jpl .nasa.gov/ home/), will explore the lunar surface beginning no later than 2008 to research and prepare for future human exploration. Using the CEV, humans will conduct extended lunar missions as early as 2015 with the goal of living and working for increasingly extended periods. The extended human presence on the moon will enable astronauts to develop new technologies and harness the moon's abundant resources to allow manned exploration of more challenging environments. NASA will increase the use of robotic exploration to maximize new knowledge about the solar system and pave the way for more ambitious manned missions using probes, landers, and similar unmanned vehicles. Astronauts will conduct cutting-edge research in astrobiology, geology, astronomy, physics, and space biology. One of the main reasons for returning to the moon is to master the technologies required for future extended-duration Mars explorations. This second Return to Flight test mission (STS-121 scheduled for Space Shuttle *Discovery* in early 2006) will carry on analysis of safety improvements that debuted on the first Return to Flight mission (STS-114) and build upon those tests, including the Multi-Purpose Logistics Module (MPLM) *Leonardo* and more than two tons of equipment and supplies.

Future Mars Missions

Future Mars missions will involve numerous launches with giant heavy-lift boosters to carry the mission's spacecraft and hardware into orbit. One of the prime objectives is

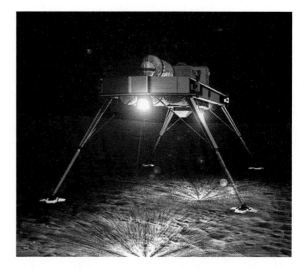

to land on the Martian surface under remote control to provide supplies for an outpost with living quarters, power, communications, and the return rocket. The voyage to Mars will require about 6 months each way. While on Mars, the crew would spend about 500 days exploring large areas of the surface, including the search for evidence of early life forms. Exploration of the Martian environment would, one hopes, confirm the presence of oxygen and water (two essential supplies), including liquid oxygen and methane—two propellants required to power the landing craft. The two NASA illustrations show two aspects of the proposed new space initiative—*above,* the robotic cargo spacecraft touching down near the planned lunar base, and on the *bottom,* the Mars Reconnaissance Orbiter (MRO) as it navigates over the Martian poles (7-month cruise to Mars and 6 months of aerobraking to reach its science orbit). The MRO will zoom in for extreme close-up photography of the Martian surface, analyze materials, look for subsurface water, trace how much dust and water are distributed in the atmosphere, and monitor daily global weather. In addition, the orbiter's telecommunications systems will establish a crucial service for future spacecraft by becoming the first link in a communications bridge back to Earth—"interplanetary Internet"—for use by international spacecraft in coming

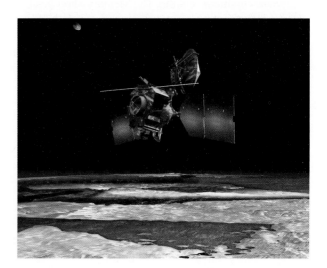

years. Testing a radio frequency called Ka-band, the MRO will demonstrate the potential for greater performance in communications using significantly less power. The orbiter also carries an experimental navigation camera. If it performs as planned, similar cameras placed on future orbiters would serve as high-precision interplanetary "eyes" to guide incoming landers to precise Mars landings, opening up exciting—but otherwise dangerous areas—for planetary exploration.[41] The orbiter's primary mission ends about 5½ years after launch on December 31, 2010 (www.marsprogram.jpl.nasa.gov/mro).

PRACTICAL BENEFITS FROM SPACE BIOLOGY RESEARCH

Of a $2.4 trillion budget, less than 0.8% is spent on the entire United States space program. That amounts to less than 1 penny for every dollar the government spends on its diverse programs. The average American spends more of their budget on a monthly cable bill or eating out at fast food restaurants. For every dollar the United States spends on research and development in the space program, seven dollars come back as corporate and personal income taxes from increased jobs and economic growth. Hundreds of companies that apply NASA technology in non–space-related areas create hundreds of thousands of jobs that ultimately affect citizens worldwide. Technologies developed over the past 35 years from NASA's current 15 centers to meet the challenges of space exploration have produced more than 30,000 secondary commercial applications in seven categories. We provide salient examples below (www.thespaceplace.com/nasa/spinoffs.html):

1. **Computer Technology**

   Ground processing scheduling system. Computer-based scheduling system uses artificial intelligence to provide real-time planning and optimization of manufacturing operations, integrated supply chains, and customer orders.

   Semiconductor cubing. The Memory Short Stack offers faster computer processing speeds, higher levels of integration, lower power requirements than conventional chip sets, and dramatic reduction in the size and weight of memory-intensive systems such as medical imaging devices.

   Virtual reality. Users with assistance from advanced technology devices can figuratively project themselves into a computer-generated environment that matches the user's head motion to create a telepresence experience.

   Other spin-offs include advanced keyboards, customer service software, database management system, laser surveying, aircraft controls, lightweight compact disk, expert system software, microcomputers, and design graphics.

2. **Consumer/Home/Recreation**

   Enriched baby food. A microalgae-based, vegetable-like oil called Formulaid contains two essential fatty acids found in human milk, believed important for mental and visual development.

   Scratch-resistant lenses. A modified version of a dual ion beam bonding process involves coating lenses with a film of diamond-like carbon that provides scratch resistance, decreases surface friction, and reduces water spots.

   Ribbed swimsuit. Riblets applied to competition swimsuits produced 10 to 15% faster speeds than any other swimsuit due to small, barely visible grooves that reduce friction and hydrodynamic drag by modifying the turbulent flow of water next to the skin.

   Athletic shoes. Moon Boot material encapsulated in running shoe midsoles improves shock absorption and provides superior stability and motion control.

   Other spin-offs include Dustbuster, shock-absorbing helmets, home security systems, smoke detectors, flat panel televisions, high-density batteries, trash compactors, food packaging and freeze-dried technology, cool sportswear, sports bras, hair-styling appliances, fogless ski goggles, self-adjusting sunglasses, composite golf clubs, hang gliders, art preservation, and quartz crystal timing equipment.

3. **Environmental and Resource Management**

   Solar energy. Photovoltaic power systems for spacecraft applications expand terrestrial applications as a viable alternative energy source.

   Forest management. A scanning system monitors and maps forestation by detecting radiation reflected and emitted from trees.

   Fire-resistant material. Materials include chemically treated fabric for sheets, uniforms for hazardous material handlers, crew's clothing, furniture, interior walls of submersibles, and auto racer and refueler suits.

   Other spin-offs include whale identification method, environmental analysis, noise abatement, pollution measuring devices, pollution control devices, smokestack monitor, radioactive leak detector, earthquake prediction system, sewage treatment, energy saving air conditioning, and air purification.

4. **Health and Medicine**

   Digital imaging breast biopsy system. The LORAD Stereo Guide Breast Biopsy system incorporates advanced Charge Coupled Devices (CCDs) to image breast tissue clearly and efficiently. This less traumatic nonsurgical system greatly reduces the pain, scarring, radiation exposure, time, and money associated with surgical biopsies.

Breast cancer detection. A solar cell sensor is positioned directly beneath x-ray film and determines when film receives sufficient radiation and has been exposed to optimum density. Reduction of mammography x-ray exposure reduces radiation hazard and doubles the number of patient examinations per machine.

Laser angioplasty. Laser angioplasty with a "cool" type of laser, called an *excimer* laser (excimer stands for excited dimer, a short-lived diatomic molecule that bonds two identical molecules only when in an electronic excited state), does not damage blood vessel walls. It offers precise nonsurgical cleanings of clogged arteries with precision and fewer complications than balloon angioplasty.

Automated urinalysis. System that automatically extracts and transfers sediment from a urine sample to an analyzer microscope that replaces the manual centrifuge method.

Other spin-offs include arteriosclerosis detection, ultrasound scanners, automatic insulin pump, portable x-ray device, invisible braces, dental arch wire, palate surgery technology, clean room apparel, implantable heart aid, MRI, bone analyzer, and cataract surgery tools.

5. **Industrial Productivity/Manufacturing**

Welding sensor system. Laser-based automated welder for industrial use incorporates a laser sensor system to track the seam where two pieces of metal are to be joined, measures gaps and minute misfits, and automatically corrects the welding torch distance and height.

Microlasers. Transmits communication signals that can drill, cut, and melt materials.

Interactive computer training. Known as Interactive Multimedia Training (IMT), trains new employees to upgrade worker skills with a computer system that uses text, video, animation, voice, sounds, and music.

Other spin-offs include gasoline vapor recovery, self-locking fasteners, machine tool software, laser wire stripper, lubricant coating process, wireless communications, engine coatings, and engine design.

6. **Public Safety**

Emergency response robot. Remotely operated robot reduces human injury levels by performing hazardous tasks that would otherwise be handled by humans.

Personal alarm system. Pen-sized ultrasonic transmitter used by prison guards, teachers, the elderly, and disabled to call for help is based on space telemetry technology. The pen transmits a silent signal to a receiver that displays the exact location of the emergency.

Firefighter's air tanks. Lighter weight firefighter's air tanks weigh only 20 pounds for a 30-minute air supply, 13 pounds less than conventional firefighting tanks. The tanks are pressurized at 4500 psi (twice current tanks). A warning device tells the firefighter when air runs out.

Personal storm warning system. Lightning detector gives 30-minute warning to golfers, boaters, homeowners, business owners, and private pilots.

Other spin-offs include storm warning services (Doppler radar), firefighters' radios, lead poison detection, fire detector, flame detector, corrosion protection coating, protective clothing, and robotic hands.

7. **Transportation**

Studless winter tires. Viking Lander parachute shroud material is adapted and used to manufacture radial tires, increasing the tire material's chainlike molecular structure to five times the strength of steel, which should increase tread life by 10,000 miles.

Better brakes. New, high-temperature composite space materials provide better brake linings. Applications include trucks, industrial equipment, and passenger cars.

Advanced lubricants. An environment-friendly lubricant provides lubricants for railroad track maintenance, electric power company corrosion prevention, and hydraulic fluid with an oxidation life of 10,000 hours.

Energy storage system. The Flywheel Energy Storage system provides a chemical-free, mechanical battery that harnesses the energy of a rapidly spinning wheel and stores it as electricity with 50 times the capacity of a lead–acid battery; very useful for electric vehicles.

Other spin-offs include safer bridges, emission testing, airline wheelchairs, electric cars, auto design, methane-powered vehicles, windshear prediction, and aircraft design analysis.

NASA maintains an active database of all its programs and technologies with commercial potential and benefits (www.sti.nasa.gov/tto/spinoff2001/cbs_div.html). TABLE 27.16 lists examples of spin-off technologies from the Apollo Space Program, and TABLE 27.17 lists spin-off contributions from the Space Shuttle Program.

TABLE 27.16 ■ EXAMPLES OF SPIN-OFF TECHNOLOGIES FROM THE APOLLO SPACE PROGRAM

SPIN-OFF DEVICE

Digital signal-processing techniques, originally developed to computer-enhance pictures of the moon for the Apollo Program, are an indispensable part of computer-aided tomography (CAT) scan and magnetic resonance imaging (MRI) technologies in hospitals worldwide

As a medical CAT scanner searches the human body for tumors or other abnormalities, the industrial version or advanced computed tomography inspection system finds imperfections in aerospace castings, rocket motors, and nozzles

Cool suits, which kept Apollo astronauts comfortable during moon walks, are worn by race car drivers, nuclear reactor technicians, shipyard workers, persons with multiple sclerosis, and children with a congenital disorder known as hypohidrotic ectodermal dysplasia

Kidney dialysis machines were developed from a NASA-developed chemical process that removed toxic waste from used dialysis fluid

A cardiovascular conditioner developed for astronauts in space led to the development of a physical therapy and athletic development machine used by football teams, sports clinics, and medical rehabilitation centers

Cordless power tools and appliances

Athletic shoe design and manufacture incorporated technology from NASA spacesuits into a shoe's external shell. A stress free "blow molding" process is used in the shoe's manufacture

Insulation barriers made of aluminum foil laid over a core of propylene or Mylar, which protected astronauts and their spacecraft's delicate instruments from radiation, protects cars and trucks and dampens engine and exhaust noise

TABLE 27.17 ■ EXAMPLES OF SPIN-OFF TECHNOLOGIES FROM THE SPACE SHUTTLE PROGRAM

SPIN-OFF DEVICE	DESCRIPTION
Artificial heart	Technology used in space shuttle fuel pumps led to the development of a miniaturized ventricular assist pump
Automotive insulation	NASCAR racing cars use materials from the space shuttle thermal protection system to protect drivers from extreme engine heat
Balance evaluation systems	Medical centers use balance systems to measure the equilibrium of space shuttle astronauts upon return from space; the balance systems diagnose and treat patients that suffer head injury, stroke, chronic dizziness, and central nervous system disorders
Bioreactor	A rotating cell culture apparatus simulates some aspects of the space environment or microgravity on the ground. Tissue samples grown in the bioreactor help to design therapeutic drugs and antibodies
Diagnostic instrument	NASA technology created a compact laboratory instrument for hospitals and doctor offices that analyzes blood in 30 seconds, which once required 20 minutes
Gas detector	Ford Motor Company uses a gas leak detection system, originally developed to monitor the shuttle's hydrogen propulsion system, to produce a natural gas–powered car
Infrared camera	A sensitive infrared hand-held camera that observes the blazing plumes from the shuttle can scan for fires. The camera localizes hot spots for firefighters
Infrared thermometer	Infrared sensors developed to remotely measure distant star and planet temperatures led to the development of the hand-held optical sensor thermometer. Placed inside the ear canal, the thermometer provides an accurate reading in two seconds or less
Land mine removal device	The same rocket fuel that helps launch the space shuttle destroys land mines. A flare device, using leftover fuel donated by NASA, is placed next to the uncovered land mine and ignited from a safe distance with a battery-triggered electric match. The explosive burns away, neutering the mine and rendering it harmless
Lifesaving light	Special lighting technology developed for plant growth experiments on space shuttle missions treats brain tumors in children. Physicians use light emitting diodes to eradicate cancerous tumors
Prosthesis material	The foam insulation to protect the shuttle's external tank replaced the heavy, fragile plaster to produce light and virtually indestructible master molds for prosthetics
Video stabilization software	Image-processing technology that analyzes space shuttle launch video and studies meteorologic images helps law enforcement agencies improve crime-solving video. The technology removes defects from image jitter, image rotation, and image zoom-in video sequences

As we close this chapter, NASA's Mars Reconnaissance Orbiter that launched August 11, 2005, is on its way to Mars for arrival in March 2006 for a mission to better understand the history and distribution of Martian water. Learning more about what has happened to the water will focus searches for possible past or present Martian life. Observations by the orbiter will also support future Mars missions by examining potential landing sites and providing a communications relay between the Martian surface and Earth. The craft will transmit 10 times as much data per minute as any previous Mars spacecraft. This will convey detailed observations of the Martian surface, subsurface, and atmosphere by the instruments on the orbiter and enable data relay to Earth from other landers currently on the Martian surface. NASA plans to launch the *Phoenix* Mars Scout in 2007 to land on the far northern side of the planet. NASA is also developing an advanced rover, the Mars Science Laboratory, for launch in 2009. This is an exciting time for NASA and future space exploration of the final frontier.

Summary

1. On Earth's surface, gravity provides an invisible attraction force that makes any mass exert downward force or have weight. Sir Isaac Newton (1642–1727) discovered the universality of the gravitational law.

2. The escape velocity of an object or celestial body depends on the mass and radius of that body. Escape velocity from Earth equals 25,039 mi $\cdot$ h^{-1}.

3. The force of gravity never reaches an absolute zero value (called zero-g) because a gravitational force still exists. The term *microgravity,* not *weightlessness* (or *zero-g*), best describes what an astronaut perceives during space flight.

4. When an elevator descends quickly, one perceives a lessening of weight because of reduced force between the feet and elevator floor. If the elevator cable suddenly snaps and the elevator plummets downward, the force against the feet equals zero until the elevator strikes bottom. If persons could lift their feet off the floor before hitting the ground, they would experience free-fall similar to space flight.

5. Two different strategies have simulated space flights' microgravity environment: (1) test equipment to create microgravity conditions for brief periods using sounding rockets and objects dropped from towers or into tubes or (2) simulated microgravity conditions using humans in head-down bed rest, wheelchair-bound individuals, water immersion, immobilization and confinement, and parabolic flights plus in vitro centrifugation, mathematical modeling, and computer simulations.

6. On October 4, 1957, the Russian's Sputnik-1 became the first Earth-orbiting satellite. One month later, Sputnik-2 remained in orbit for almost 200 days with a dog on board.

7. NASA had two main early goals: (1) launch a man into space and return him safely to Earth and (2) develop human capability to endure space missions.

8. The most significant technologic achievement of the 20th century took place when Apollo 11 astronauts Aldrin and Armstrong landed on the moon's surface.

9. During the first few days in microgravity, fluid shifts from the lower body to the upper body. Total fluid volume also decreases to reduce the heart's work effort. Continued microgravity exposure decreases overall heart size from reduced left ventricular volume, mainly left ventricular end-diastolic volume.

10. The greatest postural instability in microgravity occurs in tests that require vestibular information. Readaptation begins quickly within a few hours after landing and returns to near normal in approximately 4 days.

11. NASA's greatest biomedical concern during space missions involves the 1% per month loss in weight-bearing bone mass. This effect could compromise crew health and safety during an exploration-class mission to Mars, including performance of critical EVA tasks, landing maneuvers, and procedures for leaving orbit on return to Earth.

12. Permanent neuromuscular dysfunction has not occurred during prolonged space missions. In-flight and postflight changes during missions of nearly 1 year reveal altered muscular coordination patterns, delayed-onset muscle soreness, and generalized muscular fatigue and weakness.

13. Countermeasure strategies attempt to minimize space flight's potentially harmful deconditioning effects on crew physiologic function, performance, and overall health during mission-critical maneuvers with reentry and landing.

14. Without gravity, normal biologic functions become more susceptible to short- and longer term maladaptations such as SMS—a syndrome characterized by headache and dizziness, drowsiness, malaise, poor concentration, disorientation, nausea, pallor, and dry heaves.

15. The energy balance equation has not been satisfied successfully on most space missions because of the increased energy demands of space flight and decreased food intake.

16. Maladaptations to microgravity include decreases in lean body mass, muscle volume, and muscle strength, altered muscle fiber microarchitecture, and atrophy of skeletal muscles that support posture and locomotion.

17. Astronaut health, safety, and performance during and following long-duration missions require additional research about (1) loss of weight-bearing bone and muscle, (2) vestibular function, the vestibular ocular reflex, and sensorimotor

integration, (3) orthostatic intolerance upon return to Earth's gravity, (4) radiation hazards, and (5) stress-related physiologic effects.

18. Technologies developed by NASA over the past 35 years have produced more than 30,000 secondary commercial spinoff applications, many providing life-altering breakthroughs in computer technology, consumer/home/recreation, transportation, environmental and resource management, industrial productivity/manufacturing, health and medicine, and public safety.

References are available on the Student CD or online at http://connection.lww.com/mkk6e.

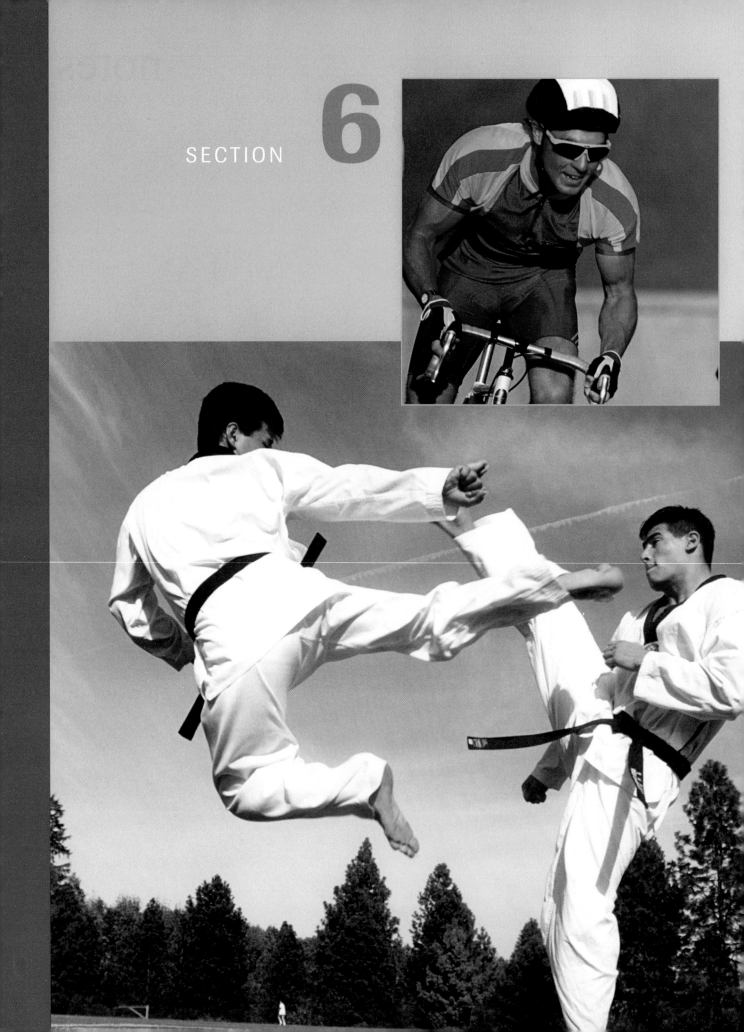

SECTION **6**

Body Composition, Energy Balance, and Weight Control

OVERVIEW

Five major reasons justify an accurate appraisal of body composition in a comprehensive program of total physical fitness:

1. It provides a starting point on which to base current and future decisions about weight loss and weight gain.
2. It provides realistic goals about how to best achieve an "ideal" balance between the body's fat and nonfat compartments.
3. It relates to general health status and plays an important role in the health and fitness goals of *all* individuals.
4. It monitors *changes* in the fat and lean components during exercise regimens of different durations and intensities.
5. It allows allied-health practitioners (sports nutritionist, dietician, personal trainer, coach, athletic trainer, physical therapist, physician, exercise leader) to interact with the individuals they deal with to provide quality information related to nutrition, weight control, and exercise.

Unfortunately, height-for-weight tables—a frequently used standard to assess overweight—serve only limited value to evaluate physique because "overweight" and "overfat" do not necessarily coincide. Athletes clearly illustrate this point; many exceed some average weight for height and gender but otherwise possess relatively low levels of body fat. Such individuals do not require weight loss, which might adversely affect their sports performance. In contrast, a prudent weight loss program would surely benefit the extreme number of overweight men and women not only in the United States but worldwide. This group spends nearly $50 billion each year to purchase diet books, products, and services at more than 1500 weight-control clinics in the hope of permanently reducing excess fat. Medicaid and Medicare finance almost one half of the nearly $100 billion spent annually on obesity-related medical spending in the United States. Worldwide, more than 300 million people fall within the definition of overweight, and this may be a conservative estimate. From antiquity to the present, regular physical activity has played an important role along with dietary restraint to maintain a healthful body composition and high level of physiologic function.

This section discusses body composition, its components and assessment, and the differences in body size and composition between sedentary and physically active men and women. We also deal with topics relevant to obesity and discuss the use of diet and exercise for weight management.

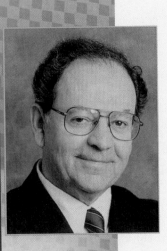

Interview *with* **Dr. Claude Bouchard**

Education: BPed (Laval University, Quebec City, Canada); MSc (University of Oregon, Eugene, OR); PhD (Population genetics, University of Texas, Austin); Postgraduate training (Deutsche Sporthochschule, Institute for Research on Circulation and Sport Medicine, Cologne; Growth Research Center, Université de Montreal)

Current Affiliation: Professor and Executive Director, George A. Bray Chair in Nutrition. Louisiana State University. Pennington Biomedical Research Center. Baton Rouge, LA.

Honors and Awards: See Appendix E, which is available on the Student CD and online at http://connection.lww.com/mkk6e.

Research Focus: Genetics of adaptation to exercise and nutritional interventions, and genetics of obesity and its comorbidities.

Memorable Publication: Bouchard C, et al. Genomic scan for maximal oxygen uptake and its response to training in the HERITAGE Family Study, J Appl Physiol 2000;88:551.

Statement of Contributions: ACSM Citation Award
In recognition of his impressive research accomplishments in exercise science, genetics, child growth and maturation, diet and exercise clinical trials, and public health.

Dr. Bouchard has made important contributions to many areas of human performance research, and has been a leader in synthesizing current knowledge to produce consensus statements in exercise science. Among other things, he has conducted innovative research on the effects of experimental manipulation of diet and exercise in monozygotic twins. He has collected more data on energy balance from carefully controlled studies in this unique population than anyone in the world. This research has led to a better understanding of the variability of responses to dietary manipulation and exercise training and to the genetics of these complex processes.

His career is characterized by high scientific standards, immense productivity, breadth of interests, creative study designs, and a willingness to collaborate with others. He serves as an ideal role model for us all.

What first inspired you to enter the exercise science field? What made you decide to pursue your advanced degree and/or line of research?

■ As a student in what was known as College Classic (the equivalent of high school, but it takes nine years and emphasizes the humanities), I became fascinated with human movement and performance. At that time, it was a very diffuse interest. That is, I was curious about the biomechanics, the exertion and the physiology, or the medical aspect, and the aesthetic of human movement. I had several career options, but came rapidly to the conclusion that I would move on to the local university, Université Laval, to learn about exercise and sports with the goal of approaching them from a scientific point of view. As you can see, even before I became a student in physical education, I was fascinated by science and human movement.

During my undergraduate studies, I was very frustrated by the poor science to which I was exposed, so I decided to go on to graduate studies. For 2 years during the summer, I traveled with friends on the East Coast of the USA and in the Midwest for the purpose of visiting universities and meeting faculty to select one for a Master's degree program. I visited at least 15 such institutions, and finally ended up at the University of Oregon, an institution that had been highly recommended to me. There, I was exposed to the teachings of Sigerseth, Clarke, Brumbach, Poley, and others.

After earning my Master's degree in Oregon, I felt that I was not quite ready to benefit from a PhD program. Following the advice of a few of my friends, I decided to go to the Sporthochschule in Cologne to work with Professor Wildor Hollmann. He was the Director of the Institute fur Kreislaufforschung und Sportmedizin, or the Institute for Research on Circulation and Sport Medicine. I knew that I could not obtain a degree there, but wanted to get more hands-on research experience. By then, my interests included not only performance but the health implications of exercise. I stayed there for 18 months and learned much.

Then I was offered a position at my alma mater, Laval University, in Quebec. I decided to accept the position with the expectation to leave after 3 years or so to obtain my PhD. If I had done so immediately, I would have entered an endocrinology PhD program, as I had made contact to be admitted in the lab of Professor Hans Selye at the Université de Montreal. But I became so involved in the development of the programs and the facilities at Laval University that it was 8 years before I left for my doctoral studies. By then, I had decided that genetics and biological individuality would be the focus of my research for the last decades of my career.

I opted to work with Professor Robert Malina, a colleague who had training in both physical education and biological anthropology, at the University of Texas. I spent 3 productive years there, which I completed with 10 months of postgraduate work at the Université de Montreal in the Human Growth and Development Center.

Obviously, mine has not been a linear career path. But I always felt that I was sharpening the focus of my research interest all along. Every phase in my career has been a useful one in the sense that it took me closer to what I am doing today—investigating the genetic and molecular basis of the response to exercise and of obesity and its comorbidities. It would have been impossible to select this line of research 35 years ago, since the field did not exist. The study of individual differences could not be even contemplated at the molecular level then.

Who were the most influential people in your career, and why?

■ Three scientists have played key roles at different times of my career. The first was Professor Fernand Landry. He was a faculty member at the University of Ottawa, but he was from the same city where I was born and went to the same colleges and community organizations that I later attended. He stimulated my interest in the biological sciences in general and the marvels of the human body's adaptation to exercise and training. He had a lasting impact on my career choices.

The second was Professor Wildor Hollmann. I got to know him very well during my stay in Cologne at his Institute. He stimulated my interest in the general topic of physical activity and health, particularly cardiovascular health. He was a very kind and patient mentor.

The last one was Professor Robert Malina. We became good friends during my doctoral studies at the University of Texas. Bob is a scholar with a strong interest in human diversity. We shared this research focus and many of the small pleasures of life.

What has been the most interesting/enjoyable aspect of your involvement in science? What was the least interesting/enjoyable aspect?

■ The most enjoyable aspect is that you always think out of the commonly accepted paradigm and look toward the future. You verify one fact only to refocus on the new questions generated by the previous experience. You also constantly meet people who are of the same mind, colleagues who are always trying to be innovative and creative in the presence of the same set of facts as you. The life of a scientist is never dull if you have the chance to interact with the best in your field.

The least enjoyable aspect is the fact that you have to hunt for research funds all the time, particularly if you run a large laboratory operation. At one point, there were 55 people working on my research projects, and I was spending at least one third of my time writing grant applications or renewals to maintain all of these positions.

What is your most meaningful contribution to the field of exercise science, and why is it so important?

■ If I have contributed anything, it is evidence for the magnitude of the individual differences in fitness and performance in the sedentary state and in the response to regular exercise. My group has also demonstrated over a period of 20 years that these individual differences were not random. They are characterized by familial clustering and are accounted for by a substantial genetic effect. We have identified some of the areas responsible for the heterogeneity in fitness and performance levels, and in trainability.

I have also spent considerable research resources investigating the genetic and molecular basis of obesity and the metabolic disturbances seen in some obese individuals, but not in others. To this end, we have used a combination of twin and family studies as well as intervention protocols to begin the dissection of the complex genotypes that predispose individuals to become overweight and then obese.

I am also proud of my contributions to the efforts undertaken over the past 15 years to arrive at evidence-based consensus concerning the role of physical activity in health and disease.

What advice would you give to students who express an interested in pursuing a career in exercise science research?

■ You will eventually need to become highly specialized in your own research pursuit, but try to acquire a broad-based understanding of the parent discipline. If you elect to become an exercise molecular biologist, you will find it useful to become an excellent biologist first. Maintaining a reasonable understanding of the changes occurring in biology in general will be a strong asset throughout your career. First, you will derive more satisfaction from your own research because you will be able to see the general implications of your work. Second, you are likely to find that a career in exercise science is more interesting if you understand what is going in the broader field of science to which you are related.

What interests have you pursued outside of your professional career?

■ At age 20, I learned to ski and enjoyed it tremendously for many years. I shifted progressively from downhill to cross-country skiing, which I still like to do. At present, my preferred activities are hiking, fly fishing for trout and salmon, working out at the gym, reading, classical music, and wine tasting. I also enjoy traveling, but these days most of my travel is for business purposes.

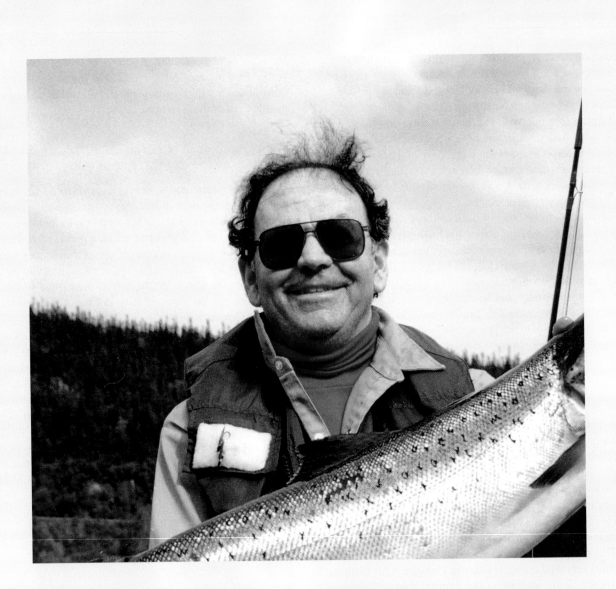

Where do you see the exercise science field (particularly your area of greatest interest) heading in the next 20 years?

■ In the next 20 years, the field of exercise science will incorporate the advances in molecular biology and genetics, something that it has failed to do in the past 10 years. The techniques of genomics and proteomics will become common technologies in our field. The benefits should be enormous, as exercise science can offer a wealth of opportunities to verify the functional consequences of DNA sequence variations in people who are not symptomatic for any disease. Such advances in the field of exercise science should make it possible for the exercise science discipline to become a significant player in preventive medicine and public health, as it will be able to develop the probes to identify those who are likely to benefit most from a physically active lifestyle. It will also change the way exercise science contributes to sports performance, as it will have the tools to identify the talented individuals at an early age.

You have the opportunity to give a "last lecture." Describe its primary focus.

■ It would be on the extent and the causes of biological individuality and its implications for human health in a Darwinian evolutionary perspective.

Body Composition Assessment

28

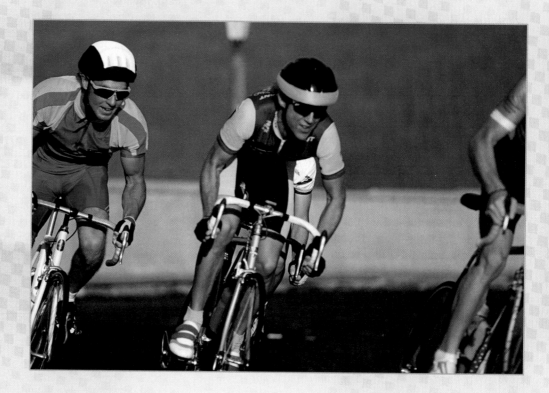

CHAPTER OBJECTIVES

- Summarize the early research on inadequacies of height–weight tables

- Outline current systems to classify overweight and obese conditions

- Delineate characteristics of the "reference man" and "reference woman," including values for storage fat, essential fat, and sex-specific essential fat

- Discuss the prevalence of menstrual irregularities within the general population and specific athletic groups, and factors associated with its occurrence

- Describe Archimedes' principle applied to human body volume measurement

- Discuss limitations in assumptions for computing percentage body fat from whole-body density

- Give the anatomic locations for six frequently measured skinfolds and girths

- Describe how skinfolds and girths provide meaningful information about body fat and its distribution

- Discuss the rationale for bioelectrical impedance analysis, and factors that affect body composition estimates with this technique

- Summarize the rationale, strengths, and weaknesses of bioelectrical impedance analysis, near-infrared interactance, ultrasound, x-ray, computed tomography, magnetic resonance imaging, dual-energy x-ray absorptiometry, and air-displacement plethysmography

- Give representative average values with variation limits for percentage body fat of typical young and older men and women

The life insurance actuarially based **height-weight tables** (weight measured with clothes and height measured with 2-inch heels) provide a popular means to assess the extent of "overweightness" on the basis of gender and bony frame size (see "In a Practical Sense," p. 778). These tables, however, provide unreliable information about the relative composition of an individual's body (muscle, bone, fat). Rather, they provide statistical landmarks based on the average ranges of body mass related to stature associated with the lowest mortality rate for persons aged 25 to 59 years. They do not consider specific causes of death or quality of health (morbidity) before death.

LIMITATIONS OF HEIGHT–WEIGHT TABLES

- Use unvalidated estimates of body frame size
- Developed from data derived primarily from white populations
- Specific focus on mortality data that may not reflect obesity-related comorbidities
- Provide no assessment of body composition

A person may weigh considerably more than the average weight-for-height standard yet still rate "underfat" for body composition; "extra" weight for this person exists as muscle mass. According to the tables, the desirable body weight (assuming a large frame size) for a professional American football player 188-cm tall and weighing 116 kg ranges between 78 and 88 kg. Similarly, body weight without regard for frame size for young adult men 188-cm tall averages 85 kg. Using either criterion, conventional standards would classify this player as overweight, implying that he should lose at least 28 kg just to achieve the upper limit of the desirable body weight range. He must lose an additional 3 kg to match his "average" American male counterpart. If the player followed these guidelines, he most likely would no longer play football and could jeopardize overall health. Body fat for the football player (even though he weighed 31 kg more than the average) was only 12.7% of body mass, compared with about 15.0% body fat for untrained young men.

Navy physician Dr. Albert Behnke (1898–1993) first observed body composition variations between elite athletes and untrained individuals in studies of football players in the early 1940s (see "Focus on Research," p. 780).[13] Careful evaluation of each player's body composition revealed that extreme muscular development primarily contributed to excess weight. These observations clearly pointed out that the term **overweight** refers only to a body mass in excess of some standard, usually the average for a given stature. Being above an average, ideal, or desirable body mass based on height–weight tables should not necessarily dictate whether someone begins a reducing regimen. A better alternative determines body composition by one of the laboratory or field techniques reviewed in this chapter. TABLE 28.1 lists terms and definitions common to the area of body composition evaluation.

THE BODY MASS INDEX: A SOMEWHAT BETTER ALTERNATIVE

Clinicians and researchers frequently use the **body mass index** (**BMI**), derived from body mass and stature, to assess "normalcy" for body weight. This measure exhibits a somewhat higher yet still moderate association with body fat and disease risk than estimates based simply on stature and body mass.

BMI Computation

BMI computes as follows:

$$BMI = Body\ mass\ (kg) \div stature\ (m^2)$$

Example

Male: stature, 175.3 cm, 1.753 m (69 in); body mass, 97.1 kg (214.1 lb)

$$BMI = 97.1 \div (1.753)^2$$
$$= 31.6\ kg \cdot m^{-2}\ or\ simply\ 31.6$$

The importance of this easily obtained index lies in its curvilinear relationship with the all-cause mortality ratio. As BMI increases throughout the range of moderate and severe overweight, so also does risk increase for cardiovascular complications (including hypertension and stroke), certain cancers, diabetes, Alzheimer's disease, gallstones, sleep apnea, osteoarthritis, and renal disease.[24,129,139,160]

A large prospective study of more than 1 million United States adults during 14 years of follow-up reveals the relationships between BMI and mortality risk. FIGURE 28.1A shows that smoking status and presence or absence of disease at time of enrollment in the study substantially modified the association between BMI and risk of premature death from all causes. Men and women who never smoked and remained disease free at the study's start *(light green lines)* experienced the greatest health risk from excess weight. Excessive leanness related to increased death risk among current and former smokers with a history of disease. In healthy people, the nadir of the curve for BMI and mortality occurred between a BMI of 23.5 and 24.9 for men (e.g.,

TABLE 28.1 ■ **TERMS FREQUENTLY USED IN DESCRIBING AND MEASURING BODY COMPOSITION**

TERM	DEFINITION
Abdominal fat	Subcutaneous and visceral fat in the abdominal region
Adipose tissue mass (ATM)	Fat (about 83%) plus its supporting structures (about 2% protein and 15% water); consists predominantly of white adipocytes (cells with a single fat droplet, mainly as triacylglycerol)
Anthropometry	Standardized techniques (e.g., calipers, tapes) to quantify (or predict) body size, proportion, and shape (*anthropo*, human; *metry*, measure)
Body density (Db)	Body mass (BM) expressed per unit body volume (body mass ÷ body volume)
Body mass index (BMI)	Ratio of BM to stature squared (body mass ÷ stature^2)
Densitometry	Archimedes' principle of water displacement to estimate whole-body density; other terms include *hydrostatic weighting, hydrodensitometry, underwater weighing*
Essential lipids	Compound lipids (phospholipids) needed for cell membrane formation—about 10% of total body fat
Fat mass (FM)	All extractable lipids from adipose and other body tissues
Fat-free body mass (FFM)	All residual lipid-free chemicals and tissues, including water, muscle, bone, connective tissue, and internal organs
Intraabdominal fat	Visceral fat in the abdominal cavity
Lean body mass (LBM)	FFM plus essential body fat
Minimal body mass	BM plus essential fat (includes sex-specific essential fat); 48.5 kg for the reference woman; computed from bone diameters, stature, and constants
Nonessential lipids	Triacylglycerols found mainly in adipose tissue—about 90% of total body fat
Reference man and reference woman	Behnke's reference standards for men and women that partition body mass into lean body mass, muscle, and bone, with fat subdivided into storage and essential fat; standards for body dimensions developed from military and anthropometric surveys
Relative body fat (%BF)	FM expressed as a percentage of total body mass
Specific gravity	Body mass in air divided by loss of weight in water (body mass ÷ [body mass − body weight in water])
Stature	Height expressed in metric units; e.g., 72 in = 182.88 cm = 1.829 m
Subcutaneous fat	Adipose tissue beneath the skin
Visceral adipose tissue (VAT)	Adipose tissue within and surrounding thoracic (e.g., heart, liver, lungs) and abdominal (e.g., liver, kidneys, intestines) cavities

5'10″ at 174 lb) and 22.0 and 23.4 for women (e.g., 5'5″ at 150 lb), with a gradient of increasing risk associated with moderate overweight. Among white men and women with the highest BMI, relative death risk equaled 2.58 (men) and 2.00 (women), compared with counterparts with a BMI of 23.5 to 24.9 (relative risk of 1.00).

Figure 28.1B shows the clear association in men and women between excess weight and a greater death risk from heart disease or cancer. A positive relationship emerged between BMI and cancer risk, with no elevation in risk among the leanest men and women. A J-shaped curve described BMI and cardiovascular disease risk, while a U-shaped curve predicted risk of death for all other causes. The authors attribute the increased death risk among the leanest men and women depicted in the J- and U-shaped curves to the presence of disease at the time of measurement.

New Standards for Overweight and Obesity

In 1998, the expert panel of the National Heart, Lung and Blood Institute lowered the BMI demarcation point for "overweight" from 27 to 25. Based on the association between excess body weight and disease, individuals with a BMI of 30 or

more were categorized as obese. Persons with a BMI of 30 average 30 pounds overweight. For example, a man 6'0″ weighing 221 pounds and a woman weighing 186 pounds at 5'6″ both have a BMI of 30, and both are approximately 30 pounds overweight. These revised standards place nearly 130 million or 62% of Americans in the overweight and obese categories—up from 72 million under the previous standard. Of this total, 30.5% (59 million people) classify as obese. For the first time, overweight persons (BMI above 25) outnumber persons of desirable weight! Analysis of available data by ethnicity and gender shows that more black, Mexican, Cuban, and Puerto Rican males and females classify as overweight than white counterparts.[138] FIGURE 28.2 shows the computed BMI and accompanying weight classifications with associated health risks.

FIGURE 28.3 presents the revised growth charts for the United States for boys and girls age 2 to 20 years. No absolute BMI standard exists to classify children and adolescents as overweight and obese.[100,119] Expert panels recommend BMI-for-age to identify the increasing number of children and adolescents at the upper end of the distribution who are either overweight (≥95th percentile) or at risk for overweight (≥85th percentile and ≤95th percentile; see Chapter 30). Less specific recommendations exist for the lower end of the distributions,

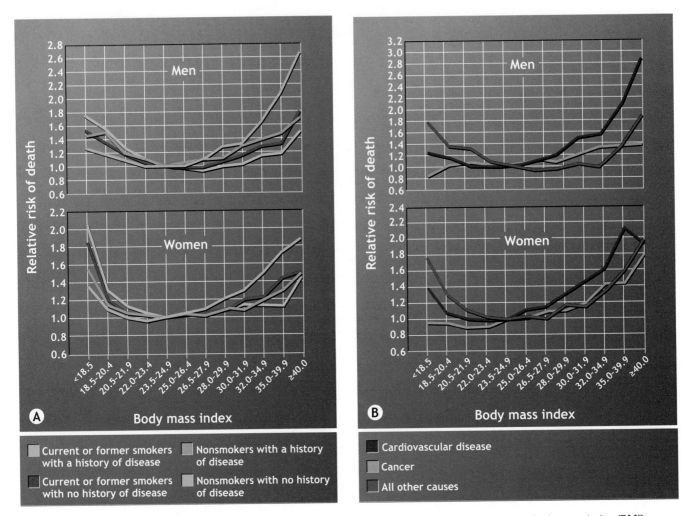

Figure 28.1   A. Multivariate relative risk of death from *all causes* among men and women according to body mass index (BMI), smoking status, and disease status. Data are from four mutually exclusive subgroups. Nonsmokers had never smoked. **B.** Multivariate relative risk of death from cardiovascular disease, cancer, and all other causes according to BMI among men and women who had never smoked and had no history of disease at enrollment. Subjects with BMIs of 23.5 to 24.9 composed the reference category in both figures. (From Calle EE, et al. Body-mass index and mortality in a prospective cohort of U.S. adults. N Engl J Med 1999;341:1097.)

but BMIs in this lower range may indicate underweight or at risk for underweight.[54,197]

BMI Limitations

Current classification for overweight (and obesity) assumes that the relationship between BMI and percentage body fat (and disease risk) remains independent of age, gender, ethnicity, and race, but this is not the case.[37,57] For example, at a given BMI level Asians have a higher body fat content than Caucasians and thus show greater risk for fat-related illness. A higher body fat percentage for a given BMI also exists among Hispanic American women compared with European American and African American women.[45] Failure to consider these sources of bias alters the proportion of individuals defined as obese by measured percentage body fat.[78,127]

The BMI, like the height-weight tables, fails to consider the body's proportional composition or the all-important com-

ponent of body fat distribution, referred to as **fat patterning**. In addition, factors other than excess body fat—bone, muscle mass, and even increased plasma volume induced by exercise training—affect the numerator of the BMI equation. A high BMI could lead to an incorrect interpretation of overfatness in lean individuals with excessive muscle mass because of genetic makeup or exercise training.

The possibility of misclassifying someone as overweight by applying BMI standards pertains particularly to large-size field athletes, bodybuilders, weight lifters, heavier wrestlers, and most professional American football players. For example, the BMI for seven defensive linemen from a former NFL Super Bowl team averaged 31.9 (team BMI averaged 28.7), clearly signaling these athletes as overweight and placing many of them in the moderate category for mortality risk. Conversely, the players' body fat percentage, 18.0% for the linemen and 12.1% for the team, indicated that they were not overfat.

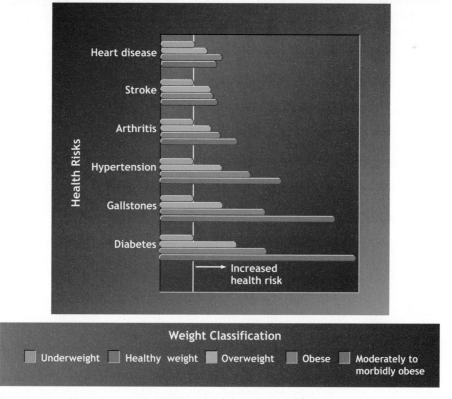

Figure 28.2 Body mass index (BMI), weight classifications, and associated health risks.

IN A PRACTICAL SENSE

DETERMINING BODY FRAME SIZE FROM STATURE AND TWO BONE DIAMETERS

■ Body frame size (BFS) becomes a useful measure for evaluating "normalcy" of body weight with standardized charts that categorize weight by frame size (bony structure). A combination of stature and bony widths (bone diameter measurements) adequately defines BFS, because BFS relates to the fat-free body mass (bone and muscle) and not body fat.

MEASUREMENTS

1. Stature (height [Ht]) measured in cm
2. Biacromial diameter (cm) measured as the distance between the most lateral projections of the acromial processes (see figure)
3. Bitrochanteric diameter (cm) measured as the distance between the most lateral projection of the greater trochanters (see figure)

CALCULATIONS

■ Regression analyses determine BFS values for women and men from Ht and sum of the biacromial and bitrochanteric bone diameters (ΣBia + Bitroc) with the following equations:

Female: BFS = Ht × 10.357 + (ΣBia + Bitroc)

Male: BFS = Ht × 8.239 + (ΣBia + Bitroc)

STEPS

1. Measure stature and biacromial and bitrochanteric diameters; use the average of two measurements.
2. Sum the average biacromial and bitrochanteric diameter measurements (ΣBia + Bitroc).
3. Compute BFS by substituting in the appropriate gender-specific formulas (example illustrated in Table 1).
4. Determine frame-size category by referring to Table 2.

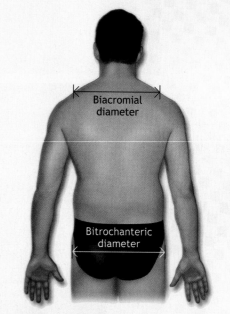

Biacromial diameter

Bitrochanteric diameter

TABLE 1 ■ EXAMPLE OF BFS CALCULATIONS FOR A MALE AND FEMALE OF DIFFERENT HEIGHTS AND BONY MEASUREMENTS

VARIABLE	SUBJECT A (MALE)	SUBJECT B (FEMALE)
Ht	167.3 cm	173.4 cm
Biacromial diameter	48.0 cm	29.8 cm
Bitrochanter diameter	35.0 cm	22.2 cm
ΣBia + Bitroc	83.0 cm	52.0 cm
BFS value	1461.4	1847.9 cm
	[BFS = Ht × 8.239 + ΣBia + Bitroc]	[BFS = Ht × 10.357 + ΣBia + Bitroc]
	[BSF = 167.3 × 8.239 + 83.0]	[BSF = 173.4 × 10.357 + 52.0]
	[BSF = 1461.4]	[BSF = 1847.9]
Frame-size category (from Table 2).	Medium	Medium

From Katch VL, Freedson PS. Body size and shape: derivation of the "HAT" frame-size model. Am J Clin Nutr 1982;36:669.

continued on page 779

Continued

TABLE 2 ■ BFS CATEGORIES

	FRAME-SIZE CATEGORY		
SEX	SMALL	MEDIUM	LARGE
Male	<1459.3	1459.4–1591.9	>1592.0
Female	<1661.9	1662.0–1850.7	>1850.8

From Katch VL, Freedson PS. Body size and shape: derivation of the "HAT" frame-size model. Am J Clin Nutr 1982;36:669.

Example

■ Table 1 shows calculations of BFS for a male and female of different heights and bony diameters. The male's height corresponds to a value below the 10th percentile for height-by-age for men in the U.S. population. This height, combined with large breadth measurements, results in a medium frame-size ranking (Table 2). In contrast, the female's height of 173.4 cm ranks above the 90th percentile for the U.S. population. However, her small breadth measurements also result in a medium frame-size ranking (Table 2).

Misclassification of body weight relative to body fat content also applies to the typical NFL player from 1920 to 1996. FIGURE 28.4 plots the average BMI for all NFL roster players at each fifth-year interval between 1920 and 1996 based on 53,333 players. Average body fat content of players measured during the late 1970s through the 1990s fell below the range typically associated with population data for men. Those with body fat evaluated by densitometry during this era included all roster players of the New York Jets, Washington Redskins, New Orleans Saints, and Dallas Cowboys (TABLE 28.2). Almost all players from 1960 onward classify as overweight based on standard height-for-weight tables. For the BMI data

up to 1989, values for linebackers, skill players, and defensive backs represent the low category for disease risk, while the BMIs for offensive and defensive linemen place them at "moderate" risk. After 1989, risk for linebackers increased from the low to moderate category. The BMIs for offensive and defensive linemen, the largest NFL players, quickly approached a high risk and remained in that category. This does not bode well from a health perspective for these large-size players, at least based on BMI risk predictions for the general population.

In contrast to professional football players, the BMI for National Basketball Association players for the 1993–1994 season averaged only 24.5. This relatively low BMI places

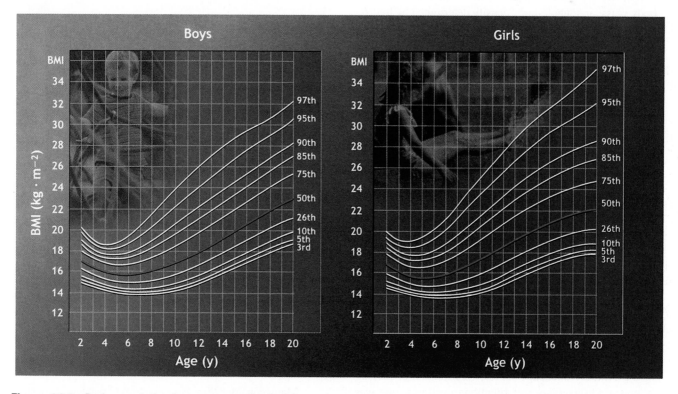

Figure 28.3 Body mass index-for-age percentiles for boys and girls ages 2 to 20 years. Developed by the National Center for Health Statistics in collaboration with the National Center for Chronic Disease Prevention and Health Promotion (2000). (From Kuczmarski RJ, et al. CDC growth charts: United States. Advance Data 2000;314. From Vital and Health Statistics of the Centers for Disease Control and Prevention/National Center for Health Statistics.)

FOCUS On Research

OVERWEIGHT BUT NOT OVERFAT

Welham WC, Behnke AR. The specific gravity of healthy men; body weight/volume and other physical characteristics of exceptional athletes and of naval personnel. JAMA 1942;18:498.

▲ The Welham and Behnke research is one of the most frequently cited studies in the body composition and exercise physiology literature. These investigators tested the hypothesis that differences in body fat among men relate chiefly to the body's specific gravity and not body mass per se. The hypothesis predicted that heavy but lean men would have higher body specific gravity values than counterparts of similar body mass, but with high body fat levels. If correct, a relatively large body mass may not always provide an appropriate measure of excessive fatness.

In 1942, the relation between the body density and estimates of body fatness remained undetermined, although scientists knew the specific gravity of the body's fat and nonfat (fat-free) components. Twenty-five professional football players, most of whom had been designated All-Americans, were classified as unfit for military service because of excessive body weight according to standard height–weight tables. Measurements included stature, body mass, and whole-body density determined by hydrostatic weighing. A unique aspect of the body density assessment corrected body volume from estimates of residual lung volume.

The *figure* shows the relationship between body density and "weight-to-height" for the athletes. The *vertical line* at a weight:height ratio of 2.65 represents the upper limit for classification as fit for military service. Men of this age who fell to the right of the vertical line did not qualify for life insurance because of their excessive body weight; 17 of the players classified as overweight. However, the high body densities of 11 of these men indicated a low percentage body fat. Body mass of all the players averaged 90.9 kg (200 lb), and body density averaged $1.080\ \mathrm{g \cdot cm^{-3}}$.

For the 6 heaviest men, body mass averaged 104.5 kg (230 lb), with body density at $1.059\ \mathrm{g \cdot cm^{-3}}$.

Welham and Behnke's research was the first to show that variations in body density related mainly to individual differences in the body's fat content. The research also pointed up the inadequacies of height–weight tables to infer body fatness or determine a desirable body weight, particularly among highly trained large athletes. The researchers suggested that a body density of $1.060\ \mathrm{g \cdot cm^{-3}}$ should serve as the demarcation for excessive fatness for men. With this criterion, 23 of the 25 lean but heavy football payers qualified as fit (and not overly fat) for military service.

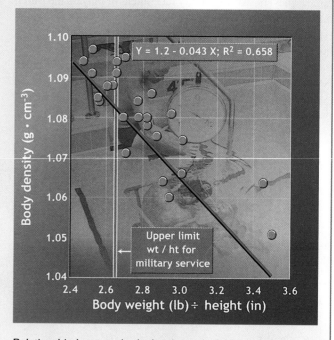

Relationship between body density and weight-to-height ratio for 25 All-American football players.

them in the very low risk category, yet height–weight standards would classify them as overweight.

Another category of world-class athletes—racing cyclists who participated in the Tour de France—had remarkably low BMIs. In the 1997 race, the BMI for 170 competitors averaged 21.5 (1.79 m stature, 68.75 kg body mass). Three years later in the 2000 race, the BMI for 162 competitors remained essentially unchanged (21.5; 1.79 m stature, 69.1 kg body mass). On average, stature among cycling teams was within 0.2 m (1.78 to 1.80 m) and body mass ranged from 66.8 kg (Swiss) to 72.1 kg (USA). The homogeneity in body size variables among these top-level performers makes it unlikely

that body composition variables per se determine individual differences in cycling performance. Instead, experiments have focused on physiologic and nutritional variables during extended-duration performance.[22,23,44,122]

Miss America and BMI—Undernourished Role Models?

Many consider Miss America beauty pageant contestants to possess the ideal combination of beauty, grace, and talent. Each competitor survives the rigors of local and state contests, thus satisfying judges that finalists have "ideal qualities"

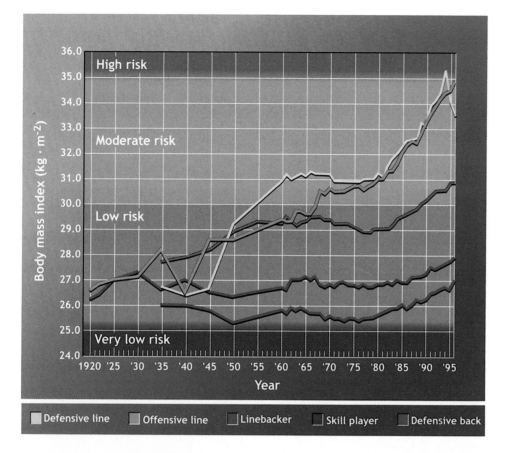

Figure 28.4 BMIs for all players in the National Football League between 1920 and 1996 ($n = 53,333$). Categories include offensive and defensive linemen, linebackers, skill players (quarterbacks, receivers, backfield), and defensive backs. (Data compiled by K. Monahan and F. Katch, Exercise Science Department, University of Massachusetts, Amherst, 1996).

TABLE 28.2 ■ PHYSIQUE AND BODY COMPOSITION OF "UNDERFAT" PROFESSIONAL FOOTBALL PLAYERS AND "OVERWEIGHT" OFFENSIVE AND DEFENSIVE PROFESSIONAL LINEMEN AND SHOT PUTTERS

VARIABLE	ALL-PRO DEFENSIVE BACKS PLAYER 1	2	3	4	DALLAS ALL-PRO OFFENSIVE BACK (*N* = 1)	DEFENSIVE LINEMEN 1977 (*N* = 10)	DALLAS LINEMEN 1977 (*N* = 5)	OLYMPIC SHOT PUTTERS (*N* = 1)
Age (y)	27.1	30.2	29.4	24.0	32	31	29	24
Stature (cm)	184.7	181.9	187.2	181.5	184.7	193.8	197.6	187.0
Mass (kg)	87.9	87.1	88.4	88.9	90.6	116.0	116.5	112.3
Relative fat (%)	3.9	3.8	3.8	2.5	1.4	18.6	13.2	14.8
Absolute fat (kg)	3.4	3.3	3.4	2.2	1.3	21.6	15.4	16.6
Fat-free body mass (kg)	84.5	83.8	85.0	86.7	89.3	94.4	101.1	95.7
Lean:fat ratio	24.85	25.39	25.00	39.41	68.69	4.37	6.57	5.77
Girth (cm)								
Shoulders	122.1	119.0	120.5	117.2	121.8	129.5	122.5	133.3
Chest	101.6	101.0	99.5	107.5	102.0	116.5	109.9	118.5
Abdomen, avg	81.8	85.5	81.0	82.6	81.7	102.0	97.0	100.3
Buttocks	98.0	99.0	101.9	102.0	96.5	112.8	111.5	112.3
Thigh	61.0	61.0	58.5	64.0	63.2	66.2	69.3	69.4
Knee	39.5	41.3	41.1	38.0	41.0	44.8	45.8	42.9
Calf	37.6	38.8	38.8	37.8	41.3	43.5	42.4	43.6
Ankle	21.8	23.1	23.5	22.4	22.7	25.8	25.7	24.7
Forearm	31.8	29.1	31.1	31.8	33.5	33.5	34.8	33.7
Biceps	38.0	35.8	37.1	37.7	40.4	41.5	41.7	42.2
Wrist	18.5	17.2	17.4	17.5	18.0	19.3	19.3	18.9

From Katch FI, Katch VL. The body composition profile: techniques of measurement and applications. Clin Sports Med 1984;3:30.

worthy of role-model status. The consummate image of the Miss America physique to some extent shapes society's generalized "ideal" for female size and shape. An important question concerns whether such images, televised worldwide to millions of viewers, reinforce an unhealthful message to those who attempt to emulate such physiques?[46]

FIGURE 28.5 shows the BMIs and accompanying anthropometric data of Miss America contestants from available data between 1922 to 1999 (excluding 1927–1933, when the pageant was not held, and from 2000 on, when data were no longer available). Also included for comparison about body size is Behnke's standard for the reference woman (Fig. 28.5C; see below). The *bottom horizontal white dashed line* in Figure 28.5A designates the World Health Organization (WHO) cutoff for undernutrition established at a BMI of 18.5.[215] The *top horizontal black dashed line* represents the

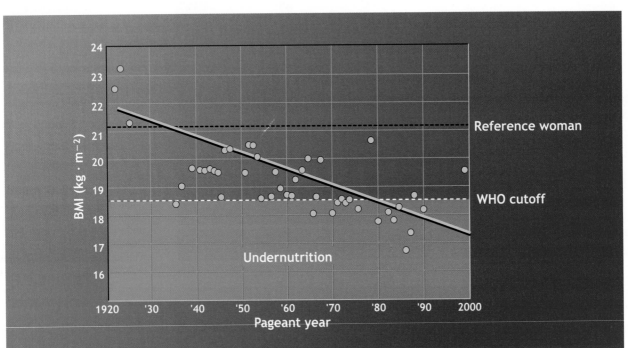

Figure 28.5   A. Body mass index (BMI) of 47 Miss America pageant contestants from 1922 to 1999. The *top horizontal black dashed line* represents the BMI for Behnke's reference woman (21.1 kg · m⁻²). The *bottom horizontal white dashed line* designates the World Health Organization's (WHO) BMI demarcation for undernutrition (18.5 kg · m⁻²). **B.** Available data for age, height (in), and weight (lb) for the contest winners. **C.** Selected girths for 24 Miss America winners from 1926 to 1965. Despite our best efforts, we were unable to locate height or weight data for Miss America winners from 2000 on.

B.

1922-1948				1951-1968				1970-1999		
	Age	Ht	Wt		Age	Ht	Wt		Age	Ht	Wt
1922	18	65	135	1951	20	65.5	119	1970	21	65.5	110
1923	19	65	140	1952	25	70	143	1971	21	68	121
1924	18	66	132	1953	19	66.5	128	1972	22	67	118
1926	18	52.5	118	1954	20	68	132	1973	23	68	120
1936	22	66	114	1955	19	68.5	124	1974	23	69	125
1937	17	66.5	120	1957	19	67	120	1976	18	70.5	128
1939	19	67	126	1958	20	68.5	130	1979	22	64	121
1941	19	65.5	120	1959	21	65	114	1980	22	67	114
1942	21	65	118	1960	21	67	120	1983	25	67	115
1943	21	68	130	1961	18	66	116	1984	20	66	110
1944	21	67	125	1962	19	65.5	118	1985	20	68	120
1945	18	70	136	1964	21	66.5	124	1986	21	69	114
1946	21	68	123	1965	22	124	124	1987	21	68.5	116
1947	21	67	130	1966	19	115	115	1988	24	70	131
1948	18	69	138	1967	19	116	116	1990	24	67.5	118
				1968	19	135	135	1999	24	69	133

C.

	Girths (inches)							
	Bust	Waist	Hips	Calf	Thigh	Ankle	Biceps	Wrist
1926	33	24.5	33.5	12.5	19.5	7	—	—
1935	33	23	35.5	—	—	—	—	—
1926	34	23.5	34.5	13	19	8.5	9.5	5.5
1941	34	24	36	14	23	8	11	6
1942	34	24	34.5	—	—	—	—	—
1943	36	23	35	—	—	—	—	—
1944	36.5	25	37.5	13	19.5	8	—	—
1945	35.5	25	35	14.5	20	8.5	—	—
1946	35.5	25.5	36	13.5	22	8.5	—	—
1947	35	35	—	—	—	—	—	—
1948	37	37	—	—	—	—	—	—
1951	35	35	—	—	—	—	—	—
1952	36	24	36	—	—	—	—	—
1953	35	23	35	—	—	—	—	—
1954	37	24	36	—	—	—	—	—
1955	34.5	22	35	—	—	—	—	—
1957	35	23	35	—	—	—	—	—
1958	35	25	36	—	—	—	—	—
1959	34	22	35	—	—	—	—	—
1960	36	24	36	—	—	—	—	—
1961	35	22	35	—	—	—	—	—
1962	35	24	35	—	—	—	—	—
1964	35	23	35	—	—	—	—	—
1965	36	24	36	—	—	—	—	—
Ref W*	36.1	30.3	36.8	14.1	21.6	8.9	12.5	6.8

Ref W* = Behnke's reference woman; stature = 163.8 cm, body mass = 56.7 kg

BMI for the reference woman (see Fig. 28.6; stature, 1.638 m; body mass, 56.7 kg; BMI, 21.1). The downward slope of the regression line from 1922 to 1999 shows a clear tendency for relative undernutrition from the mid-1960s to approximately 1990. Using the WHO cutoff, the BMIs of 30% ($n = 14$) of the 47 Miss America winners fell below 18.5. Raising the BMI cutoff to 19.0 adds another 18 women, or a total of 48% of the winners with undesirable values. Approximately 24% of contest winners had BMIs between 20.0 and 21.0, and no winner after 1924 had a BMI equaling that of the reference woman!

Interestingly, 1965 was the last year we could locate girth measurements from official press releases or newspaper coverage of the contest. We compared the percentage difference between the Miss America girth averages with the corresponding measurements for the reference woman (*bottom yellow row* of Fig. 28.5C). For the average bust, waist, and hip values (35.1, 24.0, 35.4 in, respectively), Miss America's measurement exceeded the reference woman's bust measurement by 2.6 inches (8%) but fell 7% below for the waist value (-1.8 in) and 5% (-1.7 in) for the hips. Unfortunately, no contemporary data exist from 1966 to the present, so we cannot compare the current Miss America's physique with historical data.

COMPOSITION OF THE HUMAN BODY

In 1921, Czech anthropologist J. Matiega described a four-component model consisting of the weight of the skeleton (S), skin plus subcutaneous tissue (Sk + St), skeletal muscle (M), and a remainder (R).[118] The sum of the four components equaled the body mass.

Over the past 85 years, studies have focused on body composition and how best to measure the various components. One methodology partitions the body into two distinct compartments: (1) fat-free body mass and (2) fat mass. The density of homogenized samples of fat-free body tissues in small mammals equals $1.100 \text{ g} \cdot \text{cm}^{-3}$ at 37°C.[157] Fat-free tissue maintains water content of 73.2%,[136] with potassium at 60 to 70 mmol $\cdot$ kg^{-1} in men and 50 to 60 mmol $\cdot$ kg^{-1} in women.[17] Fat stored in adipose tissue has a density of 0.900 g $\cdot$ cm^{-3} at 37°C.[128] Subsequent body composition studies expanded the two-component model to account for biologic variability in three (water, protein, fat) or four (water, protein, bone mineral, fat) distinct components.[85,211,213] Women and men differ in relative quantities of specific body composition components. Consequently, gender-specific reference standards provide a framework to evaluate "normal" body composition. Behnke's model for the reference man and reference woman proves useful for such purposes.[12]

Reference Man and Reference Woman

Figure 28.6 shows the body composition compartments for the **reference man** and **reference woman**. The schema partitions body mass into lean body mass, muscle, and bone, with total body fat subdivided into storage and essential fat components. This model integrates the average physical di-mensions from thousands of individuals measured in large-scale civilian and military anthropometric surveys with data from laboratory studies of tissue composition and structure.

The reference man is taller and heavier, his skeleton weighs more, and he possesses a larger muscle mass and lower body fat content than the reference woman. These differences exist even when expressing fat, muscle, and bone as a percentage of body mass. Just how much of the gender difference in body fat relates to biologic and behavioral factors, perhaps from lifestyle differences, remains unclear. Undoubtedly, hormonal differences play an important role. The concept of reference standards does not mean that men and women should strive to achieve this body composition or that the reference man and woman reflect some healthful standard. Instead, the reference model proves useful for statistical comparisons and interpretations of data from other studies of elite athletes, individuals involved in exercise training, different racial and ethnic groups, and the underweight and the obese.

Essential and Storage Fat

In the reference model, total body fat exists in two storage sites or depots—essential fat and storage fat. **Essential fat** consists of the fat in heart, lungs, liver, spleen, kidneys, intestines, muscles, and lipid-rich tissues of the central nervous system and bone marrow. *Normal physiologic functioning requires this fat.* In the heart, for example, dissectible fat from cadavers represents approximately 18.4 g or 5.3% of an average heart weighing 349 g in males and 22.7 g or 8.6% of a heart weighing 256 g in females.[214] Importantly, essential fat in the female includes additional **sex-specific essential fat**. Whether this fat provides reserve storage for metabolic fuel is unclear.

The **storage fat** depot includes fat primarily in adipose tissue. The adipose tissue energy reserve contains approximately 83% pure fat, 2% protein, and 15% water within its supporting structures. Storage fat includes the visceral fatty tissues that protect the organs within the thoracic and abdominal cavities from trauma, and the larger adipose tissue volume deposited beneath the skin's surface. A similar proportional distribution of storage fat exists in men and women (12% of body mass in men, 15% in women), but the total percentage of essential fat in women that includes the sex-specific fat averages four times the value in men. *The additional essential fat most likely serves biologically important functions for child bearing and other hormone-related functions.* Considering the reference body's total quantity of storage fat (approximately 8.5 kg), this depot theoretically represents 63,500 kCal of available energy, or the energy equivalent of running nonstop at a 9-minute-per-mile pace for 114 hours!

Figure 28.7 partitions the distribution of body fat for the reference woman. As part of the 5 to 9% sex-specific fat reserves, breast fat probably contributes no more than 4% of body mass for women whose total fat content ranges between 14 and 35%.[91] We interpret this to mean that other substantial sex-specific fat depots exist (e.g., pelvic, buttock, and thigh regions) that contribute to the female's body-fat stores.

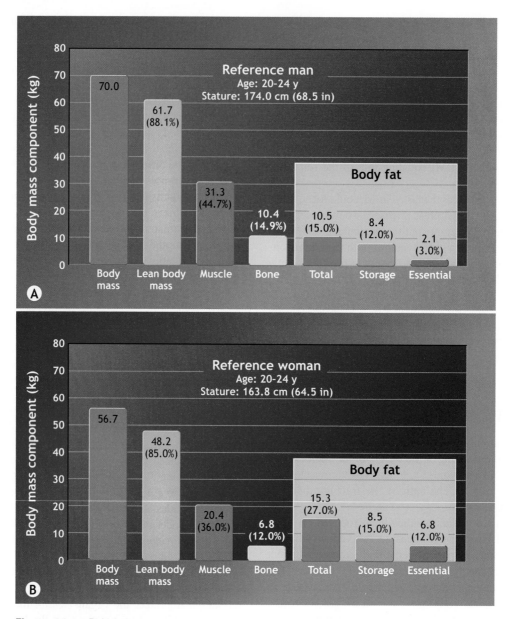

Figure 28.6   Behnke's theoretical model for the body composition of the reference man (**A**) and reference woman (**B**). Values in parenthesis indicate percentage of total body mass.

Fat-Free Body Mass and Lean Body Mass.   The terms **fat-free body mass** (**FFM**) and **lean body mass** refer to specific entities. Lean body mass contains the small percentage of non–sex-specific essential fat equivalent to approximately 3% of body mass. In contrast, FFM represents the body mass devoid of *all* extractable fat (FFM = body mass − fat mass). Behnke points out that FFM refers to an in vitro entity appropriate to carcass analysis. He considered lean body mass as an in vivo entity relatively constant in water, organic matter, and mineral content throughout the active adult's life span. *In normally hydrated, healthy adults, the FFM and lean body mass differ only in the essential fat component.*

Figure 28.6 showed that lean body mass in men and **minimal body mass** in women consist chiefly of essential fat

(plus sex-specific essential fat for women), muscle, water, and bone. The whole-body density of the reference man with 12% storage fat and 3% essential fat is $1.070 \text{ g} \cdot \text{cm}^{-3}$; the density of his FFM is $1.094 \text{ g} \cdot \text{cm}^{-3}$. If the reference man's total body fat percentage equals 15.0% (storage fat plus essential fat), the density of a hypothetical fat-free body attains the upper limit of $1.100 \text{ g} \cdot \text{cm}^{-3}$.

In the reference woman, the average whole-body density of $1.040 \text{ g} \cdot \text{cm}^{-3}$ represents a body fat percentage of 27%; of this, approximately 12% consists of essential body fat. A density of $1.072 \text{ g} \cdot \text{cm}^{-3}$ represents the minimal body mass of 48.5 kg. In actual practice, density values that exceed 1.068 for women (14.8% body fat) and $1.088 \text{ g} \cdot \text{cm}^{-3}$ for men (5% body fat) rarely occur except in young, lean athletes.

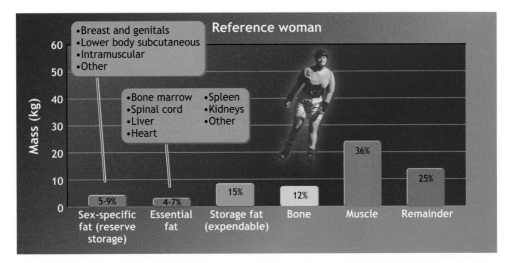

Figure 28.7 Theoretical model for body fat distribution for the reference woman with body mass of 56.7 kg, stature of 163.8 cm, and 27% body fat. (From Katch VL, et al. Contribution of breast volume and weight to body fat distribution in females. Am J Phys Anthropol 1980;53:93.)

Minimal Leanness Standards

A biologic lower limit exists beyond which a person's body mass cannot decrease without impairing health status or altering normal physiologic functions.

Men

To estimate the lower body-fat limit in men (i.e., lean body mass), subtract storage fat from body mass. For the reference man, the lean body mass (61.7 kg) includes approximately 3% (2.1 kg) essential body fat. Encroachment into this reserve may impair optimal health and capacity for vigorous exercise.

Low body fat values exist for male world-class endurance athletes and some conscientious objectors to military service who voluntarily reduced body fat stores during a prolonged experiment with semistarvation.[95] The low fat levels of marathon runners, which ranges from 1 to 8% of body mass, probably reflect adaptation to severe training for distance running. A low body fat level reduces the energy cost of weight-bearing exercise; it also provides a more effective gradient to dissipate metabolic heat generated during prolonged, intense exercise.

Considerable variation exists in the FFM of different athletes, with values ranging from a low of 48.1 kg in some jockeys to over 100 kg in football linemen and field-event athletes. Seven elite sumo wrestlers *(seki-tori)* possessed an average FFM of 109 kg.[98] Table 28.2 (p. 781) presents data on the physique status and body compositions of selected professional football players, many of whom classify as both underfat and overweight. Striking differences emerge among these athletes in body size, percentage body fat, FFM, lean:fat ratio, and a matrix of girth measures. The defensive and offensive backs in football rated underfat compared with the reference man (or any other nonathletic standard). In contrast, linemen and shot putters were clearly overweight for their statures; body mass relative to stature (mass per unit size) represented the 90th percentile for nonathletic males.

Women

In comparison to the lower limit of body mass for the reference man (with 3% essential fat), the lower limit for the reference woman includes approximately 12% essential fat. This theoretical lower limit developed by Dr. Behnke, termed *minimal body mass,* is 48.5 kg for the reference woman. Generally, the leanest women in the population do not possess less than 10 to 12% body fat, a narrow range at the lower limit for most women in good health. *Behnke's theoretical concept of minimal body mass in women that incorporates 12% essential fat, corresponds to the lean body mass in men that includes 3% essential fat.*

Five-Level Model of Body Composition

FIGURE 28.8 shows a proposed five-level model for examining the composition of the human body. Each level of the model becomes more elaborate—atoms, molecules, cells, tissue systems, whole body—as the body's complexity of biologic organization increases in accord with advances in assessment techniques. Note that subdivisions exist within each of the five levels. The model attempts to identify and then quantify each level's various components. An essential feature provides separate and distinct levels, each with measurable characteristics. Examples of measurement include the following for a reference body that weighs 70 kg:

- **Atomic level**. Body mass equals the sum of all the body's atoms (O + C + H + N + Ca + remainder). This generally represents 60% oxygen, 23% carbon, 10% hydrogen, 2.6% nitrogen, 1.4% calcium, and less than 1% for the remaining atoms. Cadaver or tissue biopsy samples determine the elemental composition. Whole-body ^{40}K counting assesses total body potassium,[137] with total body sodium, chlorine, phosphorus, and calcium determined by delayed γ neutron activation,[30] total body nitrogen by prompt γ

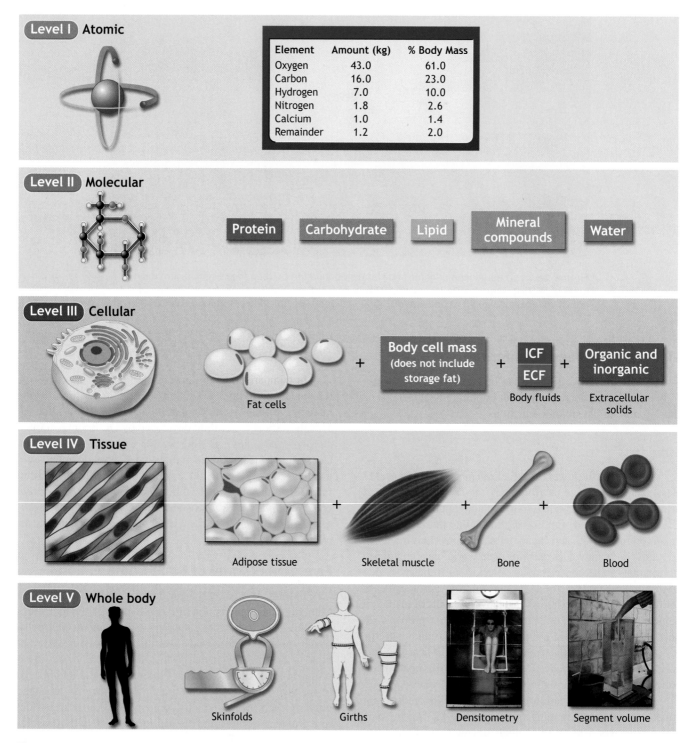

Element	Amount (kg)	% Body Mass
Oxygen	43.0	61.0
Carbon	16.0	23.0
Hydrogen	7.0	10.0
Nitrogen	1.8	2.6
Calcium	1.0	1.4
Remainder	1.2	2.0

Figure 28.8 Five-level multicomponent model to assess and interpret body composition. Each level progresses in complexity of biologic organization. Use of appropriate measurement techniques to assess the components within a particular organizational level represents the model's key feature. This allows researchers to focus on a particular body composition aspect in relation to specific and/or general biologic effects. Measurements could include changes in tissue composition from weight gain or loss or more theoretical aspects related to cellular and tissue functions. *ICF,* intracellular fluid; *ECF,* extracellular fluid. (Modified from Wang ZM, et al. The five-level model: a new approach to organizing body composition research. Am J Clin Nutr 1992;56:19.)

neutron activation,[31] and total body carbon by inelastic neutron scattering.[92]

- **Molecular level.** The body's diverse atoms form molecules that constitute more than 100,000 different chemical compounds. Water, fat (essential and storage), glycogen, protein (nitrogen-containing compounds), and minerals (metallic and nonmetallic elements) provide the major constituents. Elements can be sampled from body fluids and estimated by isotopic dilution,[53] and single[152] and dual-energy x-ray absorptiometry quantify osseous (bone containing 99% of the body's Ca and 86% of its P) and nonosseous mineral-containing compounds.[148]

- **Cellular level.** Three main compartments make up the body mass: (1) cells (cell mass = cells from muscles + connective [including fat cells], epithelial, and nervous tissues); (2) extracellular fluids (plasma + interstitial fluid); (3) extracellular solids (organic and inorganic extracellular solids). Isotopic dilution measures extracellular fluid and plasma volumes. Naturally occurring radioactive isotope of potassium (^{40}K) assesses body cell mass because more than 95% of the body's potassium remains in the intracellular fluid compartment.

- **Tissue and organ level.** The body contains 11 subsystems—circulatory, respiratory, nervous, integumentary, muscular, endocrine, respiratory, lymphatic, digestive, skeletal, and reproductive. This level of body composition evaluation groups four tissue systems to represent total body mass (adipose tissue + skeletal muscle + bone + blood). Computed tomography, magnetic resonance imaging, and ultrasound procedures estimate the volumes of subcutaneous fat, visceral adipose tissue, and segmental muscle mass.

- **Whole-body level.** Common anthropometric procedures include measurement of skinfolds, girths, bone diameters, body mass, stature, BMI, surface area, segment lengths, segmental and total body volume, and body density (hydrodensitometry).

Leanness, Regular Exercise, and Menstrual Irregularity

Physically active women, mainly participants in the "low weight" or "appearance" sports (e.g., distance running, body building, figure skating, diving, ballet, and gymnastics), increase their likelihood for one of three maladies: (1) delayed onset of menstruation, (2) irregular menstrual cycle (**oligomenorrhea**), or (3) complete cessation of menses (**amenorrhea**). Menstrual and ovarian dysfunction results largely from changes in the pituitary gland's normal pulsatile secretion of luteinizing hormone regulated by gonadotropin-releasing hormone from the hypothalamus.

Amenorrhea occurs in 2 to 5% of women of reproductive age in the general population, but it can reach 40% in some athletic groups. As a group, ballet dancers remain lean with a greater incidence of menstrual dysfunction and eating disor-

ders and a higher mean age at menarche than age-matched, nondance counterparts.[55,203] One third to one half of female endurance athletes exhibit some menstrual irregularity. In premenopausal women, irregularity or absence of menstrual function accelerates bone loss and increases risk of musculoskeletal injury during exercise and causes a longer interruption of training (see Chapter 2).[11,66,140]

A long-term high level of physical stress may disrupt the hypothalamic–pituitary–adrenal axis and modify the output of gonadotropin-releasing hormone, which results in irregular menstruation (**exercise stress hypothesis**). A concurrent hypothesis maintains that energy (fat) reserves inadequate to sustain pregnancy induce cessation of ovulation (**energy availability hypothesis**).

INTEGRATIVE QUESTION

What arguments counter the following position? No true sex difference exists in body fat level, but only a difference caused by gender-related patterns of regular physical activity and caloric intake.

Lean-to-Fat Ratio

The **lean-to-fat ratio** plays a key role in normal menstrual function, perhaps through peripheral fat's role that converts androgens to estrogens or through adipose tissue's production of leptin, a hormone intimately linked to body fat levels and appetite control (see Chapter 30) and initiation of puberty.[27,181] Thus, linkage exists between hormonal regulation of sexual maturity onset (and perhaps continued optimal sexual function) and level of stored energy from accumulated body fat.

Some researchers assert that 17% body fat represents a critical level for the onset of menstruation, with 22% fat needed to sustain a normal cycle.[55,56] They reason that lower body fat levels trigger hormonal and metabolic disturbances that affect menses. *Objective data indicate that many physically active females who are below the supposedly critical 17% body fat level have normal menstrual cycles with high levels of physiologic and exercise capacity.* Conversely, some amenorrheic athletes maintain body fat levels considered average for the population. One of our laboratories compared 30 athletes and 30 nonathletes, all with less than 20% body fat, for menstrual cycle regularity.[89] Four athletes and three nonathletes, ranging from 11 to 15% body fat, maintained regular cycles, whereas seven athletes and two nonathletes had irregular cycles or were amenorrheic. For the total sample, 14 athletes and 21 nonathletes maintained regular menstrual cycles. These data indicate that normal menstrual function *does not require* a critical body fat level of 17 to 22%.

Potential causes of menstrual dysfunction include the complex interplay of physical, nutritional, genetic, hormonal, regional fat distribution, psychologic, and environmental factors. An intense exercise bout triggers the release of an array of hormones, some of which disrupt normal reproductive function.[64,210] Intense and/or prolonged exercise that releases cortisol and other stress-related hormones also can alter ovarian function via the hypothalamic–pituitary–adrenal axis.[35,112]

Further research must determine whether regular intense exercise produces a cumulative hormonal effect or an energy deficit large enough to disrupt normal menses. Prolonged exercise does not disrupt the pulsatile release of luteinizing hormone, independent of the hormonal disturbance caused by exercise on energy and/or glucose availability.[113] Consuming well-balanced, nutritious meals prevents or reverses athletic amenorrhea without requiring the athlete to reduce exercise training volume or intensity.[111] In this regard, when injuries to young amenorrheic ballet dancers prevent them from exercising regularly, normal menstruation resumes even though body weight remains low.[80,203,218] *Proponents of this "energy deficit" explanation maintain that exercise per se exerts no deleterious effect on the reproductive system other than the potential impact of its additional energy cost on creating a negative energy balance.*[5,110,209]

The effects and risks of sustained amenorrhea on the reproductive system remain unknown. A gynecologist/endocrinologist should evaluate failure to menstruate or cessation of the normal cycle because it may reflect pituitary or thyroid gland malfunction or premature menopause.[10,109] As we point out in Chapter 2, prolonged menstrual dysfunction affects bone mass profoundly and negatively.

Delayed Onset of Menstruation and Cancer Risk

The delayed onset of menarche in chronically active young females may offer positive health benefits.[56,174] Female athletes who start training in high school or earlier show a lower lifetime occurrence of cancers of the breast and reproductive organs, and non–reproductive-system cancers than less-active counterparts. Even among older women, regular exercise protects against reproductive cancers. Swedish researchers studied the country's entire female population aged 50–74 years in 1994–1995.[135] Higher levels of occupational and leisure-time physical activity in normal-weight nonsmokers during ages 18 to 30 years related to lower postmenopausal endometrial cancer risk. Women who exercise an average of 4 hours a week after menarche reduce breast cancer risk by 50% compared with age-matched inactive women.[15] One proposed mechanism for reduced cancer risk links lower total estrogen production (or a less potent estrogen form) over the athlete's lifetime with fewer ovulatory cycles because of the delayed onset of menstruation.[105,184,204] Lower body fat levels in physically active individuals also may contribute to lowered cancer risk because peripheral fatty tissues convert androgens to estrogen.

COMMON TECHNIQUES TO ASSESS BODY COMPOSITION

Two procedures evaluate body composition:

1. Direct measurement by chemical analysis of the animal carcass or human cadaver

2. Indirect estimation by hydrostatic weighing, simple anthropometric measurements, and other clinical and laboratory procedures

Direct Assessment

Two approaches directly assess body composition. One technique dissolves the body in a chemical solution to determine its mixture of fat and fat-free components. The other physically dissects fat, fat-free adipose tissue, muscle, and bone. Considerable research has chemically assessed body composition in various animal species, but few studies have directly determined human fat content.[29,53] These labor-intensive and tedious analyses require specialized laboratory equipment and involve ethical questions and legal hurdles in obtaining cadavers for research purposes.

Direct body composition assessment suggests that while considerable individual differences exist in total body fatness, the compositions of skeletal mass and the fat-free and fat tissues remain relatively stable. Researchers have developed mathematical equations to indirectly predict the body's fat percentage on the basis of the assumed constancy of these tissues.

Indirect Assessment

Diverse indirect procedures assess body composition. One involves Archimedes' principle applied to hydrostatic weighing (also referred to as *densitometry* or *underwater weighing*). This method computes percentage body fat from body density (ratio of body mass to body volume). Other procedures predict body fat from skinfold thickness and girth measurements, x-ray, total body electrical conductivity or bioimpedance (including segmental impedance), near-infrared interactance, ultrasound, computed tomography, air plethysmography, and magnetic resonance imaging.

Hydrostatic Weighing: Archimedes' Principle

The Greek mathematician and inventor **Archimedes** (287–212 BC) discovered a fundamental principle currently applied to evaluate human body composition. An itinerant scholar of that time described the circumstances surrounding the event:

> King Hieron of Syracuse suspected that his pure gold crown had been altered by substitution of silver for gold. The King directed Archimedes to devise a method for testing the crown for its gold content without dismantling it. Archimedes pondered over this problem for many weeks without succeeding, until one day, he stepped into a bath filled to the top with water and observed the overflow. He thought about this for a moment, and then, wild with joy, jumped from the bath and ran naked through the streets of Syracuse shouting, "Eureka, Eureka! I have discovered a way to solve the mystery of the King's crown."

Archimedes reasoned that a substance such as gold must have a volume proportional to its mass; measuring the volume of an irregularly shaped object would require submersion in water with collection of the overflow. To apply his reasoning, Archimedes took lumps of gold and silver of the same mass as the crown and submerged each in a water-filled container. He discovered the crown displaced more water than the lump of gold and less than the lump of silver. This could only mean that the crown consisted of *both* silver and gold as the king suspected.

Essentially, Archimedes compared the **specific gravity** of the crown with the specific gravities for gold and silver. He probably also reasoned that an object submerged or floating in water becomes buoyed up by a counterforce that equals the weight of the volume of water it displaces. This buoyant force supports an immersed object against gravity's downward pull. Thus, an object *loses* weight in water. *Because the object's loss of weight in water equals the weight of the volume of water it displaces, its specific gravity refers to the mass of an object in air divided by its loss of weight in water.* The loss equals the weight in air minus the weight in water.

Specific gravity = Weight in air ÷ Loss of weight in water

In practical terms, suppose a crown weighed 2.27 kg in air and 0.13 kg less, or 2.14 kg, when weighed underwater (Fig. 28.9). Dividing the crown's mass (2.27 kg) by its weight loss in water (0.13 kg) yields a specific gravity of 17.5. Because this ratio differs considerably from gold's specific gravity of 19.3, we too can conclude: "Eureka, the crown is a fraud!" The physical principle Archimedes discovered allows us to use water submersion to determine the body's volume. Dividing body mass by its volume yields body density (density = mass ÷ volume), and from this, an estimate of percentage body fat.

One can think of specific gravity as an object's "heaviness" related to its volume. Objects of the same volume may vary considerably in density defined as mass per unit volume. One gram of water occupies exactly 1 cm^3 at a temperature of 39.2°F (4°C); the density equals 1 g · cm^{-3}. Water achieves its greatest density at 4°C; thus, increasing water temperature increases the volume of 1 g of water and decreases its density. One must correct the volume of an object weighed in water for water density at the weighing temperature (see Appendix A, available online at http://connection.lww.com/mkk6e). The temperature effect distinguishes density from specific gravity.

 INTEGRATIVE QUESTION

Why does a solid piece of steel or concrete sink rapidly when placed in water while a ship made of either substance readily floats?

Validity of Hydrostatic Weighing to Estimate Body Fat. Experimental evidence supports the validity of hydrostatic weighing to estimate the body's fat content. Behnke's early studies of Navy divers placed 64 subjects into two groups based on their body density. The mean difference between the groups in body mass (12.4 kg) and body volume (13.3 L) allowed Behnke to easily discern body composition differences between the groups. The ratio of the average differences (Δ mass ÷ Δ volume) equaled 0.933 g · cm^{-3}, a value within the density range of 0.92 to 0.96 g · cm^{-3} for human adipose tissue. The difference in body mass between the high- and low-density groups represented the density of adipose tissue.

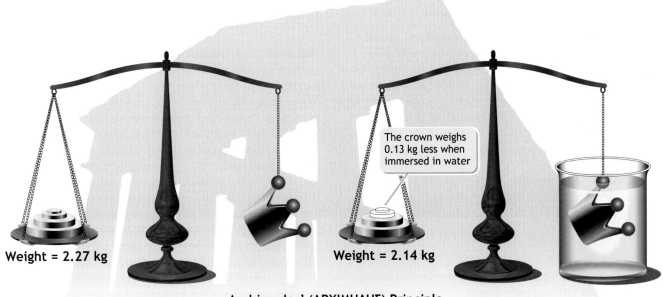

The crown weighs 0.13 kg less when immersed in water

Weight = 2.27 kg

Weight = 2.14 kg

Archimedes' (ΑΡΧΙΜΗΔΗΣ) Principle

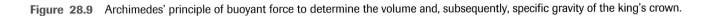

Figure 28.9 Archimedes' principle of buoyant force to determine the volume and, subsequently, specific gravity of the king's crown.

Body density for a group of heavy but lean professional football players (lean body mass 20 kg higher than the Navy divers) averaged $1.080 \ g \cdot cm^{-3}$. Behnke stated, "Here indeed was a presumptive demonstration that fat could be "separated" from bone and muscle in vivo or 'the silver from the gold' by application of a principle renowned in antiquity."[12]

The lower and upper limits of body density among humans range from $0.93 \ g \cdot cm^{-3}$ in the massively obese to nearly $1.10 \ g \cdot cm^{-3}$ in the leanest males. This coincides nicely with the 1.10 density of fat-free tissue and 0.90 for homogenized samples of fat tissue from small mammals at 37°C.

Computing Body Density.

For illustrative purposes, suppose a 50-kg person weighs 2 kg submerged in water. According to Archimedes' principle, loss of weight in water of 48 kg equals the weight of the displaced water. One can easily compute the volume of water displaced by correcting for the density of water at the weighing temperature. In this example, 48 kg of water equals 48 L, or $48,000 \ cm^3$ (1 g of water = 1 cm^3 by volume at 39.2°F [4°C]). Measuring the person at a water temperature of 39.2°F requires no density correction for water temperature. In practice, researchers use warmer water and apply the appropriate density value for water at the weighing temperature. The density of this person, computed as mass $\div$ volume, equals 50,000 g (50 kg) $\div$ 48,000 cm^3, or 1.0417 $g \cdot cm^{-3}$. The next step estimates percentage body fat and mass of the fat and fat-free tissues.

Computing Percentage Body Fat.

An equation that incorporates whole-body density estimates the body's fat percentage. The simplified equation derived by UC Berkley scientist William Siri (1919–1998) substitutes $0.90 \ g \cdot cm^{-3}$ for the density of fat and $1.10 \ g \cdot cm^{-3}$ for the density of the fat-free tissues.[169,170] The final derivation, referred to as the **Siri equation**, computes percentage body fat as:

$$\text{Percentage body fat} = (495 \div \text{body density}) - 450$$

This equation assumes the two-component model of body composition; the density of fat extracted from adipose tissue equals $0.90 \ g \cdot cm^{-3}$ and $1.10 \ g \cdot cm^{-3}$ for fat-free tissue at 37°C. The pioneer researchers in this area maintained that each of these densities remains relatively constant among individuals despite large individual variations in total fat and FFM. They also assumed that the densities of the lean tissue components of bone and muscle remained the same among individuals.

In the previous example (body mass, 50 kg and body volume, 48 L), the whole-body density of $1.0417 \ g \cdot cm^{-3}$ converted to percentage fat by the Siri equation equaled 25.2%.

$$\begin{aligned} \text{Percentage body fat} &= (495 \div 1.0417) - 450 \\ &= 25.2\% \end{aligned}$$

Several formulas other than Siri's equation also estimate percentage body fat from body density.[20,94] The basic difference among the formulas in calculating body fat generally averages less than 1% body fat units for body fat levels between 4 and 30%.

Limitations of Density Assumptions.

The generalized density values for the fat-free ($1.10 \ g \cdot cm^{-3}$) and fat ($0.90 \ g \cdot cm^{-3}$) tissue compartments represent averages for young and middle-aged adults. These "constants" vary among individuals and groups, particularly the density and chemical composition of the FFM. Such variation places some limitation in partitioning body mass into fat and fat-free components and predicting percentage body fat from whole-body density.[58] More specifically, average density of the FFM is higher for blacks and Hispanics than for whites ($1.113 \ g \cdot cm^{-3}$ blacks, $1.105 \ g \cdot cm^{-3}$ Hispanics, and $1.100 \ g \cdot cm^{-3}$ whites).[145,163,175] Racial differences also exist among adolescents.[183,216] Consequently, existing equations formulated from assumptions for whites to calculate body composition from body density in blacks or Hispanics *overestimates* FFM and *underestimates* percentage body fat. The following proposed modification of the Siri equation computes percentage body fat from body density for blacks:

$$\text{Percentage body fat} = (437.4 \div \text{body density}) - 392.8$$

Applying constant density values for the different tissues in growing children or aging adults also introduces errors in predicting body composition. For example, the water and mineral contents of the FFM continually change during the growth period including the demineralization of osteoporosis with aging. Reduced bone density makes the density of the fat-free tissue of young children and the elderly lower than the assumed $1.10 \ g \cdot cm^{-3}$ constant. This invalidates assumptions of constant densities of fat and fat-free masses in the two-compartment model and *overestimates* relative body fat calculated from densitometry. For this reason, many researchers do not convert body density to percentage body fat in children and aging adults. Others apply a multicompartment model to adjust for such factors to compute percentage body fat from body density in prepubertal children.[167,171,206] TABLE 28.3 gives equations adjusted to maturation level to predict percentage body fat from whole-body density of boys and girls ages 7 to 17.

Adjust for Large Musculoskeletal Development.

Chronic resistance training affects the density of the FFM, altering body fat estimation from whole-body density determinations.[133] White male weight lifters with considerable muscular development and nontrained controls were assessed for body density, total body water, and bone mineral content. Comparisons included estimations of percentage body fat with both the two-compartment model and a four-compartment model using the body's fat, water, mineral, and protein content and corresponding densities. Percentage body fat estimated from body density (two-compartment Siri equation) produced higher values than percentage body fat from the four-compartment model for the weight trainers but not for untrained controls. A *lower* FFM density in weight trainers than in controls (1.089 vs. $1.099 \ g \cdot cm^{-3}$) explained this discrepancy; it resulted from larger water and smaller mineral and protein fractions of the FFM in the resistance-trained men. For them, incorrect assumptions underlying the Siri equation *overestimated* percentage body fat.

TABLE 28.3 ■ PERCENTAGE BODY FAT ESTIMATED FROM BODY DENSITY (BD) USING AGE- AND GENDER-SPECIFIC CONVERSION CONSTANTS TO ACCOUNT FOR CHANGES IN THE DENSITY OF THE FAT-FREE BODY MASS AS A CHILD MATURES

AGE (YEARS)	BOYS	GIRLS
7–9	% Fat = (5.38/BD − 4.97) × 100	% Fat = (5.43/BD − 5.03) × 100
9–11	% Fat = (5.30/BD − 4.89) × 100	% Fat = (5.35/BD − 4.95) × 100
11–13	% Fat = (5.23/BD − 4.81) × 100	% Fat = (5.25/BD − 4.84) × 100
13–15	% Fat = (5.08/BD − 4.64) × 100	% Fat = (5.12/BD − 4.69) × 100
15–17	% Fat = (5.03/BD − 4.59) × 100	% Fat = (5.07/BD − 4.64) × 100

From Lohman T. Applicability of body composition techniques and constants for children and youth. Exerc Sports Sci Rev 1986;14:325.

For the weight lifters, muscularity increased disproportionately to changes in bone mass. A lower FFM density occurred because the density of their fat-free muscle (1.066 g · cm^{-3} at 37°C) was below the 1.1 g · cm^{-3} value assumed in the Siri equation. Disproportionate increases in muscle mass relative to increases in bone mass accounted for the reduced density of the FFM below 1.1 g · cm^{-3}, overpredicting percentage body fat from the two-compartment model. If resistance training does indeed progressively lower FFM density, then applying the Siri equation fails to accurately reflect true body composition changes from this training mode.

Based on revised densities of the FFM (1.089 g · cm^{-3}) and fat mass (0.9007 g · cm^{-3}), a modified equation more accurately appraises resistance-trained white males:

Percentage body fat = (521 ÷ body density) − 478

Computing Fat Mass. Using data from the example on page 790, fat mass computes by multiplying body mass by percentage body fat as follows:

Fat mass = body mass × (% fat/100)
= 50 kg × 0.252
= 12.5 kg

Further computations subdivide this person's fat mass into essential and storage fat. A female with 25.2% body fat has approximately 12% essential fat, or 6.0 kg (0.12 × 50 kg); the remaining 13.2% (6.6 kg) exists as storage fat (0.132 × 50 kg). For a male with 3% essential fat and 22.2% storage fat (based on 25.2% body fat), the corresponding values equal 1.5 kg for essential fat and 11.1 kg for storage fat. Clearly, for a man and woman with identical percentage body fat, the man rates "fatter" because storage fat represents a larger percentage of total body fat. Each gram of body fat (83% pure fat) contains approximately 7.5 kCal (7500 kCal per kg). One can compute the approximate potential energy stored in each fat depot. For storage fat in this example, the values are 49,500 kCal for the woman and 83,260 kCal for the man; for essential fat, including a female's sex-specific

fat, the values are 45,000 kCal for the woman and 11,250 kCal for the man.

Computing Fat-Free Body Mass. Compute FFM by subtracting fat mass from body mass.

Fat-free body mass = body mass − fat mass
= 50 kg − 12.5 kg
= 37.5 kg

Body Volume Measurement

The principle discovered by Archimedes applies body volume measurement in one of two ways: (1) water displacement or (2) hydrostatic weighing. Body volume requires accurate measurement because small volume variations substantially affect the density calculation and computed percentage body fat and FFM.

Water Displacement

One can measure the volume of an object submerged in water by the corresponding rise in the level of water within a container. With this technique, a finely calibrated tube secured to the side of the container that measures the rise of water permits accurate volume measurements. With this method, one must account for the volume of air remaining in the lungs during submersion. The usual protocol assesses this lung volume before the subject enters the tank and subtracts it from the total body volume determined by water displacement. **Water displacement** has proved effective in assessing arm and leg volumes and their corresponding changes with exercise training, weight gain or loss, or physical inactivity.

Hydrostatic Weighing

Hydrostatic weighing provides the most common application of Archimedes' principle to determine body volume. It computes body volume as the difference between body mass measured in air (M_a) and body weight measured during water submersion (W_w; the correct term because body mass remains unchanged under water). *Body volume equals loss of weight in water with the appropriate temperature correction for water's density.*

FIGURE 28.10 illustrates measurement of body volume by hydrostatic weighing under four different conditions. The first step in each condition accurately assesses the subject's body mass in air, usually within ±50 g. The subject, who wears a thin nylon swimsuit, sits in a lightweight, plastic tubular chair suspended from the scale and submerged beneath the water's surface. A swimming pool serves the same purpose as the tank, with the scale and chair assembly suspended from a support at the side of the pool or diving board. The tank maintains a comfortable water temperature near 95°F, similar to skin temperature. Water temperature provides the correction factor to determine water density at the weighing temperature. A diver's belt secured around the waist (or placed across the lap) stabilizes the subject from floating toward the surface during submersion. The underwater weight of this belt and chair (tare weight) is subtracted from the subject's total weight under water.

Seated with the head above water, the subject makes a forced maximal exhalation while slowly lowering the head under the water. The breath is held for 5 to 8 seconds to allow the scale pointer to stabilize before recording the reading at the midpoint of the oscillations. The subject repeats the procedure 8 to 12 times to obtain a dependable underwater weight score. Even when achieving a full exhalation, a small volume of air, the residual lung volume, remains in the lungs. Body volume calculation requires subtracting the buoyant effect of the residual lung volume measured immediately before, during, or following the underwater weighing. Failure to account for residual lung volume *underestimates* whole-body density because the lungs' air volume contributes to buoyancy. This omission creates a "fatter" person when converting body density to percentage body fat.

Variations with Menstruation. Normal fluctuations in body mass (chiefly body water) related to the menstrual cycle generally do not affect body density and body fat assessed by hydrostatic weighing. However, some females experience noticeable increases in body water (>1.0 kg) during menstru-

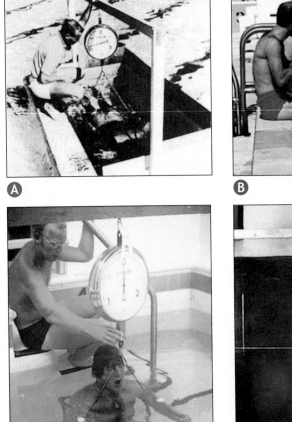

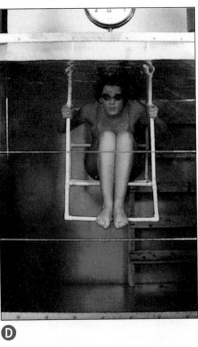

Figure 28.10 Measuring body volume by underwater weighing. Prone and supine underwater weighing methods provide the same values with residual lung volume measured before, during, or after the underwater weighing. Measurements taken (**A**) prone in a swimming pool, (**B**) seated in a swimming pool, (**C**) seated in a therapy pool, and (**D**) seated in a stainless steel tank with Plexiglas front in the laboratory. For any of the methods, subjects can use a snorkel with nose clip if they express apprehension about submersion. The final calculation of underwater weight must account for these added objects.

ation. Water retention of this magnitude affects body density and introduces a small error in computing percentage body fat.[21]

Calculating Body Composition from Body Mass, Body Volume, and Residual Lung Volume.

Data for two professional football players, an offensive guard and a quarterback, illustrate the sequence of steps in computing body density, percentage fat, fat mass, and FFM (TABLE 28.4). Mass ÷ volume is the conventional formula for computing density, with density expressed in grams per cubic centimeter ($g \cdot cm^{-3}$), mass in kilograms, and volume in liters. The difference between M_a and W_w equals body volume after applying the appropriate water temperature correction (D_w). Air remaining in the lungs and other body "spaces" (abdominal viscera, sinuses) contributes some buoyancy at the time of underwater weighing. In the extreme, consuming 800 mL of a carbonated beverage increases gastric gas volume by approximately 600 mL. This underestimates body density by hydrostatic weighing by 0.7% and overestimates percentage body fat by 11% compared with measures made before drinking the beverage.[153] In most subjects, abdominal gas and sinus air volume remain small (<100 mL) and can be ignored. *This contrasts with the relatively large and variable residual lung volume, which requires measurement and subsequent subtraction from total body volume.*

Whereas the residual lung volume decreases slightly in a person immersed in water compared with residual volume in air (from water's compressive force against the thoracic cavity), the difference exerts only a small effect on computed-percentage body fat.[73] Consequently, most laboratories measure residual lung volume in air just prior to underwater weighing.

The following formula computes body density (D_b) from underwater weighing variables:

$$D_b = mass \div volume$$

$$= M_a \div [(M_a - W_w) \div D_w] - RLV$$

For ease in computation, the following formula can be used to compute body density:

$$D_b = M_a \times D_w / (M_a - W_w - RLV \times D_w)$$

The lower part of Table 28.4 presents body composition results for the two football players based on body density.

Skinfold and Girth Measurements

In field situations, two relatively simple procedures that measure either subcutaneous fat (**skinfolds**) or circumferences (**girths**) predict body fatness with reasonable accuracy.

Subcutaneous Fat Measurement

The rationale for using skinfolds to estimate body fat comes from the interrelationships among three factors: (1) adipose tissue directly beneath the skin (subcutaneous fat), (2) internal fat, and (3) whole-body density.

The Caliper. By 1930, a pincer-type caliper accurately measured subcutaneous fat at selected anatomic sites. The three calipers shown in FIGURE 28.11 operate on a principle similar to a micrometer that measures distance between two points. Measuring skinfold thickness requires firmly grasping a fold of skin and subcutaneous fat with the thumb and forefingers, pulling it away from the underlying muscle tissue following the natural contour of the skinfold. When calibrated, the pincer jaws exert a relatively constant tension of $10 \, g \cdot mm^{-2}$ at the point of contact with the double layer of skin plus subcutaneous adipose tissue. The caliper dial indicates skinfold thickness in mm recorded within 2 seconds after applying the full force of the caliper. This time limitation avoids skinfold compression when taking the measurement. For research purposes, the investigator has considerable experience in taking measurements and demonstrates consistency in duplicating values for the same subjects on the same day, consecutive days, or weeks apart. A rule of thumb to achieve consistency requires duplicate or triplicate practice measurements on approximately 50 individuals who vary in body fat. Careful attention to detail usually ensures high measurement reproducibility.

Measurement Sites. Common anatomic sites for skinfold measurements include triceps, subscapular, suprailiac, abdominal, and upper thigh sites. The investigator should take a

TABLE 28.4 ■ MEASUREMENTS OF TWO PROFESSIONAL FOOTBALL PLAYERS FROM UNDERWATER WEIGHING			
VARIABLE	**SYMBOL**	**DEFENSIVE LINEMAN**	**RUNNING BACK**
Body mass (kg)	M_a	121.73	97.37
Net underwater weight (kg)	W_w	7.30	6.52
Water temperature correction	D_w	0.99336	0.99336
Residual lung volume (L)	RLV	1.213	1.374
Total body volume (L)	TBV	113.89	90.08
Body density ($g \cdot cm^{-3}$)	D_b	1.0688	1.0809
BODY COMPOSITION			
Relative percentage body fat (%)	%Fat	13.1	8.0
Absolute body fat (kg)	FM	15.9	7.2
Fat-free body mass (kg)	FFM	105.8	90.2

[a] Siri equation, %fat = (495/density) ÷ 450.

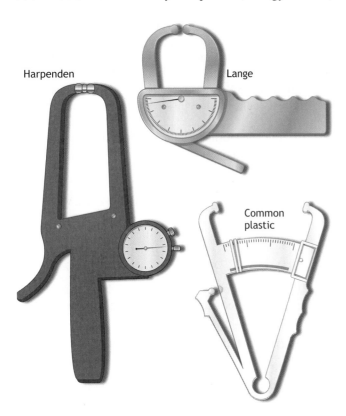

Harpenden

Lange

Common plastic

Figure 28.11 Common calipers for skinfold measurements. The Harpenden and Lange calipers provide constant tension at all jaw openings.

minimum of two or three measurements in rotational order at each site on the right side of the body with the subject standing. The average value represents the skinfold score. FIGURE 28.12 shows the anatomic location of the most frequently measured sites:

- Triceps: Vertical fold at the posterior midline of the right upper arm, halfway between the tip of the shoulder and tip of the elbow; elbow remains in an extended, relaxed position
- Subscapular: Oblique fold, just below the bottom tip of the right scapula
- Iliac (iliac crest): Slightly oblique fold, just above the right hipbone (crest of ileum); the fold follows the natural diagonal line
- Abdominal: Vertical fold 1 inch to the right of the umbilicus
- Thigh: Vertical fold at the midline of the right thigh, two thirds the distance from the middle of the patella (kneecap) to the hip

Other sites include:

- Chest (in males): Diagonal fold with long axis directed toward the right nipple; on the anterior axillary fold as high as possible
- Biceps: Vertical fold at the posterior midline of the right upper arm

Usefulness of Skinfold Scores

Skinfold measurements provide meaningful information about body fat and its distribution. We recommend two ways to use skinfolds. The first sums the skinfold scores to indicate *relative* fatness among individuals. The sum-of-skinfolds and individual values reflect either absolute or percentage body fat changes before and after an intervention program.

One can draw the following conclusions from the skinfold data in TABLE 28.5 obtained from a 22-year-old female college student before and after a 16-week aerobic exercise program:

- Largest changes in skinfold thickness occurred at the iliac and abdomen sites
- Triceps showed the largest percentage decrease and the subscapular the smallest percentage decrease
- Total reduction in subcutaneous skinfolds at the five sites was 16.6 mm or 12.6% below the "before" condition

A second use of skinfolds incorporates population-specific mathematical equations to *predict* body density or percentage body fat. The equations prove accurate for subjects similar in age, gender, training status, fatness, and race to the group from which they were derived.[18,42,142,149,191] *When meeting these criteria, predicted body fat for an individual usually ranges between 3 and 5% body fat units computed from body density with hydrostatic weighing.*

Our laboratories developed the following equations to predict percentage body fat from triceps and subscapular skinfolds in young women and men:[86–88]

Young women, ages 17 to 26 years

$$\% \text{ Body fat} = 0.55A + 0.31B + 6.13$$

Young men, ages 17 to 26 years

$$\% \text{ Body fat} = 0.43A + 0.58B + 1.47$$

In both equations, A is triceps skinfold (mm) and B is subscapular skinfold (mm).

We computed the "before" and "after" percentage body fat of the woman who participated in the 16-week physical conditioning program (Table 28.5). Percentage body fat equals 24.4% by substituting the pretraining values for triceps (22.5 mm) and subscapular (19.0 mm) skinfolds into the equation.

$$\% \text{ Body fat} = 0.55A + 0.31B + 6.13$$
$$= 0.55\,(22.5) + 0.31(19.0) + 6.13$$
$$= 12.38 + 5.89 + 6.13$$
$$= 24.4\%$$

Substituting posttraining values for triceps (19.4 mm) and subscapular (17.0 mm) skinfolds produced a body fat value of 22.1%.

$$\% \text{ Body fat} = 0.55(19.4) + 0.31(17.0) + 6.13$$
$$= 10.67 + 5.27 + 6.13$$
$$= 22.1\%$$

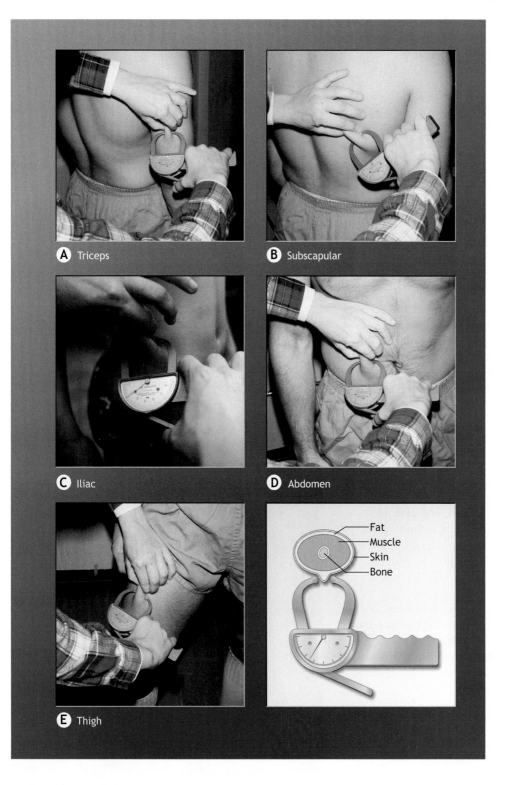

Figure 28.12 Anatomic location of five common skinfold sites: **A.** Triceps. **B.** Subscapular. **C.** Iliac. **D.** Abdomen. **E.** Thigh. Measurements taken on the right side of the body in the vertical plane except diagonally at subscapular and iliac sites.

Percentage body fat determined before and after a physical conditioning or weight-loss program provides a convenient way to evaluate alterations in body composition, independent of body weight changes.

Skinfolds and Age

In young adults, approximately one half of total fat consists of subcutaneous fat, with the remainder visceral and organ fat. With advancing age, proportionately more fat deposits in-ternally than subcutaneously. Thus, the same skinfold score reflects a *greater* total percentage of body fat as one ages. *For this reason, use age-adjusted **generalized equations** to predict body fat from skinfolds or girths in older men and women.*[76,77,154,186]

User Beware

The person taking skinfold measurements must develop expertise with the proper techniques. Also, with extremely obese people, the skinfold thickness often exceeds the width

TABLE 28.5 ■ CHANGES IN SELECTED SKINFOLDS OF A YOUNG WOMAN DURING A 16-WEEK EXERCISE PROGRAM				
SKINFOLDS (MM)	**BEFORE**	**AFTER**	**ABSOLUTE CHANGE**	**PERCENTAGE CHANGE**
Triceps	22.5	19.4	−3.1	−13.8
Subscapular	19.0	17.0	−2.0	−10.5
Suprailiac	34.5	30.2	−4.3	−12.8
Abdomen	33.7	29.4	−4.3	−12.8
Thigh	21.6	18.7	−2.9	−13.4
Sum	131.3	114.7	−16.6	−12.6

of the caliper's jaws. The particular caliper also contributes to errors of measurement.[61] It often becomes difficult to determine which sets of skinfold data provide the best comparisons because of the lack of standards for judging the results of different investigators. A prediction equation developed by one researcher (which may show high validity for the sample measured) may produce large prediction errors when another person applies the equation to skinfolds from a dissimilar group.

 INTEGRATIVE QUESTION

A friend complains that three different fitness centers determined her percentage body fat from skinfolds as follows: 25%, 29%, and 21%. How can you reconcile the differences in these values?

Measurement of Girths

Apply a linen or plastic measuring tape (not a metal tape) lightly to the skin surface so the tape remains taut but not tight. This avoids skin compression, which produces below-normal scores. Make duplicate measurements at each site and average the scores. FIGURE 28.13 shows six common anatomic landmarks for anthropometric measurement:

1. Right upper arm (biceps): Arm straight and extended in front of the body; measurement taken at midpoint between the shoulder and the elbow
2. Right forearm: Maximum girth with arm extended in front of the body
3. Abdomen: 1 inch above the umbilicus
4. Buttocks: Maximum protrusion with heels together
5. Right thigh: Upper thigh, just below the buttocks
6. Right calf: Widest girth midway between ankle and knee

Prediction equations based on girths exist for each gender and different age groups.[86,130,187] The equations for these subgroups show considerable population specificity. They do not apply to individuals who (1) appear overly thin or exces-

sively fat, (2) train regularly in strenuous endurance sports or activities with a substantial resistance-training component, and (3) differ in race from the specific group used to derive the original equations.[18,87,142]

Usefulness of Girth Scores

Girths prove most useful in ranking individuals within a group according to relative fatness. As with skinfolds, girth-based equations predict body density and/or percentage body fat. The equations and constants presented at http://connection.lww.com/mkk6e for young and older men and women predict body fat to within ± 2.5 to 4.0% body fat units of the actual value. The prediction error depends on whether the individual portrays physical characteristics similar to the original validation group. Such relatively small errors make girth predictions particularly useful in nonlaboratory settings. Specific equations based on girths also accurately estimate body composition of obese adult men and women.[186,205] Along with predicting percentage body fat, girths can analyze patterns of body fat distribution, including changes in fat pat-

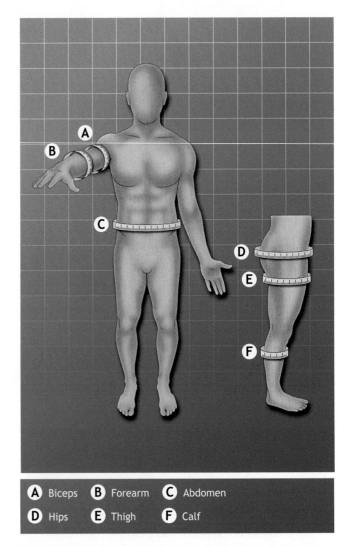

Ⓐ Biceps   **Ⓑ** Forearm   **Ⓒ** Abdomen
Ⓓ Hips   **Ⓔ** Thigh   **Ⓕ** Calf

Figure 28.13 Landmarks for measuring various girths at six common anatomic sites (see text for a description of each site).

terning during weight loss.[65,199] Not surprisingly, those equations that use the more labile sites of fat deposition (e.g., waist and hips instead of upper arm or thigh in females and abdomen in males) provide the greatest accuracy to predict *changes* in body composition.[54,84]

Body Fat Predictions from Girths

From the appropriate tables in "Body Composition," on the LWW connection website, substitute the corresponding constants *A, B,* and *C* in the formula shown at the bottom of each table. This requires one addition and two subtraction steps. The following five-step example shows how to compute percentage fat, fat mass, and FFM for a 21-year-old man who weighs 79.1 kg:

Step 1. Measure upper arm, abdomen, and right forearm girths with a cloth tape to the nearest 0.25 in (0.6 cm): upper arm = 11.5 in (29.21 cm); abdomen = 31.0 in (78.74 cm); right forearm = 10.75 in (27.30 cm)

Step 2. Determine the three constants *A, B,* and *C* corresponding to the three girths from the table: *A,* corresponding to 11.5 in = 42.56; *B,* corresponding to 31.0 in = 40.68; and *C,* corresponding to 10.75 in = 58.37.

Step 3. Compute percentage body fat by substituting the constants from step 2 in the formula for young men as follows:

$$Percentage\ fat = A + B - C - 10.2$$
$$= 42.56 + 40.68 - 58.37 - 10.2$$
$$= 83.24 - 58.37 - 10.2$$
$$= 24.87 - 10.2$$
$$= 14.7\%$$

Step 4. Determine fat mass

$$Fat\ mass = Body\ mass \times (\%fat \div 100)$$
$$= 79.1\ kg \times (14.7 \div 100)$$
$$= 79.1\ kg \times 0.147$$
$$= 11.6\ kg$$

Step 5. Determine FFM

$$FFM = Body\ mass - fat\ mass$$
$$= 79.1\ kg - 11.6\ kg$$
$$= 67.5\ kg$$

Bioelectrical Impedance Analysis

There are two modes of **bioelectrical impedance analysis (BIA)**. In single low-frequency BIA, a small alternating current flowing between two electrodes passes more rapidly through hydrated fat-free body tissues and extracellular water than through fat or bone tissues because of the greater electrolyte content (lower electrical resistance) of the fat-free component. In essence, the body's water content conducts the flow of electrical charges, so when current flows through the fluid, sensitive instrumentation can detect the water's impedance. Impedance to electric current flow, calculated by measuring current and voltage, is based on Ohm's law (R = V/I, where R = resistance, V = volume, and I = current). These relationships can quantify the volume of water within the body, and from this, percentage body fat and FFM.

Multifrequency BIA sends electric current at multiple frequencies (e.g., 5, 50, 250 kHz) to detect minute changes in the body's fluid compartments. When the body is considered a series of cylinders (e.g., trunk and right and left arm and leg), the 8-electrode system (two detector electrodes placed on each of the paired limbs) establishes the impedance of those segments separately to quantify total body water. Intracellular water is assessed by higher frequency currents (>200 mHz), and extracellular water compartments are measured by currents at 50 kHz or less. It also is possible to partition the body into segments to allow more accurate determination of tissue composition, as for example in pregnancy and aging and gastric abnormalities, edema, and other disease conditions.

FIGURE 28.14A and B shows an example for single-frequency BIA. A person lies on a flat, nonconducting surface with injector (source) electrodes attached on the dorsal surfaces of the foot and wrist and detector (sink) electrodes attached between the radius and ulna (styloid process) and at the ankle between the medial and lateral malleoli. A painless, localized electrical current (approximately 800 μA at a frequency of 50 kHz) is introduced, and the impedance (resistance) to current flow between the source and detector electrodes determined. Conversion of the impedance value to body density—adding body mass and stature; gender, age, and sometimes race; level of fatness; and several girths to the equation—computes percentage body fat from the Siri equation or other density conversion equations. Body composition prediction with such a system depends on the additional input data as part of the BIA equation. Thus, any unreliability of data input produces different output results. This becomes more pronounced for individuals at the extremes of body composition. For example, a difference of only 5 mm in a girth measurement or difference of 1.5 cm in "true" stature from measurement to measurement can produce up to a 2% change in an output variable—unrelated to any real change in a computed body composition variable such as fat mass or FFM. Figure 28.14C illustrates the segmental measurement approach including electrode configuration and how current (I) and voltage (V) are assessed for the right arm, trunk, and right leg.

Influence of Hydration Level and Ambient Temperature

Hydration level affects the accuracy of BIA and may give incorrect information about an individual's body fat content.[99,144,162] Hypohydration and hyperhydration alter the body's normal electrolyte concentrations; this in turn affects

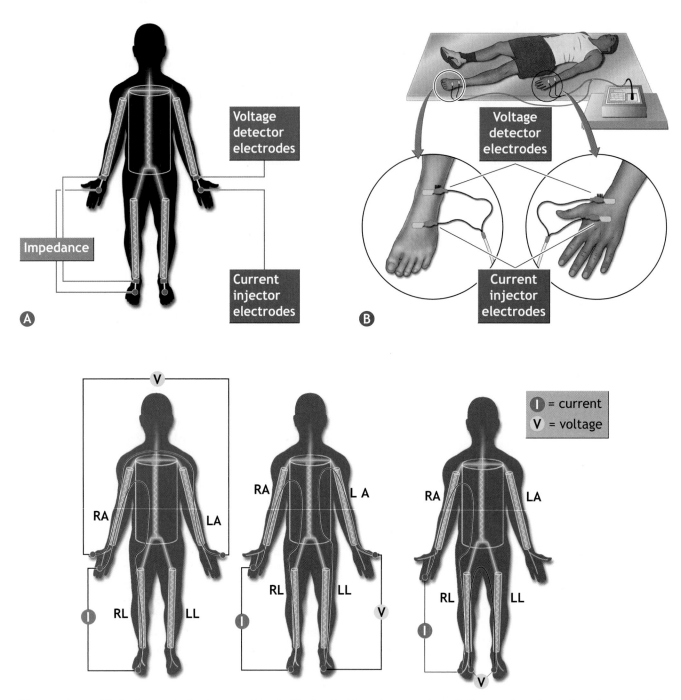

Figure 28.14 Method to assess body composition by bioelectrical impedance analysis. **A.** Four-surface electrode technique (whole-body impedance) applies current via one pair of distal (injector) electrodes, while the proximal (detector) electrode pair measures electrical potential across the conducting segment. **B.** Standard placement of electrodes and body position during whole-body impedance measurement. **C.** Segmental measurement illustrating assessment of current *(I)* and voltage *(V)* for the right arm, trunk, and right leg. The following references provide examples of the use of multifrequency BIA in humans and animals:

Bartok C, et al. The effect of dehydration on wrestling minimum weight assessment. Med Sci Sports Exerc 2004;36:160.

Buchholz AC, et al. The validity of bioelectrical impedance models in clinical populations. Nutr Clin Pract 2004;19:433.

Fielding CL, et al. Use of multifrequency bioelectrical impedance analysis for estimation of total body water and extracellular and intracellular fluid volumes in horses. Am J Vet Res 2004;65:320.

Fors H, et al. Body composition, as assessed by bioelectrical impedance spectroscopy and dual-energy x-ray absorptiometry, in a healthy paediatric population. Acta Paediatr 2002;91:755.

Kyle UG, et al. Bioelectrical impedance analysis—Part I: Review of principles and methods. Clin Nutr 2004;23:1226.

Mika C, et al. Improvement of nutritional status as assessed by multifrequency BIA during 15 weeks of refeeding in adolescent girls with anorexia nervosa. J Nutr 2004;134:3026.

current flow independent of real body composition changes. For example, voluntary fluid restriction decreases the impedance measure. This lowers the percentage body fat estimate; hyperhydration produces the opposite effect (higher body fat estimate).

Skin temperature, influenced by ambient conditions, also affects whole-body resistance and BIA prediction of body fat. Predicted body fat is lower in a warm environment (moist skin produces less impedance to electrical flow) than in a cold one.

Even with normal hydration and environmental temperature, body fat predictions with BIA prove less satisfactory than with hydrostatic weighing. BIA tends to overpredict body fat in lean and athletic subjects and underpredict body fat in obese subjects.[114,164] BIA often predicts body fat less accurately than do girths and skinfolds.[19,41,90,176] Whether BIA detects small changes in body composition during weight loss remains unclear.[102,141,151,161] Conventional BIA technology cannot determine regional fat distribution.

At best, BIA represents a noninvasive, safe, relatively easy, and reliable means to assess total body water. The technique requires that experienced personnel make measurements under standardized conditions. Particularly important are electrode placement and the subject's body position, hydration status, plasma osmolality and sodium concentration, skin temperature, recent physical activity, and previous food and beverage intake.[16,101,202] For example, ingestion of consecutive meals progressively decreases bioelectrical impedance (possibly the combined effect of increased electrolytes and a redistribution of extracellular fluid), which decreases computed percentage body fat.[168] Body fatness and racial characteristics also influence BIA's predictive accuracy.[3,146,178,200,216] The tendency to overestimate percentage body fat increases among black athletes[70,164] and lean subjects.[179] Fatness-specific BIA equations exist that predict body fat for obese and nonobese American Indian, Hispanic, and white men and women.[176] With proper measurement standardization, the menstrual cycle does not affect body composition assessment by BIA.[124]

Applicability of BIA in Sports and Exercise Training

Coaches and athletes require a safe, easily administered, and valid tool to assess body composition and detect changes with caloric restriction or exercise training. A major limitation in achieving these goals concerns BIA's lack of sensitivity to detect small body-compositional changes, particularly without appropriate control over factors that affect measurement accuracy and reliability.[141,164] For example, sweat-loss dehydration from prior exercise or reduced glycogen reserves (and associated loss of glycogen-bound water) from an intense training session reduces body resistance (impedance) to electrical current flow. This overestimates FFM and underestimates percentage body fat. Research with adequate sample sizes also must establish validity and reliability for BIA among female athletes.

Chapter 29 ("In a Practical Sense") includes BIA equations (in addition to equations using skinfolds and girths) to

estimate body density and percentage body fat for athletes in general and athletes in specific sports. Without sport-specific equations, population-based generalized equations that account for age and gender usually provide an acceptable alternative to estimate body fat.[28,76,166,182]

Near-Infrared Interactance

Near-infrared interactance (**NIR**) applies technology developed by the U.S. Department of Agriculture to assess body composition of livestock and the lipid content of various grains. The commercial versions to assess human body composition use principles of light absorption and reflection. A fiber optic probe or light wand emits a low-energy beam of near-infrared light into the single measuring site at the anterior midline surface of the dominant biceps. A detector within the same probe measures the intensity of the reemitted light, expressed as optical density. Shifts in wavelength of the reflected beam as it interacts with organic material in the arm inserted into the manufacturer's prediction equation (including adjustments for subject's body mass and stature, estimated frame size, gender, and physical activity level) computes percentage body fat and FFM. The safe, portable, lightweight equipment requires minimal training to use and necessitates little physical contact with the subject during measurement. These test administration aspects make NIR popular for body composition assessment in health clubs, hospitals, and weight-loss centers. The important question about the usefulness of NIR concerns its validity.

Questionable Validity

Early research indicated a relationship between spectrophotometric measures of light interactance at various body sites and body composition assessed by total body water.[36] Subsequent studies with humans has not confirmed NIR's validity versus hydrostatic weighing and skinfold measurements. NIR does *not* accurately predict body fat across a broad range of body fat levels; it often provides less accuracy than skinfolds.[19,28,69,177,193] It overestimates body fat in lean men and women and underestimates it in fatter subjects.[125] FIGURE 28.15 shows the inadequacy of NIR compared with skinfold measurements to predict body fat compared to hydrostatic weighing. In more than 47% of the subjects, an error greater than 4% body fat units occurred with NIR, with the largest errors at the extremes of body fatness. NIR produced large errors when estimating body fat for children[26] and youth wrestlers,[72] and underestimated body fat in collegiate football players.[71] NIR did not accurately assess body composition changes from resistance training.[19] *At this time, research does not support NIR as a robust, valid method to assess human body composition.*

Ultrasound Assessment of Fat

Ultrasound technology can assess the thickness of different tissues (fat and muscle) and image the deeper tissues such as a muscle's cross-sectional area. The method converts

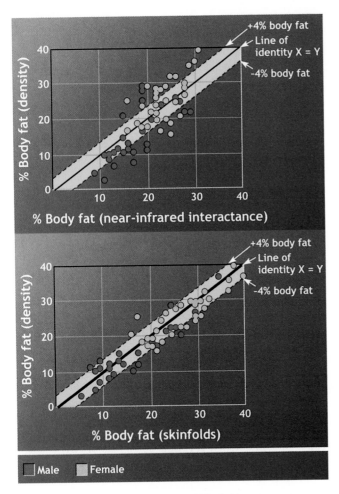

Figure 28.15 Comparison of near-infrared interactance (Futrex-5000) *(top)* and skinfolds *(bottom)* for assessing percentage body fat. *Shaded area* around line incorporates ±4% body fat units. (From McLean K, Skinner JS. Validity of Futrex-5000 for body composition determination. Med Sci Sports Exerc 1992;24:253.)

electrical energy through a probe into high-frequency (pulsed) sound waves that penetrate the skin surface into the underlying tissues. The sound waves pass through adipose tissue to penetrate the muscle layer. They then reflect from the fat–muscle interface (after reflection from a bony surface) to produce an echo, which returns to a receiver within the probe. The simplest type of ultrasound (A-mode) does not produce an image of the underlying tissues. Rather, the time required for sound wave transmission through the tissues and back to the transducer converts to a distance score that indicates fat or muscle thickness. With the more expensive and technically demanding B-mode ultrasound, a two-dimensional image provides considerable detail and tissue differentiation.

Ultrasound exhibits high reliability for repeat measurements of subcutaneous fat thickness at multiple sites in the lying and standing positions on the same day and different days.[75,82] The technique can determine total and segmental subcutaneous adipose tissue volume.[2] It proves particularly useful with obese persons who show considerable variation and compression of subcutaneous body fat with skinfold

measures. When used to map muscle and fat thickness at different body regions and quantify changes in topographic fat patterns, ultrasound serves as a valuable adjunct to body composition assessment. In hospitalized patients, ultrasonic fat and muscle thickness determinations aid in nutritional assessment during weight loss and weight gain. Ultrasonic imaging also serves a clinical role in assessing tissue growth and development, including fetal development and structure and function of the heart and other organs. With imaging devices, reflected sound waves from the soft tissues convert to a real-time image for convenient visualization or for computer digitization (area, volume, and diameter) directly from the image. Color and multiple-frequency imaging allows clinicians to trace blood flow through organs and tissues or, with the use of miniaturized probes, identify internal tissues, vessels, and organs. In consumer-oriented research, ultrasonic imaging of thigh fat depth provided evidence that treatments using two topical cream applications to the thighs and buttocks to reduce "cellulite" (dimpled fat) failed to reduce local fat thickness compared with control conditions.[34]

Arm X-Ray Assessment of Fat

X-ray technology can analyze regional body fat deposition. The thickness of fat layers at points *A, B,* and *C* in FIGURE 28.16 transforms the fat widths into a body fat value. Fat thickness from the roentgenogram substitutes for skinfold scores in the body fat prediction equation. Comparing percentage body fat from roentgenograms with body fat by hydrostatic weighing established the validity of the x-ray procedure.[83] For an individual, conversion of the x-ray widths of fat to total body fat percentage generally falls within ±3% units of body fat determined by underwater weighing, an accuracy similar to skinfolds or girths. The x-ray procedure also includes assessment of muscle size; the method contributes useful information to study body composition with training, aging, and changes in body mass.[38,84]

Computed Tomography, Magnetic Resonance Imaging, and Dual-Energy X-Ray Absorptiometry

Computed Tomography

Computed tomography (CT) generates detailed cross-sectional, two-dimensional radiographic images of body segments when an x-ray beam (ionizing radiation) passes through tissues of different densities. The CT scan produces pictorial and quantitative information about total tissue area, total fat and muscle area, and thickness and volume of tissues within an organ.[60,132,198]

FIGURE 28.17A–C shows CT scans of the upper legs and a cross section at the midthigh of a professional walker who walked 11,200 miles through the 50 United States in 50 weeks. Total cross section and muscle cross section increased and subcutaneous fat decreased correspondingly in the midthigh region in the "after" scans (not shown). Studies have demonstrated the efficacy of CT scans to establish the rela-

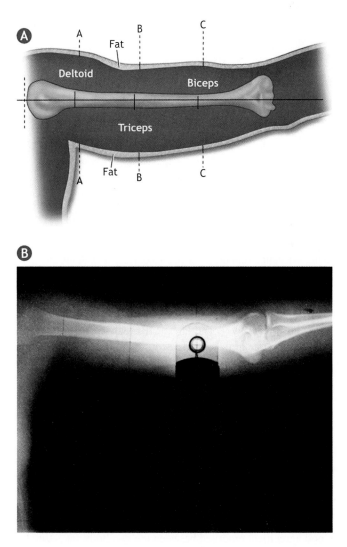

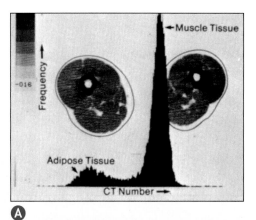

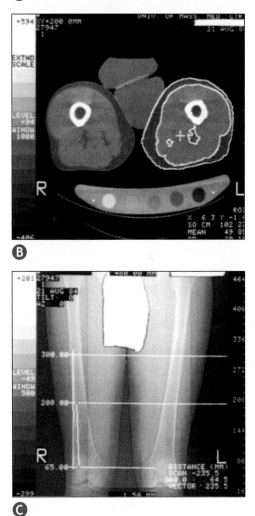

Figure 28.16 A. Schematic diagram of an arm radiograph of a 24-year-old female. *Vertical lines* perpendicular to the long axis of the humerus at points *A, B,* and *C* represent the six fat widths. Total body fat computed from the radiograph equaled 23.6%; body fat by underwater weighing equaled 23.3%. **B.** Technician uses a digitizer to calculate fat width on the radiograph. A clear demarcation between fat, muscle, and bone appears on the radiograph, which permits accurate assessment of radiographic widths. A computer processes the information from the digitizer and transmits it to a printer and graphics plotter. (Line art and photo courtesy of Dr. A. R. Behnke.)

Figure 28.17 CT scans. **A.** Plot of pixel elements (CT scan) illustrating the extent of adipose and muscle tissue in a cross section of the thigh. The two other views show (**B**) a cross section of the midthigh and (**C**) an anterior view of the upper legs prior to a 1-year walk across the United States by a champion walker. (CT scans courtesy of Dr. Steven Heymsfield, Obesity Research Center, St. Luke's-Roosevelt Hospital, Columbia University, College of Physicians and Surgeons, New York, NY.)

tionship between simple anthropometric measures (skinfolds and girths) at the abdomen and total abdominal fat volume measured from single or multiple pictorial "slices" through this region.[165] The single cut through the L4–L5 region minimizes radiation dose and provides the best view of visceral and subcutaneous fat. FIGURE 28.18 illustrates the high association between waist girth and deep **visceral adipose tissue** (**VAT**) area; men with larger waist girth also possessed greater VAT. The relationship exceeded the association between subcutaneous fat thickness (skinfolds) and VAT. An increased amount of deep abdominal adipose tissue relates to increased risk for type 2 diabetes, blood lipid profile disorders, hyper-

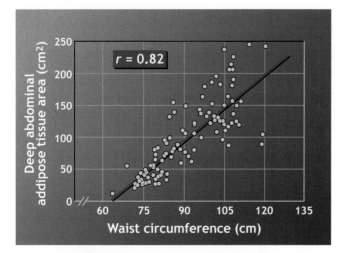

Figure 28.18   Relationship between deep visceral adipose tissue (VAT) determined by CT scanning and waist girth in 110 men, ages 18 to 42 years, who varied considerably in percentage body fat by densitometry ($\overline{X}$ = 22.9%; range, 2.2–39.9%). The best predictors of VAT included *(a)* abdominal skinfold thickness in mm, *(b)* waist girth in cm, and *(c)* waist:hip ratio. VAT (cm²) = −363.12 + (−1.113*a*) + 3.478*b* + 186.7*c*. For example, if abdominal skinfold is 23.0 mm, waist girth is 92.0 cm, and waist:hip ratio is 0.929, then by substitution in the equation, VAT = 104.7 cm². (Modified from Dépres J-P, et al. Estimation of deep abdominal adipose-tissue accumulation from simple anthropometric measurements in men. Am J Clin Nutr 1991;54:471.)

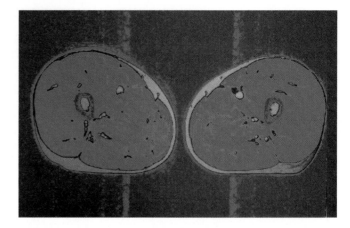

Figure 28.19   MRI scans of the midthigh of a 30-year-old male middle-distance runner. (MRI scans courtesy of J. Staab, Department of the Army, USARIEM, Natick, MA.)

tension, including the metabolic syndrome and cardiovascular disease. Chapter 30 discusses health risks from the deep type of abdominal obesity.

Magnetic Resonance Imaging

Magnetic resonance imaging (MRI), originally discovered by medical doctor and research scientist R. V. Damadian (1936–) in 1971, patented in 1974, and first constructed in 1977, provides an invaluable, noninvasive assessment of the body's tissue compartments.[1,81,104,132,180,208] FIGURE 28.19 shows a color-enhanced MRI transaxial image of the midthigh of a 30-year-old male middle-distance runner. Computer software subtracts fat and bony tissues *(lighter-colored areas)* to compute thigh muscle cross-sectional area *(red area)*. With MRI, electromagnetic radiation (not ionizing radiation as in CT scans) in a strong magnetic field excites the hydrogen nuclei of the body's water and lipid molecules. The nuclei then project a detectable signal that rearranges under computer control to visually represent the various body tissues. MRI can quantify total and subcutaneous adipose tissue in individuals of varying body fatness. Combined with muscle mass analysis, MRI assesses changes in a muscle's lean and fat components following resistance training, changes in muscle volume in and out of training, or during different stages of growth and aging.[79,185] MRI analysis has assessed postflight changes in muscle volume after a 17-day space mission and 16- to 28-week duration shuttle/MIR missions.[103] MRI has wide acceptance for diagnosis in almost all fields of medicine and related disciplines, including

muscular dystrophy.[59] The latest MRI technologies allow imaging of pacemakers with fiber optic leads rather than wire leads, MRI compatible defibrillators, and FONAR stand-up MRI that scans patients in numerous weight-bearing positions—standing, sitting, in flexion and extension, and the conventional lie-down position (http://www.invent.org/hall_of_fame/36.html; http://www.fonar.com/).

FIGURE 28.20 *(top)* shows a plot of percentage body fat determined by MRI scanning of 30 transaxial images along the length of the body and underwater weighing of 20 Swedish women, ages 23 to 40 years. Total fat from scans of the calves, thighs, lower- and upper-trunk, and lower- and upper-arms provided the basis for computing MRI percentage body fat. Good agreement emerged between the two body fat estimates ($r = 0.84$). Similar validity emerged between MRI-determined total body fat and hydrostatic weighing and total body water estimates of body fat.[126]

The *bottom of* Figure 28.20 shows the distribution of total adipose tissue, subcutaneous adipose tissue, and nonsubcutaneous adipose tissue measures from different body regions. The *bar graphs* show the smallest to the largest adipose tissue depots. Of all body regions, adipose tissue in the lower trunk (both subcutaneous and nonsubcutaneous) contained the greatest percentage of total body fat (38.5%); the lower arm region included 2.7%, the smallest amount. The *pie chart* at the *lower right* of the figure shows the relative amounts of adipose tissue in each body compartment in relation to the MRI-determined total volume of body fat. Subcutaneous fat accounted for 75.2% of the total 21.8 L of body fat. Nonsubcutaneous fat accounts for the remaining 24.8%, making it reasonable to conclude that "excess" fat deposits to the greatest extent in the subcutaneous tissues.

Comparison of Lean and Obese.   Seventeen MRI-derived tissue slices from groups of lean and obese females provided comparative data for total fat and VAT volume at four anatomic sites between the top of the patella and sternal notch. Body fat determined by densitometry for the light women

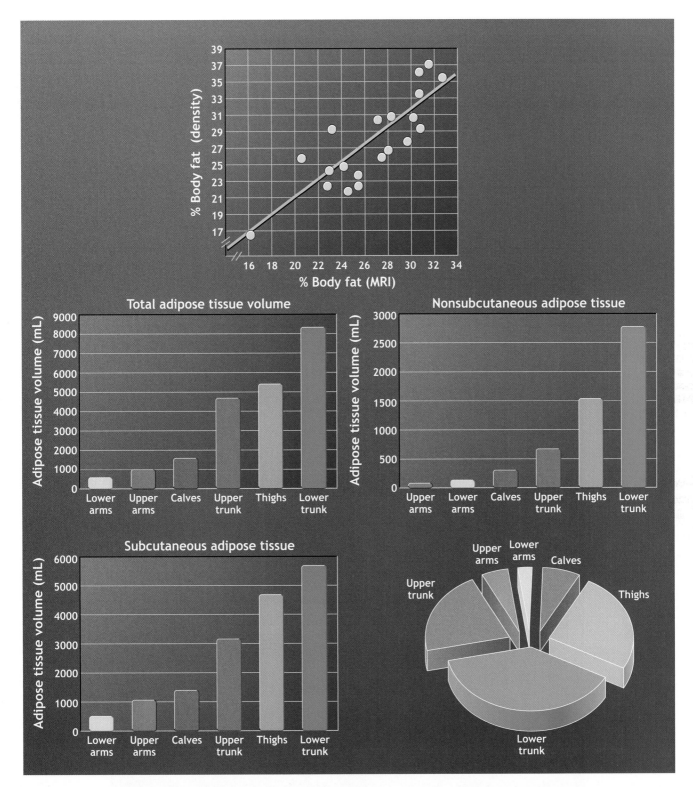

Figure 28.20 *Top.* Percentage body fat determined by hydrostatic weighing (density) and MRI scanning (graph created from individual data points presented in the original article). *Bottom bar graphs.* Distribution of adipose tissue (total, subcutaneous, and nonsubcutaneous) within the various body compartments; arrangement progresses from smallest to largest. The *right pie chart* displays the relative distribution of adipose tissue in different body regions. (Modified from Sohlstrom A, et al. Adipose tissue distribution as assessed by magnetic resonance imaging and total body fat by magnetic resonance imaging, underwater weighing, and body-water dilution in healthy women. Am J Clin Nutr 1993;58:830.)

(BMI, 20.6) averaged 25.4%; the heavy women's BMI averaged 42.4 with about 42% body fat. The three graphs in FIGURE 28.21 display differences between the relatively light and heavy groups in total body tissue (sum of fat and nonfat tissues), total adipose tissue, and subcutaneous adipose tissue at the 17 sites. The results show a fairly consistent pattern in MRI-derived adipose tissue volumes. The overfat subjects possessed 165% more subcutaneous adipose tissue and 155% more total adipose tissue. Abdominal and upper-thigh regions showed the largest fat accretion. Interestingly, the light women had a greater amount of nonfat tissue (not shown) at the upper-thorax and lower-thigh regions. The *inset graph* shows the strong relationship between MRI-determined percentage of body adipose tissue (4 instead of 17 sites) and

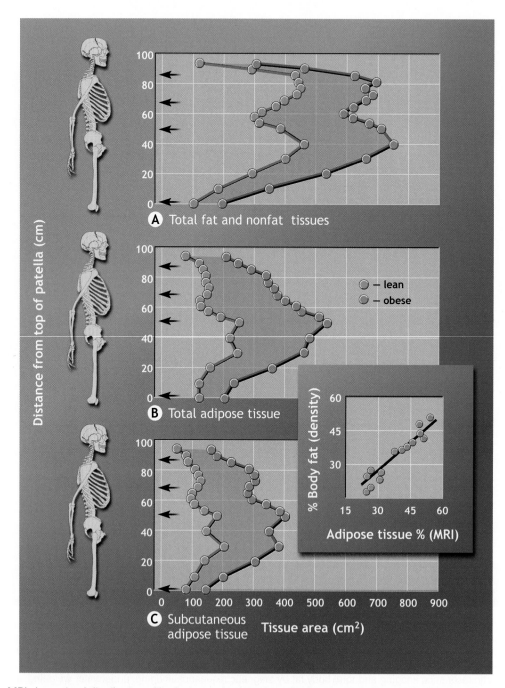

Figure 28.21   MRI-determined distribution of body tissues in seven lean *(red)* and seven obese *(blue)* females. **A.** Total body tissues (sum of fat and nonfat tissues). **B.** Total adipose tissue. **C.** Subcutaneous adipose tissue. *Arrows to the right of the* y *axis* indicate the four anatomic markers in relation to position on the skeleton. The *inset graph* displays the relationship between percentage body adipose tissue (using 4 instead of 17 MRI sites) and percentage body fat determined by hydrostatic weighing in obese and lean subjects. (Modified from Fowler PA, et al. Total and subcutaneous adipose tissue in women: the measurement of distribution and accurate prediction of quantity by using magnetic resonance imaging. Am J Clin Nutr 1991;54:18.)

percentage body fat determined by densitometry. MRI yields a wealth of useful information for accurately assessing total and regional body composition.

Exercise Training. MRI and dual-energy x-ray absorptiometry (DXA, discussed in the next section) assessed changes in regional (trunk and extremities) and whole-body fat mass, lean body mass, and bone mineral content at 3 and 6 months of periodized resistance training in 31 women.[143] MRI measured changes in thigh muscle morphology in a subset of 11 women exercisers. The women decreased fat mass by 10% and body mass and soft tissue lean mass by 2.2%, but bone mineral content did not change compared with non-training groups of men and women. Soft tissue lean mass was distributed less in women's arms than in men's both before and after training. The most striking training-induced differences occurred in the tissue composition of the women's arms (31% loss in fat mass without change in lean mass) compared with the legs (5.5% gain in lean mass without change in fat mass). Fat decreased in the trunk by 12% without change in soft tissue lean mass. The changes for fat mass by MRI and DXA showed close relationships ($r = 0.72–0.92$). Both techniques also similarly assessed increases in lean leg tissue mass. This experiment reinforced the importance of apprising changes in regional tissue morphology (including total body changes) with an experimental treatment—in this case the effects of periodized resistance training.

Dual-Energy X-Ray Absorptiometry

Dual-energy x-ray absorptiometry (DXA) reliably and accurately quantifies fat and nonbone regional lean body mass, including the mineral content of the body's deeper bony structures.[93,96,97,108,147,155,158,208] It has become the accepted clinical tool to assess spinal osteoporosis and related bone disorders.[43,152] When used for body composition assessment, DXA does not require assumptions concerning the biologic constancy of the fat and fat-free components inherent with hydrostatic weighing.

With DXA, two distinct low-energy x-ray beams (short exposure with low radiation dosage) penetrate bone and soft tissue areas to a depth of approximately 30 cm. The subject lies supine on a table so that the source and detector probes slowly pass across the body over a 12-minute period. Computer software reconstructs the attenuated x-ray beams to produce an image of the underlying tissues and quantify bone mineral content, total fat mass, and FFM. Analysis can include selected trunk and limb regions for detailed study of tissue composition and relation to disease risk, including the effects of exercise training and detraining.[14,106,116,212]

DXA shows excellent agreement with other independent estimates of bone mineral content.[152] Strong relationships also exist between DXA-determined total body fat and body fat by either densitometry,[67,120] segmental body composition (upper- and lower-extremity mass), total body potassium, or total body nitrogen[121] and abdominal adiposity.[58] Recent studies have focused on body fat estimation by DXA with other meth-

ods in young children,[40] prepubertal children,[25,74,173] younger and older men[8] and women,[7,134] the elderly,[62,172] and changes during intense resistance training.[192] FIGURE 28.22 shows the strong association between percentage body fat estimates by DXA and hydrostatic weighing over a broad age range in men and women. The strength of the prediction decreases for older and fatter subjects but remains within the typical range for comparisons among discrete methodologies. Using a more robust model of body composition assessment, the error is less than 2% body fat units between DXA and densitometry in the heterogeneous age group of adults shown in the figure.[68]

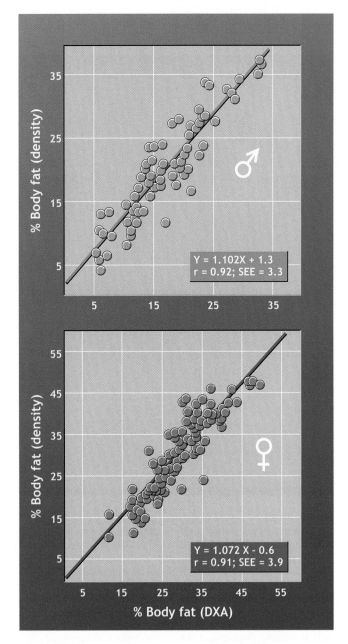

Figure 28.22 Comparison of total body fat determined by hydrostatic weighing and DXA in men *(top)* and women *(bottom)*. (Modified from Snead DB, et al. Age-related differences in body composition by hydrodensitometry and dual-energy absorptiometry. J Appl Physiol 1993;74:770.)

DXA and Body Composition in Anorectic Women.

DXA has evaluated the skeletal and regional body composition characteristics in anorexia nervosa.[156] In one study, body mass averaged 44.4 kg (97.9 lb) for 10 anorectic women. FIGURE 28.23 shows an anorectic female *(left two images)* and a typical female whose body fat percentage averaged 25% of her 56.7-kg (125-lb) body mass. Although lean body mass of the anorectic women approached the normal average of 43.0 kg, body fat equaled only 7.5%, a value more than three times less than comparison groups of typical young women. All of the women had been anorectic for at least 1 year, and the duration of amenorrhea averaged 3.1 years (range, 1–8 y). The *inset table* compares regional bone mineral densities (BMD, $g \cdot cm^{-2}$) in the anorectic females with a group of 287 normal-fat females aged 20 to 40 years. The values in the *right column* represent the percentage for BMD of the anorectic group relative to the comparison group. Total body BMD averaged 10% lower, the L2–L4 region of the lumbar spine averaged 27% less, and the femoral neck BMD fell 13% below that of the normals. Spine BMD in the anorectic women reached the identical average for 70-year-old women. Diminished BMD in anorexia nervosa, in addition to reducing skeletal size, may make these young women particularly vulnerable to osteoporotic fractures at a relatively young age.

BOD POD as a Criterion Method?

A procedure has been perfected to assess body volume and its changes for groups that range from infants to the elderly to collegiate wrestlers and exceptionally large athletes like American professional football and basketball players.[51,123,159,189,217] The method has adapted helium displacement plethysmography first reported in the late 1800s. The subject sits inside a small chamber marketed commercially as **BOD POD** (Fig. 28.24A; Life Measurement Instruments, Concord, CA). Measurement requires only 3 to 5 minutes, with high reproducibility of test scores ($r > 0.90$) within and across days. After being weighed to the nearest ±5 g on an electronic scale *(bottom left* of BOD POD illustration), the subject sits comfortably in the 750-L volume, dual-chamber fiberglass shell. The molded front seat separates the unit into front and rear chambers. The electronics, housed in the rear chamber, contain the pressure transducers, breathing circuit, and air circulation system.

The BOD POD determines body volume by measuring the initial volume of the empty chamber and then the volume with the person inside. To ensure measurement reliability and accuracy, the person wears a tight-fitting swimsuit.[49,195] Body volume represents the initial volume minus the reduced chamber volume with the subject inside. The subject breathes several breaths into an air circuit to assess pulmonary gas volume, which when subtracted from measured body volume yields body volume. Body density computes as body mass (measured in air) ÷ body volume (measured in BOD POD, including a correction for a small negative volume caused by isothermal effects related to skin surface area). The Siri equation converts body density to percentage body fat.

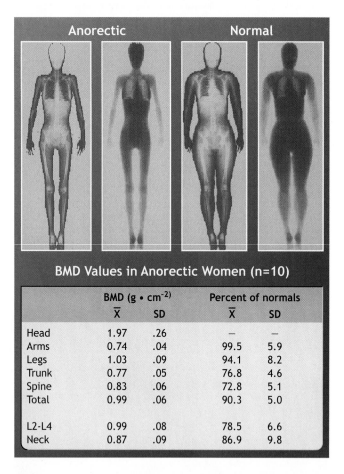

Anorectic   **Normal**

BMD Values in Anorectic Women (n=10)

	BMD ($g \cdot cm^{-2}$)		Percent of normals	
	$\overline{X}$	SD	$\overline{X}$	SD
Head	1.97	.26	—	—
Arms	0.74	.04	99.5	5.9
Legs	1.03	.09	94.1	8.2
Trunk	0.77	.05	76.8	4.6
Spine	0.83	.06	72.8	5.1
Total	0.99	.06	90.3	5.0
L2-L4	0.99	.08	78.5	6.6
Neck	0.87	.09	86.9	9.8

Figure 28.23 Example of an anorectic female *(left)* and a typical female *(right)* whose body fat percentage averaged 25% with a body mass of 56.7 kg (125 lb). The average anorectic subject weighed 44.4 kg (97.9 lb) with 7.5% body fat estimated by DXA. The *inset table* compares regional bone mineral densities (BMD) in the anorectic females with those of a group of 287 females aged 20 to 40 years with average body fat. The values in the *right columns* represent the percentage for BMD of the anorectic group relative to the comparison group. (Photo courtesy of R. B. Mazess, Department of Medical Physics, University of Wisconsin, Madison, WI, and the Lunar Radiation Corporation, Madison, WI. Data from Mazess RB, et al. Skeletal and body composition effects of anorexia nervosa. Paper presented at the international symposium on in vivo body composition studies. June 20–23, Toronto, Ontario, Canada, 1989.)

Some Discrepancies in the Literature

Figure 28.24B shows the regression of percentage body fat assessed by hydrostatic weighing versus percentage body fat assessed by BOD POD in an ethnically diverse group of adult women and men. A difference of only 0.3% (0.2% fat units) occurred between body fat determined by the two methods, with a validity coefficient of $r = 0.96$. In contrast to these rather impressive findings, BOD POD assessments of collegiate football players, although producing reliable scores, underpredicted percentage body fat compared with hydrostatic weighing and DXA.[33] Underprediction of body

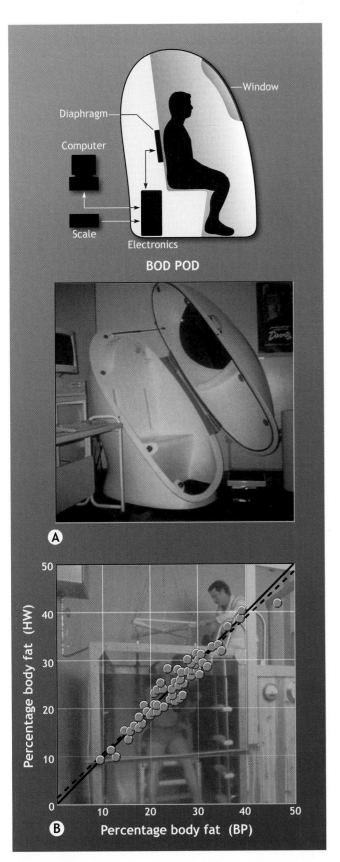

Figure 28.24 **A.** BOD POD for measuring human body volume. (Photo courtesy of Dr. Megan McCrory, Tufts University, Boston.) **B.** Regression of percentage body fat by hydrostatic weighing (HW) versus percentage body fat by BOD POD (BP). (Data from McCrory MA, et al. Evaluation of a new air displacement plethysmograph for measuring human body composition. Med Sci Sports Exerc 1995;27:1686.)

fat also occurred in a heterogeneous sample of black men who varied considerably in age, stature, body mass, percentage body fat, and self-reported physical activity level and socioeconomic status.[201] The method underpredicted percentage body fat compared with densitometry (−1.9% fat units) and DXA(−1.6% fat units). Similar underpredictions compared with DXA-derived body fat (−2.9% fat units) occurred in 54 boys and girls 10 to 18 years of age.[107] BOD POD also underestimated body fat of young adults compared with body fat predictions from a four-component model.[50,131] The method overestimated percentage body fat among lean individuals in a heterogeneous group of adults.[194] A BOD POD validation study in children ages 9 to 14 concluded that compared with DXA, total body water, and densitometry, BOD POD precisely and accurately estimated fat mass without introducing bias estimates.[47] The method has also been shown to accurately detect body composition changes from a small-to-moderate weight loss in overweight women and men.[207] Numerous studies have assessed the efficacy of BOD POD compared with other body composition methods in children; young, middle-age, and elderly adults; obese persons; and athletes.[4,6,9,32,48,52,115,117,150,171,188,196]

INTEGRATIVE QUESTION

Outline your response to a student who asks: "Why am I considered overfat by some criteria for obesity while my body fat assessment with other methods falls within normal limits?"

AVERAGE PERCENTAGE BODY FAT

TABLE 28.6 lists average values for percentage body fat in samples of men and women throughout the United States. The column headed "68% Variation Limits" indicates the range of percentage body fat that includes approximately 68 of every 100 persons measured. As an example, the average percentage body fat of 15.0% for young men from the New York sample includes the 68% variation limits from 8.9 to 21.1% body fat. This means that for every 68 of 100 young men measured, percentage fat ranges between 8.9 and 21.1%. Of the remaining 32 young men, 16 possess more than 21.1% body fat, while 16 other men have a body fat percentage below 8.9. *In general, percentage body fat for young adult men averages between 12 and 15%; the average value for women falls between 25 and 28%.*

Representative Samples Are Lacking

Considerable data describe average body composition for many groups of men and women of different ages and fitness levels and athletic specialties (see Chapter 29). No systematic evaluation exists for the body composition of a representative sample of the general population to warrant establishing norms or precise recommended values for body composition. At this time, it seems appropriate to present average values from various studies of different age groups.

TABLE 28.6 ■ AVERAGE VALUES OF BODY FAT FOR YOUNGER AND OLDER WOMEN AND MEN FROM SELECTED STUDIES

STUDY	AGE RANGE	STATURE (CM)	MASS (KG)	% FAT	68% VARIATION LIMITS
Younger women					
North Carolina, 1962	17–25	165.0	55.5	22.9	17.5–28.5
New York, 1962	16–30	167.5	59.0	28.7	24.6–32.9
California, 1968	19–23	165.9	58.4	21.9	17.0–26.9
California, 1970	17–29	164.9	58.6	25.5	21.0–30.1
Air Force, 1972	17–22	164.1	55.8	28.7	22.3–35.3
New York, 1973	17–26	160.4	59.0	26.2	23.4–33.3
North Carolina, 1975	–	166.1	57.5	24.6	–
Army Recruits, 1986	17–25	162.0	58.6	28.4	23.9–32.9
Massachusetts, 1998	17–31	165.2	57.8	21.8	16.7–27.9
Older women					
Minnesota, 1953	31–45	163.3	60.7	28.9	25.1–32.8
	43–68	160.0	60.9	34.2	28.0–40.5
New York, 1963	30–40	164.9	59.6	28.6	22.1–35.3
	40–50	163.1	56.4	34.4	29.5–39.5
North Carolina, 1975	33–50	–	–	29.7	23.1–36.5
Massachusetts, 1993	31–50	165.2	58.9	25.2	19.2–31.2
Younger men					
Minnesota, 1951	17–26	177.8	69.1	11.8	5.9–11.8
Colorado, 1956	17–25	172.4	68.3	13.5	8.3–18.8
Indiana, 1966	18–23	180.1	75.5	12.6	8.7–16.5
California, 1968	16–31	175.7	74.1	15.2	6.3–24.2
New York, 1973	17–26	176.4	71.4	15.0	8.9–21.1
Texas, 1977	18–24	179.9	74.6	13.4	7.4–19.4
Army Recruits, 1986	17–25	174.7	70.5	15.6	10.0–21.2
Massachusetts, 1998	17–31	178.1	76.4	12.9	7.8–19.0
Older men					
Indiana, 1966	24–38	179.0	76.6	17.8	11.3–24.3
	40–48	177.0	80.5	22.3	16.3–28.3
North Carolina, 1976	27–50	–	–	23.7	17.9–30.1
Texas, 1977	27–59	180.0	85.3	27.1	23.7–30.5
Massachusetts, 1993	31–50	177.1	77.5	19.9	13.2–26.5

The general trend of these data indicates a distinct tendency for percentage body fat to steadily increase with advancing age. The mechanisms that lead to increased body fat with age are poorly understood. It also remains unanswered to what extent additional fat in older age poses an increased health risk. The trend does not necessarily imply a desirable or normal aging process because participation in vigorous physical activity throughout life frequently blunts body fat accretion with age.[190] Regular physical activity maintains or increases bone mass while preserving muscle mass. A sedentary lifestyle, in contrast, increases storage fat and reduces muscle mass. This occurs even if daily caloric intake remains unchanged.

DETERMINING GOAL BODY WEIGHT

Average values for percentage body fat approximate 15% for young men and 25% for young women. In contact sports and activities that require muscular power (e.g., football, sprint swimming, and running), successful performance typically requires a large body mass with average or below-average body fat. In contrast, successful athletes in weight-bearing endurance activities generally possess a relatively light body mass with low body fat. One hopes that attaining a low body mass does not compromise the lean tissue mass and energy reserves. *Proper assessment of body composition, not body weight, determines a person's ideal body weight. For athletes,* **goal body weight** *must coincide with optimizing sport-specific measures of physiologic functional capacity and exercise performance.* The following equation computes a goal body weight based on a desired percentage body fat level:

Goal body weight = fat-free body mass

÷ 1.00 − desired %fat

Suppose a 91-kg (200-lb) man, currently with 20% body fat, wants to know how much fat weight to lose to attain a body fat composition of 15%. The computations progress as follows:

Fat mass = 91 kg × 0.20

= 18.2 kg

Fat-free body mass = 91 kg − 18.2 kg

= 72.8 kg

Goal body weight = 72.8 kg ÷ (1.00 − 0.10)

= 72.8 kg ÷ 0.90

= 80.9 kg (178 lb)

Goal fat loss = Current body weight − Goal body weight

= 91 kg − 80.9 kg

= 10.1 kg (22.2 lb)

If this athlete lost 10.1 kg of body fat, his new body weight of 80.9 kg would contain fat equal to 10% of body mass. These calculations assume no change in FFM during weight loss. Moderate caloric restriction plus increased daily energy expenditure through exercise induce fat loss and conserve the FFM. Chapter 30 discusses prudent yet effective approaches to fat loss.

Summary

1. Standard height for weight tables reveal little about body composition. Studies of athletes clearly show that overweight does not necessarily coincide with excessive body fat.

2. BMI relates more closely to body fat and health risk than simply body mass and stature. BMI still fails to consider the body's proportional composition.

3. Total body fat consists of essential fat and storage fat. Essential fat contains fat present in bone marrow, nerve tissue, and organs; it is an important component for normal biologic function. Storage fat represents the energy reserve that accumulates as adipose tissue beneath the skin and visceral depots.

4. Storage fat averages 12% of body mass for men and 15% for women. Essential fat averages 3% of body mass for men and 12% for women. The greater essential fat in females relates to childbearing and hormonal functions.

5. A person probably cannot reduce body fat below the essential fat level and still maintain optimal health.

6. Menstrual dysfunction occurs in athletes who train hard and maintain low body fat levels. This effect relates to the interaction between the physiologic and psychologic stress of regular training, hormonal balance, energy and nutrient intake, and body fat.

7. Delayed onset of menarche in chronically active young females may confer health benefits because such individuals show a lower lifetime occurrence of reproductive organ and other cancers.

8. Popular indirect methods of body composition assessment include hydrostatic weighing and prediction methods that incorporate skinfold and girth measurements.

9. Hydrostatic weighing determines body density with subsequent estimation of percentage body fat. The computation assumes a constant density for the body's fat and fat-free tissue compartments.

10. The error inherent in predicting body fat from whole-body density lies in assumptions concerning the densities of the fat and fat-free components. These densities, especially fat-free body mass, differ from assumed constants because of race, age, and athletic experience.

11. Body composition assessments that use skinfolds and girths show population specificity; they are most accurate with subjects similar to those who participated in the equations' original derivation.

12. Hydrated fat-free body tissues and extracellular water facilitate electrical flow compared with fat tissue because of the greater electrolyte content of the fat-free component. Impedance to electric current flow in BIA analysis relates to the body's fat quantity.

13. Near-infrared interactance should be used with caution to assess body composition in the exercise sciences; this methodology currently lacks verification of adequate validity.

14. Ultrasound, x-ray, CT, MRI, and DXA indirectly assesses body composition. Each has a unique application and special limitations for expanding knowledge of the compositional components of the live human body.

15. The air displacement method of BOD POD provides a reasonable alternative to hydrostatic weighing for body composition assessment.

16. Average males possess a body fat content of approximately 15% and women, 25%. These values from healthy individuals often provide a frame of reference to evaluate body fat of individual athletes and specific athletic groups.

17. Goal body weight computes as fat-free body mass ÷ 1.00 − desired %fat.

References are available on the Student CD and online at http://connection.lww.com/mkk6e.

Physique, Performance, and Physical Activity

29

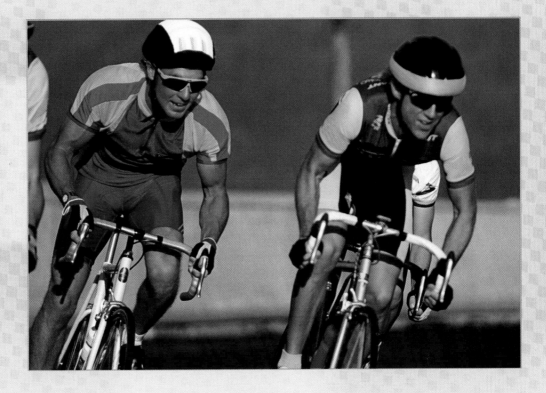

CHAPTER OBJECTIVES

- Compare body composition characteristics of average young men and women with elite competitors in endurance running, wrestling, triathlon, and weight lifting and bodybuilding

- Give examples of gender differences in world record performances for track and field, weight lifting, cycling, speed skating, and swimming

- Contrast body fat values for male and female competitive swimmers with runners and give possible reasons for the differences

- Summarize body composition characteristics, including body mass index, of early American professional football players and modern-day counterparts; compare modern professionals with current collegiate players

- Contrast body composition characteristics of elite high school wrestlers and less successful counterparts

- Contrast body composition, girths, and excess muscle mass of male and female bodybuilders

- Compare ratios of fat-free body mass (FFM) to fat mass of female bodybuilders with other elite female athletes

- Discuss the upper limit of FFM in "large-size" athletes

Body composition evaluation partitions gross size into two major structural components—body fat and fat-free body mass (FFM). In Chapter 28, we characterized the major physique differences between adult men and women. Pronounced physique differences also exist among sports participants of the same gender such as Olympic competitors, track and field specialists, wrestlers, American football players, and proficient adolescent competitors. This chapter takes a closer look at the physiques of champion athletes in different sports categories and competition levels.

Different anthropometric methodologies have quantified physique status. Visual appraisal often describes individuals as small, medium, and large or as thin (**ectomorphic**), muscular (**mesomorphic**), or fat (**endomorphic**). This older approach termed **somatotyping**, proposed by psychologist and physician William H. Sheldon (1898–1977), describes body shape by placing a person into a category such as thin or muscular. Visual appraisal quantifies neither body dimensions (e.g., size of the chest or shoulders) nor how biceps development compares with thigh or calf development. Somatotyping has been used as an adjunct method to analyze physique status of world-class athletes[7–9,14] and familial heritabilities,[35,47] but in this chapter we focus on the body fat and FFM components of body composition. Our review quantifies aspects of physique for Olympic competitors, endurance runners, collegiate and professional American football players, triathletes, high school wrestlers, champion male and female bodybuilders, collegiate gymnasts, and NBA professional basketball players.

PHYSIQUES OF CHAMPION ATHLETES

Early studies of Olympic competitors linked physique to a high level of sports achievement.[14,36] TABLES 29.1 and 29.2 list the anthropometric characteristics of male and female competitors in the 1964 Tokyo and 1968 Mexico City Olympics.[16,24] Bone diameters and stature provided estimates of lean body mass and percentage body fat. TABLE 29.3 lists anthropometric data for body mass, stature, and eight skinfolds for male and female swimmers, divers, and water polo athletes at the sixth World Championships in Perth, Australia, 1992.

Also of interest are the body size differences among different groups of athletes within a particular sport. FIGURE 29.1 *(top)* compares the body mass, stature, chest girth, upper- and lower-limb girths, and leg length for 12 male swimmers rated "best" in the 200- and 400-m free-style with less suc-

TABLE 29.1 ■ AGE, BODY SIZE, AND BODY COMPOSITION OF MALE ATHLETES WHO COMPETED IN SELECTED EVENTS IN THE TOKYO AND MEXICO CITY OLYMPICS

SPECIALTY	EVENT	OLYMPICS	N	AGE (Y)	STATURE (CM)	MASS (KG)	LBM[a] (KG)	BODY FAT[b] (%)
Sprint	100, 200 m;	Tokyo	172	24.9	178.4	72.2	64.9	10.1
	4 × 100 m; 110-m hurdles	Mexico City	79	23.9	175.4	68.4	62.8	8.2
Long-distance running	3000, 5000, 10,000 m	Tokyo	99	27.3	173.6	62.4	61.5	1.4
		Mexico City	34	25.3	171.9	59.8	60.1	−0.5[c]
Marathon	42.2 km	Tokyo	74	28.3	170.3	60.8	59.2	2.7
		Mexico City	20	26.4	168.7	56.6	58.1	2.7
Decathlon		Tokyo	26	26.3	183.2	83.5	68.5	18.0
		Mexico City	8	25.1	181.3	77.5	67.1	13.4
Jump	High, long, triple jump	Tokyo	89	25.3	181.5	73.2	67.2	8.2
		Mexico City	14	23.5	182.8	73.2	68.2	6
Weight throwing	Shot, discus, hammer	Tokyo	79	27.6	187.3	101.4	71.6	29.4
		Mexico City	9	27.3	186.1	102.3	70.7	30.9
Swimming	Free, breast, back, butterfly medley	Tokyo	450	20.4	178.7	74.1	65.1	12.1
		Mexico City	66	19.2	179.3	72.1	65.6	9.0
Basketball		Tokyo	186	25.3	189.4	84.3	73.2	13.2
		Mexico City	63	24.0	189.1	79.7	73.0	8.4
Gymnastics	All events	Tokyo	122	26.0	167.2	63.3	57.0	9.9
		Mexico City	28	23.6	167.4	61.5	57.2	7.0
Wrestling	Bantam and featherweight	Tokyo	29	27.3	163.3	62.3	54.4	12.7
		Mexico City	32	22.5	166.1	57.0	56.3	1.2
Rowing	Single and double skulls; pairs, fours, eights	Tokyo	357	25.0	186.0	82.2	70.6	14.1
		Mexico City	85	24.3	185.1	82.6	69.9	15.4

Adapted from De Garay, et al. Genetic and anthropological studies of Olympic athletes. New York: Academic Press, 1974; and Hirata K. Physique and age of Tokyo Olympic champions. J Sports Med Phys Fitness 1966;6:207.
[a] Calculated by Behnke's method: LBM (lean body mass) = h^2 × 0.204, where h = stature, dm (see reference 4).
[b] Body fat (%) = (Body mass − LBM)/Body mass × 100.
[c] Error resulting from specific prediction equation as percentage body fat cannot reach zero or a negative value.

TABLE 29.2 ■ AGE, BODY SIZE, AND BODY COMPOSITION OF FEMALE ATHLETES WHO COMPETED IN SELECTED EVENTS IN THE TOKYO AND MEXICO CITY OLYMPICS

SPECIALTY	EVENT	OLYMPICS	N	AGE (Y)	STATURE (CM)	MASS (KG)	LBM[a] (KG)	BODY FAT[b] (%)
Sprint	100, 200 m;	Tokyo	85	22.7	166.0	56.6	49.6	12.4
	100-m hurdles	Mexico City	28	20.7	165.0	56.8	49.0	13.7
Jump	High, long,	Tokyo	56	23.6	169.5	60.2	51.7	14.1
	triple jump	Mexico City	12	21.5	169.4	56.4	51.7	8.4
Weight	Shot, discus,	Tokyo	37	26.2	170.4	79.0	52.3	33.8
throwing	hammer	Mexico City	9	19.9	170.9	73.5	52.6	28.5
Swimming	Free, breast, back,	Tokyo	272	18.6	166.3	59.7	49.8	16.6
	butterfly, medley	Mexico City	28	16.3	164.4	56.9	48.6	14.5
Diving	Spring, high	Tokyo	65	18.5	160.9	54.1	46.6	13.9
		Mexico City	7	21.1	160.4	52.3	46.3	11.5
Gymnastics	All events	Tokyo	102	22.7	157.0	52.0	44.4	14.7
		Mexico City	21	17.8	156.9	49.8	44.3	11.0

Adapted from De Garay, et al. Genetic and anthropological studies of Olympic athletes. New York: Academic Press, 1974; and Hirata K. Physique and age of Tokyo Olympic champions. J Sports Med Phys Fitness 1966;6:207.
[a] Calculated by Behnke's method: LBM (lean body mass) $= h^2 \times 18$, where h $=$ stature, dm (see reference 4).
[b] Body fat (%) $=$ (Body mass $-$ LBM)/Body mass $\times$ 100.

cessful counterparts. The bottom figure also compares selected body size variables between the 12 "best" 50-, 100-, and 200-m female breaststroke swimmers with other competitors. The best male swimmers are heavier and taller and have larger chest, upper-arm, and thigh girths and upper- and lower-limb lengths than counterparts not ranking among the top 12. The best female breaststroke swimmers, also taller and heavier, possessed larger arm span, foot and arm lengths, and hand and wrist breadths than less successful competitors.

Gender

Table 29.1 indicates that for the men, basketball players, rowers, and weight throwers were tallest and heaviest; they also possessed the largest FFM and percentage body fat. For example, weight throwers in both Olympiads averaged 30% body fat, whereas 94 marathon and 133 long-distance runners averaged an exceptionally low 1.6% body fat. The largest body composition discrepancy within a sports category emerged in comparisons of the Tokyo wrestlers (12.7% body fat) and wrestlers in Mexico City (1.2% body fat). Age, stature, and FFM were similar in both groups, making this difference even more remarkable.

For female Olympians, a relatively low body fat percentage provides the most striking physique characteristic. Except for weight throwers (31% body fat), competitors in the other sports groups approximated the 13.1% average body fat for all 676 female participants in both Olympiads.

For aquatic athletes (Table 29.3), skinfolds at most sites were larger in females than in males. As noted in Chapter 10,

TABLE 29.3 ■ COMPARISON OF BODY MASS, STATURE, AND EIGHT SKINFOLDS IN MALE AND FEMALE SWIMMERS, DIVERS, AND WATER POLO ATHLETES AT THE SIXTH WORLD CHAMPIONSHIPS HELD IN PERTH, AUSTRALIA, 1992

	MASS (KG)	STATURE (CM)	TRI[a]	SCAP	SUPRA	ABD	THI	CALF	BIC	ILIAC
Males										
Swimming	78.4	183.8	7.0	7.9	6.3	9.4	9.6	6.5	3.7	9.2
Diving	66.7	170.9	6.8	7.9	6.0	9.6	9.6	6.0	3.8	8.5
Water polo	86.1	186.5	9.2	9.9	8.2	14.9	12.6	7.9	4.3	13.4
Females										
Swimming	63.1	171.5	12.1	8.8	7.3	12.1	19.1	11.4	5.9	9.8
Diving	53.7	161.2	11.4	8.5	6.8	11.1	18.2	9.7	4.9	7.9
Water polo	64.8	171.3	15.3	10.5	9.6	17.6	23.4	13.5	7.1	12.1

Modified from Mazza JC, et al. Absolute body size. In: Carter JE, Ackland TR, eds. Kinanthropometry in aquatic sports. A study of world class athletes. Human Kinetics Sport Science Monograph Series, vol 5. Champaign, IL: Human Kinetics, 1994.
[a] Abbreviations for skinfolds (mm): Tri, triceps; Scap, subscapular; Supra, supraspinale; Abd, abdomen; Calf, midcalf; Bic, biceps; Iliac, iliac crest.

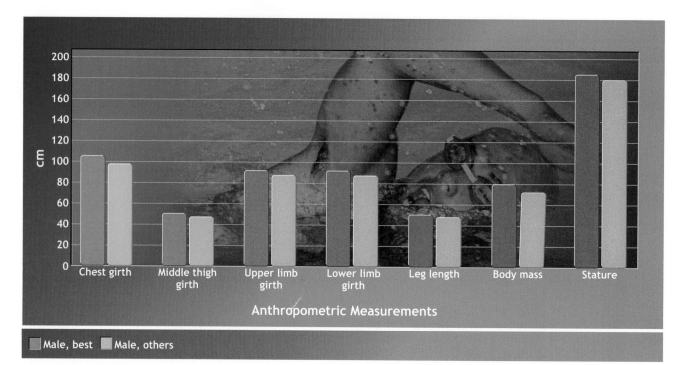

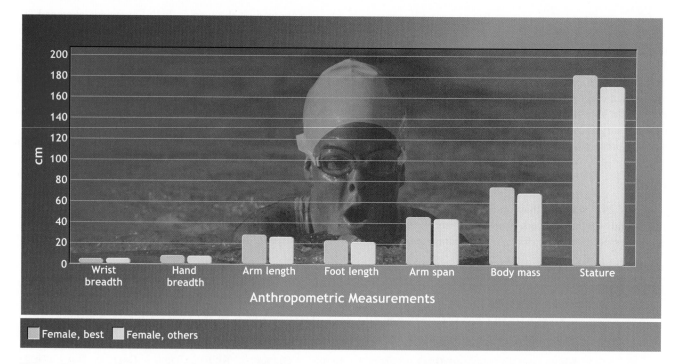

Figure 29.1 *Top.* Comparison of the body mass, stature, chest and limb girths, and leg length of the *best* (top 12 ranks) 200- and 400-m freestyle male swimmers with the remaining competitors (*others*). *Bottom.* Comparison of differences in body size variables including arm span (actual values divided by 4) between the *best* 50-, 100-, and 200-m female breaststroke swimmers (top 12 ranks) and the rest of the competitors (*others*). The *y* axis is in centimeters for all variables except body mass, which is in kilograms. (Modified from Mazza JC, et al. Absolute body size. In: Carter JE, Ackland TR, eds. Kinanthropometry in aquatic sports. A study of world-class athletes. Human Kinetics Sport Science Monograph Series, vol 5. Champaign, IL: Human Kinetics, 1994.)

a swimmer's morphology alters the horizontal components of lift and drag. Selected anthropometric variables influence the magnitude of propulsive and resistive forces that affect the swimmer's forward movement.[10,11] In well-trained freestyle swimmers, arm length, leg length, and hand and foot size—factors governed largely by genetics—influence stroke length and stroke frequency.[22] TABLE 29.4 presents additional anthropometric comparisons between male and female Olympians in five different sports (including swimming) at the 1976 Montreal Summer Olympics.

Fat–Free-to-Fat Ratio

FIGURE 29.2 compares the ratio of FFM to fat mass (FM), derived from data in the world literature for the specific sport, among male and female competitors. The *inset tables* present data for average body mass, percentage body fat, and FFM. Male marathon runners and gymnasts have the largest FFM:FM, while American football offensive and defensive linemen and shot putters show the smallest ratios. Among females, bodybuilders have the largest FFM:FM values (equal of males), while the smallest FFM:FMs emerge for field-event participants. Surprisingly, female gymnasts and ballet dancers rank intermediate compared with other female sport participants.

World Records

FIGURE 29.3 compares world records for males and females through 1991 and comparative data for 2000 for maximum running speed at distances between 100 m and 10,000 m. Essentially, percentage difference in performance between genders remained invariant over the 9-year interval. The percentage gender difference averages about 10% for all running events, including the 400-m hurdles and 400-m to 3200-m relay races (*top right figure*). The *lower left figure* shows that gender differences in world record times (expressed as maximum running speed [m · s^{-1}]) remain remarkably similar for 100-m through 10,000-m events. Males achieve identical running speeds for 100 and 200 m; speed then declines steadily for both genders as distance increases. For example, the percentage decline between 100 m and 800 m equals 29% for men and 35% for women. A lesser rate of decline occurs over the longer distances, with the cumulative decrement in maximum speed between 800 and 10,000 m averaging 28% for men and women.

Among male and female weight lifters (*top left figure*) in the same body-weight category, women in the 56-kg weight class achieved 82.0% of the men's best performance in 2000; this decreased to 70.7% in 2004, indicating that the female decreased her maximum strength relative to the male performer. The opposite occurred for women in the 82.5-kg weight category. In field events (not listed), the percentage of the men's best performance achieved by the women is as follows: long jump, 84.0%; high jump, 83.3%; javelin throw, 82.5%; and triple jump, 83.2%.

FIGURE 29.4 shows further comparisons in world record performances between males and females for swimming, speed skating, and sprint cycling. In the 400-, 800-, and 1500-m freestyle swims, females achieve times closer to males (90.7% of best male times) than in the shorter distances (88.7%). Percentage differences remain about the same in speed skating and middle-distance swimming events in 400- through 1500-m distances; in cycling from 1 km to 100 km, females achieve about 87% of males' best times.

TABLE 29.4 ■ **SELECTED ANTHROPOMETRIC MEASUREMENTS IN MALES AND FEMALES WHO COMPETED IN FIVE DIFFERENT SPORTS AT THE MONTREAL OLYMPIC GAMES**

	CANOE		GYMNASTICS		ROWING		SWIMMING		TRACK	
MEASUREMENT[a]	M	F	M	F	M	F	M	F	M	F
Stature	185.4	170.7	169.3	161.5	191.3	174.3	178.6	166.9	179.1	168.5
Upper extremity L	82.4	76.0	76.0	72.2	85.2	76.0	80.2	74.7	80.9	74.8
Lower extremity L	88.0	81.8	78.9	76.5	91.7	82.3	84.1	78.1	86.9	80.3
Biacromial D	41.4	36.8	39.0	35.9	42.5	37.4	40.8	37.1	40.2	36.3
Biiliac D	28.1	27.3	25.8	25.0	30.2	28.2	27.9	26.7	27.1	27.2
Arm relaxed G	32.2	27.6	30.7	24.3	31.7	27.6	30.6	27.3	29.1	24.5
Arm flexed G	35.3	29.6	33.9	25.9	34.9	29.3	33.3	28.2	32.2	26.4
Forearm G	29.3	25.4	27.5	23.2	30.3	25.5	27.4	23.9	27.9	23.3
Chest G	102.6	88.9	95.1	83.5	103.7	89.6	98.6	88.0	94.3	83.8
Waist G	80.6	69.8	72.8	63.2	84.0	70.8	79.3	69.4	77.7	67.4
Thigh G	54.6	54.0	51.0	49.9	60.2	57.5	55.4	52.8	56.0	53.9
Calf G	37.5	34.9	34.7	33.3	39.3	37.0	36.9	34.0	37.6	34.9

Adapted from Carter JE, et al. Anthropometry of Montreal Olympic athletes. In: Carter JEL, ed. Physical structure of Olympic athletes. Part 1: The Montreal Olympic Games Anthropological Project. Basal: Karger, 1982.
[a] L, length; D, diameter; G, girth; all values are in centimeters.

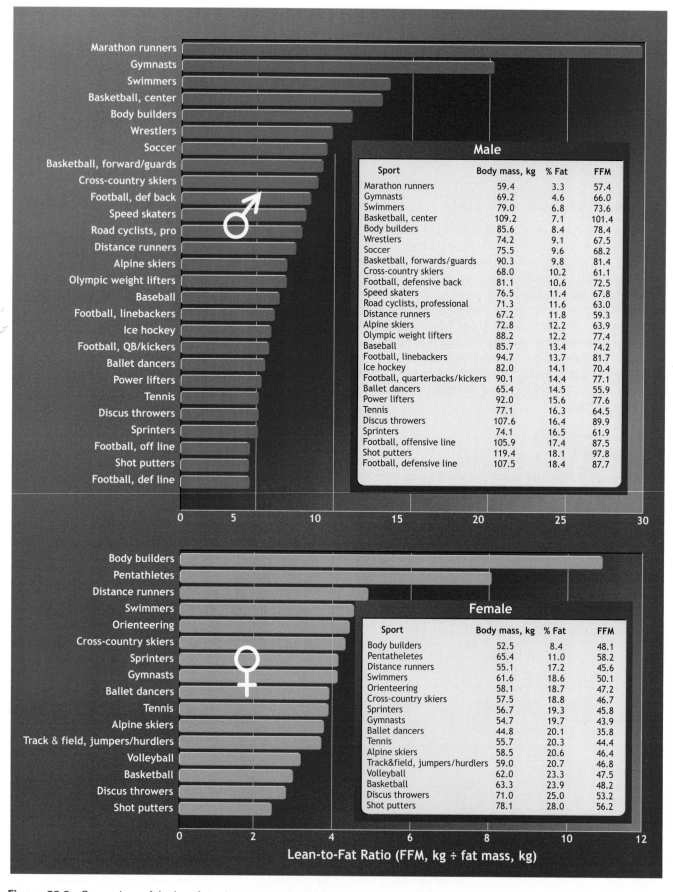

Figure 29.2 Comparison of the lean:fat ratio among male and female competitors in diverse sports. Values are based on the average body mass and percentage body fat for each sport from various studies in the literature. The lean:fat ratio is FFM (kg) ÷ fat mass (kg). Values in the *inset tables* represent averages for body composition if the literature contained two or more citations about a specific sport. The equation of Siri (Chapter 28) converted body density to percentage body fat.

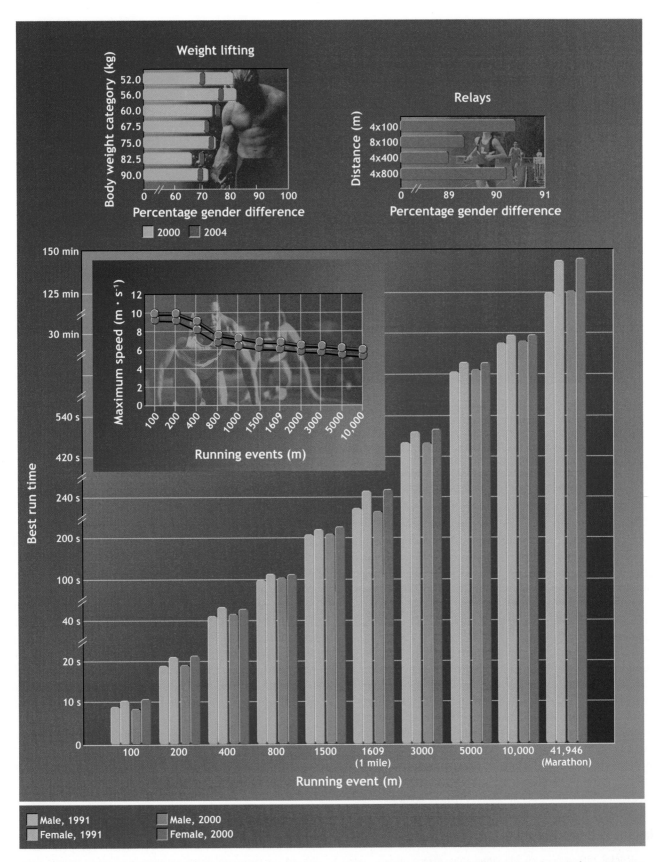

Figure 29.3 *Main figure*. World records for males and females in 1991 and 9 years later in 2000 in running events from 100 m to the marathon. Considering all events in the 1991 and 2000 data sets, women achieved between 88 and 94% of the performance of men. The *top left inset* shows percentage differences between genders (% of male values achieved by females) for total weight lifted in the snatch and clean and jerk for six weight classifications. The *top right inset* displays percentage differences in four common relay events. The *lower inset* expresses gender differences in world record times as maximum running speed (m · s^{-1}) for 100 m through 10,000 m. (Weight lifting data from the International Powerlifting Federation [www.ipf.com]).

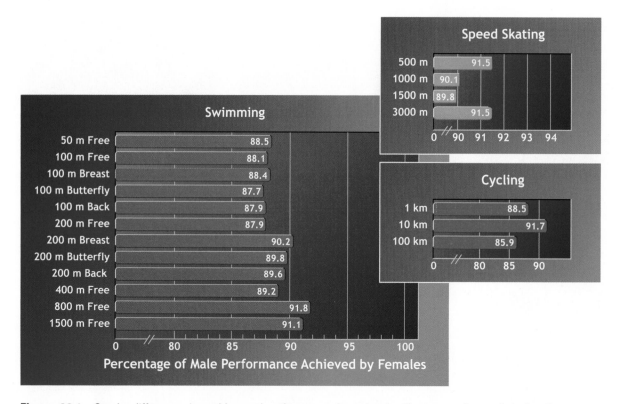

Figure 29.4   Gender differences in world-record performances for swimming (long course), speed skating (long track), and track sprint cycling. The numbers within the *purple, orange,* and *red bars* represent the percentage of the male performance achieved by females. For example, new world records for the 1500m in speed skating were established in 2005 by Chad Hendrick (United States; 3:39.02 s) and Cindy Klassen (Canada; 1:53.87 s). The female world-record performance represents 89.8% of that achieved by the male world-record holder. All world records for speed skating are as of August 16, 2005 (www.infoplease.com/ipsa/A0112783.html), and for swimming, November 3, 2005 (www.vilacom.net/swimming/men.php). Values for sprint cycling are from various web sites as of October 31, 2005.

A reasonable question concerns whether continued improvement in training methods and performance techniques can overcome apparent gender limits to maximal performance, particularly in events that require exceptional muscular strength/power and anaerobic capacity. *If gender equality in sports performance does emerge, it may occur first in middle-distance swimming events.*

Geographic Region.   FIGURE 29.5 shows gender differences in six running and two field events from five world geographic regions, including comparisons with world and Olympic records. As in Figure 29.3, percentage difference reflects the woman's record relative to the record for men. This remarkable data set reveals that similar gender differences in competition persist nearly uniformly across geographic regions. In general, more-pronounced sex differences exist in South American records than in world and Olympic records.

Racial Differences

Racial differences in physique may affect athletic performance.[54] Black sprinters and high jumpers, for example, have longer limbs and narrower hips than white counterparts. From a mechanical perspective, a black sprinter with leg and arm size identical to a white sprinter has a lighter, shorter, and

slimmer body to propel. This might confer a more favorable power-to-body mass ratio at any given body size. Greater power output provides an advantage in jumping and sprint running events where generating rapid energy for short durations remains crucial to success. The advantage diminishes somewhat in the various throwing events. Compared with whites and blacks, Asian athletes have short legs relative to upper torso components, a dimensional characteristic beneficial in short and longer distance races and in weight lifting. Successful weight lifters of all races compared with other athletic groups have relatively short arms and legs for their stature.

Percentage Body Fat of Elite Athletes

Considerable literature describes body fat levels of male and female competitive athletes in diverse sports.

By Category

FIGURE 29.6 presents six classifications of sports activities based on common characteristics and performance requirements, with percentage body fat rankings within each category for male and female competitors (where applicable). This compendium provides an overview of percentage body fat of athletes within a broad grouping of relatively similar sports.

Gender Differences (%) in "Best" Performance by World Geographic Region

Event	World record	Olympic record	African record	South American record	Nordic record	Balkan record	Commonwealth record
100 m	93.3	92.7	89.9	89.2	90.6	93.4	91.6
200 m	90.5	90.5	88.2	87.9	90.1	91.8	90.9
400 m	90.7	90.1	90.0	90.6	90.5	90.1	90.8
800 m	89.3	90.0	88.8	87.2	84.7	91.0	87.5
1500 m	89.4	90.8	88.1	87.4	87.8	91.5	87.4
5000 m	88.3	84.3	85.9	86.7	90.8	91.0	86.5
High jump	85.3	85.8	85.5	84.1	83.1	87.1	83.2
Long jump	84.0	83.1	86.1	81.2	84.8	87.9	81.7

Figure 29.5 Gender differences (% of male values achieved by females) in eight outdoor track performances grouped by five world regions, including world records and Olympic performances through March 2000.

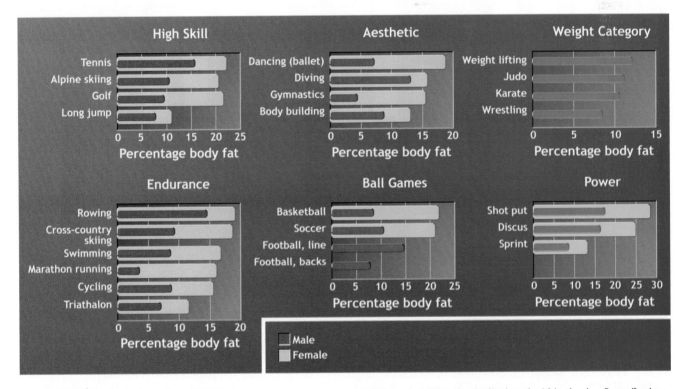

Figure 29.6 Percentage body fat in athletes grouped by sport category. The value for males is displayed within the *bar* (in red) when a corresponding value exists for females *(yellow)*. The values for percentage body fat (from body density by the Siri equation) represent averages from the literature.

Field Event Athletes

FIGURE 29.7 shows body composition obtained by hydrostatic weighing and anthropometry—percentage body fat, fat weight, FFM, and lean-to-fat ratio—for the 10 top American athletes in the discus, shot put, javelin, and hammer throw 2 years before the 1980 Moscow Olympics. Comparative data describe international elite middle- and long-distance runners (average treadmill $\dot{V}O_{2max}$ 76.9 mL · kg^{-1} · min^{-1}) and Behnke's reference man. TABLE 29.5 lists the corresponding data for girth and skinfold anthropometry. Shot putters clearly possessed the largest overall body size (body mass and girths) followed by athletes in the discus, hammer, and javelin throw.

Female Endurance Athletes

TABLE 29.6 presents body mass, stature, and body composition of 11 female long-distance runners of national and international caliber.[63] The runners averaged 15.2% body fat (hydrostatic weighing), similar to reported data for high school cross-country runners[4] but considerably lower than the 26% body fat for sedentary females of the same age, stature, and body mass.[31] Compared with other athletic groups, the runners have relatively less fat than collegiate basketball players (20.9%),[51] gymnasts (15.5%),[52] younger distance runners (18%),[36] swimmers (20.1%),[33] tennis players (22.8%),[33] or triathletes.[25]

Interestingly, the runners' average body fat equaled the 15% value generally reported for nonathletic males. The 6 to 9% body fat levels of several apparently healthy runners in Table 29.6 falls within the range for topflight male endurance athletes. The leanest women in the population, based on Behnke's reference standards, have essential fat equal to 12 to 14% of body mass. This apparent discrepancy between estimated fat content of distance runners and the theoretical lower limit for body fat in women requires further study. Note the relatively high body fat (35.4%) for one of the best runners; clearly, other factors must override limitations to distance running imposed by excess fat.

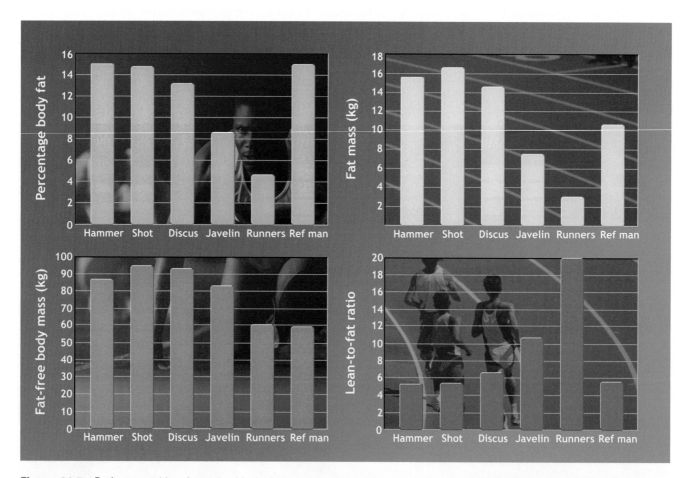

Figure 29.7   Body composition determined by hydrostatic weighing of the top 10 American male athletes in the discus, shot put, javelin, and hammer throw. Data collected by two of the authors (FK and VK) at a 1978 U.S. Olympic minicamp at the University of Houston, Houston, TX. Athletes include former gold medalist Wilkins (discus) and world record holder Powell (discus). Data for the international elite middle- and long-distance runners from Pollock ML, et al. Body composition of elite class distance runners. Ann NY Acad Sci 1977;301:361. Reference man *(Ref man)* data from Behnke's model in Chapter 28.

TABLE 29.5 ■ SKINFOLD AND GIRTH ANTHROPOMETRY OF THE TOP 10 AMERICAN ATHLETES IN THE DISCUS, SHOT PUT, JAVELIN, AND HAMMER THROW

MEASUREMENT[a]	DISCUS	SHOT PUT	JAVELIN	HAMMER	RUNNERS	REF MAN
Body mass, kg	108.2	112.3	90.6	104.2	63.1	70.0
Stature, cm	191.7	187.0	186.0	187.3	177.0	174.0
Skinfolds, mm						
Triceps	13.0	15.0	11.9	12.7	5.0	–
Scapular	18.0	23.8	12.5	21.5	6.4	–
Iliac	24.5	29.6	17.0	27.4	4.6	–
Abdomen	25.6	31.4	18.4	29.1	7.1	–
Thigh	16.4	15.7	13.3	17.3	6.1	–
Girths, cm						
Shoulders	129.8	133.3	121.5	127.4	106.1	110.8
Chest	113.5	118.5	104.6	111.3	91.1	91.8
Waist	94.1	99.1	86.6	94.8	74.6	77.0
Abdomen	97.5	101.5	87.8	98.0	74.2	79.8
Hips	110.4	112.3	102.0	108.7	87.8	93.4
Thighs	66.3	69.4	61.5	67.3	51.9	54.8
Knees	41.5	42.9	40.0	41.0	36.2[b]	36.6
Calves	42.6	43.6	39.5	41.5	35.4	35.8
Ankles	25.4	24.9	24.1	24.3	21.0	22.5
Biceps	41.8	42.2	37.7	39.9	28.2	31.7
Forearms	33.1	33.7	30.8	32.4	26.4	26.4
Wrists	18.7	18.9	18.2	18.4	16.0	17.3
Diameters, cm						
Biacromial	44.5	43.8	43.2	44.8	39.5	40.6
Chest	33.1	33.7	30.8	32.6	31.3	30.0
Bi-iliac	31.3	31.2	29.6	30.4	28.0	28.6
Bitrochanter	35.5	34.9	33.7	34.8	32.2	32.8
Knee	10.2	10.5	10.0	10.2	9.5	9.3
Wrist	6.3	6.2	6.0	6.2	5.6	5.6
Ankle	7.6	7.6	7.5	7.4	–	7.0
Elbow	7.6	7.6	7.6	7.2	–	7.0

[a] Details about measurement procedures from Katch FI, Katch VL. The body composition profile: techniques of measurement and applications. Clin Sports Med 1984;3:31. Data correspond to the athletic groups presented in Fig. 29.7.
[b] Not measured; value computed from the ratio for the reference man calf to knee.

Male Endurance Athletes

TABLE 29.7 presents body composition data for 11 male elite middle- and long-distance runners and 8 elite marathoners. The group included Steve Prefontaine, former American record holder in the 800- and 1500-m runs, and Frank Shorter, the 1976 Olympic gold medalist in the marathon. A representative sample of 95 untrained college-aged men provides comparison data.

Both groups of runners have extremely low body fat values considering that essential fat theoretically constitutes about 3% of body mass. Clearly, these competitors represent the lower end of the lean-to-fat continuum for topflight endurance athletes. This physique characteristic most likely influences success in distance running. This makes sense for several reasons. First, effective heat dissipation during running maintains thermal balance—excess fat thwarts heat dissipation. Second, excess body fat provides "dead weight"; it adds directly to exercise energy cost without contributing propulsive energy.

For body dimensions and structure, male distance runners generally have smaller girths and bone diameters than untrained males.[14] Structural differences, particularly bone diameters, reflect a genetic influence similar to the distinct anthropometric characteristics of aquatic athletes (see Fig. 29.1). The best long-distance runners inherit a slight build with well-proportioned skeletal dimensions. The prime ingredients for a champion include a genetically optimal physique profile blended with a lean body composition, highly developed aerobic system, and proper psychologic mind-set for protracted intense training.

TABLE 29.6 ■ BODY COMPOSITION OF FEMALE ENDURANCE RUNNERS

SUBJECT	AGE (Y)	STATURE (CM)	MASS (KG)	FFM (KG)	BODY FAT (KG)	BODY FAT (%)
1[a]	24	172.7	52.6	49.5	3.1	5.9
2[b]	26	159.8	71.5	46.2	25.3	35.4
3[c]	28	162.6	50.7	47.6	3.1	6.1
4	31	171.5	52.0	47.3	4.7	9.0
5	33	176.5	61.2	50.8	10.4	17.0
6	34	166.4	52.9	44.8	8.1	15.2
7	35	168.4	55.0	48.7	6.3	11.6
8	36	164.5	53.1	44.3	8.8	16.6
9	36	182.9	61.5	50.4	11.1	18.1
10	36	182.9	65.4	55.7	9.7	14.8
11	37	154.9	53.6	44.0	9.6	18.0
Average	32.4	169.4	57.2	48.1	9.1	15.2

From Wilmore JH, Brown CH. Physiological profiles of women distance runners. Med Sci Sports 1974;6:178.
[a]World's best time in marathon (2:49:40) as of 1974.
[b]World's best time in 50-mile run (7:04:31); established 18 months after the body composition evaluation.
[c]Noted U.S. distance runner. Five consecutive national and international cross-country championships.

TABLE 29.7 ■ BODY COMPOSITION CHARACTERISTICS OF ELITE MALE MIDDLE- AND LONG-DISTANCE RUNNERS AND ELITE MARATHONERS

GROUP	STATURE (CM)	MASS (KG)	DENSITY (G · CM^{-3})	BODY FAT (%)	FFM (KG)	FAT MASS (KG)	SUM 7 SKINFOLDS (MM)
Distance runners							
Brown	187.3	72.10	1.07428	10.8	64.31	7.79	53.0
Castaneda	178.6	63.34	1.09102	3.7	61.00	2.34	32.5
Crawford	171.8	58.01	1.09702	1.2	57.31	0.70	32.5
Geis	179.1	66.28	1.07551	10.2	59.52	6.76	49.0
Johnson	174.6	61.79	1.08963	4.3	59.13	2.66	35.5
Manley	177.8	69.10	1.09642	1.5	68.06	1.04	32.0
Ndoo	169.3	53.97	1.08379	6.7	50.35	3.62	33.5
Prefontaine	174.2	68.00	1.08842	4.8	64.74	3.26	38.0
Rose	175.6	59.15	1.08248	7.3	54.83	4.32	31.5
Tuttle	176.8	61.44	1.09960	0.2	61.32	0.12	31.5
Mean	170.5	60.92	1.08916	4.5	58.18	2.74	34.5
Marathon runners							
Cusack	174.6	64.19	1.08096	7.9	59.12	5.07	45.5
Galloway	180.9	65.76	1.08419	6.6	61.42	4.34	43.0
Kennedy	167.0	56.52	1.09348	2.7	54.99	1.53	37.0
Moore	184.1	64.24	1.09193	3.3	62.12	2.12	37.0
Pate	179.6	57.28	1.09676	1.3	56.54	0.74	32.5
Shorter	178.4	61.17	1.09475	2.2	59.82	1.35	45.0
Wayne	172.1	61.61	1.07859	8.9	56.13	5.48	42.5
Williams	177.2	66.07	1.09569	1.8	64.88	1.19	41.5
Mean	176.8	62.11	1.08954	4.3	59.38	2.73	40.5

Data from Pollock ML, et al. Body composition of elite class distance runners. Ann NY Acad Sci 1977;301:361.

INTEGRATIVE QUESTION

Discuss the physiologic and anthropometric characteristics necessary for successful endurance running performance.

Triathletes

The triathlon combines continuous endurance performance in swimming, bicycling, and running. The extreme triathlon, the ultraendurance Ironman competition, requires competitors to swim 3.9 km (2.4 mi), bicycle 180.2 km (112 mi), and run a standard 42.2-km (26.2-mi) marathon. The course records for the Ironman triathlon in Kailua-Kona, Hawaii, stand at 8:04:08 for men (Luc Van Lierde, 1996) and only a 10.6% slower time of 8:55:28 for women (Paula Newby-Fraser, 1992). The serious triathlete's training averages nearly 4 hours daily, covering a total of 280 miles per week by swimming 7.2 miles (30:00 min per mi pace), bicycling 227 miles (18.6 mph), and running 45 miles (7:42 min per mi pace).[24] Percentage body fat of six male and three female participants in the 1982 Ironman triathlon ranged between 5.0 and 11.3% for men and 7.4 and 17.2% for women. Body fat averaged 7.1% for the top 15 male finishers, with corresponding $\dot{V}O_{2max}$ of 72.0 mL $\cdot$ kg^{-1} $\cdot$ min^{-1}. Triathletes' body fat content and aerobic capacity is comparable to other athletes in single endurance sports,[45] with an overall physique most closely resembling that of elite cyclists[44] or swimmers[39] rather than runners. Aerobic capacity of these athletes during swimming consistently averages below values during treadmill running or stationary cycling.[37]

A longitudinal study evaluated the effects of a triathlon season on bone dynamics and hormonal status in seven male competitive triathletes at the beginning of training and 32 weeks later.[41] Total and regional bone mineral density (BMD) was determined by dual-energy x-ray absorptiometry, and specific biochemical markers assessed bone turnover. The triathlon season had a small but favorable effect on BMD at the lumbar spine and skull, but no effect on total body or proximal femur BMD. No changes occurred in hormonal levels.

Swimmers Versus Runners

Male and female competitive swimmers generally have higher body fat levels than distance runners, despite swim training's considerable energy requirement. The cool water of the training environment generally produces lower core temperatures than equivalent land exercise. A lower core temperature may prevent the depressed appetite that often accompanies intense training on land.

Limited evidence indicates similar daily energy intake for male collegiate swimmers (3380 kCal) and distance runners (3460 kCal), which balances training energy expenditure. In contrast, female swimmers averaged a higher daily energy intake of 2490 kCal, compared with 2040 kCal for running counterparts.[30] Swimmers had higher estimated daily energy expenditure than runners. The swimmers' energy expenditure surpassed energy intake placing them in a slightly *negative* energy balance. Thus, a positive energy balance (intake greater than output) does not explain typically higher body fat levels in male (12%) and female (20%) swimmers than in male (7%) and female (15%) runners. Subsequent research from the same laboratory evaluated energy expenditure and fuel use for swimmers and runners during each form of training (45 min at 75–80% $\dot{V}O_{2max}$) and 2 hours recovery.[18] The hypothesis assumed that differences in hormonal response and substrate catabolism between the two exercise modes accounted for body fat differences between groups. The results, however, indicated that the small between-group differences in energy expenditure, substrate use, and hormone levels could *not* account for body fat differences.

Future research must determine whether real differences in physiologic response to land and water training account for body composition differences between swimmers and runners. An alternative explanation suggests that self-selection causes those individuals with higher body fat levels to compete in swimming. Excess body fat presents a liability to energy cost and thermoregulation during weight-bearing exercise on land, yet contributes importantly to buoyancy and perhaps hydrodynamic economy to forward swimming movement from reduced drag forces.

American Football Players

The first detailed body composition analyses of American professional football players in the early 1940s demonstrated the inadequacy of determining a person's optimal body mass from height–weight standards (see "Focus on Research," Chapter 28).[61] The body fat content of the players averaged only 10.4% of body mass while FFM averaged 81.3 kg. Certainly these men were heavy but not fat. The heaviest lineman weighed 118 kg (17.4% body fat; 97.7 kg FFM), whereas lineman with the most body fat (23.2%) weighed 115.4 kg. Body mass of a defensive back with the least fat (3.3%) was 82.3 kg with an FFM of 79.6 kg.

TABLE 29.8 presents a clearer picture of average values for body mass, stature, percentage body fat, and FFM of college and professional football players grouped by position.[62,64] The *Pro, older* group consists of 25 players from the 1942 Washington Redskins, the first professional players measured for body composition by hydrostatic weighing. The *Pro, modern* group consists of 164 players from 14 teams in the National Football League (NFL; 69% veterans, 31% rookies). Some 107 members of the 1976 to 1978 Dallas Cowboys and New York Jets make up the third group. Four groups of collegiate players include candidates for spring practice at St. Cloud State College in Minnesota, the University of Massachusetts (U Mass), and Division III Gettysburg College and teams from the University of Southern California (USC), 1973 to 1977, national champions and participants in two Rose Bowls. Body composition measurements for this data set included hydrostatic weighing with correction for measured residual lung volume.

BODY COMPOSITION ANALYSIS BY DISSECTION

Clarys JP, et al. Gross tissue weights in the human body by cadaver dissection. Hum Biol 1984;56:459.

▲ Chemical and anatomic dissection procedures provide two *direct* methods to study human body composition. The chemical method quantifies body water, lipid, protein, and various mineral elements in different tissues and the whole body. Anatomic dissection partitions the body into components including skin, muscle, adipose tissue, bone, and whole organs. Since 1940, the body composition literature reveals only eight complete analyses of adult humans, with only three done by chemical methods.

Until the research of Clarys and colleagues, no comparisons existed between indirect (body density assessment) and direct dissection assessment of body composition. These researchers used anthropometry, radiography, photogrammetry, densitometry, and complete anatomic dissection of 25 cadavers to determine the gross tissue mass of skin, adipose tissue, muscle, bone, and vital organs (see figure). The cadavers ranged in age from 55 to 94 years and included 12 embalmed (6 male, 6 female) and 13 nonembalmed (6 male, 7 female) whites. For each cadaver, analysis included removing skeletal muscle and other major organs (brain, heart, lungs, liver, kidneys, and spleen). Bones were then separated at their articulations and scraped to leave surfaces free of muscle and adipose tissue. Muscle included the ligaments and bone retained the cartilage of any articular surface. Airtight plastic buckets stored all dissected tissues including scrapings. The tissues were weighed to within 0.1 g and their densities determined. Complete cadaver dissection took approximately 15 hours and required a team of 10 to 12 anatomists and kinesiologists.

The figure shows an average adipose tissue mass of 40.5% of total body mass in females and 28.1% in males. The researchers introduced the concept of adipose tissue-free weight (ATFW)—the whole-body mass minus the mass of all dissectible adipose tissue (adipose tissue contains about 83% pure fat). Muscle accounted for 52% of the ATFW in males and 48.1% in females, while bone constituted 19.9% of ATFW in males and 21.3% in females. Combining the data for males and females, the average proportion of the ATFW included 8.5% skin, 50.0% muscle, and 20.6% bone.

Densitometry to estimate the fat and fat-free mass (FFM) assumes a constant density for the FFM. This in turn requires that the proportions of the FFM components—fat-free muscle, fat-free adipose tissue, fat-free bone, and other fat-free tissues—remain unchanged from one person to another, including the densities for each tissue. Although Clarys' research did not include measures of whole-body fat, considerable variation existed in the ATFW. The extent of the variation challenges the important assumption of a constant density for the body's FFM when using hydrostatic weighing to assess body fat.

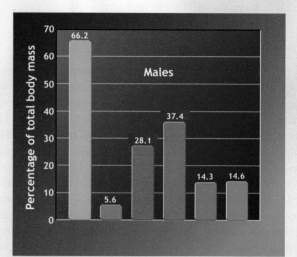

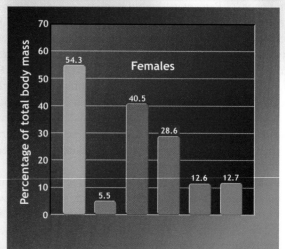

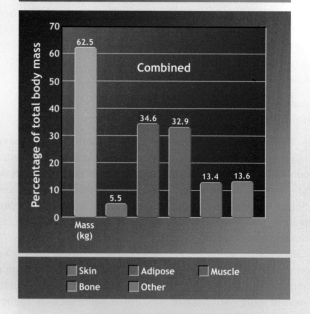

Various tissues in the adult body expressed as a percentage of total body mass. Body mass in kg.

TABLE 29.8 ■ **BODY COMPOSITIONS OF COLLEGIATE AND PROFESSIONAL FOOTBALL PLAYERS GROUPED BY POSITION**

POSITION[a]	LEVEL	N	STATURE (CM)	MASS (KG)	BODY FAT (%)	FFM (KG)
Defensive backs	St. Cloud[b]	15	178.3	77.3	11.5	68.4
	U Mass[c]	12	179.9	83.1	8.8	76.8
	USC[d]	15	183.0	83.7	9.6	75.7
	Gettysburg[e]	16	175.9	79.8	13.6	68.9
	Pro, modern[f]	26	182.5	84.8	9.6	76.7
	Pro, older[g]	25	183.0	91.2	10.7	81.4
Offensive backs and receivers	St. Cloud	15	179.7	79.8	12.4	69.6
	U Mass	29	181.8	84.1	9.5	76.4
	USC	18	185.6	86.1	9.9	77.6
	Gettysburg	18	176.0	78.3	12.9	68.2
	Pro, modern	40	183.8	90.7	9.4	81.9
	Pro, older	25	183.0	91.7	10.0	87.5
Linebackers	St. Cloud	7	180.1	87.2	13.4	75.4
	U Mass	17	186.1	97.1	13.1	84.2
	USC	17	185.6	98.8	13.2	85.8
	Gettysburg	–	–	–	–	–
	Pro, modern	28	188.6	102.2	14.0	87.6
Offensive linemen and tight ends	St. Cloud	13	186.0	99.2	19.1	79.8
	U Mass	23	187.5	107.6	19.5	86.6
	Gettysburg	15	182.6	110.4	26.2	81.0
	USC	25	191.1	106.5	15.3	90.3
	Pro, modern	38	193.0	112.6	15.6	94.7
Defensive linemen	St. Cloud	15	186.6	97.8	18.5	79.3
	U Mass	8	188.8	114.3	19.5	91.9
	USC	13	191.1	109.3	14.7	93.2
	Gettysburg	11	178.0	99.4	21.9	77.6
	Pro, modern	32	192.4	117.1	18.2	95.8
	Pro, older	25	185.7	97.1	14.0	83.5
All positions	St. Cloud	65	182.5	88.0	15.0	74.2
	U Mass	91	184.9	97.3	13.9	83.2
	USC	88	186.6	96.6	11.4	84.6
	Gettysburg	60	178.0	90.6	18.1	73.3
	Pro, modern	164	188.1	101.5	13.4	87.3
	Pro, older	25	183.1	91.2	10.4	81.3
	Dallas-Jets[h]	107	188.2	100.4	12.6	87.7

[a] Grouping according to Wilmore JH, Haskel WL. Body composition and endurance capacity of professional football players. J Appl Physiol 1972;33:564.
[b] Data from Wickkiser JD, Kelly JM. The body composition of a college football team. Med Sci Sports 1975;7:199.
[c] UMass data from Coach Robert Stull and F Katch, University of Massachusetts. Data collected during spring practice, 1985; %fat by densitometry.
[d] USC data from Dr. Robert Girandola, University of Southern California, Los Angeles, 1978, 1993.
[e] Data courtesy of Dr. Kristin Steumple, Department of Exercise and Sport Science, Gettysburg College, Gettysburg, PA, 2000.
[f] Data from Wilmore JH, et al. Football pros' strengths—and CV weakness—charted. Phys Sportsmed 1976;4:45.
[g] Data from Dr. A. R. Behnke.
[h] Data from Katch FI, Katch, VL. Body composition of the Dallas Cowboys and New York Jets football teams, unpublished, 1978.

One would generally expect modern-day professional players to have a larger body size at each position than a representative collegiate group. This occurred for comparisons with St. Cloud and U Mass players, but the USC players generally maintained a physique similar to modern professionals. With the exception of defensive linemen, the USC players at each position showed nearly the same body fat content as current professionals but they weighed less. For FFM, the USC players weighed no more than 4.4 kg less than professionals at each position. The average defensive lineman in the NFL outweighed his USC counterpart in FFM by only 1.8 kg. Total body mass of the professional linemen, however, exceeded USC counterparts, primarily because the professionals possessed 18.2% body fat versus the collegians' 14.7%. These data suggest that elite college and professional players maintain similar body size and body composition.

As a group, professional players of almost 70 years ago were lower in body fat (10.4%), were shorter, and had lower total body mass and FFM than modern professionals. The exceptions, defensive and offensive backs and receivers, were almost identical to more current players in body size and composition. The biggest differences in physique emerged for the defensive linemen; modern players were 6.7 cm taller, 20 kg heavier, fatter by 4.2 percentage points of body fat, and had 12.3 kg more FFM. Obviously, "bigness" was not an important factor in line play during the 1940s. To illustrate this point, FIGURE 29.8A shows the average body mass for all roster players in the NFL (N = 51,333) over a 76-year period.[32] From

COMPARISON OF HEIGHTS AND WEIGHTS FOR OFFENSIVE AND DEFENSIVE LINEMEN FOR COLLEGIATE 2004 ROSE BOWL PARTICIPANTS AND 2004 SUPER BOWL COMPETITORS

TEAMS, 2004	OFFENSIVE LINE		DEFENSIVE LINE	
	HEIGHT, IN	WEIGHT, LB	HEIGHT, IN	WEIGHT, LB
USC Trojans	75.6	277.5	76.2	286.2
Oklahoma Sooners	76.2	275.8	75.3	263.1
Average	75.9	276.7	75.8	274.7
BMI	33.7		33.6	
NE Patriots	75.6	295.9	75.7	299.4
Philadelphia Eagles	75.8	316.9	75.9	312.9
Average	75.7	306.4	75.8	306.2
BMI	37.6		37.5	

Comparison of team roster data for height and weight for the offensive and defensive lines for the 2004 NCAA Bowl Champion Series teams (NCAA ranked University of Southern California Trojans first and Oklahoma Sooners second) and the 2004 Super Bowl New England Patriots and Philadelphia Eagles. Contrasting the above data for the USC Trojans to corresponding values for the team's 1993 National Champion position players in Table 29.8 underscores the dramatic increases in height and weight (and BMI) for the offensive and defensive linemen. Over the 12-year period, height increased an average of about 2 inches, but weight increased 42.7 pounds for offensive linemen and 45.2 pounds for the defensive linemen.

Comparing the 2004 offensive and defensive line Super Bowl players with 1995 counterparts shows that the largest changes also occurred in body weight for both teams (refer to Figure 29.8B for 1995 values). The Eagles offensive line increased on average 21 pounds while the defensive line packed on 33 pounds; the values were less dramatic for the Patriots—a 4-pound increase for the offensive line and 24-pound increase for the defensive line. If the values for offensive and defensive line are averaged and compared to the corresponding values for all the NFL teams for 1995 (Figure 29.8A), the increase averages approximately 17 pounds for the Super Bowl 2004 offensive linemen and 31 pounds for the defensive linemen. These values are close to those predicted for 2004 using the slope of the increase for all NFL players from 1920 to 1995—without a leveling-off predicted for future years. Unfortunately, the BMI for the collegiate and pro competitors places the typical championship offensive and defensive lineman at a higher than normal health risk.

1920 to 1985, offensive linemen were the heaviest players; this changed beginning with the 1990 season, when defensive linemen achieved the same body mass as offensive linemen and then surpassed them. While the body mass for offensive linemen appeared to have leveled off at nearly 280 pounds, defensive linemen continued to increase in body weight, particularly from 1990 to 1996, when they averaged 16 pounds more (double the weight gain for offensive linemen for the comparable period). On average, offensive linemen were 1.3 pounds per year heavier from 1920 to 1995. At this rate of increase, they should attain 320 pounds by the year 2007 (with an average height of 6 ft 8 in)! At this size, BMI would be 35.2, classifying them as high for disease risk (see Fig. 28.1). Even more eye opening is the body size of the 2004 Super Bowl champion's 28 offensive and defensive linemen (New England Patriots and Philadelphia Eagles). BMI averaged 38.3 (body mass, 139.2 kg; stature, 1.947 cm), the largest yet reported except for the 2001 Super Bowl teams (38.4 BMI) and far in excess of the projected 2007 value of "only" 35.2. Research must determine if such relatively homogenous groups of elite, physically active, overweight men in fact experience greater morbidity and mortality than normal-weight peers.

The body weight of offensive linemen for each of the NFL teams during the 1994 season (Fig. 29.8B) ranged from heaviest (Kansas City Chiefs; Super Bowl 1970) to lightest (San Francisco 49ers; Super Bowls 1990 and 1995). For the 1994 season, the average body weight of the winning Super Bowl offensive line (Dallas Cowboys) ranked fifth highest of 28 teams. The heaviest defensive linemen on average played for the Baltimore Colts while the Cowboys fielded the lightest defensive line.

A recent report presented BMI data for 2168 NFL players based on 2004 team rosters.[23] The results were consistent with the data presented in Figure 29.8—almost all of the players had a BMI that exceeded 25 (97%), 56% had BMIs greater than 30, 26% had BMIs greater than 35, and 3% had BMIs greater than 40. Compared to 20- to 39-year-old men in a 1999–2002 national survey, the percentage of NFL players within the same age range with a BMI of 30 or greater was twice that of the national sample (56% v. 23%). The percentage of players with a BMI of 40 or greater was similar to that among 20- to 39-year-old men in a 1999–2002 survey (3.0% vs 3.7%). Compared to the NIH classification categories of obesity (Chapter 30), 564 players (36% of the sample) qualified as obesity class 2, with 65 players in obesity class 3. The authors concluded, as have we, that the high prevalence of obesity (overweight based on BMI) in this group of large men warrants further investigation to determine the short- and long-term health consequences of excessive weight. The data in the *unnumbered table* above

Figure 29.8 **A.** Average body weight by position for all roster players in the NFL between 1920 and 1995. **B.** Average body weight of all roster offensive and defensive linemen in the NFL in 1994. Team rankings progress from the heaviest to lightest body weight for the team's offensive linemen. (From active team rosters for 28 NFL teams as of the first regular-season weekend, September 4–5, 1994. The comparison body weight data for the pro offensive and defensive line (1977) shown in the *inset box* are combined data for the New York Jets and Dallas Cowboys football teams (collected by textbook's authors FK and VK). The 1942 data were provided by Dr. Albert Behnke from his studies of the Washington Redskins. (Data courtesy of the National Football League public relations department.)

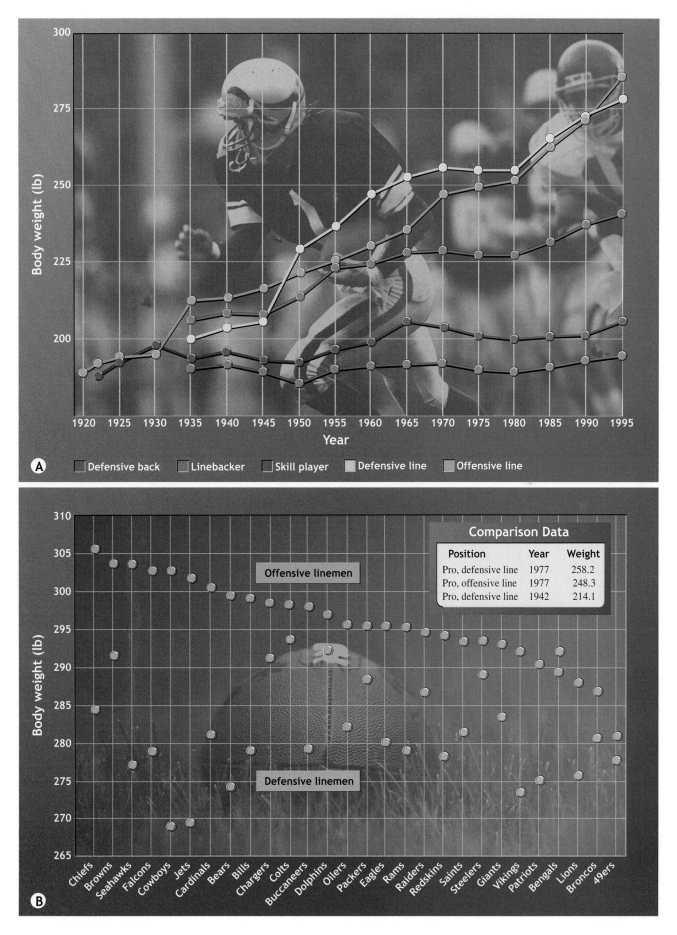

PREDICTING BODY FAT FROM SKINFOLDS, GIRTHS, AND BIA MEASUREMENTS FOR DIFFERENT ATHLETIC GROUPS

■ Appropriate assessment of body composition allows determination of optimal body weight for competition, comparisons between athletes within the same sport, and monitoring changes in the body's lean and fat components resulting from dietary modification and/or exercise training. A valid appraisal of body composition also provides an important first step in identifying potential eating disorders and formulating nutritional counseling. In the absence of body fat appraisal by hydrostatic weighing, predictions using skinfolds and/or girth measurements and bioelectric impedance analysis (BIA) have been used for diverse athletic groups.

The body's fat-free component can vary, making multicomponent models most effective to convert whole-body density to percentage body fat. The accompanying table presents population-specific skinfold, anthropometric (girth), and BIA equations for body composition assessment of athletes in general and in specific sport categories.

Method	Sport	Gender	Equation	Reference
Skinfolds	All	Women (18-29 y)	Db (g · cm^{-3})^a = 1.096095 – 0.0006952 (Σ4SKF) + 0.0000011 (Σ4SKF)^2 – 0.0000714 (age)	29
	All	Boys (14-19 y)	Db (g · cm^{-3})^a = 1.10647 – 0.00162 (subscapular SKF) – 0.00144 (abdomen SKF) – 0.00077 (triceps SKF) + 0.00071 (midaxillary SKF)	19
	All	Men (18-29 y)	Db (g · cm^{-3})^a = 1.112 – 0.00043499 (Σ7SKF) + 0.00000055 (Σ7SKF) – 0.00028826 (age)	28
	Wrestling	Boys (HS)	Db (g · cm^{-3})^a = 1.0982 – 0.000815 (Σ3SKF) – 0.00000084 (Σ3SKF)^2	55
BIA	All	Women (NR)	FFM (kg) = 0.73 (HT^2/R) + 0.23 (X$_c$) + 0.16 (BW) + 2.0	27
	All	Women (college)	FFM (kg) = 0.73 (HT^2/R) + 0.116 (BW) + 0.096 (X$_c$) – 4.03	40
	All	Men (college)	FFM (kg) = 0.734 (HT^2/R) + 0.116 (BW) + 0.096 (X$_c$) – 3.152	40
	All	Men (19-40 y)	FFM (kg) = 1.949 + 0.701 (BW) + 0.186 (HT^2/R)	43
Anthropometry (girths)	All	Women (18-23 y)	FFM (kg) = 0.757 (BW) + 0.981 (neck C) – 0.516 (thigh C) + 0.79	42
	Ballet	Females (11-25 y)	FFM (kg) = 0.73 (BW) + 3.0	23
	Wrestling	Boys (13-18 y)	Db (g · cm^{-3})^a = 1.12691 – 0.00357 (arm C) – 0.00127 (AB C) + 0.00524 (forearm C)	31
	Football	White men (18-23 y)	%BF = 55.2 + 0.481 (BW) – 0.468 (HT)	26

From Heyward VH, Stolarczyk LM. Applied body composition assessment. Champaign, IL: Human Kinetics, 1996.

4SKF (mm) = sum of four skinfolds: triceps + anterior suprailiac + abdomen + thigh; 7SKF (mm) = sum of seven skinfolds: chest + midaxillary + triceps + subscapular + abdomen + anterior suprailiac + thigh; HT = height (cm); R = resistance (Ω); Xc = reactance (Ω); BW = body weight (kg); C= circumference (cm); thigh (cm) at the gluteal fold; AB (cm): average abdominal circumference = [(AB$_1$ + AB$_2$)/2], where AB$_1$ (cm) = abdominal circumference anteriorly midway between the xyphoid process of the sternum and umbilicus, and laterally between the lower end of the rib cage and iliac crests, and AB$_2$ (cm) = abdominal circumference at the umbilicus level; NR = age not reported; HS = high school.

^{a}Use the following formulas to convert body density (Db) to % body fat (BF): Men %BF = [(4.95/Db) – 4.50] X 100; Women %BF = [(5.01/Db) – 4.57] X 100; Boys (7-12y) %BF = [(5.30/Db) – 4.89] X 100; Boys (13-16y) %BF = [(5.07/Db) – 4.64] X 100; Boys (17-19y) %BF = [(4.99/Db) – 4.55] X 100.

continued on page 829

Continued

EXAMPLE CALCULATIONS

Boy Athlete (18 y)

Data: Subscapular (SS) skinfold, 10 mm; abdominal (AB) skinfold, 18 mm; triceps (TRI) skinfold, 10 mm; midaxillary (MA) skinfold, 8 mm

$$Db = 1.10647 - (0.00162 \times SS_{SKF}) - (0.00144 \times AB_{SKF}) - (0.00077 \times TRI_{SKF}) + (0.00071 \times MA_{SKF})$$
$$= 1.10647 - (0.00162 \times 10) - (0.00144 \times 18) - (0.00077 \times 10) + (0.00071 \times 8)$$
$$= 1.10647 - 0.0162 - 0.02592 - 0.0077 + 0.00568$$
$$= 1.06233$$

$$\%BF = [(499 \div Db) - 455] \times 100$$
$$= [(499 \div 1.06233) - 455] \times 100$$
$$= 14.7\%$$

Female Ballet Dancer (20 y)

Data: Body weight, 55.0 kg
$$FFM \, (kg) = (0.73 \times BW) + 3.0$$
$$= 43.15 \, kg$$
$$\%BF = [(BW - FFM) \div BW] \times 100$$
$$= [(55 - 43.15) \div 55] \times 100$$
$$= 21.5\%$$

Male Football Player (20 y)

Data: Body weight, 105.0 kg; stature, 188 cm
$$\%BF = 55.2 + (0.481 \times BW) - (0.468 \times HT)$$
$$= 55.2 + (0.481 \times 105) - (0.468 \times 188)$$
$$= 55.2 + 50.51 - 87.98$$
$$= 17.7\%$$

---

make this very point—large-size athletes, in the short term, are at higher than normal risk for a variety of disease states.

A Worrisome Trend Even Among Less-Skilled and Younger Players. Exceptionally high BMIs also occur at less elite levels of collegiate competition. The average BMI of 33.1 for the Division III 1999 Gettysburg offensive line (*N* = 15) (29.9 for 2000 offensive line, *N* = 13),[53] and the BMI of 31.7 for other NCAA division III American football linemen (*N* = 26; 1994–1995) raises similar concern about potential health risks for such large young men (stature, 1.84 m; body mass, 107.2 kg).[49] At the high school level, the BMI of Parade Magazine's All-American football teams increased dramatically beginning in the early 1970s through 1989 and then further increased in rate of gain to the year 2004.[60] The plot in FIGURE 29.9 shows a clear shift at 1972 in the slope of the regression line (*yellow line*) relating BMI to year of competition compared with age-matched individuals from large-scale epidemiologic normative data (*red line*). This shift toward a higher BMI coincided with either improved nutrition and training and/or the emerging prevalence among high school athletes of performance-enhancing drugs (chiefly anabolic steroids),[58] a finding confirmed in a subsequent report.[5] Particularly disturbing are the most recent 2004 data for high school offensive and defensive linemen, for which the average BMI ranged between 32.3 and 40.4. For the last data point for the Parade Magazine 2004 high school football players, BMI has in just 4 years increased dramatically to 35.6 (stature, 195.9 cm; mass, 136.1 kg). Their values for stature and body mass now exceed the average values for the 2004 National Champion USC Trojan collegiate linemen (stature, 192.8 cm; body mass, 127.8 kg), runner-up Oklahoma Sooners (stature, 192.4 cm; body mass, 122.2 kg), and 2004 Super Bowl teams!

The implications of such huge body mass in terms of current health risk (e.g., high blood pressure, insulin resistance, and type 2 diabetes) and long-term outlook remain undetermined but certainly are not encouraging. Interestingly, disordered breathing problems during sleep are prevalent among Canadian professional football players.[21] The average neck girth (45.2 cm; 17.7 in) and elevated BMI (31.5) in those players predicted risk for sleep-disordered breathing and apnea (and accompanying snoring). Certainly the large-size high school players (and top college and NFL large players) are likely to have sleep-associated disorders that could affect performance and future health.

Other Longitudinal Trends in Body Size. To expand upon longitudinal trends for body size among elite athletes, we determined stature and body mass for two groups of professional athletes: (1) all National Basketball Association (NBA) players from 1970 to 1993 (*N* ranged from 156 to 400) and (2) professional major league baseball players from 28 teams during the 1986, 1988, 1990, 1992, and 1995 seasons (*N* = 5031 roster players).

For the NBA players (FIG. 29.10A), average body mass increased by 3.8 pounds (1.7 kg) or 1.8% during the 23-year interval. Stature increased more slowly; it changed by only 1 inch, or less than 1% over the same interval. The NBA players' BMI during this time remained within a narrow range of 0.8 BMI units, from 23.6 to 24.4. Major League Baseball players (shown in *red* in the same figure) show slightly higher mean values than do the basketball players. Compared with American professional and collegiate football players, baseball and basketball athletes have maintained BMIs within guidelines considered relatively healthful for minimizing mortality and disease risk.

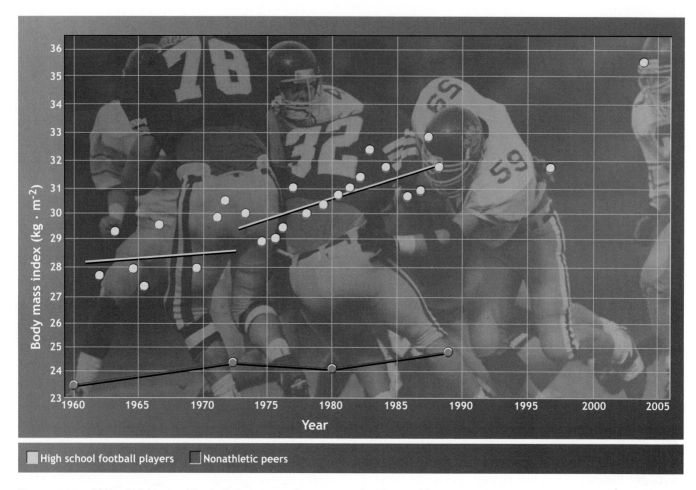

Figure 29.9 BMIs of high school football players over time compared with nonathlete counterparts.

INTEGRATIVE QUESTION

Why doesn't a singular prototype for body composition (%fat, FFM) consistently emerge when one analyzes the body composition of elite athletes in different sports?

High School Wrestlers

Wrestlers have represented a unique athletic group who train intensely and undergo repeated bouts of rapid weight loss and regain and possible chronic undernutrition.[6,15,65] Prior to recent rule changes, adolescent wrestlers would maintain long-term dietary restriction for both energy and protein during the wrestling season.[48] This pattern of food intake reduces lean tissue mass, fat stores, and muscular strength and power. In previous years, despite warnings from medical and professional groups about rapid weight loss,[2,3] most high school and college wrestlers (except heavyweights) reduced weight a few days before or on competition day. They would lose 2 to 6 kg, hoping to gain a competitive advantage by wrestling in a lower weight category.[1,66] The wrestler who "made weight" usually combined food restriction and dehydration, either through fluid and food deprivation and/or by exercising in a hot environment while wearing plastic or rubber garments. Diuretics, laxatives, extended time in a sauna or steam room, and vomiting also induced weight loss. In one study, 2% of intercollegiate wrestlers exhibited bulimic behaviors.[57] Unfortunately, the information for these athletes about how best to lose weight came from other wrestlers, not the coach, athletic trainer, or informed parents.[56] A typical wrestler experienced weight loss–weight gain from 7 to 15 times each year and repeated the cycle more than 100 times during a career.[58]

The pattern of weight loss and regain during NCAA Division I, II, and III wrestling championships remained consistent among wrestling weight categories but not levels of competition.[50] Twenty hours following the official weigh-in, wrestlers were reweighed before the first round of competition; on average, they regained 4.9% of body mass in 20 hours. The lightest-weight wrestlers gained the most relative weight (4.5 kg, or 7.8% of body mass), while heavyweights gained the least weight (0.7% of body mass). Wrestlers who advanced to the second tournament round all regained lost weight, often as much as 7 kg (15.4 lb) in a 12-hour period. To discourage rapid weight loss, the ACSM and NCAA established minimal wrestling weight standards based on body fat percentage (discussed in Chapter 14) and now holds weigh-ins immediately before competition. Chapter 30 discusses how to determine minimal weight for wrestlers and presents a prudent approach

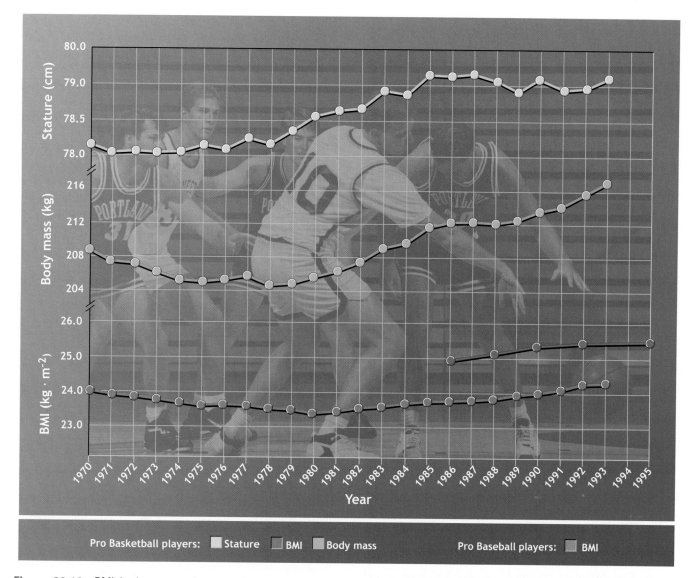

Figure 29.10   BMI, body mass, and stature of professional NBA players (1970–1993) and BMI of major league baseball players (1986–1995). (Data for NBA players from team rosters, compiled by F. Katch; major league baseball data from team rosters courtesy of Major League Baseball.)

to reduce body fat. The NCAA procedure to predict minimal wrestling weight is accurate and precise based on cross-validation methods that used diverse techniques to assess body composition.[12]

 INTEGRATIVE QUESTION

A football coach wishes to field a team whose players are not overly fat. He selects the frequently used BMI to screen out players with excessive body fat. What are the possible outcomes of his decision for football performance?

Prudent Recommendations for Wrestlers.   The Gatorade Sports Science Institute (www.qssiweb.com) presents nutrition guidelines for wrestlers. Downloads are available in PDF format. This includes general body composition and nutritional recommendations for wrestlers once the appropriate wrestling

weight has been established and achieved. Coaches should regularly assess their wrestlers' body composition and hydration and nutrition status. In response to the deaths of three collegiate wrestlers in 1997 from excessive weight loss (largely from dehydration), the NCAA introduced rule changes for the 1998–99 season to discourage dangerous weight-cutting practices and increase safe participation.[13] In addition to establishing a minimal wrestling weight, another rule change measures urine specific gravity (density of urine to the density of water). This assessment of hydration status ensures euhydration of wrestlers at weight certification. Athletes with a urine specific gravity of 1.020 or less are considered euhydrated, while those with specific gravity in excess of 1.020 cannot have body fat measured to determine minimum competitive wrestling weight for the season. Urine specific gravity reflects hydration status, but it lags behind true hydration status during rapid body fluid turnover with acute dehydration as used by wrestlers to make weight. Such a scenario would fail to detect a large number of dehydrated wrestlers.[46]

Weight Lifters and Bodybuilders

Men. Resistance-trained athletes, particularly bodybuilders, Olympic weight lifters, and power weight lifters, exhibit remarkable muscular development and FFM combined with a relatively lean physique.[34] Percentage body fat (underwater weighing) averaged 9.3% in bodybuilders, 9.1% in power weight lifters, and 10.8% in Olympic weight lifters. Considerable leanness exists for each group of athletes, even though height–weight tables classify up to 19% of these men as overweight. The groups did not differ in skeletal frame size, FFM, skinfolds, and bone diameters. The only differences occurred for shoulders, chest, biceps, and forearm girths; bodybuilders were larger at each site. The bodybuilders exhibited nearly 16 kg more muscle than predicted for their size; power weight lifters, 15 kg; and Olympic weight lifters, 13 kg.

Women. Bodybuilding gained widespread popularity among women in the United States during the late 1970s. As women aggressively undertook the vigorous demands of resistance training, competition became more intense and achievement level increased. Bodybuilding success depends upon a slim and lean appearance complemented by a well-defined yet enlarged musculature, raising interesting questions about the women's body composition. How lean do the competitors become, and does a relatively large muscle mass accompany low body-fat levels?

Body composition assessment of 10 competitive female bodybuilders averaged of 13.2% body fat (range, 8.0–18.3%) and 46.6 kg FFM.[20] Except for champion gymnasts, who also average about 13% body fat, bodybuilders were 3 to 4% shorter, 4 to 5% lighter, and had 7 to 10% lower total body fat mass than other top female athletes. The bodybuilders' most striking compositional characteristic, a dramatically large FFM:FM ratio of 7:1, nearly doubles the 4.3:1 ratio for other female athletic groups. This difference presumably occurred without steroid use. Interestingly, 8 of the 10 bodybuilders reported normal menstrual function with concurrent relatively low body fat. When female bodybuilders train for competition during a 12-week preparation period, approximately 76% of the total fat lost (−5.8 kg; from 18.3% to 12.7% body fat) occurred primarily from reduced fat mass and not fat-free mass (−1.4 kg decline).[59] Decreases in body mass and fat mass over the final 6 weeks exceeded changes over the first 6 weeks (a control group remained essentially unchanged). A 25.5-mm decline in the sum of triceps, subscapular, biceps, iliac crest, supraspinale, abdominal, front thigh, and medial calf skinfolds accompanied the body composition changes. This experiment reveals that healthy females at the lower end of the body fat continuum can still reduce fat mass over a 3-month training duration to a level that approaches the theoretical boundary for storage fat without apparent deleterious, acute health effects.

Men Versus Women. TABLE 29.9 compares body composition, girths, and excess body mass of male and female bodybuilders. Excess mass represents the difference between actual body mass and body mass-for-stature from the Metropolitan Life Insurance tables. Overweight for the men corresponded to a 14.8-kg (18%) excess; and for the women, a 1.2-kg (12%) excess. Obviously, excess body mass in these lean athletes primarily reflected FFM as increased skeletal muscle mass.

Contrasts of the girth data allow comparison of individuals (or groups) who differ in body size. The analysis shows that gender differences in girths when scaled to body size (referred to as "adjusted" in the table) do not differ as much as the uncorrected absolute girth values. Relative to body size, females exceed the male bodybuilders in 7 of 12 body areas. *Women probably can alter muscle size to almost the same relative extent as men, at least when scaled to body size.* The larger hip size in women probably reflects greater fat stores in this location.

INTEGRATIVE QUESTION

Do established gender differences in body composition justify sex-specific normative standards to evaluate different components of physical fitness and motor performance?

UPPER LIMIT FOR FAT-FREE BODY MASS

The FFM for Japanese elite sumo wrestlers *(seki-tori)* averages 109 kg.[38] These athletes share the distinction of being the world's largest with some American professional football players who weigh 159 kg (350 lb). It seems unlikely that athletes in this weight range would possess less than 15% body fat; the FFMs of the largest football players at 15% body fat theoretically corresponds to 135 kg. In reality, a football player with a body mass of 159 kg would more likely have 20 to 25% body fat. At 20% body fat, the FFM would be about 127 kg, certainly the highest value ever attained by hydrostatic weighing. But this value remains hypothetical in the absence of reliable data. Even for an exceptionally large professional basketball player (body mass, 138.3 kg [305 lb]; stature, 210.8 cm [83 in]), percentage body fat is unlikely to be less than 10% of body mass. Thus, fat mass equals 13.8 kg and FFM equals 114.2 kg—perhaps an upper limit FFM value for an athlete of such dimensions.

To gain additional insight into the question of an upper limit in FFM among athletes, we reviewed more than 30 years of body composition data from our laboratories to determine the largest FFM values determined densitometrically. Thirty-five athletes exceeded an FFM of 100 kg; the top five values were 114.3, 109.7, 108.4, 107.6, and 105.6. The three top values were larger than the two values of 106.5 kg reported for defensive football linemen from 1969–1971 data[3] and for other resistance-trained athletes.[17]

The body composition of an exceptionally large professional football player (NFL Oakland Raiders; unpublished data, Dr. Robert Girandola, Department of Kinesiology, University of Southern California) determined by repeated trials of underwater weighing exceeds values for FFM presented in research literature. The player, with a body fat content of 11.3%. (body mass, 141.4 kg; stature, 193 cm; BMI, 38.4),

TABLE 29.9 ■ BODY COMPOSITION AND ANTHROPOMETRIC GIRTHS OF MALE AND FEMALE BODYBUILDERS

SEX	AGE (Y)	MASS (KG)	STATURE (CM)	FAT (%)	FFM (KG)	EXCESS MASS[a] (KG)
Male[b] (N = 18)	27.0	82.4	177.1	9.3	74.6	14.8
Female[c] (N = 10)	27.0	53.8	160.8	13.2	46.6	1.2

	MALES		FEMALES		% DIFFERENCE (MALES VS. FEMALES)	
BODY PART (CM)	RAW	ADJUSTED[d]	RAW	ADJUSTED[d]	RAW	ADJUSTED[d]
Shoulders	123.1	37.1	101.7	36.7	17.4	1.1
Chest	106.4	32.1	90.6	32.7	14.9	−1.9
Waist	82.0	24.7	64.5	23.3	21.3	5.7
Abdomen	82.3	24.8	67.7	25.1	15.3	−1.2
Hips	95.6	28.8	87.0	31.4	9.0	−9.0
Biceps relaxed	35.9	10.8	25.8	9.3	28.1	13.9
Biceps flexed	40.4	12.2	28.9	10.4	28.5	14.8
Forearm	30.7	9.2	24.0	8.7	21.8	5.4
Wrist	17.4	5.2	15.1	5.4	13.2	−3.8
Thigh	59.6	17.9	53.0	19.1	11.1	−6.7
Calf	37.3	11.2	32.4	11.7	13.1	−4.5
Ankle	22.8	6.9	26.3	7.3	11.0	−5.8

[a] Body mass minus body mass estimated from height–weight tables.
[b] Katch VL, et al. Muscular development and lean body weight in body-builders and weight lifters. Med Sci Sports 1980;12:340..
[c] Freedson PS, et al. Physique, body composition, and psychological characteristics of competitive female bodybuilders. Phys Sportsmed 1983;11:85.
[d] Calculated as $Gi/\sqrt{mass (kg)}/stature (dm)^{0.7}$, where Gi equals any one of the girths. The term $(mass/stature^{0.7})$ is a frame structure estimate of perimetric (girth) size. The adjusted values are the perimetric equivalent adjusted girths due to sex differences, because they are corrected for whatever differences may exist as a result of differences in body size.

had a FFM of 125.4 kg, the uppermost value ever reported. With the continuing increase in the body size of pro football offensive and defensive players, this player's large FFM determined in 1997 before he turned professional will probably not remain the peak value for FFM as body composition data on other large athletes become available. In the absence of additional data, we assume that 125.4 kg represents the current upper limit of FFM in elite athletes.

Summary

1. Athletes generally have physique characteristics unique to their specific sport. Field-event athletes have a relatively large FFM and a high percentage body fat; distance runners possess the least amount of lean tissue and fat mass.
2. Champion performance blends unique physique characteristics and highly developed physiologic support systems.
3. Male and female triathletes possess a body composition and aerobic capacity most similar to elite bicyclists.
4. Body composition analyses of American football players reveal they are among the heaviest of all athletes, yet maintain a relatively lean body composition. At the highest levels of competition, Division I collegiate and professional football players show remarkable similarity in body size and composition.
5. Top-rated high school football linemen (2004) exceed the stature and body mass (and BMI) of 2004 NFL Super Bowl participants and 2004 NCAA Division I champion offensive and defensive linemen.
6. Competitive male and female swimmers generally have higher body fat levels than distance runners. The difference probably results from self-selection related to economically exercising in the different environments rather than real metabolic effects caused by the environments.
7. To discourage rapid weight loss, the ACSM and NCAA established minimal wrestling weight standards based on body fat percentage and holding weigh-ins immediately before competition.
8. Female bodybuilders alter muscle size to the same relative extent as male bodybuilders.
9. The FFM:FM ratio of competitive female bodybuilders exceeds the FFM:FM ratio of other elite female athletes.
10. A value of 125.4 kg represents the current upper limit of FFM of elite athletes.

References are available on the Student CD and online at http://connection.lww.com/mkk6e.

Overweight, Obesity, and Weight Control

30

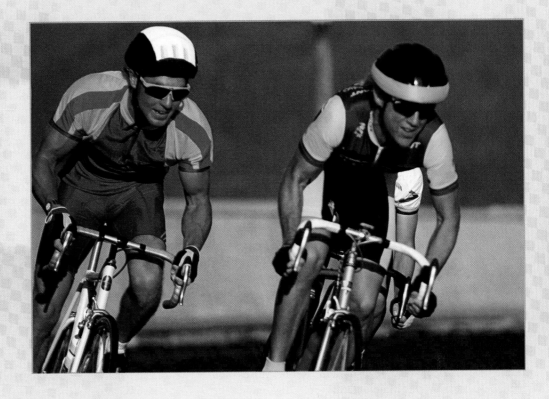

CHAPTER OBJECTIVES

- Discuss the scope of overfatness and obesity

- Distinguish between overweight, overfat, and obesity

- Evaluate the contribution of inherited factors to the development of excess body fat

- List 10 important health risks of excessive body fat

- Describe the relationship between excess body weight in childhood and adolescence and risk for obesity and poor health in adulthood

- Discuss each of the following criteria for excessive body fat: (1) percentage body fat, (2) regional fat distribution, and (3) fat cell size and number

- Compare fat cell size and number in individuals with average body fat and those massively obese

- Describe general effects of weight gain and loss on adult fat cell size and number

- Outline three approaches to "unbalance" the energy balance equation to induce weight loss

- Describe characteristics of individuals who successfully maintain prolonged weight loss

- Summarize proposed advantages and disadvantages of ketogenic diets, high-protein diets, and very low-calorie diets for reducing body fat

- Present the rationale for including regular physical activity in a prudent weight-loss program

- Review how moderate increases in physical activity for a previously sedentary, overly fat person affect (1) daily food intake and (2) energy expenditure on a short- and long-term basis

- Outline why combining regular physical activity with moderate food restriction achieves successful weight loss

- Summarize how different exercise modes affect body composition during weight loss

- Explain whether specific (target) exercises induce localized fat loss

- Give diet and exercise advice for gaining body weight to improve appearance or enhance sports performance

PART 1 • *Obesity*

HISTORICAL PERSPECTIVE

Throughout history, biblical scholars have preached against the ills of excessive food intake and sedentary living. For example, the 12th century Jewish sage, Rabbi Moses ben Maimon (also known as Maimonides;1138–1204), quotes the incomparable Greek physician Galen (AD 129–201; refer to *Roots and Historical Perspectives* in the Introduction of this text) in one of his many essays on health, that excess fat is harmful to the body and makes it sluggish, disturbs its functions, and hinders its movements. Maimonides also taught, indeed prophetically, that everyone who practices a sedentary lifestyle and does not exercise will live his or her life a painful one. He posited that excessive eating is like a deadly poison to the body and a principal cause of all illness.

Hippocrates (b. 460–377 BC), the ancient Greek physician regarded as the Father of Medicine, taught that obesity is a health risk and considered it a cause of disease that led to death. The Hippocratic texts conveyed the overarching belief that obesity deviated from the norm or ideal so essential for maintaining a healthy balance to all aspects of life. Galen and others wrote essays that extolled the virtues of walking, running, wrestling, rope climbing, and vigorous, physically active pursuits in addition to baths, massage, rest, and an "appropriate" lifestyle as antidotes to rebalance one's health. Interestingly, Hippocrates believed that one strategy for losing weight was for obese individuals to undertake exercise before eating and to eat while still breathing hard. The practice of modulating food intake for dietary control of disease conditions was made easier in the first half of the 9th century by an

ancient physician of Baghdad, Yuhanna ibn Masawayh (known in the Western world as Jean Mesue). He produced the first treatise concerning dietetics, incorporating ideas from the earlier writings of Galen. He was one of the first "medical nutritionists" to accurately describe the properties of 140 foodstuffs from the plant and animal kingdoms and their effects on the human body.

For the past 20 centuries, medical practitioners (and writers, philosophers, scientists, and theologians) throughout the world have advocated a sensible approach to healthy living, but apparently without much success. Bray in the following quote, provides a succinct summary of the historical development of scientific and cultural ideas about obesity from the ancients to the present:[19]

> Scholarly theses on this subject began to appear in the late 16th century with the first monographs published in the 18th century. The values of dietary restriction, increasing exercise, and reducing the amount of sleep were identified early in medical history dating at least from the time of Hippocrates. These concepts were often framed in a manner that implied a 'moral' weakness on the part of the overweight individual. Cases of massive obesity were identified in stone-age carvings and have been described frequently since the time of Galen and the Roman Empire. More specific types of obesity began to be identified in the 19th century. Following the identification of the cell as the basic building block of animals and plants, fat cells were described and the possibility that obesity was due to too many fat cells was suggested. After the introduction of the calorimeter by Lavoisier, the suggestion that obesity might represent a metabolic derangement has been suggested and tested. Standards for measuring body weight appeared in the 19th century. The possibility that familial factors might also be involved was clearly identified in the 18th and 19th century. Most of the concepts that are currently the basis for research in the field of obesity had their origin in the 19th century and often earlier.

Overweight, Overfat, and Obesity: No Unanimity for Terminology

Confusion surrounds the precise meaning of the terms *overweight, overfat,* and *obesity*. Each term takes on a different meaning depending on the situation and context. In most medical literature, *overweight* describes an overly fat condition, even in the absence of accompanying body fat measures, and *obesity* refers to individuals at the extreme of the overweight continuum.

Research and contemporary discussion among diverse disciplines reinforces the need to distinguish between overweight, overfat, and obesity to ensure consistency in use and interpretation. In proper context, the **overweight** condition refers to a body weight that exceeds some average for stature and perhaps age, usually by a standard deviation unit or percentage. As we discussed in Chapter 28, the overweight condition *frequently* accompanies an increase in body fat, but not always (e.g., male power athletes), and may or may not coincide with the comorbidities glucose intolerance, insulin resistance, dyslipidemia, and hypertension (e.g., physically fit over-fat men and women).

When an index of body fat is available, researchers can more accurately place body fat level on a continuum from low to high, independent of body weight. **Overfatness** then would refer to a condition where body fat exceeds an age- and/or gender-appropriate average by a predetermined amount. In most situations, "overfatness" represents the correct term when assessing individual and group body fat levels.

The term obesity refers to the overfat condition that accompanies a constellation of comorbidities that includes one or all of the following components of the "**obese syndrome**": glucose intolerance, insulin resistance, dyslipidemia, type 2 diabetes, hypertension, elevated plasma leptin concentrations, increased visceral adipose tissue, and increased risk of coronary heart disease and cancer. Limited research suggests that excess body fat, not excess body weight per se, explains the relation between above average body weight and disease risk.[209] Such findings emphasize the importance of distinguishing the composition of excess body weight to determine an overweight person's disease risk.

Many men and women may be overweight or overfat but do not exhibit components of the obese syndrome (a diseased state). In this case, we urge caution in applying the term obesity (instead of overfatness) in all cases of excessive body weight. We acknowledge the interchangeability of these terms (as we at times do in this text) to designate the same condition.

CURRENT STATUS

In our modern scientific era in which astronauts explore the weightless environment while circumventing the globe, bioengineers develop microsurgical procedures to prolong and enhance life's quality, and molecular geneticists unravel basic secrets of subcellular function, no clear answer exists to a seemingly simple question: "Why have so many people become too fat, and what can be done to reduce the problem?" A random-digit telephone survey of nearly 110,000 adults in the United States found that large numbers struggle to lose weight or just maintain body weight.[211] Only one fifth of the 45 to 50 million Americans attempting to lose weight use the recommended combination of eating fewer calories and engaging in at least 150 minutes of weekly leisure-time physical activity. Those attempting weight loss spend nearly $40 billion annually on diet books and beverages alone, often relying on potentially harmful dietary practices and drugs while ignoring sensible weight-loss programs. Each year, approximately 2 million Americans pay more than $135 million on appetite-suppressing, over-the-counter diet pills that line drugstore, health food and fitness center, and supermarket shelves, not to mention countless TV infomercials and radio direct marketing and mail order and Internet sales. Notwithstanding the upswing in attempts to lose weight, Americans are considerably more overweight than a generation ago. In the United States, 3.8 million people now exceed 300 pounds—the equivalent of the combined populations of the Bahamas, Cayman Islands, Iceland, Qatar, and the United

Arab Emirates! Obesity is an equal opportunity affliction, increasing dramatically in all regions of the United States.[160,161]

WORLDWIDE EPIDEMIC

FIGURE 30.1 compares national surveys of overweight and obesity prevalence among adults in the United States during the measurement periods 1988–1994 and 1999–2002. Current classification by the National Heart Lung and Blood Institute defines overweight as a body mass index (BMI) of 25 to 29.9 and obesity as a BMI ≥ 30. These standards place the prevalence of overweight and obesity in adults at about 130 million Americans, or 65% of the population (including 35% of college students[147]), up from 56% in 1982. Overweight occurrence is particularly high among women and minority groups (Hispanic, African American, Pacific Islanders). The major increase results from a near doubling of the obesity component to one in four Americans over the past two decades.[135,258] As of February 2006, about 31% of the adult population (60+ million people) classify as obese, compared with only 14.5% in 1980. Similar increases in obesity exist worldwide.[70,137,184,249] Such alarming rates of increase contribute to the rising onslaught of diabetes and cardiovascular disease—prompting the World Health Organization (www.who.int/en/) and the International Obesity Task Force (www.iotf.org/) to declare a global obesity epidemic. Worldwide estimates indicate that 300 million people are obese and 750 million more are overweight. Obesity is now the second leading cause of preventable deaths in the United States (300,000 deaths yearly; smoking is first), with a total upper annual cost estimated at $140 billion (www.obesity.org) or approximately 10% of the U.S.

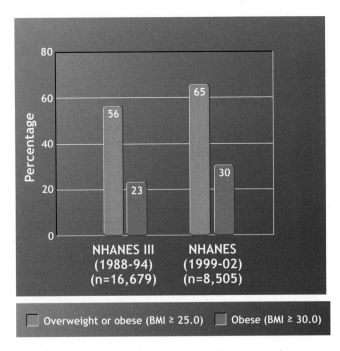

Figure 30.1 The fattening of America. Prevalence of overweight and obesity among adults in the United States during the measurement periods 1988–94 and 1999–02. NHANES, National Health and Nutrition Examination Survey.

health care expenditures.[2] FIGURE 30.2 depicts the powerful effect of excess body weight in predicting death at an older age. Overweight, but not obese, nonsmoking men and women in their mid-30s to mid-40s die at least 3 years sooner than normal-weight counterparts, a risk just as damaging to life expectancy as cigarette smoking. Obese individuals can expect about a 7-year decrease in longevity. Correctly, physicians tell us to eat less and increase the time spent exercising. In industrialized nations, economic factors operate to counter this advice: food continues to become cheaper and more fat laden, while most occupations have not changed or decreased their exertional demands.

A milestone in American governmental action took place on December 1, 2003. The United States Preventive Services Task Force, a government advisory group composed of medical experts, urged physicians to weigh and measure all patients and recommend counseling and behavior therapy for those found to be obese. Specifically, the group recommended that doctors prescribe intensive behavior therapy at least twice monthly (in indi-vidual or group sessions) for up to 3 months under supervision of a health-professional team of psychologists, registered dietitians, and exercise specialists. These guidelines, which usually become the standard of care for medical practice, represent a major shift in how the health care system treats obesity and may prompt health plans and insurers to pay for obesity treatment.

Children experience an equally depressing situation, because the prevalence of overweight in children (BMI > 95th percentile for age and sex) has attained grim proportions.[170,228] A comprehensive report released on September 30, 2004, by the National Academies of the Institutes of Medicine (www.iom.edu/) on the causes and solutions for childhood obesity in the United States indicates that in the last 30 years childhood obesity has tripled among children ages 6 to 11 (particularly in rural America), to more than 15%; rates have doubled for those aged 2 to 5 (>10%) and from 12 to 19, to more than 15%. Obesity represents childhood's most common chronic disorder, particularly prevalent among poor and minority children.[31,62,238] Part of this rise in body weight relates to the nearly

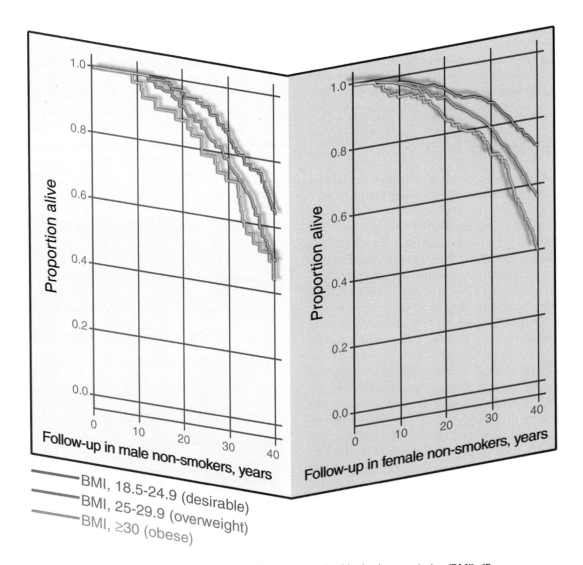

Figure 30.2 Survival estimates for women and men categorized by body mass index (BMI). (From Peeters A, et al. Obesity in adulthood and its consequences for life expectancy. Ann Intern Med 2003;138:24.)

300% increase between 1977 and 1996 in the foods that children consume from restaurants and fast-food outlets.[227] Also, soft drink consumption in young consumers accounts for an additional 188 kCal per day above energy intakes of children who do not consume these beverages.[225] Excessive fatness in youth represents an even greater adult health risk than obesity begun in adulthood. Overweight children and adolescents, regardless of final body weight as adults, exhibit higher risk of a broad range of illnesses as adults than adolescents of normal weight.[80,244]

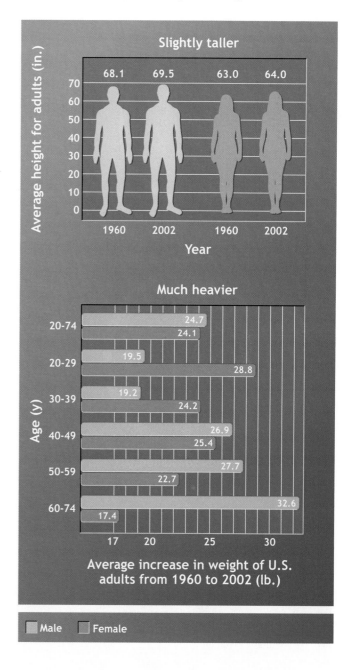

REASONS FOR CLASSIFYING OVERWEIGHT AND OBESITY
■ Provides meaningful comparisons of body weight status within and between populations
■ Identifies individuals and groups at increased risk of morbidity and mortality
■ Identifies priorities for intervention at individual and community levels
■ Establishes a firm basis for evaluating diverse intervention strategies
Source: World Health Organization

Substantial alterations in the population's gene pool (requiring millions of years of evolutionary change) cannot explain the dramatic nationwide obesity increase since 1980. Researchers maintain that if the progression of obesity continues at the current rate, the entire population will be overweight within a few generations. By 2025, 75% of the American population will classify as overweight, with about one third classified obese. More than likely, a sedentary lifestyle and ready availability of tasty, lipid- and calorie-rich foods served in increasingly larger portions remain prime culprits for expressing unhealthy patterns of preexisting susceptible genes in the fattening of Western civilization as depicted in the unnumbered figure on this page.[15,32]

A PROGRESSIVE LONG-TERM PROCESS

Excess accumulation of body fat (i.e., overfatness), represents a heterogeneous disorder in which energy intake chronically exceeds energy expenditure. Disruption in energy balance often begins in childhood, and if this occurs (particularly among older children at the upper decile for body fat), the chance for adult obesity increases considerably.[81,244] For example, obese children at ages 6 to 9 have a 55% chance of becoming obese as adults—a risk 10 times that of children of normal weight. Simply stated, a child generally does not "outgrow" the overly fat condition.

Ages 25 to 44 are the dangerous years for development of excessive fatness by adults.[36] Middle-aged men and women invariably weigh more than college-aged counterparts of the

same stature. Between ages 20 and 40, Americans gain about 2 pounds a year for a 40-pound gain in body weight. Women tend to gain the most weight; about 14% add more than 30 pounds between ages 25 and 34. The degree to which this "creeping overfatness" in adulthood reflects a normal biologic pattern remains unclear.

Generally a Nation of the Overfed

A 2004 report from the Centers for Disease Control and Prevention (www.cdc.gov/) points to a general increase in energy intake among adult Americans over a 30-year period (FIG. 30.3). Adult women now eat 335 more kCal per day than they did in 1970, while the daily intake for men has increased by 168 calories. In 2000, this translated to an average increase of 278 pounds of food, compared with 1497 pounds per capita

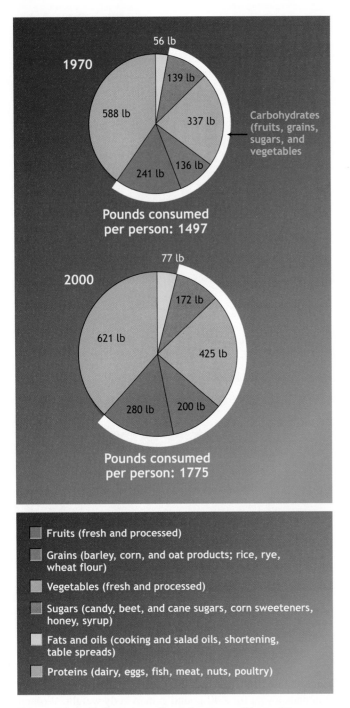

Figure 30.3 Eating more of just about everything: a 30-year comparison. (Source: USDA Economic Research Service)

intake in 1970. On the surface, some of this increase seems desirable because it includes increased vegetable intake. Nevertheless, nearly one third of these "vegetables" comprised iceberg lettuce, French fries, and potato chips. The grain component of this increase consists of processed flour-based pasta, tortillas, and hamburger buns not fiber-rich whole grain breads and cereals. Highly processed, low-fiber carbohydrates have the equivalent nutritional value of table sugar. By mid-2006, McDonald's will add nutritional data on its food wrappers that lists calories, fat, carbohydrates, protein, and sodium in the item compared to the percentage of the govern-

ment's recommended daily intakes. Hopefully, this form of communication becomes important to the consumer as they pursue balanced lifestyles between food intake and energy expenditure.

A COMPLEX INTERACTION OF MANY FACTORS

Overfatness results from a complex interaction of genetic, environmental, metabolic, physiologic, behavioral, social, and perhaps racial influences.[30,79,146,270] Individual differences in specific factors that predispose humans to excessive weight gain include eating patterns and eating environment; food packaging, body image, and variations related to resting metabolic rate; diet-induced thermogenesis; level of spontaneous activity, or "fidgeting;" basal body temperature; susceptibility to specific viral infections, levels of cellular adenosine triphosphatase, lipoprotein lipase, and other enzymes; and metabolically active brown adipose tissue.

GENETICS INFLUENCES BODY FAT ACCUMULATION

The notable interaction between genetics and environment makes it difficult to quantify the role of each in obesity development. Research with twins, adopted children, and specific segments of the population attribute up to 80% of the risk of becoming obese to genetic factors. For example, newborns with large body weights become fat adolescents only when the father or particularly the mother is overweight.[72] Little risk exists for an overweight toddler to grow into an obese adult if both parents are of normal weight. But if a child under age 10, regardless of current weight, has one or both obese parents, the child has more than twice the normal risk of becoming an obese adult.[236,257] Even for normal-weight prepubertal girls, body composition and regional fat distribution relate to the body composition characteristics of both parents.[235]

One's genetic makeup does not necessarily *cause* obesity, but it does lower the *threshold* for its development because of the impact of susceptibility genes. Researchers are only now identifying key genes and specific DNA sequence variants that relate to the molecular causes of appetite and satiety that predispose a person to obesity. A more complete understanding of the genetic role in body fat accretion requires identification of the key genes and their mutations (including the relevant proteins) that contribute to chronic energy imbalance; hopefully, unraveling this secret should occur within the next decade.

Inherited factors contribute to variability in weight gain among individuals fed an identical daily caloric excess and can contribute to the tendency to regain lost weight (see "Focus on Research," p. 842).[16,17,64] Studies of individuals who represent 9 different kinds of relatives indicate that genetic factors that affect metabolism and appetite determine about 25% of the variation among persons in percentage body fat and total fat mass. A larger percentage variation in body fat status relates to a transmissible (cultural) effect (unhealthy expression patterns of preexisting genes; FIG. 30.4). *In an obesity-producing envi-*

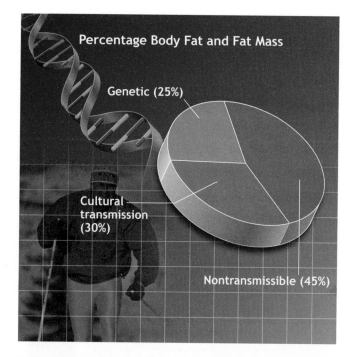

Figure 30.4 Total transmissible variance for body fat. Total body fat and percentage body fat were determined by hydrostatic weighing. (From Bouchard C, et al. Inheritance of the amount and distribution of human body fat. Int J Obes 1988; 12:205.)

ronment—sedentary and stressful, with ready access to inexpensive, large-portion, high-calorie, good-tasting food— the genetically susceptible (obesity-prone) individual gains weight and possibly lots of it. Athletes in weight-related sports with a genetic propensity for obesity must constantly battle to maintain optimal body weight and composition for competitive performance.

Mutant Gene?

Researchers now link human obesity to a mutant gene.[193,221] Studies at the University of Cambridge in England identified a specific defect in two genes that control body weight.[103,163] Two cousins from a Pakistani family in England inherited a defect in the gene that synthesizes leptin (derived from the Greek root *leptos,* meaning thin), a crucial hormonal substance produced by fat and released into the bloodstream that acts on the hypothalamus to regulate body weight. Congenital absence of leptin produced continual hunger and marked obesity in these children. The second genetic defect observed in an English patient affected the body's response to the "signal" leptin provided. The signal largely determines how much one eats, how much energy one expends, and ultimately one's body weight.

Leptin

Studies with animals provide fundamental information about the endocrine-like function of fat and genetic link to

obesity and associated diseases.[57] Research with a strain of hybrid mice that balloon up to five times the girth of normal mice supports the contention that some individuals appear genetically "predestined" to become excessively fat. Mutation in a gene called *obese,* or simply *ob*, disrupts hormonal signals that regulate metabolism, fat storage, and appetite and fundamentally change the brain's circuitry in areas that control appetite; this tips energy balance toward body fat accumulation.[270]

The model in FIGURE 30.5 proposes that the *ob* gene normally becomes activated in adipose tissue (and perhaps muscle tissue), where it encodes and stimulates production of

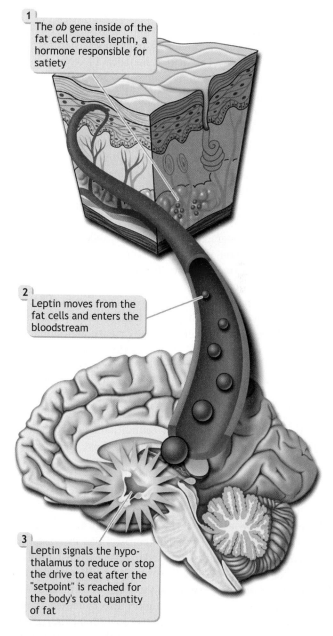

1. The *ob* gene inside of the fat cell creates leptin, a hormone responsible for satiety

2. Leptin moves from the fat cells and enters the bloodstream

3. Leptin signals the hypothalamus to reduce or stop the drive to eat after the "setpoint" is reached for the body's total quantity of fat

Figure 30.5 A genetic model for obesity. A malfunction of the satiety gene markedly affects production of the satiety hormone leptin. This disrupts events that occur in the hypothalamus, the center responsible for adjusting the body's fat level.

FOCUS On Research

GENETIC TENDENCY TO GAIN WEIGHT

Bouchard C, et al. The response to long-term feeding in identical twins. N Engl J Med 1990;322:1477.

▲ Bouchard and colleagues studied differences in body fat acquisition and its distribution from overfeeding (84,000 "extra" kCal) in 12 pairs of male monozygotic twins for 100 days. Their results provide some of the most persuasive support for an inherited tendency toward obesity.

The twin pairs (average age, 21 y; range, 19–27 y) lived in a dormitory under 24-hour supervision for 120 consecutive days. This period included 14 days of baseline testing, 3 days of testing before overfeeding, 100 days of overfeeding, and 3 days of posttesting. Subjects ate normally during baseline testing, with each meal analyzed for nutrient composition and energy content. Body mass remained stable during this time. Subjects were tested during the pre- and postoverfeeding periods for resting metabolic rate–body fat, by hydrostatic weighing; adipose tissue fat composition, by analysis of needle biopsy specimens from the abdominal (umbilicus-level) and femoral (midthigh-level) areas; trunk-fat mass by computed tomographic (CT) scans of abdominal and abdominal visceral areas; and anthropometric assessment that included five trunk and five limb skinfolds and waist and hip circumferences.

After baseline testing, the twins consumed a diet for 6 days a week containing 1000 kCal per day in excess of baseline energy requirement. Daily meal composition was 50% carbohydrate, 35% lipid, and 15% protein. On day 7, subjects consumed their baseline number of calories. The men ate three meals plus an evening snack, and daily activities included reading, playing cards and video games, watching television, and walking outdoors for 30 minutes. Measurements during overfeeding included body mass (daily), skinfolds (every 5 days), and waist and hip girths (every 25 days).

The top figure displays average percentage *changes* from before to after overfeeding. Body mass increased significantly (average 8.1-kg gain), as did fat mass and FFM. However, the 111% average gain in adipose cell mass dramatically exceeded the 5% FFM increase. The sum of skinfold thickness (used to reflect change in subcutaneous fat) increased 70%, from 76 to 129 mm. Skinfold thickness increased more on the trunk (87%) than on the limbs (50%). Waist and hip girth also increased significantly. The ratio of waist girth to hip girth increased, indicating greater fat accretion at the waist than hip. Overfeeding increased adipose tissue fat mass in all subcutaneous and visceral sections estimated from CT scans.

Importantly, considerable individual differences existed for changes in body mass and body composition with overfeeding, with greater variation between twin pairs than within pairs. The bottom figure displays within-pair differences for the changes in body mass with equivalent excess energy intake. Each colored point represents one

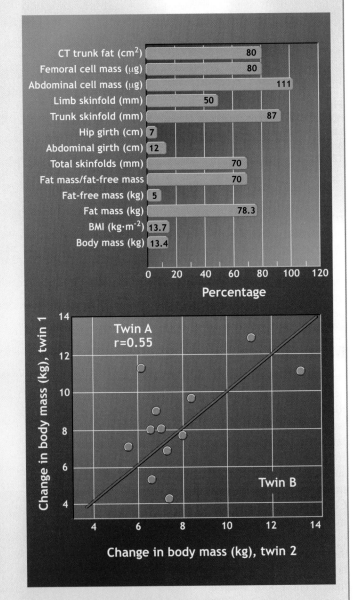

Top. Effects of 100 days of 84,000-kCal overfeeding in 12 pairs of male monozygotic twins. Values are percentage change from before to after overfeeding. *Bottom,* Similarity within twin pairs of changes in body mass in response to overfeeding.

continued on page 843

> *Continued*
>
> twin pair (A and B). The closer the points fall to the diagonal line, the more similar the twins are. The large differences between twin pairs for changes in body mass exceeded the differences within twin pairs.
>
> A threefold difference emerged for changes in body mass, body composition, trunk fat, and visceral fat between the high and low weight gainers. This clearly indicated that surplus energy intake (with other factors controlled) did not produce similar changes in the outcome variables among twin pairs. Also, neither body mass nor body fat increases predicted visceral fat accumulation. Of clinical significance was the observation that some persons store fat more readily than others on the trunk, in the abdominal cavity, or at both areas—a fat deposition pattern with increased health risk. Bouchard hypothesized that a person's genotype determines adaptations to a sustained energy surplus. More than likely, a yet-undetermined genetic characteristic produces large individual differences in the tendency toward obesity in general and the patterning of fat on the body in particular.

a body fat–signaling, hormonelike protein (**ob protein** or **leptin**), which then enters the bloodstream. This satiety signal molecule travels to the arcuate nucleus, the hypothalamic area that controls appetite and metabolism and develops soon after birth. Normally, leptin blunts the urge to eat when caloric intake maintains ideal fat stores. Leptin may affect certain neurons in the hypothalamus to stimulate production of chemicals that suppress appetite and/or reduce the levels of brain chemicals that stimulate appetite.[132] These mechanisms would explain how body fat remains intimately "connected" via a physiologic pathway to the brain for energy balance regulation. In a way, the adipocyte serves an endocrine-like function. With a gene defective for either adipocyte leptin production and/or hypothalamic leptin sensitivity (as probably exists in humans), the brain inadequately assesses the body's adipose tissue status. Thus, the urge to eat remains constant. In essence, leptin availability or its lack affects the neurochemistry of appetite and the brain's dynamic "wiring" to possibly impact appetite and obesity in adulthood.

The hormone–hypothalamic biologic control mechanism helps explain the extreme difficulty overfat persons have sustaining fat loss. In children and adults, plasma leptin circulates in direct proportion to adipose tissue mass when energy balance remains in steady state, with four times more leptin in obese than in lean individuals. Consequently, human obesity resembles a relative state of leptin resistance similar to obesity-related insulin resistance.[82,148] High blood leptin concentrations associate strongly with the combination of upper-body obesity, glucose intolerance, hypertriglyceridemia, and hypertension—core metabolic disturbances in the insulin-resistant metabolic syndrome (see Chapter 20). This unique metabolic disturbance ultimately acts as a conduit to trigger higher incidence of heart disease, stroke, and type 2 diabetes.[145]

Weight loss reduces serum leptin concentration, while weight gain increases serum leptin.[125,251] Gender, hormones, pharmacologic agents, and the body's current energy requirements also affect leptin production.[34] Neither short- nor long-term exercise meaningfully affects leptin, independent of the effects of exercise on total adipose tissue mass.[49,91,174] Subcutaneous recombinant leptin injections produced dose–response effect with body weight and body fat loss in lean and obese men and women with elevated endogenous serum leptin concentrations.[90] This suggests a potential role for leptin and related hormones in treating obesity.

The linkage of genetic and molecular abnormalities to obesity allows researchers to view overfatness as a disease rather than a psychologic flaw. Early identification of one's genetic predisposition toward obesity makes it possible to begin diet and exercise interventions before obesity sets in and fat loss becomes exceedingly difficult if not almost impossible. Pharmaceutical companies continually work to synthesize compounds that produce satiety or affect the resting rate of fat catabolism. These chemicals would facilitate weight control with a smaller caloric intake and fewer feelings of hunger and deprivation than many popular dietary regimens. The following drugs and hormonelike substances may contribute to future medical strategies against body weight-related disorders in persons with a BMI $\geq$30 (or BMI $\geq$27 for persons with comorbid conditions).

Leptin alone does not determine obesity or explain why some people eat whatever they want and gain little weight, while others become overfat with the same caloric intake. Besides defective leptin production, *defective receptor action* increases resistance to endogenous satiety chemicals. A specific gene, the uncoupling protein-2 gene *UCP2* (www.ncbi.nlm.nih.gov/entrez/dispomim.cgi?id=601693), adds another piece to the obesity puzzle. High activity of this gene activates a protein that burns excess calories as heat energy without coupling to other energy-consuming processes.[63] This **futile metabolism** blunts excess fat storage. Individual differences in gene activation and alterations in metabolic activity lend credence to the common claim "Every little bit of excess I eat turns to fat." A drug that turns on the *UCP2* gene to synthesize more of the heat-generating protein could provide a pharmacologic windfall to shed excess body fat. Other newly discovered molecules that control eating include AGRP (agouti-related protein), a protein controlled by leptin that may affect hypothalamic cells to increase caloric intake. The brain also synthesizes melanin-concentrating hormone when leptin levels increase. An excess of this protein molecule increases an animal's appetite, causing it to eat and gain weight. Drugs that inhibit or "destabilize" the action of the brain chemicals that control eating may ultimately provide the long-term "cure" for the overfat condition.

BIOCHEMICALS THAT INFLUENCE EATING BEHAVIORS: SIGNALS THAT TRAVEL AMONG THE DIGESTIVE TRACT, ADIPOSE TISSUE, AND EATING CONTROL CENTERS

- **Leptin:** Produced by adipocytes. Normal levels signal the hypothalamus to maintain food intake so body weight remains stable. Below-normal leptin levels signal the brain to increase appetite in order to increase body fat. Leptin also elevates metabolic rate.
- **Peptide YY3-36 (PYY):** A hormone released by intestinal cells in proportion to the caloric content of a meal. PYY travels to the hypothalamus to inhibit the urge to eat. Overweight persons normally make less of this satiety signal than persons of normal body weight.
- **Neuropeptide Y (NPY):** The brain's most abundant neuropeptide that acts as a potent stimulator of food intake and regulates metabolism and fat synthesis.
- **Ghrelin:** A powerful appetite-stimulating hormone (exerts effects opposite of leptin) produced in the epithelial cells that line the fundus of the stomach, with smaller amounts from the placenta, kidney, pituitary, and hypothalamus. Ghrelin increases hunger though its action on hypothalamic feeding centers. It suppresses fat utilization in adipose tissue and communicates the state of energy balance in the body to the brain.
- **Melanocortin-4 Receptor (MC4-R):** Possibly supplies a signal to stop eating. About 10% of obese patients show genetic mutations in the gene that regulates this compound. Developing an MC4-R agonist for (e.g., α-melanocyte-stimulating hormone, or α-MSH) may affect how the central nervous regulates adiposity.
- **Neuronal CB$_1$ Receptor:** The newly discovered endocannabinoid system has been shown to contribute to physiologic regulation of energy balance, food intake, and lipid and glucose metabolism through both central and peripheral effects. The system consists of endogenous ligands and two types of G-protein-coupled cannabinoid receptors: (1) CB$_1$ located in the brain and peripheral tissues, including adipose tissue, gastrointestinal tract tissue, pituitary gland, heart, liver, and bladder; and (2) CB$_2$ found in the immune system.

  The endocannabinoid system is over-activated in genetic animal models of obesity and in response to exogenous stimuli like excessive food consumption. Research has included studies with animals with genetic deletion of CB$_1$. These animals have a lean phenotype and are resistant to diet-induced obesity and associated insulin resistance produced by a high-fat diet. Blockage of CB$_1$ receptors produces weight loss and normalizes metabolic abnormalities in obese animals. Preclinical findings in humans support the role of the CB$_1$ receptor in both central and peripheral regulations of energy balance and hence body weight and fat. The drug rimonabant (Acomplia) shows promise as a selective CB$_1$-receptor antagonist (2005 Phase III clinical trials that involved 6000 obese subjects in U.S. and Europe).[243]

Influence of Racial Factors

Racial differences in food and exercise habits and cultural attitudes toward body weight help to explain the greater prevalence of obesity among black women (nearly 50%) than white women (33%). Research with obese women shows that small differences in resting energy expenditure (REE), related to racial differences in lean body mass,[25] contribute to the racial differences in obesity.[67,93,105] This "racial" effect, which also exists among children and adolescents,[77,230,234] predisposes a black female to gain weight and regain it after weight loss. On average, black women burn nearly 100 fewer kCal each day during rest than white counterparts. The slower rate of caloric expenditure persists even after adjusting for differences in body mass and body composition. A 100-kCal reduction in daily metabolism translates to nearly 1 pound of body fat gained each month. Total daily energy expenditure of black women averages 10% lower than whites, owing to a 5% lower REE and 19% lower physical activity energy expenditure.[30] Additionally, obese black women showed greater decreases in REE than white women following energy restriction and weight loss.[68] The combination of a lower initial REE and more profound depression of REE with weight loss suggests that black women (including athletes) experience greater difficulty achieving goal body weight than overweight white women.

A Word of Caution

When evaluating purported racial differences in body composition characteristics and their implications on health, one must carefully evaluate methods to explore such differences.[247] For example, interethnic and interracial differences in body size, structure, and body fat distribution can mask true differences in body fat at a given BMI. A single generalized BMI–health risk model obscures the potential to document chronic disease risks among different population groups.[74,220] As discussed in Chapter 28, the nature and magnitude of the relationship between body mass or BMI and health risk may vary among racial and ethnic groups.

PHYSICAL INACTIVITY: A CRUCIAL COMPONENT IN EXCESSIVE FAT ACCUMULATION

Regular physical activity, through either recreation or occupation, effectively impedes weight gain and adverse changes in body composition and thwarts the tendency to regain lost weight.[104,120,205,224,259] Individuals who maintain weight loss over time show greater muscle strength and engage in more physical activity than counterparts who regained lost weight.[253] Variations in physical activity alone accounted for more than 75% of regained body weight. Such findings point up the need to identify and promote strategies that increase regular exercise. Current national guidelines by the Surgeon General and Institute of Medicine recommend a minimum of 30 to 60 minutes of moderate physical activity daily. We endorse an increase to 80 minutes of daily exercise over and above regular routines to combat obesity in the U.S. population.

Physically active lifestyles lessen the "normal" pattern of fat gain in adulthood. For young and middle-aged men who exercise regularly, time spent in physical activity relates inversely to body fat level.[156] Middle-aged long-distance runners remain leaner than sedentary counterparts. Surprisingly, no relationship emerges between the runners' body fat level and caloric intake. Perhaps the relatively greater body fat among middle-aged runners results from less-vigorous training, *not* greater food intake.

From age 3 months to 1 year, the total energy expenditure of infants who later became overweight averaged 21% lower than infants with normal weight gain.[195] For children aged 6 to 9 years, percentage body fat inversely related to physical activity level in boys but not girls.[8] Obese preadolescent and adolescent children generally spend less time in physical activity or engage in lower intensity physical activity than normal-weight peers.[41,139,245] By the time young girls attain adolescence many do not engage in leisure-time physical activity. For girls, the decline in time spent in physical activity averaged nearly 100% among blacks and 64% among whites between ages 9 or 10 and 15 or 16.[119] By age 16, 56% of the black girls and 31% of the white girls reported no leisure-time physical activity.

Benefits of Increased Energy Output with Aging

A study of nearly 7000 male runners 18 years of age and older suggests that maintaining a lifestyle that includes a regular and constant level of endurance exercise does not fully forestall the tendency to add weight through middle age. Figure 30.6 shows the inverse association among distance run and BMI and waist circumference in all age categories. Active men typically remained leaner than sedentary counterparts for each age group; men who ran longer distances each week weighed less than those who ran shorter distances. The typical man who maintained a constant weekly running distance through middle age gained 3.3 pounds, and waist size increased about three fourths of an inch, regardless of distance run. Such findings suggest that by age 50, a physically active man can expect to weigh about 10 pounds more (with a 2-in larger waist) than he weighed at age 20 despite maintaining a constant level of increased physical activity. This proclivity to gain weight and girth may relate to reduced levels of testosterone and growth hormone that induce age-related changes in physique and increase abdominal and visceral fat. To counter weight gain in middle age, one should gradually increase the amount of weekly exercise 1.4 miles for each year of age starting at about age 30.

INTEGRATIVE QUESTION

What evidence documents that body fat accumulation among children and adults does not necessarily result from excessive food intake?

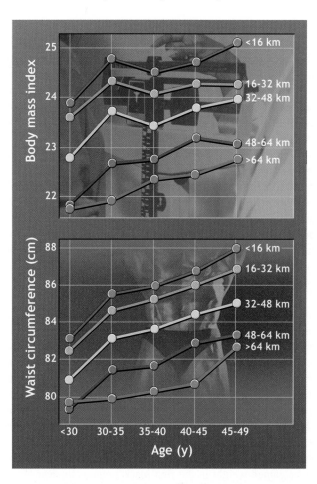

Figure 30.6 Relationship among average body mass index *(top)* and waist circumference *(bottom)* and age for men who maintained constant weekly running for varying distances (<16 to >64 km · wk⁻¹). Men who annually increase their running distance by 1.39 miles (2.24 km) per week compensate for the anticipated weight gain during middle age. (From Williams PT. Evidence for the incompatibility of age-neutral overweight and age-neutral physical activity standards from runners. Am J Clin Nutr 1997;65:1391.)

RISKS OF EXCESSIVE BODY FAT

Obesity represents an important cause of preventable death in America. The combined effects of poor diet and physical inactivity caused 400,000 deaths in the year 2000, a 33% jump over 1990. If the body weight of Americans continues to increase at its current rate, by 2020 one in five health care dollars spent on middle-aged Americans will result from obesity. Impaired glucose tolerance and overall diminished quality of life emerge even among obese children and adolescents.[208,216] Hypertension, elevated blood sugar, postmenopausal breast cancer, and elevated total cholesterol and low high-density lipoprotein-cholesterol heighten an overweight individual's risks of poor health at any given level of excess weight. The prevalence of overweight and obesity also increases musculoskeletal problems including complications from osteoarthritis.[94] Increased loads on the major joints can lead to pain and discomfort, inefficient body mechanics, and reduced mobility.

The prevalence of obesity has blunted the decline over previous years in coronary disease among middle-aged women.[99] Obese and overweight individuals with two or more heart disease risk factors should reduce weight, while overweight persons without any other risk factors should at least maintain current body weight. A modest weight reduction improves insulin sensitivity and blood lipid profile, and prevents or delays diabetes onset in high-risk individuals.[46,78]

Improved physical fitness interacts with the overfat condition to lower disease risk. For example, nearly 20,000 men age 30 to 83 years who were overweight but physically fit suffered fewer deaths from all causes than unfit but normal-weight men.[141] Unfit, lean men also show a higher risk of all-cause mortality than overfat, fit men.[140] Such findings support the strategy of increasing physical activity to improve cardiovascular fitness of overweight men and women rather than relying solely on diet to improve the health risk profile.

Despite the current obesity epidemic, weight control remains low on the list of national public health priorities; it receives far less funding from the NIH than other widely prevalent diseases.[92,102] Current direct and indirect total health-care costs of obesity have risen to nearly $117 billion, or about 10% of the more than $1 trillion dollar cost of remaining ill! Use of health-care resources also increases proportionately with excess body fat.[187] Clearly, maintaining a lean body composition throughout life reduces multiple disease risk. Whether weight loss by an already overweight or obese adult reduces health risk to the level of individuals who never gained weight in the first place remains unclear.[115,269] Research must still determine if increased death risk with obesity declines at all levels of obesity as individuals age.[14,26,164]

Excessive Fatness in Childhood and Adolescence Predicts Adverse Health Effects in Adulthood

The origin of adult obesity and its adverse health consequences often begins in childhood. Children who gain more weight than peers tend to become overweight adults with increased risk for hypertension, elevated insulin, hypercholesterolemia, and heart disease.[47,215] Being overweight during adolescence links to adverse health effects 55 years later. The Harvard Growth Study from 1922 to 1935 evaluated 3000 school children annually on a variety of health variables including triplicate measures of body mass and stature at the same time each year until they left or graduated high school.[39] Of the initial group, the researchers studied 1857 subjects for an additional 8 years. Subjects were designated either lean (in the 25th–50th percentile for BMI) or overweight (exceeding 75th percentile for BMI). Compared with leaner subjects, overweight children as adults showed a greater risk of mortality from all causes and a twofold higher coronary heart disease risk. Women overweight in adolescence were eight times more likely to report problems with personal care and routine living tasks (walking, stair climbing, lifting, and a 1.6-fold increase in arthritis) than women rated lean in adolescence.

The alarming rise in obesity during childhood and adolescence requires immediate interventions to prevent subsequent risk for disease as these children become adults. FIGURE 30.7 shows the percentile cutoffs for a two-level procedure recommended by the American Academy of Pediatrics to identify either overweight children (BMI >95th percentile; requires in-depth medical assessment) and those at risk of becoming overweight (BMI 85th–95th percentile; requires second-level screening including family history and risk factor assessment).

Defined Health Risks

Considerable information exists regarding increasing levels of body fat and defined health risks in children, adolescents, and adults. Excessive body fat relates closely to the alarming increase in type 2 diabetes among children. For adult diabetics, 70% classify as overweight and nearly 35% are obese. A moderate 4 to 10% increase in body weight after age 20 associates with 1.5 greater risk of death from coronary artery disease and nonfatal myocardial infarction.[197] Even maintaining body weight at the high end of the normal range increases heart disease risk.[151,261] An 8-year study of nearly 116,000 female nurses observed that all but the thinnest women showed increased risk for heart attack and chest pains.[150] Nurses of average body weight experienced 30% more heart attacks than the thinnest counterparts, while the risk for a moderately overweight nurse averaged 80% higher. This means that a woman who gains 9 kg from her late teens to middle age doubles her heart attack risk. A convincing argument maintains that overfatness represents an independent and powerful heart disease risk, equal to cigarette smoking, elevated blood lipids, and hypertension. Additionally, overfatness increases risk for low-grade inflammation of the inner lining of arterial vessels. In apparently healthy individuals, arterial wall inflammation can progress unnoticed for years, increasing heart attack and stroke risk. Epidemiologic evidence indicates excess body weight as an independent and powerful risk for congestive heart failure.[117]

Weight gain also increases risk for cancers of the breast, colon, esophagus, prostate, kidney, and uterus. (FIG. 30.8).[27,229,266] Maintaining a BMI below 25 could prevent one of every six cancer deaths in the United States, or about 90,000 deaths yearly.[27] Excess weight probably accounts for 14% of cancer deaths in men and 20% in women. A 16-year follow-up study of the nurses shows that even moderate weight gain after age 18 can prove deadly.[151] One half of cardiovascular deaths and one third of colon, endometrial, and breast cancer deaths linked to the overweight condition.

Researchers followed a cohort of 82,000 female nurses age 30 to 55 years every 2 years from 1976 to determine if initial BMI modifies the relation between long-term weight gain or weight loss and hypertension risk. FIGURE 30.9 depicts the relative risk for hypertension, adjusted for multiple factors linked to hypertension in three groups stratified for BMI at age 18. For women in the first and second BMI tertiles at age 18 (BMI <22.0), weight loss in later years did not reduce hypertension risk. Weight gain after age 18 markedly increased hypertension risk over that of women who maintained a stable body weight. For women whose BMI exceeded 22.0, subsequent weight loss dramatically decreased risk (relative risk of 0.72 for weight loss of 5.0–9.9 kg and 0.57 for a loss of 10 kg

A REVISED ESTIMATE: SOME UNEXPECTED FINDINGS

Being classified as overweight may not be nearly as lethal as the government thought, ranking number 7 instead of number 2 among the nation's leading preventable causes of death according to new calculations from the Centers for Disease Control and Prevention. This new analysis that controlled for the effects of smoking, age, race, and alcohol consumption, found that obesity and extreme obesity remain an indisputable death risk, but those who are modestly overweight have a lower death risk than those of normal body weight. This analysis addressed *only* the risk of death and not disability or disease because body weight increases in the overweight and obese categories associate with increased risk of diabetes, hypertension, and high cholesterol levels. Yet death from these disorders may be less prevalent, largely because of breakthrough medication. The accompanying figure indicates that obesity and extreme obesity cause about 112,000 extra deaths while overweight prevents about 86,000 deaths. No objective reasons explain the findings for this "overweight paradox"—the beneficial effect of being classified as overweight.

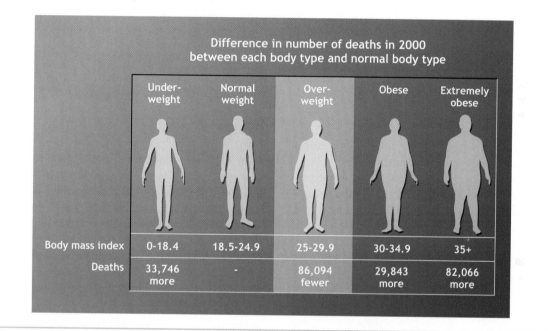

Difference in number of deaths in 2000 between each body type and normal body type

	Under-weight	Normal weight	Over-weight	Obese	Extremely obese
Body mass index	0-18.4	18.5-24.9	25-29.9	30-34.9	35+
Deaths	33,746 more	-	86,094 fewer	29,843 more	82,066 more

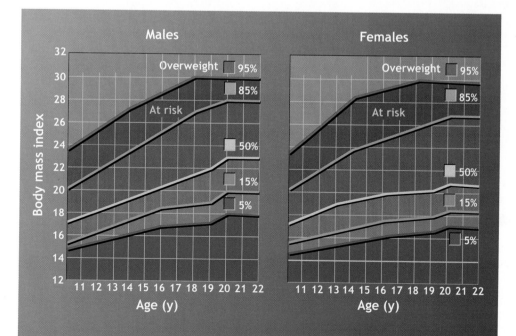

Figure 30.7 Two-level procedure using BMI to identify *overweight* adolescents and adolescents *at risk* of becoming overweight. (From Green M, ed. Bright futures: guidelines for health supervision of infants, children and adolescents. Arlington, VA: National Center for Education in Maternal and Child Health, 1994.)

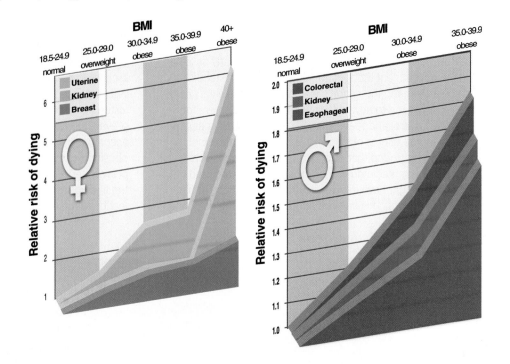

Figure 30.8 Extra weight and the risk of cancer in women and men. (From Calle EE, et al. Overweight, obesity, and mortality from cancer in a prospectively studied cohort of U.S. adults. N Engl J Med 2003;348:1625.)

or more). Weight gain increased hypertension risk in a manner similar to that of the lighter group of women.

A 5 to 10% weight loss often normalizes an obese person's serum cholesterol and triacylglycerol levels and reduces blood pressure and overall heart disease risk, including risk of congestive heart failure. The tendency to gain weight with age partially explains the relationship between age and blood pressure. After accounting for cigarette smoking and current disease status, the 27-year study of Harvard alumni showed that men with a body weight 20% or more above "desirable weight" experienced a 2.5 times greater death rate than the leanest men.[140] At all ages, the leanest men showed the least likelihood of dying. Obesity now stands on a par with high cholesterol, hypertension, cigarette smoking, and sedentary lifestyle as a *major* heart attack risk factor in contrast to its former status as a *contributing* risk factor.

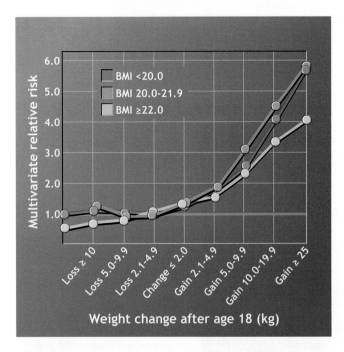

Figure 30.9 Multivariate relative risk for hypertension according to weight change after age 18 years within strata of BMI at age 18. Risk adjusted for: age, BMI at age 18, stature, family history of myocardial infarction, parity, oral contraceptive use, menopausal status, postmenopausal use of hormones, and smoking status. *Horizontal red line* indicates normal risk. (From Huang Z, et al. Body weight, weight change, and risk for hypertension in women. Ann Intern Med 1998;128:81.)

SPECIFIC HEALTH RISKS OF EXCESSIVE BODY FAT

- Impaired cardiac function from increased mechanical work and autonomic and left-ventricular dysfunction
- Hypertension, stroke, and deep-vein thrombosis
- Increased insulin resistance in children and adults and type 2 diabetes (80% of these patients are overweight)
- Renal disease
- Sleep apnea, mechanical ventilatory constraints (particularly in exercise), and pulmonary disease from impaired function because of added effort to move the chest wall
- Problems receiving anesthetics during surgery
- Osteoarthritis, degenerative joint disease, and gout
- Endometrial, breast, prostate, and colon cancers
- Abnormal plasma lipid and lipoprotein levels
- Menstrual irregularities
- Gallbladder disease
- Enormous psychologic burden and social stigmatization and discrimination

CRITERIA FOR EXCESSIVE BODY FAT: HOW FAT IS TOO FAT?

In Chapter 28, we discussed limitations of the height–weight tables and BMI to assess body composition. Three more appropriate approaches measure a person's fat content:

- Percentage of body mass composed of fat
- Distribution or patterning of fat at different anatomic regions
- Size and number of individual fat cells

Percentage Body Fat

What determines the demarcation between a normal level of body fat and an excess? In Chapter 28, we suggested a "normal" body fat range for adult men and women—the "average" percentage body fat value plus or minus one standard deviation. For men and women ages 17 to 50 years, this variation equals 5% body fat units.[13] Using this statistical boundary, overfatness then corresponds to a body fat level that exceeds the average value plus 5% body fat. For example, in young men whose body fat averages 15% of body mass, the borderline for obesity becomes 20% body fat. For older men whose fat averages 25%, obesity is body fat in excess of 30%. For young women, obesity corresponds to body fat content above 30%; for older women, borderline obesity corresponds to about 37% body fat. We emphasize that just because the average value for percentage body fat increases with age, this does *not* dictate that people should become fatter as they age. In our opinion, one criterion for determining "too fat" emerges from data for younger men and women—above 20% for men and above 30% for women. With this single gender-specific standard, average age-related population values do not become the reference standard and thus the acceptable criterion. We also recognize that this classification standard based on an average for young adults becomes extremely rigorous when applied to the entire population. It probably places more than 50% of adults in the overly fat category, a value somewhat below the data for overweight Americans presented in Figure 30.1. It also closely corresponds to proposed gender-based body fat standards computed for young adults from the relationship between BMI and four component estimates of percentage body fat for African Americans and whites.[73]

> ### STANDARDS FOR OVERFATNESS
> **Men**–above 20%; **Women**–above 30%

We consider that obesity exists along a continuum from the upper limit of normal (20% body fat for men and 30% for women) to as high as 50% and a theoretical maximum of nearly 70% of body mass in the massively obese. This latter group's weight ranges from 170 to 250 kg or higher. In this situation, body fat often exceeds lean body mass to create a life-threatening situation.

TABLE 30.1 ■ PERCENTILE RANKINGS FOR TRICEPS SKINFOLDS IN BOYS AND GIRLS AGES 6 TO 18 YEARS

| | **PERCENTILE** | | | |
AGE	**15TH**	**50TH**	**85TH**	**95TH**
Boys				
6	6.2	8.4	11.1	14.1
8	6.1	8.8	13.7	17.2
10	6.0	9.1	16.0	20.7
12	5.8	9.4	17.3	23.3
14	5.6	8.9	16.4	23.5
16	5.5	8.5	15.8	21.5
18	5.6	8.5	16.6	21.8
Girls				
6	6.8	10.1	13.4	15.6
8	7.6	11.4	16.4	20.2
10	8.4	12.7	19.0	24.4
12	9.3	14.1	21.3	28.0
14	10.4	15.5	23.3	30.9
16	11.3	26.6	25.1	33.2
18	11.7	17.0	25.8	33.8

From Must J, et al. Reference data for obesity: 85th and 95th percentiles of body mass index (wt/ht^2) and triceps skinfolds. Am J Clin Nutr 1991;53:89.

Criterion for Children

TABLE 30.1 presents percentile rankings for triceps skinfolds for boys and girls ages 6 to 18. Generally, a skinfold at or above the 85th percentile raises concern about the child's energy balance and excessive body fatness.

Regional Fat Distribution

The patterning of the body's adipose tissue, independent of total body fat, alters health risks in children, adolescents, and adults.[60,71,171,237,267] FIGURE 30.10 shows two types of regional fat distribution. Increased health risk from fat deposition in the abdominal area (**central** or **android-type obesity**), particularly internal visceral deposits, may result from this tissue's active lipolysis with catecholamine stimulation. Fat stored in this region shows greater metabolic responsiveness than fat in the gluteal and femoral regions (**peripheral** or **gynoid-type obesity**). Increases in central fat more readily support processes that cause heart disease.[218] For men, the percentage of visceral fat increases progressively with age, whereas this fat deposition in women begins to increase at menopause onset.[126]

Central fat deposition, independent of fat storage in other anatomic areas, reflects an altered metabolic profile that increases the following:

1. Hyperinsulinemia (insulin resistance)
2. Glucose intolerance

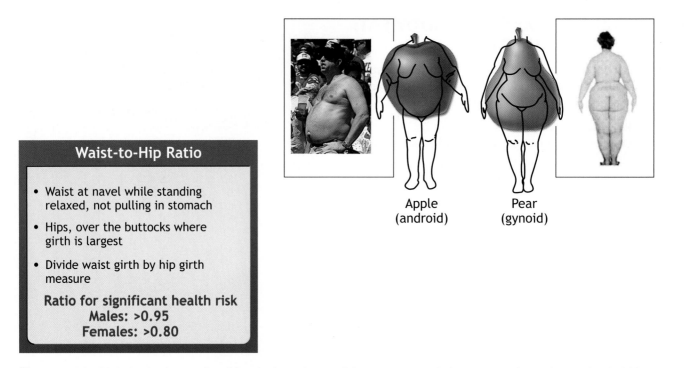

Waist-to-Hip Ratio

- Waist at navel while standing relaxed, not pulling in stomach

- Hips, over the buttocks where girth is largest

- Divide waist girth by hip girth measure

Ratio for significant health risk
Males: >0.95
Females: >0.80

Apple
(android)

Pear
(gynoid)

Figure 30.10 Male (android pattern) and female (gynoid pattern) fat patterning, including waist-to-hip girth ratio threshold for significant health risk.

3. Type 2 diabetes
4. Endometrial cancer
5. Hypertriglyceridemia
6. Hypercholesterolemia and negatively altered lipoprotein profile
7. Hypertension
8. Atherosclerosis

Waist-to-hip girth ratios that exceed 0.80 for women and 0.95 for men increase risk of death even after adjusting for BMI.[44,192,262] One limitation of the ratio is that it poorly captures the specific effects of each girth measure. Waist and hip circumferences reflect different aspects of body composition and fat distribution. Each has an independent and often opposite effect on cardiovascular disease risk. An increased waist girth is the so-called malignant form of obesity characterized by central fat deposition. This region of fat deposition provides a reasonable indication of the accumulation of intraabdominal (visceral) adipose tissue. This makes waist girth the trunk measure of clinical choice in evaluating the metabolic and health risks and accelerated mortality with obesity[97,113,165,210] when more precise assessments are impractical.[226] *Over a broad range of BMI values, men and women with high waist circumference values possess greater relative risk for cardiovascular disease, type 2 diabetes, cancer, and cataracts (the leading cause of blindness worldwide) than individuals with small waist circumference or peripheral obesity.*[108,203] Excess weight distribution in the abdominal area (and accompanying high blood insulin levels) also increases

colorectal cancer risk. For example, waist girth that exceeds 91 cm (36 in) in men and 82 cm (32 in) in women nearly doubles the risk of this cancer form.[206]

For children and adolescents, central body fat distribution associates with higher blood cholesterol, triacylglycerol, and insulin levels and lower HDL cholesterol in addition to higher blood pressure and increased left ventricular wall thickness.[37,71] Many clinicians measure waist girth before and during weight loss to gauge abdominal obesity and complement information on body fat for individuals in the normal-weight range.[59] TABLE 30.2 presents classification guidelines and associated disease risk for overweight and obesity based on BMI and waist girth. *Men with a 102-cm (40-in) or larger waist and women with waist girth above 86 cm (35 in) should reduce this excess to minimize disease risk.*

Documentation of a strong effect of regular exercise on reducing waist girth selectively in men may explain why regular physical activity reduces disease risk more effectively in men than women.

Lipoprotein Lipase Affects Body Fat Distribution

To some extent, genetic characteristics determine one's fat distribution pattern, governed by the regional activity of **lipoprotein lipase (LPL).**[176] This rate-limiting enzyme facilitates triacylglycerol uptake and storage by adipocytes. Variations in LPL activity contribute not only to interindividual differences in fat distribution, but likely change fat distri-

TABLE 30.2 ■ CLASSIFICATION OF OVERWEIGHT AND OBESITY BY BMI, WAIST CIRCUMFERENCE, AND DISEASE RISK

		DISEASE RISK[a] RELATIVE TO NORMAL WEIGHT AND NORMAL WAIST CIRCUMFERENCE	
	BMI, KG · M^{-2}	MEN ≤ 102 CM WOMEN ≤ 88 CM	MEN > 102 CM WOMEN > 88 CM
Underweight	<18.5	NR	NR
Normal[b]	18.5–24.9	NR	NR
Overweight	25.0–29.9	Increased	High
Obesity class			
I	30.0–34.9	High	Very high
II	35.0–39.9	Very high	Very high
III (extreme obesity)	≥40	Extremely high	Extremely high

[a] Disease risk for type 2 diabetes, hypertension, and cardiovascular disease. NR indicates no risk assigned at these BMI levels.
[b] Increased waist circumference can indicate increased risk even in persons of normal weight.
From Executive summary of the clinical guidelines on the identification, evaluation, and treatment of overweight and obesity in adults. Arch Intern Med 1998;158:1855.

bution in pregnancy and middle age and may cause less visceral adipose tissue in blacks than whites.[35] The gender differences in total body fat and pattern of fat distribution also relate to LPL variations; adipocytes in the hip, thigh, and breast regions produce considerable LPL in females, while abdominal adipocytes show the greatest LPL activity in males.

Adipocyte Size and Number: Hypertrophy Versus Hyperplasia

Adipocyte size and number provide another way to assess and classify obesity. Adipose tissue mass increases in two ways:

1. **Fat cell hypertrophy:** existing adipocytes enlarge or fill with fat
2. **Fat cell hyperplasia:** total adipocyte number increases

One technique for studying adipose cellularity involves sucking small fragments of subcutaneous tissue (usually from the triceps, subscapular, buttocks, and/or lower abdomen) into a syringe through a needle inserted directly into the fat depot. Chemical treatment of the tissue sample isolates the individual adipocytes for counting. Dividing fat mass in the sample by adipocyte number determines the average quantity of fat per cell. One can estimate total adipocyte number by determining total body fat by a criterion method such as hydrostatic weighing. For example, an individual who weighs 88 kg with 13% body fat has a total fat mass of 11.4 kg (0.13 × 88 kg). Dividing 11.4 kg by the average fat content per cell estimates total adipocyte number. If the average adipocyte contains 0.60 μg

of fat, then this person's body contains 19 billion adipocytes (11.4 kg ÷ 0.60 μg).

$$\text{Total adipocyte number} = \text{Mass of body fat}$$
$$\div \text{Fat content per cell}$$

In one of our laboratories, needle biopsy and photomicrographic techniques extracted fat and measured the average fat content of adipocytes at three anatomic sites. FIGURE 30.11 shows adipocytes from the upper buttocks of one of this textbook's authors whose total fat mass at the time equaled 17.02 kg (body mass, 89.1 kg; 19.1% body fat) with 0.73 μg of fat per cell; the estimated total adipocyte number was 23.3 billion (17.02 kg ÷ 0.73 μg).

Cellularity Differences Between Nonobese and Obese Persons

FIGURE 30.12 compares body mass, total fat, and adipose tissue cellularity in 25 subjects, 20 of whom classified as clinically obese (BMI about 40.0). The body mass of the obese averaged more than twice that of the nonobese, and they had nearly three times more body fat. In cellularity, adipocytes in the obese averaged 50% larger with nearly three times more cells (75 vs. 27 billion). *Cell number represents the major structural difference in adipose tissue mass between the severely obese and nonobese persons.*

Relating total body fat content to cell size and cell number further demonstrates the contribution of adipocyte number to obesity. As body fat increases, adipocytes eventually reach a biologic upper limit. Once this occurs, cell number becomes the key factor determining any further obesity. Even doubling

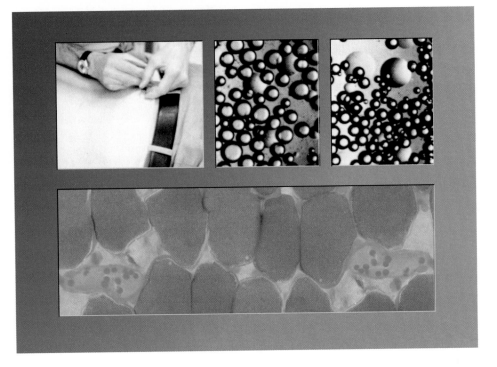

Figure 30.11 *(Upper panel)* Needle biopsy to extract adipocytes from the upper buttocks. The area is sterilized and anesthetized, and the biopsy needle is placed beneath the skin surface. Photomicrographs of the adipocytes from the buttocks of a physically active professor before *(center)* and after *(right)* 6 months of marathon training. Adipocyte diameter averaged 8.6% smaller after training. The average volume of fat in each cell decreased by 18.2%. The large spherical structures in the background are lipid droplets. *Bottom panel.* Cross section of human adipocytes ×440. (From Geneser F. Color atlas of histology. Philadelphia: Lea & Febiger, 1985. Top panel photomicrographs courtesy of P. M. Clarkson, Muscle Biochemistry Laboratory, Exercise Science Department, University of Massachusetts, Amherst, MA.)

adipocyte size does not explain the large difference in total fat mass between obese and average persons. For comparison, an average-sized person has between 25 and 30 billion adipocytes, whereas the clinically severe obese may have more than three to five times this number, particularly when obesity occurs in childhood or adolescence.

Effects of Weight Loss

FIGURE 30.13 shows a classic study of weight loss effects on adipose tissue characteristics of 19 obese adults during two stages of weight loss. During the first stage, subjects reduced body mass by 46 kg (149 to 103 kg). Adipocyte number before weight reduction averaged 75 billion; this remained unchanged even after the 46-kg reduction. In contrast, adipocyte size decreased by 33% from 0.9 to 0.6 μg of lipid per cell. When subjects attained normal body mass of 75 kg by losing an additional 28 kg, cell number still remained unchanged but cell size continued to shrink to about one third that in a nonobese comparison group. When the patients achieved a "normal" body mass and body fat level, adipocytes had become considerably smaller than the nonobese. *In adults, the major change in adipose cellularity in weight loss is shrinkage of adipocytes with no change in*

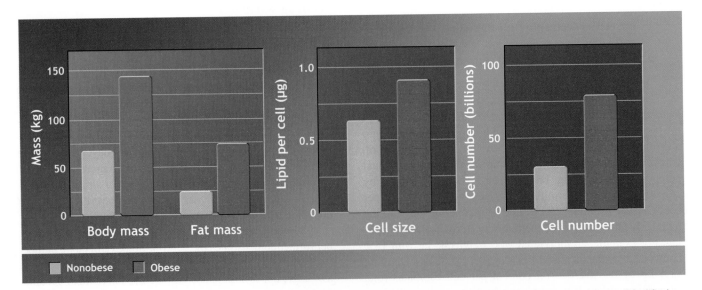

Figure 30.12 Comparison of body mass, total fat mass, and adipocyte size and number in obese and nonobese subjects. (Modified from Hirsch J, Knittle J. Cellularity of obese and non-obese human adipose tissue. Fed Proc 1970;29:1518.)

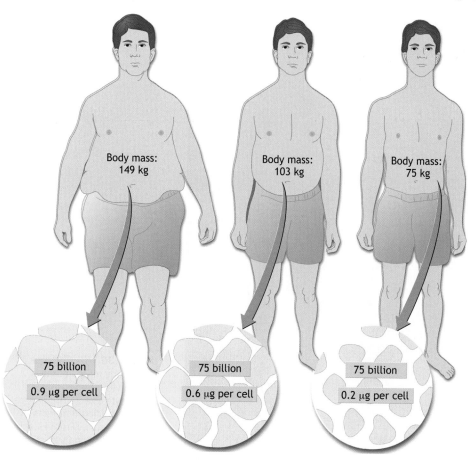

75 billion
0.9 µg per cell

75 billion
0.6 µg per cell

75 billion
0.2 µg per cell

Body mass:
149 kg

Body mass:
103 kg

Body mass:
75 kg

Figure 30.13 Changes in adipose cellularity with weight reduction in obese subjects. (Data from Hirsch J. Adipose cellularity in relation to human obesity. In: Stollerman GH, ed. Advances in internal medicine, vol 17. Chicago: Year-Book, 1971.)

cell number. These findings suggest that weight loss in obese persons does not really "cure" their obesity, at least for total adipocyte number.

Effects of Weight Gain

An interesting series of studies in the late 1960s and early 1970s evaluated the dynamics of weight gain on adipose tissue cellularity. In one study, adult male volunteers with an initial average body fat content of 15% deliberately increased daily caloric intake by three times normal to about 7000 kCal for 40 weeks.[217] For a typical subject, body mass increased 25% and percentage body fat nearly doubled from 14.6 to 28.2%. Fat deposition represented 10.5 kg of the 12.7 kg of weight gained during the overfeeding period. In a similar experiment with subjects with no personal or family history of obesity, voluntary overeating increased body mass by 16.4 kg.[200] In both experiments, adipocytes increased substantially in size with *no change* in cell number. When caloric intake decreased and subjects attained normal weight, total body fat declined and the adipocytes reverted to their original size. *In general, moderate weight gain from overeating in adults enlarges existing adipocytes rather than stimulating new adipocyte development.*

Possibility that New Adipocytes Form. Extreme accumulation of body fat in adults stimulates increased adipose

cellularity because adipocyte size reaches an upper limit of about 1.0 µg fat, beyond which no further hypertrophy occurs. At extremes of obesity, almost all adipocytes attain their hypertrophic limit. In this situation, the preadipocyte pool provides additional adipocytes to increase cell number, with a concomitant increase in the quantity of fat stored within the liver and between muscle fibers. *In maturity-onset severe obesity, in which the already obese adult gains even more body fat, hypercellularity may accompany the increasing size of existing adipocytes.* The increased number of cells at this point constitutes a failure of adipocyte regulation that unfortunately leads to further fat accumulation.

Adipocyte Development

Animal and human research provides important information about adipose tissue growth and development.

Animal Studies

Extensive studies exist on adipose cellularity in rats because these mammals live a relatively short time. This allows researchers to study diet and exercise regimens during important stages of the growth cycle. FIGURE 30.14 illustrates the general upward trend for body mass, fat mass, and adipocyte size and number in rats during the first 5 months of life. Note that cell number and cell size increase during weeks 6 through

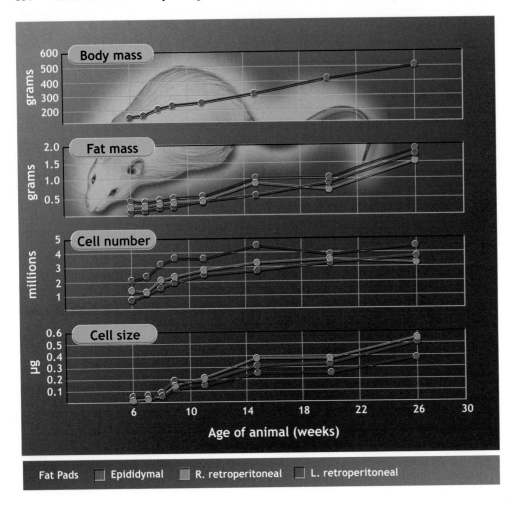

Figure 30.14   Changes in total body mass, fat mass, adipocyte number, and adipocyte size in three fat pads during the first 5 months of growth in rats. (From Hirsch J, Han PW. Cellularity of rat adipose tissue: effects of growth, starvation, and obesity. J Lipid Res 1969;10:77.)

15, after which further increases in total body fat occur primarily from increased adipocyte size, not from new adipocyte development.

Human Studies

Cell Size.   Cross-sectional studies established adipose cellularity for 34 infants and children who ranged in age from a few days to 13 years.[95] Adipocyte size in newborn infants and children up to age 1 year averaged one fourth the size in adults; cell size then tripled during the next 6 years, with little further increase to age 13. Data remain scarce concerning changes in adipocyte size between adolescence and adulthood. Adipocyte size probably increases during this growth period because adults possess larger adipocytes than adolescents.

Cell Number.   Adipocyte number increases rapidly during the first year of life to reach three times the number at birth. Most of the adipocytes before birth form during the last trimester of pregnancy. Beyond the age of 1 year, cell number increases gradually to about age 10. As with increases in cell size, significant hyperplasia takes place during the adolescent growth spurt; thereafter, cell number remains fairly stable. Percentage body fat increases from 16% at birth to about 25% over the first year.[40] By age 6, body fat decreases to 14% of body mass for girls and 11% for boys. Thereafter, percentage fat progressively increases to average 16% at age 11 years in boys and 27% in girls.

Can Body Fat Be Modified Early in Life?

Certain behaviors modify body fatness early in life. In humans, maternal nutrition during pregnancy affects body composition of the developing fetus. A mother who gains more than 18 kg generally gives birth to a baby with larger skinfold thickness than a woman that follows recommended weight gain during pregnancy.[240] Bottle-feeding and early introduction of solid food also associate with childhood obesity. Conversely, breast-feeding, which allows the infant's natural appetite to set limits on food intake, and delayed introduction of solid food may prevent overfeeding, development of poor eating habits, and subsequent obesity.[128]

Prudent caloric intake and regular physical activity during the growth stage may modify the filling of existing adipocytes and proliferation of new ones. Increased physical activity and caloric restriction begun later in life certainly can reduce body fat. As far as we know, only cell size (not cell number) decreases. *Early prevention of obesity through regular, moderate exercise and prudent diet, rather than correction of existing obesity, offers the greatest potential for curbing the overfat condition so common worldwide among children, teenagers, and adults.*

Summary

1. Obesity or excess accumulation of body fat is a heterogeneous disorder with a final common pathway where energy intake chronically exceeds energy expenditure.

2. Over the past 25 years, the average body weight of adult Americans has increased considerably. Currently, 31% of adults (60+ million) classify as obese (BMI ≥30); 65% (130 million adults) are either overweight or obese (BMI ≥25).

3. Fifteen to 20% of American children and 12% of adolescents (up from 7.6% in 1976–80) classify as overweight. Excessive body fatness, childhood's most common chronic disorder, is most prevalent among poor and minority children.

4. Genetic factors account for 25 to 30% of excessive body fat accumulation. Genetic predisposition does not necessarily cause obesity, but in the right environment, the genetically susceptible individual gains body fat.

5. Substantial alterations in the population's gene pool does not explain the dramatic worldwide obesity epidemic.

6. A defective gene for adipocyte leptin production and/or hypothalamic leptin insensitivity (plus defects in production and/or sensitivity to other chemicals) causes the brain to assess adipose tissue status improperly. Excessive food intake creates a chronic positive energy balance.

7. Excessive body fat is a leading cause of preventable death in the United States. Comorbid hypertension, elevated blood sugar level, postmenopausal breast cancer, and elevated total cholesterol and low HDL cholesterol levels increase an overweight person's risk of poor health at any level of excess weight.

8. The overfatness threshold for adult men and women should more closely reflect percentage body fat levels of younger adults—men above 20%; women above 30%.

9. Body fat patterning affects health risks independent of total body fat. Fat distributed in the abdominal region (central, or android-type, obesity) poses a greater risk than fat deposited at the thighs and buttocks (peripheral, or gynoid-type, obesity).

10. Body fat increases in two ways before adulthood: (1) enlargement of individual adipocytes (*fat cell hypertrophy*) and (2) increase in total cell number (*fat cell hyperplasia*).

11. Modest weight gain and weight loss in adults changes adipocyte size with little change in cell number. In extreme weight gain, adipocyte number increases once cell size reaches a hypertrophic limit.

12. Increases in adipocyte number involve three general time periods: last trimester of pregnancy, first year of life, and adolescent growth spurt prior to adulthood.

PART 2 • *Principles of Weight Control: Diet and Exercise*

For many adults, body weight fluctuates only slightly during the year, even though annual food intake averages more than 800 kg. This represents an impressive constancy considering that slight increases in daily food intake translate to substantial weight gain over time if unaccompanied by compensatory increases in energy expenditure. *The human body functions in accord with the laws of thermodynamics. If total food calories exceed daily energy expenditure, excess calories accumulate and store as fat in adipose tissue.*

ENERGY BALANCE: INPUT VERSUS OUTPUT

The first law of thermodynamics (often called the law of conservation of energy) posits that energy can be transferred from one system to another in many forms but cannot be created or destroyed. In human terms, this means that the energy balance equation dictates that body mass remains constant when caloric intake equals caloric expenditure. FIGURE 30.15 shows

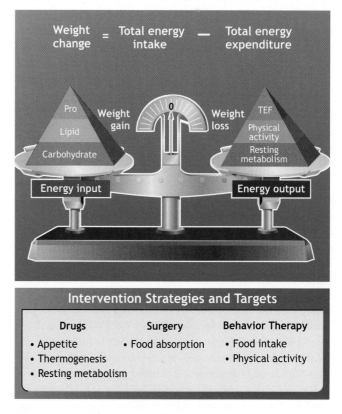

Figure 30.15 The energy balance equation plus intervention strategies and specific targets to alter energy balance in the direction of weight loss. *Pro,* protein; *TEF,* thermic effect of food.

that any chronic imbalance on the energy output or input side of the equation changes body weight.

There are three ways to unbalance the energy balance equation in order to produce weight loss:

1. Reduce caloric intake below daily energy requirements
2. Maintain caloric intake and increase energy expenditure through additional physical activity above daily energy requirements
3. Decrease daily caloric intake and increase daily energy expenditure

When considering the sensitivity of the energy balance equation, if caloric intake exceeds output by only 100 kCal per day, the surplus calories consumed in a year equal 36,500 kCal (365 days × 100 kCal). Because 0.45 kg (1.0 lb) of body fat contains 3500 kCal (each 1 lb [454 g] of adipose tissue contains about 86% fat, or 390 g × 9 kCal · g^{-1} = 3514 kCal per lb), this caloric excess causes a yearly gain of about 4.7 kg (10.3 lb) of body fat. In contrast, if daily food intake decreases by just 100 kCal and energy expenditure increases by 100 kCal (e.g., by walking or jogging one extra mile each day), then the yearly deficit equals the energy in 9.5 kg (21 lb) of body fat.

The previous arithmetic represents an overly simplistic accounting for fat accumulation because the diet's composition affects the body's efficiency in converting and storing excess calories as fat. Only about 3% of calories in ingested lipid are lost when the body converts the excess calories to stored fat. In contrast, 25% of carbohydrate calories "burn" during the conversion. Simply stated, the body synthesizes fat more efficiently from dietary lipid than from an equivalent caloric excess of carbohydrate. Whether shifting dietary composition toward higher carbohydrate content actually produces less body fat gain with a caloric excess remains unresolved.[96,260]

A Prudent Recommendation

The objective of weight-loss programs has changed dramatically since the last two editions of this text. The previous approach assigned a goal body weight that coincided with an "ideal" weight based on body mass and stature Achievement of goal body weight heralded the weight-loss program's success. Currently, the World Health Organization (www.who.int/), the Institute of Medicine of the National Academy of Sciences (www.iom.edu/), and the National Heart, Lung and Blood Institute (www.nhlbi.nih.gov/) recommend that an obese person reduce initial body weight by 5 to 15%. *This more realistic weight loss diminishes weight-related comorbidities and complications from hypertension, type 2 diabetes, and abnormal blood lipids and often exerts a positive effect on social—psychological complications.* Setting the initial weight loss goal beyond the 5 to 15% recommendation often gives patients an unrealistic and potentially unattainable target in light of current treatment methods.

DIETING FOR WEIGHT CONTROL

The first law of thermodynamics affirms that weight loss occurs whenever energy output exceeds energy intake, regardless of the diet's macronutrient mixture (despite high-profile advertising claims and celebrity testimonials). Advantages of relatively high percentages of unrefined complex carbohydrates in the reduced-calorie diet lie in their moderate-to-low glycemic index; high vitamin, mineral, and phytochemical content; low energy density; and low saturated fatty acid levels. A prudent dietary approach to weight loss unbalances the energy balance equation by reducing energy intake by 500 to 1000 kCal below daily energy expenditure. Moderately reduced food intake produces greater fat loss relative to the energy deficit than more severe energy restriction. Individuals who create larger daily deficits to lose weight more rapidly tend to regain the weight compared to those who lose weight at a slower rate.

Suppose an overfat woman who normally consumes 2800 kCal daily and maintains a body mass of 79.4 kg wishes to lose weight by caloric restriction (dieting). She maintains regular physical activity but reduces food intake to 1800 kCal to create a 1000-kCal daily deficit. In 7 days, the accumulated deficit equals 7000 kCal, or the energy equivalent of 0.9 kg of body fat. Actually, she would lose considerably more than 0.9 kg during the first week because initially the body's glycogen stores make up a large portion of the energy deficit. Stored glycogen contains fewer calories per gram and considerably more water than stored fat. For this reason, short periods of caloric restriction often encourage the dieter but produce a large percentage of water and carbohydrate loss per unit weight loss with only a small decrease in body fat. As weight loss continues, a larger proportion of body fat supports the energy deficit created by food restriction (see Fig. 30.22). To reduce body fat by an additional 1.4 kg, the dieter must maintain the reduced caloric intake of 1800 kCal for another 10.5 days;

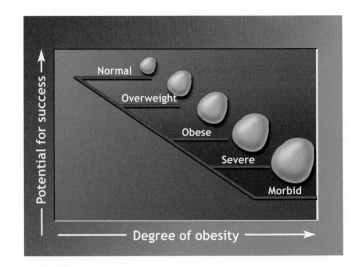

Figure 30.16 Likelihood of success in long-term maintenance of weight loss inversely relates to the level of obesity at the start of intervention.

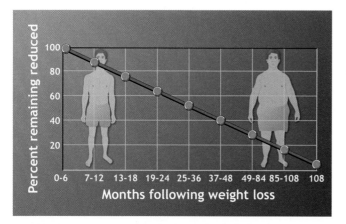

Figure 30.17 General trend for percentage of patients remaining at reduced weights at various time intervals following accomplished weight loss.

at this point, body fat theoretically decreases at a rate of 0.45 kg every 3.5 days.

Long-Term Success

The potential for successful long-term weight loss maintenance generally varies inversely with the initial degree of fatness (FIG. 30.16). For most individuals, initial success in weight loss relates poorly to long-term success. Participants in supervised weight-loss programs (pharmacologic or behavioral interventions) generally lose about 8 to 12% of their original body mass. Unfortunately, typically one to two thirds of the lost weight returns within a year, and almost all of it within 5 years.[110,158,167] Between 90 and 95% of persons who lose weight subsequently regain it. FIGURE 30.17 illustrates clearly that over a 7.3-year follow-up of 121 patients, return to original weight occurred in 50% of the dieters within 2 to 3 years, and only seven patients remained at their reduced body weights. These discouraging but typical statistics highlight the extreme difficulty of long-term maintenance of a low-calorie diet; it becomes particularly difficult in the relaxed atmosphere of one's home with ready access to food and often little emotional support.

National Weight Control Registry: Clues to Success

Many success stories exist despite difficulties usually encountered with sustaining weight loss.[89,122] Among lifetime members of a commercial weight-loss organization that promotes prudent caloric restriction, behavior modification, group support, and moderate physical activity, more than one half maintained their original weight loss goal after 2 years, and more than one third had done so after 5 years.[159] Behavior modification, a common intervention in weight loss programs, provides a set of principles and techniques to alter exercise and eating habits. The therapy increases skills for replacing existing habits with new habits associated with more healthful behav-

iors. Behavior therapy characteristics include eating well-balanced meals with reduced portion size, restricting daily caloric intake to 500 to 700 kCal, keeping meticulous records of food intake and physical activity, and increasing daily physical activity by 200 to 300 kCal.

A project recruited 784 individuals (629 women; 155 men) in the National Weight Control Registry (NWCR; www.nwcr.ws/), the largest database of individuals who successfully achieved prolonged weight loss. Criteria for NWCR membership included age 18 years or older and maintained weight loss of at least 30 pounds (13.6 kg) for 1 year or longer. Participants averaged 66 pounds (30 kg) of weight loss, and 14% lost more than 100 pounds (45.4 kg). Members maintained the required minimum 30-pound weight loss for a 5.5-year average, and 16% maintained the loss for 10 years or longer. Most participants had been overweight since childhood; nearly one half had one overweight parent, and more than 25% had both parents overweight. *Genetic background may have predisposed these persons to obesity, but an impressive weight loss and its maintenance proves that heredity alone need not predestine a person to the obese condition.*

About 55% of the NWCR members used either a formal program or professional assistance to lose weight; the rest succeeded on their own. Regarding weight-loss methods, 89% modified food intake and maintained relatively high levels of physical activity (2800 kCal weekly on average) to achieve goal weight loss. Only 10% relied solely on diet, and 1% used exercise exclusively. The diet strategy of nearly 90% of participants restricted intake of certain types and/or amounts of foods—44% counted calories, 33% limited lipid intake, and 25% restricted grams of lipid. Forty-four percent ate the same foods they normally ate but in reduced amounts (TABLE 30.3).

The registry members' belief in the importance of physical activity for weight maintenance represents a significant finding; nearly all of them exercised as part of their strategy. Many walked briskly for at least 1 hour daily. About 92% exercised at home, and one third exercised regularly with friends. Women primarily walked and did aerobic dancing, while men chose competitive sports and resistance training. The data in Table 30.3 also show that successful weight loss had far-reaching, positive effects on their lives. At least 85% improved general quality of life, level of energy, physical mobility, general mood, self-confidence, and physical health. Only 13 (1.6%) worsened in any of these areas. Such observations reaffirm that weight loss through diet and exercise can thwart a genetic predisposition to obesity. Despite the success of these individuals in maintaining a large percentage of their weight losses, small weight regains were common. Very few of these individuals were able to relose the weight after any regain.[178]

Weight Loss Improves Disease-Risk Biomarkers

Weight loss by the obese often exerts a profound effect on biologic factors related to disease risk.[50,157] FIGURE 30.18 shows the percentage changes from initial body weight and the change in biomarkers of disease risk in obese patients over

TABLE 30.3 ■ *TOP.* DIETARY STRATEGIES TO ACHIEVE WEIGHT LOSS OF PARTICIPANTS OF THE NWCR. *BOTTOM.* EFFECTS OF WEIGHT LOSS ON VARIOUS DIMENSIONS OF LIFE REPORTED BY PARTICIPANTS

	PERCENTAGE		
STRATEGY	WOMEN	MEN	TOTAL
Restricted intake of certain types or classes of food	87.8	86.7	87.6
Ate all foods but limited quantity	47.2	32.0	44.2
Counted calories	44.8	39.3	43.7
Limited % lipid intake	31.1	36.7	33.1
Counted lipid grams	25.7	21.3	25.2
Followed exchange diet	25.2	11.3	22.5
Used liquid formula	19.1	26.0	20.4
Ate only 1 or 2 food types	5.1	6.7	5.5

	PERCENTAGE		
AREA OF LIFE	IMPROVED	NO DIFFERENCE	WORSENED
Quality of life	95.3	4.3	0.4
Level of energy	92.4	6.7	0.9
Mobility	92.3	7.1	0.6
General mood	91.4	6.9	1.6
Self-confidence	90.9	9.0	0.1
Physical health	85.8	12.9	1.3
Interactions with:			
Opposite sex	65.2	32.9	0.9
Same sex	5.0	46.8	0.4
Strangers	69.5	30.4	0.1
Job performance	54.5	45.0	0.6
Hobbies	49.1	36.7	0.4
Spouse interactions	56.3	37.3	5.9

From Klem MI, et al. A descriptive study of individuals successful at long-term maintenance of substantial weight loss. Am J Clin Nutr 1997;66:239.

a 27-month period using two energy-restricting meal plans. In phase 1 during the first 3 months, group A ($N = 50$) attempted to consume an energy-restricted diet (1200–1500 kCal daily) composed of conventional, self-selected meals prepared by the subjects; group B ($N = 50$), assigned the same caloric intake, substituted two meals and two snack-replacement shakes, soups, hot chocolate, and snack bars (Slim-Fast) for self-selected foods. In phase 2 (months 4 to 27), all subjects consumed self-selected diets of equal caloric value with one meal and one shake replacement. Unequivocal results emerged from both study phases. Group B's greater weight loss during the 3-month phase 1 period was attributed to a larger caloric deficit created with this eating plan. Thereafter, both groups reduced on average an additional 0.07% of initial body weight each month (4.2 kg for group A and 3.0 kg for group B). The *bottom figure* shows absolute changes in eight disease biomarkers during phases 1 and 2. Both groups reduced systolic blood pressure and plasma insulin, glucose, and triacylglycerol concentrations over the 27-month weight-loss period. These findings support the notion that a modest but sustained weight loss produces long-term health benefits as reflected by improvement in documented risk factors.

Setpoint Theory: A Case Against Dieting

One can crash off large amounts of weight in a relatively short time by simply not eating. Unfortunately, success is short-lived, and eventually the urge to eat wins out and the lost weight returns. Some argue that the reason for this failure lies in a genetically determined "setpoint" for body weight (or body fat) that differs from what the dieter would like. The proponents of a **setpoint theory** maintain that all persons (fat or thin) have a well-regulated internal control mechanism located deep within the lateral hypothalamus that maintains with relative ease a preset level of body weight and/or body fat within a tight range. In a practical sense, this represents a person's body weight when not counting calories. Exercise and FDA-approved antiobesity drugs may lower a person's setpoint, whereas dieting exerts no effect. Each time body weight decreases below one's preestablished setpoint, internal adjustments that affect food intake and regulatory thermogenesis resist the change and conserve and/or replenish body fat. For example, resting metabolism slows and the individual becomes obsessed with food, unable to control the urge to eat. Even when persons overeat and gain body fat above their normal level, the body resists this change by increasing resting metabolism and causing the person to lose interest in food.[96]

Resting Metabolism Decreases

Resting metabolism often decreases when dieting progressively produces weight loss.[162,256] Hypometabolism with caloric deficit often exceeds the decrease attributable to the loss of body mass or FFM independent of the person's weight status or prior dieting history. A depressed metabolism conserves energy, causing the diet to become progressively less effective despite a restricted caloric intake. This produces a weight-loss plateau. Further weight loss occurs at a slower pace than predicted from the mathematics of the restricted energy intake.

FIGURE 30.19A shows the close coupling between daily total energy expenditure (TEE) required to maintain a constant FFM in obese and nonobese subjects at their usual body weights. When body weight declined by 10% below the usual weight (Fig. 30.19B), TEE declined more than explained by the normal relation between energy expenditure and FFM. Both obese and normal-weight subjects became more energy efficient, requiring disproportionately lower energy intake to maintain the lower body weight. Conversely, increasing body weight by 10% above usual weight (Fig. 30.19C) produced a

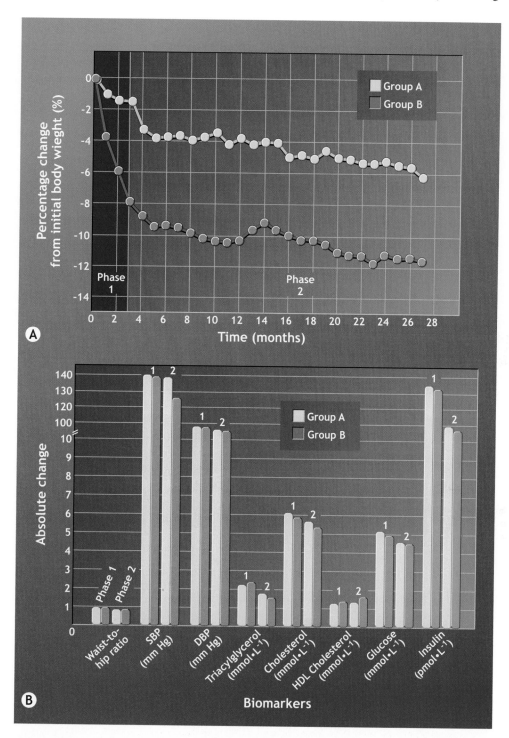

Figure 30.18   A. Average percentage change from initial body weight of obese patients during 27 months of treatment with an energy-restricted diet containing 1200–1500 kCal. **B.** Absolute changes in biomarkers for groups A (energy-restricted, self-selected, self-prepared meals) and B (Slim-Fast replacement meals) from baseline (Phase 1) to 27 months of energy restriction (Phase 2). *SBP,* systolic blood pressure; *DBP,* diastolic blood pressure. (Modified from Detschuneit HH, et al. Metabolic and weight-loss effects of a long-term dietary intervention in obese patients. Am J Clin Nutr 1999;69:198.)

15 to 20% unanticipated *increase* in energy expenditure that countered the gain in body fat. These data support the setpoint concept, or "command signal" that modulates metabolism to defend a specific level of body fat; unfortunately in the obese, regulation occurs at a higher body fat level.

FIGURE 30.20 shows further evidence of the body's "defense" against deviations in body weight. The research carefully monitored body mass, resting oxygen consumption (minimal energy requirement), and caloric intake of six obese men for 31 days. During the prediet period, body

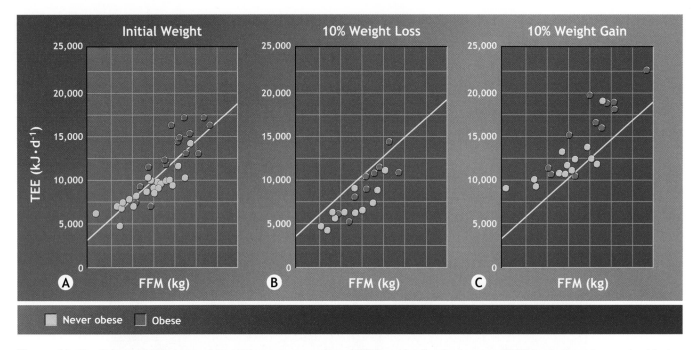

Figure 30.19   Relationship between daily total energy expenditure *(TEE)* and fat-free body mass *(FFM)* in obese and normal subjects **(A)** at their usual body weights, **(B)** after 10% weight reduction, and **(C)** after 10% weight gain. (From Leibel RL, et al. Changes in energy expenditure resulting from altered body weight. N Engl J Med 1995;332:621.)

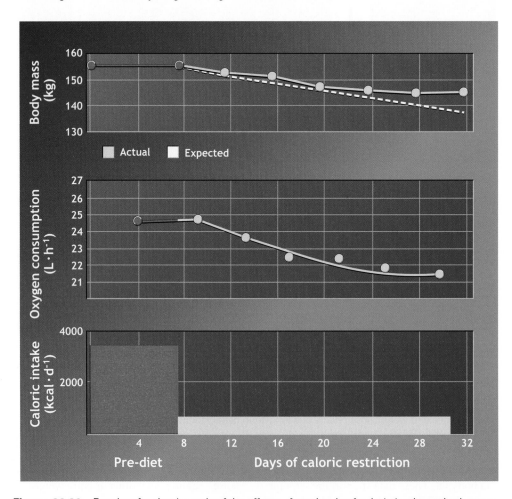

Figure 30.20   Results of a classic study of the effects of two levels of caloric intake on body mass and resting oxygen consumption. Failure of the actual weight loss to keep pace with that predicted on the basis of food restriction *(dashed line)* often leaves the dieter frustrated and discouraged. (Adapted from Bray G. Effect of caloric restriction on energy expenditure in obese subjects. Lancet 1969;2:397.)

weight and resting oxygen consumption stabilized with a daily food intake of 3500 kCal. Thereafter, daily caloric intake decreased to 450 kCal. When the subjects switched to the low-calorie diet, body weight and resting metabolism decreased, but the percentage decline in metabolism exceeded the body weight decrease. The *dashed line* (upper figure) represents the expected weight loss for the 450-kCal diet. The decline in resting metabolism (middle figure) conserved energy to make the diet progressively less effective. More than one half of the total weight loss occurred over the first 8 days of dieting; the remaining weight loss occurred during the final 16 days. A plateau in the theoretical weight-loss curve often frustrates and discourages dieters causing them to abandon the program.

Biologic Feedback Mechanism

Further disconcerting news awaits those who desire permanent fat loss. When overfat people lose weight, adipocytes increase their level of the fat-storing enzyme LPL.[118] This adaptation facilitates body fat synthesis, and the fatter the person before weight loss, the greater the LPL production with weight loss. In essence, the fatter one is at the start, the more vigorously the body attempts to regain the lost weight. This observation supports the existence of a biologic feedback mechanism between the brain and the body's fat levels and helps to explain the difficulty overfat individuals have maintaining weight loss.

The setpoint theory delivers unwelcome news for those with a setpoint "tuned" too high; encouragingly, regular exercise may lower the setpoint level. Concurrently, regular exercise conserves and even increases FFM, raises resting metabolism (if FFM increases), and induces metabolic changes that facilitate fat catabolism. These healthful adaptations all augment the weight-loss effort. On p. 867 we discuss how food intake tends to decline initially, despite the increase in energy output, for overly fat men and women who begin to exercise regularly. As a physically active lifestyle continues and body fat decreases, caloric intake balances daily energy requirements to stabilize body mass at a new, lower level.

Challenge to the Setpoint Proponents. Some research challenges the argument that individuals who lose weight necessarily *maintain* the initial depressed metabolism that predisposes them to weight regain.[252] Undoubtedly, energy restriction produces a *transient state* of hypometabolism if the dieter maintains the state of negative energy intake. This adaptive downregulation in resting metabolism does not persist when individuals lose weight but then reestablish balance where energy intake equals energy expenditure at their lower body weight. Consequently, research that fails to establish energy balance after weight loss gives the inaccurate impression that individuals who lose weight necessarily battle a prolonged overcompensating reduction in resting energy expenditure until they return to their original body weight. Replication of these findings will reinforce that downregulation of resting metabolism is not a necessary characteristic of

weight loss or a primary component to explain the tendency for weight regain.

Dieting Extremes

Professional organizations have voiced strong opposition to some dietary practices, particularly extremes of fasting and low-carbohydrate, high-fat, and high-protein diets. Dietary extremes raise concern about athletes and other adolescents and young adults who routinely engage in bizarre and often pathogenic weight-control behaviors (see "In a Practical Sense," p. 862).

Low Carbohydrate–Ketogenic Diets

Ketogenic diets emphasize carbohydrate restriction while generally ignoring total calories and the diet's cholesterol and saturated fat content. Billed as a "diet revolution" and championed by the late Dr. Robert C. Atkins,[7] the diet was first promoted in the late 1800s and has appeared in various forms since then. Long disparaged by the medical establishment, advocates maintain that restricting daily carbohydrate intake to 20 g or less for the initial 2 weeks, with some liberalization afterward, causes the body to mobilize considerable fat for energy. This generates excess plasma ketone bodies—byproducts of incomplete fat breakdown from inadequate carbohydrate catabolism; ketones supposedly suppress appetite. Theoretically, the ketones lost in the urine represent unused energy that should further facilitate weight loss. Some advocates claim that urinary energy loss becomes so great that dieters can eat all they want as long as they restrict carbohydrates.

The singular focus of the low-carbohydrate diet craze may eventually reduce caloric intake, despite claims that dieters need not consider calorie intake as long as lipid represents the excess. Initial weight loss also may result largely from dehydration caused by an extra solute load on the kidneys that increases water excretion. Water loss does *not* reduce body fat. Low-carbohydrate intake also sets the stage for lean tissue loss because the body recruits amino acids from muscle to maintain blood glucose via gluconeogenesis—an undesirable side effect for a diet designed to induce body fat loss. Although an estimated 30 to 40 million Americans attempted a low-carbohydrate diet in 2005, it remains unclear whether the ketogenic diet facilitates fat loss compared with a well-balanced, low-calorie diet rich in unrefined, fiber-rich complex carbohydrates. In general, weight loss relates principally to a diet's low caloric content and diet duration rather than reduced carbohydrate content.

Three recent controlled clinical trials compared the Atkins-type, low-carbohydrate diet with traditional low-fat diets for weight loss.[69,201,268] The low-carbohydrate diet was more effective in achieving a modest weight loss for severely overweight persons. Some measures of heart health also improved as reflected by a more favorable lipid profile and glycemic control in those who followed the low-carbohydrate diet for up to 1 year.[223] Such findings add a measure of credibility to low-carbohydrate diets and challenge conventional

RECOGNIZING WARNING SIGNS OF DISORDERED EATING

■ Disordered eating refers to a broad spectrum of complex behaviors, core attitudes, coping strategies, and conditions that share an emotionally based, inordinate, and often pathologic focus on body shape and weight.

ANOREXIA ATHLETICA

A cluster of personality traits exists among some athletes that often shares a commonality with patients with clinical eating disorders. The same traits that help an athlete excel in sports—compulsive, driven, dichotomous thinker, perfectionist, competitive, compliant and eager to please ("coachable"), and self-motivated—increase the risks for developing disordered eating patterns. This risk grows for individuals whose normal, genetically determined body size and shape deviate from the "ideal" imposed by the sport. The term **anorexia athletica** describes the continuum of subclinical eating behaviors of athletes who fail to meet the criteria for a true eating disorder but who exhibit at least one unhealthy method of weight control, including fasting, vomiting, or use of diet pills, laxatives, or diuretics ("water pills"). Clinical observations indicate a prevalence of disordered eating behaviors of 15 to 60% among athletes, depending on the sport.

For many athletes, patterns of disordered eating coincide with the competitive season and abate when the season ends. For them, the preoccupation with body weight may not reflect a true underlying pathology but a desire to achieve optimum physiologic function and competitive performance. For a small number of athletes, the season never ends and they develop a full-blown eating disorder. Anorexia nervosa and bulimia nervosa are the two most common eating disorders. A third category, binge-eating disorder, does not include purging behavior.

ANOREXIA NERVOSA

Originally described in ancient writings, anorexia nervosa is an unhealthy physical and mental state characterized by a crippling obsession with body size. A "nervous loss of appetite" reflects preoccu-

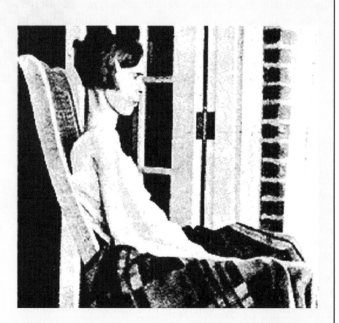

The "first published photo of an anorectic in an American medical journal. By the 1930s there were three essential techniques in the management of anorexia nervosa: change of environment, forced feeding, and psychotherapy. Severe cases were generally treated in private psychiatric hospitals." (From Fasting girls. N Engl J Med 1932;207(5):Oct.)

pation with dieting and thinness and refusal to eat enough food to maintain normal body weight. The relentless pursuit of thinness (present in about 1 to 2% of the general population) includes an intense fear of weight gain and fatness (despite a low body weight) and failure to menstruate regularly (amenorrhea). Anorectic persons have a distorted body image; they actually perceive themselves as fat despite their emaciation.

Anorexia nervosa usually begins with a normal attempt to lose weight through dieting (Table 1). With prolonged dieting, the individual continues to eat less until practically no food is consumed. Eventually, food restriction becomes an obsession, and the anorectic person achieves no sense of satisfaction despite weight loss. Eventually, the anorectic person exhibits denial of the accompanying extreme emaciation.

continued on page 863

Continued

TABLE 1 ■ WARNING SIGNS OF ANOREXIA NERVOSA

- Preoccupation with being too fat despite maintenance of normal body weight
- Loss of menstrual cycle (amenorrhea)
- Frequent commenting about body weight or shape
- Significant loss of body weight
- Weight too low for athletic performance
- Ritualistic concern and preoccupation with dieting, counting calories, cooking, and eating meals
- Excessive concern about body weight, size, and shape, even after weight loss
- Feeling of helplessness in the presence of food
- Severe shifts in mood
- Guilt about eating
- Compulsive need for continuous, vigorous physical activity that exceeds training requirements for a specific sport
- Maintenance of a skinny look (body weight less than 85% of expected weight)
- Prefers to eat in isolation
- Wears baggy clothes to disguise thin-looking appearance
- Episodes of bingeing and purging

BULIMIA NERVOSA

The term *bulimia,* literally meaning "ox hunger," refers to "gorging" or "insatiable appetite." Bulimia nervosa, far more common than anorexia nervosa, is characterized by frequent episodes of binge eating almost always followed by purging and intense feelings of guilt and shame (Table 2). Approximately 2 to 4% of all adolescents and adults in the general population (almost exclusively female, including 5% of college women) have bulimia nervosa. Unlike the continual semistarvation of anorexia nervosa, binge eating characterizes bulimia nervosa. The bulimic person consumes calorically dense food within several hours, often at night, usually containing between 1000 and 10,000 calories, followed by fasting, self-induced vomiting, taking laxatives or diuretics, or compulsive exercising solely to avoid gaining weight.

BINGE-EATING DISORDER

Episodes of bingeing, often without the subsequent purging behavior common to bulimia nervosa, characterize binge-eating disorder. Individuals eat more rapidly than normal until they can consume no additional food. Food intake greatly exceeds that determined by the physiologic hunger drive. Binge eating, done in private, occurs with feelings of guilt, depression, or self-disgust. These individuals suffer greater self-anger, shame, lack of control, and frustration than nonbingeing overfat individuals. The diagnosis of binge-eating disorder requires that the individual experiences a lack of control over eating and marked psychologic distress when it occurs. The person must binge at least an average of 2 days a week for 6 months. Binge eating differs from the overfat condition because the same level of self-anger, shame, lack of control, and frustration about binge eating does not necessarily accompany obesity. Little factual information exists about the prevalence of binge-eating disorder; it may occur in approximately 2% of the U.S. population.

TABLE 2 ■ WARNING SIGNS OF BULIMIA NERVOSA

- Excessive concern about body weight, body size, and body composition
- Frequent gains and losses in body weight
- Visits to the bathroom following meals
- Fear of not being able to stop eating
- Eating when depressed
- Compulsive dieting after binge-eating episodes
- Severe shifts in mood (depression, loneliness)
- Secretive binge eating but never overeating in front of others
- More frequent criticism of own body size and shape
- Personal or family problems with alcohol or drugs
- Irregular menstrual cycle (oligomenorrhea)

References

Agras WS, et al. Report of the National Institutes of Health workshop on overcoming barriers to treatment research in anorexia nervosa. Int J Eat Disord 2004;35:509.

Field AE, Colditz GA. Exposure to the mass media, body shape concerns, and use of supplements to improve weight and shape among male and female adolescents. Pediatrics 2005;116:214.

Hay P, Bacaltchuk J. Bulimia nervosa. Clin Evid 2004;12:1326.

Klump KL, Gobrogge KL. A review and primer of molecular genetic studies of anorexia nervosa. Int J Eat Disord 2005;37:S43.

Silber TJ. Anorexia nervosa among children and adolescents. Adv Pediatr 2005;52:49.

Striegel-Moore RH, et al. Eating disorders in white and black women. Am J Psychiatry 2003;160:1326.

Striegel-Moore RH, Franko DL. Epidemiology of binge eating disorder. Int J Eat Disord 2003;34:S19.

wisdom concerning the potential dangers from consuming a high-fat diet.

Importantly, Atkins-type, high-fat low-carbohydrate diets require systematic long-term evaluation (up to 5 years) for safety and effectiveness, particularly related to the blood lipid profile. The diet, which places no limit on the amount of meat, fat, eggs, and cheese a person consumes, poses nine potential health hazards:

1. Raises serum uric acid levels
2. Potentiates development of kidney stones
3. Alters electrolyte concentrations to initiate cardiac arrhythmias
4. Causes acidosis
5. Aggravates existing kidney problems from the extra solute burden in the renal filtrate
6. Depletes glycogen reserves, contributing to a fatigued state
7. Decreases calcium balance and increases risk for bone loss
8. Causes dehydration
9. Retards fetal development during pregnancy from inadequate carbohydrate intake

For high-performance endurance athletes who train mainly above 65% of maximum effort, switching to a high-fat diet is ill advised because of the body's need to maintain adequate glucose in the bloodstream and glycogen packed in the active muscles and liver storage depots. Fatigue during intense exercise for more than 60 minutes duration occurs more rapidly when athletes consume high-fat meals than with carbohydrate-rich meals.

High-Protein Diets

Low-carbohydrate, high-protein diets may shed pounds in the near term, but their long-term success remains questionable and may even pose health risks.[56] These diets have been promoted to the obese as "last-chance diets." Earlier versions consisted of protein in liquid form advertised as "miracle liquid." Unknown to the consumer, the liquid protein mixture often contained a blend of ground-up animal hooves and horns, with pigskin mixed in a broth with enzymes and tenderizers to "predigest" it. Collagen-based blends produced from gelatin hydrolysis (supplemented with small amounts of essential amino acids) did not contain the highest quality amino acid mixture and lacked required vitamins and minerals (particularly copper). A negative copper balance coincides with electrocardiographic abnormalities and rapid heart rate.[61] Protein-rich foods often contain high levels of saturated fat, which increase the risk for heart disease and type 2 diabetes. Diets excessively high in animal protein increase urinary excretion of oxalate, a compound that combines primarily with calcium to form kidney stones.[191] The diet's safety improves if it contains high-quality protein with ample carbohydrate, essential fatty acids, and micronutrients.[166]

Some argue that an extremely high protein intake suppresses appetite through reliance on fat mobilization and subsequent ketone formation. The elevated thermic effect of dietary protein, with its relatively low coefficient of digestibility (particularly for plant protein), reduces the net calories available from ingested protein compared with a well-balanced meal of equivalent caloric value. This point has some validity, but one must consider other factors when formulating a sound weight-loss program, particularly for physically active individuals. Four important considerations include a high-protein diet's potential for (1) strain on liver and kidney function and accompanying dehydration, (2) electrolyte imbalance, (3) glycogen depletion, and (4) lean-tissue loss.

Semistarvation Diets

A therapeutic fast or **very low-calorie diet** (**VLCD**) may benefit severe clinical obesity where body fat exceeds 40 to 50% of body mass. The diet provides between 400 and 800 kCal daily as high-quality protein foods or liquid meal replacements. Dietary prescriptions usually last up to 3 months but only as a "last resort" before undertaking more-extreme medical approaches for morbid obesity that include various surgical treatments (collectively called bariatric surgery). Surgical treatments that considerably reduce stomach size and reconfigure the small intestine induce a sustained weight loss, but they only are prescribed for patients with a BMI of at least 40, or a BMI of 35 when accompanied by other obesity-related medical conditions.

Dieting with VLCD requires close supervision, usually in a hospital setting. Proponents maintain that severe food restriction breaks established dietary habits, which in turn improves the long-term prospects for success. These diets also may depress appetite to help compliance. Daily medications that accompany a VLCD include calcium carbonate for nausea, bicarbonate of soda and potassium chloride to maintain consistency of body fluids, mouthwash and sugar-free chewing gum for bad breath (from a high level of ketones from fatty acid catabolism), and bath oils for dry skin. *For most individuals, semistarvation does not compose an "ultimate diet" or proper approach to weight control.* Because a VLCD provides inadequate carbohydrate, the glycogen-storage depots in the liver and muscles deplete rapidly. This impairs physical tasks that require either intense aerobic effort or shorter-duration anaerobic power output. The continuous nitrogen loss with fasting and weight loss reflects an exacerbated lean tissue loss. This may occur disproportionately from critical organs like the heart.[172] The success rate remains poor for prolonged fasting.

TABLE 30.4 summarizes the principles and main advantages and disadvantages of popular dietary approaches to weight loss. Most diets produce weight loss during the first several weeks, although body water makes up much of the lost weight. In addition, lean tissue loss occurs with dieting alone, particularly in the early phase of a VLCD.[119,134] An individual can certainly reduce weight through dieting alone, but few persons achieve long-term success in favorably altering body size and composition.

TABLE 30.4 ■ PRINCIPLES, ADVANTAGES, AND DISADVANTAGES OF SOME POPULAR WEIGHT LOSS METHODS

METHOD	PRINCIPLE	ADVANTAGES	DISADVANTAGES	COMMENTS
Surgical procedures	Alteration of gastrointestinal tract changes capacity or amount of absorptive surface	Caloric restriction less necessary	Risks of surgery and postsurgical complications include death[a]	Radical procedures include stomach stapling and removal of section of small intestine (jejunoileal bypass)
Fasting	No energy input ensures negative energy balance	Rapid weight loss Reduced exposure to temptation	Ketogenic Large portion of weight lost from lean body mass Nutrients lacking	Medical supervision mandatory and hospitalization recommended
Protein-sparing modified fast	Same as fasting except protein or protein with carbohydrate intake assumed to preserve lean body mass	Same as fasting	Ketogenic Nutrients lacking Some deaths reported, possibly from electrolyte depletion	Medical supervision mandatory Example: *The Last Chance Diet*
One food–centered diets	Low caloric intake favors negative energy balance	Easy to follow (initial psychologic appeal)	Too restrictive; nutrients lacking Repetitious nature causes boredom	No food or food combination "burns off" fat Examples: grapefruit diet and egg diet
Low-carbohydrate/ high-fat diets	Increased ketone excretion removes energy from the body Fat intake often voluntarily decreased; results in low caloric intake	Inclusion of rich foods has psychologic appeal Initial rapid water loss an incentive	Ketogenic High-fat intake contraindicated for heart and diabetes patients Nutrients lacking	Examples include Atkins diet and South Beach diet, and the "Mayo," "Drinking Man's," and "Air Force" diets
Low-carbohydrate/ high-protein diets	Low caloric intake favors negative energy balance	Initial rapid water loss an incentive Increased thermic effect of protein	Expense and repetitious; difficult to sustain	If meat emphasized, the diet becomes high in fat
High-carbohydrate/ low-fat diets	Low caloric intake favors negative energy balance	Wise food selections can make the diet nutritionally sound	Initial water retention (from glycogen storage) may be discouraging	Examples include the Pennington diet and the Pritikin diet

Modified and reprinted by permission from Reed PB. Nutrition: an applied science. Copyright © 1980 by West Publishing Co. All rights reserved.
[a] Zigmond DS, et al. Hospitalization before and after gastric bypass surgery. JAMA 2005;294:1918.

FACTORS THAT AFFECT WEIGHT LOSS

Hydration level and duration of the energy deficit affect the amount and composition of weight lost.

Early Weight Loss Is Largely Water

FIGURE 30.21 shows the general trend for the percentage composition of daily weight loss during 4 weeks of dieting. Water makes up about 70% of the weight lost over the first week of energy deficit. Thereafter, water loss progressively lessens, representing only about 20% of the weight lost in the second and third weeks; concurrently, body fat loss accelerates from 25 to 70%. During the fourth week of dieting, reductions in body fat produce about 85% of the weight loss without further increase in water loss. Protein's contribution

to weight loss increases from 5% initially to about 15% after the fourth week.

Hydration Level

Restricting water during the first several days of a caloric deficit increases the *proportion* of body water lost and decreases the *proportion* of fat lost. More total weight loss occurs with restricted daily water intake, but the additional weight lost comes solely from water as dehydration progresses. *Dieters lose the same quantity of body fat regardless of fluid intake level.*

Longer Term Deficit Promotes Fat Loss

FIGURE 30.22 reinforces the important concept that the caloric equivalent of the weight lost increases as duration of

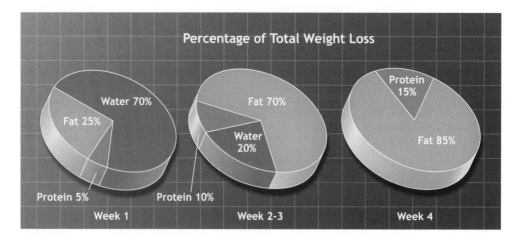

Figure 30.21   General trend for the percentage composition of the weight lost during 4 weeks of caloric restriction.

caloric restriction progresses. After 2 months on a diet, the caloric equivalent of weight loss exceeds twice that in the first week. *This points out the importance of maintaining a caloric deficit for an extended duration. Shorter periods of caloric restriction produce a larger percentage of water and carbohydrate loss per unit weight reduction with only a minimal decrease in body fat.*

EXERCISE FOR WEIGHT CONTROL

Conventional wisdom views excessive food intake as the prime cause of the overfat condition. Most persons believe that the only way to reduce unwanted body fat entails caloric restriction by dieting. This overly simplistic strategy partly accounts for the dismal success in maintaining weight loss over the long term, refocusing debate on the contribution of food intake to obesity.[86,212] Despite controversy about the precise

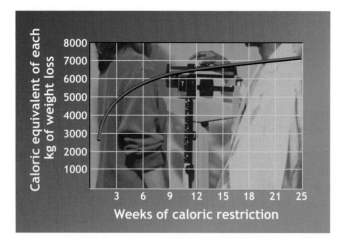

Figure 30.22   General trend for the energy (caloric) equivalent of the weight lost in relation to the duration of caloric restriction. As caloric restriction progresses, the energy equivalent per unit of weight lost increases to about 7000 kCal per kilogram after 20 weeks. This occurs because of the large initial body water loss (no calorie value) early in weight loss.

contributions of physical inactivity and excessive caloric intake to body fat accretion, a sedentary lifestyle consistently emerges as an important factor in weight gain by children, adolescents, and adults.[11,58,190,198]

Not Simply Gluttony

Excess weight gain often parallels reduced physical activity rather than increased caloric intake. Physically active individuals who eat the most often weigh the least and maintain the highest fitness levels.

Obese infants do not characteristically ingest more calories than recommended dietary standards. For children ages 4 to 6 years, daily energy expenditure averaged 25% below the current recommendation for energy intake at this age. A low level of daily physical activity primarily caused the depressed energy output.[29] More specifically, 50% of boys and 75% of girls in the United States fail to engage in even moderate physical activity three or more times weekly.[1] Physically active children tend to be leaner than less active counterparts. For preschool children, no relationship emerged between total energy intake, or the fat, carbohydrate, and protein composition of the diet and percentage body fat.[8] Excessive fatness relates directly to the number of hours spent watching television (a consistent marker of inactivity) among children, adolescents, and adults.[5,76] For example, 3 hours of television viewing a day led to a twofold increase in obesity and a 50% increase in diabetes.[100] Each 2-hour-per-day increment of TV watching coincides with a 23% increase in obesity and a 14% rise in diabetes risk. Excessive television watching, playing video games, and otherwise remaining inactive characterizes overweight minority teens. Estimates indicate that reducing the amount of time spent watching television, playing video games, or using a computer could substantially reduce the incidence of metabolic syndrome.[66] Minimizing time devoted to such behaviors can help combat childhood fat gain.[75,196]

The observation that overfat children often eat the same or even less than peers of average body weight also pertains to less physically active adults as they slowly, progressively gain weight. *Overweight individuals often do not eat more on average than persons of normal weight.* Consequently, it remains neither prudent nor justifiable to emphasize dieting alone to effectively induce long-term weight loss.[87]

Increasing Energy Output

Physically active men and women maintain a desirable body composition. An increased level of regular physical activity combined with dietary restraint maintains weight loss more effectively than long-term caloric restriction alone.[3,22,122] A negative energy balance induced by increased caloric expenditure, through either lifestyle activities or formal exercise programs, unbalances the energy balance equation for weight loss, improves physical fitness, and favorably alters body composition and body fat distribution.[128,149,177,198,241] Regular exercise produces less accumulation of central adipose tissue associated with aging.[112,124,199,239] Overweight women show a dose–response relationship between amount of exercise and long-term weight loss.[106] Obese adolescents and adults improve body composition and visceral fat distribution from both moderate physical activity or more vigorous exercise that improves cardiovascular fitness. For obese boys and girls, the most favorable body composition changes occur with (1) low-intensity, long-duration exercise; (2) aerobic exercise combined with high-repetition resistance training; and (3) exercise programs combined with a behavior-modification component.[83,144,155] Additional spin-off from regular exercise includes slowing of the age-related loss in muscle mass, possible prevention of adult-onset obesity, improvement in obesity-related comorbidities, decreased mortality, and beneficial effects on existing chronic diseases.[18,85,142,152,225,250]

Misconceptions About Exercise

Two arguments attempt to counter the exercise approach to weight loss. One maintains that exercise inevitably increases appetite to produce a proportionate increase in food intake that negates the caloric deficit exercise produces. The second argument claims that the relatively small calorie-burning effect of a normal exercise workout does not "dent" the body's fat reserves as effectively as food restriction.

Misconception 1: Exercise and Food Intake

Sedentary persons often do not balance energy intake and energy expenditure.[154,204] Failure to accurately regulate energy balance at the lower end of the physical activity spectrum contributes to the "creeping obesity" observed in highly mechanized and technically advanced societies. In contrast, regular exercisers maintain appetite control within a reactive zone where food intake more readily matches daily energy expenditure.

In considering the effects of exercise on appetite and food intake, one must distinguish exercise type and duration

and the participant's body fat status. Lumberjacks, farm laborers, and endurance athletes consume about twice as many daily calories as sedentary individuals. More specifically, marathon runners, cross-country skiers, and cyclists consume about 4000 to 5000 kCal daily, yet they are the leanest people in the population. Obviously, their large caloric intake meets the energy requirements of training while maintaining a relatively lean body composition.

For the overweight person, the extra energy required for exercise more than offsets moderate physical activity's small compensatory appetite-stimulating effect. To some extent, the large energy reserve of the overfat person makes it easier to tolerate weight loss and exercise without the obligatory increase in caloric intake typically observed for leaner counterparts.[121,207] No difference emerged in fat, carbohydrate, or protein intake or total calories consumed for overweight men and women during 16 months of supervised, moderate-intensity exercise training compared with a sedentary control group.[52] *In essence, a weak coupling exists between the short-term energy deficit induced by exercise and energy intake. Increased physical activity by overweight, sedentary individuals does not necessarily alter physiologic needs and automatically produce compensatory increases in food intake to balance additional energy expenditure.*

INTEGRATIVE QUESTION

Respond to the person who claims: "The only way to lose weight is to stop eating. It's that simple!"

Misconception 2: Caloric Stress of Physical Activity

A common misconception concerns the contribution to weight loss of the calories burned in typical exercise. Some argue correctly that it requires an inordinate amount of short-term exercise to lose just 0.45 kg of body fat: for example, chopping wood for 10 hours, playing golf for 20 hours, performing mild calisthenics for 22 hours, or playing ping pong for 28 hours or volleyball for 32 hours. Consequently, a 2- or 3-month exercise regimen produces only a small fat loss in an overfat person. From a different perspective, if one played golf (no cart) for 2 hours daily (350 kCal) 2 days per week (700 kCal), it would take about 5 weeks to lose 0.45 kg of body fat. Assuming the person plays year-round, golfing 2 days a week produces a 4.5-kg yearly fat loss provided food intake remains constant. Even an activity as innocuous as chewing gum burns an extra 11 kCal each hour, a 20% increase over normal resting metabolism. *Simply stated, the calorie-expending effects of exercise add up. A caloric deficit of 3500 kCal equals a 0.45-kg body fat loss, whether the deficit occurs rapidly or systematically over time.*

In estimating the energy cost of performing various physical activities, one assumes that exercise energy expenditure remains constant among persons of a particular body size. In Chapter 8, we noted that the energy cost data for most physical activities represent averages, often based on only a few observations. A wide range of values exists because of individual differences in performance style and technique; terrain, temperature, and wind resistance (environmental factors); and intensity of participation. Consequently, energy expenditure values for the physical activities presented in Appendix C (available online at http://connection.lww.com/mkk6e) do not represent constants. Rather, they reflect "average" values applicable under "average" conditions when applied to the "average" person of a given body mass. The data do provide useful approximations to establish the energy cost of diverse physical activities.

The Recovery "Afterglow." Controversy exists about the quantitative contribution of excess postexercise oxygen consumption to the total energy expended in physical activity. With low-to-moderate exercise, as performed by most persons who exercise for weight control, the contribution of recovery metabolism—the so-called **recovery afterglow**—to total energy expenditure remains small relative to exercise energy expenditure, ranging up to 75 kCal for exercise durations of 80 minutes.[179,188] In addition, exercise training induces faster adjustments in postexercise energetics that reduce the magnitude of the total recovery oxygen consumption.[213] *Calories burned during physical activity represent the most important factor in total exercise energy expenditure, not calories expended during recovery.*

EFFECTIVENESS OF REGULAR EXERCISE

The effectiveness of regular exercise for weight loss relates closely to the degree of excess body fat. In general, obese persons lose weight and fat more readily with exercise than normal-weight persons.[198] In addition, aerobic exercise and resistance training, even without dietary restriction, provide positive spin-off to the weight loss effort. They alter body composition favorably (reduced body fat with a small increase in FFM) for the otherwise healthy overweight person, postmenopausal woman, cardiac patient, and physically challenged individual.[127,232] Overfat children who participated in 4 months of 40-minute aerobic exercise sessions 5 days a week without dietary restriction accumulated less visceral adipose tissue than nonexercising controls.[173] The active children also gained more FFM and lost more total fat mass and percentage body fat. Adolescent males who engaged regularly in vigorous activities showed less abdominal fat than sedentary counterparts.[48] This indicates that regular exercise and improved aerobic fitness may target excess fat accumulation in the abdominal–visceral area to a greater extent than peripheral fat deposits. Even when an exercise program produces no loss in body weight, substantial reductions occur in abdominal subcutaneous and visceral fat.[199] This response certainly diminishes a tendency toward insulin resistance and resulting predisposition to type 2 diabetes.

Adding exercise to a weight-loss program favorably modifies the composition of the weight lost in the direction of greater fat loss.[9] In a pioneering study on this topic, each of three groups of adult women maintained a daily caloric deficit of 500 kCal for 16 weeks.[271] The diet group reduced daily food intake by 500 kCal, while the exercise group increased energy output by 500 kCal with a supervised walking and exercise program 5 days weekly. The women using diet plus exercise created a daily 500-kCal deficit by reducing food intake by 250 kCal and increasing energy output by 250 kCal through exercise. No difference emerged among the three groups for weight loss; each group lost approximately 5 kg. This finding shows that a caloric deficit produces body weight loss regardless of the method to create the energy imbalance. The most effective strategy to reduce body fat combined diet and exercise. FFM *increased* by 0.9 kg for the exercise group and 0.5 kg for the combination group, while dieters *lost* 1.1 kg of lean tissue.

Resistance Training. Resistance training provides an important adjunct to aerobic training for weight loss and weight maintenance. The energy expended in circuit-resistance training—continuous exercise using low resistance and high repetitions—averages about 9 kCal per minute. Consequently, this exercise mode burns substantial calories during a typical 30- to 60-minute workout. Even conventional resistance training that involves less total energy expenditure positively affects muscular strength and FFM during weight loss compared with programs that rely solely on food restriction.[10,242] Individuals who maintain high muscular strength levels tend to gain less weight than weaker counterparts.[138] Additionally, standard resistance training performed regularly reduces coronary heart disease risk, improves glycemic control, favorably modifies the lipoprotein profile, and increases resting metabolic rate (when FFM increases).[180,181,185,231]

Comparisons of conventional resistance training with endurance training indicate unique resistance-training benefits on body composition.[20,242] TABLE 30.5 summarizes the effects of 12 weeks of either endurance exercise or resistance training on nondieting, untrained young men. Endurance training reduced percentage body fat (hydrostatic weighing) from reduced fat mass (−1.6 kg; no change in FFM), while resistance training decreased body fat mass (−2.4 kg) and increased the FFM (+2.4 kg). Because FFM remains metabolically more active than body fat, conserving or increasing this tissue depot with exercise training maintains a higher level of resting metabolism, average daily metabolic rate, and possibly fat oxidation during rest, all factors that counteract the age-related increase in adiposity.[28,43,51,219]

TABLE 30.6 shows the effects of regular exercise for weight loss by six sedentary, overfat young men who exercised 5 days a week for 16 weeks by walking 90 minutes each session. The men lost nearly 6 kg of body fat, a decrease in percentage body fat from 23.5 to 18.6%. Exercise capacity also improved as did HDL cholesterol (15.6%) and the HDL-to-LDL cholesterol ratio (25.9%).

FIGURE 30.23 shows body composition changes for 40 obese women placed into one of four groups: (1) control, no exercise, and no diet; (2) diet only, no exercise (DO); (3) diet plus resistance exercise (D + E), and (4) resistance exercise

TABLE 30.5 ■ CHANGES IN BODY COMPOSITION AFTER 12 WEEKS OF EITHER RESISTANCE TRAINING OR ENDURANCE TRAINING

VARIABLE	CONTROLS		RESISTANCE TRAINED		ENDURANCE TRAINED	
	PRE-TREATMENT	POST-TREATMENT	PRE-TREATMENT	POST-TREATMENT	PRE-TREATMENT	POST-TREATMENT
Relative body fat (%)	20.1 ± 8.5	20.2 ± 8.5	21.8 ± 6.2	18.7 ± 6.6[a]	18.4 ± 7.9	16.5 ± 6.4[a]
Fat mass (kg)	16.2 ± 10.8	16.3 ± 10.5	17.2 ± 7.6	14.8 ± 6.2[a]	14.4 ± 7.9	12.8 ± 7.1[a]
Fat-free body mass (kg)	64.3 ± 5.4	64.4 ± 6.6	61.9 ± 8.3	64.4 ± 9.0[a]	64.1 ± 8.2	64.7 ± 8.6
Total body mass (kg)	80.5 ± 8.1	80.7 ± 8.5	79.1 ± 8.3	79.2 ± 7.6	78.5 ± 8.2	77.5 ± 7.9

From Broeder CE, et al. Assessing body composition before and after resistance or endurance training. Med Sci Sports Exerc 1997;29:705.
[a] Significant difference between pre- and posttest measurements ($P < .05$).
All values means ± SD.

only, no diet (EO). The women trained 3 days a week for 8 weeks. They performed 10 repetitions each of three sets of eight strength exercises. Body mass decreased for DO (−4.5 kg) and D + E (−3.9 kg), compared with EO (+0.5 kg) and controls (−0.4 kg). Importantly, FFM increased for EO (+1.1 kg), whereas the DO group lost 0.9 kg of FFM. The authors concluded that augmenting a calorie-restriction program with resistance exercise training preserves FFM better than dietary restriction alone.

Most of the health-related metabolic improvements in the obese with regular exercise relate to total exercise volume and quantity of fat loss rather than enhanced cardiorespiratory

fitness.[44,45,177] Ideal exercise consists of continuous, large-muscle activities with moderate-to-high caloric cost such as circuit resistance training, walking, running, rope skipping, stair stepping, cycling, and swimming. Many recreational sports and games also are effective in weight control, but precise quantification and regulation of energy expenditure becomes difficult. Aerobic exercise stimulates fat catabolism, establishes favorable blood pressure responses, and generally promotes cardiovascular fitness. Interestingly, aerobic exercise training may elevate resting metabolism independent of any FFM change.[265] No selective effect exists for running, walking, or bicycling; each promotes fat loss with equal effectiveness.[182] Expenditure of an extra 300 kCal daily (e.g., jogging for 30 minutes) should produce a 0.45-kg fat loss in about 12 days. This represents

TABLE 30.6 ■ EFFECTIVENESS OF A 16-WEEK WALKING PROGRAM ON BODY COMPOSITION AND BLOOD LIPID CHANGES IN SIX OVERFAT, YOUNG MEN

VARIABLE	PRE-TRAINING[a]	POST-TRAINING[a]	DIFFERENCE
Body mass (kg)	99.1	93.4	−5.7[b]
Body density, g · mL⁻¹	1.044	1.056	+0.012[b]
Body fat (%)	23.5	18.6	−4.9[b]
Fat mass (kg)	23.3	17.4	−5.9[b]
Fat-free body mass (kg)	75.8	76.0	+0.2
Sum of skinfolds (mm)	142.9	104.8	−38.1[b]
HDL cholesterol, mg · dL⁻¹	32	37	5.0[b]
HDL/LDL cholesterol	0.27	0.34	+0.07[b]

From Leon AS, et al. Effects of a vigorous walking program on body composition, and carbohydrate and lipid metabolism of obese young men. Am J Clin Nutr 1979;33:1776.
[a] Values are means.
[b] Statistically significant.

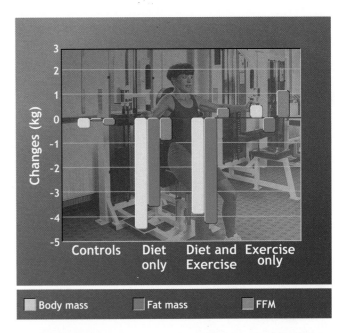

Figure 30.23 Changes in body composition with combinations of resistance exercise and/or diet in obese females. (From Ballor DL, et al. Resistance weight training during caloric restriction enhances lean body weight maintenance. Am J Clin Nutr 1988; 47:19.)

a yearly caloric deficit equivalent to the energy in 13.6 kg of body fat.

Dose–Response Relationship

The total energy expended in physical activity relates in a dose–response manner to the effectiveness of exercise for weight loss.[9,106] A reasonable goal progressively increases moderate exercise to between 60 and 90 minutes daily or a level that burns 2100 to 2800 kCal weekly.[65,111] To combat the worldwide obesity epidemic, the public health perspective must promote a population's need to increase *total* daily energy expenditure substantially and regularly rather than increase exercise intensity to induce a training response. An overly fat person who starts out with light exercise such as slow walking accrues a considerable caloric expenditure simply by extending exercise duration. The focus on exercise duration offsets the inadvisability of having a sedentary, obese individual begin a program with more strenuous exercise. Also, the energy cost of weight-bearing exercise relates directly to body mass; the overweight person expends considerably more calories in such exercise than someone of average weight.

INTEGRATIVE QUESTION

Among physically active men and women, how can individuals who consume the most calories weigh less than those who consume fewer calories?

Walking–Running for Different Durations

The duration of exercise affects fat loss. TABLE 30.7 lists changes in body fat for three groups of men who exercised for 20 weeks by walking and running for either 15, 30, or 45 minutes per workout. Data also include distance run and total duration of weekly workouts, training heart rate, body mass, sum of six skinfolds, and waist girth.

The three exercise groups decreased body fat, skinfolds, and waist girth compared with sedentary controls. Body weight also decreased with exercise, except for the 15-minute group whose weight remained stable. Comparing the three exercise groups, the 45-minute group lost more body fat than either the 30- or 15-minute group. This difference was closely linked to the greater caloric expenditure with longer exercise (i.e., a dose–response relationship).

TABLE 30.7 ■ EFFECTS OF THREE TRAINING DURATIONS OF WALKING AND RUNNING ON BODY COMPOSITION CHANGES[a]

			TRAINING GROUP					
	CONTROL (N = 16)		15 MINUTE (N = 14)		30 MINUTE (N = 17)		45 MINUTE (N = 12)	
VARIABLE	PRE	POST	PRE	POST	PRE	POST	PRE	POST
Body mass (kg)	72.1	73.2	76.9	76.3	80.6	78.9	70.9	69.9
Body fat (%)	12.5	13.0	13.7	13.2	14.2	13.6	13.2	12.0
Sum skinfolds (mm)	73.8	79.6	83.0	77.0	90.0	83.8	77.5	67.0
Waist girth (cm)	82.7	84.9	84.3	82.8	88.2	86.1	83.6	81.8
Distance run per workout (mi)	Week 4		1.56		2.89		4.13	
	8		1.54		2.95		4.46	
	13		1.79		3.19		4.82	
	17		1.75		3.24		5.06	
Total time of exercise (min:s)	Week 4		14:58		30:25		41:18	
	8		14:11		28:40		42:48	
	13		15:51		29:43		43:19	
	17		14:53		30:12		42:27	
Training heart rate (b · min^{-1})	Week 4		179		175		174	
	8		179		174		169	
	13		182		175		177	
	17		180		175		175	
Intensity (%max HR)	Week 4		89.4		83.8		84.5	
	8		89.8		73.4		81.0	
	13		94.0		90.1		89.5	
	17		92.5		90.2		88.1	

From Milesis CA, et al. Effects of different durations of physical training on cardiorespiratory function, body composition, and serum lipids. Res Q 1976;47:716.

Exercise Frequency

To determine the optimal exercise frequency for weight loss, subjects exercised for 30 to 47 minutes for 20 weeks by either running or walking, with exercise intensity maintained between 80 and 95% of maximum heart rate.[183] Training twice weekly produced no changes in body mass, skinfolds, or percentage body fat, but training 3 and 4 days weekly did. Subjects who trained 4 days a week reduced body weight and skinfolds more than subjects who trained 3 days a week. Percentage body fat decreased similarly in both groups. These findings support a recommendation to exercise a *minimum* of 3 days per week to favorably alter body composition; the additional caloric expenditure with more frequent exercise produces even greater results. The threshold exercise energy expenditure for weight loss probably remains highly individualized. The calorie-burning effect of each exercise session should eventually reach *at least* 300 kCal whenever possible. This generally occurs with 30 minutes of moderate-to-vigorous running, swimming, bicycling, or circuit-resistance training or 60 minutes of brisk walking.

INTEGRATIVE QUESTION

Why should individuals limit weight loss to no more than 2 pounds of body weight weekly?

Start Slowly and Progress Gradually

The initial stage of an exercise–weight-loss program for a previously sedentary, overly fat person should be developmental with moderate energy demands. The individual should adopt long-term goals and personal discipline and restructure eating and exercise behaviors. Unduly rapid training progressions prove counterproductive because most overfat individuals initially resist increasing their physical activity. During the first few months, intervals of faster paced walking can replace slow walking. Meaningful changes in body weight and body composition require at least 12 weeks. Most overfat persons can realistically expect to reduce body weight by 5 to 15% with programs that focus on modifying eating and exercise behaviors. Behavioral approaches to exercise should foster lifestyle changes in daily physical activity.[233] For example, walking or bicycling can replace the auto, stair climbing can replace the elevator, and manual tools can replace power tools.[4,54] Eating less and exercising more proves more effective in a group situation than going it alone. Persons who joined a weight-loss program with several friends or family members lost more weight than individuals who participated alone.[264]

Self-Selected Energy Expenditures: Mode of Exercise

No selective effect exists among diverse modes of big-muscle aerobic exercise with equivalent energy expenditures to favorably reduce body weight, body fat, skinfold thickness, and girths, yet other differences may emerge. For example,

FIGURE 30.24A shows that men and women generally self-select a higher energy expenditure level (with accompanying higher heart rates) at similar ratings of perceived exertion when running for 20 minutes on a treadmill than when performing simulated cross-country skiing (NordicTrack), cycle ergometry, or aerobic riding (HealthRider).[130] Men selected a higher absolute level of exercise intensity and oxygen consumption than women in each exercise mode (Fig. 30.24B); treadmill running generated the greatest total oxygen consumed (energy expended) for both groups. For individuals without physical activity limitations, running usually provides the most suitable exercise mode for maximizing energy expenditure during self-selected intensities of continuous exercise.

Diet Plus Exercise: The Ideal Combination

Combinations of exercise and dietary restraint offer considerably more flexibility for achieving a negative caloric imbalance than either exercise alone or diet alone.[55,136,165,189,246,263] Dietary restraint plus increased physical activity through lifestyle changes offers health and weight-loss benefits similar to those from combining dietary restraint and vigorous structured exercise.[4,23] Adding exercise to a weight-control program facilitates longer term maintenance of fat loss than total reliance on either food restriction alone or increased exercise alone.[107,122,123,175,186] Moderate regular exercise also offsets the decrement in immunoprotective natural killer cell activity associated with weight loss.[202] TABLE 30.8 summarizes the benefits of exercise to a weight-loss program.

INTEGRATIVE QUESTION

Why might large-scale studies that compare diet only and exercise plus diet often show only a small, added weight loss benefit for the exercise-plus-diet group?

How can an overfat person using exercise and dietary restraint to maintain a weight loss of about 1 pound (0.45 kg) a week reduce body mass by 20 pounds (9.1 kg)? A prudent 1-pound per week fat loss requires 20 weeks. The weekly energy deficit to achieve this goal must average 3500 kCal with a daily deficit of 500 kCal. One half-hour of moderate exercise (about 350 "extra" kCal) performed 3 days a week adds 1050 kCal to the weekly deficit. Consequently, the weekly caloric intake need only decrease by 2400 kCal (about 350 kCal a day) instead of 3500 kCal to lose the desired pound of body fat each week. If the number of exercise days increases from 3 to 5, daily food intake requires only a 250-kCal decrease. Extending the duration of the 5-day-per-week workouts from 30 minutes to 1 hour produces the desired weight loss without reducing food intake. In this case, extra physical activity creates the entire 3500 kCal deficit. If the intensity of the 1-hour exercise performed 5 days a week increases by only 10% (cycling at 22 mph instead of 20 mph; running at 6.6 mph instead of 6.0 mph), the number of calories expended each

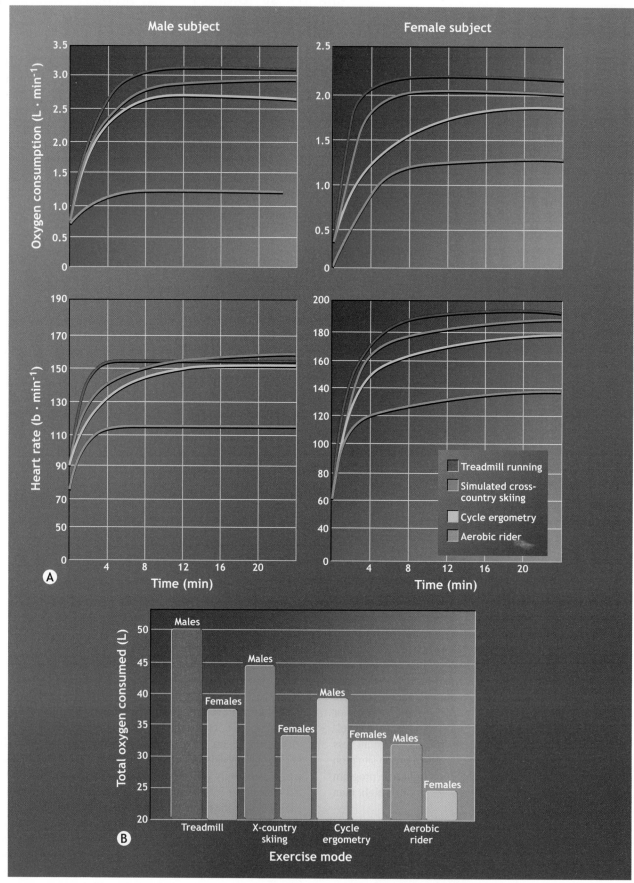

Figure 30.24 **A.** Oxygen consumption and heart rate for a representative male and female subject during 20 minutes of self-selected exercise consisting of treadmill running, leg-cycle ergometry, simulated cross-country skiing, or aerobic riding. **B.** Total oxygen consumed by males and females during 20 minutes of each form of exercise at the same rating of perceived exertion. (From Kravitz L, et al. Exercise mode and gender comparisons of energy expenditure at self-selected intensities. Med Sci Sports Exerc 1997;29:1028.)

	TABLE 30.8 ■ BENEFITS OF ADDING EXERCISE TO DIETARY RESTRICTION FOR WEIGHT LOSS

- Increases overall size of the energy deficit
- Facilitates lipid mobilization and oxidation, especially from visceral adipose tissue depots
- Increases relative body fat loss by preserving fat-free body mass
- Bunts the drop in resting metabolism that accompanies weight loss by conserving and even increasing fat-free body mass
- Requires less reliance on caloric restriction to create an energy deficit
- Contributes to long-term success of the weight-loss effort
- Provides significant health-related benefits

week through exercise increases by an additional 350 kCal (3500 kCal × 0.10). This new weekly deficit of 3850 kCal (550 kCal per day) allows the dieter to *increase* daily food intake by 50 kCal and still maintain a 1-pound weekly fat loss.

Clearly, physical activity combined with mild dietary restriction effectively *unbalances* the energy balance equation for weight loss. This approach produces less-intense feelings of hunger and less psychologic stress than one that relies exclusively on caloric restriction. Furthermore, both aerobic and resistance exercises protect against FFM loss that occurs with weight loss by diet alone. This results partly from the favorable effect of regular exercise on mobilization and use of fatty acids from adipose tissue depots.[153,194] Combining exercise with weight loss produces desirable reductions in blood pressure at rest and in situations that typically elevate blood pressure such as intense physical activity and emotional distress.[222] Exercise also facilitates protein retention in skeletal muscle and retards its rate of breakdown. *The fat-burning, protein-sparing benefits of regular exercise contribute to facilitated fat loss in a weight-loss program.*

Reality Check. Regardless of the approach to weight loss, a statement from the National Task Force on the Prevention and Treatment of Obesity best sums up the difficulty in solving the overly fat condition on a long-term basis: "Obese individuals who undertake weight loss efforts should be ready to commit to lifelong changes in their behavioral patterns, diet, and physical activity."[168]

The benefits of regular physical activity in weight loss and weight maintenance outlined in Table 30.8 come primarily from highly structured experimental research on relatively small numbers of subjects who significantly increased physical activity with high compliance. On the other hand, large-scale intervention studies (randomized clinical trials) that compare diet only with a combination of diet and regular exercise produce generally less remarkable results. In some cases, adding exercise did not augment weight loss; when a benefit did occur, the extra weight loss remained small. Clearly, the relatively modest amount of extra physical activity in the exercise group combined with high noncompliance to the exercise regimen in large-scale studies accounts for some blunting of an exercise effect. The key to unlocking the benefits of regular exercise for weight control in the general population lies in effective implementation of psychologic–behavioral factors that favor increased *regular* physical activity.

INTEGRATIVE QUESTION

Outline a prudent, effective plan for a middle-aged woman who wants to shed 10 kg of excess weight. Provide the rationale for each recommendation.

Spot Reduction Does Not Work

The notion of spot reduction emanates from the belief that an increase in a muscle's metabolic activity stimulates relatively greater fat mobilization from the adipose tissue in proximity to the active muscle. As such, exercising a specific body area region to "sculpt" it should selectively reduce more fat from that area than exercising a different muscle group at the same metabolic intensity. Advocates of spot reduction recommend performing large numbers of sit-ups or side-bends to reduce excessive abdominal and hip fat. The promise of spot reduction with exercise seems attractive from an aesthetic and health risk standpoint—unfortunately, critical evaluation of the research evidence does not support its use.[133,169]

INTEGRATIVE QUESTION

How can small adjustments in daily energy expenditure and daily food intake alter body fat content over time? Use specific examples.

To examine claims for spot reduction, researchers compared the girths and subcutaneous fat stores of the right and left forearms of high-caliber tennis players.[84] As expected, the girth of the dominant or playing arm exceeded the nondominant arm because of a modest muscular hypertrophy from the exercise overload of tennis. Measurements of skinfold thickness, however, clearly showed that regular and prolonged tennis exercise did not reduce subcutaneous fat in the playing arm. Another study evaluated fat biopsy specimens from abdominal, subscapular, and buttock sites before and after 27 days of sit-up exercise training.[116] The number of sit-ups increased from 140 at the end of the first week to 336 on day 27. Despite the considerable amount of localized exercise, adipocytes in the abdominal region were no smaller than adipocytes in the unexercised buttocks or subscapular control regions.

Undoubtedly, the negative energy balance created through regular exercise contributes to reducing total body fat. Exercise stimulates the mobilization of fatty acids via hormones and enzymes that act on fat depots throughout the body. Body areas of greatest fat concentration and/or lipid-mobilizing enzyme activity supply the greatest amount of this energy. *Exercise does not cause greater fatty acid release from the fat pads directly over the active muscle.*

> ## WHERE ON THE BODY DOES FAT LOSS OCCUR?
>
> Decreases in body fat with exercise training and/or caloric restriction preferentially mobilize and reduce upper-body subcutaneous and deep abdominal fat rather than the more "resistant" fat depots in gluteal and femoral regions.[42,124]

Possible Gender Difference

An interesting question concerns the possibility of a gender difference in the responsiveness of weight loss to regular exercise. A meta-analysis of 53 research studies on this topic concluded that men generally respond more favorably than women to the effects of exercise on weight loss.[9] One possible explanation involves the gender difference in body fat distribution. As discussed previously, fat distributed in the upper body and abdominal regions (central fat) shows active lipolysis to sympathetic nervous system stimulation and becomes preferentially mobilized for energy during exercise.[6,248] Consequently, the greater upper-body fat distribution in men may contribute to a greater sensitivity to lose fat in the abdominal region with regular exercise. Women also may more effectively preserve energy balance with increased physical activity.[54,255] Men often reduce energy intake with exercise training, whereas the depression of food intake with exercise may be less for women. The final answer to this intriguing question awaits further research.

WEIGHT LOSS RECOMMENDATIONS FOR WRESTLERS AND OTHER POWER ATHLETES

Weight lifters, gymnasts, and other athletes in sports that require a high level of muscular strength and power per unit of body mass often must reduce body fat without compromising exercise performance. Any increase in relative muscular strength and short-term power output capacity should improve competitive performance. The following discussion focuses on wrestlers, but applies to all physically active individuals who desire to reduce body fat without negatively affecting health, safety, and exercise capacity.

To reduce injury and medical complications from short- and longer-term periods of weight loss and dehydration, the ACSM, NCAA, and AMA recommend assessing each wrestler's body composition. The National Federation of State High School Associations required the adoption of weight certification beginning with the 2005 season. This assessment takes place several weeks prior to the competitive season to determine a **minimal wrestling weight** based on

percentage body fat. *Five percent body fat (determined using hydrostatic weighing or population-specific skinfold equations) represents the lowest acceptable level for safe wrestling competition.* The hydrostatic weighing or skinfold assessment of body fat recommended by the NCAA has been cross-validated by the more rigorous four-component body composition assessment and found to be acceptable for accuracy and precision.[33] For wrestlers under age 16, 7% body fat level represents the recommended lower limit. Importantly, percentage body fat must be determined in the euhydrated state because dehydration of between 2 and 5% body weight through fluid restriction and exercise in a hot environment (techniques commonly used by wrestlers) violates the assumptions necessary for accurate and precise prediction of minimal wrestling weight.[12] TABLE 30.9 outlines a practical application to determine minimal wrestling weight and an appropriate competitive weight class. The ACSM also recommends that legitimate weight loss should progress gradually and not exceed a 1- to 2-pound reduction per week. At the same time, the athlete should continue to consume a well-balanced, nutritious diet.

GAINING WEIGHT: THE COMPETITIVE ATHLETE'S DILEMMA

Gaining weight to enhance body composition and exercise performance in activities that require muscular strength and power or aesthetic appearance poses a unique problem not easily resolved. Most persons focus on weight loss to reduce excess body fat and improve overall health and appearance. Weight (fat) gain per se occurs all too readily by tilting the body's energy balance to favor greater caloric intake. Weight gain for athletes should represent muscle mass and accompanying connective tissue. Generally, this form of weight gain occurs if increased caloric intake—carbohydrate for adequate energy and protein sparing, plus the amino acid building blocks of protein for tissue synthesis—accompanies a balanced, progressive resistance exercise regimen.

Unsupported Hype

Athletes attempting to increase muscle mass often fall easy prey to health food and diet supplement manufacturers who market "high-potency, tissue-building" substances—chromium, boron, vanadyl sulfate, β-hydroxy-β-methyl butyrate, and various protein and amino acid mixtures, none of which reliably increases muscle mass. Concerning protein supplementation, no evidence indicates that commercially prepared mixtures of powdered protein, predigested amino acids, or special high-protein "cocktails" promote muscle growth any more effectively than protein consumed in a well-balanced diet (see Chapter 23).[131]

Increase the Lean, Not the Fat

Endurance exercise training usually increases FFM only slightly, but the overall effect reduces body weight because of

---

TABLE 30.9 ■ USING ANTHROPOMETRIC EQUATIONS TO PREDICT A MINIMAL WRESTLING WEIGHT AND TO SELECT A COMPETITIVE WEIGHT CLASS

A. To predict body density (BD), use one of the following equations. (For each skinfold, record the average of at least three trials in mm.)
  1. Lohman equation[a]
     BD = 1.0982 − (0.00815 × [triceps + subscapular + abdominal skinfolds])
        + (0.00000084 × [triceps + subscapular + abdominal skinfolds]^2)
  2. Katch and McArdle equation[b]
     BD = 1.09448 − (0.00103 × triceps skinfold) − (0.00056 × subscapular skinfold) − (0.00054 × abdominal skinfold)
  3. Behnke and Wilmore equation[c]
     BD = 1.05721 − (0.00052 × abdominal skinfold) + (0.00168 × iliac diameter) + (0.00114 × neck circumference)
        + (0.00048 × chest circumference) + (0.00145 × abdominal circumference)
  4. Thorland equation[d]
     BD = 1.0982 − (0.000815 × [triceps + abdominal skinfolds]) + (0.00000084 × [triceps + abdominal skinfolds])

B. To determine fat percentage, use the Brožek equation:
  % Fat = [4.570 ÷ BD − 4.142] × 100

C. To determine fat-free weight and to identify a minimum weight class, follow the examples below:
  1. Fifteen-year-old wrestler who weighs 132 lb, has a body density of 1.075 g · cc^{-1}, and hopes to compete in the 119-lb weight class.
  2. Percentage fat is (4.570 ÷ 1.075 − 4.142) × 100 = 10.9%
  3. Fat weight and fat-free weight are:
     a. 132.0 lb × 0.109 = 14.4 lb fat
     b. 132.0 lb − 14.4 lb fat = 117.6 lb fat-free weight

D. To calculate a minimal wrestling weight:
  1. Realize that the recommended minimum body weight for those 15 years and younger contains 93% (0.93) fat-free weight and 7% fat (0.07)
  2. Divide the wrestler's calculated fat-free weight by the greatest allowable fraction of fat-free weight to estimate minimal wrestling weight:
     117.6 ÷ (93/100) = 117.6 ÷ 0.93 = 126.5 lb

E. To allow for a 2% error, perform the following calculations:
  1. 126.5 minimal weight × 0.02 = 2.5 lb error allowance
  2. 126.5 lb − 2.5 lb = 124.0 lb minimum wrestling weight

F. Conclusion: This boy cannot wrestle in the 119-pound weight class; rather he must compete in the 125-pound class.

From Tipton CM. Making and maintaining weight for interscholastic wrestling. Gatorade Sports Science Exchange. 1990;2(22).
[a] Lohman TG. Skinfolds and body density and their relationship to body frames: a review. Hum Biol 1981;53:181.
[b] Katch FI, McArdle WD. Prediction of body density from simple anthropometric measurements in college-age men and women. Hum Biol 1973;l45:445.
[c] Behnke AR, Wilmore JH. Evaluation and regulation of body build and composition. Englewood Cliffs, NJ: Prentice Hall, 1974.
[d] Thorland W, et al. New equations for prediction of a minimal weight in high school wrestlers. Med Sci Sports Exerc 1989;21:S72.

---

fat loss from the calorie-burning and possible appetite-depressing effects of this exercise mode. In contrast, muscular overload through resistance training, supported by adequate energy and protein intake (with sufficient recovery), increases muscle mass and strength. Adequate energy intake ensures that no catabolism of protein available for muscle growth occurs from an energy deficit. *Thus, intense aerobic training should not coincide with resistance training to increase muscle mass.*[88,129] More than likely, the added energy (and perhaps protein) demands of concurrent resistance and aerobic exercise training impose a limit on muscle growth and responsiveness to resistance training. A prudent recommendation increases daily protein intake to about 1.6 g per kg of body mass during the resistance-training period.[143] The individual should consume a variety of plant and animal proteins; relying solely on animal protein (high in saturated fatty acids and cholesterol) potentially increases heart disease risk.

If all calories consumed in excess of the energy requirement during resistance training sustained muscle growth, then 2000 to 2500 extra kCal could supply each 0.5-kg increase in lean tissue. In practical terms, 700 to 1000 kCal added to the well-balanced daily meal plan supports a weekly 0.5- to 1.0-kg

gain in lean tissue and additional energy needs for training. This ideal situation presupposes that all extra calories synthesize lean tissue. In Chapter 23, we give specific recommendations for nutrient timing to optimize muscle responsiveness to resistance training.

How Much Gain to Expect

A 1-year program of heavy resistance training for young, athletic men increases body mass by about 20%, mostly from lean tissue accrual. The rate of lean tissue gain rapidly plateaus as training progresses beyond the first year. For athletic women, first-year gains in lean tissue mass average 50 to 75% of the absolute values for men, probably from the women's smaller initial lean body mass. Individual differences in the daily quantity of nitrogen incorporated into body protein (and protein incorporated into muscle) also limit and explain differences among persons in muscle mass increases with resistance training. FIGURE 30.25 lists eight specific factors that affect the responsiveness of lean tissue synthesis to resistance training.

Individuals with relatively high androgen-to-estrogen ratios and greater percentages of fast-twitch muscle fibers

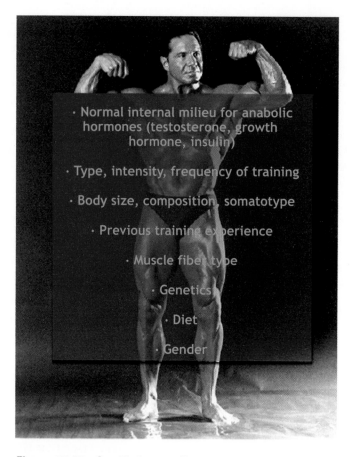

Figure 30.25 Specific factors affecting the magnitude of lean tissue synthesis with resistance training. (Photo of Bill Pearl courtesy of Bill Pearl.)

probably increase lean tissue to the greatest extent. Muscle mass increases most at the start of training in individuals with the largest relative FFM (FFM corrected for stature and body fat).[242] Regularly monitoring body mass and body fat verifies whether the combination of training and additional food intake increases lean tissue and not body fat. This requires an accurate (valid) appraisal of body composition at regular intervals throughout the training period.

INTEGRATIVE QUESTION

Outline recommendations to a high school student who wishes to increase body weight to improve physical appearance and sports performance.

Summary

1. Three ways unbalance the energy-balance equation to produce weight loss: (1) reduce energy intake below energy expenditure, (2) maintain normal energy intake and increase energy expenditure, and (3) decrease energy intake and increase energy expenditure.

2. Long-term maintenance of weight loss through dietary restriction has a success rate less than 20%. Typically, one to two thirds of the lost weight returns within a year and almost all of it within 5 years.

3. A caloric deficit of 3500 kCal, created through either diet or exercise, represents the equivalent of the calories in 0.45 kg of adipose tissue.

4. Prudent dieting effectively promotes weight loss. Disadvantages of extremes of caloric restriction include loss of FFM, lethargy, malnutrition, and depressed resting metabolism. Some of these factors conserve energy and reduce the diet's effectiveness.

5. Reduced resting metabolism represents a well-documented response to weight loss through dieting.

6. Rapid weight loss during the first few days of caloric deficit mainly reflects loss of body water and stored glycogen; greater fat loss occurs per unit of weight lost as caloric restriction continues.

7. The calories burned in exercise accumulate. Over time, regular extra physical activity creates a considerable energy deficit.

8. The precise role of exercise in appetite suppression or stimulation remains unclear, but moderate increases in physical activity may depress appetite and energy intake of a previously sedentary, overweight person. Most athletes eventually consume enough calories to counterbalance training's added caloric expenditure.

9. Exercise combined with caloric restriction offers a flexible and effective way to achieve weight loss. Exercise enhances fat mobilization and catabolism to accelerate body fat loss.

10. Regular aerobic exercise retards lean tissue loss while resistance training increases FFM.

11. Selective exercise of specific body regions by "spot exercise" proves no more effective for localized fat loss than more general physical activity of equivalent caloric expenditure.

12. Differences in body fat distribution partially explain gender difference in responsiveness to exercise-induced weight loss.

13. Athletes should gain weight as lean body tissue (muscle mass and connective tissue). Modest increases in caloric intake with systematic resistance training effectively produce this effect.

14. Ideally, 700 to 1000 extra kCal per day supports a weekly 0.5- to 1.0-kg gain in lean tissue and resistance training energy requirements.

References are available on the Student CD and online at http://connection.lww.com/mkk6e.

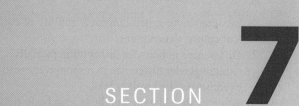

Exercise, Successful Aging, and Disease Prevention

OVERVIEW

The physiologic and exercise capacities of older persons usually rate below those of younger peers. It remains uncertain whether these differences reflect true biologic aging or the effect of disuse from alterations in lifestyle and reduced physical activity as people age. Encouraging news reveals that older men and women no longer conform to a sedentary stereotype with little or no initiative for active pursuits. A meaningful upswing currently exists in participation of senior citizens in a broad range of physical activities and exercise programs. Research clearly demonstrates that maintenance of an active lifestyle into later years helps older adults retain a relatively high level of functional capacity. In addition, regular exercise offers significant protection against and rehabilitation from a variety of disabilities, diseases, and risk factors, particularly those related to cardiovascular health. Within this framework, the exercise physiologist provides considerable skills and contributions through the prudent use of regular exercise in the clinical setting.

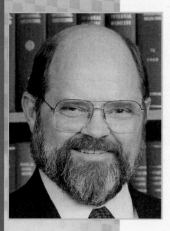

Interview *with* Dr. Steven N. Blair

Education: BA (Kansas Wesleyan University, Salina, KS); MS and PED (Indiana University, Bloomington, IN); Postgraduate training (Scholar in Preventive Cardiology, Stanford University School of Medicine, Palo Alto, CA)

Current Affiliation: Director of Epidemiology and Clinical Applications, and Director of Research, The Cooper Institute for Aerobics Research, Dallas, TX.

Honors and Awards: See Appendix E, which is available on the Student CD and online at http://connection.lww.com/mkk6e.

Research Focus: My research has two major foci: (1) The Aerobics Center Longitudinal Study, an investigation of the relation of physical activity, cardiorespiratory fitness, and health outcomes and (2) randomized clinical trials of physical activity interventions and their health-related outcomes.

Memorable Publication: Blair SN, et al. Physical fitness and all-cause mortality: a prospective study of healthy men and women. JAMA 1989;262:2395.

Statement of Contributions: ACSM Citation Award

In recognition of his outstanding contributions to the body of knowledge concerning the health implications of a physically active lifestyle.

Dr. Blair is recognized for his insightful, skillful, and persistent application of epidemiological research techniques in the exploration of the health effects of physical activity and physical fitness. His studies of the Cooper Clinic population have markedly advanced our knowledge of the association between physical activity and risk of chronic disease morbidity and mortality. These studies, by demonstrating that moderate levels of physical activity and fitness provide important health benefits, have had a critical impact on public health policy.

Through his research, through his extensive service to the American College of Sports Medicine, and through his highly effective communication with health professionals and with the public, Dr. Blair has made an enormous contribution to exercise science.

What first inspired you to enter the exercise science field? What made you decide to pursue your advanced degree and/or line of research?

■ I participated in sports in high school and college, and decided during my college career that I wanted to be a physical education teacher and athletic coach.

What influence did your undergraduate education have on your final career choice?

■ My physical education teachers and coaches encouraged and influenced me to continue my education with graduate school. I had conducted a small, independent research project as an undergraduate and found that I liked defining a problem, collecting data, and trying to make sense of the results. In graduate school, I developed an interest in an academic research career, but I think it was the solid foundation in the liberal arts and specific areas of physical education that influenced my career direction.

Who were the most influential people in your career, and why?

■ Gene Bissell was a strong early mentor. He is a man of uncompromising principles, dedication, and genuine concern for his students. He once forfeited a win in football when, after the game was over, he realized that an official had missed a call. When Coach Bissell pointed out the infraction, the league office replied that, sometimes calls are missed and that is just one of the breaks of the game. Coach Bissell refused to accept that ruling and insisted that his team be declared the loser.

I had several influential mentors at Indiana University. Karl and Carolyn Bookwalter gave me a research assistantship, helped me with my first publication, and generally introduced me to the world of scientific writing. Arthur Slater-Hammel introduced me to the scientific process, taught me about experimental design, and was the director of my doctoral dissertation. George Cousins was inquisitive and skeptical—two traits I consider essential for a scientist.

My first academic job was at the University of South Carolina. My interests soon turned to preventive cardiology, with a specific interest in exercise as a preventive and therapeutic modality. In the early 1970s I wrote an application for the Multiple Risk Factor Intervention Trial (MRFIT), and we received a grant to serve as one of the 20 MRFIT clinical centers. I learned much from leaders of the MRFIT, including Professors Jerry Stamler, Henry Taylor, Paul Ogelsby, Henry Blackburn, Steve Hulley, Mark Kjelsburg, Lew Kuller, and many others.

In 1978, I had an opportunity to work with Bill Haskell and Peter Wood at the Stanford University Heart Disease Prevention Program. I have had literally hundreds of hours of discussion with them over the years about various issues in exercise science and public health, and I continue to learn from their work and examples.

I also had the great opportunity to develop a relationship with Dr. Ralph S. Paffenbarger, who has considerably influenced my research over the past 20 years. "Paff" has made enormous contributions to the epidemiology of physical activity and health. His work is a model of rigorous methodology, clear thinking, poetic writing, and carefully drawn conclusions. He continues to be a good friend, research collaborator, mentor, and inspiration.

Last, I will mention colleagues at the Cooper Institute. I feel very fortunate that Dr. Cooper had the vision to establish the database for the Aerobics Center Longitudinal Study. My many colleagues at the Cooper Institute have been instrumental in our work over the past 20 years. I have learned much from them, and any success we have had is due in large part to their hard work, dedication, and scientific expertise.

What has been the most interesting/enjoyable aspect of your involvement in science? What was the least interesting/enjoyable aspect?

■ The most interesting/enjoyable aspect of science for me is the discovery that accompanies research. Nothing is more exciting than seeing the results of an analysis that yield something new and perhaps unexpected.

The least desirable aspects of my scientific life are the constant scrambling for funds to support our research activities and the routine administrative tasks that are inherent in managing an enterprise of 25 to 30 people.

What is your most meaningful contribution to the field of exercise science, and why is it so important?

■ I think that our work on low cardiorespiratory fitness as a predictor of morbidity and mortality in middle-aged and older women and men is a meaningful contribution to exercise science. Our report on fitness and mortality that was published in the Journal of the American Medical Association in 1989 seemed to come at the right time and struck a responsive chord in both the scientific and lay communities. This research helped influence several statements on the significance of physical inactivity on public health, which have had a substantial effect on exercise science, public health, and clinical medicine.

I also am proud of our research on lifestyle physical activity interventions. Our epidemiological studies revealed a curvilinear, dose–response relation between cardiorespiratory fitness and mortality, with the steepest part of the curve at the low end of the fitness continuum. Moderate levels of fitness are associated with reduced risk, and moderate amounts and intensities of physical activity can produce these moderate levels of fitness. We designed a randomized clinical trial to test the hypothesis that behaviorally based lifestyle physical activity intervention would be as effective as a traditional, structured exercise program in increasing physical activity, improving cardiorespiratory fitness, and improving other health parameters. I am pleased that this work is leading to greater flexibility and more options for exercise programming to achieve health benefits.

What advice would you give to students who express an interest in pursuing a career in exercise science research?

■ Obtain a strong foundation in science as an undergraduate. Read widely in your area of interest and become familiar with the leading researchers in this area of investigation. Talk to your professors about your plans and seek their advice. Do not be afraid to approach well-known researchers and ask for their advice in making your career choices. Most of them are very nice people and will be flattered if you come well prepared with good questions. As you begin to narrow your choice of institutions for graduate school, make up a visitation schedule and try to visit at least three or four programs that you think match your needs. Go to the very best program that will accept you.

What interests have you pursued outside your professional career?

■ I like to garden, and my wife and I are proud of our landscaping and flowers. We have season tickets to the symphony, opera, summer musicals, and one of the Dallas theaters. We both use running as our main form of exercise, and we run nearly every day and have over the past 30 years. We like to travel and feel fortunate that my work has afforded us many opportunities to travel in the United States and abroad.

Where do you see the exercise science field (particularly your area of greatest interest) heading in the next 30 years?

■ Genetic epidemiology will make important contributions to our understanding of which individuals are at greatest risk of a sedentary way of life. We will work out in much greater detail the specific types, amounts, and intensities of activity that prevent or delay specific diseases or conditions. We will finally establish appropriate public health surveillance systems to monitor accurately patterns and trends of physical activity and physical fitness in people of all ages. Physical inactivity will be recognized as the major and most expensive public health problem in the U.S.

We will learn much more about how to help sedentary individuals adopt and maintain physical activity. These advances, however, may not be sufficient to overcome the ever more toxic environment in which we live, as indicated by our continuing to engineer physical activity out of daily life. The threat posed to our public health and well-being by an increase in the prevalence of sedentary habits may finally cause us to seriously consider, develop, and implement policy and legislative solutions to encourage more physical activity.

You have the opportunity to give a "last lecture." Describe its primary focus.

■ I would describe the joys of scientific discovery and the pleasure of collaborating with colleagues to address important public health issues. I would illustrate how hazardous it is to be sedentary and unfit, and how a fit and active way of life can bring benefits to virtually all demographic groups. I would outline the seriousness of the public health problem of inactivity and try to issue a rousing call to action to encourage all to help address this problem. After accepting sustained applause, and even standing ovations and shouts of "Bravo," I would exit the stage and leave the work to the younger generation.

Physical Activity, Health, and Aging

31

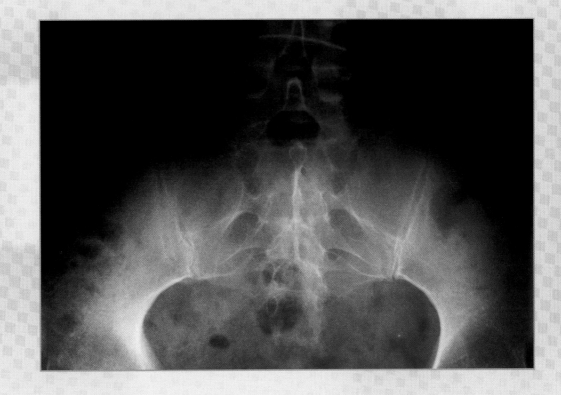

CHAPTER OBJECTIVES

- Summarize aging trends in the American population

- Describe the physical activity level of typical adult American men and women

- Outline the major findings of the Surgeon General's report on the population's physical activity participation

- Answer the question: "How safe is exercising?"

- List factors that increase the likelihood of experiencing an exercise catastrophe

- Contrast physiologic responses to exercise of children and adults and their implications for evaluating physiologic function and exercise performance

- List important age-related changes in (1) muscular function, (2) nervous system function, (3) cardiovascular function, (4) pulmonary function, and (5) body composition components

- Summarize the potential benefits of moderate resistance training for the elderly

- Discuss the following statement: "A sedentary lifestyle causes losses in functional capacity at least as great as the effects of aging itself"

- Describe research about the role of regular physical activity in coronary heart disease prevention and life extension

■ Indicate the types and levels of physical activity that induce the greatest improvement in risk-factor profile and overall health

■ Describe vulnerable plaque and its proposed role in sudden death

■ List the major modifiable heart disease risk factors and how regular physical activity affects each

■ Outline the normal dynamics of homocysteine, its proposed role in coronary heart disease, and factors that affect plasma levels

■ Discuss the prevalence of heart disease risk factors in children

THE GRAYING OF AMERICA

Elderly persons—those 85 and older—make up the fastest growing segment of American society. Thirty years ago, age 65 represented the onset of old age. Gerontologists now consider 85 the demarcation of "oldest-old" and age 75, "young-old." Currently, nearly 13% or approximately 38 million exceed age 65, and by the year 2030, 20% or 70 million will exceed age 85. Assuming consistent mortality rates, the number of Americans over the age of 85 will more than triple over the next four decades, reaching 15 million by 2040. While the life expectancy for men is less than women, the gap has begun to narrow; for white males and females, it has declined from 7.5 years in 1980, 5.5 years in 2001, and to 5.1 years in 2005 (www.cdc.gov). For black males and females in 2005, the gap is somewhat larger at 6.9 years. Some demographers project that one half of the girls and one third of the boys born in developed countries near the end of the 20th century will live in three centuries. In the short term, disease prevention, water purification and better sanitation, improved nutrition and health care, and more effective treatment of age-related heart disease and osteoporosis help people live longer. Far fewer persons now die from infectious childhood diseases, so those with the genetic potential actualize their proclivity for longevity.[73] On a different but parallel front, anticipated breakthroughs in genetic therapies may slow the aging of individual cells. Gene therapies could boost human life spans to a much greater extent than improved medical treatment or even eradication of some diseases.

FIGURE 31.1A shows that, proportionately, centenarians are the fastest growing age group in the United States. In 2005, there were 71,000 centenarians, up from the estimate of 15,000 in 1980 and almost none at the beginning of the 20th century. According to the U.S. Census Bureau (www.census.gov), this number will swell to 114,000 by 2010 and then exceed 241,000 by 2020. No longer viewed as a quirk of nature, 2 in 10,000 Americans now lives to age 100. Demographers project that by the middle of this century, more than 800,000 Americans will exceed age 100, with many maintaining relatively good health. Figures 31.1B–D depict longevity statistics retirement-pension organizations use to calculate the payout of annuity dividends. For example, a 55-year-old person today can expect to live on average an additional 31.4 years for a life span of 86 years (Fig. 31.1B). But if this 55-year-old lives an additional 15 years to age 70, life expectancy extends to almost 89 years. Figure 31.1C indicates the proportion of individuals aged 65 years who survive to specified ages. Among current 65-year-olds, 95.5% will live to age 70, 63.3% to age 85, and nearly 10% will achieve 100 years. Web sites that offer life-expectance calculators include the National Center for Health Statistics (www.cdc.gov/nchs/fastats/lifexpec.htm) and Northwestern Mutual Life Insurance Company (www.nmfn.com/tn/learnctr-lifeevents-longevity).

Physical inactivity causes nearly 30% of all deaths from heart disease, colon cancer, and diabetes.[94,158] Lifestyle changes could reduce mortality from these ailments and greatly improve cardiovascular and muscular functional capacities, quality of life, and independent living.[32,98,125] The greatest health benefits would come from strategies that promote regular physical activity.[2,3,6,185,216,271] At any age, behavioral changes—becoming more physically active, quitting cigarette smoking, and controlling body weight and blood pressure—act independently to delay all-cause mortality and extend life.[181,225] Persons with more healthful lifestyles survive longer, and the risk of disability and the necessity to seek home health care is postponed and compressed into fewer years at the end of life.[263,264] The increased number of 65-and-over participants in marathons (and even ultramarathons) aptly illustrates the exercise capacities of active older individuals. For example, the male winner of the 2004 New York City Marathon in the 80- to 89-year-old age group achieved a time of 5:05:30, while the female winner in the 75- to 79-year-old group completed the race in 5:24:09.

The New Gerontology

Many gerontologists maintain that research on aging should focus not simply on increasing life span but rather on improving "**healthspan,**" or the total number of years a person remains in excellent health. The "**new gerontology**" addresses areas beyond age-related diseases and their prevention to recognize that *successful aging* requires maintenance of enhanced physiologic function and physical fitness. Vitality, not longevity per se remains a primary goal. Researchers now view much of the physiologic deterioration previously considered "normal aging" dependent on lifestyle and environmental influences subject to considerable modification with proper diet and exercise.[68,133,225] For those achieving older age, low muscular strength, diminished cardiovascular function, and poor joint range of motion, as well as sleep disturbances, relate directly to functional limitations regardless of disease status.[98,163,164,217] Gerontologists consider that successful aging includes four main components: (1) physical health, (2) spirituality, (3) emotional and educational health, and (4) social satisfaction. Maintaining and even enhancing physical

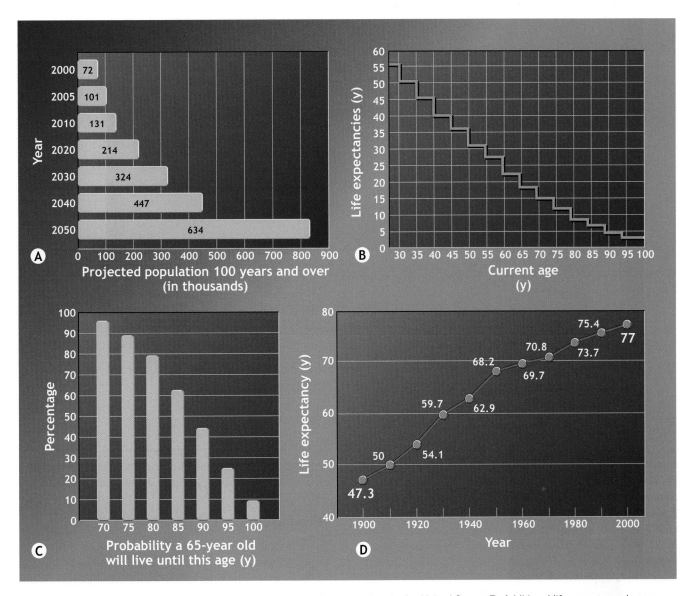

Figure 31.1 The graying of America. **A.** Growth in number of centenarians in the United States. **B.** Additional life expectancy in years for individuals currently at a specific age. **C.** Probability that a current 65-year-old will live to a certain age. **D.** Average life expectancy at birth has increased by more than 60% since 1900. (Data from U.S. Bureau of the Census, National Center for Health Statistics, Centers for Disease Control and Prevention: Washington, DC, and actuarial tables from insurance companies.)

and cognitive functions, fully engaging in life, and participating in productive activities and interpersonal relations contribute to achieving these goals.

Healthy Life Expectancy: A New Concept

Life expectancy estimates determine the overall length of life based on mortality data without considering the quality of life as aging progresses. At some point during the life span, some level of disability detracts from longevity. The Centers for Disease Control and Prevention (CDC) reports that nearly 1 in 10 Americans over age 70 needs help with daily activities such as bathing, and 4 in 10 use assistive walkers or hearing aids. Approximately one half of men and two thirds of women

above age 70 have arthritis; one third of all Americans in this age group also have high blood pressure and 11% have diabetes. Of all seniors, women over age 85 are the most likely to need everyday help; 23% require assistance with at least one basic activity (e.g., dressing or going to the toilet).

To estimate healthful longevity, the World Health Organization (WHO [www.who.int/whr/]) has introduced the concept of **healthy life expectancy**—the expected number of years a person might live in the equivalent of full health. This involves **disability-adjusted life expectancy** (**DALE**), which considers the years of ill health, weighted according to severity and subtracted from expected overall life expectancy to compute the equivalent years of healthy life. The WHO rankings by country show substantially more years lost to disability in poorer countries from the impact of injury, blindness,

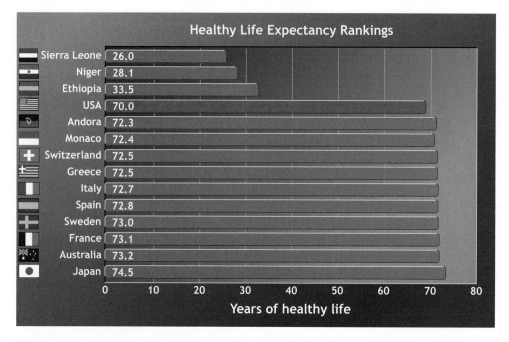

Figure 31.2 Disability-adjusted life expectancy rankings (DALE; an estimate of healthy life expectancy) of populations of selected countries as assessed by the World Health Organization. Of all countries surveyed, the United States ranked 24th, with Japan ranked at the top.

and paralysis and because the debilitating effects of tropical diseases such as malaria strike children and young adults more frequently. FIGURE 31.2 shows the DALE for a sample of 14 countries. Of the 191 countries evaluated, DALE estimates reached 70 years in 24 countries and 60 years in more than one half. Thirty-two countries fell at the lower extreme, where DALE estimates were less than 40 years. Many of these countries experience major epidemics of HIV/AIDS including other causes of death and disability.

Japanese citizens experience the longest healthy life expectancy of 74.5 years. Surprisingly, the United States rates 24th, with 70.0 years of healthy life for babies born in 1999 (72.6 y for females and 67.5 y for males). Native Americans, rural African Americans, and inner-city poor experience the poor health characteristics of underdeveloped countries. The HIV/AIDS epidemic, tobacco-related diseases, violent deaths, and prevalence of CHD all contribute to the United States' lower ranking than other industrialized nations.

PART 1 • *Physical Activity in the Population*

PHYSICAL ACTIVITY EPIDEMIOLOGY

Epidemiology involves quantifying factors that influence the occurrence of illness to better understand, modify, and/or control a disease pattern in the general population. The specific field of **physical activity epidemiology** applies the general research strategies of epidemiology to study physical activity as a health-related behavior linked to disease and other outcomes.

Terminology

Physical activity epidemiology applies specific definitions to characterize behavioral patterns and outcomes of the group(s) under investigation. Relevant terminology includes the following:

- **Physical activity**: Body movement produced by muscle action that increases energy expenditure
- **Exercise**: Planned, structured, repetitive, and purposeful physical activity
- **Physical fitness**: Attributes related to how well one performs physical activity
- **Health**: Physical, mental, and social well-being, not simply absence of disease
- **Health-related physical fitness**: Components of physical fitness associated with some aspect of good health and/or disease prevention
- **Longevity**: Length of life

Within this framework, physical activity becomes a generic term with exercise its major component. Similarly, the definition of health focuses on the broad spectrum of well-being that ranges from complete absence of health (near death) to the highest levels of physiologic function. Such definitions often challenge how we measure and quantify health and physical activity objectively. They provide a broad perspective to study the role of physical activity in health and disease.

The trend in physical fitness assessment during the past 35 years deemphasizes tests that stress motor performance and athletic fitness (i.e., speed, power, balance, and agility). Instead, current assessment focuses on functional capacities related to overall good health and disease prevention. The four most common components of **health-related physical fitness** are aerobic and/or cardiovascular fitness, body composition, abdominal muscular strength and endurance, and lower back and hamstring flexibility (FIG. 31.3; see "In a Practical Sense," p. 888).

Physical Activity Participation

More than 30 different methods assess physical activity. They include direct and indirect calorimetry, self-reports and questionnaires, job classifications, physiologic markers, behavioral observations, mechanical or electronic monitors, and activity surveys. Each approach offers unique advantages but also has disadvantages depending on the situation and population studied. Obtaining valid estimates of physical activity of large groups is difficult because such studies, by necessity, apply self-reports of daily activity and exercise participation rather than direct monitoring or objective measurement.

Despite limitations in assessment, a discouraging picture of physical activity participation worldwide, both of work/occupational and of leisure-time activity, emerges consistently as emphasized for United States citizens in the Surgeon General's report on physical activity and data provided by others:[38,175,186,242,251,253]

Adults

- Only about 15% engage in vigorous physical activity during leisure time, 3 times a week for at least 30 minutes
- More than 60% do not engage in physical activity regularly
- Twenty-five percent lead sedentary lives (i.e., do not exercise at all)

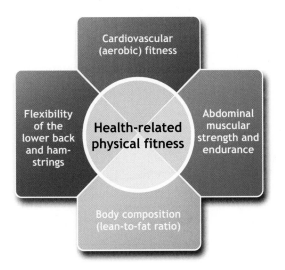

Figure 31.3 Health-related physical fitness components.

- Walking, gardening, and yard work are the most popular leisure-time activities
- Twenty-two percent engage in light-to-moderate physical activity regularly during leisure time (5 times/week for at least 30 min)
- Physical inactivity occurs more among women than men, blacks and Hispanics than whites, older than younger adults, and less-affluent than wealthier persons
- Physical inactivity contributes to 300,000 preventable deaths a year in the United States. Moderate daily physical activity can substantially reduce the risk of developing or dying from cardiovascular disease, type 2 diabetes, and some cancers. Daily physical activity lowers blood pressure and cholesterol levels, retards osteoporosis, and reduces obesity, symptoms of anxiety and depression, and arthritis.
- Participation in fitness activities declines with age; a large number of older citizens have such poor functional capacity they cannot rise from a chair or bed, walk to the bathroom, or climb a single stair without assistance

Children and Teenagers

- Nearly one half of those between ages 12 and 21 do not exercise vigorously on a regular basis; a sharp decline in physical activity occurs during adolescence regardless of gender
- Fourteen percent report no recent physical activity—more prevalent among females, particularly black females
- Twenty-five percent engage in light-to-moderate physical activity (e.g., walk or bicycle) nearly every day
- Participation in all types of physical activity declines strikingly with increasing age and school grade
- More males participate in vigorous physical activity, strengthening activities, and walking or bicycling than females
- Daily attendance in school physical education programs declined from 42% in early 1990 to less than 25% in 2005

ACTIVITIES OF THOSE AMERICANS WHO REPORT EXERCISING REGULARLY

	PERCENTAGE	
ACTIVITY	MALE	FEMALE
Walking	39	48
Resistance training	20	9
Cycling	16	15
Running	12	6
Stair climbing	10	12
Aerobics	3	10

IN A PRACTICAL SENSE

ASSESSING LOWER BACK, HAMSTRING, AND SHOULDER–WRIST FLEXIBILITY

■ Two types of flexibility include (1) **static flexibility**, full range of motion (ROM) of a specific joint and (2) **dynamic flexibility**, torque or resistance encountered as the joint moves through its ROM. Field tests commonly assess static flexibility indirectly through linear measurement of ROM.

FIELD TESTS OF HIP-AND-TRUNK AND SHOULDER–WRIST STATIC FLEXIBILITY
■ Administer a minimum of three trials following a standardized warm-up.

TEST 1: HIP-AND-TRUNK FLEXIBILITY (MODIFIED SIT-AND-REACH TEST)

Starting Position
■ Sit on the floor with the back and head against a wall, legs fully extended, with the bottoms of the feet against the sit-and-reach box. Place hands on top of each other, stretching the arms forward while keeping the head and back against the wall. Measure the distance from the fingertips to the box edge with a yardstick. This represents the zero, or starting, point (FIG. A).

Movement
■ Slowly bend and reach forward as far as possible (move head and back away from the wall), sliding the fingers along the yardstick; hold the final position for 2 seconds (FIG. B).

Score
■ Total distance reached to the nearest 1/4 inch represents the final score.

MODIFIED SIT-AND-REACH RATINGS

| | MEN | | | WOMEN | |
AGE RANGE (Y)	≤35	36–49	RATING	≤35	36–49
	>17.9	>16.1	**Excellent**	>17.9	>17.4
	17.0–17.9	14.6–16.1	**Good**	16.7–17.9	16.2–17.4
	15.8–17.0	13.9–14.6	**Average**	16.2–16.7	15.2–16.2
	15.0–15.8	13.4–13.9	**Fair**	15.8–16.2	14.5–15.2
	<15.0	<13.4	**Poor**	<15.4	<14.5

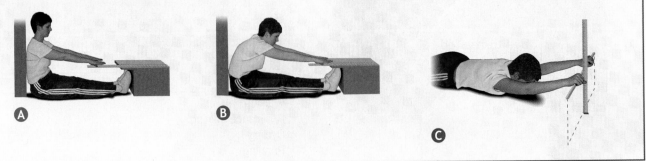

Test 1: Hip-and-trunk flexibility (modified sit-and-reach test)

Test 2: Shoulder-wrist flexibility (shoulder-and-wrist elevation test)

Ⓐ   Ⓑ   Ⓒ

continued on page 889

Continued

TEST 2: SHOULDER–WRIST FLEXIBILITY (SHOULDER-AND-WRIST ELEVATION TEST)

Starting Position
■ Lie prone on the floor with the arms fully extended overhead; grasp a yardstick with the hands shoulder-width apart.

Movement
■ Raise the stick as high as possible (FIG. C).

• Measure the vertical distance (nearest 0.5 in) the yardstick rises from the floor.
• Measure arm length from the acromial process to the tip of longest finger.
• Subtract the average vertical score from arm length.

Score
■ Arm length–average vertical score (nearest 0.25 in)

SHOULDER-AND-WRIST ELEVATION RATINGS

MEN	RATING	WOMEN
6.00 or less	**Excellent**	5.50 or less
8.25–6.25	**Good**	7.50–5.75
11.50–8.50	**Average**	10.75–7.75
12.50–11.75	**Fair**	11.75–11.00
12.75 or more	**Poor**	12.00 or more

Modified from Johnson BL, Nelson JK. Practical measurements for evaluation in physical education. 4th ed. New York: Macmillan, 1986.

Healthy People 2000

At best, no more than 20% and possibly less than 10% of adults in the United States, Australia, Canada, and England obtain sufficient regular physical activity at an intensity that imparts discernible health and fitness benefits. Among Americans, a widespread erosion of physical activity patterns becomes particularly apparent with increasing age among adolescents and adults; the decline is greater for adolescent and adult females than for males.[39] The age-related decline in physical activity among humans has a biologic basis that relates to altered neurotransmission involving the central dopamine system, the system that regulates motivation for locomotion.[104] Regardless of the cause for progressive inactivity as adults age, *increased* levels of physical activity predict *decreased* levels of morbidity and mortality.[28]

In July, 1996, the Surgeon General of the United States acknowledged the importance of physical activity to the nation with the release of the first *Surgeon General's Report on Physical Activity and Health*. This wide-ranging report, now updated to include good nutrition (www.cdc.gov/nccdphp/aag/aag_dnpa.htm), summarized the benefits of regular physical activity in disease prevention. The Surgeon General proposed a national agenda, a call to action that urged the nation to adopt and maintain a physically active lifestyle to combat ailments associated with the country's generally low level of energy expenditure. The following represent major conclusions from that first report:

• Men and women of all ages benefit from regular physical activity.
• Significant health benefits accrue from including moderate physical activity (e.g., 30 min of brisk walking or raking leaves, 15 min of running, or 45 min of playing volleyball) on most, if not all days of the week.[14,18,58,237]

The *"Physical Activity Pyramid"* illustrated in FIGURE 31.4 summarizes major goals for increasing the level of regular physical activity in the general population and emphasizes diverse forms of behavioral and lifestyle options.

Healthy People 2010

The **Healthy People 2010** initiative, launched on January 25, 2000, builds on the initiatives of the previous two decades as an instrument to improve national health for the first decade of the 21st century. Healthy People 2010 outlines a comprehensive, nationwide health promotion and disease prevention agenda as a roadmap to promote health and prevent illness, disability, and premature death among all persons in the United States.[222]

Healthy People 2010 is designed to achieve two primary goals:

1. Increase quality and years of healthy life
2. Eliminate health disparities among the nation's citizens

Progress will be monitored through achievements within 467 objectives in the 28 focus areas. Many goals and objectives—several of which either directly or indirectly involve upgrading the national level of regular physical activity—converge on interventions designed to reduce or eliminate illness, disability, and premature death among individuals and communities. Other objectives focus on broader issues, such as improving access to quality health care, strengthening public

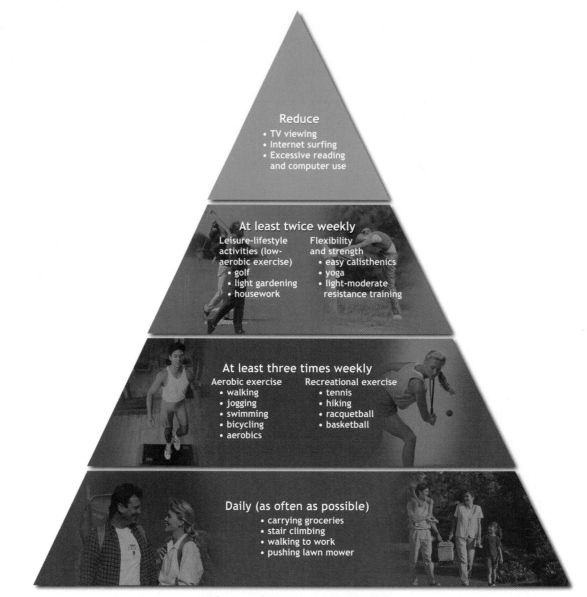

Physical Activity Pyramid

Figure 31.4 The Physical Activity Pyramid: Prudent goals for increasing daily physical activity.

health services, and improving availability and dissemination of health-related information. Each objective has a target for specific improvements and explicit guidelines on how to achieve the stated goal by 2010.

Safety of Exercising

Several well-publicized reports of sudden death during exercise raised the question of exercise safety.[129,220] Actually, the death rate during exercise has declined over the past 25 years despite an overall increase in exercise participation. In one report of cardiovascular episodes over a 65-month period, 2935 exercisers recorded 374,798 hours of exercise that included 2,726,272 km of running and walking. No deaths occurred during this time, with only two nonfatal cardiovascular complications. This amounted to two complications per 100,000 hours of exercise for women and three complications for men.

Intense physical exertion does raise a small risk of sudden death (e.g., 1 sudden death per 1.51 million episodes of exertion) during the activity (compared with resting an equivalent time), particularly for sedentary persons with a genetic predisposition to sudden death. Nonetheless, the longer term reduction in overall death risk from regular exercise outweighs any small potential for acute cardiovascular complications.[141,215] Regular exercisers have considerably less risk of death during physical activity. A 12-year follow-up of more than 21,000 male physicians showed that men who exercised at least five times a week had a much lower sudden death risk during vigorous exertion—about sevenfold less—than those who exercised only once weekly.[9] The likelihood of an exercise catastrophe—cerebrovascular accident, aortic dissection and rupture, lethal arrhythmias, myocardial infarction—increases under the following conditions:

- Genetic predisposition (family history of sudden death at a relatively young age)
- History of fainting or chest pain with exercise
- Unaccustomed vigorous exercise
- Exercise performed with accompanying psychologic stress
- Extremes of environmental temperature
- Straining-type exercise that requires a considerable static muscle-action component (e.g., shoveling wet snow)
- Exercise during viral infection or when feeling ill
- Co-mingling of prescription drugs or dietary supplements (e.g., ephedra)

Musculoskeletal injuries represent the most prevalent exercise complications. A longitudinal study of aerobic dance injuries in 351 participants and 60 instructors during nearly 30,000 hours of activity reported 327 medical complaints.[76] Just 84 of the injuries caused disability (2.8 per 1000 person-hours of participation) and only 2.1% required medical attention. National estimates from self-reported frequency and severity of injuries in five common physical activities—walking, gardening, weight lifting, outdoor bicycling, and aerobics—report relatively low injury rates.[191] Most injuries required no treatment or reduction in physical activity. Age does not affect incidence of orthopedic problems for exercise of moderate intensity and duration.[150] For activities that involve running, the greatest orthopedic injury risk exists in individuals who exercise for prolonged durations.[11]

Prospective epidemiologic research evaluated clinically significant medical incidents and emergencies for 7725 low-risk, apparently healthy corporate fitness enrollees in a supervised facility at a major medical center.[165] Two and one-half years of surveillance reported 15 medically significant events (0.048 per 1000 participant-hours) and two medical emergencies (both recovered), which equaled a rate of 0.0063 per 1000 participant-hours. Such a low rate of medical incidents in a supervised health-fitness facility illustrates convincingly that the health-related fitness benefits outweigh any small risk of participation.

The most recently published report (July 2000–June 2001) from the National Electronic Injury Surveillance System All Injury Program (NEISS-AIP) that characterizes sports- and recreation-related injuries among the U.S. population revealed 4.3 million nonfatal injuries were treated in U.S. hospital emergency departments (comprising 6% of all unintentional injury-related emergency room visits).[168] Injury rates varied by sex and age and were highest for persons aged 10 to 14 years (51.5% for boys, 38% for girls) and lowest for persons over age 45 (6.4% for men, 3.1% for women.) The overall rate of sports- and recreation-related injuries was 15.4 per 1000 population. For persons 20 to 24 years, basketball- and bicycle-related injuries ranked among the three leading types of injury. Basketball-related injuries

ranked highest for men aged 25 to 44 years. Exercise (e.g., weight lifting, aerobics, stretching, walking, jogging, and running) was the leading injury-related activity for women over age 20 and ranked among the top four types of injuries for men over age 20. The most frequent injury diagnosis included strains/sprains (29.1%), fractures (20.5%), contusions/abrasions (20.1%), and lacerations (13.8%). The body parts injured most commonly were ankles (12.2%), fingers (9.5%), face (9.2%), head (8.2%), and knees (8.1%). Overall, hospitalizations included 2.3% of persons with sports- and recreation-related injuries.

Sedentary Death Syndrome (SeDS)

A review of the world literature over the last 50 years has concluded that inactivity alone results in a constellation of problems and conditions eventually leading to premature death. The term **sedentary death syndrome (SeDS)** identifies this condition.[28] Recent research evidence reveals the following:

- SeDS will cause 2.5 million Americans to die prematurely in the next decade.
- SeDS will cost $2 to 3 trillion in health care expenses in the United States in the next decade.
- Chronic diseases have increased because of physical inactivity. In the United States, type 2 diabetes has increased 9-fold since 1958, obesity has doubled since 1980, and heart disease remains the number one cause of death.
- U.S. children are now getting SeDS-related diseases—they are increasingly overweight, showing fatty streaks in their arteries, and developing type 2 diabetes (a disease formerly restricted to adults).
- SeDS relates to 23 conditions: high blood triacylglycerol, high blood cholesterol, high blood glucose, type 2 diabetes, hypertension, myocardial ischemia, arrhythmias, congestive heart failure, obesity, breast depression, chronic back pain, spinal cord injury, stroke, disease cachexia, debilitating illnesses, fall resulting in broken hips, vertebral/femoral fractures.
- Efforts to lessen the time adults spend watching television or videos or using a computer, if coupled with increases in physical activity above daily routines, could substantially decrease the prevalence of metabolic syndrome. Individuals who do not engage in any moderate or vigorous physical activity during leisure time have about twice the odds of having metabolic syndrome as those who exercise up to 150 minutes a week or more.

Summary

1. Physical activity epidemiology evaluates the nature, extent, and demographics of exercise participation in a large population. Such data often reflect disease occurrence and other health-related outcomes.

2. A discouraging picture exists about physical activity participation by adult Americans. Only 10 to 15% of adults in the United States obtain enough regular physical activity of adequate intensity to impart health and fitness benefits.

3. Health benefits accrue from including a moderate amount of physical activity on most if not all days of the week.

4. Intense physical effort raises a small risk of sudden death during the activity compared with resting for an equivalent time, particularly for sedentary people. The longer term health benefits of regular exercise far outweigh the risk of acute cardiovascular complications.

5. The current Healthy People 2010 goals and objectives for the nation include 226 targeted health objectives in 28 focus areas. Several of these either directly or indirectly aim at increasing regular physical activity among all citizens.

6. For activities that involve running, the greatest orthopedic injury potential exists among individuals who exercise for extended durations.

7. Physical inactivity promotes unhealthy gene expression; increasing regular exercise in the population must become a top public health priority.

PART 2 • *Aging and Physiologic Function*

AGE TRENDS

Physiologic and performance measures improve rapidly during childhood and reach a maximum between late adolescence and approximately age 30. Functional capacity declines thereafter, with deterioration varying at any age depending on lifestyle and genetic characteristics.

Differences in Exercise Physiology Between Children and Adults

One must consider the interaction between physical activity and aging when evaluating physiologic responses and exercise performance across a broad age span. The distinct differences between children and adults can be summarized as follows:

- During weight-bearing walking and running, oxygen consumption ($mL \cdot kg^{-1} \cdot min^{-1}$) of children averages 10 to 30% higher than adults at a designated submaximal pace.[266] The lower exercise economy from children's lower ventilatory efficiency, greater body surface area:mass ratio, shorter stride length, and greater stride frequency, makes a standard walking or running pace physiologically more stressful and performance scores poorer.

- Exercise performance disadvantages exist even though children typically maintain equal or somewhat higher aerobic capacities than adults. Also, walking and running economy and percentage $\dot{V}O_{2max}$ sustainable during exercise at the lactate threshold continually improve as children age, independent of aerobic capacity changes. This limits the usefulness of a single walking or running performance test to predict $\dot{V}O_{2max}$ throughout childhood and adolescence.[49]

- Children exhibit lower absolute aerobic capacity values ($L \cdot min^{-1}$) than adults from a smaller fat-free body mass (FFM; FIG. 31.5). Consequently, children are disadvantaged when exercising against a standard external resistance (unadjusted for body size) in stationary cycling and arm cranking. The fixed oxygen cost ($L \cdot min^{-1}$) of such exercise represents a greater percentage of a child's smaller absolute aerobic capacity. During weight-bearing exercise, energy cost relates directly to body mass, so children are not disadvantaged by a smaller body size.

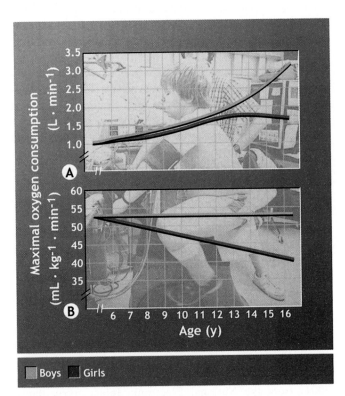

Figure 31.5   A. $\dot{V}O_{2max}$ ($L \cdot min^{-1}$) for boys and girls remains similar until 12 years of age; $\dot{V}O_{2max}$ at age 14 averages 25% higher in boys, and by age 16 the difference exceeds 50%. The differences largely reflect greater muscle mass development in boys and gender differences in daily physical activity. **B.** For boys, $\dot{V}O_{2max}$ ($mL \cdot kg^{-1} \cdot min^{-1}$) averages about 52 mL $\cdot$ kg^{-1} $\cdot$ min^{-1} from age 6 to 16; for females, the line slopes downward with age, reaching approximately 40 mL $\cdot$ kg^{-1} $\cdot$ min^{-1} at age 16, a value 32% below male counterparts. This difference closely parallels the greater accumulation of body fat in females; extra fat increases the energy cost of exercise but does not increase capacity for aerobic metabolism. (From Krahenbuhl GS, et al. Developmental aspects of maximal aerobic power in children. Exerc Sport Sci Rev 1985;13:503.)

- Children do less well than adults on sprint tests of anaerobic power capacity because they cannot generate a high level of blood lactate during maximal exercise. Lower intramuscular levels of the glycolytic enzyme phosphofructokinase may contribute to children's poorer anaerobic exercise performance.
- Children breathe relatively larger air volumes (greater ventilatory equivalent) than adults at any level of submaximal exercise oxygen consumption.
- Perception of effort (rating of perceived exertion, or RPE) is higher in children than adults when both exercise at equivalent percentages of aerobic capacity. Greater pulmonary discomfort owing to the higher respiratory rate and ventilatory equivalent of children may produce this effect.[244]
- Children and adults increase muscle strength with resistance training. Prepubescent children, unlike pubescent children and adults, have limited ability to increase muscle mass presumably from their relatively low androgen levels.

 INTEGRATIVE QUESTION

What factors would explain the relatively poor performances of children in a 10-K run compared with adults of equal aerobic capacity?

Muscular Strength

Age and gender affect muscular strength and muscular power, with the magnitude of each effect influenced by the muscle group studied and the type of muscle action. Some general trends in muscular strength and power of adults with increasing age can be summarized as follows:

- Men and women attain their highest strength levels between ages 20 and 40, the time when muscle cross-sectional area is largest. Thereafter, concentric strength of most muscle groups declines, slowly at first and then more rapidly after middle age.
- Accelerated strength loss in middle age coincides with weight loss and increase in chronic diseases such as stroke, diabetes, arthritis, and CHD.[198]
- The capacity for power generation declines faster than that for maximal strength.[105]
- Declines in eccentric strength begin at a later age and progress more slowly than for concentric strength. Strength loss begins at a later age for women than for men.[145]
- Arm strength for men and women deteriorates more slowly than leg strength.[148]
- Rate of decline in muscular power with aging is similar among male and female weight lifters as well as world record holders, elite master athletes, and healthy, untrained individuals.[239]
- Strength loss among the elderly directly relates to limited mobility and fitness status and the potential for increased incidence of accidents from muscle weakness, fatigue, and poor balance.[112,238]

Age Trends Among Elite Weight Lifters and Power Lifters

Master athletes more accurately reflect the effects of physiologic aging because these healthy, motivated athletes maintain a rigorous training schedule to compete at the highest level. FIGURE 31.6 illustrates age trends for weight lifting and power lifting records of the U.S. Weightlifting and U.S. Powerlifting Organizations. These findings indicate the following:

- Peak lifting performance declines for men and women with advancing age. Weight lifting performance follows a curvilinear trend, while power lifting performance declines linearly with age.

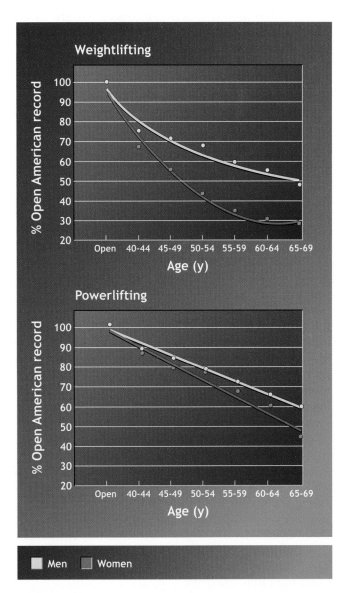

Figure 31.6 Age-related sex differences in (**A**) weight lifting (average snatch and clean and jerk scores) and (**B**) power lifting (average deadlift, squat, and bench press scores) based on analysis of top age-group records of the U.S. Weightlifting and U.S. Powerlifting Organizations. (From Anton MA, et al. Age-related declines in anaerobic muscular performance: weightlifting and powerlifting. Med Sci Sports Exerc 2004;36:143.)

- The rate and overall magnitude of decline in performance with age are markedly greater in weight lifting than in power lifting.
- The magnitude of decline in peak muscular power is greater in lifting tasks that require more omplex and explosive power movements (weight lifting).
- Sex differences in age-related performance decrements emerge only in events that require more complex and explosive power movements with performance declining in women to a greater extent than in men.

These findings indicate a gender- and task-specific influence of age on muscular performance among elite resistance-trained athletes. More powerful and complex tasks undergo greater decline with age than tasks that require simpler movement patterns; women experience greater age-related declines in such tasks.

Muscle Mass Decrease

Motor unit remodeling represents a normal, continual process that involves motor endplate repair and reconstruction. Remodeling progresses by selective denervation of muscle fibers, followed by terminal sprouting of axons from adjacent motor units. Motor unit remodeling gradually deteriorates in old age. This leads to **denervation muscle atrophy**, an irreversible degeneration of muscle fibers, particularly type II fibers, and associated with reduction in circulating growth hormone (GH), insulin-like growth factor-1 (IGF-1), muscle-specific isoforms of IGF, and endplate structures.[35,54,78,83,84] This deterioration progressively reduces muscle cross section and mass (termed **sarcopenia**), even after adjustment for changes in body mass and stature.[29,75,109] Muscle fibers also tend to "type group," in that fast- and slow-twitch fibers lose their typical chessboard distribution and cluster within groups of similar type—perhaps from denervation and subsequent fiber death. Older adults have more than twice the noncontractile content in locomotor muscles as younger adults.[118] Impaired neural drive does not produce the decline in muscle strength with age because older adults achieve full muscle activation during a maximal voluntary muscle action.[51]

The primary cause of reduced strength with aging is the 40 to 50% reduction in muscle mass from muscle fiber atrophy and loss of motor units between ages 25 and 80, even among healthy, physically active adults. FIGURE 31.7A shows that muscle-fiber loss appears near ages 50 to 60. The reduction in total muscle area (Fig. 31.7B) usually parallels reduced fiber size, particularly fast-twitch fibers in the lower extremities. This proportionately increases the area occupied by slow-twitch (type I) muscle fibers.

In a longitudinal study of age-related declines in muscular strength, 9 of 12 men initially evaluated for muscular strength and muscle fiber composition 12 years earlier were remeasured.[74] Knee and elbow extensor and flexor strengths tested at slow and fast angular velocities decreased by 20 to 30%. Muscle cross-sectional area for the same muscle groups

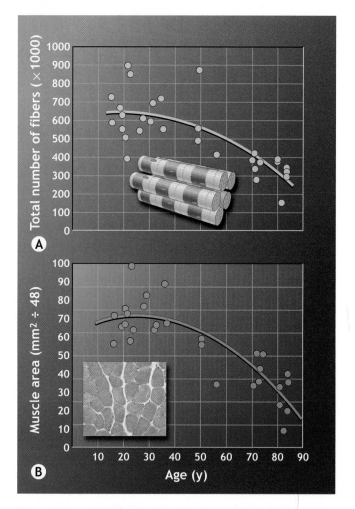

Figure 31.7 Relationship between age and (**A**) total number of muscle fibers and (**B**) muscle cross-sectional area. Muscle size begins to decrease at approximately age 30, decreasing 10% by age 50. Thereafter, muscle area declines more precipitously, largely from decreased total number of muscle fibers. (From Lexell J, et al. What is the cause of the ageing atrophy? Total number, size, and proportion of different fiber types studied in whole vastus lateralis muscle from 15- to 83-year-old men. J Neurol Sci 1988;84:275.)

evaluated by CT scans decreased between 13 and 16%. Muscle biopsies from the vastus lateralis muscle showed a 42% reduction in type I fibers without changes in mean fiber type area. Capillary-to-fiber ratio decreased with aging (0.31 units lower after 12 y). The researchers concluded that changes in muscle cross-sectional area largely contributed to the strength decline from age 65 to 77.

Resistance Training Among the Elderly

Sarcopenia and strength loss with aging reflect the combined effects of progressive neuromotor deterioration and chronic decrease in regular muscle loading. Moderate resistance training provides a remarkably safe way to augment protein synthesis and retention and slow the "normal" and somewhat inevitable loss of muscle mass and strength with aging.[3,103,149,160,189,199] Older men typically demonstrate

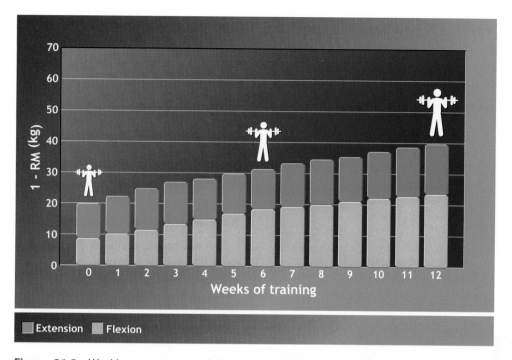

Figure 31.8 Weekly measurements of dynamic muscle strength (1-RM) in left knee extension *(green)* and flexion *(orange)* during resistance training in older men. (From Frontera WR, et al. Strength conditioning in older men: skeletal muscle hypertrophy and improved function. J Appl Physiol 1988;64:1038.)

greater absolute gains in muscle size and strength than female counterparts, but they are similar in percentage improvements.[248] Healthy men between ages 60 and 72 years who trained for 12 weeks with standard-resistance exercise at loads equivalent to 80% of 1-RM demonstrate how well the elderly respond to resistance training. FIGURE 31.8 shows that muscle strength increased progressively throughout training. At week 12, knee extension strength increased by 107% and knee flexion strength by 227%. Improvement rate of 5% per training session matched similar increases reported for young adults. Fast- and slow-twitch muscle fiber hypertrophy accompanied the dramatic strength improvements. In other research, muscle cross-sectional area and strength in 70-year-olds who had resistance trained since age 50 equaled values for a group of 28-year-old students.[121] Older individuals possess impressive plas-

ticity in physiologic, structural, and performance characteristics. Muscle responds to vigorous training with rapid improvement into the ninth decade of life (FIG. 31.9).[67] Improved muscle strength, bone density, dynamic balance, and overall functional status with regular exercise can minimize or reverse the syndrome of physical frailty. Regular exercise provides the most effective way to reduce orthopedic injury (e.g., high prevalence of falls) in older men and women.[196] Even for older persons disabled with osteoarthritis of the knee, regular aerobic or resistance exercises induce beneficial effects on measures of disability, pain, and physical performance.[63] For disabled older female cardiac patients, a 6-month program of resistance training improved muscular strength and physical capacity over a wide range of household physical activities and also improved endurance, balance, coordination, and flexibility.[7]

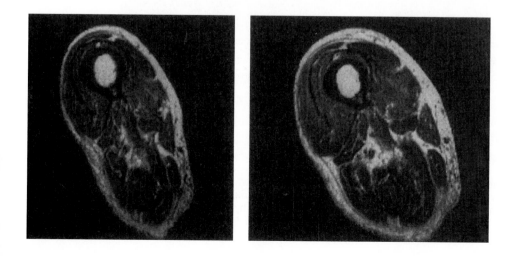

Figure 31.9 Plasticity in physiologic response to resistance training among the elderly. Magnetic resonance images taken at the midthigh region of a male subject 92 years of age before *(left)* and after *(right)* 112 weeks of resistance training of the knee extensor and flexor muscles. Quadriceps lean cross-sectional area increased by 44% in this individual. (From Harridge SD, et al. Knee extensor strength, activation, and size in very elderly people following strength training. Muscle Nerve 1999;22:831.)

TABLE 31.1 ■ STUDIES OF RESISTANCE TRAINING IN OLDER INDIVIDUALS

Study	Age (y)	Gender	Training Type	Strength Gain (%)	Hypertrophy (%)
1	62–84	MF	RT	57	NM
2	18–26	M	RT	30	9
	67–72	M	RT	22	NC
3	69–74	M	CT	9–22	NC
4	22–65	M	CT	3–8	19–20
5	63–84	F	RT	7–13	10
6	60–72	M	RT	9–19	9–12
1	62–84	MF	Iso	45.8	N
7	41–80	M	Iso	12–24	NM
8	20–26	F	Iso	95	NM
	65–73	F	Iso	72	NM
9	55–78	MF	CV	1.9–13.4	NM
10	51–87	M	CV (6 wk)	6.4	NC
		M	CV (42 wk)	11.9	1.0
11	65	MF	CV	5–13	NM
12	65	M	Hdr	15–132	NC

RT, resistance training; CT, circuit training; Iso, isometric training; CV, cardiovascular endurance training; Hdr, hydraulic resistance training; NC, no change; NM, not measured.

1. Perkins LC, Kaiser H. Phys Ther Rev 1961;41:633.
2. Moritaini T, deVries HA. J Gerontol 1980;35:672.
3. Aniansson A, Gustafsson E. Clin Physiol 1981;1:87.
4. Larsson L. Med Sci Sports Exerc 1982;19:203.
5. Aniansson A, et al. Arch Gerontol Geriatr 1984;3:229.
6. Frontera WF, et al. J Appl Physiol 1988;64:1038.
7. Liemohm WP. Int J Aging Hum Dev 1975;6:347.
8. Kauffman TL. Arch Phys Med Rehab 1985;66:223.
9. Barry AJ, et al. J Gerontol 1966;21:192.
10. deVries HA, J Gerontol 1970;25:325.
11. Sidney LH, et al. Am J Clin Nutr 1977;30:326.
12. Becque MD. PhD dissertation, University of Michigan, 1989.

TABLE 31.1 summarizes relevant literature on changes in muscle strength and size in older adults who participated in resistance training programs. Most programs produced positive responses, with strength improvements ranging between 1.9 and 132% in individuals older than age 60. Mechanisms that explain how middle-aged and elderly persons respond to resistance training include enhanced motor unit recruitment and innervation patterns and muscular hypertrophy discussed in Chapter 22. As with younger adults, the number of sets and repetitions and intensity, duration, and frequency of training determine the magnitude of strength adaptations.

Neural Function

A nearly 40% decline in the number of spinal cord axons and a 10% decline in nerve conduction velocity reflect the cumulative effects of aging on central nervous system function. These changes likely contribute to the age-related decrement in neuromuscular performance assessed by simple and complex reaction and movement times. Partitioning reaction time into central processing time and muscle action time, aging most adversely affects the time to detect a stimulus and process the information to produce the response. Knee-jerk reflexes do not involve processing in the brain, so aging affects them less than voluntary responses that involve reaction and movement. FIGURE 31.10 shows slower movement times for simple and complex tasks by older subjects than by younger subjects of similar physical activity levels. *In all instances, the young or old active groups moved considerably faster than the less-active age group.* A physically active lifestyle affects neuromuscular functions positively at any age to slow the age-related decline in cognitive performance associated with speed of information processing.[258] Older individuals who remain physically active for 20 years or longer show reaction speeds that equal or exceed inactive individuals in their 20s.

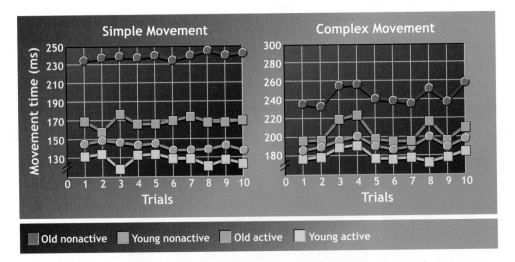

Figure 31.10 Simple and complex movement time in subjects classified as young active, old active, young nonactive, and old nonactive. Note the slower movement times (higher scores) in simple and complex tasks by the old and young nonactive subjects than by their active counterparts. (From Spirduso WW. Reaction and movement time as a function of age and physical activity level. J Gerontol 1975;30:435.)

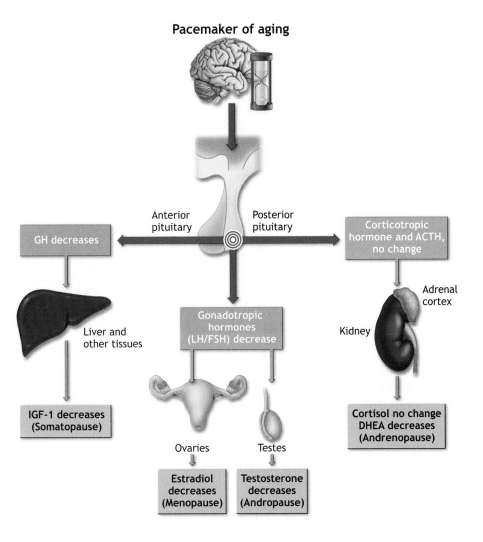

Pacemaker of aging

Anterior pituitary   Posterior pituitary

GH decreases

Corticotropic hormone and ACTH, no change

Adrenal cortex

Liver and other tissues

Gonadotropic hormones (LH/FSH) decrease

Kidney

IGF-1 decreases (Somatopause)

Ovaries   Testes

Cortisol no change DHEA decreases (Andrenopause)

Estradiol decreases (Menopause)

Testosterone decreases (Andropause)

Figure 31.11 Age-related decline in three hormone systems that affect the rate of biologic aging. *Left.* Decreased growth hormone (GH) release by the anterior pituitary depresses production of IGF-1 by the liver and other tissues, which inhibits cellular growth (a condition of aging termed *somatopause*). *Middle.* Decreased output of gonadotropic luteinizing hormone (LH) and follicle-stimulating hormone (FSH) by the anterior pituitary, coupled with reduced estradiol secretion from the ovaries and testosterone from the testes, causes *menopause* (females) and *andropause* (males). *Right.* Adrenocortical cells responsible for DHEA production decrease their activity (termed *adrenopause*) without clinically evident changes in this gland's corticotropin (ACTH) and cortisol secretion. A central pacemaker in the hypothalamus and/or higher brain areas mediates these processes to produce aging-related changes in peripheral organs (ovaries, testicles, and adrenal cortex).

These findings reinforce that regular physical activity slows the biologic aging of select neuromuscular functions. The potential magnitude of these changes and amount of physical activity required to induce meaningful responses remain controversial.[219]

Endocrine Changes

Endocrine function, particularly of the pituitary, pancreas, adrenal, and thyroid glands, changes with age.[133] Approximately 40% of individuals ages 65 and 75 years and 50% of those older than age 80 have impaired glucose tolerance that leads to the most common form of the disease—type 2 diabetes (see Chapter 20).

Increased disease prevalence among the elderly largely relates to controllable factors such as poor diet quality, inadequate physical activity, and increased body fat, particularly in the visceral–abdominal region.[4]

Thyroid dysfunction among the elderly primarily occurs from lowered pituitary gland release of the thyroid-stimulating hormone thyrotropin (and reduced output of thyroxine). Thyroid dysfunction directly affects metabolic function including decreased glucose metabolism and protein synthesis.

FIGURE 31.11 depicts changes in three other hormonal systems associated with aging: (1) hypothalamic–pituitary–gonadal axis, (2) adrenal cortex, and (3) GH/IGF axis.

Hypothalamic–Pituitary–Gonadal Axis

In females, alteration in the interaction between stimulating hormones from the hypothalamus and anterior pituitary gland and gonads decreases estradiol output from the ovaries. This effect probably initiates the permanent cessation of menses (**menopause**) in the aging female. Changes in hypothalamic–pituitary–gonadal axis activity in males occur more slowly and subtly. Serum total and free testosterone, for example, gradually decline with aging in males. Age-related decreases in gonadotropic secretions from the anterior pituitary gland characterize male **andropause**.

Adrenal Cortex

Adrenopause refers to the reduced adrenal cortex output of dehydroepiandrosterone (DHEA) and its sulfated ester DHEAS. In contrast to the glucocorticoid and mineralocorticoid adrenal steroids whose plasma levels remain relatively high with aging, DHEA exhibits a long, progressive decline after age 30. By age 75, the plasma level is only 20 to 30% of the value in young adults. This has evoked speculation that plasma DHEA levels might serve as a biochemical marker of biologic aging and disease susceptibility. Research with animals suggests that exogenous DHEA protects against cancer, atherosclerosis, viral infections, obesity, and diabetes; enhances immune function; and even extends life. Despite its quantitative significance as a hormone in humans, researchers know little about DHEA's (1) role in health and aging, (2) cellular or molecular mechanism(s) of action, (3) possible receptor sites, or (4) potential for adverse effects from supplemental use among young adults with normal DHEA levels. Chapter 23 discusses the case for ergogenic effects of DHEA supplements (and potential risks) on adult men and women.

Growth Hormone/Insulin-Like Growth Factor Axis

Mean pulse amplitude, duration, and fraction of secreted GH gradually decrease with aging, a condition termed **somatopause**. A parallel decrease also occurs in circulating levels of IGF-1, produced by the liver and other cells. IGF-1 stimulates tissue growth and protein synthesis. The interaction between the hypothalamus and anterior pituitary gland probably triggers the age-related GH decrease.

The extent to which changes in gonadal function (menopause and andropause) contribute to adrenopause and somatopause (present in both sexes) remains uncertain. Evidence indicates that muscle size and strength, body composition and bone mass alterations, and progression of atherosclerosis relate directly to hormonal changes with aging. Hormonal replacement therapy, nutritional supplementation, and regular physical activity can delay or even prevent aspects of hormone-related aging dysfunction.

Pulmonary Function

Mechanical constraints on the pulmonary system progress with age to cause deterioration in static and dynamic lung function.[16] Also, pulmonary ventilation and gas exchange kinetics during the transition from rest to submaximal exercise slow substantially.[48] In elderly men, aerobic training increases the kinetics of gas exchange to levels that approach values for fit young adults.[17] Likewise, older endurance-trained athletes demonstrate greater pulmonary functional capacity than sedentary peers. Values for vital capacity, total lung capacity, residual lung volume, maximum voluntary ventilation, $FEV_{1.0}$, and $FEV_{1.0}/FVC$ in athletes above age 60 remain higher than predicted from body size and higher than values for sedentary, healthy individuals.[79] Such findings indicate that regular exercise retards the pulmonary function decline associated with aging.

Cardiovascular Function

Cardiovascular function and aerobic capacity do not escape age-related decrements.

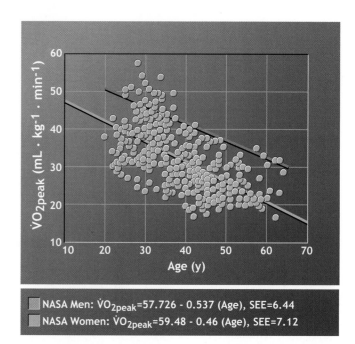

Figure 31.12 Linear regression lines from a cross-sectional assessment of the decline in $\dot{V}O_{2peak}$ with age for a large group of female *(individual green data points)* and male *(purple regression line only)* employees at the National Aeronautics and Space Administration (NASA)/Johnson Space Center (JSC). *SEE,* standard error of estimate. (Modified from Jackson AS, et al. Changes in aerobic power of women, ages 20–64 yr. Med Sci Sports Exerc 1996;28:884.)

Aerobic Capacity

The precise effect of regular aerobic training on the age-related decline in aerobic capacity remains unresolved. Cross-sectional data reveal that $\dot{V}O_{2max}$ declines between 0.4 and 0.5 mL $\cdot$ kg^{-1} each year (approximately 1% per year) in adult men and women (FIG. 31.12).[107,272] Extrapolating this average rate of decline reduces aerobic capacity by age 100 to a level that equals the resting oxygen consumption. This represents a somewhat severe estimate because differences exist in the age-related rate of decline in $\dot{V}O_{2max}$ in sedentary and active individuals.[80,107,207] Decline in $\dot{V}O_{2max}$ with advancing age occurs nearly twice as fast in sedentary men and women as in individuals who maintain exercise training throughout life. A study of a large cohort of men who varied considerably in age, aerobic capacity, body composition, and lifestyle revealed that maintaining relatively stable physical activity and body composition levels over time produced an average yearly decline in $\dot{V}O_{2max}$ of 0.25 mL $\cdot$ kg^{-1} $\cdot$ min^{-1}. No decline in aerobic capacity occurred in individuals who maintained constant training during a 10-year period.[115,187]

For most individuals, regular aerobic exercise cannot fully prevent the decline in aerobic capacity with aging.[69,233,249] For example, aerobic capacity of 50-year-old endurance athletes decreased between 8 and 15% per decade despite continued exercise over a 20-year period.[188] Changes in the volume and intensity of exercise training over time likely account for discrepancies in the $\dot{V}O_{2max}$ decline among physically active individuals. *Despite this disparity, research consistently shows that physically active older men and women maintain a 10 to 50% higher aerobic capacity than sedentary counterparts.*

Factors other than physical activity level influence the age-related decline in $\dot{V}O_{2max}$. Heredity undoubtedly plays a crucial role, as does the well-documented increase in body fat and decrease in skeletal muscle mass.[207] Aging also relates to a decline in a muscle's oxidative function from reduced synthesis of mitochondrial and other proteins.[218] An analysis of aerobic capacity of young and older endurance-trained men and women (FIG. 31.13) indicates an average $0.5 \text{ L} \cdot \text{min}^{-1}$ lower $\dot{V}O_{2max}$ per kilogram of limb (appendicular) muscle mass for the older athletes, independent of age-associated decreases in muscle and increases in fat. No clear answer exists as to how much the lower aerobic capacity per kilogram of limb muscle mass in the older subjects reflects reduced oxygen extraction by the active muscles and/or reduced oxygen delivery via decreased cardiac output and/or active muscle blood flow. However, leg blood flow and vascular conductance during cycle ergometer exercise averaged 20 to 30% lower in older endurance-trained men than in younger peers at similar submaximal oxygen consumptions.[193] Consequently, older athletes achieve an equivalent submaximal oxygen consumption at reduced leg blood flows from an increased local oxygen extraction (a-v O_2 difference) from the available blood supply. For a group of older untrained women, a diminished leg blood flow during peak exercise contributed considerably to their lower $\dot{V}O_{2peak}$ than untrained younger counterparts. The diminished leg blood flow occurred from both central (cardiac output) and peripheral (reduced vascular conductance) limitations.[194]

Central and Peripheral Functions

Decrements in central and peripheral functions linked to oxygen transport and use influence the age-related decline in aerobic capacity.

Heart Rate. *A decline in maximum exercise heart rate represents a well-documented change in cardiovascular function with age.* It typically decreases in accord with the following equation, although this provides only a reasonable approximation:

$$HR_{max} = 220 - \text{age (y)}$$

This age effect reflects reduced medullary outflow of sympathetic activity (depressed β-adrenergic stimulation), which occurs similarly in men and women. Several longitudinal studies of elite athletes reveal that decreases in maximum heart rate over a 20-year period (from age 50 to 70 y) are smaller than predicted from the equation typically used to predict maximum heart rate in nonathletes.[188] For untrained older persons, maximum heart rate may be higher than predicted by 220 − age (y) and, more accurately predicted by the formula:[236]

$$HR_{max} = 208 - 0.7 \times \text{age (y)}$$

Age exerts no meaningful effect on resting heart rate.

Cardiac Output. *Maximum cardiac output typically decreases with age in trained and untrained men and women because of a lower maximum heart rate.* A reduction in the heart's stroke volume also contributes up to 50% of the age-related reduced capacity for blood flow and oxygen consumption. The stroke volume decline reflects the combined effects of reduced left ventricular systolic and diastolic myocardial performance, although some physically active individuals maintain contractile function.[132] Healthy elderly individuals often compensate for a diminished maximum heart rate with increased cardiac filling (end-diastolic volume), which subsequently increases stroke volume by the Frank-Starling mechanism.[70,272]

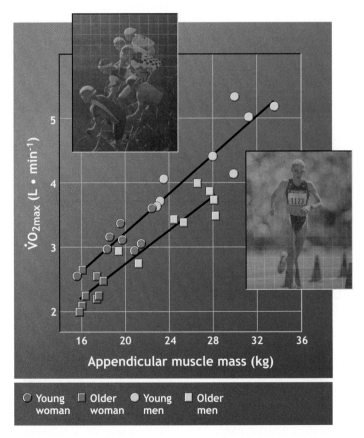

Figure 31.13 Individual maximal oxygen consumption values ($\dot{V}O_{2max}$) related to appendicular muscle mass in young *(top line)* and older *(bottom line)* endurance-trained women and men. For an equivalent appendicular muscle mass, $\dot{V}O_{2max}$ averaged 0.5 $L \cdot min^{-1}$ less for older subjects. These data suggest that aerobic capacity per kilogram of appendicular muscle mass decreases with age in highly trained men and women. (From Procter DN, Joyner MJ. Skeletal muscle mass and the reduction of $\dot{V}O_{2max}$ in trained older subjects. J Appl Physiol 1997;82:1411.)

Large Artery Compliance. Compliance of the large arteries in the cardiothoracic circulation declines with age from changes in the arterial wall's structural and nonstruc-

Within figure:
Young woman | Older woman | Young men | Older men

$\dot{V}O_{2max}$ (L · min⁻¹)

Appendicular muscle mass (kg)

tural properties.[131,213] The inability of the internal diameter of an artery to expand and recoil in response to fluctuations in intravascular pressure during the cardiac cycle associates with impaired cardiovascular function and elevated heart disease risk factors—hypertension, stroke, atherosclerosis, thrombosis, myocardial infarction, and congestive heart failure. Regular endurance exercise slows or prevents the "stiffening" of the large arteries with advancing age[229,234,235,256] and slows the decline in limb vasodilator capacity with healthy aging.[195]

Peripheral Factors. Reduced peripheral blood flow capacity accompanies age-related decreases in muscle mass. A decrease in the capillary-to-muscle fiber ratio and reduced arterial cross-sectional area produces lower blood flow to active muscle.[223] Yet to be determined is how aging and regular exercise interact to affect a muscle's oxidative enzymes.[95,192]

Lifestyle or Aging?

Sedentary living produces losses in functional capacity at least as great as the effects of aging. A high degree of trainability exists among older men and women; positive training-induced adaptations in skeletal muscle structure and function, substrate metabolism, and cardiovascular function often equal those for younger individuals.[36,231] Both low- and higher intensity exercise enable older individuals to retain cardiovascular functions at a higher level than age-paired sedentary subjects. Active middle-aged men who endurance trained over a 10-year period forestalled the usual 9 to 15% decline in aerobic capacity.[114] At age 55, the men maintained the same values for blood pressure, body mass, and $\dot{V}O_{2max}$ as 10 years earlier.

Endurance Performance

Comparing the endurance performance of athletes of different ages provides further evidence for the impressive effects of regular exercise on preservation of cardiovascular function throughout life. FIGURE 31.14A shows age-group, world-record times for 50-, 100-, and 200-km runs for men and women of different ages. The world record at each ultra-distance (always recorded by the youngest age group) corresponds to an average running pace of approximately 5 minutes 38 seconds per mile for the 50-km run; 6 minutes 33 seconds per mile for the 100-km run, and 7 minutes 28 seconds per mile for the 200-km run. Figure 31.14B presents world-record marathon times, beginning at age 4 for males and at age 5 for females and up to age 86 years for men and age 80 years for women. The world record marathon for men set on 9/28/03 of 2 hours, 4 minutes, 15 seconds by Paul Tergat of Kenya (age, 34 y; first person to run under 2 h, 5 min) corresponds to a running speed of 4 minutes 44.3 seconds per mile. The world record marathon for women set by Paula Radcliff (age 31 y) of Great Britain of 2 hours, 15 minutes, 25 seconds also in

2003 corresponds to an average running speed of 5 minutes 9.9 seconds per mile.

Considerable performance decrements occur after age 40, yet a remarkable number of individuals above age 70 now participate in long-distance running. Among marathon finishers in 2003, nearly 500 were age 70 or older compared with about 100 fifteen years ago. The run times for the marathons are particularly noteworthy for the older runners. Not until age 80 to 84 and older does a noticeable drop-off occur in run times. The data for the 70- to 74-year-old group are illustrative; the record—2 hours, 54 minutes, 49 seconds (6:40 per mile pace), set in 2003 by 73-year old Canadian Ed Whitlock—was the first time anyone over age 70 ran a sub-3 hour marathon. This time would have placed him 306th in the New York City Marathon, or among the top 1% of the 33,000 finishers; only 480 runners bettered 3 hours in this marathon. That individuals in their eighth and ninth decade of life successfully run for 12 or 14 hours (Fig 31.13B) affirms the tremendous cardiovascular potential of older men and women who continue vigorous training as they age. The similarity in ultraendurance performance times of older men and women for the 50- and 100-km distances suggests similar cardiovascular fitness levels between genders among elite athletes as they age.

Sprint Performance

FIGURE 31.15 illustrates the relationship between age and 100-m sprint performance in male and female master sprinters ages 35 to 88 years. Performance declined in both groups of athletes with age, the decreases becoming more evident after age 60. Remarkable similarities exist for age-related decrements in running velocity between sexes. Running velocity during the different phases of the run declined from 5 to 6% per decade in men and 5 to 7% per decade for women. Reduced stride length and increase in contact time of the foot with the ground primarily accounted for the overall performance deterioration with age.

Body Composition

After age 18, men and women progressively gain body fat until their fifth or sixth decade at which time total body mass decreases despite increasing body fat. This results partly from a disproportionately greater death rate among the obese in the upper age group, leaving fewer of these individuals to measure.

Most age-trend studies do not track the same subjects over time; instead, they evaluate different subjects in different age categories at the same time. From such **cross-sectional data**, one attempts to generalize about an individual's expected age-related changes, but sometimes this creates misleading generalizations. For example, today's 70- and 80-year-olds typically are shorter than 20-year-old college students. This observation does not necessarily mean that individuals become shorter with age (although this does happen to

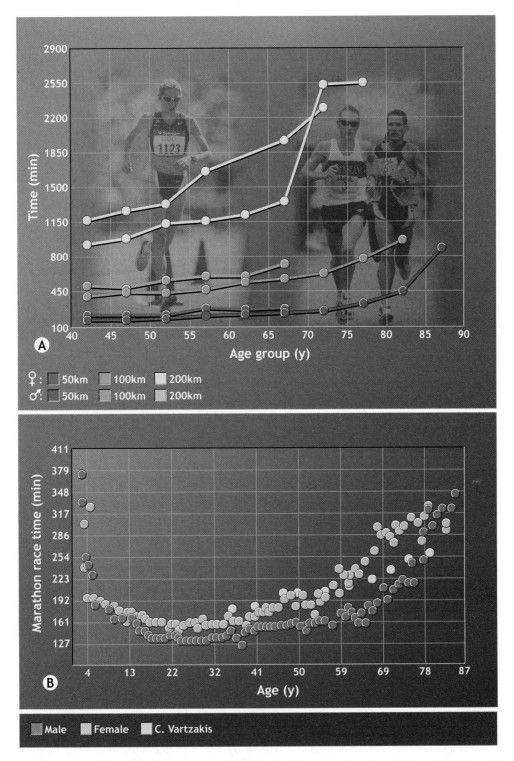

Figure 31.14   A. Ultradistance world records by age for men and women. **B.** Plot of world record marathon run times for men and women of different ages. The *yellow data points* represent the remarkable marathon achievements of the Greek runner Christos Vartzakis from age 36 to 79 years. Over a 43-year span, his average speed decreased by 30% from 13.9 km · h^{-1} at age 36 to 9.73 km · h^{-1} at 79 years of age. Interestingly, his marathon time of 3 hours 56 minutes at age 72 bettered the average speed of master's runners 40 years younger competing in the Basa Marathon Race. (Data on Vartzakis courtesy of Dr. George Rontoyannis, Hellenic Sports Research Institute, Athens, Greece. Data originally published in Rontoyannis G. Sixty-three years of competitive sport activity. Case study. J Sports Med Phys Fitness 1992;32:331.)

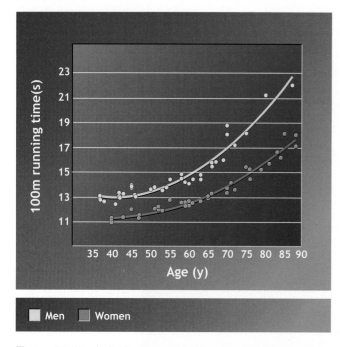

Figure 31.15 Individual values of 100-m running time as a function of age in male and female sprinters. (From Korhonen MT, et al. Age-related differences in 100-m sprint performance in male and female master runners. Med Sci Sports Exerc 2003;35:1419.)

some extent). Instead, the young adults of the current generation receive better nourishment than 80-year-olds received at age 20.

The limited **longitudinal data** (collected on the same subjects over time) show trends in body fat changes similar to data in cross-sectional studies.[43] It is not known if the body fat increases during adulthood represent a normal biologic pattern or simply reflect sedentary lifestyle choices. Longitudinal observations of individuals who maintain a physically active lifestyle support a biologic tendency to gain fat as one ages. FIGURE 31.16 shows body composition changes for 21 endurance athletes who continued to train over a 20-year period starting at age 50. Despite maintaining a relatively constant body mass during the prolonged period of exercise training, gains occurred in body fat and indicators of abdominal obesity while FFM declined. The roughly 3% body fat unit increase per decade paralleled increases in waist girth. The magnitude of increase in body fat and decrease in FFM, while discouraging to some, average at least 20% less than reported for nonathletes. Habitual endurance exercise confers at least some "protection" from the effects of aging on body composition.

Individuals who train regularly for many years with resistance exercise often demonstrate increased FFM and decreased body fat. FIGURE 31.17 shows an older resistance-trained athlete; these photos illustrate the impressive potential to increase and then maintain a large muscle mass into late middle age. Individuals who begin resistance training in late adolescence seem to "defy" certain aspects of typical aging.

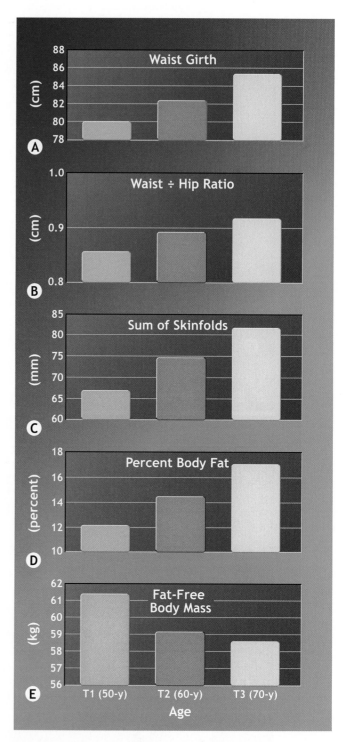

Figure 31.16 Changes in (**A**) waist girth, (**B**) waist:hip girth ratio, (**C**) sum of skinfolds, (**D**) percentage body fat, and (**E**) FFM for 21 endurance athletes who continued to train over a 20-year period, starting at age 50. (From Pollock ML, et al. Twenty-year follow-up of aerobic power and body composition of older track athletes. J Appl Physiol 1997;82:1508.)

Bone Mass

Osteoporosis poses a major problem with aging, particularly among postmenopausal women. This condition produces loss of bone mass as the aging skeleton demineralizes and becomes porous. Bone mass can decrease by 30 to 50% in

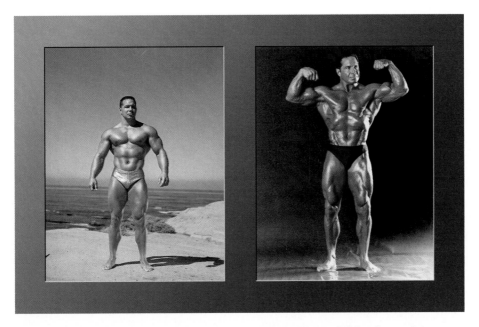

Figure 31.17   Fifty-six consecutive years of resistance training. Bill Pearl, one of the greatest bodybuilding champions of all time. Holder of four Mr. Universe titles (1956, 1961, 1967, 1971), he still trains 2.5 hours daily beginning at 4:30 AM. *Left.* 1967 Mr. Universe, age 37. *Right.* Formal pose at age 59. (Photos courtesy of Bill Pearl.)

persons above age 60. As emphasized in Chapter 2, regular weight-bearing exercise and resistance exercise not only retard bone loss but often increase bone mass in elderly men and women.[5,135] In postmenopausal women, regular exercise augments hormone replacement therapy to increase total bone mineral density and preserve these gains.[123]

TRAINABILITY AND AGE

Exercise training improves physiologic responses at any age. Several factors affect the magnitude of the training response, including initial fitness status, genetics, and specific type of training.

Research over the past 30 years has modified the classic view of the diminished improvements from physical conditioning as a person ages (FIG. 31.18). The current view maintains that over a broad age range, improvements in physiologic function result from an appropriate training stimulus, often at a rate and magnitude *independent* of the person's age.[35,45] Older men and women and younger adults show similar adaptations of muscle fiber size, capillarization, and glycolytic and respiratory enzymes to specific endurance or resistance-training exercise. These adaptations emerge most readily with relatively intense exercise that continuously adjusts to training improvements.

Aerobic Trainability Among the Elderly: Perhaps a Gender Difference

Exercise training for healthy elderly men enhances the heart's systolic and diastolic properties and increases aerobic capacity to the same relative extent (15–30%) as in younger adults.[31,60,143,212] Research has evaluated the contribution of training-induced increases in stroke volume and a-$\bar{v}O_2$ difference to aerobic fitness improvements in healthy older men and women. Nine to 12 months of endurance training increased $\dot{V}O_{2max}$ by 19% in men and 22% in women (TABLE 31.2). These values represent the high end of improvement typically observed for younger adults. Gender differences emerged in certain aspects of the training response. For men, improved aerobic capacity associated with a 15% larger maximum stroke

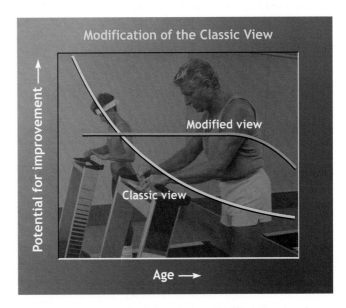

Figure 31.18   New view of old beliefs. Traditional versus the more current view of the expected improvements from physical training with aging.

TABLE 31.2 ■ **EFFECTS OF 9 MONTHS OF ENDURANCE TRAINING ON MAXIMAL OXYGEN CONSUMPTION AND CARDIOVASCULAR FUNCTION IN 15 MEN (AGE, 63 ± 3 Y) AND 16 WOMEN (64 ± 3 Y)**

	$\dot{V}O_{2MAX}$ L · MIN^{-1}	$\dot{Q}_{MAX}$ L · MIN^{-1}	HR_{MAX} B · MIN^{-1}	SV_{MAX} mL	$A\bar{V}O_2DIFF$ mL · dL^{-1}
Men					
Before	2.35	17	170	101	13.8
After	2.8[a]	19[a]	164[a]	116[a]	14.8[a]
Women					
Before	1.36	11.2	161	70	12.2
After	1.66[a]	11.5	164	70	14.4[a]

From Spina RJ, et al. Differences in cardiovascular adaptations to endurance exercise training between older men and women. J Appl Physiol 1993;75:849.

Values are means; $\dot{V}O_{2max}$, maximal O_2 consumption; $\dot{Q}_{max}$, maximal cardiac output; HR_{max}, maximal heart rate; SV_{max}, stroke volume at maximal exercise; $a\bar{v}O_2$diff, arteriovenous O_2 content difference at maximal exercise.

[a] $P ± 0.01$ vs. before training.

volume (corresponding cardiac output increase represented two thirds of the $\dot{V}O_{2max}$ increase) and 7% greater maximum a-$\bar{v}O_2$ difference (representing one third of the $\dot{V}O_{2max}$ increase).

For the women, the a-$\bar{v}O_2$ difference explained the *total* $\dot{V}O_{2max}$ increase, with no change in left ventricular performance at maximal exercise. This indicates that the training-induced increase in aerobic capacity for older women depends on peripheral adaptations in trained muscle and suggests that sex hormones influence gender-related adaptations to endurance training.[120,223] The lack of a stroke volume increase among older women with training may result from (1) blunting of the normal increase in plasma volume, (2) depression of cardiopulmonary baroreflex sensitivity, and (3) estrogen deficiency–related decrease in vascular compliance (i.e., increased vascular stiffness).[223,224,226] These apparent gender differences in physiology do not impair endurance performance in older women as reflected by male–female similarities in ultradistance running performance (Fig. 31.13A).

Summary

1. Physiologic and performance capabilities usually decline after age 30. Many factors, including diminished physical activity level, affect the rate of decline.

2. Regular physical activity and exercise training enable older persons to retain higher levels of functional capacity, notably cardiovascular and muscular function.

3. Biologic aging relates to changes in three hormonal systems: hypothalamic–pituitary–gonadal axis, adrenal cortex, and growth hormone/insulin-like growth factor axis.

4. Four factors are important when evaluating physiologic and performance differences between children and adults: (1) exercise economy, (2) FFM, (3) anaerobic power capacity, and (4) anabolic hormone levels.

5. The primary cause of the age-associated reduction in muscle strength between ages 25 and 80 is a 40 to 50% reduction in muscle mass from a loss of motor units and muscle fiber atrophy.

6. Considerable plasticity exists in physiologic, structural, and performance characteristics among older individuals that enable marked and rapid strength improvement with training into the ninth decade of life.

7. A physically active lifestyle affects neuromuscular functions positively at any age and possibly slows the age-related decline in cognitive performance associated with speed of information processing.

8. VO_{2max} declines approximately 1% each year in adult men and women. Physically active older men and women maintain a higher aerobic capacity than sedentary peers at any age.

9. Sedentary living causes losses in functional capacity at least as great as aging itself. Regular exercise improves physiologic function at any age; initial fitness, genetics, and type and amount of training control the magnitude of change.

10. Active older athletes average at least 20% less body fat and 20% more FFM than nonathletic peers; this suggests that habitual physical activity confers some protection from the negative effects of aging on body composition.

PART 3 • *Physical Activity, Health, and Longevity*

Older fit individuals possess many characteristics of younger persons. One might therefore argue that improved physical fitness retards aging and offers health protection and possible longevity. Exercise may not necessarily represent a "fountain of youth," yet the preponderance of evidence shows that regular physical activity retards the decline in functional capacity associated with aging and disuse. Exercise participation can reverse the loss of function regardless of when a person becomes more physically active.

CAUSES OF DEATH IN THE UNITED STATES

Substantial changes in lifestyle during the last two to three decades have led to variations in causes of death in the United States. Mortality rates from heart disease, stroke, and cancer have declined. Concurrently, behavioral changes have increased the prevalence of obesity and type 2 diabetes. TABLE 31.3 summarizes the ten leading causes of death in the United States in the year 2002. Diseases of the heart (696,947), malignant neoplasm–cancers (557,271), and cerebrovascular disease (162,672) account for the vast majority of the deaths.

TABLE 31.4 compares the causal factors of death in the U.S. in 1990 and 2000. The most striking finding is the substantial increase in the number of estimated deaths attributable to poor diet and physical inactivity. Approximately one half of

TABLE 31.3 ■ TEN LEADING CAUSES OF DEATH IN THE UNITED STATES IN 2002

CAUSE OF DEATH	NUMBER OF DEATHS
Heart disease	696,947
Malignant neoplasm	557,271
Cerebrovascular disease	162,672
Chronic lower respiratory tract disease	124,816
Unintentional injuries	106,742
Diabetes mellitus	73,249
Influenza and pneumonia	65,681
Alzheimer's disease	58,866
Nephritis, nephritic syndrome, nephrosis	40,974
Septicemia (bacterial infections)	33,865
Total	1,921,083

From: National Center for Injury Prevention and Control. Leading causes of death reports, 1999–2002. CDC.

TABLE 31.4 ■ ACTUAL CAUSES OF DEATH IN THE UNITED STATES IN 1990 AND 2000

ACTUAL CAUSE	NUMBER (%) 1990[a]	NUMBER (%) 2000
Tobacco	400,000 (19%)	435,000 (18.1%)
Poor diet and physical inactivity	300,000 (14%)	400,000 (16.6%)
Alcohol consumption	100,000 (5%)	85,000 (3.5%)
Microbial agents	90,000 (4%)	75,000 (3.1%)
Toxic agents	60,000 (3%)	55,000 (2.3%)
Motor vehicle	25,000 (1%)	43,000 (1.8%)
Firearms	35,000 (2%)	29,000 (1.2%)
Sexual behavior	30,000 (1%)	20,000 (0.8%)
Illicit drug use	20,000 (<1%)	17,000 (0.7%)

[a] Data from McGinnis JM, Foege WH. JAMA 1993;270:2207.
From Mokdad AH, et al. Actual causes of death in the United States. JAMA 2004;291:1238.

all deaths in 2000 can be attributed to a limited number of largely preventable behaviors and exposures, most of which relate directly to physical inactivity and overweight and obesity.

EXERCISE, HEALTH, AND LONGEVITY

In one of the first studies of the possibility that sport and regular exercise prolongs life, former Harvard oarsmen exceeded their predicted longevity by 5.1 years per man.[91] Other early studies showed similar but more modest life span extension.[12] Methodologic problems that plagued this research included inadequate record keeping, small sample size, improper statistical procedures to estimate expected longevity, and no accounting for socioeconomic status, body type, tobacco use, and family background.

Subsequent findings showed that participation in athletics as a young adult does *not* ensure good health and longevity later in life.[197] In contrast, maintaining increased physical activity and fitness *throughout life* provides significant health and longevity benefits.[25,64,88,166,210,243] A continuing longitudinal study of the health consequences of different fitness levels in 25,341 men and 7080 women shows low aerobic fitness to be a more important precursor of all cause mortality than any of the other risk factors (FIG. 31.19). In addition, inverse risk gradients emerged across categories of low, moderate, and high fitness, with a lower death rate among moderately fit individuals than those in the low-fitness group. The least fit men and women were nearly twice as likely to die from all causes as the most fit counterparts during an 8-year follow-up period. Increased physical fitness countered the negative effects of other important risk factors. Moderately fit smokers with hypertension and high cholesterol lived longer than healthy but sedentary nonsmokers. *Low physical fitness emerged as a more powerful risk factor than high blood pressure, high cholesterol, obesity, and family history.*

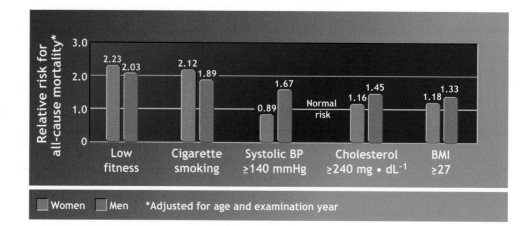

Figure 31.19 Comparative influence of low physical fitness as a precursor of all-cause mortality in men and women. (From Blair S, et al. Influences of cardiorespiratory fitness and other precursors on cardiovascular disease and all-cause mortality in men and women. JAMA 1996;276:205.)

Enhanced Quality to a Longer Life: The Harvard Alumni Study

The lifestyles and exercise habits of 17,000 Harvard alumni who entered college between 1916 and 1950 provide evidence that *moderate* aerobic exercise equivalent to jogging 3 miles daily promotes good health and adds several years to life. The results of these long-term studies showed that:

- Regular exercise countered the life-shortening effects of cigarette smoking and excess body weight.
- Individuals with hypertension who exercised regularly reduced death rate by one half.
- Regular exercise countered genetic tendencies toward early death. Individuals with one or both parents who died before age 65 (a significant health risk) reduced death risk by 25% with a lifestyle of regular exercise.
- Mortality rate decreased by 50% for physically active men whose parents lived beyond 65 years.

FIGURE 31.20 illustrates that persons who do more exercise further reduce their risk of dying. For example, men who walked 9 or more miles each week showed a 21% lower mortality rate than men who walked 3 miles or less. Life expectancy was higher for men who exercised at the equivalent of light sport activity than sedentary men. Life expectancy of Harvard alumni increased steadily from a weekly exercise energy expenditure of 500 kCal up to 3500 kCal, a value equivalent to 6 to 8 hours of strenuous exercise. The active men lived an average of 1 to 2 years longer than sedentary classmates. Weekly exercise beyond 3500 kCal offered no additional health or longevity benefits.

Vigorous Exercise and Longevity

The previously discussed research with Harvard alumni examined only the total amount of weekly physical activity, not its intensity, in relation to heart disease and mortality. Ensuing research with the same group indicates that vigorous regular exercise exerts the greatest effect on extending life.[137] Men who expended at least 1500 kCal weekly in vigorous exercise—equivalent to 6 METs or more, as in jogging or walking briskly, lap swimming, singles tennis, fast cycling, or heavy yard chores for an hour, three or four times weekly—during the 20-year study showed a 25% lower death rate than the most sedentary men. The most active men showed the greatest life expectan-

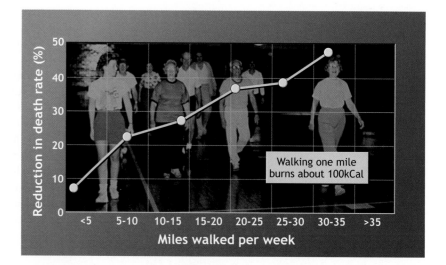

Figure 31.20 Reduced death risk for individuals who participate in regular exercise. (Adapted from Paffenbarger RS Jr, et al. Physical activity, all-cause mortality, and longevity of college alumni. N Engl J Med 1986;314:605.)

cies, largely from reduced deaths from cardiovascular disease. The benefits of vigorous exercise also extended to overweight smokers. Risk associated with a sedentary lifestyle equaled the risk of smoking one pack of cigarettes daily or being 20% overweight. Subsequent research with these men (and others[8]) showed that the exercise equivalent of a 1-hour brisk walk 5 days weekly or a vigorous workout at least once weekly cut stroke risk almost in half; brisk walking for 30 minutes 5 days weekly reduced stroke risk by 24%.[138,139] Other stroke-protective activities included stair climbing or participating in moderate activities as gardening, dancing, and bicycling. An intensive poststroke exercise program also facilitates the stroke survivor's recovery of motor skills.[57]

Epidemiologic Evidence

A critique of 43 studies of the relationship between physical inactivity and CHD concluded that lack of regular exercise contributes to heart disease in a *cause-and-effect* manner; the sedentary person runs almost twice the risk of developing heart disease as the most active individual.[190] *The strength of the association between lack of exercise and heart disease risk equals that for hypertension, cigarette smoking, and high serum cholesterol. This makes physical inactivity the greater heart disease risk because more people lead sedentary lifestyles than possess one or more other primary risks.* The life-protecting benefits of exercise link more with preventing early mortality than extending life span. Surprisingly, only light-to-moderate regular walking, gardening, stair climbing, and household chores produce health benefits for previously sedentary middle-aged and older men and women.[23,122,205,250,269] These sedentary citizens represent the largest percentage of the population at greatest risk for chronic disease.

 INTEGRATIVE QUESTION

Discuss whether physical activity benefits a person's health profile even if exercise intensity does not produce a training effect?

REGULAR MODERATE EXERCISE PROVIDES SIGNIFICANT BENEFITS

A sedentary lifestyle represents an independent and powerful predictor of CHD risk and mortality.[64,162] Encouraging the most sedentary 25% of the American adult population to become only moderately active yields substantial public health benefits.[14,24,58,130,200] For postmenopausal women, walking briskly for 2.5 hours weekly (about 30 min a day 5 days a week) reduced heart disease risk by 30%—a reduction comparable to that achieved with cholesterol-lowering drugs—regardless of race, age, or how much the women weighed.[155] Women who did the most exercise reduced risk by 63%. FIGURE 31.21 further illustrates the health-related benefits of regular physical activity.[81] The analysis assessed the effect of miles walked each day on overall mortality rate in 707 nonsmoking men ages 61 to 81 years. An inverse relationship

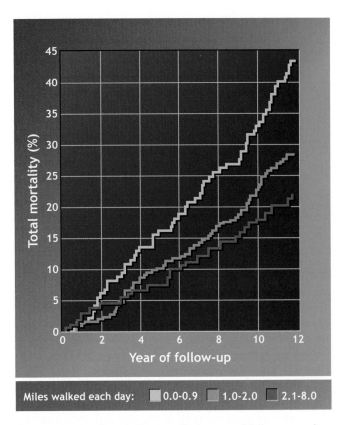

Figure 31.21 Cumulative mortality by year of follow-up and distance walked per day. (To convert distances to kilometers, multiply by 1.609.) (From Hakim AA, et al. Effects of walking on mortality among nonsmoking retired men. N Engl J Med 1998;338:94.)

between distance walked and mortality emerged after adjusting for overall physical activity and other risk factors. Men who walked less than 1 mile daily had a cumulative death incidence in 7 years that required 12 years for the most active men who walked at least 2 miles daily. Over 7 years, 43.1% of the less active men died compared with 21.5% of the most active walkers.

TABLE 31.5 presents corroborative research findings for leisure-time physical activity of 333 patients ages 25 to 74 years who suffered a first heart attack and 503 control subjects without a heart attack selected randomly and matched for age and gender. After adjustments for heart disease risks (age, smoking, diabetes, hypertension), regular walkers reduced cardiac arrest risk by 73%, and those who gardened regularly reduced risk by 66% compared with sedentary peers (risk ratio set at 1.00). Walking exercise or gardening for more than 60 minutes a week reduced risk similarly to high-intensity leisure-time physical activity. The benefits of walking also applied to women who regularly walked 3 mph or faster for at least 3 hours per week; cardiac arrest risk decreased up to 40% below the risk for sedentary women. Risk reduced by one half for women who walked briskly (≥3.0 mph) for 5 hours a week.[154] These findings complement and further support exercise recommendations from the CDC and ACSM to accumulate 30 minutes or more of moderate-intensity physical activity on most days of the week.

TABLE 31.5. ■ MODERATE- AND HIGH-INTENSITY LEISURE-TIME PHYSICAL ACTIVITY (LTPA) AND RISK OF PRIMARY CARDIAC ARREST

	CASE		ODDS RATIO CARDIAC ARREST RISK	
TYPE OF LTPA	PATIENTS, NO. (%)	CONTROLS, NO. (%)	UNADJUSTED	ADJUSTED[a]
No activity	45 (14)	18 (4)	1.0 (Reference)	1.0 (Reference)
Moderate intensity	160 (48)	192 (38)	0.36	0.36
High intensity	128 (38)	293 (58)	0.19	0.36

From Lemaitre RN, et al. Leisure-time physical activity and the risk of primary cardiac arrest. Arch Intern Med 1999;159:686.
[a]Adjusted for age, smoking, education, diabetes, hypertension, and health status.

Influence of Physical Fitness

A low-level of cardiorespiratory fitness (including low exercise capacity, low $\dot{V}O_{2max}$, low heart rate recovery, and failure to achieve target heart rate) provides a strong independent predictor of increased risk for cardiovascular disease and all-cause mortality.[1,42,275] The predictive effect equals that of diabetes mellitus and other heart disease risks.[59,268] One study directly examined aerobic fitness (rather than verbal or written reports of physical activity habits) and heart disease risk in more than 13,000 men and women observed for an average of 8 years. To isolate the effect of physical fitness, the study accounted for cigarette smoking, high cholesterol and blood sugar levels, hypertension, and family history of heart disease. Based on age-adjusted death rates per 10,000 person-years, the least fit group averaged more than three times the death rate of the most fit individuals (FIG. 31.22). The greatest health benefits emerged for the group rated just above the most sedentary category. For men, the decrease in death rate from the least fit category to the next category exceeded 38 (64.0 vs. 25.5 deaths per 10,000 person-years), whereas the drop in mortality between the second group and most fit group was only 7. Enhanced aerobic fitness benefits women to a similar if not greater extent.[174] For every increased score of 1 MET in exercise capacity, the risk of death from all causes decreased by 17%.[155] To move from the most sedentary category to the next highest group—the change that produced the greatest health benefits—requires

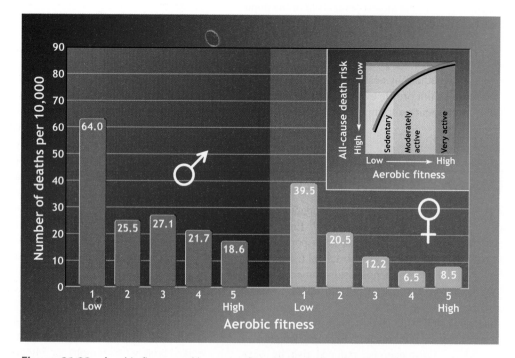

Figure 31.22 Aerobic fitness and longevity. Going from the low fitness category to a moderate level produces the greatest reduction in death risk with only a small added benefit from further fitness improvements. *Inset figure* shows a generalized curve that depicts health benefits from increased daily physical activity and aerobic fitness. (Modified from Blair SN, et al. Physical fitness and all-cause mortality: a prospective study of healthy men and women. JAMA 1989;262:2395.)

only such moderate-intensity exercise as walking briskly for 30 minutes several times weekly.

Studies of Finnish men complement the above findings. Aerobic capacity and leisure-time physical activity showed an inverse, graded, independent association with risk for acute myocardial infarction.[113] Even after adjusting for genetic effects and other familial factors that predict mortality, current aerobic fitness and physical activity level offered significant protection from death.[128] Physical fitness also counters the negative impact of existing disease. For example, an inverse and independent relationship emerged between aerobic capacity and incidence of fatal and nonfatal cardiovascular events and all-cause mortality in male and female hypertensives followed over 16.5 years.[183]

TABLE 31.6 summarizes 30 years of research relating physical activity level or physical fitness to chronic disease or medical conditions. *Clearly, a strong inverse association exists between regular exercise and level of aerobic fitness and all causes of death. Moderate-intensity regular exercise substantially reduces the risk of dying from heart disease, cancer, and other causes.*[22,37,116,267]

TABLE 31.6. ■ GENERAL TREND FOR EFFECTS OF REGULAR PHYSICAL ACTIVITY AND/OR INCREASED PHYSICAL FITNESS AND RISK FOR CHRONIC DISEASE CONDITIONS

DISEASE OR CONDITION	TRENDS ACROSS ACTIVITY OR FITNESS CATEGORIES AND STRENGTH OF EVIDENCE[a]
All-cause mortality	↑↑↑
Coronary artery disease	↑↑↑
Hypertension	↑↑
Obesity	↑↑↑
Stroke	↑
Peripheral vascular disease	→
Cancer	
Colon	↑↑
Rectum	→
Stomach	→
Breast	↑
Prostate	↑
Lung	↑
Pancreas	→
Type 2 diabetes	↑↑↑
Osteoarthritis	→
Osteoporosis	↑↑

[a] →, No apparent difference in disease rates across activity or fitness categories; ↑, *some* evidence of reduced disease rates across activity or fitness categories; ↑↑, *good* evidence of reduced disease rates across activity or fitness categories, control of potential confounders, good methods, some evidence of biologic mechanisms; ↑↑↑, *excellent* evidence of reduced disease rates across activity or fitness categories, good control of potential confounders, excellent methods, extensive evidence of biologic mechanisms, relationship is considered causal.

Structured Exercise Not Necessary

Researchers monitored two groups of 116 sedentary men and 119 women ages 35 to 60 years during a 2-year randomized clinical trial.[58] One group spent 20 to 60 minutes exercising vigorously by swimming, stair stepping, walking, or biking up to 5 days a week at a fitness center. The other group incorporated 30 minutes a day of "lifestyle" exercises such as extra walking, raking leaves, stair climbing, walking around the airport while waiting for a plane, and participating in a walking club most days of the week. The lifestyle participants also learned cognitive and behavioral strategies to increase daily physical activity.[156] The intervention consisted of 6 months of intensive exercise followed by 18 months of maintenance for each of the programs. At the end of 24 months, *both* groups showed similar improvements in physical activity, cardiorespiratory fitness, systolic and diastolic blood pressure, and body fat percentage. These findings show that the health-derived benefits from regular exercise do not require structured or vigorous exercise.

 INTEGRATIVE QUESTION

Respond to the statement: "The fact that overwhelming epidemiologic evidence links on-the-job or leisure-time physical activity to reduced CHD risk does not necessarily prove that exercise *causes* improved cardiovascular health."

CAN CHANGING ACTIVITY LEVEL IMPROVE HEALTH AND EXTEND LIFE?

Current level of physical activity and physical fitness relates to health risk, but an important question concerns whether a sustained increase in regular activity can reduce disease risk. To answer this question, previously sedentary, apparently healthy male Harvard alumni reported whether they changed their typical physical activity and other lifestyle habits over an 11- to 15-year period. FIGURE 31.23 relates changes in health-related lifestyle characteristics to changes in mortality risk. Regardless of age, sedentary men who adopted a more moderate to vigorous level of regular activity had a 51% lower risk of dying than men who remained sedentary. For lifestyle change and heart disease mortality risk, becoming more physically active on a regular basis provided risk reduction benefits equivalent to quitting cigarette smoking, reducing body weight, or controlling blood pressure.

Summary

1. Vigorous physical activity early in life contributes little to increased longevity or health in later life. A physically active lifestyle throughout life confers significant health benefits.

2. Regular, moderate exercise counters the life-shortening effects of CHD risks that include cigarette

Figure 31.23 Adjusted relative risks for CHD mortality from changes in lifestyle characteristics. Each relative risk is adjusted for age and all other variables in the figure. *First bar* of each pair represents men with initial unfavorable characteristics (in 1962 or 1966) and at follow-up in 1977. The *second bar* of the pair shows adjusted relative risks for men who achieved favorable changes in the variable of interest between baseline and 1977 follow-up. *BMI,* body mass index; *Yes* and *No* refer to presence or absence of trait at date indicated. (Modified from Blair SN. Physical activity, physical fitness, and health. Res Q Exerc Sport 1993;64:365. Data from Paffenbarger RS Jr, et al. The association between changes in physical-activity level and other lifestyle characteristics with mortality among men. N Engl J Med 1993;328:538.)

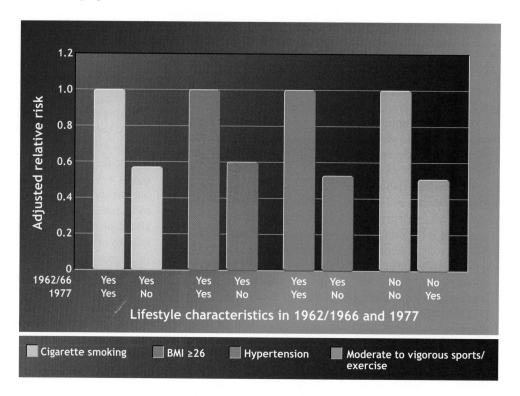

smoking and excess body weight. A sedentary person runs almost twice the risk of developing heart disease as the most active individuals.

3. The risk of CHD from sedentary living equals that for hypertension, cigarette smoking, and high serum cholesterol. The life-protecting benefits of exercise relate more to preventing early mortality than to extending overall life span.

4. A moderate amount of regular exercise substantially reduces the risk of dying from heart disease, cancer, and other medically related maladies. The greatest health benefits emerge when a person alters a sedentary lifestyle and becomes just moderately physically active.

5. Strategies that modify lifestyle toward increased daily physical activity beneficially alter factors associated with CHD risk.

PART 4 • *Coronary Heart Disease*

Coronary heart disease involves degenerative changes in the intima or inner lining of the larger arteries that supply the myocardium.

CHANGES ON THE CELLULAR LEVEL

Damage to arterial walls begins as a multifactorial largely immunologically mediated inflammatory response to injury, perhaps from hypertension, cigarette smoking, infection, homo-

cysteine, elevated cholesterol, or free radicals. One response triggers the chemical modification of various compounds, which includes oxidation of low-density lipoprotein cholesterol (LDL-C). This initiates a complex series of changes that produce lesions that sometimes bulge into the vessel lumen or protrude outward into the arterial wall. Lesions initially take the form of fatty streaks, the first signs of atherosclerosis. With further inflammatory damage from continued lipid deposition and proliferation of smooth muscle cells and connective tissue, the vessel congests with lipid-filled plaques, fibrous scar tissue, or both. Progressive occlusion gradually reduces blood flow capacity with ensuing myocardial ischemia (reduced supply of oxygen).

C-Reactive Protein: An Indication of Arterial Inflammation

About one half of persons with heart disease have normal or just moderately elevated cholesterol levels, which has led researchers to consider other factors in the heart disease process. Guidelines issued by the AHA and the CDC propose an important role for inflammation testing to judge whether persons need aggressive treatment to protect their hearts and vascular system. Mounting evidence indicates that painless chronic low-grade arterial inflammation, including that of the coronary arteries, is central to every stage of atherosclerotic disease and a major trigger for heart attack—more substantial even than high cholesterol. The inflammation produces heart attacks by weakening the walls of blood vessels, making plaque burst, and interfering with substances that increase myocardial circulation. **C-reactive protein (CRP)**, a natural chemical produced by the liver and necessary for fighting injury, inflammation, and infection, indicates the degree of inflammation. This compound may be just as important an independent coronary artery disease risk factor as elevated LDL-cholesterol. In fact, CRP reduction with statin drugs (and associated reduction in plaque size) is at least as crucial as cholesterol reduction in preventing heart attacks.[173,202] CRP frequently rises when arteries begin to accumulate plaque. High CRP levels also associate with the development of hypertension,[214] a finding that suggests that hypertension is part of an inflammatory disorder. Normal CRP levels average 1.5 mg · dL^{-1} of blood. Individuals with abnormally high CRP levels (>3.0 to 4.0 mg · dL^{-1}) are four times more likely to experience impaired blood flow to the heart. They also are twice as likely to die from heart attacks and strokes as individuals with high cholesterol—a finding that explains why some persons with low cholesterol develop heart disease or why lowering cholesterol sometimes fails to prevent serious heart problems.

Guidelines suggest limiting CRP testing to those already judged to be at intermediate risk (10–20% risk of heart disease over the next 10 years; about 40% of the U.S. adults), based on risk factors of age, cholesterol level, and blood pressure. Individuals with CRP levels above 1.0 mg · dL^{-1} should take aggressive action to reduce the level, which is also elevated in children and adolescents with the metabolic syndrome.[71] Strategies to lower CRP include weight loss, abstinence from cigarette smoking, consuming a healthful diet, and regular exercise.[108]

Vulnerable Plaque: Difficult to Detect Yet Lethal

Vulnerable plaque, a soft type of metabolically active, unstable plaque, does not necessarily produce coronary artery narrowing but tends to fissure and burst. The rupture of unstable plaque—the sudden breakdown of fatty plaques in the lining of coronary arteries—exposes the blood to thrombogenic compounds. This triggers a cascade of chemical events that can produce clot formation (**thrombus**) and subsequent myocardial infarction and possible death. The sudden, complete obstruction of a coronary artery frequently occurs in blood vessels with only mild-to-moderate obstructions ($<70\%$ blockage). Arterial blockage often occurs before the coronary vessel has narrowed enough to produce angina symptoms or electrocardiographic (ECG) abnormalities or to indicate the need for revascularization procedures (e.g., coronary bypass surgery or balloon angioplasty). Acute disruption and rupture of arterial plaque provides a plausible explanation for sudden death from acute physical and emotional exertion in middle-aged men with coronary artery disease compared with sudden death under resting conditions.[34] The beneficial effects of cholesterol-lowering strategies on heart disease risk do not always improve coronary blood flow. Stability of vulnerable plaque may improve with reduction in overall blood cholesterol.[142] This stabilizing effect would reduce the likelihood of rupture of existing coronary artery plaque.

Vascular Degeneration Begins Early in Life

Landmark studies of atherosclerosis in young American soldiers killed in Korea showed advanced lesions in men whose age averaged 22 years.[62] These surprising findings focused attention on the possible childhood origins of atherosclerosis. We now know that fatty streaks and clinically significant fibrous plaques develop rapidly during adolescence through the third decade of life.[232] Autopsies of 93 young persons aged 2 to 39 years, most of whom died from trauma, revealed that fatty streaks and fibrous plaques in the aorta and coronary arteries appear early and progress in severity with aging.[20] Body mass index, systolic and diastolic blood pressure, and total serum cholesterol, triacylglycerols, and LDL-C strongly and positively related to the extent of vascular lesions in the deceased young people (high-density lipoprotein cholesterol [HDL-C] related negatively). History of cigarette smoking magnified the vascular damage, a disconcerting fact in light of data that indicate tobacco use is common and on the increase among college students.[204] As the number of risk factors increased, so also did the severity of atherosclerosis in these asymptomatic individuals. Analyses of microscopic qualities of coronary atherosclerosis in 760 teenagers and young adults who died from accidents, suicide, and murder indicated that many had arteries so clogged that they could suffer a myocardial infarction.[161] Two percent of those ages 15 to 19 and 20% of those 30 to 34 had advanced plaque formation, the blockages considered most likely to break off and precipitate a heart attack or stroke. Collectively, the autopsy findings support the wisdom of primary prevention of atherosclerosis through risk factor identification *and* intervention early in childhood or adolescence.

FIGURE 31.24 shows the progressive occlusion of an artery from a buildup of calcified fatty substances in atherosclerosis. The first overt sign of atherosclerotic change occurs when lipid-laden macrophage cells cluster under the endothelial lining in the artery to form a bulge (fatty streak). Over time, proliferating smooth muscle cells migrate to the inner endothelial layer and accumulate to narrow the lumen (center) of the artery. A thrombus forms and plugs the artery, depriving the myocardium of normal blood flow and oxygen supply. When the thrombus blocks one of the smaller coronary vessels, a portion of the heart muscle dies (necrosis) and the person suffers a heart attack or **myocardial infarction** (**MI**). MIs are caused by blockage in one or more arteries that supply the heart, cutting off myocardial blood supply or sudden spasms (constrictions) of a coronary vessel that causes tissue necrosis from oxygen deprivation. MI contrasts with **cardiac arrest** from irregular neural–electrical transmission within the myocardium. Cardiac arrest results from chaotic, unregulated beating of the heart's upper chambers (atrial fibrillation) or lower chambers (ventricular fibrillation).

If coronary artery narrowing progresses to cause brief periods of inadequate myocardial perfusion, the person may experience temporary chest pains termed **angina pectoris** (see Chapter 32). These pains usually emerge during exertion because physical activity increases demand for myocardial

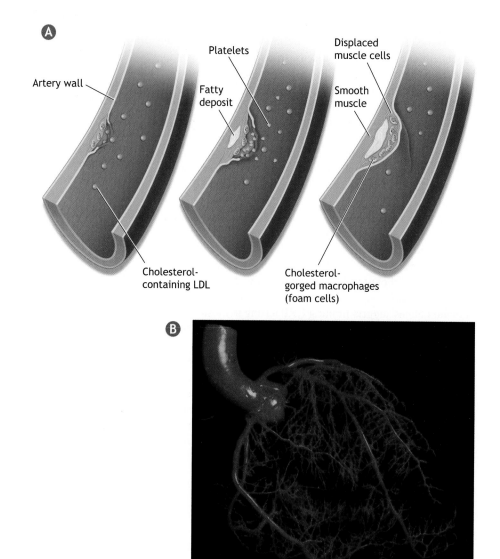

Figure 31.24   A. Deterioration of a coronary artery from deposits of fatty substances that roughen the vessel's center. When α thrombus (blood clot) forms above the plaque, complete blockage of the artery produces a myocardial infarction or heart attack. A coronary artery bypass graft (CABG) creates a new "transportation route" around the blocked region to allow the required blood flow to deliver oxygen and nutrients to the previously "starved" surrounding heart muscle. The saphenous vein from the leg is the most commonly used bypass vessel. CABG involves sewing the graft vessels to the coronary arteries beyond the narrowing or blockage, with the other end of the vein attached to the aorta. Medications (statins) lower total and LDL-cholesterol, and daily low-dose aspirin (81 mg) reduces post-CABG artery narrowing beyond the insertion site of the graft. Repeat CABG surgical mortality averages 5 to 10%. **B.** Cast of coronary artery vasculature.

blood flow. Anginal attacks provide painful, dramatic evidence of the importance of adequate myocardial oxygen supply.

INTEGRATIVE QUESTION

Design an experiment to evaluate the effects of (1) aerobic exercise training and (2) standard resistance exercise training on cardiovascular risk factors in middle-aged women. Indicate controls, measurement variables, and tests to show a training effect.

Cardiovascular Disease Epidemic

Currently, cardiovascular disease ranks second only to cancer as the leading health problem and the primary cause of death among Americans younger than age 85. The primary reason for this reversal in rank is that while the number of deaths from both causes has fallen, the detection and treatment improvements have been more dramatic for heart disease. Heart disease is an expensive condition to treat and a resource-intensive chronic condition. Consider the most recent (2001–2002) statistics released by the AHA in 2005:

- At least 64.4 million people (one person in four) in the United States suffer from some form of cardiovascular disease.
- Cardiovascular disease is a major killer of women and men. Diseases of the cardiovascular system claim the lives of more than 500,000 females every year or about one death a minute.
- Cardiovascular disease accounts for almost 1 of every 2.4 deaths.
- Since 1900, cardiovascular disease was the leading cause of death in every year but 1918 and 2005; it caused more deaths than the next seven causes combined.

- Every 34 seconds an American suffers a coronary event; each minute someone dies from one.
- No previous symptoms of the disease existed in 57% of men and 64% of women who died suddenly from cardiovascular disease.
- Coronary heart disease alone caused 502,189 deaths—or one in five deaths—in 2001. Another 13.2 million Americans that year survived heart attacks, chest pains, and other aliments caused by coronary heart disease.
- In 2004, cardiovascular disease produced an economic burden on society that cost an estimated $368.4 billion.

Despite these rather discouraging statistics, age-adjusted death rate from cardiovascular disease since 1950 has decreased by approximately 60%. Still, heart diseases account for approximately 32% of the total mortality in the United States.[40,41,254] When a heart attack does strike, its severity has decreased over the past decade. A large portion of the decline in incidence and severity relates to risk factor reduction (e.g., 25% of adults smoking now vs. 42% 30 years ago, better pharmacologic control of high blood pressure and cholesterol levels, improved exercise behaviors), more effective pharmacologic therapies, and more-intense treatment immediately after a heart attack. Survival rates can reach 96% for those who receive immediate hospital treatment.[77,102,206]

CORONARY HEART DISEASE RISK FACTORS

Research over the past 50 to 60 years has identified various personal characteristics, behaviors, and environmental factors linked to increased CHD susceptibility. Although many of these factors relate strongly to CHD risk, the associations do not necessarily imply a causal relationship (e.g., male-pattern baldness[146]). In some instances, it remains unclear whether risk-factor modification offers effective disease protection.

Until definite proof emerges, it seems prudent to assume that elimination or reduction of one or more of the modifiable risk factors reduces the likelihood of CHD and cumulative disability in later years. For example, a radical heart risk-reduction program that requires a vegetarian diet that limits fat intake to no more than 10% of total calories and includes regular exercise, stress-management training, and support meetings substantially reduces subsequent heart attack rate and other adverse heart events (e.g., bypass operations and angioplasty procedures).[179] In contrast, patients in conventional care steadily worsened over the same 5-year period. The following lists contain the most frequently implicated **CHD risk factors**:[72,87,96,170,225]

Modifiable risk factors

- Diet
- Elevated blood lipids
- Hypertension
- Personality and behavior patterns
- Cigarette smoking

- High serum uric acid
- Sedentary lifestyle
- Pulmonary function abnormalities
- Excessive body fat
- Diabetes mellitus
- ECG abnormalities
- Tension and stress
- Poor education
- Elevated homocysteine

Nonmodifiable risk factors

- Age
- Gender
- Ethnic background
- Male-pattern baldness, particularly lack of hair on the crown of the head; possibly from raised androgen levels
- Family history

Determining the quantitative importance of any single CHD risk factor remains difficult because of the interrelationships among blood lipid abnormalities, type 2 diabetes, heredity (gene polymorphism), and obesity.[27,262]

Age, Gender, and Heredity

Age represents a CHD risk factor largely because of its association with hypertension, elevated blood lipid levels, and glucose intolerance. After age 35 in men and age 45 in women, the chances of dying from CHD increase progressively and dramatically.

In contrast to the beliefs of many physicians who still adhere to the antiquated notion that cardiovascular disease is primarily a man's illness, FIGURE 31.25 shows that as of 1984, women show greater risk of death from cardiovascular diseases (heart disease, stroke, hypertension) than men. Women also have more lethal and severe first-time heart attacks and suffer a 70 to 100% greater risk of dying within months of a first heart attack than men, particularly women under age 50 (approximately 6% of all heart attacks in women).[30,93,157,255] Specifically, 17% of women who suffer heart attacks die while still in the hospital compared with 12% of men, and 38% of women die within a year compared with 25% of men. Yet there remains a troubling and enduring gap in treatment for women. Women account for about one half of the coronary artery disease deaths in the United States, yet receive only about one third of the nearly 1 million annual intervention procedures. To close this gap, the AHA has issued new gender-specific guidelines that encourage doctors to make greater use of new cardiac imaging tests in women (as high a diagnostic accuracy as in men), which includes single photon emission computed tomography and stress echocardiography (see Chapter 32).[106] Also recommended is an increase in the application of life-saving procedures as balloon angioplasty and drug-coated stents to open blocked arteries. Special attention should be paid to women with diabetes who have particularly high heart disease risk, as do women with metabolic syndrome and polycystic ovary syndrome (hormonal disorder among women of repro-

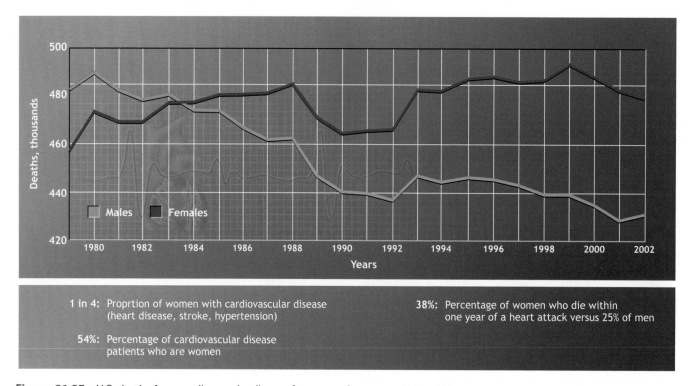

Figure 31.25   U.S. deaths from cardiovascular disease for men and women: 1979 to 2002.

ductive age). The pattern of coronary artery blockage may also differ between sexes. Men exhibit discrete blockages at distinct focal points, making them more amenable to stenting, while women show a more diffuse blockage that occupies a longer segment of the vessel. The good news is that current trends in smoking reduction (smoking among American adults fell sharply between 1965 and 2000, to 22% from 42%), diet improvement, and increase in postmenopausal hormone use largely account for the current decline in coronary artery disease in middle-aged women.[97]

Heart attacks that strike at an early age tend to run in families. Familial predisposition relates to a genetic role in determining risk of heart disease. In the following sections we examine blood lipid abnormalities, obesity, cigarette smoking, and physical inactivity related to CHD (Chapters 15 and 32 discuss hypertension). These modifiable factors represent the "big five" heart disease risks proposed by the AHA. Each exists as a potent, independent CHD risk that can change considerably with lifestyle modification.

 INTEGRATIVE QUESTION

Explain how risk factor modification can affect change in disease risk.

Blood Lipid Abnormalities

Serum cholesterol levels in adults have declined substantially in the United States over the past 35 years, a decline that coincides with a decreased national incidence of CHD.

Despite this support for the effectiveness of public health programs geared to lowering heart disease risks, nearly 30% of adults still require intervention for high cholesterol levels.[111] Unfortunately, data from the CDC indicate that approximately 60% of persons with high cholesterol levels did not know they were high. Of those who knew, only 14% were taking a cholesterol-lowering drug. An abnormal blood lipid level or **hyperlipidemia** is a crucial component in the genesis of atherosclerosis.

AHA Recommendations for Cholesterol and Triacylglycerol

FIGURE 31.26 shows the rate of increase in death risk from CHD related to total serum cholesterol. The *inset table* presents AHA serum cholesterol and lipoprotein and triacylglycerol level classifications for adults (www.americanheart.org). Recommendations also include that individuals above age 20 have a fasting "lipoprotein profile" every 5 years (9 to 12 h following the last meal and without liquids or pills). Current guidelines focus less on total cholesterol and more on its lipoprotein components. The new guidelines, based on findings concerning the effects of the powerful cholesterol-lowering statin drugs on heart health (i.e., reduced risk of heart attack, bypass surgery, plaque growth in coronary vessels, angioplasty),[26,172,211] are more stringent than prior recommendations. Adherence to the guidelines will nearly triple the number of adults taking cholesterol-lowering drugs to 36 million Americans and raise by 25% the number who should be on a cholesterol-lowering diet.[134] Early treatment becomes crucial because of a strong association between high serum cholesterol

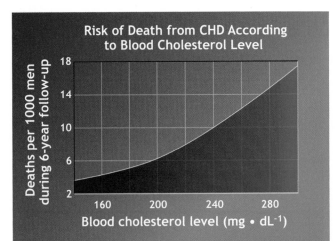

Risk of Death from CHD According to Blood Cholesterol Level

x-axis: Blood cholesterol level (mg · dL⁻¹)
y-axis: Deaths per 1000 men during 6-year follow-up

American Heart Association Recomendations and Classifications for Total Cholesterol and HDL and LDL cholesterol and Triacylglycerol	
Total cholesterol level*	**Category**
≥ 240	High blood cholesterol. A person with this level has more than twice the risk of heart disease as someone with cholesterol below 200.
200 to 239	Borderline high
≤ 200	Desirable level that puts you at a lower risk for heart disease. Cholesterol level of 200 or higher raises risk.
HDL cholesterol level	**Category**
< 40	Low HDL cholesterol. A major risk factor for heart disease.
40 to 59	Higher HDL levels are better.
≥ 60	High HDL cholesterol. An HDL of 60 mg · dL⁻¹ and above is considered protective against heart disease.
LDL cholesterol level	**Category**
> 190	Very high; cholesterol-lowering drug therapies even if no heart disease and no risk factors.**
160-189	High; cholesterol-lowering drug therapies even if there is no heart disease but 2 or more risk factors present.
130-159	Borderline high; cholesterol-lowering drug therapies if heart disease is present.
100-129	Near optimal; doctor may consider cholesterol-lowering drug therapies plus dietary modification if heart disease is present.
< 100	Optimal; no therapy needed.
Triacylglycerol level	**Category**
< 150	Normal
150-199	Borderline high
200-499	High
≥ 500	Very high

* All levels in mg · dL⁻¹.
** In men under age 35 and premenopausal women with LDL cholesterol levels of 190 to 219 mg · dL⁻¹, drug therapy should be delayed except in high-risk patients like those with diabetes.

as a young adult and cardiovascular disease in middle age. A cholesterol level of 200 mg · dL⁻¹ or lower is usually desirable, although risk for a fatal heart attack begins to rise at 150 mg · dL⁻¹. A cholesterol level of 230 mg · dL⁻¹ increases heart attack risk to about twice that of 180 mg · dL⁻¹, and 300 mg · dL⁻¹ increases the risk fourfold. For triacylglycerol, 150–199 mg · dL⁻¹ is considered as an upper-limit normal level, with 200 to 499 considered high. The latter requires changes in exercise, diet, and possibly drug intervention if accompanied by other CHD risk factors.

Lipids do not circulate freely in blood plasma; they combine with a carrier protein to form lipoproteins composed of a hydrophobic cholesterol core and a coat of free cholesterol, phospholipid, and regulatory protein (**apolipoprotein [Apo]**). TABLE 31.7 lists the four different lipoproteins, their approximate gravitational densities, and percentage composition in the blood. *Serum cholesterol is a composite of the total cholesterol contained in each of the different lipoproteins.* Discussions commonly refer to hyperlipidemia, but the more meaningful focus addresses the different types of **hyperlipoproteinemia**.

Cholesterol distribution among the various lipoproteins provides a more powerful predictor of heart disease risk than total blood cholesterol. Specifically, elevated HDL-C levels relate causally with a lower heart disease risk even among individuals with total cholesterol below 200 mg · dL⁻¹. Overwhelming evidence links high LDL-C and apolipoprotein (B) levels with increased CHD risk.[132] A more effective evaluation of heart disease risk than either total cholesterol or LDL-C levels divides total cholesterol by HDL-C. *A ratio greater than 4.5 indicates high heart disease risk; a ratio of 3.5 or lower represents a more desirable risk level.*

LDL-C (synthesized in the liver) and very low-density lipoprotein cholesterol (VLDL-C) transport fats to cells, including the smooth muscle walls of arteries. Upon oxidation, LDL-C participates in artery-clogging, plaque-forming atherosclerosis by stimulating monocyte–macrophage infiltration and lipoprotein deposition.[228] LDL-C's surface coat contains the specific apolipoprotein (Apo B) that facilitates cholesterol removal from the LDL-C molecule by binding to LDL-C receptors of specific cells. Prevention of LDL-C oxidation, in contrast, slows CHD progression. In this case, any potential benefit of dietary antioxidants such as vitamins C and E and β-carotene on heart disease risk may lie in their ability to blunt LDL-C oxidation (see Chapter 2).[53,85,127,144]

Whereas LDL-C targets peripheral tissue and contributes to arterial damage, HDL-c (also produced in the liver and whose levels relate to genetic factors[110]) facilitates **reverse**

Figure 31.26 *Top.* Death risk from coronary heart disease (CHD) in relation to total serum cholesterol level in middle-age men. *Inset table.* The American Heart Association recommendations and classifications for serum cholesterol, lipoproteins, and triacylglycerol levels for adults.

TABLE 31.7. ■ APPROXIMATE COMPOSITION OF SERUM LIPOPROTEINS

	CHYLOMICRONS	VERY LOW-DENSITY LIPOPROTEINS (VLDL:PREBETA)	LOW-DENSITY LIPOPROTEINS (LDL:BETA)	HIGH-DENSITY LIPOPROTEINS (HDL:ALPHA)
Density (g · cm^{-3})	0.95	0.95–1.006	1.006–1.019	1.063–1.210
Protein (%)	0.5–1.0	5–15	25	45–55
Lipid (%)	99	95	75	50
Cholesterol (%)	2–5	10–20	40–45	18
Triacylglycerol (%)	85	50–70	5–10	2
Phospholipid (%)	3–6	10–20	20–25	30

cholesterol transport. HDL-C promotes surplus cholesterol removal from peripheral tissues (including arterial walls) for transport to the liver for bile synthesis and subsequent excretion via the digestive tract. The apolipoprotein A-1 (Apo A-1) in HDL-C activates **lecithin acetyl transferase (LCAT)**. This enzyme converts free cholesterol into cholesterol esters, facilitating cholesterol removal from lipoproteins and diverse tissues.[180]

Factors That Affect Blood Lipids

Six behaviors that favorably affect cholesterol and lipoprotein levels include:

1. Weight loss
2. Regular aerobic exercise (independent of weight loss)
3. Increased dietary intake of water-soluble fibers (fibers in beans, legumes, and oat bran)
4. Increased dietary intake of polyunsaturated-to-saturated fatty acid ratio and monounsaturated fatty acids
5. Increased dietary intake of unique polyunsaturated fatty acids in fish oils (omega-3 fatty acids) and elimination of *trans* fatty acids
6. Moderate alcohol consumption

Four variables that adversely affect cholesterol and lipoprotein levels include:

1. Cigarette smoking
2. Diet high in saturated fatty acids and preformed cholesterol and *trans* fatty acids
3. Emotionally stressful situations
4. Oral contraceptives

Specific Exercise Effects

Short-Term Effects. Reaching the threshold that changes blood lipid and lipoprotein levels in a single exercise session requires considerable physical activity. For example, healthy trained men needed to expend 1100 kCal in one exercise bout to elevate HDL-C, 1300 kCal of exercise to lower LDL-C, and 800 kCal of exercise to decrease triacylglycerol levels.[65]

Long-Term Effects. A single exercise session produces only transient favorable changes in lipid and apolipoprotein concentrations, yet the change persists with exercising at least every other day.[47]

LDL-C. Exercising regularly usually produces only small reductions in LDL-C level when controlling for serum cholesterol-related factors of body fat and dietary lipid and cholesterol intake. Regular exercise may improve the quality of this circulating lipoprotein by promoting a less-oxidized form of LDL-C to reduce atherosclerosis risk.[260] In addition, regular aerobic exercise increases the success of dietary efforts to favorably alter high-risk lipoprotein profiles.[227]

HDL-C. Endurance athletes usually maintain relatively high HDL-C levels, and favorable alterations occur for sedentary men and women of all ages who engage in regular moderate-to-vigorous aerobic exercise.[55,58,273] To some extent, exercise intensity and duration exert independent effects in modifying specific CHD risk factors. In general, exercise duration exerts the greatest effect on HDL-C while exercise intensity most favorably modifies blood pressure and waist girth.[274] In most cases, a favorable change in lipoprotein profile does not require exercise intensity to improve cardiovascular fitness. With the exception of triacylglycerols, exercise-induced lipid alterations usually progress independent of body weight changes.[136] For overweight individuals, the typical increase in HDL-C with exercise training diminishes without concomitant weight loss.[169,241] Favorable exercise-related lipoprotein changes probably result from enhanced triacylglycerol clearance from plasma in response to exercise.

Protection from Gallstones. The benefits of regular aerobic exercise on modifying cholesterol and lipoprotein profiles extend to protection against painful gallstones and accompanying gallbladder removal (the usual treatment for 500,000 Americans yearly, of whom two thirds are women). The NIH reports that gallstone formation and its consequences are the most common and costly ($5 billion yearly) digestive disease requiring hospitalization and surgery. Overall, women who exercised 30 minutes daily reduced their need for gallbladder surgery by 31%.[140] Physical activity increases the movement of the large intestine and improves blood glucose and insulin regulation; both factors reduce gallstone risk. Regular exercise also may reduce the cholesterol content of bile, the digestive juice stored in the gallbladder. Eight percent of gallstones are solid cholesterol.

Other Influences

Even trained endurance athletes exhibit considerable variability in HDL-C levels, with some elite runners' values approaching the median value for the general population. No single factor—nutrition, body composition, or training status—distinguishes runners with high HDL-C values from runners with lower values. This suggests that genetic factors exert a strong influence on the blood lipid profile. In fact, a specific gene produces endothelial lipase (EL), an enzyme that may affect HDL-C production.[110] Excessive activity (turning on) of this gene increases EL synthesis, which may lower HDL-C and subsequently increase cardiovascular risk.

Standard resistance training exerts little or no effect on serum levels of triacylglycerol, cholesterol, or lipoproteins. From a dietary perspective, substituting soy-derived protein for protein from animal sources improves the cholesterol and lipoprotein profile, particularly in persons with high blood cholesterol.[13] A moderate daily alcohol intake—2 oz or 30 mL of 90-proof alcohol, three 6-oz glasses of wine, or slightly less than three 12-oz beers—reduces an otherwise healthy person's risk of heart attack and stroke independent of their physical activity level.[44,209,273] The heart-protective benefit of alcohol consumption also applies to individuals with type 2 diabetes.[257] The mechanism for the benefit remains elusive, yet a moderate alcohol intake increases HDL-C and its subfractions HDL_2 and HDL_3. The polyphenols in red wine may inhibit LDL-C oxidation, thus blunting a critical step in plaque formation.[171,203] Moderate wine intake also tends to associate with more heart-healthy dietary choices with a positive impact on plasma lipids.[245] Excessive alcohol consumption offers no lipoprotein benefit and increases liver disease and cancer risk.

Lipoprotein(a). **Lipoprotein(a) [Lp(a)]** represents a diverse class of protein particles formed in the liver when two distinct apolipoproteins unite. Lp(a) structurally resembles LDL-C but contains an additional unique apolipoprotein(a) coat. Heredity determines elevated Lp(a) levels, which occur in approximately 20% of the population. The independent risk for atherosclerosis, thrombosis, and acute MI increases when Lp(a) levels exceed 25 to 30 mg $\cdot$ dL^{-1} with raised LDL-C levels.[21] Dietary changes and either short- or long-term exercise exert little or no effect on serum Lp(a) concentrations.[82,100,101,151]

Dietary Fiber, Insulin, and CHD Risk. Insulin resistance and associated hyperinsulinemia relate to CHD risk factors of age, obesity, central body fat distribution, smoking, physical inactivity, hypertension, dyslipidemia, and abnormalities in blood-clotting factors. Many researchers and clinicians now consider insulin resistance and consequent hyperinsulinemia as independent CHD risk factors.[208]

The combined effects of established CHD risk factors account for approximately 50% of the observed variability in insulin resistance and hyperinsulinemia within the population. The question then is what other factors might contribute to excessive insulin output and, by implication, increased CHD risk. Perhaps total lipid or saturated fatty acid intake and dietary carbohydrates are possible causal factors. Dietary fiber also may play a key role in optimizing insulin response.[147] For example, dietary fiber reduces insulin secretion by slowing the rate of nutrient digestion and glucose absorption following a meal. Because of its inherently high glycemic index, a low-fiber meal stimulates relatively more insulin secretion than a high-fiber meal of equivalent carbohydrate content. Thus, dietary fiber can serve a dual role in heart-disease prevention by (1) attenuating the insulin response to a carbohydrate-containing meal and (2) reducing the tendency to accumulate body fat from insulin's facilitatory role in fat synthesis. Excessive body fat increases insulin resistance, which ultimately leads to hyperinsulinemia.

Immunologic Factors. An immune response is a likely trigger for plaque development within arterial walls. During this process, mononuclear immune cells produce proteins called *cytokines,* some of which stimulate plaque buildup while others inhibit plaque formation. Regular exercise may stimulate the immune system to inhibit agents that facilitate arterial disease. For example, 2.5 hours of weekly exercise for 6 months decreased cytokine production that aids in plaque development by 58%, while cytokines that inhibit plaque formation increased by nearly 36%.[221]

Beyond Cholesterol: Homocysteine and Coronary Heart Disease

Homocysteine, a highly reactive, sulfur-containing amino acid, forms as a byproduct of methionine metabolism. Researches in the 1960 and 1970s described three different inborn errors of homocysteine metabolism that involved B-vitamin enzymes. High levels of homocysteine in the blood and urine were common to all three disorders of the afflicted individuals, and one half of these persons developed arterial or venous thrombosis by age 30. It was postulated that moderate elevation of homocysteine in the general population predisposes individuals to atherosclerosis in a manner similar to elevated cholesterol concentration.

Numerous studies have shown a nearly lockstep association between plasma homocysteine levels and heart attack and mortality in men and women.[61,201,265,270] This metabolic abnormality occurs in nearly 30% of CHD patients and 40% of patients with cerebrovascular disease. Excessive homocysteine causes blood platelets to clump, fostering blood clots and deterioration of smooth muscle cells that line the arterial wall. Chronic homocysteine exposure eventually scars and thickens arteries and provides a fertile medium for circulating LDL-C to initiate damage. In the presence of other conventional CHD risks (e.g., smoking and hypertension), synergistic effects magnify the negative impact of homocysteine on cardiovascular health.[152,277] Resting homocysteine levels exerted an independent increased risk on a continuum for vascular disease similar to that of smoking and hyperlipidemia. A powerful multiplicative interaction effect also emerged in the presence of other risks, particularly cigarette smoking and hypertension. In general, persons in the highest quartile for homocysteine levels experience nearly twice the risk of heart attack or stroke of those in the lowest quartile. Why some persons accumulate homocysteine is uncertain, but the evidence points to a deficiency of B vitamins (B_6, B_{12}, and particularly folic acid; FIG. 31.27B); lifestyle factors of cigarette smoking and coffee and high meat intake also associate with elevated homocysteine concentrations.[33,153,167,177,178,230]

Figure 31.27A proposes a mechanism for homocysteine's negative impact on cardiovascular health. The homocysteine model helps explain why some persons with low-to-normal cholesterol levels contract heart disease. Figure 31.27C gives the relative risk for vascular disease in groups defined by the presence or absence of classic risk factors and elevated plasma homocysteine levels adjusted for age, gender, and research center.

No clear standard currently exists for normal or desirable homocysteine levels, although most evidence indicates that the current "normal range" of 8 to 20 μmol per liter of plasma is too high. Evidence suggests as little as 12 μmol can double heart disease risk. Until recently, debate has focused on whether normalizing homocysteine reduces risk of arterial occlusive disease that precipitates heart attack and stroke. Consequently, little is known regarding whether an elevated homocysteine level is simply a CHD risk factor or an actual cause (not an effect) of CHD.[159,176] The first study of its kind, a double-blind, randomized, controlled trial, determined whether once-daily high doses of folic acid (2.5 mg), vitamin B_6 (25 mg), and vitamin B_{12} (0.4 mg) over a 2-year period lowered homocysteine levels and reduced recurrent stroke risk in patients with ischemic stroke.[247] Reduction of total homo-

cysteine averaged 2.0 μmol · L^{-1} greater in the group that received the high-dose supplement than in the group receiving lower doses. The moderate homocysteine reduction produced no effect on vascular outcomes during a 2-year follow-up. The researchers concluded that the consistent findings of other researchers of an association of total homocysteine with vascular risk justified longer trials in different populations with elevated homocysteine.

Research on the effects of exercise on homocysteine levels remains inconclusive. Intense exercise training may increase homocysteine levels accompanied by changes in vitamin B_{12} and folate status.[56,89,90] Other data indicate that individuals who engage in long-term exercise (and who exhibit higher plasma folate levels) show reduced homocysteine levels.[86,124,126,182] Also, resistance training reduced homocysteine in the elderly.[261]

INTEGRATIVE QUESTION

If regular physical activity contributes little to extending life span, what other reasons make sense for maintaining a physically active lifestyle throughout middle and older age?

CHD Risk Factor Interactions

Many risk factors interact with each other and with CHD.[117] FIGURE 31.28 shows that the presence of three primary CHD risk factors in the same person magnify individual effects. With one risk factor, a 45-year-old man's chance of CHD during the year averages twice the risk for a man without risk factors. With three risk factors, this man's chance for angina, heart attack, or sudden death increases to nearly 10 times the level for those without risk factors.

The four major modifiable cardiovascular risk *factors—cigarette smoking, diabetes mellitus, hypertension,* and *hypercholesterolemia*—account for only about 50% of individuals who subsequently develop CHD. Thus, researchers have investigated novel markers and other nontraditional risk factor candidates to increase cardiovascular risk predictability.[27,262] TABLE 31.8 presents different novel risk factors that independently associate with atherosclerotic vascular disease.

Several reports directly challenge this "only 50%" claim for the aforementioned four risk factors. Analysis of data from 14 randomized clinical trials ($N = 122{,}458$) and three observational studies ($N = 386{,}915$) showed that in contrast to previous belief, 80 to 90% of patients who developed clinically significant CHD and more than 95% of patients who experienced a fatal CHD event had at least one of the four traditional major risk factors, including overweight/obesity. Remarkably, these finding may even underestimate the true extent of the relationship, given the self-report design of the observational studies and number of patients unaware or not

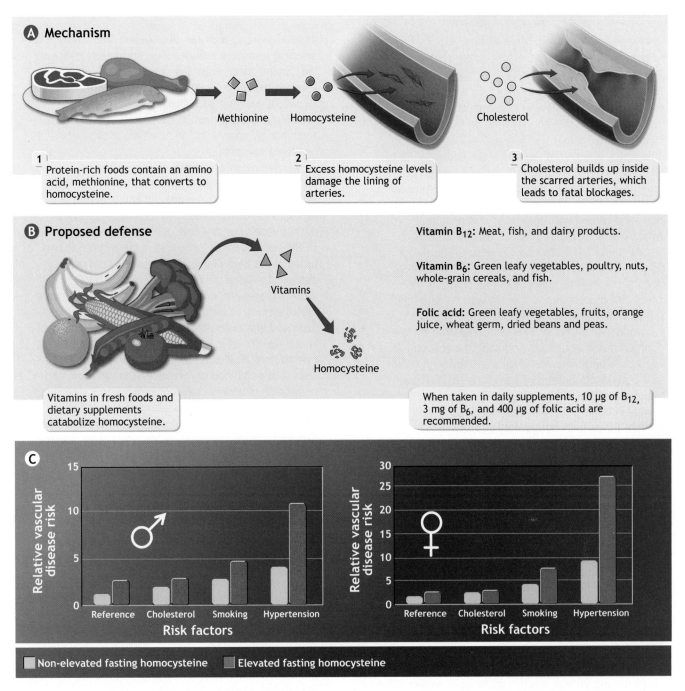

Figure 31.27 **A.** Proposed mechanism for how the amino acid homocysteine damages the lining of arteries and sets the stage for cholesterol infiltration into a vessel. **B.** Proposed defense against the possible harmful effects of elevated homocysteine levels. **C.** Relative risk of all vascular diseases defined by the presence of classic risk factors with and without elevated plasma total homocysteine levels adjusted for age, gender, and research center. (Graphs from Graham IM, et al. Plasma homocysteine as a risk factor for vascular disease: The European Concerted Action Project. JAMA 1997;277:1775.)

diagnosed as having risk factors at the time of evaluation. These findings have enormous public health implications for targeting a large segment of the population at risk of developing CHD. Smoking is arguably the single most important modifiable and preventable cardiovascular disease risk factor and one of the strongest predictors of premature CHD. Obesity and physical inactivity are equally important CHD predictors.

Many CHD risks link in common to behavioral patterns; they become influenced by similar and, in some cases, identical interventions. For example, regular exercise exerts a positive influence on obesity, hypertension, type 2 diabetes, stress, and elevated blood lipid profile. No other modifiable behavior exerts such a potent positive effect for the greatest number of persons, causing many to argue that regular physical activity constitutes the most important behavioral intervention to reduce CHD.

AN UNDERDIAGNOSED AND UNDERTREATED CDH RISK FACTOR: SLEEP DISORDERS

The prevalence of sleeping disorders worldwide continues to increase (www.wrongdiagnosis.com/s/sleep_disorders/stats-country.htm). In the United States, approximately 1 in 6 individuals, or 43 million Americans, suffer from sleep loss (an additional 20 to 30 million experience intermittent sleep-related problems) that directly or indirectly impacts CHD—insulin resistance and hypertension,[b] obesity and diabetes,[c] increased carotid wall thickness,[a] and nocturnal myocardial ischemia from apnea-associated oxygen desaturation.[d,e] The National Commission on Sleep Disorders Research (www.nhlbi.nih.gov/health/prof/sleep/reschpln.htm) attributed $15.9 billion as the direct cost of sleeping conditions, with an estimated $50 to $100 billion in indirect and related costs. All of the world's countries in 2004 were impacted by sleep-disordered consequences (including unnecessary automobile accidents and deaths and spiraling health care costs) from Belize (7%) to China (8%). The NIH's National Institute of Neurological Disorders and Stroke (www.ninds.nih.gov/); National Heart, Lung, and Blood Institute (www.nhlbi.nih.gov/health/prof/sleep/); National Center on Sleep Disorders Research (www.nhlbi.nih.gov/about/ncsdr/index.htm); National Sleep Foundation (www.sleepfoundation.org/); and Patient Education Institute (www.nlm.nih.gov/medlineplus/sleepdisorders.html) provide excellent resources about sleep disorders that explain the sleep apneas (complications from repeated, interrupted breathing during sleep that can be life threatening if untreated) and other sleep disorder-related restless leg syndrome (RLS), insomnia (inability to fall asleep or remain asleep), and narcolepsy (neurological disorder from failure to regulate sleep-wake cycles normally and characterized by excessive daytime sleepiness and dramatic decrease in muscle tone and loss of reflexes or cateplexy). Sleep disorders also afflict between 80 and 90% of mostly middle-aged women diagnosed with fibromyalgia. Their sleep problems and chronic daytime fatigue occur in addition to pain and muscle and joint stiffness. A common characteristic of sleeping disorders includes loud and intermittent snoring. During these episodes, the blood's oxygen saturation can decrease to 80% or less. In severe cases, the individual spends more time not breathing than breathing—placing them at increased risk for death (common symptoms include daytime drowsiness and nighttime insomnia).

Treatments for sleep disorders include continuous positive airway pressure (CPAP; a mask system that regulates the amount and pressure of air sent into the nose to keep the nasal passages open during sleep), surgery (uvulopalatopharyngoplasty, or UPPP; removal of the back part of the soft palate and tissue at the back of the throat to open up more airspace to widen the passageway at the back of the throat), oral appliance that repositions the jaw forward while sleeping to maintain a more open airway, pharmacologic interventions, and cognitive/behavioral strategies. The objective in all the procedures is to restore normal sleep patterns (without snoring), stabilization of blood oxygen levels during sleep, and restoration of normal daily functions without sleepiness. The NIH has identified 30 research issues critical to understanding the effects of sleep disorders and sleep restriction related to cardiovascular and other disease treatment regiments (www.nhlbi.nih.gov/about/ncsdr/research/research-a.htm); considerably more research is required to better understand all of the correlates among sleep disorders and their underlying mechanisms.

[a]Altin R, et al. Evaluation of carotid artery wall thickness with high-resolution sonography in obstructive sleep apnea syndrome. J Clin Ultrasound 2005;33:80.
[b]Harsch IA, et al. Insulin resistance and other metabolic aspects of the Obstructive Sleep Apnea Syndrome. Med Sci Monit 2005 Feb 25;11(3):RA70–75.
[c]Kiely JL, McNicholas WT. Cardiovascular risk factors in patients with obstructive sleep apnoea syndrome. Eur Respir J 2000;16:128.
[d]Schafer H, et al. Sleep-related myocardial ischemia and sleep structure in patients with obstructive sleep apnea and coronary heart disease. Chest 1997;111:387.
[e]Wieber SJ. The cardiac consequences of the obstructive sleep apnea-hypopnea syndrome. Mt Sinai J Med 2005;72:10.

Risk Factors in Children

The frequent occurrence of multiple CHD risk factors in young children emphasizes the need for early CHD initiatives to reduce atherosclerosis risk later in life.[52,246,275] For example, risk factors measured in childhood and adolescence were associated with the thickness of the carotid artery later in life. As with adults, the association between body fat and serum lipid levels becomes readily apparent in overfat children; the fattest children usually have the highest levels of serum cholesterol and triacylglycerols. General adiposity and visceral adipose tissue also relate to unfavorable hemostatic factors that increase CHD morbidity and mortality in adulthood.[66] Of 62 overfat children aged 10 to 15 years, only one child had just one CHD risk factor.[19] Of the remaining children, 14% had two risk factors, 30% three, 29% four, 18% had five, and the remaining five children, or 8%, had six. A subsample then enrolled in a 20-week program to evaluate the effects on the risk profile of either diet plus behavior therapy or regular exercise plus diet plus behavior therapy.

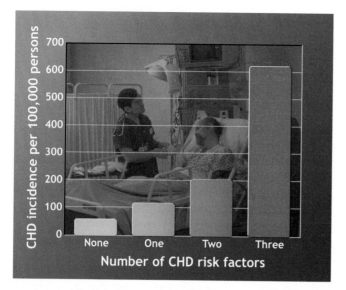

Figure 31.28 General relation between a combination of abnormal risk factors (cholesterol ≥ 250 mg · dL^{-1}; systolic blood pressure ≥ 160 mm Hg; smoking ≥ 1 pack of cigarettes per day) and incidence of coronary heart disease (CHD).

No changes resulted in multiple-risk reduction in either the control group or those receiving diet plus behavior treatment. In contrast, children undergoing exercise plus diet plus behavior therapy dramatically reduced multiple risks (FIG. 31.29). These encouraging findings demonstrate that a supervised program of moderate food restriction and exercise with behavior modification reduces CHD risk factors in obese adolescents. Adding regular exercise augmented the effectiveness of risk-factor intervention.

Autopsy evidence and prevalence of CHD risk factors among preadolescents and adolescents indicate that heart disease begins in childhood. Usually, the most sedentary children (e.g., those who watch the most TV) have more body fat and a higher BMI than physically active peers.[15] School-based programs that increase the level of daily physical activity and/or reduce risk factors increase students' knowledge about risk factors and benefits of physical activity without impairing academic performance.[117] Such programs can produce a long-term positive effect on exercise habits and overall health.[119,252] If regular physical activity upgrades or stabilizes a poor risk factor profile, then school curricula at all grade levels (especially kindergarten and elementary grades) should strongly encourage more physically active lifestyles. Not implementing required daily physical education seems counterproductive from a public health policy standpoint.

Calculating CHD Risk

Risk inventories assess an individual's susceptibility to CHD. Several different quantitative methods estimate CHD risk. The Framingham Risk Score derived from the Framingham Heart Study Cohort predicts 10-year risk of mortality from CHD and nonfatal myocardial infarction.[50,240] The Framingham Risk Scores take into account age, gender, smoking status, total cholesterol, high-density lipoprotein cholesterol, systolic blood pressure, and diabetes.

An alternative risk scoring method, the European SCORE, was developed by the European Society of Cardiology in 2003 to estimate 10-year risk of fatal cardiovascular disease in European nations in primary prevention.[46] SCORE estimates total cardiovascular risk rather than risk of CHD alone by totaling calculated coronary and noncoronary com-

TABLE 31.8 ■ NOVEL RISK FACTORS FOR ATHEROSCLEROTIC VASCULAR DISEASE

INFLAMMATORY MARKERS	HEMOSTATIC/THROMBOSIS MARKERS	PLATELET-RELATED FACTORS	LIPID-RELATED FACTORS	OTHER FACTORS
• C-reactive protein • Interleukins (e.g., IL-6) • Serum amyloid A • Vascular and cellular adhesion molecules • Soluble CD40 ligand • Leukocyte count	• Fibrinogen • von Willebrand factor antigen • Plasminogen activator inhibitor 1 (PAI-1) • Tissue-plasminogen activator • Factors V, VII, VIII • D-dimer • Fibrinopeptide A • Prothrombin fragment 1 +2	• Platelet aggregation • Platelet activity • Platelet size and volume	• Low-density lipoprotein (LDL) • Lipoprotein (a) • Remnant lipoproteins • Apolipoproteins A1 and B • High-density lipoprotein subtypes • Oxidized LDL	• Homocysteine • Lipoprotein-associated phospolipase A(2) • Microalbuminuria • Insulin resitance • PAT-1 genotype • Angiotensin-converting enzyme genotype • ApoE genotype • Infectious agents: cytomegalovirus, *Chlamydia pneumonia*, *Helicobacter pylori*, herpes simplex virus • Psychosocial factors

PHYSICAL INACTIVITY: A SIGNIFICANT CORONARY HEART DISEASE RISK

Morris JN, et al. Coronary heart disease and physical activity of work. Lancet 1953;265:1053.

▲ Epidemiologists of the1940s and 1950s did not consider regular exercise a way to protect against early development of coronary heart disease (CHD). Morris and colleagues demonstrated an impressive link between physical activity in specialized occupations and reduced CHD risk. The researchers compiled statistics on CHD incidence for two groups of workers. One group consisted of 31,000 men aged 35 to 64 years employed by the London Transport Authority. Job classifications included *drivers* and *conductors* of trams and trolley buses and *motormen* and *guards* on the underground railway system. Drivers and motormen classified as sedentary, while a conductor represented a more physically demanding occupation (e.g., walking through a double-decker bus collecting tickets). The second work group consisted of 110,000 *postal workers* and *civil servants*. Physical activity level composed the basic differences between these workers in job requirements: postmen maintained a moderate physical activity level walking delivering mail, while civil servants (postal and telegraph officers, telephone operators, clerks) remained sedentary in office jobs.

The figure shows the CHD incidence (rate per 1000 per age group determined from medical records) for the first clinical episode of CHD—angina pectoris, myocardial infarction, or death directly attributable to CHD. The London Transport workers exhibited 119 total CHD episodes (3.8% per 1000). In 25% of these episodes, death occurred within 3 days (34 of 119 cases); in 40%, death ensued within 3 months

(49 of 119 cases). Nonetheless, the pattern of CHD incidence differed between conductors and drivers. Drivers contracted the disease at a younger age and had a higher incidence (2.7 vs. 1.9) than conductors; also, drivers showed a rate of immediate mortality twice that of conductors. In contrast, angina occurred twice as frequently in the conductors (0.8 vs. 0.4 per 1000). Overall, conductors exhibited less CHD than drivers and the disease appeared at a later age. Like the transport workers, the physically active postmen averaged a substantially lower total incidence of CHD and mortality than sedentary clerks. The physically active group experienced less CHD; when disease did occur, it remained less severe.

Morris offered three possible explanations for the findings:

1. Differences in constitution (e.g., CHD susceptibility) affected existing health status, causing the men to self-select a job category based on its physical requirements.
2. Differences in mental strains from a specific job affected the progression of CHD.
3. Differences in job-related physical activity *caused* group differences in CHD incidence.

While all three explanations seemed plausible, the researchers suggested that differences in on-the-job physical effort provided protection against CHD. More than 50 years of subsequent cross-sectional and longitudinal research confirms that increased physical activity confers a protective effect against CHD.

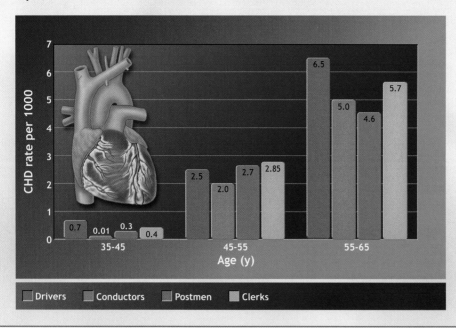

Coronary heart disease (CHD) incidence per 1000 persons for drivers, conductors, postmen, and clerks. Note that within each age and job classification, the most-active workers (conductors and postmen) exhibit the lowest CHD incidence.

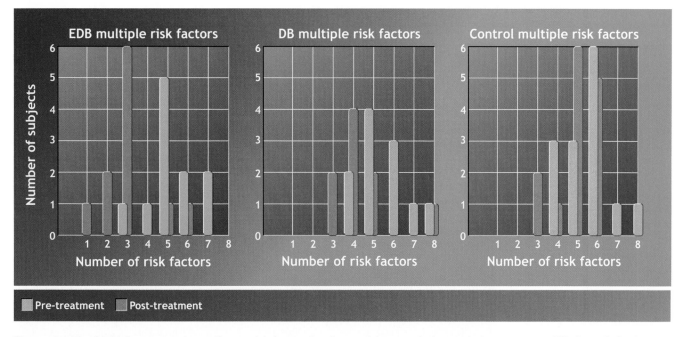

Figure 31.29 Multiple coronary heart disease risk factors for obese adolescents before and after treatment. *DB,* diet + behavior change group; *EDB,* exercise + diet + behavior change group. (From Becque DB, et al. Coronary risk incidence of obese adolescents: reduction by exercise plus diet intervention. Pediatrics 1988;81:605.)

ponents. The variables used for SCORE include age, gender, total cholesterol, systolic blood pressure, and smoking status.

FIGURE 31.30 presents a popular risk inventory developed by the AHA. To determine risk profile, review each risk factor and accompanying numerical value that best describes a person's status. Find the applicable box and circle the number in it. For example, a 19-year-old person circles the number 1 in the box labeled 10 to 20 years. After checking all the rows, add the circled numbers. The total number of points represents the risk score; see the table in the footnote for relative risk category.

Summary

1. CHD represents the most prevalent cause of death in the Western world. Its pathogenesis involves degenerative changes in the inner lining of the arterial wall that progressively occlude blood vessels.

2. Major risk CHD factors include age and gender, blood lipid abnormalities, hypertension, cigarette smoking, obesity, physical inactivity, diet, family history, and ECG abnormalities during rest and exercise. Prudent treatment attempts to eliminate or reduce "modifiable" CHD risk factors.

3. A serum cholesterol level of 200 mg · dL^{-1} or lower is desirable, although experts recommend lower values to achieve the lowest CHD risk.

4. Treatment of elevated cholesterol should begin early in life because of a strong association between serum cholesterol level as a young adult and cardiovascular disease in middle age.

5. The distribution of HDL-C and LDL-C provides a more powerful predictor of heart disease risk than total serum cholesterol concentration alone.

6. LDL-C upon oxidation participates in atherosclerosis by stimulating monocyte–macrophage infiltration and lipoprotein deposition.

7. HDL-C facilitates reverse cholesterol transport by removing surplus cholesterol from peripheral tissues (including arterial walls) for transport to the liver for bile synthesis and excretion via the small intestine.

8. Favorable alterations in HDL-C occur in sedentary men and women of all ages who regularly participate in moderate to intense aerobic exercise.

9. A high level of homocysteine exerts a powerful independent risk for vascular disease.

10. Dietary fiber exerts a dual role to prevent hyperinsulinemia by decreasing circulating insulin levels directly and thwarting obesity with its associated insulin resistance.

11. Cigarette smokers experience almost twice the risk of death from heart disease as nonsmokers. One mechanism for risk involves the adverse effects of smoking on lipoprotein levels.

12. Sedentary men and women face approximately

Age: Men
0 pts: <35 y
1 pt: 35 to 39 y
2 pts: 40 to 48 y
3 pts: 49 to 53 y
4 pts: 54+

☐

Smoking
1 pt: I am a smoker

☐

Age: Women
0 pts: <42 y
1 pt: 42 to 44 y
2 pts: 45 to 54 y
3 pts: 55 to 73 y
4 pts: 73+

☐

Diabetes
1 pt: Male diabetic
2 pts: Female diabetic

☐

Family History
2 pts: My family has a
       history of heart
       disease or heart
       attacks before
       age 60

☐

Total Cholesterol Level
0 pts: <240 mg · dL^{-1}
1 pt: 240 to 315 mg · dL^{-1}
2 pts: >315 mg · dL^{-1}

☐

Inactive Lifestyle
1 pt: I rarely exercise
       or do anything
       physically
       demanding

☐

HDL (Good Cholesterol) Level
0 pts: 39 to 59 mg · dL^{-1}
1 pt: 30 to 38 mg · dL^{-1}
2 pts: Under 30 mg · dL^{-1}
-1 pt: Over 60 mg · dL^{-1}

☐

Body Weight
1 pt: I am ≥20 pounds
       over ideal weight

☐

Blood Pressure (BP)
I do not take BP medication.
My BP is: (use top or higher BP number)
0 pts: <140 mm Hg
1 pt: 140 to 170 mm Hg
2 pts: >140 to 170 mm Hg
          or
1 pt: I am currently taking BP medication

☐

TOTAL POINTS = ☐

If you scored 4 points or more, you could be at above average risk for a first heart attack compared to the general adult population. The more points you score, the greater your risk.

If you have already had a heart attack or have heart disease, your heart attack risk is significantly higher. Your doctor may perform additional tests to assess your risk for heart disease. Only your doctor can evaluate your risk and recommend treatment plans to reduce your risk. If you don't know your cholesterol level or blood pressure, ask your doctor if your levels should be checked.

Figure 31.30 American Heart Association's checklist to evaluate coronary heart disease risk.

twice the risk of a fatal heart attack than more physically active counterparts. Maintenance of a physically active lifestyle throughout life lowers CHD risk factors and disease occurrence.

13. The interaction of CHD risk factors magnifies their individual effects on overall disease risk.

14. Nutrition, exercise, and weight control programs favorably alter CHD risk factors and usually improve an individual's health outlook.

References are available on the Student CD and online at *http://connection.lww.com/mkk6e.*

Clinical Exercise Physiology for Cancer, Cardiovascular, and Pulmonary Rehabilitation

32

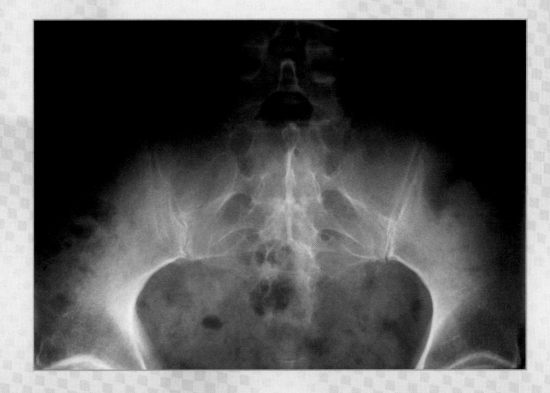

CHAPTER OBJECTIVES

- Discuss the role of the exercise physiologist/ health–fitness professional in the clinical setting

- Summarize the exercise benefits for cancer prevention and rehabilitation and make exercise recommendations for persons with cancer

- Review the potential benefits of aerobic exercise for moderate hypertension

- Discuss the role of regular exercise in congestive heart failure

- Discuss the general components in the clinical assessment for cardiac disease

- Summarize noninvasive and invasive procedures to identify specific cardiac dysfunctions

- Describe three phases of cardiac rehabilitation, including objectives, required levels of supervision, and prudent physical activities

- Give three important reasons to include graded exercise stress testing for coronary heart disease screening

- Describe objective indicators of coronary heart disease during an exercise stress test

- List 10 reasons to stop a stress test

- Define the following terms for stress test results: *true positive, false positive, true negative,* and *false negative*

- Outline an approach to individualize an exercise prescription

- Discuss the heart transplant patient's responses and adaptations to regular aerobic exercise and resistance training

- Categorize and describe five diseases that affect the pulmonary system

- Outline two proposed mechanisms for exercise-induced bronchospasm and factors that modify its severity

- Describe the different neuromuscular diseases and the role that physical activity plays in their rehabilitation

- Describe the major classifications of cognitive/emotional diseases and the potential for exercise as adjunctive therapy

THE EXERCISE PHYSIOLOGIST IN THE CLINICAL SETTING

Regular exercise participation is widespread and increasing in the global prevention of disease, in rehabilitation from injury, and as adjunctive therapy for medically related disorders.

Attention now focuses on understanding the mechanisms by which exercise improves health, physical fitness, and rehabilitation potential of patients challenged by chronic disease and disability. TABLE 32.1 lists several clinical applications of exercise interventions for some of the medical/health conditions that exercise influences positively.

The clinical exercise physiologist becomes an integral component in the team approach to health and total patient care. In the clinical setting, the exercise physiologist focuses primarily on restoring patient mobility and functional capacity while working closely with physical therapists, occupational therapists, and physicians. The exercise physiologist has an expanded role in clinical practice because of fundamental relationships among measures of functional capacity, physical fitness, and overall good health. The World Health Organization (WHO) defines health as *"a state of complete physical, mental and social well-being, not merely the absence of disease and infirmity."* This definition considers good health the ability to complete physical tasks successfully and maintain functional independence. Functional capacity measurement as depicted in the unnumbered figure provides an objective assessment of a person's current status and quantifies changes from diverse strategies to improve fitness, health, and well-being.

Vital Link Between Sports Medicine and Exercise Physiology

One traditional view of sports medicine concerns rehabilitating athletes from sports-related injuries. In its broader context, **sports medicine** relates to scientific and medical aspects of physical activity, physical fitness, health, and sports performance. Indeed, the WHO defines physical fitness as the ability to perform muscular work satisfactorily. This definition encompasses one's capacity to perform physical activity at work, at home, or on the athletic field. Sports medicine thus becomes closely linked to clinical exercise physiology because the sports medicine profession encompasses a broad spectrum of individuals. Patients with low functional capacity recover-

---

TABLE 32.1 ■ **CLINICAL AREAS AND CORRESPONDING DISEASES AND DISORDERS WHERE REGULAR PHYSICAL ACTIVITY APPLIES**

CLINICAL AREAS	DISEASES AND DISORDERS
Cardiovascular Diseases and Disorders	Ischemia; Chronic heart failure; Dyslipidemia; Cardiomyopathies; Cardiac valvular disease; Heart transplantation; Congenital
Pulmonary Diseases and Disorders	Chronic obstructive pulmonary disease; Cystic fibrosis; Asthma and exercise-induced asthma
Neuromuscular Diseases and Disorders	Stroke; Multiple sclerosis; Parkinson's diseases; Alzheimer's disease; Polio; Cerebral palsy
Metabolic Diseases and Disorders	Obesity (adult and pediatric); Diabetes; Renal disease; Menstrual dysfunction
Immunologic and Hematologic Diseases and Disorders	Cancer; Breast cancer; Immune deficiency; Allergies; Sickle cell disease; HIV and AIDS
Orthopedic Diseases and Disorders	Osteoporosis; Osteoarthritis and rheumatoid arthritis; Back pain; Sports injuries
Aging	Sarcopenia
Cognitive and Emotional Disorders	Anxiety and stress disorders; Mental retardation; Depression

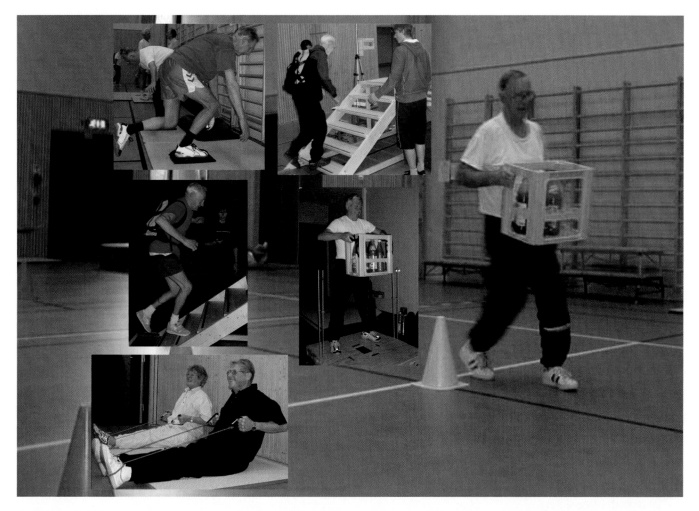

Exercise physiologists work in cooperation with local community groups to determine the effects of arm and leg strength training combined with static and dynamic balance and kinesthetic training in a large cohort of men and women above age 65. The ongoing studies include force platform analysis and EMG with load and photo cells to quantify balance and kinesthetic awareness and dynamic strength assessments using isoinertial lifting tasks. Photos courtesy of Hilde Lohne Seiler, Agder University College, Faculty of Health and Sport, Kristiansand, Norway.

ing from injury, disease, and medical interventions comprise one end of the continuum; the other extreme encompasses healthy, able-bodied and disabled athletes with well-developed levels of physical fitness. Carefully prescribed physical activity contributes to overall good health and quality of life (TABLE 32.2).[19,79] To this end, exercise physiologists assume an important clinical role in sports medicine by evaluating and reconditioning individuals with acute and chronic diseases and physical disabilities.

TRAINING AND CERTIFICATION PROGRAMS FOR PROFESSIONAL EXERCISE PHYSIOLOGISTS

During the past 30 years, regular exercise has gained widespread acceptance as an integral part of rehabilitative programs of care and health maintenance for a growing list of chronic diseases and disabling conditions. Likewise, expanding public interest in exercise for health promotion has stimulated a parallel need to certify qualified professionals

to provide sound advice and supervision regarding physical activities for preventive and rehabilitative purposes. In 1975, the American College of Sports Medicine (ACSM; www.acsm.org) initiated the first ACSM Clinical Track certification program with a Health/Fitness Track begun in the early 1980s. More than 20,000 certificates have been awarded since 1975; the ACSM continues to be the preeminent organization to offer certification programs, newsletters, and continuing education credits (CEUs or CECs) to support the professional growth of health and fitness professionals. The sports nutrition and body composition certifications offered by the International Society of Sports Nutrition (ISSN;www.sportsnutritionsociety.org) incorporate important concepts about exercise, fitness, and health; natural historical and contemporary ties exist between sports nutrition and exercise physiology.

The ACSM certifications consist of two different tracks: (1) *Health/Fitness Track* for those who want to provide leadership in fitness assessment and exercise programming of a preventive nature for apparently healthy individuals and for controlling diseases in corporate, commercial, and community

TABLE 32.2 ■ HEALTH BENEFITS OF REGULAR PHYSICAL ACTIVITY[a]

PHYSICAL ACTIVITY BENEFIT	SURETY RATING	PHYSICAL ACTIVITY BENEFIT	SURETY RATING
FITNESS OF BODY		**CIGARETTE SMOKING**	
Improves heart and lung function	****	Improves success in quitting	**
Improves muscular strength/size	****	**DIABETES**	
CARDIOVASCULAR DISEASE		Prevention of type 2	****
Coronary heart disease prevention	****	Treatment of type 2	***
Regression of atherosclerosis	**	Treatment of type 1	*
Treatment of heart disease	***	Improvement in diabetic's life quality	***
Prevention of stroke	**	**INFECTION AND IMMUNITY**	
CANCER		Prevention of the common cold	**
Prevention of colon cancer	****	Improves overall immunity	**
Prevention of breast cancer	**	Slows progression of HIV to AIDS	*
Prevention of uterine cancer	**	Improves life quality of HIV-infected persons	****
Prevention of prostate cancer	**	**ARTHRITIS**	
Prevention of other cancer	*	Prevention of arthritis	*
Treatment of cancer	*	Treatment/cure of arthritis	*
OSTEOPOROSIS		Improvement life quality/fitness	****
Helps increase bone mass and density	****	**HIGH BLOOD PRESSURE**	
Prevention of osteoporosis	***	Prevention of high blood pressure	****
Treatment of osteoporosis	**	Treatment of high blood pressure	****
BLOOD CHOLESTEROL/LIPOPROTEINS		**ASTHMA**	
Lowers blood total cholesterol	*	Prevention/treatment of asthma	*
Lowers LDL cholesterol	*	Improvement in asthmatic's life quality	***
Lowers triacylglycerols	***	**SLEEP**	
Raises HDL cholesterol	***	Improvement in sleep quality	***
LOW BACK PAIN		**PSYCHOLOGIC WELL-BEING**	
Prevention of low back pain	**	Elevation in mood	****
Treatment of low back pain	**	Buffers effects of mental stress	***
NUTRITION AND DIET QUALITY		Alleviates/prevents depression	****
Improvement in diet quality	**	Anxiety reduction	****
Increase in total energy intake	***	Improves self-esteem	****
WEIGHT MANAGEMENT		**SPECIAL ISSUES FOR WOMEN**	
Prevention of weight gain	****	Improves total body fitness	****
Treatment of obesity	**	Improves fitness while pregnant	****
Helps maintain weight loss	***	Improves birthing experience	**
CHILDREN AND YOUTH		Improves health of fetus	**
Prevention of obesity	***	Improves health during menopause	***
Controls disease risk factors	***		
Reduction of unhealthy habits	**		
Improves odds of adult activity	**		
ELDERLY AND THE AGING PROCESS			
Improvement in physical fitness	****		
Counters loss in heart/lung fitness	**		
Counters loss of muscle	***		
Counters gain in fat	***		
Improvement in life expectancy	****		
Improvement in life quality	****		

> ****   Strong consensus with little or no conflicting data
> ***   Most data supportive, but more research required for clarification
> **   Some supportive data, but much more research needed
> *   Little or no data to support

[a]Based on a total physical fitness program that includes physical activity to improve aerobic and musculoskeletal fitness. From Newman CC. The human body. ACSM's Health Fitness J 1998;2(3):30.

settings and (2) *Clinical Track* for professionals who work with groups at high risk or with existing disease in addition to apparently healthy individuals. The accompanying *inset table* on the facing page shows the different levels of certification within each track.

Certification at a given level requires a knowledge and skill base commensurate with that specific certification. Additionally, each level has a minimum requirement for experience, level of education, or other ACSM certifications.

Certification programs continually undergo review and revision to ensure the highest level of professionalism. Over 400 groups and organizations offer different types of "certifications" for interested individuals, some without undergraduate degree requirements or some requiring a short examination or "experience" in place of core content. These so-called certifications, without approved standards and exclusions, confuse the public about the level of competence or care provided by a "certified" exercise professional. TABLE 32.3 lists nine organ-

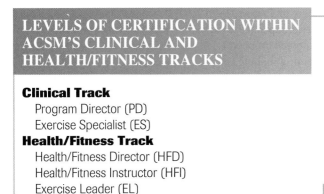

LEVELS OF CERTIFICATION WITHIN ACSM'S CLINICAL AND HEALTH/FITNESS TRACKS

Clinical Track
    Program Director (PD)
    Exercise Specialist (ES)
Health/Fitness Track
    Health/Fitness Director (HFD)
    Health/Fitness Instructor (HFI)
    Exercise Leader (EL)

izations that offer related training and/or certification programs that deal with personal training.

Currently, no universally recognized certification, licensure, or accreditation exists to become a "professional exercise physiologist" except that offered by the American Society of Exercise Physiologists (ASEP; www.asep.org/index.htm). This organization represents and promotes the *profession* of exercise physiology. ASEP has modeled its exercise physiologist licensure program around successful unified health care professionals such as nurses, dietitians, physical therapists, and occupational therapists. These organizations all have clearly defined standards of professional practice, a code of ethics, a scope of practice, accred-

ited academic program guidelines, and a recognized Board Certified Examination.

CLINICAL APPLICATIONS OF EXERCISE PHYSIOLOGY TO ONCOLOGY, CARDIOVASCULAR DISEASES, PULMONARY DISEASES, NEUROMUSCULAR DISEASES, RENAL DISEASE, AND COGNITIVE/EMOTIONAL DISEASES AND DISORDERS

The following sections present clinical applications of exercise physiology for the major areas of oncology, cardiovascular diseases, pulmonary system disabilities, neuromuscular diseases and disorders, renal disease, and psychologic disorders. We focus on these disabilities because they currently receive the greatest involvement from the clinical exercise physiologist.

ONCOLOGY

Cancer represents a group of diseases collectively characterized by uncontrolled growth of abnormal cells. More than 100 different types of cancers exist, mostly in adults. **Carcinomas** develop from epithelial cells that line the surface of the body, glands, and internal organs. They account for 80 to 90% of all cancers that include prostate, colon, lung, cervical, and breast cancer. Cancers also can arise from cells of the blood

---

TABLE 32.3 ■ ORGANIZATIONS THAT OFFER TRAINING/CERTIFICATION PROGRAMS RELATED TO PHYSICAL ACTIVITY

ORGANIZATION	AREAS OF SPECIALIZATION AND CERTIFICATION
Aerobics and Fitness Association of America (AFAA) www.afaa.com	Aerobics Fitness Practitioner, Primary Aerobics Instructor, Personal Trainer & Fitness Counselor, Step Reebok Certification, Weight Room/Resistance Training Certification, Emergency Response Certification
American College of Sports Medicine (ACSM) www.acsm.org	Exercise Leader, Health/Fitness Instructor, Exercise Test Technologist, Health/Fitness Director, Exercise Specialist, Program Director
American Council on Exercise (ACE) www.acefitness.com	Group Fitness Instructor, Personal Trainer, Lifestyle & Weight Management Consultant
Canadian Personal Trainers Network (CPTN) www.cptn.com	CPTN/OFC Certified Personal Trainer, CPTN Certified Specialty Personal Trainer, CPTN/OFC Assessor of Personal Trainers, CPTN/OFC Course Conductor for Personal Trainers
Canadian Society for Exercise Physiology www.csep.ca	CFC-Certified Fitness Consultant, PFLC-Professional Fitness and Lifestyle Consultant, AFAC-Accredited Fitness Appraisal Center
Cooper Institute for Aerobics Research www.cooperinst.org	Certifications in Physical Fitness Specialist, Master Fitness Specialist, Biomechanics of Resistance Training Specialty, Providing Dietary Guidance: Nutrition Specialty, Fitness Specialist for Older Adults Specialty, Special Populations Specialty, Martial Arts Specialist, Group Exercise Leadership, Indoor Cycling Specialty, Aquatics Specialty, Health Promotion Director, Developing Lifestyle Physical Activity Programs, Physical Fitness Specialist, Master Fitness Specialist
National Academy of Sports Medicine (NASM) www.nasm.org	Certified Personal Trainer (NASM-CPT), Performance Enhancement Specialist (NASM-PES)
National Strength & Conditioning Association (NSCA) www.ncsa.com	Certified Strength and Conditioning Specialist (CSCS), Certified Personal Trainer (NSCA-CPT)
UCLA Certificate Program in Fitness Instruction www.uclaextension.edu/	Exercise and Fitness, Exercise Science and Nutrition, Continuing Education for Fitness Professionals

(**leukemias**), the immune system (**lymphomas**), and connective tissues such as bones, tendons, cartilage, fat, and muscle (**sarcomas**).

The current population of more than eight million cancer survivors (many initially diagnosed in the 1970s and 1980s) illustrates the ongoing need for rehabilitative and maintenance options in this expanding area of medicine. The most serious outcomes for current cancer patients and survivors include loss of body mass and functional status. Depressed functional status includes difficulty walking (even short distances) and serious fatigue that limits completion of simple household chores. Approximately 75% of cancer survivors report extreme fatigue during and following radiotherapy or chemotherapy treatment. These decrements are accompanied by weight loss, decreased muscular strength, and suboptimal cardiovascular endurance. Maintaining and restoring functional capacity challenges the cancer survivor, even those considered "cured." Sufficient rationale now justifies exercise intervention for cancer patients during and following different treatment modalities.

Cancer Statistics

Cancer has currently replaced heart disease as the top killer of Americans younger than age 85, and approximately one third of the population have some type of cancer (www.cancer.gov/cancerinformation). Highlights from the American Cancer Society's 2004 annual statistical report indicate the following:

- An estimated 1,372,910 new cancer cases and 570,260 cancer deaths are expected in 2005. Five-year survival rates have risen to 74% from 50% in the 1970s.
- Lung cancer remains the biggest killer, projected to claim 163,510 lives in 2005. Smoking accounts for more than 85% of all lung cancer deaths, and smoking tobacco, chewing smokeless tobacco, and regular exposure to environmental tobacco account for one third of all cancer deaths in the United States annually. After lung cancer, prostate and colorectal cancers kill men the most often.[170]
- Prostate cancer will be diagnosed in about 232,000 men in 2005, and it will kill 30,350.
- Breast cancer will be diagnosed in 211,240 women and it will kill 40,410.

Cancer death rates, particularly striking for colon cancer and lung cancer, have declined about 1% per year since 1999 owing to earlier detection, prevention efforts, and better treatments. The biggest reason for the drop in deaths is that fewer persons now smoke—one third of all cancers relate to smoking and another one third to obesity, poor diet, and lack of regular exercise.

In 2005, the nation's leading cancer organizations reported that Americans' risk of getting and dying from cancer continued to decline, and survival rates for many cancers continued to improve. The Annual Report to the Nation on the Status of Cancer, 1975–2001,[92] shows that cancer incidence rates dropped 0.5% per year, while death rates from all cancers combined dropped 1.1% per year from 1993 to 2001. The first ever drop in lung cancer incidence in women, indicating early detection and newer treatments, exerted a significant effect on reduced death rates.

The percentage of patients who survive more than 5 years following cancer diagnosis increased over the past two decades. Death rates from all cancers combined have been decreasing since the early 1990s. Among men, cancer incidence rates have declined for 7 of the top 15 cancer sites: lung, colon, oral cavity, leukemia, stomach, pancreas, and larynx. Incidence rates increased only for melanoma and cancers of the prostate, kidney, and esophagus. Incidence rates decreased for five of the top 15 cancers in women (colon, cervix, pancreas, ovary, and oral cavity). Only breast, thyroid, bladder, and kidney cancer and melanoma rates continue to increase.

TABLE 32.4 summarizes the estimated number of cancer cases and actual cancer deaths in the United States for year 2001. Also included are changes in cancer incidence and mortality from 1950 to 2001 (the latest statistics available) and 5-year relative survival rates for 1995 to 2000 for each of the primary cancer sites.

For men, greater than 10% gains in 5-year survival rates occurred for cancers of the prostate, colon, and kidney, and non-Hodgkin lymphoma, melanoma, and leukemia. Modest gains (5–10%) occurred for cancers of the bladder, stomach, liver, brain, and esophagus. For women, there were gains in survival rates for cancers of the colon, kidney, and breast and for non-Hodgkin lymphoma. Modest gains occurred for bladder, oral cavity, stomach, brain, esophageal, and ovarian cancers and melanoma and leukemia.

Clinical Features

Clinical features of cancer relate to the effects of the three primary cancer treatment modalities: surgery, radiation, and systemic (pharmacologic) therapy (this includes application of proteonomics that use proteins as biomarkers for clinical diagnosis). Surgery represents the oldest and most common modality in cancer therapy. Surgeries include operations to remove high-risk tissues to prevent cancer development, biopsies of abnormal tissue to diagnose cancer, excision of tumors with curative intent, insertion of central venous catheters to support chemotherapy infusions, reconstruction after definitive surgery, and palliative or symptom relief for incurable disease (e.g., partial bowel removal or resection). Radiation treatment occurs in over 50% of all cancer survivors. It involves photon penetration into a specific tissue to produce an ionized (electrically charged) particle that damages DNA to inhibit cell replication and produce cell death. Daily radiation treatment typically lasts between 5 and 8 weeks. Pharmacologic therapy is prescribed for many advanced solid tumors if cancer cells are suspected of metastasizing beyond the primary site and regional lymph nodes. Chemotherapy, endocrine therapy, and bio-

TABLE 32.4 ■ CANCER INCIDENCE AND MORTALITY (1950–2001) AND FIVE-YEAR RELATIVE SURVIVAL RATES (1995-2000)

	ALL RACES		PERCENTAGE CHANGE 1950–2001 (WHITES ONLY)		
PRIMARY SITE	ESTIMATED CANCER CASES, 2001	ACTUAL CANCER DEATHS, 2001	TOTAL U.S. MORTALITY	ANNUAL CHANGE	5-YR RELATIVE SURVIVAL RATES 1995–2000 (%)
Oral cavity, Pharynx	30,100	7,701	−48.9	−1.2	60.9
Esophagus	13,200	12,529	27.2	0.6	15.8
Stomach	21,700	12,319	−84.0	−3.5	21.5
Colon, Rectum	135,400	56,887	−40.9	−1.0	64.1
Liver	16,200	16,952	27.4	0.6	8.0
Pancreas	29,200	29,802	21.2	0.1	4.2
Larynx	10,000	3,797	−25.8	−0.5	67.4
Lung, Bronchus	169,500	156,380	265.4	2.2	15.4
Males	90,700	90,660	197.5	1.6	13.7
Females	78,800	65,720	608.1	4.3	17.4
Skin Melanoma	51,400	41,394	−22.2	−0.3	88.9
Breast (females)	192,200	41,394	−22.2	−0.3	88.9
Cervix uteri (females)	12,900	4,092	−79.5	−3.5	74
Corpus and Uterus (females)	38,300	6,783	−68.0	−2.0	86.1
Ovary (female)	23,400	14,800	3.8	−0.2	44.0
Prostate (male)	198,100	30,719	−8.8	0.3	100.0
Testis (male)	7,200	335	−73.3	−3.0	96.2
Urinary bladder	54,300	12,538	−31.6	−0.9	82.7
Kidney, Renal	30,800	12,372	42.8	0.7	63.9
Brain, Other nervous	17,200	12,609	54.9	0.8	32.2
Thyroid	19,500	1,354	−44.3	−1.5	96.8
Hodgkin lymphoma	7,400	1,323	−75.3	−3.3	85.9
Non-Hodgkin lymphoma	56,200	22,123	140.9	1.7	60.3
Myeloma	14,400	10,795	252.0	1.9	31.9
Leukemia	31,500	21,451	7.9	−0.2	47.8
Childhood (0–14 y)	8,600	1,494	−70.0	−2,8	80.1
All Sites	1,268,000	5553,760	−1.5	0.1	65.5

From: National Cancer Institute: SEER Cancer Statistics Review, 1975–2001.

logic therapy represent the three major types of systemic therapy. TABLE 32.5 presents common clinical symptoms, effects, and outcome from surgery, radiation therapy, and systemic therapy interventions.

Cancer Rehabilitation Through Exercise

Regular physical activity helps cancer patients recuperate and return to a normal lifestyle with greater independence and functional capacity. For most cancer survivors, loss of body mass and decreased energy level and functional status are the most serious outcomes, particularly following surgery and during chemotherapy and radiation therapy.[27,43,63,132,179] Loss of functional status includes difficulty walking more than one block and chronic fatigue that limits completion of routine household chores. Approximately 75% of cancer survivors report extreme fatigue during radiation therapy or chemotherapy, probably from weight loss and decreased muscular strength and cardiovascular endurance.[197] Home-based exercise regimens reduce feelings of fatigue[180,181] and enhance life quality and other biosocial outcomes following cancer diagnosis.[38] Maintaining and restoring function presents challenges to the cancer survivor. Evidence justifies exercise intervention for breast cancer survivors,[82,132,163,182,208] and nutrition intervention plus regular exercise reduces risk of contracting additional cancers.[154,172,196,201]

TABLE 32.6 lists 10 general preventive and intervention goals for patients who face sustained periods of inactivity, disuse, and bed rest. *The overall goal of the health-care team is to rehabilitate the patient to a level of function that allows return to work and pursuit of normal recreational activities.* FIGURE 32.1 shows the effects of a 6-week exercise rehabilitation program of treadmill walking weekdays at 80% of peak heart rate during a stress test for five cancer patients suffering severe fatigue. During the first 3 weeks, each patient walked five intervals of 3 minutes with 3 minutes of

TABLE 32.5 ■ CANCER THERAPIES AND THEIR COMPLICATIONS

TYPE OF TREATMENT	DESCRIPTION AND EFFECTS/OUTCOME
Surgery	**Lung:** reduced lung capacity, dyspnea, deconditioning **Neck:** reduced range of motion, muscle weakness, occasional cranial nerve palsy **Pelvic region:** urinary incontinence, erectile dysfunction, deconditioning **Abdomen:** deconditioning, diarrhea **Limb amputation:** chronic pain, deconditioning
Radiation Therapy	**Skin:** redness, pain, dryness, peeling, sloughing, reduced elasticity **Brain:** nausea, vomiting, fatigue, memory loss **Thorax:** some degree of irreversible lung fibrosis, heart may receive radiation causing pericardial inflammation or fibrosis, premature atherosclerosis, cardiomyopathy **Abdomen:** vomiting, diarrhea **Pelvis:** diarrhea, pelvic pain, bladder scarring, occasional incontinence, sexual dysfunction **Joints:** connective tissue and joint capsule fibrosis; possible decreased range of motion
Systemic Therapy	**Chemotherapies** [Depending on type and amount]: extreme fatigue, anorexia, nausea, anemia, neutropenia, muscle pain, sensory and motor peripheral neuropathy, ataxia, anemia, vomiting, loss of muscle mass, deconditioning, infection **Endocrine Therapies** [Depending on type and amount]: fat redistribution (truncal and facial obesity), proximal muscle weakness, osteoporosis, edema, infection, weight gain, extreme fatigue, hot flashes, loss of muscle mass **Biologic Therapies** [Depending on type and amount]: Fevers or allergic reactions, chills, fever, headache, extreme fatigue, low blood pressure, skin rash, anemia

From Courneya KS, et al. In Myers J (Ed). ACSM's resource manual for clinical exercise physiology for special populations. Baltimore: Lippincott Williams & Wilkins, 2002.

active recovery. Exercise duration increased weekly, with the number of exercise intervals reduced until the patient could complete one continuous 30- to 35-minute bout during week 6. Submaximal exercise heart rate and blood lactate concentration decreased during exercise (Fig. 32.1A), while walking speed and distance and maximal performance on the stress test increased (Fig. 32.1B). All subjects increased daily physical activity level without substantial limitations and each reported increased daily vigor. This clinical investigation did not meet the rigors of experimental research design (e.g., it lacked nonexercise control patients); nevertheless, the results highlight the positive potential of regular exercise for the physical and emotional rehabilitation of cancer patients.

Protective Effects of Exercise on Cancer Occurrance

Firm epidemiologic evidence shows an inverse relation between amount of occupational or leisure-time physical activity and reduction in all-cause cancer risk. For example, one review concludes "the magnitude of the protective effect of physical activity on estrogen-dependent cancer warrants including low-to-moderate exercise as a prudent preventive strategy."[107] Other large-scale, community-based studies of colorectal and prostatic hyperplasia indicate that increased physical activity reduces cancer risk and mortality.[87,115,124,125,159] A study of nearly 122,000 women found that exercising at least 1 hour daily reduced breast cancer risk by 20%.[172] The benefits may differ depending on menopausal status, with a greater risk reduction for postmenopausal women.[61] The proportion of men at high risk for colon cancer would decrease considerably if men eliminated the modifiable risk factors of physical inactivity and excessive red meat consumption, obesity,

TABLE 32.6 ■ TEN GENERAL TREATMENT GOALS OF THE CLINICAL EXERCISE PHYSIOLOGIST FOR PATIENTS WITH DECONDITIONING, IMMOBILITY, OR DISUSE SYNDROMES

1. Improve overall functional status
2. Improve active motion for nonrestrictive segments and joints
3. Prevent loss of flexibility by active motion and passive movements
4. Stimulate peripheral and central circulation through active motion exercise based on current functional level
5. Increase ventilatory function with systematic breathing exercises
6. Prevent thrombosis through physical activities
7. Prevent loss of motor control and muscle strength and endurance with resistance exercises
8. Reduce rate of bone loss through weight-bearing aerobic and muscle-strengthening exercises
9. Through active aerobic and resistance exercise, slow the loss of fat-free body mass and subsequent reduction of BMR that accompanies deconditioning
10. Monitor signs of increased fatigue or weakness, lethargy, dyspnea, pallor, dizziness, claudication, or cramping during or following exercise

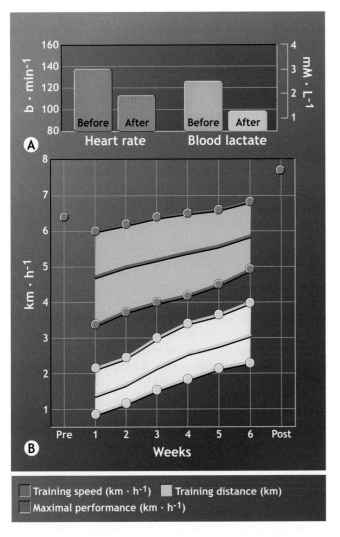

Figure 32.1 A. Reduction in heart rate and blood lactate concentration during submaximal walking at 5 km · h⁻¹ following 6 weeks of exercise rehabilitation in five cancer patients suffering severe fatigue. **B.** Weekly changes in training speed (km · h⁻¹) and daily distance walked (km) and pre- and posttraining maximal exercise performance. (From Dimeo F, et al. Aerobic exercise as therapy for cancer fatigue. Med Sci Sports Exerc 1998;30:475.)

alcohol consumption, cigarette smoking, and low folic acid intake.[160]

Several hypotheses explain how exercise reduces cancer risk. The mechanism for breast cancer risk reduction may involve the lowering effect of exercise on estrogen that stimulates breast cell growth. Regular physical activity also exerts the following effects that thwart cancerous tumor formation:

- Lowers circulating levels of blood glucose and insulin
- Increases corticosteroid hormones
- Increases antiinflammatory cytokines
- Augments insulin-receptor expression in cancer-fighting T cells
- Promotes interferon production
- Stimulates glycogen synthetase

- Enhances leukocyte function
- Improves ascorbic acid metabolism
- Exerts beneficial effects on provirus or oncogene activation

Exercise Prescription and Cancer

Research evidence from exercising animals, former athletes, persons in active occupations, and those with active recreational lifestyles justifies an important role for physical activity in cancer rehabilitation. Less certainty exists regarding the proper exercise prescription for patients, and little research has addressed the timing of exercise relative to the various phases of cancer treatment. Thus, determining the best time to initiate exercise intervention in the recovery process remains problematic, but results have been encouraging. Thirty-five stomach cancer patients were placed in an exercise or control group immediately following curative surgery.[137] From postoperative day 2, patients performed arm and leg ergometer exercise twice daily, 5 days weekly for 14 days at 60% of maximal heart rate. The early exercise intervention increased natural killer cell cytotoxic activity in the exercise group compared with the control group. No information exists regarding the proper dose of exercise or corresponding response of specific cancers to exercise intervention among patients of different ages. In light of limited information, exercise prescription recommendations for cancer rehabilitation generally include symptom-limited, progressive, and individualized physical activities. Ambulation of any kind as soon as practical becomes important for the most sedentary and deconditioned patients. *Emphasis should focus on intervals of low-to-moderate aerobic activity performed several times daily rather than one relatively strenuous bout of continuous exercise.* A dose–response relationship seems to emerge between increased physical activity and improved health and functional capacity.[82] Most sedentary patients derive clinically significant benefits by accumulating up to 30 minutes of daily walking (or equivalent energy expenditure in other activities). Health benefits accrue whether activity takes the form of structured exercise, home-based programs, or sport, household, occupational, or recreational activities.

Cancer patients initially receive a symptom-limited, graded exercise test (GXT) on a treadmill or cycle ergometer to form their exercise prescription. Testing procedures remain the same as for healthy individuals except the patient receives greater attention about their sensations of fatigue. Generally, patients should not exercise to maximum. The exercise prescription initially aims to produce ambulation if no specific contraindications exist. The prescription also provides for range-of-motion movements and other exercises to improve muscular strength, augment fat-free body mass (FFM), and improve overall mobility (e.g., submaximal static exercises of the antigravity muscles, deep breathing exercises, and dynamic trunk rotation movements). Exercise progression and intensity are individualized, with initial work:rest ratios of 1:1 increasing to 2:1. Eventually, continuous exercise for up to 15 minutes can replace intermittent exercise bouts. TABLE 32.7 presents special

TABLE 32.7 ■ **SPECIAL PRECAUTIONS FOR TESTING THE FUNCTIONAL CAPACITY OF CANCER PATIENTS**

COMPLICATION	PRECAUTION
Ataxia/dizziness/peripheral sensory neuropathy	Avoid tests that require balance and coordination (treadmill; weights)
Bone pain	Avoid high-impact tests that increase risk of fracture (treadmill; weights)
Low blood count (hemoglobin ≤8.0 g · dL^{-1}; neutrophil count ≤0.5 x 10^9 · L^{-1})	Avoid tests that require high oxygen consumption or high impact (risk of bleeding); ensure proper sterilization of equipment
Dyspnea	Avoid maximal tests
Fever ≥38°C	May indicate systemic infection; avoid exercise testing
Mouth sores/ulcerations	Avoid mouthpieces; use face masks
Low functional status	Avoid exercise testing
Surgical wounds/tenderness	Avoid pressure/trauma to surgical site
Severe nausea/vomiting	Avoid/postpone exercise testing

Modified from Courneya KS, et al., Coping with cancer: can exercise help? Phys Sportsmed 2000;28(5):49.

precautions to consider when testing the functional capacity of cancer patients. TABLE 32.8 presents general aerobic exercise guidelines for otherwise healthy cancer survivors.

Breast Cancer Rehabilitation and Exercise

Carcinoma of the breast, the most common form of cancer in white females aged 40 years and older, causes the greatest number of deaths in women between the ages of 40 and 55 years. In 2001, 192,200 new invasive breast cancer cases were diagnosed (see Table 32.4) and almost 22% of those died. This means that one of every nine females contracts breast cancer at some time during her life with a high rate of reoccurrence.[3] By age 30, the chance of being diagnosed with breast cancer is 1 in 2000; by age 40, the chances increase considerably to 1 in 233 and 1 in 22 by age 60. *Risk factors for breast cancer include family history and/or personal history of cancer, first menstrual period at an early age, menopause at a late age, first child born after age 30 or no childbirth, and high-fat diet.*

Most studies of exercise for cancer patients have demonstrated physiologic and psychologic benefits. Unfortunately, most of this research is limited because it did not involve randomized controlled trials and/or it used small sample sizes. Research with breast cancer patients has mainly used aerobic training rather than resistance exercise as the exercise modality. Recent evidence, however, supports resistance exercise during cancer management as an effective exercise mode to counteract disease and treatment side effects.

In a study from one of our laboratories, 28 patients recovering from breast cancer surgery enrolled in a 10-week program of circuit-resistance training to evaluate the effects of exercise on depression, self-esteem, and anxiety.[183] Patients performed hydraulic resistance exercises in a 14-station aerobic exercise circuit 4 days per week with a self-paced, individualized program adjusted to meet patient needs and fitness levels. FIGURE 32.2 shows that exercisers exhibited a 38% decrease in depression compared with a 13% increase for nonexercising counterparts recovering from breast cancer surgery. The exercisers also

TABLE 32.8 ■ **GENERAL AEROBIC EXERCISE GUIDELINES FOR OTHERWISE HEALTHY CANCER SURVIVORS**

PRESCRIPTION VARIABLE	GUIDELINES
Frequency	At least 3–5 times per week; daily activity may be optimal for deconditioned patients
Intensity	Depends on fitness status and GXT results; usually 50–70% $\dot{V}O_{2peak}$; or 60%–80% HR_{max}; or RPE = 11 to 14
Type (mode)	Large muscle group activity, particularly walking and cycling in some cases
Time (duration)	20 to 30 continuous minutes per session; this goal may have to be achieved through multiple intermittent shorter sessions with adequate rest intervals
Progression	May not always be linear; rather it may be cyclical with periods of regression, depending on treatments, etc.

Modified from Courneya KS, et al. Coping with cancer: can exercise help? Phys Sportsmed 2000;28(5):49.

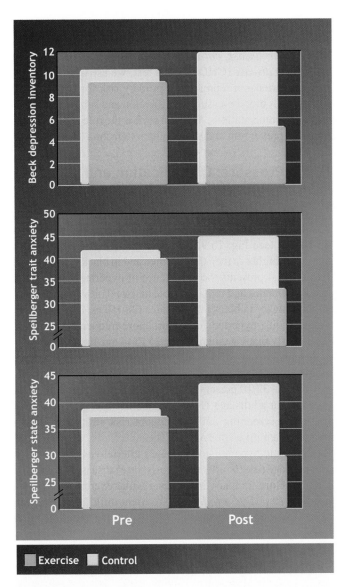

Figure 32.2 Effects of 10 weeks of moderate aerobic exercise on depression *(top)*, trait *(middle)*, and state *(bottom)* anxiety in 28 women recovering from breast cancer surgery. (From Segar ML, et al. The effect of aerobic exercise on self-esteem and depressive and anxiety symptoms among breast cancer survivors. Oncol Nurs Forum 1998;25:107.)

showed a 16% decrease in trait anxiety and 20% reduction in state anxiety whereas increases in both variables occurred for the nonexercising patients. These results demonstrate a potent effect of regular exercise on psychosocial variables during breast cancer rehabilitation. Such findings certainly support structured, moderate exercise in a comprehensive program for breast cancer rehabilitation. Unfortunately, most breast cancer survivors do not meet the physical activity recommendations for the general adult population.[91]

Nutrition and Cancer

Many dietary factors affect cancer risk; this includes type of food, its preparation, portion sizes, diversity, and overall energy balance. Diets with a high proportion of fruits, vegetables, grains, and beans and limited amounts of meat, dairy products, and other high-fat foods may reduce cancer risk.[132,144.188]

Based on a review of scientific evidence, the American Cancer Society's (www.cancer.org) current recommendations agree in principle with the USDA Dietary Guidelines for Americans released January 2005 (www.health.gov/dietaryguidelines/) and dietary recommendations of other agencies that promote healthful behaviors to prevent coronary heart disease, type 2 diabetes, and other diet-related chronic conditions.[30]

CARDIOVASCULAR DISEASE

Chapter 21 examines the effects of regular exercise on cardiovascular function, aerobic capacity, and exercise performance. We examine the prevalence of different diseases of the cardiovascular system, possible causes and diagnosis of the disease, and the specific application of exercise in rehabilitating patients with cardiovascular disease.

Overview and Scope of Cardiovascular Disease

FIGURE 32.3 presents the prevalence of cardiovascular diseases (coronary heart disease, congestive heart failure, stroke, and hypertension) in Americans age 20 and older for

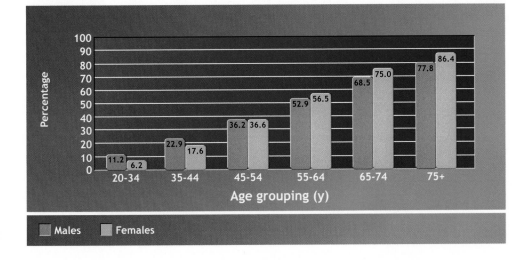

Figure 32.3 Prevalence of cardiovascular diseases (coronary heart disease, congestive heart failure, stroke, and hypertension) in Americans age 20 and older for the period 1999–2002. (From NHANES 1999–2002.)

TABLE 32.9 ■ CARDIAC DISEASES THAT CAUSE FUNCTIONAL IMPAIRMENT

DISEASES AFFECTING THE HEART MUSCLE	DISEASES AFFECTING HEART VALVES	DISEASES AFFECTING THE CARDIAC NERVOUS SYSTEM
CHD	Rheumatic fever	Arrhythmias
Angina	Endocarditis	Tachycardia
Myocardial infarction	Mitral valve	Bradycardia
Pericarditis	prolapse	
Congestive	Congenital	
heart failure	deformations	
Aneurysms		

the period of 1999–2002. Nearly one in four Americans will experience some form of cardiovascular disease in their lifetime.[6] Fortunately, disease and death rates have declined (in males) since the late 1970s and early 1980s. This has occurred partly from aggressive efforts to reduce risk factors through early screening and implementation of heart disease prevention and rehabilitation programs.[67,173,207]

Aerobic exercise programs for cardiac patients consider the specific pathophysiology of the disease, the mechanisms that may limit exercise performance, and individual differences in functional capacity. TABLE 32.9 lists three general categories of heart disease that cause functional impairment. Diseases of the myocardium predominate, particularly with advancing age. Any one of the following terms indicates myocardial disease: *degenerative heart disease* (DHD), *atherosclerotic cardiovascular disease, arteriosclerotic cardiovascular disease, coronary artery disease* (CAD), or *coronary heart disease* (CHD). In this text, we use CHD.

Hypertension represents a primary risk for CHD, so we first discuss blood pressure stratification and subsequent treatment recommendations. We then review the role of regular exercise in preventing and treating hypertension.

Blood Pressure: Classification and Risk Stratification

Hypertension (www.bloodpressure.com) afflicts between 33 and 57% of men and 25 and 60% of women between ages 45 and 74 (see Fig. 15.9). Prevalence increases sharply with age and is higher in men than women and in blacks than whites. FIGURE 32.4 presents the prevalence of hypertension in black and white males and females. Note that total prevalence is only slightly higher in blacks than whites (28.1% vs. 23.2%), yet in young adults, hypertension occurs more frequently in blacks, particularly black women. In the 35 to 44 age range, hypertension occurs in one third as many white women (8.5%) as black women (22.9%).

TABLE 32.10 presents the standard classification of blood pressure for adults age 18 years and older. Recommendations for initial screening and subsequent risk stratification and treatment are given in TABLE 32.11.

Chronic hypertension damages arterial vessels; it serves as a primary risk for arteriosclerosis, heart disease, stroke, and kidney failure. In many instances, regular exercise provides a prudent *first line of defense* to treat mild hypertension (140–159 mm Hg systolic; 90–99 mm Hg diastolic) and

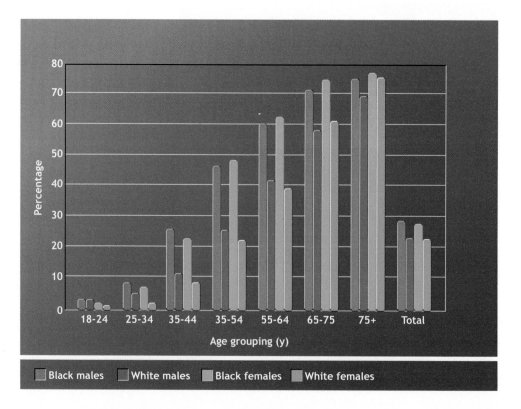

Figure 32.4 Blood pressure differences for blacks versus whites for both males and females or different age groupings. (From Wolz M, et al. Statement from the National High Blood Pressure Education Program: prevalence of hypertension. Am J Hypertens 2000;13:103.)

TABLE 32.10 ■ CLASSIFICATION OF BLOOD PRESSURE FOR ADULTS AGE 18 YEARS AND OLDER

CATEGORY	SYSTOLIC (MM HG)		DIASTOLIC (MM HG)
Optimal	<120	and	<80
Normal	120–129	and	80–84
High normal	130–139	or	85–89
Hypertension			
Stage 1	140–159	or	90–99
Stage 2	160–179	or	100–109
Stage 3	≥180	or	≥110

From the sixth report of the Joint Committee on Prevention, Detection, Evaluation, and Treatment of High Blood Pressure (JNVI), Public Health Service, National Institutes of Health, National Heart, Lung and Blood Institute, NIH Publ. no. 98-4080, Nov 1997. This classification should be used with individuals not taking antihypertensive medication and not acutely ill. When systolic and diastolic blood pressures fall into different categories, the higher category should be used to classify status. For example, 160/92 mm Hg would be stage 2 and 174/120 mm Hg, stage 3.

moderate hypertension (160–179 mm Hg systolic; 100–109 mm Hg diastolic).

Exercise Training and Hypertension

Systolic and diastolic blood pressures decrease by 6 to 10 mm Hg with aerobic exercise training in previously sedentary men and women regardless of age. Beneficial results occur with normotensive and hypertensive subjects during rest and exercise.[42,70,106,206] Regular exercise as preventive therapy also controls the tendency for blood pressure to increase over time in individuals at risk for hypertension.[153]

Patients with mild hypertension respond favorably to exercise training.[4,34,72,105,140] TABLE 32.12 shows that average resting systolic blood pressure in seven middle-aged male patients decreased from 139 to 133 mm Hg following 4 to 6 weeks of interval training. During submaximal exercise, systolic pressure decreased from 173 to 155 mm Hg, while diastolic pressure decreased from 92 to 79 mm Hg. Consequently, training produced approximately a 14% decrease in mean arterial exercise blood pressure. Similar results occurred for an apparently healthy yet borderline hypertensive group of 37 middle-aged men following 6 months of regular aerobic exercise.[31] For hypertensive older men and women, 9 months of low-intensity, aerobic exercise lowered systolic blood pressure by 20 mm Hg and diastolic pressure by 12 mm Hg.[72] FIGURE 32.5 shows changes in resting blood pressure with aerobic training and 1 month of detraining in elderly hypertensive men and women who trained at the lactate threshold three to six times a week for 9 months. Baseline values 3 months prior to training indicate subjects' blood pressures with normal antihypertensive drug therapy. Regular exercise (with continued medication) produced decreases of 15 mm Hg in systolic blood pressure, 11 mm Hg in mean arterial pressure, and 9 mm Hg in diastolic blood pressure. Blood pressure returned to pretraining levels within 1 month for the five subjects who discontinued training. The ACSM's "Position Stand on Physical Activity, Physical Fitness, and Hypertension" can be accessed at www.acsm-msse.org/.

TABLE 32.11 ■ RISK STRATIFICATION AND RECOMMENDED TREATMENT FOR HYPERTENSION

BLOOD PRESSURE STAGES (MM HG)[a]	RISK GROUP A (NO RISK FACTORS; NO TOD[b] OR CCD[c])	RISK GROUP B (ONE RISK FACTOR NOT INCLUDING DIABETES; NO TOD OR CCD)	RISK GROUP C (TOD AND/OR CCD AND/OR DIABETES, WITH OR WITHOUT OTHER RISK FACTORS)
High-normal 130–139/85–89	Lifestyle modification	Lifestyle modification	Drug therapy
Stage 1 140–159/90–99	Lifestyle modification (up to 12 months)	Lifestyle modification (up to 6 months)	Drug therapy
Stages 2 and 3 ≥160/≥100	Drug therapy	Drug therapy	Drug therapy

[a]See Table 32.10.
[b]TOD, target organ disease.
[c]CCD, clinical cardiovascular disease.
A person with diabetes, blood pressure of 142/94 mm Hg, and left ventricular hypertrophy classifies as having stage 1 hypertension with target organ disease (left ventricular hypertrophy) and another major risk factor (diabetes). This patient would be classified as stage 1, risk group C, and recommended for immediate drug therapy.
From the sixth report of the Joint Committee on Prevention, Detection, Evaluation, and Treatment of High Blood Pressure (JNVI), Public Health Service, National Institutes of Health, National Heart, Lung and Blood Institute, NIH Publication no. 98-4080, Nov, 1997.

TABLE 32.12 ■ BLOOD PRESSURE DURING REST AND SUBMAXIMAL EXERCISE BEFORE AND AFTER 4 TO 6 WEEKS OF TRAINING IN SEVEN MIDDLE-AGED CHD PATIENTS

| | REST | | | SUBMAXIMAL EXERCISE | | |
| | AVERAGE VALUE | | | AVERAGE VALUE | | |
MEASURE[a]	BEFORE	AFTER	DIFFERENCE (%)	BEFORE	AFTER	DIFFERENCE (%)
Systolic blood pressure (mm Hg)	139	133	−4.3	173	155	−10.4
Diastolic blood pressure (mm Hg)	78	73	−6.4	92	79	−14.1
Mean blood pressure (mm Hg)	97	92	−5.2	127	109	−14.3

Modified from Clausen JP, et al. Physical training in the management of coronary artery disease. Circulation 1969;40:143.
[a]Intraarterial catheter.

The precise mechanism(s) for how regular exercise lowers blood pressure remains unknown. Contributing factors include the following:

- Reduced sympathetic nervous system activity with training and possible normalization of arteriole

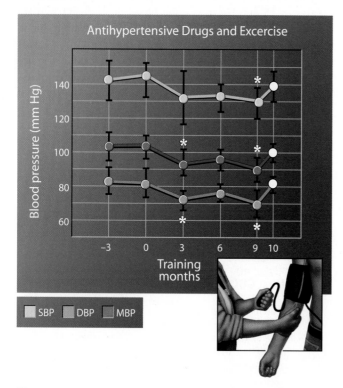

Figure 32.5 Blood pressure changes in elderly subjects who received hypertensive medication following 9 months of exercise training at the lactate threshold and after 1 month of detraining (five subjects). Baseline values 3 months before training (−3) indicate subjects' blood pressures with their normal antihypertensive drug therapy only. SBP, systolic blood pressure; MBP, mean blood pressure; DBP, diastolic blood pressure; *, statistically significant from baseline value. (From Motoyama M, et al. Blood pressure lowering effect of low intensity aerobic training in elderly hypertensive patients. Med Sci Sports Exerc 1998;30:818.)

morphology decrease peripheral resistance to blood flow to lower blood pressure.[2,47,150]

- Altered renal function facilitates the kidneys' elimination of sodium, which subsequently reduces fluid volume and hence blood pressure.

Not all research supports exercise as a way to treat hypertension.[36,60] Even when research shows that regular exercise lowers blood pressure in humans, the studies often have methodologic shortcomings and inadequate design, particularly the lack of appropriate control subjects who have their blood pressure measured but do not exercise. *Despite these limitations, it remains prudent to recommend regular aerobic exercise (and proper diet to induce weight loss when necessary) as a first line of defense to manage borderline hypertension.*[4,80,96,190]

Improved fitness often neutralizes increased mortality associated with elevated blood pressure. Even if regular exercise does not return elevated blood pressure to a normal level, aerobic training confers important independent health benefits. Aerobically fit individuals with hypertension had a 60% lower mortality rate than unfit normotensive peers.[18] More severe elevations in blood pressure require pharmacologic intervention (more than 60 drugs and 30 pill combinations are available for treatment; see Fig. 15.10).

Chronic Resistance Training Effects on Blood Pressure

Despite the relatively large rise in blood pressure during resistance exercise, long-term resistance training does *not* elevate resting blood pressure.[35,49,73,155] In fact, resistance training lessens the typical short-term blood pressure increases during this exercise mode. Trained bodybuilders, for example, show smaller increases in systolic and diastolic blood pressures with resistance exercise than novice bodybuilders and untrained individuals.[49,176] The diminished blood pressure response posttraining becomes most evident when a person exercises at the same absolute load during pretraining and posttraining measurements.[129] Some resistance training protocols lower resting blood pressure,[71,205] but aerobic exercise training (not standard resistance training) confers the greater blood pressure–lowering benefits for hypertensives.[97,98,148] *As a general guideline, resistance training should not serve as the sole exercise mode to lower blood pressure in hypertensive individuals.*

Diseases of the Myocardium

Recent advances in molecular biology have isolated a possible genetic link to CHD. The gene, termed the **atherosclerosis susceptibility (*ATHS*) gene** (www.hgmp.mrc.ac.uk), appears on chromosome 19 near the gene that regulates the receptor that removes low-density lipoprotein cholesterol (LDL-C) from the blood.[194] The *ATHS* gene accounts for nearly 50% of the 13.5 million cases of CHD in the United States.[142] It apparently expresses a set of characteristics—abdominal obesity, low levels of high-density lipoprotein cholesterol (HDL-C), and high levels of LDL-C—that triple a person's risk of myocardial infarction (MI) or heart attack.

Symptoms rarely present in the early stages of CHD. As the disease progresses and coronary arteries narrow, clinical symptoms become evident and advance with increasing severity. The first sign of CHD is often slight angina pain accompanied by decreased functional capacity. This eventually leads to ischemia (reduced blood flow) and possible myocardial tissue necrosis. In severe cases, the person experiences persistent chest pain, anxiety, nausea, vomiting, and dyspnea. Chronic, untreated angina weakens the myocardium and eventually produces heart failure as cardiac output fails to meet metabolic demands. Pulmonary congestion (with a persistent cough) often accompanies heart failure. At this stage, the patient becomes dyspneic even when sitting at rest and can suffer a sudden MI.

CHD pathogenesis progresses in five stages as follows:

1. Injury to the endothelial cell wall of the coronary artery
2. Fibroblastic proliferation of the inner lining (intima) of the artery
3. Further obstruction of blood flow as fat accumulates at the junction of the arterial intima and middle lining
4. Cellular degeneration and subsequent formation of hyalin (a clear, homogeneous substance produced in degeneration) within the arterial intima
5. Calcium deposition at the edges of hyalinated area

The major disorders caused by reduced myocardial blood supply in CHD include angina pectoris, MI, and congestive heart failure.

Angina Pectoris

Chest-related pain called **angina pectoris** *occurs in approximately 30% of initial manifestations of CHD. This temporary but painful condition indicates that coronary blood flow (and thus oxygen supply) momentarily reaches inadequate levels.* Current theory suggests that metabolites within an

TABLE 32.13 ■ COMPARISON OF SYMPTOMS OF ANGINA PECTORIS AND HEARTBURN	
ANGINA PECTORIS	**HEARTBURN**
• Gripping, viselike feelings of pain or pressure behind the breast bone • Pain that radiates to the neck, jaw, back, shoulders, or arms (usually left) • Toothache • Burning indigestion • Shortness of breath • Nausea • Frequent belching	• Frequent feeling of heartburn • Frequent use of antacids to relieve pain • Heartburn that wakes person up at night • Acid or bitter taste in mouth • Burning chest sensation • Discomfort after eating spicy food • Difficulty swallowing

ischemic segment of the heart muscle stimulate myocardial pain receptors. The sensation of angina pectoris includes squeezing, burning, and pressing or choking in the chest region, sensations that often mimic the discomforts of benign heartburn (TABLE 32.13). Anginal pain usually lasts 1 to 3 minutes. Approximately one third of individuals who experience recurring anginal episodes die suddenly from an MI. Chronic stable angina (often called *walk-through* angina) occurs at a predictable level of physical exertion. Drugs that promote coronary artery vasodilation and reduce systemic peripheral vascular resistance (e.g., nitroglycerin) commonly treat this condition. FIGURE 32.6 illustrates the usual pain pattern with an acute episode of angina pectoris. Pain generally appears in the left shoulder along the arm to the elbow or occasionally in the midback region near the left scapula along the spinal cord.

Myocardial Infarction

Between 1999 and 2002, 1.78 million **myocardial infarctions** occurred per year with more than 500,000 fatalities. An MI can result from sudden insufficiency in myocardial blood flow, usually from coronary artery occlusion. A prior clot (thrombus) formed from plaque accumulation in

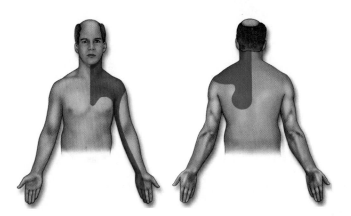

Figure 32.6 Locations for pain generally associated with angina pectoris.

one or more coronary vessels (see Chapter 31) can trigger sudden occlusion. Severe fatigue for several days without specific pain frequently precedes the onset of MI. FIGURE 32.7 shows the varied locations for pain and discomfort that represent early warning of an MI. During the infarction, severe, unrelenting chest pain can persist for more than 1 hour.

Congestive Heart Failure

In **congestive heart failure** (**CHF**, chronic decompensation or heart failure), the heart fails to pump adequately to meet other organ needs. CHF results from one or all of the following:

- Narrowed arteries from CHD that limit myocardial blood supply
- Past MI with accompanying scar tissue (necrosis) that diminishes myocardial pumping efficiency
- Chronic hypertension
- Heart valve disease from past rheumatic fever or other pathology

- Primary disease of the myocardium, called *cardiomyopathy*
- Defects present in the heart at birth (congenital heart disease)
- Infection of heart valves and/or myocardium (endocarditis or myocarditis)

A "failing" heart keeps pumping but inefficiently. Heart failure produces shortness of breath and fatigue upon minimal exertion. As blood flowing from the heart slows, blood returning to the heart through the veins backs up, causing fluid to accumulate in the lungs and edema in legs and ankles. When fluid collects in the lungs, it interferes with breathing and causes shortness of breath, especially when lying supine. CHF also affects the kidneys' disposal of sodium and water, further accentuating edema.

CHF, the only form of heart disease on the increase, afflicts more than 5 million Americans (550,000 new cases diagnosed and 52,828 deaths recorded in 2002; data reported in early 2005). CHF is the most common cause for hospitaliza-

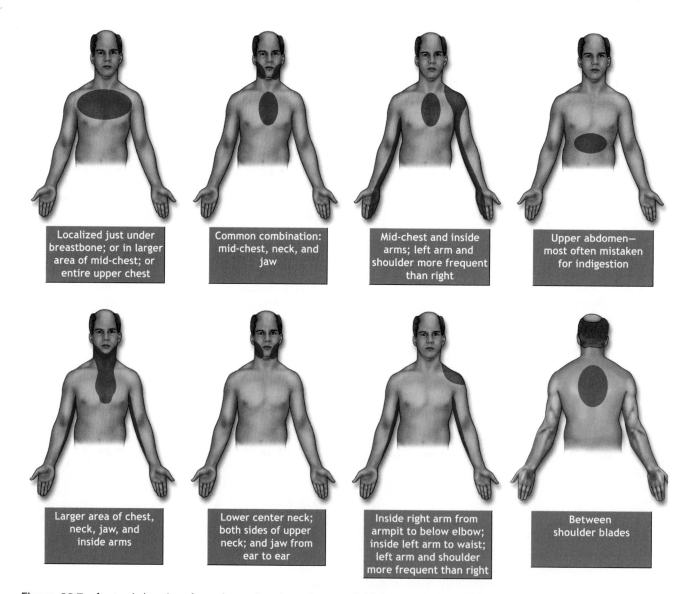

Figure 32.7   Anatomic locations for early warning signs of myocardial infarction. Note the diverse locations for pain.

tion of persons older than age 65. It is responsible for more than 800,000 hospital stays including many repeat visits. FIGURE 32.8 shows the consequences of CHF when the heart fails to pump adequately. The figure illustrates that nearly one third (1.4 million) of CHF patients contract the disease before age 60; 20% of patients die within 1 year of diagnosis, and nearly one half die within 5 years.

CHF usually develops slowly as the heart gradually weakens and performs less effectively. Primary causes of CHF include (1) chronic hypertension, (2) intrinsic myocardial disease, or (3) structural defects (e.g., diseased heart valves). These conditions produce an oversized, misshapen heart with inadequate pump performance reflected by a low resting left ventricular ejection fraction (LVEF)—a marker of life-threatening heart dysfunction—and failure to increase heart rate with exercise.[54,94] Associated risk factors include diabetes, alcoholism, and chronic lung diseases such as emphysema. CHF symptoms produce extreme disability, but symptom intensity frequently bears little relation to disease severity.[8,152] Patients with a low LVEF may not exhibit symptoms, while individuals whose hearts demonstrate normal pump function can experience severe disability. Heart disease and chronic hypertension contribute to disease progression. At the extreme stage, cardiac output from the left and/or right ventricles decreases to an extent that blood accumulates in the abdomen and lungs and sometimes in legs and feet. This stage of CHF produces fatigue, shortness of breath, and eventual flooding of the alveoli with blood, a condition termed *pulmonary congestion.* Impaired blood flow may also damage other organs, particularly kidneys. Nearly 70,000 CHF patients qualify yearly for heart transplantation.

CHF Treatment and Rehabilitation. Before the 1980s, treatment for all stages of CHF advocated rest as the immediate treatment to reduce stress on the compromised cardiovascular system. Until recently, patients routinely received drugs aimed primarily at easing symptoms (e.g., digitalis to increase the heart's pumping function [inotropic effect]). Current recommendations promote a four-drug regimen with two traditional drugs, digitalis and a diuretic (to increase fluid excretion by kidneys), with newer angiotensin-converting enzyme (ACE) inhibitors and β-blockers. These two latter drugs lower CHF death rates because they block hormones believed to promote disease progression. Dramatic improvement has occurred in survival, hospitalization, and symptoms in patients with standard therapy who also received Aldactone (known generically as spironolactone), a relatively inexpensive drug used routinely for heart

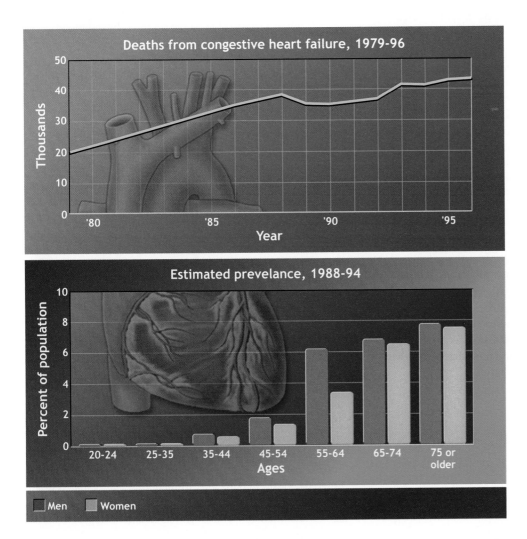

Figure 32.8 Consequences of congestive heart failure (CHF) from impaired pumping ability of either the right or left heart or both. Although the prevalence of and deaths from CHF increase with age, nearly one third (1.4 million) contract the disease before age 60 years. (Sources: National Center for Health Statistics and American Heart Association, 2000.)

failure and hypertension. This drug blocks the fluid-conserving action of aldosterone to a greater extent than ACE inhibitors.[158]

Surgical treatment replaces damaged heart valves or repairs myocardial aneurysms—bulging areas that form on the myocardial wall. Cardiac transplantation represents the extreme treatment of progressive disability from CHF, although the shortage of donor organs persists. For patients awaiting a transplant, electrically powered pump implants placed in the abdomen below the heart mechanically assist ventricular function.

Clinicians have reevaluated the role of regular exercise because many of the functional deteriorations in CHF duplicate those that accompany extreme physical deconditioning. Reduced physical fitness and intrinsic changes in skeletal muscle exacerbate the patient's physical incapacity.[68] Current therapy advocates regular exercise as an effective adjunct in CHF rehabilitation.[74,120]

CHF and Exercise Training. Clinical practice indicates that regular moderate exercise formulated from a symptom-limited GXT and prescribed medications benefits relatively low-risk, stable, compensated patients.[22,45,100,135,168,169,209] These benefits include improvements in functional capacity, exercise tolerance, muscle metabolism, level for dyspnea and ventilatory response to exercise, risk for arrhythmias, quality of life, and shift toward greater dominance of vagal (parasympathetic) tone.

It remains controversial whether the benefits of exercise rehabilitation for CHF link directly to enhanced central circulatory function—either improved myocardial performance per se or disease reversal reflected by reduced heart size.[15,54,74] To a large extent, peripheral adaptations with regular exercise enhance function and symptomatic improvements.

The clinician supervises an exercise program (commencing with medical supervision) for compensated patients with controlled fluid volume status and absence of unstable or exercise-induced ventricular arrhythmias. The GXT provides the basis for the exercise prescription. For patients with marked exercise intolerance, relatively brief exercise intervals afford benefits (2–5 min of light exercise with 1–3 min of recovery). The prescription also includes multiple exercise sessions interspersed throughout the day. Because of the usually abnormal heart-rate response in CHF patients, exercising at between 40 and 60% $\dot{V}O_{2peak}$ provides a more objective standard to establish initial exercise intensity. Alternatively, a rating of perceived exertion (RPE) on the Borg scale of "light" to "somewhat hard" (see Fig. 21.19) and/or 2 on the dyspnea scale ("mild, some difficulty;" see Fig. 32.18) generally proves effective. Supervisory personnel should recognize the six warning symptoms of cardiac decompensation:

1. Dyspnea
2. Hypotension
3. Cough
4. Angina
5. Lightheadedness
6. Arrhythmias

After the patient begins to increase physical activity, exercise duration can increase to 20 to 40 minutes at least three times weekly. Following 6 to 12 weeks of supervised exercise, patients usually can undertake an unsupervised home exercise program.

Aneurysm

Aneurysm describes an abnormal dilation in the wall of an artery, vein, or cardiac chamber. Vascular aneurysms develop when a vessel wall weakens from trauma, congenital vascular disease, infection, or atherosclerosis. Aneurysms are either arterial or venous and classify according to their specific regions of origin (e.g., thoracic aneurysm). Most aneurysms develop without symptoms and often are discovered during a routine x-ray. The most common symptoms include chest pain with a specific palpable, pulsating mass in the chest, abdomen, or lower back.

Heart Valve Diseases

Medical conditions that relate to heart valve abnormalities include:

- **Stenosis**: Narrowing or constriction that prevents heart valves from opening fully; may result from growths, scars, or abnormal calcified deposits
- **Insufficiency** (also called *regurgitation*): Occurs when a heart valve closes improperly and blood moves back into a heart chamber
- **Prolapse**: Occurs when enlarged valve leaflets in the mitral valve bulge backward into the left atrium during ventricular systole

Valvular abnormalities increase the heart's workload, causing it to pump harder to propel blood through a stenosed valve or to maintain cardiac output if blood seeps backward into one of its chambers in diastole. Rheumatic fever, a serious group A streptococcal bacterial infection, causes valvular scarring and heart valve deformity. The most common symptoms include fever and joint pain. Penicillin or other antibiotics treat this inflammatory condition, which usually occurs in children 5 to 15 years old. In 1997, rheumatic fever and rheumatic heart disease afflicted 1.8 million Americans, and in 2002, killed 3579 individuals. From 1992 to 2002, the death rate from rheumatic fever and rheumatic heart disease fell 23.5% and actual deaths declined 39.1%.

Mitral Valve Prolapse. **Mitral valve prolapse (MVP)** occurs in 10% of the population, predominately in females. First described in the 1600s, MVP has been known as irritable heart, soldier's heart, floppy valve syndrome, Barlow's syndrome, and Da Costa's syndrome. MVP diagnoses increased in the 1990s because of its association with endocarditis, atherosclerosis, and muscular dystrophy. MVP probably results from connective tissue abnormalities in the mitral valve leaflets, which deform the valve's shape or structure (enlarged valve leaflets bulge backward into the left atrium during ventricular systole). This valvular "billowing" or "stretchiness" creates a clicking sound identified by stethoscope examination. Regurgitation of blood into the heart's upper chamber occasionally occurs (which can be heard as a murmur). Sixty percent of patients exhibit no symptoms; 40% experience profound fatigue during mild physical activity.

Inflammation Conditions: Endocarditis and Pericarditis

Endocarditis, predominantly of bacterial origin, inflames the cardiac endothelium and damages the tricuspid, aortic, or mitral valves. Patients initially experience musculoskeletal symptoms that include arthritis, low back pain, and general joint weakness. Antibiotic drugs usually treat this disease.

Pericarditis, classified as either acute or chronic (recurring or constrictive pericarditis), presents as inflammation of the heart's outer pericardial lining. Symptoms of acute pericarditis vary; they include chest pain, dyspnea, and increased resting heart rate and body temperature. Over time, the inflammation causes extreme chest pain from fluid accumulation in the pericardial sac that inhibits full myocardial expansion during diastole. The prognosis for acute viral pericarditis remains excellent; chronic pericarditis of bacterial origin represents a more dire condition.

Congenital Malformations

Congenital heart malformations appear in one of every 100 births. They include ventricular or atrial septal defects (hole between the ventricles and atria) and patent ductus arteriosus (shunt caused by an opening between the descending aorta and left pulmonary artery). These defects require surgical repair during childhood.

Cardiac Nervous System Diseases

Cardiac diseases that affect the heart's electrical conduction system include the following: **dysrhythmias (arrhythmias)** that cause the heart to beat too rapidly (**tachycardia**), too slowly (**bradycardia**), or with extra contractions (**ectopic, extrasystole,** or **premature ventricular contractions [PVCs]**) that possibly lead to fibrillation. Dysrhythmias can produce changes in circulatory dynamics that cause hypotension (extremely low blood pressure), heart failure, and shock. They often occur after a stroke induced by increased physical exertion or other stressful conditions.

Sinus tachycardia describes a resting heart rate above $100 \, \mathrm{b} \cdot \mathrm{min}^{-1}$; *bradycardia* describes a resting heart rate below $60 \, \mathrm{b} \cdot \mathrm{min}^{-1}$. Sinus bradycardia occurs frequently in endurance athletes and young adults and generally represents a benign dysrhythmia; it may benefit cardiac function by producing a longer ventricular filling time during the cardiac cycle.

CARDIAC DISEASE ASSESSMENT

Before initiating an exercise intervention program, the healthcare team decides the extent of health screening. This may include a medical history, physical examination, laboratory assessments, and pertinent physiologic testing.

Purpose of Health Screening and Risk Stratification

Optimizing safety during exercise testing and program participation requires health screening and risk stratification. Assessment of specific risk factors and/or symptoms for chronic cardiovascular, pulmonary, and metabolic diseases optimizes safety during exercise testing and program participation. Proper preparticipation screening accomplishes the following:

- Identifies and excludes persons with medical contraindications to exercise
- Identifies persons who require in-depth medical evaluation because of age, symptoms, and/or risk factors
- Identifies persons with clinically significant disease who require medical supervision when exercising

Before beginning an exercise program, the ACSM recommends that age, health status, symptoms, and risk factor information classify individuals into one of three risk strata to ensure their safety (see ACSM Risk Stratification inset below).[5] Proper risk stratification provides a basis to recommend further testing, medical assessment, or diagnostic interventions before exercise participation. "In a Practical Sense," p. 944, provides the **Physical Activity Readiness Questionnaire (Par-Q)** commonly used as a minimal first-pass, preparticipation screening tool.

ACSM RISK STRATIFICATION

Low risk
Men <45 years; women <55 years, asymptomatic with ≤1 risk factor[a,b]

Moderate risk
Men ≥45 years; women ≥55 years, or with ≥2 risk factors[a,b]

High risk
Individuals with ≥1 sign/symptom of cardiovascular or pulmonary disease[c] or known cardiovascular (cardiac, peripheral vascular, or cerebrovascular), pulmonary (obstructive pulmonary disease, asthma, cystic fibrosis), or metabolic (diabetes, thyroid disorder, renal or liver) disease

From Franklin BA, et al. ACSM's guidelines for exercise testing and prescription. 6th ed. Baltimore, Lippincott Williams & Wilkins, 2000.
[a] Risk factors: family history of heart disease; cigarette smoking; hypertension; hypercholesterolemia; impaired fasting glucose; obesity; sedentary lifestyle.
[b] HDL ≥60 mg · dL^{-1} (subtract 1 risk factor from the sum of other risk factors because high HDL decreases CHD risk).
[c] Signs/symptoms of cardiovascular and pulmonary disease: pain, discomfort in chest, neck, jaw, left arm; shortness of breath at rest or with mild exertion; dizziness or syncope; orthopnea or paroxysmal nocturnal dyspnea; ankle edema; tachycardia; intermittent claudication; heart murmur; unusual fatigue or shortness of breath with mild activity.

IN A PRACTICAL SENSE

PAR-Q TO ASSESS READINESS FOR PHYSICAL ACTIVITY

ORIGINAL PAR-Q

Common sense is your best guide in answering these questions. Please read each question carefully and check *yes* or *no* if it applies to you.

The Physical Activity Readiness Questionnaire (Par-Q) has been recommended as *minimal* screening for entry into moderate-intensity exercise programs. Par-Q was designed to identify the small number of adults for whom physical activity might be inappropriate or those who should receive medical advice concerning the most suitable type of activity.

YES ___ NO ___ 1. Has your doctor ever said that you have a heart trouble?

YES ___ NO ___ 2. Do you frequently have pains in your heart and chest?

YES ___ NO ___ 3. Do you often feel faint or have spells of severe dizziness?

YES ___ NO ___ 4. Has a doctor ever said your blood pressure was too high?

YES ___ NO ___ 5. Has your doctor told you that you have a bone or joint problem that has been aggravated by exercise or might be made worse with exercise?

YES ___ NO ___ 6. Is there a good physical reason not mentioned here why you should not follow an activity program even if you wanted to?

YES ___ NO ___ 7. Are you over age 65 and not accustomed to vigorous exercise?

IF YOU ANSWERED YES TO ONE OR MORE QUESTIONS:

If you have not recently done so, consult with your personal physician by telephone or in person BEFORE increasing your physical activity and/or taking a fitness test. Show your doctor a copy of this quiz. After medical evaluation, seek advice from your physician as to your suitability for:

- Unrestricted physical activity, probably on a gradually increasing basis
- Restricted or supervised activity to meet your specific needs, at least on an initial basis; check in your community for special programs or services

IF YOU ANSWERED NO TO ALL QUESTIONS:

If you answered NO honestly to all Par-Q questions, you have reasonable assurance of your present suitability for:

- *A graduated exercise program*—a gradual increase in proper exercise promotes good fitness development while minimizing or eliminating discomfort
- *An exercise test*—simple tests of fitness (such as the Canadian Home Fitness Test) or more complex types may be undertaken if you so desire
- *Postpone exercising*—if you have a temporary minor illness, such as a common cold, postpone any exercise program

rPAR-Q (REVISED 1994)

One limitation of the original Par-Q was that about 20% of potential exercisers failed the test—many of these exclusions were unnecessary because subsequent evaluations showed that the individuals were apparently healthy. The revised Par-Q (rPar-Q) was developed to reduce the number of unnecessary exclusions (false positives). The revision can determine the exercise readiness of apparently healthy middle-aged adults with no more than one major risk factor for coronary heart disease.

YES ___ NO ___ 1. Has your doctor ever said that you have a heart condition and recommended only medically supervised activity?

YES ___ NO ___ 2. Do you have chest pain brought on by physical activity?

YES ___ NO ___ 3. Have you developed chest pain in the past month?

continued on page 945

Continued

YES ___ NO ___ 4. Do you lose your balance because of dizziness, or do you ever lose consciousness?

YES ___ NO ___ 5. Do you have a bone or joint problem that could be worsened by a change in your physical activity?

YES ___ NO ___ 6. Is your doctor currently prescribing drugs (for example, water pills) for high blood pressure or a heart condition?

YES ___ NO ___ 7. Do you know of any other reason why you should not do physical activity?

Note: Postpone testing if you have a temporary illness such as a common cold or are not feeling well.

IF YOU ANSWERED YES TO ONE OR MORE QUESTIONS:

Talk with your doctor by phone or in person BEFORE you start becoming much more physically active or BEFORE you have a fitness appraisal. Tell your doctor about the rPar-Q and which questions you answered YES.

• You may be able to do any activity you want—as long as you start slowly and build up gradually. Or, you may need to restrict your activities to those that are safe for you. Talk with your doctor about the kinds of activities you wish to participate in and follow his or her advice.

• Find out which community programs are safe and helpful for you.

IF YOU ANSWERED NO TO ALL QUESTIONS:

If you answered NO honestly to all rPar-Q questions, you can be reasonably sure that you can:

• Start becoming much more physically active— begin slowly and build up gradually; this is the safest and easiest way to go

• Take part in a fitness appraisal—this is an excellent way to determine your basic fitness so that you can plan the best way for you to live actively

Delay becoming much more active:

• If you are not feeling well because of a temporary cold or fever—wait until you feel better, or

• If you are or may be pregnant—talk to your doctor before you start becoming more active

Please note: If your health changes so that you then answer YES to any of the above questions, tell your fitness or health professional. Ask whether you should change your physical activity plan.

From Par-Q and You. Gloucester, Ontario: Canadian Society for Exercise Physiology, 1994.

Patient History

A thorough patient history, including past and current medical problems, documents the most common patient complaints and establishes the CHD risk profile. Most CHD symptoms include chest pain, so the differential diagnosis of this pain is a primary focus. TABLE 32.14 lists symptoms, possible causes, and related pathology of chest pain. A patient history typically includes the following entries:

• Medical diagnosis of diseases
• Previous physical examination findings to uncover abnormalities
• Recent illnesses, hospitalizations, or surgical procedures
• History of significant symptoms
• Orthopedic problems
• Medications
• Work record
• Family background
• Psychologic record

Physical Examination

The physician usually conducts the physical examination. This includes vital signs (body temperature, heart rate, breathing rate, and blood pressure) and possible indications of problems. Assessments encompass auscultation of lungs; palpation and inspection of lower extremities for edema; tests of neurologic function that include reflexes and cognition; and inspection of the skin, especially of the lower extremities in diabetics. Resting cardiorespiratory variables sometimes provide indirect, noninvasive clues to cardiovascular dysfunction. For example, sinus tachycardia or abnormal bradycardia and increased breathing rate and systolic blood pressure can contraindicate exercise without further evaluation.

The clinical exercise physiologist must know the patient's heart rate and blood pressure response to graded exercise to prescribe exercise and identify early warning signs. For example, a systolic blood pressure increase of 20 mm Hg or more with low-intensity exercise (2 to 4 METs) can reflect abnormal myocardial oxygen demand and signal cardiovascular

TABLE 32.14 ■ DIAGNOSIS OF CHEST PAIN

PAIN/COMPLAINT/FINDINGS	POSSIBLE CAUSES	STIMULI	POSSIBLE PATHOLOGY
Pressure, ache, tightness or burning in midsternum, left shoulder, arm; sweating; nausea; vomiting; S-T segment changes	MI	Exertion; cold; smoking; heavy meal; fluid overload	CHD
Sharp pain worsens with inspiration, improves with sitting	Inflammation	Acute MI	Pericarditis
Chest tightness with breathlessness; low-grade fever	Infection	IV drug use; microbes	Myocarditis; endocarditis
Sharp, stabbing pain; breathlessness; cough; loss of consciousness	Pulmonary	Recent surgery	Pulmonary embolism
Burning pain; indigestion relieved by antacids	Referred pain	Heavy meal, spicy food	Esophageal reflux
Angina pain; breathlessness; wide pulse pressure; ventricular hypertrophy on ECG	Ventricular outflow tract obstruction	Exertion; CHD	Aortic stenosis; mitral valve prolapse

impairment. Similarly, failure of systolic blood pressure to increase (hypotensive response) may indicate blunted ventricular function; a depressed response with high-intensity exercise (e.g., failure to achieve systolic blood pressures above 140 mm Hg) frequently reflects dormant cardiac disease.

Heart Auscultation

Listening to sounds (**auscultation**) during the cardiac cycle can assess cardiac performance. The exercise physiologist should become familiar with the different abnormal heart sounds and learn to identify heart murmurs (www.wilkes.med.ucla.edu/intro.html). Auscultation can uncover valvular conditions (e.g., MVP, diagnosed by *click-murmur* sounds) and congenital heart abnormalities (regurgitation sounds in ventricular septal defects; egeneralmedical.com/egeneralmedical/listohearmur.html).

Laboratory Tests

Laboratory studies with chest x-ray, electrocardiogram (ECG), blood lipid and lipoprotein analyses, and serum enzyme testing contribute to assessing the extent of CHD.

The chest x-ray reveals the size and shape of the heart and lungs, whereas resting and exercise ECGs assess myocardial electrical conductivity and degree of oxygenation. Clinical exercise physiologists require considerable experience reading and interpreting ECGs. TABLE 32.15 lists six different categories of ECG measurements and interpretations. Chapter 31 discusses various ECG abnormalities and atypical physiologic responses to exercise. Careful ECG monitoring during a GXT provides more extensive evaluation to target individuals with possible CHD. TABLE 32.16 presents common ECG changes during exercise and anomalies associated with CHD.

Alterations in serum enzymes often confirm the existence of an acute MI. With myocardial cell death (necrosis) or prolonged ischemia, the following cardiac muscle enzymes leak into the blood from increased plasma membrane permeability: (1) creatine phosphokinase (CPK), (2) lactate dehydrogenase (LDH), and (3) serum glutamic oxaloacetic transaminase (SGOT). Elevated CPK levels reflect either skeletal or cardiac muscle fiber damage. To pinpoint the source of the enzyme leak, electrophoresis or radioimmunoassay analysis separates CPK into three different isoenzymes: MM-isoenzyme, unique to skeletal muscle; BB-isoenzyme, specific to brain tissue; and MB-isoenzyme, specific for cardiac muscle necrosis. Like CPK, LDH fractionates into different isoenzymes, one of which increases during an MI. An acute MI also raises SGOT. Additional blood tests for CHD diagnosis include serum homocysteine (see Chapter 31),

TABLE 32.15 ■ ECG INTERPRETATION USES ONE OF SIX DIFFERENT CRITERIA

1. Measurements
   - Heart rate (atrial and ventricular)
   - P-R interval (0.12–0.20 s)
   - QRS duration (0.06–0.10 s)
   - Q-T interval (HR dependent)
   - Frontal plane QRS axis (30–90°)
2. Rhythm diagnosis
3. Conduction diagnosis
4. Wave form description
   - P wave (atrial enlargement)
   - QRS complex (ventricular hypertrophy, infarction)
   - S-T segment (elevated or depressed)
   - T wave (flattened or inverted)
   - U wave (prominent or inverted)
5. ECG diagnosis
   - Within normal limits
   - Borderline abnormal
   - Abnormal
6. Comparison with previous ECG

From Fardy P, Yanowitz FG. Cardiac rehabilitation, adult fitness and exercise testing. Baltimore: Williams & Wilkins, 1996.

TABLE 32.16 ■ NORMAL AND ABNORMAL ECG CHANGES DURING EXERCISE

NORMAL ECG RESPONSE IN HEALTHY INDIVIDUALS	ABNORMAL ECG RESPONSE WITH CHD
1. Slight increase in P wave amplitude 2. Shortening of P-R interval 3. Shift to the right of QRS axis 4. S-T segment depression <1.0 mm 5. Decreased T wave amplitude 6. Single or rare PVCs during exercise and recovery 7. Single or rare PVCs or PACs	1. Appearance of bundle branch block at a critical HR 2. Recurrent or multifocal PVCs during exercise and recovery 3. Ventricular tachycardia 4. Appearance of bradyarrhythmias, tachyarrhythmias 5. S-T segment depression/ elevation of ≥1.0 mm 0.08 s after J point 6. Exercise bradycardia 7. Submaximal exercise tachycardia 8. Increase in frequency or severity of any known arrhythmia

PVC, premature ventricular contraction; PAC, premature atrial contraction.

lipoprotein (a), fibrinogen, tissue-type plasminogen activator (tPA), and C-reactive protein.

Invasive Physiologic Tests

Invasive cardiovascular testing provides information unattainable through noninvasive procedures. This includes the extent, severity, and location of coronary atherosclerosis, degree of ventricular dysfunction, and specific cardiac abnormalities.

Radionuclide Studies. Radionuclide studies require injecting a radioactive isotope (e.g., mostly manmade technetium-99) into the circulation during rest and exercise. Two examples include:

1. **Thallium imaging**: Evaluates areas of myocardial blood flow and tissue perfusion to differentiate between a true-positive and false-positive S-T segment depression obtained by ECG evaluation during a GXT
2. **Nuclear ventriculography**: Radiographic imaging procedure that analyzes regional left ventricular contractility following injection of radioactive isotope contrast material

Pharmacologic Stress Testing. A **pharmacologic stress test** benefits individuals unable to undergo routine exercise stress testing because of extreme deconditioning, peripheral vascular disease, orthopedic disabilities, neurologic disease, or other health problems. This test involves systematic intravenous drug infusion (e.g., dobutamine, dipyridamole, or adenosine) every 3 minutes until the patient receives the ap-

propriate dosage. Echocardiography and/or thallium scanning then monitor for changes in wall motion abnormalities or coronary perfusion limitations, respectively. Heart rate response, arrhythmias, angina symptoms, S-T segment depression, and blood pressure dynamics also reflect myocardial viability during a pharmacologic stress test.

Cardiac Catheterization. A fine tube (catheter) inserted into a vein or artery passes into the heart's right or left side. The intracardiac catheter can sample blood, assess pressure differences within the heart's chambers or vessels, and add contrast media to evaluate cardiac function.

Coronary Angiography. Radiography images the coronary circulation by injecting a contrast medium that flows into the coronary vasculature. The technique, highly effective to evaluate the extent of coronary atherosclerosis, serves as the gold standard to assess coronary blood flow and provides the baseline for other test comparisons. Unlike thallium imaging, angiography cannot determine how easily blood flows within portions of the myocardium and cannot be applied during exercise. The accompanying angiogram (FIG. 32.9) pinpoints

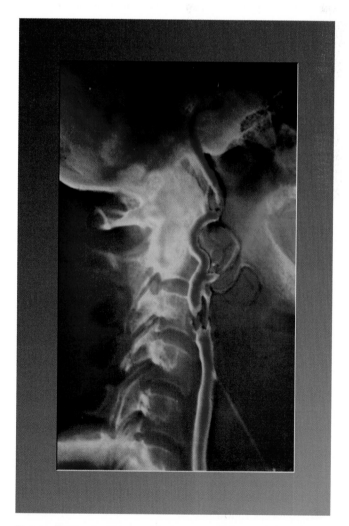

Figure 32.9 Angiogram showing constriction and absence of blood flow through the right carotid artery (*in red*). (Courtesy of Dr. Barry Franklin, Beaumont Hospital, Birmingham, MI.)

impaired blood flow in the carotid artery (shown in *red*). Resectioning a vessel or removing its atherosclerotic plaques improves blood flow to reduce stroke occurrence.

Noninvasive Physiologic Tests

Echocardiography. Pulses of reflected ultrasound (echo) assess the functional and structural characteristics of the myocardium.[51] Ultrasound (high-frequency sound waves) identifies the heart's anatomic components during a cardiac cycle and measures their distances from the echo transducers to accurately estimate heart chamber and vessel size and myocardial wall thickness. Echocardiograms diagnose heart murmurs, evaluate valvular lesions, and quantify congenital defects and myopathies. The echocardiogram is preferred to the ECG in recognizing chamber enlargement, inefficient ventricular contractility, myocardial hypertrophy, and other structural abnormalities.

Ultrafast CT Scan. This 10-minute, noninvasive test uses a rapid (ultrafast) electron beam computed tomographic (EBCT) scan to assess calcium deposition within plaque in coronary artery linings. Test results determine how aggressively to treat blood lipid abnormalities (e.g., diet and exercise vs. drug therapy) and other CHD risk factors. Testing to detect coronary calcium deposition with EBCT is highly sensitive in men and women with coronary disease validated by coronary angiography.[69] Exclusion of coronary calcium buildup helps to characterize individuals with a low probability of significant stenosis.

Graded Exercise Stress Testing. *The graded exercise stress test (GXT) evaluates the ECG under conditions that exceed resting requirements in defined, progressive increments to increase myocardial workload.* The GXT also objectifies the functional capacity of patients with known disease and evaluates progress after surgery or other therapeutic interventions.

TABLE 32.17 presents subjective and objective information obtained during a GXT for designing an exercise prescription. The cardiologist and exercise physiologist supervise the exercise test, interpret the data, and prepare the exercise prescription.

Prudent Preexercise Evaluation

Aerobic exercise serves important protective and rehabilitative functions to battle heart disease and improve cardiovascular functional capacity.[187] One should view the potential therapeutic benefits of regular exercise in proper perspective. For a sedentary person with undetected CHD, a sudden burst of strenuous exercise can inordinately strain cardiovascular function. Medical evaluation before initiating an exercise program reduces this risk considerably. A GXT provides a crucial component of the medical evaluation.

The term GXT generally describes the systematic use of exercise for the following:

1. ECG observations
2. Evaluating patients with exertional discomfort

TABLE 32.17 ■ DATA FROM AN EXERCISE STRESS TEST TO DIAGNOSE AND FORMULATE THE EXERCISE PRESCRIPTION
Subjective data
Angina pain
Dyspnea ratings
Fatigue and weakness
Leg discomfort
Dizziness
Rating of perceived exertion (RPE)
Objective data
• **Physical examination data**
Breathing sounds
Murmurs and gallops
Blood pressure
Pulmonary function tests (before or after exercise)
Heart rate response
Blood gas parameters
Rate-pressure product (RPP = HR × systolic blood pressure)
• **Physical performance data**
Time on treadmill/cycle ergometer
Maximum work or power output
• **Electrocardiogram data**
S-T segment changes
Rate responses
Dysrhythmias
Conduction abnormalities
• **Cardiorespiratory data**
Lactate threshold
Carbon dioxide output
Minute ventilation
Oxygen consumption
Respiratory exchange ratio (R)

3. Assessing pharmacologic and therapeutic treatment strategies
4. Evaluating physiologic adjustments to increasing metabolic demands to objectify physical activity recommendations.

Multistage bicycle and treadmill tests are the most common exercise stress testing modes. These tests, graded for exercise intensity, usually include several levels of 3 to 5 minutes of submaximal effort that bring the person to a self-imposed fatigue level or end point. The graded nature of testing allows exercise intensity to increase in small increments to pinpoint ischemic manifestations and rhythm disorders (e.g., anginal pain or ECG abnormalities). With heart disease, exercise testing provides a reliable, quantitative index of the person's functional impairment; this objectifies the diagnosis and subsequent exercise prescription.[56,75] Testing generally does not require maximal effort but the person should exercise to at least 85% of age-predicted maximum heart rate.

A resting ECG precedes the exercise test to provide the important comparative baseline and to certify a person's safety in subsequent graded exercise testing. Unfortunately, exercise stress testing cannot show the extent of CHD or its specific location. Twenty-five to 40% of people with relatively advanced CHD (significant blockage in one or more coronary arteries) achieve a normal GXT evaluation. Interestingly, an abnormal heart rate recovery (i.e., failure of heart rate to decrease by more than 12 b · min^{-1} in the first minute after peak exercise) predicts, independent of ECG assessment, subsequent mortality in patients referred specifically for exercise electrocardiography.[141] This indicates that recovery heart rate provides additional prognostic information to complement interpretation of the exercise stress test.

Reasons for Stress Testing

Stress testing serves the following six functions in a CHD evaluation:

1. *Diagnoses overt heart disease and screens for "silent" coronary disease in seemingly healthy adults.* Approximately 30% of persons with confirmed CHD have a normal resting ECG. Graded exercise testing generally uncovers 70% of the abnormalities.
2. *Assesses exercise-related chest symptoms.* Individuals older than age 40 suffer chest or related pain in the left shoulder or arm during physical exertion. ECG analysis identifies myocardial abnormalities and more precisely diagnoses exercise-induced pain.
3. *Screens candidates for entry into preventive and cardiac rehabilitative exercise programs.* Test results provide an objective framework to design a program based on current functional capacity and health status. Repeat testing assesses progress and adaptations to regular exercise and provides for program modification.
4. *Uncovers abnormal blood pressure responses.* Individuals with normal resting blood pressure sometimes show greater-than-normal increases in systolic blood pressure during mild-to-moderate exercise, which may signify developing cardiovascular complications.
5. *Monitors effectiveness of therapeutic interventions (drug, surgical, dietary) to improve heart disease status and cardiovascular function.* A patient's capacity to achieve a target heart rate without complications often confirms success of coronary bypass surgery.
6. *Quantifies functional aerobic capacity ($\dot{V}O_{2peak}$) to evaluate its deviation from normal standards.*

INTEGRATIVE QUESTION

Give recommendations for a middle-aged man who experiences breathlessness and chest discomfort while walking the golf course yet wants to begin an aerobic exercise program.

Who Requires Stress Testing?

TABLE 32.18 outlines screening and supervisory procedures for exercise testing that conform to policies and practices of the ACSM and the AMA.

RISK CATEGORY	MEDICAL EXAMINATION AND GXT	M.D. SUPERVISION
TABLE 32.18 ■ ACSM RECOMMENDATIONS FOR CURRENT MEDICAL EXAMINATION AND EXERCISE STRESS TESTING (GXT) AND PHYSICIAN SUPERVISION OF GXT PRIOR TO PARTICIPATION IN EXERCISE PROGRAM		
Low risk Men <45 years Women <55 years; asymptomatic with ≤1 risk factor[a,b]	Moderate exercise; not necessary Vigorous exercise; not necessary	Moderate exercise; not necessary Vigorous exercise; not necessary
Moderate risk Men HDL-C ≤45 mg · dL^{-1} Women HDL-C ≤55 mg · dL^{-1}, with ≥2 risk factors[a,b]	Moderate exercise; not necessary Vigorous exercise; recommended	Moderate exercise; not necessary Vigorous exercise; recommended
High risk Individuals with ≥1 sign/symptom of cardiovascular or pulmonary disease[c] or known cardiovascular (cardiac, peripheral vascular, or cerebrovascular), pulmonary (obstructive pulmonary disease, asthma, cystic fibrosis), or metabolic (diabetes, thyroid disorder, renal or liver) disease	Moderate exercise; recommended Vigorous exercise; recommended	Moderate exercise; recommended Vigorous exercise; recommended

Modified from Franklin BA, et al. ACSM's guidelines for exercise testing and prescription. 6th ed. Baltimore: Lippincott Williams & Wilkins, 2000.
[a] Risk factors: family history of heart disease; cigarette smoking; hypertension; hypercholesterolemia; impaired fasting glucose; obesity; sedentary lifestyle.
[b] HDL >60 mg · dL^{-1} (subtract 1 risk factor from the sum of other risk factors because high HDL decreases CHD risk).
[c] Signs and symptoms of cardiovascular and pulmonary disease: pain, discomfort in chest, neck, jaw, left arm; shortness of breath at rest or with mild exertion; dizziness or syncope; orthopnea or paroxysmal nocturnal dyspnea; ankle edema; tachycardia; intermittent claudication; heart murmur; unusual fatigue or shortness of breath with mild activity.

Informed Consent

All testing and exercise training must be performed on "informed" volunteers. **Informed consent** should raise the individual's awareness about all potential participation risks. It must include a written statement that the person had an opportunity to ask questions about the procedures, with sufficient information clearly stated so that consent occurs from a knowledgeable (informed) perspective. A legal guardian or parent must sign the consent form for minors. Individuals need assurance that test results remain confidential and that they can terminate testing or training at any time and for any reason. TABLE 32.19 presents a sample consent form to obtain before administering a health-related exercise test.

Stress Testing Contraindications

Absolute contraindications

A stress test should not take place without direct medical supervision if the following contraindications exist:

- Resting ECG suggesting acute cardiac disease
- Recent complicated MI

- Unstable angina pectoris
- Uncontrolled ventricular arrhythmias
- Uncontrolled atrial arrhythmias that compromise cardiac function
- Third-degree AV heart block without pacemaker
- Acute CHF
- Severe aortic stenosis
- Active or suspected myocarditis or pericarditis
- Recent systemic or pulmonary embolism
- Acute infections
- Acute emotional distress

Relative contraindications

A GXT can be administered with caution *and with medical personal in the test area* under the following conditions:

- Resting diastolic blood pressure ≤115 mm Hg or systolic blood pressure ≤200 mm Hg
- Moderate valvular disease
- Electrolyte abnormalities
- Frequent or complex ventricular ectopy
- Ventricular aneurysm

TABLE 32.19 ■ **SAMPLE INFORMED CONSENT FOR A HEALTH-RELATED EXERCISE STRESS TEST**

Patient/Subject Name _____

1. *Explanation of the exercise test*
   You will perform an exercise test on a cycle ergometer or a motor-driven treadmill. The exercise intensity begins at a level you can easily accomplish and will advance in stages depending on your fitness level. We may stop the test at any time because of signs of fatigue, or you may stop the test when you wish because of feelings of fatigue or discomfort.

2. *Risks and discomforts*
   The possibility exists that certain abnormal physiologic changes can occur during the test. These include abnormal blood pressure, fainting, disorder of heart beat, and in rare instances heart attack, stroke, or death. Every effort will be made to minimize these risks by evaluating preliminary information related to your health and fitness and by observations during testing. Emergency equipment and available trained personnel can deal with unusual situations that may arise.

3. *Responsibilities of the participant*
   Information you possess about your health status or previous experiences of unusual feelings with physical effort may affect the safety and value of your exercise test. Your prompt reporting of how you feel during the exercise test is also important. You are responsible for fully disclosing such information when requested to do so by the testing staff.

4. *Expected benefits from the test*
   The results obtained from the exercise test may assist in diagnosing an illness or evaluating what type of physical activities you might do with low risk of harm.

5. *Questions*
   We encourage you to ask any questions about the procedures used in the exercise test or in the estimation of functional capacity. If you have doubts or questions, please ask us for further explanations.

6. *Freedom of consent*
   Your permission to perform this exercise test is voluntary. You are free to deny consent or stop the test at any point.

   I have read this form and all procedures, risks, and potential benefits have been explained. I voluntarily consent to participate in this test.

   Date: _____
   Signature of Patient: _____
   Signature of Witness: _____
   Questions: _____
   _____

   Responses: _____
   Signature of Physician or Authorized Delegate: _____ Date: _____

- Uncontrolled metabolic disease (diabetes, thyrotoxicosis)
- Chronic infectious disease (hepatitis, mononucleosis, AIDS)
- Neuromuscular or musculoskeletal disorders
- Pregnancy (complicated or in the last trimester)
- Psychologic distress and/or apprehension about taking the test

GXT Termination

Graded exercise testing is generally safe when following recognized guidelines and taking proper precautions. TABLE 32.20 lists reasons why test termination may be required before the person attains maximum volitional fatigue.

Stress Test Outcomes

The clinical success of the GXT depends on its predictive outcome; this means how effectively the test correctly diagnoses a person with heart disease.

Four possible GXT outcomes include:

1. **True positive** (successful test): The GXT correctly identifies a person with heart disease
2. **True negative** (successful test): The GXT correctly identifies a person without heart disease
3. **False positive** (unsuccessful test): The GXT incorrectly identifies a normal person as having heart disease
4. **False negative** (unsuccessful test): The GXT incorrectly identifies a person with heart disease as normal

---

TABLE 32.20 ■ CRITERIA FOR TERMINATING A GRADED EXERCISE TEST BY APPARENTLY HEALTHY ADULTS

- Onset of angina or angina-like symptoms
- Significant drop of 20 mm Hg in systolic blood pressure or failure of systolic blood pressure to rise with an increase in exercise intensity
- Excessive rise in blood pressure: systolic pressure >260 mm Hg or diastolic pressure >115 mm Hg
- Signs of poor perfusion: light-headedness, confusion, ataxia, pallor, cyanosis, nausea, or cold and clammy skin
- Failure of heart rate to increase with increasing exercise intensity
- Noticeable change in heart rhythm
- Subject requests to stop
- Physical or verbal manifestations of severe fatigue
- Failure of testing equipment
- Early-onset horizontal or downsloping S-T segment depression or elevation (>4 mm)
- Increasing ventricular ectopy; multiform PVCs
- Sustained supraventricular tachycardia

A test's **sensitivity** refers to the percentage of persons for whom the test detects an abnormal (positive) response. This represents a true-positive condition that only subsequent follow-up can verify. False-negative results (unsuccessful test) occur 25% of the time, and false-positive (unsuccessful test) results approximately 15%. Factors that contribute to false-negative results include the patient's failure to reach an ischemic threshold, failure to recognize non-ECG signs and symptoms associated with underlying CHD, and technical or observer errors. Various drugs and conditions also increase the probability of false-negative results, particularly if the person takes β-blockers, nitrates, and calcium channel blocking agents.

Test **specificity** refers to the number of true-negative test results—correctly identifying someone without CHD. More false-positive results occur under the influence of the drug digitalis and hypokalemia (low blood potassium levels), mitral valve prolapse, pericardial disorders, and anemia.

Stress Testing the "Oldest Old"

The stress testing guidelines in Table 32.18 do not apply to individuals 75 years and older, those considered among the "oldest-old."[66] Only a small, highly select subgroup of these individuals participates in vigorous exercise or can successfully complete a stress test. For example, approximately 30% of persons aged 75 to 79 years can achieve a maximal exercise effort, 25% of those aged 80 to 84 years, and only 9% of those 85 years or older.[83] The oldest-old differ markedly from younger persons in two key areas relative to stress testing: (1) high prevalence of asymptomatic CHD and (2) coexistence of other chronic conditions and physical limitations. Elderly, asymptomatic men and women exhibit increased ECG abnormalities, many of which diminish the diagnostic accuracy of the GXT. The prevalence of asymptomatic ischemic episodes uncovered by the exercise ECG increases dramatically among the elderly with no history of MI or ECG abnormalities. Given the large reservoir of asymptomatic CHD among older persons, routine exercise stress testing would likely initiate a cascade of requirements for follow-up invasive cardiac procedures.[203] In the absence of strong evidence to support aggressive evaluation in the elderly, this practice would place many at unnecessary risk for complications from invasive assessment. For this reason, empirical screening for the elderly prescribes physical activity based on the person's previous exercise experiences and overall sense of well-being. This approach to exercise testing, training, and safety monitoring observes the widely accepted geriatric dictum, *"start low and go slow."*

Exercise-Induced Indicators of CHD

Physical activity creates the greatest demand for coronary blood flow, thus making exercise testing an effective means of probing for CHD.

Angina Pectoris

Myocardial ischemia—usually from restricted coronary circulation caused by atherosclerosis—stimulates sensory nerves in the walls of the coronary arteries and myocardium. Pain or discomfort generally manifests in the upper chest region, although it frequently feels like increased pressure or constriction in the left shoulder or arm, neck, or jaw (see Figs. 32.6 and 7). Impaired cardiac performance—reduced stroke volume and cardiac output and generally diminished left ventricular contractility—also accompanies angina. The pain usually subsides after a few minutes of inactivity without permanent myocardial damage. Physical activity frequently precipitates an angina episode, yet angina also can occur at rest (called *Prinzmetal's angina* or *variant angina*) with attacks usually occurring in the late evening or nighttime through early morning. In variant angina, caused by a coronary artery spasm, approximately two thirds of people with it have severe blockage in at least one major coronary vessel. Stable angina indicates predictable chest pain on exertion or under mental or emotional stress. According to 2005 data from the AHA, in 2002, 3.8% of the population (6,400,000 total cases; 3,100,000 males and 3,300,000 females) were diagnosed with angina, with 400,000 reported additional cases of stable angina.

Electrocardiographic Abnormalities

Alterations in the heart's normal pattern of electrical activity often indicate insufficient myocardial oxygen supply. Such electrical "clues" rarely emerge unless myocardial metabolic and blood flow requirements exceed resting conditions.

FIGURE 32.10A shows a tracing of the dynamic electrical activity of the myocardium throughout the cardiac cycle. Standard ECG paper contains 1-mm and 5-mm squares. Horizontally, each small square represents 0.04 seconds (with normal paper speed of 25 mm · s^{-1}); each large square represents 0.2 seconds. On the vertical axis, a small square indicates a 0.1-mV deflection with a calibration of 10 mm · mV^{-1}. One normal heartbeat (cardiac cycle) consists of five major electrical waves labeled P, Q, R, S, and T. The P wave indicates the electrical impulse (wave of depolarization) before atrial contraction. The Q, R, and S waves, collectively known as the **QRS complex**, represent depolarization of the ventricles immediately before their contraction. Ventricular repolarization generates the T wave. The cause of **S-T segment depression** (Fig. 32.10B) remains unknown, yet this abnormal deviation correlates with other CHD indicators that include coronary artery narrowing. *Individuals with significant S-T segment depression usually have severe, extensive obstruction in one or more coronary arteries.* The amount of S-T segment depression relates directly to the chances of dying from CHD. Generally, persons with 1- to 2-mm S-T segment depression during exercise exhibit a nearly 5-fold increase in CHD mortality. The death risk increases approximately 20-fold for those with more than 2-mm depression. Current opinion advocates including nonspecific ECG findings in the overall heart disease risk assessment.[40] Even nonspecific minor S-T segment or T-wave abnormalities or both (termed *ST-T abnormalities*) provide a disquieting hint of increased long-term risk of mortality from cardiovascular disease.

During a standard ECG-monitored treadmill test, special electrodes can identify extremely subtle electrical patterns to predict a patient's risk for ventricular fibrillation. The test, termed the **alternans test**, identifies electrical alternation of the heart. Specifically, it uses a device to analyze T-wave alternans, which represent beat-to-beat electrical fluctuations of just one millionth of a volt. T-wave alternans reflect abnormalities in the way myocardial cells recover after transmitting the heart's electrical impulse. Oscillation of the cells' impulse can initiate a chain reaction that produces arrhythmias, fibrillation, and subsequent cardiac arrest in some 350,000 individuals in the United States. Predicting risk for sudden death via T-wave alternans gives high-risk patients medical protection that might include an implanted defibrillator (placed beneath the skin of the chest) to automatically correct abnormal cardiac electrical activity. The defibrillator activates a built-in pacemaker to restabilize the heart's rhythm if it detects minor arrhythmias. If that fails, the pacemaker delivers a small defibrillating electrical jolt that resets the rhythm.

Cardiac Rhythm Abnormalities

Graded exercise testing uncovers abnormalities in the pattern of the heart's electrical activity. A PVC (Fig. 32.10C) during exercise often reflects abnormal alteration in cardiac rhythm or **arrhythmia**. In this case, the normal depolarization wave through the atrioventricular node does not stimulate the ventricles. Instead, portions of the ventricle spontaneously depolarize. This disorganized electrical activity produces an "extra" ventricular beat (QRS complex) without the P wave (atrial depolarization) that normally precedes it.

PVCs in exercise generally herald the presence of severe ischemic atherosclerotic heart disease that often involves two or more major coronary vessels. This specific myocardial electrical instability with exercise has greater predictive value than S-T segment depression for CHD diagnosis. Patients with exercise-induced PVCs have a 6- to 10-times greater risk of sudden death from abnormal course or fine rapid movements of the ventricles (**ventricular fibrillation**) than patients without this instability. Fibrillation risk becomes more prevalent for individuals with family history of this occurrence. With fibrillation, the ventricles do not contract in a unified manner, and cardiac output falls dramatically. Sudden death ensues unless normal ventricular rhythm returns. One way to reduce this risk requires implanting an electrical stimulator to correct the abnormal myocardial electrical conductance pattern.

Other Exercise-Induced CHD Indicators

Blood pressure and heart rate responses to exercise provide three useful non-ECG indices of possible CHD:

1. **Hypertensive exercise response:** Normally, systolic blood pressure progressively increases during graded exercise from approximately 120 mm Hg at rest to

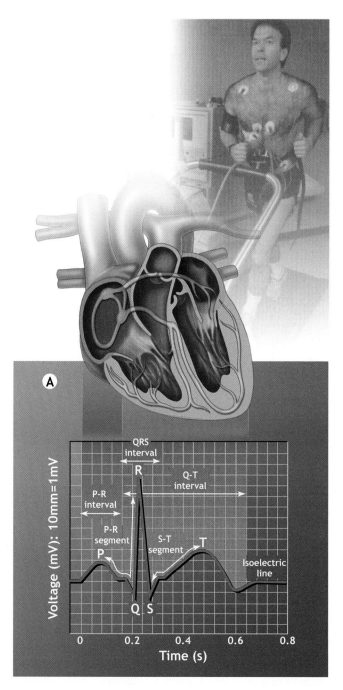

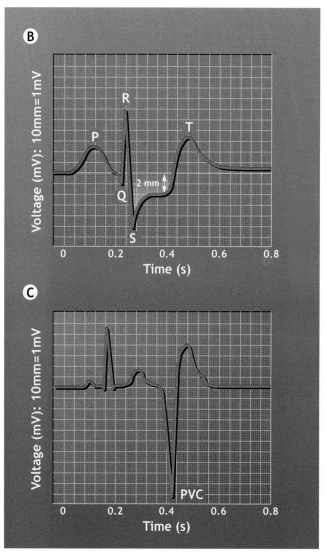

Figure 32.10 **A.** Normal ECG tracing with an upward-sloping S-T segment. **B.** ECG tracing showing an abnormal horizontal S-T segment depression *(shaded area)* of 2 mm, measured from a stable baseline. **C.** ECG tracing illustrating a premature ventricular contraction *(PVC)*.

160 to 190 mm Hg during peak-intensity exercise. The change in diastolic pressure is generally less than 10 mm Hg. In exercise, systolic blood pressure can rise to well above 200 mm Hg, whereas the diastolic pressure can approach 150 mm Hg. This abnormal hypertensive response provides a significant clue to the presence of cardiovascular disease.

2. **Hypotensive exercise response:** Inability for blood pressure to increase during graded exercise reflects cardiovascular malfunction. For example, failure of systolic blood pressure to increase by at least 20 or 30 mm Hg often results from diminished cardiac reserve.

3. **Heart rate response:** A rapid, large increase in heart rate (tachycardia) early in graded exercise often

indicates cardiac dysfunction. Likewise, abnormally low exercise heart rates (bradycardia) in non–endurance-trained individuals may reflect unhealthy function of the heart's SA node. Inability of heart rate to increase during graded exercise (**chronotropic incompetence**), particularly when accompanied by extreme fatigue indicates cardiac strain and CHD. An attenuated maximal exercise heart rate in apparently healthy men and women raises cardiovascular disease mortality risk.[104,113] Specifically, failure to achieve at least 85% of age-predicted maximum heart rate during exercise predicts eventual all-cause mortality, independent of any exercise-induced myocardial perfusion defects.[114]

STRESS TEST PROTOCOLS

A survey in 2000, based on 75,828 exercise tests performed at Veterans Affairs Medical Centers with cardiology divisions, reported that 78% used the treadmill (82% of those used the Bruce or Modified Bruce protocol). Four major cardiac events occurred (3 MIs and one sustained ventricular tachycardia) representing an event rate of 1.2 per 10,000 exercise tests.[136]

Bruce and Balke Treadmill Tests

Chapter 11 outlines protocols for the Bruce and Balke GXTs. Each test has distinct advantages and disadvantages. For example, the Bruce test provides more abrupt increases in exercise intensity between stages. This may improve sensitivity to detect ischemic ECG responses, but the patient must possess adequate fitness to tolerate increased exercise levels. Both protocols begin at relatively high levels of exercise for cardiac patients and older individuals and thus often require modification. The Bruce protocol incorporates lower initial exercise levels, whereas the Balke test includes a preliminary 2- to 3-minute initial stage at 2 mph and 0% grade.

Choice of a specific exercise test should consider overall health, age, and the person's fitness status. A stress test generally begins at a low level with increments in exercise intensity every several minutes. A warm-up, either separately or incorporated within the test protocol, eases the patient into exercise. Total exercise duration should average at least 8 minutes. A test much longer than 15 minutes adds little additional information because the most meaningful cardiac and physiologic data emerge within this time interval.

Bicycle Ergometer Tests

Bicycle ergometers have distinct advantages for exercise stress testing. In contrast to the treadmill, power output on the ergometer is readily computed and remains independent of the person's body mass. Most bicycle ergometers are portable, safe, and relatively inexpensive. Generally, two types of ergometers have application for graded exercise testing: (1) electrically braked ergometers and (2) weight-loaded, friction-type ergometers. With electrically braked ergometers, the preselected power output remains fixed within a range of pedaling frequencies. With weight-loaded ergometers, power output, usually expressed in $kg\text{-}m \cdot min^{-1}$ or watts (1 W = 6.12 $kg\text{-}m \cdot min^{-1}$), relates directly to frictional resistance and pedaling rate.

The general guidelines for treadmill testing also apply to testing with the bicycle ergometer. Test protocols provide 2- to 4-minute stages of graded exercise with an initial resistance between 0 and 15 or 30 watts; power output generally increases in 15- to 30-watt increments per stage. The subject usually pedals the weight-loaded ergometer at either 50 or 60 revolutions per minute.

Arm-Crank Ergometer Tests

Arm cranking has application for graded exercise testing in special situations (e.g., cardiac assessment during upper-body effort) and for disabled individuals. Chapters 15 and 17 point out that arm exercise lowers $\dot{V}O_{2peak}$ up to 30%, and maximum heart rate generally averages 10 to 15 $b \cdot min^{-1}$ lower than with treadmill or bicycle exercise. Blood pressure is also difficult to measure during arm-crank exercise. Furthermore, *submaximal* arm cranking produces higher blood pressure, heart rate, and oxygen consumption values than the same power output with leg exercise.[156] Nevertheless, graded exercise protocols similar to those developed for leg cycling tests apply to evaluating a patient's response to upper-body exercise. The initial frictional resistance remains lower in arm exercise with smaller increments in power output adjusted accordingly.

INTEGRATIVE QUESTION

What type of exercise prescription most benefits a patient with CHD who experiences angina during upper-body work in his job as a plasterer or paperhanger?

Stress Testing Safety

The safety of stress testing largely depends on knowing who not to test (prescreening health histories reveal noncandidates for testing), knowing when to terminate a test, and preparing for emergencies. TABLE 32.21 summarizes the results of 12 reports about exercise stress testing complications (morbidity and mortality during and after the test) involving 2 million exercise tests with different supervision levels.[10,28,57,102,117,191]

Only 16 high-risk but apparently healthy patients suffered coronary episodes in approximately 170,000 submaximal and maximal stress tests. This represents about one person per 10,000 or approximately 0.01% of the total group. For more than 9000 stress tests, no cardiovascular episodes occurred for subjects with increased heart disease risk. In other reports, risk of coronary episodes for healthy, middle-aged adults during a maximum stress test equaled about 1 in 3000.[58] Test risk in most middle-aged men and women generally increases about 6 to 12 times more than for young adults. For patients with documented CHD (including previous myocardial infarction or episodes of angina), risk of cardiovascular incident in stress testing increases 30 to 60 times above normal. Based on total risk analyses, many experts believe that a *lower* "overall risk" exists for those who take a GXT and then initiate a regular exercise program than for those who take no GXT and remain sedentary.

Despite differences in testing techniques, purposes, safety precautions, type, and mode of testing, three conclusions about risk during or immediately following a GXT appear warranted:

1. Low risk of death ($\leq 0.01\%$)
2. Low risk of an acute MI ($\leq 0.04\%$)
3. Low risk of complications that require hospitalization including acute MI or serious arrhythmias ($\leq 0.2\%$)

TABLE 32.21 ■ SUMMARY REPORTS OF INCIDENCE OF MORBIDITY AND/OR MORTALITY DURING OR FOLLOWING A GRADED EXERCISE TEST (1969–1995)

STUDY	GXT TESTS	TYPE OF SUBJECT	MORBIDITY RATE (PER 10,000)	MORTALITY RATE (PER 10,000)	TOTAL COMPLICATIONS[b] (PER 10,000)
1	50,000[a]	Variety	5.2	0.4	5.6
2	18,707	Variety	3.8	0.9	4.7
3					
4	>12,000	Variety	—	2.5	—
5	58,047	Variety	2.1	0.3	2.4
6	71,914[a]	Variety	0.7	0.1	0.8
7	28,133	Variety	3.2	0	3.2
8	4,050	Variety	0.3	0	0.3
9	170,000[a]	Variety	2.4	1.0	3.4
10	353,638[a]	Athlete	0	0	0
	712,285[a]	CHD patients	1.4	0.2	1.6
11	518,448[a]	Variety	8.4	0.5	8.9
12	1377[a]	Severe CHD	232	0	232

From Franklin BA, et al. ACSM's guidelines for exercise testing and prescription. 6th ed. Baltimore: Lippincott Williams & Wilkins, 2000.
[a] Direct physician supervision of GXT.
[b] Complications defined as the occurrence of serious arrhythmias during exercise testing (i.e., ventricular fibrillation, ventricular tachycardia, or bradycardia) that mandated immediate medical treatment (cardioversion, use of intravenous drugs, or closed-chest compression).
  1. Atterhog JH, et al. Am Heart J 1979;98:572.
  2. Cahalin LP, et al. J Cardiopulm Rehabil 1987;7:269.
  3. Blessey RL. Exercise Standards and Malpractice Reporter 1989;3:69.
  4. DeBrusk RF. Exercise Standards and Malpractice Reporter 1988;2:65.
  5. Franklin BA, et al. Chest 1997;111:262.
  6. Gibbons L, et al. Circulation 1989;80:846.
  7. Knight JA, et al. Am J Cardiol 1995;75:390.
  8. Lem V, et al. Heart Lung 1985;14:280.
  9. Rochmis P, Blackburn H. JAMA 217:1971;1061.
  10. Scherer D, Kaltenbach M. Dtsch Med Wochenschr 1979;33:1161.
  11. Stuart RJ Jr, Ellestad MH. Chest 1980;77:94.
  12. Young, et al. Circulation 1984;70:184.

Clearly, the risk–benefit ratio favors GXT testing as part of the medical evaluation process.

PRESCRIBING EXERCISE

An exercise prescription should improve fitness, promote overall health by reducing risk factors, and ensure a safe and enjoyable exercise experience.[59] *Prescribing exercise involves successful integration of exercise science with behavioral objectives to enhance patient compliance and goal attainment.*

Heart rate and oxygen consumption (or exercise intensity) measured during the stress test provide the basis for the exercise prescription. The prescription individualizes exercise based on current fitness and health status, with emphasis on intensity, frequency, duration, and exercise type.

Initiating an exercise program at the proper level takes on added importance for CHD patients because beginners do not often recognize their limitations.

Practical Illustration

FIGURE 32.11 illustrates a practical approach that permits functional translation of treadmill or bicycle exercise test responses to the exercise prescription. The figure depicts data for a male cardiac patient generated from an algorithm of responses from the Bruce treadmill protocol for level-ground ambulation. Heart rate *(A)* was plotted as a function of time, with a mathematical line of best fit *(B)* applied to the data points. A target zone for heart rate *(shaded portion, C)* represented approximately 75 to 85% of the maximum heart rate of 170 b · min^{-1}. The individualized prescription is then detailed for pace (13.8 to 15.4 mi · min^{-1}, *D*) and/or METs (4.1 to 5.9, *E*). The acceptable exercise intensity range in area *C,* based on heart rate response during the exercise test, includes the following recreational activities: aerobics, bicycling, canoeing, light-to-moderate volleyball, skating, skiing, tennis and badminton, swimming, skating, touch football, and water-skiing. This practical approach to prescribing exercise may improve the prescription's effectiveness and adherence for the healthy, previously sedentary individual and CHD patient.

Improvements in CHD Patients

A properly prescribed and monitored exercise program safely improves a cardiac patient's functional capacity. Clinical symptoms (e.g., ECG abnormalities) often improve or disappear. This occurs partly from structural and func-

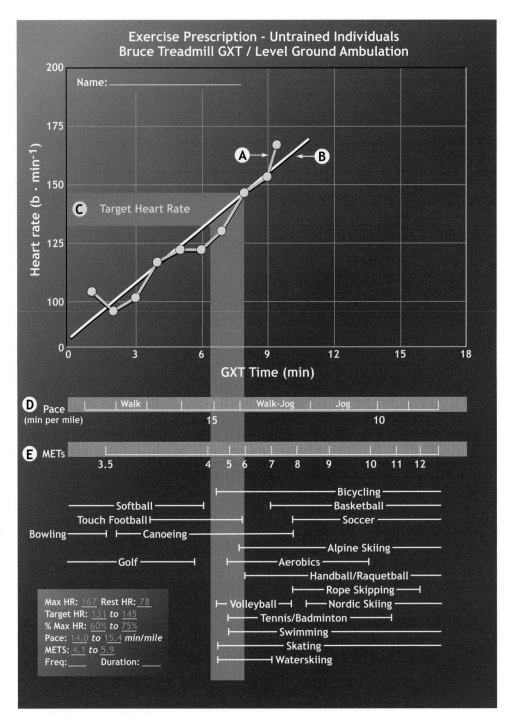

Figure 32.11 Exercise prescription based on functional translation algorithm for level-ground ambulation. Letters in figure identified in text. (Used with permission of Dr. Carl Foster, University of Wisconsin-LaCrosse, LaCrosse, WI.)

tional changes in the myocardium. Cardiac patients and normals respond to exercise training with physiologic adjustments that reduce cardiac work at any given external exercise load. For example, reduced exercise heart rate and blood pressure (two major determinants of myocardial workload and oxygen consumption) reduce myocardial effort. The reduced rate– pressure product (HR × SBP) delays the onset of anginal pain and allows exercise of greater intensity and duration. For individuals whose occupations predominantly require arm exercise, training (and testing) should emphasize this musculature because physical conditioning

benefits are highly specific and generally not transferable among muscle groups.[128]

The Program

The following website provides joint recommendations of the ACSM and AHA for cardiovascular screening of children, adolescents, and adults before enrollment or participation in activities at health/fitness facilities: www. acsmmsse.org/pt/pt-core/template-journal/msse/media/ 0698c.htm. The recommendations also discuss staff qualifications and emergency policies related to cardiovascular safety.

The most effective preventive and rehabilitative exercise programs focus on individual needs. Low- to moderate-intensity exercise regimens evoke greater adherence than intense physical activity.[127] Prescribed exercises usually include rhythmic big-muscle movements that stimulate cardiovascular improvement; examples include walking, jogging, cycling, rope skipping, swimming, stair-climbing and cross-country ski simulation, dynamic calisthenics, and higher intensity interval training, even among the elderly and patients with congestive heart failure.[1,133,134,187] On an outpatient basis, less restricted activities such as mountain biking serve as a recreational adjunct to rehabilitate regularly exercising MI patients with stable CHD.[88]

Chapter 21 discussed guidelines for decision making concerning training frequency, duration, and intensity. Ideally, the personalized exercise prescription should include a recommendation for weight loss and dietary modification (if necessary), warm-up and cool-down exercises, and a developmental flexibility and strength program. Some heart disease patients exhibit a reduced exercise heart rate response with correspondingly reduced maximum heart rate. In such cases, target heart rates based on age-predicted maximum for the general, healthy population grossly overestimate the appropriate training intensity. This supports the wisdom of exercise stress testing each patient to *symptom-limited maximum* and then formulating the exercise prescription from the test's heart rate data.

Supervision Level

The ACSM has categorized several types of exercise programs with specific criteria for entry and supervision (TABLE 32.22). These programs are either *unsupervised* or *supervised*, with four subdivisions in the supervised category. Unsupervised programs meet the needs of asymptomatic participants of any age with functional capacities of at least 8 METs without known major risk factors. The supervised exercise programs focus on patients with specific needs. These include asymptomatic physically active or inactive persons of any age with CHD risk factors but no known disease (B4) and symptomatic individuals, including individuals with recent onset of CHD and those with a changed disease status (B1 to B3).

Resistance Exercise Provides Benefits

Resistance exercises added to a cardiac rehabilitation program restore muscular strength, promote preservation of FFM, improve psychologic status and quality of life, and increase glucose tolerance and insulin sensitivity.[59,129,130] For patients with advanced heart disease, no adverse effects occur while performing weightlifting arm exercise at 50, 65, and 85% of 1-RM.[101] In comparisons of resting and exercise responses, no changes occurred in pulmonary wedge pressures, S-T segment of the ECG, or incidence of dysrhythmias. Contraindications to resistance training for cardiac patients parallel those for aerobic training.[162] The following conditions preclude cardiac patients from participating in resistance training:

- Unstable angina
- Uncontrolled arrhythmias
- Left ventricular outflow obstruction (e.g., hypertrophic cardiomyopathy with obstruction)
- Recent history of CHF without follow-up and treatment
- Severe valvular disease, hypertension (systolic blood pressure >160 mm Hg and/or diastolic blood pressure >105 mm Hg)
- Poor left ventricular function and exercise capacity below 5 METs with anginal symptoms or ischemic S-T segment depression

Resistance Training Prescription. Cardiac patients should exercise with light resistance (range of 30 to 50% of 1-RM) because of exaggerated blood pressure responses with straining-type exercise. In the absence of contraindications, elastic bands, light (1–5 lb) cuff and hand weights, light free weights, and wall pulleys can be applied at entrance to an outpatient program. Do not initiate low-level resistance training until 2 to 3 weeks post-MI. Introduce barbells and/or weight machines after 4 to 6 weeks of convalescence.

TABLE 32.22 ■ **ACSM CATEGORIES FOR EXERCISE PROGRAMS RELATED TO PATIENT SYMPTOMS**

TYPE	PARTICIPANTS	ENTRY MET LEVEL	SUPERVISION
A. Unsupervised	Asymptomatic	8+	None
B. Supervised			
1. Inpatient	All symptomatics—post-myocardial infarction, postoperative, pulmonary disease	3	Supervised ambulatory therapy
2. Outpatient	All symptomatics—post-myocardial infarction, postoperative, pulmonary disease	3+	Exercise specialist, physician on call
3. In home	Symptomatic + asymptomatic	>3-5	Unsupervised; periodic hospital reevaluation
4. Community	Symptomatic + asymptomatic, 6-8 weeks postinfarct, 4-8 weeks postoperative	>5	Exercise program director + exercise specialist

Most cardiac patients begin range-of-motion exercises using relatively light weights for the lower and upper extremities. In accordance with AHA recommendations, they should perform one set of 10 to 15 repetitions to moderate fatigue, using 8 to 10 different exercises (e.g., chest press, shoulder press, triceps extension, biceps curl, lat pull-down, lower back extension, abdominal crunch/curl-up, quadriceps extension or leg press, leg curl, calf raise). Exercises performed 2 to 3 days a week produce favorable adaptations.[162] The RPE should range from 11 to 14 on the Borg scale ("fairly light" to "somewhat hard"). To minimize dramatic blood pressure fluctuations during lifting, patients should be warned to avoid straining, performing the Valsalva maneuver, and gripping weight handles or bars tightly.

Cardiac Medications and Exercise Response

Knowledge of the physiologic effects of drug intervention allows the clinical exercise physiologist to properly assess patient response during physical activity. TABLE 32.23 presents six classifications of common cardiac drugs along with trade names, side effects, and possible effects on exercise responses.

INTEGRATIVE QUESTION

Why would participating in a weightlifting competition pose a risk to a person with advanced CHD?

CARDIAC REHABILITATION

A comprehensive **cardiac rehabilitation program** should focus on improving longevity and quality of life,[46] in addition to risk factor modification to reduce mortality.[147,187] After diagnosis and intervention (e.g., aggressive risk factor reduction, bypass surgery, angioplasty), the exercise physiologist evaluates the cardiac patient for functional capacity and ensuing classification and rehabilitation.[48] TABLE 32.24 outlines functional and therapeutic classifications of heart disease from the New York Heart Association and guidelines for risk stratification from the AHA (www.americanheart.org) to categorize patients for subsequent rehabilitation. Patients differ greatly in symptoms, functional capacities, and rehabilitation strategies. The rehabilitation program incorporates stringent guidelines to promote low-risk treatment.[50,52,77,198] CHD patients with mild ischemia tolerate steady-rate exercise at intensities consistent for aerobic training without progressive deterioration in left ventricular function. For patients without ischemia, left ventricular function in prolonged exercise remains similar to healthy controls.[53] Five important aspects of a successful cardiac rehabilitation program include:

1. Appropriate patient selection
2. Concurrent medical, surgical, and pharmacologic therapies
3. Comprehensive patient education
4. Appropriate exercise prescription
5. Careful patient monitoring during rehabilitation

Traditional cardiac rehabilitation programs consist of three distinct phases with different objectives, physical activities, and required supervision. More contemporary programs have changed on the basis of new theories of risk stratification, exercise safety data, and changes in the health-care industry. Current programs recognize individual differences in rehabilitation when determining program length, degree of supervision, and required ECG monitoring.

Contemporary cardiac rehabilitation includes inpatient and outpatient programs and services, with emphasis on outcome measures. Almost all postsurgery patients benefit from inpatient exercise intervention, risk factor assessment, lifestyle activity and dietary counseling, and patient and family education. Patients stay at the hospital an average of 3 to 5 days postsurgery before release.

Inpatient Programs

Inpatient cardiac rehabilitation focuses on the following four objectives:

1. Medical surveillance
2. Identification of patients with significant impairments before discharge
3. Rapid patient return to daily activities
4. Preparation of patient and family to optimize recovery upon discharge

In-hospital physical activity during the first 48 hours following an MI and/or cardiac surgery is restricted to self-care movements, including arm and leg range of motion and intermittent sitting and standing to maintain cardiovascular reflexes. After several days, patients usually sit and stand without assistance, perform self-care activities, and walk independently up to six times daily, provided none of the following contraindications exist:

- Unstable angina
- Elevated resting blood pressure
- Orthostatic systolic blood pressure above 200 mm Hg with symptoms
- Critical aortic stenosis
- Acute systemic illness or fever
- Uncontrolled atrial or ventricular arrhythmias
- Uncontrolled sinus tachycardia above 120 b · min^{-1}
- Uncompensated CHF
- Active pericarditis or myocarditis
- Recent embolism or thrombophlebitis
- Resting S-T segment displacement of 2 mm or more
- Severe orthopedic conditions

Outpatient Programs

Upon discharge, the patient should know appropriate and inappropriate physical activities and dietary guidelines and have a prudent and progressive plan of risk reduction with specific exercise prescription. Enrollment in an outpa-

TABLE 32.23 ■ CARDIAC MEDICATIONS: THEIR USE, SIDE EFFECTS, AND EFFECTS ON EXERCISE RESPONSE

TYPE/TRADE NAME	USE	SIDE EFFECTS	EFFECTS ON EXERCISE RESPONSE
I. Antianginal agents			
A. Nitroglycerin compounds [*Amyl nitrate; Isordil; Nitrostat*]	Smooth muscle relaxation; decrease cardiac output	Headache, dizziness, hypotension	Hypotension; increase exercise capacity
B. β-Blockers [*Inderal; propranolol; Lopressor; Corgard; Biocadren*]	Block β receptors; decrease sympathetic tone; decrease HR, myocardial contractility, BP	Bradycardia, heart block, insomnia, weakness, nausea, fatigue, increased cholesterol and blood sugar	Decrease HR; hypotension; decrease cardiac contractility
C. Calcium antagonists [*Verapamil; nifedipine; Procardia*]	Block influx of calcium; dilate coronary arteries; suppress dysrhythmias	Dizziness, syncope, flushing, hypotension, headache, fluid retention	Hypotension
II. Antihypertensive agents			
A. Diuretics [*Thiazides, Lasix, Aldactone*]	Inhibit Na^+ and Cl^- in kidney; increase excretion of sodium and water, and control high BP and fluid retention	Drowsiness, dehydration, electrolyte imbalance; gout, nausea, pain, hearing loss, elevated cholesterol and lipoproteins	Hypotension
B. Vasodilators [*Hydralazine, Captopril, Apresoline, Loniten, Minoxidil*]	Dilate peripheral blood vessels; used in conjunction with diuretics; decrease BP	Increase HR and contractility; headache, drowsiness, nausea, vomiting, diarrhea	
C. Drugs interfering with sympathetic nervous system [*Reserpine, propranolol, Aldomet, Catapres, Minipress*]	Decrease BP, HR, and cardiac output by dilating blood vessels	Drowsiness, depression, sexual dysfunction, fatigue, dry mouth, stuffy nose, fever, upset stomach, fluid retention, weight gain	Hypotension
III. Digitalis glycosides, derivatives [*Digoxin, Lonoxin, digitoxin*]	Strengthen heart's pumping force and decrease electrical conduction	Arrhythmias, heart block, altered ECG, fatigue, weakness, headache, nausea, vomiting	Increase exercise capacity; increase myocardial contractility
IV. Anticoagulant agents [*Coumadin, sodium heparin, aspirin, Persantine*]	Prevent blood clot formation	Easy bruising, stomach irritation, joint or abdominal pain, difficulty swallowing, unexplained swelling, uncontrolled bleeding	
V. Antilipidemic agents [*Cholestyramine, Lopid, niacin, Atromid-S, Mevacor, Questran, Zocor, Lipitor*]	Interfere with lipid metabolism and lower cholesterol and low-density lipoproteins	Nausea, vomiting, diarrhea, constipation, flatulence, abdominal discomfort, glucose intolerance, myalgia, liver dysfunction, muscle fatigue	
VI. Antiarrhythmic agents [*Cardioquin, procaine, quinidine, lidocaine, Dilantin, propranolol, bretylium tosylate, verapamil*]	Alter conduction patterns throughout the myocardium	Nausea, palpitations, vomiting, rash, insomnia, dizziness, shortness of breath, swollen ankles, coughing up blood, fever, psychosis, impotence	Hypotension; decrease HR; decrease cardiac contractility

TABLE 32.24 ■ **A. FUNCTIONAL AND THERAPEUTIC CLASSIFICATIONS OF HEART DISEASE FROM THE NEW YORK HEART ASSOCIATION. B. GUIDELINES FOR RISK STRATIFICATION FROM THE AHA WHEN CONSIDERING AN EXERCISE PROGRAM**

A. NEW YORK HEART ASSOCIATION

Functional Capacity Classification

Class I: No limitation of physical activity. Ordinary physical activity does not cause undue fatigue, palpitation, dyspnea, or anginal pain

Class II: Slight limitation of physical activity. Comfortable at rest, but ordinary physical activity results in fatigue, palpitation, dyspnea, or anginal pain

Class III: Marked limitation of physical activity. Comfortable at rest, but less than ordinary activity causes fatigue, palpitation, dyspnea, or anginal pain

Class IV: Unable to carry on any physical activity without discomfort. Symptoms of cardiac insufficiency or of the anginal syndrome may be present even at rest; any physical activity increases discomfort

Therapeutic Classification

Class A: Physical activity need not be restricted

Class B: Ordinary physical activity need not be restricted, but unusually severe or competitive efforts should be avoided

Class C: Ordinary physical activity should be moderately restricted, and more strenous efforts should be discontinued

Class D: Ordinary physical activity should be markedly restricted

Class E: Patient should be at complete rest and confined to bed or chair

B. AMERICAN HEART ASSOCIATION

AHA CLASSIFICATION	NYHA[a] CLASS	EXERCISE CAPACITY	ANGINA/ISCHEMIA AND CLINICAL CHARACTERISTICS	ECG MONITORING
A. Apparently healthy			Less than 40 years of age; without symptoms, no major risk factors, and normal GXT	No supervision or monitoring required
B. Known stable CHD, low risk for vigorous exercise	I or II	5–6 METs	Free of ischemia or angina at rest or on the GXT; EF = 40 to 60%	Monitored and supervised only during prescribed sessions (6–12 sessions); light resistance training may be included in comprehensive rehabilitation programs
C. Stable CHD with low risk for vigorous exercise but unable to self-regulate activity	I or II	5–6 METs	Same disease states and clinical characteristics as class B but without the ability to self-monitor exercise	Medical supervision and ECG monitoring during prescribed sessions; nonmedical supervision of other exercise sessions
D. Moderate-to-high risk for cardiac complications during exercise	≥III	<6 METs	Ischemia (≥4.0 mm S-T depression) or angina during exercise; two or more previous MIs; EF < 30%	Continuous ECG monitoring during rehabilitation until safety established; medical supervision during all exercise sessions until safety established
E. Unstable disease with activity restriction	≥III	<6 METs	Unstable angina; uncompensated heart failure; uncomfortable arrhythmias	No activity recommended for conditioning purposes; attention directed to restoring patient to class D or higher

Adapted from American College of Sports Medicine. Guidelines for exercise testing and prescription. 6th ed. Baltimore: Williams & Wilkins, 2000.
[a]NYHA, New York Heart Association; EF, ejection fraction; CHD, coronary heart disease; GXT, graded exercise test.

tient exercise program is the ideal. Four goals for **outpatient cardiac rehabilitation** include:

1. Monitoring and supervising patient to detect changes in clinical status
2. Returning patient to premorbid/vocational/recreational activities
3. Assisting patient to implement at-home, unsupervised exercise program
4. Providing family support and education

Most outpatient program sites encourage multiple physical activities that include resistance exercise and walking, cycling, and swimming. Supervision should include personnel trained in CPR and advanced life support, and in some cases, home defibrillators.

REHABILITATION FOLLOWING HEART TRANSPLANTATION

Chapter 16 (Fig. 16.11) shows that cardiac transplantation improved peak oxygen consumption, which remained elevated for up to 9 years. Transplant patients generally respond positively to aerobic exercise training,[11,22,99] with some patients achieving exercise performance comparable to or even exceeding values of healthy subjects.[161] Debate concerns whether general improvements exceed those of coronary artery bypass surgery patients.[39,149] Generally, heart transplant recipients achieve 55 to 60% of predicted $\dot{V}O_{2max}$ during a GXT. In addition to improvements in $\dot{V}O_{2peak}$, training improves blood lactate kinetics. This lowers blood lactate concentration during exercise and recovery in part from improved lactate removal efficiency.[112] Graded exercise to fatigue does not pose an oxidative-stress risk to exercise-trained heart transplant patients despite immunosuppressive drug use.[93]

TABLE 32.25 summarizes a randomized, controlled prospective trial of exercise rehabilitation initiated shortly after heart transplantation.[103] Twenty-seven patients discharged within 2 weeks after receiving a heart transplant participated in either a 6-month structured cardiac rehabilita-

tion program or unstructured home therapy. Exercise consisted of a supervised indivualized resistance training and aerobic training (walking); control patients received no formal exercise training. All subjects received graded exercise testing within 1 month of heart transplantation (baseline) and 6 months later. Both groups improved functional capacity from baseline to 6-month follow-up. The exercise-trained group improved more than controls in $\dot{V}O_{2peak}$ (49% vs. 18%) and total work output (59% vs. 18%). From a practical perspective, transplant patients respond positively to regular exercise training and improve physical activity capacity.

Similar guidelines apply to training the transplant recipient and any postcardiac surgery patient.[95] However, training heart rate guidelines (see Chapter 21) do not apply to the transplant patient because of the blunted heart rate responses of a denervated transplanted organ (neural regulation of heart rate absent, hormonal regulation dominant; see Chapter 16). As an alternative, the RPE scale can gauge exercise intensity for ratings between "fairly light" to "somewhat hard" (RPE between 11 and 14). The inordinately slow heart rate response at the onset of exercise requires a longer, graded warm-up takes on added importance. The transplanted heart does not connect to the afferent nervous system so a patient with advanced CHD with a transplanted heart does not experience the painful warnings of exercise-induced angina pectoris.

TABLE 32.25 ■ **EFFECTS OF A SIX-MONTH CARDIAC REHABILITATION PROGRAM BEGUN WITHIN ONE MONTH AFTER HEART TRANSPLANTATION (BASELINE) ON CARDIOPULMONARY EXERCISE TEST RESULTS**

VARIABLE	EXERCISE GROUP (N = 14)			CONTROL GROUP (N = 13)		
	BASELINE	6 MONTHS	DIFFERENCE (% CHANGE)[a]	BASELINE	6 MONTHS	DIFFERENCE (% CHANGE)[a]
Peak oxygen consumption ($mL \cdot kg^{-1} \cdot min^{-1}$)	9.2	13.6	+4.4 (+49)	10.4	12.3	+1.9 (+18)
Workload (W)	59	94	+35 (+59)	66	78	+12 (+18)
Ventilatory equivalent for carbon dioxide ($\dot{V}E/\dot{V}CO_2$)	66	53	−13 (−20)	54	48	−6 (−11)
Ventilatory equivalent for oxygen ($\dot{V}E/\dot{V}O_2$)	79	67	−12 (−15)	64	60	−4 (−6)
Exercise duration (min)	6.9	9.0	+2.1 (+30)	7.2	8.3	+1.1 (+15)
Time to estimated lactate threshold (min)	1.8	3.3	+1.5 (83)	2.3	2.3	0
Resting heart rate ($b \cdot min^{-1}$)	90	100	+10 (11)	91	109	+18 (+20)
Peak heart rate ($b \cdot min^{-1}$)	102	125	+23 (+23)	107	134	+27 (+25)
Systolic blood pressure at rest (mm Hg)	126	121	−5 (−4)	130	114	−16 (−12)
Peak systolic blood pressure (mm Hg)	141	148	+7 (+5)	139	148	+9 (+6)
Minute ventilation ($L \cdot min^{-1}$)	38	45	+7 (+18)	46	62	+16 (+35)
Sitting-to-standing rate ($\# \cdot min^{-1}$)[b]	10.6	23.9	+13.3 (+125)	12.3	17.9	+5.6 (+46)

From Kobashigawa JA, et al. A controlled trial of exercise rehabilitation after heart transplantation. N Engl J Med 1999;340:272.
[a] Plus sign denotes increase, and minus sign, a decrease.
[b] The sitting-to-standing rate is the number of times per minute a patient could rise from a sitting position to a standing position.

Transplant Patients Experience Unique Benefits from Resistance Training

Chronic glucocorticoid therapy to combat tissue rejection causes muscle wasting, strength losses, and reduced bone mineral density and generally hinders a transplant patient's overall recovery and rehabilitation.[23,24] Steroid-induced muscle atrophy and weakness also affect lifestyle negatively. This includes the patient's recreational pursuits and range of occupational physical tasks. FIGURE 32.13 shows that a 6-month monitored resistance exercise program for major muscle groups slows the negative alterations in body composition from exogenous glucocorticoid therapy following transplantation.[26] Fourteen heart transplant patients were randomly assigned prior to surgery to either no exercise or resistance training that began 2 months after transplantation and immunosuppressive glucocorticoid therapy. Exercise training consisted of lumbar extensor exercise 1 day a week and upper- and lower-body resistance training 2 days weekly. Initial resistance set at 50% of 1-RM consisted of one set of 10 to 15 repetitions. Resistance increased 5 to 10% with completion of 15 repetitions. Fat mass increased and FFM decreased equally for both groups during glucocorticoid treatment following transplantation (Fig. 32.12A). Six months of resistance training restored FFM to higher levels than before transplantation, while the control group's FFM progressively decreased. Muscular strength increased for both groups during the posttransplant period (Fig.

32.12B), but improvements were four to six times greater for the training group. Additional research indicates that regular resistance exercise restores bone mineral density toward pretransplant levels despite continued immunosuppression with glucocorticoids.[25] Three recommendations help to sustain venous return and prevent blood pooling and accompanying hypotension in heart transplant patients during resistance training:[22]

1. Alternate between upper- and lower-body exercises during the workout
2. Walk for 2 minutes between exercises or perform standing calf raises
3. End each training session with a 5-minute, low-intensity cool-down walk

PULMONARY DISEASES

The clinical exercise physiologist's involvement in treating patients with pulmonary disease focuses on improving ventilatory capacity, decreasing the energy cost of breathing, and increasing overall level of physiologic function.[37] The personal history, physical examination, pertinent laboratory data, and imaging studies provide important background information. Cardiovascular system disorders almost always affect pulmonary function, which eventually leads to varying degrees of pulmonary disability. Conversely, pulmonary disease intimately relates to cardiovascular complications.

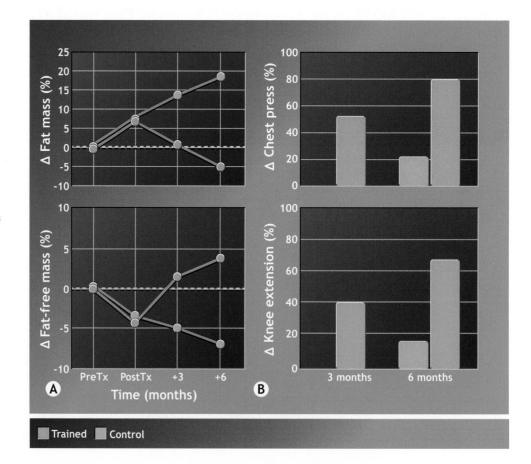

Figure 32.12 **A.** Changes (Δ) in fat mass and fat-free body mass (FFM) at 2 months posttransplantation and after 3 and 6 months of resistance exercise training or no training. Points represent average values for 14 heart transplant patients randomly assigned before surgery to a control group or resistance training.
B. Changes (Δ) in chest press strength and bilateral knee extension strength after 3 and 6 months of resistance exercise training or no training. The nontraining control group was not tested at 3 months. (From Braith RW, et al. Resistance exercise prevents glucocorticoid-induced myopathy in heart transplant recipients. Med Sci Sports Exerc 1998;30:483.)

Patients with pulmonary disease and disabilities often benefit from exercise rehabilitation. Pulmonary abnormalities classify as either obstructive (normal airflow impeded) or restrictive (lung volume dimensions reduced). Despite the convenience of this classification system, pulmonary disorders often reflect both restrictive and obstructive impairment.

Restrictive Lung Dysfunction

Abnormal reduction in pulmonary ventilation, along with diminished lung expansion, decreased tidal volume, and loss of functioning alveolar–capillary units, characterize a large and diverse group of pulmonary disorders collectively termed **restrictive lung disease**, or **RLD**.

The genesis of RLD involves pathophysiology of three aspects of pulmonary ventilation: (1) lung compliance, (2) lung volumes and capacities, and (3) work of breathing. **Lung compliance**, a measure of lung and/or chest wall distensibility, refers to the change in lung volume in relation to transpulmonary pressure differentials. In RLD, the chest and lung tissues stiffen and resist expansion under the normal pressure differentials of breathing. The additional resistance to lung expansion requires greater pulmonary force to maintain adequate alveolar ventilation. This increases the energy cost of normal ventilation and accounts for up to 50% of the total oxygen requirement during physical activity.[86] Eventually, the progression of RLD negatively affects all lung volumes and capacities. FIGURE 32.13 provides examples of typical lung volumes in different conditions associated with RLD. Diminished inspiratory and expiratory reserve volumes occur consistently under all conditions.

TABLE 32.26 lists major RLD conditions, along with their causes, signs and symptoms, and suggested treatments. Known causes of RLD include rheumatoid arthritis, immuno-logic pathology, massive obesity, diabetes mellitus, trauma from injury, penetrating wounds, radiation, burns, other inhalation injuries, poisoning, and complications from drug therapy (including reactions to antibiotics and antiinflammatory drugs).

Chronic Obstructive Pulmonary Disease

Chronic obstructive pulmonary disease (**COPD**), also termed *chronic airflow limitations* (*CAL*), comprises several respiratory tract diseases that obstruct airflow (e.g., emphysema, asthma, and chronic bronchitis). The disease destroys lung parenchyma, causing a mismatch between regional alveolar air and blood flow. This ultimately affects the lung's mechanical function to compromise gas exchange (ventilation:perfusion ratio) at the alveolar level. *A dramatic decrease in exercise tolerance almost always accompanies COPD.* The disease afflicts 15 to 25 million Americans and ranks as the fourth leading cause of death and second leading cause of morbidity in the United States. The natural history of COPD spans 20 to 50 years and closely parallels a history of chronic cigarette smoking. The Heart, Blood, and Lung Institute (NHBLI; www.nhlbi.nih.gov) projects that COPD will be the third leading cause of death by the year 2020. In 2001, the NHBLI reported 12.1 million U.S. adults 25 and older had COPD, with an additional 14 million or more still undiagnosed (or underdiagnosed; beginning stages with minimal symptoms without health care claims).

Changes in pulmonary function measures, most notably decreased expiratory flow rate and increased residual lung volume, usually form the diagnosis of COPD. The classic disease symptoms include spontaneous spasms of bronchial smooth muscle that produce chronic cough, increased mucus production, inflammation and thickening of the mucosal

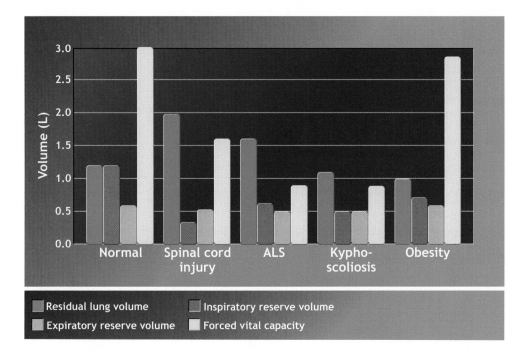

Figure 32.13 Values for lung volumes in different conditions that cause restrictive lung disease. *ALS,* amyotrophic lateral sclerosis.

TABLE 32.26 ■ **RESTRICTIVE LUNG DISEASES**^{a}

CAUSES/TYPE	ETIOLOGY	SIGNS AND SYMPTOMS	TREATMENT
I. Maturational			
a. Abnormal fetal lung development	Premature birth (hypoplasia-reduced lung tissue)	Asymptomatic; pulmonary insufficiency	No specific treatment
b. Respiratory distress syndrome (hyaline membrane disease)	Insufficient maturation of lungs due to premature birth	↑ Respiration rate; ↓ lung volumes; ↓ PaO₂; acidemia; rapid and labored respiration pressure	Treat mother prior to birth (corticosteroids); hyperalimentation; continuous positive airway
c. Aging	Aging and cumulative effects of pollution, noxious gas, inhaled drug use, and cigarette smoking	↑ Residual volume; ↓ vital capacity; repetitive periodic apnea	No specific treatment; increase physical activity
II. Pulmonary			
a. Idiopathic pulmonary fibrosis	Unknown origin (perhaps viral or genetic)	↓ Lung volumes; pulmonary hypertension; dyspnea; cough; weight loss, fatigue	Corticosteroids; maintain adequate nutrition and ventilation
b. Coal workers' pneumoconiosis	Repeated inhalation of coal dust over 10–12 years	↓ TLC, VC, FRC; ↓ lung compliance; dyspnea; ↓ PaO₂; pulmonary hypertension; cough	Nonreversible, no known cure
c. Asbestosis	Long-term exposure to asbestos	↓ Lung volumes; abnormal x-ray; ↓ PaO₂; dyspnea on exertion, shortness of breath	Nonreversible, no known cure
d. Pneumonia	Inflammatory process caused by various bacteria microbes, viruses	↓ Lung volumes; abnormal x-ray; tachypneic dyspnea; high fever, chills, cough; pleuritic pain	Drug therapy (antibiotic)
e. Adult respiratory distress syndrome	Acute lung injury (fat emboli, drowning, drug-induced, shock, blood transfusion, pneumonia)	Abnormal lung function tests; PaO₂ <60 mm Hg; extreme dyspnea; cyanotic; headache; anxiety	Intubation and mechanical ventilation
f. Bronchogenic carcinoma	Tobacco use	Variable, depending on type and location of growth	Surgery, radiation, chemotherapy; specific drainage
g. Pleural effusions	Accumulation of fluid within pleural space; heart failure; cirrhosis	Shortness of breath; pleuritic chest pain; ↓ PaO₂	
III. Cardiovascular			
a. Pulmonary edema	↑ Pulmonary capillary hydrostatic pressure secondary to left ventricular failure	↑ Respiration rate; ↓ lung volumes; ↓ PaO₂; arrhythmias; report feelings of suffocation, shortness of breath, cyanotic, cough	Drug therapy, diuretics; supplemental oxygen
b. Pulmonary emboli	Complications of venous thrombosis	↓ Lung volumes; ↓ PaO₂; tachycardia; acute dyspnea, shortness of breath; syncope	Heparin therapy; mechanical ventilation
IV. Neuromuscular			
a. Spinal cord injury	Trauma paralysis of respiratory muscle	↓ Lung volumes; hypoxemia; fatigue; shortness of breath; inability to cough; ↓ voice volume	Active and passive chest wall stretching
b. Amyotrophic lateral sclerosis	Degenerative disease of nervous system	↓ Lung volumes; ↓ maximum voluntary volume	No treatment except supportive therapy
c. Poliomyelitis	Viral infectious disease that attacks motor nerves	Paralysis of diaphragm; shortness of breath	No treatment except supportive therapy
d. Guillain-Barré syndrome	Demyelinating disease of motor neurons	Profound muscular weakness; ↓ lung volumes	Passive range-of-motion exercises; active exercise
e. Neuromuscular diseases (myasthenia gravis, tetanus, muscular dystrophy)	Diseases of neuromuscular system, genetic or other cause resulting in chronic muscular weakness and wasting	Weakness, fatigue, loss of muscle function and strength, paralysis affects pulmonary system with eventual loss of function	Drugs; passive and active exercise; supportive therapy

continued on page 965

TABLE 32.26 ■ *continued*

CAUSES/TYPE	ETIOLOGY	SIGNS AND SYMPTOMS	TREATMENT
V. Musculoskeletal			
a. *Diaphragmatic paralysis*	Loss or impairment of motor function of diaphragm muscle due to specific lesion	↓ Lung volumes; dyspnea, shortness of breath	Not needed
b. *Kyphoscoliosis*	Excessive anteroposterior and lateral curvature of thoracic spine (cause unknown)	↓ Lung volumes; exertional dyspnea	Use of orthotic devices; active exercise
c. *Ankylosing spondylitis*	Chronic inflammatory disease of spine (inherited)	Exertional dyspnea	No treatment

ªwww.nlm.nih.gov/medlineplus/; www.cvm.msu.edu/RESEARCH/PULMON/site/respiratory_diseases/diseases/Heaves/mainFrame.html

lining of the bronchi and bronchioles, wheezing, and dyspnea upon exertion. TABLE 32.27 summarizes differences in anatomic location and pathology among major COPD conditions. Factors predisposing to COPD include chronic cigarette smoking (greater effect in women than men; particularly on the increase among college students[171]), air pollution, occupational exposure to irritating dusts or gases, heredity, infection, allergies, aging, and drugs. *COPD rarely occurs in nonsmokers*. The airways narrow to obstruct pulmonary airflow in all forms of COPD. Airway narrowing hinders ventilation by trapping air in the bronchioles and alveoli; in essence, the disease increases pulmonary physiologic dead space. The obstruction also increases resistance to airflow (chiefly in expiration), hinders normal gas exchange, and reduces exercise performance by increasing the energy cost of breathing. The latter reduces ventilatory capacity to hinder full arterial oxygen saturation and carbon dioxide elimination. Patients with severe COPD exhibit decreased whole-body mechanical efficiency during exercise.[166] This suggests that factors associated with the respiratory effort also magnify the energy requirements of whole-body exercise to further negatively impact exercise capacity.

Interestingly, poor exercise tolerance and early onset of lactate accumulation in COPD patients do not always link closely to limitations in pulmonary ventilation and gas exchange during exercise. Rather, peripheral skeletal muscle performance deteriorates in COPD reflected by decreased muscle mass and strength, and reduced skeletal muscle oxidative capacity from marked decrease in type I and increase in type IIb muscle fiber proportions and reduced mitochondrial enzyme activities. Detraining with a sedentary lifestyle probably accounts for the loss of peripheral function.[121,122] Exercise intervention can sometimes reverse peripheral abnormalities associated with COPD.[204]

The following sections focus on the major COPD diseases—chronic bronchitis, emphysema, cystic fibrosis, and exercise-induced bronchospasm (asthma).

Chronic Bronchitis

Acute bronchitis, an inflammation of the trachea and bronchi, usually is self-limiting and of short duration. In contrast, prolonged exposure to nonspecific irritants produces **chronic bronchitis**. Over time, the swollen mucous membranes and increased mucus production obstruct airways, causing wheezing and chronic coughing. Partial or complete airway blockage from mucus secretion produces inadequate arterial oxygen saturation, diminished carbon

TABLE 32.27 ■ DIFFERENCES AMONG MAJOR COPD DISEASES

NAME	AREA AFFECTED	RESULT
Bronchitis	Membrane lining bronchial tubes	Inflammation of bronchial lining
Bronchiectasis	Bronchial tubes (bronchi or air passages)	Breakdown of alveolar walls; air spaces enlarged
Emphysema	Air spaces beyond terminal bronchioles (alveoli)	Bronchial dilation with inflammation
Asthma	Bronchioles (small airways)	Bronchioles obstructed by muscle spasm; swelling of mucosa; thick secretions
Cystic fibrosis	Bronchioles	Bronchioles become obstructed and obliterated; plugs of mucus cling to airway walls, leading to bronchitis, atelectasis, pneumonia, or pulmonary abscess

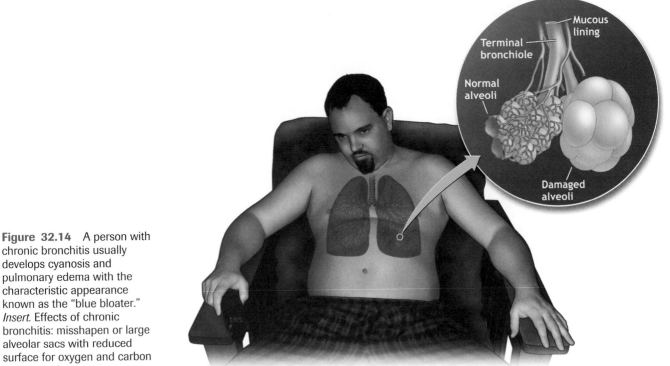

Figure 32.14 A person with chronic bronchitis usually develops cyanosis and pulmonary edema with the characteristic appearance known as the "blue bloater." *Insert.* Effects of chronic bronchitis: misshapen or large alveolar sacs with reduced surface for oxygen and carbon dioxide exchange.

dioxide elimination, and pulmonary edema. Eventually, the patient develops the characteristic look of a "blue bloater" (FIG. 32.14). Chronic bronchitis develops slowly and worsens over time. Patients usually have a history of cigarette smoking for decades. Functional capacity decreases considerably, and fatigue occurs readily with mild exercise. If left untreated, this disease leads to premature death.

Emphysema

An abnormal, permanent enlargement of air spaces distal to the terminal bronchioles characterizes **emphysema**. The disease occurs most frequently among chronic cigarette smokers. It develops as a consequence of chronic bronchitis; its symptoms include dyspnea, hypercapnea, persistent cough, cyanosis, and digital clubbing (evidence of chronic hypoxemia; FIG. 32.15). Emphysemic patients consistently demonstrate low exercise capacity and extreme dyspnea with exertion; patients appear thin and often lean forward with arms braced on the knees to support the shoulders and chest to ease breathing. The chronic effects of trapped air and alveolar distension change the size and shape of the chest, causing the characteristic emphysemic "barrel chest" appearance (FIG. 32.16). Regular exercise does not improve pulmonary function of individuals with emphysema, but it enhances cardiovascular fitness, strengthens both respiratory and nonrespiratory musculature, and improves psychologic status.[16,29] In selected patients with severe emphysema, lung-volume reduction surgery has improved pulmonary function, exercise capacity, and quality of life. Its effects on longevity remain uncertain.[64]

Cystic Fibrosis

The term **cystic fibrosis** (**CF**; www.cff.org) originates from the diagnosis of cysts and scar tissue observed on the pancreas during autopsy. Pancreatic cysts and scar tissue often exist but do not reflect the primary characteristics of the dis-

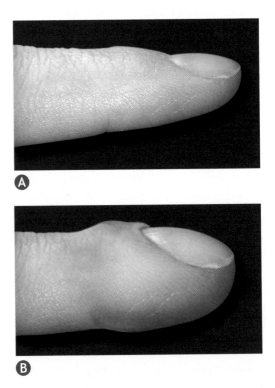

Figure 32.15 Normal digit configuration (**A**) and digital clubbing (**B**). Club fingers and toes indicate chronic tissue hypoxia, a common diagnosis in emphysema.

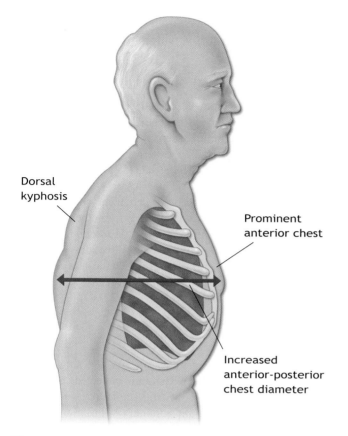

Dorsal
kyphosis

Prominent
anterior chest

Increased
anterior-posterior
chest diameter

Figure 32.16 Emphysema traps air in the lungs, making exhalation difficult. With time, changes occur in the physical features of the patient, hence the name "pink puffer."

TABLE 32.28 ■ CLINICAL SIGNS AND SYMPTOMS OF CYSTIC FIBROSIS AND RELATED PULMONARY INVOLVEMENT
Early stage clinical signs and symptoms of cystic fibrosis   • Persistent cough and wheezing   • Recurrent pneumonia   • Excessive appetite but poor weight gain   • Salty skin or sweat   • Bulky, foul-smelling stools (undigested lipids)
Late stage clinical signs and symptoms of cystic fibrosis with pulmonary involvement   • Tachypnea (rapid breathing)   • Sustained chronic cough with mucus production on vomiting   • Barrel chest   • Cyanosis and digital clubbing   • Exertional dyspnea with decreased exercise capacity   • Pneumothorax   • Right heart failure secondary to pulmonary hypertension

ease.[151] TABLE 32.28 lists clinical signs and symptoms of this inherited and always fatal disease characterized by thickening secretions of all exocrine glands (e.g., pancreatic, pulmonic, gastrointestinal). Glandular secretions ultimately lead to pulmonary obstruction, mainly in lung tissue. CF, the most common inherited disease (both parents must carry the recessive trait) in whites, afflicts approximately 1 in 2000 infants in the United States. Approximately 5% (12 million) of Americans carry the gene for CF located on chromosome 7, first identified in 1985. CF currently afflicts about 30,000 children and adults in the United States.

A positive sweat electrolyte (chloride) test result diagnoses CF. Patients possess a faulty copy of the gene that allows cells to construct a channel for the passage of chloride ions. Consequently, salt accumulates in the cells that line the lungs and digestive tissues making the surrounding mucus thicker and salty. These mucous secretions, the critical feature of CF, obstruct ducts and passages in the pancreas, liver, and lungs.

Pulmonary impairment represents the most common and severe manifestation of CF. Airway obstruction leads to chronic lung hyperinflation. Over time, RLD superimposes on the obstructive disease that leads to chronic hypoxia, hypercapnia, and acidosis. These three maladies increase the risk of arterial desaturation during exercise. The disease progresses to pneumothorax and pulmonary hypertension and eventually death.

Treatment of CF includes antibiotics, the FDA-approved mucus-thinning drug Pulmozyme, TOBI (tobramycin) solution

for inhalation, high dosages of ibuprofen, enzyme supplements, nutritional intervention, and frequent mucous secretion removal. Assessments of physical capacity of children with CF suggest a positive role for regular physical activity. For example, aerobic fitness correlates inversely with 8-year mortality.[143] The anaerobic power of children with CF is lower than healthy counterparts, although CF patient rely more on anaerobic pathways during strenuous exercise.[20,21] The kinetics of oxygen uptake slow in cystic fibrosis patients.[80] Increased minute ventilation with aerobic exercise helps to clear airways of excessive secretions.[177,210] For example, 20 to 30 minutes of aerobic exercise replaces one session of secretion removal for some children. Thus, increasing physical fitness can delay CF's crippling effects. An abnormally high NaCl loss in the sweat increases the likelihood of plasma hypoosmolality with a concomitant reduction in thirst drive. A flavored drink with relatively high salt content (e.g., 50 mmol $\cdot$ L^{-1}) enhances drinking and reduces exercise dehydration risk in CF patients.[108]

Pulmonary Assessments

Exercise physiologists do not diagnose pulmonary disease, but understanding the different tests and their results assists in planning and implementing exercise interventions. Pulmonary disease diagnosis involves several different objective measures that include chest imaging, flow and volume tests, blood gas analyses, and cytologic and hematologic evaluations.

X-Ray

Chest and lung imaging are the most popular pulmonary assessment techniques. These include the conventional x-ray in which roentgen rays (named after German physicist and

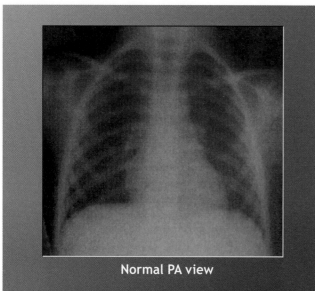

Normal PA view

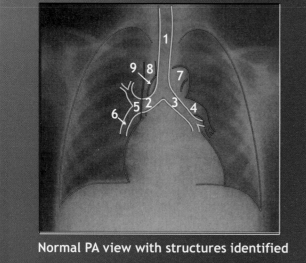

Normal PA view with structures identified

Figure 32.17   Chest x-ray. The *top* radiograph shows a normal chest x-ray in the posteroanterior (PA) view. The *bottom* radiograph shows labeling of the normal anatomic structures. *1,* trachea; *2,* right mainstem bronchus; *3,* left mainstem bronchus; *4,* left pulmonary artery; *5,* pulmonary vein to the right upper lobe; *6,* right interlobular artery; *7,* aortic knob; *8,* superior vena cava; *9,* ascending aorta.

1901 Nobel laureate in physics Wilhelm Konrad Roentgen [1845–1923]) penetrate the body to provide an image of the chest's anatomy on film (radiograph or roentgenogram). This standard diagnostic tool screens for abnormalities, provides a baseline for subsequent assessments, and monitors disease progression. A chest radiograph shows body fat, water, tissue, bone, and air space. The low density of air in the lungs allows greater roentgen ray penetration, which produces a dark image. Relatively dense bone represents the other extreme; it allows fewer roentgen rays to penetrate its tissue, thus producing a white image. The *top* of FIGURE 32.17 illustrates a normal chest radiograph taken in the posteroanterior (PA) position. The *bottom* of the figure shows the same radiograph

with the normal anatomic structures labeled. Abnormal radiographic densities identify specific lung lesions.

Computed Tomography

Most clinical radiologists consider computed tomography (CT) scanning, invented in 1972, the single greatest advance in radiography of anatomic structures since the discovery of roentgen rays (1979 Nobel Prizes were awarded in Physiology or Medicine to Godfrey N. Hounsfield [1919–2004] and Allan M. Cormack [1924–1998]). CT uses a narrow x-ray beam that moves across the body to define adjacent cross-sectional columns of tissue known as a *translation.* Another pass of the beam progresses at a different angle or *rotation.* Repeated translations and rotations in different directions in a given plane with subsequent digitization produces a clear computer-summated image of x-ray transmission data for diagnostic interpretation.

Other Measures

Chapter 12 discusses static and dynamic lung function tests with simple spirometry. Carefully collected spirometric forced vital capacity (FVC), forced expiratory volume in 1 second ($FEV_{1.0}$), maximum voluntary ventilation (MVV), peak expiratory flow (PEF), and lung compliance provide crucial diagnostic information. To measure compliance, the patient swallows a balloon catheter. The technician positions the catheter in the lower third of the esophagus and connects it to a manometer to measure esophageal pressure. The relation of lung volume change to any change in pressure within the catheter then establishes the curve for lung compliance.

Other useful functional tests include pulmonary diffusing capacity (DL or DLCO, expressed in mL $\cdot$ min^{-1} $\cdot$ mm Hg^{-1}), which measures how much gas enters pulmonary blood per unit time per unit pressure differential across the alveolar–capillary membrane. Flow-volume loops provide graphic representations of events occurring during forced inspiration and expiration. Recording the flow versus volume in an X–Y presentation diagnoses central or peripheral airway obstructions.

Blood gas analyses provide important information to assess problems related to acid–base balance, alveolar ventilation, and level of arterial oxygen saturation and carbon dioxide elimination. Cytologic and hematologic tests identify microorganisms that cause pulmonary disease.

Pulmonary Rehabilitation and Exercise Prescription

Pulmonary rehabilitation programs receive considerably less attention than programs for cardiovascular and musculoskeletal diseases. The lack of emphasis on pulmonary rehabilitation stems from a failure of rehabilitation to improve pulmonary function significantly or "cure" these potentially deadly diseases. Nevertheless, successful pulmonary rehabilitation places central focus on exercise training because of its positive impact on exercise capacity, respiratory and nonrespiratory muscle functions, ventilatory equivalents for oxygen, psychologic status, quality-of-life variables (e.g., self-esteem and self-efficacy), frequency of hospitalization, and disease progression.[16,33] The spiral of progressive physical deconditioning from a sedentary lifestyle (as patients attempt to avoid dyspnea) is not *just* the direct effect of COPD.[29,164,185] Peripheral and respiratory muscle weakness frequently contribute to the COPD patients' poor exercise performance and physiologic incapacity.[78,184] Within this framework, the major goals for pulmonary rehabilitation include:

- Improving health status
- Improving respiratory symptoms (shortness of breath and cough)
- Recognizing early signs that require medical intervention
- Decreasing frequency and severity of respiratory problems

TABLE 32.29 ■ COMPONENTS OF THE COPD EXERCISE PRESCRIPTION

Evaluation
- Assess cardiac risk
- Assess exercise capacity with Naughton-type protocol (see Fig. 11.10) using a treadmill or stationary cycle, starting at a low workload and increasing slowly, and monitoring desaturation with pulse oximeter
- Determine appropriate exercise levels to prevent arrhythmias or hypoxia in cardiac-impaired patients
- Determine amount of supplemental oxygen needed during exercise
- Determine need for bronchodilators during exercise
- Assess side effects of β-agonist inhalers or aminophylline derivatives during exercise

Supervised exercise
- Direct patient to supervised rehabilitation if disease is significant
- Set goal of eventually graduating to independent exercise (many patients can do this in about 6 weeks)

Independent exercise
- Suggest appropriate training mode: stationary cycling, bicycling, treadmill walking, outdoor walking, stair climbing, or arm ergometry
- Set goal of 60 to 80% of HR_{max} for 20 to 30 minutes, 3 days per week (build on individual ability)
- Expect 70 to 80% increase over initial work capacity within 6 weeks
- Provide active encouragement and reassurance (especially at first) to overcome anxiety associated with dyspnea

Exercise aids
- Supplemental oxygen
- Bronchodilators (adrenergic agonists and/or aminophylline derivatives)
- Mucolytics
- Corticosteroids (inhaled or oral)
- Monitoring

From Mink BD. Exercise and chronic obstructive pulmonary disease: modest fitness gains pay big dividends. Phys Sportsmed 1997;25(11):43.

- Maximizing arterial oxygen saturation and carbon dioxide elimination
- Enhancing daily functional capacity through improved muscular strength, joint flexibility, and cardiorespiratory endurance
- Modifying body composition to enhance functional capacity
- Optimizing nutritional status

The overall pulmonary rehabilitation program emphasizes general patient care, pulmonary respiratory care, exercise and functional training, education about the disease, and psychosocial management. Table 32.29 outlines the important components of an exercise prescription for COPD patients. The training aspects of rehabilitation take on importance for patients with weakness, fatigue, and severe dyspnea that profoundly limit physical activity. Physiologic monitoring during exercise rehabilitation includes measurement of heart rate, blood pressure, respiratory rate, arterial oxygen saturation by pulse oximetry, and dyspnea. Dyspnea monitoring as a target for exercise training involves a perceived **dyspnea scale** (FIG. 32.18) similar to the ratings of perceived exertion scale.[55,85] The dyspnea scale emphasizes symptoms of breathing difficulty rather than perceptions of whole-body physical distress, which the RPE measures. Self-monitoring exercise intensity in this manner has two inherent advantages because (1) respiratory disease usually impairs exercise pulmonary function rather than cardiovascular response and (2) target heart rate for training healthy individuals usually exceeds the peak heart rate achieved when stress testing pulmonary patients. The most common reasons for

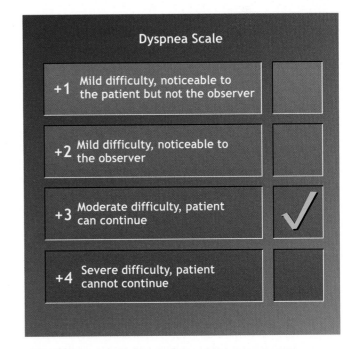

Figure 32.18 Dyspnea scale. Subjective ratings of dyspnea on a scale of 1 to 4 during graded exercise testing. Dyspnea usually accompanies poor exercise capacity and an impaired systolic blood pressure response.

stopping exercise include extreme shortness of breath, fatigue, palpitations, chest discomfort, and a 3 to 5% decrease in pulse oximetry.

The pretraining GXT and spirometric analyses form the basis for the exercise prescription.[41] Interpretation of the exercise stress test includes determining the following:

1. Whether the test terminated because of cardiovascular or ventilatory end points
2. The difference between pre- and postexercise pulmonary function (e.g., a decrease of 10% in $FEV_{1.0}$ indicates the need for bronchodilator therapy before exercise)
3. Need for supplemental oxygen during exercise (e.g., a pre- to posttest decrease in PaO_2 of more than 20 mm Hg or a PaO_2 below 55 mm Hg)

Exercise prescription (cycling, walking, treadmill exercise, and stair climbing) for patients with **mild lung disease**—shortness of breath with intense exercise—remains similar to requirements for healthy subjects. Exercise for patients with **moderate lung disease**—shortness of breath with normal daily activities or clinical symptoms of RLD or COPD—typically achieves an intensity no greater than 75% of the ventilatory reserve or the point where the patient becomes noticeably dyspneic. For most patients, this exercise intensity usually falls in the middle of the calculated training heart rate range—50–70% of age-predicted maximum with a goal of 60–80% of maximum—and corresponds to 40 to 85% of maximum MET level on the GXT. In this case, exercise duration averages 20 minutes, 3 times weekly. If the patient can exercise only for a shorter duration (e.g., 5–15 min per session), exercise frequency can increase to 5 to 7 days weekly.

Patients with **severe lung disease**—shortness of breath during most daily activities and FVC and $FEV_{1.0}$ below 55% of predicted values—require a modified approach to exercise testing and prescription. Low-level, discontinuous testing usually begins at 2 to 3 METs with increments every 2 to 3 minutes. Exercise prescription relies on symptom-limited walking speeds and distances. Brief bouts of interval exercise also provide an option. The low level of the initial training prescription means that patients should exercise a minimum of once daily. Even small gains in exercise tolerance add to improving daily function and quality of life.

General exercise and specific expiratory muscle training effectively improve respiratory muscle function and reduce sensations of respiratory effort during exercise in nearly all patients with pulmonary disease.[32,110,193] Two approaches achieve this goal:

1. Resistance training of the ventilatory musculature with a continuous positive airway pressure (CPAP) device; this specifically overloads the respiratory muscles similarly to progressive resistance exercise for nonrespiratory skeletal muscles
2. Increasing respiratory muscle force and endurance capacity through regular aerobic exercise training

INTEGRATIVE QUESTION

Why might regular exercise prove more effective for coronary heart disease patients than patients with pulmonary disease?

Pulmonary Medications

Pulmonary medications include bronchodilators, antiinflammatory agents, decongestants, antihistamines, mucokinetic agents, respiratory stimulants, depressants, and paralyzing and antimicrobial agents. The drugs promote bronchodilation, facilitate removal of lung secretions, improve alveolar ventilation and arterial oxygenation, and optimize breathing patterns. TABLE 32.30 lists the most commonly administered pulmonary drugs.

EXERCISE AND ASTHMA

Asthma Statistics

The latest available statistics indicate that asthma has increased in severity and scope (www.aafa.org).[9,192] Hyperirritability of the pulmonary airways followed by bronchial spasm, edema, and mucus secretion characterize this obstructive pulmonary disease (FIG. 32.19). Common asthma symptoms include chest tightness, coughing, wheezing, and/or shortness of breath.

A high level of physical fitness does not confer immunity from asthma.[145,200] U.S. women's basketball player Tamika Catchings, an asthma sufferer, won a gold medal in the 2004 Olympic games, and 21% of British athletes in these games were confirmed asthmatics. Studies of Finnish elite track and field athletes report physician-diagnosed asthma in 17% of long-distance runners, 8% of power athletes, and 3% of nonathletic controls,[81] while 35% of figure skaters showed a significant increase in airway resistance following skating routines.[123]

For nearly 90% of persons with asthma and 30 to 50% of those suffering from allergic rhinitis and hay fever, exercise provides a potent stimulus for bronchoconstriction termed **exercise-induced bronchospasm**. Reduced vagal tone and increased catecholamine release from the sympathetic nervous system during exercise *normally* relax pulmonary airway smooth muscle.[14,119,189] Figure 32.19A shows that initial bronchodilation with exercise occurs in healthy persons and asthmatics. For the asthmatic, bronchospasm accompanied by excessive mucus secretion follow initial bronchodilation. An acute episode of airway obstruction often occurs within 5 to 15 minutes postexercise (Fig. 32.19B); recovery usually occurs spontaneously within 30 to 90 minutes. One useful technique to detect an exercise-induced asthmatic response applies progressive exercise increments. A spirometric evaluation of FVC and $FEV_{1.0}$ takes place after each exercise period and during 10 to 20 minutes of recovery. *A 10 to 15% reduction in preexercise $FEV_{1.0}/FVC$ confirms the diagnosis of exercise-induced bronchospasm.*[84,109,131] For elite athletes who perform in

TABLE 32.30 ■ MAJOR PULMONARY BRONCHODILATOR DRUGS: THEIR USES AND SIDE EFFECTS

DRUG/NAME	ACTION AND CLINICAL USES	SIDE EFFECTS
Sympathomimetics Isoproterenol, ephedrine, Bronkosol, Alupent, Brethine, Proventil, Ventolin (Albuterol inhaler)	Decrease intracellular calcium; smooth muscle relaxation; bronchodilation	Tachycardia, palpitations, GI distress, nervousness, headache, dizzines
Methylxanthines Amnodur, Elixophyllin, Theo-dur, Choladril	Increase cAMP; block cAMP decrease	Agitation, hypotension, chest pain, nausea, tachycardia, palpitations, GI distress, nervousness, headache, dizziness
α-Sympatholytics	Block cAMP decrease; bronchodilation	Agitation, hypotension, chest pain, nausea, tachycardia, palpitations, GI distress, nervousness, headache, dizziness
Parasympatholytics Atrovent, atropine sulfate	Block parasympathetic stimulation and prevents increases in cGMP; prevents bronchoconstriction	Central nervous system stimulation with low doses and depression with high doses; delirium, hallucinations, decreased GI activity
Glucocorticoids Prednisone, Cortisol, Azmacort, Vanceril	Decrease inflammatory response; bronchodilation	Obesity, growth suppression, hyperglycemia and diabetes, mood changes, irritability or depression, thinning of skin, muscle wasting
Cromolyn sodium Intal, Fivent	Prevents influx of calcium ions, thus blocking mast cell release of mediators responsible for bronchoconstriction; bronchodilation	Throat irritation, hoarseness, dry mouth, cough, chest tightness, bronchospasm

cold-weather sports (e.g., biathlon, canoe/kayak, cross-country skiing, ice hockey, Nordic combined, and speed skating), combining pulmonary function testing with near-maximal sport-specific exercise testing, preferably in a cold, dry environment, provides greater sensitivity for screening than laboratory-based (warm air environment) challenges[174] or self-reported symptoms.[175]

Sensitivity to Thermal Gradients and Fluid Loss

Several mechanisms help to explain bronchospastic responses to exercise.[7,65,199] An attractive theory relates to how ventilation in exercise and recovery alters the rate and magnitude of heat and water exchange in the tracheobronchial tree. As the incoming breath of air moves down the respiratory tract, heat and water move away from the airway lining as the air warms and humidifies. The conditioning of inspired air ultimately cools and dries the respiratory mucosa. Drying increases mucosal lining osmolality with accompanying mast cell degranulation. This in turn releases powerful proinflammatory mediators that trigger bronchoconstriction (e.g., leukotrienes, histamine, and prostaglandins).[116] Rewarming the airways following exercise dilates the bronchial microcirculation to increases blood flow. Bronchial vasculature engorgement precipitates edema that constricts the airway, independent of any constrictive action of bronchial smooth muscle. Bronchial cooling during exercise and rewarming in recovery also stimulate chemical mediator release that induces bronchoconstriction.

Regardless of the precise mechanism, the large volume of incompletely conditioned inspired air taxes the tracheobronchial tree's smaller airways, causing mucosal temperature to decrease. Heat loss from the airways during exercise relates directly to the degree of bronchoconstriction. In susceptible individuals, the thermal gradient generated by the combination of airway cooling during exercise and subsequent rewarming in recovery intensifies bronchospastic processes.

Environmental Impact

Figure 32.19C shows that a warm–humid (summer) environment suppresses the magnitude of exercise-induced bronchospasm regardless of air temperature.[12,131] Inhaling ambient air fully saturated with water vapor often abolishes an asthmatic's bronchospastic exercise response. This explains why persons with asthma tolerate walking or jogging on a warm, humid day or swimming in an indoor pool, in contrast to outdoor winter sports that typically trigger an asthmatic attack.[90,178]

Benefits of Warm-Up and Medication

Fifteen to 30 minutes of a light-to-moderate, continuous warm-up or repeat several-minute warm-up intervals initiate a **refractory period** where subsequent intense exercise does not trigger as severe a bronchoconstrictive response.[14,17,165] The warm-up benefit continues for up to 2 hours, perhaps from prostaglandin release. Prolonging the cool-down period also reduces the severity of postexercise bronchoconstriction; this could occur by slowing airway rewarming and subsequent bronchiole vascular dilation and edema.

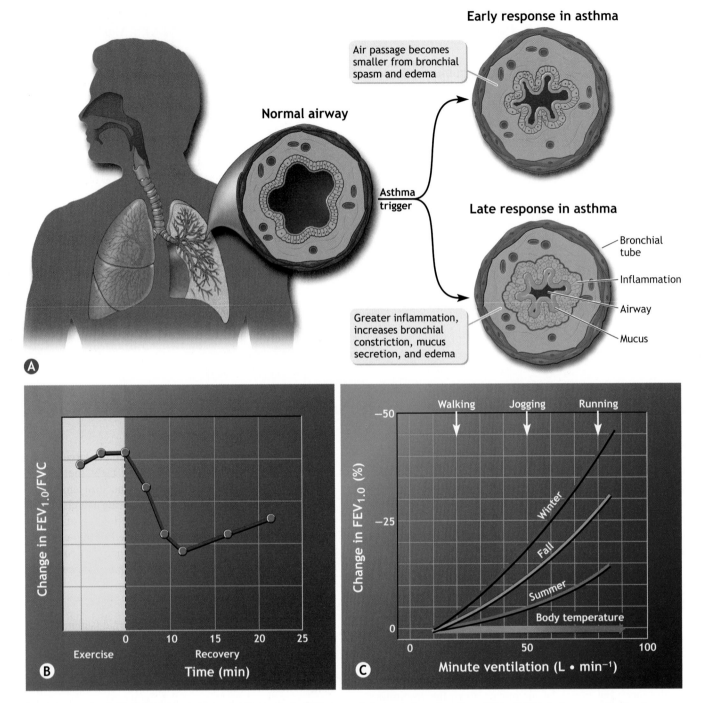

Figure 32.19 **A.** Typical response to an asthma attack. **B.** Pattern of dynamic lung function *(FEV$_{1.0}$/FVC)* during an episode of exercise-induced bronchospasm. **C.** Interaction between exercise intensity (walking, jogging, running) and environmental characteristics. Note that maximal obstruction occurs when inhaling dry air at low temperature (e.g., winter) and minimal obstruction occurs when breathing warm, humid air (e.g., summer). (*C.* modified from McFadden ER Jr, Gilbert IA. Current concepts in exercise-induced asthma. N Engl J Med 1994;330:1362.)

Effective preexercise medications limit bronchoconstriction for those desiring to exercise regularly without adversely affecting exercise performance.[89,111,146] Medications include (1) bronchodilators such as theophylline or the leukotriene-receptor antagonist montelukast[44,116,167] or β$_2$-agonists (salmeterol)[139] and (2) inhaled heparin therapy or antiinflammatory corticosteroids or cromolyn sodium.

Exercise training does not eliminate or cure an asthmatic condition; instead, it increases pulmonary airflow reserve and reduces ventilatory work by potentiating exercise bronchodilation. This lets asthmatics maintain higher airflow and sustain relatively intense exercise despite impaired pulmonary function. For asthmatic children, aerobic exercise training (swimming and cycle ergometry) improves $\dot{V}O_{2max}$ and suppresses asthmatic symptoms.[126,138]

NEUROMUSCULAR DISEASES, DISABILITIES, AND DISORDERS

Neuromuscular diseases and disabilities affect the brain in specific ways. Progressive degeneration or trauma to specific brain neurons induces distinct impairment that ranges from simple to complex. The economic costs of brain dysfunction are enormous but pale in comparison with the staggering emotional toll on victims and their families (www.mdausa.org/index.html).

Stroke

Stroke refers to a potentially fatal reduction in the brain's blood flow from restricted blood flow (ischemia) or bleeding (hemorrhage). The resulting brain injury affects multiple systems depending on injury site and amount of damage sustained. Effects include motor and sensory impairment and language, perception, and affective and cognitive dysfunction. Strokes cause severe limitations in mobility and cognition or can be less severe with short-term, nonpermanent consequences (www.strokeassociation.org/presenter.jhtml?identifier=1200037).

Clinical Features

Clinical features of stroke depend on location and severity of injury. Signs of a hemorrhagic stroke include altered levels of consciousness, severe headache, and elevated blood pressure. Cerebellar hemorrhage usually occurs unilaterally and associates with disequilibrium, nausea, and vomiting. TABLE 32.31 presents the typical physical and psychologic conditions and comorbidities associated with a stroke.

Cerebral blood flow (CBF) represents the primary marker to assess ischemic strokes. When CBF drops below 10 mL · 100 g · min^{-1} of brain tissue (normal CBF = 50–55 mL · 100 g · min^{-1}) synaptic transmission failure occurs; cell death results at a CBF of ≤8 mL · 100 g · min^{-1}).

Stroke produces physical and cognitive damage. Left-hemisphere lesions typically associate with expressive and receptive language deficits compared with right-hemisphere lesions. Motor impairment from a stroke usually triggers hemiplegia (paralysis) or hemiparesis (weakness). Damage to descending neural pathways produces abnormal regulation of spinal motor neurons. This adversely changes postural and stretch reflexes and produces difficulty with voluntary movement. Deficits in motor control involve muscle weakness, abnormal synergistic organization of movement, impaired regulation of force, decreased reaction times, abnormal muscle tone, and loss of active range of joint motion.

Exercise Prescription

The emphasis for stroke survivors centers on rehabilitation of movement (passive and active-assisted flexibility and muscle strength) during the first 6 months of recovery. The few exercise–training studies with stroke patients support exercise to improve mobility and functional independence and prevent or reduce further disease and functional impairment.[13,118,202]

Stroke survivors vary widely in age, degree of disability, motivational level, and number and severity of comorbidities, secondary conditions, and associated circumstances. The specific exercise prescription focuses on reducing these conditions and to improve functional capacity.

Multiple Sclerosis

Multiple sclerosis (MS) represents a chronic, often disabling disease characterized by destruction of the myelin sheath (demyelination) that surrounds CNS nerve fibers. Lesions of inflammatory demyelination can be present in any part of the brain and spinal cord.

Clinical Features

Two or more areas of demyelination confirm the diagnosis of MS. This disease usually develops between ages 20 and 40. Frequently a history emerges of transient neurologic deficits that include extremity numbness, weakness, blurred vision, and diplopia (double vision) in childhood or adolescence prior to more persistent neurologic deficits that lead to the definitive diagnosis. Fatigue is the most common symptom of MS. MS occurs worldwide at a higher frequency in latitudes further from the equator (40°). For unknown reasons, MS prevalence in the United States below the 37th parallel is 57 to 78 cases per 100,000, whereas the prevalence rate above the 37th parallel averages 140 cases per 100,000. Patients with a definite MS diagnoses often have a variety of other autoimmune illnesses such as systemic lupus erythematosus, rheumatoid arthritis, polymyositis, and myasthenia gravis. A first-degree relative with MS has a 12- to 20-fold increased chance of developing MS.

TABLE 32.31 ■ PHYSICAL AND PSYCHOLOGIC CONDITIONS AND COMORBIDITIES IN STROKE PATIENTS		
PHYSICAL CONDITIONS	**PSYCHOLOGIC CONDITIONS**	**COMORBIDITIES**
Aphasia	Cognitive impairment	Coronary heart
Balance	Emotional instability	disease
problems	Cognitive impairment	Diabetes mellitus
Falls	Depression	Hypertension
Fatigue	Memory loss	Hyperlipidemia
Muscle	Low self esteem	Obesity
weakness	Social isolation	Peripheral vascular
Obesity		disease
Paralysis		
Paresis		
Spasticity		
Visual		
impairments		

Exercise Prescription

MS patients benefit from a comprehensive health prescription that involves aerobic, strength, balance, and flexibility exercises. About 80% of MS patients report adverse effects to heat exposure. This occurs whether generated environmentally by outside climatic changes or internally via fever or exercise-induced thermogenesis. This effect makes continuous exercise training difficult and not well tolerated. Nevertheless, MS patients still can improve cardiovascular function. Stationary cycling, walking, and low-impact chair or water aerobics provide excellent training choices depending on personal interest and level and nature of physical impairment. Ideal exercise consists of walking in a climate-controlled area that provides stable temperatures, a level surface, and opportunity to rest frequently. Controlling body temperature is a primary consideration in the exercise prescription. A realistic and achievable goal for structured exercise provides training three times a week for a minimum of 30 minutes each session placed into three 10-minute periods.

Parkinson Disease

Parkinson disease (**PD**) is a common neurodegenerative disease with a prevalence of 60 to 187 per 100,000 persons worldwide (all populations are at risk for the disease). The risk of developing PD increases with age; 10% of patients become symptomatic before age 40; 30% before age 50; and 40% between 50 and 60 years. (www.parkinson.org).

Clinical Features

Clinical symptoms of PD include (1) varying degrees of tremor, (2) decrease in spontaneity and movement (bradykinesia), (3) rigidity, and (4) impaired postural reflexes. These conditions produce extreme gait and postural instability that increases falling episodes and difficulty walking. Some patients exhibit a complete lack of movement (akinesia). Functional problems hinder getting out of bed or a car and rising from a chair. Other problems include difficulties dressing, writing, talking, and swallowing. A person with PD generally experiences difficulty with more than one task at a time. As the disease progresses, these problems become more pronounced, and the person eventually loses ability to perform activities of daily living. In the last stage of the disease, the person becomes wheelchair and/or bed bound.

Exercise Prescription

Most exercise prescriptions for PD patients are individualized and directed toward interventions that affect associated motor control problems. They emphasize slow, controlled movements for specific tasks through various ranges of motion while lying, sitting, standing, and walking. Treatment protocols include range-of-motion exercises that emphasize slow static stretches for all major muscle/joint areas, balance and gait training, mobility, and/or coordination exercises.

RENAL DISEASE

Treatment modalities for the major metabolic diseases of obesity, diabetes, and renal dysfunction use regular exercise as adjunctive therapy. Diabetes and obesity are discussed in Chapters 20 and 30, respectively, of this text. This section reviews aspects of renal disease related to exercise physiology.

Renal Disease

Chronic renal disease occurs when kidneys no longer adequately carry out their filtering functions. Acute renal failure occurs from a toxin (e.g., drug allergy or poison) or severe blood loss or trauma. Diabetes is the primary cause of kidney disease, responsible for about 40% of all kidney failures; hypertension is the second cause, responsible for about 25%. Genetic diseases, autoimmune diseases, and birth defects most commonly cause kidney ailments.

Clinical Features

Common symptoms of chronic kidney disease, sometimes referred to as **uremia** (retention in the blood of waste products normally excreted in urine), include the following characteristics:

- *Changes in urination:* Making more or less urine than usual, feeling pressure when urinating, changes in the color of urine, foamy or bubbly urine, or having to get up frequently at night to urinate.
- *Swelling of the feet, ankles, hands, or face:* Fluid the kidneys are unable to remove stays in the tissues.
- *Fatigue or weakness:* Build-up of wastes or a shortage of red blood cells (anemia) causes these problems as the kidneys begin to fail.
- *Shortness of breath:* Kidney failure is sometimes confused with asthma or heart failure because fluid builds up in the lungs.
- *Ammonia breath or an ammonia or metal taste in the mouth:* Waste build-up causes bad breath, changes in taste, or an aversion to protein foods such as meat.
- *Back or flank pain:* The kidneys are located on either side of the spine in the back.
- *Itching:* Waste accumulation causes severe itching, especially of the legs.
- *Loss of appetite*
- *Nausea and vomiting*
- *Increased hypoglycemic episodes, if diabetic*

Chronic uremia eventually progresses to **end-stage renal disease** (**ESRD**) that requires life-long dialysis or kidney transplant. The number of renal transplants has increased steadily worldwide in the last decade and generally offers a more normal lifestyle and full rehabilitation. Nearly 80% of transplant patients function at near normal levels compared with 40 to 60% of those treated with dialysis. Almost 75% of transplant patients resume work compared with 50 to 60% of patients who receive dialysis.

Exercise Prescription

Regular exercise is important in rehabilitating dialysis and transplant patients to better adapt to their illness. The rehabilitation program should begin prior to the start of dialysis to optimize beneficial effects. Normal low-level endurance training (following ACSM guidelines) reduces muscle protein degradation in moderate renal insufficiency, reduces resting blood pressure in some hemodialysis patients, and modestly improves aerobic capacity in patients who undergo hemodialysis.

No longitudinal data exist about aerobic training effects or more physically active lifestyle on patient survival with chronic uremia or kidney transplants. Uremic patients who maintain diverse physical activity report enhanced quality of life. Despite lack of quantitative, long-term quality of life and survival data, more than 23 years have passed since initiation of the first U.S. Transplant Games (www.kidney.org/recips/athletics/tgames/index.cfm). Participants in these games, open to recipients of a currently functioning solid organ or tissue transplant, train daily and perform at near world record levels.

COGNITIVE/EMOTIONAL DISEASES AND DISORDERS

The National Institutes of Mental Health (www.nimh.nih.gov/) reports that 22.1% of Americans ages 18 and older—about 1 in 5 adults—suffer from a diagnosable mental disorder in a given year. When applied to the 2002 U.S. Census residential population estimates, this translates to about 44.5 million people. In addition, 4 of the 10 leading causes of disability in the United States and other developed countries are mental disorders—major depression, bipolar disorder, schizophrenia, and obsessive-compulsive disorder. Suicide, closely linked to depression, represents the third leading cause of death among 10- to 24-year-olds. Also, 6 to 8% of all outpatients in primary care settings suffer major depression. The National Ambulatory Medical Care Survey indicates that more than 7 million primary care visits were made annually in the early 1990s to treat depression, double the number 10 years earlier. In 2004, the number of individuals seeking treatment for depression reached an all-time high. Despite the large numbers of depressed patients, the disease remains underdiagnosed; only about one-third of those diagnosed receive treatment.

The five major classifications of cognitive/emotional diseases include:

1. **Major depressive disorder**—commonly referred to as "depression."
2. **Dysthymia**—mildly depressed on most days over a period of at least 2 years.
3. **Seasonal affective disorder**—recurrence of the depressive symptoms during certain seasons (e.g., winter).
4. **Postpartum depression**—in women who have recently given birth; typically occurs in the first few months after delivery, but can happen within the first year after giving birth.
5. **Bipolar disorder** (previously known as manic-depressive illness)—characterized by extremes in mood and behavior that lasts for at least 2 weeks.

Clinical Features

Depression has no single cause, but often results from a combination of factors or events. Whatever its cause, depression is not just a "state of mind." Depression relates to physical changes in the brain and a chemical imbalance of neurotransmitters.

Women are almost twice as likely to become depressed as men, partly because of hormonal changes from puberty, menstruation, menopause, and pregnancy. Although the risk for depression is lower, men more likely go undiagnosed and are less likely to seek help. Men may show the typical symptoms of depression, but tend to be angry and hostile or mask their condition with alcohol or drug abuse. Suicide remains a serious risk for depressed men who are four times more likely than women to kill themselves. Depression among the elderly poses a unique situation. Older persons often lose loved ones and have to adjust to living alone. Physical illness depresses normal levels of physical activity. Such changes all contribute to depression. Loved ones may attribute signs of depression to normal aging, and many older persons are reluctant to talk about their symptoms. As such, older persons may not receive proper treatment for depression.

Common factors in depression include:

- **Family situation**—trauma and stress from financial problems, breakup of a relationship, death of a loved one, other major life changes
- **Pessimistic personality**—higher risk for individuals who have low self-esteem and a negative outlook
- **Health status**—medical conditions such as heart disease, cancer, and HIV contribute to depression
- **Other psychologic disorders**—anxiety disorders, eating disorders, schizophrenia, and substance abuse often appear with depression

TABLE 32.32 presents common signs and symptoms of depression.

TABLE 32.32 ■ **COMMON SIGNS AND SYMPTOMS OF DEPRESSION**

- Loss of enjoyment from things that were once pleasurable
- Loss of energy
- Feelings of hopelessness or worthlessness
- Difficulty concentrating
- Difficulty making decisions
- Insomnia or excessive sleep
- Stomachache and digestive problems
- Decreased sex drive
- Aches and pains (e.g., recurrent headaches)
- Change in appetite causing weight loss or gain
- Thoughts of death or suicide
- Attempting suicide

FOCUS On Research

PHYSICAL FITNESS PROTECTS AGAINST DEATH

Blair S, et al. Physical fitness and all-cause mortality: a prospective study of healthy men and women. JAMA 1989;262:2395.

▲ A 1998 report by the Centers for Disease Control and Prevention stated that "physical inactivity is one of the major underlying causes of premature mortality in the United States" (Centers for Disease Control and Prevention. Self-reported physical inactivity by degree of urbanization—United States. MMWR 1998;47:1097.) This assertion confirmed that sedentary living causes about one third of deaths from coronary heart disease, colon cancer, and type 2 diabetes. Increasing the nation's collective level of regular physical activity would therefore reduce the rate of premature deaths from these diseases by two thirds.

The 1989 study by Blair and associates was the first to reveal the striking relationship between all-cause mortality and physical fitness in a healthy group of 10,224 men and 3120 women. Measurements included maximal treadmill testing for aerobic capacity, including extensive follow-up of large enough samples of both men *and* women to permit meaningful statistical analyses. The research focused on physical fitness—a biologic attribute as an objective marker for habitual physical activity—rather than physical activity, a behavior subject to measurement and interpretation difficulties. The dependent variable comprised all-cause and cause-specific mortality followed for up to 110,482 person-years, or an average of more than 8 years. This research and subsequent studies by the same investigators formed the basis for renewed interest and research support about the role of regular physical activity in overall health and disease prevention.

Participants underwent baseline measurements that included personal and family history, physical examination, a questionnaire on demographic characteristics and health habits (including cigarette smoking), anthropometry, resting ECG, blood chemistry, blood pressure, and a maximal treadmill exercise test. Subjects had no known heart problems, hypertension, stroke, diabetes, and resting or exercise ECG abnormalities. Total treadmill test time quantified physical fitness level; treadmill time correlated highly ($r \geq 0.92$) with $\dot{V}O_{2max}$ in men and women. Initial test results placed subjects into one of five aerobic fitness categories (1, low fitness; 5, high fitness) based on gender and age to assess the link between physical fitness and all-cause and cause-specific mortality.

Figure 1 shows age-specific, all-cause death rates for men *(top)* and women *(bottom)* categorized by fitness level. For both groups, the decline in death rate with higher fitness

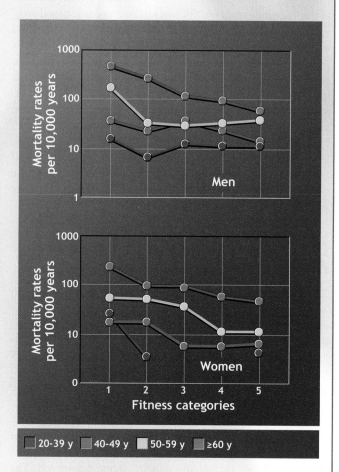

Figure 1 Age-specific, all-cause death rates per 10,000 person-years of follow-up in 10,224 men and 3,120 women by physical fitness quintiles as determined by maximal treadmill exercise testing.

became more pronounced with aging. Table 1 shows the age-adjusted all-cause death rates per 10,000 person-years of follow-up (1970–1985) by fitness grouping. Clearly, less fit women and men experienced higher death risk than more fit counterparts. Significantly higher relative risk for all-cause mortality emerged for the least fit quintile of men and for the two least fit quintiles of women.

Figure 2 shows age-adjusted mortality per 10,000 person-years as a function of metabolic equivalents (METs) and estimated $\dot{V}O_{2max}$ from maximal treadmill testing. The lower limit for mortality risk for men *(orange bars)* and women *(yellow bars)* asymptotes at about the same point for each age grouping—9 METs ($\dot{V}O_{2max} = 31.5$ mL · kg^{-1} · min^{-1}) for women and 10 METs ($\dot{V}O_{2max} = 35.0$ mL · kg^{-1} · min^{-1}) for men. These MET values and corresponding $\dot{V}O_{2max}$ values objectify a lower-limit aerobic fitness cutoff below which health risk increases. Individuals

continued on page 977

Continued

TABLE 1 ■ AGE-ADJUSTED, ALL-CAUSE DEATH RATES PER 10,000 PERSON-YEARS OF FOLLOW-UP (1970–1985) BY AEROBIC FITNESS CATEGORIES IN WOMEN AND MEN

FITNESS GROUP	PERSON-YEARS OF FOLLOW-UP	NUMBER OF DEATHS	AGE-ADJUSTED RATES PER 10,000 PERSON-YEARS	RELATIVE RISK
Men				
1 (low)	14,515	75	64.0	3.44
2	16,898	40	25.5	1.37
3	17,287	47	27.1	1.46
4	18,792	43	21.7	1.17
5 (high)	17,557	35	18.6	1.0
Women				
1 (low)	4916	18	39.5	4.65
2	5329	11	20.5	2.42
3	5053	6	12.2	1.43
4	5522	4	6.5	0.76
5 (high)	4613	4	8.5	1.00

who regularly engage in moderate exercise generally achieve a fitness level above that associated with increased death risk. Brisk walking for 30 to 60 minutes daily provides sufficient exercise overload to sustain a threshold aerobic fitness standard of 9 METs for women and 10 METs for men.

The data showed a clear, strong, and graded inverse relationship between aerobic fitness and mortality from all causes. The finding remained consistent for men and women, even after adjustment for age, serum cholesterol level, blood pressure, smoking habit, fasting blood glucose level, family history of CHD, and length of follow-up. The strength of the associations and the high prevalence of sedentary habits and low fitness levels produce high attributable risk estimates for the general population.

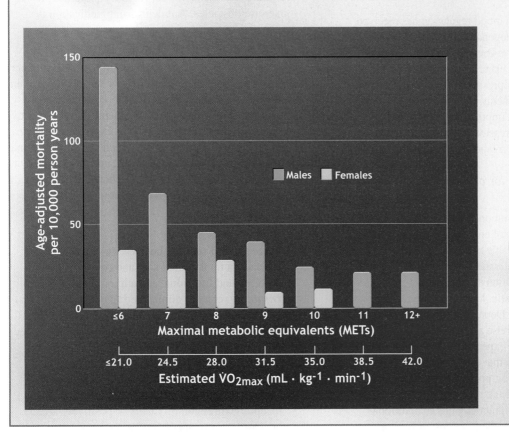

Figure 2 Age-adjusted, all-cause death rates per 10,000 person-years of follow-up by aerobic fitness categories in 3120 women and 10,224 men. Fitness categories expressed as maximal metabolic equivalents (METs) achieved during the maximal treadmill test. Estimated $\dot{V}O_{2max}$ $(mL \cdot kg^{-1} \cdot min^{-1})$ for each category is presented along the bottom axis.

Exercise Prescription

Exercise studies in clinically depressed populations include both hospitalized and ambulatory patients. Overall, the data support the positive effects of regular physical activity on depressive symptoms. In most, but not all studies, exercising patients had significantly decreased depression scores.

No one kind of exercise has the greatest impact on depression, yet most studies have used running or other aerobic-type activities. Interestingly, positive psychologic outcomes do not depend on achieving physical fitness, although such fitness-related indicators as lower blood pressure and increased aerobic capacity frequently do improve.

How exercise alleviates depression remains unclear. Different psychologic and physiologic mechanisms have been suggested. Psychologically, exercise enhances one's sense of mastery and self-esteem, which is important for depressed individuals who feel a loss of control over their lives. Exercise also provides a therapeutic distraction that diverts a patient's attention from areas of worry, concern, and guilt. Improving one's health, physique, flexibility, and body weight also can enhance mood. Large-muscle activity in exercise may help to discharge feelings of pent-up frustration, anger, and hostility.

Researchers continue to study exercise effects on the neurochemistry of mood regulation, specifically turnover of monoamines and other central neurotransmitters at presynaptic and postsynaptic sites. Antidepressant medications, including the selective serotonin reuptake inhibitors, exert their effect by increasing the availability of neurotransmitters at receptor sites. Exercise may exert its beneficial effect on mood by influencing the metabolism and availability of these central neurotransmitters.

The role of β-endorphins in mood regulation has received considerable attention. These endogenous chemicals that reduce pain and can induce euphoria have been linked to the "runner's high" experienced by committed exercisers (see Chapter 20).

Because disturbed sleep represents both a symptom of depression and an aggravating factor, the beneficial effects of exercise on sleep take on added importance. Controlled clinical trials in individuals with depression demonstrate improved subjective sleep quality and corresponding improvement in depression measures.

The exercise prescription for patients with depression considers the following:

- **Anticipate barriers**. Common symptoms of depression—fatigue, lack of energy, and psychomotor retardation—pose formidable barriers to physical activity. Feelings of hopelessness and worthlessness also interfere with motivation to exercise.
- **Keep expectations realistic**. Make exercise recommendations with caution. Depressed patients often self-blame and may view exercise as another occasion for failure. Do not raise false expectations that can arouse anxiety and guilt. Explain that exercise provides an adjunct to, not a substitute for, primary treatment.
- **Design a feasible plan**. Make the exercise prescription realistic and practical, not an additional burden to compound the patient's sense of futility.

Consider the individual's background and history. For severely depressed patients, postpone exercise until medication and psychotherapy alleviate symptoms. Previously sedentary patients should start with a light exercise schedule; for example, just a few minutes of walking each day.

- **Accentuate pleasurable aspects**. Guide the choice of exercise by the patient's preferences and circumstances. Use pleasurable activities that are easily added to the patient's schedule.
- **Include group activities**. Depressed, isolated, and withdrawn patients are most likely to benefit from increased social involvement. The stimulation of being outdoors in a pleasant setting may enhance mood; exposure to light exerts therapeutic effects for seasonal depression.
- **State specifics**. Walking is almost universally acceptable, carries minimal risk of injury, and benefits mood enhancement. In keeping with recent ACSM recommendations for healthy adults, a goal of 20 to 60 minutes of walking or other aerobic exercise, three to five times a week, remains reasonable. The ACSM also recommends resistance and flexibility training 2 to 3 days per week.
- **Encourage compliance**. Improved fitness may be a valuable consequence of exercise participation but is not necessary to produce an antidepressant effect. Compliance increases with less physically demanding exercise programs.
- **Integrate exercise with other treatments**. The primary treatments for depression should not present exercise obstacles. Antidepressant medication is frequently prescribed when depression impairs a patient's ability to function.

The spectrum of brief and longer term psychotherapies is widely used for depression, either alone or with antidepressant medication. An exercise prescription complements psychotherapy when the goal increases the patient's overall activity level and adds pleasurable, satisfying experiences. The patient's difficulties with exercise, such as motivational problems, fear of interpersonal situations, and/or a tendency to transform exercise into a burdensome chore, may shed light on dysfunctional attitudes that psychotherapy can explore.

Summary

1. In the clinical setting, the exercise physiologist focuses on total patient care and restoring patient mobility and functional capacity.
2. *Disability* refers to diminished functional capacity, compounded by an inactive lifestyle. *Handicapped* denotes a physical performance frame of reference defined by society.
3. Exercise plays an important role in cancer risk reduction, perhaps by increasing levels of antiinflammatory cytokines. These augment insulin receptor expression in T cells or positively affect provirus and oncogene activation.

4. The exercise prescription for cancer patients is symptom-limited, progressive, and individualized, with improved ambulation the primary goal.

5. A carefully planned, circuit-resistance exercise program decreases depression and state and trait anxieties for women recovering from breast cancer surgery.

6. Cardiovascular disease affects the heart muscle directly, the heart valves, or neural regulation of cardiac function. Each disorder has its specific pathogenesis and intervention strategy.

7. Myocardial pathologies include angina pectoris, myocardial infarction, pericarditis, congestive heart failure (CHF), and aneurysm. Moderate-intensity exercise and prescribed medications provide benefits with relatively low risk for stable, compensated CHF patients.

8. Heart valve diseases include stenosis, insufficiency (regurgitation), prolapse, and endocarditis. Congenital malformations include ventricular or atrial septal defects and patent ductus arteriosus. Dysrhythmias (bradycardia, tachycardia, and premature ventricular contractions) are diseases of the heart's nervous system.

9. Cardiac patient assessment includes medical history, physical examination, heart auscultation to uncover murmurs and valvular problems, and laboratory tests (chest x-ray, ECG, blood lipid analyses, serum enzyme testing).

10. Physiologic assessments for CHD include noninvasive tests (echocardiography, exercise stress testing, and ECG analysis). Invasive testing includes radionuclide (thallium) imaging, cardiac catheterization, and coronary angiography.

11. Resistance exercise in cardiac rehabilitation restores and maintains muscular strength, promotes preservation of FFM, improves psychologic status and quality of life, and increases glucose tolerance and insulin sensitivity.

12. Graded exercise stress testing provides low-risk screening for CHD preventive and rehabilitative exercise programs. Stress-test results provide the objective framework to design an exercise program within a person's current functional capacity and health status.

13. Multistage bicycle and treadmill tests usually include several levels of 3 to 5 minutes of submaximal exercise to a self-imposed fatigue level.

14. Alterations in the heart's normal electrical activity pattern often indicate insufficient myocardial oxygen supply. Significant S-T segment depression heralds severe, extensive obstruction in one or more coronary arteries.

15. PVCs in exercise generally indicate severe atherosclerotic heart disease, often involving two or more major coronary vessels. Sudden death from ventricular fibrillation averages 6 to 10 times higher in patients with frequent PVCs.

16. Significant deviations from normal blood pressure and heart rate responses during graded exercise testing often indicate underlying cardiovascular pathology.

17. Stress tests have four possible outcomes: true positive (test successful); false negative (person with CHD misdiagnosed); true negative (test successful); false positive (healthy person misdiagnosed).

18. With a properly prescribed and monitored exercise program, cardiac patients improve functional capacity to the same extent as healthy counterparts.

19. Heart transplant patients respond positively to regular exercise training by improving capacity for physical activity. Adding resistance training diminishes negative effects of immunosuppressive therapy on body composition and muscular strength.

20. RLD and COPD are the two major categories of pulmonary disease. RLD increases chest–lung resistance to inflation. COPD affects expiratory flow capacity and ultimately impedes aeration of alveolar blood.

21. Regular exercise can effectively manage various pulmonary diseases, providing that exercise intensity, patient monitoring, and exercise progression receive close attention.

22. Exercise-induced bronchospasm is associated with ambient temperature and humidity and their drying effects on the respiratory mucosa. Drying increases mucosal lining osmolality, which stimulates release of powerful mediators that trigger broncho-constriction.

23. Exercise training does not "cure" asthma; instead, it increases airflow reserve and reduces breathing work during exercise.

24. The few exercise-training studies with stroke patients support the use of exercise to improve mobility and functional independence and reduce further disease and functional impairment.

25. Fatigue is the most common symptom of MS; other symptoms include muscle weakness in the extremities, clumsiness, and numbness and tingling. Patients benefit from a comprehensive health prescription that involves aerobic, strength, balance, and flexibility exercises.

26. Clinical symptoms of Parkinson's disease (PD) include varying degrees of tremor, decreased spontaneity and movement (bradykinesia), rigidity, and impaired postural reflexes.

27. Exercise prescriptions for PD are individualized and directed toward interventions that affect associated motor control problems. They emphasize slow, controlled movements for specific tasks through various ranges of motion while lying, sitting, standing, and walking.

References are available on the Student CD and online at http://connection.lww.com/mkk6e.

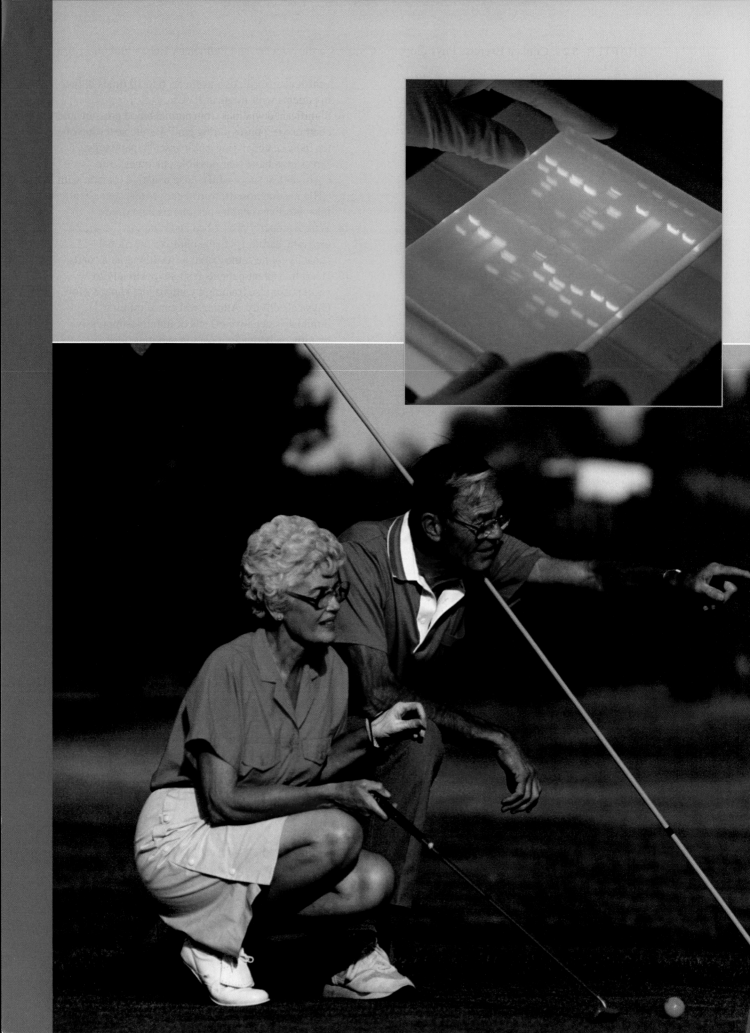

On the Horizon

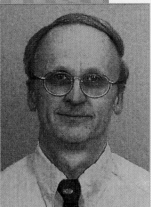

Interview *with* **Frank Booth**

Education: BS (Denison University, Granville, OH); PhD (Exercise Physiology, University of Iowa, Ames, IA); Postgraduate Studies; School of Aerospace Medicine, Brooks Air Force Base, San Antonio, TX. Department of Preventive Medicine, Washington University School of Medicine, St. Louis, MO.

Current Affiliation: Professor, Department of Veterinary Biomedical Sciences, College of Veterinary Medicine; Department of Physiology, and Dalton Cardiovascular Research Institute, University of Missouri, Columbia, MO.

Honors and Awards: See Appendix E, which is available on the Student CD and online at http://connection.lww.com/mkk6e.

Research Focus: Molecular basis of how physical inactivity increases the risk of unhealthy syndromes and diseases in humans and companion animals.

Memorable Publication: Booth FW. Perspectives on molecular and cellular exercise physiology. J Appl Physiol 1988;65:1461.

Statement of Contributions: ACSM Citation Award

In recognition of outstanding contributions in the basic and applied sciences related to exercise physiology and biochemistry.

Dr. Booth is recognized for his innovation and quantitative and integrative investigations on the cellular and molecular mechanisms in skeletal muscles associated with the conditions of immobilization, simulated microgravity, acute exercise, and training. His findings have given a new meaning and interpretation for the adaptive response of muscle.

Dr. Booth is also deserving of citation for his dedicated leadership and his outstanding example in bringing the discipline of exercise physiology into the realm of molecular biology.

What first inspired you to enter the exercise science field? What made you decide to pursue your advanced degree and/or line of research?

■ My biology advisor at Denison University, Dr. Robert Haubrich, also was the assistant swim coach. Because I was on the swim team, he and I had many talks together, not only about swimming but science in general, including discussions about exercise and training methods. Dr. Haubrich knew of my interest in biology and sports, and one day after practice gave me a flyer advertising a new graduate program in exercise physiology at the University of Iowa. As soon as I finished reading it, I knew graduate school was what I wanted to pursue, so I applied to the program.

What influence did your undergraduate education have on your final career choice?

■ The courses I took as part of my biology program, along with Dr. Haubrich's encouragement, were the two primary influences. I loved my comparative anatomy class, where we did animal dissections. This caused me to think about how things worked in humans. My favorite course was philosophy of religion, a course that really made me think.

Who were the most influential people in your career, and why?

■ Four individuals exerted a profound effect on my thinking about my career. First, Dr. Haubrich made me think critically about the science of exercise, although I didn't think of it as a "real" science back then. On team bus trips, or when I would speak with him in his office, we would discuss science in general. I always wondered what was happening to my body during all those hours in the pool. I recall writing a paper for one of my classes about "metabolic pathways" that really turned me on about the topic.

Second, Dr. Charles Tipton (see "Interview" in the front matter) at the University of Iowa taught me to explore mechanisms of exercise adaptations. He stressed honesty, as he was a real "straight shooter." Dr. Tipton encouraged me to convey what was on my mind and not simply to tell people what they wanted to hear. He was instrumental in getting me to communicate precisely what I thought and to be human yet honest in doing so. From a physiological—metabolic perspective, Dr. Tipton consistently tried to uncover why something occurred. I've never lost that burning desire to seek out basic explanations.

The third person was Dr. James Barnard, a fellow graduate student and now a professor at UCLA. Jim was an exemplary student (perhaps the smartest I've met), always getting "A"s in the hardest courses. His ability and enthusiasm for knowledge motivated me to push myself intellectually, both in coursework and in the laboratory. Jim was a great role model for me.

The fourth person, Dr. John Holloszy (see "Interview" in Section 2), mentored my postdoctoral work and taught me to think more critically. As I was continually around other "post-docs" and scientists who were trying to devise creative ways to explain biologic phenomena, there was no way to "hide" from contributing. More than any person I know, Dr. Holloszy possessed the most amazing intuitive "feel" for which experimental procedures would work and which would not. He taught me the basic tenets about how to do science. My interactions with Dr. Holloszy and the other postdoctoral students in conducting various experiments and writing up the results of our work were invaluable in shaping my career in science.

What has been the most interesting/enjoyable aspect of your involvement in science? What was the least interesting/enjoyable aspect?

■ I cherish the camaraderie of exercise science colleagues, particularly those with whom I have in-depth discussions about various science topics. The individuals who open up and share the truth about their research are the ones I truly enjoy knowing and relating to. The ideal and most enjoyable environment enables one to speak freely, to really express truthful opinions about a topic. I do not enjoy people who tell you what they want you to hear or know for purposes of personal gain (i.e., to build their own ego or self-promote) instead of communicating with respect for the purity of scientific discovery.

What is your most meaningful contribution to the field of exercise science, and why is it so important?

■ This is a very difficult question, for which I have no answer. I suspect that the answer will emanate from the judgments of others. However, I do love applying cutting-edge technology to try to answer mechanistic questions concerning exercise. It is important to try to get to the bottom of things, and using new techniques often provides the key to unlocking the required information. Sometimes, it takes months to perfect the procedure you need for an experiment, and then months more to finally get it to work properly.

What advice would you give to students who express an interest in pursuing a career in exercise science research?

■ It is important for the student to be excited by a course or topic in a course. Sometimes, undergraduate students have difficulty making a decision about their future. I encourage students with an interest in discovering new insights about any exercise-related topic to become involved with a professor's research projects. Even in graduate school, there is a wide range of "true" desire to continue to pursue research interests. However, those students who experience joyous feelings when searching for the unknown will know deep down they have found a suitable path to follow. If a student can find a mentor, then by all means take advantage of the situation, and do whatever it takes to become deeply involved in the intellectual pursuit.

What interests have you pursued outside your professional career?

■ I am basically a big-time workaholic. Except for evening runs with my dog Swim, I pretty much start in the lab early and end late. I love vigorous exercise and try to do as much as I can when time permits.

Where do you see the exercise science field (particularly your area of greatest interest) heading in the next 20 years?

■ Our field needs to produce the very best science to counter the cultural trends that have created a sedentary society with all of its ailments and diseases. Discovering the benefits of exercise and conveying those benefits to the public, from the broadest possible topic areas to the molecular basis of disease, remains our best chance to prevent many diseases and upgrade the nation's health. The field needs to cooperate with multiple partners in a major public health effort to convince the world about the long-term health benefits of regular exercise. We as scientists must systematically provide the medical evidence and cross-disciplinary connections to show that exercise, not drugs, exerts the greatest impact on disease to improve health. All of us must become strong advocates, using education and laboratory-based research to convince people everywhere to pursue a healthy lifestyle.

You have the opportunity to give a "last lecture." Describe its primary focus.

■ The basis of my talk would involve how regular exercise affects daily living. I would focus not just on the physiologic function and performance aspects, but on exercise's effects on chronic ills like diabetes, pulmonary and kidney diseases, heart disease, and cancer. For the ever-increasing number of American citizens living in nursing homes, I would discuss the profound effect of sedentary living on muscular atrophy and reduced strength, two factors that limit these individual's ability to carry out even the simplest tasks of daily living. I would emphasize that relying on pills to tackle disease contributes relatively little to a happy and healthy life. I would also hope to convince the audience that the exercise biologists' role is not simply to study the effects of physical activity or enhance sport performance. The "new" exercise physiologist must reintroduce regular physical activity into an unhealthy, overweight, and sedentary population that is genetically programmed to expect physical activity. I refer to this unhealthy state as SeDS, an abbreviation for sedentary death syndrome.

Achievement of a future, healthy world must involve cooperative effort among diverse public and private organizations that invest enough money in fundamental research to make a real difference. Talking a good game simply will not do it; putting sufficient resources to work will create newer and better opportunities for success through proper research.

Molecular Biology— A New Vista for Exercise Physiology

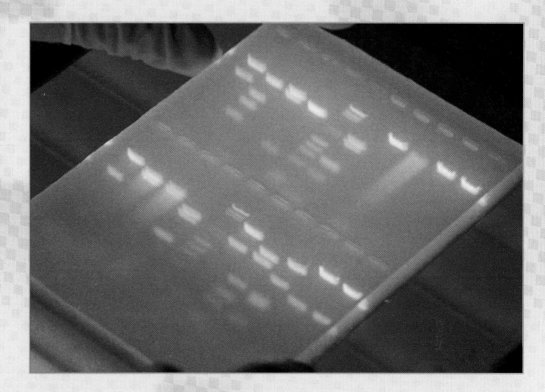

The most sensible way to prepare for the challenges and opportunities arising from progress in the identification of the genetic and molecular basis of health and disease is to become familiar with this field and to learn its tools.

Claude Bouchard, Robert Malina, and Louis Pérusse. *Genetics of Fitness and Physical Performance*. Champaign, IL: Human Kinetics, 1997.

Gene: segment of DNA with an ordered nucleotide sequence for encoding a specific functional substance (i.e., a protein or RNA molecule)

Molecular biology: study of the molecular basis of life

Molecular genetics: study of the structure and sequence of the molecules that carry genetic information

Pharmacogenetics: genetic engineering to design specific drugs to target specific disease conditions of an individual's genetic code; this field investigates how genetic diversity affects the efficacy and side effects of targeted drugs

Pharmacogenomics: application of genomic methods and perspectives to study drug-responsive genes

Bioinformatics: understanding the underlying chemical codes of organisms by interpreting gene sequences, converting primary linear code into complex three-dimensional structures, managing automated screens, and running combinatorial chemistry syntheses

Protein: relatively large molecule composed of one or more chains of amino acids in a specific order (determined by the base sequence of nucleotides in the gene coding for the protein); proteins (perhaps up to 140,000 different structures in the body) provide for unique structure, function, and regulation of cells, tissues, and organs; examples include hormones, enzymes, and antibodies

Gene expression: converting a gene's coded information by transcription and translation into cellular structures; expressed genes include those transcribed (copied) from DNA nucleotide sequences into mRNA and then translated by ribosomes into specific nucleotide sequences to form protein

Transcription: RNA polymerase assembles an mRNA molecule complementary to the gene's nucleotide (making an RNA copy of a gene)

Messenger RNA (mRNA): molecule that carries genetic information (complementary copy of one of the two DNA strands) between a gene and the ribosomes that translate the genetic information into proteins

The early 1950s ushered in the dawn of the modern age of molecular biology, and the past 15 years of exercise physiology research has, albeit slowly, embraced this field. And so it should. Techniques now available to study how genetic characteristics shape human behavior will revolutionize almost every facet of human physical activity and sports medicine. The new generation of exercise physiologists has a wonderful opportunity to study the molecular world of **genes** and their role in human exercise performance and health and disease. Today's exercise physiology students often cooperate in research projects from basic science, clinical and environmental medicine, chemistry, **molecular biology** and **molecular genetics**, **pharmacogenetics**, **pharmacogenomics**, **bioinformatics**, and other newly emerging disciplines in the physical and life sciences.

Many exercise physiology laboratories have well-funded research programs to study the genetic basis of increased physical activity (and inactivity) related to diseases and dysfunctions. This spans the gamut from the role of genetics in training and exercise performance to skeletal muscle adaptations to prolonged microgravity exposure. Occupational, physical, and rehabilitation medicine anticipate the use of gene therapy as a way to transfer genetic material to enhance the patient's production of growth factors. These small **protein** molecules stimulate cell proliferation, migration, and differentiation; promote matrix synthesis to facilitate healing of injured or surgically repaired tissues with limited blood supply and slowed cell growth that can impair normal processes of tissue repair.[85] In addition to delivering therapeutic proteins to injured tissues, molecular biology provides a way to potentially engineer new tissues. These biologic substitutes—exogenous structures and/or tissue scaffolding—may eventually link with gene therapy procedures to support tissue regeneration and healing from athletic trauma. Current interest in molecular biology also focuses on how short-term and chronic physical activity act and interact to induce structural and functional adaptations that enhance exercise performance and produce desirable health outcomes.

Booth and colleagues[22,23] assert that future exercise physiology research should emphasize primary disease prevention, with focus on uncovering environmental roots of modern chronic diseases such as type 2 diabetes almost entirely preventable with increased physical activity.[80] These maladies annually cause 250,000 premature deaths and play a role in $1 trillion dollars in health care costs for conditions associated with sedentary living, not to mention the toll on human suffering. Dr. Frank Booth, whose contributions we chronicled on pages 982 to 983; coined the term *SEDS* (sedentary death syndrome) to characterize the effects of a sedentary lifestyle on unhealthy outcomes.[21]

The related fields of molecular biology offer novel ways to study disease mechanisms and the strategies that best combat them. Research challenges also emerge in the exercise biology sciences. More specifically, six questions have been posed concerning molecular biology's role in prospective exercise physiology research:[20]

1. How does endurance training coregulate **gene expression** of most mitochondrial proteins in trained skeletal muscle?
2. Which enzymes trigger the shift in the metabolic fuel mixture that occurs with endurance training?
3. What chemical signal(s) induced by resistance training cause skeletal muscle hypertrophy?
4. What DNA regulatory sequences alter **transcription** of a **messenger RNA (mRNA)**?
5. What proteins regulate skeletal muscle function?
6. What important factors affect differential gene expression that occurs in response to changes in a muscle's contractile activity?

Fifteen years ago, Baldwin made a compelling case that the membership of the American College of Sports Medicine should exploit new fields and technologies involved with "molecular exercise sciences."[9] The views of Booth and Baldwin, not unlike our own, maintain that exercise physiology and sports medicine have progressed over the past decade from an organismal focus, to exercise biochemistry at the organ level, to a current emphasis on molecular dynamics. These scientists posit that our field has already shifted to the molecular age, as evidenced by research emphasis in integrative biology and **proteomics**. In the 5th edition of this text, a literature search on PubMed (www.ncbi.nlm.nih.gov:80/entrez) reinforced their point. For the 3-month period between January 1, 2001 and April 1, 2001, almost one fourth of the citations to the term "muscle" were linked to the term gene (502 citations), and 72 articles concerned genes and human muscle. Not surprisingly, a search for the term "**genome**" yielded 64,112 entries through March 2001, most occurring from 1998 to 2001.

Compared with the 2001 citation search, a tremendous proliferation has occurred in molecular biology research in the ensuing 4 years related to the exercise sciences as illustrated in FIGURE 1. As of May 9, 2005, 102,150 articles were tagged to "genome" (a 59.3% increase over 2001), while citations with the terms *muscle* and *genes* increased from 502 in 2001 to 16,184 in 2005! We have included other combinations of terms to use as a frame of comparison in future editions of the text.

Proteomics: systematic analysis of the protein expression of healthy and unhealthy genomes at the molecular level by identifying, characterizing, and quantifying proteins

Genome: an organism's complete genetic information (DNA and RNA)

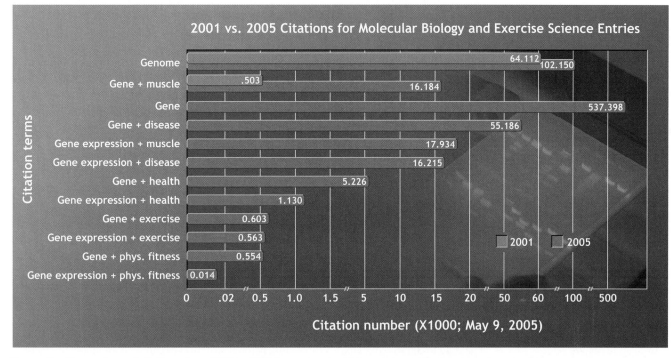

Figure 1   Comparison of citations from 2001 to 2005 for molecular biology terms with exercise science entries.

Funding for research in the genomics area has also increased dramatically. FIGURE 2 shows that in 1988, the Department of Energy (DOE) and the National Institutes of Health (NIH) spent a combined $27.9 million for their human genomic programs; in 2000, that amount increased nearly 13-fold to $360.6 million and continued to climb steadily, reaching 437 million in 2003–2004. One hopes that funding will continue to increase in the many disciplines related to molecular medicine despite the fact the Human Genome Project was officially completed in 2003. The range of scientific activities related to genomics includes studies of human diseases, experimental organisms (e.g., bacteria, yeast, worms, flies, mice, rats); development of emerging technologies for biologic and medical research; computational methods to analyze genomes; and ethical, legal, and social issues related to genetics.

In this chapter, we introduce molecular biology in general, with specific emphasis on gene expression and **protein synthesis**. Where possible, we link applications to human exercise performance, exercise testing, and sports medicine. Our tour begins with background information about Watson and Crick's

Human genome project budget (values in $ millions)			
Fiscal year	DOE*	NIH*	US total
1988	10.7	17.2	27.9
2000	88.9	271.7	360.6
2001	86.4	308.4	394.8
2002	90.1	346.7	434.3
2003	64.2	372.8	437.0
2004	64.2	372.8	437.0

*DOE = Department of Energy;
*NIH = National Institutes of Health

Figure 2   DOE and NIH budget from 1988 to 2004. Note level funding for 2003–2004. Data unavailable for 2005.

Protein synthesis: process of creating a protein from amino acid subunits

Deoxyribose nucleic acid (DNA): double-helix molecule (two complementary chains of nucleotides) containing an organism's total hereditary information

pioneering 1953 achievement in deciphering the three-dimensional molecular structure of the **deoxyribonucleic acid (DNA)** molecule.[136] Their seminal publication, included with the reference materials on the website for this textbook, immediately thrust research in molecular biology to the forefront of scientific exploration worldwide. Their solving the puzzle of the DNA structure led to new techniques and models of how organisms transmit genetic information from parent to offspring and ultimately to successive generations. The spectacular growth of molecular biology affects almost every facet of biomedical research and has forever changed the face of hereditary science. Research in molecular biology will surely fundamentally impact human exercise performance.

In all likelihood, future limits to athletic performance will be determined less by an athlete's innate physiology and anatomy (and commitment to training) and more by surgical enhancement (e.g., more flexible tendons) and genetic interventions engineered for faster-acting, more powerful muscles, greater oxygen transport, and more rapid circulation. The continuing use of banned substances made public at the 2000 Sydney Olympic Games and 27th Athens Olympiad in 2004 highlights challenges facing the new, independent drug-testing agency to confront the consequences of illegal drug use in the 2008 Beijing Games. It would not surprise us if breakthroughs in gene therapy techniques in the coming years infiltrate the athlete's arsenal of "tricks" in time for this Olympiad. This will cause both students and an educated general public to confront specialists in exercise physiology concerning the implications of the molecular biology of gene therapy and "genetic ergogenics," as increasing numbers of athletes cheat with these techniques to gain a competitive edge.

A new feature of this chapter includes supplementary material on the web page dedicated to this textbook (http://connection.lww.com/mkk6e). This website includes (1) readings related to molecular biology and **genetics**, twins, and human performance, (2) excellent texts that devote hundreds of pages to the intricacies of the molecular biology of gene transcription and protein synthesis, (3) articles from *Scientific American* that concern molecular biology, (4) useful molecular biology Internet sites, and (5) a reprint of Watson and Crick's one-page classic paper in *Nature* about their discovery of DNA's structure, which 50 years later unraveled the pieces to the primordial jigsaw puzzle of the **Human Genome Project**.

Genetics: branch of science that studies patterns of inheritance of specific traits in successive generations

Human Genome Project: government-sponsored project (Department of Energy and National Institutes of Health) to (1) create an ordered set of DNA segments from known chromosomal locations, (2) develop new computational methods to analyze genetic maps and DNA sequence data, and (3) develop new techniques and instruments for detecting and analyzing DNA (i.e., deciphering the complete sequence of genetic instructions in humans). Hundreds of robotic sequencing machines work around the clock to analyze nucleotide sequences using the Sanger-Coulson dideoxy DNA sequencing method to map different genomes

Nucleus: structure that contains the cell's genetic material (chromosomal DNA)

Natural selection: Darwin's basic idea that species survive because more favorable phenotypic traits pass down through successive generations

BRIEF HISTORY TOUR OF MOLECULAR BIOLOGY

The road to uncovering DNA's three-dimensional structure began with an innocent discovery by Swiss physiologist Friedrich Miescher (1844–1895), Professor of Physiology at the University of Basel, Switzerland, and charter member of the 1889 First International Congress of Physiologists. In 1869, Miescher identified what he considered a new biologic substance. Cells from fish sperm and human tissue cells obtained from pus in discarded surgical bandages contained unusual proportions of nitrogen and phosphorus in their **nucleus**. Miescher called the substance *nuclein,* which one of his students, Richard Altman, in 1899 termed *nucleic acid* because of its slightly acidic properties.

As late as the second half of the 19th century, chemists and biologists did not know what role if any genes played in transmitting hereditary information in plants or animals. But this would change when English naturalist, geologist, and biologist, Charles Robert Darwin (1809–1882) (www.bbc.co.uk/education/darwin/biblio/links.htm) proposed a theory of evolution based on **natural selection** of random variation.[38] Darwin developed his theory gradually after many years of geologic and biologic observations on native lands, particularly along the western coast of South America including the Galapagos Islands. Darwin's insightful observations about the distribution and continuation of animal and plant phenotypic traits were first published on November 26, 1859, 10 years before Miescher discovered nuclein.

Researchers at Brandeis University, Boston, have used Darwin's basic ideas about natural selection to create the GOLEM project (Genetically Organized Lifelike Electro Mechanics; http://demo.cs.brandeis.edu/golem/). They success-

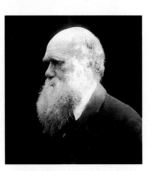

Charles Darwin

fully created artificial locomoting machines that mimicked biologic life forms (e.g., robots that design and build other robots without human assistance). The simulations demonstrated the feasibility of creating successively more complex entities from proceeding generations to solve more difficult simulation tasks. The implications of such "biologic" simulations may have a bearing on the role of natural selection on intelligence and memory.

Another English naturalist, Alfred Russel Wallace (1823–1913; www.wku.edu/~smithch/index1.htm), had independently formed his own views regarding natural selection at about the same time Darwin completed his work dealing with evolution theory. Except for sharing his thoughts with selected colleagues in various disciplines, Darwin had not yet made them widely known in formal publications. Darwin's reading of Wallace's 1855 paper about natural selection, *On the Tendency of Varieties to Depart Indefinitely From the Original Type* (reprinted in reference 130) no doubt accelerated his pace to publish the single-volume discourse on evolutionary theory that remains an enduring legacy, forever changing our view about human evolutionary progression through the ages. It was Wallace who encouraged Darwin to use the phrase "survival of the fittest" (coined by British sociologist and philosopher Herbert Spencer [1820–1903]), to convey the basic idea about natural selection to the general public.

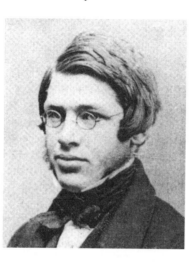

Alfred Russel Wallace, age 25

Darwin's carefully crafted, thought-provoking treatise, *On the Origin of Species by Means of Natural Selection, or The Preservation of Favoured Races in the Struggle for Life*,[37] indirectly provided empirical "data" on how environmental pressures selected for the survival of a species' observable characteristics (traits) from one generation to the next. His ideas about evolution emerged mainly from insightful observations of subtle differences among plant and animal species during his 4-year, 9-month, and 2-day voyage around the world, begun in 1831 aboard the survey ship HMS *Beagle*.[36] Darwin's theory explained how adaptive modifications to environmental stressors impacted the common descent of current animal and plant species and how natural selection preserved a species' survival.

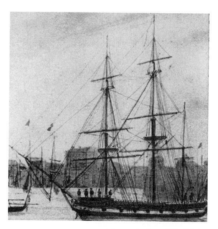

HMS *Beagle*

Interestingly, Miescher's discovery of nuclein came 4 years after Austrian monk Gregor Johann Mendel's (1822–1884) elegant 25-year breeding experiments with 10,000 varieties of edible pea plants *Pisum sativum*. Mendel vigilantly tracked the pea's inherited characteristics and submitted his findings in 1865, "Versuche über Pflanzen-Hybriden," to an obscure natural history society journal. The work appeared in 1866 and in 1950 was translated into English by William Bateson (1861–1926).[14] Darwin's unifying evolution theory and Mendel's experiments on heredity formed "scientific pillars" of insights embraced by a relatively new field of study—molecular biology—that would subsequently dominate fundamental discoveries in biology, chemistry, genetics, nutrition,

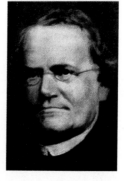

Gregor Johann Mendel

and medicine for years to come. The importance of Darwin's contributions is reflected in a Google search on Charles Darwin (May 2005) that references 3,470,000 websites! Interestingly, British scientists using molecular biology methods in 2005 unraveled the cause of Darwin's 40 years of suffering from long bouts of vomiting, gut pain, headaches, severe tiredness, skin problems, and depression.[27] Darwin's family history revealed a major inherited component of predisposed hypolactasia (aversion to milk and cream). The authors concluded that Darwin's multifold symptoms and illness highlights a missed observation—the importance of lactose in mammalian and human evolution.

Mendel's meticulous scientific insights remained relatively obscure for nearly three decades until three scientists (Correns, De Vries, van Tschermak-Seysenegg) rediscovered his research in about 1900. It would take nearly 65 years after Mendel's initial publication (and enormous progress in biochemical techniques) to unravel further secrets highlighting the mysteries of hereditary transmission in human cells. In 1929, Phoebus A. T. Levene (1869–1940) discovered that the essential components of the nucleic acids DNA and **ribonucleic acid (RNA)** were long chains of repeating **nucleotides**. It remained unclear to Levene and others how these molecules assembled. If the genes indeed contained the hereditary information, scientists needed to know the process involved. Twenty-five years later, a major breakthrough occurred (discussed in the next section) that delivered the biggest biologic thunderbolt since Darwin stirred a revolution in scientific thinking concerning evolutionary theory. This breakthrough impacted at least eight other crucial scientific milestones:

1. 1966—cracking the DNA genetic code
2. 1972–1973—start of tremendous advances in biotechnology by splicing pieces of DNA together to form genes (called *recombinant molecules*) that were inserted into bacteria to produce human proteins
3. 1977—elucidating the complete genetic information of a microorganism, paving the way for the Human Genome Project
4. 1981—creating the first **transgenic** animal by inserting a viral gene into the DNA of a mouse, permitting such animals to serve as models for the study of human diseases
5. 1984—devising the **polymerase chain reaction** (**PCR**), an ingenious method of sequencing DNA from minute samples of DNA
6. 1997—cloning the first mammal, the lamb Dolly, from an adult cell
7. 2000–2004—deciphering the human genome; sequencing the genome of the fruit fly *Drosophila melanogaster;* DNA of rice sequenced (first decoding of a crop); initial sequencing and comparative analysis of the mouse and brown Norway rat genomes; somatic cell nuclear transfer (SCNT) technology produces a single embryonic stem cell line from a human blastocyst, representing the first published report of cloned human stem cells
8. 2005—creating 11 human stem cell lines from human embryos by cloning and then extracting patient-specific, immune-matched human embryonic stem cells to create genetic matches in patients with disease or injury

REVOLUTION IN THE BIOLOGIC SCIENCES

In 1953, James D. Watson (1928–), an American postdoctoral student who earned a PhD in genetics from Indiana University at age 22, teamed with English physicist Francis H. C. Crick (1916–2004) who was pursuing a PhD in x-ray studies of protein in the Cavendish Laboratory, Cambridge, England. Watson and Crick's breakthrough, deduced from other scientists' research, published and unpublished, posited that the DNA molecule consisted of two polynucleotide linear strands coiled around each other to form a **double helix**.[134]

Future Nobel laureate James D. Watson said at the time of the discovery, "We used to think our fate was in our stars. Now we know our fate, in large measure, is in our genes. Never will a more important set of instruction manuals be made available."

The young researchers constructed a ball-and-wire model of DNA, proposing that the two helical strands connected like the steps of a spiral staircase by nucleotide **base pairs** held together by **hydrogen bonds**. Their eventual Nobel Prize rewarded their contribution

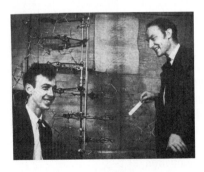

James D. Watson *(left)* and Francis H. C. Crick *(right)* at the Cavendish Laboratory next to their DNA ball and wire model. May, 1953.

Ribonucleic acid (RNA): nucleic acid that contains the sugar ribose; usually single stranded

Nucleotide: segment of a nucleic acid containing a 5-carbon sugar, phosphate group, and nitrogen-containing base

Transgenic: transforming genes from one species into another

Polymerase chain reaction (PCR): technique for artificially amplifying the number of copies of a target DNA sequence, usually by 106- to 109-fold, during repeated cycles of denaturation, annealing with primer, and extension with DNA polymerase

Double helix: two DNA strands twisted in a spiral around each other

Base pairs: two complementary nucleotide bases (G-C or A-T) in a double-stranded DNA molecule held together by hydrogen bonds

Hydrogen bonds: weak, interactive bonding from simultaneous attraction of a positive hydrogen atom to other atoms with negative charges

about DNA's architecture and the three-dimensional fit of its molecular components (fueled in part by substantial theoretical contributions about DNA's helical structure from Kings College, London, colleague Rosalind Franklin (1920–1957; see "Introduction").

In their 1953 landmark publication in *Nature* that described DNA's molecular structure, Watson and Crick state that their research efforts were stimulated by "a knowledge of the general nature of the unpublished experimental results and ideas of Drs. M. H. F. Wilkins and R. E. Franklin and coworkers at King's College, London." This statement, interpreted with the hindsight of many years of investigative efforts by historians and researchers, paints quite a different picture of Rosalind E. Franklin's prior discoveries about DNA's structure, which eventually led Watson and Crick to deduce DNA's final configuration correctly. Franklin's sophisticated x-ray diffraction photo reflecting her expertise with x-ray crystallography (shown to Watson and Crick surreptitiously without Franklin's knowledge) provided the missing pieces about DNA's double helix that empowered Watson and Crick to decipher the puzzle quickly. Interestingly, unlike many biologists, Watson and Crick did not conduct experiments. Their technique was thinking, arguing, and rethinking ideas and concepts about how to put together pieces of a puzzle with many components. On this front (for the structure of the DNA molecule), they scored a home run!

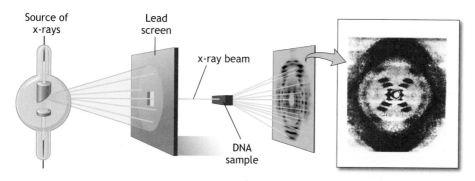

Figure 3   The technique of x-ray crystallography bombards crystals with thin x-ray beams of single (monochromatic) wavelength to determine a substance's three-dimensional crystal structure. The right photo shows Franklin's x-ray photograph of DNA; she focused the x-ray beam on extra-wet DNAB fibers for a longer-than-usual time, with a 62-hour exposure to obtain the vivid photo of DNA's cruciform pattern. Without her knowledge or permission, this recent x-ray photograph was shown to Watson and Crick, and along with knowledge about base-pairing, they correctly deduced that DNA must have originated from a helix-shaped molecule.

For historic perspective, we recommend two books with different views about how the DNA puzzle was solved. First, read Watson's colorful personal interpretation of one of the most important discoveries in all of science by one of the scientists who made the discovery.[132] Then read Sayre's compelling and insightful first full account of Rosalind Franklin's previously unacknowledged major contribution to discovering DNA's structure.[110]

Since Watson and Crick's decisive discovery, we know that DNA's helical structure carries the biologic blueprint for specifying the *order* in which the body's twenty amino acids assemble to create a protein. Each protein has its own unique amino acid sequence; this sequence ultimately dictates the protein molecule's final shape and distinctive chemical and functional characteristics. We also know that each double-helix strand provides a **template** for synthesizing a new strand, something Watson and Crick had hinted at

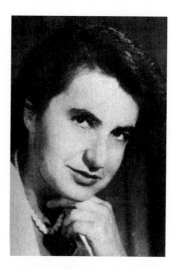

Dr. Rosalind Franklin

Template: copy, replica, or pattern; sequence of nucleotides from which a complementary DNA or RNA strand forms

TABLE 1 ■ NOBEL PRIZES AWARDED IN RESEARCH RELATED TO CELL AND MOLECULAR BIOLOGY FROM 1958 TO 2005

YEAR	SCIENTIST	PRIZE[a]	RESEARCH	YEAR	SCIENTIST	PRIZE[a]	RESEARCH
2005				1983	**Barbara McClintock**	P or M	Mobile elements in the genome
2004	Richard Axel **Linda B. Buck**	P or M	Odorant receptors and the organization of the olfactory system	1982	Aaron Klug	Chemistry	Structure of nucleic acid-protein complexes
2003	Paul C. Lauterbur Sir Peter Mansfield	P or M	Magnetic resonance imaging	1980	Paul Berg	Chemistry	Recombinant DNA technology
2002	Sydney Brenner H. Robert Horvitz John E. Sulston	P or M	Genetic regulation of organ development and programmed cell death		Walter Gilbert Frederick Sanger		DNA-sequencing technology
2001	Leland H. Hartwell R. Timothy Hunt Sir Paul M. Nurse	P or M	Identified key molecular regulators of the cell cycle in all eukaryotic organisms, including yeasts, plants, animals, and humans		Baruj Benacerraf Jean Dausset George D. Snell	P or M	Major histocompatibility complex
2000	Arvid Carlsson Paul Greengard Eric Kandel	P or M	Slow synaptic neural transmission among neural cells, biology of memory, and development of selective serotonin reuptake inhibitors	1978	Werner Arber Daniel Nathans Hamilton Smith	P or M	Restriction endonuclease technology
					Peter Mitchell	Chemistry	Chemiosmotic mechanism of oxidative phosphorylation
1999	Günter Blobel	P or M	Proteins' intrinsic signals govern cell transport and localization	1976	D. Carleton Gajdusek	P or M	Prion-based diseases
1998	Robert F. Furchgott Louis J. Ignarro Ferid Murad	P or M	Nitric acid as a signaling molecule in cardiovascular regulation	1975	David Baltimore Renato Dulbecco Howard M. Temin	P or M	Reverse transcriptase and tumor virus activity
1997	Rolf M. Zinkernagel Peter C. Doherty	P or M	Immune system recognition of virus-infected cells	1974	Albert Claude Christian de Duve George E. Palade	P or M	Structure and function of internal components of cells
1996	Jens C. Skou Paul Boyer John Walker	Chemistry	Na+/K+-ATPase	1972	Gerald Edelman Rodney R. Porter	P or M	Immunoglobulin structure
	Stanley B. Prusiner	P or M	Protein structure of prions		Christian B. Anfinsen	Chemistry	Relationship between primary and tertiary structure of proteins
1995	Edward B. Lewis **Christiane Nüsslein-Volhard** Eric Wieschaus	P or M	Genetic control of embryonic development	1971	Earl W. Sutherland Jr.	P or M	Mechanism of hormone action and cyclic AMP
1994	Alfred Gilman Martin Rodbell	P or M	Structure and function of GTP-binding (G) proteins	1970	Bernard Katz Ulf S. von Euler	P or M	Nerve impulse propagation and transmission
1993	Richard Roberts Philip Sharp	P or M	Split genes and RNA processing		Luis F. Leloir	Chemistry	Role of sugar nucleotides in carbohydrate synthesis
	Kary Mullis	Chemistry	Polymerase chain reaction (PCR)	1969	Max Delbrück Alfred D. Hershey Salvador E. Luria	P or M	Genetic structure of viruses
	Michael Smith		Site-directed mutagenesis (SDM)				
1992	Edmond Fisher Edwin Kerbs	P or M	Alteration of enzyme activity by phosphorylation/ dephosphorylation	1968	H. Gobind Khorana Marshall W. Nirenberg Robert W. Holley	P or M	Genetic code
1991	Erwin Neher Bert Sakmann	P or M	Measurement of ion flux by patch-clamp recording	1966	Peyton Rous	P or M	Tumor viruses
1989	J. Michael Bishop Harold Varmus	P or M	Cellular genes capable of causing malignant transformation	1965	F. Francois Jacob Andres M. Lwoff Jacques L. Monod	P or M	Bacterial operons and messenger RNA
	Thomas R. Cech Sidney Altman	Chemistry	Ability of RNA to catalyze reactions	1964	**Dorothy C. Hodgkin**	Chemistry	Structure of complex organic molecules
1988	Johann Deisenhofer Robert Huber Hartmut Michel	Chemistry	Bacterial photosynthetic reaction center	1963	John C. Eccles Alan L. Hodgkin Andrew F. Huxley	P or M	Ionic basis of nerve membrane potentials
1987	Susumu Tonegawa	P or M	DNA rearrangements responsible for antibody diversity	1962	Francis H. C. Crick Maurice H. F. Wilkins	P or M	Three-dimensional structure of DNA
1986	**Rita Levi-Montalcini** Stanley Cohen	P or M	Factors that affect nerve outgrowth		John C. Kendrew Max F. Perutz	Chemisty	Three-dimensional structure of globular proteins
1985	Michael S. Brown Joseph L. Goldstein	P or M	Regulation of cholesterol metabolism and endocytosis	1961	Melvin Calvin	Chemistry	Biochemistry of CO_2 assimilation during photosynthesis
1984	Georges Köhler César Milstein	P or M	Monoclonal antibodies	1960	F. MacFarlane Burnet Peter B. Medawar	P or M	Clonal selection theory of antibody formation
	Niels K. Jerne		Antibody formation	1959	Arthur Kornberg Severo Ochoa	P or M	Synthesis of DNA and RNA
				1958	George W. Beadle Joshua Lederberg Edward L. Tatum	P or M	Gene expression
					Frederick Sanger	Chemistry	Primary structure of proteins

[a]P or M, physiology or medicine. *Note:* corecipients for some awards were excluded if their primary research did not involve molecular and cell biology. Frederic Sanger won two Nobels (1958, 1980); his important contributions helped to pave the way for future human genome research.
Bold type identifies females.

in their seminal *Nature* paper. A **template strand** represents an original DNA strand. Once faithfully copied, each newly created double-helix strand is a duplicate of its predecessor, with its genetic code sequence preserved. This mechanism of self-replication preserves the genetic flow of information to ensure that successive generations receive the same coded DNA "messages." In fact, all living things on Earth share a common molecular plan. Each of a human's trillions of cells relies on four basic molecular building blocks—nucleic acid, protein, lipid, and polysaccharide—along with other nano-sized biomolecules, to perform their functions efficiently. In addition, all living cells shuttle the flow of information from DNA to RNA to protein. We cannot overstate the full impact of what Watson and Crick deduced about DNA's structural configuration. Their contribution and subsequent years of investigation have affected every facet of biomedical science, from how primordial DNA formed and survived to the nature of deadly diseases and the all-out search for their eventual cure. Their unraveling of DNA's structure also profoundly affected all of science, particularly subsequent discoveries about the human, plant, and animal genomes (see next section).

The field of molecular biology has shown explosive growth during the past 45 years. Discoveries have been so startling that almost every year since 1958 a Nobel Prize has been awarded for research related to molecular biology. TABLE 1 lists the Nobel Prize winners in the fields of chemistry and physiology or medicine. Note that since its 1901 inception, 4 of the only 10 women awarded a Nobel Prize in science won for molecular biology-related research.[88] Marie Curie won in both physics (1903) and chemistry (1911). TABLE A at the end of this chapter (page 1063) presents a timeline for "genetics" from before Mendel to salient discoveries in genetics and molecular biology, culminating with elucidation of the genetic sequence of the fruit fly *Drosophila melanogaster* in September 1999, the first human genome in June 2000, more than 95% of the genetic code of the laboratory mouse 4 months later in October 2000, the complete genome sequence of the dimorphic bacterium *Caulobacter crescentus* in 2001,[95] rice (2002), and the rat genome in 2004.

HUMAN GENOME

The **human genome** represents the full complement of genetic material in a human cell. A private company, Celera Genomics (www.celera.com/), and the publicly funded National Human Genome Research Institute (www.nhgri.nih.gov/) announced on June 26, 2000, their completion of the first assembly draft of the human genome. Different organizations disagree about the genome's full size and the number of human genes. However, scientists know for sure that the total number of base pairs determines **genome** size. The genome, distributed among 23 pairs of **chromosomes**, each repeated over and over like a genetic stutter without interruption, imparts our individual uniqueness. At conception, one complete chromosome set from the father (22 plus an **X** or **Y sex chromosome**) joins with one complete set from the mother (22 plus an X sex chromosome) to give each human offspring 46 chromosomes. The helical DNA structures (**genotype**) contain the genetic blueprint or "roadmap" of instructions for almost every aspect of our being (**phenotype**).

The phenotype reflects the expression of our gene pool from the physical dimensions, texture, color, composition, and shape of every internal and external body part to our personalities with all their idiosyncrasies. The human genome greatly exceeds the genome size of other organisms. For example, the bacterium *Escherichia coli* shown at *right* (*E. coli*; primary member of the large bacterial family *Enterobacteriaceae*) contains 4.6 million base pairs,

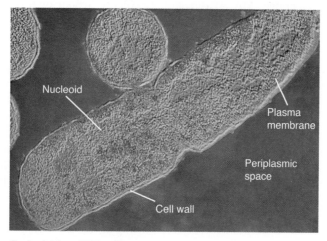

Escherichia coli (*E. coli*)

Template strand: original DNA strand that guides the synthesis of a new DNA strand by complementary base pairing

Human genome: the full complement of genetic material in a human cell; contains about 80,000 to 140,000 genes and from 3.12 (Celera Genomics estimate) to 3.15 (National Human Genome Research Institute estimate) billion nucleotide base pairs

X chromosome: sex chromosome present in two copies in female animals

Y chromosome: sex chromosome present in one copy in male animals

Genotype: the individual's genetic makeup at the molecular level comprising the entire set of genes

Phenotype: observable characteristics or attributes resulting from the expression of genes

Escherichia coli (E. coli): rod-like anaerobic bacterium with 4.6 million base pairs, found in the colon of humans and other mammals; studied in many disciplines for its genetic characteristics

while yeast contains 15 million base pairs. In contrast, the smallest human chromosome (the so-called male or Y chromosome) consists of 50 million base pairs, and the largest human chromosome contains 250 million base pairs. For some idea of the enormity of the genetic structures, consider the following analogy:

A double-spaced 8.5 × 11–inch page of text using normal margins contains about 3000 letters or roughly 250 words. Porting the human genome to pages would equal the number of letters in 1000 copies of the Sunday *New York Times* or 1200 copies of the 4th edition of our 900-page *Exercise Physiology* text. Stated another way, reading one letter of code every second would require about 100 years without a break to peruse the entire genome! A single DNA strand in one **diploid** human cell with 23 pairs of chromosomes, if unwound and stacked end to end, would stretch to the height of a person 60 inches tall, yet it occupies a width of only 50 trillionths of an inch; and it is not only DNA's remarkably large size but also its relative molecular weight. For example, the chromosome of *Escherichia coli* has a molecular weight of 2500 × 10^6, contrasted with a molecular weight of only 180 for the monosaccharide glucose.

To unravel the submicroscopic secrets of genetic material, sophisticated detection techniques help scientists "decode" the human genome. Most of the DNA sequences never become part of the final transcript that ultimately directs protein synthesis. In 2003, the Human Genome Project (www.ornl.gov/TechResources/Human_Genome/home.html) achieved its major objective of sequencing the total DNA of the human genome. By November 2000, more than one half of the genome had been identified, sequenced, and recorded in public databases (e.g., www.acedb.org/). The December 1999 issue of *Nature* featured a milestone scientific achievement—the sequence or "genetic map" for 12 contiguous segments of human chromosome 22, the second smallest of the 23 chromosomes (chromosome 22 contains about 1.6 to 1.8% of the total genomic DNA).[45] The DNA sequence includes the longest, continuous stretch of DNA ever deciphered and assembled. It contains over 23 million letters. The sequencing of chromosome 22 allowed scientists for the first time to view the entire DNA of a chromosome. At least 27 human disorders link to chromosome 22 genes, including ovarian, colon, and breast cancers; cataracts; congenital heart disease; schizophrenia; **neurofibromatosis**; mental retardation; and disorders of the nervous system and fetal development (www.ornl.gov/sci/techresources/Human_Genome/launchpad/chrom22.shtml).

Scientists view this monumental genomic accomplishment as somewhat like completing an intricately detailed inaugural chapter in the human genetic instruction book composed of many complex chapters. An international collaboration from eight laboratories in the United Kingdom, Japan, the United States, Canada, and Sweden disclosed that chromosome 22 contained at least 545 genes (and 134 **pseudogenes**) in its 33.4-**megabase** structure. Through July 2001, sequencing of chromosomes 1 to 22 was nearly complete (100%); for chromosome Y, it is 62.4% complete, and 85.2% for chromosome X. Five large science centers currently work on about 85% of the Human Genome Project: the Whitehead Institute in Cambridge, MA; Washington University School of Medicine in St. Louis, MO; Baylor College of Medicine in Houston, TX; the Joint Genome Institute in Walnut Creek, CA; and the Sanger Center in Cambridge, England. Government-supported laboratories in France, Germany, Japan, and China also support genome research. The research teams discovered 160 human genes that have comparable sequences in the mouse. Examining the chromosomal locations of the mouse genes with counterparts on human chromosome 22 showed that the order of the genes along the chromosome in the two species is genetically conserved, although the mouse homologues of human genes on chromosome 22 were dispersed to eight different mouse chromosomal regions. Determining the way genes are arranged along a strip of DNA has paved the way for major advances in disease diagnosis and treatment. Knowing the identity and order of the chemical components of the DNA of the 23 pairs of chromosomes found in almost every human cell has provided an important tool to determine the basis of health and disease.

In a material sense, a relatively few discrete genetic instructions ultimately determine all of the subtlety of our species, including the thousands of years of accomplishment in fields of

Diploid: having two representatives of every chromosome (i.e., two copies of each gene)

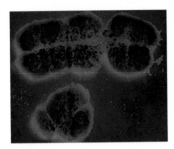

Figure 4 Human males have X (larger; top) and Y (smaller; bottom) chromosomes.

Neurofibromatosis: hereditary disorder characterized clinically by the combination of patches of hyperpigmentation in both cutaneous and subcutaneous tumors over the entire body

Pseudogene: stretch of DNA similar in nucleotide sequence to normal DNA but containing defective (mutated) genes, rendering it nonfunctional for transcription and translation

Megabase: one billion base pairs

study from architecture to poetry and medicine to computer science and zoology. Anatomic and psychologic differences between any two unrelated individuals really reflect relatively few differences in their genomic blueprint—perhaps one or two gene sequences out of thousands. For example, the person next door, the golf champion Tiger Woods, and the brilliant Austrian physicist Lise Meitner (1878–1968[113]; deprived of a Nobel Prize for contributing to the discovery of nuclear fission because of her religion and professional animosities) are far more *alike* than different, yet the variety among individuals approaches infinity!

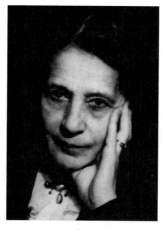

Dr. Lise Meitner

NUCLEIC ACIDS

FIGURE 5 shows the central configurational differences between the two nucleic acids, DNA and RNA; the three *yellow text boxes* highlight the important differences. Both structures carry and then transmit the hereditary information among the same type of cells when they divide (i.e., liver cells produce liver cells) and from generation to generation through reproductive cells. Within all living cells, genes encode the hereditary set of instructions that determine an organism's unique characteristics, from a simple bacterium such as *Streptococcus pneumoniae* to the complex multicellular organism *Homo sapiens*. As organisms within a species increase in complexity, the total information stored within the genome also increases tremendously. In subsequent sections, we describe just how much encoded information must be transcribed and translated to ultimately create proteins, which characterize thousands of unique cells, tissues, and organs that define the organism. Think of DNA as the raw material or building blocks of genes, and RNA as the link or intermediary to protein synthesis. Two excellent Internet sites provide a starting point for the study of DNA and the revolution it spawned (www.dnai.org/index.htm; www.dnaftb.org/dnaftb/), including an excellent website devoted to animations about most of the key processes involved in DNA and associated activities (highered.mcgraw-hill.com/sites/dl/free/0072437316/120060/ravenanimation.html).

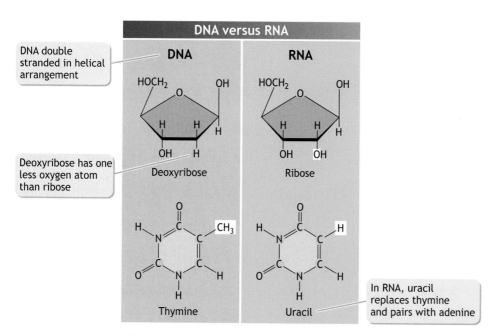

Figure 5   Differences in molecular configuration between DNA and RNA.

Nucleic acid: large molecule containing nucleotide subunits

Polymer: high-molecular-weight substance linked together by repeating similar or identical subunits (e.g., glucose polymer starch); long-chain molecule linkage forms a two- and three-dimensional network

Polynucleotide: two or more nucleotides joined together; the phosphate at carbon 5′ of one sugar combines at the 3′ position of another sugar

Deoxyribose: sugar with five carbon atoms

Metaphase: step in mitosis (or meiosis) in which micro-tubules organize into a spindle and chromosomes move to the cell's equator to align in pairs but have not yet migrated to the poles

DNA and RNA

The **nucleic acids** DNA and RNA consist of polarized **polymers** of repeating subunits or nucleotides. A nucleotide consists of a nitrogen-containing organic base having 6 carbon atoms, a 5-carbon sugar, and a phosphate molecule (FIG. 6). A nucleotide's main support structure (backbone) consists of the sugar and phosphate molecules. The sugar-phosphate backbone lies on the outside of the helix, with the amine bases on the inside. In this configuration, a base on one strand points at a base on the second strand. When nucleotides join to form **polynucleotides**, they link at specific carbon locations on the sugar molecule. These locations, numbered, in the *red circles* from 1′ to 5′, begin with 1′ to the right of the oxygen (O) atom in the ring. The "prime" symbol (′) distinguishes the carbons in the sugar from carbons in the base. Note from Figure 5 that RNA has one additional O atom in its sugar. Thus, the ribose sugar in RNA differs from the **deoxyribose** sugar in DNA. Nucleotides link when the phosphate at carbon 5′ of one sugar combines at the carbon 3′ position of another sugar. The phosphate group attaches to the 5′ carbon; the base attaches to the 1′ carbon. DNA and RNA synthesis always proceeds in the 5′ to 3′ direction.

The *top* of FIGURE 7 shows the successive levels (stages) of DNA packaging in a chromosome, proceeding from condensed **metaphase** *(upper left)* to supercoiled *(middle right),* loosely condensed, and uncondensed chromatin fiber stages. The negatively charged

Nucleotide components

Numbering

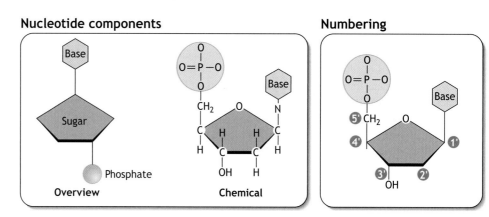

Joining

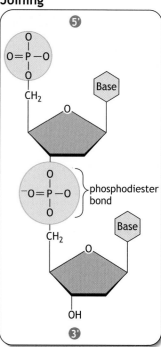

Figure 6 The components of a nucleotide, nucleotide-numbering nomenclature, and how nucleotides join together by phosphodiester bonding.

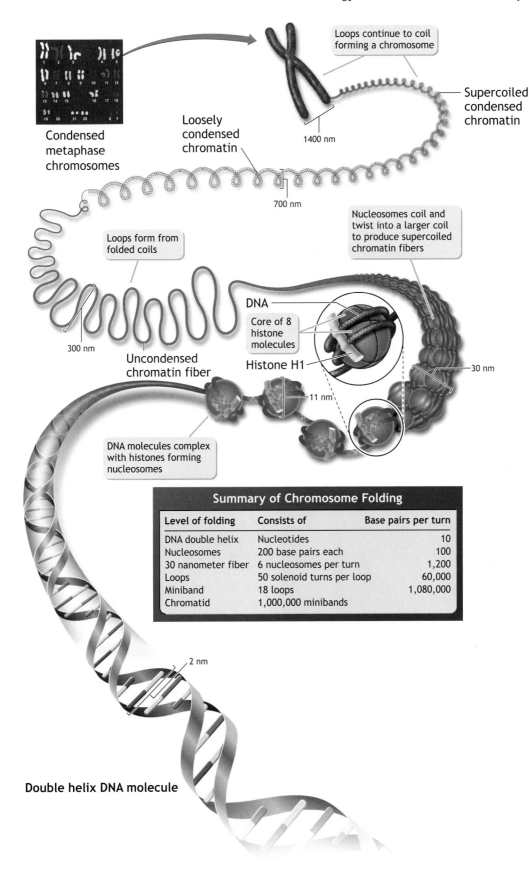

Loops continue to coil forming a chromosome

Supercoiled condensed chromatin

1400 nm

Condensed metaphase chromosomes

Loosely condensed chromatin

700 nm

Nucleosomes coil and twist into a larger coil to produce supercoiled chromatin fibers

Loops form from folded coils

DNA

Core of 8 histone molecules

Histone H1

30 nm

300 nm

Uncondensed chromatin fiber

11 nm

DNA molecules complex with histones forming nucleosomes

Summary of Chromosome Folding

Level of folding	Consists of	Base pairs per turn
DNA double helix	Nucleotides	10
Nucleosomes	200 base pairs each	100
30 nanometer fiber	6 nucleosomes per turn	1,200
Loops	50 solenoid turns per loop	60,000
Miniband	18 loops	1,080,000
Chromatid	1,000,000 minibands	

2 nm

Double helix DNA molecule

Figure 7 Double-helix DNA molecule packaged in a chromosome from the condensed metaphase stage, to supercoiled stage, to loosely condensed stage, and uncondensed chromatin fiber stage. The *inset table* provides details about chromosome folding from the DNA double helix to the chromatid. nm (nanometer), one-millionth mm.

Histone: positively charged small nuclear protein molecule cluster that binds to DNA (DNA winds around it) before it uncoils at the replication site; histones neutralize negatively charged DNA

Nucleosome: DNA coiled around a cluster of histone proteins; linked nucleosomes form chromatin

Electron microscope: electron beams with wavelengths thousands of times shorter than visible light replace light, allowing significantly higher resolution and magnification; the electrons pass through an ultrathin, specially prepared stained section of an embedded and dehydrated specimen maintained in a vacuum

Chromatid: one of the two double-stranded DNA daughter molecules of a duplicated, mitotic chromosome joined by a centromere

Mitosis: separation of duplicated chromosomes to create identical daughter cells with mirror-image (genetically identical) chromosomes; prophase, metaphase, anaphase, and telophase are the four phases of mitosis

Centromere: region of a mitotic chromosome (indentation) before replication where two daughter chromatids join

Daughter chromosome: descendent chromosome following replication of the original (mother) chromosome

DNA molecule encircles and binds to a cluster of positively charged eight **histone** proteins. The histone (purple ball-like structure) clamps the DNA to the core of the molecule. The term **nucleosome** describes DNA wrapped around the puck-shaped histone proteins. Examining this region by **electron microscopy** reveals that one beadlike nucleosome contains 146 nucleotide base pairs wound twice like a rope around one cluster of the eight histones. The cluster contains two each of four different protein subunits (H2A, H2B, H3, H4), with each specific subunit having a different molecular mass. A DNA strand with about 60 base pairs and a ninth histone molecule links each cluster to the next one. During replication, the DNA uncoils from the histone core. The DNA molecule shown at the *bottom* of the figure eventually packs into the single metaphase chromosome displayed at the *top left* of the figure. The *inset table* of Figure 7 provides relevant information about chromosome folding in the DNA double helix, nucleosomes, 30-nm fiber, loops, minibands, and **chromatids**.

The packaging of DNA within cells reflects a remarkable architectural accomplishment. The *inset table* summarizes DNA folding and how compacting the molecule enhances the efficiency of replication. In the compacted configuration as chromosomes, no transcription takes place, to ensure that DNA remains intact to survive **mitosis**. The chromatids (listed in the *last line of the table*) with 1 million minibands represent duplicate strands of DNA held together by a **centromere** just before the DNA separates into two **daughter chromosomes**. FIGURE 8 shows the details for chromosome 2 and the general nomenclature for identifying specific genes on the short p and long q arms of a chromosome. The *right* of the figure reveals the architectural details of a condensed metaphase chromosome.

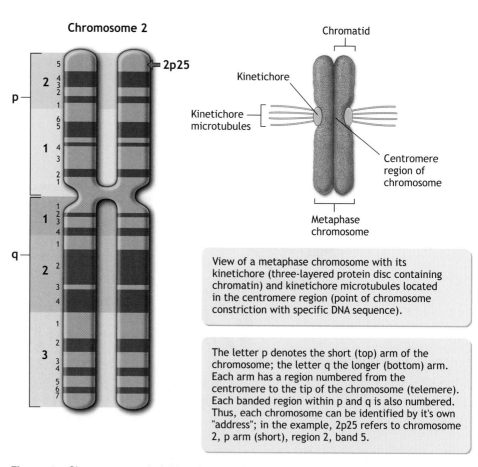

View of a metaphase chromosome with its kinetichore (three-layered protein disc containing chromatin) and kinetichore microtubules located in the centromere region (point of chromosome constriction with specific DNA sequence).

The letter p denotes the short (top) arm of the chromosome; the letter q the longer (bottom) arm. Each arm has a region numbered from the centromere to the tip of the chromosome (telemere). Each banded region within p and q is also numbered. Thus, each chromosome can be identified by it's own "address"; in the example, 2p25 refers to chromosome 2, p arm (short), region 2, band 5.

Figure 8 Chromosome 2. *Left.* Identification of gene *2p25* on chromosome 2. *Right.* Metaphase chromosome.

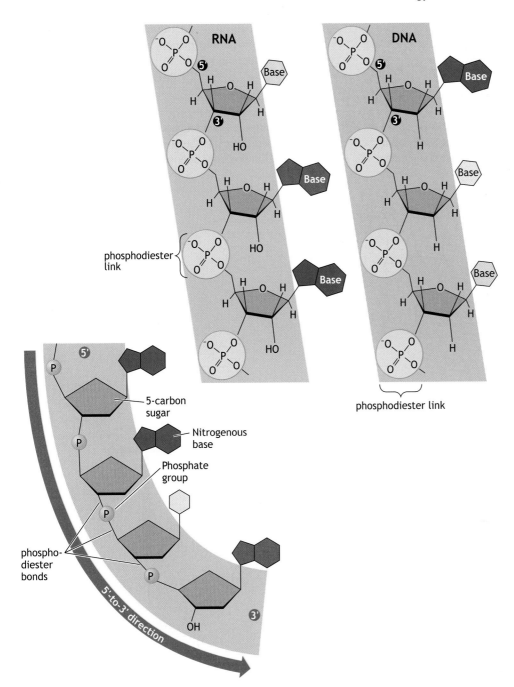

Figure 9 Linking of nucleotides by phosphodiester bonding in RNA and DNA. The general schema shown at the *bottom left* illustrates the relative position of the sugar, base, and phosphate groups within a nucleotide along the 5′ to 3′ direction, including phosphodiester bonding.

Linking Nucleotides: Phosphodiester Bonding

The chemical reaction when two nucleotides link together eliminates a water molecule, a process termed **dehydration synthesis**; it involves the phosphate molecule from one nucleotide and the hydroxyl (OH) molecule of another nucleotide. The resultant **phosphodiester bond** (FIG. 9) shown for RNA and DNA is a relatively strong **covalent bond**. The new polymer, now two units long, still has free phosphate and OH groups for linking to other nucleotides. This linkage forms an incredibly long chain with thousands of nucleotides, although the example shows only a few. In DNA measurement, the term **kilobase (kb)** represents a unit of DNA fragment length equal to 1000 nucleotides. Another nucleic acid,

Dehydration synthesis: removal of the equivalent of a water molecule from two subunit molecules that form a new, larger molecule

Phosphodiester bond: strong covalent bond formed when two nucleotides link together eliminating a water molecule; bonding involves the phosphate molecule from one nucleotide and the hydroxyl (OH) molecule of another nucleotide

Covalent bond: sharing one or more pairs of electrons between two atoms

Kilobase (kb): a unit of length for DNA fragments equal to 1000 nucleotides

Adenine: one of the four bases in DNA; always pairs with thymine

adenosine triphosphate (ATP), contains a 5-carbon sugar base (**adenine**) and three phosphate groups. Unlike DNA and RNA that transfer genetic information, ATP continually transfers *chemical energy* to power the body's cells throughout life.

Structure of DNA

FIGURE 10 shows the DNA molecule composed of a sequence of sugar phosphate chains with hydrogen bonding between the nitrogenous bases. In the double-stranded DNA molecule the strands are not identical. They lie parallel but line up in opposite directions. One strand runs

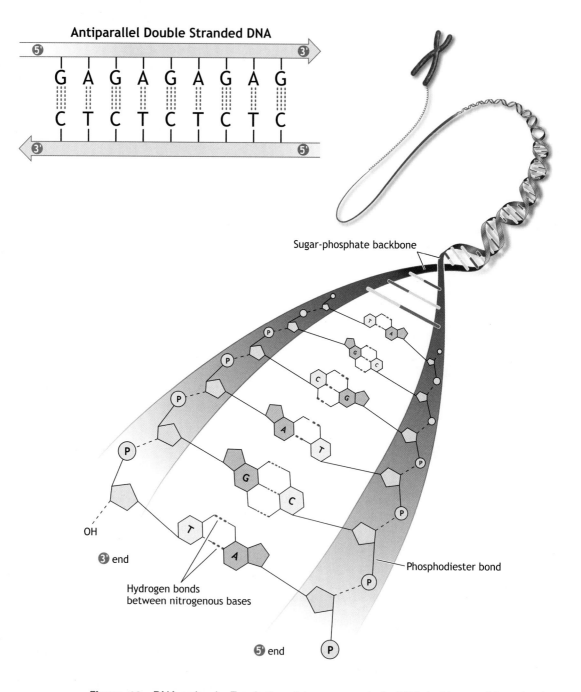

Figure 10 DNA molecule. *Top.* Antiparallel arrangement of a DNA double strand from the 5′ to 3′ and 3′ to 5′ directions. Note the hydrogen bonding between G and C and A and T. *Bottom.* DNA molecule with its sequence of sugar-phosphate chains and hydrogen bonding between nitrogenous bases. The specific sequence of base pairs ultimately determines every protein's specific characteristics. Adenine *always* binds with thymine.

in the 5′ to 3′ direction, and its **complementary strand** runs from 3′ to 5′ The *top left* of the figure illustrates the **antiparallel** arrangement of the DNA strands, including a close-up view of the hydrogen bonding between the base pairs that holds the parallel spiral ribbons together. The deduction by Watson and Crick of the antiparallel nature of the DNA strands resolved one of the remaining mysteries about DNA's structure and ultimately how replication proceeds.

Base Pairing

One of the "golden rules" of DNA's molecular arrangement displayed in FIGURE 11 relates to the pairing of the four bases, the letters of the DNA alphabet. **Guanine (G)** always links with **cytosine (C)** and **adenine (A)** always links with **thymine (T)** in the same proportions within all DNA molecules. Stated somewhat differently, whenever a G base occurs in one of the strands, a C base occurs opposite it in the opposing strand. Likewise, when an A base occurs in one strand, a T base occurs in the other strand. The proportionality of the four bases was confirmed in 1950 by Erwin Chargaff (1905–2002) of Columbia University who determined the relative amounts of each base in DNA. **Chargaff's rule** determined regularities among the four chemical bases of DNA—the molar amount of thymine always equaled the molar amount of adenine, and similarly, molar amounts of guanine always equaled cytosine on one DNA strand ([T] = [A]; [G] = [C]). Watson and Crick relied on this information to piece together DNA's structure. In their model, each rung of the DNA ladder consists of a purine connected to a pyrimidine. The term *base pairing* refers to the joining of **complementary bases** (G with C or A with T). The G and A nitrogenous bases consist of two rings (called a **purine**), while the two other bases C and T have a single ring (called a **pyrimidine**). Thus, each base pair consists of one larger purine base mated to a smaller pyrimidine base. Adenine and thymine form two strong hydrogen bonds between the base pairs, but not with G or C. Similarly, G and C form three strong hydrogen bonds to keep the C–G base pair intact, but not with A or T. The additive effect of millions of relatively weak hydrogen bonds within the DNA molecule keeps the helix from separating. Applying Chargaff's rule within an organism, the pyrimidine content (TC) equals the purine content (AG); however, the relative amounts of pyrimidines and purines differ among organisms.

The *top* of Figure 11 illustrates the DNA double-helix molecule, with the base pairing and hydrogen bonding for A–T and G–C. Precise x-ray measurements have determined that the DNA double helix has a width of 2.0 nm (nanometers; 10^{-9} m (or 10 Å) = one-millionth millimeter, or 1000 nm = 1 μm), with exactly 10 base pairs in each full turn, with the height of each turn equal to 3.4 nm. The *bottom* of the figure shows the five bases classified as either a purine or pyrimidine. Note the pyrimidine base **uracil**. In RNA (next section), uracil replaces thymine, so that adenine pairs with uracil as A–U. The inclusion of uracil helps to distinguish RNA from DNA—besides RNA's extra oxygen atom in the ribose sugar and usually single-strand configuration. The simple mnemonic "cut the pie" helps to associate the pyrimidine or purine bases: **CUT** represents **c**ytosine, **u**racil, and **t**hymine, with the **py**rimidines represented by **pie**.

The heat required to dissociate the H bonds between two strands of DNA determines the DNA molecule's melting temperature. Proportionality exists between the number of bonds in the base pair and the energy required to break the bonds. Thus, the three hydrogen bonds holding C and G together require more heat to break (higher melting point) than the two hydrogen bonds between A and T.

Forms of RNA

The three forms of RNA include:

1. Messenger RNA (mRNA) molecules, which serve as a template for protein synthesis, based on the molecular sequence from a small section of the DNA molecule
2. **Transfer RNA(tRNA)** molecules, which, as the name implies, transfer amino acids to the growing peptide chain on the ribosome
3. **Ribosomal RNA(rRNA)** molecules, which account for about 50% of the mass of ribosomes; the structures aid in assembling amino acids into polypeptides

Each of the three RNA forms has its own **polymerase** or complex enzyme: polymerase I is associated with rRNA, polymerase II with mRNA, and polymerase III with tRNA. RNA

Complementary strand: when one DNA strand runs in the 5′ to 3′ direction, the complementary strand runs oppositely from 3′ to 5′

Antiparallel: arranged in parallel but with opposite orientation as in DNA

Guanine: one of the four bases in DNA; always pairs with cytosine

Cytosine: one of the four bases in DNA; always pairs with guanine

Thymine: one of the four bases in DNA; always pairs with adenine

Chargaff's rule: pyrimidine content (T + C) equals purine content (A + G), where ([T] = [A]; [G] = [C]); (A + T)/(G + C) varies between different organisms but is constant within an organism

Complementary: pairing in DNA between bases A-T or T-A, and C-G or G-C

Purine: nitrogen-containing, double-ring basic compound in nucleic acids; purines in DNA and RNA include adenine and guanine

Pyrimidine: nitrogen-containing, single-ring basic compound in nucleic acids; pyrimidines include cytosine and thymine in DNA and cytosine and uracil in RNA

Uracil: base that replaces thymine in RNA that pairs with the adenine base

Transfer RNA (tRNA): RNA molecules that transport a specific amino acid to ribosomes; translating information in the mRNA nucleotide into the amino acid sequence of a polypeptide

Ribosomal RNA (rRNA): structural part of a ribosome that contains RNA molecules

Polymerase (DNA or RNA): enzyme that catalyzes nucleic acid synthesis on preexisting nucleic acid templates; assembles RNA from ribonucleotides or DNA from deoxyribonucleotides

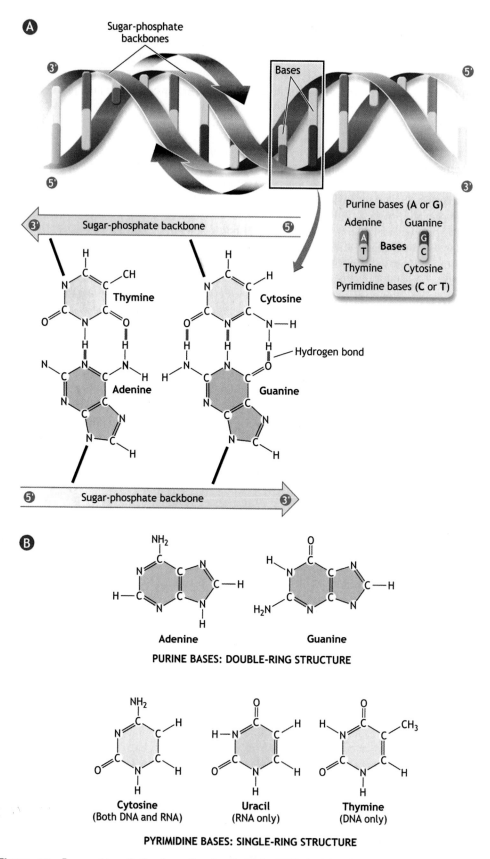

Figure 11   Base pairing. **A**. Configuration details of the DNA double helix molecule with base pairing and hydrogen bonding for adenine (A)–thymine (T) and guanine (G)–cytosine (C). The two spiral ribbons represent the sugar (deoxyribose)-phosphate backbone of DNA. Note that two hydrogen bonds shown in *dark red* form between A and T and three form between G and C. This happens because the two polynucleotide chains that contain them lie antiparallel to each other. **B**. The five bases classified as purines (A and G) or pyrimidines (C, uracil, T).

polymerases, unlike their DNA counterparts, do not require a **primer** to initiate RNA chain synthesis. The term **primase** refers to the RNA polymerase that produces the primer for DNA synthesis. The three RNA polymerases have between 6 and 10 protein subunits that differ in molecular structure and regulatory function. About 97% of cellular RNA exists as rRNA; mRNA accounts for about 2%, and tRNA less than 1%. Compared with the DNA in a single chromosome that contains up to 250 million base pairs, RNA contains no more than a few thousand, which makes an RNA molecule considerably shorter. This makes sense because RNA carries only part of the information from one segment of the DNA molecule that it copied. In a subsequent section on protein synthesis, beginning on page 1007, we discuss how mRNA duplicates DNA's genetic information and the roles of rRNA and tRNA in protein synthesis.

Primer: a short nucleotide segment that pairs with a single DNA strand at a free 3′-OH end (template strand) so DNA polymerase can synthesize a DNA chain; cells use RNA primers, while the PCR method uses DNA primers

Primase: enzyme that synthesizes the RNA primer to initiate DNA synthesis

Codons and Nature's Genetic Code

First presented by Marshall Nirenberg (1968 Nobel Prize in Physiology or Medicine; interpretation of the genetic code and its function in protein synthesis) and Johann Matthaei (best known for discovering that the RNA sequence "UUU" directs the addition of phenylalanine to any growing protein chain) of the NIH in 1961 at the International Congress of Biochemistry in Moscow (and 3 years later by Philip Leder and Marshall Nirenberg), the coded message carried by the mRNA molecule exists as a series of three bases or **codons**. Each three-letter codon block of information corresponds to one of the body's 20 amino acids. A codon codes for one amino acid, but most amino acids are represented by more than one codon. If only one base coded for an amino acid, only four amino acids could be coded instead of 20. Even if two adjacent bases coded for an amino acid, there would still not be enough combinations to make 20 amino acids. Fortunately, scientists deduced that three bases coding for an amino acid ($4^3 = 64$ combinations) met the requirement to include all the amino acids. For example, the triplet sequence A-U-G on mRNA displayed in FIGURE 12 *(green box within yellow panel)* refers to a specific code for the amino acid **methionine**. The A (adenine) is called the first letter, U (uracil), the second letter,

Codon: sequence of three DNA or RNA bases (nucleotides) that encode (specify) a single amino acid

Methionine: nutritionally essential amino acid; most natural source of active methyl groups in the body. The triplet sequence A-U-G on mRNA codes this amino acid

First base (First letter) DNA	mRNA	Second base (Second letter): DNA A / mRNA U	DNA G / mRNA C	DNA T / mRNA A	DNA C / mRNA G	Third base (Third letter) mRNA	DNA
A	U	UUU Phenylalanine	UCU Serine	UAU Thyrosine	UGU Cysteine	U	A
		UUC Phenylalanine	UCC Serine	UAC Thyrosine	UGC Cysteine	C	G
		UUA Leucine	UCA Serine	UAA STOP Codon	UGA STOP Codon	A	T
		UUG Leucine	UCG Serine	UAG STOP Codon	UGG Tryptophan	G	C
G	C	CUU Leucine	CCU Proline	CAU Histidine	CGU Arginine	U	A
		CUC Leucine	CCC Proline	CAC Histidine	CGC Arginine	C	G
		CUA Leucine	CCA Proline	CAA Glutamine	CGA Arginine	A	T
		CUG Leucine	CCG Proline	CAG Glutamine	CGG Arginine	G	C
T	A	AUU Isoleucine	ACU Thereonine	AAU Asparagine	AGU Serine	U	A
		AUC Isoleucine	ACC Thereonine	AAC Asparagine	AGG Serine	C	G
		AUA Isoleucine	ACA Thereonine	AAA Lysine	AGA Arginine	A	T
		AUG START Methionine	ACG Thereonine	AAG Lysine	AGG Arginine	G	C
C	G	GUU Valine	GCU Alanine	GAU Aspartic acid	GGU Glycine	U	A
		GUC Valine	GCC Alanine	GAC Aspartic acid	GGC Glycine	C	G
		GUA Valine	GCA Alanine	GAA Glutamic acid	GGA Glycine	A	T
		GUG Valine	GCG Alanine	GAG Glutamic acid	GGG Glycine	G	C

Figure 12 The codon table–the alphabet of the universal genetic code. From the time that Watson and Crick correctly deduced DNA's helical structure in 1953, different coding schemes attempted to explain DNA's alphabetic configuration (including imaginative proposals by physicists George Gamow, Richard Feynman, and Edward Teller[58]); in 1964, Paul Leder and Marshall Nirenberg established the final code-breaking sequences for RNA synthesis.[79] The three-letter codon "word" in mRNA is complementary to the corresponding three-letter codon within DNA from which it was transcribed.

and G (guanine), the third letter. With only 20 amino acids and 64 codons, several codons code for more than one amino acid. In fact, as mentioned, most amino acids have more than one codon or sequence of letters, with no intervening code disrupting the sequence.

Sequencing of Codons

The amino acid serine exemplifies a four-codon sequence that differs only in the base occupying the third nucleotide or letter. The sequence is U-C-U, U-C-C, U-C-A, and U-C-G, with identical first two letters. The first two bases are the defining letters of the codon sequence. Reading from the 5′ end of each codon, the first and second letters remain generally constant for each amino acid, while the base in the third position "wobbles." Thus, for example, the codon for phenylalanine contains a U or C as the third letter. Because both U-U-U and U-U-C code for phenylalanine, phenylalanine is inserted into a newly synthesized polypeptide if U-U-U or U-U-C were "read" during **translation** or protein synthesis.

Codon Table. Similar to the English alphabet with its 26 letters, the *codon table* in Figure 12 provides the genetic code "alphabet," but with only four distinct letters—the code words in the analogy. When we exclude the three **stop codons** (*red boxes*) that signal termination of linkages in polypeptide chains, the remaining 61 codons represent the useful information for protein synthesis. The stop codons, U-A-A, U-A-G, and U-G-A, signal the end of a genetic message (i.e., termination of protein synthesis), like periods at the end of a sentence. When the translation machinery encounters one of these chain terminators, translation halts, releasing the polypeptide from the translation complex. Recall that the start codon for methionine (A-U-G) initiates polypeptide formation; it also can code for methionine within peptide chains.

HOW DNA REPLICATES

A **DNA replication fork** refers to the Y-shaped region of replicating DNA molecules. As the double helix unwinds, nucleotide duplication occurs on both strands at a rate of about 50 nucleotide additions per second. Each strand serves as a template to create two new daughter strands by complementary base pairing. This mechanism provides each daughter helix with one intact strand from the parent (original strand) and one newly synthesized strand. Each strand, a complementary mirror image of the other, can serve as a template to reconstruct the other strand. FIGURE 13 presents a schematic overview of DNA replication. Replication begins with the untwisted, unzipped appearance of two DNA strands (the helicase unwinds a segment of the DNA) on the *top,* where replication starts at specific zones called **origins of replication** and ends where **RNA primers** (*green*) start new DNA chains on the leading strand. Unwinding a segment of DNA breaks the hydrogen bonds between the two complementary strands of DNA. Several origins of replication exist along a chromosome, replicating simultaneously in *opposite* directions. Multiple replications reduce the time to propagate DNA by an order of magnitude, since complete duplication of one strand of human DNA takes approximately 6 hours. The number of base pairs along the chromosome's replication region ranges from 10,000 up to 1 million, with an average of about 100,000 base pairs.

Stages of DNA Replication

FIGURE 14 amplifies the three stages of DNA replication illustrated in Figure 13. In stage 1, helicase enzymes *(orange)* unwind the molecule's double helix. This stabilizes the strands, while **single-strand binding protein** (SSB) maintains separation between the two DNA strands. In stage 2, **DNA polymerase** *(purple sphere)* immediately acts on DNA's **leading strand** to add nucleotides *toward* the strand's 3′ end *(red)*. The process of creating the strand, called **continuous synthesis**, proceeds uninterrupted. The other DNA strand, known as a **lagging strand**, is created in shorter segments, with gaps in its structure *away* from the replication fork, compared with the leading strand. In stage 3 **discontinuous synthesis**, a 10-nucleotide RNA primer, under the influence of **DNA polymerase I**, adds 1000 nucleotides ahead of the lagging strand's 5′ end

Translation: polypeptide formation (protein synthesis) on a ribosome using the amino acid sequence specified by an mRNA nucleotide sequence

Stop codon: 3 of the 64 codon combinations that terminate a polypeptide assembly

DNA replication fork: Y-shaped region of replicating DNA molecules where the enzymes replicating a DNA molecule bind to an untwisted, single DNA strand

Origins of replication: sites on DNA where replication begins

RNA primer: small segment of 10 RNA nucleotides complementary to the parent DNA template that adds DNA nucleotides to it to synthesize a new DNA strand

Single-strand binding protein (SSB): protein that keeps separated strands of DNA from rejoining

DNA polymerase: enzyme responsible for creating new DNA strands during replication or repair

Leading strand: new DNA daughter strand formed during continuous synthesis of DNA

Continuous synthesis: process of creating a DNA strand

Lagging strand: new shorter DNA strand formed during discontinuous synthesis; joined end to end by DNA ligase away from the replication fork

Discontinuous synthesis: RNA primer 10 nucleotides long under the influence of DNA polymerase I that adds 1000 nucleotides ahead of the lagging strand's 5′ end until its gap fills

DNA polymerase I: enzyme that makes small bits of DNA to fill in gaps between Okazaki fragments during stage 3 discontinuous synthesis

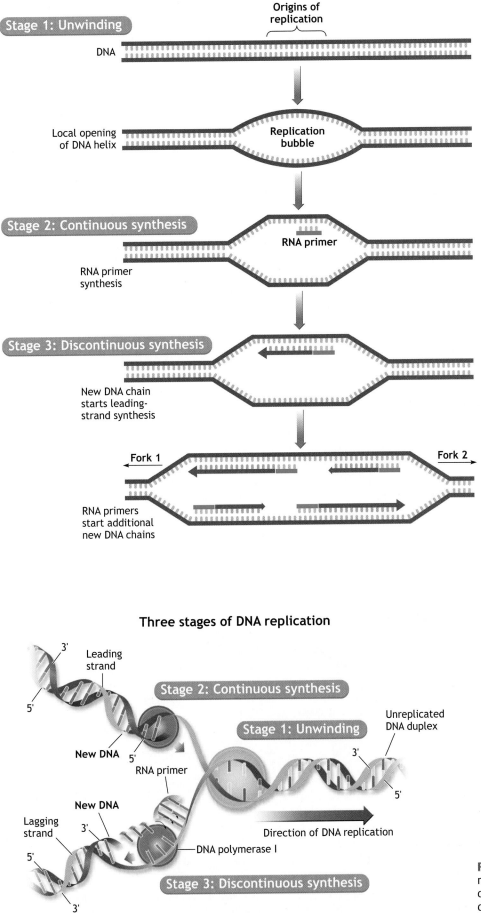

Stage 1: Unwinding

Origins of replication

DNA

Local opening of DNA helix

Replication bubble

Stage 2: Continuous synthesis

RNA primer

RNA primer synthesis

Stage 3: Discontinuous synthesis

New DNA chain starts leading-strand synthesis

Fork 1   Fork 2

RNA primers start additional new DNA chains

Figure 13 Replication bubble and DNA replication. Note the straight (not helical) double strands of DNA in stage 1 after untwisting by DNA gyrase and unwinding by helicase. The DNA resembles an elongated bubble as the double strand opens and DNA begins to divide (stage 2, continuous synthesis). In stage 3 (discontinuous synthesis), replication proceeds in opposite directions along each end of the Y-shaped replication forks.

Three stages of DNA replication

3'

Leading strand

Stage 2: Continuous synthesis

5'

Stage 1: Unwinding

New DNA

5'

Unreplicated DNA duplex

RNA primer

3'

New DNA

5'

Lagging strand

3'

Direction of DNA replication

5'

DNA polymerase I

3'

Stage 3: Discontinuous synthesis

3'

Figure 14 Three stages of DNA replication. Stage 1, unwinding; stage 2, continuous synthesis; stage 3, discontinuous synthesis.

DNA ligase: enzyme that binds short Okazaki fragments of the lagging strand into a continuous strand in DNA replication during stage 3 discontinuous synthesis

Okazaki fragments: short DNA segments 100–200 nucleotides long assembled by discontinuous replication in the 5′ to 3′ direction away from the replication fork; forms the lagging strand

until its gap fills. Thus, new DNA nucleotides replace the existing RNA nucleotides. **DNA ligase** then affixes the newly created, smaller **Okazaki fragments,** 100–200 nucleotides long, to the lagging strand in the 5′ to 3′ direction to make a complete DNA strand.

Pivotal Role for DNA Polymerase

DNA polymerase plays the central role in life's processes because this enzyme consistently duplicates the genetic information from generation to generation. The rich instructional bank of DNA information has been modified and improved over more than 3 billion years to build proteins and other molecules atom by atom according to selective molecular directions. For every cell that divides, DNA polymerase duplicates its entire DNA, so that cells transfer one copy to each daughter cell. DNA polymerase can be considered the most accurate of the thousands of enzymes because it creates an exact DNA copy, transmitting less than one "error" in a billion bases. Stated another way, one might find only one grammatical mistake in a thousand novels. The excellent match of C to G and A to T provides much of the specificity needed for this high accuracy, but DNA polymerase adds an extra step. After it copies each base, it "proofreads" it and deletes any wrong base sequence from its grasp. Polymerases can vary in structure from relatively "simple" to complex. In humans, polymerases are complex structures that unwind the helix, build an RNA primer, and construct a new strand. Some even have a ring-shaped structure that clamps the polymerase to the DNA strand. Polymerase function varies from day-to-day DNA repair and maintenance to the complex task of DNA replication when the cell divides. Here, we discuss the important role of DNA polymerase in forensic medicine in building a large quantity of identical DNA strands from a miniscule amount of DNA from a crime scene or paternity case.

Control of DNA Synthesis

Cell cycle: four stages of a cell's life cycle

Several molecular control mechanisms trigger DNA synthesis in cells. The **cell cycle** illustrated in FIGURE 15 depicts the four phases of a cell's life. Like a clock or thermostat, each phase has defined "on" and "off" periods regulated by enzymes that start and terminate a particular stage. DNA replication (synthesis) occurs in the S phase, which lasts approximately 6 hours. The three checkpoints identified by the *stars* serve as the thermostat's sensors, each

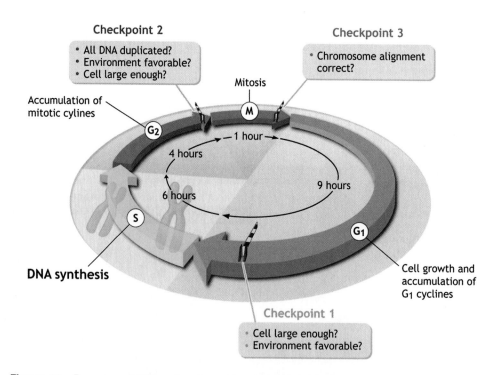

Figure 15 Four stages of the cell cycle and its molecular control mechanisms. Note the three checkpoints and the question(s) posed prior to DNA synthesis during the S phase.

with specific regulator enzymes called **cyclins** governing a specific function. Toward the end of the G_1 (growth) stage, cyclin enzymes achieve a critical activity level that triggers a response when the cell achieves adequate size within a favorable environment. If cell size and environment prove satisfactory, the cell proceeds to S phase for DNA synthesis. Following DNA synthesis, the G_1 cyclins degrade as the cell prepares to enter mitosis (M phase). The next checkpoint occurs between the G_2 and M phases, a crucial time in the cell cycle. When the DNA has been replicated without error, the cell enters mitosis and then progresses to complete **telophase**. Mitosis produces two cells genetically identical to the original parent cell.

Cell Life Cycle Controllers

Figure 15 provides details of the workings of cell life cycle controllers. Cyclin-dependent **kinases** (cdk_1 and cdk_2) activate specific cyclins. Once this occurs, the complex of the two **protein kinases** regulates how the cell proceeds through its cycle. After each stage, cyclin degradation temporarily halts cdk activity. With mitosis complete, the process begins again, accumulating cyclins for the next initial G_1 growth stage.

The cdk_2 protein "turns on" in the transition between the G_1 and S stages; cdk_1 drives the cell cycle from stage G_2 to M stage. In other words, the cyclin-dependent protein kinases phosphorylate their target cyclin proteins through the different stages of the cell cycle. Signaling proteins called growth factors operate in concert during the cycle. For example, mitosis-promoting factor (MPF) governs the sequence of events between the G_1 and M phases of the cell cycle. Other growth factors also exert their effect. For example, the hormone **erythropoietin** produced by the kidneys (see Chapters 20, 23, and 24) initiates proliferation of red blood cell precursors and their maturation to erythrocytes. Nerve growth factor (NGF) modulates neuronal cell growth during development of the nervous system, interleukin-2 participates in immune cell proliferation, and **insulin-like growth factor** (IGF) facilitates many metabolic events related to cellular growth and development. A unique feature of growth factors relates to how they control the transition stages during cellular growth and differentiation. Failure to work in concert with cyclins and kinases during cellular proliferation terminates control of cellular proliferation, causing cells to continue to divide unchecked. This can serve both positive and negative functions. The latter produce lethal effects because DNA synthesis would progress to the M stage by successfully reproducing a mutant **cancer** gene. If highly specialized genes called tumor suppressors (e.g., the *p53* gene) cannot halt the cell cycle long enough for DNA repair enzymes to function, then cell growth proceeds rapidly and unchecked to produce tumors. Also, deleterious mutations can pass to progeny cells; the successive buildup of mutations in all likelihood ultimately develops into cancer.

PROTEIN SYNTHESIS: TRANSCRIPTION AND TRANSLATION

Protein synthesis involves two prominent events:

1. Transcription in the cell nucleus that creates a single-stranded RNA copy of the genetic information stored in the double-stranded DNA molecule
2. RNA translation in the cell cytoplasm to form proteins

In essence, the DNA molecule's nucleotide base sequence defines the protein's ultimate three-dimensional shape. Our tour of protein synthesis begins by considering a "roadmap" of the prominent events in assembling proteins from precursor biomolecules. The story originates in the cell's ribosomes and ends with creation of a fully **functional protein**—a unique molecule whose structure dictates its operation and specific mode of action.

Generalized Overview

FIGURE 16 provides a generalized overview of six stages in protein synthesis. Prior to stage 1, the DNA under enzyme control "untwists" to expose its code. Before DNA's hydrogen bonds break, DNA topoisomerase enzymes (e.g., **DNA gyrase**) "relaxes" the **supercoiled DNA** by literally cutting the DNA to create a double-stranded break, but maintains hold of

Cyclins: specific cell-regulator enzymes that activate and de-activate protein kinases in the cell cycle and help to control progression from one stage in the cycle to the next. They are destroyed after their function by a ubiquitin-signaled process

G_1: period within the cell cycle preceding DNA synthesis

G_2: period within the cell cycle from the end of DNA synthesis and start of the M phase

Telophase: final stage in mitosis (or meiosis); the spindle disappears and daughter sets of separated chromosomes decondense, the cytoplasm splits, a nuclear envelope resurrounds the chromosomes, and nucleoli appear

Kinase: enzyme that shuttles a phosphate group (PO_4) from ATP or another nucleoside triphosphate to a different molecule

Protein kinase: enzyme that transfers phosphate groups to other proteins, changing their activity

Insulin-like growth factor (IGF): small protein hormone with the potent effect of increasing aspects of cellular growth and development; IGF-1 (also known as somatomedin C) controls the general effects of growth hormone on growth

Cancer: accelerated, unplanned growth and division of mutant cells that form larger-than-normal cell clusters that become tumors

Functional protein: protein with its own set of genetically determined information to carry out specific function(s)

DNA gyrase: enzyme that relaxes supercoiled DNA

Supercoiled DNA: configuration of twisted DNA packed into a cell prior to replication

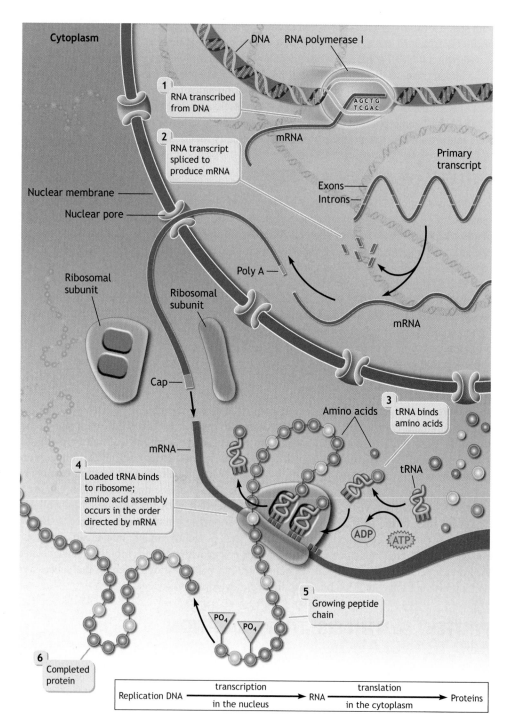

Figure 16 Generalized overview of six stages (*numbered yellow boxes*) in protein synthesis. Notable features include the schematic depiction of events during *transcription* (stages labeled *1* and *2* within the cell's nucleus) and *translation* (stages labeled *3* to *6* in the cell's cytoplasm). The *bottom inset box* summarizes the two principle aspects of protein synthesis (transcription and translation) following replication of the DNA molecule.

Labels in figure:

Cytoplasm
DNA   RNA polymerase I
1 RNA transcribed from DNA
2 RNA transcript spliced to produce mRNA
mRNA
Primary transcript
Exons
Introns
Nuclear membrane
Nuclear pore
Poly A
mRNA
Ribosomal subunit
Ribosomal subunit
Cap
Amino acids
3 tRNA binds amino acids
tRNA
mRNA
4 Loaded tRNA binds to ribosome; amino acid assembly occurs in the order directed by mRNA
ADP
ATP
5 Growing peptide chain
PO₄   PO₄
6 Completed protein

Replication DNA → (transcription in the nucleus) → RNA → (translation in the cytoplasm) → Proteins

DNA helicase: enzyme that catalyzes the unwinding of double-helical DNA by using energy released from ATP hydrolysis

DNA polymerase III (Pol III): enzyme involved in making DNA when chromosomes replicate

Replication bubble: site where DNA divides

RNA polymerase 1: enzyme that synthesizes RNA from a DNA template

both ends of the DNA. The two halves of the molecule then rotate relative to each other (they untwist) before rejoining. Once the strand untwists, **DNA helicase** unwinds the helical DNA molecule by separating the hydrogen bonds between the base pairs. The single-strand binding protein (SSB) binds to one of the unpaired DNA strands to inhibit its reemerging with its neighbor (complementary) strand. This prevents the strands from recoiling and re-forming the double helix. **DNA polymerase III (Pol III)** serves as a "verifier" to ensure that the bases pair correctly. If they do, the enzyme joins the nucleotides together. If not, the mismatched base pair is rejected. A previous section ("How DNA Replicates") provides further details about the DNA **replication bubble** and three stages of DNA replication.

Stage 1 signifies the start of transcription. This involves copying a discrete section of the genetic sequence directly from the DNA template to the growing RNA strand. The enzyme **RNA polymerase 1** (referred to as "I" because it was discovered before the other polymerases) in

Figure 16 binds to the specific **promoter** (initiator) region at the beginning of a gene. Linking to a specific nitrogenous base sequence, it "alerts" transcription to initiate formation of the complementary RNA strand. When RNA polymerase arrives at the end of the gene, it receives a "stop" signal from one of three nucleotide sequences (U-A-A, U-A-G, U-G-A; see Fig. 12) and disengages from the DNA. The newly assembled RNA strand, called the **primary RNA transcript** of the gene (stage 2), is processed and eventually exits the nucleus to the cytoplasm through the octagon disk-shaped **nuclear pore complex**. This complex selectively transports proteins across the nuclear envelope after specific protein receptors dock with the protein, allowing it to enter its channel and pass to the cytoplasm. Note that once mRNA leaves the nucleus in stage 2, it links to the ribosome's poly A site and waits to bind to the appropriately coded amino acid floating freely in the cytoplasm. A specific orientation of mRNA on the ribosome exposes only one codon at a time to match and bind with its anticodon contained on a tRNA.

Within the cytoplasm, translation proceeds through stage 3 (tRNA binds amino acids), stage 4 (tRNA binds to a ribosome, signifying the start of amino acid assembly), and stage 5 (the peptide chain increases in length), until stage 6, when a fully functional protein forms. The *inset box at the bottom* of Figure 16 summarizes the two key aspects of protein synthesis following DNA molecule **replication**:

1. Transcription of information in the genetic code from DNA molecules to RNA molecules in the nucleus (RNA synthesis) for decoding
2. Translation of genetic information in the cytoplasm to synthesize proteins

Transcription of the Genetic Code: RNA Synthesis and Gene Expression

A **gene**, located along a specific chromosome at a specific site, contains the sequence (code or "plan") required to synthesize a protein. The gene within the DNA molecule ranges from several thousand to millions of bases. Unlocking the regulation of a particular gene provides the driving force for many molecular biologists' passion for the field.

The *left side* of FIGURE 17 highlights the five stages of gene expression in human cells. The same two basic sequences of molecular events occur whether in the simplest **bacteria (prokaryotes)** that dominated Earth during its first 2 billion or so years of evolution or in **eukaryotes** that evolved about 1.5 billion years ago. The eukaryotes include thousands of uni- and multicellular organisms (including humans) with membrane-bound **organelles**. The cells of these organisms include a true nucleus with chromosomes. In contrast, prokaryotes have no defined nucleus and generally have no membrane-bound organelles, the DNA remains single stranded, and the main events—transcription and translation—occur coupled, not separately in the nucleus and cytoplasm, respectively. In eukaryotes, in contrast, translating the code for protein synthesis does not occur until the RNA strand exits the nucleus. The *right side* of the figure illustrates the proposed flow of genetic information that Francis Crick in 1956 termed the **central dogma**.

The Watson and Crick hypothesis posited that chromosomal DNA functions as the template for RNA molecules. These molecules then move to the cytoplasm to dictate a protein's amino acid arrangement. The *down arrow* (Fig. 17, *right*) from DNA emphasizes the proposition that DNA provides the template for self-replication. The next phase emphasizes that all cellular RNA molecules were made on (transcribed from) DNA templates. Concomitantly, RNA templates determined (translated) the proteins. The unidirectionality of the *two arrows* between stages 3 and 4 and 4 and 5 indicates that protein templates would never determine RNA sequences, nor would RNA templates create DNA. With few exceptions, the central dogma has stood the test of time and remains essentially valid. Except in some instances in which the reproductive cycle of **retroviruses** adds a step using a reverse transcriptase enzyme, proteins almost never serve as templates for RNA. If they did, the arrows would go bidirectionally between DNA and RNA. Interestingly, at the time Crick proposed the central dogma, little direct experimental support existed for this mechanistic concept that RNA serves as the template for DNA.

Examples of Gene Expression

Beginning with conception, gene expression lays the eventual groundwork for each person's diverse cells, tissues, organs, and systems. Gene expression explains why no two people match exactly in any outer or even inner physical traits. No two hearts, livers, kidneys, brains,

---

Promoter: site on DNA where RNA polymerase binds and initiates transcription (promotes gene expression); required for expression and regulation of gene transcription

Primary RNA transcript: mRNA molecule transcribed as an exact complement to a gene

Nuclear pore complex: octagonal, disk-shaped structure that allows proteins to cross the nuclear envelope into the cytoplasm after protein receptors dock with the protein

Replication: duplication of DNA prior to cell division

Bacteria: primitive, single-celled organisms used to study genetic characteristics and to clone mammalian genes

Prokaryote: cell or organism lacking a structurally discrete nucleus or nuclear membrane; contains a single circular chromosome

Eukaryotes: multicellular organisms with membrane-bound organelles and a true nucleus containing multiple linear chromosomes (Greek; from *eu-karyon* or true nucleus)

Organelle: intracellular structure within a cell that carries out specialized functions (e.g., mitochondrion)

Central dogma: Crick's belief that the genetic information flow creates proteins from DNA (transcription in the nucleus) and RNA (translation in the cytoplasm) to protein

Retrovirus: RNA virus that can enter a cell using reverse transcriptase to reproduce a copy of itself into the genome; a retrovirus carrying an oncogene can transform a host cell into a cancerous cell

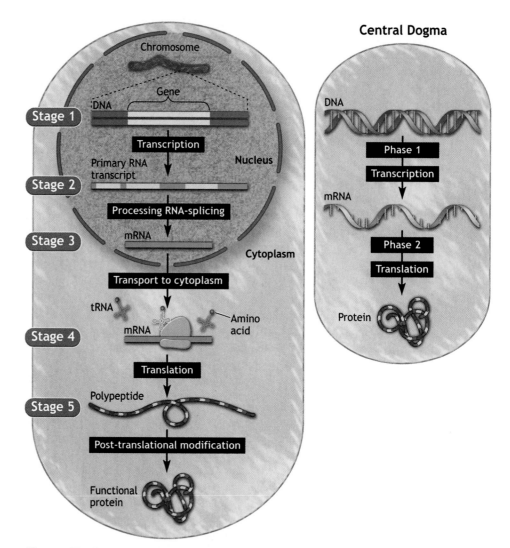

Figure 17   Gene expression and translation. *Left.* Five stages of gene expression in eukaryotes. Transcription (stage 1) produces an mRNA copy of the gene. In translation (stage 4), the information in mRNA molecules "directs" which amino acid to produce and where to position the amino acids when the ribosomes synthesize polypeptides. Translation refers to the creation (assembly) of a protein on the ribosome; mRNA copies the specific coded information from the DNA strand. Posttranslational modifications can alter polypeptides in their transition to a functional protein (stage 5). *Right.* Crick's 1956 working hypothesis (central dogma) posits that two distinct phases play the defining role in expressing the genetic information encoded in DNA molecules. In phase 1 (transcription), RNA polymerase enzyme assembles a mRNA molecule with its nucleotide sequence complementary to the gene's nucleotide sequence. In phase 2 (translation), a ribosome assembles a polypeptide (protein) in which mRNA's nucleotide sequence specifies the final amino acid configuration.

vertebrae, adrenal glands, intraabdominal fat distributions, teeth, nostrils, ears, or fingerprints match precisely. Even identical twins with the same starting genetic machinery have unique and subtle outward physical characteristics and often not-so-subtle distinctive personalities. At times, some aspect of gene expression remains repressed or "off," no longer needing to remain active or "on." Most of the time, gene expression "fits" or modulates to the body's current metabolic state, persisting throughout the individual's life span. The biologic catalysts—the enzymes containing a minimum of 100 amino acid residues—effectively control the genetic machinery and subsequent transformation and control of different energy forms. Six potential regions within the nucleus and cytoplasm shown in FIGURE 18 regulate gene expression. When the mRNA travels to the cytoplasm from the nucleus, protein regulation via translation in the cytoplasm at sites 3 to 6 can begin, as can further modifications once a protein forms as indicated at site 6.

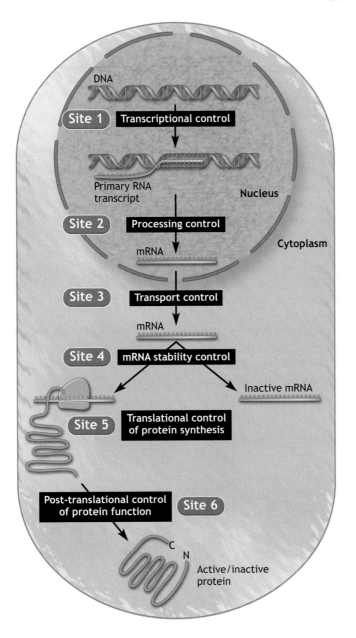

Figure 18   Six potential sites regulate gene expression.

Protein Enzymes

Acting as biomolecular switches, enzymes selectively regulate thousands of cellular activities, coupling some and uncoupling others, all orchestrated in fractions of a second throughout an organism's life. To categorize different kinds of enzymes, the Enzyme Commission (EC) of the International Union of Biochemistry and Molecular Biology (ICBMB) devised a nomenclature and numbering system for enzymes described in detail at www.iubmb.unibe.ch/. The following six major classes of enzymes exist, each with subgroups and sub-subgroups:

1. *Oxidoreductases:* catalyze oxidation–reduction reactions
2. *Transferases:* catalyze transfer of functional groups between molecules
3. *Hydrolases:* catalyze hydrolytic cleavage
4. *Lyases:* catalyze removal of a group from or addition of a group to a double bond, or other changes involving electron rearrangement
5. *Isomerases:* catalyze intramolecular rearrangement
6. *Ligases:* catalyze reactions that join two molecules

Transcription Control

Activator protein: binds to DNA at enhancer sites to position RNA polymerase correctly on the gene

Repressor protein: blocks action of RNA polymerase on DNA that turns genes "off"

Factors that affect gene expression during transcription include diverse "switches" or regulator enzyme **activator proteins** and **repressor proteins**. These operate at the site of the active gene and also at sites thousands of nucleotides away from the starting site. This geography of operation provides great regulatory freedom in how genes initially switch on and off prior to and during transcription. For example, some enzymes accelerate the capture of RNA polymerase to enhance transcription, while others repress transcription by delaying different sequences of events. In essence, activator and repressor proteins control transcription rate in the following two ways:

1. Activator proteins bind to DNA at sites called *enhancer sites*. FIGURE 19 shows the transcription complex (proteins involved in transcription) correctly positioning RNA polymerase at the proper gene location. The folding of the DNA strand brings the **enhancer site** into close proximity to the transcription complex. This increases communication between the activator proteins and the transcription complex. Another group of proteins, termed **coactivator proteins**, transmits signals from activator proteins to other factors (called *basal factors*) close to the DNA strand, helping to position RNA polymerase correctly at the precise location in DNA's **coding region**.

Enhancer site: where gene expression increases from contact with the transcription complex

Coactivator protein: transmits signals from activator proteins to basal factors

Coding region: location on the DNA strand where transcription occurs

2. Repressor proteins bind to "silencer" protein binding sites along the DNA strand. The silencer sequence, adjacent to or overlapping the enhancer region, can prevent an activator protein from binding to a neighboring enhancer site. This delays or cancels transcription from initiating at a discrete mRNA coding sequence.

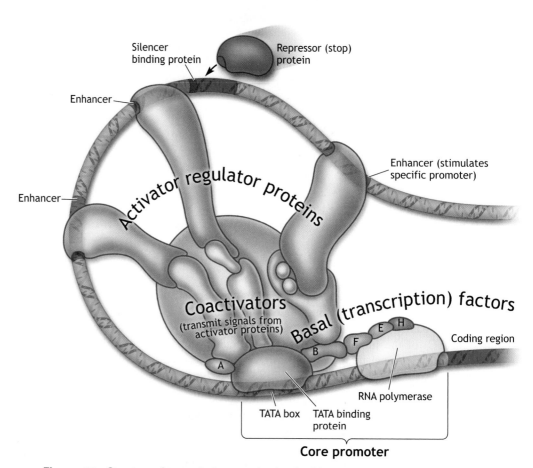

Figure 19   Structure of transcription complex involved in transcriptional control. At the start of the coding sequence along DNA's double helix *(purple ropelike structure)*, the basal (transcription) factors labeled (from *left to right*) *A,* TATA binding protein, *B, F, E,* and *H* correctly position RNA polymerase and then release it to transcribe mRNA.

Enzyme Turnover Number

Some enzymes fulfill their functions more quickly than others. An important way to measure an enzyme's performance relates to how quickly it binds to and releases from its substrate(s) during biomolecular reactions; that is, its turnover rate or number. To encourage a reaction, an enzyme must correctly position or orient itself with its substrate. The electrical properties of a substrate change depending in part on its correct spatial arrangement with the substrate. In essence, the enzyme's positive and negative charges align with the substrate's positive and negative charges to favorably continue a chemical reaction.

The *top* of FIGURE 20 shows an enzyme arranging to link up with its intended substrate to create an enzyme–substrate complex. Once the enzyme fulfills its function, the complex breaks down, releasing its product. The enzyme then almost instantaneously catalyzes another reaction. The rate of end-product formation depends on two factors: (1) the concentration of substrate, and (2) the nature of the enzyme–substrate complex. As the concentration of substrate increases, the reaction rate moves toward its maximum. At this point, all of the enzymes' active sites fully engage the substrate's active sites. Continued new product formation now depends only on the rapidity of substrate processing, referred to as **turnover number**. This can vary tremendously, from 1 to 10,000 molecules per second, but a turnover number of 1000 substrate molecules per second characterizes many enzymes. A high turnover ensures that enzymes remain "turned on" at their optimal concentration during gene expression.

The enzyme's binding sites, while they remain in the "on" position with their substrate for extremely brief periods, may do so more dynamically than previously believed. Instead of remaining coupled for the entire period, other similar binding sites may switch places with the originally bound site (analogous to "hit-join-and-run"), suggesting that enzyme molecules maintain more mobility than previously thought. Future research will determine whether changes in binding site cycling will allow other proteins in the signaling chain to participate in still other gene-regulating pathways. If so, then the elaborate nature of enzyme turnover rates and unique protein–receptor interactions take on even greater complexity than previously believed.

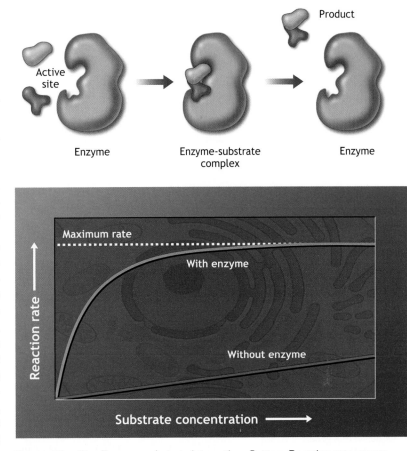

Figure 20   *Top.* Enzyme–substrate interaction. *Bottom.* Reaction rate versus substrate concentration with and without enzyme action.

Turnover number: units of enzyme activity per mole of enzyme (μmol $\cdot$ min^{-1} $\cdot$ mol^{-1} of enzyme); the turnover number (also called catalytic constant) allows relative catalytic comparisons among enzymes; for example, catalase (5 $\times$ 104) is about 2500 times more active than amylase (1.9 $\times$ 104)

Gene Expression and Human Exercise Performance

The next decades in exercise physiology research will build upon the rapidly developing knowledge base about gene expression and the human gene map for exercise performance and health-related phenotypes (see *Medicine and Science in Sports and Exercise* 2001;33:885; with annual updates through 2006, and the obesity gene map database; http://obesitygene.pbrc.edu/, with access to 1999 to 2006 publications from the Human Genomics Laboratory). In the not-too-distant future, sport scientists will routinely incorporate simplified molecular biologic techniques to assess an individual's potential for strength, speed, endurance, and other traits that can be "turned on" to selectively enhance exercise performance. While it might seem far-fetched now, choosing astronauts for extended-duration missions to other planets may rely on molecular biology to "select" candidates with more resistant genes to protect against bone loss or spatial disorientation with prolonged microgravity exposure. Coaches and trainers in future decades will undoubtedly apply technologies from molecular medicine to genetically screen young children for gene clusters that indicate potential for desirable athletic traits (and traits related to training responsiveness), such as predominance of a specific muscle fiber type, abundance of targeted aerobic enzymes, muscle capillaries, or left ventricular cavity size. Today, sports scientists use laboratory and field testing to screen athletes for performance and physiologic capacities. Similar application and acceptance of molecular genetics will require mastery of the new technologies with ethical issues considered.

Gene expression is tightly controlled. When muscle tissue rebuilds, gene expression for actin and myosin protein filament enlargement remains "on," while gene expression for generating new muscle cells remains "off" because cellular hypertrophy not hyperplasia usually prevails. These "on–off" genes are referred to as "**housekeeping genes.**" In bodily processes such as coding for the proteins involved in aerobic metabolism, gene expression does not shut down but remains continually on until death. The same applies to all cell and tissue metabolic activities controlled by enzymes that dominate cellular and subcellular events. Organisms from bacteria to humans use the same two basic principles of gene expression. First, an RNA duplicate is made of a particular gene with its unique coding sequence on a DNA template that represents some combination in succession of G, C, T, A. Second, the RNA copy containing the sequence of the **genetic code** on the **ribosome** (located outside the nucleus) orchestrates the sequential construction of amino acids into a protein possessing unique biomolecular characteristics.

Exons and Introns

The RNA primary transcript molecule contains all of the information needed from the gene to create a protein. The RNA primary transcript structure discovered by Crick,[135] called a coding region or **exon**, shown in the green primary transcript within the purple nucleus in FIGURE 21, also contains additional, unwanted stretches of nucleotide "spacers" or noncoding regions termed **introns** (five introns also shown in *pink* within the primary transcript of Fig. 21). In fact, 97% of DNA consists of introns. An example of just three exons and two introns shows the individual numbering for the base pair sequences within each exon and intron. For example, the numbers 1–30 designate the base pairs for the first exon along the RNA strand, while 105–146 signify the base pairs for the last exon. The two introns with their base pairs have the numbers 30–31 and 104–105. During transcription, note the removal of intron links 30–31 and 104–105, leaving the remaining three exons that splice together (their base pairs now numbered 1–146) to create the final mRNA transcript. This must occur before the mRNA strand leaves the nucleus and enters the cytoplasmic space (cytosol).

The cytoplasm cannot receive partially processed transcripts. Intron removal likely occurs because these structures provide no known usable code for any part of the polypeptide initially specified by the gene. These clusters of repeated, apparently nonfunctional and random DNA sequences scattered throughout the genome exist as either short interspersed elements of 500 or fewer base pairs (called SINEs) or long interspersed elements of more than 1000 base pairs (LINEs) in length. The mature mRNA transcript displayed at the *bottom* of Figure 21 contains the correct sequence of codes to create proteins. The example shows the specified order for seven amino acids inserted into the elongating polypeptide chain, determined originally during translation based on codon sequence.

RNA Splicing

RNA splicing removes unwanted intron sequences from the primary transcript before it is translated, allowing translation to avoid those sequences. Introns usually occupy an area 10 to 30 times greater than exons. Small nuclear RNA (snRNA; composed of proteins and a special type of RNA), play a contributing role in RNA splicing. Another protein (small nuclear ribonucleoprotein, or snRNP) contains snRNA. This structure can bind to the 5′ end of an intron, while a different snRNP binds to the intron's 3′ end. Introns interact to form a loop that joins the free ends of the intron. A collection of snRNPs is known as a spliceosome. Its function is to excise the intron (allowing the entron to join it but without the snRNPs). The final, mature mRNA strand is shorter than the primary transcript owing to the excision of about 90% of the introns in the primary transcript prior to translation. Consider exon splicing a unique

Housekeeping genes: genes automatically switched "on" all the time to maintain essential cell functions

Genetic code: sequence of nucleotides, coded in triplets (codons) along the mRNA that determine the amino acid sequence in protein synthesis; the gene's DNA sequence can predict the mRNA sequence; the genetic code in turn predicts the amino acid sequence

Ribosome: small cellular component (organelle) composed of specialized ribosomal RNA; site of polypeptide (protein)

Exon: protein-coding DNA sequence of a gene

Intron: DNA base noncoding sequence that interrupts a gene's protein-coding sequence; the sequence transcribes into RNA, but gets excised from the "message" before it translates into protein

RNA splicing: excision of unwanted sequence of introns from the primary transcript so the exons fuse together

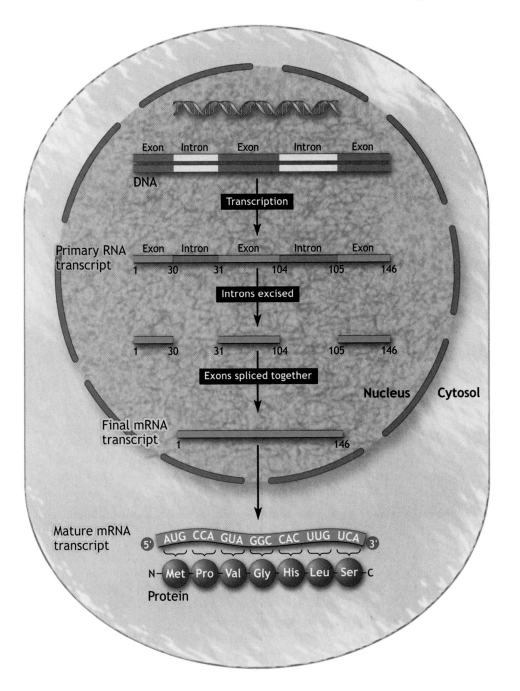

Exon   Intron   Exon   Intron   Exon

DNA

Transcription

Primary RNA transcript

Exon   Intron   Exon   Intron   Exon

1   30   31   104   105   146

Introns excised

1   30   31   104   105   146

Exons spliced together

Nucleus   Cytosol

Final mRNA transcript

1   146

Mature mRNA transcript

5'   AUG CCA GUA GGC CAC UUG UCA   3'

N— Met –Pro –Val –Gly –His –Leu –Ser —C

Protein

Figure 21 Example of exons and introns, individual numbering for the base pair sequences, and intron excision and exon splicing to form the final (mature) mRNA transcript. For this structure, note the three-letter codons shown in *white lettering* along the *green* mRNA, and the corresponding amino acids listed in the *blue circles* below. The codon table in Figure 12 (page 1003) lists the full names of these amino acids.

phase of protein construction at the start of protein assembly. Splicing manipulates intron sequencing in many ways to form **polypeptides**. The hemoglobin (Hb) molecule, for example, requires 432 nucleotides to encode its 144 amino acids, yet before intron excision, 1356 nucleotides exist in the primary mRNA transcript of the *Hb* gene. Regulation of gene expression occurs by changes in how splicing takes place during different stages of a cell's development and the type of cell involved.

mRNA Packaging: Polyadenylic Acid and Guanosine Triphosphate—Tails and Caps

Before the RNA transcript migrates through the nuclear pore as the final transcribed mRNA, a **polyadenylic acid (poly [A]) tail**, 100–200 adenine nucleotides long, joins one end at the 3′ region via the action of the enzyme poly(A) polymerase, and a terminal portion or "cap" (methylated **guanosine triphosphate** or **GTP**) joins near the 5′ end. Much as a college

Polypeptide: unbranched string of amino acids linked by peptide bonds formed during gene translation

Polyadenylic acid [poly (A)] tail: chain 100–200 adenine nucleotides long; joins one end at the 3′ region of the final transcribed mRNA before the RNA transcript migrates through the nuclear pore

Guanosine triphosphate (GTP): initiates translation when it binds mRNA at the 5′ end of the molecule to the smaller of the ribosome's two subunits; referred to as the "cap" on the final transcribed mRNA

student wears a cap and gown during the graduation ceremony before entering the "real" world, so mRNA must be "capped and tailed" to prepare the transcribed molecule for translation before it exits the nucleus to participate in subsequent protein synthesis. The newly formed cap performs the important function of initiating translation when it binds the mRNA to the smaller of the ribosome's two subunits.

The *top* of FIGURE 22 shows how the GTP cap and poly(A) tail join to RNA. Note that the capping enzyme (symbolized by the *shorter curved purple arrow*) cleaves two phosphates (*circles enclosed in red*) from GTP and one phosphate from the mRNA strand. In forming the cap, the GTP now attaches near the end of the first base of the mRNA. The *bottom* of Figure 22 illustrates the addition of the poly(A) tail when a specific endonuclease enzyme (*orange*) recognizes the sequence A-A-U-A-A-A on the mRNA and snips the strand near that point. This permits a tail of 100–200 adenine residues to affix to the 3′ end of the mRNA strand. The

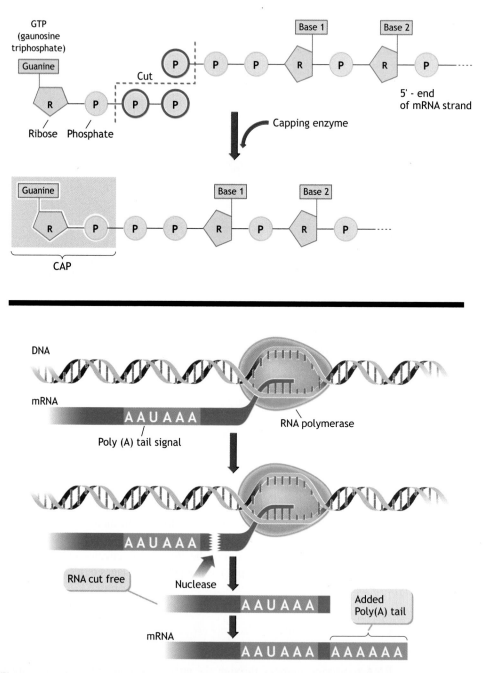

Figure 22   Caps and tails. *Top.* Addition of a guanosine triphosphate (GTP) cap to mRNA. The red dashes indicate where the "cut" occurs by the action of the capping enzyme. *Bottom.* Addition of a poly (A) tail to mRNA. The mRNA molecule exits the nucleus once capping and tailing occurs, carrying the "coded message" for the upcoming translation phase in protein synthesis.

addition of poly(A) promotes mRNA stability. It permits the mRNA molecule to maintain translation for up to several weeks, sometimes producing 100,000 protein molecules. Recall that transcription that uses DNA occurs inside the cell's nucleus, whereas ribosomal assembly takes place in the cytoplasm. The capping and tailing function enables the mRNA to exit the nucleus to begin the next phase of protein synthesis.

Exiting the Nucleus

The mRNA now contains a copy of the specific nucleotide sequence from the DNA gene. The mRNA then shuttles the "coded message," after the transcription stage, through the nuclear membrane into the cytoplasm where protein synthesis (translation) begins. Translation includes three main stages: (1) initiation, (2) elongation, and (3) termination. Using high-resolution x-ray crystallography, researchers have determined that a tunnellike groove runs through the middle of the larger 50S subunit, providing the location that links amino acids together.[96] Thirty-one separate proteins affix to the outside of the subunit where they also reach inside the ribosome. Because a protein needs to be within a 3 Å distance to induce any effect and because the proteins on the surface and those that reach around the surface remain within 18 Å, the source of any protein interaction must be RNA. In this case, adenosine 2486 is the nucleotide in question with an associated nitrogen atom. Therefore, the RNA gives the catalytic power to protein synthesis—in essence, ribosomes serve as ribozymes. This finding helps to explain why some bacteria remain resistant to antibiotics. A mutation on one of the ribosomal proteins within the ribosomal groove locks up with part of the antibiotic molecule, preventing the peptide from exiting the region and thus stopping further antibiotic binding and subsequent damage to the bacterium.

Translation of the Genetic Code: Ribosomal Assembly of Polypeptides

Translation initiates protein construction. Once the mRNA enters the cytoplasm through the nuclear pore, it seeks out a ribosome with which to bind. The nucleus is the original source of the millions of ribosomes in the cell's cytoplasm. A ribosome consists of a large and a small subunit, the latter fitting into a depression on the ribosome's larger surface. A ribosome has three sites that associate with mRNA: (1) A-site (A for attachment), (2) P-site (P for polypeptide), and (3) E-site (E for exit).

Ribosomes and Polypeptide Synthesis: Initiation of Protein Construction

The cell's ribosomes provide the catalysts for initiating protein synthesis and serve as submicroscopic factories to produce polypeptides. FIGURE 23 illustrates a four-step sequence of a ribosome binding to one end of an mRNA molecule and the subsequent three nucleotide increments down the mRNA molecule. Decoding of genetic information occurs when the ribosomes bound to mRNA translate a genetic code sequence. The tRNA then interacts with a specific amino acid, adding one at

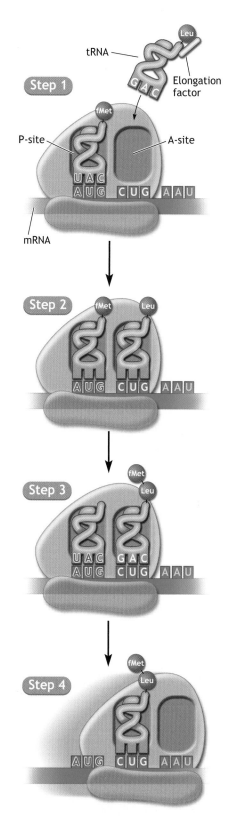

Figure 23 Ribosomes, the initiators for protein synthesis. Polypeptide synthesis proceeds from the top in *step 1* with the anticodon of tRNA complementary to the mRNA codon. The tRNA occupies the ribosome's A-site, with an anticodon complementary to the mRNA's codon at the opposite A-site. The ribosome translocates down the mRNA one codon at a time. *Step 2*. The lengthening polypeptide chain *fMet* (f, formyl-methionyl; Met, amino acid methionine) is transferred to *Leu* (leucine), the incoming amino acid. The ribosome ejects the original tRNA *(step 3)* with its amino acid, exposing the next codon on the mRNA chain. When the tRNA molecule recognizes the next exposed codon, it binds to that codon, thus lengthening the growing peptide chain *(step 4)*. fMet represents an addition to the lengthening polypeptide chain already occupied by *Leu*.

Polypeptide chain: repeated polypeptide units

Peptide bonding: chemical linking that binds amino acids in a protein; formed when the carboxyl group of one amino acid reacts with a second amino acid's amino group

Anticodon: three complementary bases at the end of a tRNA molecule that recognize and bind to an mRNA codon

Aminoacyl-tRNA synthetase: activating enzyme that covalently links amino acids to the 3′ ends of their cognate tRNA

a time to the end of the progressively elongating **polypeptide chain**. Sequential linking of amino acids by **peptide bonding** ultimately forms the specific protein with its unique genetically determined information to achieve its specific function(s).

Role of tRNA

The tRNA molecule shown in FIGURE 24 has a three-dimensional structure resembling a cloverleaf, with an amino acid at one end and three nitrogenous bases that match the mRNA's codon (called an **anticodon**) at the other end. The tRNA with matching codon serves as a relay or go-between in protein synthesis. In effect, the tRNA acts as a "personal shuttle" to deliver a specific free-floating amino acid to the ribosome's A-site. For example, the triplet U-A-C represents the codon for the amino acid methionine. When the tRNA with the matching U-A-C anticodon (it carries no other amino acid) interacts with the free-floating U-A-C amino acid, it binds to it by action of the activating enzyme **aminoacyl-tRNA synthetase**. Each amino acid's specific activating enzyme serves two purposes: (1) it deciphers and then binds (couples) to a specific amino acid, and (2) it identifies the anticodon on the tRNA molecule. Some activating enzymes decipher the sequence of one anticodon and thus only one tRNA, while others recognize multiple tRNA molecules. Thus, the activating enzyme "reads" the genetic code on both the particular amino acid, such as tryptophan, and its tRNA tryptophan anticodon sequence A-C-C. Figure 24 shows three views of tRNA: (1) a computer-generated model, (2) a three-dimensional representation that highlights internal base pairing with hydrogen bonding, and (3) two-dimensional cloverleaf model with the tRNA anticodon shown in *blue*. This example represents the complementary three-nucleotide sequence C-A-U matching mRNA's codon G-U-A.

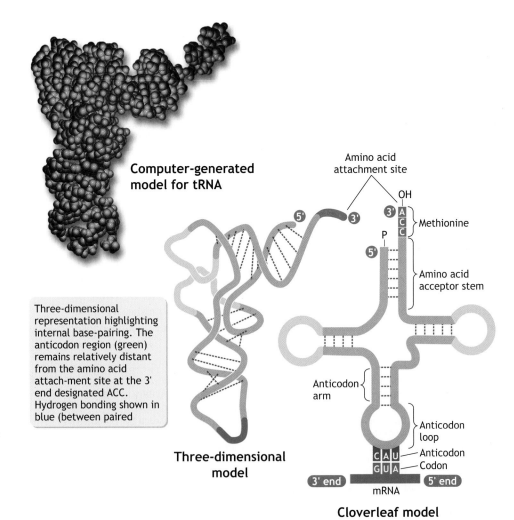

Figure 24 Three views of tRNA: computer-generated model, three-dimensional model, and cloverleaf model. Note that the anticodon displayed in the cloverleaf model (complementary three-nucleotide sequence) matches up with the mRNA codon using complementary (antiparallel) binding between the anticodon *(blue)* and codon *(green)*.

Computer-generated model for tRNA

Three-dimensional representation highlighting internal base-pairing. The anticodon region (green) remains relatively distant from the amino acid attach-ment site at the 3′ end designated ACC. Hydrogen bonding shown in blue (between paired

Three-dimensional model

Amino acid attachment site

OH

A C C — Methionine

P

Amino acid acceptor stem

Anticodon arm

Anticodon loop

Anticodon

Codon

C A U
G U A

3′ end   5′ end

mRNA

Cloverleaf model

Polypeptide Elongation and Termination

The polypeptide chain increases in length when an amino acid from tRNA **translocates** to it. The A-U-G codon shown in Figure 23 within the mRNA message initiates the "start" signal for peptide elongation. The same A-U-G sequence that encodes tryptophan also encodes methionine. The first A-U-G message "sensed" in the mRNA molecule initiates translation. The ribosome translocates down the mRNA a distance of three nucleotide blocks (one codon) at a time. After each third nucleotide, the ribosome ejects the original tRNA with its amino acid, exposing the next codon on the mRNA chain. When the tRNA molecule recognizes the next exposed codon, it binds to it, thus lengthening the growing peptide chain. The elongation procedure for building the polypeptide continues repeatedly until a stop codon terminates the process.

FIGURE 25 schematically illustrates the three stages in polypeptide termination. The three "stop" codons, or base sequences, include U-A-A, U-A-G, and U-G-A. These codons "turn off" the signal in the mRNA message, preventing addition of another amino acid sequence to the chain. Stage 1 shows the stop codon U-A-A on the mRNA strand

Translocation: describes movement along the ribosome by an mRNA molecule a distance of three nucleotide blocks (one codon) at a time

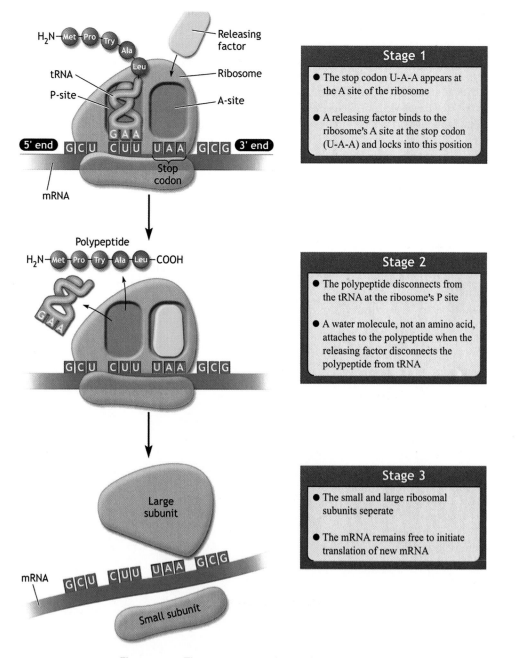

Figure 25   Three stages in polypeptide termination.

within the A-site of the ribosome, where one of three kinds of releasing factors—eRF1, eRF2, or eRF3—locks into position to split apart the linking covalent bond. In stage 2, the polypeptide chain releases from tRNA at the ribosome's P-site, to effectively end protein synthesis. Once the polypeptide and tRNA uncouple from the termination complex, the small and large ribosomal units recycle along with mRNA in stage 3 for further mRNA translation.

Protein Delivery System: The Golgi Complex

Golgi complex: stack of membrane-bound vesicles between the endoplasmic reticulum and plasma membrane; involved in posttranslational modification of proteins, and sorting and delivering them to different intracellular compartments

Endoplasmic reticulum: tubules, vesicles, and flattened sac structures of the cell's endomembrane system; ribosomes cover its outer rough, granular surface

Glycoprotein: protein complexed with a polysaccharide

Glycolipid: polysaccharide bound to a lipid

Once the ribosome produces its polypeptide, newly formed strands can exit a cell through its outer membrane into the external interstitial fluid environment. The highly membranous **Golgi complex** structures within the cell provide the transfer mechanism for moving materials from the cell to its external environment. Italian physiologist and microscopist Camillo Golgi (1843–1926), who shared the 1906 Nobel Prize in physiology or medicine for his work on nervous system anatomy, first called attention in 1898 to these minute intracellular structures using the light microscope. Many biologists of his time doubted the existence of such structures; 60 years later, the electron microscope confirmed their existence in exquisite detail.

The Golgi complex receives a polypeptide from the cell's **endoplasmic reticulum**. FIGURE 26 shows polypeptide transport into the Golgi complex where this molecule may become a **glycoprotein**. When a polysaccharide binds to a lipid it forms a **glycolipid**. Glycoproteins or glycolipids then collect within the flattened, membranous sacs called the *cisternae region of the Golgi complex,* where specialized enzymes modify the protein component. The transport vesicles that hold proteins that pass from the endoplasmic reticulum pinch off and break away from the roughened endoplasmic surfaces. The tiny vesicles attached to the cell's outer membrane expel their contents to the extracellular spaces via secretory vesicles. In essence (but not always), the Golgi complex takes up the polypeptide on one of its surfaces and then modifies and repackages it into molecules that leave the Golgi complex via a transport vesicle at its other membrane.

Termination of Protein Synthesis

The end-point of protein synthesis creates one of thousands of completed or functional proteins, each with a specific function and mode of action depending in part on its structure. TABLE 2 shows eight categories of proteins and their biologic functions.

Figure 26 Polypeptide transport into the Golgi complex. The Golgi complex accepts polypeptides on one of its surfaces after the ribosomes release them, repackaging them as glycoproteins, and expels them contained in secretory vesicles for final expulsion through the plasma membrane or delivery to another cell area. The Golgi structures modify proteins within their lumen for use within cells or outside of cells once they pass through the plasma membrane.

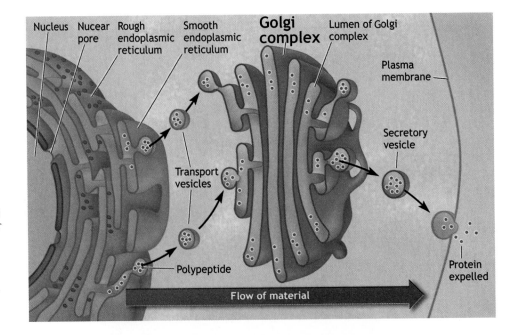

TABLE 2 ■ EIGHT CATEGORIES OF PROTEINS AND THEIR BIOLOGIC FUNCTIONS

PROTEIN CATEGORY	FUNCTION	EXAMPLE
1. Contractile	Form muscles	Actin, myosin
2. Enzyme	Catalyze biological processes	Protease
3. Hormone	Regulate body functions	Cortisol
4. Protective	Fight infection	Antibodies
5. Storage	Store nutrients	Calcium within bone
6. Structural	Form structures	Endoplasmic reticulum
7. Transport	Deliver substances among cells, tissues, organs	Hemoglobin
8. Toxic	Defense mechanism	Snake venom (disintegrins)

It usually takes between 20 seconds and 2 minutes to synthesize most proteins, depending on the protein's complexity. The Hb molecule and its amino acid sequence serves as an excellent example of the four levels of protein structure (FIG. 27). This generalized example begins with the linear sequence of amino acids from the amino acid at the amino-terminal end through to the carboxyl-terminal residue. The polypeptide strand formed when peptide linkages join amino acid monomers represents protein's **primary structure**. In a **secondary structure**, the protein can twist into a three-dimensional form known as an **α helix**. It can also fold back onto itself to give a flat look (β-pleated sheets), with regular repeating interactions using hydrogen bonding among closely linked residues in the primary sequence. Interactions among residues farther apart in the primary structure determine a **tertiary structure**, such as disulfide bond formation between two cysteine residues. In this conformation, the protein literally folds up on itself, much like a roll of pretzel dough twisting into a pretzel. The topology of the α helices and β-pleated sheets play important roles in determining the final shape assumed by a protein.[34] The complex Hb molecule consists of two α subunits and two β subunits (tetramer). The term **quaternary structure** refers to protein's subunit structure; Hb contains multiple subunits.

Hemoglobin and the Evolutionary Tree

Figure 27 shows that the Hb molecule contains two α and two β chains; the heme group is associated with each chain. The central iron atom (shown in *red*) binds with one oxygen molecule and acts as a magnet to attract and hold it. Interestingly, our closest blood relative, the chimpanzee, has an identical α chain. The Hb amino acid sequence in cows and pigs diverges from that of humans by about 12%, while for chickens the divergence increases to 25%. Molecular biologists have constructed an evolutionary tree for many proteins (e.g., the iron-containing mitochondrial cytochromes) as a way of tracking evolution.

Some proteins change relatively slowly, taking hundreds of millions of years to evolve. Histones change at a rate of 0.25 mutations per 100 amino acids per 100 million years. In contrast, other proteins such as neurotoxins and immunoglobulins mutate more rapidly (rates of 110 to 140). Variation in the resistance to change makes "sense" because crucial cellular functions like energy generation in the citric acid cycle or correct folding of DNA requires that gene sequences remain almost invariant. Proteins sensitive to relatively large variations in their operational properties sustain faster evolutionary changes.

Proteolysis: The Ultimate Fate of Proteins

Protein synthesis from amino acids and degradation into amino acid constituents progresses unabated throughout life. The rates of protein synthesis and degradation, a process called **proteolysis**, regulate the organism's total protein content at any given time, independent of the proteins' structural configurations (bone or muscle) or functions (metabolic

Primary structure: specific linear sequence of amino acids determined by the nucleotide sequence of the gene that encodes the protein

Secondary structure: coiled protein similar to the pairing of strands in DNA or folded back onto itself to give a flat look; formed from regular repeating interactions among closely linked residues in the primary sequence using hydrogen bonding

α Helix: one possible secondary structure of polypeptides; right-handed peptide chain maintained by hydrogen (H) bonds between carbon (C) and oxygen (O) atoms of every fifth amino acid along the chain. The degree of rotation remains regular for bonds on either side of the α carbon (with nitrogen, C, H, and amino side chain attached to it) along the polypeptide chain

Tertiary structure: final 3-dimensional folding of a polymer chain; interactions between residues remain farther apart

Quaternary structure: highly complex, 3-dimensional structure or functional protein formed by joining two or more polypeptides

Proteolysis: protein degradation

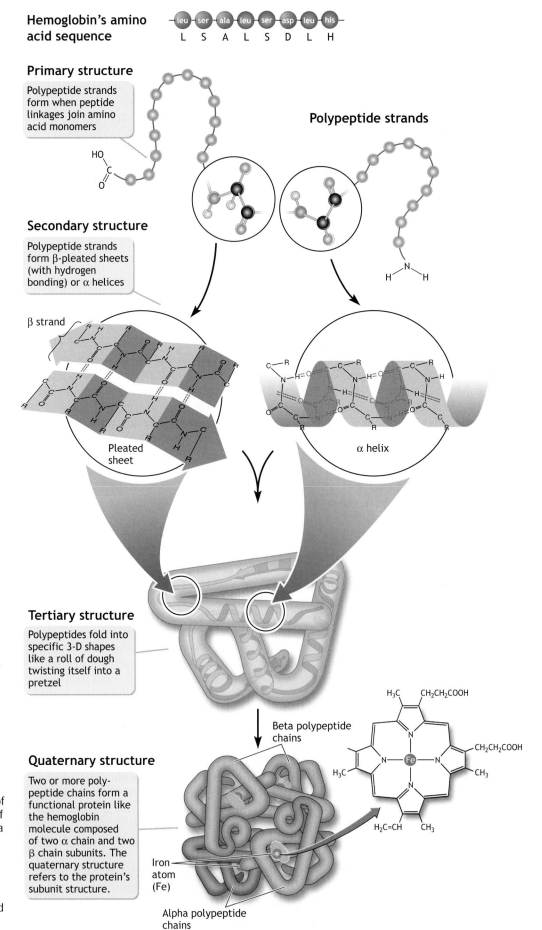

Hemoglobin's amino acid sequence

leu – ser – ala – leu – ser – asp – leu – his
L   S   A   L   S   D   L   H

Primary structure

Polypeptide strands form when peptide linkages join amino acid monomers

Polypeptide strands

Secondary structure

Polypeptide strands form β-pleated sheets (with hydrogen bonding) or α helices

β strand

Pleated sheet

α helix

Tertiary structure

Polypeptides fold into specific 3-D shapes like a roll of dough twisting itself into a pretzel

Beta polypeptide chains

Quaternary structure

Two or more poly-peptide chains form a functional protein like the hemoglobin molecule composed of two α chain and two β chain subunits. The quaternary structure refers to the protein's subunit structure.

Iron atom (Fe)

Alpha polypeptide chains

Figure 27 Four protein structures (primary, secondary, tertiary, quaternary) in the synthesis of the complex hemoglobin molecule first deciphered by Max Perutz in 1960 and published in *Nature* (1960;185:416). The purified molecule's precise arrangement was calculated from the way its crystals diffracted a beam of x-rays. Hemoglobin's tertiary structure contains eight α-helical regions; the quaternary structure contains four polypeptide chains (two α and two β). Knowledge of the configuration of new protein structures has increased exponentially since Perutz first worked out the details of hemoglobin's structure; as of July 9, 2001, the Protein Data Bank (www.rcsb.org/pdb/) contained 15,531 unique structures into which proteins can fold. Of these, x-ray diffraction identified 12,817 unique structures and NMR, identified 2384.

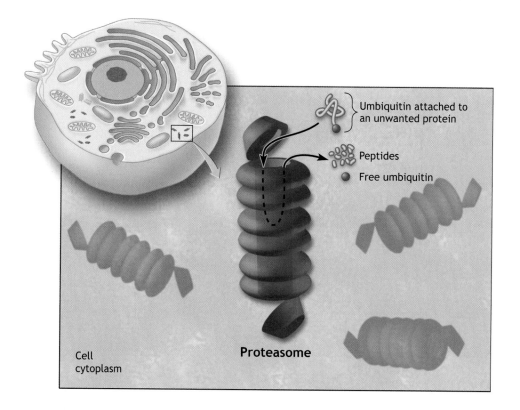

Umbiquitin attached to an unwanted protein

Peptides

Free umbiquitin

Proteasome

Cell cytoplasm

Figure 28 Proteosomes in the cell cytoplasm maintain a balance between protein synthesis and protein degradation. The free ubiquitin tag (displayed in *red*) attaches to an active site on the designated protein, identifying it for degradation to its peptide components within the proteosome's cylindrical structure. Once ejected, the ubiquitin recycles to another unwanted protein.

and intracellular enzymes). For example, the structural proteins[a] in bone may not decay significantly for months or years, while enzyme proteins in intermediary metabolism or those that regulate cell growth may survive for only minutes or fractions of a second. The enzymes that control proteolysis (proteases) hydrolyze the amino acids' peptide bonds, splitting them into their constituent molecules. A relatively large trash can–shaped **proteosome** formed from protease enzymes degrades the unwanted proteins in the cell's cytoplasm (FIG. 28). These cylindrical structures capture proteins destined for destruction by recognizing a small marker or tag protein (**ubiquitin**) that attaches by covalent bonding to an active site on the protein. Once tagged, the ubiquinated protein enters the proteosome, which degrades it to smaller peptide units before expelling it along with the ubiquitin tag. Proteosomes degrade many types of proteins, from denatured or misfolded ones to misformed or oxidized amino acids.

Proteosome: proteolytic enzyme that degrades unwanted proteins in the cytoplasm of eukaryotic cells

Ubiquitin: small protein that attaches by covalent bonding to a protein "marked" for destruction by proteosomes

Summary of Main Sequence of Events in Protein Synthesis

TABLE 3 charts the sequence of key events in the flow of genetic information in living cells from DNA → RNA → protein.

---

[a]Collagen, the most plentiful structural protein, accounts for about one fourth of the body's protein. In essence, it forms molecular cables that strengthen the tendons and plentiful, resilient sheets that support the skin and internal organs. This simple protein, composed of three chains wound together in a tight triple helix, contains more than 1400 amino acids in each chain. Collagen forms from a repeated sequence of three amino acids; every third amino acid is glycine, a small amino acid that fits perfectly inside the helix. Many of the remaining positions in the chain are filled by two amino acids, proline and hydroxyproline, the latter a modified version of proline. Hydroxyproline formation involves modifying normal proline amino acids after building the collagen. The reaction requires vitamin C to assist in the addition of oxygen. Unfortunately, vitamin C deficiency slows hydroxyproline production and stops new collagen construction, ultimately causing scurvy. When heated, collagen's triple helix unwinds and the chains separate. When the denatured mass of tangled chains cools down, it soaks up the surrounding water like a sponge to form gelatin used commonly in cooking.

TABLE 3 ■ ESSENTIAL CONCEPTS AND SEQUENCE OF EVENTS IN PROTEIN SYNTHESIS

- A nucleotide sequence from DNA provides the genetic information required to begin transcription into RNA
- The enzyme RNA polymerase binds to the specific promoter region of a gene; nucleotide sequences in the DNA indicate where to begin and end transcription
- RNA polymerase manufactures messenger RNA (mRNA) molecules to mirror the base sequence of DNA; transcription copies a sequence of the genetic code direction from DNA to an mRNA strand; this includes both coding and noncoding segments of genetic information
- The RNA transcript contains the information it needs to create a protein; RNA splicing removes random, intervening sequences of unwanted "junk" nucleotides (introns) from mRNA
- The mRNA strand (linked entrons) carrying a duplicate copy of the genetic code shuttles the "coded message" (sequence of codons), exiting the nucleus and entering the cytoplasm to begin protein synthesis
- Translation initiates protein construction; the A-U-G codon acts as the "start" signal
- In the cytoplasm, the mRNA molecule searches to bind with a ribosome (ribonucleoprotein, a "protein-manufacturing machine"
- The anticodon of transfer RNA (tRNA) positions itself to match up with a three-nucleotide sequence of codons, each codon corresponding to one amino acid; the codon contains a copy or transcription of the DNA code
- With the four RNA nucleotides, 64 different codons in the genetic code exist, with each amino acid having at least one (and usually more than one) codon
- Binding takes place at the ribosome's attachment site between the tRNA molecule (carrying the same genetic sequence on its anticodon) and the complementary base sequence of the mRNA codon (e.g., G-A-C with C-U-G)
- The ribosome, coupled to one end of the mRNA molecule, shifts (translocates) over one codon (three nucleotide blocks) to the polypeptide site, allowing exposure of a new codon; a new incoming tRNA (with its amino acid) links to the ribosome's attachment site; the amino acid at the ribosome's polypeptide region releases and binds to a new amino acid on tRNA at the ribosome's attachment site; thus, the tRNA with one amino acid now gains another amino acid, then another one, and so on; successive addition of new amino acids elongates the peptide chain
- Protein synthesis terminates when a chain-terminating nonsense "stop" codon (UAA, UAG, UGA) turns off the signal for adding more amino acids to the peptide chain
- A complete (fully assembled) protein exists in one of four geometric configurations (primary, secondary, tertiary, quaternary) shown in Figure 27

MUTATIONS

The slightest aberration in the sequence of the 3 billion letters of the genome can produce catastrophic effects on health and well-being. Fortunately, an exquisite array of internal repair mechanisms (specialized protein complexes) correct mismatches along the double helix, thus avoiding a phalanx of dreadful, life-altering genetic disorders. On a daily basis, factors in the external environment continually threaten the body's DNA from cosmic and ultraviolet radiation bombardment to radioactive decay and gamma waves, including dangerously reactive free radical species (see page 1029). A **mutation** results from a minor alteration or "misspelling" in DNA sequence that cripples the corresponding RNA or protein. **Sickle cell anemia** provides a salient example when an abnormality occurs in the hemoglobin molecule as illustrated in the second row of the inset table below:

Mutation: gene with permanently altered or defective genetic information that causes heritable changes

Sickle cell anemia: usually fatal hereditary disease affecting hemoglobin; develops when the amino acid valine substitutes for glutamic acid because of a change in its codon nucleotide sequence from G-A-A to G-U-A; the disease afflicts 2 of every 1000 African Americans; the erythrocyte becomes irregular, thin, elongated, and crescent-shaped, severely affecting oxygen-transport capacity

Junk DNA: DNA sequences that perform no currently known useful purpose but still remain part of chromosomes

Normal hemoglobin β-chain amino acids						
Valine	Histidine	Leucine	Threonine	Proline	Glutamic acid	Glutamic acid

					↓	
Sickle cell anemia hemoglobin β-chain amino acids						
Valine	Histidine	Leucine	Threonine	Proline	Valine	Glutamic acid

In the sickle cell condition, the amino acid valine shown in *red* substitutes for glutamic acid and alters hemoglobin's β chain because of a codon change from G-A-A to G-U-A. Many human diseases generally form from protein abnormalities caused by a change in the sequence of only one of the 3×10^9 or more DNA nucleotide pairs in the human genome. Not all of the coding sequences in amino acids make "sense." The term **junk DNA** (also called *noncoding DNA*) describes such DNA sequences. These inherited sequences perform no currently known "genetically useful" purpose,[16,128] yet they remain part of the chromosomes. Junk DNA replicates inside a cell the same way any other DNA molecule replicates, but without gene expression. In this sense, it too is considered defective.

Varieties of Mutations

The guiding principle of the central dogma discussed earlier implicitly states that any change in the inherited genetic material produces a ripple effect on replication, transcription, and translation. This ultimately means that a mutation in the original daughter chromosomes passes on sets of characteristics to the next generation so the offspring inherits the mutation. One can accomplish little short of a temporary, stop-gap measure using **genetic engineering** to replace the defective sequences or arrest their development a distance far removed from the gene. For example, small deletions hundreds of thousands of bases away from a particular gene *(PAX6)* can alter the gene's expression and actually cause a mutation in which a typical characteristic (e.g., iris in the eye) fails to develop, producing a developmental syndrome called aniridia (www.aniridia.org/). Poorly understood processes can *silence* genes up to 90 million bases down the chromosome. Once transcription uses the DNA template to make an RNA copy of the inherited mutated sequences, the altered RNA translates the defective code during protein synthesis. All of the body's vital processes depend on proteins for their intended functions; mutated genes pose a health hazard.

The doggerel below provides eight examples of different types of mutations and what can happen to disrupt the orderly sequence in the genetic code:

Genetic engineering: laboratory-altered DNA that changes its characteristics, usually in four stages that involve: (1) cleaving the source DNA, (2) creating recombinants, (3) cloning copies of recombinants, and (4) locating cloned copies for the desired gene; screening makes the desired clones resistant to antibiotics and gives them different properties for easy identification

MUTATION TYPE	EXAMPLE OF DISRUPTION IN THE CODING SEQUENCE
Wild type	The cat sat on the mat
Substitution	The rat sat on the mat
Insertion (single)	The cat spat on the mat
Insertion (multiple)	The cattle sat on the mat
Deletion (single)	The c-t sat on the mat
Deletion (multiple)	The cat --- — the mat
Inversion (small)	The tac sat on the mat
Inversion (large)	Tam echt no tas tac echt

A graphic example points out the probability for "errors" to creep into a DNA sequence. If the total DNA compacted in the body's 10 trillion cells was laid end to end like a long link of sausages, it would stretch from Earth to the sun 667 times—not a trivial length because of the 93-million mile one-way distance to the sun! Thus, a single genetic code mismatch can wreak havoc on the "normal" sequence of DNA nucleotides and hence genes. A defect in code sequence often remains quiescent for nearly a lifetime before it emerges. For example, it may take 60 years before a seemingly minor misalignment in a receptor gene devastates heart function, causing congestive heart failure within a few months. When researchers identify this human gene variant years before its expression, as discussed below, they will prescribe highly specific drugs to combat the defect. Within the next decade, new classes of drugs will target specific mutated cells instead of the current "shot-gun" approach that attempts to cripple just about all cells with a massive pharmacologic overdose. A case in point concerns a stretch of genes along chromosome 21 where mutations give rise to Alzheimer's disease, amyotrophic lateral sclerosis (ALS; known as Lou Gehrig's disease), epilepsy, deafness, autoimmune disease, birth defects, and manic depression. For Down syndrome (named after English physician John Langdon Down [1828–1896] who observed individuals in a British asylum in 1866 and published *Observations on an Ethnic Classification of Idiots*), researchers have been on a quest to develop animal models of this genetic form of mental insufficiency and other genetic abnormalities in hopes of developing genetically engineered strategies to eradicate them. Gene testing may also prove useful for patients who often respond differently to warfarin (Coumadin), a widely prescribed anti-blood-clotting drug because of newly identified genetic variations. Misjudgments in drug doses can critically affect the clotting mechanism to potentially cause fatal bleeding. One gene, known as vitamin K epoxide reductase gene *(VKORC1)* makes the enzyme that destroys warfarin in the body. DNA variations responsible for changing the gene's activity and the amount of protein it makes account for 25% of the overall variation in warfarin dosage; patients with a particular variation of the gene usually took similar doses of warfarin.

Single Nucleotide Polymorphisms

Pharmaceutical and computer chip manufacturers have partnered to develop techniques to identify specific molecular markers called **single nucleotide polymorphisms**, or **SNPs** (pronounced *snips*), thousands of which reside within each person's genetic code. Most of these tiny nucleotide genetic code "snippets" are normally configured with no deviant code. Some, however, have a single "mismatch" in the nucleotide sequence that predisposes an individual to a particular disease or injury (e.g., ligament tear in football or gymnastics) or renders their immune system resistant to drug treatment. Identifying a specific gene variant allows appropriate lifestyle changes (e.g., nutrition, weight loss, exercise training) or introduction of a particular class of drugs to prevent emergence of the disease or disability, or delay its onset. Thirteen major multinational companies have formed a nonprofit alliance (SNP Consortium LTD: snp.cshl.org) to identify 300,000 variants on human chromosomes and develop drugs that target the disease by its genetic profile. A new Entrez database, dbSNP (www.ncbi.nlm.nih.gov/entrez/query.fcgi?db= snp), similar in operation to PubMed (www.ncbi.nlm.nih.gov/entrez/query.fcgi?DB= pubmed), and GenBank (NIH genetic database of nucleotide sequences; http://www.ncbi. nlm.nih.gov/), also have been created.

SNP assessment (FIG. 29) uses microarrays of chips (biochips) and a "library" of artificial DNA to compare the individual's DNA sample with the chips' existing gene sequences. A microarray (DNA chip) is a spatial array of oligonucleotide probes arranged on a tiny supporting surface. The probe (representing sequences of nucleotides in known genes) is synthesized on the support surface. This allows the researcher to know the position and sequence of each probe. With this information, the DNA chip can identify organisms and select genes by hybridization of the source DNA to the oligonucleotide probes on the chip. One of the hallmarks of this process is to achieve 100% accuracy because even a small error (incorrect identification) could prove disastrous from a worldwide health standpoint.[30] For example, 99.9% accuracy in matching the 300,000 biochip SNPs for only 1000 people would create 300,000 errors! As of May 11, 2005, researchers had identified and published on the Internet the code for 1.8 million mapped SNPs (http://snp.cshl.org/). Once SNP biochips become widely available, the next step requires development of technologies that follow the trail from where the gene gives its instructions to create a specific protein to where the proteins reside in the body. The technique of **photolithography** involves a combination of etching, chemical deposition, and chemical treatments in repeated steps on an initially flat substrate or wafer. Etching microcircuits on a silicon chip could also encode a single biochip containing the entire human genome. Within this decade, disposable, microfabricated "lab-on-a-chip" technologies will enable widespread, less expensive assay techniques. Figure 29 illustrates the four-step procedure to identify SNPs and their specific genetic sequences or anomalies. The challenge to molecular biologists is to map as many SNP genotypes as possible (hence the need for faster sequencers) for purposes of analyzing an individual's genome, since the latter is linked to the predisposition/susceptibility to many diseases.[29,31,52,104]

Cancer

The body's defense mechanisms include "error-correcting" proteins that literally "erase" an apparent aberration in DNA sequencing. Unfortunately, the external effects of ionizing and ultraviolet radiation and chemical and pharmacologic **mutagens** exert catastrophic effects on genetic machinery, specifically the code sequence in DNA. In extreme cases of mutations, structural defects in embryos produce gross deformities such as missing limbs and multiple organs. In these cases, the extreme form of chemical mutagen known as a **teratogen** (*teras* in Greek means monster) produces the effect.

The term **carcinogen** refers to any agent that causes cancer. In cancer, cell growth proceeds unchecked, forming larger-than-normal cell clusters that become tumors. A **benign tumor** remains in one location; cells from a **malignant tumor** migrate to invade

---

Single nucleotide polymorphism (SNP): polymorphism due to variation at a single nucleotide

Allele: abbreviation for "allelomorph"; refers to a gene's different DNA forms or sequences

Locus: location of a specific gene on a chromosome

Photolithography: optimal technology for etching (transferring) electrical circuits on suitable media (silicon wafer with silicon dioxide)

Mutagen: ionizing radiation, ultraviolet radiation, or a chemical agent that disrupts the genetic machinery (sequence of DNA code) and causes mutations

Teratogen: agent that causes extreme mutations

Carcinogen: any agent that causes cancer; for example, smoke from cigarettes contains known carcinogenic agents (e.g., carbon monoxide, formaldehyde, and the metals aluminum, copper, lead, mercury, zinc)

Benign tumor: tumor that remains in one location; it no longer responds to normal growth control and lacks the capacity to invade distant sites

Malignant tumor: tumor that invades other tissues and forms secondary or tertiary cancers

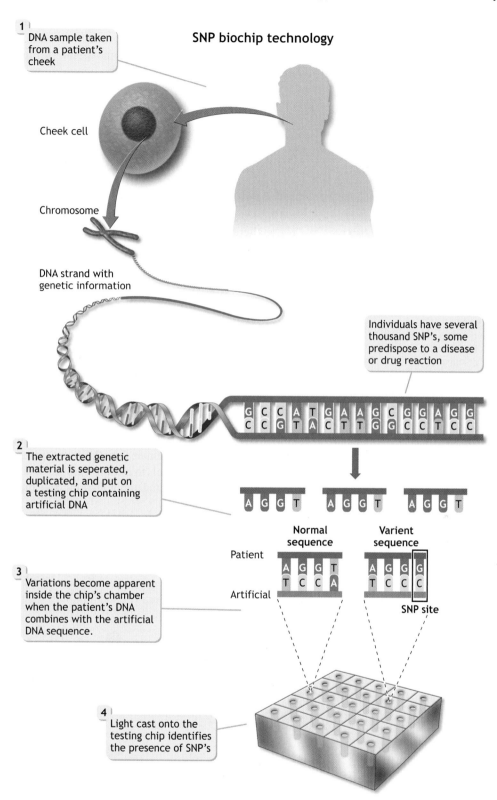

SNP biochip technology

1 DNA sample taken from a patient's cheek

Cheek cell

Chromosome

DNA strand with genetic information

Individuals have several thousand SNP's, some predispose to a disease or drug reaction

2 The extracted genetic material is seperated, duplicated, and put on a testing chip containing artificial DNA

Normal sequence   Varient sequence

Patient

3 Variations become apparent inside the chip's chamber when the patient's DNA combines with the artificial DNA sequence.

Artificial

SNP site

4 Light cast onto the testing chip identifies the presence of SNP's

Figure 29 Four main stages in SNP biochip technology that looks at many genes at once to determine which are expressed in a particular cell type. Thousands of individual genes can be spotted on a single square-inch slide. Note the relative size of the SNP biochip made possible by barcode scanning the microarrays on the biochip. Rapidly identifying the microarrays allows them to link to genes, probe samples, reagents, and experimental protocols.[89] Consult www.lab-on-a-chip.com for research links about microarray technology, and Agilent Technologies for new products and specifications (www.agilent.com).

Sarcoma: cancers forming from connective, muscle, or bone tissue

Carcinoma: cancers formed from epithelial tissue

Metastasize: spread of cancerous cells from the original tumor mass to form secondary cancers (metastases) elsewhere in the body

Oncogene: mutant gene that promotes the loss of cellular growth control, transforming a cell to a malignant state; many oncogenes directly or indirectly control a cell's growth rate

Protooncogene: gene that produces a protein that regulates cell growth; altering a protooncogene can transform it to a cancer-causing oncogene

Vasculogenesis: in vivo formation of blood vessels by differentiation of vascular precursor cells; in implanted bioartificial organs, molecular biology techniques can stimulate the growth of new blood vessels or treat peripheral vascular diseases, wounds, and ulcers from compromised microvasculature

Angiogenesis: new blood vessel formation, usually during embryo development but can also occur abnormally around malignant tumors

other tissues and form secondary cancers. Cancers that form from connective tissue, muscle, or bone are called **sarcomas**; the most prevalent cancers (breast, lung), called **carcinomas**, originate from epithelial tissue. Malignant tumors tend to **metastasize** or spawn cells that invade healthy tissue when they travel via the lymphatic or vascular circulation to form new secondary cancers termed *metastases*. Mutation of a gene into an **oncogene** (cancer-causing gene) often produces numerous cancers, many of which cannot be eradicated by surgery and/or drugs that target specific cells or tissues. Cancer occurs from a failure to "turn on" specific genes that code nucleotide sequences to repress uncontrolled cell division. A tumor cell can develop from a mutation in any of the stages that regulate cell growth and differentiation. In colon cancer, for example, loss of the *APC* gene (adenomatous polyposis coli) on chromosome 5q alters the gut's normal epithelial tissue lining. This leads to abnormal alterations in DNA, activation of the *k-ras* **protooncogene** on chromosome 12q, and loss of two other genes (*DCC* on chromosome 18q and *p53* on chromosome 17p). These alterations induce malignant colon carcinoma and metastasis. A new cell imaging technology (imaging mass spectrometry) can pinpoint the exact location in tissues that produce high levels of the protein thyosin beta-4 believed to trigger tumor growth.[116] Digital computer images that identify the location of specific tissue proteins allow researchers to determine when new proteins invade tumor cells or when normally produced proteins disappear. Protein imaging opens a new vista in cancer screening for searching out specific molecules for comparison between normal and disease states, and developing strategies to arrest existing cancers.

Researchers know that as some cancerous cells become more lethal, they form into primitive channels to create blood vessels (**vasculogenesis**). The new blood vessels eventually connect with preexisting vessels at the edge of the tumor. This process, completely independent of **angiogenesis**, may explain why therapies that attack angiogenesis may not treat some cancers effectively. The figure *below* shows angiogenesis and subsequent vascularization of tumors. First, the tumor proliferates as it forms a small mass of cells. Note the lack of blood vessels in *A*. Without blood vessels the tumor remains small. Second, protein factors in *B* stimulate the endothelial cells of nearby blood vessels to grow toward the tumor cells. Third, blood vessels in *C* proliferate, creating almost unlimited tumor growth. Note the approximate quadrupling of tumor cells.

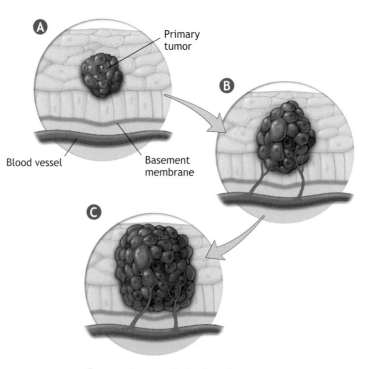

Progressive vascularization of a tumor.

Researchers have developed **gene therapy** strategies to attack tumor growth (e.g., angiogenesis inhibitors) in clinical trials (www.cancer.gov/clinicaltrials/developments/anti-angio-table). For example, Millennium Pharmaceuticals, Inc., in cooperation with the National Cancer Institute in 2003, received approval from the FDA to market the drug Velcade (bortezomib) to treat multiple myeloma patients who received at least two prior therapies and demonstrated disease progression on the last therapy. This new class of drugs targets the proteosome to remove abnormal, aged, or damaged proteins. By blocking the activity of the proteosome, Velcade causes a buildup of proteins in the cell. One of these proteins, BAX, promotes cell suicide or programmed cell death (**apoptosis;**[74] *apopt*, falling off, *osis,* process), by blocking the activity of an antiapoptosis protein. As BAX levels increase in response to Velcade, BAX inhibition of *bcl-2* also increases, and the cell ultimately undergoes apoptosis.

The new anticancer approach uses a peptide that targets tumor blood vessels, invades cells, and literally "tricks" cancer cells into killing themselves. The peptide contains two domains: (1) one that seeks out tumor blood vessels, and (2) one that triggers apoptosis. This normally occurring process in both invertebrate and vertebrate biology should be considered one of nature's defensive mechanisms to purge the organism of cells damaged by mutation, viral invasion, external radiation, malignancy, and other deleterious cellular events (not always abnormalities).

Researchers are studying four main areas of apoptosis:[1,74,100,106,108] (1) molecular mechanisms involved in apoptosis induction, (2) control of intracellular protease pathways responsible for induction, (3) biochemical events during apoptosis, particularly events that mediate cell death, and (4) role of mechanisms in normal development and disease.

Anticancer drugs foster eradication of specific cancers once SNPs or a related technology identifies them. A subsequent section discusses the fight against mutation-caused diseases with a new generation of genetically engineered vaccines.

Mitochondrial DNA Mutations and Diseases

Normally, scientists view the chromosomes as the sole repository for DNA. However, DNA also exists in mitochondria. The complete human mitochondrial genome (www.mitomap.org/) consists of 16,569 base pairs, with the genetic blueprint for 37 molecules that produce about 90 % of the body's energy needs. In Chapters 5 and 6, we described energy release during cellular respiration when electron transfer ultimately produces water by uniting oxygen and hydrogen in the synthesis of significant quantities of energy-rich ATP. Researchers have determined the mitochondrial DNA (mtDNA) codes for 13 proteins that regulate respiratory chain oxidation and for 24 RNA molecules (2 tRNAs, 22 rRNAs) that manufacture subunits of respiratory chain proteins.[131–133] Thus, a defect (mutation) in mtDNA can induce devastating and unpredictable effects on basic cellular metabolic processes, in neural, muscular, renal, and endocrine tissues. FIGURE 30 lists 12 diseases from mutations in mtDNA. The ring of DNA displayed in the schematic view shows different base pairs of mtDNA, numbered counterclockwise from the top center position labeled *OH in white*. Mitochondrial DNA mutations also may be implicated in aging, affecting the impact of **free radicals** on tissues of the cardiovascular system.[65,130] In addition to studying serious human diseases caused by deleterious mutations, other uses of mtDNA fall into two additional categories: (1) forensic medicine, and (2) molecular anthropology. In **forensic medicine**, mtDNA analysis proves particularly useful because the high number of nucleotide polymorphisms (sequence variants) allow discrimination among individuals and/or biologic samples. Even when degraded by environmental insult or time, minute samples of body fluids or fragments of hair, skin, muscle, bone, and blood may yield enough material for typing the mtDNA locus.[7,69,82,117] The likelihood of recovering mtDNA in small or degraded biologic samples exceeds that for nuclear DNA. Mitochondrial DNA molecules exist in hundreds to thousands of copies per cell compared with only two nuclear copies per cell. Also, because mtDNA is inherited only from the mother, any maternally related individual can provide a reference sample in situations where an individual's DNA cannot be directly compared with a biologic sample. In **molecular anthropology**, mtDNA analysis examines the extent of genetic variation in humans and the relatedness of world popula-

Gene therapy: introducing genes into cells (genetic surgery) to alter phenotype (i.e., cure diseases like cystic fibrosis using engineered adenovirus carrying a "good" gene to replace the crippled cystic fibrosis gene); gene therapy cures symptoms but cannot correct the genetic defect in next-generation germ cells

Apoptosis: death of a cell following preprogrammed "instructions." The dead cell is eventually removed by phagocytosis; a small family of proteases called caspases transmit the apoptotic death signal

Free radical: highly reactive ionized atom or molecule with a single unpaired electron in the outer orbit; can cause a mutation by reacting violently with DNA

Forensic medicine: branch of medicine concerned with the uses of medical knowledge applied to the law

Molecular anthropology: application of molecular biology and genetics to contemporary populations and origins of ancient specimens

Disease	Features
Alzheimer's disease	Progressive loss of cognitive capacity
CPEO (chronic progressive external ophthalmoplegia)	Paralysis of eye muscles and mitochondrial myopathy
Diabetes mellitus	High blood glucose levels; numerous complications
Dystonia	Abnormal movements involving muscular rigidity; degeneration of brain's basal ganglia
KSS (Kearns-Sayre syndrome)	CPEO combined with retinal degeneration, heart disease, hearing loss, diabetes, kidney failure
Leigh's syndrome	Progressive motor and verbal skill loss and degeneration of basal ganglia (potentially lethal childhood disease)
LHON (Leber's hereditary optic neuropathy)	Permanent or temporary blindness stemming from optic nerve damage

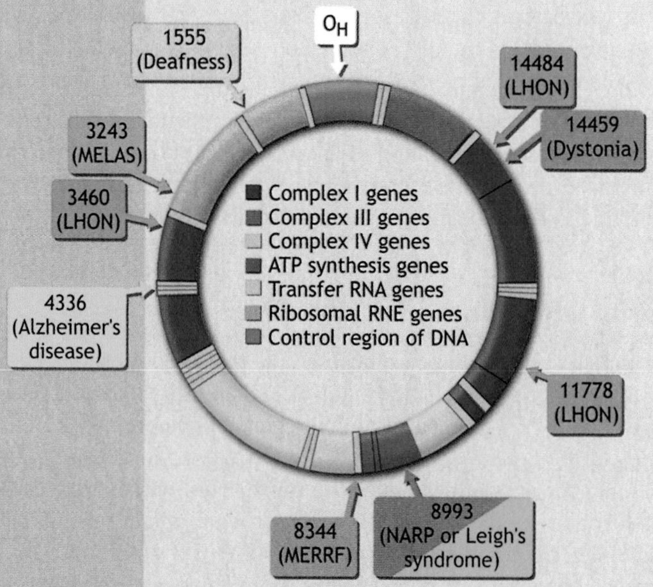

Figure 30 Mitochondrial DNA diseases. The ring of DNA displayed in the *central schematic view* shows the genes associated with a particular disorder. Many of the mitochondrial DNA diseases are inherited, but they also can occur spontaneously in the developing embryo and become widespread during fetal development. The mutations also can form in different tissues (at different times during the life span), often taking years to become fully expressed and often potentially lethal or severely debilitating. (Adapted from Wallace DC, et al. Report of the committee on human mitochondrial DNA. In: Cuticchia AJ, ed. Human gene mapping: a compendium. Baltimore: Johns Hopkins University Press, 1995:910–954. Also available at (www.gen.emory.edu/mitomap.html).

Disease	Features
MELAS (mitochondrial encephalomyopathy, lactic acidosis and strokelike episodes)	Dysfunction of brain tissue (often causing seizures, transient regional paralysis, and dementia) with mitochondrial myopathy and toxic blood acidity
MERRF (myoclonic epilepsy and ragged red fibers)	Seizures combined with mitochondrial myopathy, hearing loss, and dementia
Mitochondrial myopathy	Deterioration of muscle; poor exercise tolerance; muscle often displays ragged red fibers filled with abdormal mitochondria
NARP (neurogenic muscle weakness, ataxia and retinitis pigmentosa)	Muscle strength and coordination loss; regional brain degeneration and retinal deterioration
Pearson's syndrome	Childhood bone marrow dysfunction (leading to loss of blood cells) and pancreatic failure; survivors often progress to KSS

tions.[29,104,107] Because of its unique mode of maternal inheritance, mtDNA can reveal ancient population histories to delineate migration patterns, expansion dates, and geographic homelands (www.talkorigins.org/faqs/homs/mtDNA.html). Mitochondrial DNA has been extracted and sequenced from Neanderthal skeletons, providing evidence that modern humans do *not* share a close relationship with Neanderthals in the human evolutionary tree. The Neandertal mtDNA studies strengthen the arguments that Neandertals should be considered a separate species that did not contribute significantly to the modern gene pool.[102] The FBI laboratory (www.fbi.gov/hq/lab/labhome) began conducting mtDNA analysis for human identity testing in the late 1980s, and its various laboratories currently conduct more than one million examinations yearly.

NEW HORIZONS IN MOLECULAR BIOLOGY

Watson and Crick's pioneering achievements in deciphering the molecular structure of DNA ushered in a new era. Currently, various microscopic and genetic engineering techniques affect not only medically related research but also strategies involving human exercise performance. The successful sequencing of the human genome, announced on June 26, 2000, was one of the most remarkable scientific feats in the history of medical science. Understanding the genetic blueprint of human life will speed the discovery of innovative new drugs to battle existing diseases.

Microscope Technologies

To provide insight into the capabilities of microscopic technologies germane to molecular biology, we compare four procedures, three of which have helped to unravel the secrets locked within the chemical configuration of structures that house the genetic code. Before presenting the different technologies, consider units of measurement and how they relate to what the human eye can observe and what the most powerful microscopes can reveal. FIGURE 31 displays nine different sublevels of organization, ranging from the minimum resolvable minute cellular structures revealed by electron microscopy of 0.2 nm to what the unaided eye observes by just looking at a small piece of skin at the outer region of the biceps.

The examples show each succeeding sublevel of detail using a multiplier of 10. Even with the most powerful electron microscopes individual atoms cannot yet be seen. Single molecules of labeled ATP (and other molecules) have been imaged using total internal reflection **fluorescence microscopy** (TIRFM). The technique to assess single molecules has broad application in studies of the mechanism of molecular motors (motility.york.ac.uk/).[35,73,125]

Fluorescence microscope: microscope shown in Figure 26B that illuminates fluorescent-stained objects

Light Microscope

The **light microscope** shown FIGURE 32A magnifies the interior of cells 1000 times. This represents a quantum leap in technology from the primitive microscope first used in 1655 by British experimental physicist Robert Hooke (1635–1703) to describe what he termed "cells" in sections of cork, and Dutch microscopist Anton van Leeuwenhoek's (1632–1723) 1674 discovery of the single-celled protozoa and later observations of bacteria. The images at the right of the microscope represent the same structure viewed by three different light microscopes, each with a more complex lens system. Each microscope uses a different system of interchangeable lenses to exploit how light travels when it passes through the cell's interior to give a different portrayal of the image. A standard light microscope, in which a bright light focuses on the specimen through lenses in the condenser, provided the three images involved in cell division including a more detailed view shown in color. The **phase-contrast light microscope** uses a different optical system than that shown in *panel A,* as does the **interference-contrast light microscope** that obtained the close-up image in *panel C.* In the fluorescence microscope shown in Figure 32B, light passes through two filters labeled *1* and *2* in the illustration. The first filters any light within the specimen except wavelengths that "excite" a previously applied fluores-

Light microscope: microscope shown in Figure 26A that uses light, fixation of an object, and suitable lens that magnifies objects up to 1000 times with a resolution of 0.2 μm
Phase-contrast light microscope: category of light microscope
Interference-contrast light microscope: category of light microscope

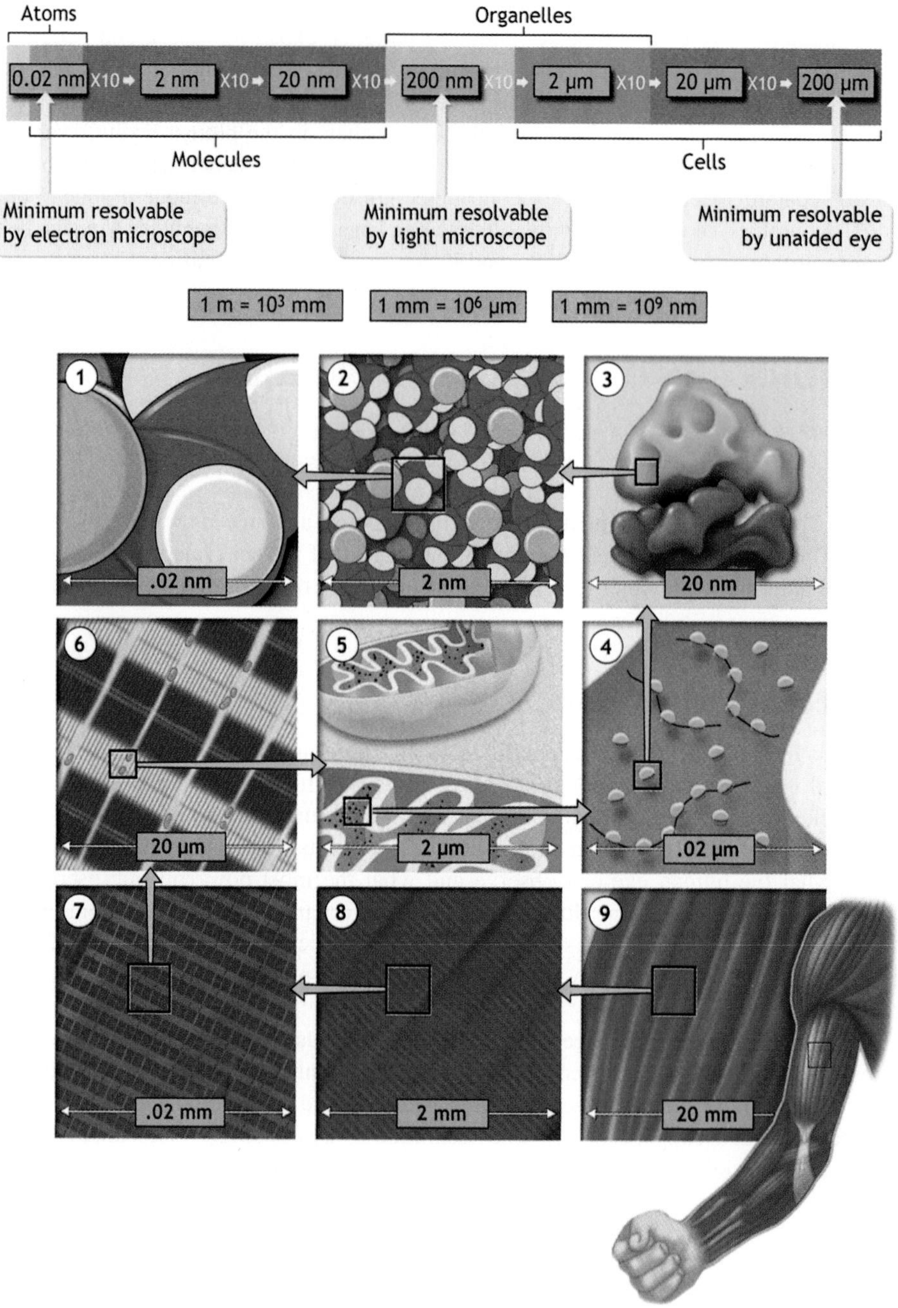

Figure 31 *Top.* Units of measurement for revealing the size of cellular structures from the minimum resolvable distance viewing an object directly (0.2 mm) or through the light (200 nm) and electron (0.2 nm; 200 μm) microscopes. *Bottom.* Nine different sublevels of organization from the macro level at the biceps to the atomic level.

Fluorescence: a molecule absorbs light of one wavelength and then emits light of another longer, lower energy wavelength

cent dye. The second blocks the wavelength of the excited **fluorescent** dye but allows only those wavelengths emitted from the fluorescent dye to pass. Fluorescent dyes absorb light at one wavelength and emit light at longer wavelengths. In staining for DNA in the mitotic spindle *(green dye),* the fluorescent dye "tags" a particular protein molecule within the cell to reveal its structure and location. Another example of fluorescence dye technology shown in FIGURE 33 clearly identifies the human karyotype with its 22 pairs of chromosomes and X and Y sex chromosomes.

The development of precise technologies (e.g., dynamic molecular combing and gel stretching) enables researchers to analyze DNA molecules for genetic abnormalities and patterns. This makes pinpointing disease-related genes an easier task and, consequently, development of new drugs to eradicate inborn or environmentally induced errors within the genetic alphabet.

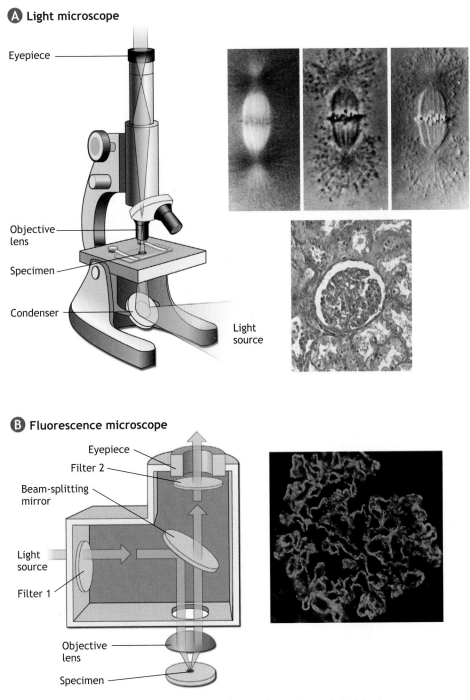

A Light microscope

Eyepiece

Objective lens

Specimen

Condenser

Light source

B Fluorescence microscope

Eyepiece

Filter 2

Beam-splitting mirror

Light source

Filter 1

Objective lens

Specimen

Figure 32 Four different microscopes evaluate cell structures. **A.** Light microscope. **B.** Fluorescence microscope. (Continued on p. 1034.)

C Scanning electron microscope

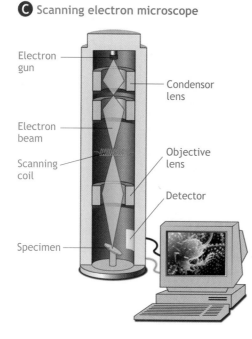
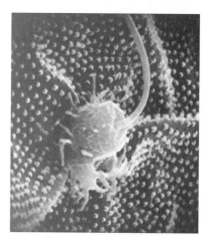

D Transmission electron microscope

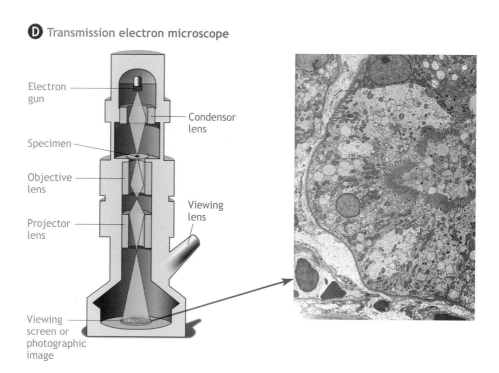

Figure 32 *(continued)* **C.** Scanning electron microscope (SEM). **D.** Transmission electron microscope (TEM).

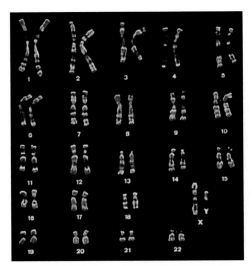

Figure 33 Human karyotype (photomicrograph of an individual's chromosomes arranged in a standard format showing the number, size, and shape of each chromosome type) prepared by 24-color FISH (fluorescent in situ hybridization) uniquely identifies each of the 22 pairs of chromosomes and one sex chromosome (total of 46 chromosomes at conception). Recent advances in fluorescence in situ imaging technology have improved the resolution from 1 million to 10 million bases.

Electron Microscopes

The first electron microscopes invented in the early 1930s represented a technologic advance for unraveling the innermost secrets about cell structures and functions. One half of the 1986 Nobel Prize in Physics was awarded to Ernst Ruska (1906–1988) for his fundamental work in electron optics and design of the first electron microscope, and the other half of the Nobel Prize went to Heinrich Rohrer (1933–) and Gerd Binnig (1947–) for their design of the powerful and precise scanning tunneling microscope that gives 3-D images of objects down to the atomic level. Many pioneers in muscle contraction theory relied on data from electron microscopy to elucidate structural components of a muscle's intricate protein filament structures during contraction and relaxation.[17] In 1964, H. E. Huxley proposed his sliding-filament mechanism of muscle contraction from studies using electron microscopy.[67]

Scanning Electron Microscope. The **scanning electron microscope (SEM)** shown in Figure 32C uses electron beams with wavelengths thousands of times shorter than those of visible light. These waves replace light, allowing considerably greater resolution and magnification. Electromagnetic coils focus the beam on the specimen, similar to the lens of a light microscope. The electrons pass through an ultrathin, stained specimen coated with a thin film of a heavy metal. The detector measures the electrons scattered or emitted by the beam as it passes through the dehydrated specimen and provides a highly detailed image magnified 1 million times (resolution of 2 nm). To prepare the sample, the tissue enters a fixing solution and then is washed and dehydrated in successively higher acetone or alcohol concentrations. The tissue then is placed into a dilute solution of plastic embedding medium, then into a specimen vial, and a final embedding mixture for polymerization in an oven. The hard, plastic-containing specimen is then set in an **ultramicrotome** (FIGURE 34) for slicing with a glass or diamond knife. The ultrathin sections are lifted from the surface with a copper grid, dried, and stained with the electron-dense, heavy metal solution (salts of uranium and lead) in preparation for viewing. The scanned images have a resolution between 3 and 20 nm and provide exquisite, detailed three-dimensional images.

Transmission Electron Microscope. Figure 32D shows an extremely thin slice of a prepared substance (biopsy of lung tissue) within the vacuum of the transmission electron microscope (TEM). Multiple stains reveal different parts of a structure because each stain clings to a different structural part.

Laser Scanning Confocal Microscopy. In **laser scanning confocal microscopy** (LSCM; also known as confocal scanning laser microscopy or CSLM; FIGURE 35), an expanded laser light beam creates high-resolution images and three-dimensional reconstructions of biologic

Scanning electron microscope (SEM): uses electron beams with wavelengths thousands of times shorter than visible light to produce significantly higher resolution and magnification

Ultramicrotome: microtome that cuts specimen sections 0.01 μm thick or less for electron microscopy

Laser scanning confocal microscopy (LSCM): laser light beam creates high resolution images and 3-D reconstructions of biologic specimens

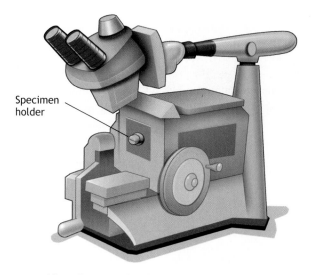

Figure 34 Ultramicrotome for ultrathin slicing of specimen sections.

specimens (www.loci.wisc.edu/confocal/confocal.html). The projected beam becomes a scanning beam with an objective lens that focuses a small spot onto a fluorescent specimen. After conversion into a static beam, the reflected and emitted fluorescent light mixture focuses onto a photodetector (photomultiplier) via a dichroic mirror (beam splitter). The dichroic mirror splits the reflected light, while emitted fluorescent light passes through to the photomultiplier. A confocal aperture (pinhole) placed in front of the photodetector selectively allows fluorescent light to pass from points on the specimen not within the focal plane. This greatly reduces out-of-focus information (both above and below the focal plane). The spot focused on the pinhole center is known as the "confocal spot." Most confocal microscopes are coupled to a conventional microscope. Advanced software now permits four-dimensional microscopy to study three-dimensional specimens as they grow or change over time (www.loci.wisc.edu/); additional techniques include multiple-photon excitation fluorescence (www.its.caltech.edu/~pinelab/2photon.html) and computational optical scanning, and a variety of optimal techniques for experimental intervention into living specimens.

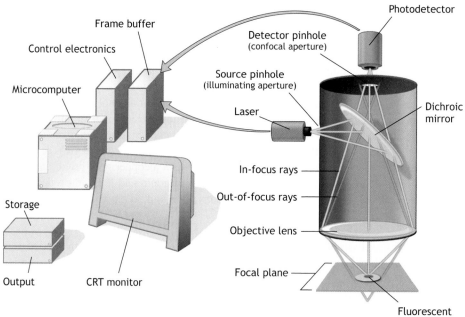

Figure 35 Laser scanning confocal microscopy. The image shown on the CRT monitor, a virus-infected cell structure, was the fluorescent specimen scanned by the microscope.

Positron Emission Tomography (PET). The **PET scanner** (FIGURE 36) provides detailed images of biochemical activity in the body without surgery for diagnosing heart disease, stroke, epilepsy, Parkinson's disease, and cancer. Patients are injected with a low dose of a short-lived radioactive sugar. Detectors assess release of gamma rays from the sugar, which concentrates in the tissues under study. The tomographic images of the brain on the *top* of Figure 36, taken with a 32-ring PET scanner, clearly show areas of interest detected by differ-

PET scanner: provides detailed images of biochemical activity in the body without surgery. Patients are injected with a low dose of a short-lived radioactive sugar that concentrates in tissues for easy visualization

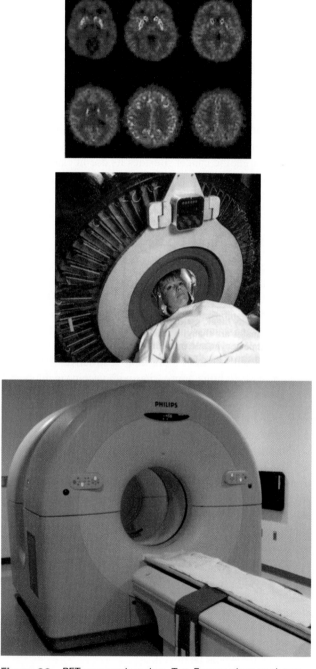

Figure 36   PET scanner imaging. *Top.* Excess glucose shows as yellow colored region in the brain PET scan. *Middle.* Patient undergoing brain scan with the 32-ring PET scanner. *Bottom.* PET/CT scanner allows a full-body scan that averages about 30 minutes duration. The hybrid PET/CT scan detects minute changes in the body's metabolism caused by abnormal cell growth (PET), while CT simultaneously pinpoints the exact size, shape, and location of diseased tissue. Bottom photo courtesy of United Medical Systems.

ent colored radiopharmaceuticals. In this example, the image shows glucose *(bright yellow)* used in excess of normal requirements, as in a growing tumor. Unlike magnetic resonance imaging (MRI), which primarily examines *anatomy* in detail, the PET scan can visualize body *functions* during the course of a disease like cancer and accurately show its extent (i.e., whether it is malignant or benign and treatment effects). In Alzheimer's disease, for example, a PET scan can recognize abnormal brain patterns years before a physician can confirm the disease. In Parkinson's disease, the presence of a labeled amino acid (F-DOPA) quantifies a deficiency in dopamine synthesis. Early confirmation of the deficiency leads to a different treatment modality than is used if the deficiency cannot be established. Several web sites provide excellent information about PET scanning (www.muc.ucla.edu/; www.laxm.nuc.ucla.edu:8000/lpp/).

The latest PET scanners now link with CT scanners, called *PT/CT scanners,* offer improved diagnostic imaging. The hybrid technology combines the strengths of two well-established imaging modalities in a single imaging session to more accurately diagnose and locate the following types of cancers: breast, colon, esophageal, head and neck, lung, lymphoma, and melanoma. The PET/CT scan overlays the metabolic data of the PET scan with the detailed anatomic data of the CT scan to pinpoint the location and stage of tumors. Compared with individual PET and CT scans, the new hybrid technology alters a patient's treatment plan to better target the cancer. Besides its use in cancer diagnosis and treatment, the PET/CT scanner has applications in cardiology and brain imaging, including epilepsy and Parkinson's disease.

Medically Related Research

Almost every aspect of medicine now benefits from molecular biology/molecular genetics research. Within the past 20 years, researchers have developed new strategies to fight many diseases, including cancer, AIDS, asthma, diabetes, influenza, heart and vascular disease, rheumatic fever, and malaria. The new disease fighters use genetic engineering to improve the immunologic antigen defense machinery against viral, bacterial, fungal, or parasitic **pathogens**. All pathogens contain antigens in their structure, so a new generation of genetically engineered vaccines will severely blunt their destructive effects. FIGURE 37 provides a capsule view of four disease-fighting approaches with vaccine techniques that manipulate the genetic code.

1. *Live vector vaccines* (www.niaid.nih.gov/daids/vaccine/live.htm). Genes from a dangerous virus such as HIV are inserted into a **virus** that is harmless to humans. When injected, the altered virus prompts a strong **immune response** to combat the pathogen.
2. *Reassortment virus vaccines* (http://virology-online.com/viruses/Influenza.htm). Combining genes from different pathogenic strains creates a decoy virus that looks dangerous to the pathogen but remains harmless while triggering an appropriate immune response.
3. *Naked DNA vaccines* (www.niaid.nih.gov/daids/vaccine/dna.htm). A pathogen's DNA is injected directly into the body. The cells incorporate the DNA, using the preprogrammed specific genetic "instructions" to create antigens to fight offending pathogens or existing tumors.
4. *Recombinant subunit vaccines* (www.niaid.nih.gov/daids/vaccine/recombinant.htm). Culturing a pathogen's genetic code (genes) produces massive quantities of a specific antigen. The disease-fighting vaccine is made from the cultured antigens rather than from the whole pathogen.

Some genetically engineered vaccines trick the immune system into creating antibodies to seek out and destroy undesirable molecules before they cross the blood–brain barrier. For example, small cocaine molecules escape the body's protein antibody defenses without mechanisms to stop them. Engineered vaccines can create a larger cocaine derivative, which the immune system can then recognize and disarm. This aspect of genetic design, although currently more expensive than cloning to make drug therapies, offers new hope in battling addictive diseases.

Pathogen: any virus, microorganism, or other substance that causes disease; *Streptococcus* bacteria cause scarlet fever, rheumatic fever, and pneumonia in humans; in plants, destructive diseases caused by bacteria (mostly pseudomonads) include blights, soft rots, and wilts. Viruses cannot replicate independently; they exist only within the cells of other organisms. Viruses usually contain a protein coating (capsid) and lipid-rich protein envelope around the capsid ("a piece of bad news wrapped up in a protein") and reproduce using the metabolic apparatus of their host

Vector: plasmid, retrovirus, or bacterial or yeast artificial chromosome used to transfer a segment of foreign DNA among cells or species to produce more end product; the vector represents the genome that transports alien DNA into a host cell

Virus: small structure that grows by infecting other cells; adenovirus, retrovirus, and adeno-associated viruses are the most commonly used viral gene vectors

Immune response: immediate defensive reaction of the immune system upon encountering an invasion by a foreign substance such as a pathogen

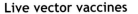

Live vector vaccines

Reassortment vaccines

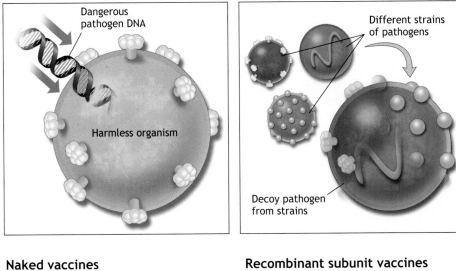

Naked vaccines

Recombinant subunit vaccines

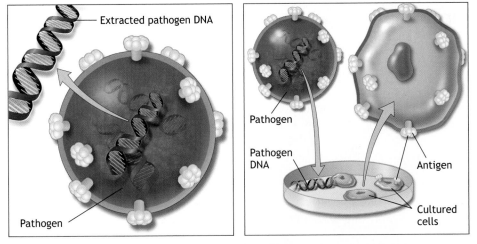

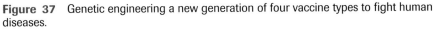

Figure 37 Genetic engineering a new generation of four vaccine types to fight human diseases.

FIGURE 38 lists the body's 22 numbered chromosomes, including X and Y chromosomes, and specific genes on each chromosome linked to cancers and metabolic/endocrine, neurologic/psychiatric, and cardiovascular disorders. The *right side* of Figure 38 profiles chromosome 17 on which seven deadly cancers have already been identified. The *bottom* of Figure 38 shows the mechanism of action of different chemical carcinogens on this particular nucleotide sequence of the tumor suppressor gene *p53*. About 50% of human cancers occur from inactivating this gene. Each carcinogen produces a distinctive nucleotide substitution. Note the C or G substitution that displaces six T nucleotides.

Many areas of medicine other than cancer benefit from new findings in molecular biology.[103] Individuals with advanced sleep-phase syndrome (ASPS) cannot resist the urge either to sleep or to wake up early. Research indicates that ASPS does not reflect a learned behavior or some other factor but follows a specific inherited pattern. Eventually, researchers may tie disorders to a single gene, opening new vistas to the genetics of the biologic clock in humans,[72,119,120] with potential applications to many aspects of human exercise performance. Some of the same medical research techniques have found their way into the arsenal of technologies to probe secrets about topics of interest to exercise physiologists. These include blood pressure control, endurance and strength training adaptations, maturational shifts related to caloric input and output, hormonal balance with exercise, and pulmonary, cardiovascular, and body weight regulation (including anorexia nervosa[54]).

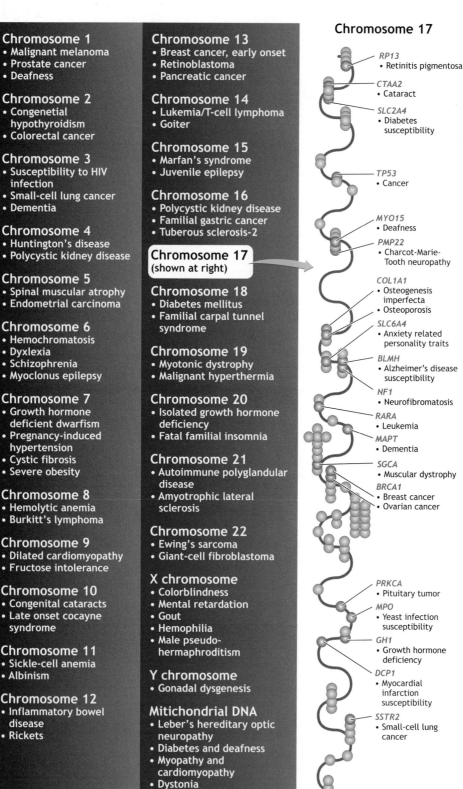

Chromosome 1
- Malignant melanoma
- Prostate cancer
- Deafness

Chromosome 2
- Congenetial hypothyroidism
- Colorectal cancer

Chromosome 3
- Susceptibility to HIV infection
- Small-cell lung cancer
- Dementia

Chromosome 4
- Huntington's disease
- Polycystic kidney disease

Chromosome 5
- Spinal muscular atrophy
- Endometrial carcinoma

Chromosome 6
- Hemochromatosis
- Dyxlexia
- Schizophrenia
- Myoclonus epilepsy

Chromosome 7
- Growth hormone deficient dwarfism
- Pregnancy-induced hypertension
- Cystic fibrosis
- Severe obesity

Chromosome 8
- Hemolytic anemia
- Burkitt's lymphoma

Chromosome 9
- Dilated cardiomyopathy
- Fructose intolerance

Chromosome 10
- Congenital cataracts
- Late onset cocayne syndrome

Chromosome 11
- Sickle-cell anemia
- Albinism

Chromosome 12
- Inflammatory bowel disease
- Rickets

Chromosome 13
- Breast cancer, early onset
- Retinoblastoma
- Pancreatic cancer

Chromosome 14
- Lukemia/T-cell lymphoma
- Goiter

Chromosome 15
- Marfan's syndrome
- Juvenile epilepsy

Chromosome 16
- Polycystic kidney disease
- Familial gastric cancer
- Tuberous sclerosis-2

Chromosome 17
(shown at right)

Chromosome 18
- Diabetes mellitus
- Familial carpal tunnel syndrome

Chromosome 19
- Myotonic dystrophy
- Malignant hyperthermia

Chromosome 20
- Isolated growth hormone deficiency
- Fatal familial insomnia

Chromosome 21
- Autoimmune polyglandular disease
- Amyotrophic lateral sclerosis

Chromosome 22
- Ewing's sarcoma
- Giant-cell fibroblastoma

X chromosome
- Colorblindness
- Mental retardation
- Gout
- Hemophilia
- Male pseudo-hermaphroditism

Y chromosome
- Gonadal dysgenesis

Mitichondrial DNA
- Leber's hereditary optic neuropathy
- Diabetes and deafness
- Myopathy and cardiomyopathy
- Dystonia

Chromosome 17

RP13
- Retinitis pigmentosa

CTAA2
- Cataract

SLC2A4
- Diabetes susceptibility

TP53
- Cancer

MYO15
- Deafness

PMP22
- Charcot-Marie-Tooth neuropathy

COL1A1
- Osteogenesis imperfecta
- Osteoporosis

SLC6A4
- Anxiety related personality traits

BLMH
- Alzheimer's disease susceptibility

NF1
- Neurofibromatosis

RARA
- Leukemia

MAPT
- Dementia

SGCA
- Muscular dystrophy

BRCA1
- Breast cancer
- Ovarian cancer

PRKCA
- Pituitary tumor

MPO
- Yeast infection susceptibility

GH1
- Growth hormone deficiency

DCP1
- Myocardial infarction susceptibility

SSTR2
- Small-cell lung cancer

Figure 38 Links on the body's chromosomes to specific cancer, metabolic/endocrine, neurologic/psychiatric, and cardiovascular disorders. *Right.* Close-up of disorders found on chromosome 17. On this chromosome, *red* designates the specific gene name and its location. (Continued on p. 1041.)

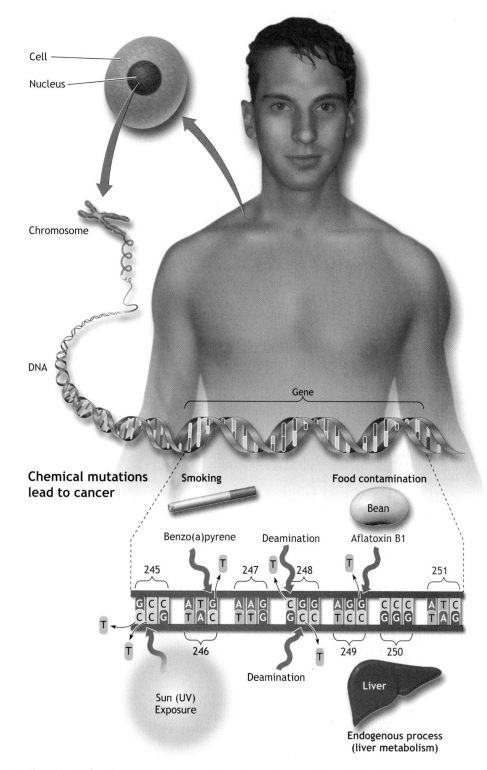

Figure 38 *(continued)* Graphic illustrating how different carcinogens (chemical and other) affect the nucleotide sequence of the *p53* gene responsible for about 50% of human cancers. The *p53* gene's name comes from the product it encodes, a polypeptide with a molecular mass of 53,000 daltons (1 dalton equals one twelfth the mass of carbon 12; for comparison, a water molecule weighs 18 daltons, and hemoglobin weighs 64,500 daltons).

DNA Technologies

By isolating a small fragment of DNA from a chromosome in an animal species (including humans), scientists can "remake" an exact copy of the DNA segment in a test tube to preserve the precise sequence of its nucleotide base pairs. Researchers use several terms to describe this process of eventual gene reconfiguration or manipulation on chromosomes—genetic engineering, **gene splicing**, or **recombinant DNA**.

A crucial step along the path to genetic engineering occurred in 1967 when Dr. Arthur Kornberg synthesized biologically active DNA (1959 Nobel Prize in physiology or medicine; discovered the mechanisms in the biologic synthesis of DNA and RNA). This was followed in 1970 in classic experiments by Drs. David Baltimore, Renato Dulbecco, and Howard Temin who won the 1975 Nobel Prize in physiology or medicine for discoveries concerning the interaction between tumor viruses and a cell's genetic material. They discovered that a specific enzyme tumor virus (**reverse transcriptase**) made a DNA copy from RNA. The researchers used purified mRNA from muscle or liver tissue to show that this enzyme interacts with the mRNA. Reverse transcriptase duplicates the mRNA to the specific sequence of complementary DNA (**cDNA**). DNA polymerase can then convert the single-stranded DNA to a double strand for eventual cloning into a **bacteriophage** or other vector. These experiments proved transfer of the content stored in the genetic material to DNA; subsequent experiments also proved that purified DNA from one cell introduced into other cells produce new particles of RNA tumor virus.

In 1973, two American researchers Stanford's Stanley Cohen, cofounder of Genentech (www.gene.com/), one of the first biotechnology corporations, and Herbert Boyer (1986 Nobel Prize in physiology or medicine with Rita Levi-Montalcini for discovering cell growth factors) at the University of California, San Francisco, built upon the research described above. They introduced the recombinant DNA technique shown schematically in FIGURE 39. They successfully cut DNA from an amphibian gene (primitive frog *Xenopus*) into segments,

Gene splicing: attaching a fragment of DNA from one species (e.g., mammal) to another species (e.g., bacterium) to clone mammalian DNA

Recombinant DNA: forming a hybrid DNA molecule by fusing DNA fragments from different species; attaching a segment of DNA from one species to a second species, followed by inserting the hybrid molecule into a host organism such as a bacterium

Reverse transcriptase: enzyme that allows a single-stranded RNA template to synthesize a double-stranded DNA copy for insertion elsewhere in the genome

cDNA: single-stranded DNA complementary to an RNA and synthesized from it using reverse transcriptase; this kind of DNA only codes exons

Bacteriophage: any virus that infects bacteria

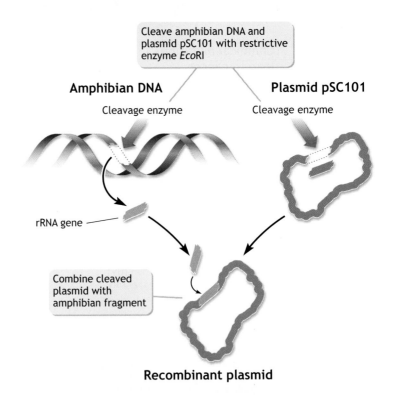

Figure 39 Drs. Stanley Cohen and Herbert Boyer produce the first recombinant DNA organism in 1973. Their pioneering experiment combined the cleaved plasmid vector (pSC101 shown at the *right*) with a fragment of amphibian DNA (shown at the top *left*) using restriction endonuclease enzyme (*Eco*R1) to produce the recombinant plasmid shown at the *bottom*. The cells that contained the plasmid that carried the tetracycline gene grew and formed a cell colony (containing the frog ribosomal RNA gene).

using a **restriction endonuclease** enzyme (*Eco*RI) to cut the plasmid. They then rejoined the 9000-nucleotide segment to form a circular plasmid called pSC101, so-named by Cohen because it was the 101st plasmid he isolated.

Their experimental procedure (explained further in the section on RNA cloning) produced the first plasmid to clone a vertebrate gene. In essence, the frog–bacterial molecule represented recombinant DNA using gene splicing to rejoin the two ends of the pSC101 plasmid. This technique can be likened to "cutting" and "pasting" text or images from one section of a document to another in a computer software program. The endonuclease first cleaves the amphibian DNA, setting it free. The two ends of the rRNA gene now join the pSC101 plasmid cleaved by *Eco*R1. Fundamentally, gene splicing creates a new genetic blueprint in a test tube that leapfrogs nature's own genetic engineering methods based on natural selection—a process that normally comingles genes within Earth's plant and animal species over tens of millions of years of evolution.

With the opening of trade routes and exploration in the ancient world, different sizes, shapes, and characteristics of plant and animal species from one location gained options to "share" their genetic code with similar species in other more distant locations thousands of miles away. Unknowingly, humans helped to selectively breed (genetically engineer) plants and animals, in effect revising and updating the original gene pool that now forms the great variety of flowers, vegetables, and animals around us. What took nature millions of years to accomplish, scientists can now duplicate in a day and produce thousands of copies of DNA's exact nucleotide sequence from a particular gene in a given genome. By manipulating DNA's configuration, a newly created gene can be inserted into cells of plants and animals, creating new cells or species with unique characteristics expressed by the new genetic instructions.

DNA Cloning Isolates Human Genes

DNA **cloning** progresses in several stages. The first involves mechanically breaking the genetic material within a DNA sample or, alternatively, using restriction endonucleases that precisely cut the nucleotide sequence along DNA's double helix into smaller segments to facilitate manipulation. The collection of DNA pieces formed by endonuclease cleavage represents single, random segments of the organism's entire DNA, which includes all of the genetic material. The term **genomic library** describes the collection of cloned fragments. Many genomic libraries exist in the public domain (e.g., www.gdb.org), so researchers can use them without having to reduplicate the particular DNA sequences of interest. FIGURE 40 shows formation of a genomic library.

A restriction endonuclease cleaves a short strand of human double helix chromosomal DNA, usually four to six base pairs in length, into millions of fragments. Restriction endonucleases have become a fundamental tool in molecular biology research because treatment of DNA with the same restriction endonuclease allows any two DNA fragments to join together—providing for an essentially endless supply of DNA for further experimentation. One of the most widely used chemical techniques, **gel electrophoresis** (Greek *phoresis*, "to be carried"), perfected by 1948 Chemistry Nobel laureate Arne Wilhelm Tiselius (1902–1971; for research on electrophoresis and adsorption analysis, and discoveries concerning the complex nature of the serum proteins), separates DNA fragments within an electric field. The DNA strands inserted into a circular plasmid carrier molecule recombine the DNA (hence the term *recombinant DNA*). This occurs when the enzyme DNA ligase with addition of ATP covalently links the DNA fragment to the previously opened **plasmid** composed of several thousand nucleotide pairs. Once inserted, the ligase rejoins the ends of the plasmid to produce the new recombinant plasmid molecule known as a vector. Recombinant plasmids are then inserted into bacteria (e.g., *E. coli*) to ensure that only one bacterium receives one plasmid. At this stage, the total culture of bacteria represents the genomic library illustrated in Figure 40.

The next stage of DNA cloning grows the bacterium in a nutrient-rich broth that sustains cell multiplication that doubles its number every hour. This therefore doubles the number of recombinant DNA copies. By simple multiplication, doubling the number of DNA copies each hour over 24 hours produces almost 17 million new copies from a single bacterium! The bacteria are then broken apart (lysed), and the millions of DNA copies culled from the larger bacterial chromosome and other cellular contents to provide pure replicas of the original DNA

Restriction endonuclease: enzyme that cleaves a specific short DNA nucleotide sequence whenever it occurs at a target site

Cloning: creating a cell(s) or molecule(s) from a single ancestral cell or molecule

Genomic library: collection of DNA fragments from an organism's genome; a library includes noncoding DNA and cDNA

Gel electrophoresis: separation of electrically charged substances (e.g., proteins) through a gel mesh according to size; smaller substances migrate faster than larger substances when they pass through the electric field from the top (negative) to bottom (positive) electrode through a slab of agarose gel, a polysaccharide extracted from seaweed

Plasmid: small circular molecule in bacteria without chromosomal DNA; serves as a vector for transferring genes among cells

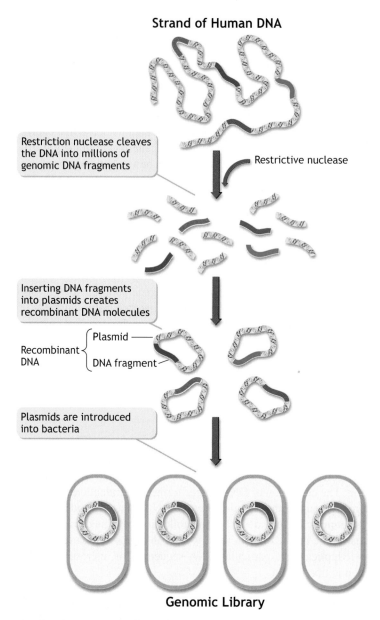

Strand of Human DNA

Restriction nuclease cleaves the DNA into millions of genomic DNA fragments

Restrictive nuclease

Inserting DNA fragments into plasmids creates recombinant DNA molecules

Recombinant DNA { Plasmid — DNA fragment —

Plasmids are introduced into bacteria

Genomic Library

Figure 40   Creating a genomic library from human DNA. The library consists of bacteria with specific DNA fragments contained in carrier substances such as plasmids. Note in the example how four different-colored DNA segments (red, blue, purple, green) from the original human DNA shown at the top end up within the bacterial host. The rest of the DNA fragments also can make clones.

Restriction enzyme: cuts DNA at precise locations, and with DNA ligase, reassembles the pieces into a desired order. Cutting between G and A leaves overhanging "sticky end" chains because base pairs formed between the two overhanging portions "glue" the two strands together where the sticky ends match, assembling them into customized genomes (e.g., designer bacteria that make insulin or growth hormone, or genes for disease resistance added to agricultural plants)

segment. Recovering this segment occurs after the specific **restriction enzyme** isolates the segment from plasma DNA for separation by gel electrophoresis (see Fig. 43).

Practical Application in Bioremediation

Implementation of bacterial cloning has practical applications in the field of bioremediation, which uses bacteria to degrade dangerous compounds. For example, the pink-colored, bacteria that smell like rotten cabbage, *Deinococcus radiodurans (D. radi),* shown in FIGURE 41 have been genetically cloned from strains of *E. coli* previously made resistant to toxic wastes. *D. radi* was isolated in 1956 from a can of ground beef that had been "sterilized" by gamma radiation but still spoiled. Researchers determined that *D. radi* survived approximately 17 kGy (1.7 million rads), a value equal to 3000 times the lethal dose of radiation for humans. The economic value of *D. radi* is straightforward; easily producing trillions of copies of the new bacterium will save hundreds of billions of dollars in biohazard cleanup. For example, because *D. radi* con-

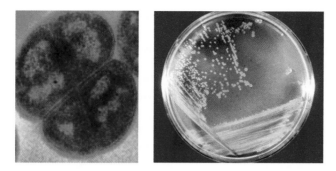

Figure 41   Bioremediation. *Left.* Electron photomicrograph of *D. radi* (sequenced in the DOE Microbial Genome Program as a cluster of four cells or tetrad). *D. radi* and related species have been identified worldwide,[83] including in Antarctic granite and in tanks of powerful cobalt-60 irradiators in Denmark. *Right. D. radi* growing on a nutrient agar plate; the orange color is from carotenoid pigment. (Images from the Uniformed Services University of the Health Sciences, Bethesda, MD; www.usuhs.mil/).

sumes heavy metals and radioactive wastes, it can scavenge toxic wastes buried at 1000 sites throughout the United States and other sites worldwide, a legacy from nuclear weapons production between 1945 and 1986. Researchers have also fused a gene that encodes toluene dioxygenase (the enzyme that decomposes toluene) to a *D. radi* promoter (site that activates the gene) and then inserted it into one of the bacterium's chromosomes. The resulting recombinant bacterium "upgraded" *D. radi* for degrading toluene and other organic compounds at levels exceeding those at radioactive waste sites. *D. radi* not only survives high radiation doses, but also long periods of dehydration and ultraviolet irradiation. *D. radi* apparently repairs its radiation-damaged DNA base pairs by use of redundant genetic "signals." The 2 billion-year-old microbe has from 4 to 10 DNA molecules. The protein, RecA, matches the damaged DNA base pairs and splices them together. During the repair process, cell-building activities shut down and the broken DNA pieces stay in place. The complete genome of *D. radi* has been decoded (see Timeline, 1999; TABLE A, p. 1063) and can be accessed from the TIGR web site, www.tigr.org/. The DNA of *D. radi* consists of 3.3 million chemical base units. The genome contains two circular chromosomes, one of about 2.6 million and the other 400,000 base pairs, and two smaller circular molecules (megaplasmid of 177,000 base pairs and plasmid of 45,000 base pairs). Despite its high tolerance for radioactivity, *D. radi* decomposes at 45°C.

Locating Specific Genes with Plasmids

Creating cloned DNA involves locating a specific gene within the plasmid or viral culture. Consider the analogy of entering a five-story department store without signs or a computer database to search for a single unmarked item. One could begin searching on the first floor, proceeding to every shelf and cupboard of every floor until finding the item, but the inefficiency of this strategy seems obvious. To facilitate locating a specific gene, a specific **DNA probe** of known nucleotide sequence, labeled with colored fluorescent markers or radioisotopes, searches the pool of millions of copies of DNA fragments. The probes used in **hybridization** reactions capture a single DNA or RNA strand to form another nucleic acid with a complementary nucleotide sequence. The probe searches the genomic library until it locates a matching code on a specific chromosomal gene or a specific RNA sequence in cells or tissues.

Searching for a single gene remains complicated because the gene can contain both coding exons and noncoding introns. If the clone with its isolated sequences contains only exons (i.e., only the uninterrupted coding sequences), then the new genomic library is called a **cDNA library** (the *c* refers to a copy or complementary DNA). Different cDNA libraries reflect different tissues because the libraries contain the specifically transcribed mRNA from the original source tissue. A cDNA library contains the gene's coding regions, often including the

DNA probe: radioactive or fluorescent-labeled nucleotide that identifies, isolates (targets), or binds to a gene or gene product

Hybridization: selective binding of two complementary nucleic acid strands (DNA or RNA) to detect specific nucleotide sequences

cDNA library: contains the genes' coding regions, including leading and trailing mRNA sequences

leading and trailing sequences of the mRNA. The absence of chromosomal DNA serves as a cDNA clone's most distinguishing feature. The enzyme reverse transcriptase uses the source cell or tissue mRNA to construct DNA. Cloning cDNA molecules is similar to cloning genomic DNA fragments. Each different type of tissue (e.g., heart, liver, kidney) has a different cDNA library associated with it. Cloned DNA makes it possible to manufacture exact copies of "pure" genetic material relatively quickly from among millions of nucleotide sequences. The uninterrupted coding sequence for a particular gene gives the cDNA clone a clear advantage for duplicating the gene in bulk or deducing a protein's amino acid sequence. Like genomic libraries, cDNA libraries exist in the public domain for sharing among researchers; commercial vendors also make them available for purchase. Many Internet sites provide valuable links to databases (e.g.,www.ddbj.nig.ac.jp/) for mammals and other vertebrates, fungi, plants, eukaryotes, prokaryotes, viruses, specific gene groups, and large-scale genome sequencing centers. FIGURE 42 illustrates the basic difference in creating genomic DNA and cDNA libraries. In both cases, fragments of digested DNA (shown as *purple* fragments) are inserted into cloning vectors such as phage.

Electrophoresis and Gel Transfer Methods

The electrophoresis technique moves charged particles such as proteins through an electrically charged supporting medium. The negatively charged phosphate groups of DNA molecules migrate to the positive pole (anode) of the apparatus. FIGURE 43 shows two ways of separating DNA fragments. The top example *(A)* shows cutting the same DNA molecule from the

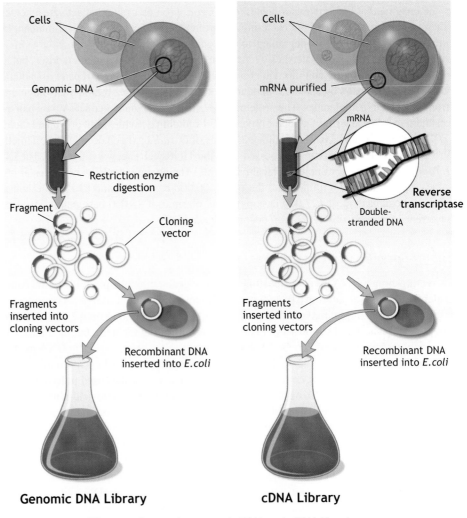

Genomic DNA Library   **cDNA Library**

Figure 42   Basic differences in creating genomic DNA and cDNA libraries.

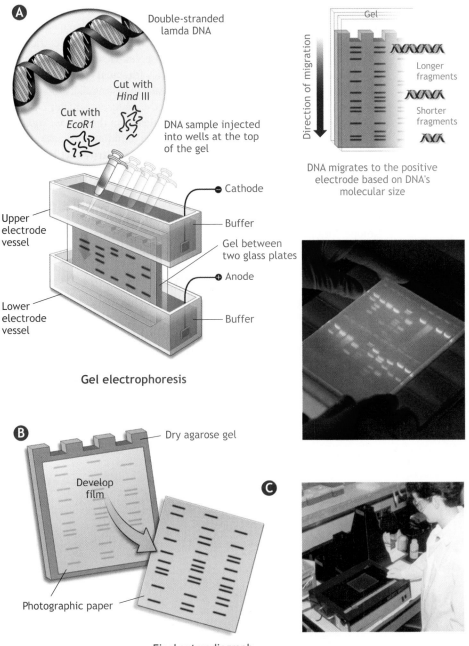

Gel electrophoresis

Final autoradiograph

Figure 43   Gel electrophoresis: separating DNA fragments by molecular size. **A.** Two restriction endonucleases cleave DNA into two segments for placement at the top of a thin agarose gel slab supported in a vertical position. An electric current separates the DNA fragments as they pass through the hydrated gel according to their mobility; small fragments move more quickly through the electric current and fixate at the bottom of the gel at the positive electrode. Larger fragments settle nearer to the top. The *top right photo* reveals the DNA bands fluoresced under ultraviolet light. Note: The restriction enzyme takes the initials of the bacterial type and strain from its source; *Eco*R1 refers to *E. coli* strain RY13, and the 1 means this restriction enzyme was found first in the strain. The cleavage site is 5′–GAATTC–3′ and 3′–CTTAAG–5′; the *Hind*III source is *Haemophilus influenzae* R_d. The cleavage site is 5′–AAGCTT–3′ and 3′–TTCGAA–5′. **B.** Autoradiography technique displays radioisotope ^{32}P-labeled DNA bands on exposed photographic paper placed over the agarose gel. **C.** Dr. Kristin Stuempfle, Department of Health and Exercise Sciences, Gettysburg College, reviewing the film of a sequencing gel on a light box.

Ultraviolet light: electromagnetic rays at higher frequencies than the violet end of the visible spectrum

Radioisotope: isotope that becomes more stable by emitting radiation

Southern blotting: technique that detects single-stranded DNA from transferring DNA fragments to nylon paper with a DNA-binding probe

Northern blotting: hybridization technique that binds a DNA probe to a target RNA molecule; the technique detects a specific RNA sequence in a cell

Western blotting: technique for separating genetic fragments using a probe (usually an antibody) that binds to a target protein

In vitro: in an artificial environment such as a test tube or culture medium

λ (bacteriophage) genome with two different restriction endonucleases, *Eco*R1 and *Hind*III (hundreds of other enzymes with distinct specificity have been isolated). Small fragments migrate faster than large fragments when they pass through the electric field from top (negative) to bottom (positive) through a slab of agarose gel. Heating the gel causes its protein fibers to congeal and form a grid through which DNA fragments pass. Separating DNA fragments by size in an electric field makes it relatively easy to distinguish among DNA segments. Note the bands at the *lower right panel* of the gel. These represent smaller DNA fragments than the upper longer fragments. The DNA shows up clearly in the *bottom right* photo because soaking the medium with a DNA- or RNA-specific dye (ethidium bromide) stains DNA orange (pinkish in photo), which becomes clearly visible under **ultraviolet light**. Extraction of DNA provides samples of pure DNA fragments. Purified DNA can be used in cloning experiments or for matching in size to other DNA fragments.[75,121]

Figure 43B shows an alternative technique using the labeled **radioisotope** [32]P to expose DNA bands when photographic paper placed over the gel reveals β particles emitted from the isotope. FIGURE 44 illustrates three gel transfer methods to separate fragments of genetic material and proteins: **Southern blotting**, **Northern blotting**, and **Western blotting**.

DNA Amplification with the Polymerase Chain Reaction

The polymerase chain reaction (PCR) method developed in 1987 by Dr. Kerry Mullis (1993 Nobel Prize in chemistry; invention of the PCR method) represents a milestone in molecular biology.[92] The PCR method, carried out **in vitro** without prior transfer in living cells, artificially amplifies an extremely small amount of DNA and rapidly creates billions of copies of a specific region of a single DNA molecule. FIGURE 45 illustrates the basic concept of the PCR, in which purified DNA polymerase copies a DNA template in three cycles of replication. In the first step of the initial cycle, a minute amount of double-stranded DNA

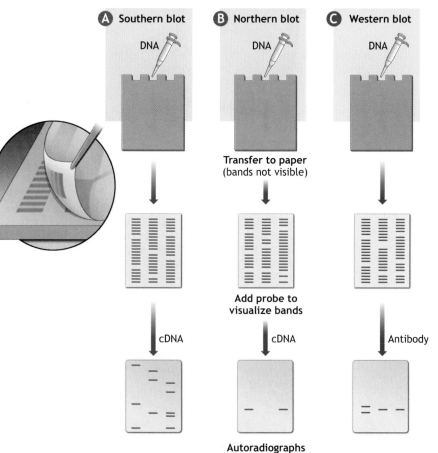

Gel electrophoresis

Figure 44 Identifying DNA sequences by three gel transfer methods. **A.** Southern blot (named for Dr. E. M. Southern) produced when single-stranded DNA on a sheet of nitrocellulose is placed in a tray of buffer atop a sponge. The pattern on the gel is copied or "blotted" to the nitrocellulose and then incubated with radioactively labeled nucleic acids. This process produces radioactive bands, which means that nucleic acid bands hybridize with those labeled by radioactivity. **B.** Northern blots are produced when RNA on a nitrocellulose blot hybridizes with a single-stranded DNA probe without using alkali (alkali hydrolyzes RNA). **C.** Western blot gel electrophoresis separates proteins using antibody probes to target specific proteins.

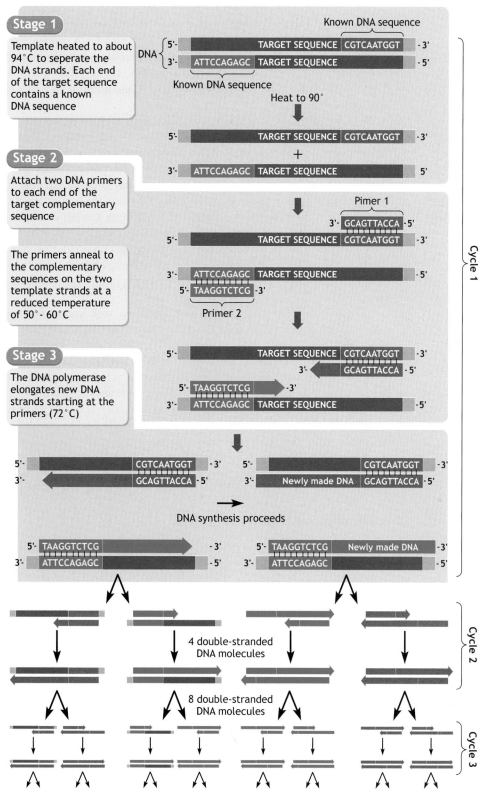

Figure 45 Artificial DNA amplification using the PCR method. *Cycle 1.* Three stages during the first PCR cycle. *Cycle 2.* Second PCR cycle produces four double strands of DNA. *Cycle 3.* Third cycle produces eight double-stranded DNA molecules. Each succeeding cycle produces twice as much DNA as was produced in the previous cycle. Thirty cycles produce more than 1 billion DNA fragments. Several hours of production creates hundreds of billions of copies. The thermocycler PCR apparatus controls reaction temperature to ensure that repeated replication cycles and separation occur systematically on a preset schedule. The Internet site (www.info.med.yale.edu/genetics/ward/tavi/Guide.html) provides a step-by-step protocol guide for standard PCR and a variant termed multiplex PCR (for downloading as a PDF document).

Anneal: rejoin separated single complementary strands of DNA to form a double helix

is heated to about 94°C for several minutes to denature (separate) the strands. Each strand has a known sequence of nucleotides on either side of the target nucleotides. Next, two short, specifically designed synthetic primers of known DNA sequence (shown in *green* and *red*) hybridize or **anneal** to one of the two separated strands at the exact beginning and ending position of the target DNA nucleotide sequence. In other words, only the target sequence, bracketed by the primers, duplicates because no primers attach elsewhere along the DNA fragment.

The annealing process cannot withstand the initial high temperature required to separate the double helix, so it occurs at a lower 54°C. At this temperature, the single-stranded DNA fragments match complementary nucleotide sequences at the ends of the target DNA sequence. DNA synthesis would not proceed without appropriate primers. Adding a heat-resistant DNA polymerase to the reaction in step 3 synthesizes a new DNA strand, now creating two strands. The most widely used polymerase (Taq) is isolated from the heat-resistant bacterium ***Thermus aquaticus***. The temperature, now increased to 70°C for another minute or two, lets the polymerase elongate new DNA strands that begin at the primers. Because the PCR technique requires that reactants cycle through a varied temperature profile during incubation, the PCR apparatus (thermocycler) automatically progresses through a preset thermal sequence. This first cycle, repeated 20 to 40 times, doubles the amount of DNA synthesized in each succeeding cycle.

Thermus aquaticus: thermally stable bacterium that survives at very high temperatures found in hot springs and geysers. The bacterium provides the important *Taq* DNA-replicating polymerase; voted 1989 "Molecule of the Year" by the prestigious journal *Science*

The PCR method only clones DNA fragments with known beginning and ending sequences. With prior knowledge of the code, it takes only 20 repeat cycles to duplicate enough target DNA to produce 1,048,536 copies (2^{20}) of the original sequence. The second and third cycles displayed in Figure 45 show how the PCR method eventually copies millions (or billions) of the original DNA sequence. The second cycle repeats the first cycle. It progresses through each temperature change, first to separate strands at about 94°C, then to anneal the primers at a cooler 54°C, and finally through polymerase action to make two additional DNA strands at 72°C. Note that the third cycle produces eight double-stranded DNA molecules; after seven cycles, the newly created DNA consists of double strands with flush ends (same length) uniquely identical to the original target sequence. The next 17 cycles produce the additional 1,048,528 copies, and just 10 more cycles produce one thousand million more target molecules!

Applications of PCR

The PCR technique has impacted numerous fields besides molecular biology;[78] they include biotechnology, entomology and the environmental sciences, molecular epidemiology, forensic science, genetic engineering, most medical specialties, microbiology, proteomics, the food industry, and even apparel manufacturing. For the 2000 Sydney Olympic Games, a special ink containing a small DNA snippet from a saliva swab from two Australian athletes was affixed to labels, tags, pins, and stickers of official Olympic merchandise to thwart counterfeiters. An electronic scanner could check the invisible ink to verify an item's authenticity. The same DNA-marking strategy, impossible to reverse-engineer, can verify rare and one-of-a-kind objects from premium grade oil to fine wine. PCR also can identify diverse viruses and bacteria or any DNA extracted from a current or ancient plant or animal organism. It identifies the unique sequence of a miniscule amount of DNA nucleotide material, even in substances millions of years old.

The amplification potential for PCR remains truly awesome. It requires only one tenth of one millionth of a liter (0.1 μL) of a substance such as saliva or another body fluid or tissue to prove that the genetic sample's sequence originated from a specific person or species. The PCR method can easily produce 1 μg of substance (about 500 base pairs long), equal to one millionth of a gram (10^{-6}), enough to completely sequence or clone DNA. In fact, beginning with less than a picogram (0.000 000 000 001 or 10^{-12} g) of DNA with a chain length of 10,000 nucleotides (about 100,000 molecules), in several hours PCR can produce several micrograms of DNA (10^{11} molecules). Interestingly, scientists have identified the genetic blueprint of insects trapped within 80 million–year-old amber (fossilized pine resin) from a miniscule amount of DNA, using present-day insects to "match" the DNA sequences. In a controversial report published in *Nature*, (October 2000), scientists reported reviving a bacterium (spore) from a drop of fluid trapped for 250 million years in a crystal of rock salt excavated 1850 feet below the earth's surface. In extinct fossils, on the other hand, not enough DNA sequences exist for cloning because the DNA decomposes significantly every 5000 years. While some gene fragments may survive, cloning a "Jurassic Park" prehistoric monster falls outside the realm of possibility with today's available molecular archeology technologies.

In forensic medicine, a single hair salvaged from a crime scene can be matched for its DNA sequence to hair samples from a suspect or victim. When a PCR-generated DNA sequence matches the original DNA template strand sequence, chances of misidentifying the true suspect become almost infinitesimal against a coincidental DNA match. In fact, if an individual's known DNA profile matches the DNA profile from the crime scene, the probability is 82 billion to 1 that the crime scene DNA comes from that person!

Paternity cases routinely involve DNA analysis using PCR techniques such as DNA fingerprinting **autoradiography** to identify parental offspring correctly (see Fig. 46). In the figure's example, the DNA from suspected fathers 1 and 2 did not match the known marker DNA from the child; thus father 3, with an exact banding match, was deemed the biologic father. The control DNA from a known source verifies the validity of the test procedures. The many variations of the PCR method allow researchers to produce hybrid genes with desirable (or undesirable) traits. Fusing DNA segments from different biologic specimens opens a tremendous avenue to study genetic variation in cells and tissues. It also elucidates how "errors" in specific gene sequences relate to diseases and how genetic engineering can combat them.

Paternity: fatherhood

Autoradiography: process that produces an image (autoradiograph) on a photographic film placed flat on an electrophoresis gel; shows the position of radioactive molecules "transferred" to the gel

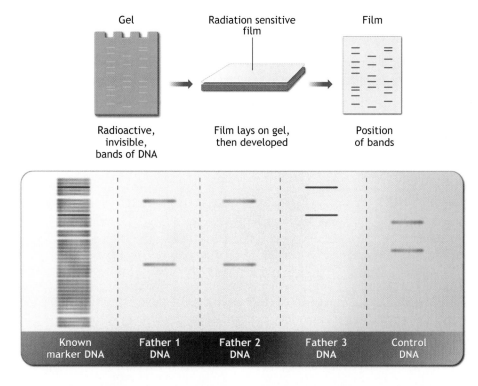

Figure 46 DNA fingerprinting autoradiography compares DNA fragments after their separation by gel electrophoresis to identify the child's father. Matched patterns of DNA banding from different tissues or body fluids confirm the original DNA source. Specific restriction enzymes sever the DNA fragments at precise sites in the chain. Thus, snippets of DNA, known as RFLPs (**r**estriction **f**ragment **l**ength **p**olymorphisms), have different lengths and hence different molecular weights. A match between the known marker DNA and the sample (e.g., father 3) provides prima facie direct evidence that father 3 is the biologic father. By the end of the year 2000, 43 previously convicted criminals were exonerated on the basis of DNA analysis of forensic evidence, often years following incarceration. Several hundred more criminal cases based on DNA analysis are currently pending. We recommend the following book for its riveting (but disturbing), frank discussion about the criminal justice system and the important role DNA fingerprinting should play to ensure that the accused have the opportunity to present objective evidence (data) about criminal wrongdoing: Scheck, B et al. *Active Innocence, and Other Dispatches from the Wrongly Convicted.* New York: Doubleday, 2000.

Injection Experiments

Transfection: introduction of an external donor source of DNA into a recipient host

Injection **transfection** performed in cultured cells refers to a microtechnique for introducing an outside (exogenous) DNA donor source into a recipient host. Injection of purified DNA with a known sequence of nucleotides for a particular gene presents a potentially desirable strategy for expressing an outcome trait in the host. Injection strategies have been useful in exercise physiology-related animal research. By injecting a gene with a particular trait into the egg of a mother, the new trait can be "turned on" in the offspring. This allows researchers to observe the effects of "knocking out" a section of one gene and replacing it with another segment to glean insight into the functional role of that gene product.

Gamete: egg or sperm

Transgene: genetic engineering technique that places a foreign gene in the cells of a different species

Pronucleus: fertilized egg containing the haploid egg or sperm nucleus

Founder mice: original engineered mice (with one copy of a transgene) bred together to create transgenic animals

Heterozygous: having two different copies (alleles) of the same gene

Homozygous: having two identical copies (alleles) of the same gene

Knockin animal model: harbors a specific mutation in a predetermined gene created and subsequently analyzed for altered drug responses

Consider the example in FIGURE 47 that illustrates the basic principle of microinjection applied to a rodent (mouse) model. Immediately after the **gametes** join (one egg and one sperm), a microinjection technique using a thin glass needle inserts a target gene (**transgene**) into the larger male **pronucleus** just before the cells fuse into a single egg. The egg(s) is then surgically harvested and implanted into the womb of a female rodent who serves as the "foster" mother. When the mother produces progeny, the newborns, referred to as **founder mice**, should carry a copy of the transgene on a single chromosome (i.e., be **heterozygous** for the transgene). When two founder mice breed, 25% of the progeny receive two copies of the transgene (i.e., are **homozygous** for the transgene), 50% have one transgene, and 25% have no transgenes. These percentages follow basic laws of inheritance discovered by geneticist Gregor Mendel (see p. 989). Researchers have used hundreds of strains of transgenic organisms created with the above procedures to study the metabolic and developmental characteristic of many diseases.

Working with transgenic organisms has proved beneficial for experimenting with different genetic manipulations (including mutated genes) to shed light on possible mechanisms for disease conditions. Consider the following four ways researchers carry out such experiments:

1. Replacing a normal gene with a mutant gene ("trading places") and observing effects on the offspring (a **knockin animal model**)

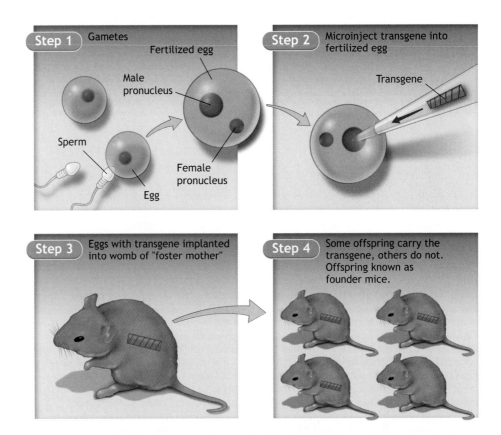

Figure 47   Generalized procedure for creating transgenic offspring by injecting a target gene (transgene) into a fertilized egg. Some of the progeny, called *founder mice,* carry the transgene in their chromosomes, but the process may fail in others.

2. Inactivating or interrupting a normal gene's function and observing effects on the offspring (a **knockout animal model**)

3. Adding a mutant gene and observing the combined effects of the mutant gene *and* normal gene on the offspring

4. Increasing the expression of a given protein by increasing the number of copies of a gene

Because of its relevance to exercise physiology, we take a closer look on p. 1056 at strategies for disabling genes related to obesity using the knockout technique elegantly described in 1994 by University of Utah researchers.

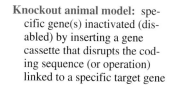

Knockout animal model: specific gene(s) inactivated (disabled) by inserting a gene cassette that disrupts the coding sequence (or operation) linked to a specific target gene

Cloning a Mammal

Genetics researchers use three methods to clone a mammal: (1) somatic cell nuclear transfer (SCNT), (2) Roslin technique, and (3) Honolulu technique.

SCNT Method. FIGURE 48 illustrates the eight-step SCNT technology (also called therapeutic cloning) to create stem cells from somatic cells (cells other than a sperm or egg cell). This modern technique had its genesis when experimental embryologist Hans Spemann (1869–1938; 1935 Nobel Prize in physiology or medicine for discovering the organizer effect in embryonic development at the gastrula stage) with codiscoverer Hilde Mangold (1898–1924) pioneered microsurgical techniques while working with embryos. Spemann and Mangold's histologic evidence from experiments with five manipulated embryos proved the reality of the concept of induction (interaction between two groups of cells, in which one

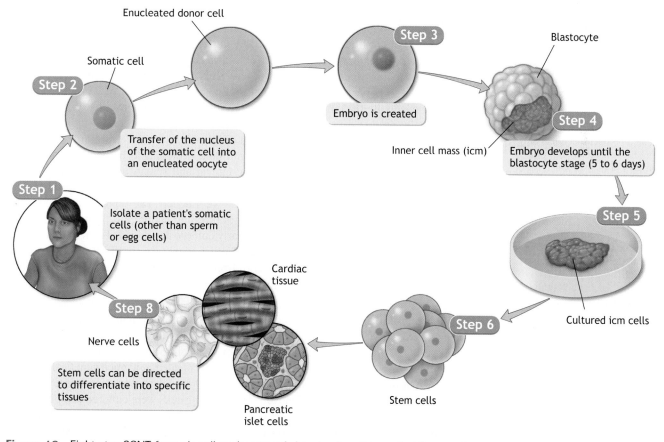

Figure 48 Eight-step SCNT (somatic cell nuclear transfer) technology (also called therapeutic cloning) to create stem cells from somatic cells. Tissue rejection is eliminated with SCNT because the new grafts (tissues) are autologous (donor and host are the same individual). SCNT is not reproductive cloning because it uses only unfertilized egg cells to generate stem cells.[87] The International Society for Stem Cell Research provides additional details about SCNT (www.isscr.org/public/therapeutic.htm).

group directly influences the developmental fate of the other). In the SCNT technique, two cells are required—a donor cell and an oocyte (an unfertilized egg cell early in development). Somatic cells are secured from the patient and prepared for the next step, which transfers the nucleus of the cell (with its DNA) into an enucleated oocyte (not having a nucleus eliminates most of the genetic information). This process (step 3) prompts the cell to begin forming an embryo (a fertilized egg that can begin cell division). In step 4, the embryo undergoes cell division until it develops into the blastocyte stage, a mass of about 100 cells. At this stage of development, the mass remains a group of undifferentiated cells. The next phase of the process (step 5) separates the inner cell mass (ICM) from the cell by a microchemical technique called immunosurgery (using different chemicals to dislodge the ICM from the cell wall). The cultured ICMs produce pluripotent stem cells (step 6), the most versatile kinds of cells, with the potential to become different types of tissues (i.e., skin, brain, heart, muscle, kidney, bone, pancreas, intestine). In essence, stem cells are relatively unspecialized cells that have not yet differentiated into any specific type of tissue. Once the cells become differentiated (e.g., acquire the features of a specialized cell and develop into specific tissues) as shown in step 7, the new line of specialized cell types can be reintroduced into the patient. This begins the process of creating new tissues to replace or repopulate damaged or diseased tissues.

Roslin Method. Scientists at the Roslin Institute, Scotland, in 1997 tapped the complete genetic library contained within the zygote (i.e., cell **totipotent** potentiality) to clone the Dorset sheep "Dolly." This milestone represented the first such viable intact donor derived from adult mammalian cells.[140] The researchers removed an unfertilized oocyte from an adult ewe and replaced its nucleus with the nucleus from a mammary gland cell of an adult sheep. They then implanted this egg in another ewe, producing the healthy offspring sheep. The idea behind the **nuclear transfer** experiment was to produce genetically engineered transgenic mammals inexpensively that could reliably produce large quantities of pharmaceuticals in their milk. A likely benefit would be large quantities of human proteins for drug synthesis to treat diseases such as cystic fibrosis, hemophilia, and emphysema, with potential benefits toward aging and cancer research. Milk produced from transgenic sheep, goats, and cattle can yield up to 40 g of protein per liter at relatively low cost. This circumvents the need to use purified, expensive blood to harvest protein, with risk of contamination from AIDS or hepatitis C. Proteins produced in human cell cultures have high cost and relatively low yields. Transgenetically produced proteins have application in the **nutraceutical** industry, **xenotransplantation**, animal models of disease, and cell therapy.

The first Dolly experiments represented a milestone in cloning technology, but not before unleashing a firestorm of criticism concerning ethical and scientific issues related to the possibilities of eventual experiments with human cloning. FIGURE 49 shows that Dolly possesses the same genes as the cells from the ewe's udder. The reproductive cell cycle developed normally following intermediate stages (keeping donor cells "**quiescent**" so that their DNA did not replicate or divide) until the early embryo developed. The researchers then transplanted the embryo into a receptive ewe (Scottish blackface sheep). Following several hundred unsuccessful implants, Dolly was born from the implanted ewe and survived. Dolly subsequently gave birth through normal mating to produce three additional, healthy lambs.

Honolulu Technique. This cloning technique developed by Hawaiian researchers[129] differs substantially from SNCT and the Roslin methods. The Honolulu technique does not generate clones either by injection or fusion of embryonic or fetal cells or by fusion of adult cells (how sheep Dolly was created). In contrast, adult mouse cells created new mice genetically identical to the parent mouse. Using a special pipette, the donor nucleus was microinjected into an egg whose nucleus was previously removed. The resulting cells were cultured and placed into a surrogate mouse, allowing the clone to develop. By repeating the procedure, the team created second and third generations of cloned mice that genetically matched their sister/parent, sister/grandparent, and sister/great grandparent. The research succeeded in cloning mice from adult cells by using (1) a new method, and (2) a new cell type able to repeat the procedure to produce clones of clones of clones—essentially creating identical mice born a generation or more apart. The Honolulu technique, in contrast to SNCT and Roslyn methods, allows researchers to manipulate adult donor nuclei. The same Honolulu technique also produced three

Totipotent: the cell possesses the required genetic information or "blueprint" to form an intact organism

Nuclear transfer: DNA removed from an unfertilized egg and introduced into the nucleus of a specially prepared cell by an electrical pulse or chemical to fuse the two substances together to initiate their development

Nutriceutical: genetically engineered product that alters or modifies characteristics of a product or its byproduct

Xenotransplantation: transfer of organs or tissues from a donor of one species to a recipient of another. Successful transplants require that the immune system of the recipient accept the donor organ successfully

Quiescent: having all but the most fundamental functions of a cell or group of cells stopped; in essence, with switched-off genes that define the special functions of the cell (i.e., restricting food supply or creating an unfavorable internal cellular environment)

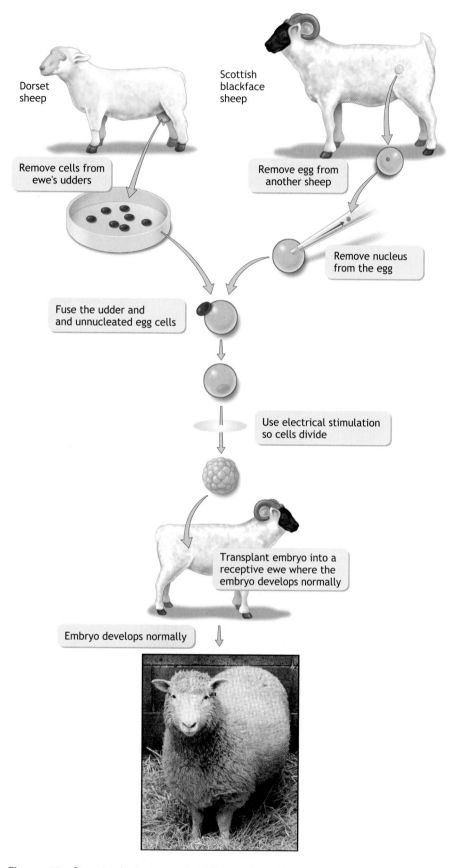

Dorset sheep

Scottish blackface sheep

Remove cells from ewe's udders

Remove egg from another sheep

Remove nucleus from the egg

Fuse the udder and and unnucleated egg cells

Use electrical stimulation so cells divide

Transplant embryo into a receptive ewe where the embryo develops normally

Embryo develops normally

Figure 49 Steps in cloning a mammal. Dorset sheep Dolly *(bottom photo)* has genes identical to those of the ewe that donated the original genes (Dorset sheep, *upper left*).

live male offspring from tail-tip cells. Two died shortly after birth, but the surviving clone developed normally and mated successfully, producing two healthy litters. The Honolulu technique shows that animals of either sex can be cloned with somatic cells used in the process. The technique offers hope in preserving endangered species and transgenic animals.

Gene Knockout Technique

Mice provide a useful model to study genetic manipulations because of control afforded the experimental subjects and the environment, and the animal's shorter life span. Researchers can study a strain of normal-sized mice with black fur, obese mice with black fur, obese mice with white fur, and so on. Genetic "tampering" could verify whether the gene actually modulated the specific effect, independent of its influence on fur color. Deactivating a gene(s) within the DNA known to produce an obese strain of mice should produce litters of normal-weight mice.

FIGURE 50 illustrates the experimental strategy for creating a transgenic mouse with a knocked-out gene.

Gene cassette: artificially constructed DNA segment containing a genetic marker with restriction sites at both ends of the nucleotide segment

Pseudopregnant: ovulation induced by sterile copulation

- A DNA fragment receives a genetically modified gene (**gene cassette** shown in *purple*), thus altering the target gene's usual nucleotide sequence.
- Growth of the cell culture produces one or more cell colonies containing the altered gene. Finding such a colony means the mutant gene altered the DNA fragment.
- Inject the genetically altered cells into the developing embryo of a previously mated female mouse.
- Place the developing embryo into a normal **pseudopregnant** mouse that gives birth to a litter in which most progeny possess cells with the altered gene.
- Mating two offspring with the mutant gene can produce an offspring with the mutant gene on each of two chromosomes. The grafted transgene can also be incorporated into the mice from another strain of mouse into a totally different organism.

Germ line: cell lineage consists of mature reproductive germ cells (sperm, egg)

If the original gene alteration inactivated the function of one of the genes, then the transgenic mouse inherits the mutant gene that replaced or "knocked out" the primary target gene. This strain of mice can be reliably bred to produce progeny with the foreign gene now permanently part of their **germ line** DNA. In studying the etiology of cancer, for example, two transplanted oncogenes (*ras* and *myc*) remain dominant in the host and always produce a mouse with cancer. The same strategy can apply to study mechanisms of obesity described below.

Knockout Mice to Study Mechanisms of Obesity

Proopiomelanocortin (POMC): precursor of neurotransmitters (β-endorphin) and hormones (melanocortin peptides), whose roles include pigmentation, adrenocortical function, food intake and fat storage, and immune and neural functions

Neurohormone: hormone formed by neurosecretory cells and liberated by nerve impulses (e.g., norepinephrine)

Researchers have developed transgenic mice that lack the gene that encodes for the complex molecule **proopiomelanocortin** (**POMC**) produced mainly in the brain and skin.[142] POMC, a precursor of melanocortin peptides, possesses a wide range of physiologic properties that include roles in food intake and body fat accumulation. The researchers originally intended to study POMC-deficient mice to evaluate **neurohormone** signaling and CNS functioning. Their strain of transgenic mutant mice overate and became obese, with altered pigmentation that produced yellowish fur on their abdomen instead of typical brownish-black fur. They also showed significantly less adrenal tissue than littermates of normal size and color. FIGURE 51A shows that after 1 month of age, the body weight of the mutant mice steadily increased to twice the weight of normal littermates.

These findings coincided with a previous report describing a rare genetic disease in two children caused by a mutant *Pomc* gene.[76] These red-haired children had no melanocortins, and they developed severe obesity soon after birth and suffered adrenal insufficiency. *Panel D* in Figure 51 shows the rapid weight gain of this young girl and boy whose weight far exceeded typical age standards. The connection between the mice and children was striking; functional characteristics caused by the *Pomc* gene mutation in humans paralleled those in the transgenic mice with yellow pigmentation and obesity.

Injecting the obese, POMC-deficient mice with the melanocortin peptide, α-melanocyte-stimulating-hormone agonist (α-MSH) produced a significant body weight loss within 1 day; within 1 week, body weight decreased by about 38% and declined further to 48% after the second week (Fig. 51B). A reversal also occurred in the pigmentation of the mice, and their fur lost its yellowish tinge. Within 10 days of terminating α-MSH "therapy," the mice began to regain

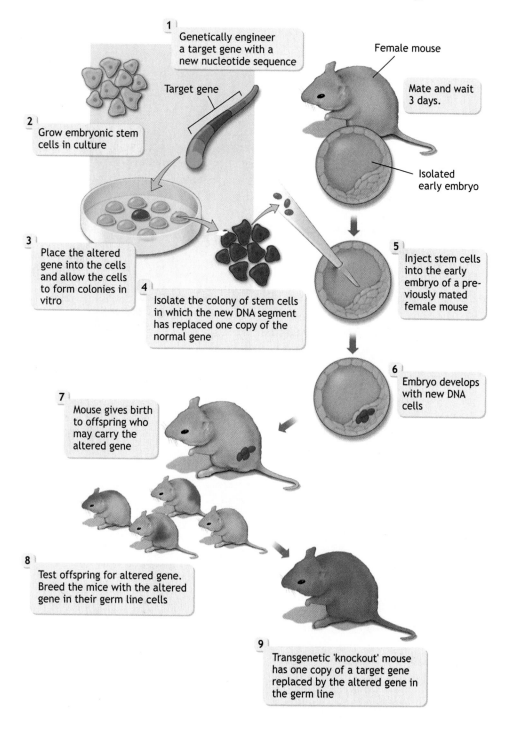

Figure 50 Creating a transgenic mouse with a knocked-out gene.

lost weight, reaching preinjection weight in another 14 days. Their yellow fur color in the ventral and dorsal sites also reappeared. In contrast, α-MSH injections and subsequent cessation of treatment produced no effect on body mass or fur pigmentation in normal control littermates. The researchers explained that weight loss during treatment exceeded expectations from the energy-balance equation. This occurred although the mutant mice ate significantly more food daily than the control mice (35.7 vs. 24.2 g; Fig. 51C). Because fat cells contain melanocortin receptors, and these receptors induce **lipolysis**, melanocortin-based drugs may eventually prove helpful as therapeutic agents to combat obesity. Interestingly, injections of MSH analogues also reduced excess body fat in another strain of obese transgenic mice, deficient in the

Lipolysis: splitting up (hydrolysis) or chemical decomposition of triglyceride

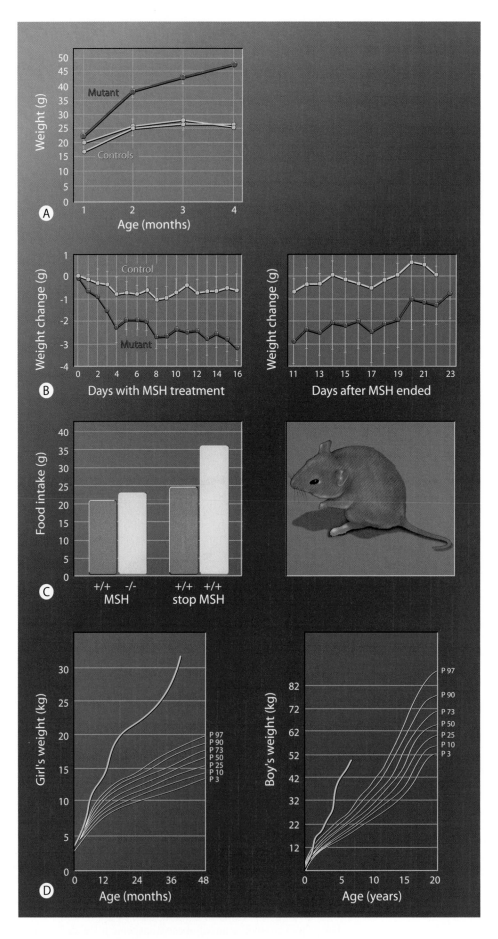

Figure 51 POMC-deficient transgenic mice provide new clues to obesity. **A.** Body weight gain in mutant and control mice. **B.** Change in body weight with and without treatment. **C.** Differences in food intake with and without treatment. **D.** Extreme weight gain in a young boy and girl with the POMC mutation. The *white lines* represent growth curves for children representing the 3rd through 97th percentile (p). (Data from *A, B,* and *C* modified from Yaswen L, et al. Obesity in the mouse model of pro-opiomelanocortin deficiency responds to peripheral melanocortin. Nat Med 1999;5:1066. Data in *D* from Krude H, et al. Severe early-onset obesity, adrenal insufficiency and red hair pigmentation caused by POMC mutations in humans. Nat Genet 1998;19:155.)

hormone **leptin**.[61] In studies of 87 unrelated Italian obese children and adolescents, three new mutations were identified within the POMC signal peptide (substitution of Ser with Thr at codon 7; Ser with Leu at codon 9; Arg with Gly at codon 236).[40] The researchers believe that the mutations in codons 7 and 9 of the signal peptide alter the translocation of pre-POMC into the endoplasmic reticulum and, therefore, explain the linkage between POMC and the genetic predisposition to obesity, a view shared by others studying this association. Further studies of genetic variations in the POMC coding region should provide new insights concerning the etiology of obesity.[41,47,77] On-going experiments with transgenic animal and human models will help researchers understand the etiology of obesity and its treatment.[97,144] Extremes in obesity have been linked to DNA polymorphisms in the translated portion of the leptin *(LEP)* gene.[84] Leptin-regulated endocannabinoids (marijuana-like substances naturally produced in the brain) stimulate appetite and play a role in food regulation as a component in the leptin signaling cascades.[43] In the not-too-distant future, excess body fat may provide a ready source of stem cells from which to create replacement tissues (e.g., bone, muscle, cartilage) for diseased or damaged ones.[147] Incorporating a person's own stem cells would avoid rejection of transplanted tissue and circumvent moral objections concerning the use of human embryonic stem cells.

Newer approaches also apply genetic techniques using **antisense RNA** to suppress expression of a target gene as a way to assess gene function. By incompletely blocking the function of knockout genes, researchers should be able to uncover unexpected roles for sequenced genes.[44] The field of proteomics (using sophisticated imaging software and molecular scanners integrated with protein chemistry techniques) also offers a new approach to study how proteins expressed in a genome act in complex, biologic processes.[63] For example, scientists have developed an ion channel "nanopore" technique that discriminates among almost identical DNA molecules that differ by only one base pair or one nucleotide.[126] This level of differentiation permits highly accurate molecular identification to unscramble intricacies of gene expression and ultimately to develop strategies that target mutagens.

HUMAN PERFORMANCE RESEARCH

Molecular biologists studying physical activity and exercise training seek to decipher signaling pathways by which genes transcribe the effects of a mechanical stressor and resultant phenotypic expression. For example, resistance training applies muscular overload of the biceps as a mechanical stressor,[98,127] while increasing upper-arm strength and size represent expression of a phenotype characteristic. Crucial, unanswered questions concern "where" and "how" skeletal overload translates into newly acquired "strength" and muscle hypertrophy. The answers likely reside within signal transduction pathways leading from cell surface receptors to the nucleus, resulting in transcription of genes and subsequent protein synthesis.[13,60] Little doubt remains that scientists will progressively uncover the secrets of the genome as they learn more about the intricacies of how different signaling processes interact, integrate, and differentiate to produce function and consequences, and possibly even share common intermediates.[15,60]

Consider a seemingly simple series of movements such as releasing the bowstring when shooting an arrow and the highly complex maneuvers of a triple back summersault from a 10-m diving platform. The movement patterns of both activities require precise coordination and integration of neural stimulation and muscular action. In turn, each component of the movement demands specific timing and force requirements to achieve a desired outcome. At the molecular level, thousands of enzymes govern such precision requirements, each turning on and off at precisely the right time and in the correct sequence to make the movement successful (or unsuccessful). A better understanding of signaling processes governing enzyme activity between stressors and genes may someday explain the how and why of individual differences in human movement capacities. For example, why does one identical twin perform better than the other twin does in a particular activity? Identical twins come from the same genetic pool, so one would expect few differences in performance between them, but this is not the case. Even if twins had identical experiences in mastering the mechanics of an activity, from practice time to coaching, their performance levels would differ. Fractions of a second or tenths of a centimeter often mean the difference between victory and second place—whether the performers are twins or Olympic-caliber athletes. A combination of biochemical individuality and known allelic variations should enable researchers to determine optimal nutritional profiles

Leptin: protein hormone involved with appetite and fat storage

Antisense RNA: RNA complementary in sequence to mRNA, thus capable of base pairing with it by using the nontemplate strand of DNA to transcribe RNA from it. Analogous to two original strands in DNA base pairing with each other. In practice, synthesis of an oligonucleotide hybridizes a mutant mRNA sequence, stopping its translation into protein

(i.e., targeted doses of vitamins, minerals, and other nutrients) to create personalized comprehensive lifestyle prescriptions tailored to the needs of each person.[48] A tremendous challenge also exists among the disciplines to determine the molecular basis of disease expression, as for example, for type 2 diabetes that increased 39% in the United States from 1990 to 1999.[3,90]

When reduced to the most fundamental level, all physical activities, or aspects of all life, ultimately depend on the multiplicity of molecular events that turn genes on and off. The new generation of molecular exercise scientists must expand research to uncover how different signaling mechanisms regulate transcriptional, translational, and posttranslational events. Elucidation of these mechanisms will enable scientists to manipulate experimental variables to answer questions related to our field. For example, how does long-term exercise intensity and duration alter levels of a specific mRNA or an upstream signaling molecule such as Ca^{+2}, an intermediary involved in multiple signal transduction cascades?[49] A simple muscle contraction corresponds to a 100-fold increase in intramuscular Ca^{+2} concentration (from 10^{-7} to 10^{-5} M). Some researchers believe that the huge Ca^{+2} influx, which coincides with myofilament cross-bridge cycling (see Chapter 18), serves as an important signaling messenger that links a muscle's function to transcriptional dynamics.[6] Other exercise-related physiologic regulators of transcription include hypoxia and cellular oxidative stress (or redox). The hypoxic state affects production of erythropoietin (*EPO* gene) and **glucose transporter-1 (GLUT-1)**.[46] Understanding the functional characteristics of how genes operate under hypoxic conditions will provide key information about oxygen delivery to cells and ultimately its use via citric acid cycle reactions, electron transport, and ATP synthesis associated with oxidative energy transformations.[64,146]

Oxygen free radicals and reducing agents (i.e., antioxidants) also modulate transcription.[115] In Chapter 6, we discuss how the mitochondrion's reduction of oxygen to form water serves as the final common step in ATP synthesis. Imprecise coupling of this pathway forms free radicals of oxygen. Diverse antioxidants within skeletal muscle then scavenge and quench most of these **reactive oxygen species (ROS)**.[112] However, during high-intensity endurance exercise when aerobic metabolism increases 15- to 20-fold, ROS form in greater numbers to possibly produce damaging effects similar to those produced by lipid peroxidation.[39,91,141,142] The protein **thioredoxin**, which reduces oxidized proteins, helps to balance a cell's redox state during energy metabolism and also appears to affect transcriptional activity.[62,66] Determining how ROS influence transcription will pave the way for improved understanding of long-term health effects (or potential risks) of aerobic-type activities. Researchers have discovered that endurance training nearly doubles mitochondrial protein and mitochondrial mass.[65,93] This means that having a robust experimental model (endurance exercise/training) from which to study gene expression will surely lead to important discoveries about the essence of endurance exercise effects and adaptations per se. In fact, experiments have already described alterations in mRNA gene expression with long-term electrical stimulation,[145] including exercise effects related to muscle mitochondrial and overall cellular activity[23,28,51,57,68,70,94,99,122,123,132,143] and molecular-related alterations in skeletal muscle and muscle fiber type.[15,18,19,50,111,119] Microgravity's effects on gene expression in skeletal muscle provide a fruitful area for further study.[2,8,10–12,25–26,39,42,55,56,58,101,118,137,146] Studies of identical twins attempt to explain why one individual tends to participate regularly in sports and physical activities while the other twin shows little inclination to remain physically active. As part of the Heritage Family Study,[32,71,105,109,114,136–139] a search for genes related to body composition changes following 20 weeks of exercise training from 364 sib-pairs from 99 Caucasian families provided evidence of linkage of fat-free mass and insulin-like growth factor 1 genes, including gene sites for BMI and fat mass, and plasma leptin levels with the low-density lipoprotein receptor gene.[32] Further study of the genomic basis of training-induced changes in body composition with systematic endurance-type training will help to enlighten mechanisms in body weight regulation.

Another viable area for application of molecular biology research to the sport sciences involves various gene therapy techniques (viral and nonviral delivery strategies) (1) to treat acute and chronic musculoskeletal injuries such as muscle tears, cartilage defects, and tendon ruptures; (2) to reconstruct ligaments, osseous nonunions, and meniscus tears; and (3) to transplant tissue or genetic material. One hopes that inserting relevant genes directly into target tissues or systemically via vectors into the bloodstream will increase the probability of successful therapy and accelerated recuperation.[86] Researchers in the molecular biology sciences are just now beginning to track down the flaws in human DNA that cause debilitating musculoskeletal disease, as for example, those involved with lumbar disks.[5,81,85,124] One must

Glucose transporter-1 (GLUT-1): facilitates glucose transport across the plasma membrane independently of the hormone insulin

Reactive oxygen species (ROS): oxygen free radical formed from imprecise coupling during oxygen's reduction to water in the final stage of electron transport–oxidative phosphorylation

Thioredoxin: protein involved in oxidation–reduction reactions to balance the cell's redox state

temper such expectations by perhaps justifiable concerns that genetic engineering's potential benefits could also result in "tinkering" with issues related to doping and drug testing.

New techniques of molecular and cell biology such as nuclear magnetic resonance-- detected carbon-14, nitrogen-15, and hydrogen exchange now make it possible to study aspects of protein structure and functions.[53] For example, the computer-generated structural model of a protein in FIGURE 52 shows color-coded regions of high- and low-stability constants when binding to another molecule such as **monoclonal antibody** D1.3. The *red region* that interacts directly with D1.3 shows the highest stability; the *yellow* and *blue regions* remain unaffected by D1.3 binding. Thus, high and low regions of stability within a protein molecule may relate differently to its functional associations with other molecules. The important implication for protein synthesis is that sites within the conformational structure of a molecule may serve dual functions, depending on the molecule's configuration and structural residues.

As far as we know, no research in exercise molecular biology has studied whether exercise training might induce changes in a protein's structure. Will these changes alter the region(s) within the molecule for cooperative binding or interactions among binding pathways with other molecules?

Crucial questions concern what "signals" control cooperation among different molecules, and whether changes occur selectively in some proteins (in certain regions within the molecule) and not others. A question such as the following, for example, requires an answer: "What contribution do both genetics and environmental factors have in affecting the complex etiology of many common and debilitating diseases?"[24] The model describing gene–exercise interaction (FIG. 53) affects health status indirectly by altering gene expression that itself affects intermediate phenotypes and disease outcome. In addition, increased physical activity (exercise) and training influence health. Often, indirect evidence can link a particular disease state with an outcome variable. Consider the known association and linkage studies of Parkinson's disease that have led to the discovery of eleven genetic regions involved in parkinsonism (mayoresearch.mayo.edu/mayo/research/mcj/PDMolecular.cfm). In four of these regions, the genes and the proteins they encode have been identified. Now consider the following results that offer a connection between Parkinson's disease and physical activity.

In the first comprehensive examination of strenuous physical activity and the risk of developing Parkinson's disease,[33] Harvard researchers reported that men who exercised regularly and vigorously early in their adult life had a lower risk for developing Parkinson's

Monoclonal antibody: pure antibody of a single type that only recognizes a single antigen; produced in cell culture as a fusion product from a cancer cell and an antibody-producing cell

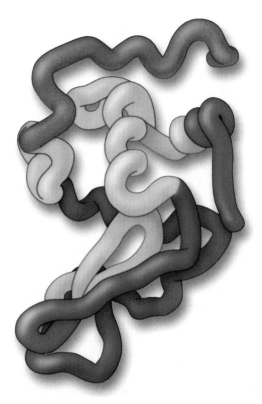

Figure 52 Computer-generated model of hen egg white **lysozyme** (HEWL) color coded to show regions of high *(red)* and lower *(blue and yellow)* stability constants when binding to monoclonal antibody D1.3 (along the *red* area). Lysozyme, discovered by Sir Alexander Fleming (1881–1955) 5 years before he discovered penicillin, protects against bacterial infection. This small enzyme, the first ever to have its structure solved, attacks the bacterial protective cell wall. Some bacteria build a protective outer layer of carbohydrate chains interlocked by short peptide strands, which brace their delicate plasma membranes against their high intracellular osmotic pressure. Lysozyme breaks these carbohydrate chains, destroying the cell membrane's structural integrity, and the bacteria burst under their own internal pressure. The lysozyme from hen egg whites protects proteins and fats that nourish the developing chick. (Figure constructed using program GRASP [trantor.bioc.columbia .edu/grasp/]. Dr. Ernesto Freire. Professor of Biology and Biophysics. Director of the Biocalorimetry Center. The Johns Hopkins University, Baltimore.)

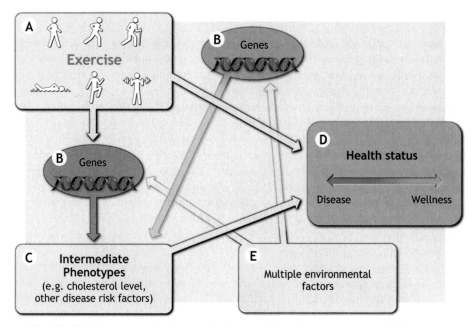

Figure 53   Model of gene–exercise interaction, intermediate phenotype, and multiple environmental factor interactions in determining health status along the disease–wellness continuum. (Adapted from Bray MS. Genomics, genes, and environmental interaction: the role of exercise. J Appl Physiol 2000;88:788.) Note: The journal *Medicine & Science in Sports & Exercise* now publishes an annual update of the human gene map for performance and health-related fitness phenotypes. The inaugural issue (Rankinen T, et al. Med Sci Sports Exerc 2001;33:855) contains specific reference to genes and their location published through December 2000. The initial work was a collaboration among scientists at five laboratories who have worked in the area relating genetics of fitness and performance.

disease than men who did not. The most physically active men at the start of the study cut their risk of developing Parkinson's by 50% compared with male study participants who were the least physically active. Men who reported regularly having engaged in strenuous physical activity in early adult life cut their risk by 60% compared with those who did not. Among women, strenuous activity in the early adult years was linked to a lower risk of Parkinson's, but the relationship was not statistically significant, and no clear relationship existed between physical activity later in life and Parkinson's risk.

A crucial challenge to this kind of information requires resolution: scientists must connect the evidence about the interaction of the genes in Parkinson's with *physical inactivity* throughout life. This is true for all of the other major diseases and the possible role for a genetic basis of physical activity.

We hope that during the last half of this decade of the third millennium, researchers from varied disciplines will continue to cross boundaries to solve challenging questions in exercise physiology. Many PhD programs now require students to complete course work in molecular biology as part of the required core curriculum (e.g., www.uiowa.edu/~exsci/Graduate/PhDexphy.htm), and many graduate programs affiliated with exercise science programs offer interdisciplinary graduate study in molecular biology, genetics, biochemistry, and physiology (http://programs.gradschools.com/). Working together, exercise physiologists trained in molecular biology (or molecular biologists with training in exercise physiology) can profit from the insights of biologists, geneticists, pharmacologists, and chemists who study human physical activity at the molecular level. Their shared explorations will benefit all humanity.

There can be no doubt that this treasure of genetic information will irrevocably change our view of our place in the world. Our children will be diagnosed for diseases they have not even developed and treated with drugs that match their body chemistry. Our grandchildren may be plucked from a pool of cells bathing in a petri dish after being screened for hidden flaws in their DNA. And our great-grandchildren will have dominion over the generations to come, with the capability to engineer traits into the genetic material as easily as sewing a button on a shirt.

KEVIN DAVIES. *Cracking the Genome.* NEW YORK: THE FREE PRESS, 2001.

TABLE A ■ TIMELINE OF EVENTS ABOUT "GENETICS" BEFORE MENDEL, FOLLOWED BY NOTABLE EVENTS IN GENETICS AND MOLECULAR BIOLOGY TO THE PRESENT

DATE	EVENT
Before Mendel	
420 BC	Socrates speculated about why children and parents seemed to differ in so many physical and psychologic characteristics
400 BC	Hippocrates believed that semen contributed to a child's physical and mental characteristics and that a woman passed on physical and mental traits via an analogous fluid
320 BC	Aristotle denounced Hippocrates's ideas believing a father's semen contributes a child's inherited characteristics; he taught that mothers provided the raw materials to create the child and that a "force" in mother's blood creates female babies
AD 1000	Hindu philosophers teach that parents pass on all their characteristics to offspring—"A man of base descent can never escape his origins"
1100–1700	Spontaneous generation remains the governing theory that organisms arise from nonliving matter, and how traits pass to new generation
1630	William Harvey deduces that males contribute sperm or pollen and females contribute eggs to reproduce their kind by sexual means
1655	Englishman Robert Hooke designs a microscope to examine thin slices of cork, observing honeycomb compartments he calls *cellulae* (Latin for "small rooms," known now as cells)
1657	Dutch naturalist Antonie van Leeuwenhoek observed the first living cells; he called them *animalcules* (little animals; protozoa and bacteria) and believed they played a role in fermentation
1724	Cross-fertilization of corn discovered
1838	Mathias Schleiden studied plants, observing that all plants "are aggregates of fully individualized, independent, separate beings, namely the cells themselves"
1839	Theodor Schwann developed the cell theory—cells serve as the basic building units of all animal tissues
1858	Naturalists Charles Darwin and Alfred Wallace independently propose their ideas about natural section—animal populations that survive adapt their hereditary characteristics and variations (see pages xxx–xxx)
1859	Charles Darwin publishes *On the Origin of Species by Means of Natural Selection, or The Preservation of Favoured Races in the Struggle for Life*
1865	Gregor Mendel, Austrian botanist and monk, presents his "Laws of Heredity" to the Natural Science Society, based on his 25-year cross-breeding experiments with 10,000 varieties of edible pea plants
After Mendel	
1868	Swiss biologist Friedrich Miescher isolates "nuclein" (now called DNA) from cells of open wounds and fish sperm
1882	German embryologist Walther Fleming discovers thin threads in nuclei (known now as chromosomes) that divide lengthwise in salamander larvae; he names mitosis; Robert Koch discovers the cause (bacterium) of a human microbial disease
1883	German physiologist August Weismann proposes the germ plasm theory that both parents contribute chromosomes equally to transmit hereditary characteristics to offspring
1900	Hugo De Vries, Carl Correns, and Erich van Tschermak-Seysenegg independently rediscover Mendel's classic cross-breeding experiments in the late 1860s
1902	American geneticist Walter Sutton develops chromosomal theory of heredity (similar chromosomes pair with one another during meiosis, each going to a different cell); he called Mendel's "factors" *genes*. British pediatric physician Sir Archibald Garrod (1857–1936) describes inborn errors of metabolism, recognizing that an inherited disease (alkaptonuria) might reflect genetic enzyme deficiencies
1907	Thomas Hunt Morgan proves with fruit flies that chromosomes play a role in heredity
1910	T. H. Morgan proves that chromosomes carry genes, and "crossing-over" experiments determine gene location (Principle of Linkage)
1911	T. H. Morgan maps gene location on fruit fly chromosomes
1912	Lawrence Bragg discovers that x-rays elucidate the molecular structure of crystalline substances, leading to x-ray crystallography and Rosalind Franklin's discovery of DNA's helical structure in the early 1950s
1915–1917	J. Frederick Twort (1915) first isolates viruses that infect bacteria; K. Felix d'Herelle (1917) establishes the existence of viruses that infect bacteria and invents a method to culture them; he also demonstrates that a virus (which he named *bacteriophage* or devourer of bacteria) reproduces only in live bacteria
1916	Publication of journal *Genetics*
1917–1918	Sewell Wright shows that enzymes mediate discrete biochemical steps determining coat colors in guinea pigs, mice, rats, rabbits, and large mammals
1926	T. H. Morgan publishes the influential *The Theory of the Gene*; Hermann Muller discovers that x-rays produce mutations in fruit flies, paving the way for future discoveries in genetics
1927	Herman Muller (1946 Nobel Prize for production of mutations by x-ray irradiation) treats sperm with heavy doses of x-rays and induces true "gene mutations" in germ cells (mutagenesis)
1928	British microbiologist Frederick Griffith proposes that an unknown "factor" transformed the harmless R strain of diplococcus to the virulent or pathogenic S strain *(Streptococcus pneumoniae)*; mice injected with R lived; mice injected with S died; adding both S and R killed the mice, proving that one strain passed to the other strain

continued on page 1064

TABLE A ■ *continued*

DATE	EVENT
1929	Phoebus Levine discovers the sugar deoxyribose
1931	Harriet Creighton and Barbara McClintock (future Nobel Prize winner) were first to discover that genetic recombination or "crossing over" (in maize) was caused by physical crossing over of the chromosomes (exchange of genes with breakage and chromosome rearrangement). German *Drosophila* geneticist Curt Stern independently verified Creighton and McClintock's findings of "crossing over" in flies
1935	Wendell Stanley crystallizes tobacco mosaic virus; Andrie Belozersky isolates pure DNA
1937	Frederick Bawden discovers that tobacco mosaic virus contains RNA
1938	The term "molecular biology" comes into use
1941	George Beadle and Edward Tatum use the bread mold *Neurospora* to confirm the "one gene–one enzyme" hypothesis (one gene–one polypeptide)—each gene determined a specific enzyme that performs a specific metabolic task
1944	Oswald Avery, Colin MacLeod, and Maclyn McCarty at Rockefeller Institute confirm that DNA, not proteins, serves as the hereditary material in bacteria ("transforming principle"); if proteins were involved, proteases would block transformation, but they did not; Frederick Sanger uses chromatography to determine the amino acid sequence of insulin
1945	Salvador Luria and Max Delbrück develop a phage model to study how genetic information transfers to host bacterial cells
1946	Edward Tatum and Joshua Lederberg discover that bacteria can exchange genetic material directly by plasma conjugation
1947	Barbara McClintock first reports on "transposable elements" (known today as jumping genes or transposons)
1950	Erwin Chargaff discovers that in DNA the number of thymines always equaled the number of adenines, and the number of guanines always equaled the number of cytosines ($[T] = [A]$; $[G] = [C]$) (known as "Chargaff's rule")
1952	Joshua Lederberg discovers bacterial structures (plasmids) that contain extrachromosomal genetic material; Lederberg and Norton Zinder prove that bacterial genes can infiltrate more than one cell (transduction)—a virus takes DNA from one bacterial cell and transports the genes to another cell it infects; Alfred Hershey (early 1960s Director of the Cold Spring Harbor Genetics Research Unit with members Nobel laureate Barbara McClintock and John Cairns [1969 Nobel Prize laureate for the genetic structure of viruses]) and assistant Martha Chase "tag" the DNA (^{32}P) and protein (^{35}S) in bacteriophage T2 (which attacks bacteria) to determine their roles during replication—that phage DNA, not its protein component, contains the phage genes; only the viral DNA (not viral protein) entered the cell in significant amounts to produce new viruses, which verified its role as the genetic carrier; electron microscopy verifies the structure of ribosomes; William Hayes discovers conjugation; Jean Brachet shows that protein synthesis involves RNA
1953	James Watson and Francis Crick publish their landmark paper in *Nature* (see page 1068) concerning their deduction about the 3-D, helical, complementary, antiparallel configuration of DNA; W. Hayes discovers that plasmids can transfer genetic markers among bacteria
1956	Francis Fraenkel-Conrat demonstrates genetic "self-assembly" by reassembling the tobacco mosaic virus from its constituent elements; Francis Crick and George Gamow (physicist) propose the "central dogma"—genetic information flows unidirectionally from DNA to mRNA to protein
1958	Arthur Kornberg purifies the enzyme DNA polymerase I from *E. coli* and uses it to create DNA in a test tube; Jérôme Lejeune discovers that children with Down syndrome contained a forty-seventh chromosome (trisomy)
1959	Francois Jacob and Jacques Monod discover repressors and operons—clusters of controlling genes in DNA that regulate "on" and "off" transcriptional control functions
1961	Marshall Nirenberg and Johann Matthaei use the base uracil to create mRNA (poly-U), the UUU codon for phenylalanine—a step toward cracking the DNA code
	Sydney Brenner, François Jacob, and Matthew Meselson provide biochemical proof using density-gradient centrifugation that genes code for proteins through messenger RNA
1964	Paul Leder and M. Nirenberg crack the genetic code, interpreting the triplet mRNA codons that specify each of the 20 amino acids; geneticist Charles Yanofsky and colleagues at Stanford, studying the mold *Neurospora crassa*, discover that suppressor mutations restored a mutant's active enzyme that previously produced an inactive protein.
1965	Alfred Hershey and Elizabeth Burgi demonstrate that bacteriophage λ DNA has 20 base, single-stranded tails at each end. The tails' base sequences were complementary, allowing their "sticky ends" to find each other and form circular DNA molecules; Ruth Sager and Zenta Ramanis discover intragenic recombination in nonchromosomal genes due to DNA in the cellular organelles
1967	Mary Weiss and Howard Green join human and mouse cells together (somatic cell fusion) to add the gene for thymidine kinase to chromosome 17 (forming a hybrid cell); this powerful technique assists in gene mapping and other human genetic analyses
1970	Peter Duesberg and Peter Vogt discover the first oncogene from experiments with retroviruses and map the genetic structure of these viruses; David Baltimore and Howard Temin independently purify reverse transcriptase restriction enzyme that cuts DNA at specific locations; Swedish scientists stain mammalian chromosomes that show a banding pattern
1972	Hugh McDevitt observes that specific genes control immune responses, suggesting heritability of acquired diseases
1973	Stanley Cohen, Ann Chang, and Herbert Boyer produce the first recombinant DNA organism (created DNA using *E. coli* restriction enzyme to splice genomes into a novel combination); Paul Berg suggests the NIH establish guidelines about DNA splicing techniques; Bruce Ames develops a test to identify DNA damaged by unwanted chemicals; improved method developed for DNA electrophoresis using agarose gel and ethidium bromide staining

continued on page 1065

TABLE A ■ *continued*

DATE	EVENT
1975	At an international conference, scientists call for establishing guidelines for recombinant-DNA research
1976	Venture capitalist Robert Swanson with biochemist H. Boyer form Genentech, Inc. whose mission is to develop, manufacture, and market pharmaceuticals
1977	Genentech scientists first use *E. coli* to produce a human protein—somatostatin (growth hormone–releasing factor); this milestone, using a recombinant gene to clone a protein, unleashed a biotechnologic revolution that continues today; Bill Rutter and Howard Goodman isolate the rat gene for insulin; Fred Sanger (Nobel Prize in Chemistry 1980) developed new methods for amino acid sequencing to deduce the complete sequence of insulin
1978	Genentech scientists with the City of Hope National Medical Center use recombinant DNA technology to produce human insulin; Stanford scientists transplant a mammalian gene; David Botstein and colleagues discover restriction fragment length polymorphisms (RFLPs—genetic variation in the length of mutant regions of DNA fragments produced by interaction with restriction enzymes; used in "genetic fingerprinting"); Steen Willadsen performs the first successful embryo splitting, dividing sheep embryos in two
1979	John Baxter clones the human growth hormone gene; Arnold Levine and David Lane discover the *p53* gene
1980	U.S. Supreme Court (Diamond *v.* Chakrabarty, 447 U.S. 303, 1980) upholds a patent for inventing a human-made, genetically created bacterium capable of breaking down crude oil, opening up commercialization of genetic engineering; researchers, using a bacterium, insert a gene that codes for the protein interferon; Martin Cline and colleagues create a transgenic mouse; Christiane Nüsslein-Volhard and Eric Wieschaus first report mutations in each of three major classes of genes in *Drosophila* concerned with early embryonic development (awarded Nobel Prize in 1995 honoring their work)
1981	Mary Harper and colleagues use in situ hybridization to map the insulin gene
1982	FDA approves Genentech's application to market genetically engineered human insulin (licensed to Eli Lilly and Company)
1983	Kery Mullis at Cetus Corporation develops the polymerase chain reaction (PCR) technique, which can make almost unlimited copies of specific regions of DNA from a tiny sample, amplifying it to a large enough quantity for analysis, revolutionizing molecular biology research (see Fig. 45); Jay Levy isolates the AIDS virus almost simultaneously with the Pasteur Institute and NIH
1984	Chiron Corporation clones and sequences the HIV genome; Richard Seed successfully transplants a human embryo from one woman to a surrogate mother who suffered from infertility problems; Alec Jeffreys discovers genetic "fingerprinting" that revolutionizes forensic medicine (confirmed the skeletal remains of Nazi war criminal Josef Mengele) and validity of paternity and immigration cases; Steen Willadsen (1944–), a Danish scientist at the Institute of Animal Physiology, Cambridge, England, creates the first verified cloned farm animal (a sheep) using the method of nuclear transfer from immature sheep embryo cells (and coating the embryo with agar)
1985	Axel Ullrich and his team at Genentech sequence the human insulin receptor, leading to diabetes treatment with human insulin; NIH approves guidelines for human gene therapy experiments; Cal Bio clones the gene that encodes human lung surfactant protein; biotechnology companies field test genetically engineered plants resistant to insects, bacteria, and viruses; Steen Willadsen successfully clones cattle from differentiated week-old embryo cells, proving that the DNA of specialized cells can be returned to their original state
1986	Peter Schultz combines antibodies and enzymes (catalytic antibodies) to produce pharmaceuticals by cutting, splicing, and modifying biologic molecules at specific points; the Health and Environmental Research Advisory Committee of the Department of Energy prepare an initial report about the possibility of initiating the human genome project; Yuri Dubrova and colleagues (including Sir Alec Jeffreys) present the first direct evidence that radiation from Chernobyl causes heritable mutations in humans (*Nature* 1996 25;380:683); the Food and Drug Administration (FDA) approves Hepatitis B, the first genetically engineered human vaccine
1987	Genentech receives FDA approval to market Activase (Alteplase, recombinant), a tissue plasminogen activator (t-PA), to dissolve blood clots in patients with coronary disease; David Burke, Georges Carle, and Maynard Olson develop a high-capacity cloning system using in vitro construction of linear DNA transformed into a yeast plasmid and maintained as artificial chromosome vectors (maintained as yeast artificial chromosomes or YACs)
1988	Philip Leder and Timothy Stewart patent the first genetically altered transgenic mouse ("Harvard Mouse" susceptible to breast cancer); genetic engineering companies begin cross-licensing agreements for products with parallel products (e.g., Hoffman-LaRoche, Inc. and Cetus Corporation cross-license Interleukin-1 and Polyethylene Glycol Modified IL-2); the DOE and the NIH signed a memorandum of understanding to "coordinate research and technical activities related to the human genome" (www.nhgri.nih.gov/HGP/#When); (www.nhgri.nih.gov/HGP_goals/5yrplan.html)
1989	UC Davis scientists develop a recombinant vaccine against the rinderpest virus; National Center for Human Genome Research founded with James Watson first director (now called the National Human Genome Research Institute [NHGRI: www.nhgri.nih.gov/])

continued on page 1066

TABLE A ■ *continued*

DATE	EVENT
1990	Mary-Claire King at UC Berkeley proves that the *BRCA1* breast cancer gene on chromosome 17 has a familial basis and that the gene can stop (suppress) and reverse several types of cancers; biotechnology companies receive patents for genetically engineered pharmaceuticals; the Human Genome Project to map and sequence the genomes of model organisms officially begins with a multiphase, $200 million budget for 15 years; formal launch of the International Human Genome Project; Calgene Inc., successfully field tests genetically engineered cotton plants; scientists introduce the bioluminescent gene *Agrobacterium tumefaciens* from the firefly into tobacco plant cells, producing a tobacco plant that glows green after receiving the catalyst luciferin; geneticist W. French Anderson successfully uses gene therapy for the first time in a 4-year-old girl with the rare autosomal recessive diseases adenosine deaminase (ADA) deficiency; Alan Handyside and Robert Winston at London's Hammersmith Hospital pioneer in vitro fertilization
1991	The online *Mendelian Inheritance in Man* database publishes a catalog of genetic diseases and their cytogenetic map locations (www.ncbi.nlm.gov/omim/); scientists begin the full-scale genome sequencing of *E. coli*
1992	U.S. Army institutes program to collect blood and tissue samples from new recruits (genetic "dog tag" surveillance) to better identify soldiers killed in action; British and American researchers discover a technique for vitro testing of embryos for genetic disorders (e.g., hemophilia, cystic fibrosis)
1993	Daniel Cohen and an international team of scientists produce a rough map of the 23 pairs of human chromosomes.
1994	The FDA approves Calgene Inc.'s Flavr-Savr tomato for sale in the United States, the first genetically engineered food product (designed to stay firm after harvest and remain on the vine longer to ripen to full flavor); the *BRCA1* gene, implicated in familial breast cancer, also plays a role in noninherited breast cancers; scientists worldwide discover many genes linked to inherited and noninherited diseases (hearing loss, sudden infant death syndrome, cerulean cataracts, melanoma, dyslexia, thyroid cancer, dwarfism, prostate cancer, bipolar disorder); first nonvirus genome reported in *Science* (1994;265:)[1132] for the bacterium *Haemophilus influenzae* clone calves from embryos that have grown to at least 120 cells
1995	Duke researchers transplant hearts from genetically altered pigs into baboons, proving the feasibility of cross-species transplants; leptin, a protein product of the obesity *(ob)* gene triggers weight loss in experimental animals; scientists develop the STS gene mapping technique; scientists develop a transgenic mouse carrying a gene for a form of inherited Alzheimer's disease characterized by more brain amyloid protein (APP)
1996	The FDA approves Biogen's recombinant interferon drug Avonex for treating multiple sclerosis; scientific collaboration sequences the entire genome of the most complex organism yet studied, *Saccharomyces cerevisiae* (baker's yeast), with 12 million base pairs; scientists sequence the genome of the ancient organism archaea, neither a eukaryote or prokaryote; researchers determine the 3-D structure of T cells; the FDA develops an inexpensive diagnostic biosensor test for the toxic strain of *E. coli;* scientists discover a gene involved with Parkinson's disease
1997	Charles Roberts, Gary Silberstein, and Charles Daniel discover the *WT1* tumor suppressor gene implicated in breast cancer; Ian Wilmut and Keith Campbell (Roslin Institute, Edinburgh) clone "Dolly" the sheep, the first mammal successfully cloned from an adult cell; scientists develop the first artificial human chromosome; Japanese researchers configure bits of DNA as "logic" elements (instructions) for a computer; scientists sequence the genomes of *E. coli, H. pylori,* and *B. burgdorferi* (Lyme disease pathogen); Azim Surani merged mouse thymocytes (type of white blood cells) with mouse embryonic germ cells—stem cells that develop into sperm or egg cells. The reprogrammed cells wouldn't form embryos, but instead develop directly into needed cells or tissues (*EMBO* 1997;16:6510)
1998	Scientists successfully grow embryonic stem cells; Japanese scientists clone eight calves using cells from a single adult cow; John Sulston (Sanger Center, Cambridge, England) and Robert Waterston (Washington University, St. Louis, MO) sequence the complete genome for the worm *C. elegans* (*Science* 1998;282:2012); Rod MacKinnon and associates of Rockefeller University determine the first crystal structure of a membrane channel (*Cell* 1998;95:649). FDA grants marketing clearance to Remicade (infliximab), a monoclonal antibody, to treat Crohn's disease; scientists develop a new cloning technique with a mouse model that creates three generations of cloned clones
1999	An international collaboration of scientists determines the DNA sequence of human chromosome 22 (*Nature* 1999;402:489); whole-genome shotgun optional mapping of *D. radi* (*Science* 1999;285:1558)
2000	FDA approves the drug Taxol for treating early stage breast cancer; researchers discover that existing AIDS patients can become infected with a stronger form of the virus; Gerald Schatten and colleagues subdivide the embryos of primates, producing a live offspring (107 rhesus monkey embryos divided into two to nine pieces to form 368 embryos; one survived, producing a baby monkey); CuraGen Corporation announces the first functional genomics map of an entire genome (yeast); Celera Corporation and the Human Genome Project announce the deciphering of the human genome (June 26, 2000); Celera estimates 3.12 billion bases for the human genome, 30 million fewer that the public consortium estimate; the Celera estimate includes 26.4 million DNA segments of about 500 letters (14.5 billion letters); this requires more than 500 million trillion DNA comparisons using 20,000 hours on Celera's super-computer (800 Alpha EV6 and EV67 processors with 64-bit architecture and 80 terabytes of memory, equivalent to about 5 to 6 times the Library of Congress); Craig Venter and Gerald Rubin sequence the genome of the fruit fly *Drosophila melanogaster*

continued on page 1067

TABLE A ■ *continued*

DATE	EVENT
2001	William Nierman and colleagues complete the genomic sequence of *Caulobacter crescentus*; Richard Peek and associates at Vanderbilt University use whole-genome microarrays to determine how genetic differences between strains of *Helicobacter pylori* influence gastric cancer type and the severity; American and Japanese researchers characterize gene expression in 49 embryonic and adult mouse tissues using DNA microarrays with 13,600 genes; University of Buffalo researchers demonstrate horizontal gene transfer between different families of mouth bacteria; Arnold Levine receives the first Albany Medical Center Prize in Medicine and Biomedical Research for discovering the *p53* gene that normally protects against cancer but causes cancer when it mutates (single mutation in the 135th position of the gene's 393 amino acids); *Science* (2001;291:1304–1351) and *Nature* (2001;409:860–921) simultaneously publish the sequence of the human genome; the research finds that humans have approximately 30,000 genes that carry within them the instructions for making the body's diverse collection of proteins; federal funding is allowed for 64 existing human embryonic stem cell lines; the Centers for Disease Control and Prevention (CDC) awards funding to schools of public health at the Universities of Michigan, North Carolina, and Washington to establish the first "Centers for Genomics and Public Health"
2002	DNA of rice sequenced (first decoding of a crop). Scientists publish the initial sequencing and comparative analysis of the mouse genome (*Nature* 2002;420:520–562)
2003	Human Genome Project (HGP) completed (13-year project coordinated by U.S. Department of Energy and NIH); Michael Gould and colleagues create the first "knockout" rats, a genetic trick that allows scientists to disrupt specific genes (screening for the *BRACA1 BRACA2* suppressor genes) to study how these genes function in rats; random mutations were introduced into male rats; these rats were then bred with females to create thousands of pups, which were screened for specific mutations; researchers identify a gene crucial to gene silencing; researchers show that bacteria exchange genetic material with totally unrelated species, called *lateral gene transfer*
2004	The same research group that published the sequencing of the mouse genome publish about 90% of the genome sequence of the brown Norway rat (*Nature* 2004;428: 493–521)—the rat genome is smaller than the human genome but larger than the mouse version; all three species—the first mammals to be sequenced—have roughly the same number of genes—between 25,000 and 30,000; California voters on November 2, 2004, approve a $6 billion bond measure over a 30-year period to establish a publicly funded stem cell research program (California Institute for Regenerative Medicine); scientists discover that gene function in mammals can be quickly and reliably predicted using a high-throughput analysis of patterns of RNA expression; researchers discover that changes in gene expression scale closely with initial expression levels in most organisms; highly expressed genes change in a dynamic way, while genes with lower expression levels show less variability; Korean researchers Woo Suk Hwang and coworkers at Seoul National University used 248 human eggs via somatic cell nuclear transfer (SCNT) technology to produce a single embryonic stem cell line from a human blastocyst; the researchers created 30 cloned embryos that grew to about 100 cells in size—further than any verified experiment thus far—confirming that they could harvest embryonic stem cells (ESC) from one of the embryos and that ESC could develop into different tissue types; this breakthrough experiment represents the first published report of cloned human stem cells (*Science* 2004;303(5664):1669–1674).
2005	UC Riverside researchers discover a way that yeast governs genetic expression and repression, findings that could be repeated in cells of other organisms; Brown University scientists Leon Cooper and John Sedivy develop a correlation-based statistical method (in contrast to a linear model) as a more reliable way to map complex gene interactions and pinpoint genes as potential cancer treatment targets; researchers in California, Israel, and Germany compared three distantly related species—baker's yeast, a worm, and fruit fly—and found that protein "wiring" connections in one species were often conserved in all three; the research supports both the concept of a basic wiring diagram for all eukaryotic cells and that more-selective pharmaceuticals could be designed to tweak the wiring plan of human cells to more effectively treat diseases while also generating fewer side effects; University of Arizona researchers establish that bacteria acquire up to 90% of their genetic material from distantly related bacterial species; determination of the chimpanzee genome reveals similarities in gene expression and coding sequences with human brain, heart, liver, kidney, and testis; a soluble form of the activin type IIB receptor (ACVR2B) dramatically increased muscle mass up to 60% in 2 weeks by blocking the myostatin signaling pathway (genetic evidence that the receptors can regulate muscle growth—potentially useful in disease prevention and athletic endeavors; *Proc. Natl Acad Sci* 2005;102:18117).

FIRST PUBLISHED REPORT OF THE DNA STRUCTURE*

MOLECULAR STRUCTURE OF NUCLEIC ACIDS

A Structure for Deoxyribose Nucleic Acid

We wish to suggest a structure for the salt of deoxyribose nucleic acid (D.N.A.). This structure has novel features which are of considerable biological interest.

A structure for nucleic acid has already been proposed by Pauling and Corey[1]. They kindly made their manuscript available to us in advance of publication. Their model consists of three intertwined chains, with the phosphates near the fibre axis, and the bases on the outside. In our opinion, this structure is unsatisfactory for two reasons: (1) We believe that the material which gives the X-ray diagrams is the salt, not the free acid. Without the acidic hydrogen atoms it is not clear what forces would hold the structure together, especially as the negatively charged phosphates near the axis will repel each other. (2) Some of the van der Waals' distances appear to be too small.

Another three-chain structure has also been suggested by Frasser (in the press). In his model the phosphates are on the outside and the bases on the inside, linked together by hydrogen bonds. This structure as described is rather ill-defined, and for this reason we shall not comment on it.

We wish to put forward a radically different structure for the salt of deoxyribose nucleic acid. This structure has two helical chains each coiled round the same axis (see diagram). We have made the usual chemical assumptions, namely, that each chain consists of phosphate diester groups joining β-D-deoxyribofuranose residues with 3',5' link-

This figure is purely diagrammatic. The two ribbons symbolize the two phosphate–sugar chains, and the horizontal rods the pairs of bases holding the chains together. The vertical line marks to fibre axis.

ages. The two chains (but not their bases) are related by a dyad perpendicular to the fibre axis. Both chains follow right-handed helices, but owing to the dyad the sequences of the atoms in the two chains run in opposite directions. Each chain loosely resembles Furberg's[2] model No. 1; that is, the bases are on the inside of the helix and the phosphates on the outside. The configuration of the sugar and the atoms near it is close to Furberg's 'standard configuration', the sugar being roughly perpendicualr to the attached base. There is a residue on each chain every 3 · 4A. In the z-direction. We have assumed an angle of 36° between adjacent residues in the same chain, so that the structure repeats after 10 residues on each chain, that is, after 34A. The distance of a phosphorus atom from the fibre axis is 10A. As the phosphates are on the outside, cations have easy access to them.

The structure is an open one, and its water content is rather high. At lower water contents we would expect the bases to tilt so that the structure could become more compact.

The novel feature of the structure is the manner in which the two chains are held together by the purine and pyrimidine bases. The planes of the bases are perpendicular to the fibre axis. They are joined together in pairs, a single base from one chain being hydrogen-bonded to a single base from the other chain, so that the two lie side by side with identical z-co-ordinates. One of the pair must be a purine and the other a pyrimidine for bonding to occur. The hydrogen bonds are made as follows: purine position 1 to pyrimidine position 1; purine position 6 to pyrimidine position 6.

If it is assumed that the bases only occur in the structure in the most plausible tautomeric forms (that is, with the keto rather than the enol configurations) it is found that only specific pairs of bases can bond together. These pairs are: adenine (purine) with thymine (pyrimidine), and guanine (purine) with cytosine (pyrimidine).

In other words, if an adenine forms one member of a pair, on either chain, then on these assumptions the other member must be thymine; similarly for guanine and cytosine. The sequence of bases on a single chain does not appear to be restricted in any way. However, if only specific pairs of bases can be formed, it follows that if the sequence of bases on one chain is given, then the sequence on the other chain is automatically determined.

It has been found experimentally[3,4] that the ratio of the amounts of adenine to thymine, and the ratio of guanine to cytosine, are always very close to unity for deoxyribose nucleic acid.

It is probably impossible to build this structure with a ribose sugar in place of the deoxyribose, as the extra oxygen atom would make too close a van der Waals contact.

The previously published X-ray data[5,6] on deoxyribose nucleic acid are insufficient for a rigorous test of our structure. So far as we can tell, it is roughly compatible with the experimental data, but it must be regarded as unproved until it has been checked against more exact results. Some of these are given in the following communications. We were not aware of the details of the results presented there when we devised our structure, which rests mainly though not entirely on published experimental data and stereochemical arguments.

It has not escaped our notice that the specific pairing we have postulated immediately suggests a possible copying mechanism for the genetic material.

Full details of the structure, including the conditions assumed in building it, together with a set of co-ordinates for the atoms, will be published elsewhere.

We are much indebted to Dr. Jerry Donohue for constant advice and criticism, especially on interatomic distances. We have also been stimulated by a knowledge of the general nature of the unpublished experimental results and ideas of Dr. M. H. F. Wilkins, Dr. R. E. Franklin and their co-workers at King's College, London. One of us (J. D. W.) has been aided by a fellowship from the National Foundation for Infantile Paralysis.

J.D. Watson
F.H.C. Crick

Medical Research Council Unit for the
Study of the Molecular Structure of
Biological Systems,
Cavendish Laboratory, Cambridge,
April 2.

[1]Pauling, L., and Corey, R.B., *Nature*, 171, 346 (1953); *Proc. U.S. Nat. Acad Sci.*, 39, 84(1953).

[2]Furberg, S., *Acta Chem. Scand*, 6, 634 (1952).

[3]Chargaff, E., for references see Zamenhof, S., Brawerman, G. and Chargaff, E., *Biochim. et Biophys. Acta*, 9, 402 (1952).

[4]Wyatt, G. R., *J. Gen. Physiol.*, 36, 201 (1952).

[5]Astbury, W. T., Symp. Soc. Exp. Biol. 1, Nucleic Acid, 66 (Camb. Univ. Press, 1947).

[6]Wilkins, M.H.F., and Randall, J. T., *Biochim. et Biophys. Acta,* 10, 192 (1953).

*Reprinted by permission from *Nature*, April 25, 1953, p. 737.

Page numbers in italics denote figures. Those followed by (t) denote tables.